IV Compa
Incompat
important i
IV drugs.

rigidity, peripheral circulatory collapse, cardiac arrest, anaphylactoid effects).
Storage • Store at room temperature.

Epidural, Liposomal
• May give either diluted or undiluted. • Do not use an in-line filter. • Store solution in refrigerator; do not freeze. May store at room temperature for 7 days. • Following withdrawal from vial, use within 4 hrs. • Gently invert vial to resuspend drug; avoid aggressive agitation.

IV INCOMPATIBILITIES

Amphotericin B complex (Abelcet, AmBisome, Amphotec), cefepime (Maxipime), doxorubicin (Doxil), lipids, phenytoin (Dilantin), thiopental.

IV COMPATIBILITIES

Amiodarone (Cordarone), atropine, bumetanide (Bumex), bupivacaine (Marcaine, Sensorcaine), diltiazem (Cardizem), diphenhydramine (Benadryl), dobutamine (Dobutrex), dopamine (Intropin), glycopyrrolate (Robinul), heparin, hydroxyzine (Vistaril), lidocaine, lorazepam (Ativan), magnesium, midazolam (Versed), milrinone (Primacor), nitroglycerin, potassium, propofol (Diprivan), total parenteral nutrition (TPN).

INDICATIONS/ROUTES/DOSAGE

ALERT Dosage should be titrated to desired effect.

Analgesia
PO (IMMEDIATE-RELEASE): ADULTS, ELDERLY: 10–30 mg q3–4h as needed. **CHILDREN:** 0.15–0.3 mg/kg q3–4h as needed.
PO (EXTENDED-RELEASE [AVINZA]): ADULTS, ELDERLY: Dosage requirement should be established using prompt-release formulations and is based on total daily dose. Avinza is given once a day only.
PO (EXTENDED-RELEASE [KADIAN]): ADULTS, ELDERLY: Dosage requirement should be established using prompt-release formulations and is based on total daily dose. Dose is given once a day or divided and given q12h.

Patient-Controlled Analgesia (PCA)
IV: ADULTS, ELDERLY: Loading dose: 5–10 mg. **Intermittent bolus:** 0.5–3 mg. **Lockout interval:** 5–12 min. **Continuous infusion:** 1–10 mg/hr. **4-hr limit:** 20–30 mg.

SIDE EFFECTS

Frequent: Sedation, decreased B/P (including orthostatic hypotension), diaphoresis, facial flushing, constipation, dizziness, drowsiness, nausea, vomiting. **Occasional:** Allergic reaction (rash, pruritus), dyspnea, confusion, palpitations, tremors, urinary retention, abdominal cramps, vision changes, dry mouth, headache, decreased appetite, pain/burning at injection site. **Rare:** Paralytic ileus.

ADVERSE EFFECTS/ TOXIC REACTIONS

Overdose results in respiratory depression, skeletal muscle flaccidity, cold/clammy skin, cyanosis, extreme drowsiness progressing to seizures, stupor, coma. Tolerance to analgesic effect, physical dependence may occur with repeated use.

NURSING CONSIDERATIONS

BASELINE ASSESSMENT
Pt should be in recumbent position before drug is given by parenteral route. Assess onset, type, location, duration of pain.

INTERVENTION/EVALUATION
Monitor vital signs 5–10 min after IV administration, 15–30 min after subcutaneous, IM. Be alert for decreased respirations, B/P. Check for adequate voiding. Monitor daily pattern of bowel activity and stool consistency. Avoid constipation.

PATIENT/FAMILY TEACHING
• Discomfort may occur with injection. • Change positions slowly to avoid orthostatic hypotension. • Avoid tasks that require alertness, motor skills until response to drug is established. • Avoid alcohol, CNS depressants.

Side Effects section in each drug monograph specifies the frequency of particular side effects.

Adverse Reactions highlight the particularly dangerous side effects.

High Alert drugs are shaded in purple for easy identification.

New to this Edition!
- 20 drugs recently approved by the FDA
- Hundreds of updates and revisions
- More than 275 Black Box Warnings

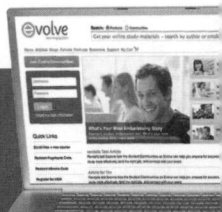

CONTENTS

DRUGS BY DISORDER xiv

DRUG CLASSIFICATIONS 1C

A–Z DRUG ENTRIES 1

APPENDIXES 1239

A. Calculation of Doses 1240
B. Controlled Drugs (United States) 1241
C. Drip Rates for Critical Care Medications 1242
D. Drugs of Abuse 1248
E. Equianalgesic Dosing 1255
F. FDA Pregnancy Categories 1256
G. Herbal Therapies and Interactions 1257
H. Lifespan, Cultural Aspects, and Pharmacogenomics of Drug Therapy 1270
I. Non-Crushable Drugs 1274
J. Normal Laboratory Values 1280
K. Orphan Drugs 1282
L. Cytochrome P450 (CYP) Enzymes 1284
M. Poison Antidote Chart 1287
N. Preventing Medication Errors and Improving Medication Safety 1291
O. Recommended Childhood and Adult Immunizations 1294
P. Signs and Symptoms of Electrolyte Imbalance 1301
Q. Parenteral Fluid Administration 1302
R. Spanish Phrases Often Used in Clinical Settings 1304
S. Techniques of Medication Administration 1312
T. Chronic Wound Care 1320
U. QT-Interval Prolongation and Medication Safety 1324

GENERAL INDEX 1325

Saunders Nursing Drug Handbook 2012

BARBARA B. HODGSON, RN, OCN
Morton Plant Mease Northbay Hospital
Former Staff Nurse
New Port Richey, Florida;
St. Joseph's Hospital
Former Staff Nurse in the Cancer Institute
Tampa, Florida

ROBERT J. KIZIOR, BS, RPh
Education Coordinator
Department of Pharmacy
Alexian Brothers Medical Center
Elk Grove Village, Illinois

ELSEVIER
SAUNDERS

ELSEVIER
SAUNDERS

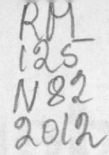

3251 Riverport Lane
St. Louis, Missouri 63043

SAUNDERS NURSING DRUG HANDBOOK 2012

ISBN: 978-1-4377-2334-2
ISSN: 1098-8661

NOTICES

Knowledge and best practice in this field are constantly changing. As new research and experience broaden our understanding, changes in research methods, professional practices, or medical treatment may become necessary.

Practitioners and researchers must always rely on their own experience and knowledge in evaluating and using any information, methods, compounds, or experiments described herein. In using such information or methods they should be mindful of their own safety and the safety of others, including parties for whom they have a professional responsibility.

With respect to any drug or pharmaceutical products identified, readers are advised to check the most current information provided (i) on procedures featured or (ii) by the manufacturer of each product to be administered, to verify the recommended dose or formula, the method and duration of administration, and contraindications. It is the responsibility of practitioners, relying on their own experience and knowledge of their patients, to make diagnoses, to determine dosages and the best treatment for each individual patient, and to take all appropriate safety precautions.

To the fullest extent of the law, neither the Publisher nor the authors, contributors, or editors, assume any liability for any injury and/or damage to persons or property as a matter of products liability, negligence or otherwise, or from any use or operation of any methods, products, instructions, or ideas contained in the material herein.

ISBN: 978-1-4377-2334-2

Acquisitions Editor: Sandra E. Clark
Senior Developmental Editor: Charlene Ketchum
Publishing Services Manager: Pat Joiner-Myers
Senior Project Manager: Joy Moore
Designer: Amy Buxton

Printed in the United States of America

Last digit is the print number: 9 8 7 6 5 4 3 2 1

I dedicate this work to my daughter Lauren, a true friend, for her unconditional love; my daughter Kathryn, always supportive, always encouraging; and my son, Keith, a source of great pride to us all. This is also dedicated to my sons-in-law, Jim and Andy, who have added so very much to my family, and to my granddaughters, Jaime, Sarah, Andrea, and Katie, and the smallest members of my family, my granddaughter, Paige Olivia, and my grandsons, Logan James, Ryan James, and Dylan Boyd. I couldn't love you more.

Barbara B. Hodgson, RN, OCN

To all health care professionals, who in the expectation of little glory or material reward dedicate themselves to the art and science of healing.

Robert J. Kizior, BS, RPh

AUTHOR BIOGRAPHIES

Barbara B. Hodgson, RN, OCN

Born and raised in Michigan, Barbara was married and raising a young family in Chicago when she decided to fulfill a lifelong dream and become a nurse. After graduation, she started her own business as author and publisher of **Medcards, The Total Medication Reference Guide**, the first of its kind. These drug cards were designed to assist nursing students in understanding drug information to give knowledgeable care to their patients.

In 1981, she met co-author Robert (Bob) Kizior, who was teaching a pharmacology class. After class, Barbara approached him and asked if he would be interested in working on **Medcards** with her. He agreed, and together they became so successful that a few years later Barbara was able to fulfill another dream and move to Florida.

By 1987, Barbara was approached by W.B. Saunders and asked to author the **Saunders Nursing Drug Handbook.** Since then, Barbara and Bob have worked together on this handbook and on two more drug resources, the **Saunders Electronic Nursing Drug Cards** and the **Saunders Drug Handbook for Health Professions.**

Barbara specialized in oncology at the Cancer Institute, St. Joseph's Hospital, in Tampa, Florida, and at Morton Plant Mease Northbay Hospital in New Port Richey, Florida. Barbara's daughter Lauren is a nurse manager, and her daughter Kathryn, her son Keith, and her son-in-law Jim are all nurses, working in their respective fields of patient care.

Barbara's favorite interests are spending time with her very busy, tight-knit family and, when she has a rare moment, getting her hands full of dirt working in her garden.

Robert (Bob) J. Kizior, BS, RPh

Bob graduated from the University of Illinois School of Pharmacy and is licensed to practice in the state of Illinois. He has worked as a hospital pharmacist for more than 40 years at Alexian Brothers Medical Center in Elk Grove Village, Illinois—a suburb of Chicago. Bob is the Education Coordinator for the Department of Pharmacy, where he participates in educational programs for pharmacists, nurses, physicians, and patients. He plays a major role in conducting Drug Utilization Reviews and is a member of the Infection Control Committee and the Bariatric Committee. His hospital experience is diverse and includes participation in clinical pharmacy initiatives on inpatient units and in the surgical pharmacy satellite. Bob is a former adjunct faculty member at William Rainey Harper Community College in Palatine, Illinois. It was there that Bob first met Barbara and commenced their long-standing professional association.

An avid fan of Big Ten college athletics, Bob also has eclectic tastes in music that range from classical, big band, rock 'n' roll, and jazz to country and western. Bob spends much of his free time reviewing the professional literature to stay current on new drug information. He and his wife, Marcia, and their two Labrador retrievers—Zak and Callie—enjoy escape weekends at their year-round lake house in central Wisconsin.

CONSULTANTS

Katherine B. Barbee, MSN, ANP, F-NP-C
Kaiser Permanente
Washington, District of Columbia

Lisa Brown
Jackson State Community College
Jackson, Tennessee

Marla J. DeJong, RN, MS, CCRN, CEN, Capt
Wilford Hall Medical Center
Lackland Air Force Base, Texas

Diane M. Ford, RN, MS, CCRN
Andrews University
Berrien Springs, Michigan

Denise D. Hopkins, PharmD
College of Pharmacy
University of Arkansas
Little Rock, Arkansas

Barbara D. Horton, RN, MS
Arnot Ogden Medical Center School of Nursing
Elmira, New York

Mary Beth Jenkins, RN, CCRN, CAPA
Elliott One Day Surgery Center
Manchester, New Hampshire

Kelly W. Jones, PharmD, BCPS
McLeod Family Medicine Center
McLeod Regional Medical Center
Florence, South Carolina

Autumn E. Korson
Western Michigan University Bronson School of Nursing
Kalamazoo, Michigan

Linda Laskowski-Jones, RN, MS, CS, CCRN, CEN
Christiana Care Health System
Newark, Delaware

Jessica K. Leet, RN, BSN
Cardinal Glennon Children's Hospital
St. Louis, Missouri

Denise Macklin, BSN, RNC, CRNI
President, Professional Learning Systems, Inc.
Marietta, Georgia

Nancy L. McCartney
Valencia Community College
Orlando, Florida

Judith L. Myers, MSN, RN
Health Sciences Center
St. Louis University School of Nursing
St. Louis, Missouri

Kimberly R. Pugh, MSEd, RN, BS
Nurse Consultant
Baltimore, Maryland

Regina T. Schiavello, BSN, RNC
Wills Eye Hospital
Philadelphia, Pennsylvania

Gregory M. Susla, PharmD, FCCM
National Institutes of Health
Bethesda, Maryland

Elizabeth Taylor
Tennessee Wesleyan College of Nursing
Fort Saunders Regional
Knoxville, Tennessee

REVIEWERS

Joy Chih-Ting Lai, PharmD
Pharmacist
St. Louis Psychiatric Rehabilitation Center
St. Louis, Missouri

April Iris Holmes, PharmD
Pharmacist
Wal-Mart Pharmacy
Fenton, Missouri

James E. Tisdale, PharmD
Professor
Perdue University
Indianapolis, Indiana

PREFACE

Nurses are faced with the ever-challenging responsibility of ensuring safe and effective drug therapy for their patients. Not surprisingly, the greatest challenge for nurses is keeping up with the overwhelming amount of new drug information, including the latest FDA-approved drugs and changes to already approved drugs, such as new uses, dosage forms, warnings, and much more. Nurses must integrate this information into their patient care quickly and in an informed manner.

Saunders Nursing Drug Handbook 2012 is designed as an easy-to-use source of current drug information to help the busy nurse meet these challenges. What separates this book from others is that it guides the nurse through patient care to better practice and better care.

This handbook contains the following:

1. **An IV Compatibility Chart.** This handy chart is bound into the handbook to prevent accidental loss.
2. **The Classification Section.** The action and uses for some of the most common clinical and pharmacotherapeutic classes are presented. Unique to this handbook, each class provides an at-a-glance table that compares all the generic drugs within the classification according to product availability, dosages, side effects, and other characteristics. Its purple full-page color tab ensures you can't miss it!
3. **An alphabetical listing of drug entries by generic name.** Purple letter thumb tabs help you page through this section quickly. Information on medications that contain a Black Box Alert is an added feature of the drug entries. This alert identifies those medications for which the FDA has issued a warning that the drugs may cause serious adverse effects. Tall Man lettering, with emphasis on certain syllables to avoid confusing similar sounding/looking medications, is shown in slim purple capitalized letters (e.g., *aceta**ZOLAMIDE**). High Alert drugs with a purple icon HIGH ALERT are considered dangerous by The Joint Commission and the Institute for Safe Medication Practices (ISMP) because if they are administered incorrectly, they may cause life-threatening or permanent harm to the patient. The entire High Alert generic drug entry sits on a purple-shaded background so it's easy to spot! To make scanning pages easier, each new entry begins with a shaded box containing the generic name, pronunciation, trade name(s), fixed-combination(s), and classification(s).
4. **Herbal entries.** Included in this edition are 16 of the most commonly used herbs, each indicated with a purple leaf. In this edition, each herb is cross-referenced to Herbal Therapies and Interactions (Appendix G) so that you have the most comprehensive view of herbal therapies related to patient care.
5. **Trade name cross-references in the A to Z section of the book.** These entries are shaded in gray for easy identification.
6. **A comprehensive reference section.** Appendixes include vital information on calculation of doses, controlled drugs, drip rates for critical care medications, drugs of abuse, equianalgesic dosing, FDA pregnancy categories, herbal therapies and interactions, lifespan, cultural aspects, and pharmacogenomics of drug therapy, non-crushable drugs, normal laboratory values, orphan drugs, cytochrome P450 enzymes, poison antidotes, preventing medication errors, recommended childhood and adult immunizations, signs and symptoms of electrolyte imbalance, parenteral

fluid administration, Spanish phrases often used in clinical settings, techniques of medication administration, chronic wound care, and QT-interval prolongation and medication safety.

7. **Drugs by Disorder.** You'll find Drugs by Disorder in the front of the book for easy reference. It lists common disorders and the drugs most often used for treatment.
8. **The index.** The comprehensive index is located at the back of the book on light purple pages. Undoubtedly the best tool to help you navigate the handbook, the comprehensive index is organized by showing generic drug names in **bold**, trade names in regular type, classifications in *italics,* and the page number of the main drug entry listed first and in **bold.**

A DETAILED GUIDE TO THE SAUNDERS NURSING DRUG HANDBOOK

An intensive review by Consultants and Reviewers helped us to revise the **Saunders Nursing Drug Handbook** so that it is most useful in both educational and clinical practice. The main objective of the handbook is to provide essential drug information in a user-friendly format. The bulk of the handbook contains an alphabetical listing of drug entries by generic name.

To maintain the portability of this handbook and meet the challenge of keeping content current, we have also included additional information for some medications on the Evolve® Internet site. Users can also choose from 200 monographs for the most commonly used medications and customize and print drug cards. Evolve® also includes drug alerts (e.g., medications removed from the market) and drug updates (e.g., new drugs, updates on existing entries). Information is periodically added, allowing the nurse to keep abreast of current drug information.

You'll also notice that some entries for infrequently used medications are condensed to reflect only the absolutely essential points the nurse should know when called on to administer them.

We have incorporated the IV Incompatibilities/Compatibilities heading. The drugs listed in this section are not compatible with the generic drug when administered directly by IV push, via Y-site, or via IV piggyback. We have highlighted the intravenous drug administration and handling information with a special heading icon and have broken it down by Reconstitution, Rate of Administration, and Storage.

We present entries in an order that follows the logical thought process the nurse undergoes whenever a drug is ordered for a patient:

- What is the drug?
- How is the drug classified?
- What does the drug do?
- What is the drug used for?
- Under what conditions should you **not** use the drug?
- How do you administer the drug?
- How do you store the drug?
- What is the dose of the drug?
- What should you monitor the patient for once he or she has received the drug?
- What do you assess the patient for?
- What interventions should you perform?
- What should you teach the patient?

The following are included within the drug entries:

Generic Name, Pronunciation, Trade Names. Each entry begins with the generic name and pronunciation, followed by the U.S. and Canadian trade names. Exclusively Canadian trade names are followed by a purple maple leaf ✤. Trade names that were most prescribed in the year 2010 are underlined in this section.

Black Box Alert. This feature highlights drugs that carry a significant risk of serious or life-threatening adverse effects. Black box alerts are ordered by the FDA.

Do Not Confuse With. Drug names that sound similar to the generic and/or trade names are listed under this heading to help you avoid potential medication errors.

Fixed-Combination Drugs. Where appropriate, fixed-combinations, or drugs made up of two or more generic medications, are listed with the generic drug.

Pharmacotherapeutic and Clinical Classification Names. Each full entry includes both the pharmacotherapeutic and clinical classifications for the generic drug. The page number of the classification description in the front of the book is provided in this section as well.

Action/Therapeutic Effect. This section describes how the drug is predicted to behave, with the expected therapeutic effect(s) under a separate heading.

Pharmacokinetics. This section includes the absorption, distribution, metabolism, excretion, and half-life of the medication. The half-life is bolded in purple for easy access.

Uses/Off-Label. The listing of uses for each drug includes both the FDA uses and off-label uses. The off-label heading is shown in bold purple for emphasis.

Precautions. This heading incorporates a discussion about when the generic drug is contraindicated or should be used with caution. The cautions warn the nurse of specific situations in which a drug should be closely monitored.

Lifespan Considerations ⌛. This section includes the pregnancy category and lactation data and age-specific information concerning children and the elderly.

Interactions. This heading enumerates drug, food, and herbal interactions with the generic drug. As the number of medications a patient receives increases, awareness of drug interactions becomes more important. Also included is information about therapeutic and toxic blood levels in addition to the altered lab values that show what effects the drug may have on lab results.

Product Availability. Each drug monograph gives the form and availability of the drug. The icon identifies non-crushable drug forms.

Administration/Handling. Instructions for administration are given for each route of administration (e.g., IV, IM, PO, rectal). Special handling, such as refrigeration, is also included where applicable. The routes in this section are always presented in the order IV, IM, Subcutaneous, and PO, with subsequent routes in alphabetical order (e.g., Ophthalmic, Otic, Topical). **IV administration** is broken down by reconstitution, rate of administration (how fast the IV should be given), and storage (including how long the medication is stable once reconstituted).

IV Compatibilities/IV Incompatibilities . These sections give the nurse the most comprehensive compatibility information possible when administering medications by direct IV push, via a Y-site, or via IV piggyback. This edition includes information about lipids.

Indications/Routes/Dosage. Each full entry provides specific dosing guidelines for adults, the elderly, children, and patients with renal and/or hepatic impairment. Dosages are clearly indicated for each approved indication and route.

Side Effects. Side effects are defined as those responses that are usually predictable with the drug, are **not** life-threatening, and may or may not require discontinuation of the drug. Unique to this handbook, side effects are grouped by frequency listed from highest occurrence percentage to lowest so that the nurse can focus on patient care without wading through myriad signs and symptoms of side effects.

Adverse Effects/Toxic Reactions. Adverse effects and toxic reactions are very serious and often life-threatening undesirable responses that require prompt intervention from a health care provider.

Nursing Considerations. Nursing considerations are organized as care is organized. That is:

- What needs to be assessed or done before the first dose is administered? (Baseline Assessment)
- What interventions and evaluations are needed during drug therapy? (Intervention/Evaluation)
- What explicit teaching is needed for the patient and family? (Patient/Family Teaching)

Saunders Nursing Drug Handbook is an easy-to-use source of current drug information for nurses, students, and other health care providers. It is our hope that this handbook will help you provide quality care to your patients.

We welcome any comments you may have that would help us to improve future editions of the handbook. Please contact us via the publisher at *http://evolve.elsevier.com/SaundersNDH.*

Barbara B. Hodgson, RN, OCN
Robert J. Kizior, BS, RPh

ACKNOWLEDGMENTS

I offer a special heartfelt thank you to my co-author, Bob Kizior, for his continuing, superb work. Without Bob's effort in this major endeavor, this book would not have reached the par excellence it has achieved. Bob and I particularly and especially thank Sandra Clark, our Acquisitions Editor, for her total dedication to making this edition one of Saunders' finest works. We gratefully acknowledge Charlene Ketchum, our Senior Developmental Editor, in helping ease our workload. Our thanks also go to Dan Fitzgerald and the staff at Graphic World Publishing Services for their tenacious detail work. It takes many eyes to transform a book into a work of art. Without their efforts, this would not have happened. I thank Jane Sperry and Milt, Bruce, Rich, Vance, Greg Boyd, Carolyn Steele, Jim Witmer, BSN, CEN, and Keith Hodgson, RN, BSN, for their unending help, encouragement, and support, and Andrew Ross, who enlightens my family so dearly.

Barbara B. Hodgson, RN, OCN

BIBLIOGRAPHY

Briggs GG, Freeman RK, Yaffe SJ: *Drugs in Pregnancy and Lactation: A Reference Guide to Fetal and Neonatal Risk,* ed 8, Philadelphia, 2008, Lippincott Williams & Wilkins.

Drug Facts and Comparisons 2010, Philadelphia, 2010, Lippincott Williams & Wilkins.

Generali J, Paxton L: *Black Box Warnings Study Guide 2010,* Black Box Rx LLC.

Lacy CF, Armstrong LL, Goldman MP, Lance LL: *Lexi-Comp's Drug Information Handbook,* ed 19, Hudson, OH, 2010–2011, Lexi-Comp.

Lexi-Comp's Drug Information Handbook for Oncology, ed 8, Hudson, OH, 2010, Lexi-Comp.

Natural Medicines Comprehensive Database, 2009.

Takemoto CK, Hodding JH, Kraus DM: *Lexi-Comp's Pediatric Dosage Handbook,* ed 17, Hudson, OH, 2010–2011, Lexi-Comp.

Trissel LA: *Handbook of Injectable Drugs,* ed 15, Bethesda, MD, 2008, American Society of Health-System Pharmacists.

ILLUSTRATION CREDITS

Kee JL, Hayes ER, McCuiston LE (eds): *Pharmacology: A Nursing Process Approach,* ed 6, Philadelphia, 2009, Saunders.

Mosby's GenRx, ed 12, St. Louis, 2004, Mosby.

NEWLY APPROVED MEDICATIONS

Name	Indication
Alglucosidase alfa (Lumizyme)	An enzyme needed for muscle function with late-onset Pompe disease (Evolve site only)
Alpha$_1$-proteinase inhibitor (Glassia)	Replacement therapy for patients with emphysema due to deficiency of alpha$_1$-proteinase inhibitor (Evolve site only)
Cabazitaxel (Jevtana)	A microtubule inhibitor for prostate cancer
Carglumic acid (Carbaglu)	An enzymatic activator for elevated ammonia levels due to *N*-acetylglutamate synthase deficiency (Evolve site only)
Ceftaroline (Teflaro)	An IV cephalosporin antibiotic for pneumonia and skin infectins (including MRSA)
Collagenase clostridium histolyticum (Xiaflex)	A proteolytic enzyme for treatment of Dupuytren's contracture (a progressive hand disease that affects connective tissue in the palm of the hand) (Evolve site only)
Dabigatran (Pradaxa)	A direct thrombin inhibitor indicated to reduce the risk of stroke and systemic embolism in patients with nonvalvular atrial fibrillation
Dalfampridine (Ampyra)	A potassium channel blocker to improve walking in patients with multiple sclerosis
Denosumab (Prolia)	A RANK ligand inhibitor for treatment of postmenopausal osteoporosis
Eribulin (Halaven)	A microtubule inhibitor for metastatic breast cancer
Fingolimod (Gilenya)	An oral sphingosine-1-phosphate receptor modulator to reduce relapses and delay disability progression in certain patients with multiple sclerosis
Incobotulinum toxin A (Xeomin)	An acetylcholine release inhibitor and neuromuscular blocking agent for cervical dystonia and blepharospasm (Evolve site only)
Liraglutide (Victoza)	A GLP-1 agonist to improve glucose control in type 2 diabetes
Lurasidone (Latuda)	An atypical antipsychotic agent for treatment of schizophrenia in adults
Pegloticase (Krystexxa)	A uric acid-specific enzyme for chronic refractory gout

Name	Indication
Polidocanol (Asclera)	An injectable agent for small varicose veins (spider veins and reticular veins) (Evolve site only)
Sipuleucel-T (Provenge)	Autologous cellular immunotherapy for treatment of advanced prostate cancer
Tesamorelin (Egrifta)	A growth hormone-releasing factor for HIV-associated lipodystrophy (Evolve site only)
Tocilizumab (Actemra)	An interleukin-6 inhibitor for moderate to severe rheumatoid arthritis
Velaglucerase alfa (VPRIV)	An enzyme replacement therapy for type 1 Gaucher disease (Evolve site only)

DRUGS BY DISORDER

Note: Not all medications appropriate for a given condition are listed, nor are those not listed inappropriate.
Generic names appear first, followed by brand names in parentheses.

Alcohol dependence
Acamprosate (Campral)
Disulfiram (Antabuse)
Naltrexone (Depade, ReVia, Vivitrol)

Allergic rhinitis
Azelastine (Astepro)
Beclomethasone (Beconase AQ)
Budesonide (Rhinocort Aqua)
Ciclesonide (Omnaris)
Flunisolide (Nasarel)
Fluticasone (Flonase)
Mometasone (Nasonex)
Olapatadine (Patanase)
Triamcinolone (Nasacort)

Allergy
Beclomethasone (Beclovent, Vanceril)
Betamethasone (Celestone)
Brompheniramine (Dimetane)
Budesonide (Pulmicort, Rhinocort)
Cetirizine (Zyrtec)
Chlorpheniramine (Chlor-Trimeton)
Clemastine (Tavist)
Cyproheptadine (Periactin)
Desloratadine (Clarinex)
Dexamethasone (Decadron)
Dimenhydrinate (Dramamine)
Diphenhydramine (Benadryl)
Epinephrine (Adrenalin)
Fexofenadine (Allegra)
Flunisolide (AeroBid, Nasalide)
Fluticasone (Flovent)
Hydrocortisone (Solu-Cortef)
Levocetirizine (Xyzal)
Loratadine (Claritin)
Prednisolone (Prelone)
Prednisone (Deltasone)
Promethazine (Phenergan)
Triamcinolone (Kenalog)

Alzheimer's disease
Donepezil (Aricept, Aricept ODT)
Galantamine (Razadyne, Razadyne ER)
Memantine (Namenda)
Rivastigmine (Exelon, Exelon Patch)
Tacrine (Cognex)

Angina
Amlodipine (Norvasc)
Atenolol (Tenormin)
Diltiazem (Cardizem, Dilacor)
Isosorbide (Imdur, Isordil)
Metoprolol (Lopressor)
Nadolol (Corgard)
Nicardipine (Cardene)
Nifedipine (Adalat, Procardia)
Nitroglycerin
Propranolol (Inderal)
Verapamil (Calan, Isoptin)

Anxiety
Alprazolam (Xanax)
Buspirone (BuSpar)
Diazepam (Valium)
Hydroxyzine (Atarax, Vistaril)
Lorazepam (Ativan)
Oxazepam (Serax)
Paroxetine (Paxil)
Trazodone (Desyrel)
Venlafaxine (Effexor)

Arrhythmias
Acebutolol (Sectral)
Adenosine (Adenocard)
Amiodarone (Cordarone, Pacerone)
Digoxin (Lanoxin)
Diltiazem (Cardizem, Dilacor)
Disopyramide (Norpace)
Dofetilide (Tikosyn)
Dronedarone (Multaq)

Esmolol (Brevibloc)
Flecainide (Tambocor)
Ibutilide (Corvert)
Lidocaine
Magnesium sulfate
Metoprolol (Lopressor)
Mexiletine (Mexitil)
Procainamide (Procan, Pronestyl)
Propafenone (Rythmol)
Propranolol (Inderal)
Quinidine
Sotalol (Betapace)
Tocainide (Tonocard)
Verapamil (Calan, Isoptin)

Arthritis, rheumatoid (RA)
Abatacept (Orencia)
Adalimumab (Humira)
Anakinra (Kineret)
Aspirin
Auranofin (Ridaura)
Aurothioglucose (Solganal)
Azathioprine (Imuran)
Capsaicin (Zostrix)
Celecoxib (Celebrex)
Certolizumab (Cimzia)
Cyclosporine (Sandimmune)
Diclofenac (Cataflam, Voltaren)
Diflunisal (Dolobid)
Etanercept (Enbrel)
Golimumab (Simponi)
Hydroxychloroquine (Plaquenil)
Infliximab (Remicade)
Leflunomide (Arava)
Methotrexate
Penicillamine (Cuprimine)
Prednisone (Deltasone)
Rituximab (Rituxan)
Sulfasalazine (Azulfidine-EN)
Tocilizumab (Actemra)

Asthma
Albuterol (Proventil, Ventolin)
Aminophylline (Theophylline)
Arformoterol (Brovana)
Beclomethasone (Beclovent, Vanceril)
Budesonide (Pulmicort)
Ciclesonide (Alvesco)
Cromolyn (Crolom, Intal)
Epinephrine (Adrenalin)
Flunisolide (AeroBid)
Fluticasone (Flovent)
Formoterol (Foradil)
Hydrocortisone (Solu-Cortef)
Ipratropium (Atrovent)
Levalbuterol (Xopenex)
Metaproterenol (Alupent)
Methylprednisolone (Solu-Medrol)
Mometasone (Asmanex)
Montelukast (Singulair)
Nedocromil (Tilade)
Prednisolone (Prelone)
Prednisone (Deltasone)
Salmeterol (Serevent)
Terbutaline (Brethine)
Theophylline (SloBid)
Zafirlukast (Accolate)
Zileuton (Zyflo, Zyflo CR)

Attention-deficit hyperactivity disorder (ADHD)
Atomoxetine (Strattera)
Bupropion (Wellbutrin)
Clonidine (Catapres)
Desipramine (Norpramin)
Dexmethylphenidate (Focalin, Focalin XR)
Dextroamphetamine (Dexedrine, Dextrostat)
Guanfacine (Intuniv)
Imipramine (Tofranil)
Lisdexamphetamine (Vyvanse)
Methylphenidate (Concerta, Daytrana, Focalin, Methylin, Ritalin)
Mixed amphetamine (Adderall, Adderall XR)
Modafinil (Provigil)
Nortriptyline (Aventyl, Pamelor)
Venlafaxine (Effexor)

Benign prostatic hypertrophy (BPH)
Alfuzosin (UroXatral)
Doxazosin (Cardura)
Dutasteride (Avodart)
Finasteride (Proscar)
Tamsulosin (Flomax)
Terazosin (Hytrin)

Bladder hyperactivity
Darifenacin (Enablex)
Oxybutynin (Ditropan, Gelnique)

Solifenacin (VESIcare)
Tolterodine (Detrol)
Trospium (Sanctura)

Bronchospasm
Albuterol (Proventil, Ventolin)
Bitolterol (Tornalate)
Levalbuterol (Xopenex)
Metaproterenol (Alupent)
Salmeterol (Serevent)
Terbutaline (Brethine)

Cancer
Abarelix (Plenaxis)
Aldesleukin (Proleukin)
Alemtuzumab (Campath)
Alitretinoin (Panretin)
Altretamine (Hexalen)
Anastrozole (Arimidex)
Arsenic trioxide (Trisenox)
Asparaginase (Elspar)
Azacitadine (Vidaza)
BCG (TheraCys, Tice BCG)
Bendamustine (Treanda)
Bevacizumab (Avastin)
Bexarotene (Targretin)
Bicalutamide (Casodex)
Bleomycin (Blenoxane)
Bortezomib (Velcade)
Busulfan (Myleran)
Cabazitaxel (Jevtana)
Capecitabine (Xeloda)
Carboplatin (Paraplatin)
Carmustine (BiCNU)
Cetuximab (Erbitux)
Chlorambucil (Leukeran)
Cisplatin (Platinol)
Cladribine (Leustatin)
Clofarabine (Clolar)
Cyclophosphamide (Cytoxan)
Cytarabine (Ara-C, Cytosar)
Dacarbazine (DTIC)
Dactinomycin (Cosmegen)
Dasatinib (Sprycel)
Daunorubicin (Cerubidine, DaunoXome)
Degarelix (Firmagon)
Denileukin (Ontak)
Docetaxel (Taxotere)
Doxorubicin (Adriamycin, Doxil)
Epirubicin (Ellence)
Eribulin (Halaven)
Erlotinib (Tarceva)
Estramustine (Emcyt)
Etoposide (VePesid)
Everolimus (Afinitor)
Fludarabine (Fludara)
Fluorouracil
Flutamide (Eulexin)
Fulvestrant (Faslodex)
Gefitnib (Iressa)
Gemcitabine (Gemzar)
Goserelin (Zoladex)
Hydroxyurea (Hydrea)
Ibritumomab (Zevalin)
Idarubicin (Idamycin)
Ifosfamide (Ifex)
Imatinib (Gleevec)
Interferon alfa-2a (Roferon A)
Interferon alfa-2b (Intron A)
Irinotecan (Camptosar)
Ixabepilone (Ixempra)
Lapatinib (Tykerb)
Letrozole (Femara)
Leuprolide (Lupron)
Lomustine (CeeNU)
Mechlorethamine (Mustargen)
Megestrol (Megace)
Melphalan (Alkeran)
Mercaptopurine (Purinethol)
Methotrexate
Mitomycin (Mutamycin)
Mitotane (Lysodren)
Mitoxantrone (Novantrone)
Nelarabine (Arranon)
Nilotinib (Tasigna)
Nilutamide (Nilandron)
Ofatumumab (Arzerra)
Oxaliplatin (Eloxatin)
Paclitaxel (Taxol)
Panitumumab (Vectibix)
Pazopanib (Votrient)
Pemetrexed (Alimta)
Pentostatin (Nipent)
Plicamycin (Mithracin)
Pralatrexate (Folotyn)
Procarbazine (Matulane)
Rituximab (Rituxan)
Romidepsin (Istodax)
Sipuleucel-T (Provenge)
Sorafenib (Nexavar)
Streptozocin (Zanosar)
Sunitinib (Sutent)

Tamoxifen (Nolvadex)
Temozolomide (Temodar)
Temsirolimus (Torisel)
Teniposide (Vumon)
Thioguanine
Thiotepa (Thioplex)
Tipifarnib (Zarnestra)
Topotecan (Hycamtin)
Toremifene (Fareston)
Tositumomab (Ber)
Trastuzumab (Herceptin)
Tretinoin (ATRA, Vesanoid)
Valrubicin (Valstar)
Vinblastine (Velban)
Vincristine (Oncovin)
Vinorelbine (Navelbine)
Vorinostat (Zolinza)

Cerebrovascular accident (CVA)
Aspirin
Clopidogrel (Plavix)
Heparin
Nimodipine (Nimotop)
Prasugrel (Effient)
Ticlopidine (Ticlid)
Warfarin (Coumadin)

Chronic obstructive pulmonary disease (COPD)
Albuterol (Proventil HFA, Ventolin HFA)
Aminophylline (Theophylline)
Arformoterol (Brovana)
Budesonide (Pulmicort)
Budesonide/formoterol (Symbicort)
Formoterol (Foradil)
Ipratropium (Atrovent HFA)
Levalbuterol (Xopenex)
Pirbuterol (Maxair)
Salmeterol (Serevent)
Salmeterol/fluticasone (Advair)
Theophylline (Theochron, Theo ZY)
Tiotropium (Spiriva)

Congestive heart failure (CHF)
Bisoprolol (Zebeta)
Bumetanide (Bumex)
Candesartan (Atacand)
Captopril (Capoten)
Carvedilol (Coreg)
Digoxin (Lanoxin)
Dobutamine (Dobutrex)
Dopamine (Intropin)
Enalapril (Vasotec)
Eplerenone (Inspra)
Fosinopril (Monopril)
Furosemide (Lasix)
Hydralazine (Apresoline)
Isosorbide (Isordil)
Lisinopril (Prinivil, Zestril)
Losartan (Cozaar)
Metoprolol (Lopressor)
Milrinone (Primacor)
Nitroglycerin
Quinapril (Accupril)
Ramipril (Altace)
Spironolactone (Aldactone)
Torsemide (Demadex)
Valsartan (Diovan)

Constipation
Bisacodyl (Dulcolax)
Docusate (Colace)
Lactulose (Kristalose)
Lubriprostone (Amitiza)
Methylcellulose (Citrucel)
Milk of magnesia (MOM)
Polyethylene glycol (Miralax)
Psyllium (Metamucil)
Senna (Senokot)
Tegaserod (Zelnorm)

Crohn's disease
Adalimumab (Humira)
Azathioprine (Azasan)
Budesonide (Entocort EC)
Certolizumab (Cimzia)
Hydrocortisone (Cortenema)
Infliximab (Remicade)
Mesalamine (Asacol, Pentasa)
Natalizumab (Tysabri)
Sulfasalazine (Azulfidine)

Deep vein thrombosis (DVT)
Dalteparin (Fragmin)
Enoxaparin (Lovenox)
Heparin
Tinzaparin (Innohep)
Warfarin (Coumadin)

Depression
Amitriptyline (Elavil, Endep)
Bupropion (Wellbutrin)

Citalopram (Celexa)
Clomipramine (Anafranil)
Desipramine (Norpramin)
Desvenlafaxine (Pristiq)
Doxepin (Sinequan)
Duloxetine (Cymbalta)
Escitalopram (Lexapro)
Fluoxetine (Prozac)
Fluvoxamine (Luvox)
Imipramine (Tofranil)
Maprotiline (Ludiomil)
Mirtazapine (Remeron)
Nortriptyline (Aventyl, Pamelor)
Paroxetine (Paxil)
Phenelzine (Nardil)
Selegiline (Emsam)
Sertraline (Zoloft)
Tranylcypromine (Parnate)
Trazodone (Desyrel)
Venlafaxine (Effexor)

Diabetes mellitus
Acarbose (Precose)
Bromocriptine (Cycloset)
Exenatide (Byetta)
Glimepiride (Amaryl)
Glipizide (Glucotrol)
Glyburide (Micronase)
Insulin preparations
Liraglutide (Victoza)
Metformin (Glucophage)
Miglitol (Glyset)
Nateglinide (Starlix)
Pioglitazone (Actos)
Pramlintide (Symlin)
Repaglinide (Prandin)
Rosiglitazone (Avandia)
Saxagliptin (Onglyza)
Sitagliptin (Januvia)

Diabetic peripheral neuropathy
Amitriptyline (Elavil)
Bupropion (Wellbutrin)
Capsaicin (Zostrix)
Carbamazepine (Tegretol)
Citalopram (Celexa)
Desipramine (Norpramin)
Duloxetine (Cymbalta)
Gabapentin (Neurontin)
Lamotrigine (Lamictal)
Lidocaine patch (Lidoderm)
Nortriptyline (Pamelor)
Oxcarbazepine (Trileptal)
Oxycodone (Oxycontin)
Paroxetine (Paxil)
Pregabalin (Lyrica)
Tramadol (Ultram)
Venlafaxine (Effexor)

Diarrhea
Bismuth subsalicylate (Pepto-Bismol)
Diphenoxylate and atropine (Lomotil)
Kaolin-pectin (Kaopectate)
Loperamide (Imodium)
Octreotide (Sandostatin)
Rifaximin (Xifaxan)

Duodenal, gastric ulcer
Cimetidine (Tagamet)
Esomeprazole (Nexium)
Famotidine (Pepcid)
Lansoprazole (Prevacid)
Misoprostol (Cytotec)
Nizatidine (Axid)
Omeprazole (Prilosec)
Pantoprazole (Protonix)
Rabeprazole (Aciphex)
Ranitidine (Zantac)
Sucralfate (Carafate)

Edema
Amiloride (Midamor)
Bumetanide (Bumex)
Chlorthalidone (Hygroton)
Ethacrynic acid (Edecrin)
Furosemide (Lasix)
Hydrochlorothiazide (HydroDIURIL)
Indapamide (Lozol)
Metolazone (Zaroxolyn)
Spironolactone (Aldactone)
Torsemide (Demadex)
Triamterene (Dyrenium)

Epilepsy
Acetazolamide (Diamox)
Carbamazepine (Tegretol)
Clonazepam (Klonopin)
Clorazepate (Tranxene)
Diazepam (Valium)
Fosphenytoin (Cerebyx)
Gabapentin (Neurontin)
Lamotrigine (Lamictal, Lamictal ODT, Lamictal XR)

Levetiracetam (Keppra)
Lorazepam (Ativan)
Oxcarbazepine (Trileptal)
Phenobarbital
Phenytoin (Dilantin)
Primidone (Mysoline)
Tiagabine (Gabitril)
Topiramate (Topamax)
Valproic acid (Depakene, Depakote)
Vigabatrin (Sabril)
Zonisamide (Zonegran)

Esophageal reflux, esophagitis
Cimetidine (Tagamet)
Dexlausoprazole (Kapidex)
Esomeprazole (Nexium)
Famotidine (Pepcid)
Lansoprazole (Prevacid)
Nizatidine (Axid)
Omeprazole (Prilosec)
Pantoprazole (Protonix)
Rabeprazole (Aciphex)
Ranitidine (Zantac)

Fever
Acetaminophen (Tylenol)
Aspirin
Ibuprofen (Advil, Caldolor, Motrin)
Naproxen (Aleve, Anaprox, Naprosyn)

Fibromyalgia
Acetaminophen (Tylenol)
Amitriptyline (Elavil)
Carisoprodol (Soma)
Citalopram (Celexa)
Cyclobenzapine (Flexeril)
Duloxetine (Cymbalta)
Fluoxetine (Prozac)
Gabapentim (Neurontin)
Minacipran (Savella)
Paroxetine (Paxil)
Pregabalin (Lyrica)
Tramadol (Ultram)
Venlafaxine (Effexor)

Gastritis
Cimetidine (Tagamet)
Famotidine (Pepcid)
Nizatidine (Axid)
Ranitidine (Zantac)

Gastroesophageal reflux disease (GERD)
Cimetidine (Tagamet)
Dexlansoprazole (Kapidex)
Esomeprazole (Nexium)
Famotidine (Pepcid)
Lansoprazole (Prevacid)
Metoclopramide (Metozolv ODT, Reglan)
Nizatidine (Axid)
Omeprazole (Prilosec)
Pantoprazole (Protonix)
Rabeprazole (Aciphex)
Ranitidine (Zantac)

Glaucoma
Acetazolamide (Diamox)
Apraclonidine (Iopidine)
Betaxolol (Betoptic)
Bimatoprost (Lumigan)
Brimonidine (Alphagan)
Brinzolamide (Azopt)
Carbachol
Carteolol (Ocupress)
Dipivefrin (Propine)
Dorzolamide (Trusopt)
Echothiophate iodide (Phospholine)
Latanoprost (Xalatan)
Levobunolol (Betagan)
Metipranolol (OptiPranolol)
Pilocarpine (Isopto Carpine)
Timolol (Timoptic)
Travoprost (Travatan)
Unoprostone (Rescula)

Gout
Allopurinol (Zyloprim)
Colchicine (Colcrys)
Febuxostat (Uloric)
Ibuprofen (Motrin)
Indomethacin (Indocin)
Naproxen (Naprosyn)
Pegloticase (Krystexxa)
Piroxicam (Feldene)
Probenecid (Benemid)
Sulindac (Clinoril)

Hepatitis B
Adefovir (Hepsera)
Entecavir (Baraclude)
Lamivudine (Epivir)
Pegylated interferon alpha 2a (Pegasys)

Telbivudine (Tyzeka)
Tenofovir (Viread)

Human immunodeficiency virus (HIV)
Abacavir (Ziagen)
Atazanavir (Reyataz)
Darunavir (Prezista)
Delavirdine (Rescriptor)
Didanosine (Videx)
Efavirenz (Sustiva)
Emtricitabine (Emtriva)
Enfuvirtide (Fuzeon)
Etravirine (Intelence)
Fosamprenavir (Lexiva)
Indinavir (Crixivan)
Lamivudine (Epivir)
Lopinavir/ritonavir (Kaletra)
Maraviroc (Selzentry)
Nelfinavir (Viracept)
Nevirapine (Viramune)
Raltegravir (Isentress)
Ritonavir (Norvir)
Saquinavir (Invirase)
Stavudine (Zerit)
Tenofovir (Viread)
Tesamorelin (Egrifta)
Tipranavir (Aptivus)
Zidovudine (AZT, Retrovir)

Hypercholesterolemia
Atorvastatin (Lipitor)
Cholestyramine (Questran)
Colesevelam (Welchol)
Colestipol (Colestid)
Ezetimibe (Zetia)
Fenofibrate (Antara, Lofibra, Tricor)
Fish oil (Lovaza)
Fluvastatin (Lescol)
Gemfibrozil (Lopid)
Lovastatin (Altoprev, Mevacor)
Niacin (Niaspan, Slo-Niacin)
Pitavastatin (Livalo)
Pravastatin (Pravachol)
Rosuvastatin (Crestor)
Simvastatin (Zocor)

Hyperphosphatemia
Aluminum salts
Calcium salts
Lanthanum (Fosrenol)
Sevelamer (Renagel)

Hypertension
Aliskiren (Tekturna)
Amlodipine (Norvasc)
Atenolol (Tenormin)
Benazepril (Lotensin)
Bisoprolol (Zebeta)
Candesartan (Atacand)
Captopril (Capoten)
Clevidipine (Cleviprex)
Clonidine (Catapres)
Diltiazem (Cardizem, Dilacor)
Doxazosin (Cardura)
Enalapril (Vasotec)
Eplerenone (Inspra)
Eprosartan (Teveten)
Felodipine (Plendil)
Fosinopril (Monopril)
Hydralazine (Apresoline)
Hydrochlorothiazide (HydroDIURIL)
Indapamide (Lozol)
Irbesartan (Avapro)
Isradipine (DynaCirc)
Labetalol (Normodyne, Trandate)
Lisinopril (Prinivil, Zestril)
Losartan (Cozaar)
Methyldopa (Aldomet)
Metolazone (Diulo, Zaroxolyn)
Metoprolol (Lopressor)
Minoxidil (Loniten)
Moexipril (Univasc)
Nadolol (Corgard)
Nebivolol (Bystolic)
Nicardipine (Cardene)
Nifedipine (Adalat, Procardia)
Nitroglycerin
Nitroprusside (Nipride)
Olmesartan (Benicar)
Perindopril (Aceon)
Pindolol (Visken)
Prazosin (Minipress)
Propranolol (Inderal)
Quinapril (Accupril)
Ramipril (Altace)
Spironolactone (Aldactone)
Telmisartan (Micardis)
Terazosin (Hytrin)
Timolol (Blocadren)
Trandolapril (Mavik)
Valsartan (Dovan)
Verapamil (Calan, Isoptin)

Hypertriglyceridemia
Atorvastatin (Lipitor)
Fenofibrate (Tricor)
Fluvastatin (Lescol)
Gemfibrozil (Lopid)
Lovastatin (Mevacor)
Niacin (Niaspan)
Omega-3 acid ethyl esters (Lovaza)
Pravastatin (Pravachol)
Rosuvastatin (Crestor)
Simvastatin (Zocor)

Hyperuricemia
Allopurinol (Zyloprim)
Febuxostat (Uloric)
Pegloticase (Krystexxa)
Probenecid (Benemid)

Hypotension
Dobutamine (Dobutrex)
Dopamine (Intropin)
Ephedrine
Epinephrine
Norepinephrine (Levophed)
Phenylephrine (Neo-Synephrine)

Hypothyroidism
Levothyroxine (Levoxyl, Synthroid)
Liothyronine (Cytomel)
Thyroid

Idiopathic thrombocytopenic purpura (ITP)
Cyclophosphamide (Cytoxan)
Dexamethasone (Decadron)
Hydrocortisone (SoluCortef)
Immune globulin intravenous
Methylprednisolone (SoluMedrol)
Prednisone
Rh_0(D) immune globulin (RhoGam)
Rituximab (Rituxan)

Insomnia
Diphenhydramine (Benadryl)
Estazolam (ProSom)
Eszopiclone (Lunesta)
Flurazepam (Dalmane)
Ramelteon (Rozerem)
Temazepam (Restoril)
Zaleplon (Sonata)
Zolpidem (Ambien, Edluar)

Migraine headaches
Almotriptan (Axert)
Amitriptyline (Elavil, Endep)
Diclofenac (Cambia)
Dihydroergotamine
Eletriptan (Relpax)
Ergotamine (Ergomar)
Frovatriptan (Frovan)
Naratriptan (Amerge)
Propranolol (Inderal)
Rizatriptan (Maxalt)
Sumatriptan (Imitrex)
Zolmitriptan (Zomig)

Multiple sclerosis (MS)
Dalfampridine (Ampyra)
Fingolimod (Gilenya)
Glatiramer (Copaxone)
Interferon beta-1a (Avonex, Rebif)
Interferon beta-1b (Betaseron)
Mitoxantrone (Novantrone)
Natalizumab (Tysabri)

Myelodysplastic syndrome
Azacitidine (Vidaza)
Clofarabine (Clolar)
Decitabine (Dacagen)
Lenalinomide (Revlimid)

Myocardial infarction (MI)
Alteplase (Activase)
Aspirin
Atenolol (Tenormin)
Captopril (Capoten)
Clopidogrel (Plavix)
Dalteparin (Fragmin)
Diltiazem (Cardizem, Dilacor)
Enalapril (Vasotec)
Enoxaparin (Lovenox)
Heparin
Lidocaine
Lisinopril (Prinivil, Zestril)
Metoprolol (Lopressor)
Morphine
Nitroglycerin
Propranolol (Inderal)
Quinapril (Accupril)
Ramipril (Altace)
Reteplase (Retavase)
Streptokinase
Timolol (Blocadren)
Warfarin (Coumadin)

Nausea
Aprepitant (Emend)
Chlorpromazine (Thorazine)
Dexamethasone (Decadron)
Dimenhydrinate (Dramamine)
Dolasetron (Anzemet)
Dronabinol (Marinol)
Droperidol (Inapsine)
Fosaprepitant (Emend)
Granisetron (Kytril)
Hydroxyzine (Vistaril)
Lorazepam (Ativan)
Meclizine (Antivert)
Metoclopramide (Reglan)
Nabilone (Cesamet)
Ondansetron (Zofran)
Palonosetron (Aloxi)
Prochlorperazine (Compazine)
Promethazine (Phenergan)
Trimethobenzamide (Tigan)

Obesity
Benzphetamine (Didrex)
Bupropion (Wellbutrin)
Diethylpropion (Tenuate)
Methamphetamine (Desoxyn)
Orlistat (Xenical)
Phendimetrazine (Bontril)
Phentermine (Ionamin)

Obsessive-compulsive disorder (OCD)
Citalopram (Celexa)
Clomipramine (Anafranil)
Fluoxetine (Prozac)
Fluvoxamine (Luvox)
Paroxetine (Paxil)
Sertraline (Zoloft)

Organ transplant, rejection prophylaxis
Azathioprine (Imuran)
Basilixumab (Simulect)
Cyclophosphamide (Cytoxan, Neosar)
Cyclosporine (Sandimmune)
Daclizumab (Zenapax)
Everolimus (Zortress)
Mycophenolate (CellCept)
Sirolimus (Rapamune)
Tacrolimus (Prograf)

Osteoarthritis
Acetaminophen (Tylenol)
Celecoxib (Celebrex)
Diclofenac (Cataflam, Pennsaid, Voltaren)
Etodolac (Lodine)
Flavocoxid (Limbrel)
Flurbiprofen (Ansaid)
Ibuprofen (Motrin)
Ketoprofen (Orudis)
Meloxicam (Mobic)
Nabumetone (Relafen)
Naproxen (Naprosyn)
Oxaprozin (Daypro)
Piroxicam (Feldene)
Salicylates (Aspirin)
Sulindac (Clinoril)
Tramadol (Ultram)

Osteoporosis
Alendronate (Fosamax)
Calcitonin (Miacalcin)
Calcium salts
Conjugated estrogens (Premarin)
Denosumab (Prolia)
Estradiol (Estrace)
Ibandronate (Boniva)
Raloxifene (Evista)
Risedronate (Actonel)
Teriparatide (Forteo)
Vitamin D
Zoledronic acid (Reclast)

Paget's disease
Alendronate (Fosamax)
Calcitonin (Miacalcin)
Etidronate (Didronel)
Pamidronate (Aredia)
Risedronate (Actonel)
Tiludronate (Skelid)
Zoledronic acid (Reclast)

Pain, mild to moderate
Acetaminophen (Tylenol)
Aspirin
Celecoxib (Celebrex)
Codeine
Diclofenac (Cataflam, Voltaren, Zipsor)
Diflunisal (Dolobid)
Etodolac (Lodine)
Flurbiprofen (Ansaid)

Ibuprofen (Advil, Caldolor, Motrin)
Ketorolac (Toradol)
Naproxen (Anaprox, Naprosyn)
Salsalate (Disalcid)
Tramadol (Ultram)

Pain, moderate to severe
Butorphanol (Stadol)
Fentanyl (Onsolis, Sublimaze)
Hydromorphone (Dilaudid)
Meperidine (Demerol)
Methadone (Dolophine)
Morphine (MS Contin)
Morphine/naltrexone (Embeda)
Nalbuphine (Nubain)
Oxycodone (OxyFast, Roxicodone)
Oxymorphone (Oprana)
Ziconotide (Prialt)

Panic attack disorder
Alprazolam (Xanax)
Clonazepam (Klonopin)
Paroxetine (Paxil)
Sertraline (Zoloft)
Venlafaxine (Effexor)

Parkinsonism
Amantadine (Symmetrel)
Apomorphine (Apokyn)
Bromocriptine (Parlodel)
Carbidopa/levodopa (Sinemet, Sinemet CR)
Diphenhydramine (Benadryl)
Entacapone (Comtan)
Pramipexole (Mirapex)
Rasagiline (Azilect)
Ropinirole (Requip)
Rotigotine (Neupro)
Selegiline (Eldepryl, Zelapar)
Tolcapone (Tasmar)

Peptic ulcer disease
Cimetidine (Tagamet)
Esomeprazole (Nexium)
Famotidine (Pepcid)
Lansoprazole (Prevacid)
Misoprostol (Cytotec)
Nizatidine (Axid)
Omeprazole (Prilosec)
Pantoprazole (Protonix)
Rabeprazole (Aciphex)
Ranitidine (Zantac)
Sucralfate (Carafate)

Pneumonia
Amoxicillin (Amoxil)
Amoxicillin/clavulanate (Augmentin)
Ampicillin (Polycillin)
Azithromycin (Zithromax)
Cefaclor (Ceclor)
Cefpodoxime (Vantin)
Ceftriaxone (Rocephin)
Cefuroxime (Kefurox, Zinacef)
Clarithromycin (Biaxin)
Co-trimoxazole (Bactrim, Septra)
Erythromycin
Gentamicin (Garamycin)
Levofloxacin (Levaquin)
Linezolid (Zyvox)
Moxifloxacin (Avelox)
Piperacillin/tazobactam (Zosyn)
Tobramycin (Nebcin)
Vancomycin (Vancocin)

Pneumonia, *Pneumocystis jiroveci*
Atovaquone (Mepron)
Clindamycin (Cleocin)
Co-trimoxazole (Bactrim, Septra)
Pentamidine (Pentam)
Trimethoprim (Proloprim)

Post-traumatic stress disorder
Amitriptyline (Elavil)
Aripiprazole (Abilify)
Citalopram (Celexa)
Escitalopram (Lexapro)
Fluoxetine (Prozac)
Imipramine (Tofranil)
Lamotrigine (Lamictal)
Olanzapine (Zyprexa)
Paroxetine (Paxil)
Phenelzine (Nardil)
Propranolol (Inderal)
Quetiapine (Seroquel)
Risperidone (Risperdol)
Sertraline (Zoloft)
Topiramate (Topamax)
Valproic acid (Depakote)
Venlafaxine (Effexor)
Ziprasidone (Geodon)

Pruritus
Amcinonide (Cyclocort)
Brompheniramine (Dimetane)
Cetirizine (Zyrtec)
Chlorpheniramine (Dimetane)
Clemastine (Tavist)
Clobetasol (Temovate)
Cyproheptadine (Periactin)
Desloratadine (Clarinex)
Desonide (Tridesilon)
Desoximetasone (Topicort)
Diphenhydramine (Benadryl)
Fluocinolone (Synalar)
Fluocinonide (Lidex)
Halobetasol (Ultravate)
Hydrocortisone (Cort-Dome, Hytone)
Hydroxyzine (Atarax, Vistaril)
Prednisolone (Prelone)
Prednisone (Deltasone)
Promethazine (Phenergan)

Psychosis
Aripiprazole (Abilify)
Asenapine (Saphris)
Chlorpromazine (Thorazine)
Clozapine (Clozaril)
Fluphenazine (Prolixin)
Haloperidol (Haldol)
Iloperidone (Fanapt)
Lurasidone (Latuda)
Olanzapine (Zyprexa)
Perphenazine (Trilafon)
Quetiapine (Seroquel, Seroquel XR)
Risperidone (Risperdal)
Thioridazine (Mellaril)
Thiothixene (Navane)
Ziprasidone (Geodon)

Pulmonary arterial hypertension
Ambrisentan (Letairis)
Bosentan (Tracleer)
Epoprostenol (Flolan)
Iloprost (Ventavis)
Sildenafil (Revatio)
Tadalafil (Adcirca)
Treprostinil (Remodulin, Tyvaso)

Respiratory distress syndrome (RDS)
Beractant (Survanta)
Calfactant (Infasurf)
Poractant alfa (Curosurf)

Restless legs syndrome
Cabergoline (Dostinex)
Carbidopa/levodopa (Sinemet)
Clonazepam (Klonopin)
Gabapentin (Neurontin)
Pramipexole (Mirapex)
Ropinirole (Requip)
Zolpidem (Ambien)

Schizophrenia
Aripiprazole (Abilify)
Asenapine (Saphris)
Chlorpromazine (Thorazine)
Clozapine (Clozaril)
Fluphenazine (Prolixin)
Haloperidol (Haldol)
Iloperidone (Fanapt)
Lurasidone (Latuda)
Olanzapine (Zyprexa)
Paliperidone (Invega, Invega Sustenna)
Perphenazine (Trilafon)
Quetiapine (Seroquel, Seroquel XR)
Risperidone (Risperdal)
Thioridazine (Mellaril)
Thiothixene (Navane)
Ziprasidone (Geodon)

Smoking cessation
Bupropion (Zyban)
Clonidine (Catapres)
Nicotine (Nicoderm, Nicotrol)
Nortriptyline (Pamelor)
Varenicline (Chantix)

Thrombosis
Dalteparin (Fragmin)
Enoxaparin (Lovenox)
Fondaparinux (Arixtra)
Heparin
Tinzaparin (Innohep)
Warfarin (Coumadin)

Thyroid disorders
Levothyroxine (Levoxyl, Synthroid)
Liothyronine (Cytomel)
Thyroid

Transient ischemic attack (TIA)
Aspirin
Clopidogrel (Plavix)
Prasugrel (Effient)

Ticlopidine (Ticlid)
Warfarin (Coumadin)

Tremor
Atenolol (Tenormin)
Chlordiazepoxide (Librium)
Diazepam (Valium)
Lorazepam (Ativan)
Metoprolol (Lopressor)
Nadolol (Corgard)
Propranolol (Inderal)

Tuberculosis (TB)
Cycloserine (Seromycin)
Ethambutol (Myambutol)
Isoniazid (INH)
Pyrazinamide
Rifabutin (Mycobutin)
Rifampin (Rifadin)
Rifapentine (Priftin)
Streptomycin

Urticaria
Cetirizine (Zyrtec)
Cimetidine (Tagamet)
Clemastine (Tavist)
Cyproheptadine (Periactin)
Diphenhydramine (Benadryl)
Hydroxyzine (Atarax, Vistaril)
Loratadine (Claritin)
Promethazine (Phenergan)
Ranitidine (Zantac)

Vertigo
Dimenhydrinate (Dramamine)
Diphenhydramine (Benadryl)
Meclizine (Antivert)
Scopolamine (Trans-Derm Scop)

Vomiting
Aprepitant (Emend)
Chlorpromazine (Thorazine)
Dexamethasone (Decadron)
Dimenhydrinate (Dramamine)
Dolasetron (Anzemet)
Dronabinol (Marinol)
Droperidol (Inapsine)
Fosaprepitant (Emend)
Granisetron (Kytril)
Hydroxyzine (Vistaril)
Lorazepam (Ativan)
Meclizine (Antivert)
Metoclopramide (Reglan)
Nabilone (Cesamet)
Ondansetron (Zofran)
Palonosetron (Aloxi)
Prochlorperazine (Compazine)
Promethazine (Phenergan)
Scopolamine (Trans-Derm Scop)
Trimethobenzamide (Tigan)

Zollinger-Ellison syndrome
Aluminum salts
Cimetidine (Tagamet)
Esomeprazole (Nexium)
Famotidine (Pepcid)
Lansoprazole (Prevacid)
Omeprazole (Prilosec)
Pantoprazole (Protonix)
Rabeprazole (Aciphex)
Ranitidine (Zantac)

Drug Classification Contents

allergic rhinitis nasal preparations
anesthetics: general
anesthetics: local
anesthetics: local topical
angiotensin-converting enzyme (ACE) inhibitors
angiotensin II receptor antagonists
antacids
antianxiety agents
antiarrhythmics
antibiotics
antibiotic: aminoglycosides
antibiotic: cephalosporins
antibiotic: fluoroquinolones
antibiotic: macrolides
antibiotic: penicillins
anticoagulants/antiplatelets/thrombolytics
anticonvulsants
antidepressants
antidiabetics
antidiarrheals
antifungals: systemic mycoses
antifungals: topical
antiglaucoma agents
antihistamines
antihyperlipidemics
antihypertensives
antimigraine (triptans)
antipsychotics
antivirals
beta-adrenergic blockers
bronchodilators
calcium channel blockers
chemotherapeutic agents
cholinergic agonists/anticholinesterase
contraception
corticosteroids
corticosteroids: topical
diuretics
fertility agents
H_2 antagonists
hematinic preparations
hormones
human immunodeficiency virus (HIV) infection
immunosuppressive agents
laxatives
neuromuscular blockers
nitrates
nonsteroidal anti-inflammatory drugs (NSAIDs)
nutrition: enteral
nutrition: parenteral
obesity management
ophthalmic medications for allergic conjunctivitis
opioid analgesics
osteoporosis
Parkinson's disease treatment
proton pump inhibitors
sedative-hypnotics
skeletal muscle relaxants
smoking cessation agents
sympathomimetics
thyroid
vitamins

Allergic Rhinitis Nasal Preparations

USES

Relieves symptoms associated with allergic rhinitis. These symptoms include rhinorrhea, nasal congestion, pruritus, sneezing, postnasal drip, nasal pain.

Allergic rhinitis or hay fever is an inflammation of the nasal airways occurring when an allergen (e.g., pollen) is inhaled. This triggers antibody production. The antibodies bind to mast cells, which contain histamine. Histamine is released, causing symptoms of allergic rhinitis.

ACTION

Intranasal corticosteroids: Decrease inflammation associated with allergic rhinitis by decreasing and preventing tissue from responding processes.

Intranasal antihistamines: Reduces histamine mediated symptoms of allergic rhinitis, including pruritus, sneezing, rhinorrhea, watery eyes.

Intranasal mast cell stabilizers: Inhibits the mast cell release of histamine and other inflammatory mediators.

Intranasal anticholinergics: Blocks acetylcholine in the nasal mucosa. Effective in treating rhinorrhea associated with allergic rhinitis.

Intranasal decongestants: Vasoconstricts the respiratory mucosa, provides short-term relief of nasal congestion.

CORTICOSTEROIDS

Generic (Brand)	Adult Dose	Pediatric Dose	Side Effects
Beclomethasone (p. 113) (Beconase AQ)	1–2 sprays in each nostril 2 times/day	5–11 yrs: 1 spray in each nostril 2 times/day	Altered taste and smell, epistaxis, burning, stinging, headache, nasal septum perforation
Budesonide (p. 145) (Rhinocort Aqua)	1–4 sprays in each nostril daily	6–11 yrs: 1–2 sprays in each nostril daily	Same as beclomethasone
Ciclesonide (p. 232) (Omnaris)	2 sprays in each nostril daily	6–11 yrs: (only seasonal allergic rhinitis) 2 sprays in each nostril daily	Same as beclomethasone
Flunisolide (p. 493) (Nasarel)	2 sprays in each nostril 2 or 3 times/day (maximum: 8 sprays in each nostril daily)	6–14 yrs: 2 sprays in each nostril 2 times/day or 1 spray in each nostril 3 times/day (maximum: 4 sprays in each nostril daily)	Same as beclomethasone
Fluticasone (p. 505) (Flonase)	1–2 sprays in each nostril daily	4–17 yrs: 1–2 sprays in each nostril daily	Same as beclomethasone

Fluticasone (p. 505) (Veramyst)	1–2 sprays in each nostril daily	2–11 yrs: 1–2 sprays in each nostril daily	Same as beclomethasone
Mometasone (p. 787) (Nasonex)	2 sprays in each nostril daily	2–11 yrs: 1 spray in each nostril daily	Same as beclomethasone
Triamcinolone (p. 1171) (AllerNaze, Nasacort AQ)	1–2 sprays in each nostril daily	6–11 yrs: 1–2 sprays in each nostril daily	Same as beclomethasone

ANTIHISTAMINES

Generic (Brand)	Adult Dose	Pediatric Dose	Side Effects
Azelastine (p. 102) (Astelin)	1–2 sprays in each nostril 2 times/day	5–11 yrs: 1 spray in each nostril 2 times/day	Sedation, epistaxis, nasal irritation
Olopatadine (Patanase)	2 sprays in each nostril 2 times/day	Not approved for children 12 yrs and under	Same as azelastine

MAST CELL STABILIZERS

Generic (Brand)	Adult Dose	Pediatric Dose	Side Effects
Cromolyn (p. 282) (Nasalcrom)	1 spray in each nostril 3–6 times/day	2–11 yrs: 1 spray in each nostril 3–6 times/day	Nasal irritation, unpleasant taste

ANTICHOLINERGICS

Generic (Brand)	Adult Dose	Pediatric Dose	Side Effects
Ipratropium (p. 628) (Atrovent) 0.03%	2 sprays in each nostril 2–3 times/day	6–11 yrs: 2 sprays in each nostril 2–3 times/day	Nasal irritation, epistaxis, dizziness, headache, blurry vision

(continued)

Allergic Rhinitis Nasal Preparations *(continued)*

ANTICHOLINERGICS

Generic (Brand)	Adult Dose	Pediatric Dose	Side Effects
Ipratropium (p. 628) (Atrovent) 0.06%	2 sprays in each nostril 4 times/day	5–11 yrs: 2 sprays in each nostril 4 times/day	Same as ipratropium 0.03%

DECONGESTANTS

Generic (Brand)	Adult Dose	Pediatric Dose	Side Effects
Oxymetazoline (Afrin)	2–3 drops or sprays 2 times/day	2–3 drops or sprays 2 times/day	Insomnia, tachycardia, nervousness, nausea, vomiting, transient burning, headache, rebound congestion if used longer than 72 hrs
Phenylephrine (Neo-Synephrine)	2–3 drops or 1–2 sprays q4h as needed (0.25% or 0.5%)	6–11 yrs: 2–3 drops (0.25%) q4h as needed 1–5 yrs: 2–3 drops (0.125%) q4h as needed	Restlessness, nervousness, headache, rebound nasal congestion, burning, stinging, dryness

Anesthetics: General

USES

IV anesthetic agents are used to induce general anesthesia. The general anesthetic state consists of unconsciousness, amnesia, analgesia, immobility, and attenuation of autonomic responses to noxious stimuli.

Volatile inhalation agents produce all the components of the anesthetic state but are administered through the lungs via an anesthesia machine. Agents for use include desflurane, sevoflurane, isoflurane, enflurane, and halothane.

General anesthetics are medications producing unconsciousness and a lack of response to all painful stimuli.

ACTION

IV anesthetic agents: Most agents produce CNS depression by action on the gamma-aminobutyric acid (GABA) receptor complex. GABA is the primary inhibitory neurotransmitter in the CNS. Ketamine produces dissociation between the thalamus and the limbic system.

Volatile inhalation agents: The action of these agents is not fully understood but they may disrupt neuronal transmission throughout the CNS. These agents may either block excitatory or enhance inhibitory transmission through axons or synapses.

ANESTHETICS: GENERAL

Name	Availability	Uses	Dosage Range	Side Effects
Etomidate (Amidate)	**I:** 2 mg/ml	IV induction	0.2–0.6 mg/kg	Myoclonus, pain on injection, nausea, vomiting, respiratory depression
Ketamine (p. 647) (Ketalar)	**I:** 10 mg/ml, 50 mg/ml, 100 mg/ml	Analgesia, sedation, IV induction	1–4.5 mg/kg	Delirium, euphoria, nausea, vomiting
Methohexital (Brevital)	**Powder for injection:** 500 mg	IV induction, sedation	50–120 mg	Cardiovascular depression, myoclonus, nausea, vomiting, respiratory depression
Midazolam (p. 767) (Versed)	**I:** 1 mg/ml, 5 mg/ml	Anxiolytic, amnesic, sedation	1–5 mg titrated slowly	Respiratory depression
Propofol (p. 976) (Diprivan)	**I:** 10 mg/ml	Sedation IV induction Maintenance	0.5 mg/kg 2–2.5 mg/kg 100–200 mcg/kg/min	Cardiovascular depression, delirium, euphoria, pain on injection, respiratory depression
Thiopental (Pentothal)	**Powder for injection:** 2.5% (25 mg/ml)	IV induction	Titrate vs. pt response **Average:** 50–75 mg	Cardiovascular depression, nausea, vomiting, respiratory depression

I, Injection.

Anesthetics: Local

USES	ACTION
Local anesthetics suppress pain by blocking impulses along axons. Suppression of pain does not cause generalized depression of the entire nervous system. Local anesthetics may be given topically and by injection (local infiltration, peripheral nerve block [axillary], IV regional [Bier block], epidural, and spinal).	Most local anesthetics fall into one of two groups: esters or amides. Both provide anesthesia and analgesia by reversibly binding to and blocking sodium (Na) channels. This slows the rate of depolarization of the nerve action potential; thus, propagation of the electrical impulses needed for nerve conduction is prevented.

ANESTHETICS: LOCAL

Name	Uses	Onset (min)	Duration (hrs)	Side Effects
Esters				
Chloroprocaine (Nesacaine)	Local infiltrate, nerve block, spinal	6–12	0.5–1	Seizures, bradycardia, cardiac arrest, hypotension, arrhythmias, anxiety, dizziness, restlessness, erythema, pruritus, urticaria, blurred vision, allergic reaction
Procaine (Novocaine)	Local infiltrate, nerve block, spinal	2–5	0.5–1.5	Burning sensation/pain at site of injection, tissue irritation, CNS stimulation followed by CNS depression, chills
Amides				
Bupivacaine (Marcaine, Sensorcaine)	Local infiltrate, nerve block, epidural, spinal	5	2–9	Cardiac arrest, hypotension, bradycardia, palpitations, seizures, restlessness, anxiety, dizziness, nausea, vomiting, blurred vision, weakness, tinnitus, apnea

Lidocaine (p. 689)	Local infiltrate, nerve block, spinal, epidural, topical, IV regional	Less than 2	0.5–1	Bradycardia, hypotension, arrhythmias, agitation, anxiety, dizziness, seizures, pruritus, rash, nausea, vomiting, altered taste, visual changes, tinnitus, respiratory depression, allergic reaction
Mepivacaine (Carbocaine, Polocaine)	Local infiltrate, nerve block, epidural	3–20	2–2.5	Bradycardia, syncope, arrhythmias, anxiety, seizures, dizziness, restlessness, chills, pruritus, urticaria, nausea, vomiting, incontinence, blurred vision, tinnitus, allergic reaction
Ropivacaine (Naropin)	Local infiltrate, nerve block, epidural, spinal	1–15	3–15	Hypotension, bradycardia, headache, pruritus, nausea, vomiting, dizziness, anxiety, tinnitus, dyspnea, cardiac arrest, arrhythmias, seizures, syncope, chills

Note: Most side effects are manifestations of excessive plasma concentrations.

Anesthetics: Local Topical

ANESTHETICS: LOCAL TOPICAL

Name	Indications	Peak Effect (min)	Duration (min)
Amides			
Dibucaine (Nupercainal)	Skin	Less than 5	15–45
Lidocaine (p. 689)	Skin, mucous membranes	2–5	15–45

(continued)

ANESTHETICS: LOCAL TOPICAL *(continued)*

Name	Indications	Peak Effect (min)	Duration (min)
Esters			
Benzocaine	Skin, mucous membranes	Less than 5	15–45
Cocaine	Mucous membranes	2–5	30–60
Tetracaine (Pontocaine)	Skin, mucous membranes	3–8	30–60

Angiotensin-Converting Enzyme (ACE) Inhibitors

USES

Treatment of hypertension (HTN), adjunctive therapy for CHF.

ACTION

Antihypertensive: Exact mechanism unknown. May be related to competitive inhibition of angiotensin I converting enzyme (ACE) activity causing decreased conversion of angiotensin I to angiotensin II, a potent vasoconstrictor. Reduces peripheral arterial resistance.

Congestive heart failure: Decreases peripheral vascular resistance (afterload), pulmonary capillary wedge pressure (preload), improves cardiac output, exercise tolerance.

ACE INHIBITORS

Name	Availability	Uses	Dosage Range (per day)	Side Effects
Benazepril (p. 114) (Lotensin)	**T:** 5 mg, 10 mg, 20 mg, 40 mg	HTN	**HTN:** 5–30 mg	Headaches, dizziness, fatigue, cough
Captopril (p. 172) (Capoten)	**T:** 12.5 mg, 25 mg, 50 mg, 100 mg	HTN CHF	**HTN:** 50–450 mg **CHF:** 12.5–450 mg	Insomnia, headaches, dizziness, fatigue, GI complaints, cough, rash
Enalapril (p. 407) (Vasotec)	**T:** 2.5 mg, 5 mg, 10 mg, 20 mg **IV:** 1.25 mg/ml	HTN CHF	**HTN:** 10–40 mg; (**IV:** 1.25 mg q6h) **CHF:** 5–20 mg	Chest pain, hypotension, headaches, fatigue, dizziness
Fosinopril (p. 519) (Monopril)	**T:** 10 mg, 20 mg, 40 mg	HTN CHF	**HTN:** 10–80 mg **CHF:** 20–40 mg	Hypotension, nausea, vomiting, cough
Lisinopril (p. 696) (Prinivil, Zestril)	**T:** 2.5 mg, 5 mg, 10 mg, 20 mg, 40 mg	HTN CHF	**HTN:** 10–40 mg **CHF:** 5–20 mg	Chest pain, hypotension, headaches, dizziness, fatigue, diarrhea
Moexipril (p. 786) (Univasc)	**T:** 7.5 mg, 15 mg	HTN	**HTN:** 7.5–30 mg	Dizziness, fatigue, diarrhea, cough
Perindopril (Aceon)	**T:** 2 mg, 4 mg, 6 mg	HTN	**HTN:** 4–16 mg	Hypotension, dizziness, fatigue, syncope, cough
Quinapril (p. 991) (Accupril)	**T:** 5 mg, 10 mg, 20 mg, 40 mg	HTN CHF	**HTN:** 10–80 mg **CHF:** 10–40 mg	Chest pain, hypotension, headaches, dizziness, fatigue, diarrhea, nausea, vomiting, cough
Ramipril (p. 1001) (Altace)	**C:** 1.25 mg, 2.5 mg, 5 mg, 10 mg	HTN CHF	**HTN:** 2.5–20 mg **CHF:** 1.25–10 mg	Hypotension, headaches, dizziness, cough
Trandolapril (p. 1160) (Mavik)	**T:** 1 mg, 2 mg, 4 mg	HTN CHF	**HTN:** 1–4 mg **CHF:** 1–4 mg	Dizziness, dyspepsia, cough, asthenia, syncope, myalgia

C, Capsules; ***CHF,*** congestive heart failure; ***HTN,*** hypertension; ***IV,*** intravenous; ***T,*** tablets.

Angiotensin II Receptor Antagonists

USES

Treatment of hypertension (HTN) alone or in combination with other antihypertensives. Treatment of heart failure (HF).

ACTION

Angiotensin II receptor antagonists (AIIRA) block vasoconstrictor and aldosterone-secreting effects on angiotensin II by selectively blocking the binding of angiotensin II to AT_1 receptors in vascular smooth muscle and adrenal gland, causing vasodilation and a decrease in aldosterone effects.

ANGIOTENSIN II RECEPTOR ANTAGONISTS

Name	Availability	Uses	Dosage Range (per day)	Side Effects
Candesartan (p. 169) (Atacand)	**T:** 4 mg, 8 mg, 16 mg, 32 mg	HTN HF	2–32 mg 4–32 mg	Headaches, upper respiratory tract infection, pain, dizziness
Eprosartan (p. 424) (Teveten)	**T:** 400 mg, 600 mg	HTN	400–800 mg	Headaches, upper respiratory tract infection, myalgia
Irbesartan (p. 629) (Avapro)	**T:** 75 mg, 150 mg, 300 mg	HTN	75–300 mg	Headaches, upper respiratory tract infection
Losartan (p. 708) (Cozaar)	**T:** 25 mg, 50 mg, 100 mg	HTN	25–100 mg	Dizziness, headaches, upper respiratory tract infection, diarrhea, fatigue, cough
Olmesartan (p. 860) (Benicar)	**T:** 5 mg, 20 mg, 40 mg	HTN	20–40 mg	Headaches, upper respiratory tract infection, flu-like symptoms, dizziness, bronchitis, rhinitis, back pain, pharyngitis, sinusitis, diarrhea, peripheral edema
Telmisartan (p. 1099) (Micardis)	**T:** 40 mg, 80 mg	HTN	20–80 mg	Upper respiratory tract infection, dizziness, back pain, sinusitis, diarrhea
Valsartan (p. 1190) (Diovan)	**T:** 80 mg, 160 mg	HTN HF	80–320 mg 80–320 mg	Dizziness, headaches, upper respiratory tract infection, diarrhea, fatigue

HF, Heart failure; ***HTN,*** hypertension; ***T,*** tablets.

Antacids

USES

Relief of symptoms associated with hyperacidity (e.g., heartburn, acid indigestion, sour stomach), hyperacidity associated with gastric/duodenal ulcers, treatment of pathologic gastric hypersecretion associated with Zollinger-Ellison syndrome, symptomatic treatment of gastroesophageal reflux disease (GERD), prevention and treatment of upper GI stress-induced ulceration and bleeding (esp. in ICU).

Aluminum hydroxide in conjunction with a low-phosphate diet to reduce elevated phosphate in pts with renal insufficiency. Calcium for calcium deficiency, magnesium for magnesium deficiency.

ACTION

Antacids act primarily in the stomach to neutralize gastric acid (increase pH). Antacids do not have a direct effect on acid output. The ability to increase pH depends on the dose, dosage form used, presence or absence of food in the stomach, and acid-neutralizing capacity (ANC). ANC is the number of mEq of hydrochloric acid that can be neutralized by a particular weight or volume of antacid.

Antacids reduce elevated phosphate by binding with phosphate in the intestine to form an insoluble complex, which is then eliminated.

ANTACIDS

Antacid	Brand Names	Availability	Dosage Range	Side Effects
Aluminum				
Hydroxide	Amphojel, Alu-Tab, Dialume	**T:** 300 mg, 500 mg, 600 mg **C:** 500 mg	500–1,500 mg 3–6 times/day	Chalky taste, mild constipation, abdominal cramps *Long-term use:* Neurotoxicity in dialysis pts, hypercalcemia, osteoporosis *Large doses:* Fecal impaction, peripheral edema

(continued)

ANTACIDS ***(continued)***

Antacid	Brand Names	Availability	Dosage Range	Side Effects
Calcium				
Carbonate (p. 163)	Tums, Caltrate 600, Oyst-Cal 500	**T (chewable):** 500 mg, 750 mg, 1,000 mg **T:** 1,250 mg	500–1,500 mg as needed (**Maximum:** 7,000 mg in 24 hrs)	Chalky taste *Large doses:* Fecal impaction, peripheral edema, metabolic alkalosis *Long-term use:* Difficult/painful urination
Magnesium				
Hydroxide (p. 715)	Milk of Magnesia	**T (chewable):** 311 mg **L:** 400 mg/5 ml, 800 mg/5 ml	**T:** 622–1,244 mg up to 4 times/day **L:** 2.5–7.5 ml up to 4 times/day	Chalky taste, diarrhea, laxative effect, electrolyte imbalance (dizziness, irregular heartbeat, fatigue)
Oxide (p. 715)	Mag-Ox 400	**T:** 400 mg, 420 mg, 500 mg	400–800 mg/day	Same as above

C, Capsules; ***L,*** liquid; ***T,*** tablets.

Antianxiety Agents

USES

Treatment of anxiety including generalized anxiety disorder (GAD), panic disorder, obsessive-compulsive disorder (OCD), social anxiety disorder (SAD), posttraumatic stress disorder (PTSD), and acute stress disorder. In addition, some benzodiazepines are used as hypnotics, anticonvulsants to prevent delirium tremors during alcohol withdrawal, and as adjunctive therapy for relaxation of skeletal muscle spasms. Midazolam, a short-acting benzodiazepine, is used for preop sedation and relief of anxiety for short diagnostic/endoscopic procedures (see individual monograph for midazolam).

ACTION

Benzodiazepines are the largest and most frequently prescribed group of antianxiety agents. The exact mechanism is unknown but may increase the inhibiting effect of gamma-aminobutyric acid (GABA), which inhibits nerve impulse transmission by binding to specific benzodiazepine receptors in various areas of the central nervous system (CNS).

◀ALERT▶ Refer to individual entries of nonbenzodiazepine drugs for more information on uses and actions.

ANTIANXIETY AGENTS

Name	Availability	Uses	Dosage Range (per day)	Side Effects
Benzodiazepine				
Alprazolam (p. 38) (Xanax)	**T:** 0.25 mg, 0.5 mg, 1 mg, 2 mg **S:** 0.5 mg/5 ml, 1 mg/ml	Anxiety, panic disorder	0.75–10 mg	Drowsiness, weakness, fatigue, ataxia, slurred speech, confusion, lack of coordination, impaired memory, paradoxical agitation, dizziness, nausea
Chlordiazepoxide (p. 226) (Librium)	**C:** 5 mg, 10 mg, 25 mg **T:** 10 mg, 25 mg **I:** 100 mg	Anxiety, alcohol withdrawal	5–300 mg	Same as alprazolam
Clorazepate (p. 264) (Tranxene)	**C:** 3.75 mg, 7.5 mg, 15 mg **SD:** 11.25 mg, 22.5 mg	Anxiety, alcohol withdrawal, anticonvulsant	7.5–90 mg	Same as alprazolam
Diazepam (p. 342) (Valium)	**T:** 2.5 mg, 5 mg, 10 mg **S:** 5 mg/5 ml, 5 mg/ml **I:** 5 mg/ml	Anxiety, alcohol withdrawal, anticonvulsant, muscle relaxant	2–40 mg	Same as alprazolam

(continued)

ANTIANXIETY AGENTS ***(continued)***

Name	Availability	Uses	Dosage Range (per day)	Side Effects
Lorazepam (p. 706) (Ativan)	**T:** 0.5 mg, 1 mg, 2 mg **S:** 2 mg/ml **I:** 2 mg/ml, 4 mg/ml	Anxiety	0.5–10 mg	Same as alprazolam
Oxazepam (Serax)	**C:** 10 mg, 15 mg, 30 mg **T:** 15 mg	Anxiety, alcohol withdrawal	30–120 mg	Same as alprazolam
Nonbenzodiazepine				
Buspirone (p. 154) (BuSpar)	**T:** 5 mg, 10 mg, 15 mg, 30 mg	Anxiety	7.5–60 mg	Dizziness, light-headedness, headaches, nausea, restlessness
Hydroxyzine (p. 584) (Atarax, Vistaril)	**T:** 10 mg, 25 mg, 50 mg, 100 mg	Anxiety, rhinitis, pruritus, urticaria, nausea or vomiting	100–400 mg	Drowsiness; dry mouth, nose, and throat
Paroxetine (p. 899) (Paxil)	**S:** 10 mg/5 ml **T:** 10 mg, 20 mg, 30 mg, 40 mg **T (CR):** 12.5 mg, 25 mg, 37.5 mg	Anxiety, depression, obsessive-compulsive disorder, panic disorder	10–50 mg	Drowsiness; dry mouth, nose, and throat; dizziness; diarrhea; diaphoresis; constipation; vomiting; tremors
Trazodone (p. 1166) (Desyrel)	**T:** 50 mg, 100 mg, 150 mg, 300 mg	Anxiety, depression	100–400 mg	Drowsiness, dizziness, headaches, dry mouth, nausea, vomiting, unpleasant taste
Venlafaxine (p. 1198) (Effexor)	**C:** 37.5 mg, 75 mg, 150 mg	Anxiety, depression	37.5–225 mg	Drowsiness, nausea, headaches, dry mouth

C, Capsules; ***CR,*** controlled-release; ***I,*** injection; ***S,*** solution; ***SD,*** single dose; ***T,*** tablets.

Antiarrhythmics

USES	ACTION
Prevention and treatment of cardiac arrhythmias, such as premature ventricular contractions, ventricular tachycardia, premature atrial contractions, paroxysmal atrial tachycardia, atrial fibrillation and flutter.	The antiarrhythmics are divided into four classes based on their effects on certain ion channels and/or receptors located on the myocardial cell membrane. Class I is further divided into three subclasses (IA, IB, IC) based on electrophysiologic effects. *Class I:* Block cardiac sodium channels and slow conduction velocity, prolonging refractoriness and decreasing automaticity of sodium-dependent tissue. *Class IA:* Block sodium and potassium channels. *Class IB:* Shorten the repolarization phase. *Class IC:* No effect on repolarization phase, but slow conduction velocity. *Class II:* Slow sinus and atrioventricular (AV) nodal conduction. *Class III:* Block cardiac potassium channels, prolonging the repolarization phase of electrical cells. *Class IV:* Inhibit the influx of calcium through its channels, causing slower conduction through the sinus and AV nodes.

ANTIARRHYTHMICS

Name	Availability	Uses	Dosage Range	Side Effects
Class IA				
Disopyramide (p. 365) (Norpace, Norpace CR)	**C:** 100 mg, 150 mg **C (ER):** 100 mg, 150 mg	AF, WPW, PSVT, PVCs, VT	400–800 mg/day	Dry mouth, blurred vision, urinary retention, CHF, proarrhythmia, heart block, nausea, vomiting, diarrhea, hypoglycemia, nervousness
Procainamide (p. 965) (Procan-SR, Pronestyl)	**T:** 250 mg, 375 mg, 500 mg **C:** 250 mg, 375 mg, 500 mg **T (SR):** 250 mg, 500 mg, 750 mg, 1,000 mg **I:** 100 mg/ml, 500 mg/ml	AF, WPW, PVCs, VT	**A (PO):** 250–500 mg q3h; **(ER):** 250–750 mg q6h	Hypotension, fever, agranulocytosis, SLE, headaches, proarrhythmia, confusion, disorientation, GI symptoms, hypotension
Quinidine (p. 993) (Quinaglute, Quinidex)	**T:** 200 mg, 300 mg **T (ER):** 300 mg, 324 mg **I:** 80 mg/ml	AF, WPW, PVCs, VT	**A:** 200–600 mg q2–4h; **(ER):** 300–600 mg q8h	Diarrhea, hypotension, nausea, vomiting, cinchonism, fever, bitter taste, heart block, thrombocytopenia, proarrhythmia
Class IB				
Lidocaine (p. 689) (Xylocaine)	**I:** 300 mg for IM **IV Infusion:** 2 mg/ml, 4 mg/ml	PVCs, VT, VF	**IV:** 50–100 mg bolus, then 1–4 mg/min infusion	Drowsiness, agitation, muscle twitching, seizures, paresthesias, proarrhythmia, slurred speech, tinnitus, cardiac depression, bradycardia, asystole
Mexiletine (Mexitil)	**C:** 150 mg, 200 mg, 250 mg	PVCs, VT, VF	**A:** 600–1,200 mg/day	Drowsiness, agitation, muscle twitching, seizures, paresthesias, proarrhythmia, nausea, vomiting, blood dyscrasias, hepatitis, fever
Tocainide (Tonocard)	**T:** 400 mg, 600 mg	PVCs, VT, VF	**A:** 1,200–1,800 mg/day	Drowsiness, agitation, muscle twitching, seizures, paresthesias, proarrhythmia, nausea, vomiting, diarrhea, agranulocytosis

Class IC				
Flecainide (Tambocor)	**T:** 50 mg, 100 mg, 150 mg	AF, PSVT, life-threatening ventricular arrhythmias	**A:** 200–400 mg/day	Dizziness, tremors, light-headedness, bradycardia, heart block, heart failure, GI upset, neutropenia, flushing, blurred vision, metallic taste, proarrhythmia
Propafenone (p. 975) (Rythmol)	**T:** 150 mg, 225 mg, 300 mg	PAF, WPW, life-threatening ventricular arrhythmias	**A:** 450–900 mg/day	Dizziness, blurred vision, altered taste, nausea, exacerbation of asthma, proarrhythmia, bradycardia, heart block, heart failure, GI upset, bronchospasm, hepatotoxicity
Class II (Beta-Blockers)				
Acebutolol (Sectral)	**C:** 200 mg, 400 mg	AF, A flutter, PSVT, PVCs	**A:** 600–1,200 mg/day	Bradycardia, hypotension, depression, nightmares, fatigue, sexual dysfunction, SLE, arthritis, myalgia
Esmolol (p. 437) (Brevibloc)	**I:** 10 mg/ml, 20 mg/ml	AF, A flutter, PSVT, PVCs	**A:** 50–200 mcg/kg/min	Hypotension, heart block, heart failure, bronchospasm
Propranolol (p. 978) (Inderal)	**T:** 10 mg, 20 mg	AF, A flutter, PSVT, PVCs	**A:** 10–30 mg 3–4 times/day	Bradycardia, hypotension, depression, nightmares, fatigue, sexual dysfunction, heart block, bronchospasm
Class III				
Amiodarone (p. 51) (Cordarone, Pacerone)	**T:** 200 mg, 400 mg **I:** 50 mg/ml	AF, PAF, PSVT, life-threatening ventricular arrhythmias	**A (PO):** 800–1,600 mg/day for 1–3 wks, then 600–800 mg/day **(IV):** 150 mg bolus, then IV infusion	Blurred vision, photophobia, constipation, ataxia, proarrhythmia, pulmonary fibrosis, bradycardia, heart block, hyperthyroidism or hypothyroidism, peripheral neuropathy, GI upset, blue-gray skin, optic neuritis, hypotension

(continued)

ANTIARRHYTHMICS *(continued)*

Name	Availability	Uses	Dosage Range	Side Effects
Dofetilide (p. 372) (Tikosyn)	**C:** 125 mcg, 250 mcg, 500 mcg	AF, A flutter	**A:** Individualized	Torsade de pointes, hypotension
Dronedarone (Multaq)	**T:** 400 mg	AF, A flutter	**A (PO):** 400 mg 2 times/day	Diarrhea, nausea, abdominal pain, vomiting, asthenia
Ibutilide (Corvert)	**I:** 0.1 mg/ml	AF, A flutter	**A (greater than 60 kg):** 1 mg over 10 min; **(less than 60 kg):** 0.01 mg/kg over 10 min	Torsade de pointes
Sotalol (p. 1076) (Betapace)	**T:** 80 mg, 120 mg, 160 mg, 240 mg	AF, PAF, PSVT, life-threatening ventricular arrhythmias	**A:** 160–640 mg/day	Fatigue, dizziness, dyspnea, bradycardia, proarrhythmia, heart block, hypotension, bronchospasm
Class IV (Calcium Channel Blockers)				
Diltiazem (p. 354) (Cardizem)	**I:** 25 mg/ml vials **Infusion:** 1 mg/ml	AF, A flutter, PSVT	**A (IV):** 20–25 mg bolus, then infusion of 5–15 mg/hr	Hypotension, bradycardia, dizziness, headaches, heart block, asystole, heart failure
Verapamil (p. 1200) (Calan, Isoptin)	**I:** 5 mg/2 ml	AF, A flutter, PSVT	**A (IV):** 5–10 mg	Hypotension, bradycardia, dizziness, headaches, constipation, heart block, heart failure, asystole, fatigue, edema, nausea

A, Adults; ***AF,*** atrial fibrillation; ***A flutter,*** atrial flutter; ***C,*** capsules; ***CHF,*** congestive heart failure; ***ER,*** extended-release; ***I,*** injection; ***PAF,*** paroxysmal atrial fibrillation; ***PSVT,*** paroxysmal supraventricular tachycardia; ***PVCs,*** premature ventricular contractions; ***SLE,*** systemic lupus erythematosus; ***SR,*** sustained-release; ***T,*** tablets; ***VT,*** ventricular tachycardia; ***WPW,*** Wolff-Parkinson-White syndrome.

Antibiotics

USES

Treatment of wide range of gram-positive or gram-negative bacterial infections, suppression of intestinal flora before surgery, control of acne, prophylactically to prevent rheumatic fever, prophylactically in high-risk situations (e.g., some surgical procedures or medical conditions) to prevent bacterial infection.

ACTION

Antibiotics (antimicrobial agents) are natural or synthetic compounds that have the ability to kill or suppress the growth of microorganisms.

One means of classifying antibiotics is by their antimicrobial spectrum. Narrow-spectrum agents are effective against few microorganisms (e.g., aminoglycosides are effective against gram-negative aerobes), whereas broad-spectrum agents are effective against a wide variety of microorganisms (e.g., fluoroquinolones are effective against gram-positive cocci and gram-negative bacilli).

Antimicrobial agents may also be classified based on their mechanism of action.

- Agents that inhibit cell wall synthesis or activate enzymes that disrupt the cell wall, causing a weakening in the cell, cell lysis, and death. Include penicillins, cephalosporins, vancomycin, imidazole antifungal agents.
- Agents that act directly on the cell wall, affecting permeability of cell membranes, causing leakage of intracellular substances. Include antifungal agents amphotericin and nystatin, polymyxin, colistin.
- Agents that bind to ribosomal subunits, altering protein synthesis and eventually causing cell death. Include aminoglycosides.
- Agents that affect bacterial ribosome function, altering protein synthesis and causing slow microbial growth. Do not cause cell death. Include chloramphenicol, clindamycin, erythromycin, tetracyclines.
- Agents that inhibit nucleic acid metabolism by binding to nucleic acid or interacting with enzymes necessary for nucleic acid synthesis. Inhibit DNA or RNA synthesis. Include rifampin, metronidazole, fluoroquinolones (e.g., ciprofloxacin).
- Agents that inhibit specific metabolic steps necessary for microbial growth, causing a decrease in essential cell components or synthesis of nonfunctional analogues of normal metabolites. Include trimethoprim, sulfonamides.
- Agents that inhibit viral DNA synthesis by binding to viral enzymes necessary for DNA synthesis, preventing viral replication. Include acyclovir, vidarabine.

Antibiotics *(continued)*

SELECTION OF ANTIMICROBIAL AGENTS

The goal of therapy is to achieve antimicrobial action at the site of infection sufficient to inhibit the growth of the microorganism. The agent selected should be the most active against the most likely infecting organism, least likely to cause toxicity or allergic reaction. Factors to consider in selection of an antimicrobial agent include the following:

- Sensitivity pattern of the infecting microorganism
- Location and severity of infection (may determine route of administration)
- Pt's ability to eliminate the drug (status of renal and hepatic function)
- Pt's defense mechanisms (includes both cellular and humoral immunity)
- Pt's age, pregnancy status, genetic factors, allergies, CNS disorder, preexisting medical problems

CATEGORIZATION OF ORGANISMS BY GRAM STAINING

Gram-Positive Cocci	Gram-Negative Cocci	Gram-Positive Bacilli	Gram-Negative Bacilli
Aerobic	**Aerobic**	**Aerobic**	**Aerobic**
Staphylococcus aureus	*Neisseria gonorrhoeae*	*Listeria monocytogenes*	*Escherichia coli*
Staphylococcus epidermidis	*Neisseria meningitidis*	*Bacillus anthracis*	*Klebsiella pneumoniae*
Streptococcus pneumoniae	*Moraxella catarrhalis*	*Corynebacterium diphtheriae*	*Proteus mirabilis*
Streptococcus pyogenes		**Anaerobic**	*Serratia marcescens*
Viridans streptococci		*Clostridium difficile*	*Acinetobacter* spp.
Enterococcus faecalis		*Clostridium perfringens*	*Pseudomonas aeruginosa*
Enterococcus faecium		*Clostridium tetani*	*Enterobacter* spp.
Anaerobic		*Actinomyces* spp.	*Haemophilus influenzae*
Peptostreptococcus spp.			*Legionella pneumophila*
Peptococcus spp.			**Anaerobic**
			Bacteroides fragilis
			Fusobacterium spp.

Antibiotic: Aminoglycosides

USES

Treatment of serious infections when other less toxic agents are not effective, are contraindicated, or require adjunctive therapy (e.g., with penicillins or cephalosporins). Used primarily in the treatment of infections caused by gram-negative microorganisms, such as those caused by *Proteus, Klebsiella, Pseudomonas, Escherichia coli, Serratia, and Enterobacter*. Inactive against most gram-positive microorganisms. Not well absorbed systemically from GI tract (must be administered parenterally for systemic infections). Oral agents are given to suppress intestinal bacteria.

ACTION

Bactericidal. Transported across bacterial cell membrane; irreversibly binds to specific receptor proteins of bacterial ribosomes. Interfere with protein synthesis, preventing cell reproduction and eventually causing cell death.

ANTIBIOTIC: AMINOGLYCOSIDES

Name	Availability	Dosage Range	Side Effects
Amikacin (p. 48) (Amikin)	**I:** 50 mg/ml, 250 mg/ml	**A:** 15 mg/kg/day **C:** 15 mg/kg/day	Nephrotoxicity, neurotoxicity, ototoxicity (both auditory and vestibular), hypersensitivity (skin itching, redness, rash, swelling)
Gentamicin (p. 540) (Garamycin)	**I:** 10 mg/ml, 40 mg/ml	**A:** 3–5 mg/kg/day **C:** 6–7.5 mg/kg/day	Same as amikacin
Neomycin	**T:** 500 mg	**A:** 1 g for 3 doses as preop	Nausea, vomiting, diarrhea
Streptomycin	**I:** 1 g	**A:** 15 mg/kg/day **C:** 20–40 mg/kg/day **Maximum:** 1 g	Same as amikacin Peripheral neuritis (numbness), optic neuritis (any vision loss)
Tobramycin (p. 1141) (Nebcin)	**I:** 40 mg/ml, 10 mg/ml	**A:** 3–5 mg/kg/day **C:** 6–7.5 mg/kg/day	Same as amikacin

A, Adults; ***C** (dosage),* children; ***I,*** injection; ***T,*** tablets.

Antibiotic: Cephalosporins

USES

Broad-spectrum antibiotics, which, like penicillins, may be used in a number of diseases, including respiratory diseases, skin and soft tissue infection, bone/joint infections, GU infections, prophylactically in some surgical procedures.

First-generation cephalosporins have activity against gram-positive organisms (e.g., streptococci and most staphylococci) and activity against most gram-negative organisms, including *Escherichia coli, Klebsiella pneumoniae, Proteus mirabilis, Salmonella,* and *Shigella.*

ACTION

Second-generation cephalosporins have same effectiveness as first-generation and increased activity against gram-negative organisms, including *H. influenzae, Neisseria, Enterobacter,* and several anaerobic organisms.

Third-generation cephalosporins are less active against gram-positive organisms but more active against the Enterobacteriaceae with some activity against *Pseudomonas aeruginosa, Serratia* spp., and *Acinetobacter* spp.

Fourth-generation cephalosporins have good activity against gram-positive organisms (e.g., *Staphylococcus aureus*) and gram-negative organisms (e.g., *Pseudomonas aeruginosa, E. coli, Klebsiella,* and *Proteus*).

Cephalosporins inhibit cell wall synthesis or activate enzymes that disrupt the cell wall, causing cell lysis and cell death. May be bacteriostatic or bactericidal. Most effective against rapidly dividing cells.

ANTIBIOTIC: CEPHALOSPORINS

Name	Availability	Dosage Range	Side Effects
First-Generation			
Cefadroxil (p. 188) **(Duricef)**	**C:** 500 mg **T:** 1 g **S:** 125 mg/5 ml, 250 mg/5 ml, 500 mg/5 ml	**A:** 1–2 g/day **C:** 30 mg/kg/day	Abdominal cramps/pain, fever, nausea, vomiting, diarrhea, headaches, oral/vaginal candidiasis
Cefazolin (p. 190) **(Ancef)**	**I:** 500 mg, 1 g, 2 g	**A:** 0.75–6 g/day **C:** 25–100 mg/kg/day	Same as cefadroxil

Cephalexin (p. 216) **(Keflex, Keftab)**	**C:** 250 mg, 500 mg **T:** 250 mg, 500 mg, 1 g	**A:** 1–4 g/day **C:** 25–100 mg/kg/day	Same as cefadroxil
Second-Generation			
Cefaclor (p. 187) **(Ceclor)**	**C:** 250 mg, 500 mg **T (ER):** 500 mg **S:** 125 mg/5 ml, 187 mg/5 ml, 250 mg/5 ml, 375 mg/5 ml	**A:** 250–500 mg q8h **C:** 20–40 mg/kg/day	Same as cefadroxil May have serum sickness–like reaction
Cefotetan	**I:** 1 g, 2 g	**A:** 1–6 g/day	Same as cefadroxil May cause unusual bleeding/ecchymoses
Cefoxitin (p. 199) **(Mefoxin)**	**I:** 1 g, 2 g	**A:** 3–12 g/day	Same as cefadroxil
Cefprozil (p. 203) **(Cefzil)**	**T:** 250 mg, 500 mg **S:** 125 mg/5 ml, 250 mg/5 ml	**A:** 0.5–1 g/day **C:** 30 mg/kg/day	Same as cefadroxil
Cefuroxime (p. 212) **(Ceftin, Kefurox, Zinacef)**	**T:** 125 mg, 250 mg, 500 mg **S:** 125 mg/5 ml, 250 mg/5 ml **I:** 750 mg, 1.5 g	**A (PO):** 0.25–1 g/day; **(IM/IV):** 2.25–9 g/day **C (PO):** 250–500 mg/day; **(IM/IV):** 50–100 mg/kg/day	Same as cefadroxil

(continued)

ANTIBIOTIC: CEPHALOSPORINS ***(continued)***

Name	Availability	Dosage Range	Side Effects
Third-Generation			
Cefdinir (p. 192) (Omnicef)	**C:** 300 mg **S:** 125 mg/5 ml	**A:** 600 mg/day **C:** 14 mg/kg/day	Same as cefadroxil
Cefditoren (Spectracef)	**T:** 200 mg	**A:** 400–800 mg/day	Same as cefadroxil
Cefotaxime (p. 197) (Claforan)	**I:** 500 mg, 1 g, 2 g	**A:** 2–12 g/day **C:** 100–200 mg/kg/day	Same as cefadroxil
Cefpodoxime (p. 201) (Vantin)	**T:** 100 mg, 200 mg **S:** 50 mg/5 ml, 100 mg/5 ml	**A:** 200–800 mg/day **C:** 10 mg/kg/day	Same as cefadroxil
Ceftazidime (p. 206) (Fortaz, Tazicef, Tazidime)	**I:** 500 mg, 1 g, 2 g	**A:** 0.5–6 g/day **C:** 90–150 mg/kg/day	Same as cefadroxil
Ceftibuten (p. 208) (Cedax)	**C:** 400 mg **S:** 90 mg/5 ml, 180 mg/5 ml	**A:** 400 mg/day **C:** 9 mg/kg/day	Same as cefadroxil
Ceftizoxime (Cefizox)	**I:** 500 mg, 1 g, 2 g	**A:** 1–12 g/day **C:** 150–200 mg/kg/day	Same as cefadroxil
Ceftriaxone (p. 210) (Rocephin)	**I:** 250 mg, 500 mg, 1 g, 2 g	**A:** 1–4 g/day **C:** 50–100 mg/kg/day	Same as cefadroxil
Fourth-Generation			
Cefepime (p. 194) (Maxipime)	**I:** 500 mg, 1 g, 2 g	**A:** 1–6 g/day	Same as cefadroxil

A, Adults; ***C,*** capsules; ***C (dosage),*** children; ***ER,*** extended-release; ***I,*** injection; ***S,*** suspension; ***T,*** tablets.

Antibiotic: Fluoroquinolones

USES

Fluoroquinolones act against a wide range of gram-negative and gram-positive organisms. They are used primarily in the treatment of lower respiratory infections, skin/skin structure infections, UTIs, and sexually transmitted diseases.

ACTION

Bactericidal. Inhibit DNA gyrase in susceptible microorganisms, interfering with bacterial DNA replication and repair.

ANTIBIOTIC: FLUOROQUINOLONES

Name	Availability	Dosage Range	Side Effects
Ciprofloxacin (p. 240) (Cipro)	**T:** 250 mg, 500 mg, 750 mg **S:** 5 g/100 ml **I:** 200 mg, 400 mg	**A (PO):** 250–750 mg q12h; **(IV):** 200–400 mg q12h	Dizziness, headaches, anxiety, drowsiness, insomnia, abdominal pain, nausea, diarrhea, vomiting, phlebitis (parenteral)
Gemifloxacin (p. 538) (Factive)	**T:** 320 mg	**A:** 320 mg/day	Same as ciprofloxacin
Levofloxacin (p. 684) (Levaquin)	**T:** 250 mg, 500 mg, 750 mg **I:** 250 mg, 500 mg, 750 mg	**A (PO/IV):** 250–750 mg/day as single dose	Same as ciprofloxacin
Moxifloxacin (p. 794) (Avelox)	**T:** 400 mg **I:** 400 mg	**A:** 400 mg/day	Same as ciprofloxacin; may prolong QT interval
Norfloxacin (p. 847) (Noroxin)	**T:** 400 mg	**A:** 400 mg q12h	Same as ciprofloxacin
Ofloxacin (p. 856) (Floxin)	**T:** 200 mg, 300 mg, 400 mg	**A:** 200–400 mg q12h	Same as ciprofloxacin

A, Adults; ***I,*** injection; ***S,*** suspension; ***T,*** tablets.

Antibiotic: Macrolides

USES	ACTION
Macrolides act primarily against most gram-positive microorganisms and some gram-negative cocci. Azithromycin and clarithromycin appear to be more potent than erythromycin. Macrolides are used in the treatment of pharyngitis/tonsillitis, sinusitis, chronic bronchitis, pneumonia, uncomplicated skin/skin structure infections.	Bacteriostatic or bactericidal. Reversibly bind to the P site of the 50S ribosomal subunit of susceptible organisms, inhibiting RNA-dependent protein synthesis.

ANTIBIOTIC: MACROLIDES

Name	Availability	Dosage Range	Side Effects
Azithromycin (p. 104) (Zithromax)	**T:** 250 mg, 600 mg **S:** 100 mg/5 ml, 200 mg/5 ml, 1-g packet **I:** 500 mg	**A (PO):** 500 mg once, then 250 mg on days 2–5; **(IV):** 500 mg/day **C (PO):** 10 mg/kg once, then 5 mg/kg/day on days 2–5	**PO:** Nausea, diarrhea, vomiting, abdominal pain **IV:** Pain, redness, swelling at injection site
Clarithromycin (p. 248) (Biaxin)	**T:** 250 mg, 500 mg **T (XL):** 500 mg **S:** 125 mg/5 ml	**A:** 250–500 mg q12h **C:** 7.5 mg/kg q12h	Headaches, loss of taste, nausea, vomiting, diarrhea, abdominal pain/discomfort
Erythromycin (p. 433) (EES, Eryc, EryPed, Ery-Tab, Erythrocin, PCE)	**T:** 200 mg, 250 mg, 333 mg, 400 mg, 500 mg **C:** 250 mg **S:** 125 mg/5 ml, 200 mg/5 ml, 250 mg/5 ml, 400 mg/5 ml, 100 mg/2.5 ml	**A (PO):** 250–500 mg q6h **C (PO):** 30–50 mg/kg/day **A, C (IV):** 15–20 mg/kg/day **Maximum:** 4 g/day	**PO:** Nausea, vomiting, diarrhea, abdominal pain **IV:** Inflammation, phlebitis at injection site

A, Adults; ***C,*** capsules; ***C (dosage),*** children; ***I,*** injection; ***S,*** suspension; ***T,*** tablets; ***XL,*** long acting.

Antibiotic: Penicillins

USES

Penicillins (also referred to as beta-lactam antibiotics) may be used to treat a large number of infections, including pneumonia and other respiratory diseases, UTIs, septicemia, meningitis, intra-abdominal infections, gonorrhea and syphilis, bone/joint infection.

Penicillins are classified based on an antimicrobial spectrum:

Natural penicillins are very active against gram-positive cocci but ineffective against most strains of *Staphylococcus aureus* (inactivated by enzyme penicillinase).

Penicillinase-resistant penicillins are effective against penicillinase-producing *Staphylococcus aureus* but are less effective against gram-positive cocci than the natural penicillins.

Broad-spectrum penicillins are effective against gram-positive cocci and some gram-negative bacteria (e.g., *Haemophilus influenzae, Escherichia coli, Proteus mirabilis, Salmonella,* and *Shigella*).

Extended-spectrum penicillins are effective against gram-negative organism, including *Pseudomonas aeruginosa, Enterobacter, Proteus* spp., *Klebsiella, Serratia* spp., and *Acinetobacter* spp.

ACTION

Penicillins inhibit cell wall synthesis or activate enzymes, which disrupt the bacterial cell wall, causing cell lysis and cell death. May be bacteriostatic or bactericidal. Most effective against bacteria undergoing active growth and division.

ANTIBIOTIC: PENICILLINS

Name	Availability	Dosage Range	Side Effects
Natural			
Penicillin G benzathine (p. 914) (Bicillin, Bicillin LA)	**I:** 600,000 units, 1.2 million units, 2.4 million units	**A:** 1.2 million units/day **C:** 0.3–1.2 million units/day	Mild diarrhea, nausea, vomiting, headaches, sore mouth/tongue, vaginal itching/discharge, allergic reaction (including anaphylaxis, skin rash, urticaria, pruritus)
Penicillin G potassium (p. 915) (Pfizerpen)	**I:** 1, 2, 3, 5 million-unit vials	**A:** 2–24 million units/day **C:** 100,000–250,000 units/kg/day	Same as penicillin G benzathine
Penicillin V potassium (p. 916) (Apo-Pen-VK)	**T:** 250 mg, 500 mg **S:** 125 mg/5 ml, 250 mg/5 ml	**A:** 0.5–2 g/day **C:** 25–50 mg/kg/day	Same as penicillin G benzathine
Penicillinase-Resistant			
Cloxacillin (Tegopen)	**C:** 250 mg, 500 mg **S:** 125 mg/5 ml	**A:** 1–2 g/day **C:** 50–100 mg/kg/day	Same as penicillin G benzathine Increased risk of hepatotoxicity
Dicloxacillin (Dynapen, Pathocil)	**C:** 125 mg, 250 mg, 500 mg **S:** 62.5 mg/5 ml	**A:** 1–2 g/day **C:** 12.5–25 mg/kg/day	Same as penicillin G benzathine Increased risk of hepatotoxicity
Nafcillin (p. 804) (Unipen)	**C:** 250 mg **I:** 500 mg, 1 g, 2 g	**A (PO):** 1–6 g/day; **(IV):** 2–6 g/day **C (PO):** 25–50 mg/kg/day; **(IV):** 50 mg/kg/day	Same as penicillin G benzathine Increased risk of interstitial nephritis
Oxacillin (Bactocill)	**C:** 250 mg, 500 mg **S:** 250 mg/5 ml **I:** 250 mg, 500 mg, 1 g, 2 g	**A (PO/IV):** 2–6 g/day **C (PO/IV):** 50–100 mg/kg/day	Same as penicillin G benzathine Increased risk of hepatotoxicity, interstitial nephritis

Broad-Spectrum			
Amoxicillin (p. 57) **(Amoxil, Trimox)**	**T**: 125 mg, 250 mg, 500 mg, 875 mg **C**: 250 mg, 500 mg **S**: 50 mg/ml, 125 mg/5 ml, 250 mg/5 ml	**A**: 0.75–1.5 g/day **C**: 20–40 mg/kg/day	Same as penicillin G benzathine
Amoxicillin/clavulanate (p. 59) **(Augmentin)**	**T**: 250 mg, 500 mg, 875 mg **T (chewable)**: 125 mg, 200 mg, 250 mg, 400 mg **S**: 125 mg/5 ml, 200 mg/5 ml, 250 mg/5 ml, 400 mg/5 ml	**A**: 0.75–1.5 g/day **C**: 20–40 mg/kg/day	Same as penicillin G benzathine
Ampicillin (p. 63) **(Principen)**	**C**: 250 mg, 500 mg **S**: 125 mg/5 ml, 250 mg/5 ml **I**: 125 mg, 250 mg, 500 mg, 1 g, 2 g	**A**: 1–12 g/day **C**: 50–200 mg/kg/day	Same as penicillin G benzathine
Ampicillin/sulbactam (p. 65) **(Unasyn)**	**I**: 1.5 g, 3 g	**A**: 6–12 g/day **C**: 100–200 mg/kg/day	Same as penicillin G benzathine
Extended-Spectrum			
Piperacillin/tazobactam (p. 935) **(Zosyn)**	**I**: 2.25 g, 3.375 g, 4.5 g	**A**: 2.25–4.5 g q6–8h **C**: 200–400 mg/kg/day	Same as penicillin G benzathine
Ticarcillin/clavulanate **(Timentin)**	**I**: 3.1 g	**A**: 3.1 g q4–6h **C**: 200–300 mg/kg/day	Same as penicillin G benzathine

A, Adults; ***C,*** capsules; ***C** (dosage),* children; ***I,*** injection; ***S,*** suspension; ***T,*** tablets.

Anticoagulants/Antiplatelets/Thrombolytics

USES

Treatment and prevention of venous thromboembolism, acute MI, acute cerebral embolism; reduce risk of acute MI; reduce total mortality in pts with unstable angina; prevent occlusion of saphenous grafts following open heart surgery; prevent embolism in select pts with atrial fibrillation, prosthetic heart valves, valvular heart disease, cardiomyopathy. Heparin also used for acute/chronic consumption coagulopathies (disseminated intravascular coagulation).

ACTION

Anticoagulants: Inhibit blood coagulation by preventing the formation of new clots and extension of existing ones *but do not dissolve formed clots.* Anticoagulants are subdivided into three classes. *Heparin* (including low molecular weight heparin): Indirectly interferes with blood coagulation by blocking the conversion of prothrombin to thrombin and fibrinogen to fibrin. *Coumarin:* Acts indirectly to prevent synthesis in the liver of vitamin K–dependent clotting factors. *Direct Thrombin Inhibitors:* Inhibits thrombin from converting fibrinogen to fibrin.

Antiplatelets: Interfere with platelet aggregation. Effects are irreversible for life of platelet. Medications in this group act by different mechanisms. Aspirin irreversibly inhibits cyclooxygenase, irreversibly inhibits formation of thromboxane A_2. Clopidogrel, dipyridamole, prasugrel, and ticlopidine have similar effects as aspirin and are known as adenosin diphosphate (ADP) inhibitors. Abciximab, eptifibatide, and tirofiban block binding of fibrinogen to the glycoprotein IIb/IIIa receptor on platelet surface (known as platelet glycoprotein IIb/IIIa receptor antagonists).

Thrombolytics: Act directly or indirectly on fibrinolytic system to dissolve clots (converting plasminogen to plasmin, an enzyme that digests fibrin clot).

ANTICOAGULANTS/ANTIPLATELETS/THROMBOLYTICS

Name	Availability	Uses	Side Effects
Anticoagulants			
Direct Thrombin Inhibitors			
Argatroban (p. 74)	**I:** 100 mg/ml	Prevent/treat VTE in pts with HIT or at risk for HIT undergoing PCI	Bleeding, hypotension

Bivalirudin (p. 133) (Angiomax)	**I:** 250-mg vials	Pts with unstable angina undergoing PTCA	Bleeding, hypotension, pain, headache, nausea
Lepirudin (p. 673) (Refludan)	**I:** 50-mg vials	Prevent VTE in pts with HIT	Anemia
Heparin, Low Molecular Weight Heparins			
Dalteparin (p. 299) (Fragmin)	**I:** 2,500 units, 5,000 units, 7,500 units, 10,000 units	Hip surgery; abdominal surgery; unstable angina or non–Q-wave MI	Bleeding, hematoma, increased ALT, AST, pain at injection site
Enoxaparin (p. 410) (Lovenox)	**I:** 30 mg, 40 mg, 60 mg, 80 mg, 100 mg, 120 mg, 150 mg	Hip surgery; knee surgery; abdominal surgery; unstable angina or non–Q-wave MI; acute illness	Bleeding, thrombocytopenia, hematoma, increased ALT, AST, nausea, bruising
Fondaparinux (p. 511) (Arixtra)	**I:** 2.5 mg	Hip surgery; knee surgery	Bleeding, thrombocytopenia, hematoma, fever, nausea, anemia
Heparin (p. 566)	**I:** 1,000 units/ml, 2,500 units/ml, 5,000 units/ml, 7,500 units/ml, 10,000 units/ml, 20,000 units/ml	Prevent/treat VTE	Bleeding, thrombocytopenia, skin rash, itching, burning
Tinzaparin (p. 1136) (Innohep)	**I:** 20,000 units/ml vials	Treatment of VTE (with warfarin)	Bleeding, thrombocytopenia, increased ALT, injection site hematoma

HIT, Heparin-induced thrombocytopenia; ***I,*** injection; ***MI,*** myocardial infarction; ***PCI,*** percutaneous coronary intervention; ***PO,*** oral; ***PTCA,*** percutaneous transluminal coronary angioplasty; ***VTE,*** venous thromboembolism.

(continued)

ANTICOAGULANTS/ANTIPLATELETS/THROMBOLYTICS *(continued)*

Name	Availability	Uses	Side Effects
Coumarin			
Warfarin (p. 1221) (Coumadin)	**PO:** 1 mg, 2 mg, 2.5 mg, 3 mg, 4 mg, 5 mg, 6 mg, 7.5 mg, 10 mg **I:** 2 mg/ml	Prevent/treat VTE in pts; prevent systemic embolism in pts with heart valve replacement, valve heart disease, MI, atrial fibrillation	Bleeding, skin necrosis, anorexia, nausea, vomiting, diarrhea, rash, abdominal cramps
Antiplatelets			
Abciximab (p. 4) (ReoPro)	**I:** 2 mg/ml	Adjunct to PCI to prevent acute cardiac ischemic complications (with heparin and aspirin)	Bleeding, hypotension, nausea, vomiting, back pain, allergic reactions, thrombocytopenia
Aspirin (p. 86)	**PO:** 81 mg, 165 mg, 325 mg, 500 mg, 650 mg	TIA in males; MI prophylaxis; cardiac vascular disease	Tinnitus, dizziness, hypersensitivity, dyspepsia, minor bleeding, GI ulceration
Clopidogrel (p. 263) (Plavix)	**PO:** 75 mg	Reduce risk of atherothrombotic events in pts with unstable angina, non–Q-wave MI, recent myocardial infarction, CVA	Bleeding
Dipyridamole (p. 364) (Persantine)	**PO:** 25 mg, 50 mg, 75 mg	Prevent postop thromboembolic complications following cardiac valve replacement	Dizziness, GI distress

Eptifibatide (p. 425) (Integrilin)	**I:** 0.75 mg/ml, 2 mg/ml	Treatment of acute coronary syndrome	Bleeding, hypotension
Prasugrel (Effient)	**PO:** 5 mg, 10 mg	Reduce thrombotic cardiovascular events in pts with ACS to be managed with PCI	Bleeding, hypotension
Ticlopidine (p. 1129) (Ticlid)	**PO:** 250 mg	Reduce risk stroke in pts with CVA precursors, TIA	Neutropenia, agranulocytosis, thrombocytopenia, aplastic anemia, increased serum cholesterol/triglycerides, rash, diarrhea, nausea, vomiting, GI pain
Tirofiban (Aggrastat)	**I:** 50 mcg/ml, 250 mcg/ml	Treatment of acute coronary syndrome	Bleeding, thrombocytopenia
Thrombolytics			
Alteplase (p. 41) (Activase)	**I:** 50 mg, 100 mg	Acute MI, acute ischemic stroke, pulmonary embolism	Bleeding, cholesterol embolism, arrhythmias
Reteplase (p. 1010) (Retavase)	**I:** 10.4 units	Acute MI	Bleeding, cholesterol embolism, arrhythmias
Tenecteplase (p. 1105) (TNKase)	**I:** 50 mg	Acute MI	Bleeding, cholesterol embolism, arrhythmias

ACS, Acute coronary syndrome; ***CVA,*** cerebrovascular attack; ***I,*** injection; ***MI,*** myocardial infarction; ***PCI,*** percutaneous coronary intervention; ***PO,*** oral; ***TIA,*** transient ischemic attack.

Anticonvulsants

USES

Anticonvulsants are used to treat seizures. Seizures can be divided into two broad categories: partial seizures and generalized seizures. *Partial seizures* begin focally in the cerebral cortex, undergoing limited spread. Simple partial seizures do not involve loss of consciousness but may evolve secondarily into generalized seizures. Complex partial seizures involve impairment of consciousness.

Generalized seizures may be convulsive or nonconvulsive and usually produce immediate loss of consciousness.

ACTION

Anticonvulsants can prevent or reduce excessive discharge of neurons with seizure foci or decrease the spread of excitation from seizure foci to normal neurons. The exact mechanism is unknown but may be due to (1) suppressing sodium influx, (2) suppressing calcium influx, or (3) increasing the action of gamma-aminobutyric acid (GABA), which inhibits neurotransmitters throughout the brain.

ANTICONVULSANTS

Name	Availability	Uses	Dosage Range	Side Effects
Carbamazepine (p. 174) (Carbatrol, Tegretol, Tegretol XR)	**S:** 100 mg/5 ml **T (chewable):** 100 mg **T:** 200 mg **T (ER):** 100 mg, 200 mg, 400 mg **C (ER):** 200 mg, 300 mg	Complex partial, tonic-clonic, mixed seizures; trigeminal neuralgia	**A:** 800–1,200 mg/day **C:** 400–800 mg/day	Dizziness, diplopia, leukopenia, drowsiness, blurred vision, headache, ataxia, nausea, vomiting, hyponatremia
Clonazepam (p. 259) (Klonopin)	**T:** 0.5 mg, 1 mg, 2 mg	Petit mal, akinetic, myoclonic, absence seizures	**A:** 1.5–20 mg/day	CNS depression, sedation, ataxia, confusion, depression, behavior disorders

Fosphenytoin (p. 520) (Cerebyx)	**I:** 50 mg PE/ml	Status epilepticus, seizures occurring during neurosurgery	**A:** 15–20 mg PE/kg bolus, then 4–6 mg PE/kg/day maintenance	Burning, itching, paresthesia, nystagmus, ataxia
Gabapentin (p. 528) (Neurontin)	**C:** 100 mg, 300 mg, 400 mg	Partial seizures with and without secondary generalization	**A:** 900–1,800 mg/day	CNS depression, fatigue, drowsiness, dizziness, ataxia, nystagmus, blurred vision, confusion
Lamotrigine (p. 661) (Lamictal)	**T:** 25 mg, 100 mg, 150 mg, 200 mg **T (ER):** 25 mg, 50 mg, 100 mg, 200 mg **T (ODT):** 25 mg, 50 mg, 100 mg, 200 mg	Partial seizures Primary generalized tonic-clonic seizures Generalized seizures of Lennox-Gastaut syndrome	**A:** 100–600 mg/day	Dizziness, ataxia, drowsiness, diplopia, nausea, rash, headache, vomiting, insomnia, incoordination
Levetiracetam (p. 681) (Keppra)	**T:** 250 mg, 500 mg, 750 mg, 2,000 mg **S:** 100 mg/ml	Adjunctive therapy, partial seizures, primary tonic-clonic seizures, myoclonic seizures	**A:** 1,000–3,000 mg/day	Dizziness, drowsiness, weakness, irritability, hallucinations, psychosis
Oxcarbazepine (p. 877) (Trileptal)	**T:** 150 mg, 300 mg, 600 mg	Partial seizures	**A:** 900–1,800 mg/day	Drowsiness, dizziness, headaches, diplopia, ataxia, nausea, vomiting
Phenobarbital (p. 923)	**T:** 30 mg, 60 mg, 100 mg **I:** 65 mg, 130 mg	Tonic-clonic, partial seizures; status epilepticus	**A (PO):** 100–300 mg/day; **(IM/IV):** 200–600 mg **C (PO):** 3–5 mg/kg/day; **(IM/IV):** 100–400 mg	CNS depression, sedation, paradoxical excitement and hyperactivity, rash
Phenytoin (p. 929) (Dilantin)	**C:** 100 mg **T (chewable):** 50 mg **S:** 125 mg/5 ml **I:** 50 mg/ml	Tonic-clonic, psychomotor seizures	**A (PO):** 300–600 mg/day; **IV:** 150–250 mg **C (PO):** 4–8 mg/kg/day; **(IV):** 10–15 mg/kg	Nystagmus, ataxia, hypertrichosis, gingival hyperplasia, rash, osteomalacia, lymphadenopathy
Pregabalin (p. 960) (Lyrica)	**C:** 25 mg, 50 mg, 75 mg, 100 mg, 150 mg, 200 mg, 225 mg, 300 mg	Adjunctive therapy, partial seizures	**A:** 150–600 mg/day	Confusion, drowsiness, dizziness, ataxia, weight gain, dry mouth, blurred vision, peripheral edema

(continued)

ANTICONVULSANTS *(continued)*

Name	Availability	Uses	Dosage Range	Side Effects
Primidone (p. 962) (Mysoline)	**T:** 50 mg, 250 mg **S:** 250 mg/5 ml	Complex partial, akinetic, tonic-clonic seizures	**A:** 750–2,000 mg/day **C:** 10–25 mg/kg/day	CNS depression, sedation, paradoxical excitement and hyperactivity, rash, dizziness, ataxia
Tiagabine (p. 1128) (Gabitril)	**T:** 4 mg, 12 mg, 16 mg, 20 mg	Partial seizures	**A:** Initially, 4 mg up to 56 mg **C:** Initially, 4 mg up to 32 mg	Dizziness, asthenia, nervousness, anxiety, tremors, abdominal pain
Topiramate (p. 1149) (Topamax)	**T:** 25 mg, 100 mg, 200 mg	Partial seizures	**A:** 25–400 mg/day **C:** 1–9 mg/kg/day	Drowsiness, dizziness, headache, ataxia, confusion, weight loss, diplopia
Valproic acid (p. 1187) (Depakene, Depakote)	**C:** 250 mg **S:** 250 mg/5 ml **Sprinkles:** 125 mg **T:** 125 mg, 250 mg, 500 mg **T (ER):** 500 mg **I:** 100 mg/ml	Complex partial, absence seizures	**A, C:** 15–60 mg/kg/day	Nausea, vomiting, tremors, thrombocytopenia, hair loss, hepatic dysfunction, weight gain, decreased platelet function
Vigabatrin (Sabril)	**T:** 500 mg **PS:** 500 mg	Infantile spasms, refractory complex partial seizures	**A:** 1,000–4,000 mg/day **C:** 40–100 mg/kg/day	Vision changes, eye pain, abdominal pain, agitation, confusion, mood/mental changes, abnormal coordination
Zonisamide (p. 1237) (Zonegran)	**C:** 100 mg	Partial seizures	**A:** 500 mg/day	Drowsiness, dizziness, anorexia, diarrhea, weight loss, agitation, irritability, rash, nausea

A, Adults; ***C,*** capsules; ***C** (dosage),* children; ***ER,*** extended-release; ***I,*** injection; ***ODT,*** orally-disintegrating tablets; ***PE,*** phenytoin equivalent; ***PS,*** powder sachet; ***R,*** rectal; ***S,*** suspension; ***T,*** tablets.

Antidepressants

USES

Used primarily for the treatment of depression. Depression can be chronic or recurrent mental disorder presenting with symptoms such as depressed mood, loss of interest or pleasure, guilt feelings, disturbed sleep/appetite, low energy, and difficulty in thinking. Depression can also lead to suicide.

ACTION

Antidepressants include tricyclics, monoamine oxidase inhibitors (MAOIs), selective serotonin reuptake inhibitors (SSRIs), serotonin-norepinephrine reuptake inhibitors (SNRIs), and other antidepressants. Depression may be due to reduced functioning of monoamine neurotransmitters (e.g., norepinephrine, serotonin [5-HT], dopamine) in the CNS (decreased amount and/or decreased effects at the receptor sites). Antidepressants block metabolism, increase amount/effects of monoamine neurotransmitters, and act at receptor sites (change responsiveness/sensitivities of both presynaptic and postsynaptic receptor sites).

ANTIDEPRESSANTS

Name	Availability	Uses	Dosage Range (per day)	Side Effects
Tricyclics				
Amitriptyline (p. 54) (Elavil)	**T:** 10 mg, 25 mg, 50 mg, 75 mg, 100 mg, 150 mg	Depression, neuropathic pain	40–300 mg	Drowsiness, blurred vision, constipation, confusion, postural hypotension, cardiac conduction defects, weight gain, seizures
Clomipramine (p. 258) (Anafranil)	**C:** 25 mg, 50 mg, 75 mg	OCD	25–250 mg	Same as amitriptyline
Desipramine (p. 325) (Norpramin)	**T:** 10 mg, 25 mg, 50 mg, 75 mg, 100 mg, 150 mg	Depression, neuropathic pain	25–100 mg	Same as amitriptyline

(continued)

ANTIDEPRESSANTS ***(continued)***

Name	Availability	Uses	Dosage Range (per day)	Side Effects
Doxepin (p. 382) (Sinequan)	**C:** 10 mg, 25 mg, 50 mg, 75 mg, 100 mg, 150 mg **OC:** 10 mg/ml	Depression, anxiety, neuropathic pain	25–300 mg	Same as amitriptyline
Imipramine (p. 603) (Tofranil)	**T:** 10 mg, 25 mg, 50 mg **C:** 75 mg, 100 mg, 125 mg, 150 mg	Depression, enuresis, neuropathic pain, panic disorder, ADHD	30–300 mg	Same as amitriptyline
Nortriptyline (p. 848) (Aventyl, Pamelor)	**C:** 10 mg, 25 mg, 50 mg, 75 mg **S:** 10 mg/5 ml	Depression, neuropathic pain, smoking cessation	25–100 mg	Same as amitriptyline
Monoamine Oxidase Inhibitors				
Phenelzine (p. 922) (Nardil)	**T:** 15 mg	Depression	15–90 mg	Sedation, hypertensive crisis, weight gain, orthostatic hypotension
Tranylcypromine (p. 1162) (Parnate)	**T:** 10 mg	Depression	30–60 mg	Same as phenelzine

Selective Serotonin Reuptake Inhibitors

Citalopram (p. 245) (Celexa)	**T:** 20 mg, 40 mg **S:** 10 mg/5 ml	Depression, OCD, panic disorder	25–60 mg	Insomnia or sedation, nausea, agitation, headaches
Escitalopram (p. 436) (Lexapro)	**T:** 5 mg, 10 mg, 20 mg	Depression, GAD	10–20 mg	Insomnia or sedation, nausea, agitation, headaches
Fluoxetine (p. 497) (Prozac)	**C:** 10 mg, 20 mg, 40 mg **T:** 10 mg **S:** 20 mg/5 ml	Depression, OCD, bulimia, panic disorder, anorexia, bipolar disorder, premenstrual syndrome	10–80 mg	Akathisia, sexual dysfunction, skin rash, urticaria, pruritus, decreased appetite, asthenia, diarrhea, drowsiness, headaches, diaphoresis, insomnia, nausea, tremors
Fluvoxamine (p. 508) (Luvox, Luvox CR)	**T:** 25 mg, 50 mg, 100 mg **C (SR):** 100 mg, 150 mg	OCD, SAD	100–300 mg	Sexual dysfunction, fatigue, constipation, dizziness, drowsiness, headaches, insomnia, nausea, vomiting
Paroxetine (p. 899) (Paxil)	**T:** 10 mg, 20 mg, 30 mg, 40 mg **S:** 10 mg/5 ml	Depression, OCD, panic attack, SAD	20–50 mg	Asthenia, constipation, diarrhea, diaphoresis, insomnia, nausea, sexual dysfunction, tremors, vomiting, urinary frequency or retention
Sertraline (p. 1052) (Zoloft)	**T:** 25 mg, 50 mg, 100 mg **S:** 20 mg/ml	Depression, OCD, panic attack	50–200 mg	Sexual dysfunction, dizziness, drowsiness, anorexia, diarrhea, nausea, dry mouth, abdominal cramps, decreased weight, headaches, increased diaphoresis, tremors, insomnia

(continued)

ANTIDEPRESSANTS ***(continued)***

Name	Availability	Uses	Dosage Range (per day)	Side Effects
Serotonin-Norepinephrine Reuptake Inhibitors				
Desvenlafaxine (p. 330) (Pristiq)	**T:** 50 mg, 100 mg	Depression	50–100 mg	Nausea, dizziness, insomnia, hyperhidrosis, constipation, drowsiness, decreased appetite, anxiety, male sexual function disorders
Duloxetine (p. 394) (Cymbalta)	**C:** 20 mg, 30 mg, 60 mg	Depression, fibromyalgia, neuropathic pain	40–60 mg	Nausea, dry mouth, constipation, decreased appetite, fatigue, diaphoresis
Venlafaxine (p. 1198) (Effexor)	**T:** 25 mg, 37.5 mg, 50 mg, 75 mg, 100 mg **T (ER):** 37.5 mg, 75 mg, 150 mg	Depression, anxiety	75–375 mg	Increased blood pressure, agitation, sedation, insomnia, nausea
Other				
Bupropion (p. 151) (Wellbutrin)	**T:** 75 mg, 100 mg **SR:** 100 mg, 150 mg	Depression, smoking cessation, ADHD, bipolar disorder	150–450 mg	Insomnia, irritability, seizures
Mirtazapine (p. 778) (Remeron)	**T:** 15 mg, 30 mg, 45 mg	Depression	15–45 mg	Sedation, dry mouth, weight gain, agranulocytosis, hepatic toxicity
Trazodone (p. 1166) (Desyrel)	**T:** 50 mg, 100 mg, 150 mg, 300 mg	Depression	50–600 mg	Sedation, orthostatic hypotension, priapism

ADHD, Attention deficit hyperactivity disorder; ***C,*** capsules; ***ER,*** extended-release; ***GAD,*** generalized anxiety disorder; ***OC,*** oral concentrate; ***OCD,*** obsessive-compulsive disorder; ***S,*** suspension; ***SAD,*** social anxiety disorder; ***SR,*** sustained-release; ***T,*** tablets.

Antidiabetics

USES

Insulin: Treatment of insulin-dependent diabetes (type 1) and non–insulin-dependent diabetes (type 2). Also used in acute situations such as ketoacidosis, severe infections, major surgery in otherwise non–insulin-dependent diabetics. Administered to pts receiving parenteral nutrition. Drug of choice during pregnancy. All insulins, including long-acting insulins, can cause hypoglycemia and weight gain.

Sulfonylureas: Adjunct to diet and exercise for management of type 2 diabetes mellitus.

Alpha-glucosidase inhibitors: Adjunct to diet and exercise for management of type 2 diabetes mellitus.

Biguanides: Adjunct to diet and exercise for management of type 2 diabetes mellitus.

Thiazolinediones: Adjunct to diet and exercise for management of type 2 diabetes mellitus.

Dipeptidyl Peptidase 4 inhibitors (DPP-4): Adjunct to diet and exercise for management of type 2 diabetes mellitus.

Meglitinide: Adjunct to diet and exercise for management of type 2 diabetes mellitus.

ACTION

Insulin: A hormone synthesized and secreted by beta cells of Langerhans' islet in the pancreas. Controls storage and utilization of glucose, amino acids, and fatty acids by activated transport systems/enzymes. Inhibits breakdown of glycogen, fat, protein. Insulin lowers blood glucose by inhibiting glycogenolysis and gluconeogenesis in liver; stimulates glucose uptake by muscle, adipose tissue. Activity of insulin is initiated by binding to cell surface receptors.

Sulfonylureas: Stimulate release of insulin from beta cells of the pancreas.

Alpha-glucosidase inhibitors: Work locally in small intestine, slowing carbohydrate breakdown and glucose absorption.

Biguanides: Inhibit hepatic gluconeogenesis, glycogenolysis; enhance insulin sensitivity in muscle and fat.

Thiazolinediones: Enhance insulin sensitivity in muscle and fat.

DPP-4: Inhibits degradation of endogenous incretins, which increases insulin secretion, decreases glucagon secretion.

Meglitinide: Stimulates pancreatic insulin secretion.

Antidiabetics *(continued)*

ANTIDIABETICS

INSULIN (p. 615)

Type	Onset	Peak	Duration	Comments
Rapid Acting				
Apidra, glulisine	10–15 min	1–1.5 hrs	3–5 hrs	Stable at room temp for 28 days Can mix with NPH
Humalog, lispro	15–30 min	0.5–2.5 hrs	6–8 hrs	Stable at room temp for 28 days Can mix with NPH
Novolog, aspart	10–20 min	1–3 hrs	3–5 hrs	Stable at room temp for 28 days Can mix with NPH
Short Acting				
Humulin R, Novolin R, regular	30–60 min	1–5 hrs	6–10 hrs	Stable at room temp for 28 days Can mix with NPH
Intermediate Acting				
Humulin N, Novolin N, NPH	1–2 hrs	6–14 hrs	16–24 hrs	Stable at room temp for 28 days Can mix with aspart, lispro, glulisine
Long Acting				
Lantus, glargine	1.1 hrs	No significant peak	24 hrs	Do NOT mix with other insulins Stable at room temp for 28 days
Levemir, detemir	0.8–2 hrs	Relatively flat	12–24 hrs (dose dependent)	Do NOT mix with other insulins Stable at room temp for 42 days

Oral Agents

Name	Availability	Dosage Range	Side Effects
Sulfonylureas			
Chlorpropamide (Diabinese)	**T:** 100 mg, 250 mg	100–500 mg/day	Hypoglycemia, weight gain, skin rash, hemolytic anemia, GI distress, cholestasis
Glimepiride (p. 547) (Amaryl)	**T:** 1 mg, 2 mg, 4 mg	1–8 mg/day	Hypoglycemia, weight gain
Glipizide (p. 548) (Glucotrol)	**T:** 5 mg, 10 mg **T (XL):** 5 mg	**T:** 2.5–40 mg/day **XL:** 5–20 mg/day	Same as glimepiride
Glyburide (p. 552) (DiaBeta, Micronase)	**T:** 1.25 mg, 2.5 mg, 5 mg **PT:** 1.5 mg, 3 mg	**T:** 1.25–20 mg/day **PT:** 1–12 mg/day	Same as glimepiride
Alpha-Glucosidase Inhibitors			
Acarbose (p. 8) (Precose)	**T:** 25 mg, 50 mg, 100 mg	75–300 mg/day	Flatulence, diarrhea, abdominal pain, increased risk of hypoglycemia when used with insulin or sulfonylureas
Miglitol (Glyset)	**T:** 25 mg, 50 mg, 100 mg	75–300 mg/day	Same as acarbose
Dipeptidyl Peptidase Inhibitors			
Saxagliptin (Onglyza)	**T:** 2.5 mg, 5 mg	2.5–5 mg/day	Upper respiratory tract infection, urinary tract infection, headache
Sitagliptin (p. 1063) (Januvia)	**T:** 25 mg, 50 mg, 100 mg	25–100 mg/day	Nasopharyngitis, upper respiratory infection, headaches, modest weight gain, increased incidence of hypoglycemia when added to a sulfonylurea
Biguanides			
Metformin (p. 741) (Glucophage)	**T:** 500 mg, 850 mg **XR:** 500 mg	**T:** 0.5–2.5 g/day **XR:** 1,500–2,000 mg/day	Nausea, vomiting, diarrhea, loss of appetite, metallic taste, lactic acidosis (rare but potentially fatal complication)

(continued)

ANTIDIABETICS ***(continued)***

Name	Availability	Dosage Range	Side Effects
Glucagon-Like Receptor Agonists			
Liraglutide (Victoza)	**I:** 0.6 mg, 1.2 mg, 1.8 mg (6 mg/ml)	0.6–1.8 mg/day	Headache, nausea, diarrhea
Meglitinides			
Nateglinide (p. 815) (Starlix)	**T:** 60 mg, 120 mg	60–120 mg 3 times/day	Hypoglycemia, weight gain
Repaglinide (p. 1009) (Prandin)	**T:** 0.5 mg, 1 mg, 2 mg	0.5–1 mg with each meal (**Maximum:** 16 mg/day)	Same as nateglinide
Thiazolidinediones			
Pioglitazone (p. 934) (Actos)	**T:** 15 mg, 30 mg, 45 mg	15–45 mg/day	Mild to moderate peripheral edema, weight gain, increased risk of CHF, associated with reduced bone mineral density and increased incidence of fractures
Rosiglitazone (p. 1036) (Avandia)	**T:** 2 mg, 4 mg, 8 mg	4–8 mg/day	Same as pioglitazone
Miscellaneous			
Bromocriptine (Cycloset)	**T:** 0.8 mg	1.6–4.8 mg/day	Nausea, fatigue, dizziness, vomiting
Exenatide (p. 459) (Byetta)	**I:** 5 mcg, 10 mcg	5–10 mcg 2 times/day	Diarrhea, dizziness, dyspnea, headaches, nausea, vomiting
Pramlintide (p. 951) (Symlin)	**I:** 0.6 mg/ml	15–60 mcg immediately prior to meals	Abdominal pain, anorexia, headaches, nausea, vomiting, severe hypoglycemia may occur when used in combination with insulin (reduction in dosages of short-acting, including premixed, insulins recommended)

CHF, Congestive heart failure; ***I,*** injection; ***PT,*** Prestab; ***T,*** tablets; ***XL,*** extended-release; ***XR,*** extended-release.

Antidiarrheals

USES	ACTION	
Acute diarrhea, chronic diarrhea of inflammatory bowel disease, reduction of fluid from ileostomies.	*Systemic agents:* Act as smooth muscle receptors (enteric) disrupting peristaltic movements, decreasing GI motility, increasing transit time of intestinal contents.	*Local agents:* Adsorb toxic substances and fluids to large surface areas of particles in the preparation. Some of these agents coat and protect irritated intestinal walls. May have local anti-inflammatory action.

ANTIDIARRHEALS

Name	Availability	Type	Dosage Range
Bismuth (p. 130) (Pepto-Bismol)	**T**: 262 mg **C**: 262 mg **L**: 130 mg/15 ml, 262 mg/15 ml, 524 mg/15 ml	Local	**A**: 2 **T** or 30 ml **C (9–12 yrs)**: 1 **T** or 15 ml **C (6–8 yrs)**: 2/3 **T** or 10 ml **C (3–5 yrs)**: 1/3 **T** or 5 ml
Diphenoxylate with atropine (p. 362) (Lomotil)	**T**: 2.5 mg **L**: 2.5 mg/5 ml	Systemic	**A**: 5 mg 4 times/day **C**: 0.3–0.4 mg/kg/day in 4 divided doses **(L)**
Kaolin (with pectin) (Kaopectate)	**S**: 262 mg/15 ml, 525 mg/15 ml	Local	**A**: 60–120 ml after each bowel movement **C (6–12 yrs)**: 30–60 ml **C (3–5 yrs)**: 15–30 ml
Loperamide (p. 701) (Imodium)	**C**: 2 mg **T**: 2 mg **L**: 1 mg/5 ml, 1 mg/ml	Systemic	**A**: Initially, 4 mg (**Maximum:** 16 mg/day) **C (9–12 yrs)**: 2 mg 3 times/day **C (6–8 yrs)**: 2 mg 2 times/day **C (2–5 yrs)**: 1 mg 3 times/day **(L)**

A, Adults; ***C,*** capsules; ***C** (dosage),* children; ***L,*** liquid; ***S,*** suspension; ***T,*** tablets.

Antifungals: Systemic Mycoses

Systemic mycoses are subdivided into opportunistic infections (*candidiasis*, *aspergillosis*, *cryptococcosis*, and *mucomycosis*) that are seen primarily in debilitated or immunocompromised hosts and nonopportunistic infections (*blastomycosis*, *histoplasmosis*, and *coccidioidomycosis*) that occur in any host. Treatment can be difficult because these infections often resist treatment and may require prolonged therapy.

ANTIFUNGALS: SYSTEMIC MYCOSES

Name	Indications	Side Effects
Amphotericin B (p. 61)	Potentially life-threatening fungal infections, including aspergillosis, blastomycosis, coccidioidomycosis, Cryptococcus, histoplasmosis, systemic candidiasis	Fever, chills, headache, nausea, vomiting, nephrotoxicity, hypokalemia, hypomagnesemia, hypotension, dyspnea, arrhythmias, abdominal pain, diarrhea, increased hepatic function tests
Amphotericin B lipid complex (Abelcet) (p. 61)	Invasive fungal infections	Same as amphotericin B
Amphotericin B liposomal (AmBisome) (p. 61)	Empiric therapy for presumed fungal infections in febrile neutropenic pts, treatment of cryptococcal meningitis in HIV-infected pts, treatment of aspergillosis, candida, Cryptococcus infections, treatment of visceral leishmaniasis	Same as amphotericin B
Amphotericin colloidal dispersion (Amphotec) (p. 61)	Invasive aspergillosis	Same as amphotericin B

Anidulafungin (Eraxis) (p. 69)	Candidemia, esophageal candidiasis	Diarrhea, hypokalemia, increased hepatic function tests, headache
Caspofungin (Cancidas) (p. 185)	Candidimia, invasive aspergillosis, empiric therapy for presumed fungal infections in febrile neutropenic pts	Headache, nausea, vomiting, diarrhea, increased hepatic function tests
Fluconazole (Diflucan) (p. 487)	Treatment of vaginal candidiasis, oropharyngeal, esophageal candidiasis and cryptococcal meningitis. Prophylaxis to decrease incidence of candidiasis in pts undergoing bone marrow transplant receiving cytotoxic chemotherapy and/or radiation	Nausea, vomiting, abdominal pain, diarrhea, dysgeusia, increased hepatic function tests, liver necrosis, hepatitis, cholestasis, headache, rash, pruritus, eosinophilia, alopecia
Itraconazole (Sporanox) (p. 642)	Blastomycosis, histoplasmosis, aspergillosis, onychomycosis, empiric therapy of febrile neutropenic pts with suspected fungal infections, treatment of oropharyngeal and esophageal candidiasis	Congestive heart failure, peripheral edema, nausea, vomiting, abdominal pain, diarrhea, increased hepatic function tests, liver necrosis, hepatitis, cholestasis, headache, rash, pruritus, eosinophilia
Ketoconazole (Nizoral) (p. 648)	Candidiasis, chronic mucocutaneous candidiasis, oral thrush, candiduria, blastomycosis, coccidiodomycosis	Nausea, vomiting, abdominal pain, diarrhea, gynecomastia, increased hepatic function tests, liver necrosis, hepatitis, cholestasis, headache, rash, pruritus, eosinophilia
Micafungin (Mycamine) (p. 765)	Esophageal candidiasis, candida infections, prophylaxis in pts undergoing hematopoietin stem cell transplantation	Fever, chills, hypokalemia, hypomagnesemia, hypocalcemia, myelosuppression, thrombocytopenia, nausea, vomiting, abdominal pain, diarrhea, increased hepatic function tests, dizziness, headache, rash, pruritus, pain or inflammation at injection site, fever
Posaconazole (Noxafil) (p. 944)	Prevent invasive aspergillosis and candida infections in pts 13 yrs and older who are immunocompromised, treatment of oropharyngeal candidiasis	Fever, headaches, nausea, vomiting, diarrhea, abdominal pain, hypokalemia, cough, dyspnea
Voriconazole (Vfend) (p. 1218)	Invasive aspergillosis, candidemia, esophageal candidiasis, serious fungal infections	Visual disturbances, nausea, vomiting, abdominal pain, diarrhea, increased hepatic function tests, liver necrosis, hepatitis, cholestasis, headache, rash, pruritus, eosinophilia

Antifungals: Topical

USES

Treatment of tinea infections, cutaneous candidiasis (moniliasis) due to *Candida albicans.*

ACTION

Exact mechanism unknown. May deplete essential intracellular components by inhibiting transport of potassium, other ions into cells; alter membrane permeability, resulting in loss of potassium, other cellular components.

ANTIFUNGALS: TOPICAL

Name	Availability	Dosage Range	Side Effects
Butenafine (Mentax)	**C:** 1%	2 times/day	Burning, stinging, pruritus, contact dermatitis, erythema
Ciclopirox (Loprox)	**C:** 1% **L:** 1%	2 times/day	Irritation, pruritus, redness
Clioquinol (Vioform)	**C:** 3% **O:** 3%	2–3 times/day	Irritation, stinging, swelling
Clotrimazole (p. 266) (Lotrimin, Mycelex)	**C:** 1% **L:** 1% **S:** 1%	2 times/day	Erythema, stinging, blistering, edema, pruritus
Econazole (Spectazole)	**C:** 1%	1–2 times/day	Burning, stinging, irritation, erythema
Ketoconazole (p. 648) (Nizoral)	**C:** 2%	1–2 times/day	Irritation, pruritus, stinging
Miconazole (p. 766) (Micatin, Monistat)	**C:** 2% **P:** 2%	2 times/day	Irritation, burning, allergic contact dermatitis

Nystatin (p. 850) (Mycostatin, Nilstat)	**C:** 100,000 g **O:** 100,000 g **P:** 100,000 g	2–3 times/day	Irritation
Oxiconazole (Oxistat)	**C:** 1% **L:** 1%	1–2 times/day	Pruritus, burning, stinging, irritation, pain, tingling
Sertaconazole (Ertaczo)	**C:** 2%	2 times/day	Dry skin, burning, pruritus, erythema
Terbinafine (p. 1109) (Lamisil)	**C:** 1% **G:** 10 mg	1–2 times/day	Irritation, burning, pruritus, dryness
Tolnaftate (Tinactin)	**C:** 1% **G:** 1% **S:** 1%	2 times/day	Mild irritation
Triacetin (Fungoid)	**C:** 1% **S:** 1%	3 times/day	Irritation
Undecylenic acid (Caldesene, Cruex, Desenex)	**C:** 8%, 20% **P:** 10%, 12%, 15%, 19%, 25% **O:** 25%	As needed	None significant

C, Cream; ***G,*** gel; ***L,*** lotion; ***O,*** ointment; ***P,*** powder; ***S,*** solution.

Antiglaucoma Agents

USES

Reduction of elevated intraocular pressure (IOP) in pts with open-angle glaucoma and ocular hypertension.

ACTION

Medications decrease IOP by two primary mechanisms: decreasing aqueous humor (AH) production or increasing AH outflow.

- *Miotics (direct acting and indirect acting):* Constrict pupils, opening channels in the trabecular meshwork, reducing resistance to outflow of AH.
- *Alpha$_2$-agonists:* Activate receptors in ciliary body, inhibiting aqueous secretion and increasing uveoscleral aqueous outflow.
- *Beta-blockers:* Reduce production of aqueous humor.
- *Carbonic anhydrase inhibitors:* Decrease production of AH by inhibiting enzyme carbonic anhydrase.
- *Prostaglandins:* Increase outflow of aqueous fluid through uveoscleral route.

ANTIGLAUCOMA AGENTS

Name	Availability	Dosage Range	Side Effects
Miotics			
Carbachol (Miostat)	**S:** 0.01%	1 ml to anterior chamber of eye	Ciliary or accommodative spasm, blurred vision, reduced night vision, diaphoresis, increased salivation, urinary frequency, nausea, diarrhea
Echothiophate (Phospholine Iodide)	**S:** 0.03%, 0.06%, 0.125%, 0.25%	1 drop 2 times/day	Headaches, accommodative spasm, diaphoresis, vomiting, nausea, diarrhea, tachycardia
Pilocarpine (Pilipine HS)	**G:** 4%	½ inch ribbon on lower conjunctiva at bedtime	Same as carbachol

Alpha$_2$-Agonists			
Apraclonidine (Iopidine)	**S:** 0.5%	1–2 drops 3 times/day	Hypersensitivity reaction, change in visual acuity, lethargy
Brimonidine (Alphagan)	**S:** 0.1%, 0.15%, 0.2%	1 drop 2–3 times/day	Hypersensitivity reaction, headaches, drowsiness, fatigue
Prostaglandins			
Bimatoprost (Lumigan)	**S:** 0.03%	1 drop daily in evening	Ocular hyperemia, eyelash growth, pruritus
Latanoprost (Xalatan)	**S:** 0.005%	1 drop daily in evening	Burning, stinging, iris pigmentation
Travoprost (Travatan)	**S:** 0.004%	1 drop daily in evening	Ocular hyperemia, eye discomfort, foreign body sensation, pain, pruritus

(continued)

ANTIGLAUCOMA AGENTS ***(continued)***

Name	Availability	Dosage Range	Side Effects
Beta-Blockers			
Betaxolol (Betoptic, Betoptic-S)	**Suspension (Betoptic-S):** 0.25% **S: (Betoptic)** 0.5%	Betoptic-S: 1 drop 2 times/day Betoptic: 1–2 drops 2 times/day	Transient irritation, burning, tearing, blurred vision
Carteolol (Ocupress)	**S:** 1%	1 drop 2 times/day	Mild, transient ocular stinging, burning, discomfort
Levobunolol (Betagan)	**S:** 0.25%, 0.5%	1–2 drops 1–2 times/day	Local discomfort, conjunctivitis, brow ache, tearing, blurred vision, headaches, anxiety
Metipranolol (OptiPranolol)	**S:** 0.3%	1 drop 2 times/day	Transient irritation, burning, stinging, blurred vision
Timolol (p. 1133) (Betimol, Istalol, Timoptic, Timoptic XE)	**S:** 0.25%, 0.5% **G, Timoptic XE:** 0.25%, 0.5%	**S:** 1 drop 2 times/day (Istalol): 1 drop daily **G:** 1 drop daily	Drowsiness, difficulty sleeping, fatigue, weakness
Carbonic Anhydrase Inhibitors			
Acetazolamide (p. 12) (Diamox)	**T:** 250 mg **C:** 500 mg	0.25–1 g/day	Diarrhea, loss of appetite, metallic taste, nausea, paresthesia
Brinzolamide (Azopt)	**Suspension:** 1%	1 drop 3 times/day	Blurred vision, bitter taste
Dorzolamide (Trusopt)	**S:** 2%	1 drop 3 times/day	Burning, stinging, blurred vision, bitter taste

C, Capsules; ***G,*** gel; ***O,*** ointment; ***S,*** solution; ***T,*** tablets.

Antihistamines

USES

Symptomatic relief of upper respiratory allergic disorders. Allergic reactions associated with other drugs respond to antihistamines, as do blood transfusion reactions. Used as a second-choice drug in treatment of angioneurotic edema. Effective in treatment of acute urticaria and other dermatologic conditions. May also be used for preop sedation, Parkinson's disease, and motion sickness.

ACTION

Antihistamines (H_1 antagonists) inhibit vasoconstrictor effects and vasodilator effects on endothelial cells of histamine. They block increased capillary permeability, formation of edema/wheal caused by histamine. Many antihistamines can bind to receptors in CNS, causing primarily depression (decreased alertness, slowed reaction times, drowsiness) but also stimulation (restlessness, nervousness, inability to sleep). Some may counter motion sickness.

ANTIHISTAMINES

Name	Availability	Dosage Range	Side Effects
Azatadine (Optimine)	**T:** 1 mg	**A:** 1–2 mg q12h **C:** 0.05 mg/kg/day	Dry mouth, urinary retention, blurred vision, sedation, dizziness, paradoxical excitement
Brompheniramine (Brovex)	**T:** 4 mg **T (SR):** 4 mg, 6 mg **S:** 2 mg/5 ml	**A:** 4–8 mg q4–6h or **T (SR):** 8–12 mg q12–24h **C:** 0.5 mg/kg/day	Dry mouth, urinary retention, blurred vision
Cetirizine (p. 219) (Zyrtec)	**T:** 5 mg, 10 mg **S:** 5 mg/5 ml	**A:** 5–10 mg/day **C (6–12 yrs):** 5–10 mg/day **C (2–5 yrs):** 2.5–5 mg/day	Minimal CNS and anticholinergic side effects

(continued)

ANTIHISTAMINES *(continued)*

Name	Availability	Dosage Range	Side Effects
Chlorpheniramine (Chlor-Trimeton)	**T:** 4 mg **T (chewable):** 2 mg **T (SR):** 8 mg, 12 mg **S:** 2 mg/5 ml	**A:** 2–4 mg q4–6h or **SR:** 8–12 mg q12–24h **C:** 0.35 mg/kg/day	Same as brompheniramine
Clemastine (p. 250) (Tavist Allergy)	**T:** 1.34 mg, 2.68 mg **S:** 0.67 mg/5 ml	**A:** 1.34–2.68 mg q8–12h **C (6–12 yrs):** 0.67–1.34 mg q8–12h	Same as azatadine
Cyproheptadine (Periactin)	**T:** 4 mg **S:** 2 mg/5 ml	**A:** 4 mg q8h **C:** 0.25 mg/kg/day	Same as azatadine
Dexchlorpheniramine (Polaramine)	**T:** 2 mg **S:** 2 mg/5 ml	**A:** 2 mg q4–6h **C:** 0.5–1 mg q4–6h	Same as brompheniramine
Dimenhydrinate (p. 357) (Dramamine)	**T:** 50 mg **L:** 12.5 mg/5 ml	**A:** 50–100 mg q4–6h **C:** 12.5–50 mg q6–8h	Same as azatadine
Diphenhydramine (p. 360) (Benadryl)	**T:** 25 mg, 50 mg **C:** 25 mg, 50 mg **L:** 6.25 mg/5 ml, 12.5 mg/5 ml	**A:** 25–50 mg q6–8h **C (6–11 yrs):** 12.5–25 mg q4–6h **C (2–5 yrs):** 6.25 mg q4–6h	Same as azatadine
Fexofenadine (p. 480) (Allegra)	**T:** 30 mg, 60 mg, 180 mg	**A:** 60 mg q12h or 180 mg/day **C (6–11 yrs):** 30 mg q12h	Same as cetirizine
Hydroxyzine (p. 584) (Atarax)	**T:** 10 mg, 25 mg, 50 mg, 100 mg **C:** 25 mg, 50 mg, 100 mg **S:** 10 mg/5 ml, 25 mg/5 ml	**A:** 25 mg q6–8h **C:** 2 mg/kg/day	Same as azatadine
Levocetirizine (p. 683) (Xyzal)	**T:** 5 mg	**A, C (12 yrs and older):** 5 mg once daily in evening **C (6–11 yrs):** 2.5 mg once daily in evening	Same as cetirizine

Loratadine (p. 705) **(Claritin)**	**T**: 10 mg **S**: 1 mg/ml	**A**: 10 mg/day **C (6–12 yrs)**: 10 mg/day	Same as cetirizine
Promethazine (p. 972) **(Phenergan)**	**T**: 12.5 mg, 25 mg, 50 mg **S**: 6.25 mg/5 ml, 25 mg/5 ml	**A**: 25 mg at bedtime or 12.5 mg q8h **C**: 0.5 mg/kg at bedtime or 0.1 mg/kg q6–8h	Same as azatadine

A, Adults; ***C,*** capsules; ***C (dosage),*** children; ***L,*** liquid; ***S,*** syrup; ***SR,*** sustained-release; ***T,*** tablets.

Antihyperlipidemics

USES	ACTION
Cholesterol management.	*Bile acid sequestrants:* Bind bile acids in the intestine; prevent active transport and reabsorption and enhance bile acid excretion. Depletion of hepatic bile acid results in the increased conversion of cholesterol to bile acids. *HMG-CoA reductase inhibitors (statins):* Inhibit HMG-CoA reductase, the last regulated step in the synthesis of cholesterol. Cholesterol synthesis in the liver is reduced. *Niacin (nicotinic acid):* Reduces hepatic synthesis of triglycerides and secretion of VLDL by inhibiting the mobilization of free fatty acids from peripheral tissues. *Fibric acid:* Increases the oxidation of fatty acids in the liver, resulting in reduced secretion of triglyceride-rich lipoproteins, and increases lipoprotein lipase activity and fatty acid uptake. *Cholesterol absorption inhibitor:* Acts in the gut wall to prevent cholesterol absorption through the intestinal villi.

Antihyperlipidemics *(continued)*

ANTIHYPERLIPIDEMICS

Name	Primary Effect	Dosage	Comments/Side Effects
Bile Acid Sequestrants			
Cholestyramine (Prevalite, Questran) (p. 230)	Decreases LDL	4 g once or twice daily	May bind drugs given concurrently. Take at least 1 hr before or 4–6 hrs after cholestyramine. **Side Effects:** Constipation, heartburn, nausea, vomiting, stomach pain
Colesevelam (Welchol)	Decreases LDL	6–7 625-mg tablets once daily or 2 divided doses with meals	Take with food. **Side Effects:** Constipation, dyspepsia, weakness, myalgia, pharyngitis
Colestipol (Colestid)	Decreases LDL	**T:** 2–16 g daily **G:** 5–30 g daily	Do not crush tablets. May bind drugs given concurrently. Take at least 1 hr before or 4–6 hrs after colestipol. **Side Effects:** Constipation, headache, dizziness, anxiety, vertigo, drowsiness, nausea, vomiting, diarrhea, flatulence
Cholesterol Absorption Inhibitor			
Ezetimibe (Zetia) (p. 460)	Decreases LDL	10 mg once daily	Administer at least 2 hrs before or 4 hrs after bile acid sequestrants. **Side Effects:** Dizziness, headache, fatigue, diarrhea, abdominal pain, arthralgia, sinusitis, pharyngitis
Fibric Acid			
Fenofibrate (Antara, Lofibra, Tricor, Triglide) (p. 467)	Decreases TG	**Antara:** 43–130 mg/day **Lofibra:** 67–200 mg/day **Tricor:** 48–145 mg/day **Triglide:** 50–160 mg/day	May increase levels of ezetimibe. Concomitant use of statins may increase rhabdomyolysis, elevate CPK levels, and cause myoglobinuria. **Side Effects:** Abdominal pain, constipation, diarrhea, respiratory complaints, headache, fever, flu-like syndrome, asthenia

Fenofibric acid (Trilipix)	Decreases TG, LDL Increases HDL	45–135 mg/day	May give without regard to meals. Concomitant use of statins may increase rhabdomyolysis. **Side Effects:** Headache, upper respiratory tract infection pain, nausea, dizziness, naopharyngitis
Gemfibrozil (Lopid) (p. 537)	Decreases TG	600 mg 2 times/day	Give 30 min before breakfast and dinner. Concomitant use of statins may increase rhabdomyolysis, elevate CPK levels, and cause myoglobinuria. **Side Effects:** Fatigue, vertigo, headache, rash, eczema, diarrhea, abdominal pain, nausea, vomiting, constipation
Niacin			
Niacin, nicotinic acid (Niacor, Niaspan) (p. 825)	Decreases LDL, TG Increases HDL	**Regular-release (Niacor):** 1.5–6 g/day in 3 divided doses **Extended-release (Niaspan):** 375 mg to 2 g once daily at bedtime	Diabetics may experience a dose-related elevation in glucose. **Side Effects:** Increased hepatic function tests, hyperglycemia, dyspepsia, itching, flushing, dizziness, insomnia
Statins			
Atorvastatin (Lipitor) (p. 93)	Decreases LDL, TG Increases HDL	10–80 mg/day	May interact with CYP3A4 inhibitors (e.g., amiodarone, diltiazem, cyclosporine, grapefruit juice) increasing risk of myopathy. **Side Effects:** Myalgia, myopathy, rhabdomyolysis, headache, chest pain, peripheral edema, dizziness, rash, abdominal pain, constipation, diarrhea, dyspepsia, nausea, flatulence, increased hepatic function tests, back pain, sinusitis

(continued)

ANTIHYPERLIPIDEMICS *(continued)*

Name	Primary Effect	Dosage	Comments/Side Effects
Fluvastatin (Lescol) (p. 507)	Decreases LDL, TG Increases HDL	20–80 mg/day	Primarily metabolized by CYP2C9 enzyme system. May increase levels of phenytoin, rifampin. May lower fluvastatin levels. **Side Effects:** Headache, fatigue, dyspepsia, diarrhea, nausea, abdominal pain, myalgia, myopathy, rhabdomyolysis
Lovastatin (Mevacor) (p. 710)	Decreases LDL, TG Increases HDL	10–80 mg/day	May interact with CYP3A4 inhibitors (e.g., amiodarone, diltiazem, cyclosporine, grapefruit juice) increasing risk of myopathy. **Side Effects:** Increased CPK levels, headache, dizziness, rash, constipation, diarrhea, abdominal pain, dyspepsia, nausea, flatulence, myalgia, myopathy, rhabdomyolysis
Pitavastatin (Livalo)	Decreases LDL, TG Increases HDL	1–4 mg/day	Erythromycin, rifampin may increase concentration. **Side Effects:** Myalgia, back pain, diarrhea, constipation, pain in extremities.
Pravastatin (Pravachol) (p. 954)	Decreases LDL, TG Increases HDL	10–80 mg/day	May be less likely to be involved in drug interactions. Cyclosporine may increase pravastatin levels. **Side Effects:** Chest pain, headache, dizziness, rash, nausea, vomiting, diarrhea, increased hepatic function tests, cough, flu-like symptoms, myalgia, myopathy, rhabdomyolysis
Rosuvastatin (Crestor) (p. 1037)	Decreases LDL, TG Increases HDL	5–40 mg/day	May be less likely to be involved in drug interactions. Cyclosporine may increase rosuvastatin levels. **Side Effects:** Chest pain, peripheral edema, headache, rash, dizziness, vertigo, pharyngitis, diarrhea, nausea, constipation, abdominal pain, dyspepsia, sinusitis, flu-like symptoms, myalgia, myopathy, rhabdomyolysis
Simvastatin (Zocor) (p. 1059)	Decreases LDL, TG Increases HDL	5–80 mg/day	May interact with CYP3A4 inhibitors (e.g., amiodarone, diltiazem, cyclosporine, grapefruit juice) increasing risk of myopathy. **Side Effects:** Constipation, flatulence, dyspepsia, increased hepatic function tests, increased CPK, upper respiratory tract infection

Antihypertensives

USES

Treatment of mild to severe hypertension.

ACTION

Many groups of medications are used in the treatment of hypertension.

ACE inhibitors: Decrease conversion of angiotensin I to angiotensin II, a potent vasoconstrictor, reducing peripheral vascular resistance and B/P.

Alpha-agonists (central action): Stimulate $alpha_2$-adrenergic receptors in the cardiovascular centers of the CNS, reducing sympathetic outflow and producing an antihypertensive effect.

Alpha-antagonists (peripheral action): Block $alpha_1$-adrenergic receptors in arterioles and veins, inhibiting vasoconstriction and decreasing peripheral vascular resistance, causing a fall in B/P.

Angiotensin receptor blockers: Block vasoconstrictor effects of angiotensin II by blocking the binding of angiotensin II to AT1 receptors in vascular smooth muscle, helping blood vessels to relax and reduce B/P.

Beta-blockers: Decrease B/P by inhibiting $beta_1$-adrenergic receptors, which lowers heart rate, heart workload, and the heart's output of blood.

Calcium channel blockers: Reduce B/P by inhibiting flow of extracellular calcium across cell membranes of vascular tissue, relaxing arterial smooth muscle.

Diuretics: Inhibit sodium (Na) reabsorption, increasing excretion of Na and water. Reduce plasma, extracellular fluid volume, and peripheral vascular resistance.

Renin inhibitors: Directly inhibits renin decreasing plasma renin activity (PRA), inhibiting conversion of angiotensinogen to angiotensin, producing antihypertensive effect.

Vasodilators: Directly relax arteriolar smooth muscle, decreasing vascular resistance. Exact mechanism unknown.

ANTIHYPERTENSIVES

Name	Availability	Dosage Range	Side Effects
(ACE) Inhibitors			
Benazepril (Lotensin)	T: 5 mg, 10 mg, 20 mg, 40 mg	10–40 mg/day	Same as enalapril

(continued)

ANTIHYPERTENSIVES *(continued)*

Name	Availability	Dosage Range	Side Effects
Enalapril (Vasotec)	**T:** 2.5 mg, 5 mg, 10 mg, 20 mg	2.5–10 mg/day	Cough, rash, hyperkalemia, hypotension (volume-depleted pts), acute renal failure, angioedema
Lisinopril (Prinivil, Zestril)	**T:** 2.5 mg, 5 mg, 10 mg, 20 mg, 30 mg, 40 mg	10–40 mg/day	Same as enalapril
Quinapril (Accupril)	**T:** 5 mg, 10 mg, 20 mg, 40 mg	10–40 mg/day	Same as enalapril
Ramipril (Altace)	**T or C:** 1.25 mg, 2.5 mg, 5 mg, 10 mg	2.5–20 mg/day	Same as enalapril
Alpha-Agonists: Central Action			
Clonidine (p. 261) (Catapres)	**T:** 0.1 mg, 0.2 mg, 0.3 mg **P:** 0.1 mg/hr, 0.2 mg/hr, 0.3 mg/hr	**PO:** 0.2–0.8 mg/day **Topical:** 0.1–0.6 mg/wk	Sedation, dry mouth, constipation, sexual dysfunction, bradycardia
Methyldopa (Aldomet)	**T:** 125 mg, 250 mg, 500 mg	**PO:** 0.5–3 g/day	Same as clonidine Impaired memory, depression, nasal congestion
Alpha-Agonists: Peripheral Action			
Doxazosin (p. 380) (Cardura)	**T:** 1 mg, 2 mg, 4 mg, 8 mg	**PO:** 2–16 mg/day	Dizziness, vertigo, headaches
Prazosin (p. 956) (Minipress)	**C:** 1 mg, 2 mg, 5 mg	**PO:** 6–20 mg/day	Dizziness, light-headedness, headaches, drowsiness
Terazosin (p. 1107) (Hytrin)	**C:** 1 mg, 2 mg, 5 mg, 10 mg	**PO:** 1–20 mg/day	Dizziness, headaches, asthenia
Angiotensin Receptor Blockers			
Candesartan (Atacand)	**T:** 4 mg, 8 mg, 16 mg, 32 mg	8–32 mg/day	Same as losartan
Losartan (Cozaar)	**T:** 25 mg, 50 mg, 100 mg	25–100 mg/day	Headache, dizziness, hyperkalemia, hypotension (volume-depleted pts), angioedema (very rare)

Olmesartan (Benicar)	**T:** 5 mg, 20 mg, 40 mg	20–40 mg/day	Same as losartan
Valsartan (Diovan)	**T:** 80 mg, 160 mg, 320 mg	80–320 mg/day	Same as losartan
Beta Blockers			
Atenolol (Tenormin)	**T:** 25 mg, 50 mg, 100 mg	25–100 mg/day	Fatigue, bradycardia, reduced exercise tolerance, increased triglycerides, bronchospasm, sexual dysfunction, masked hypoglycemia
Metoprolol (Lopressor)	**T:** 25 mg, 50 mg, 100 mg	50–200 mg/day	Same as atenolol
Metoprolol XL (Toprol XL)	**T:** 25 mg, 50 mg, 100 mg, 200 mg	50–300 mg/day	Same as atenolol
Calcium Channel Blockers			
Amlodipine (Norvasc)	**T:** 2.5 mg, 5 mg, 10 mg	2.5–10 mg/day	Headache, fatigue, peripheral edema, flushing, worsening heart failure
Diltiazem CD (Cardizem CD)	**C:** 120 mg, 180 mg, 240 mg, 300 mg	180–420 mg/day	Dizziness, headache, bradycardia, heart block, worsening heart failure, edema, constipation
Felodipine (Plendil)	**T:** 2.5 mg, 5 mg, 10 mg	2.5–20 mg/day	Same as amlodipine
Nifedipine XL (Adalat CC, Procardia XL)	**T:** 30 mg, 60 mg, 90 mg	30–120 mg/day	Same as amlodipine
Verapamil SR (Calan SR, Isoptin SR)	**T:** 120 mg, 180 mg, 240 mg	120–480 mg/day	Same as diltiazem CD
Diuretics			
Chlorthalidone (Hygroton)	**T:** 25 mg, 50 mg, 100 mg	6.25–25 mg/day	Same as hydrochlorothiazide
Hydrochlorothiazide (Hydrodiuril)	**T:** 25 mg, 50 mg	12.5–50 mg/day	Hypokalemia, hyperuricemia, hypomagnesemia, hyperglycemia

(continued)

ANTIHYPERTENSIVES ***(continued)***

Name	Availability	Dosage Range	Side Effects
Renin Inhibitor			
Aliskiren (p. 33) (Tekturna)	**T:** 150 mg, 300 mg	**PO:** 150–300 mg/day	Diarrhea, dyspepsia, headache, dizziness, fatigue, upper respiratory tract infection
Vasodilators			
Hydralazine (p. 569) (Apresoline)	**T:** 10 mg, 25 mg, 50 mg, 100 mg	**PO:** 40–300 mg/day	Anorexia, nausea, diarrhea, vomiting, headaches, palpitations
Minoxidil (p. 776) (Loniten)	**T:** 2.5 mg, 10 mg	**PO:** 10–40 mg/day	Rapid/irregular heartbeat, hypertrichosis, peripheral edema

C, Capsules; ***P,*** patch; ***T,*** tablets.

Antimigraine (Triptans)

USES

Treatment of migraine headaches with or without aura in adults 18 yrs and older.

ACTION

Triptans are selective agonists of the serotonin (5-HT) receptor in cranial arteries, which cause vasoconstriction and reduce inflammation associated with antidromic neuronal transmission correlating with relief of migraine headache.

TRIPTANS

Name	Availability	Dosage Range	Contraindications	Side Effects
Almotriptan (p. 36) (Axert)	**T:** 6.25 mg, 12.5 mg	6.25–12.5 mg; may repeat after 2 hrs	Ischemic heart disease, angina pectoris, arrhythmias, previous MI, uncontrolled hypertension	Drowsiness, dizziness, fatigue, hot flashes, chest pain/discomfort, paresthesia, nausea, vomiting
Eletriptan (p. 403) (Relpax)	**T:** 20 mg, 40 mg	**A:** 20–40 mg; may repeat after 2 hrs	Same as almotriptan	Asthenia, nausea, dizziness, drowsiness
Frovatriptan (p. 523) (Frova)	**T:** 2.5 mg	2.5 mg; may repeat after 2 hrs; no more than 3 **T**/day	Same as almotriptan	Hot/cold sensations, dizziness, fatigue, headaches, chest pain, skeletal pain, dry mouth, dyspepsia, flushing
Naratriptan (p. 813) (Amerge)	**T:** 1 mg, 2.5 mg	2.5 mg; may repeat once after 4 hrs	Same as almotriptan	Atypical sensations, pain, nausea
Rizatriptan (p. 1030) (Maxalt, Maxalt-MLT)	**T:** 5 mg, 10 mg **DT:** 5 mg, 10 mg	5 or 10 mg; may repeat after 2 hrs	Same as almotriptan	Atypical sensations, pain, nausea, dizziness, drowsiness, asthenia, fatigue
Sumatriptan (p. 1087) (Imitrex, Sumavel DosePro)	**T:** 25 mg, 50 mg **NS:** 5 mg, 20 mg **I:** 4 mg, 6 mg	**PO:** 25–100 mg; may repeat after 2 hrs **NS:** 5–20 mg; may repeat after 2 hrs **Subcutaneous:** 4–6 mg; may repeat after 1 hr	Same as almotriptan	*Oral:* Atypical sensations, pain, malaise, fatigue *Injection:* Atypical sensations, flushing, chest pain/discomfort, injection site reaction, dizziness, vertigo *Nasal:* Discomfort, nausea, vomiting, altered taste
Zolmitriptan (p. 1234) (Zomig, Zomig ZMT)	**T:** 2.5 mg, 5 mg **DT:** 2.5 mg, 5 mg	2.5–5 mg; may repeat after 2 hrs	Same as almotriptan	Atypical sensations, pain, nausea, dizziness, asthenia, drowsiness

A, Adults; ***DT,*** disintegrating tablets; ***I,*** injection; ***NS,*** nasal spray; ***T,*** tablets.

Antipsychotics

USES

Primarily used in managing psychotic illness (esp. in pts with increased psychomotor activity). Also used to treat the manic phase of bipolar disorder, behavioral problems in children, nausea and vomiting, intractable hiccups, anxiety and agitation, as adjunct in treatment of tetanus, and to potentiate effects of narcotics.

ACTION

Effects of these agents occur at all levels of the CNS. Antipsychotic mechanism unknown but may antagonize dopamine action as a neurotransmitter in basal ganglia and limbic system. Antipsychotics may block postsynaptic dopamine receptors, inhibit dopamine release, increase dopamine turnover. These medications can be divided into the phenothiazines and nonphenothiazines (miscellaneous). In addition to their use in the symptomatic treatment of psychiatric illness, some have antiemetic, antinausea, antihistamine, anticholinergic, and/or sedative effects.

ANTIPSYCHOTICS

			Relative Side Effect Profile			
Name	Availability	Dosage	EPS	Anticholinergic	Sedation	Hypotension
Aripiprazole (p. 76) (Abilify)	**T:** 5 mg, 10 mg, 15 mg **DT:** 10 mg, 15 mg **I:** 9.75 mg	**PO:** 15–30 mg/day **I:** Up to 30 mg/day	Low	Very low	Very low	Low
Asenapine (Saphris)	**TSL:** 5 mg, 10 mg	10 mg/day	Low	Very low	Moderate	Low/moderate
Chlorpromazine (p. 227) (Thorazine)	**T:** 10 mg, 25 mg, 50 mg, 100 mg, 200 mg **SR:** 30 mg, 75 mg, 100 mg **OC:** 30 mg/ml, 100 mg/ml	50–2,000 mg/day	Moderate	Moderate	High	High
Clozapine (p. 268) (Clozaril, FazaClo)	**T:** 25 mg, 100 mg **DT:** 25 mg, 100 mg	75–900 mg/day	Very low	High	High	High

Fluphenazine (p. 499) (Prolixin)	**T:** 1 mg, 2.5 mg, 5 mg, 10 mg **I:** 25 mg/ml **OC:** 5 mg/ml	**PO:** 2–40 mg/day **I:** 12.5–75 mg q2wk	High	Low	Low	Low
Haloperidol (p. 564) (Haldol)	**T:** 0.5 mg, 1 mg, 2 mg, 5 mg, 10 mg, 20 mg **I:** 5 mg/ml **OC:** 2 mg/ml	2–40 mg/day	High	Low	Low	Low
Iloperidone (Fanapt)	**T:** 1 mg, 2 mg, 4 mg, 6 mg, 8 mg, 10 mg, 12 mg	12–24 mg/day	Low	Very low	Low	Low/moderate
Loxapine (Loxitane)	**C:** 5 mg, 10 mg, 25 mg, 50 mg **OC:** 25 mg/ml **I:** 50 mg/ml	20–250 mg/day	Moderate	Low	Moderate	Low
Mesoridazine (Serentil)	**T:** 10 mg, 25 mg, 50 mg, 100 mg **I:** 25 mg/ml **OC:** 25 mg/ml	100–400 mg/day	Low	High	High	High
Olanzapine (p. 858) (Zyprexa)	**T:** 2.5 mg, 5 mg, 7.5 mg, 10 mg, 15 mg, 20 mg **DT:** 5 mg, 10 mg **I:** 10 mg	10–20 mg/day	Low	Moderate	Moderate/high	Moderate
Paliperidone (Invega)	**T:** 1.5 mg, 3 mg, 6 mg, 9 mg **I:** 39 mg, 78 mg, 117 mg, 234 mg	3–12 mg/day **IM:** Initially, 234 mg once, then 156 mg 1 wk later, then 39–234 mg monthly	Low	Very low	Low/moderate	Moderate
Quetiapine (p. 989) (Seroquel)	**T:** 25 mg, 100 mg, 200 mg, 300 mg	100–800 mg/day	Very low	Moderate	Moderate/high	Moderate

(continued)

ANTIPSYCHOTICS ***(continued)***

Name	Availability	Dosage	Relative Side Effect Profile			
			EPS	Anticholinergic	Sedation	Hypotension
Risperidone (p. 1023) (Risperdal)	**T:** 0.25 mg, 0.5 mg, 1 mg, 2 mg, 3 mg, 4 mg **OC:** 1 mg/ml **I:** 25 mg, 37.5 mg, 50 mg	2–6 mg/day **IM:** 25–50 mg q2wk	Low	Very low	Low/moderate	Moderate
Thioridazine (p. 1123) (Mellaril)	**T:** 10 mg, 15 mg, 25 mg, 50 mg, 100 mg, 150 mg, 200 mg **OC:** 30 mg/ml, 100 mg/ml	50–800 mg/day	Low	High	High	Moderate/high
Thiothixene (p. 1127) (Navane)	**C:** 1 mg, 2 mg, 5 mg	5–60 mg/day	High	Low	Low	Low/moderate
Trifluoperazine (p. 1175) (Stelazine)	**T:** 1 mg, 2 mg, 5 mg, 10 mg **I:** 5 mg/ml **OC:** 2 mg/ml	5–80 mg/day	High	Low	Low	Low
Ziprasidone (p. 1231) (Geodon)	**C:** 20 mg, 40 mg, 60 mg, 80 mg **I:** 20 mg	40–160 mg/day	Low	Very low	Low to moderate	Low to moderate

C, Capsules; ***DT,*** disintegrating tablets; ***EPS,*** extrapyramidal symptoms; ***I,*** injection; ***OC,*** oral concentrate; ***SR,*** sustained-release; ***T,*** tablets; ***TSL,*** sublingual tablets.

Antivirals

USES

Treatment of HIV infection. Treatment of cytomegalovirus (CMV) retinitis in pts with AIDS, acute herpes zoster (shingles), genital herpes (recurrent), mucosal and cutaneous herpes simplex virus (HSV), chickenpox, and influenza A viral illness.

ACTION

Effective antivirals must inhibit virus-specific nucleic acid/protein synthesis. Possible mechanisms of action of antivirals used for non-HIV infection may include interference with viral DNA synthesis and viral replication, inactivation of viral DNA polymerases, incorporation and termination of the growing viral DNA chain, prevention of release of viral nucleic acid into the host cell, or interference with viral penetration into cells.

ANTIVIRALS

Name	Availability	Uses	Side Effects
Abacavir (p. 1) (Ziagen)	**T:** 300 mg **OS:** 20 mg/ml	HIV infection	Nausea, vomiting, loss of appetite, diarrhea, headaches, fatigue
Acyclovir (p. 16) (Zovirax)	**T:** 400 mg, 800 mg **C:** 200 mg **I:** 50 mg/ml	Mucosal/cutaneous HSV-1 and HSV-2, varicella-zoster (shingles), genital herpes, herpes simplex, encephalitis, chickenpox	Malaise, anorexia, nausea, vomiting, light-headedness
Adefovir (p. 20) (Hepsera)	**T:** 10 mg	Chronic hepatitis B	Asthenia, headaches, abdominal pain, nausea, diarrhea, flatulence, dyspepsia
Amantadine (p. 45) (Symmetrel)	**C:** 100 mg **S:** 50 mg/5 ml	Influenza A	Anxiety, dizziness, light-headedness, headaches, nausea, loss of appetite
Cidofovir (p. 234) (Vistide)	**I:** 75 mg/ml	CMV retinitis	Decreased urination, fever, chills, diarrhea, nausea, vomiting, headaches, loss of appetite

(continued)

ANTIVIRALS *(continued)*

Name	Availability	Uses	Side Effects
Darunavir (p. 308) (Prezista)	**T:** 300 mg	HIV infection	Diarrhea, nausea, vomiting, headaches, skin rash, constipation
Delavirdine (p. 320) (Rescriptor)	**T:** 100 mg, 200 mg	HIV infection	Diarrhea, fatigue, rash, headaches, nausea
Didanosine (p. 349) (Videx)	**T:** 25 mg, 50 mg, 100 mg, 150 mg, 200 mg **C:** 125 mg, 200 mg **Powder for suspension:** 100 mg, 167 mg, 250 mg	HIV infection	Peripheral neuropathy, anxiety, headaches, rash, nausea, diarrhea, dry mouth
Efavirenz (p. 401) (Sustiva)	**C:** 50 mg, 100 mg, 200 mg	HIV infection	Diarrhea, dizziness, headaches, insomnia, nausea, vomiting, drowsiness
Etravirine (p. 454) (Intelence)	**T:** 100 mg	HIV infection	Rash, nausea, abdominal pain, vomiting
Famciclovir (p. 461) (Famvir)	**T:** 125 mg, 250 mg, 500 mg	Herpes zoster, genital herpes	Headaches
Foscarnet (p. 516) (Foscavir)	**I:** 24 mg/ml	CMV retinitis, HSV infections	Decreased urination, abdominal pain, nausea, vomiting, dizziness, fatigue, headaches
Ganciclovir (p. 531) (Cytovene)	**C:** 250 mg, 500 mg **I:** 500 mg	CMV retinitis, CMV disease	Sore throat, fever, unusual bleeding/bruising
Indinavir (p. 610) (Crixivan)	**C:** 200 mg, 400 mg	HIV infection	Blood in urine, weakness, nausea, vomiting, diarrhea, headaches, insomnia, altered taste

Lamivudine (p. 659) (Epivir)	**T:** 100 mg, 150 mg **OS:** 5 mg/ml, 10 mg/ml	HIV infection	Nausea, vomiting, abdominal pain, paresthesia
Lopinavir/ritonavir (p. 703) (Kaletra)	**C:** 133/33 mg **OS:** 80/20 mg	HIV infection	Diarrhea, nausea
Maraviroc (p. 721) (Selzentry)	**T:** 150 mg, 300 mg	HIV infection	Cough, pyrexia, upper respiratory tract infection, rash, musculoskeletal symptoms, abdominal pain, dizziness
Nelfinavir (p. 820) (Viracept)	**T:** 250 mg **Powder:** 50 mg/g	HIV infection	Diarrhea
Oseltamivir (p. 872) (Tamiflu)	**C:** 75 mg **S:** 12 mg/ml	Influenza	Diarrhea, nausea, vomiting
Raltegravir (p. 999) (Isentress)	**T:** 400 mg	HIV infection	Nausea, headache, diarrhea, pyrexia
Ribavirin (p. 1014) (Virazole)	**Aerosol:** 6 g	Lowers respiratory infections in infants, children due to respiratory syncytial virus (RSV)	Anemia
Ritonavir (p. 1025) (Norvir)	**C:** 100 mg **OS:** 80 mg/ml	HIV infection	Weakness, diarrhea, nausea, decreased appetite, vomiting, altered taste
Saquinavir (p. 1042) (Invirase)	**C:** 200 mg	HIV infection	Weakness, diarrhea, nausea, oral ulcers, abdominal pain
Stavudine (p. 1081) (Zerit)	**C:** 15 mg, 20 mg, 30 mg, 40 mg **OS:** 1 mg/ml	HIV infection	Paresthesia, decreased appetite, chills, fever, rash
Tenofovir (p. 1106) (Viread)	**T:** 300 mg	HIV infection	Diarrhea, nausea, pharyngitis, headaches

(continued)

ANTIVIRALS *(continued)*

Name	Availability	Uses	Side Effects
Valacyclovir (p. 1183) (Valtrex)	**T:** 500 mg	Herpes zoster, genital herpes	Headaches, nausea
Valganciclovir (p. 1186) (Valcyte)	**T:** 450 mg	CMV retinitis	Anemia, abdominal pain, diarrhea, headaches, nausea, vomiting, paresthesia
Zalcitabine (Hivid)	**T:** 0.375 mg, 0.75 mg	HIV infection	Paresthesia, arthralgia, rash, nausea, vomiting
Zanamivir (p. 1226) (Relenza)	**Inhalation:** 5 mg	Influenza	Cough, diarrhea, dizziness, headaches, nausea, vomiting
Zidovudine (p. 1227) (Retrovir)	**T:** 300 mg **C:** 100 mg **S:** 50 mg/5 ml	HIV infection	Fatigue, fever, chills, headaches, nausea, muscle pain

C, Capsules; ***I,*** injection; ***OS,*** oral solution; ***S,*** syrup; ***T,*** tablets.

Beta-Adrenergic Blockers

USES

Management of hypertension, angina pectoris, arrhythmias, hypertrophic subaortic stenosis, migraine headaches, MI (prevention), glaucoma.

ACTION

Beta-adrenergic blockers competitively block $beta_1$-adrenergic receptors, located primarily in myocardium, and $beta_2$-adrenergic receptors, located primarily in bronchial and vascular smooth muscle. By occupying beta-receptor sites, these agents prevent naturally occurring or administered epinephrine/norepinephrine from exerting their effects. The results are basically opposite to those of sympathetic stimulation.

Effects of $beta_1$-blockade include slowing heart rate, decreasing cardiac output and contractility; effects of $beta_2$-blockade include bronchoconstriction, increased airway resistance in pts with asthma or COPD. Beta-blockers can affect cardiac rhythm/automaticity (decrease sinus rate, SA/AV conduction; increase refractory period in AV node). Decrease systolic and diastolic B/P; exact mechanism unknown but may block peripheral receptors, decrease sympathetic outflow from CNS, or decrease renin release from kidney. All beta-blockers mask tachycardia that occurs with hypoglycemia. When applied to the eye, reduce intraocular pressure and aqueous production.

BETA-ADRENERGIC BLOCKERS

Name	Availability	Indication	Dosage Range	Selectivity
Acebutolol (Sectral)	**C:** 200 mg, 400 mg	HTN, Arrhythmias	200–1,200 mg/day	$Beta_1$
Atenolol (p. 90) (Tenormin)	**T:** 25 mg, 50 mg, 100 mg	HTN, Angina, MI	50–100 mg/day	$Beta_1$
Betaxolol (Kerlone)	**T:** 10 mg, 20 mg	HTN	10–20 mg/day	$Beta_1$
Bisoprolol (p. 131) (Zebeta)	**T:** 5 mg, 10 mg	HTN	2.5–20 mg/day	$Beta_1$

(continued)

BETA-ADRENERGIC BLOCKERS *(continued)*

Name	Availability	Indication	Dosage Range	Selectivity
Carvedilol (p. 183) (Coreg)	**T:** 3.125 mg, 6.25 mg, 12.5 mg, 25 mg **C (SR):** 10 mg, 20 mg, 40 mg, 80 mg	HF, LVD after MI, HTN	12.5–100 mg/day	Alpha$_1$, Beta$_1$, Beta$_2$
Esmolol (p. 437) (Brevibloc)	**I:** 10 mg/ml, 20 mg/ml	HTN, arrhythmias	50–200 mcg/kg/min	Beta$_1$
Labetalol (Trandate)	**T:** 100 mg, 200 mg, 300 mg **I:** 5 mg/ml	HTN	200–2,400 mg/day **I:** 20–80 mg at 10-min intervals (**Maximum:** 300 mg)	Alpha$_1$, Beta$_1$, Beta$_2$
Metoprolol (p. 760) (Lopressor)	**T:** 50 mg, 100 mg/ml **I:** 1 mg/ml **T (SR):** 25 mg, 50 mg	HTN, angina, HF, MI	**T:** 50–450 mg/day **I:** 1.25–5 mg q6–12 h **SR:** Up to 200 mg/day	Beta$_1$
Nadolol (p. 801) (Corgard)	**T:** 20 mg, 40 mg, 80 mg, 120 mg, 160 mg	HTN, angina	40–320 mg/day	Beta$_1$, Beta$_2$
Nevibolol (Bystolic)	**T:** 2.5 mg, 5 mg, 10 mg	HTN	5–40 mg/day	Beta$_1$
Pindolol (Visken)	**T:** 5 mg, 10 mg	HTN	10–60 mg/day	Beta$_1$, Beta$_2$
Propranolol (p. 978) (Inderal)	**T:** 10 mg, 20 mg, 40 mg, 60 mg, 80 mg, 90 mg **C (SR):** 60 mg, 80 mg, 120 mg, 160 mg **S:** 4 mg/ml, 8 mg/ml **I:** 1 mg/ml	HTN, angina, MI, arrhythmias, migraine, essential tremor, hypertrophic subaortic stenosis	80–320 mg/day	Beta$_1$, Beta$_2$
Sotalol (p. 1076) (Betapace)	**T:** 80 mg, 120 mg, 160 mg, 240 mg	Arrhythmias	160–640 mg/day	Beta$_1$, Beta$_2$
Timolol (p. 1133) (Blocadren)	**T:** 5 mg, 10 mg, 20 mg	HTN, migraine	10–60 mg/day	Beta$_1$, Beta$_2$

C, Capsules; ***HF,*** heart failure; ***HTN,*** hypertension; ***I,*** injection; ***LVD,*** left ventricular dysfunction; ***MI,*** myocardial infarction; ***S,*** solution; ***SR,*** sustained-release; ***T,*** tablets.

Bronchodilators

USES

Relief of bronchospasm occurring during anesthesia and in bronchial asthma, bronchitis, emphysema.

ACTION

Inhaled corticosteroids: Exact mechanism unknown. May act as anti-inflammatories, decrease mucus secretion.

Beta$_2$-adrenergic agonists: Stimulate beta-receptors in lung, relax bronchial smooth muscle, increase vital capacity, decrease airway resistance.

Anticholinergics: Inhibit cholinergic receptors on bronchial smooth muscle (block acetylcholine action).

Leukotriene modifiers: Decrease effect of leukotrienes, which increase migration of eosinophils, producing mucus/edema of airway wall, causing bronchoconstriction.

Methylxanthines: Directly relax smooth muscle of bronchial airway, pulmonary blood vessels (relieve bronchospasm, increase vital capacity). Increase cyclic 3,5-adenosine monophosphate.

BRONCHODILATORS

Name	Availability	Dosage Range	Side Effects
Anticholinergics			
Ipratropium (p. 628) (Atrovent)	**Neb:** 0.02% **MDI:** 18 mcg/actuation	**A (Neb):** 0.02% q3–4h **A (MDI):** 2 puffs 4 times/day	Upper respiratory tract infection, bronchitis, sinusitis, headache, dyspnea
Tiotropium (p. 1137) (Spiriva)	**Inhalation powder:** 18 mcg/capsule	**A:** Once/day	Xerostomia, upper respiratory tract infection, sinusitis, pharyngitis

(continued)

BRONCHODILATORS ***(continued)***

Name	Availability	Dosage Range	Side Effects
Bronchodilators			
Albuterol (p. 25) (AccuNeb, ProAir HFA, Proventil HFA, Ventolin HFA)	**MDI:** 90 mcg/actuation **NEB:** 2.5 mg/3 ml, 2.5 mg/0.5 ml, ***(AccuNeb):*** 0.63–1.25 mg/3 ml	**MDI:** 2 inhalations q4–6h as needed **NEB:** 2.5 mg q6–8h as needed	Tachycardia, skeletal muscle tremors, muscle cramping, palpitations, insomnia, hypokalemia, increased serum glucose
Albuterol/ipratropium (pp. 25, 628) (Combivent, DuoNeb)	**MDI:** 90 mcg albuterol/ 18 mcg ipratropium/ actuation **NEB:** 2.5 mg albuterol/ 0.5 mg ipratropium/3 ml	**MDI:** 2 inhalations 4 times/day as needed **NEB:** 2.5 mg/0.5 mg 4 times/day as needed	Same as individual listing for albuterol and ipratropium
Arformoterol (Brovana)	**NEB:** 15 mcg/2 ml	**NEB:** 15 mcg 2 times/day	Same as formoterol
Formoterol (p. 512) (Foradil, Perforomist)	**DPI:** 12 mcg/capsule **NEB:** 20 mcg/2 ml	**DPI:** 12 mcg 2 times/day **NEB:** 20 mcg 2 times/day	Diarrhea, nausea, asthma exacerbation, bronchitis, infection
Formoterol/budesonide (pp. 145, 512) (Symbicort)	**MDI:** 80, 160 mcg/ 4.5 mcg/inhalation	**MDI:** 2 inhalations 2 times/day	Same as individual listing for formoterol and budesonide
Levalbuterol (p. 679) (Xopenex)	**MDI:** 45 mcg/actuation **NEB:** 0.31, 0.63, 1.25 mg/3 ml	**MDI:** 2 inhalations q4–6h as needed **NEB:** 0.63–1.25 mg q6-8h	Tremor, rhinitis, viral infection, headache, nervousness, asthma, pharyngitis, rash
Salmeterol (p. 1041) (Serevent Diskus)	**DPI:** 50 mcg/blister	**DPI:** 50 mcg 2 times/day	Headache, pain, throat irritation, nasal congestion, bronchitis, pharyngitis

Salmeterol/fluticasone (pp. 505, 1041) (Advair Diskus, Advair HFA)	**DPI**: 100, 250, 500 mcg/50 mcg/blister **MDI**: 45, 115, 230 mcg/21 mcg/inhalation	**DPI**: 1 inhalation 2 times/day **MDI**: 2 inhalations 2 times/day	Same as individual listing for salmeterol and fluticasone
Inhaled Corticosteroids			
Beclomethasone (p. 113) (Qvar)	**MDI**: 40, 80 mcg/inhalation	**MDI**: 40–320 mcg 2 times/day	Cough, hoarseness, headache, pharyngitis
Budesonide (p. 145) (Pulmicort Flexhaler, Pulmicort Respules)	**DPI: (Flexhaler)**: 90, 180 mcg/inhalation **DPI: (Turbuhaler)**: 200 mcg/inhalation **NEB: (Respules)**: 0.25, 0.5 mg/2 ml	**DPI: (Flexhaler)**: 360–720 mcg 2 times/day **DPI: (Turbuhaler)**: 200–800 mcg 2 times/day **NEB: (Respules)**: 250–500 mcg 1–2 times/day or 1 mg once daily	Headache, nausea, respiratory infection, rhinitis
Ciclesonide (p. 232) (Alvesco HFA)	**HFA**: 80 mcg/inhalation	**HFA**: 160–320 mcg 2 times/day	Headache, nasopharyngitis, upper respiratory infection, epistaxis, nasal congestion, sinusitis
Flunisolide (p. 493) (AeroBid)	**MDI: (Aerobid)**: 250 mcg/inhalation **MDI: (Aerospan HFA)**: 80 mcg/inhalation	**MDI: (Aerobid)**: 500–1,000 mcg 2 times/day **MDI: (Aerospan HFA)**: 160–320 mcg 2 times/day	Headache, nasal congestion, pharyngitis, upper respiratory infections
Fluticasone (p. 505) (Flovent Diskus, Flovent HFA)	**DPI: (Flovent Diskus)**: 50, 100, 250 mcg/blister **MDI: (Flovent HFA)**: 44, 110, 220 mcg/inhalation	**DPI: (Flovent Diskus)**: 100–500 mcg 2 times/day **MDI: (Flovent HFA)**: 88–440 mcg 2 times/day	Headache, nasal congestion, pharyngitis, sinusitis, respiratory infections
Formoterol/budesonide (pp. 145, 512) (Symbicort)	**MDI**: 80, 160 mcg/4.5 mcg/inhalation	**MDI**: 2 inhalations 2 times/day	Same as individual listing for formoterol and budesonide

(continued)

BRONCHODILATORS *(continued)*

Name	Availability	Dosage Range	Side Effects
Mometasone (p. 787) (Asmanex Twisthaler)	**DPI:** 220 mcg/inhalation	**DPI:** 220–440 mcg 1–2 times/day	Same as beclomethasone
Salmeterol/fluticasone (pp. 505, 1041) (Advair Diskus, Advair HFA)	**DPI:** 100, 250, 500 mcg/ 50 mcg/blister **MDI:** 45, 115, 230 mcg/ 21 mcg/inhalation	**DPI:** 1 inhalation 2 times/day **MDI:** 2 inhalations 2 times/day	Same as individual listing for salmeterol and fluticasone
Triamcinolone (p. 1171) (Azmacort)	**MDI:** 75 mcg/inhalation	**MDI:** 150 mcg 3–4 times/day or 300 mcg 2 times/day	Headache, pharyngitis, sinusitis, cough, flu-like syndrome
Leukotriene Modifiers			
Montelukast (p. 789) (Singulair)	**T:** 4 mg, 5 mg, 10 mg	**A:** 10 mg/day **C (6–14 yrs):** 5 mg/day **C (2–5 yrs):** 4 mg/day	Dyspepsia, increased hepatic function tests, cough, nasal congestion, headache, dizziness, fatigue
Zafirlukast (p. 1224) (Accolate)	**T:** 10 mg, 20 mg	**A, C (12 yrs and older):** 20 mg 2 times/day **C (5–11 yrs):** 10 mg 2 times/day	Headache, nausea, diarrhea, infection
Zileuton (p. 1229) (Zyflo CR)	**T:** 600 mg **SR:** 600 mg	**A, C (12 yrs and older):** **T:** 600 mg 4 times/day **SR:** 1,200 mg 2 times/day	Increased hepatic function tests

A, Adults; ***C** (dosage),* children; ***DPI,*** dry powder inhaler; ***HFA,*** hydrofluoroalkane; ***MDI,*** metered dose inhaler; ***Neb,*** nebulization; ***SR,*** sustained-release; ***T,*** tablets.

Calcium Channel Blockers

USES

Treatment of essential hypertension, treatment of and prophylaxis of angina pectoris (including vasospastic, chronic stable, unstable), prevention/control of supraventricular tachyarrhythmias, prevention of neurologic damage due to subarachnoid hemorrhage.

ACTION

Calcium channel blockers inhibit the flow of extracellular Ca^{2+} ions across cell membranes of cardiac cells, vascular tissue. They relax arterial smooth muscle, depress the rate of sinus node pacemaker, slow AV conduction, decrease heart rate, produce negative inotropic effect (rarely seen clinically due to reflex response). Calcium channel blockers decrease coronary vascular resistance, increase coronary blood flow, reduce myocardial oxygen demand. Degree of action varies with individual agent.

CALCIUM CHANNEL BLOCKERS

Name	Availability	Dosage Range	Side Effects	Indications
Amlodipine (p. 56) (Norvasc)	**T:** 2.5 mg, 5 mg, 10 mg	2.5–10 mg/day	Abdominal pain, flushing, headaches, peripheral edema	HTN, angina
Diltiazem (p. 354) (Cardizem)	**T:** 30 mg, 60 mg, 90 mg **T (SR):** 120 mg, 180 mg, 240 mg **C (SR):** 60 mg, 90 mg, 120 mg, 180 mg, 240 mg, 300 mg, 360 mg **I:** 5 mg/ml	**PO:** 120–360 mg/day **I:** 20–25 mg IV bolus, then 5–15 mg/hr infusion	Dizziness, drowsiness, edema, headache	**PO:** HTN **IV:** Arrhythmias
Felodipine (p. 466) (Plendil)	**T:** 2.5 mg, 5 mg, 10 mg	5–10 mg/day	Peripheral edema, headaches	HTN
Isradipine (p. 641) (DynaCirc)	**T:** 5 mg, 10 mg **C:** 2.5 mg, 5 mg	5–20 mg/day	Headaches	HTN

(continued)

CALCIUM CHANNEL BLOCKERS *(continued)*

Name	Availability	Dosage Range	Side Effects	Indications
Nicardipine (p. 827) (Cardene)	**C**: 20 mg, 30 mg **C (ER)**: 30 mg, 45 mg, 60 mg **I**: 2.5 mg/ml	**PO**: 60–120 mg/day	Flushing, peripheral edema, headache, dizziness	HTN, angina
Nifedipine (p. 831) (Adalat, Procardia)	**C**: 10 mg, 20 mg **T (ER)**: 30 mg, 60 mg, 90 mg	30–120 mg/day	Peripheral edema, dizziness, flushed face, headaches, nausea	HTN, angina
Nimodipine (p. 835) (Nimotop)	**C**: 30 mg	60 mg q4h for 21 days	Nausea, reduced B/P, headache, rash, diarrhea	Prevent neurologic damage following subarachnoid hemorrhage
Verapamil (p. 1200) (Calan, Isoptin)	**T**: 40 mg, 80 mg, 120 mg **T (SR)**: 120 mg, 180 mg, 240 mg	120–480 mg/day	Nausea, gingival hyperplasia, headache, fatigue, dizziness	HTN, angina, arrhythmias

C, Capsules; ***ER,*** extended-release; ***HTN,*** hypertension; ***I,*** injection; ***SR,*** sustained-release; ***T,*** tablets.

Chemotherapeutic Agents

USES

Treatment of a variety of cancers; may be palliative or curative. Treatment of choice in hematologic cancers. Often used as adjunctive therapy (e.g., with surgery or irradiation); most effective when tumor mass has been removed or reduced by radiation. Often used in combinations to increase therapeutic results, decrease toxic effects. Certain agents may be used in nonmalignant conditions: polycythemia vera, psoriasis, rheumatoid arthritis, or immunosuppression in organ transplantation (used only in select cases that are severe and unresponsive to other forms of therapy). Refer to individual monographs.

ACTION

Most antineoplastics can be divided into alkylating agents, antimetabolites, anthracyclines, plant alkaloids, and topoisomerase inhibitors. These agents affect cell division or DNA synthesis. Newer agents (monoclonal antibodies and tyrosine kinase inhibitors) directly target a molecular abnormality in certain types of cancer. Hormones modulate tumor cell behavior without directly attacking those cells. Some agents are classified as miscellaneous.

CHEMOTHERAPEUTIC AGENTS

Name	Availability	Category	Side Effects
Aldesleukin (pp. 27, 625) (Proleukin)	**I:** 22 million units	Biologic response modifier	Hypotension, sinus tachycardia, nausea, vomiting, diarrhea, renal impairment, anemia, rash, fatigue, agitation, pulmonary congestion, dyspnea, fever, chills, oliguria, weight gain, dizziness
Alemtuzumab (p. 28) (Campath)	**I:** 30 mg/3 ml	Monoclonal antibody	Rigors, fever, fatigue, hypotension, neutropenia, anemia, sepsis, dyspnea, bronchitis, pneumonia, urticaria
Alitretinoin (Panretin)	**Gel:** 0.1%	Retinoic acid derivative	Burning, pain, edema, dermatitis, rash, skin disorders

(continued)

CHEMOTHERAPEUTIC AGENTS *(continued)*

Name	Availability	Category	Side Effects
Altretamine (Hexalen)	**C:** 50 mg	Miscellaneous	Nausea, vomiting, myelosuppression, peripheral neuropathy, altered mood, ataxia, dizziness, anxiety, vertigo
Anastrozole (p. 68) (Arimidex)	**T:** 1 mg	Aromatase inhibitor	Peripheral edema, chest pain, nausea, vomiting, diarrhea, constipation, abdominal pain, anorexia, pharyngitis, vaginal hemorrhage, anemia, leukopenia, rash, weight gain, diaphoresis, increased appetite, pain, headaches, dizziness, depression, paresthesias, hot flashes, increased cough, dry mouth, asthenia, dyspnea, phlebitis
Arsenic trioxide (p. 79) (Trisenox)	**I:** 10 mg/ml	Miscellaneous	AV block, GI hemorrhage, hypertension, hypoglycemia, hypokalemia, hypomagnesemia, neutropenia, oliguria, prolonged QT interval, seizures, sepsis, thrombocytopenia
Asparaginase (p. 84) (Elspar)	**I:** 10,000 units	Miscellaneous	Anorexia, nausea, vomiting, hepatic toxicity, pancreatitis, nephrotoxicity, clotting factor abnormalities, malaise, confusion, lethargy, EEG changes, respiratory distress, fever, hyperglycemia, depression, stomatitis, allergic reactions, drowsiness
Azacitidine (p. 99) (Vidaza)	**I:** 100 mg	DNA methylation inhibitor	Edema, hypokalemia, weight loss, myalgia, cough, dyspnea, upper respiratory tract infection, back pain, pyrexia, weakness
BCG (TheraCys, Tice BCG)	**I:** 50 mg, 81 mg	Biologic response modulator	Nausea, vomiting, anorexia, diarrhea, dysuria, hematuria, cystitis, urinary urgency, anemia, malaise, fever, chills
Bendamustine (p. 116) (Treanda)	**I:** 100 mg	Alkylating agent	Neutropenia, pyrexia, thrombocytopenia, nausea, anemia, leukopenia, vomiting
Bevacizumab (p. 124) (Avastin)	**I:** 25 mg/ml	Monoclonal antibody	Increased B/P, fatigue, blood clots, diarrhea, decreased WBCs, headaches, decreased appetite, stomatitis
Bexarotene (p. 126) (Targretin)	**C:** 75 mg **Gel:** 1%	Miscellaneous	Anemia, dermatitis, fever, hypercholesterolemia, infection, leukopenia, peripheral edema

Bicalutamide (p. 127) (Casodex)	**T:** 50 mg	Antiandrogen	Gynecomastia, hot flashes, breast pain, nausea, diarrhea, constipation, nocturia, impotence, pain, muscle pain, asthenia, abdominal pain
Bleomycin (p. 135) (Blenoxane)	**I:** 15 units, 30 units	Antibiotic	Nausea, vomiting, anorexia, stomatitis, hyperpigmentation, alopecia, pruritus, hyperkeratosis, urticaria, pneumonitis progression to fibrosis, weight loss, rash
Bortezomib (p. 137) (Velcade)	**I:** 3.5 mg	Proteasome inhibitor	Anxiety, dizziness, headaches, insomnia, peripheral neuropathy, pruritus, rash, abdominal pain, decreased appetite, constipation, diarrhea, dyspepsia, nausea, vomiting, arthralgia, dyspnea, asthenia, edema, pain
Busulfan (p. 155) (Myleran)	**T:** 2 mg	Alkylating agent	Nausea, vomiting, hyperuricemia, myelosuppression, skin hyperpigmentation, alopecia, anorexia, weight loss, diarrhea, stomatitis
Cabazitaxel (Jevtana)	**I:** 60 mg/1.5 ml	Microtubule inhibitor	Neutropenia, anemia, leukopenia, thrombocytopenia, diarrhea, fatigue, nausea, vomiting, constipation, asthenia, abdominal pain, hematuria, anorexia, peripheral neuropathy, dyspnea, alopecia
Capecitabine (p. 170) (Xeloda)	**T:** 150 mg, 300 mg	Antimetabolite	Nausea, vomiting, diarrhea, stomatitis, myelosuppression, palmoplantar erythrodysesthesia syndrome, dermatitis, fatigue, anorexia
Carboplatin (p. 178) (Paraplatin)	**I:** 50 mg, 150 mg, 450 mg	Alkylating agent	Nausea, vomiting, nephrotoxicity, myelosuppression, alopecia, peripheral neuropathy, hypersensitivity, ototoxicity, asthenia, diarrhea, constipation
Carmustine (p. 182) (BiCNU)	**I:** 100 mg	Alkylating agent	Anorexia, nausea, vomiting, myelosuppression, pulmonary fibrosis, pain at injection site, diarrhea, skin discoloration
Cetuximab (p. 220) (Erbitux)	**I:** 2 mg/ml	Monoclonal antibody	Dyspnea, hypotension, acne-like rash, dry skin, weakness, fatigue, fever, constipation, abdominal pain
Chlorambucil (p. 224) (Leukeran)	**T:** 2 mg	Alkylating agent	Myelosuppression, dermatitis, nausea, vomiting, hepatic toxicity, anorexia, diarrhea, abdominal discomfort, rash
Cisplatin (p. 243) (Platinol-AQ)	**I:** 50 mg, 100 mg	Alkylating agent	Nausea, vomiting, nephrotoxicity, myelosuppression, neuropathies, ototoxicity, anaphylactic-like reactions, hyperuricemia, hypomagnesemia, hypophosphatemia, hypokalemia, hypocalcemia, pain at injection site

(continued)

CHEMOTHERAPEUTIC AGENTS *(continued)*

Name	Availability	Category	Side Effects
Cladribine (p. 247) (Leustatin)	**I:** 1 mg/ml	Antimetabolite	Nausea, vomiting, diarrhea, myelosuppression, chills, fatigue, rash, fever, headaches, anorexia, diaphoresis
Cyclophosphamide (p. 287) (Cytoxan)	**I:** 100 mg, 200 mg, 500 mg, 1 g, 2 g **T:** 25 mg, 50 mg	Alkylating agent	Nausea, vomiting, hemorrhagic cystitis, myelosuppression, alopecia, interstitial pulmonary fibrosis, amenorrhea, azoospermia, diarrhea, darkening skin/fingernails, headaches, diaphoresis
Cytarabine (p. 291) (Ara-C, Cytosar)	**I:** 100 mg, 500 mg, 1 g, 2 g	Antimetabolite	Anorexia, nausea, vomiting, stomatitis, esophagitis, diarrhea, myelosuppression, alopecia, rash, fever, neuropathies, abdominal pain
Dacarbazine (p. 295) (DTIC)	**I:** 200 mg	Alkylating agent	Nausea, vomiting, anorexia, hepatic necrosis, myelosuppression, alopecia, rash, facial flushing, photosensitivity, flu-like symptoms, confusion, blurred vision
Dasatinib (p. 310) (Sprycel)	**T:** 20 mg, 50 mg, 70 mg	Tyrosine kinase inhibitor	Pyrexia, pleural effusion, febrile neutropenia, GI bleeding, pneumonia, thrombocytopenia, dyspnea, anemia, cardiac failure, diarrhea
Daunorubicin (p. 311) (Cerubidine)	**I:** 20 mg	Anthracycline	CHF, nausea, vomiting, stomatitis, mucositis, diarrhea, hematuria, myelosuppression, alopecia, fever, chills, abdominal pain
Daunorubicin (p. 311) (DaunoXome)	**I:** 50 mg	Anthracycline	Nausea, diarrhea, abdominal pain, anorexia, vomiting, stomatitis, myelosuppression, rigors, back pain, headaches, neuropathy, depression, dyspnea, fatigue, fever, cough, allergic reactions, diaphoresis
Denileukin (p. 322) (Ontak)	**I:** 300 mcg/2 ml	Miscellaneous	Hypersensitivity reaction, back pain, dyspnea, rash, chest pain, tachycardia, asthenia, flu-like symptoms, chills, nausea, vomiting, infection
Docetaxel (p. 368) (Taxotere)	**I:** 20 mg, 80 mg	Antimicrotubular	Hypotension, nausea, vomiting, diarrhea, mucositis, myelosuppression, rash, paresthesia, hypersensitivity, fluid retention, alopecia, asthenia, stomatitis, fever
Doxorubicin (p. 384) (Adriamycin)	**I:** 10 mg, 20 mg, 50 mg, 75 mg, 150 mg, 200 mg	Anthracycline	Cardiotoxicity, including CHF; arrhythmias, nausea, vomiting, stomatitis, esophagitis, GI ulceration, diarrhea, anorexia, hematuria, myelosuppression, alopecia, hyperpigmentation of nail beds and skin, local inflammation at injection site, rash, fever, chills, urticaria, lacrimation, conjunctivitis

Doxorubicin (p. 384) (Doxil)	**I:** 20 mg, 50 mg	Anthracycline	Neutropenia, palmoplantar erythrodysesthesia syndrome, cardiomyopathy, CHF
Epirubicin (p. 418) (Ellence)	**I:** 2 mg/ml	Anthracycline	Anemia, leukopenia, neutropenia, infection, mucositis
Erlotinib (p. 430) (Tarceva)	**T:** 25 mg, 100 mg, 150 mg	Tyrosine kinase inhibitor	Diarrhea, rash, nausea, vomiting
Estramustine (p. 444) (Emcyt)	**C:** 140 mg	Alkylating agent	Increased risk of thrombosis, gynecomastia, nausea, vomiting, diarrhea, thrombocytopenia, peripheral edema
Etoposide (p. 452) (VePesid)	**I:** 20 mg/ml **C:** 50 mg	Podophyllotoxin derivative	Nausea, vomiting, anorexia, myelosuppression, alopecia, diarrhea, drowsiness, peripheral neuropathies
Everolimus (Afinitor)	**T:** 5 mg, 10 mg	mTOR kinase inhibitor	Stomatitis, infections, asthenia, fatigue, cough, diarrhea
Exemestane (p. 457) (Aromasin)	**T:** 25 mg	Aromatase inactivator	Dyspnea, edema, hypertension, mental depression
Fludarabine (p. 489) (Fludara)	**I:** 50 mg	Antimetabolite	Nausea, diarrhea, stomatitis, bleeding, anemia, myelosuppression, skin rash, weakness, confusion, visual disturbances, peripheral neuropathy, coma, pneumonia, peripheral edema, anorexia
Fluorouracil (p. 495) (Adrucil, Efudex)	**I:** 50 mg/ml **Cream:** 1%, 5% **Solution:** 1%, 2%, 5%	Antimetabolite	Nausea, vomiting, stomatitis, GI ulceration, diarrhea, anorexia, myelosuppression, alopecia, skin hyperpigmentation, nail changes, headaches, drowsiness, blurred vision, fever
Flutamide (p. 503) (Eulexin)	**C:** 125 mg	Antiandrogen	Hot flashes, nausea, vomiting, diarrhea, hepatitis, impotence, decreased libido, rash, anorexia
Fulvestrant (p. 525) (Faslodex)	**I:** 125 mg/2.5 ml, 250 mg/5 ml syringes	Estrogen receptor antagonist	Asthenia, pain, headaches, injection site pain, flu-like symptoms, fever, nausea, vomiting, constipation, anorexia, diarrhea, peripheral edema, dizziness, depression, anxiety, rash, increased cough, UTI

(continued)

CHEMOTHERAPEUTIC AGENTS *(continued)*

Name	Availability	Category	Side Effects
Gefitinib (Iressa)	**T:** 250 mg	Tyrosine kinase inhibitor	Diarrhea, rash, acne, nausea, dry skin, vomiting, pruritus, anorexia
Gemcitabine (p. 535) (Gemzar)	**I:** 200 mg, 1 g	Antimetabolite	Increased hepatic function tests, nausea, vomiting, diarrhea, stomatitis, hematuria, myelosuppression, rash, mild paresthesias, dyspnea, fever, edema, flu-like symptoms, constipation
Gemtuzumab (Mylotarg)	**I:** 5 mg/20 ml	Monoclonal antibody	Anemia, hematuria, hepatotoxicity, pneumonia, herpes simplex, nausea, vomiting, dyspnea, headaches, hypotension, hypoxia, mucositis, myelosuppression, peripheral edema, tachycardia, thrombocytopenia
Goserelin (p. 557) (Zoladex)	**I:** 3.6 mg, 10.8 mg	Hormone agonist	Hot flashes, sexual dysfunction, erectile dysfunction, gynecomastia, lethargy, pain, lower urinary tract symptoms, headaches, nausea, depression, diaphoresis
Hydroxyurea (p. 582) (Hydrea)	**C:** 500 mg	Antimetabolite	Anorexia, nausea, vomiting, stomatitis, diarrhea, constipation, myelosuppression, fever, chills, malaise
Ibritumomab (p. 589) (Zevalin)	Injection kit	Monoclonal antibody	Neutropenia, thrombocytopenia, anemia, infection, asthenia, abdominal pain, fever, pain, headaches, nausea, peripheral edema, allergic reaction, GI hemorrhage, apnea
Idarubicin (p. 593) (Idamycin PFS)	**I:** 5 mg, 10 mg, 20 mg	Anthracycline	CHF, arrhythmias, nausea, vomiting, stomatitis, myelosuppression, alopecia, rash, urticaria, hyperuricemia, abdominal pain, diarrhea, esophagitis, anorexia
Ifosfamide (p. 595) (Ifex)	**I:** 1 g, 3 g	Alkylating agent	Nausea, vomiting, hemorrhagic cystitis, myelosuppression, alopecia, lethargy, drowsiness, confusion, hallucinations, hematuria
Imatinib (p. 599) (Gleevec)	**C:** 100 mg	Tyrosine kinase inhibitor	Nausea, fluid retention, hemorrhage, musculoskeletal pain, arthralgia, weight gain, pyrexia, abdominal pain, dyspnea, pneumonia

Interferon alfa-2b (p. 619) (Intron-A)	**I:** 3 million units, 5 million units, 10 million units, 18 million units, 25 million units, 50 million units	Miscellaneous	Mild hypotension, hypertension, tachycardia with high fever, nausea, diarrhea, altered taste, weight loss, thrombocytopenia, myelosuppression, rash, pruritus, myalgia, arthralgia associated with flu-like symptoms
Irinotecan (p. 631) (Camptosar)	**I:** 40 mg, 100 mg	Camptothecin	Diarrhea, nausea, vomiting, abdominal cramps, anorexia, stomatitis, increased AST, severe myelosuppression, alopecia, diaphoresis, rash, weight loss, dehydration, increased serum alkaline phosphatase, headaches, insomnia, dizziness, dyspnea, cough, asthenia, rhinitis, fever, back pain, chills
Ixabepilone (p. 644) (Ixempra)	**I:** 15 mg, 45 mg	Antimicrotubular	Peripheral sensory neuropathy, fatigue, myalgia, alopecia, nausea, vomiting, stomatitis, diarrhea, anorexia, abdominal pain
Lapatinib (p. 668) (Tykerb)	**T:** 250 mg	Tyrosine kinase inhibitor	Diarrhea, palmar-plantar erythrodysesthesia, nausea, rash, vomiting, fatigue
Letrozole (p. 674) (Femara)	**T:** 2.5 mg	Aromatase inhibitor	Hypertension, nausea, vomiting, constipation, diarrhea, abdominal pain, anorexia, rash, pruritus, musculoskeletal pain, arthralgia, fatigue, headaches, dyspnea, coughing, hot flashes
Leuprolide (p. 677) (Lupron)	**I:** 3.75 mg, 5 mg, 7.5 mg, 11.25 mg, 15 mg, 22.5 mg, 30 mg	Hormone agonist	Hot flashes, gynecomastia, nausea, vomiting, constipation, anorexia, dizziness, headaches, insomnia, paresthesias, bone pain
Lomustine (p. 700) (CeeNU)	**C:** 10 mg, 40 mg, 100 mg	Alkylating agent	Anorexia, nausea, vomiting, stomatitis, hepatotoxicity, nephrotoxicity, myelosuppression, alopecia, confusion, slurred speech
Mechlorethamine (Mustargen)	**I:** 10 mg/ml	Alkylating agent	Severe nausea and vomiting, metallic taste, diarrhea, myelosuppression, alopecia, phlebitis, vertigo, tinnitus, hyperuricemia, infertility, azoospermia, anorexia, headaches, drowsiness, fever

(continued)

CHEMOTHERAPEUTIC AGENTS *(continued)*

Name	Availability	Category	Side Effects
Megestrol (p. 725) (Megace)	**T:** 20 mg, 40 mg **Suspension:** 40 mg/ml	Hormone	Deep vein thrombosis, Cushing-like syndrome, alopecia, carpal tunnel syndrome, weight gain, nausea
Melphalan (p. 729) (Alkeran)	**T:** 2 mg	Alkylating agent	Anorexia, nausea, vomiting, myelosuppression, diarrhea, stomatitis
Mercaptopurine (Purinethol)	**T:** 50 mg	Antimetabolite	Anorexia, nausea, vomiting, stomatitis, hepatic toxicity, myelosuppression, hyperuricemia, diarrhea, rash
Methotrexate (p. 747) (Rheumatrex)	**T:** 2.5 mg, 5 mg, 7.5 mg, 10 mg, 15 mg **I:** 5 mg, 50 mg, 100 mg, 200 mg, 250 mg	Antimetabolite	Nausea, vomiting, stomatitis, GI ulceration, diarrhea, hepatic toxicity, renal failure, cystitis, myelosuppression, alopecia, urticaria, acne, photosensitivity, interstitial pneumonitis, fever, malaise, chills, anorexia
Mitomycin (p. 781) (Mutamycin)	**I:** 20 mg, 40 mg	Antibiotic	Anorexia, nausea, vomiting, stomatitis, diarrhea, renal toxicity, myelosuppression, alopecia, pruritus, fever, hemolytic uremic syndrome, weakness
Mitotane (Lysodren)	**T:** 500 mg	Miscellaneous	Anorexia, nausea, vomiting, diarrhea, skin rashes, depression, lethargy, drowsiness, dizziness, adrenal insufficiency, blurred vision, impaired hearing
Mitoxantrone (p. 783) (Novantrone)	**I:** 20 mg, 25 mg, 30 mg	Anthracenedione	CHF, tachycardia, ECG changes, chest pain, nausea, vomiting, stomatitis, mucositis, myelosuppression, rash, alopecia, urine discoloration (bluish green), phlebitis, diarrhea, cough, headaches, fever
Nelarabine (p. 818) (Arranon)	**I:** 5 mg/ml	Antimetabolite	Anemia, neutropenia, thrombocytopenia, nausea, vomiting, diarrhea, fatigue, fever, dyspnea, severe neurologic events (convulsions, peripheral neuropathy)
Nilotinib (p. 833) (Tasigna)	**C:** 200 mg	Tyrosine kinase inhibitor	Rash, pruritis, nausea, fatigue, headache, constipation, diarrhea, vomiting, thrombocytopenia, neutropenia

Nilutamide (p. 834) (Nilandron)	**T:** 50 mg	Antiandrogen	Hypertension, angina, hot flashes, nausea, anorexia, increased hepatic enzymes, dizziness, dyspnea, visual disturbances, impaired adaptation to dark, constipation, decreased libido
Oxaliplatin (p. 873) (Eloxatin)	**I:** 50 mg, 100 mg	Alkylating agent	Fatigue, neuropathy, abdominal pain, dyspnea, diarrhea, nausea, vomiting, anorexia, fever, edema, chest pain, anemia, thrombocytopenia, thromboembolism, altered hepatic function tests
Paclitaxel (p. 886) (Taxol)	**I:** 30 mg, 100 mg	Antimicrotubular	Hypertension, bradycardia, ECG changes, nausea, vomiting, diarrhea, mucositis, myelosuppression, alopecia, peripheral neuropathies, hypersensitivity reaction, athralgia, myalgia
Panitumumab (p. 896) (Vectibix)	**I:** 20 mg/ml	Monoclonal antibody	Pulmonary fibrosis, severe dermatologic toxicity, infusion reactions, abdominal pain, nausea, vomiting, constipation, skin rash, fatigue
Pegaspargase (Oncaspar)	**I:** 750 international units/ml	Miscellaneous	Hypotension, anorexia, nausea, vomiting, hepatotoxicity, pancreatitis, depression of clotting factors, malaise, confusion, lethargy, EEG changes, respiratory distress, hypersensitivity reaction, fever, hyperglycemia, stomatitis
Pemetrexed (p. 910) (Alimta)	**I:** 500 mg	Antimetabolite	Anorexia, constipation, diarrhea, neuropathy, anemia, chest pain, dyspnea, rash, fatigue
Pentostatin (Nipent)	**I:** 10 mg	Antibiotic	Nausea, vomiting, hepatic disorders, elevated hepatic function tests, leukopenia, anemia, thrombocytopenia, rash, fever, upper respiratory infection, fatigue, hematuria, headaches, myalgia, arthralgia, diarrhea, anorexia
Procarbazine (p. 967) (Matulane)	**C:** 50 mg	Alkylating agent	Nausea, vomiting, stomatitis, diarrhea, constipation, myelosuppression, pruritus, hyperpigmentation, alopecia, myalgia, paresthesias, confusion, lethargy, mental depression, fever, hepatic toxicity, arthralgia, respiratory disorders
Rituximab (p. 1027) (Rituxan)	**I:** 100 mg, 500 mg	Monoclonal antibody	Hypotension, arrhythmias, peripheral edema, nausea, vomiting, abdominal pain, leukopenia, thrombocytopenia, neutropenia, rash, pruritus, urticaria, angioedema, myalgia, headaches, dizziness, throat irritation, rhinitis, bronchospasm, hypersensitivity reaction

(continued)

CHEMOTHERAPEUTIC AGENTS *(continued)*

Name	Availability	Category	Side Effects
Sipuleucel-T (Provenge)	**I:** Minimum of 50 million autologous $CD54^+$ cells in lactated Ringer's	Miscellaneous	Chills, fatigue, fever, back pain, nausea, headache, joint ache
Sorafenib (p. 1075) (Nexavar)	**T:** 200 mg	Tyrosine kinase inhibitor	Fatigue, alopecia, nausea, vomiting, anorexia, constipation, diarrhea, neuropathy, dyspnea, cough, asthenia, pain
Streptozocin (Zanosar)	**I:** 1 g	Alkylating agent	May lead to insulin-dependent diabetes, nausea, vomiting, nephrotoxicity, renal tubular acidosis, myelosuppression, lethargy, diarrhea, confusion, depression
Sunitinib (p. 1088) (Sutent)	**C:** 12.5 mg, 25 mg, 50 mg	Tyrosine kinase inhibitor	Hypotension, edema, fatigue, headache, fever, dizziness, rash, hyperpigmentation, diarrhea, nausea, dyspepsia, altered taste, vomiting, neutropenia, thrombocytopenia, increased ALT/AST
Tamoxifen (p. 1094) (Nolvadex-D)	**T:** 10 mg, 20 mg	Estrogen receptor antagonist	Skin rash, nausea, vomiting, anorexia, menstrual irregularities, hot flashes, pruritus, vaginal discharge or bleeding, myelosuppression, headaches, tumor or bone pain, ophthalmic changes, weight gain, confusion
Temozolomide (p. 1102) (Temodar)	**C:** 5 mg, 20 mg, 100 mg, 250 mg	Alkylating agent	Amnesia, fever, infection, leukopenia, neutropenia, peripheral edema, seizures, thrombocytopenia
Temsirolimus (p. 1103) (Torisel)	**I:** 25 mg/ml	mTOR kinase inhibitor	Rash, asthenia, mucositis, nausea, edema, anorexia, thrombocytopenia, leukopenia
Teniposide (Vumon)	**I:** 50 mg/5 ml	Miscellaneous	Hypotension with rapid infusion, diarrhea, nausea, vomiting, mucositis, myelosuppression, alopecia, anemia, rash, hypersensitivity reaction
Thioguanine	**T:** 40 mg	Antimetabolite	Anorexia, stomatitis, myelosuppression, hyperuricemia, nausea, vomiting, diarrhea
Thiotepa (p. 1125) (Thioplex)	**I:** 15 mg	Alkylating agent	Anorexia, nausea, vomiting, mucositis, myelosuppression, amenorrhea, reduced spermatogenesis, fever, hypersensitivity reactions, pain at injection site, headaches, dizziness, alopecia

Topotecan (p. 1151) (Hycamtin)	**I:** 4 mg	Camptothecin	Nausea, vomiting, diarrhea, constipation, abdominal pain, stomatitis, anorexia, neutropenia, leukopenia, thrombocytopenia, anemia, alopecia, headaches, dyspnea, paresthesia
Toremifene (p. 1153) (Fareston)	**T:** 60 mg	Estrogen receptor antagonist	Elevated hepatic function tests, nausea, vomiting, constipation, skin discoloration, dermatitis, dizziness, hot flashes, diaphoresis, vaginal discharge or bleeding, ocular changes, cataracts, anxiety
Tositumomab (p. 1156) (Bexxar)	**I:** 14 mg/ml	Monoclonal antibody	Headaches, rash, pruritus, abdominal pain, anorexia, diarrhea, nausea, vomiting, arthralgia, myalgia, cough, dyspnea, asthenia, chills, fever, infection
Trastuzumab (p. 1164) (Herceptin)	**I:** 440 mg	Monoclonal antibody	CHF, heart murmur (S3 gallop), nausea, vomiting, diarrhea, abdominal pain, anorexia, rash, peripheral edema, back or bone pain, asthenia, headaches, insomnia, dizziness, cough, dyspnea, rhinitis, pharyngitis
Tretinoin (p. 1169) (Vesanoid)	**C:** 10 mg	Miscellaneous	Flushing, nausea, vomiting, diarrhea, constipation, dyspepsia, mucositis, leukocytosis, dry skin/mucous membranes, rash, pruritus, alopecia, dizziness, anxiety, insomnia, headaches, depression, confusion, intracranial hypertension, agitation, dyspnea, shivering, fever, visual changes, earaches, hearing loss, bone pain, myalgia, arthralgia
Valrubicin (Valstar)	**I:** 200 mg/5 ml	Anthracycline	Dysuria, hematuria, urinary frequency/incontinence/urgency
Vinblastine (p. 1204) (Velban)	**I:** 10 mg	Vinca alkaloid	Nausea, vomiting, stomatitis, constipation, myelosuppression, alopecia, peripheral neuropathy, loss of deep tendon reflexes, paresthesias, diarrhea
Vincristine (p. 1206) (Oncovin)	**I:** 1 mg, 2 mg, 3 mg	Vinca alkaloid	Nausea, vomiting, stomatitis, constipation, pharyngitis, polyuria, myelosuppression, alopecia, numbness, paresthesias, peripheral neuropathy, loss of deep tendon reflexes, headaches, abdominal pain
Vinorelbine (p. 1208) (Navelbine)	**I:** 10 mg, 50 mg	Vinca alkaloid	Elevated hepatic function tests, nausea, vomiting, constipation, ileus, anorexia, stomatitis, myelosuppression, alopecia, vein discoloration, venous pain, phlebitis, interstitial pulmonary changes, asthenia, fatigue, diarrhea, peripheral neuropathy, loss of deep tendon reflexes
Vorinostat (p. 1220) (Zolinza)	**C:** 100 mg	Histone deacetylase inhibitor	Diarrhea, fatigue, nausea, thrombocytopenia, anorexia, dysgeusia

C, Capsules; ***I,*** injection; ***T,*** tablets.

Cholinergic Agonists/Anticholinesterase

USES

Paralytic ileus and atony of urinary bladder. Myasthenia gravis (weakness, marked fatigue of skeletal muscle). Terminates, reverses effects of neuromuscular blocking agents.

ACTION

Cholinergic agonists: Referred to as *muscarinics* or *parasympathetics* and consist of two basic drug groups: choline esters and cholinomimetic alkaloids. Primary action mimics actions of acetylcholine at postganglionic parasympathetic nerves. Primary properties include the following:

Cardiovascular system: Vasodilation; decreased cardiac rate; decreased conduction in SA, AV nodes; decreased force of myocardial contraction.

Gastrointestinal: Increased tone, motility of GI smooth muscle, increased secretory activity of GI tract.

Urinary tract: Increased contraction of detrusor muscle of urinary bladder, resulting in micturition.

Eye: Miosis, contraction of ciliary muscle.

Anticholinesterase (anti-ChE), also known as *cholinesterase inhibitors:* Inactivates cholinesterase, which prevents acetylcholine breakdown, causing acetylcholine to accumulate at cholinergic receptor sites. These agents can be considered indirect-acting cholinergic agonists. Primary properties include action of cholinergic agonists just noted.

Skeletal neuromuscular junction: Effects are dose dependent. At therapeutic doses, increases force of skeletal muscle contraction; at toxic doses, reduces muscle strength.

CHOLINERGIC AGONISTS/ANTICHOLINESTERASE

Name	Availability	Uses	Dosage Range	Side Effects
Bethanechol (p. 123) (Urecholine)	**T:** 5 mg, 10 mg, 25 mg, 50 mg **I:** 5 mg/ml	Nonobstructive urinary retention	**PO:** 10–50 mg 3–4 times/day **Subcutaneous:** 2.5–5 mg 3–4 times/day	Increased urinary frequency, salivation, belching, nausea, dizziness

Edrophonium (Tensilon)	**I:** 10 mg/ml	Diagnosis of myasthenia gravis, reverses tubocurarine	**IV:** 10 mg over 30 sec up to 40 mg	Bradycardia, nausea, vomiting, diarrhea, urinary frequency
Neostigmine (p. 821) (Prostigmin)	**T:** 15 mg **I:** 0.25 mg/ml, 0.5 mg/ml, 1 mg/ml	Symptomatic control of myasthenia gravis, neuromuscular blocker	**PO:** 15–365 mg/day **Subcutaneous, IM:** 0.5 mg **IV:** 0.5–2 mg	Diarrhea, diaphoresis, nausea, vomiting, abdominal cramps
Pyridostigmine (p. 987) (Mestinon)	**T:** 60 mg **T (ER):** 180 mg **S:** 60 mg/5 ml **I:** 5 mg/ml	Treats myasthenia gravis, reverses tubocurarine	**PO:** 60–1,500 mg/day **IM:** 0.5–1.5 mg/kg **IV:** 0.1–0.25 mg/kg	Diarrhea, diaphoresis, nausea, vomiting, abdominal cramps

ER, Extended release; ***I,*** injection; ***S,*** suspension; ***T,*** tablets.

Contraception

ACTION

Combination oral contraceptives decrease fertility primarily by inhibition of ovulation. In addition, they can promote thickening of the cervical mucus, thereby creating a physical barrier for the passage of sperm. Also, they can modify the endometrium, making it less favorable for nidation.

CLASSIFICATION

Oral contraceptives either contain both an estrogen and a progestin (combination oral contraceptives) or contain only a progestin (progestin-only oral contraceptives). The combination oral contraceptives have three subgroups:

Monophasic: Daily estrogen and progestin dosage remains constant.

Biphasic: Estrogen remains constant, but the progestin dosage increases during the second half of the cycle.

Triphasic: Progestin changes for each phase of the cycle.

Over the past several years, options have expanded to include a combined hormonal patch (Ortho Evra), vaginal ring (NuvaRing), and extended cycle contraceptives (e.g., Loestrin-24 FE, Seasonale, Seasonique, Yaz). The latest oral contraceptive, Natazia, is a four-phase dosing regimen (estradiol steps down and dienogest, a progestin, steps up during the cycle to help avoid breakthrough bleeding).

(continued)

COMMON COMPLAINTS WITH ORAL CONTRACEPTIVES

Too much estrogen	Nausea, bloating, breast tenderness, increased B/P, melasma, headache
Too little estrogen	Early or mid-cycle breakthrough bleeding, increased spotting, hypomenorrhea
Too much progestin	Breast tenderness, headache, fatigue, changes in mood
Too little progestin	Late breakthrough bleeding
Too much androgen	Increased appetite, weight gain, acne, oily skin, hirsutism, decreased libido, increased breast size, breast tenderness, increased LDL cholesterol, decreased HDL cholesterol

CONTRACEPTIVES

Name	Estrogen Content	Progestin Content
Low-Dose Monophasic Pills		
Aviane-28 Lessina Lutera Sronyx	EE 20 mcg	Levonorgestrel 0.1 mg
Junel 1/20 Junel Fe 1/20 Loestrin Fe 1/20 Microgestin Fe 1/20	EE 20 mcg	Norethindrone 1 mg
Levora Nordette-28 Portia-28	EE 30 mcg	Levonorgestrel 0.15 mg
Cryselle-28 Lo/Ovral-28 Low-Ogestrel-21, -28	EE 30 mcg	Norgestrel 0.3 mg

Junel 1.5/30 Junel Fe 1.5/30 Loestrin Fe 1.5/30 Microgestin 1.5/30 Microgestin Fe 1.5/30	EE 30 mcg	Norethindrone acetate 1.5 mg
Apri Desogen Ortho-Cept Reclipsen Solia	EE 30 mcg	Desogestrel 0.15 mg
Yasmin Ocella	EE 30 mcg	Drospirenone 3 mg
Kelnor 1/35 Zovia 1/35	EE 35 mcg	Ethynodiol diacetate 1 mg
Ortho-Cyclen-28 Mononessa Previfem Sprintec	EE 35 mcg	Norgestimate 0.25 mg
Necon 1/50 Norinyl 1+50	Mestranol 50 mcg	Norethindrone 1 mg
Balziva Femcon Fe Ovcon-35 Zenchent	EE 35 mcg	Norethindrone 0.4 mg
Brevicon-28 Modicon-28 Necon 0.5/35 Nortrel 0.5/35	EE 35 mcg	Norethindrone 0.5 mg (total of 10.5 mg/cycle)

(continued)

CONTRACEPTIVES *(continued)*

Name	Estrogen Content	Progestin Content
Necon 1/35-28 Norinyl 1+35-28 Nortrel 1/35-28 Ortho-Novum 1/35-28	EE 35 mcg	Norethindrone 1 mg (total of 21 mg/cycle)
High-Dose Monophasic Pills		
Zovia 1/50-28	EE 50 mcg	Ethynodiol diacetate 1 mg
Ogestrel 0.5/50-28	EE 50 mcg	Norgestrel 0.5 mg
Ovcon-50	EE 50 mcg	Norethindrone 1 mg
Biphasic Pills		
Azurette Kariva Mircette	EE 20 mcg × 21 days, placebo × 2 days, 10 mcg × 5 days	Desogestrel 0.15 mg × 21 days
Necon 10/11	EE 35 mcg	Norethindrone 0.5 mg × 10 days, 1 mg × 11 days
Triphasic Pills		
Estrostep Fe Tilia Tilia Fe Tri-Legest Fe	EE 20 mcg × 5 days, 30 mcg × 7 days, 35 mcg × 9 days	Norethindrone 1 mg × 21 days
Ortho Tri-Cyclen Lo Tri Lo Spriutec	EE 25 mcg × 21 days	Norgestimate 0.18 mg × 7 days, 0.215 mg × 7 days, 0.25 mg × 7 days

Caziant Cesia Cyclessa Velivet	EE 25 mcg × 21 days	Desogestrel 0.1 mg × 7 days, 0.125 mg × 7 days, 0.15 mg × 7 days
Enpresse Trivora	EE 30 mcg × 6 days, 40 mcg × 5 days, 30 mcg × 10 days	Levonorgestrel 0.05 mg × 6 days, 0.075 mg × 5 days, 0.125 mg × 10 days
Ortho Tri-Cyclen Trinessa Tri-Previfem Tri-Sprintec	EE 35 mcg × 21 days	Norgestimate 0.18 mg × 7 days, 0.215 mg × 7 days, 0.25 mg × 7 days
Aranelle Leena Tri-Norinyl	EE 35 mcg × 21 days	Norethindrone 0.5 mg × 7 days, 1 mg × 9 days, 0.5 mg × 5 days
Ortho-Novum 7/7/7 Nortrel 7/7/7 Necon 7/7/7	EE 35 mcg × 21 days	Norethindrone 0.5 mg × 7 days, 0.75 mg × 7 days, 1 mg × 7 days
Four Phasic		
Natazia	Estradiol 3 mg × 2 days, then 2 mg × 22 days, then 1 mg × 2 days, then 2-day pill-free interval	Dienogest none × 2 days, then 2 mg × 5 days, then 3 mg × 17 days, then none for 4 days
Extended-Cycle Pills		
Loestrin-24 FE	EE 20 mcg × 24 days	Norethindrone 1 mg × 24 days
Jolessa Quasense Seasonale	EE 30 mcg × 84 days	Levonorgestrel 0.15 mg × 84 days
Seasonique	EE 30 mcg × 84 days, 10 mcg × 7 days	Levonorgestrel 0.15 mg × 84 days

(continued)

CONTRACEPTIVES *(continued)*

Name	Estrogen Content	Progestin Content
Yaz Gianvi	EE 20 mcg × 24 days	Drospirenone 3 mg × 24 days
Continuous Cycle Pill		
Lybrel	EE 20 mcg	Levonorgestrel 90 mcg
Progestin-Only Pills		
Camilia Errin Jolivette Micronor Nor-QD Nora-BE	N/A	Norethindrone 0.35 mg
Emergency Contraception		
Plan B Next chance	N/A	Levonorgestrel 0.75-mg tablets × 2
Ella (Ulipristal)	N/A	Ulipristal 30 mg × 1 within 5 days after unprotected intercourse
Hormonal Alternative to Oral Contraception		
Depo-Provera CI Medroxyprogesterone Acetate	None	Medroxyprogesterone 150 mg
Depo-SubQ Provera 104	None	Medroxyprogesterone 104 mg
Implanon	None	Etonogestrel (release rate varies over time)
Mirena	None	Levonorgestrel 20 mcg/day for 5 yrs
NuvaRing	Ethinyl estradiol 15 mcg/day	Etonogestrel 0.12 mg/day
Ortho Evra	Ethinyl estradiol 20 mcg/day	Norelgestromin 150 mcg/day

Corticosteroids

USES	ACTION
Replacement therapy in adrenal insufficiency, including Addison's disease. Symptomatic treatment of multi-organ disease/conditions. Rheumatoid arthritis (RA), osteoarthritis, severe psoriasis, ulcerative colitis, lupus erythematosus, anaphylactic shock, acute exacerbation of asthma, status asthmaticus, organ transplant.	Suppress migration of polymorphonuclear leukocytes (PML) and reverse increased capillary permeability by their anti-inflammatory effect. Suppress immune system by decreasing activity of lymphatic system.

CORTICOSTEROIDS

Name	Availability	Route of Administration	Side Effects
Beclomethasone (p. 113) (Beconase)	**Inhalation, nasal:** 42 mcg/spray, 84 mcg/spray	Inhalation, intranasal	**I:** Cough, dry mouth/throat, headaches, throat irritation **Nasal:** Headaches, sore throat, intranasal ulceration
Betamethasone (p. 121) (Celestone, Diprolene)	**I:** 4 mg/ml	IV, intralesional, intra-articular	Nausea, vomiting, increased appetite, weight gain, insomnia
Budesonide (p. 145) (Pulmicort, Rhinocort)	**Nasal:** 32 mcg/spray	Intranasal	Headaches, sore throat, intranasal ulceration
Cortisone (p. 277) (Cortone)	**T:** 5 mg, 10 mg, 25 mg	PO	Insomnia, nervousness, increased appetite, indigestion
Dexamethasone (p. 331) (Decadron)	**T:** 0.5 mg, 1 mg, 4 mg, 6 mg **OS:** 0.5 mg/5 ml **I:** 4 mg/ml	PO, parenteral	Insomnia, weight gain, increased appetite

(continued)

CORTICOSTEROIDS ***(continued)***

Name	Availability	Route of Administration	Side Effects
Fludrocortisone (Florinef)	**T:** 0.1 mg	PO	Edema, headache, peptic ulcer
Flunisolide (p. 493) (AeroBid, Nasalide)	**Inhalation, nasal:** 25 mcg/spray	Inhalation, intranasal	Headache, nasal congestion, pharyngitis, upper respiratory infections, altered taste/smell
Fluticasone (p. 505) (Flonase, Flovent)	**Inhalation:** 44 mcg, 110 mg, 220 mcg **Nasal:** 50 mg, 100 mcg	Inhalation, intranasal	Headache, burning/stinging, nasal congestion, upper respiratory infections
Hydrocortisone (p. 575) (Solu-Cortef)	**T:** 5 mg, 10 mg, 25 mg **I:** 100 mg, 250 mg, 500 mg, 1 g	PO, parenteral	Insomnia, headache, nausea, vomiting
Methylprednisolone (p. 754) (Solu-Medrol)	**T:** 4 mg **I:** 40 mg, 125 mg, 500 mg, 1 g, 2 g	PO, parenteral	Headache, insomnia, nervousness, increased appetite, nausea, vomiting
Prednisolone (p. 957) (Prelone)	**T:** 5 mg **OS:** 5 mg/5 ml, 15 mg/5 ml	PO	Headache, insomnia, weight gain, nausea, vomiting
Prednisone (p. 959)	**T:** 1 mg, 2.5 mg, 5 mg, 10 mg, 20 mg, 50 mg	PO	Headache, insomnia, weight gain, nausea, vomiting
Triamcinolone (p. 1171) (Azmacort, Kenalog)	**T:** 4 mg, 8 mg **Inhalation:** 100 mcg	PO, inhalation	**PO:** Insomnia, increased appetite, nausea, vomiting **I:** Cough, dry mouth/throat, headaches, throat irritation

I, Injection; ***OS,*** oral suspension; ***T,*** tablets.

Corticosteroids: Topical

USES

Provide relief of inflammation/pruritus associated with corticosteroid-responsive disorders (e.g., contact dermatitis, eczema, insect bite reactions, first- and second-degree localized burns/sunburn).

ACTION

Diffuse across cell membranes, form complexes with cytoplasm. Complexes stimulate protein synthesis of inhibitory enzymes responsible for anti-inflammatory effects (e.g., inhibit edema, erythema, pruritus, capillary dilation, phagocytic activity).

Topical corticosteroids can be classified based on potency:

May use for facial and intertriginous application for only limited time.

High potency: For more severe inflammatory conditions (e.g., lichen simplex chronicus, psoriasis). May use for facial and intertriginous application for short time only. Used in areas of thickened skin due to chronic conditions.

Low potency: Modest anti-inflammatory effect, safest for chronic application, facial and intertriginous application, with occlusion, for infants/young children.

Medium potency: For moderate inflammatory conditions (e.g., chronic eczematous dermatoses).

Very high potency: Alternative to systemic therapy for local effect (e.g., chronic lesions caused by psoriasis). Increased risk of skin atrophy. Used for short periods on small areas. Avoid occlusive dressings.

CORTICOSTEROIDS: TOPICAL

Name	Availability	Potency	Side Effects
Alclometasone (Aclovate)	**C, O:** 0.05%	Low	Skin atrophy, contact dermatitis, stretch marks on skin, enlarged blood vessels in the skin, hair loss, pigment changes, secondary infections
Amcinonide (Cyclocort)	**C, O, L:** 0.1%	High	Same as alclometasone
Betamethasone dipropionate (p. 121)	**C, O, G, L:** 0.05%	High	Same as alclometasone

(continued)

CORTICOSTEROIDS: TOPICAL *(continued)*

Name	Availability	Potency	Side Effects
Betamethasone valerate (p. 121)	**C:** 0.01%, 0.05%, 0.1% **O:** 0.1% **L:** 0.1%	High	Same as alclometasone
Clobetasol (Temovate)	**C, O:** 0.05%	High	Same as alclometasone
Desonide (Tridesilon)	**C, O, L:** 0.05%	Low	Same as alclometasone
Desoximetasone (Topicort)	**C:** 0.25%, 0.5% **O:** 0.25% **G:** 0.05%	High	Same as alclometasone
Dexamethasone (p. 331) (Decadron)	**C:** 0.1%	Medium	Same as alclometasone
Fluocinolone (Synalar)	**C:** 0.01%, 0.025%, 0.2% **O:** 0.025%	High	Same as alclometasone
Fluocinonide (Lidex)	**C, O, G:** 0.05%	High	Same as alclometasone
Flurandrenolide (Cordran)	**C, O, L:** 0.025%, 0.05%	Medium	Same as alclometasone
Fluticasone (p. 505) (Cutivate)	**C:** 0.05% **O:** 0.005%	Medium	Same as alclometasone
Halobetasol (Ultravate)	**C, O:** 0.05%	High	Same as alclometasone
Hydrocortisone (p. 575) (Hytone)	**C, O:** 0.5%, 1%, 2.5%	Medium	Same as alclometasone
Mometasone (p. 787) (Elocon)	**C, O, L:** 0.1%	Medium	Same as alclometasone
Prednicarbate (Dermatop)	**C:** 0.1%	—	Same as alclometasone
Triamcinolone (p. 1171) (Aristocort, Kenalog)	**C, O, L:** 0.025%, 0.1%, 0.5%	Medium	Same as alclometasone

C, Cream; ***G,*** gel; ***L,*** lotion; ***O,*** ointment.

Diuretics

USES

Thiazides: Management of edema resulting from a number of causes (e.g., CHF, hepatic cirrhosis); hypertension either alone or in combination with other antihypertensives.
Loop: Management of edema associated with CHF, cirrhosis of the liver, and renal disease. Furosemide used in treatment of hypertension alone or in combination with other antihypertensives.
Potassium-sparing: Adjunctive treatment with thiazides, loop diuretics in treatment of CHF and hypertension.

ACTION

Act to increase the excretion of water/sodium and other electrolytes via the kidneys. Exact mechanism of antihypertensive effect unknown; may be due to reduced plasma volume or decreased peripheral vascular resistance. Subclassifications of diuretics are based on their mechanism and site of action.
Thiazides: Act at the cortical diluting segment of nephron, block reabsorption of Na, Cl, and water; promote excretion of Na, Cl, K, and water. *Loop:* Act primarily at the thick ascending limb of Henle's loop to inhibit Na, Cl, and water absorption.
Potassium-sparing: Spironolactone blocks aldosterone action on distal nephron (causes K retention, Na excretion). Triamterene, amiloride act on distal nephron, decreasing Na reuptake, reducing K secretion.

DIURETICS

Name	Availability	Dosage Range	Side Effects
Thiazide, Thiazide-related			
Chlorothiazide (Diuril)	**T:** 250 mg, 500 mg **S:** 250 mg/5 ml **I:** 500 mg	5–20 mg/day	Confusion, fatigue, muscle cramps, abdominal discomfort
Chlorthalidone (Hygroton)	**T:** 15 mg, 25 mg, 50 mg, 100 mg	25–200 mg/day	Same as chlorothiazide

(continued)

DIURETICS *(continued)*

Name	Availability	Dosage Range	Side Effects
Hydrochlorothiazide (p. 571) (HydroDIURIL)	**T:** 25 mg, 50 mg, 100 mg **C:** 12.5 mg **Solution:** 50 mg/15 ml	25–100 mg/day	Orthostatic hypotension, photosensitivity, hypokalemia, anorexia, epigastric distress
Indapamide (p. 608) (Lozol)	**T:** 1.25 mg, 2.5 mg	2.5–5 mg/day	Loss of appetite, diarrhea, headaches, dizziness, light-headedness, insomnia, upset stomach
Metolazone (p. 758) (Zaroxolyn)	**T:** 2.5 mg, 5 mg, 10 mg	2.5–10 mg/day	Orthostatic hypotension, dizziness, hypokalemia, nausea, diarrhea, abdominal pain
Loop			
Bumetanide (p. 147) (Bumex)	**T:** 0.5 mg, 1 mg, 2 mg **I:** 0.25 mg/ml	**HTN:** 5–10 mg/day **Edema:** 1–10 mg/day	Orthostatic hypotension, cramps or pain, hypokalemia (dry mouth, fatigue, muscle cramps), blurred vision, headaches
Furosemide (p. 526) (Lasix)	**T:** 20 mg, 40 mg, 80 mg **OS:** 10 mg/ml, 40 mg/5 ml **I:** 10 mg/ml	**HTN:** 40–80 mg/day **Edema:** Up to 600 mg/day	Orthostatic hypotension, cramps or pain, hypokalemia (dry mouth, fatigue, muscle cramps), blurred vision, headaches
Torsemide (p. 1154) (Demadex)	**T:** 5 mg, 10 mg, 20 mg, 100 mg **I:** 10 mg/ml	**Edema:** 10–200 mg/day **HTN:** 5–10 mg/day up to 200 mg/day	Constipation, dizziness, upset stomach, headache, hypokalemia (dry mouth, fatigue, muscle cramps)
Potassium-sparing			
Amiloride (Midamor)	**T:** 5 mg	5–20 mg/day	Hyperkalemia, nausea, abdominal pain, diarrhea
Spironolactone (p. 1078) (Aldactone)	**T:** 25 mg, 50 mg, 100 mg	25–100 mg/day	Hyperkalemia, nausea, vomiting, abdominal cramps, diarrhea
Triamterene (p. 1173) (Dyrenium)	**C:** 50 mg, 100 mg	Up to 300 mg/day	Same as amiloride

C, Capsules; ***HTN,*** hypertension; ***I,*** injection; ***OS,*** oral solution; ***S,*** suspension; ***T,*** tablets.

Fertility Agents

Infertility is defined as unsuccessful conception after 12 months of attempting to conceive, as opposed to *sterility,* the inability to reproduce. Infertility may be due to reproduction dysfunction of the male, female, or both.

Female infertility can be due to disruption of any phase of the reproductive process. The most critical phases include follicular maturation, ovulation, transport of the ovum through the fallopian tubes, fertilization of the ovum, nidation, and growth/development of the conceptus. Causes of infertility include the following:

Anovulation, failure of follicular maturation: Absence of adequate hormonal stimulation; ovarian follicles do not ripen, and ovulation will not occur.

Unfavorable cervical mucus: Normally the cervical glands secrete large volumes of thin watery mucus, but if the mucus is unfavorable (scant, thick, or sticky), sperm is unable to pass through to the uterus.

Hyperprolactinemia: Excessive prolactin secretion may cause amenorrhea, galactorrhea, and infertility.

Luteal phase defect: Progesterone secretion by the corpus luteum is insufficient to maintain endometrial integrity.

Endometriosis: Endometrial tissue is implanted in abnormal locations (e.g., uterine wall, ovary, extragenital sites).

Androgen excess: May decrease fertility (most common condition is polycystic ovary).

Male infertility is due to decreased density or motility of sperm or semen of abnormal volume or quality. The most obvious manifestation of male infertility is impotence (inability to achieve erection). Whereas in female infertility an identifiable endocrine disorder can be found, most cases of male infertility are not associated with an identifiable endocrine disorder.

ACTION

Antiestrogens: Nonsteroidal estrogen antagonist that increases follicle-stimulating hormone (FSH) and leutinizing hormone (LH) levels by blocking estrogen-negative feedback at the hypothalamus.

Gonadotropins: Produce ovulation induction in women with hypogonadotropic hypogonadism and polycystic ovarian syndrome (PCOS). Ovaries must be able to respond normally to FSH and LH stimulation.

Gonadotropin-releasing hormone (GnRH) agonists: Causes down-regulation of endogenous FSH and LH levels. GnRH agonists stimulate release of pituitary gonadotropins. Suppression of endogenous LH can decrease number of oocytes released prematurely, improve oocyte quality, and increase pregnancy rates.

Gonadotropin-releasing hormone (GnRH) antagonists: Suppress endogenous LH surges during ovarian stimulation. GnRH antagonists avoid initial flare-up seen with GnRH agonists, shortening the number of days needed for LH suppression and allowing ovarian stimulation to begin within the spontaneous cycle.

MEDICATIONS TO INDUCE OVULATION

Name	Category	Availability	Uses	Side Effects
Cetrorelix (Cetrotide)	GnRH antagonist	**I:** 0.25 mg, 3 mg	Inhibition of premature LH surges in women undergoing ovarian hyperstimulation	OHSS (ovarian hyperstimulation syndrome): Abdominal pain, indigestion, bloating, decreased urinary output, nausea, vomiting, diarrhea, rapid weight gain, shortness of breath, peripheral/dependent edema; headaches, pain/redness at injection site, mood swings, hot flashes, insomnia, vaginal dryness
Chorionic gonadotropin (p. 231) (Novarel, Ovidrel, Pregnyl)	Gonadotropin	**I:** 5,000 units, 10,000 units, 20,000 units	In conjunction with clomiphene, human menotropins or urofolitropin to stimulate ovulation	OHSS (ovarian hyperstimulation syndrome): Abdominal pain, indigestion, bloating, decreased urinary output, nausea, vomiting, diarrhea, rapid weight gain, shortness of breath, peripheral/dependent edema; ovarian enlargement, ovarian cyst formation, headache, pain at injection site
Clomiphene (Clomid, Milophene, Serophene)	Antiestrogen	**T:** 50 mg	Anovulation, oligo-ovulation with intact pituitary/ovarian response and endogenous estrogen	Ovarian cyst formation, ovarian enlargement visual disturbances, premenstrual syndrome, hot flashes, headaches, blurred vision, nausea, breast tenderness
Follitropin alpha (Gonal-F)	Gonadotropin	**I:** 37.5 international units FSH, 75 international units FSH, 150 international units FSH	In conjunction with human chorionic gonadotropin to stimulate ovarian follicular development in pts with ovulatory dysfunction not due to primary ovarian failure (e.g., anovulation, oligo-ovulation)	OHSS (ovarian hyperstimulation syndrome): Abdominal pain, indigestion, bloating, decreased urinary output, nausea, vomiting, diarrhea, rapid weight gain, shortness of breath, peripheral/dependent edema; flu-like symptoms, upper respiratory tract infections, bleeding between menstrual periods, nausea, ovarian enlargement, ovarian cysts, acne, breast pain/tenderness, mood swings

Follitropin beta (Follistim AQ)	Gonadotropin	**I:** 75 international units FSH	In conjunction with human chorionic gonadotropin to stimulate ovarian follicular development in patients with ovulatory dysfunction not due to primary ovarian failure (e.g., anovulation, oligo-ovulation)	OHSS (ovarian hyperstimulation syndrome): Abdominal pain, indigestion, bloating, decreased urinary output, nausea, vomiting, diarrhea, rapid weight gain, shortness of breath, peripheral/dependent edema; flu-like symptoms, breast tenderness, dry skin, rash, dizziness, fever, headaches, nausea, fatigue, mood swings
Ganirelex (Antagon)	GnRH antagonist	**I:** 250 mcg/0.5 ml	Inhibition of premature LH surges in women undergoing ovarian hyperstimulation	OHSS (ovarian hyperstimulation syndrome): Abdominal pain, indigestion, bloating, decreased urinary output, nausea, vomiting, diarrhea, rapid weight gain, shortness of breath, peripheral/dependent edema; headaches, nausea, pain/redness at injection site, mood swings, hot flashes, insomnia, vaginal dryness
Goserelin (p. 557) (Zoladex)	GnRH agonist	**Implant:** 3.6 mg, 10.8 mg	Endometriosis, adjunct to menotropins for ovulation induction	Hot flashes, amenorrhea, blurred vision, edema, headaches, nausea, vomiting, breast tenderness, weight gain, mood swings, insomnia, vaginal dryness
Leuprolide (p. 677) (Lupron)	GnRH agonist	5 mg/ml for subcutaneous injection	Endometriosis, adjunct to menotropins/human chorionic gonadotropin for ovulation induction	Hot flashes, amenorrhea, blurred vision, edema, headaches, nausea, vomiting, breast tenderness, weight gain, mood swings, insomnia, vaginal dryness

(continued)

MEDICATIONS TO INDUCE OVULATION *(continued)*

Name	Category	Availability	Uses	Side Effects
Menotropins (Menopur, Repronex)	Gonadotropin	75 units FSH, 75 units LH activity; 150 units FSH, 150 units LH activity	In conjunction with chorionic gonadotropin for ovulation stimulation in pts with ovulatory dysfunction due to primary ovarian failure	OHSS (ovarian hyperstimulation syndrome): Abdominal pain, indigestion, bloating, decreased urinary output, nausea, vomiting, diarrhea, rapid weight gain, shortness of breath, edema of lower extremities; ovarian enlargement, ovarian cyst formation, breast tenderness, mood swings
Nafarelin (p. 803) (Synarel)	GnRH	2 mg/ml nasal spray	Endometriosis, adjunct to menotropins/human chorionic gonadotropin for ovulation induction	Loss of bone mineral density, breast enlargement, bleeding between regular menstrual periods, acne, mood swings, seborrhea, hot flashes, headache, insomnia, vaginal dryness
Urofollitropin (Bravelle)	Gonadotropin	75 units FSH activity, 150 units FSH activity	In conjunction with human chorionic gonadotropin for ovulation stimulation in pts with polycystic ovary syndrome who have elevated LH:FSH ratio and have failed clomiphene therapy	OHSS (ovarian hyperstimulation syndrome): Abdominal pain, indigestion, bloating, decreased urinary output, nausea, vomiting, diarrhea, rapid weight gain, shortness of breath, edema of lower extremities; ovarian enlargement, ovarian cyst formation, pain/redness at injection site, breast tenderness, nausea, vomiting, diarrhea, mood swings

I, Injection; ***T,*** tablets.

H_2 Antagonists

USES

Short-term treatment of duodenal ulcer (DU), active benign gastric ulcer (GU), maintenance therapy of DU, pathologic hypersecretory conditions (e.g., Zollinger-Ellison syndrome), gastroesophageal reflux disease (GERD), and prevention of upper GI bleeding in critically ill pts.

ACTION

Inhibit gastric acid secretion by interfering with histamine at the histamine H_2 receptors in parietal cells. Also inhibit acid secretion caused by gastrin. Inhibition occurs with basal (fasting), nocturnal, food-stimulated, or fundic distention secretion. H_2 antagonists decrease both the volume and H_2 concentration of gastric juices.

H_2 ANTAGONISTS

Name	Availability	Dosage Range	Side Effects
Cimetidine (p. 237) (Tagamet)	**T:** 200 mg, 300 mg, 400 mg, 800 mg **L:** 300 mg/5 ml **I:** 150 mg/ml	**Treatment of DU:** 800 mg/at bedtime, 400 mg 2 times/day or 300 mg 4 times/day **Maintenance of DU:** 400 mg/at bedtime **Treatment of GU:** 800 mg/at bedtime or 300 mg 4 times/day **GERD:** 1,600 mg/day **Hypersecretory:** 1,200–2,400 mg/day	Headaches, fatigue, dizziness, confusion, diarrhea, gynecomastia

(continued)

H_2 ANTAGONISTS *(continued)*

Name	Availability	Dosage Range	Side Effects
Famotidine (p. 463) (Pepcid)	**T:** 10 mg, 20 mg, 40 mg **T (chewable):** 10 mg **DT:** 20 mg, 40 mg **Gelcap:** 10 mg **OS:** 40 mg/5 ml **I:** 10 mg/ml	**Treatment of DU:** 40 mg/day **Maintenance of DU:** 20 mg/day **Treatment of GU:** 40 mg/day **GERD:** 40–80 mg/day **Hypersecretory:** 80–640 mg/day	Headaches, dizziness, diarrhea, constipation, abdominal pain, tinnitus
Nizatidine (p. 844) (Axid)	**T:** 75 mg **C:** 150 mg, 300 mg	**Treatment of DU:** 300 mg/day **Maintenance of DU:** 150 mg/day	Fatigue, urticaria, abdominal pain, constipation, nausea
Ranitidine (p. 1003) (Zantac)	**T:** 75 mg, 150 mg, 300 mg **C:** 150 mg, 300 mg **Syrup:** 15 mg/ml **Granules:** 150 mg **I:** 0.5 mg/ml, 25 mg/ml	**Treatment of DU:** 300 mg/day **Maintenance of DU:** 150 mg/day **Treatment of GU:** 300 mg/day **GERD:** 300 mg/day **Hypersecretory:** 0.3–6 g/day	Blurred vision, constipation, nausea, abdominal pain

C, Capsules; ***DT,*** disintegrating tablets; ***I,*** injection; ***L,*** liquid; ***OS,*** oral suspension; ***T,*** tablets.

Hematinic Preparations

USES

Prevention or treatment of iron deficiency resulting from improper diet, pregnancy, impaired absorption, or prolonged blood loss.

ACTION

Iron supplements are provided to ensure adequate supplies for the formation of hemoglobin, which is needed for erythropoiesis and O_2 transport.

HEMATINIC (IRON) PREPARATIONS

Name	Availability	Elemental Iron	Side Effects
Ferrous fumarate (p. 475) (Femiron, Feostat)	**T:** 63 mg, 200 mg, 324 mg **S:** 100 mg/5 ml **D:** 45 mg/0.6 ml	33	Constipation, nausea, vomiting, diarrhea, abdominal pain/cramps
Ferrous gluconate (p. 475) (Fergon)	**T:** 240 mg, 325 mg	12	Same as ferrous fumarate
Ferrous sulfate (p. 475) (Fer-In-Sol)	**T:** 325 mg **Syrup:** 90 mg/5 ml **E:** 220 mg/5 ml **D:** 75 mg/0.6 ml	20	Same as ferrous fumarate
Ferrous sulfate exsiccated (p. 475) (Slow-Fe)	**T:** 187 mg, 200 mg **T (SR):** 160 mg **C (ER):** 160 mg	30	Same as ferrous fumarate

C, Caplets; ***D,*** drops; ***E,*** elixir; ***ER,*** extended-release; ***S,*** suspension; ***SR,*** sustained-release; ***T,*** tablets.

Hormones

USES

Functions of the body are regulated by two major control systems: the nervous system and the endocrine (hormone) system. Together they maintain homeostasis and control different metabolic functions in the body.

Hormones are concerned with control of different metabolic functions in the body (e.g., rates of chemical reactions in cells, transporting substances through cell membranes, cellular metabolism [growth/secretions]). By definition, a hormone is a chemical substance secreted into body fluids by cells and has control over other cells in the body.

Hormones can be local or general:

- *Local hormones* have specific local effects (e.g., acetylcholine, which is secreted at parasympathetic and skeletal nerve endings).

Hormones (continued)

ACTION

- *General hormones* are mostly secreted by specific endocrine glands (e.g., epinephrine/norepinephrine are secreted by the adrenal medulla in response to sympathetic stimulation), transported in the blood to all parts of the body, causing many different reactions.

Some general hormones affect all or almost all cells of the body (e.g., thyroid hormone from the thyroid gland increases the rate of most chemical reactions in almost all cells of the body); other general hormones affect only specific tissue (e.g., ovarian hormones are specific to female sex organs and secondary sexual characteristics of the female).

Endocrine hormones almost never directly act intracellularly affecting chemical reactions. They first combine with hormone receptors either on the cell surface or inside the cell (cell cytoplasm or nucleus). The combination of hormone and receptors alters the function of the receptor, and the receptor is the direct cause of the hormone effects. Altered receptor function may include the following:

Altered cell permeability, which causes a change in protein structure of the receptor, usually opening or closing a channel for one or more ions. The movement of these ions causes the effect of the hormone.

Activation of intracellular enzymes immediately inside the cell membrane (e.g., hormone combines with receptor that then becomes the activated enzyme adenyl cyclase, which causes formation of cAMP).
◀**ALERT**▶ cAMP has effects inside the cell. It is not the hormone but cAMP that causes these effects.
Regulation of hormone secretion is controlled by an internal control system, the negative feedback system:

- Endocrine gland oversecretes.
- Hormone exerts more and more of its effect.
- Target organ performs its function.
- Too much function in turn feeds back to endocrine gland to decrease secretory rate.

The endocrine system contains many glands and hormones. A summary of the important glands and their hormones secreted are as follows:

The pituitary gland (hypophysis) is a small gland found in the sella turcica at the base of the brain. The pituitary is divided into two portions physiologically: the anterior pituitary (adenohypophysis) and the posterior pituitary (neurohypophysis). Six important hormones are secreted from the anterior pituitary and two from the posterior pituitary.

Anterior pituitary hormones:

- Growth hormone (GH)
- Adrenocorticotropin (corticotropin)
- Thyroid-stimulating hormone (thyrotropin) (TSH)
- Follicle-stimulating hormone (FSH)
- Luteinizing hormone (LH)
- Prolactin

ACTION *(cont.)*

Posterior pituitary hormones:

- Antidiuretic hormone (vasopressin)
- Oxytocin

Almost all secretions of the pituitary hormones are controlled by hormonal or nervous signals from the hypothalamus. The hypothalamus is a center of information concerned with the well-being of the body, which in turn is used to control secretions of the important pituitary hormones just listed. Secretions from the posterior pituitary are controlled by nerve signals originating in the hypothalamus; anterior pituitary hormones are controlled by hormones secreted within the hypothalamus. These hormones are as follows:

- Thyrotropin-releasing hormone (TRH) releasing thyroid-stimulating hormone
- Corticotropin-releasing hormone (CRH) releasing adrenocorticotropin
- Growth hormone-releasing hormone (GHRH) releasing growth hormone and growth hormone inhibitory hormone (GHIH) (same as somatostatin)
- Gonadotropin-releasing hormone (GnRH) releasing the two gonadotropic hormones LH and FSH
- Prolactin inhibitory factor (PIF) causing inhibition of prolactin and prolactin-releasing factor

Anterior Pituitary Hormones

All anterior pituitary hormones (except growth hormone) have as their principal effect stimulating target glands.

Growth Hormone (GH)

Growth hormone affects almost all tissues of the body. GH (somatopropin) causes growth in almost all tissues of the body (increases cell size, increases mitosis with increased number of cells, and differentiates certain types of cells). Metabolic effects include increased rate of protein synthesis, mobilization of fatty acids from adipose tissue, decreased rate of glucose utilization.

Thyroid-Stimulating Hormone (TSH)

Thyroid-stimulating hormone controls secretion of the thyroid hormones. The thyroid gland is located immediately below the larynx on either side of and anterior to the trachea and secretes two significant hormones, thyroxine (T_4) and triiodothyroxine (T_3), which have a profound effect on increasing the metabolic rate of the body. The thyroid gland also secretes calcitonin, an important hormone for calcium metabolism. Calcitonin promotes deposition of calcium in the bones, which decreases calcium concentration in the extracellular fluid.

Adrenocorticotropin

Adrenocorticotropin causes the adrenal cortex to secrete adrenocortical hormones. The adrenal glands lie at the superior poles of the two kidneys. Each gland is composed of two distinct parts: the adrenal medulla and the cortex. The adrenal medulla, related to the sympathetic nervous system, secretes the hormones epinephrine and norepinephrine. When stimulated, they cause constriction of blood vessels, increased activity of the heart, inhibitory effects on the GI tract, and dilation of the pupils. The adrenal cortex secretes corticosteroids, of which there are two major types: mineralocorticoids and glucocorticoids. Aldosterone, the principal mineralocorticoid, primarily affects electrolytes of the extracellular fluids. Cortisol, the principal glucocorticoid, affects glucose, protein, and fat metabolism.

Luteinizing Hormone (LH)

Luteinizing hormone plays an important role in ovulation and causes secretion of female sex hormones by the ovaries and testosterone by the testes.

Follicle-Stimulating Hormone (FSH)

Follicle-stimulating hormone causes growth of follicles in the ovaries before ovulation and promotes formation of sperm in the testes.

Hormones *(continued)*

ACTION *(cont.)*

Ovarian sex hormones are estrogens and progestins. Estradiol is the most important estrogen; progesterone is the most important progestin.

Estrogens mainly promote proliferation and growth of specific cells in the body and are responsible for development of most of the secondary sex characteristics. Primarily cause cellular proliferation and growth of tissues of sex organs/other tissue related to reproduction. Ovaries, fallopian tubes, uterus, vagina increase in size. Estrogen initiates growth of breast and milk-producing apparatus, external appearance.

Progesterone stimulates secretion of the uterine endometrium during the latter half of the female sexual cycle, preparing the uterus for implantation of the fertilized ovum. Decreases the frequency of uterine contractions (helps prevent expulsion of the implanted ovum). Progesterone promotes development of breasts, causing alveolar cells to proliferate, enlarge, and become secretory in nature.

Testosterone is secreted by the testes and formed by the interstitial cells of Leydig. Testosterone production increases under the stimulus of the anterior pituitary gonadotropic hormones. It is responsible for distinguishing characteristics of the masculine body (stimulates the growth of male sex organs and promotes the development of male secondary sex characteristics, e.g., distribution of body hair, effect on voice, protein formation, and muscular development).

Prolactin

Prolactin promotes the development of breasts and secretion of milk.

POSTERIOR PITUITARY HORMONES

Antidiuretic Hormone (ADH) (Vasopressin)

ADH can cause antidiuresis (decreased excretion of water by the kidneys). In the presence of ADH the permeability of the renal-collecting ducts and tubules to water increases, which allows water to be absorbed, conserving water in the body. ADH in higher concentrations is a very potent vasoconstrictor, constricting arterioles everywhere in the body, increasing B/P.

Oxytocin

Oxytocin contracts the uterus during the birthing process, esp. toward the end of the pregnancy, helping expel the baby. Oxytocin also contracts myoepithelial cells in the breasts, causing milk to be expressed from the alveoli into the ducts so that the baby can obtain it by suckling.

PANCREAS

The pancreas is composed of two tissue types: *acini* (secrete digestive juices in the duodenum) and *islets of Langerhans* (secrete insulin/glucagons directly into the blood). The islets of Langerhans contain three cells: alpha, beta, and delta. Alpha cells secrete glucagon, beta cells secrete insulin, and delta cells secrete somatostatin.

Insulin promotes glucose entry into most cells, thus controlling the rate of metabolism of most carbohydrates. Insulin also affects fat metabolism.

Glucagon effects are opposite those of insulin, the most important of which is increasing blood glucose concentration by releasing it from the liver into the circulating body fluids.

Somatostatin (same chemical as secreted by the hypothalamus) has multiple inhibitory effects: depresses secretion of insulin and glucagon, decreases GI motility, decreases secretions/absorption of the GI tract.

Human Immunodeficiency Virus (HIV) Infection

USES

Antiretroviral agents are used in the treatmentof HIV infection.

ACTION

Seven classes of antiretroviral agents are used in the treatment of HIV disease. *Nucleoside reverse transcriptase inhibitors (NRTIs)* compete with natural substrates for formation of proviral DNA by reverse transcriptase inhibiting viral replication.

Nucleotide reverse transcriptase inhibitors (*NtRTIs*) inhibit reverse transcriptase by competing with the natural substrate deoxyadenosine triphosphate and by DNA chain termination.

Nonnucleoside reverse transcriptase inhibitors (NNRTIs) directly bind to reverse transcriptase and block RNA-dependent and DNA-dependent DNA polymerase activities by disrupting the enzyme's catalytic site.

Protease inhibitors (PIs) bind to the active site of HIV-1 protease and prevent the processing of viral gag and gag-pol polyprotein precursors resulting in immature, noninfectious viral particles.

Fusion inhibitors interfere with the entry of HIV-1 into cells by inhibiting fusion of viral and cellular membranes.

CCR5 co-receptor antagonist selectively binds to human chemokine receptor CCR5 present on cell membrane preventing HIV-1 from entering cells.

Integrase inhibitor inhibits catalytic activity of HIV-1 integrase, an HIV-1 encoded enzyme required for viral replication.

Human Immunodeficiency Virus (HIV) Infection *(continued)*

ANTIRETROVIRAL AGENTS FOR TREATMENT OF HIV INFECTION

Name	Availability	Dosage Range	Side Effects
Nucleoside Analogues			
Abacavir (p. 1) (Ziagen)	**T:** 300 mg **OS:** 20 mg/ml	**A:** 300 mg 2 times/day	Nausea, vomiting, malaise, rash, fever, headaches, asthenia, fatigue
Abacavir/lamivudine (Epzicom)	**T:** 600 mg abacavir/ 300 mg lamivudine	**A:** once/day	Allergic reaction, insomnia, headaches, depression, dizziness, fatigue, diarrhea, fever, abdominal pain, anxiety
Didanosine (p. 349) (Videx)	**T:** 25 mg, 50 mg, 100 mg, 150 mg, 200 mg **C:** 125 mg, 200 mg, 250 mg, 400 mg **OS:** 100 mg, 167 mg, 250 mg	**T (weighing more than 60 kg):** 200 mg 2 times/day; **(weighing less than 60 kg):** 125 mg 2 times/day **OS (weighing more than 60 kg):** 250 mg 2 times/day; **(weighing less than 60 kg):** 167 mg 2 times/day	Peripheral neuropathy, pancreatitis, diarrhea, nausea, vomiting, headaches, insomnia, rash, hepatitis, seizures
Emtricitabine (p. 405) (Emtriva)	**C:** 200 mg	**A:** 200 mg/day	Headaches, insomnia, depression, diarrhea, nausea, vomiting, rhinitis, asthenia, rash
Emtricitabine/efavirenz/ tenofovir (Atripla)	**T:** 200 mg emtricitabine/ 600 mg efavirenz/ 300 mg tenofovir	**A:** once/day	Lactic acidosis, headaches, dizziness, abdominal pain, nausea, vomiting, rash

Emtricitabine/tenofovir (Truvada)	**T:** 200 mg emtricitabine/ 300 mg tenofovir	**A:** once/day	Dizziness, diarrhea, headaches, rash, belching/ flatulence, skin discoloration
Lamivudine (p. 659) (Epivir)	**T:** 100 mg, 150 mg **OS:** 5 mg/ml, 10 mg/ml	**A:** 150 mg 2 times/day **C:** 4 mg/kg 2 times/day	Diarrhea, malaise, fatigue, headaches, nausea, vomiting, abdominal pain, peripheral neuropathy, arthralgia, myalgia, skin rash
Stavudine (p. 1081) (Zerit)	**C:** 15 mg, 20 mg, 30 mg, 40 mg **OS:** 1 mg/ml	**A:** 40 mg 2 times/day (20 mg 2 times/ day if peripheral neuropathy occurs)	Peripheral neuropathy, anemia, leukopenia, neutropenia
Zalcitabine (Hivid)	**T:** 0.375 mg, 0.75 mg	**A (weighing more than 60 kg):** 0.75 mg 3 times/day; **(weighing less than 60 kg):** 0.375 mg 3 times/day	Peripheral neuropathy, stomatitis, granulocytopenia, leukopenia
Zidovudine (p. 1227) (Retrovir)	**C:** 100 mg **T:** 300 mg **Syrup:** 50 mg/5 ml, 10 mg/ml	**A:** 500–600 mg/day (100 mg 5 times/ day or 300 mg 2 times/day)	Anemia, granulocytopenia, myopathy, nausea, malaise, fatigue, insomnia
Zidovudine/lamivudine (AZT/3TC) (Combivir)	**C:** 300 mg AZT/150 mg 3TC	**A:** 1 capsule 2 times/day	Myelosuppression, peripheral neuropathy, pancreatitis
Zidovudine/lamivudine/ abacavir (AZT/3TC/ABC) (Trizivir)	**C:** 300 mg AZT/150 mg 3TC/ 300 mg ABC	**A:** 1 capsule 2 times/day	Myelosuppression, peripheral neuropathy, anaphylactic reaction

(continued)

ANTIRETROVIRAL AGENTS FOR TREATMENT OF HIV INFECTION *(continued)*

Name	Availability	Dosage Range	Side Effects
Nucleotide Analogues			
Tenofovir (p. 1106) (Viread)	**T:** 300 mg	**A:** 300 mg/day	Nausea, vomiting, diarrhea
Nonnucleoside Analogues			
Delavirdine (p. 316) (Rescriptor)	**T:** 100 mg, 200 mg	**A:** 200 mg 3 times/day for 14 days, then 400 mg 3 times/day	Rash, nausea, headaches, elevated hepatic function tests
Efavirenz (p. 401) (Sustiva)	**C:** 50 mg, 100 mg, 200 mg	**A:** 600 mg/day **C:** 200–600 mg/day based on weight	Headaches, dizziness, insomnia, fatigue, rash, nightmares
Etravirine (p. 454) (Intelence)	**T:** 100 mg	**A:** 200 mg 2 times/day	Skin reactions (e.g., Stevens-Johnson syndrome, erythema multiforme), nausea, abdominal pain, vomiting
Nevirapine (p. 824) (Viramune)	**T:** 200 mg	**A:** 200 mg/day for 14 days, then 200 mg 2 times/day	Rash, nausea, fatigue, fever, headaches, abnormal hepatic function tests
Protease Inhibitors			
Atazanavir (p. 88) (Reyataz)	**C:** 100 mg, 150 mg, 200 mg, 300 mg	**A:** 400 mg/day	Headaches, diarrhea, abdominal pain, nausea, rash
Darunavir (p. 308) (Prezista)	**T:** 300 mg	**A:** 600 mg 2 times/day	Diarrhea, nausea, vomiting, headaches, skin rash, constipation

Fosamprenavir (p. 514) (Lexiva)	**T:** 700 mg	**A:** 1,400–2,800 mg/day	Headaches, fatigue, rash, nausea, diarrhea, vomiting, abdominal pain
Indinavir (p. 610) (Crixivan)	**C:** 200 mg, 400 mg	**A:** 800 mg q8h	Nephrolithiasis, hyperbilirubinemia, abdominal pain, asthenia, fatigue, flank pain, nausea, vomiting, diarrhea, headaches, insomnia, dizziness, altered taste
Lopinavir/ritonavir (p. 703) (Kaletra)	**C:** 133/33 mg **OS:** 80/20 mg	**A:** 400/100 mg/day **C (4–12 yrs):** 10–13 mg/kg 2 times/day	Diarrhea, nausea, vomiting, abdominal pain, headaches, rash
Nelfinavir (p. 820) (Viracept)	**T:** 250 mg **Oral Powder:** 50 mg/g	**A:** 750 mg q8h **C:** 20–25 mg/kg q8h	Diarrhea, fatigue, asthenia, headaches, hypertension, impaired concentration
Ritonavir (p. 1025) (Norvir)	**C:** 100 mg **OS:** 80 mg/ml	**A:** Titrate up to 600 mg 2 times/day	Nausea, vomiting, diarrhea, altered taste, fatigue, elevated hepatic function tests and triglyceride levels
Saquinavir (p. 1042) (Invirase)	**C:** 200 mg	**A:** 600 mg 3 times/day	Diarrhea, elevated hepatic function tests, hypertriglycerides, cholesterol, abnormal fat accumulation, hyperglycemia
Tipranavir (p. 1138) (Aptivus)	**C:** 250 mg	**A:** 500 mg (with 200 mg ritonavir) 2 times/day	Diarrhea, nausea, fatigue, headaches, vomiting
Fusion Inhibitors			
Enfuvirtide (p. 409) (Fuzeon)	**I:** 108 mg (90 mg when reconstituted)	**Subcutaneous:** 90 mg 2 times/day	Insomnia, depression, peripheral neuropathy, decreased appetite, constipation, asthenia, cough

(continued)

ANTIRETROVIRAL AGENTS FOR TREATMENT OF HIV INFECTION *(continued)*

Name	Availability	Dosage Range	Side Effects
CCR5 Antagonists			
Maraviroc (p. 721) (Selzentry)	**T:** 150 mg, 300 mg	**A:** 150–600 mg/day	Cough, pyrexia, upper respiratory tract infections, rash, musculoskeletal symptoms, abdominal pain, dizziness
Integrase Inhibitor			
Raltegravir (p. 999) (Isentress)	**T:** 400 mg	**A:** 400 mg 2 times/day	Nausea, headache, diarrhea, pyrexia

A, Adults; ***C,*** capsules; ***C (dosage),*** children; ***I,*** injection; ***OS,*** oral solution; ***T,*** tablets.

Immunosuppressive Agents

USES

Improvement of both short- and long-term allograft survivals.

ACTION

Basiliximab: An interleukin-2 (IL-2) receptor antagonist inhibiting IL-2 binding. This prevents activation of lymphocytes, and the response of the immune system to antigens is impaired.

Cyclosporine: Inhibits production and release of IL-2.

Daclizumab: An IL-2 receptor antagonist inhibiting IL-2 binding.

Mycophenolate: A prodrug that reversibly binds and inhibits inosine monophosphate dehydrogenase (IMPD), resulting in inhibition of purine nucleotide synthesis, inhibiting DNA and RNA synthesis and subsequent synthesis of T and B cells.

Sirolimus: Inhibits IL-2–stimulated T-lymphocyte activation and proliferation, which may occur through formation of a complex.

Tacrolimus: Inhibits IL-2–stimulated T-lymphocyte activation and proliferation, which may occur through formation of a complex.

IMMUNOSUPPRESSIVE AGENTS

Name	Availability	Dosage	Side Effects
Basiliximab (p. 111) (Simulect)	**I:** 20 mg	20 mg for 2 doses	Abdominal pain, asthenia, cough, dizziness, dyspnea, dysuria, edema, hypertension, infection, tremors
Cyclosporine (p. 289) (Neoral, Sandimmune)	**C:** 25 mg, 50 mg, 100 mg **S:** 100 mg/ml **I:** 50 mg/ml	7–10 mg/kg/day	Hypertension, hyperkalemia, nephrotoxicity, coarsening of facial features, hirsutism, gingival hyperplasia, nausea, vomiting, diarrhea, hepatotoxicity, hyperuricemia, hypertriglyceridemia, hypercholesterolemia, tremors, paresthesia, seizures, risk of infection/malignancy
Daclizumab (p. 296) (Zenapax)	**I:** 25 mg/5 ml	1 mg/kg (**Maximum:** 100 mg)	Dyspnea, fever, hypertension, nausea, peripheral edema, tachycardia, tremors, vomiting, weakness, wound infection
Mycophenolate (p. 797) (CellCept)	**C:** 250 mg **I:** 500 mg **S:** 200 mg/ml **T:** 500 mg	1 g 2 times/day	Diarrhea, vomiting, leukopenia, neutropenia, infections
Sirolimus (p. 1062) (Rapamune)	**S:** 1 mg/ml **T:** 1 mg	2–10 mg/day	Dyspnea, leukopenia, thrombocytopenia, hyperlipidemia, abdominal pain, acne, arthralgia, fever, diarrhea, constipation, headaches, vomiting, weight gain
Tacrolimus (p. 1090) (Prograf)	**C:** 0.5 mg, 1 mg, 5 mg **I:** 5 mg/ml	0.1–0.15 mg/kg/day	Nephrotoxicity, neurotoxicity, hyperglycemia, nausea, vomiting, photophobia, infections, hypertension, hyperlipidemia

C, Capsules; ***I,*** injection; ***S,*** oral solution or suspension; ***T,*** tablets.

Laxatives

USES

Short-term treatment of constipation; colon evacuation before rectal/bowel examination; prevention of straining (e.g., after anorectal surgery, MI); to reduce painful elimination (e.g., episiotomy, hemorrhoids, anorectal lesions); modification of effluent from ileostomy, colostomy; prevention of fecal impaction; removal of ingested poisons.

ACTION

Laxatives ease or stimulate defecation. Mechanisms by which this is accomplished include (1) attracting, retaining fluid in colonic contents due to hydrophilic or osmotic properties; (2) acting directly or indirectly on mucosa to decrease absorption of water and NaCl; or (3) increasing intestinal motility, decreasing absorption of water and NaCl by virtue of decreased transit time.

Bulk-forming: Act primarily in small/large intestine. Retain water in stool, may bind water, ions in colonic lumen (soften feces, increase bulk); may increase colonic bacteria growth (increases fecal mass). Produce soft stool in 1–3 days.

Osmotic agents: Act in colon. Similar to saline laxatives. Osmotic action may be enhanced in distal ileum/colon by bacterial metabolism to lactate, other organic acids. This decrease in pH increases motility, secretion. Produce soft stool in 1–3 days.

Saline: Acts in small/large intestine, colon (sodium phosphate). Poorly, slowly absorbed; causes hormone cholecystokinin release from duodenum (stimulates fluid secretion, motility); possesses osmotic properties; produces watery stool in 2–6 hrs (small doses produce semifluid stool in 6–12 hrs).

Stimulant: Acts in colon. Enhances accumulation of water/electrolytes in colonic lumen, enhances intestinal motility. May act directly on intestinal mucosa. Produces semifluid stool in 6–12 hrs.

◀**ALERT**▶ Bisacodyl suppository acts in 15–60 min.

Stool softener: Acts in small/large intestine. Hydrates and softens stools by its surfactant action, facilitating penetration of fat and water into stool. Produces soft stool in 1–3 days.

LAXATIVES

Name	Onset of Action	Uses	Side Effects/Precautions
Bulk-forming			
Methylcellulose (Citrucel)	12–24 hrs up to 3 days	Treatment of constipation for postpartum women, elderly, pts with diverticulosis, irritable bowel syndrome, hemorrhoids	Gas, bloating, esophageal obstruction, colonic obstruction, calcium and iron malabsorption
Psyllium (p. 984) (Metamucil)	Same as methylcellulose	Treatment of chronic constipation and constipation associated with rectal disorders; management of irritable bowel syndrome	Diarrhea, constipation, abdominal cramps, esophageal/colon obstruction, bronchospasm
Stool Softener			
Docusate (p. 371) (Colace, Surfak)	1–3 days	Treatment of constipation due to hard stools, in painful anorectal conditions, and for those who need to avoid straining during bowel movements	Stomachache, mild nausea, cramping, diarrhea, irritated throat (with liquid and syrup dose forms)
Saline			
Magnesium hydroxide (p. 715)	30 min–3 hrs	Short-term treatment of occasional constipation	Electrolyte abnormalities can occur; use caution in pts with renal or cardiac impairment; diarrhea, abdominal cramps, hypotension
Magnesium citrate (p. 715) (Citrate of Magnesia, Citro-Mag)	30 min–3 hrs	Bowel evacuation prior to certain surgical and diagnostic procedures	Hypotension, abdominal cramping, diarrhea, gas formation, electrolyte abnormalities

(continued)

LAXATIVES *(continued)*

Name	Onset of Action	Uses	Side Effects/Precautions
Sodium phosphate (Fleets Phospho Soda)	2–15 min	Relief of occasional constipation; bowel evacuation prior to certain surgical and diagnostic procedures	Electrolyte abnormalities; do not use for pts with CHF, severe renal impairment, ascites, GI obstruction, active inflammatory bowel disease
Osmotic			
Lactulose (p. 658) (Kristalose)	24–48 hrs	Short-term relief of constipation	Nausea, vomiting, diarrhea, abdominal cramping, bloating, gas
Polyethylene glycol (p. 941) (MiraLax)	24–48 hrs	Short-term relief of constipation	Bitter taste, diarrhea
Stimulant			
Bisacodyl (p. 129) (Dulcolax)	**PO:** 6–12 hrs **Rectal:** 15–60 min	Short-term relief of constipation	Elecrolyte imbalance, abdominal discomfort, gas, potential for overuse/abuse
Senna (p. 1051) (Senokot)	6–12 hrs	Short-term relief of constipation	Abdominal discomfort, cramps

Neuromuscular Blockers

USES

Adjuvant in surgical anesthesia to relax skeletal muscle (esp. abdominal wall) for surgery (allows lighter level of anesthesia; valuable in orthopedic procedures). Neuromuscular blocking agents of short duration often used to facilitate endotracheal intubation, laryngoscopy, bronchoscopy, and esophagoscopy in combination with general anesthetics. Provide muscle relaxation in pts undergoing mechanical ventilation, muscle relaxation in diagnosis of myasthenia gravis. Prevent convulsive movements during electroconvulsive therapy.

ACTION

Paralysis results from blocking of normal neuromuscular transmission. Succinylcholine, a depolarizing agent, attaches to the acetylcholine (ACh) receptor on the motor end plate, causing depolarization. It prevents the binding of ACh to the receptor. Nondepolarizing agents also bind to the receptor at the motor end plate but competitively block ACh from attaching to the receptor. These agents also block presynaptic channels that cause the release of ACh.

NEUROMUSCULAR BLOCKERS

Name	Class	Intubation Dose	ICU Dose	Side Effects
Cisatracurium (Nimbex)	Intermediate	0.15–2 mg/kg	0.10–0.2 mg/kg bolus, then 2.5–3 mcg/kg/min	Skin rash, flushing
Doxacurium (Nuromax)	Long	0.05 mg/kg	0.025–0.05 mg/kg bolus, then 0.3–0.5 mg/kg/min	Injection site reaction, urticaria
Mivacurium (Mivacron)	Short	0.15–0.2 mg/kg	0.15–0.25 mg/kg bolus, then 9–10 mcg/kg/min	Flushing, hypotension, dizziness, muscle spasm

(continued)

NEUROMUSCULAR BLOCKERS ***(continued)***

Name	Class	Intubation Dose	ICU Dose	Side Effects
Pancuronium (Pavulon)	Long	0.06–0.1 mg/kg	0.05–0.1 mg/kg bolus, then 1–2 mcg/kg/hr	Increased B/P, increased salivation, pruritus
Rocuronium (Zemuron)	Intermediate	0.45–1.2 mg/kg	0.15–0.25 mg/kg bolus, then 10–12 mcg/kg/min	Pain at injection site, hypertension, hypotension
Succinylcholine (Anectine, Quelicin)	Ultrashort	1–2 mg/kg	NA	Increased intracranial pressure, increased intra-ocular pressure, postop muscle pain, weakness, increased salivation, bradycardia, cardiac arrhythmias
Tubocurarine	Intermediate	0.5–0.6 mg/kg	NA	Decreased B/P
Vecuronium (Norcuron)	Intermediate	0.08–0.1 mg/kg	0.08–0.1 mg/kg bolus, then 0.8–1.2 mcg/kg/min	Skeletal muscle weakness with prolonged use

Nitrates

USES	ACTION
Sublingual: Acute relief of angina pectoris. *Oral, topical:* Long-term prophylactic treatment of angina pectoris. *Intravenous:* Adjunctive treatment in CHF associated with acute MI. Produce controlled hypotension during surgical procedures; control B/P in perioperative hypertension, angina unresponsive to organic nitrates or beta-blockers.	Relax most smooth muscles, including arteries and veins. Effect is primarily on veins (decrease left/right ventricular end-diastolic pressure). In angina, nitrates decrease myocardial work and O_2 requirements (decrease preload by venodilation and afterload by arteriodilation). Nitrates also appear to redistribute blood flow to ischemic myocardial areas, improving perfusion without increase in coronary blood flow.

NITRATES

Name	Availability	Dosage Range	Side Effects
Isosorbide (p. 637) **(Isordil)**	**T:** 5 mg, 10 mg, 20 mg, 30 mg, 40 mg **T (ER):** 30 mg, 40 mg, 60 mg, 120 mg **SL:** 2.5 mg, 5 mg **T (chewable):** 5 mg, 10 mg **C (SR):** 40 mg	**SL:** 2.5–10 mg q2–3h **PO:** 10–40 mg q6h **PO (SR):** 40–80 mg q8–12h	Flushing, headaches, nausea, vomiting, orthostatic hypotension, restlessness, tachycardia

(continued)

NITRATES ***(continued)***

Name	Availability	Dosage Range	Side Effects
Nitroglycerin (p. 839) (Minitran, Nitro-Bid, Nitro-Dur, Nitrostat)	**SL:** 0.4 mg **T (SR):** 2.6 mg, 6.5 mg, 9 mg **C (SR):** 2.5 mg, 6.5 mg, 9 mg, 13 mg **Topical:** 2% ointment **Trans:** 0.1 mg/hr, 0.2 mg/hr, 0.3 mg/hr, 0.4 mg/hr, 0.6 mg/hr, 0.8 mg/hr **I:** 0.5 mg/ml, 5 mg/ml **Infusion:** 100 mcg/ml, 200 mcg/ml	**SL:** 0.4 mg up to 3 times q15min **SR:** 2.5–26 mg 3–4 times/day **Trans:** 0.1–0.8 mg/hr **T:** 1–2 inches up to 4–5 inches q4h	Same as isosorbide

C, Capsules; ***ER,*** extended-release; ***I,*** injection; ***SL,*** sublingual; ***SR,*** sustained-release; ***T,*** tablets; ***Trans,*** transdermal.

Nonsteroidal Anti-Inflammatory Drugs (NSAIDs)

USES

Provide symptomatic relief from *pain/inflammation* in the treatment of musculoskeletal disorders (e.g., rheumatoid arthritis [RA], osteoarthritis, ankylosing spondylitis), *analgesic* for low to moderate pain, *reduction in fever* (many agents not suited for routine/prolonged therapy due to toxicity). By virtue of its action on platelet function, aspirin is used in treatment or prophylaxis of diseases associated with hypercoagulability (reduces risk of stroke/heart attack).

ACTION

Exact mechanism for anti-inflammatory, analgesic, antipyretic effects unknown. Inhibition of enzyme cyclooxygenase, the enzyme responsible for prostaglandin synthesis, appears to be a major mechanism of action. May inhibit other mediators of inflammation (e.g., leukotrienes). Direct action on hypothalamus heat-regulating center may contribute to antipyretic effect.

NSAIDs

Name	Availability	Dosage Range	Side Effects
Aspirin (p. 86)	**T:** 81 mg, 160 mg, 325 mg **Supplement:** 300 mg, 600 mg	**P (A):** 325–650 mg q4h as needed **C:** Up to 60–80 mg/kg/day **Arthritis:** 3.2–6 g/day **JRA:** 60–110 mg/kg/day **RF (A):** 5–8 g/day **C:** 75–100 mg/kg/day **TIA:** 1,300 mg/day **MI:** 81–325 mg/day	GI discomfort, dizziness, headaches
Celecoxib (p. 214) (Celebrex)	**C:** 100 mg, 200 mg	**OA:** 200 mg/day **RA:** 100–200 mg 2 times/day **FAP:** 400 mg 2 times/day	Diarrhea, back pain, dizziness, heartburn, headaches, nausea, abdominal pain
Diclofenac (p. 344) (Voltaren)	**T:** 25 mg, 50 mg, 75 mg, 100 mg	**Arthritis:** 100–200 mg/day	Indigestion, constipation, diarrhea, nausea, headaches, fluid retention, abdominal cramps
Diflunisal (Dolobid)	**T:** 250 mg, 500 mg	**Arthritis:** 0.5–1 g/day **P:** 0.5 g q8–12h	Headaches, abdominal cramps, indigestion, diarrhea, nausea
Etodolac (p. 450) (Lodine)	**T:** 400 mg, 500 mg **T (ER):** 400 mg, 500 mg, 600 mg **C:** 200 mg, 300 mg	**Arthritis:** 600–800 mg/day **P:** 200–400 mg q6–8h	Indigestion, dizziness, headaches, bloated feeling, diarrhea, nausea, weakness, abdominal cramps
Fenoprofen (Nalfon)	**C:** 200 mg, 300 mg **T:** 600 mg	**Arthritis:** 300–600 mg 3–4 times/day **P:** 200 mg q4–6h as needed	Nausea, indigestion, anxiety, constipation, shortness of breath, heartburn

(continued)

NSAIDs *(continued)*

Name	Availability	Dosage Range	Side Effects
Flurbiprofen (p. 502) (Ansaid)	**T:** 50 mg, 100 mg	**Arthritis:** 200–300 mg/day	Indigestion, nausea, fluid retention, headaches, abdominal cramps, diarrhea
Ibuprofen (p. 590) (Advil, Caldolor, Motrin)	**I:** 100 mg/ml **T:** 100 mg, 200 mg, 400 mg, 600 mg, 800 mg **T (chewable):** 50 mg, 100 mg **C:** 200 mg **S:** 100 mg/5 ml, 100 mg/2.5 ml **Drops:** 40 mg/ml	**Arthritis:** 1.2–3.2 g/day **P: (PO):** 400 mg q4–6h as needed **(I):** 400–800 mg q6h as needed **Fever (PO):** 200 mg q4–6h as needed **(I):** 400 mg q4–6h as needed or 100–200 mg q4h as needed **JA:** 30–40 mg/kg/day	Dizziness, abdominal cramps, abdominal pain, heartburn, nausea
Indomethacin (p. 611) (Indocin)	**C:** 25 mg, 50 mg **C (SR):** 75 mg **S:** 25 mg/5 ml **Supplement:** 50 mg	**Arthritis:** 50–200 mg/day **Bursitis/tendonitis:** 75–150 mg/day **GA:** 150 mg/day	Fluid retention, dizziness, headaches, abdominal pain, indigestion, nausea
Ketoprofen (p. 650) (Orudis KT)	**T:** 12.5 mg **C:** 25 mg, 50 mg, 75 mg **C (ER):** 100 mg, 150 mg, 200 mg	**Arthritis:** 150–300 mg/day **P:** 25–50 mg q6–8h as needed	Headaches, anxiety, abdominal pain, bloated feeling, constipation, diarrhea, nausea
Ketorolac (p. 652) (Toradol)	**T:** 10 mg **I:** 15 mg/ml, 30 mg/ml	**P (PO):** 10 mg q4–6h as needed; **(IM/IV):** 60–120 mg/day	Fluid retention, abdominal pain, diarrhea, dizziness, headaches, nausea
Meloxicam (p. 727) (Mobic)	**C:** 7.5 mg	**Arthritis:** 7.5–15 mg/day	Heartburn, indigestion, nausea, diarrhea, headaches

Nabumetone (p. 800) (Relafen)	**T:** 500 mg, 750 mg	**Arthritis:** 1–2 g/day	Fluid retention, dizziness, headaches, abdominal pain, constipation, diarrhea, nausea
Naproxen (p. 811) (Anaprox, Naprosyn)	**T:** 200 mg, 250 mg, 375 mg, 500 mg **T (CR):** 375 mg **S:** 125 mg/5 ml	**Arthritis:** 250–550 mg/day **P:** 250 mg q6–8h **JA:** 10 mg/kg/day **GA:** 750 mg once, then 250 mg q8h	Tinnitus, fluid retention, shortness of breath, dizziness, drowsiness, headaches, abdominal pain, constipation, heartburn, nausea
Oxaprozin (p. 875) (Daypro)	**C:** 600 mg	**Arthritis:** 600–1,800 mg/day	Constipation, diarrhea, nausea, indigestion
Piroxicam (p. 937) (Feldene)	**C:** 10 mg, 20 mg	**Arthritis:** 20 mg/day	Abdominal pain, stomach pain, nausea
Sulindac (p. 1085) (Clinoril)	**T:** 150 mg, 200 mg	**Arthritis:** 300 mg/day **GA:** 400 mg/day	Dizziness, abdominal pain, constipation, diarrhea, nausea
Tolmetin (Tolectin)	**T:** 200 mg, 600 mg **C:** 400 mg	**Arthritis:** 600–1,800 mg/day **JA:** 15–30 mg/kg/day	Fluid retention, dizziness, headaches, weakness, abdominal pain, diarrhea, indigestion, nausea, vomiting

A, Adults; ***C,*** capsules; ***C** (dosage),* children; ***CR,*** controlled-release; ***ER,*** extended-release; ***FAP,*** familial adenomatous polyposis; ***GA,*** gouty arthritis; ***I,*** injection; ***JA,*** juvenile arthritis; ***JRA,*** juvenile rheumatoid arthritis; ***MI,*** myocardial infarction; ***OA,*** osteoarthritis; ***P,*** pain; ***RA,*** rheumatoid arthritis; ***RF,*** rheumatic fever; ***S,*** suspension; ***SR,*** sustained-release; ***T,*** tablets; ***TIA,*** transient ischemic attack.

Nutrition: Enteral

	INDICATIONS	ROUTES OF ENTERAL NUTRITION DELIVERY
Enteral nutrition (EN), also known as *tube feedings,* provides food/nutrients via the GI tract using special formulas, delivery techniques, and equipment. All routes of EN consist of a tube through which liquid formula is infused.	Tube feedings are used in pts with major trauma, burns; those undergoing radiation and/or chemotherapy; pts with hepatic failure, severe renal impairment, physical or neurologic impairment; preop and postop to promote anabolism; prevention of cachexia, malnutrition.	**NASOGASTRIC (NG):** **INDICATIONS:** Most common for short-term feeding in pts unable or unwilling to consume adequate nutrition by mouth. Requires at least a partially functioning GI tract. **ADVANTAGES:** Does not require surgical intervention and is fairly easily inserted. Allows full use of digestive tract. Decreases abdominal distention, nausea, vomiting that may be caused by hyperosmolar solutions. **DISADVANTAGES:** Temporary. May be easily pulled out during routine nursing care. Has potential for pulmonary aspiration of gastric contents, risk of reflux esophagitis, regurgitation. **NASODUODENAL (ND), NASOJEJUNAL (NJ):** **INDICATIONS:** Pts unable or unwilling to consume adequate nutrition by mouth. Requires at least a partially functioning GI tract. **ADVANTAGES:** Does not require surgical intervention and is fairly easily inserted. Preferred for pts at risk for aspiration. Valuable for pts with gastroparesis.

ROUTES OF ENTERAL NUTRITION DELIVERY *(cont.)*

DISADVANTAGES: Temporary. May be pulled out during routine nursing care. May be dislodged by coughing, vomiting. Small lumen size increases risk of clogging when medication is administered via tube, more susceptible to rupturing when using infusion device. Must be radiographed for placement, frequently extubated.

GASTROSTOMY:
INDICATIONS: Pts with esophageal obstruction or impaired swallowing; pts in whom NG, ND, or NJ not feasible; when long-term feeding indicated.
ADVANTAGES: Permanent feeding access. Tubing has larger bore, allowing noncontinuous (bolus) feeding (300–400 ml over 30–60 min q3–6h). May be inserted endoscopically using local anesthetic (procedure called *percutaneous endoscopic gastrostomy* [PEG]).
DISADVANTAGES: Requires surgery; may be inserted in conjunction with other surgery or endoscopically (see **ADVANTAGES**). Stoma care required. Tube may be inadvertently dislodged. Risk of aspiration, peritonitis, cellulitis, leakage of gastric contents.

JEJUNOSTOMY:
INDICATIONS: Pts with stomach or duodenal obstruction, impaired gastric motility; pts in whom NG, ND, or NJ not feasible; when long-term feeding indicated.
ADVANTAGES: Allows early postop feeding (small bowel function is least affected by surgery). Risk of aspiration reduced. Rarely pulled out inadvertently.
DISADVANTAGES: Requires surgery (laparotomy). Stoma care required. Risk of intraperitoneal leakage. Can be dislodged easily.

INITIATING ENTERAL NUTRITION

With continuous feeding, initiation of isotonic (about 300 mOsm/L) or moderately hypertonic feeding (up to 495 mOsm/L) can be given full strength, usually at a slow rate (30–50 ml/hr) and gradually increased (25 ml/hr q6–24h). Formulas with osmolality greater than 500 mOsm/L are generally started at half strength and gradually increased in rate, then concentration. Tolerance is increased if the rate and concentration are not increased simultaneously.

Nutrition: Enteral *(continued)*

SELECTION OF FORMULAS

Protein: Has many important physiologic roles and is the primary source of nitrogen in the body. Provides 4 kcal/g protein. Sources of protein in enteral feedings: sodium caseinate, calcium caseinate, soy protein, dipeptides.

Carbohydrate (CHO): Provides energy for the body and heat to maintain body temperature. Provides 3.4 kcal/g carbohydrate. Sources of CHO in enteral feedings: corn syrup, cornstarch, maltodextrin, lactose, sucrose, glucose.

Fat: Provides concentrated source of energy. Referred to as *kilocalorie dense* or *protein sparing.* Provides 9 kcal/g fat. Sources of fat in enteral feedings: corn oil, safflower oil, medium-chain triglycerides.

Electrolytes, vitamins, trace elements: Contained in formulas (not found in specialized products for renal/hepatic insufficiency).

All products containing protein, fat, carbohydrate, vitamin, electrolytes, trace elements are nutritionally complete and designed to be used by pts for long periods.

COMPLICATIONS

MECHANICAL: Usually associated with some aspect of the feeding tube.

Aspiration pneumonia: Caused by delayed gastric emptying, gastroparesis, gastroesophageal reflux, or decreased gag reflex. May be prevented or treated by reducing infusion rate, using lower-fat formula, feeding beyond pylorus, checking residuals, using small-bore feeding tubes, elevating head of bed 30°–45° during and for 30–60 min after intermittent feeding, and regularly checking tube placement.

Esophageal, mucosal, pharyngeal irritation, otitis: Caused by using large-bore NG tube. Prevented by use of small bore whenever possible.

Irritation, leakage at ostomy site: Caused by drainage of digestive juices from site. Prevented by close attention to skin/stoma care.

Tube, lumen obstruction: Caused by thickened formula residue, formation of formula-medication complexes. Prevented by frequently irrigating tube with clear water (also before and after giving formulas/medication), avoiding instilling medication if possible.

GASTROINTESTINAL: Usually associated with formula, rate of delivery, unsanitary handling of solutions or delivery system.

Diarrhea: Caused by low-residue formulas, rapid delivery, use of hyperosmolar formula, hypoalbuminemia, malabsorption, microbial contamination, or rapid GI transit time. Prevented by using fiber supplemented formulas, decreasing rate of delivery, using dilute formula, and gradually increasing strength.

Cramps, gas, abdominal distention: Caused by nutrient malabsorption, rapid delivery of refrigerated formula. Prevented by delivering formula by continuous methods, giving formulas at room temperature, decreasing rate of delivery.

Nausea, vomiting: Caused by rapid delivery of formula, gastric retention. Prevented by reducing rate of delivery, using dilute formulas, selecting low-fat formulas.

COMPLICATIONS (cont.)

Constipation: Caused by inadequate fluid intake, reduced bulk, inactivity. Prevented by supplementing fluid intake, using fiber-supplemented formula, encouraging ambulation.

METABOLIC: Fluid/serum electrolyte status should be monitored. Refer to monitoring section. In addition, the very young and very old are at greater risk of developing complications such as dehydration or overhydration.

MONITORING

Daily: Estimate nutrient intake, fluid intake/output, weight of pt, clinical observations.

Weekly: Serum electrolytes (potassium, sodium, magnesium, calcium, phosphorus) blood glucose, BUN, creatinine, hepatic function tests (e.g., AST, alkaline phosphatase), 24-hr urea and creatinine excretion, total iron-binding capacity (TIBC) or serum transferrin, triglycerides, cholesterol.

Monthly: Serum albumin.

Other: Urine glucose, acetone (when blood glucose is greater than 250), vital signs (temperature, respirations, pulse, B/P) q8h.

DRUG THERAPY: DOSAGE FOR SELECTION/ADMINISTRATION:
Drug therapy should not have to be compromised in pts receiving enteral nutrition:

- Temporarily discontinue medications not immediately necessary
- Consider an alternate route for administering medications (e.g., transdermal, rectal, intravenous)
- Consider alternate medications when current medication is not available in alternate dosage forms

ENTERAL ADMINISTRATION OF MEDICATIONS:
Medications may be given via feeding tube with several considerations:

- Tube type
- Tube location in the GI tract
- Site of drug action
- Site of drug absorption
- Effects of food on drug absorption
- Use of liquid dosage forms preferred whenever possible, many tablets may be crushed, contents of many capsules may be emptied and given through large-bore feeding tubes
- Many oral products should not be crushed (e.g., sustained-release, enteric coated)
- Some medications should not be given with enteral formulas because they form precipitates that may clog the feeding tube and reduce drug absorption
- Feeding tube should be flushed with water before and after administration of medications to clear any residual medication

Nutrition: Parenteral

Parenteral nutrition (PN), also known as *total parenteral nutrition* (TPN) or *hyperalimentation* (HAL), provides required nutrients to pts by IV route of administration. The goal of PN is to maintain or restore nutritional status caused by disease, injury, or inability to consume nutrients by other means.

INDICATIONS

Conditions when pt is unable to use alimentary tract via oral, gastrostomy, or jejunostomy route. Impaired absorption of protein caused by obstruction, inflammation, or antineoplastic therapy. Bowel rest necessary because of GI surgery or ileus, fistulas, or anastomotic leaks. Conditions with increased metabolic requirements (e.g., burns, infection, trauma). Preserve tissue reserves (e.g., acute renal failure). Inadequate nutrition from tube feeding methods.

COMPONENTS OF PN

To meet IV nutritional requirements, six essential categories in PN are needed for tissue synthesis and energy balance.

Protein: In the form of crystalline amino acids (CAA), primarily used for protein synthesis. Several products are designed to meet specific needs for pts with renal failure (e.g., NephrAmine), hepatic disease (e.g., HepatAmine), stress/trauma (e.g., Aminosyn HBC), use in neonates and pediatrics (e.g., Aminosyn PF, TrophAmine). Calories: 4 kcal/g protein.

Energy: In the form of dextrose, available in concentrations of 5%–70%. Dextrose less than 10% may be given peripherally; concentrations greater than 10% must be given centrally. Calories: 3.4 kcal/g dextrose.

IV fat emulsion: Available in 10% and 20% concentrations. Provides a concentrated source of energy/calories (9 kcal/g fat) and is a source of essential fatty acids. May be administered peripherally or centrally.

COMPONENTS OF PN (cont.)

Electrolytes: Major electrolytes (calcium, magnesium, potassium, sodium; also acetate, chloride, phosphate). Doses of electrolytes are individualized, based on many factors (e.g., renal/hepatic function, fluid status).

Vitamins: Essential components in maintaining metabolism and cellular function; widely used in PN.

Trace elements: Necessary in long-term PN administration. Trace elements include zinc, copper, chromium, manganese, selenium, molybdenum, iodine.

Miscellaneous: Additives include insulin, albumin, heparin, and histamine$_2$ blockers (e.g., cimetidine, ranitidine, famotidine). Other medication may be included, but compatibility for admixture should be checked on an individual basis.

ROUTE OF ADMINISTRATION

PN is administered via either peripheral or central vein.

Peripheral: Usually involves 2–3 L/day of 5%–10% dextrose with 3%–5% amino acid solution along with IV fat emulsion. Electrolytes, vitamins, trace elements are added according to pt needs. Peripheral solutions provide about 2,000 kcal/day and 60–90 g protein/day.

ADVANTAGES: Lower risks vs. central mode of administration.

DISADVANTAGES: Peripheral veins may not be suitable (esp. in pts with illness of long duration); more susceptible to phlebitis (due to osmolalities over 600 mOsm/L); veins may be viable only 1–2 wks; large volumes of fluid are needed to meet nutritional requirements, which may be contraindicated in many pts.

Central: Usually utilizes hypertonic dextrose (concentration range of 15%–35%) and amino acid solution of 3%–7% with IV fat emulsion. Electrolytes, vitamins, trace elements are added according to pt needs. Central solutions provide 2,000–4,000 kcal/day. Must be given through large central vein with high blood flow, allowing rapid dilution, avoiding phlebitis/thrombosis (usually through percutaneous insertion of catheter into subclavian vein then advancement of catheter to superior vena cava).

ADVANTAGES: Allows more alternatives/flexibility in establishing regimens; allows ability to provide full nutritional requirements without need of daily fat emulsion; useful in pts who are fluid restricted (increased concentration), those needing large nutritional requirements (e.g., trauma, malignancy), or those for whom PN indicated more than 7–10 days.

DISADVANTAGES: Risk with insertion, use, maintenance of central line; increased risk of infection, catheter-induced trauma, and metabolic changes.

Nutrition: Parenteral (continued)

MONITORING

May vary slightly from institution to institution.

Baseline: CBC, platelet count, PT, weight, body length/head circumference (in infants), serum electrolytes, glucose, BUN, creatinine, uric acid, total protein, cholesterol, triglycerides, bilirubin, alkaline phosphatase, LDH, AST, albumin, other tests as needed.

Daily: Weight, vital signs (temperature, pulse, respirations [TPR]), nutritional intake (kcal, protein, fat), serum electrolytes (potassium, sodium chloride), glucose (serum, urine), acetone, BUN, osmolarity, other tests as needed.

2–3 times/wk: CBC, coagulation studies (PT, PTT), serum creatinine, calcium, magnesium, phosphorus, acid-base status, other tests as needed.

Weekly: Nitrogen balance, total protein, albumin, prealbumin, transferrin, hepatic function tests (AST, ALT), serum alkaline phosphatase, LDH, bilirubin, Hgb, uric acid, cholesterol, triglycerides, other tests as needed.

COMPLICATIONS

Mechanical: Malfunction in system for IV delivery (e.g., pump failure; problems with lines, tubing, administration sets, catheter). Pneumothorax, catheter misdirection, arterial puncture, bleeding, hematoma formation may occur with catheter placement.

Infectious: Infections (pts often more susceptible to infections), catheter sepsis (e.g., fever, shaking chills, glucose intolerance where no other site of infection is identified).

Metabolic: Includes hyperglycemia, elevated serum cholesterol and triglycerides, abnormal serum hepatic function tests.

Fluid, electrolyte, acid-base disturbances: May alter serum potassium, sodium, phosphate, magnesium levels.

Nutritional: Clinical effects seen may be due to lack of adequate vitamins, trace elements, essential fatty acids.

DRUG THERAPY/ADMINISTRATION METHODS: Compatibility of other intravenous medications pts may be administered while receiving parenteral nutrition is an important concern.

Intravenous medications usually are given as a separate admixture via piggyback to the parenteral nutrition line, but in some instances may be added directly to the parenteral nutrition solution. Because of the possibility of incompatibility when adding medication directly to the parenteral nutrition solution, specific criteria should be considered:

- Stability of the medication in the parenteral nutrition solution
- Properties of the medication, including pharmacokinetics that determine if the medication is appropriate for continuous infusion
- Documented chemical and physical compatibility with the parenteral nutrition solution

In addition, when medication is given via piggyback using the parenteral nutrition line, important criteria should include:

- Stability of the medication in the parenteral nutrition solution
- Documented chemical and physical compatibility with the parenteral nutrition solution

Obesity Management

USES

Adjunct to diet and physical activity in the treatment of chronic, relapsing obesity.

ACTIONS

Two categories of medications are used for weight control.

Appetite suppressants: Blocks neuronal uptake of norepinephrine, serotonin, dopamine causing a feeling of fullness or satiety.

Digestion inhibitors: Reversible lipase inhibitors that block the breakdown and absorption of fats, decreasing appetite and reducing calorie intake.

ANOREXIANTS

Name	Type	Availability	Dosage	Side Effects
Benzphetamine (Didrex)	AS	**T:** 50 mg	25–50 mg 1–3 times/day	Headaches, insomnia, nervousness, anxiety, irritability, dry mouth, constipation, euphoria, palpitations, hypertension
Diethylpropion (Tenuate)	AS	**T:** 25 mg, 75 mg	25 mg 3 times/day or 75 mg once/day	Headaches, insomnia, nervousness, anxiety, irritability, dry mouth, constipation, euphoria, palpitations, hypertension
Orlistat (p. 871) (Xenical)	DI	**C:** 120 mg	120 mg 3 times/day before meals	Flatulence, rectal incontinence, oily stools
Phendimetrazine (Bontril)	AS	**C:** 105 mg **T:** 35 mg	17.5–70 mg 2–3 times/day or 105 mg once/day	Headaches, insomnia, nervousness, anxiety, irritability, dry mouth, constipation, euphoria, palpitations, hypertension
Phenteramine (Ionamin)	AS	**C:** 15 mg, 30 mg, 37.5 mg	15–37.5 mg once/day	Headaches, insomnia, nervousness, anxiety, irritability, dry mouth, constipation, euphoria, palpitations, hypertension
Sibutramine (Meridia)	AS	**C:** 5 mg, 10 mg, 15 mg	Initially, 10 mg, then increase to 15 mg/day or decrease to 5 mg/day	Hypertension, tachycardia, headaches, dry mouth, loss of appetite, insomnia, constipation

AS, Appetite suppressant; ***C,*** capsules; ***DI,*** digestion inhibitor; ***T,*** tablets.

Ophthalmic Medications for Allergic Conjunctivitis

Ophthalmic products used for allergic conjunctivitis include antihistamines, mast cell stabilizing agents, combination antihistamine/decongestants, and corticosteroids. **Antihistamines** selectively inhibit the H_1 histamine receptor, thus antagonizing histamine-stimulated vascular permeability in the conjunctiva. **Mast cell stabilizing agents** block the release of mediators of hypersensitivity reactions from mast cells, eosinophils, neutrophils, macrophages, monocytes, and platelets. They inhibit the release of histamine from mast cells. **Combination antihistamine/decongestants** are used only for a short time because the regular use of a decongestant may cause rebound congestion. **Mast cell stabilizers/antihistamine** combinations provide both the quick action of the antihistamine and more delayed action of the mast cell stabilizer. This latter combination is used for mild to moderately severe allergic conjunctivitis. **Corticosteroids,** although having no definite mechanism of action, exert their effect by controlling the biosynthesis of potent mediators of inflammation.

ANTIHISTAMINE

Names	Dosage	Comments/Side Effects
Alcaftadine 0.25% (Lastacaft)	One drop each eye once daily	Eye irritation, burning/stinging on instillation, eye redness/pruritus, nasopharyngitis, headache, influenza

ANTIHISTAMINE/DECONGESTANTS

Names	Dosage	Comments/Side Effects
Naphazoline/pheniramine (Naphcon-A, Opcon-A, Visine-A)	One or two drops into affected eye(s) up to 4 times/day	Remove contact lenses prior to using Do not use for more than 3 days Not for use in pts with heart disease, enlarged prostate, high blood pressure, and/or glaucoma Side effects: headache, mydriasis, pain in eye

MAST CELL STABILIZER

Names	Dosage	Comments/Side Effects
Cromolyn 4% (p. 282) (Crolom)	One to two drops in affected eye(s) 4–6 times/day	Avoid wearing contact lenses during treatment Side effects: allergic reaction, dryness around eye, eye irritation, inflammation of eyelids, itchy eyes, watery eyes
Lodoxamine 0.1% (Alomide)	One to two drops in affected eye(s) 4 times/day	Avoid wearing contact lenses during treatment Side effects: burning, stinging, or irritation of eyes, watery, itching eyes, blurred vision, headache, dizziness, nausea or stomach discomfort
Nedocromil 2% (Alocril)	One or two drops in affected eye(s) 2 times/day	Remove contact lenses prior to using; may reinsert after 15 min if eyes are not red Side effects: headache, dizziness, blurring sensation in eye, light intolerance
Pemirolast 0.1% (Alamast)	One or two drops in affected eye(s) 4 times/day	Avoid wearing contact lenses if eyes are red Remove contact lenses prior to using; may reinsert after 10 min if eyes are not red Side effects: foreign body sensation, headache, dry eyes, burning sensation

ANTIHISTAMINE/MAST CELL STABILIZER

Names	Dosage	Comments/Side Effects
Azelastine 0.05% (p. 102) (Optivar)	One drop in affected eye(s) 2 times/day	Avoid wearing contact lenses if eyes are red Remove soft contact lenses prior to using; may reinsert after 10 min if eyes are not red Side effects: headache, drowsiness, burning sensation in eye
Epinastine 0.05% (Elestat)	One drop in affected eye(s) 2 times/day	Avoid wearing contact lenses if eyes are red Remove soft contact lenses prior to using; may reinsert after 10 min if eyes are not red Side effects: headache, burning sensation in eye
Ketotifen 0.025% (Alaway, Zaditor)	One drop in affected eye(s) 2 times/day	Avoid wearing contact lenses if eyes are red Remove soft contact lenses prior to using; may reinsert after 10 min if eyes are not red Side effects: headache, dry eyes, eye irritation, pain in eye

(continued)

ANTIHISTAMINE/MAST CELL STABILIZER *(continued)*

Names	Dosage	Comments/Side Effects
Olopatadine 0.1% (Patanol)	One drop in affected eye(s) 2 times/day	Avoid wearing contact lenses if eyes are red Remove soft contact lenses prior to using; may reinsert after 10 min if eyes are not red Side effects: headache, burning sensation in eye

CORTICOSTEROIDS

Names	Dosage	Comments/Side Effects
Loteprednol 0.2% (Alrex)	One drop in affected eye(s) 4 times/day	Recommended for short-term use only Remove soft contact lenses prior to using; may reinsert after 10 min if eyes are not red Side effects: abnormal vision, blurred vision, burning sensation in eye, itching in eye, light intolerance
Loteprednol 0.5% (Lotemax)	One or two drops in affected eye(s) 4 times/day	Recommended for short-term use only Remove soft contact lenses prior to using; may reinsert after 10 min if eyes are not red Side effects: abnormal vision, blurred vision, burning sensation in eye, itching in eye, light intolerance
Prednisolone 1% (p. 957) (AK-Pred)	Two drops in affected eye(s) 2–4 times/day	Recommended for short-term use only Remove soft contact lenses prior to using; may reinsert after 10 min if eyes are not red Side effects: blurred vision, burning sensation or irritation in eye, pain in eye

Opioid Analgesics

USES

Relief of moderate to severe pain associated with surgical procedures, MI, burns, cancer, or other conditions. May be used as an adjunct to anesthesia, either as a preop medication or intraoperatively as a supplement to anesthesia. Also used for obstetric analgesia. Codeine and hydrocodone have an antitussive effect. Opium tinctures, such as paregoric, are used for severe diarrhea. Methadone relieves severe pain but is used primarily as part of heroin detoxification.

ACTION

Opioids refer to all drugs having actions similar to morphine and to receptors combining with these agents. Major effects are on the CNS (produce analgesia, drowsiness, mood changes, impaired concentration, analgesia without loss of consciousness, nausea and vomiting) and GI tract (decrease HCl secretion; diminish biliary, pancreatic, and intestinal secretions; diminish propulsive peristalsis). Also affects respiration (depressed) and cardiovascular system (peripheral vasodilation, decrease peripheral resistance, inhibit baroreceptor reflexes).

OPIOID ANALGESICS

Names	Equianalgesic Dose	Analgesic Effect			Dosage Range
		Onset (min)	Peak (min)	Duration (hrs)	
Butorphanol (p. 157) (Stadol)	**IM:** 2 mg **IV:** —	**IM:** 10–30 **IV:** 2–3	**IM:** 30–60 **IV:** 30	**IM:** 3–4 **IV:** 2–4	**IM:** 1–4 mg q3–4h **IV:** 0.5–2 mg q3–4h
Codeine (p. 269)	**IM:** 15–30 mg **PO:** 15–30 mg	**IM:** 10–30 **PO:** 30–45	**IM:** 30–60 **PO:** 60–120	**IM/PO:** 4–6	**IM/PO (A):** 15–60 mg q4–6h; **(C):** 0.5 mg/kg q4–6h
Fentanyl (p. 472) (Sublimaze)	**IM:** 0.1–0.2 mg **IV:** —	**IM:** 7–15 **IV:** 1–2	**IM:** 20–30 **IV:** 3–5	**IM:** 1–2 **IV:** 0.5–1	**IM:** 50–100 mcg q1–2h

(continued)

OPIOID ANALGESICS *(continued)*

Names	Equianalgesic Dose	Analgesic Effect: Onset (min)	Analgesic Effect: Peak (min)	Analgesic Effect: Duration (hrs)	Dosage Range
Hydrocodone (p. 573)	**PO:** 5–10 mg	10–30	30–60	4–6	5–10 mg q4–6h
Hydromorphone (p. 578) (Dilaudid)	**PO:** 7.5 mg **IM:** 1.5 mg	**PO:** 30 **IM:** 15 **IV:** 10–15	**PO:** 90–120 **IM:** 30–60 **IV:** 15–30	**PO:** 4–5 **IM:** 4–5 **IV:** 4	**PO:** 1–4 mg q3–6h **IM:** 1–4 mg q3–6h **IV:** 0.5–1 mg q3h **R:** 3 mg q4–8h
Levorphanol (Levo-Dromoran)	**PO:** 4 mg **IM:** 2 mg	**PO:** 10–60 **IM:** —	**PO:** 90–120 **IM:** 60	4–5	**PO:** 2–4 mg q4h **IM:** 2–3 mg q4h
Meperidine (p. 732) (Demerol)	**PO:** 300 mg **IM:** 75 mg **IV:** —	**PO:** 15 **IM:** 10–15 **IV:** 1	**PO:** 60–90 **IM:** 30–60 **IV:** 5–7	2–4	**PO, IM (A):** 50–150 mg q3–4h; **(C):** 1–1.8 mg/kg q3–4h
Methadone (p. 743) (Dolophine)	**PO:** 10–20 mg **IM:** 10 mg	**PO:** 30–60 **IM:** 10–20 **IV:** —	**PO:** 90–120 **IM:** 60–120 **IV:** 15–30	**PO:** 4–6 **IM:** 4–5 **IV:** 3–4	**IM, PO:** 2.5–10 mg q3–4h
Morphine (p. 791) (MS Contin, Roxanol)	**PO:** 30 mg **IM:** 10 mg **IV:** —	**PO:** 30–60 **IM:** 10–30 **IV:** —	**PO:** 90 **IM:** 30–60 **IV:** 20	**PO:** 4 **IM/IV:** 4–5	**PO:** 10–30 mg q4h **IM:** 5–20 mg q4h **IV:** 0.05–0.1 mg/kg q4h
Nalbuphine (p. 805) (Nubain)	**IM:** 10 mg **IV:** —	**IM:** 2–15 **IV:** 2–3	**IM:** 60 **IV:** 30	**IM:** 3–6 **IV:** 3–4	**IM/IV:** 10–20 mg q3–6h
Oxycodone (p. 880) (Roxicodone)	**PO:** 20–30 mg	30	60	3–4	5–15 mg or 5 ml q4–6h **(ER):** q12h (dose titrated)
Oxymorphone (p. 882) (Opana, Opana ER)	N/A	N/A	N/A	N/A	**PO:** 10–20 mg q4–6h **ER:** Half PO total daily dose q12h

A, Adults; ***C,*** children; ***ER,*** extended-release

Osteoporosis

HISTORY

Osteoporosis is a bone disease that can lead to fractures. Bone mineral density (BMD) is reduced, bone microarchitecture is disrupted, and the amount and variety of proteins in bone are altered. Osteoporosis primarily affects women after menopause (postmenopausal osteoporosis) but may develop in men, in anyone in the presence of particular hormonal disorders (e.g., parathyroid glands), after overconsumption of dietary proteins, or as a result of medications (e.g., glucocorticoids). Several pharmacologic options, along with lifestyle changes, that can be used to prevent and/or treat osteoporotic fractures include bisphosphonates, selective estrogen receptor modulator (SERM), parathyroid hormone (PTH), calcitonin, and monoclonal antibodies.

ACTION

Bisphosphonates: Inhibit bone resorption via actions on osteoclasts or osteoclast precursors, decrease the rate of bone resorption, leading to an indirect increase in BMD.

Selective estrogen receptor modulator (SERM): Decreases bone resorption, increasing BMD and decreasing the incidence of fractures.

Parathyroid hormone: Stimulates osteoblast function, increasing gastrointestinal calcium absorption and increasing renal tubular reabsorption of calcium. This increases BMD, bone mass, and strength, resulting in a decrease in osteoporosis-related fractures.

Calcitonin: Inhibitor of bone resorption. Efficacy not observed in early postmenopausal women and is used only in women with osteoporosis who are at least 5 yrs beyond menopause.

Monoclonal antibody: Inhibits the RANK ligand (RANKL), a cytokine member of the tumor necrosis factor family. This inhibits osteoclast formation, function, and survival, which decreases bone resorption and increases bone mass and strength in cortical and trabecular bone.

BISPHOSPHONATES

Name	Availability	Dosage	Side Effects
Alendronate (Fosamax)	**T:** 5 mg, 10 mg, 35 mg, 40 mg, 70 mg **S:** 70 mg/75ml	**Prevention:** 5 mg/day or 35 mg/wk **Treatment:** 10 mg/day or 70 mg/wk	Transient, mild hypocalcemia, hypophosphatemia, dysphagia, esophagitis, esophageal and gastric ulcer
Ibandronate (Boniva)	**T:** 2.5 mg, 150 mg **I:** 1 mg/ml	**Prevention and treatment:** 2.5 mg/day or 150 mg/month **IV Injection: Treatment:** 3 mg/3 months	Dyspepsia, back pain, dysphagia, esophagitis, esophageal and gastric ulcer

I, injection; ***IM,*** intramuscular; ***IV,*** intravenous; ***S,*** solution (oral); ***T,*** tablet

(continued)

BISPHOSPHONATES *(continued)*

Name	Availability	Dosage	Side Effects
Risedronate (Actonel)	**T:** 5 mg, 30 mg, 35 mg, 150 mg	**Prevention and treatment:** 5 mg/day, 35 mg/wk, or 150 mg/month	Hypertension, headache, rash, dysphagia, esophagitis, esophageal and gastric ulcer
Zoledronic acid (Reclast)	**I:** 5 mg	**Prevention: IV:** 5 mg every 2 yrs **Treatment: IV:** 5 mg every yr	Hypertension, pain, fever, headache, chills, fatigue, nausea

SERM

Name	Availability	Dosage	Side Effects
Raloxifene (Evista)	**T:** 60 mg	**Prevention and treatment:** 60 mg/day	Peripheral edema, hot flashes, arthralgia, leg cramps, muscle spasms, flu syndrome, infection

PARATHYROID HORMONE

Name	Availability	Dosage	Side Effects
Teriparatide (Forteo)	**I:** 250 mcg/ml syringe delivers 20 mcg/dose	**Treatment:** 20 mcg subcutaneously once daily	Hypercalcemia, muscle cramps, nausea, dizziness

CALCITONIN

Name	Availability	Dosage	Side Effects
Calcitonin (Fortical, Miacalcin)	**I (Miacalcin):** 200 units/ml **Nasal (Fortical, Miacalcin):** 200 units/activation	**Treatment: IM/Subcutaneous (Miacalcin):** 100 units every other day. **Nasal:** 200 units in 1 nostril daily	Rhinitis, local nasal irritation. **Injection:** nausea, local inflammation, flushing of face, hands

MONOCLONAL ANTIBODY

Name	Availability	Dosage	Side Effects
Denosumab (Prolia)	**I:** 60 mg/ml	**Subcutaneous:** 60 mg once every 6 mos	Back pain, pain in extremity, hypercholesterolemia, musculoskeletal pain, cystitis

I, injection; ***IM,*** intramuscular; ***IV,*** intravenous; ***S,*** solution (oral); ***T,*** tablet

Parkinson's Disease Treatment

USES	ACTION
To slow or stop clinical progression of Parkinson's disease and to improve pt function and quality of life in those with Parkinson's disease, a progressive neurodegenerative disorder.	Normal motor function is dependent on the synthesis and release of dopamine by neurons projecting from the substantia nigra to the corpus striatum. In Parkinson's disease, disruption of this pathway results in diminished levels of the neurotransmitter dopamine. Medication is aimed at providing improved function using the lowest effective dose.

TYPES OF MEDICATIONS FOR PARKINSON'S DISEASE

DOPAMINE PRECURSOR

Levodopa/carbidopa:

Levodopa: Dopamine precursor supplementation to enhance dopaminergic neurotransmission. A small amount of levodopa crosses the blood-brain barrier and is decarboxylated to dopamine, which is then available to stimulate dopaminergic receptors.

Carbidopa: Inhibits peripheral decarboxylation of levodopa, decreasing its conversion to dopamine in peripheral tissues, which results in an increased availability of levodopa for transport across the blood-brain barrier.

COMT INHIBITORS

Entacapone, tolcapone: Reversible inhibitor of catechol-*O*-methyltransferase (COMT). COMT is responsible for catalyzing levodopa. In the presence of a decarboxylase inhibitor (carbidopa), COMT becomes the major metabolizing enzyme for levodopa in the brain and periphery. By inhibiting COMT, higher plasma levels of levodopa are attained, resulting in more dopaminergic stimulation in the brain and lessening the symptoms of Parkinson's disease.

DOPAMINE RECEPTOR AGONISTS

Bromocriptine: Stimulates postsynaptic dopamine type 2 receptors in the neostriatum of the CNS.

Pramipexole: Stimulates dopamine receptors in the striatum of the CNS.

Ropinirole: Stimulates postsynaptic dopamine D2 type receptors within the caudate putamen in the brain.

MONOAMINE OXIDASE B INHIBITORS

Rasagiline, Selegiline: Increases dopaminergic activity due to irreversible inhibition of monoamine oxidase type B (MAO B). MAO B is involved in the oxidative deamination of dopamine in the brain.

Parkinson's Disease Treatment

MEDICATIONS FOR TREATMENT OF PARKINSON'S DISEASE

Name	Type	Availability	Dosage	Side Effects
Bromocriptine (p. 144) (Parlodel)	Dopamine agonist	**T:** 2.5 mg **C:** 5 mg	15–45 mg/day in 2–3 divided doses	Nausea, drowsiness, lower extremity edema, postural hypotension, confusion, toxic psychosis (avoid use in pts with dementia)
Carbidopa/levodopa (p. 176) (Parcopa, Sinemet, Sinemet CR)	Dopamine precursor	**Orally-disintegrating (Parcopa):** 10/100 mg, 25/100 mg, 25/250 mg **Immediate release (Sinemet):** 10/100 mg, 25/100 mg, 25/250 mg **Controlled release (Sinemet CR):** 25/100 mg, 50/200 mg	**Parcopa:** 300–1,500 mg levodopa in divided doses **Sinemet:** 300–1,500 mg levodopa in divided doses **Sinemet CR:** 400–2,200 mg levodopa in divided doses	Anorexia, nausea, vomiting, orthostatic hypotension initially; vivid dreams, hallucinations, delusions, confusion, and sleep disturbances with chronic use
Entacapone (p. 412) (Comtan)	COMT inhibitor	**T:** 200 mg	200 mg 3–4 times/day	Dyskinesias, nausea, diarrhea, urine discoloration
Pramipexole (p. 949) (Mirapex)	Dopamine agonist	**T:** 0.125 mg, 0.25 mg, 0.5 mg, 1 mg, 1.5 mg	0.5–1.5 mg 3 times/day	Nausea, drowsiness, lower extremity edema, postural hypotension, confusion, toxic psychosis (avoid use in pts with dementia)
Rasagiline (p. 1007) (Azilect)	MAO B inhibitors	**T:** 0.5 mg, 1 mg	0.5–1 mg once daily	Nausea, orthostatic hypotension
Ropinirole (p. 1034) (Requip)	Dopamine agonist	**T:** 0.25 mg, 0.5 mg, 1 mg, 2 mg, 3 mg, 4.5 mg	3–8 mg 3 times/day	Nausea, drowsiness, lower extremity edema, postural hypotension, confusion, toxic psychosis (avoid use in pts with dementia)

Selegiline (p. 1049) (Eldepryl, Zelapar)	MAO B inhibitor	**C: (Eldepryl):** 5 mg **OD: (Zelapar):** 1.25 mg	**C:** 5 mg with breakfast and lunch **OD:** 1.25–2.5 mg daily in the morning	Nausea, orthostatic hypotension
Tolcapone (Tasmar)	COMT inhibitor	**T:** 100 mg, 200 mg	100 mg 3 times/day	Dyskinesias, nausea, diarrhea, urine discoloration

C, Capsules; ***COMT,*** catechol-*O*-methyltransferase; ***I,*** injection; ***MAO B,*** monoamine oxidase B; ***OD,*** orally-disintegrating; ***T,*** tablets.

Proton Pump Inhibitors

USES

Treatment of various gastric disorders, including gastric and duodenal ulcers, gastroesophageal reflex disease (GERD), pathologic hypersecretory conditions.

ACTION

Suppress gastric acid secretion by specific inhibition of the hydrogen-potassium-adenosine triphosphatase (H^+/K^+ ATPase) enzyme system, which transports the acid at the gastric parietal cells. These agents do not have anticholinergic or histamine receptor antagonistic properties.

PROTON PUMP INHIBITORS

Name	Availability	Indications	Usual Dosage	Side Effects
Deslansoprazole (Kapidex)	**C**: 30 mg, 60 mg	Erosive esophagitis, heartburn associated with nonerosive GERD	30 mg/day	Diarrhea, abominal pain, nausea, upper respiratory tract infection, vomiting, flatulence
Esomeprazole (p. 439) (Nexium)	**C**: 20 mg, 40 mg **I**: 20 mg	*H. pylori* eradication, GERD, erosive esophagitis	20–40 mg/day	Headaches, diarrhea, abdominal pain, nausea
Lansoprazole (p. 665) (Prevacid)	**C**: 15 mg, 30 mg **I**: 30 mg	Duodenal ulcer, gastric ulcer, NSAID-associated gastric ulcer, hypersecretory conditions, *H. pylori* eradication, GERD, erosive esophagitis	15–30 mg/day	Diarrhea, skin rash, pruritus, headaches
Omeprazole (p. 866) (Prilosec)	**C**: 10 mg, 20 mg, 40 mg	Duodenal ulcer, gastric ulcer, hypersecretory conditions, *H. pylori* eradication, GERD, erosive esophagitis	20–40 mg/day	Headaches, diarrhea, abdominal pain, nausea
Omeprazole and Sodium Bicarbonate (Zegerid)	**C**: 20 mg, 40 mg **P**: 20 mg, 40 mg	Duodenal ulcer, benign gastric ulcer, GERD, erosive esophagitis	20–40 mg/day	Headaches, abdominal pain, diarrhea, nausea
Pantoprazole (p. 898) (Protonix)	**T**: 20 mg, 40 mg **I**: 40 mg	Erosive esophagitis, hypersecretory conditions	40 mg/day	Diarrhea, headaches
Rabeprazole (p. 996) (Aciphex)	**T**: 20 mg	Duodenal ulcer, hypersecretory conditions, *H. pylori* eradication, GERD, erosive esophagitis	20 mg/day	Headaches

C, Capsules; ***GERD,*** gastroesophageal reflux disease; ***I,*** injection; ***NSAID,*** nonsteroidal anti-inflammatory drug; ***P,*** powder for suspension; ***T,*** tablets.

Sedative-Hypnotics

USES

Treatment of insomnia (i.e., difficulty falling asleep initially, frequent awakening, awakening too early).

ACTION

Benzodiazepines are the most widely used agents and largely replace barbiturates due to greater safety, lower incidence of drug dependence. Benzodiazepines nonselectively bind to at least three receptor subtypes accounting for sedative, anxiolytic, relaxant, and anticonvulsant properties. Benzodiazepines enhance the effect of the inhibitory neurotransmitter gamma-aminobutyric acid (GABA), which inhibits impulse transmission in the CNS reticular formation in brain. Benzodiazepines decrease sleep latency, number of nocturnal awakenings, and time spent in awake stage of sleep; increase total sleep time. The *nonbenzodiazepines* zaleplon and zolpidem preferentially bind with one receptor subtype, reducing sleep latency and nocturnal awakenings and increasing total sleep time.

SEDATIVE-HYPNOTICS

Name	Availability	Dosage Range	Side Effects
Benzodiazepines			
Estazolam (ProSom)	**T:** 1 mg, 2 mg	**A:** 1–2 mg **E:** 0.5–1 mg	Daytime sedation, memory and psychomotor impairment, tolerance, withdrawal reactions, rebound insomnia, dependence
Flurazepam (p. 500) (Dalmane)	**C:** 15 mg, 30 mg	**A/E:** 15–30 mg	Headaches, unpleasant taste, dry mouth, dizziness, anxiety, nausea
Quazepam (Doral)	**T:** 7.5 mg, 15 mg	**A:** 7.5–15 mg **E:** 7.5 mg	Same as flurazepam
Temazepam (p. 1100) (Restoril)	**C:** 7.5 mg, 15 mg, 30 mg	**A:** 15–30 mg **E:** 7.5–15 mg	Same as flurazepam

(continued)

SEDATIVE-HYPNOTICS ***(continued)***

Name	Availability	Dosage Range	Side Effects
Triazolam (Halcion)	**T:** 0.125 mg, 0.25 mg	**A:** 0.125–0.25 mg **E:** 0.125 mg	Same as flurazepam
Nonbenzodiazepines			
Eszopiclone (p. 446) (Lunesta)	**T:** 1 mg, 2 mg, 3 mg	**A:** 2–3 mg **E:** 1–2 mg	Headaches, unpleasant taste, dry mouth, dizziness, anxiety, nausea
Ramelteon (p. 1000) (Rozerem)	**T:** 8 mg	**A, E:** 8 mg	Headaches, dizziness, fatigue, nausea
Zaleplon (p. 1225) (Sonata)	**C:** 5 mg, 10 mg	**A:** 5–10 mg **E:** 5 mg	Headaches, dizziness, myalgia, drowsiness, asthenia, abdominal pain
Zolpidem (p. 1235) (Ambien, Ambien CR, Edluar)	**T:** 5 mg, 10 mg **CR:** 6.25 mg, 12.5 mg **SL:** 5 mg, 10 mg	**A:** 10 mg, 12.5 mg **E:** 5 mg, 6.25 mg	Dizziness, daytime drowsiness, headaches, confusion, depression, hangover, asthenia

A, Adults; ***C,*** capsules; ***CR,*** controlled-release; ***E,*** elderly; ***SL,*** sublingual; ***T,*** tablets.

Skeletal Muscle Relaxants

USES

Central acting muscle relaxants: Adjunct to rest, physical therapy for relief of discomfort associated with acute, painful musculoskeletal disorders (i.e., local spasms from muscle injury).

Baclofen, dantrolene, diazepam: Treatment of spasticity characterized by heightened muscle tone, spasm, loss of dexterity caused by multiple sclerosis, cerebral palsy, spinal cord lesions, CVA.

ACTION

Central acting muscle relaxants: Exact mechanism unknown. May act in CNS at various levels to depress polysynaptic reflexes; sedative effect may be responsible for relaxation of muscle spasm.

Baclofen, diazepam: May mimic actions of gamma-aminobutyric acid on spinal neurons; does not directly affect skeletal muscles.

Dantrolene: Acts directly on skeletal muscle, relieving spasticity.

SKELETAL MUSCLE RELAXANTS

Name	Indication	Dosage Range	Side Effects/Comments
Baclofen (p. 109) (Lioresal)	Spasticity associated with multiple sclerosis, spinal cord injury	Initially 5 mg 3 times/day Increase by 5 mg 3 times/day q3days **Maximum:** 20 mg 4 times/day	Drowsiness, dizziness, GI effects Caution with renal impairment, seizure disorders Withdrawal syndrome (e.g., hallucinations, psychosis, seizures)

(continued)

SKELETAL MUSCLE RELAXANTS *(continued)*

Name	Indication	Dosage Range	Side Effects/Comments
Carisoprodol (Rela)	Discomfort due to acute, painful, musculoskeletal conditions	250–350 mg 4 times/day	Drowsiness, dizziness, GI effects Hypomania at higher than recommended doses Withdrawal syndrome Hypersensitivity reaction (skin reaction, bronchospasm, weakness, burning eyes, fever) or idiosyncratic reaction (weakness, visual or motor disturbances, confusion) usually occurring within first 4 doses
Chlorzoxazone (Parafon Forte)	Discomfort due to acute, painful, musculoskeletal conditions	Initially 250–500 mg 3–4 times/day **Maximum:** 750 mg 3–4 times/day	Drowsiness, dizziness, GI effects; rare hepatotoxicity Hypersensitivity reaction (urticaria, itching) Urine discoloration to orange, red, or purple
Cyclobenzaprine (p. 285) (Flexeril)	Muscle spasm, pain, tenderness, restricted movement due to acute, painful, musculoskeletal conditions	Initially 5–10 mg 3 times/day **Maximum:** 20 mg 3 times/day	Drowsiness, dizziness, GI effects Anticholinergic effects (dry mouth, urinary retention) Quinidine-like effects on heart (QT prolongation) Long half-life
Dantrolene (p. 302) (Dantrium)	Spasticity associated with multiple sclerosis, cerebral palsy, spinal cord injury	Initially 25 mg/day for 1 week, then 25 mg 3 times/day for 1 week, then 50 mg 3 times/day for 1 week, then 100 mg 3 times/day **Maximum:** 100 mg 4 times/day	Drowsiness, dizziness, GI effects Contraindicated with hepatic disease Dose-dependent hepatotoxicity Diarrhea that is dose dependent and may be severe, requiring discontinuation

Diazepam (p. 342) (Valium)	Spasticity associated with cerebral palsy, spinal cord injury; reflex spasm due to muscle, joint trauma or inflammation	2–10 mg 3–4 times/day	Drowsiness, dizziness, GI effects Abuse potential
Metaxalone (Skelaxin)	Discomfort due to acute, painful, musculoskeletal conditions	800 mg 3–4 times/day	Drowsiness (low risk), dizziness, GI effects Paradoxical muscle cramps Mild withdrawal syndrome Contraindicated in serious hepatic or renal disease
Methocarbamol (Robaxin)	Discomfort due to acute, painful, musculoskeletal conditions	Initially 1,500 mg 4 times/day **Maintenance:** 1,000 mg 4 times/day	Drowsiness, dizziness, GI effects Urine discoloration to brown, brown-black, or green
Orphenadrine (Norflex)	Discomfort due to acute, painful, musculoskeletal conditions	100 mg 2 times/day	Drowsiness, dizziness, GI effects Long half-life Anticholinergic effects (dry mouth, urinary retention) Rare aplastic anemia Some products may contain sulfites
Tizanidine (p. 1140) (Zanaflex)	Spasticity	Initially 4 mg q6–8h (**Maximum** 3 times/day), may increase by 2–4 mg as needed/tolerated **Maximum:** 36 mg (limited information on doses greater than 24 mg)	Drowsiness, dizziness, GI effects Hypotension (20% decrease in B/P) Hepatotoxicity (usually reversible) Withdrawal syndrome (hypertension, tachycardia, hypertonia) Effect is short lived (3–6 hrs) Dose cautiously with creatinine clearance less than 25 ml/min

Smoking Cessation Agents

Tobacco smoking is associated with the development of lung cancer and chronic obstructive pulmonary disease. Smoking is harmful not just to the smoker but also to family members, coworkers, and others breathing cigarette smoke.

Quitting smoking decreases the risk of developing lung cancer, other cancers, heart disease, stroke, and respiratory illnesses. Several medications have proved useful as smoking cessation aids. Nausea and light-headedness are possible signs of overdose of nicotine warranting a reduction in dosage.

SMOKING CESSATION AGENTS

Name	Availability	Dose Duration	Cautions/Side Effects	Comments
Bupropion (p. 151) (Zyban)	**T:** 150 mg	150 mg every morning for 3 days, then 150 mg 2 times/day Start 1–2 wks before quit date **Duration:** 7–12 wks up to 6 mos for maintenance	History of seizure, eating disorder, use of MAOI within previous 14 days, bipolar disorder **Side effects:** Insomnia, dry mouth, tremor, rash	Stop smoking during second wk of treatment and use counseling support services along with medication
Clonidine (p. 261) (Catapres, Catapres-TTS)	**T:** 0.1 mg, 0.2 mg **Patch:** 0.1 mg/24 hrs, 0.2 mg/24 hrs, 0.3 mg/24 hrs	**Oral:** 0.15–0.75 mg/day **Patch:** 0.1–0.2 mg daily **Duration:** 3–10 weeks	Rebound hypertension. **Side effects:** Dry mouth, drowsiness, dizziness, sedation, constipation	Abrupt discontinuation can result in anxiety, agitation, headaches, tremors accompanied or followed by rapid rise in B/P

Nicotine gum (p. 829) (Nicorette, Thrive)	**Squares:** 2 mg, 4 mg	1 gum q1–2h for 6 wks, then q2–4h for 3 wks **Maximum:** 24 pieces/day **Duration:** up to 12 wks	Recent MI (within 2 wks), serious arrhythmias, serious or worsening angina pectoris **Side effects:** Dyspepsia, mouth soreness, hiccups	2 mg recommended for pts smoking less than 25 cigarettes/day, 4 mg for pts smoking 25 or more cigarettes/day Chew until a peppery or minty taste emerges and then "park" between cheek and gums to facilitate nicotine absorption through oral mucosa Chew slowly and intermittently to avoid jaw ache and achieve maximum benefit Only water should be taken 15 min before and during chewing
Nicotine inhaler (p. 829) (Nicotrol)	**Cartridge:** 10 mg (delivers 4 mg nicotine)	6–16 cartridges daily; taper frequency of use over the last 6–12 wks **Duration:** up to 6 mos	Recent MI (within 2 wks), serious arrhythmias, serious or worsening angina pectoris **Side effects:** Local irritation of mouth and throat, coughing, rhinitis	Use at or above room temperature (cold temperatures decrease amount of nicotine inhaled)
Nicotine lozenge (p. 829) (Commit)	**Lozenges:** 2 mg, 4 mg	One lozenge q1–2h for 6 wks, then q2–4h for 3 wks, then q4–8h for 3 wks **Duration:** 12 wks	Recent MI (within 2 wks), serious arrhythmias, serious or worsening angina pectoris **Side effects:** Local skin reaction, insomnia, nausea, sore throat	First cigarette smoked within 30 min of waking, use 4 mg; after 30 min of waking, use 2 mg Use at least 9 lozenges/day first 6 wks Only 1 lozenge at a time, 5 per 6 hrs and 20 per 24 hrs Do not chew or swallow

(continued)

SMOKING CESSATION AGENTS *(continued)*

Name	Availability	Dose Duration	Cautions/Side Effects	Comments
Nicotine nasal spray (p. 829) (Nicotrol NS)	10 mg/ml (delivers 0.5 mg/spray)	8–40 doses/day A dose consists of one 0.5 mg delivery to each nostril; initial dose is 1–2 sprays/hr, increasing as needed **Duration:** 3–6 mos	Recent MI (within 2 wks), serious arrhythmias, serious or worsening angina pectoris **Side effects:** Nasal irritation	Do not sniff, swallow, or inhale through nose while administering nicotine doses (may increase irritation) Tilt head back slightly for best results
Nicotine patch (p. 829) (NicoDerm CQ)	**Nicoderm CQ:** 7 mg/24 hrs, 14 mg/24 hrs, 21 mg/24 hrs **Nicotrol:** 5 mg/16 hrs, 10 mg/16 hrs, 15 mg/16 hrs	Apply upon waking on quit date: **Nicoderm CQ:** 21 mg/24 hrs for 4 wks, then 14 mg/24 hrs for 2 wks, then 7 mg/24 hrs for 2 wks **Nicotrol:** 15 mg/16 hrs for 6 wks, then 10 mg/16 hrs for 2 wks, then 5 mg/16 hrs for 2 wks	Recent MI (within 2 wks), serious arrhythmias, serious or worsening angina pectoris **Side effects:** Local skin reaction, insomnia	The 16- and 24-hr patches are of comparable efficacy Begin with a lower-dose patch in pts smoking 10 or fewer cigarettes/day Place new patch on relatively hair-free location, usually between neck and waist, in the morning If insomnia occurs, remove the 24-hr patch prior to bedtime or use the 16-hr patch Rotate patch site to diminish skin irritation
Nortriptyline (p. 848) (Pamelor)	**T:** 25 mg, 50 mg, 75 mg, 100 mg	Initially 25 mg/day, increasing gradually to target dose of 75–100 mg/day **Duration:** up to 12 wks	Risk of arrhythmias **Side effects:** Sedation, dry mouth, blurred vision, urinary retention, light-headedness, shaky hands	Initiate therapy 10–28 days before the quit date to allow steady state of nortriptyline at target dose

Varenicline (p. 1195) (Chantix)	**T:** 0.5 mg, 1 mg	**Days 1–3:** 0.5 mg daily; **days 4–7:** 0.5 mg 2 times/day; **day 8 to end of treatment:** 1 mg 2 times/day **Duration:** begin 1 wk before set quit date continue for 12 wks. May use additional 12 wks if failed to quit after first 12 wks	**Side effects:** Nausea; sleep disturbances; headaches; may impair ability to drive, operate machinery; depressed mood; altered behavior; suicidal ideation reported	Use lower dosage if not able to tolerate nausea and vomiting Use counseling support services along with medication

MAOI, Monoamine oxidase inhibitor; ***MI,*** myocardial infarction; ***T,*** tablets.

Sympathomimetics

USES

Stimulation of alpha$_1$-receptors: Induce vasoconstriction primarily in skin and mucous membranes, nasal decongestion; combine with local anesthetics to delay anesthetic absorption; increases B/P in certain hypotensive states; produce mydriasis, facilitating eye exams, ocular surgery.
Stimulation of beta$_1$-receptors: Treatment of cardiac arrest, heart failure, shock, AV block.
Stimulation of beta$_2$-receptors: Treatment of asthma.
Stimulation of dopamine receptors: Treatment of shock.

ACTION

The sympathetic nervous system (SNS) is involved in maintaining homeostasis (involved in regulation of heart rate, force of cardiac contractions, B/P, bronchial airway tone, carbohydrate, fatty acid meters [primarily norepinephrine, epinephrine, and dopamine]), which act on adrenergic receptors. These receptors include beta$_1$, beta$_2$, alpha$_1$, alpha$_2$, and dopaminergic. Sympathomimetics differ widely in their actions based on their specificity to affect these receptors.

- *Alpha$_1$:* Causes mydriasis, constriction of arterioles, veins.
- *Alpha$_2$:* Inhibits transmitter release.
- *Beta$_1$:* Increases rate, force of contraction, conduction velocity of heart; releases renin from kidney.
- *Beta$_2$:* Dilates arterioles, bronchi, relaxes uterus.
- *Dopaminergic:* Dilates kidney vasculature.

Sympathomimetics *(continued)*

SYMPATHOMIMETICS

Name	Availability	Receptor Specificity	Uses	Dosage Range
Dobutamine (p. 367) (Dobutrex)	**I:** 12.5 mg/ml, 500 mg/250 ml	$Beta_1$, $beta_2$, $alpha_1$	Inotropic support in cardiac decompensation	**IV infusion:** 2.5–10 mcg/kg/min
Dopamine (p. 377) (Intropin)	**I:** 40 mg/ml, 80 mg/ml, 160 mg/ml vials, 800 mcg/ml, 1,600 mcg/ml	$Beta_1$, $alpha_1$, dopaminergic	Vasopressor, cardiac stimulant	**Dopaminergic:** 0.5–3 mcg/kg/min **$Beta_1$:** 2–10 mcg/kg/min **$Alpha_1$:** more than 10 mcg/kg/min
Ephedrine	**I:** 50 mg/ml	Alpha, $beta_1$, $beta_2$	Acute hypotensive states, esp. with spinal anesthesia	**IV:** 5–25 mg
Epinephrine (p. 415) (Adrenalin)	**I:** 0.1 mg/ml, 1 mg/ml	$Beta_1$, $beta_2$, $alpha_1$	Cardiac arrest, anaphylactic shock	**Vasopressor:** 1–10 mcg/min **Cardiac arrest:** 1 mg q3–5min during resuscitation
Norepinephrine (p. 845) (Levophed)	**I:** 1 mg/ml	$Beta_1$, $alpha_1$	Vasopressor	**IV:** 0.5–1 mcg/min up to 2–12 mcg/min
Phenylephrine (p. 927) (Neo-Synephrine)	**I:** 10 mg/ml	$Alpha_1$	Vasopressor	**IV:** Initially, 10–180 mcg/min, then 40–60 mcg/min

I, Injection.

Thyroid

USES

Treatment of hypothyroidism, a common endocrine disorder in which the thyroid fails to release sufficient amounts of thyroid hormones.

ACTION

Thyroid hormones are necessary for proper metabolism, growth, and homeostasis. Thyroid hormone regulates energy and heat production; facilitates development of the CNS, growth, and puberty. Regulates the synthesis of proteins that are important in hepatic, cardiac, neurologic, and muscular functions.

THYROID

Name	Availability	Dosage Average	Side Effects
Levothyroxine (p. 687) (Levothroid, Levoxyl, Synthroid, Unithroid)	**T:** 25 mcg, 50 mcg, 75 mcg, 88 mcg, 100 mcg, 112 mcg, 125 mcg, 137 mcg, 150 mcg, 175 mcg, 200 mcg, 300 mcg	75–100 mcg/day	Side effects are due to excessive amounts of medication, including diarrhea, heat intolerance, palpitations, tremors, tachycardia, vomiting, weight loss, increased B/P
Liothyronine (Cytomel, Triostat)	**T:** 5 mcg, 25 mcg, 50 mcg	25–50 mcg/day	Same as levothyroxine
Liotrix (Thyrolar)	**T:** ¼ grain, ½ grain, 1 grain, 2 grains, 3 grains	½–1 grain/day	Same as levothyroxine
Thyroid dessicated (Armour Thyroid Nature Throid, Wes Throid)	**T:** 15 mg, 30 mg, 60 mg, 90 mg, 120 mg, 180 mg, 240 mg, 300 mg	60–120 mg/day	Same as levothyroxine

T, Tablets.

Vitamins

INTRODUCTION	WATER SOLUBLE	FAT SOLUBLE
Vitamins are organic substances required for growth, reproduction, and maintenance of health and are obtained from food or supplementation in small quantities (vitamins cannot be synthesized by the body or the rate of synthesis is too slow/inadequate to meet metabolic needs). Vitamins are essential for energy transformation and regulation of metabolic processes. They are catalysts for all reactions using proteins, fats, carbohydrates for energy, growth, and cell maintenance.	Water-soluble vitamins include vitamin C (ascorbic acid), B_1 (thiamine), B_2 (riboflavin), B_3 (niacin), B_5 (pantothenic acid), B_6 (pyridoxine), folic acid, B_{12} (cyanocobalamin). Water-soluble vitamins act as coenzymes for almost every cellular reaction in the body. B-complex vitamins differ from one another in both structure and function but are grouped together because they first were isolated from the same source (yeast and liver).	Fat-soluble vitamins include vitamins A, D, E, and K. They are soluble in lipids and are usually absorbed into the lymphatic system of the small intestine and then into the general circulation. Absorption is facilitated by bile. These vitamins are stored in the body tissue when excessive quantities are consumed. May be toxic when taken in large doses (see sections on individual vitamins).

VITAMINS

Name	Uses	RDA	Side Effects
Vitamin A (p. 1211) (Aquasol A)	Required for normal growth, bone development, vision, reproduction, maintenance of epithelial tissue	**M:** 1,000 mcg **F:** 800 mcg	**High dosages:** Hepatotoxicity, cheilitis, facial dermatitis, photosensitivity, mucosal dryness
Vitamin B_1 (p. 1122) (thiamine)	Important in red blood cell formation, carbohydrate metabolism, neurologic function, myocardial contractility, growth, energy production	**M:** 1.5 mg **F:** 1.1 mg	**Large parenteral doses:** May cause pain on injection
Vitamin B_2 (riboflavin)	Necessary for function of coenzymes in oxidation-reduction reactions, essential for normal cellular growth, assists in absorption of iron and pyridoxine	**M:** 1.7 mg **F:** 1.3 mg	Orange-yellow discoloration in urine
Vitamin B_3 (p. 825) (niacin)	Coenzyme for many oxidation-reduction reactions	**M:** 19 mg **F:** 15 mg	**High dosage (over 500 mg):** Nausea, vomiting, diarrhea, gastritis, hepatotoxicity, skin rash, facial flushing, headaches
Vitamin B_5 (pantothenic acid)	Precursor to coenzyme A, important in synthesis of cholesterol, hormones, fatty acids	**M:** 4–7 mg **F:** 4–7 mg	Occasional GI disturbances (e.g., diarrhea)
Vitamin B_6 (p. 988) (pyridoxine)	Enzyme cofactor for amino acid metabolism, essential for erythrocyte production, Hgb synthesis	**M:** 2 mg **F:** 1.6 mg	**High dosages:** May cause sensory neuropathy

(continued)

VITAMINS *(continued)*

Name	Uses	RDA	Side Effects
Vitamin B_{12} (p. 284) (cyanocobalamin)	Coenzyme in cells, including bone marrow, CNS, and GI tract, necessary for lipid metabolism, formation of myelin	**M:** 2.4 mcg **F:** 2.4 mcg	Skin rash, diarrhea, pain at injection site
Vitamin C (p. 81) (ascorbic acid)	Cofactor in various physiologic reactions, necessary for collagen formation, acts as antioxidant	**M:** 90 mg **F:** 75 mg (increased with smoking, pregnancy, lactation)	**High dosages:** May cause calcium oxalate crystalluria, esophagitis, diarrhea
Vitamin D (p. 1212) (Calciferol)	Necessary for proper formation of bone, calcium, mineral homeostasis, regulation of parathyroid hormone, calcitonin, phosphate	**M:** 200–400 units **F:** 200–400 units	Hypercalcemia, kidney stones, renal failure, hypertension, psychosis, diarrhea, nausea, vomiting, anorexia, fatigue, headaches, altered mental status
Vitamin E (p. 1216) (Aquasol E)	Antioxidant	**M:** 15 mg **F:** 15 mg	**High dosages:** GI disturbances, malaise, headaches

F, Females; ***M,*** males.

abacavir

ah-bah-**kay**-veer
(Ziagen)

BLACK BOX ALERT Serious, sometimes fatal hypersensitivity reactions, lactic acidosis, severe hepatomegaly with steatosis (fatty liver) have occurred.

FIXED-COMBINATION(S)

Epzicom: abacavir/lamivudine (antiretroviral): 600 mg/300 mg. **Trizivir:** abacavir/lamivudine (antiretroviral)/zidovudine (antiretroviral): 300 mg/150 mg/300 mg.

◆ CLASSIFICATION

PHARMACOTHERAPEUTIC: Antiretroviral agent. **CLINICAL:** Antiviral (see pp. 67C, 114C).

ACTION

Inhibits activity of HIV-1 reverse transcriptase by competing with natural substrate dGTP and by its incorporation into viral DNA. **Therapeutic Effect:** Inhibits viral DNA growth.

PHARMACOKINETICS

Rapidly and extensively absorbed after PO administration. Protein binding: 50%. Widely distributed, including to cerebrospinal fluid (CSF) and erythrocytes. Metabolized in liver to inactive metabolites. Primarily excreted in urine. Unknown if removed by hemodialysis. **Half-life:** 1.5 hrs.

USES

Treatment of HIV infection, in combination with other agents.

PRECAUTIONS

Contraindications: Moderate or severe hepatic impairment. **Cautions:** Mild hepatic disease.

⌛ LIFESPAN CONSIDERATIONS

Pregnancy/Lactation: Unknown if excreted in breast milk. Breast-feeding not recommended (may increase potential for HIV transmission, adverse effects). **Pregnancy Category C. Children:** Safety and efficacy not established in those less than 3 mos of age. **Elderly:** No age related precautions noted.

INTERACTIONS

DRUG: **Alcohol** may increase concentration, risk of toxicity. **HERBAL:** None significant. **FOOD:** None known. **LAB VALUES:** May increase serum AST, ALT, GGT, blood glucose, triglycerides. May decrease Hgb, leukocytes, lymphocytes.

AVAILABILITY (Rx)

Solution, Oral: 20 mg/ml. **Tablets:** 300 mg.

ADMINISTRATION/HANDLING

PO

• May give without regard to food. • Oral solution may be refrigerated. Do not freeze.

INDICATIONS/ROUTES/DOSAGE

HIV Infection (in Combination with Other Antiretrovirals)

PO: ADULTS: 300 mg twice a day or 600 mg once a day. **CHILDREN 3 MOS–16 YRS:** 8 mg/kg twice a day. **Maximum:** 300 mg twice a day.

Dosage in Hepatic Impairment

Mild impairment: 200 mg twice a day (oral solution recommended). **Moderate to severe impairment:** Not recommended.

SIDE EFFECTS

ADULT: **Frequent:** Nausea (47%), nausea with vomiting (16%), diarrhea (12%), decreased appetite (11%). **Occasional:** Insomnia (7%). CHILDREN: **Frequent:** Nausea with vomiting (39%), fever (19%), headache, diarrhea (16%), rash (11%). **Occasional:** Decreased appetite (9%).

ADVERSE EFFECTS/ TOXIC REACTIONS

Hypersensitivity reaction may be life-threatening. Signs and symptoms include fever, rash, fatigue, intractable nausea/

vomiting, severe diarrhea, abdominal pain, cough, pharyngitis, dyspnea. Life-threatening hypotension may occur. Lactic acidosis, severe hepatomegaly may occur.

NURSING CONSIDERATIONS

BASELINE ASSESSMENT

Question for possibility of pregnancy. Obtain baseline laboratory testing, esp. hepatic function tests, before beginning therapy and at periodic intervals during therapy. Offer emotional support.

INTERVENTION/EVALUATION

Assess for nausea, vomiting. Monitor daily pattern of bowel activity and stool consistency. Assess eating pattern; monitor for weight loss. Monitor lab values carefully, particularly hepatic function. Stop abacavir if 3 or more of the following occur: rash, fever, GI disturbances (diarrhea, nausea, vomiting), flu-like symptoms, respiratory difficulty.

PATIENT/FAMILY TEACHING

• Do not take any medications, including OTC drugs, without consulting physician. • Small, frequent meals may offset anorexia, nausea. • Abacavir is not a cure for HIV infection, nor does it reduce risk of transmission to others. • Pt must continue practices to prevent HIV transmission.

abatacept

ah-**bah**-tah-cept
(Orencia)
Do not confuse Orencia with Oracea.

CLASSIFICATION

PHARMACOTHERAPEUTIC: Selective T-cell co-stimulation modulator. **CLINICAL:** Rheumatoid arthritis agent.

ACTION

Inhibits T-lymphocyte activation, necessary in the inflammatory cascade leading to joint inflammation and destruction. **Therapeutic Effect:** Induces major clinical response to adult pts with moderate to severely active rheumatoid arthritis (RA).

PHARMACOKINETICS

Higher clearance with increasing body weight. Age, gender do not affect clearance. **Half-life:** 8–25 days.

USES

Reduces signs and symptoms, progression of structural damage in adults with moderate to severe rheumatoid arthritis (RA) unresponsive to other disease-modifying antirheumatic drugs. Treatment of moderate to severe active polyarticular juvenile idiopathic arthritis in pts 6 yrs and older. May use alone or in combination (do not use with anakinra or tumor necrosis factor (TNF) antagonists).

PRECAUTIONS

Contraindications: None known. **Cautions:** Chronic, latent, or localized infection, COPD, elderly.

LIFESPAN CONSIDERATIONS

Pregnancy/Lactation: Crosses placenta; unknown if distributed in breast milk. **Pregnancy Category C. Children:** Safety and efficacy not established. **Elderly:** Cautious use due to increased risk of serious infection and malignancy.

INTERACTIONS

DRUG: May increase risk of infection, decrease efficacy of immune response associated with **live vaccines. Tumor necrosis factor (TNF) antagonists (adalimumab, etanercept, infliximab)** may increase levels, effects of abatacept. **HERBAL:** Avoid **echinacea** (possesses immunostimulant properties). **FOOD:** None known. **LAB VALUES:** None significant.

AVAILABILITY (Rx)

Injection, Powder for Reconsitution: 250 mg.

ADMINISTRATION/HANDLING

IV

Reconstitution • Reconstitute powder in each vial with 10 ml Sterile Water for Injection using the silicone-free syringe provided with each vial and an 18–21-gauge needle. • Rotate solution gently to prevent foaming until powder is completely dissolved. • From a 100 ml 0.9% NaCl infusion bag, withdraw and discard an amount equal to the volume of the reconstituted vials (for 2 vials remove 20 ml, for 3 vials remove 30 ml, for 4 vials remove 40 ml). • Slowly add the reconstituted solution from each vial into the infusion bag using the same syringe provided with each vial. • Concentration in the infusion bag will be 10 mg/ml or less abatacept.

Rate of administration • Infuse over 30 min using a low-protein binding filter.

Storage • Store vials in refrigerator. • Any reconstitution that has been prepared by using siliconized syringes will develop translucent particles and must be discarded. • Solution should appear clear and colorless to pale yellow. Discard if solution is discolored or contains precipitate. • Solution is stable for up to 24 hrs after reconstitution. • Reconstituted solution may be stored at room temperature or refrigerated.

IV INCOMPATIBILITIES

Do not infuse concurrently in same IV line as other agents.

INDICATIONS/ROUTES/DOSAGE

Rheumatoid Arthritis (RA)

IV: BODY WEIGHT 101 KG OR MORE: 1 g (4 vials) given as a 30-min infusion. Following initial therapy, give at 2 wks and 4 wks after first infusion, then q4wk thereafter. **BODY WEIGHT 60–100 KG:** 750 mg (3 vials) given as a 30-min infusion. Following initial therapy, give at 2 wks and 4 wks after first infusion, then q4wk thereafter. **BODY WEIGHT 59 KG OR LESS:** 500 mg (2 vials) given as a 30-min infusion. Following initial therapy, give at 2 wks and 4 wks after first infusion, then q4wk thereafter.

Juvenile Idiopathic Arthritis

IV: CHILDREN 6 YRS AND OLDER, WEIGHING LESS THAN 75 KG: 10 mg/kg. **CHILDREN WEIGHING 75 KG OR MORE:** Refer to adult dosing. **Maximum:** 1,000 mg. Following initial therapy, give 2 wks and 4 wks after first infusion, then q4wk thereafter.

SIDE EFFECTS

Frequent (18%): Headache. **Occasional (9%–6%):** Dizziness, cough, back pain, hypertension, nausea.

ADVERSE EFFECTS/ TOXIC REACTIONS

Upper respiratory tract infection, nasopharyngitis, sinusitis, UTI, influenza, bronchitis occur in 5% of pts. Serious infections manifested as pneumonia, cellulitis, diverticulitis, acute pyelonephritis occur in 3% of pts. Hypersensitivity reaction (rash, urticaria, hypotension, dyspnea) occurs rarely.

NURSING CONSIDERATIONS

BASELINE ASSESSMENT

Assess onset, type, location, duration of pain/inflammation. Inspect appearance of affected joint for immobility, deformities, skin condition.

INTERVENTION/EVALUATION

Assess for therapeutic response: relief of pain, stiffness, swelling, increased joint mobility, reduced joint tenderness, improved grip strength. Monitor for hypersensitivity reaction (headache, B/P change, lightheadedness).

PATIENT/FAMILY TEACHING

• Consult physician or nurse if infection, hypersensitivity reaction, infusion-related reaction occur. • Do not receive live vaccines during treatment or within 3 mos of its discontinuation. • COPD pts to report worsening of respiratory symptoms.

abciximab

HIGH ALERT

ab-**six**-ih-mab
(c7E3 Fab, ReoPro)

CLASSIFICATION

PHARMACOTHERAPEUTIC: Glycoprotein IIb/IIIa receptor inhibitor. **CLINICAL:** Antiplatelet; antithrombotic (see p. 32C).

ACTION

Rapidly inhibits platelet aggregation by preventing the binding of fibrinogen to GP IIb/IIIa receptor sites on platelets. **Therapeutic Effect:** Prevents occlusion of treated coronary arteries. Prevents acute cardiac ischemic complications.

PHARMACOKINETICS

Rapidly cleared from plasma. Initial-phase half-life is less than 10 min; second-phase half-life is 30 min.

USES

Adjunct to aspirin and heparin therapy to prevent cardiac ischemic complications in pts undergoing percutaneous coronary intervention (PCI) and those with unstable angina not responding to conventional medical therapy when PCI is planned within 24 hrs. **OFF-LABEL:** Treatment of acute MI.

PRECAUTIONS

Contraindications: Active internal bleeding, arteriovenous malformation or aneurysm, CVA with residual neurologic deficit, history of CVA (within the past 2 yrs) or oral anticoagulant use within the past 7 days unless PT is less than 1.2× control, history of vasculitis, hypersensitivity to murine proteins, intracranial neoplasm, prior IV dextran use before or during percutaneous transluminal coronary angioplasty (PTCA), recent surgery or trauma (within the past 6 wks), recent GI or GU bleeding (within the past 6 wks), thrombocytopenia (less than 100,000 cells/mcl), and severe uncontrolled hypertension. **Cautions:** Pts who weigh less than 75 kg; those older than 65 yrs; those with history of GI disease; those receiving thrombolytics, heparin, aspirin, PTCA in less than 12 hrs of onset of symptoms for acute MI, prolonged PTCA (longer than 70 min), failed PTCA.

LIFESPAN CONSIDERATIONS

Pregnancy/Lactation: Unknown if distributed in breast milk. **Pregnancy Category C. Children:** Safety and efficacy not established. **Elderly:** Increased risk of major bleeding.

INTERACTIONS

DRUG: **Antiplatelet medications, heparin, other anticoagulants, thrombolytics** may increase risk of bleeding. **HERBAL:** None significant. **FOOD:** None known. **LAB VALUES:** Increases activated clotting time (ACT), prothrombin time (PT), activated partial thromboplastin time (aPTT); decreases platelet count.

AVAILABILITY (Rx)

Injection Solution: 2 mg/ml (5-ml vial).

ADMINISTRATION/HANDLING

IV

Reconstitution • Use 0.2- to 0.22-micron filter; filtering may be done during preparation or at administration. • Bolus dose may be given undiluted. • Withdraw desired dose and further dilute in 250 ml of 0.9% NaCl or D_5W (e.g., 10 mg in 250 ml equals concentration of 40 mcg/ml).

Rate of administration • See Indications/Routes/Dosage.

Administration precautions • Give in separate IV line; do not add any other medication to infusion. • For bolus injection and continuous infusion, use sterile, nonpyrogenic, low protein-binding 0.2- or 0.22-micron filter. • While vascular sheath is in position, maintain pt on complete bed rest with head of bed elevated at 30°. • Maintain affected limb in straight position. • After sheath removal, apply femoral pressure for 30 min, either manually or mechanically, then apply pressure dressing. **Storage** • Store vials in refrigerator. • Solution appears clear, colorless. • Do not shake. • Prepared solution is stable for 12 hrs. Discard any unused portion left in vial or if preparation contains *any* opaque particles.

IV INCOMPATIBILITY

Administer in separate line; no other medication should be added to infusion solution.

IV COMPATIBILITIES

Adenosine (Adenocard), atropine sulfate, bivalirudin (Angiomax), diphenhydramine (Benadryl), fentanyl (Sublimaze), midazolam (Versed).

INDICATIONS/ROUTES/DOSAGE

Percutaneous Coronary Intervention (PCI)

IV BOLUS: ADULTS: 0.25 mg/kg 10–60 min before PCI, then 12-hr IV infusion of 0.125 mcg/kg/min. **Maximum:** 10 mcg/min.

PCI (Unstable Angina)

IV BOLUS: ADULTS: 0.25 mg/kg, followed by 18- to 24-hr infusion of 10 mcg/min, ending 1 hr after procedure.

SIDE EFFECTS

Frequent: Nausea (16%), hypotension (12%). **Occasional (9%):** Vomiting. **Rare (3%):** Bradycardia, confusion, dizziness, pain, peripheral edema, UTI.

ADVERSE EFFECTS/ TOXIC REACTIONS

Major bleeding complications may occur; stop infusion immediately. Hypersensitivity reaction (rash, urticaria, hypotension, dyspnea) may occur. Atrial fibrillation or flutter, pulmonary edema, complete AV block occur occasionally.

NURSING CONSIDERATIONS

BASELINE ASSESSMENT

Heparin should be discontinued 4 hrs before arterial sheath removal. Maintain pt on bed rest for 6–8 hrs following sheath removal or drug discontinuation, whichever is later. Check platelet count, PT, aPTT before infusion (assess for preexisting blood abnormalities), 2–4 hrs following treatment, and at 24 hrs or before discharge, whichever is first. Check insertion site, distal pulse of affected limb while femoral artery sheath is in place, and then routinely for 6 hrs following femoral artery sheath removal. Minimize need for injections, blood draws, catheters, other invasive procedures.

INTERVENTION/EVALUATION

Stop abciximab and/or heparin infusion if serious bleeding occurs that is uncontrolled by pressure. Observe for mental status changes. Assess skin for ecchymosis, petechiae, particularly at femoral arterial access, also at catheter insertion, arterial and venous puncture, cutdown, needle sites. Handle pt carefully and as infrequently as possible to prevent bleeding. Do not obtain B/P in lower extremities (possible deep vein thrombi). Assess for decrease in B/P, increase in pulse rate, complaint of abdominal or back pain, severe headache, evidence of GI hemorrhage. Monitor ACT, PT, aPTT, platelet counts, Hgb, Hct. Question for increase in discharge during menses. Assess urinary output for hematuria. Monitor for hematoma. Use care in removing any dressing, tape.

PATIENT/FAMILY TEACHING

• Assess skin for bruising up to 3 days after infusion. • Report signs of bleeding.

Abelcet, *see amphotericin B*

Abilify, *see aripiprazole*

abobotulinum toxin A

aye-bow-**botch**-you-lin-em tocks-inn (Dysport)

BLACK BOX ALERT Effects may spread beyond treatment area; may occur hrs to wks after injection. Dysphagia, breathing difficulties, including fatalities, asthenia, diplopia, blurred vision, ptosis, have been reported. Risk greatest in children treated for spasticity.

Do not confuse abobotulinum toxin A with botulinum toxin A or botulinum toxin B.

CLASSIFICATION

PHARMACOTHERAPEUTIC: Acetylcholine release inhibitor. **CLINICAL:** Neuromuscular conduction blocker.

ACTION

Blocks neuromuscular conduction by binding to receptor sites on motor nerve endings, inhibiting release of acetylcholine, resulting in muscle denervation. **Therapeutic Effect:** Reduces neuromuscular transmission, local muscle activity.

PHARMACOKINETICS

Minimal to no systemic absorption. **Half-life:** N/A.

USES

Treatment of cervical dystonia in adults to reduce severity of abnormal head position and neck pain. Temporary improvement of brow furrow lines in those 65 yrs and younger. **OFF-LABEL:** Treatment of blepharospasm, spasmodic torticollis, hemifacial spasm in adults, equinus foot deformity in children with cerebral palsy. Symptomatic treatment of excessive axillary sweating.

PRECAUTIONS

Contraindications: Infection at proposed injection sites, hypersensitivity to milk proteins, albumin. **Cautions:** Those with neuromuscular junctional disorders (amyotrophic lateral sclerosis, motor neuropathy, myasthenia gravis, Lambert-Eaton syndrome) may experience significant systemic effects (severe dysphagia, respiratory compromise), previous surgical alterations of facial anatomy, excessive weakness or atrophy in target muscles, marked facial asymmetry, ptosis, deep dermal scarring, thick sebaceous skin, diabetes mellitus.

LIFESPAN CONSIDERATIONS

Pregnancy/Lactation: Unknown if crosses placenta or is distributed in breast milk. **Pregnancy Category C. Children:** Safety and efficacy not established. **Elderly:** No age-related precautions noted.

INTERACTIONS

DRUG: Aminoglycoside antibiotics, neurologic blocking agents may potentiate effects. **HERBAL:** None significant. **FOOD:** None known. **LAB VALUES:** None significant.

AVAILABILITY (Rx)

Injection: 300 units/vial, 500 units/vial.

ADMINISTRATION/HANDLING

IM

Reconstitution • For treatment of glabellar lines, reconstitute 300-unit vial with 2.5 ml of 0.9% NaCl to yield solution containing 10 units of Dysport per 0.08 ml. • Slowly and gently inject diluent into vial. Prevent bubble formation; rotate vial gently to mix. • For treatment of cervical dystonia, reconstitute 500-unit vial with 1.5 ml of 0.9% NaCl for solution containing 10 units per 0.05 ml.

Rate of administration • Inject into affected muscle using 25-, 27-, or 30-gauge needle for superficial muscles or 22-gauge needle for deeper musculature.

Storage • Store in refrigerator. • Administer within 4 hrs after reconstitution; store reconstituted solution in refrigerator until administered. • Reconstituted solution should appear clear, colorless, without particulate matter.

INDICATIONS/ROUTES/DOSAGE

◀ALERT▶ Noninterchangeable forms; potency units of botulinum toxin products may not be compared or converted to units of any other botulinum toxin product. To be administered into affected muscle by physician.

Glabellar Lines

IM: ADULTS, ELDERLY: Dosage is dependent on severity of lines and specific muscle being treated. For corrugator and procerus muscles, 40–60 units divided between injection sites as follows: 8–12 units in each of 5 sites, 2 in each corrugator muscle, and 1 in procerus muscle for total dose of 60 units.

Cervical Dystonia

IM: ADULTS, ELDERLY: 500 units as divided dose among affected muscles with retreatment every 12–16 wks or longer, as needed. Administer doses between 250 and 1,000 units to optimize clinical benefit. Titrate in 250-unit steps according to pt response.

SIDE EFFECTS

Frequent (16%–11%): Muscular weakness, dysphagia, injection site discomfort, dry mouth, fatigue, headache. **Occasional (7%–4%):** Musculoskeletal pain, blurred/double vision, reduced visual acuity, dry eye, blepharoptosis with glabellar line treatment. **Rare (2.5%–1%):** Facial pain, erythema, local muscle weakness, ecchymosis, skin tightness, paresthesia, nausea.

ADVERSE EFFECTS/ TOXIC REACTIONS

Mild to moderate dysphagia occurs in 15%–39% of pts treated for cervical dystonia. Overdose produces systemic weakness, muscle paralysis.

NURSING CONSIDERATIONS

BASELINE ASSESSMENT

Assess onset, type, location, duration of dystonia.

INTERVENTION/EVALUATION

Improvement of severity of glabellar lines generally occurs within 72 hrs after treatment and persists for 3–6 mos. Peak effect in cervical dystonia occurs in 2–4 wks. Re-treatment, if needed, should not occur in intervals of less than 12 wks.

PATIENT/FAMILY TEACHING

• Resume activities slowly and carefully. • Seek medical attention immediately if swallowing, speech, or respiratory difficulties occur. • Avoid driving or engaging in potentially hazardous activities if loss of strength, muscle weakness, blurred vision, or drooping eyelids occur.

acamprosate

ah-**cam**-pro-sate
(Campral)

◆CLASSIFICATION

CLINICAL: Alcohol abuse deterrent.

ACTION

Appears to interact with glutamate and gamma-aminobutyric acid neurotransmitter systems centrally, restoring their balance. **Therapeutic Effect:** Reduces alcohol dependence.

PHARMACOKINETICS

Slowly absorbed from GI tract. Protein binding: Negligible. Does not undergo metabolism. Excreted in urine. **Half-life:** 20–33 hrs.

USES

Maintenance of alcohol abstinence in pts with alcohol dependence who are abstinent at treatment initiation.

PRECAUTIONS

Contraindications: Severe renal impairment (creatinine clearance 30 ml/min or less). **Cautions:** Mental depression, renal impairment.

LIFESPAN CONSIDERATIONS

Pregnancy/Lactation: Unknown if distributed in breast milk. **Pregnancy Category C. Children:** Safety and efficacy not established. **Elderly:** Age-related renal impairment may require dosage adjustment.

INTERACTIONS

DRUG: None significant. HERBAL: None significant. FOOD: None known. LAB VALUES: None significant.

AVAILABILITY (Rx)

Tablets (Enteric-Coated, Extended-Release): 333 mg.

ADMINISTRATION/HANDLING

PO

• Do not crush, chew, break enteric-coated tablets. • Give without regard to meals; however, giving with food may aid in compliance of pts who regularly eat three meals daily.

INDICATIONS/ROUTES/DOSAGE

Alcohol Abstinence

PO: ADULTS, ELDERLY: Two tablets 3 times a day. Lower dose may be effective in some pts. (Lower dose of 4 tablets/day may be considered in pts with low body wgt.)

Dosage in Renal Impairment

Creatinine clearance 30–49 ml/min: Decrease dosage to 1 tablet 3 times a day. Contraindicated in pts with severe renal impairment (creatinine clearance less than 30 ml/min).

SIDE EFFECTS

Frequent (17%): Diarrhea. **Occasional (6%–4%):** Insomnia, asthenia, fatigue, anxiety, flatulence, nausea, depression, pruritus. **Rare (3%–1%):** Dizziness, anorexia, paresthesia, diaphoresis, dry mouth.

ADVERSE EFFECTS/ TOXIC REACTIONS

Acute renal failure has been reported.

NURSING CONSIDERATIONS

BASELINE ASSESSMENT

Obtain BUN, serum creatinine before treatment. Assess motor responses (agitation, trembling, tension), autonomic responses (cold and clammy hands, diaphoresis).

INTERVENTION/EVALUATION

Monitor daily pattern of bowel activity and stool consistency. Assess sleep pattern and provide environment conducive to sleep (quiet environment, low lighting). Offer emotional support to anxious pt. Assist with ambulation if dizziness occurs.

PATIENT/FAMILY TEACHING

• Medication does not eliminate or diminish withdrawal symptoms. • Avoid tasks that require alertness, motor skills until response to drug is established. • Medication helps maintain abstinence only when used as a part of a treatment program that includes counseling and support.

acarbose

HIGH ALERT

ah-**car**-bose
(Glucobay, Precose)
Do not confuse Precose with PreCare.

CLASSIFICATION

PHARMACOTHERAPEUTIC: Alpha glucosidase inhibitor. **CLINICAL:** Antidiabetic: Oral (see p. 43C).

ACTION

Delays glucose absorption and digestion of carbohydrates, resulting in a smaller rise in blood glucose concentration after meals. **Therapeutic Effect:** Lowers postprandial hyperglycemia.

USES

Adjunctive therapy to diet in treatment of pts with type 2 diabetes. Primarily used to reduce postprandial rise in blood glucose. May be used alone or in combination with other antidiabetic agents (sulfonylurea, metformin, insulin).

PRECAUTIONS

Contraindications: Chronic intestinal diseases associated with marked disorders of digestion or absorption, cirrhosis, colonic ulceration, conditions that may deteriorate as a result of increased gas formation in intestine, diabetic ketoacidosis, hypersensitivity to acarbose, inflammatory bowel disease, partial intestinal obstruction or predisposition to intestinal obstruction, significant renal dysfunction (serum creatinine level greater than 2 mg/dl). **Cautions:** Fever, infection, surgery, trauma (may cause loss of glycemic control). **Pregnancy Category B.**

INTERACTIONS

DRUG: **Digestive enzymes, intestinal absorbents (e.g., charcoal)** reduce acarbose effect. Do not use concurrently. May increase levels/effects of **hypoglycemic agents,** decrease levels/effects of **digoxin.** **HERBAL:** None significant. **FOOD:** None known. **LAB VALUES:** May increase serum transaminase levels.

AVAILABILITY (Rx)

Tablets: 25 mg, 50 mg, 100 mg.

ADMINISTRATION/HANDLING

PO

• Give with the first bite of each main meal.

INDICATIONS/ROUTES/DOSAGE

Diabetes Mellitus

PO: ADULTS, ELDERLY: Initially, 25 mg 3 times a day with first bite of each main meal. May increase at 4- to 8-wk intervals. **Maximum:** For pts weighing more than 60 kg, 100 mg 3 times a day; for pts weighing 60 kg or less, 50 mg 3 times a day.

SIDE EFFECTS

Side effects diminish in frequency and intensity over time. **Frequent:** Transient GI disturbances: flatulence (77%), diarrhea (33%), abdominal pain (21%).

ADVERSE EFFECTS/ TOXIC REACTIONS

None known.

NURSING CONSIDERATIONS

BASELINE ASSESSMENT

Check blood glucose level. Discuss lifestyle to determine extent of learning, emotional needs.

INTERVENTION/EVALUATION

Monitor blood glucose, glycosylated hemoglobin, transaminase values, food intake. Assess for hypoglycemia (cool/wet skin, tremors, dizziness, anxiety, headache, tachycardia, numbness in mouth, hunger, diplopia) or hyperglycemia (polyuria, polyphagia, polydipsia, nausea, vomiting, dim vision, fatigue, deep/rapid breathing). Be alert to conditions that alter glucose requirements: fever, increased activity/stress, surgical procedure.

PATIENT/FAMILY TEACHING

• Do not skip or delay meals. • Check with physician when glucose demands are altered (e.g., fever, infection, trauma, stress, heavy physical activity). • Limit alcoholic beverages. • Weight control, exercise, hygiene (including foot care), nonsmoking are essential parts of therapy.

Accupril, *see quinapril*

Accutane, *see isotretinoin*

acetaminophen

ah-see-tah-**min**-oh-fen

(Abenol ✤, Acephen, Apo-Acetaminophen ✤, Atasol ✤, Feverall, Genapap, Genapap Infant, Mapap, Ofirmev, Tempra ✤, Tylenol, Tylenol Arthritis Pain, Tylenol Children's

Meltaways, Tylenol Junior Meltaways, Tylenol Extra Strength)
Do not confuse Acephen with Aciphex, Feverall with Fiberall, Fioricet with Fiorinal, Percocet with Percodan, Tylenol with timolol, Tylenol PM, or Tylox, or Vicodin with Hycodan.

FIXED-COMBINATION(S)

Balacet 325: acetaminophen/propoxyphene napsylate: 325 mg/100 mg. **Capital with Codeine, Tylenol with Codeine:** acetaminophen/codeine: 120 mg/12 mg per 5 ml. **Darvocet-N:** acetaminophen/propoxyphene: 325 mg/50 mg, 650 mg/100 mg. **Endocet:** acetaminophen/oxycodone: 325 mg/5 mg, 325 mg/7.5 mg, 325 mg/10 mg, 500 mg/7.5 mg, 650 mg/10 mg. **Fioricet:** acetaminophen/caffeine/butalbital: 325 mg/40 mg/50 mg. **Hycet:** acetaminophen/hydrocodone: 325 mg/7.5 mg per 15 ml. **Lortab:** acetaminophen/hydrocodone: 500 mg/5 mg, 500 mg/7.5 mg. **Lortab Elixir:** acetaminophen/hydrocodone: 167 mg/2.5 mg per 5 ml. **Magnacet:** acetaminophen/oxycodone: 400 mg/2.5 mg, 400 mg/5 mg, 400 mg/7.5 mg, 400 mg/10 mg. **Norco:** acetaminophen/hydrocodone: 325 mg/5 mg, 325 mg/7.5 mg, 325 mg/10 mg. **Percocet, Roxicet:** acetaminophen/oxycodone: 325 mg/5 mg. **Tylenol with Codeine:** acetaminophen/codeine: 300 mg/15 mg, 300 mg/30 mg, 300 mg/60 mg. **Tylox:** acetaminophen/oxycodone: 500 mg/5 mg. **Ultracet:** acetaminophen/tramadol: 325 mg/37.5 mg. **Vicodin:** acetaminophen/hydrocodone: 500 mg/5 mg. **Vicodin ES:** acetaminophen/hydrocodone: 750 mg/7.5 mg. **Vicodin HP:** acetaminophen/hydrocodone: 660 mg/10 mg. **Xodol:** acetaminophen/hydrocodone: 300 mg/5 mg, 300 mg/7.5 mg, 300 mg/10 mg. **Zydone:** acetaminophen/hydrocodone: 400 mg/5 mg, 400 mg/7.5 mg, 400 mg/10 mg.

◆CLASSIFICATION

PHARMACOTHERAPEUTIC: Central analgesic. **CLINICAL:** Non-narcotic analgesic, antipyretic.

ACTION

Appears to inhibit prostaglandin synthesis in the CNS and, to a lesser extent, block pain impulses through peripheral action. Acts centrally on hypothalamic heat-regulating center, producing peripheral vasodilation (heat loss, skin erythema, diaphoresis). **Therapeutic Effect:** Results in antipyresis. Produces analgesic effect.

PHARMACOKINETICS

Route	Onset	Peak	Duration
PO	Less than 60 min	1–3 hrs	4–6 hrs

Rapidly, completely absorbed from GI tract; rectal absorption variable. Protein binding: 20%–50%. Widely distributed to most body tissues. Metabolized in liver; excreted in urine. Removed by hemodialysis. **Half-life:** 1–4 hrs (increased in those with hepatic disease, elderly, neonates; decreased in children).

USES

Relief of mild to moderate pain, fever.

PRECAUTIONS

Contraindications: Active alcoholism, hepatic disease, viral hepatitis, all of which increase the risk of hepatotoxicity. **Cautions:** Sensitivity to acetaminophen, severe renal impairment, phenylketonuria, G6PD deficiency. Limit dose to less than 4g/day.

⌛ LIFESPAN CONSIDERATIONS

Pregnancy/Lactation: Crosses placenta; distributed in breast milk. Routinely used in all stages of pregnancy, appears safe for short-term use. **Pregnancy Category B. Children/Elderly:** No age-related precautions noted.

INTERACTIONS

DRUG: **Alcohol** (chronic use), **hepatotoxic medications (e.g., phenytoin), liver enzymes inducers (e.g., cimetidine)** may increase risk of hepatotoxicity with prolonged high dose or single toxic dose. May increase risk of bleeding with **warfarin** with chronic, high-dose use. HERBAL: **St. John's wort** may decrease blood levels. FOOD: None known. LAB VALUES: May increase serum AST, ALT, bilirubin, prothrombin levels (may indicate hepatotoxicity). **Therapeutic serum level:** 10–30 mcg/ml; **toxic serum level:** greater than 200 mcg/ml.

AVAILABILITY (OTC)

Caplets (Genapap, Tylenol): 500 mg. Elixir: 160 mg/5 ml. Injection, Solution: 1,000 mg/100 ml glass vial. Liquid (Oral [Tylenol Extra Strength]): 160 mg/5 ml, 500 mg/5 ml, 500 mg/15 ml. Solution (Oral Drops [Genapap Infant]): 80 mg/0.8 ml. Suppository (Acephen, Feverall): 120 mg, 325 mg, 650 mg. Suspension (Mapap): 160 mg/5 ml. Tablets (Genapap, Mapap, Tylenol): 325 mg, 500 mg. Tablets (Chewable [Mapap]): 80 mg. Tablets (Orally-Disintegrating): 80 mg, 160 mg.

Caplets: (Extended-Release [Tylenol Arthritis Pain]): 650 mg.

ADMINISTRATION/HANDLING

IV

Reconstitution • Does not require further dilution. • Store at room temperature. • Withdraw doses less than 1,000 mg. • Place in separate empty, sterile container.

Rate of administration • Infuse over 15 min.

Stability • Once opened or transferred, stable for 6 hrs at room temperature.

PO

• Give without regard to meals. • Tablets may be crushed. • Do not crush extended-release caplets. • Suspension: Shake well before use. • Take with full glass of water.

Rectal

• Moisten suppository with cold water before inserting well up into rectum.
• Do not freeze suppositories.

INDICATIONS/ROUTES/DOSAGE

Analgesia and Antipyresis

IV: ADULTS, ADOLESCENTS WEIGHING 50 KG OR MORE: 1,000 mg q6h or 650 mg q4h. ADULTS, ADOLESCENTS WEIGHING LESS THAN 50 KG: 15 mg/kg q6h or 12.5 mg/kg q4h. CHILDREN 2–12 YRS: 15 mg/kg q6h or 12.5 mg/kg q4h. **Maximum:** 75 mg/kg/day.
PO: ADULTS, ELDERLY, CHILDREN 13 YRS AND OLDER: 325–650 mg q4–6h or 1 g 3–4 times a day. **Maximum:** 4 g/day. CHILDREN 12 YRS AND YOUNGER: 10–15 mg/kg/dose q4–6h as needed. **Maximum:** 5 doses/24 hrs. NEONATES: 10–15 mg/kg/dose q6–8h as needed.
RECTAL: ADULTS: 325–650 mg q4–6h. **Maximum:** 4 g/24 hrs. CHILDREN: 10–15 mg/kg/dose q4–6h as needed. **Maximum:** 5 doses/24 hrs. NEONATES: 10–15 mg/kg/dose q6–8h as needed. **Maximum:** 90 mg/kg/day.

Dosage in Renal Impairment

Creatinine Clearance	Frequency
10–50 ml/min	q6h
Less than 10 ml/min	q8h

SIDE EFFECTS

Rare: Hypersensitivity reaction.

ADVERSE EFFECTS/ TOXIC REACTIONS

Early Signs of Acetaminophen Toxicity: Anorexia, nausea, diaphoresis, fatigue within first 12–24 hrs. **Later Signs of Toxicity:** Vomiting, right upper quadrant tenderness, elevated hepatic function tests within 48–72 hrs after ingestion. **Antidote:** Acetylcysteine (see Appendix M for dosage).

NURSING CONSIDERATIONS

BASELINE ASSESSMENT

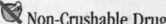

If given for analgesia, assess onset, type, location, duration of pain. Effect of medication is reduced if full pain response recurs prior to next dose. Assess for fever. Assess alcohol usage.

INTERVENTION/EVALUATION

Assess for clinical improvement and relief of pain, fever. **Therapeutic serum level:** 10–30 mcg/ml; **toxic serum level:** greater than 200 mcg/ml. Do not exceed maximum daily recommended dose: 4 g/day.

PATIENT/FAMILY TEACHING

• Consult physician for use in children younger than 2 yrs; oral use longer than 5 days (children) or longer than 10 days (adults), or fever longer than 3 days. • Severe/recurrent pain or high/continuous fever may indicate serious illness. • Advise not to take more than 4 g/24-hr period. Many nonprescription combination products contain acetaminophen. Avoid alcohol use.

*acetaZOLAMIDE

ah-seat-ah-**zole**-ah-myd
(Apo-Acetazolamide 🍁, Diamox, Diamox Sequels)
Do not confuse Diamox with Trimox.

◆CLASSIFICATION

PHARMACOTHERAPEUTIC: Carbonic anhydrase inhibitor. **CLINICAL:** Antiglaucoma, anticonvulsant, diuretic, urinary alkalinizer (see p. 52C).

ACTION

Reduces formation of hydrogen and bicarbonate ions by inhibiting the enzyme carbonic anhydrase. **Therapeutic Effect:** Increases excretion of sodium, potassium, bicarbonate, water in kidney; decreases formation of aqueous humor in eye; retards abnormal discharge from CNS neurons.

PHARMACOKINETICS

Well absorbed from GI tract. Protein binding: 90%. Excreted unchanged in urine. **Half-life:** (Tablets) 10–15 hrs.

USES

Treatment of glaucoma, control of IOP before surgery, adjunct in management of seizures, edema, decreases incidence/severity of symptoms associated with acute altitude sickness. **OFF-LABEL:** Lowers IOP in treatment of malignant glaucoma, treatment of toxicity of weakly acidic medications, prevents uric acid/renal calculi by alkalinizing the urine, respiratory stimulant in COPD, metabolic acidosis.

PRECAUTIONS

Contraindications: Hypersensitivity to sulfonamides, severe renal disease, adrenal insufficiency, hypochloremic acidosis. **Cautions:** History of hypercalcemia, diabetes mellitus, gout, concurrent digoxin therapy, obstructive pulmonary disease. **Pregnancy Category C.**

INTERACTIONS

DRUG: May increase **digoxin** levels (due to hypokalemia). May increase effects/toxicity of **amphetamines;** may decrease effects of **methenamine. HERBAL:** None significant. **FOOD:** None known. **LAB VALUES:** May increase serum ammonia, bilirubin, glucose, chloride, uric acid, calcium; may decrease serum bicarbonate, potassium.

AVAILABILITY (Rx)

Injection, Powder for Reconstitution: 500 mg. **Tablets (Diamox):** 125 mg, 250 mg.

Capsules (Extended-Release [Diamox Sequels]): 500 mg.

ADMINISTRATION/HANDLING

IV

Reconstitution • Reconstitute with at least 5 ml Sterile Water for Injection to provide concentration not more than 100 mg/ml.

Rate of administration • Maximum rate: 500 mg/min.

Storage • Following reconstitution, stable for 12 hrs at room temperature, 1 wk if refrigerated.

PO

• Give with food. • May crush tablets. • Do not crush, chew extended-release capsule. • May open, sprinkle on food.

IV INCOMPATIBILITY

Diltiazem (Cardizem).

IV COMPATIBILITIES

Cimetidine (Tagamet), pantoprazole (Protonix), ranitidine (Zantac).

INDICATIONS/ROUTES/DOSAGE

Glaucoma

IV: ADULTS, ELDERLY: 250–500 mg; may repeat in 2–4 hrs, then continue with oral therapy. **CHILDREN:** 5–10 mg/kg q6h. **Maximum:** 1 g a day.

PO: ADULTS, ELDERLY: 250 mg 1–4 times a day. **CHILDREN:** 8–30 mg/kg/day in divided doses q8h.

PO (EXTENDED-RELEASE): ADULTS, ELDERLY: 500 mg twice a day.

Edema

PO, IV: ADULTS: 250–375 mg once daily. **CHILDREN:** 5 mg/kg/dose once a day.

Epilepsy

PO: ADULTS, ELDERLY, CHILDREN: 8–30 mg/kg/day in up to 4 divided doses. **Maximum:** 1 g/day. Extended-release formulation not recommended for epilepsy.

Altitude Sickness

PO: ADULTS: 250 mg q8–12h or 500 mg extended-release capsule q12–24h. Begin 24–48 hrs before and continue during ascent and for at least 48 hrs following arrival at high altitude.

Dosage in Renal Impairment

Creatinine Clearance	Dosage Interval
10–50 ml/min	q12h
Less than 10 ml/min	Not recommended

SIDE EFFECTS

Frequent: Fatigue, diarrhea, increased urination/frequency, decreased appetite/weight, altered taste (metallic), nausea, vomiting, paresthesia, circumoral numbness. **Occasional:** Depression, drowsiness. **Rare:** Headache, photosensitivity, confusion, tinnitus, severe muscle weakness, loss of taste.

ADVERSE EFFECTS/ TOXIC REACTIONS

Long-term therapy may result in acidotic state. Nephrotoxicity/hepatotoxicity occurs occasionally, manifested as dark urine/stools, pain in lower back, jaundice, dysuria, crystalluria, renal colic/calculi. Bone marrow depression may occur manifested as aplastic anemia, thrombocytopenia, thrombocytopenic purpura, leukopenia, agranulocytosis, hemolytic anemia.

NURSING CONSIDERATIONS

BASELINE ASSESSMENT

Glaucoma: Assess affected pupil for dilation, response to light. Question potential for eye discomfort, decrease in visual acuity. **Epilepsy:** Obtain history of seizure disorder (length, intensity, duration of seizure, presence of aura, level of consciousness [LOC]).

INTERVENTION/EVALUATION

Monitor for acidosis (headache, lethargy progressing to drowsiness, CNS depression, Kussmaul's respiration).

PATIENT/FAMILY TEACHING

• Report tingling/tremor in hands or feet, unusual bleeding or bruising, unexplained fever, sore throat, flank pain. • Avoid tasks that require alertness, motor skills until response to drug is established. • Use sunscreen, wear protective clothing.

acetylcysteine (*N*-acetylcysteine)

ah-seat-il-**sis**-teen

(Acetadote, Mucomyst, Parvolex ✤)

Do not confuse acetylcysteine with acetylcholine, or Mucomyst with Mucinex.

CLASSIFICATION

PHARMACOTHERAPEUTIC: Respiratory inhalant, intratracheal. **CLINICAL:** Mucolytic, antidote.

ACTION

Splits linkage of mucoproteins, reducing viscosity of pulmonary secretions. **Therapeutic Effect:** Facilitates removal of pulmonary secretions by coughing, postural drainage, mechanical means. Protects against acetaminophen overdose-induced hepatotoxicity.

USES

Inhalation: Adjunctive treatment for abnormally viscid mucous secretions present in acute and chronic bronchopulmonary disease and pulmonary complications of cystic fibrosis and surgery, diagnostic bronchial studies. **Injection, PO:** Antidote in acute acetaminophen toxicity. **OFF-LABEL:** Prevention of contrast-induced nephropathy from dyes given during certain diagnostic tests (such as CT scans). Treatment of *H. pylori* infection, distal obstruction syndrome.

PRECAUTIONS

Contraindications: None known. **Cautions:** Bronchial asthma, elderly, debilitated with severe respiratory insufficiency. **Pregnancy Category B.**

INTERACTIONS

DRUG: None significant. **HERBAL:** None significant. **FOOD:** None known. **LAB VALUES:** None significant.

AVAILABILITY (Rx)

Inhalation Solution (Mucomyst): 10% (100 mg/ml), 20% (200 mg/ml). **Injection Solution (Acetadote):** 20% (200 mg/ml).

ADMINISTRATION/HANDLING

IV

Acetadote is hyperosmolar (2,600 mOsm/l) and is compatible with 5% Dextrose (D_5W) or ½ Normal Saline (0.45% Sodium Chloride Injection). The total dose is 300 mg/kg administered over 21 hrs. Dose preparation is based upon pt weight. Total volume administered should be adjusted for pts less than 40 kg and for those requiring fluid restriction.

Three-Bag Method: Loading, Second, and Third Doses

Pts Greater Than or Equal to 40 kg:
Loading Dose: 150 mg/kg in 200 ml of diluent administered over 60 min.
Second Dose: 50 mg/kg in 500 ml of diluent administered over 4 hrs.
Third Dose: 100 mg/kg in 1,000 ml of diluent administered over 16 hrs.

Pts Greater Than 20 kg but Less Than 40 kg:
Loading Dose: 150 mg/kg in 100 ml of diluent administered over 60 min.
Second Dose: 50 mg/kg in 250 ml of diluent administered over 4 hrs.
Third Dose: 100 mg/kg in 500 ml of diluent administered over 16 hrs.

Pts Less Than or Equal to 20 kg:
Loading Dose: 150 mg/kg in 3 ml/kg of body weight of diluent administered over 60 min.
Second Dose: 50 mg/kg in 7 ml/kg of body weight of diluent administered over 4 hrs.
Third Dose: 100 mg/kg in 14 ml/kg of body weight of diluent administered over 16 hrs.

PO

- For treatment of acetaminophen overdose. • Give as 5% solution. • Dilute 20% solution 1:3 with cola, orange juice, other soft drink. • Give within 1 hr of preparation.

Inhalation, Nebulization

- May administer either undiluted or diluted with 0.9% NaCl.

IV COMPATIBILITIES

Cefepime (Maxipime), ceftazidime (Fortaz).

INDICATIONS/ROUTES/DOSAGE

Bronchopulmonary Disease

INHALATION, NEBULIZATION

◄ALERT► Bronchodilators should be given 10–15 min before acetylcysteine. **ADULTS, ELDERLY, CHILDREN:** 3–5 ml (20% solution) 3–4 times a day or 6–10 ml (10% solution) 3–4 times a day. Range: 1–10 ml (20% solution) q2–6h or 2–20 ml (10% solution) q2–6h. **INFANTS:** 1–2 ml (20%) or 2–4 ml (10%) 3–4 times a day.

INTRATRACHEAL: ADULTS, CHILDREN: 1–2 ml of 10% or 20% solution instilled into tracheostomy q1–4h.

Acetaminophen Overdose

PO (ORAL SOLUTION 5%): ADULTS, ELDERLY, CHILDREN: Loading dose of 140 mg/kg, followed in 4 hrs by maintenance dose of 70 mg/kg q4h for 17 additional doses (or until acetaminophen assay reveals nontoxic level). Repeat dose if emesis occurs within 1 hr of administration.

IV: ADULTS, ELDERLY, CHILDREN: 150 mg/kg infused over 60 min, then 50 mg/kg infused over 4 hrs, then 100 mg/kg infused over 16 hrs (see Administration/Handling). Duration of administration may vary depending upon acetaminophen levels and hepatic function tests obtained during treatment. Pts who still have detectable levels of acetaminophen or elevated hepatic function test results continue to benefit from additional acetylcysteine administration beyond 24 hrs.

Prevention of Contrast-Induced Nephropathy

PO: ADULTS, ELDERLY: 600–1,200 mg twice a day for 4 doses starting the day before the procedure. Hydrate pt with 0.9% NaCl concurrently.

Diagnostic Bronchial Studies

INHALATION, NEBULIZATION: ADULTS: 1–2 ml of 20% solution or 2–4 ml of 10% solution 2–3 times before the procedure.

SIDE EFFECTS

IV: (7%–6%): Acute flushing, erythema. **(4%):** Pruritus. **Frequent: Inhalation:** Stickiness on face, transient unpleasant odor. **Occasional: Inhalation:** Increased bronchial secretions, throat irritation, nausea, vomiting, rhinorrhea. **Rare: Inhalation:** Rash. **PO:** Facial edema, bronchospasm, wheezing.

ADVERSE EFFECTS/ TOXIC REACTIONS

Large doses may produce severe nausea/vomiting. **(Less than 2%):** Serious anaphylactoid reactions including cough, wheezing, stridor, respiratory distress, bronchospasm, hypotension, and death have been known to occur with IV administration.

NURSING CONSIDERATIONS

BASELINE ASSESSMENT

Mucolytic: Assess pretreatment respirations for rate, depth, rhythm. **IV Antidote:** Obtain baseline labs, including serum AST, ALT, bilirubin, PT/INR, BUN, creatinine, glucose, and drug screen. Obtain acetaminophen level to determine need for treatment with acetylcysteine.

INTERVENTION/EVALUATION

If bronchospasm occurs, discontinue treatment, notify physician; bronchodilator may be added to therapy. Monitor rate, depth, rhythm, type of respiration (abdominal, thoracic). Check sputum for color, consistency, amount. **IV Antidote:** Administer within 8 hrs of acetaminophen ingestion for maximal hepatic protection; ideally, within 4 hrs after immediate-release and 2 hrs after liquid formulations.

PATIENT/FAMILY TEACHING

• Slight, disagreeable odor from solution may be noticed during initial administration but disappears quickly. • Adequate hydration is important part of therapy. • Follow guidelines to proper coughing and deep breathing techniques.

AcipHex, *see rabeprazole*

Actiq, *see fentanyl*

Activase, *see alteplase*

Actonel, *see risedronate*

Actos, *see pioglitazone*

acyclovir

aye-**sigh**-klo-veer
(Apo-Acyclovir, Zovirax)
Do not confuse acyclovir with ganciclovir, Retrovir, or valacyclovir, or Zovirax with Valtrex, Zithromax, Zyloprim, Zostrix, or Zyvox.

FIXED-COMBINATION(S)

Lipsovir: acyclovir/hydrocortisone (a steroid): 5%/1%.

◆CLASSIFICATION

PHARMACOTHERAPEUTIC: Synthetic nucleoside. **CLINICAL:** Antiviral (see p. 67C).

ACTION

Converts to acyclovir triphosphate, becoming part of DNA chain. **Therapeutic Effect:** Interferes with DNA synthesis and viral replication. Virustatic.

PHARMACOKINETICS

Poorly absorbed from GI tract; minimal absorption following topical application. Protein binding: 9%–36%. Widely distributed. Partially metabolized in liver. Excreted primarily in urine. Removed by hemodialysis. **Half-life:** 2.5 hrs (increased in renal impairment).

USES

Treatment of genital herpes simplex virus (HSV), herpes labialis (cold sores), herpes zoster (shingles), HSV encephalitis, neonatal HSV, mucocutaneous HSV in immunocompromised pts, varicella-zoster (chickenpox). **OFF-LABEL: PO, parenteral:** Prophylaxis of herpes simplex and herpes zoster infections, infectious mononucleosis. Prevents HSV reactivation in HIV positive pts, hematopoietic stem cell transplant recipients and during periods of neutropenia in pts with acute leukemia. **Topical:** Treatment adjunct for herpes zoster infections.

PRECAUTIONS

Contraindications: Use in neonates when acyclovir is reconstituted with Bacteriostatic Water for Injection containing benzyl alcohol. **Cautions:** Renal/hepatic impairment, dehydration, fluid/electrolyte imbalance, concurrent use of nephrotoxic agents, neurologic abnormalities, immunocompromised pts.

⌛ LIFESPAN CONSIDERATIONS

Pregnancy/Lactation: Crosses placenta; distributed in breast milk. **Pregnancy Category B. Children:** Safety and efficacy not established in those younger than 2 yrs (younger than 1 yr for IV use). **Elderly:** Age-related renal impairment may require decreased dosage. May experience more neurologic effects (e.g., agitation, confusion, hallucinations).

INTERACTIONS

DRUG: Nephrotoxic medications (e.g., aminoglycosides) may increase nephrotoxicity. **HERBAL:** None significant. **FOOD:** None known. **LAB VALUES:** May increase BUN, serum creatinine concentrations, hepatic function tests.

AVAILABILITY (Rx)

Cream: 5%. **Injection, Powder for Reconstitution:** 500 mg, 1,000 mg. **Injection, Solution:** 50 mg/ml. **Ointment:** 5%. **Suspension, Oral:** 200 mg/5 ml. **Tablets:** 400 mg, 800 mg.

Capsules: 200 mg.

ADMINISTRATION/HANDLING

IV

Reconstitution • Add 10 ml Sterile Water for Injection to each 500-mg vial (50 mg/ml). Do not use Bacteriostatic Water for Injection containing benzyl alcohol or parabens (will cause precipitate). • Shake well until solution is clear. • Further dilute with at least 100 ml D_5W or 0.9 NaCl. Final concentration should be 7 mg/ml or less. (Concentrations greater than 10 mg/ml increase risk of phlebitis.)
Rate of administration • Infuse over at least 1 hr (renal tubular damage may occur with too rapid rate). • Maintain adequate hydration during infusion and for 2 hrs following IV administration.
Storage • Store vials at room temperature • Solutions of 50 mg/ml stable for 12 hrs at room temperature; may form precipitate if refrigerated. Potency not affected by precipitate and redissolution. • IV infusion (piggyback) stable for 24 hrs at room temperature. Yellow discoloration does not affect potency.

PO

• May give without regard to food. • Do not crush/break capsules. • Store capsules at room temperature.

Topical

• Avoid eye contact. • Use finger cot/rubber glove to prevent autoinoculation.

IV INCOMPATIBILITIES

Aztreonam (Azactam), cefepime (Maxipime), diltiazem (Cardizem), dobutamine (Dobutrex), dopamine (Intropin), levofloxacin (Levaquin), lipids, meropenem (Merrem IV), ondansetron (Zofran), piperacillin and tazobactam (Zosyn), total parenteral nutrition (TPN).

IV COMPATIBILITIES

Allopurinol (Alloprim), amikacin (Amikin), ampicillin, cefazolin (Ancef), cefotaxime (Claforan), ceftazidime (Fortaz), ceftriaxone (Rocephin), cimetidine (Tagamet), clindamycin (Cleocin), diphenhydramine (Benadryl), famotidine (Pepcid), fluconazole (Diflucan), gentamicin, heparin, hydromorphone (Dilaudid), imipenem (Primaxin), lorazepam (Ativan), magnesium sulfate, meperidine (Demerol), methylprednisolone (SoluMedrol), metoclopramide (Reglan), metronidazole (Flagyl), morphine, multivitamins, potassium chloride, propofol (Diprivan), ranitidine (Zantac), vancomycin.

INDICATIONS/ROUTES/DOSAGE

Genital Herpes (Initial Episode)

IV: ADULTS, ELDERLY, CHILDREN 12 YRS AND OLDER: 5 mg/kg q8h for 5–7 days.
PO: ADULTS, ELDERLY, CHILDREN 12 YRS AND OLDER: 200 mg q4h 5 times a day for 10 days or 400 mg 3 times a day for 5–10 days. **CHILDREN YOUNGER THAN 12 YRS:** 40–80 mg/kg/day in 3–4 divided doses for 5–10 days. **Maximum:** 1 g/day.
TOPICAL: ADULTS: (Ointment) ½ inch for 4-inch square surface q3h (6 times a day) for 7 days.

Genital Herpes (Recurrent)

Intermittent Therapy

PO: ADULTS, ELDERLY, CHILDREN 12 YRS AND OLDER: 200 mg q4h 5 times a day for 5 days or 400 mg 3 times a day for 5–10 days.

Chronic Suppressive Therapy

PO: ADULTS, ELDERLY, CHILDREN 12 YRS AND OLDER: 400 mg twice a day or 200 mg 3–5 times a day for up to 12 mos. **CHILDREN YOUNGER THAN 12 YRS:** 80 mg/kg/day in 3 divided doses. **Maximum:** 1 g/day.

Herpes Simplex Mucocutaneous

PO: ADULTS, ELDERLY: 400 mg 5 times a day for 7–14 days.
IV: ADULTS, ELDERLY, CHILDREN 12 YRS AND OLDER: 5 mg/kg/dose q8h for 7–14 days. **CHILDREN YOUNGER THAN 12 YRS:** 10 mg/kg q8h for 7 days.
TOPICAL: ADULTS (Ointment) ½ inch for 4-inch square surface q3h (6 times a day) for 7 days.

A

Herpes Simplex Neonatal
IV: CHILDREN YOUNGER THAN 4 MOS: 10 mg/kg q8h for 10 days.

Herpes Simplex Encephalitis
IV: ADULTS, ELDERLY, CHILDREN 12 YRS AND OLDER: 10 mg/kg q8h for 10 days. **CHILDREN 3 MOS–YOUNGER THAN 12 YRS:** 20 mg/kg q8h for 10 days.

Herpes Zoster (Shingles)
IV: ADULTS, CHILDREN 12 YRS AND OLDER: (immunocompromised) 10 mg/kg/dose q8h for 7 days. **CHILDREN YOUNGER THAN 12 YRS:** (immunocompromised) 20 mg/kg/dose q8h for 7 days.
PO: ADULTS, ELDERLY, CHILDREN 12 YRS AND OLDER: 800 mg q4h 5 times a day for 7–10 days.

Herpes Labialis (Cold Sores)
TOPICAL: ADULTS, ELDERLY, CHILDREN 12 YRS AND OLDER: Apply to affected area 5 times a day for 4 days.

Varicella-Zoster (Chickenpox)
◀ALERT▶ Begin treatment within 24 hrs of onset of rash.
PO: ADULTS, ELDERLY, CHILDREN OLDER THAN 12 YRS AND CHILDREN 2–12 YRS, WEIGHING 40 KG OR MORE: 800 mg 4 times a day for 5 days. **CHILDREN 2–12 YRS, WEIGHING LESS THAN 40 KG:** 20 mg/kg 4 times a day for 5 days. **Maximum:** 800 mg/dose.

Dosage in Renal Impairment
Dosage and frequency are modified based on severity of infection and degree of renal impairment.
PO: Normal dose 200 mg q4h, 200 mg q8h, or 400 mg q12h.
Creatinine clearance 10 ml/min and less: 200 mg q12h.
PO: Normal dose 800 mg q4h.
Creatinine clearance greater than 25 ml/min: Give usual dose and at normal interval, 800 mg q4h. **Creatinine clearance 10–25 ml/min:** 800 mg q8h. **Creatinine clearance less than 10 ml/min:** 800 mg q12h.

IV:

Creatinine Clearance	Dosage
Greater than 50 ml/min	100% of normal q8h
25–50 ml/min	100% of normal q12h
10–24 ml/min	100% of normal q24h
Less than 10 ml/min	50% of normal q24h

SIDE EFFECTS

Frequent: Parenteral (9%–7%): Phlebitis or inflammation at IV site, nausea, vomiting. **Topical (28%):** Burning, stinging. **Occasional: Parenteral (3%):** Pruritus, rash, urticaria. **PO (12%–6%):** Malaise, nausea. **Topical (4%):** Pruritus. **Rare: PO (3%–1%):** Vomiting, rash, diarrhea, headache. **Parenteral (2%–1%):** Confusion, hallucinations, seizures, tremors. **Topical (less than 1%):** Rash.

ADVERSE EFFECTS/ TOXIC REACTIONS

Rapid parenteral administration, excessively high doses, or fluid and electrolyte imbalance may produce renal failure (abdominal pain, decreased urination, decreased appetite, increased thirst, nausea, vomiting). Toxicity not reported with oral or topical use.

NURSING CONSIDERATIONS

BASELINE ASSESSMENT

Question for history of allergies, esp. to acyclovir. Assess herpes simplex lesions before treatment to compare baseline with treatment effect.

INTERVENTION/EVALUATION

Assess IV site for phlebitis (heat, pain, red streaking over vein). Evaluate cutaneous lesions. Ensure adequate ventilation. Manage chickenpox and disseminated herpes zoster with strict isolation. Provide analgesics and comfort measures; esp. exhausting to elderly. Encourage fluids.

PATIENT/FAMILY TEACHING

• Drink adequate fluids. • Do not touch lesions with fingers to prevent spreading infection to new site. • **Genital Herpes:** Continue therapy for full length of treatment. • Space doses evenly. • Use finger cot/rubber glove to apply topical ointment. • Avoid sexual intercourse during duration of lesions to prevent infecting partner. • Acyclovir does not cure herpes infections. • Pap smear should be done at least annually due to increased risk of cervical cancer in women with genital herpes.

Adalat, *see nifedipine*

adalimumab

ah-dah-**lim**-you-mab
(Humira)

BLACK BOX ALERT Tuberculosis, invasive fungal infections, other opportunistic infections have occurred. Test for tuberculosis prior to and during treatment.

Do not confuse Humira with Humalog or Humulin.

CLASSIFICATION

PHARMACOTHERAPEUTIC: Monoclonal antibody. **CLINICAL:** Rheumatoid arthritis agent.

ACTION

Binds specifically to tumor necrosis factor (TNF) alpha cell, blocking its interaction with cell surface TNF receptors. **Therapeutic Effect:** Reduces inflammation, tenderness, swelling of joints; slows or prevents progressive destruction of joints in rheumatoid arthritis (RA).

PHARMACOKINETICS

Half-life: 10–20 days.

USES

Reduces signs/symptoms, progression of structural damage and improves physical function in adults with moderate to severe RA unresponsive to other disease-modifying antirheumatic drugs. First-line treatment of moderate to severe RA, treatment of psoriatic arthritis, treatment of ankylosing spondylitis, to induce/maintain remission of moderate to severe active Crohn's disease, moderate to severe plaque psoriasis, reduce signs and symptoms of moderate to severe active polyarticular juvenile rheumatoid arthritis in pts 4 yrs and older.

PRECAUTIONS

Contraindications: Active infections. **Cautions:** History of sensitivity to monoclonal antibodies, cardiovascular disease, pregnancy, preexisting or recent-onset CNS demyelinating disorders, elderly.

LIFESPAN CONSIDERATIONS

Pregnancy/Lactation: Unknown if distributed in breast milk. **Pregnancy Category B. Children:** Safety and efficacy not established. **Elderly:** Cautious use due to increased risk of serious infection and malignancy.

INTERACTIONS

DRUG: **Abatacept, anakinra, immunosuppressive therapy** may increase risk of infections. May decrease efficacy of immune response with **live vaccines. Methotrexate** reduces absorption of adalimumab by 29%–40%, but dosage adjustment is unnecessary if given concurrently. **HERBAL: Echinacea** may decrease effects. **FOOD:** None known. **LAB VALUES:** May increase levels of serum cholesterol, other lipids, alkaline phosphatase.

AVAILABILITY (Rx)

Injection Solution: 20 mg/0.4 ml, 40 mg/0.8 ml in prefilled syringes.

ADMINISTRATION/HANDLING

Subcutaneous

• Refrigerate; do not freeze. • Discard unused portion. • Rotate injection sites. Give new injection at least 1 inch from an old site and never into area where skin is tender, bruised, red, or hard.

INDICATIONS/ROUTES/DOSAGE

Rheumatoid Arthritis (RA)

SUBCUTANEOUS: ADULTS, ELDERLY: 40 mg every other wk. Dose may be increased to 40 mg/wk in those not taking methotrexate.

Ankylosing Spondylitis, Psoriatic Arthritis

SUBCUTANEOUS: ADULTS, ELDERLY: 40 mg every other wk.

Crohn's Disease

SUBCUTANEOUS: ADULTS, ELDERLY: Initially, 160 mg given as 4 injections on day 1 or over 2 days, then 80 mg 2 wks later (day 15). Maintenance: 40 mg every other wk beginning at wk 4.

Plaque Psoriasis

SUBCUTANEOUS: ADULTS, ELDERLY: Initially, 80 mg, then 40 mg every other week starting one week after initial dose.

Juvenile Rheumatoid Arthritis

SUBCUTANEOUS: CHILDREN 4 YRS AND OLDER, WEIGHING 15–29 KG: 20 mg every other week. **WEIGHING 30 KG OR MORE:** 40 mg every other week.

SIDE EFFECTS

Frequent (20%): Injection site erythema, pruritus, pain, swelling. **Occasional (12%–9%):** Headache, rash, sinusitis, nausea. **Rare (7%–5%):** Abdominal or back pain, hypertension.

ADVERSE EFFECTS/ TOXIC REACTIONS

Hypersensitivity reactions (rash, urticaria, hypotension, dyspnea), infections (primarily upper respiratory tract, bronchitis, urinary tract) occur rarely. More serious infections (pneumonia, tuberculosis, cellulitis, pyelonephritis, septic arthritis) also occur rarely.

NURSING CONSIDERATIONS

BASELINE ASSESSMENT

Assess onset, type, location, duration of pain or inflammation. Inspect appearance of affected joints for immobility, deformities, skin condition. If pt is to self-administer, instruct on subcutaneous injection technique, including areas of the body acceptable for injection sites.

INTERVENTION/EVALUATION

Monitor lab values, particularly CBC. Assess for therapeutic response: relief of pain, stiffness, swelling; increased joint mobility; reduced joint tenderness; improved grip strength.

PATIENT/FAMILY TEACHING

• Injection site reaction generally occurs in first month of treatment and decreases in frequency during continued therapy. • Do not receive live vaccines during treatment. Report rash, nausea.

adefovir

add-eh-**foe**-vir
(Hepsera)

BLACK BOX ALERT May cause HIV resistance in unrecognized or untreated HIV infection. Lactic acidosis, severe hepatomegaly with steatosis (fatty liver), acute exacerbation of hepatitis have occurred. Use with caution in pts with renal dysfunction or in pts at risk for renal toxicity.

◆CLASSIFICATION

PHARMACOTHERAPEUTIC: Antiviral.
CLINICAL: Hepatitis B agent.

ACTION

Inhibits DNA polymerase, an enzyme, causing DNA chain termination after its incorporation into viral DNA. **Therapeutic Effect:** Prevents cell replication.

PHARMACOKINETICS

Rapidly converted to adefovir in intestine. Binds to proteins after PO administration. Protein binding: less than 4%. Excreted in urine. **Half-life:** 7 hrs (increased in renal impairment).

USES

Treatment of chronic hepatitis B in adults with evidence of active viral replication based on persistent elevations of serum AST or ALT or histologic evidence.

PRECAUTIONS

Contraindications: None known. **Cautions:** Pts with known risk factors for hepatic disease, renal impairment, elderly.

LIFESPAN CONSIDERATIONS

Pregnancy/Lactation: Unknown if drug crosses placenta or is distributed in breast milk. **Pregnancy Category C. Children:** Safety and efficacy not established. **Elderly:** Age-related renal impairment, decreased cardiac function requires cautious use.

INTERACTIONS

DRUG: Nephrotoxic agents (aminoglycosides, cyclosporin, NSAIDs, tacrolimus, vancomycin) may increase risk of nephrotoxicity. **HERBAL:** None significant. **FOOD:** None known. **LAB VALUES:** May increase serum ALT, AST, amylase.

AVAILABILITY (Rx)

Tablets: 10 mg.

ADMINISTRATION/HANDLING

PO

- Give without regard to food.

INDICATIONS/ROUTES/DOSAGE

Chronic Hepatitis B (Normal Renal Function)

PO: ADULTS, ELDERLY: 10 mg once a day.

Chronic Hepatitis B (Impaired Renal Function)

PO: ADULTS, ELDERLY WITH CREATININE CLEARANCE 30–49 ML/MIN: 10 mg q48h. **ADULTS, ELDERLY WITH CREATININE CLEARANCE 10–29 ML/MIN:** 10 mg q72h. **ADULTS, ELDERLY ON HEMODIALYSIS:** 10 mg every 7 days following dialysis.

SIDE EFFECTS

Frequent (13%): Asthenia. **Occasional (9%–4%):** Headache, abdominal pain, nausea, flatulence. **Rare (3%):** Diarrhea, dyspepsia.

ADVERSE EFFECTS/ TOXIC REACTIONS

Nephrotoxicity, characterized by increased serum creatinine and decreased serum phosphorus levels, is treatment-limiting toxicity of adefovir therapy. Lactic acidosis, severe hepatomegaly occur rarely, particularly in female pts.

NURSING CONSIDERATIONS

BASELINE ASSESSMENT

Obtain baseline renal function lab values before therapy begins and routinely thereafter. Those with renal insufficiency, preexisting or during treatment, may require dose adjustment. HIV antibody testing should be performed before therapy begins (unrecognized or untreated HIV infection may result in emergence of HIV resistance).

INTERVENTION/EVALUATION

Monitor I&O, serum creatinine; AST, ALT, alkaline phosphatase levels. Closely monitor for adverse reactions in those taking other medications that are excreted renally or with other drugs known to affect renal function.

PATIENT/FAMILY TEACHING

- Report nausea, vomiting, abdominal pain.

adenosine

ah-**den**-oh-seen
(Adenocard, Adenoscan)

CLASSIFICATION

PHARMACOTHERAPEUTIC: Cardiac agent, diagnostic aid. **CLINICAL:** Antiarrhythmic.

ACTION

Slows impulse formation in SA node and conduction time through AV node. Acts as a diagnostic aid in myocardial perfusion imaging or stress echocardiography. **Therapeutic Effect:** Depresses left ventricular function, restores normal sinus rhythm.

USES

Adenocard: Treatment of paroxysmal supraventricular tachycardia (PSVT), including those associated with accessory bypass tracts (Wolff-Parkinson-White syndrome). **Adenoscan:** Adjunct in diagnosis in myocardial perfusion imaging or stress echocardiography.

PRECAUTIONS

Contraindications: Atrial fibrillation or flutter, second- or third-degree AV block or sick sinus syndrome (with functioning pacemaker), ventricular tachycardia. **Cautions:** Heart block, arrhythmias at time of conversion, asthma, hepatic/renal failure. **Pregnancy Category C.**

INTERACTIONS

DRUG: **Methylxanthines (e.g., theophylline)** may decrease effect. **Dipyridamole** may increase effect. **Carbamazepine** may increase degree of heart block caused by adenosine. **HERBAL:** None significant. **FOOD:** Avoid **caffeine** (may decrease effect). **LAB VALUES:** None significant.

AVAILABILITY (Rx)

Injection Solution (Adenocard): 3 mg/ml in 2-ml, 4-ml vials. **Injection Solution (Adenoscan):** 3 mg/ml in 20-ml, 30-ml vials.

ADMINISTRATION/HANDLING

IV

Rate of administration • Administer very rapidly (over 1–2 sec) undiluted directly into vein, or if using IV line, use closest port to insertion site. If IV line is infusing any fluid other than 0.9% NaCl, flush line first. • After rapid bolus injection, follow with 0.9% NaCl flush.

Storage • Store at room temperature. Solution appears clear. • Crystallization occurs if refrigerated; if crystallization occurs, dissolve crystals by warming to room temperature. • Discard unused portion.

IV INCOMPATIBILITIES

Any drug or solution other than 0.9% NaCl, D_5W, or Ringer's lactate.

INDICATIONS/ROUTES/DOSAGE

Paroxysmal Supraventricular Tachycardia (PSVT)

RAPID IV BOLUS: ADULTS, ELDERLY, CHILDREN WEIGHING 50 KG OR MORE: Initially, 6 mg given over 1–2 sec. If first dose does not convert within 1–2 min, give 12 mg; may repeat 12-mg dose in 1–2 min if no response has occurred. **CHILDREN WEIGHING LESS THAN 50 KG:** Initially 0.05–0.1 mg/kg. If first dose does not convert within 1–2 min, may increase dose by 0.05–0.1 mg/kg. May repeat until sinus rhythm is established or up to a maximum single dose of 0.3 mg/kg or 12 mg.

Diagnostic Testing

IV INFUSION: ADULTS: 140 mcg/kg/min for 6 min. **Total dose:** 0.84 mg/kg. Thallium is injected at midpoint (3 min) of infusion.

SIDE EFFECTS

Frequent (18%–12%): Facial flushing, dyspnea. **Occasional (7%–2%):** Headache, nausea, light-headedness, chest pressure. **Rare (1% or less):** Paresthesias, dizziness, diaphoresis, hypotension, palpitations; chest, jaw, or neck pain.

ADVERSE EFFECTS/ TOXIC REACTIONS

May produce short-lasting heart block.

NURSING CONSIDERATIONS

BASELINE ASSESSMENT

Identify arrhythmia per cardiac monitor and assess apical pulse.

INTERVENTION/EVALUATION

Assess cardiac performance per continuous EKG. Monitor B/P, apical pulse (rate, rhythm, quality). Auscultate pt breath sounds for clarity. Monitor respiratory rate. Monitor I&O; assess for fluid retention. Check electrolytes.

PATIENT/FAMILY TEACHING

- Flushing/headache may occur temporarily following drug administration.
- Report chest pain, light-headedness, head or neck pain, difficulty breathing.

Advair, *see fluticasone*

Advair Diskus, *see fluticasone and salmeterol*

Aggrenox, *see aspirin and dipyridamole*

albumin, human

al-**byew**-min

(Albumarc, Albuminar-5, Albuminar-25, AlbuRx, Albutein, Buminate, Flexbumin, Plasbumin)

Do not confuse albumin with albuterol.

◆ CLASSIFICATION

PHARMACOTHERAPEUTIC: Plasma protein fraction. **CLINICAL:** Blood derivative.

ACTION

Blood volume expander. **Therapeutic Effect:** Provides temporary increase in blood volume, reduces hemoconcentration and blood viscosity.

PHARMACOKINETICS

Route	Onset	Peak	Duration
IV	15 min (in well-hydrated pt)	N/A	Dependent on initial blood volume

Distributed throughout extracellular fluid. **Half-life:** 15–20 days.

USES

Used for plasma volume expansion, maintenance of cardiac output in treatment of shock or impending shock. May be useful in treatment of severe burns, neonatal hyperbilirubinemia, adult respiratory distress syndrome (ARDS), cardiopulmonary bypass, ascites, acute nephrosis or nephrotic syndrome, hemodialysis, pancreatitis, intra-abdominal infections, acute hepatic failure. **OFF-LABEL:** Plasmapheresis (5% concentration). In cirrhotics, with diuretics to help facilitate diuresis; volume expansion in dehydrated, mildly hypotensive cirrhotics; renal impairment, phlebitis.

PRECAUTIONS

Contraindications: Heart failure, history of allergic reaction to albumin level, hypervolemia, normal serum albumin, pulmonary edema, severe anemia. **Cautions:** Hypertension, normal serum albumin concentration, low cardiac reserve, pulmonary disease, hepatic/renal failure.

⧗ LIFESPAN CONSIDERATIONS

Pregnancy/Lactation: Unknown if drug crosses placenta or is distributed in breast milk. **Pregnancy Category C. Children/Elderly:** No age-related precautions noted.

INTERACTIONS

DRUG: None significant. **HERBAL:** None significant. **FOOD:** None known. **LAB VALUES:** May increase serum alkaline phosphatase concentration.

AVAILABILITY (Rx)

Injection Solution: **(5%):** 50 ml, 250 ml, 500 ml. **(25%):** 20 ml, 50 ml, 100 ml.

ADMINISTRATION/HANDLING

IV

Reconstitution • A 5% solution may be made from 25% solution by adding 1 volume 25% to 4 volumes 0.9% NaCl (NaCl preferred). Do not use Sterile Water for Injection (life-threatening hemolysis, acute renal failure can result). Do not dilute in D_5W.
Rate of administration • Give by IV infusion. Rate is variable, depending on use, blood volume, concentration of solute. 5%: Do not exceed 2–4 ml/min in pts with normal plasma volume, 5–10 ml/min in pts with hypoproteinemia. 25%: Do not exceed 1 ml/min in pts with normal plasma volume, 2–3 ml/min in pts with hypoproteinemia. 5% is administered undiluted; 25% may be administered undiluted or diluted with 0.9% NaCl. • May give without regard to pt blood group or Rh factor.
Storage • Store at room temperature. Appears as clear, brownish, odorless, moderately viscous fluid. • Do not use if solution has been frozen, appears turbid, contains sediment, or if not used within 4 hrs of opening vial.

IV INCOMPATIBILITIES

Lipids, midazolam (Versed), vancomycin (Vancocin), verapamil (Isoptin).

IV COMPATIBILITIES

Diltiazem (Cardizem), lorazepam (Ativan).

INDICATIONS/ROUTES/DOSAGE

◄ALERT► 5% should be used in hypovolemic or intravascularly depleted pts. 25% should be used in pts in whom fluid and sodium intake must be minimized.

Usual Dosage

IV: ADULTS, ELDERLY: Initially, 25 g; may repeat in 15–30 min. **Maximum:** 250 g within 48 hrs.

Hypovolemia

IV: ADULTS, ELDERLY: 5% albumin: 0.5–1 g/kg/dose, repeat as needed. **CHILDREN:** 0.5–1 g/kg/dose (10–20 ml/kg/dose of 5% albumin). **Maximum:** 6 g/kg/day.

Hypoproteinemia

IV: ADULTS, ELDERLY, CHILDREN: 0.5–1 g/kg/dose, repeat every 1–2 days as needed to replace ongoing losses.

Hemodialysis

IV: ADULTS, ELDERLY: 50–100 ml (12.5–25 g) of 25% albumin as needed.

Hyperbilirubinemia, Erythroblastosis Fetalis

IV: INFANTS: 1 g/kg of 25% solution prior to or during exchange transfusion.

SIDE EFFECTS

Occasional: Hypotension. **Rare:** High dose in repeated therapy: altered vital signs, chills, fever, increased salivation, nausea, vomiting, urticaria, tachycardia.

ADVERSE EFFECTS/ TOXIC REACTIONS

Fluid overload may occur, marked by increased B/P, distended neck veins. Pulmonary edema may occur, evidenced by rapid respirations, rales, wheezing, coughing. Neurologic changes that may occur include headache, weakness, blurred vision, behavioral changes, incoordination, isolated muscle twitching.

NURSING CONSIDERATIONS

BASELINE ASSESSMENT

Obtain B/P, pulse, respirations immediately before administration. Adequate hydration required before albumin is administered.

INTERVENTION/EVALUATION

Monitor B/P for hypotension/hypertension. Monitor Hgb, Hct, urine specific gravity. Assess frequently for evidence of fluid overload, pulmonary edema (see Adverse Effects/Toxic Reactions). Check skin for flushing, urticaria. Monitor I&O ratio (watch for decreased output). Assess for therapeutic response (increased B/P, decreased edema).

albuterol

ale-**but**-er-all
(AccuNeb, Airomir ✤, Apo-Salvent ✤, PMS-Salbutamol ✤, ProAir HFA, Proventil HFA, Ventolin HFA, VoSpire ER)
Do not confuse albuterol with Albutein or atenolol, Proventil with Bentyl, Prilosec, or Prinivil, or Ventolin with Benylin or Vantin.

FIXED-COMBINATION(S)

Combivent: albuterol/ipratropium (a bronchodilator): 103 mcg/18 mcg per actuation. **DuoNeb:** albuterol/ipratropium 3 mg/0.5 mg.

◆ CLASSIFICATION

PHARMACOTHERAPEUTIC: Sympathomimetic (adrenergic agonist). **CLINICAL:** Bronchodilator (see p. 74C).

ACTION

Stimulates beta_2-adrenergic receptors in lungs, resulting in relaxation of bronchial smooth muscle. **Therapeutic Effect:** Relieves bronchospasm and reduces airway resistance.

PHARMACOKINETICS

Route	Onset	Peak	Duration
PO	15–30 min	2–3 hrs	4–6 hrs
PO (extended-release)	30 min	2–4 hrs	12 hrs
Inhalation	5–15 min	0.5–2 hrs	2–5 hrs

Rapidly, well absorbed from GI tract; rapidly absorbed from bronchi after inhalation. Metabolized in liver. Primarily excreted in urine. **Half-life:** 3.8–6 hrs.

USES

Relief of bronchospasm due to reversible obstructive airway disease, prevention of exercise-induced bronchospasm.

PRECAUTIONS

Contraindications: History of hypersensitivity to sympathomimetics. **Cautions:** Hypertension, cardiovascular disease, hyperthyroidism, diabetes mellitus.

⌛ LIFESPAN CONSIDERATIONS

Pregnancy/Lactation: Appears to cross placenta; unknown if distributed in breast milk. May inhibit uterine contractility. **Pregnancy Category C. Children:** Safety and efficacy not established in those younger than 2 yrs (syrup) or younger than 6 yrs (tablets). **Elderly:** May be more sensitive to tremor or tachycardia due to age-related increased sympathetic sensitivity.

INTERACTIONS

DRUG: **Beta-adrenergic blocking agents (beta-blockers)** antagonize effects. May increase risk of arrhythmias with **digoxin. MAOIs, tricyclic antidepressants** may potentiate cardiovascular effects. **Thyroid hormones** may increase effect, enhance risk of coronary insufficiency in pts with coronary artery disease (CAD). **HERBAL: St. John's wort** may decrease levels/effects. **Ephedra, yohimbe** may cause CNS stimulation. **FOOD:** None known. **LAB VALUES:** May increase blood glucose level. May decrease serum potassium level.

AVAILABILITY (Rx)

Inhalation Aerosol (Proair HFA, ProventilHFA, Ventolin HFA): 90 mcg/spray. **Solution for Nebulization: Accuneb:** 0.63 mg/3 ml (0.021%), 1.25 mg/3 ml (0.042%). **Proventil:** 2.5 mg/3 ml (0.084%). **Syrup:** 2 mg/5 ml. **Tablets (Proventil, Ventolin):** 2 mg, 4 mg.

Tablets (Extended-Release [Vospire ER]): 4 mg, 8 mg.

ADMINISTRATION/HANDLING

PO

• Do not crush/break extended-release tablets. • Administer with water 1 hr before or 2 hrs after meals.

Inhalation

• Shake container well before inhalation. • Wait 2 min before inhaling second dose (allows for deeper bronchial penetration). • Rinse mouth with water immediately after inhalation (prevents mouth/throat dryness).

Nebulization

• Administer over 5–15 min. • Nebulizer should be used with compressed air or O_2 at rate of 6–10 L/min.

INDICATIONS/ROUTES/DOSAGE

Acute Bronchospasm

INHALATION: ADULTS, ELDERLY, CHILDREN OLDER THAN 12 YRS: 4–8 puffs q20min up to 4 hrs, then q1–4h as needed. **CHILDREN 12 YRS AND YOUNGER:** 4–8 puffs q20min for 3 doses, then q1–4h as needed.
NEBULIZATION: ADULTS, ELDERLY, CHILDREN OLDER THAN 12 YRS: 2.5–5 mg q20min for 3 doses, then 2.5–10 mg q1–4h or 10–15 mg/hr continuously. **CHILDREN 12 YRS AND YOUNGER:** 0.15 mg/kg q20min for 3 doses (minimum: 2.5 mg), then 0.15–0.3 mg/kg q1–4h as needed. **Maximum:** 10 mg q1–4h as needed or 0.5 mg/kg/hr by continuous infusion.

Chronic Bronchospasm

PO: ADULTS, CHILDREN OLDER THAN 12 YRS: 2–4 mg 3–4 times a day. **Maximum:** 8 mg 4 times a day. **ELDERLY:** 2 mg 3–4 times a day. **Maximum:** 8 mg 4 times a day. **CHILDREN 6–12 YRS:** 2 mg 3–4 times a day. **Maximum:** 24 mg/day. **CHILDREN 2–5 YRS:** 0.1–0.2 mg/kg/dose 3 times a day. **Maximum:** 4 mg 3 times a day.
PO (EXTENDED-RELEASE): ADULTS, CHILDREN OLDER THAN 12 YRS: 4–8 mg q12h. **Maximum:** 32 mg/day. **CHILDREN 6–12 YRS:** 4 mg q12h. **Maximum:** 24 mg/day.
NEBULIZATION: ADULTS, ELDERLY, CHILDREN OLDER THAN 12 YRS: 2.5 mg q4–8h as needed. **CHILDREN 12 YRS AND YOUNGER:** 0.63–1.25 mg q4–6h as needed.
INHALATION: ADULTS, ELDERLY, CHILDREN 4 YRS AND OLDER: 1–2 puffs q4–6h. **Maximum:** 12 puffs per day.

Exercise-Induced Bronchospasm

INHALATION: ADULTS, ELDERLY, CHILDREN OLDER THAN 12 YRS: 2 puffs 5–30 min before exercise. **CHILDREN 12 YRS AND YOUNGER:** 1–2 puffs 5 min before exercise.

SIDE EFFECTS

Frequent: Headache (27%); restlessness, nervousness, tremors (20%); nausea (15%); dizziness (less than 7%); throat dryness and irritation, pharyngitis (less than 6%); B/P changes, including hypertension (5%–3%); heartburn, transient wheezing (less than 5%). **Occasional (3%–2%):** Insomnia, asthenia, altered taste. **Inhalation:** Dry, irritated mouth or throat; cough; bronchial irritation. **Rare:** Drowsiness, diarrhea, dry mouth, flushing, diaphoresis, anorexia.

ADVERSE EFFECTS/ TOXIC REACTIONS

Excessive sympathomimetic stimulation may produce palpitations, extrasystole, tachycardia, chest pain, slight increase in B/P followed by substantial decrease, chills, diaphoresis, blanching of skin. Too-frequent or excessive use may lead to decreased bronchodilating effectiveness and severe, paradoxical bronchoconstriction.

NURSING CONSIDERATIONS

BASELINE ASSESSMENT

Assess lung sounds, pulse, B/P, color, character of sputum noted. Offer emotional support (high incidence of anxiety due to difficulty in breathing and sympathomimetic response to drug).

INTERVENTION/EVALUATION

Monitor rate, depth, rhythm, type of respiration; quality and rate of pulse; EKG; serum potassium, glucose, ABG determinations. Assess lung sounds for wheezing (bronchoconstriction), rales.

PATIENT/FAMILY TEACHING

• Follow guidelines for proper use of inhaler. • Increase fluid intake (decreases lung secretion viscosity). • Do not take more than 2 inhalations at any one time (excessive use may produce paradoxical bronchoconstriction or decreased bronchodilating effect). • Rinsing mouth with water immediately after inhalation may prevent mouth/throat dryness. • Avoid excessive use of caffeine derivatives (chocolate, coffee, tea, cola, cocoa).

aldesleukin HIGH ALERT

all-des-**lyew**-kin
(Interleukin-2, IL-2, Proleukin)
See Interleukin-2, pp. 79C, 625.

alefacept

ale-fah-cept
(Amevive)

◆ CLASSIFICATION

PHARMACOTHERAPEUTIC: Immunologic agent. **CLINICAL:** Immunosuppressive.

ACTION

Interferes with activation of T-lymphocytes by binding to the lymphocyte antigen, inhibiting their interaction. **Therapeutic Effect:** Reduces number of circulating total lymphocytes, predominant in chronic plaque psoriasis.

PHARMACOKINETICS

Half-life: 270 hrs.

USES

Treatment of adults with moderate to severe chronic plaque psoriasis who are candidates for systemic therapy or phototherapy.

PRECAUTIONS

Contraindications: History of systemic malignancy, concurrent use of immunosuppressive agents or phototherapy. Do not administer to pts infected with HIV (reduces $CD4^+$ T-lymphocyte count, which may accelerate disease progression or increase disease complications). **Cautions:** Those at high risk for malignancy, chronic infections, history of recurrent infection, elderly.

⌛ LIFESPAN CONSIDERATIONS

Pregnancy/Lactation: Unknown if drug crosses placenta or is distributed in breast milk. **Pregnancy Category B.** **Children:** Safety and efficacy not established. **Elderly:** Cautious use due to higher incidence of infections and certain malignancies.

INTERACTIONS

DRUG: **Immunosuppressive agents, methotrexate** may increase possibility of excessive immunosuppression. **HERBAL:** **Echinacea** may decrease effects. **FOOD:** None known. **LAB VALUES:** Decreases serum T-lymphocyte levels. May increase serum AST, ALT levels.

AVAILABILITY (Rx)

Injection, Powder for Reconstitution: 15 mg for IM administration.

ADMINISTRATION/HANDLING

◀ALERT▶ Withdraw 0.6 ml of the supplied diluent and with the needle pointed at the side wall of the vial, slowly inject the diluent into the vial of alefacept. Prevent excessive foaming by swirling gently to dissolve.

IM

Reconstitution • Reconstitute 15 mg with 0.6 ml of supplied diluent (Sterile

Water for Injection); 0.5 ml of reconstituted solution contains 15 mg alefacept. • Inject the full 0.5 ml of solution. • Use a different IM site for each new injection. Give new injections at least 1 inch from the old site. Avoid areas where the skin is tender, bruised, red, or hard.

Storage • Store unopened vials at room temperature. • Following reconstitution, use immediately, or if refrigerated, within 4 hrs. • Discard unused portion within 4 hrs of reconstitution. • Reconstituted solution should be clear and colorless to slightly yellow. • Do not use if discolored or cloudy or if undissolved material remains.

INDICATIONS/ROUTES/DOSAGE

Plaque Psoriasis

IM: ADULTS, ELDERLY: 15 mg once weekly for 12 wks.

SIDE EFFECTS

Frequent (16%): Injection site pain and inflammation (with IM administration). **Occasional (5%):** Chills. **Rare (2% or less):** Pharyngitis, dizziness, cough, nausea, myalgia.

ADVERSE EFFECTS/ TOXIC REACTIONS

Hypersensitivity reaction (rash, urticaria, hypotension, dyspnea), lymphopenia, malignancies, serious infections requiring hospitalization (abscess, pneumonia, postop wound infection) occur rarely. Coronary artery disease and MI occur in less than 1% of pts.

NURSING CONSIDERATIONS

BASELINE ASSESSMENT

Obtain baseline $CD4^+$ T-lymphocyte levels before treatment and weekly during the 12-wk dosing period.

INTERVENTION/EVALUATION

Closely monitor $CD4^+$ T-lymphocyte levels. Withhold dose if $CD4^+$ T-lymphocyte levels are below 250 cells/mcl. If levels remain below 250 cells/mcl for 1 mo, discontinue treatment.

PATIENT/FAMILY TEACHING

• Regular monitoring of WBC count during therapy is necessary. • Promptly report any signs of infection or evidence of malignancy.

alemtuzumab

HIGH ALERT

ah-lem-**two**-zoo-mab
(Campath, MabCampath)

BLACK BOX ALERT Serious infections (bacterial, viral, fungal, protozoal) have been reported. Potentially fatal infusion-related reactions (respiratory distress, cardiac arrest, hypotension) may occur. Profound myelosuppression (anemia, thrombocytopenia) has occurred.

CLASSIFICATION

PHARMACOTHERAPEUTIC: Monoclonal antibody. **CLINICAL:** Antineoplastic (see p. 79C).

ACTION

Binds to CD52, cell surface glycoprotein, found on surface of all B- and T-lymphocytes, most monocytes, macrophages, natural killer cells, granulocytes. **Therapeutic Effect:** Produces cytotoxicity, reducing tumor size.

PHARMACOKINETICS

Half-life: About 12 days. Peak and trough levels rise during first few wks of therapy and approach steady state by about wk 6.

USES

Treatment of B-cell chronic lymphocytic leukemia (B-CLL) in pts who have been treated with alkylating agents and who have failed fludarabine (Fludara) therapy. **OFF-LABEL:** Treatment of refractory T-cell leukemia, rheumatoid arthritis, multiple myeloma, autoimmune cytopenia; preconditioning regimen for stem cell transplantation, renal and liver transplantation.

PRECAUTIONS

Contraindications: Active systemic infections, history of hypersensitivity or anaphylactic reaction to alemtuzumab, other monoclonal antibodies, immunosuppression. **Cautions:** None known.

LIFESPAN CONSIDERATIONS

Pregnancy/Lactation: Has potential to cause fetal B- and T-lymphocyte depletion. Breast-feeding not recommended during treatment and for at least 3 mos after last dose. **Pregnancy Category C. Children:** Safety and efficacy not established. **Elderly:** No age-related precautions noted.

INTERACTIONS

DRUG: Concurrent use with **live virus vaccines** may potentiate virus replication, increase side effects, or decrease pt's antibody response. **Immunosuppressive agents** causing blood dyscrasias may have additive effects. **HERBAL:** **Echinacea** may decrease effect. **FOOD:** None known. **LAB VALUES:** May decrease Hgb level, platelet count, WBC count.

AVAILABILITY (Rx)

Injection Solution: 30 mg/ml.

ADMINISTRATION/HANDLING

IV

ALERT Do not give by IV push or bolus.

Reconstitution • Withdraw needed amount from ampule into a syringe. • Using a low-protein binding, non–fiber-releasing 5-micron filter, inject into 100 ml 0.9% NaCl or D_5W. • Invert bag to mix; do not shake.

Rate of administration • Give the 100-ml solution as a 2-hr IV infusion.

Storage • Refrigerate undiluted ampules; do not freeze. • Use within 8 hrs after dilution. Diluted solution may be stored at room temperature or refrigerated. • Discard if particulate matter is present or if solution is discolored.

IV INCOMPATIBILITIES

Do not mix with any other medications.

INDICATIONS/ROUTES/DOSAGE

ALERT Pretreatment with acetaminophen 650 mg and diphenhydramine 50 mg before each infusion may prevent infusion-related side effects.

Chronic Lymphocytic Leukemia

ALERT Dose escalation required. Do not exceed single doses greater than 30 mg or cumulative doses more than 90 mg/wk.

IV: ADULTS, ELDERLY: Initially, 3 mg/day as a 2-hr infusion. When tolerated (with only low-grade or no infusion-related toxicities), increase daily dose to 10 mg. When the 10 mg/day dose is tolerated, maintenance dose may be initiated. Maintenance: 30 mg/day 3 times a wk on alternate days (such as Monday, Wednesday, and Friday or Tuesday, Thursday, and Saturday) for up to 12 wks. The increase to 30 mg/day is usually achieved in 3–7 days. Adjust dosage for hematologic toxicity (severe neutropenia or thrombocytopenia).

SIDE EFFECTS

Frequent: Rigors, tremors (86%), fever (85%), nausea (54%), vomiting (41%), rash (40%), fatigue (34%), hypotension (32%), urticaria (30%), pruritus, skeletal pain, headache (24%), diarrhea (22%), anorexia (20%). **Occasional (less than 10%):** Myalgia, dizziness, abdominal pain, throat irritation, vomiting, neutropenia, rhinitis, bronchospasm, urticaria.

ADVERSE EFFECTS/ TOXIC REACTIONS

Neutropenia occurs in 85% of pts, anemia occurs in 80% of pts, and thrombocytopenia occurs in 72% of pts. Rash occurs in 40% of pts. Respiratory toxicity, manifested as dyspnea, cough, bronchitis, pneumonitis, and pneumonia, occurs in 26%–16% of pts. Serious, sometimes fatal bacterial, viral, fungal, and protozoan infections have been reported.

NURSING CONSIDERATIONS

BASELINE ASSESSMENT

Pretreatment with acetaminophen and diphenhydramine before each infusion may prevent infusion-related side effects. CBC, platelet count should be obtained frequently during and after therapy to assess for neutropenia, anemia, thrombocytopenia.

INTERVENTION/EVALUATION

Monitor for infusion-related symptoms complex consisting mainly of rigors, fever, chills, hypotension, generally occurring within 30 min–2 hrs of beginning of first infusion. Slowing infusion rate resolves symptoms. Monitor for hematologic toxicity (fever, sore throat, signs of local infection, unusual bleeding/bruising from any site), symptoms of anemia (excessive fatigue, weakness).

PATIENT/FAMILY TEACHING

• Avoid crowds, those with known infection. • Avoid contact with those who recently received live virus vaccine; do not receive vaccinations. • Report dyspnea, fever, chills, rash, nausea.

alendronate

ah-**len**-dro-nate
(Apo-Alendronate ✱, Fosamax, Novo-Alendronate ✱)
Do not confuse alendronate with risedronate, or Fosamax with Flomax.

FIXED-COMBINATION(S)

Fosamax Plus D: alendronate/cholecalciferol (vitamin D analog): 70 mg/2,800 international units, 70 mg/5,600 international units.

◆CLASSIFICATION

PHARMACOTHERAPEUTIC: Bisphosphonate. **CLINICAL:** Bone resorption inhibitor, calcium regulator.

ACTION

Inhibits normal and abnormal bone resorption, without retarding mineralization. **Therapeutic Effect:** Leads to significantly increased bone mineral density; reverses progression of osteoporosis.

PHARMACOKINETICS

Poorly absorbed after PO administration. Protein binding: 78%. After PO administration, rapidly taken into bone, with uptake greatest at sites of active bone turnover. Excreted in urine, feces (as unabsorbed drug). **Terminal half-life:** Greater than 10 yrs (reflects release from skeleton as bone is resorbed).

USES

Treatment of osteoporosis in men. Treatment adjunct in glucocorticoid-induced osteoporosis in men and women, treatment and prevention of osteoporosis in postmenopausal women, treatment of Paget's disease. **OFF-LABEL:** Treatment of breast cancer.

PRECAUTIONS

Contraindications: GI disease, including dysphagia, frequent heartburn, GI reflux disease, hiatal hernia, ulcers, inability to stand or sit upright for at least 30 min; renal impairment; sensitivity to alendronate. **Cautions:** Hypocalcemia, vitamin D deficiency.

⌛ LIFESPAN CONSIDERATIONS

Pregnancy/Lactation: Possible incomplete fetal ossification, decreased maternal weight gain, delay in delivery. Unknown if distributed in breast milk. Breast-feeding not recommended. **Pregnancy Category C. Children:** Safety and efficacy not established. **Elderly:** No age-related precautions noted.

INTERACTIONS

DRUG: **IV ranitidine** may double drug bioavailability. **Aspirin** may increase GI disturbances. **HERBAL:** None significant. **FOOD:** Concurrent **beverages, dietary**

supplements, food may interfere with alendronate absorption. **Caffeine** may reduce efficacy. **LAB VALUES:** Reduces serum calcium, phosphate concentrations. Significant decrease in serum alkaline phosphatase noted in those with Paget's disease.

AVAILABILITY (Rx)

Solution, Oral: 70 mg/75 ml. **Tablets:** 5 mg, 10 mg, 35 mg, 40 mg, 70 mg.

ADMINISTRATION/HANDLING

PO

• Give at least 30 min before first food, beverage, or medication of the day. • Give with 6–8 oz plain water only (mineral water, coffee, tea, juice will decrease absorption). • Instruct pt **not** to lie down or eat for at least 30 min after administering medication (allows medication to reach stomach quickly, minimizing esophageal irritation).

INDICATIONS/ROUTES/DOSAGE

Osteoporosis (in Men)

PO: ADULTS, ELDERLY: 10 mg once a day in the morning or 70 mg weekly.

Glucocorticoid-Induced Osteoporosis

PO: ADULTS, ELDERLY: 5 mg once a day in the morning. **POSTMENOPAUSAL WOMEN NOT RECEIVING ESTROGEN:** 10 mg once a day in the morning.

Postmenopausal Osteoporosis

PO (TREATMENT): ADULTS, ELDERLY: 10 mg once a day in the morning or 70 mg weekly.

PO (PREVENTION): ADULTS, ELDERLY: 5 mg once a day in the morning or 35 mg weekly.

Paget's Disease

PO: ADULTS, ELDERLY: 40 mg once a day in the morning for 6 mos.

Dosage in Renal Impairment

Not recommended with creatinine clearance less than 35 ml/min.

SIDE EFFECTS

Frequent (8%–7%): Back pain, abdominal pain. **Occasional (3%–2%):** Nausea, abdominal distention, constipation, diarrhea, flatulence. **Rare (less than 2%):** Rash, severe bone, joint, muscle pain.

ADVERSE EFFECTS/ TOXIC REACTIONS

Overdose produces hypocalcemia, hypophosphatemia, significant GI disturbances. Esophageal irritation occurs if not given with 6–8 oz of plain water or if pt lies down within 30 min of administration.

NURSING CONSIDERATIONS

BASELINE ASSESSMENT

Hypocalcemia, vitamin D deficiency must be corrected before therapy. Check electrolytes (esp. calcium and alkaline phosphatase serum levels).

INTERVENTION/EVALUATION

Monitor electrolytes (esp. serum calcium, phosphorus, and alkaline phosphatase levels).

PATIENT/FAMILY TEACHING

• Expected benefits occur only when medication is taken with full glass (6–8 oz) of plain water, first thing in the morning and at least 30 min before first food, beverage, or medication of the day is taken. Any other beverage (mineral water, orange juice, coffee) significantly reduces absorption of medication. • Do not lie down for at least 30 min after taking medication (potentiates delivery to stomach, reducing risk of esophageal irritation). • Consider weight-bearing exercises, modify behavioral factors (e.g., cigarette smoking, alcohol consumption).

alfuzosin

ale-few-**zoe**-sin
(Apo-Alfuzosin ✦, Uroxatral, Xatral ✦)

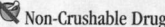

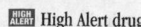

◆CLASSIFICATION

PHARMACOTHERAPEUTIC: Alpha$_1$-adrenergic blocker. **CLINICAL:** Benign prostatic hyperplasia agent.

ACTION

Targets receptors around bladder neck and prostate capsule. **Therapeutic Effect:** Relaxes smooth muscle, improves urinary flow, symptoms of prostatic hyperplasia.

PHARMACOKINETICS

Readily absorbed (decreased under fasting conditions). Protein binding: 90%. Extensively metabolized in liver. Primarily excreted in urine. **Half-life:** 10 hrs.

USES

Treatment of signs and symptoms of benign prostatic hyperplasia (BPH).

PRECAUTIONS

Contraindications: None known. **Cautions:** Coronary artery disease, hepatic disease, orthostatic hypotension, general anesthesia.

⌛ LIFESPAN CONSIDERATIONS

Pregnancy/Lactation: Not indicated for use in this pt population. **Pregnancy Category B. Children:** Not indicated for use in this pt population. **Elderly:** No age-related precautions noted.

INTERACTIONS

DRUG: **Atenolol, diltiazem** blood levels may be increased with concomitant use. **Other alpha-blocking agents (doxazosin, prazosin, tamsulosin, terazosin)** may have additive effect. **Cimetidine** may increase alfuzosin concentration. **Itraconazole, ketoconazole, ritonavir** increase blood levels. **HERBAL:** None significant. **FOOD:** **Food** increases absorption. **LAB VALUES:** None significant.

AVAILABILITY (Rx)

Tablets (Extended-Release): 10 mg.

ADMINISTRATION/HANDLING

PO

• Give immediately after the same meal each day. • Do not chew/crush extended-release tablets.

INDICATIONS/ROUTES/DOSAGE

Benign Prostatic Hyperplasia

PO: ADULTS: 10 mg once a day, after same meal each day.

SIDE EFFECTS

Frequent (7%–6%): Dizziness, headache, malaise. **Occasional (4%):** Dry mouth. **Rare (3%–2%):** Nausea, dyspepsia (heartburn, epigastric discomfort), diarrhea, orthostatic hypotension, tachycardia, drowsiness.

ADVERSE EFFECTS/ TOXIC REACTIONS

Ischemia-related chest pain may occur rarely (2%). Priapism has been reported.

NURSING CONSIDERATIONS

BASELINE ASSESSMENT

Question for sensitivity to alfuzosin, use of other alpha-blocking agents (doxazosin, prazosin, tamsulosin, terazosin). Obtain B/P.

INTERVENTION/EVALUATION

Assist with ambulation if dizziness occurs. Report headache. Monitor for hypotension. Question improvement in urine flow, hesitancy.

PATIENT/FAMILY TEACHING

• Take after the same meal each day. • Avoid tasks that require alertness, motor skills until response to drug is established. • Do not chew/crush extended-release tablets.

Alimta, *see pemetrexed*

aliskiren

HIGH ALERT

ah-lis-**kye**-ren
(Rasilez ✤, Tekturna)

BLACK BOX ALERT May cause fetal injury, mortality if used during second or third trimester of pregnancy.

Do not confuse Tekturna with Valturna.

FIXED-COMBINATION(S)

Amturnide: aliskiren/amlodipine (a calcium channel blocker)/hydrochlorothiazide (a diuretic): 150 mg/5 mg/12.5 mg, 300 mg/5 mg/12.5 mg, 300 mg/5 mg/25 mg, 300 mg/10 mg/12.5 mg, 300 mg/10 mg/25 mg. **Tekamlo:** aliskiren/amlodipine (a calcium channel blocker): 150 mg/5 mg, 150 mg/10 mg, 300 mg/5 mg, 300 mg/10 mg. **Tekturna HCT:** aliskiren/hydrochlorothiazide (a diuretic): 150 mg/12.5 mg, 150 mg/25 mg, 300 mg/12.5 mg, 300 mg/25 mg. **Valturna:** aliskiren/valsartan (an angiotensin II receptor antagonist): 150 mg/160 mg, 300 mg/320 mg.

CLASSIFICATION

PHARMACOTHERAPEUTIC: Renin-angiotensin system antagonist. **CLINICAL:** Antihypertensive.

ACTION

Direct renin inhibitor. Decreases plasma renin activity (PRA), inhibiting the conversion of angiotensinogen to angiotensin I, blocking the effect of increased renin levels. Therapeutic Effect: Reduces B/P.

PHARMACOKINETICS

Peak plasma concentration reached within 1–3 hrs. Protein binding: 49%. Metabolized in liver. Minimally excreted in urine. Half-life: 24 hrs. Peak plasma steady-state levels reached in 7–8 days.

USES

Treatment of hypertension. May be used alone or in combination with other antihypertensives. OFF-LABEL: Treatment of persistent proteinuria in pts with type 2 diabetes, hypertension, nephropathy.

PRECAUTIONS

Contraindications: None known. Cautions: Renal impairment.

LIFESPAN CONSIDERATIONS

Pregnancy/Lactation: Carcinogenic potential to fetus. May cause fetal/neonatal morbidity, mortality. Unknown if distributed in breast milk. **Pregnancy Category C (D if used in second or third trimester). Children:** Safety and efficacy not established. **Elderly:** No age-related precautions noted.

INTERACTIONS

DRUG: May reduce effect of **furosemide.** HERBAL: **Ephedra, ginseng, yohimbe** may increase hypertension. **Garlic** may increase antihypertensive effect. FOOD: **High-fat meal** substantially decreases absorption. LAB VALUES: May increase BUN, serum creatinine, uric acid, creatinine kinase, potassium. May decrease Hgb, Hct.

AVAILABILITY (Rx)

Tablets, Film-Coated: 150 mg, 300 mg.

ADMINISTRATION/HANDLING

PO

• High-fat meal substantially decreases absorption. • Do not crush film-coated tablets.

INDICATIONS/ROUTES/DOSAGE

Hypertension:

PO: ADULTS, ELDERLY: Initially, 150 mg/day. May increase to 300 mg/day.

SIDE EFFECTS

Rare (2%–1%): Diarrhea, particularly in women, elderly (older than 65 yrs), gastroesophageal reflux, cough, rash.

ADVERSE EFFECTS/ TOXIC REACTIONS

Angioedema, periorbital edema, edema of hands and entire body have been reported.

NURSING CONSIDERATIONS

BASELINE ASSESSMENT

Correct hypovolemia in pts on concurrent diuretic therapy. Obtain B/P and apical pulse immediately before each dose, in addition to regular monitoring (be alert to fluctuations). If excessive reduction in B/P occurs, place pt in supine position, feet slightly elevated.

INTERVENTION/EVALUATION

Assess for edema. Monitor I&O, volume status; weigh daily. Monitor daily pattern of bowel activity and stool consistency. Monitor B/P, renal function tests, potassium, Hgb, Hct.

PATIENT/FAMILY TEACHING

• Pregnant pts should avoid second- and third-trimester exposure to aliskiren. • Inform physician if diarrhea, swelling of face/lips/tongue, difficulty breathing occurs. • Avoid exercising during hot weather (risk of dehydration, hypotension).

Alkeran, *see melphalan*

Allegra, *see fexofenadine*

Allegra-D, *see fexofenadine and pseudoephedrine*

allopurinol

al-low-**pure**-ih-nal
(Aloprim, Apo-Allopurinol ✤, Zyloprim)

Do not confuse allopurinol with Apresoline or haloperidol, or Zyloprim with Zorprin or Zovirax.

◆CLASSIFICATION

PHARMACOTHERAPEUTIC: Xanthine oxidase inhibitor. **CLINICAL:** Antigout.

ACTION

Decreases uric acid production by inhibiting xanthine oxidase, an enzyme. **Therapeutic Effect:** Reduces uric acid concentrations in serum and urine.

PHARMACOKINETICS

Route	Onset	Peak	Duration
PO, IV	2–3 days	1–3 wks	1–2 wks

Well absorbed from GI tract. Widely distributed. Protein binding: less than 1%. Metabolized in liver to active metabolite. Excreted primarily in urine. Removed by hemodialysis. **Half-life:** 1–3 hrs; metabolite, 12–30 hrs.

USES

PO: Prevents attacks of gouty arthritis, nephropathy. Treatment of secondary hyperuricemia that may occur during cancer treatment. Prevents recurrent uric acid and calcium oxalate calculi. **Injection:** Management of elevated uric acid in cancer pts unable to tolerate oral therapy. **OFF-LABEL:** In mouthwash following fluorouracil therapy to prevent stomatitis.

PRECAUTIONS

Contraindications: Asymptomatic hyperuricemia. **Cautions:** Renal/hepatic impairment, CHF, diabetes mellitus, hypertension.

⌛ LIFESPAN CONSIDERATIONS

Pregnancy/Lactation: Unknown if drug crosses placenta or is distributed in breast milk. **Pregnancy Category C. Children/Elderly:** No age-related precautions noted.

INTERACTIONS

DRUG: **Thiazide diuretics** may decrease effect. May increase effect of **oral anticoagulants.** May increase effect, toxicity of **azathioprine, mercaptopurine. Amoxicillin, ampicillin** may increase incidence of rash. **HERBAL:** None significant. **FOOD:** None known. **LAB VALUES:** May increase serum alkaline phosphatase, AST, ALT, BUN, creatinine.

AVAILABILITY (Rx)

Injection, Powder for Reconstitution (Aloprim): 500 mg. **Tablets (Zyloprim):** 100 mg, 300 mg.

ADMINISTRATION/HANDLING

IV

Reconstitution • Reconstitute 500-mg vial with 25 ml Sterile Water for Injection, giving a clear, almost colorless solution (concentration of 20 mg/ml). • Further dilute with 0.9% NaCl or D_5W (19 ml of added diluent yields 1 mg/ml, 9 ml yields 2 mg/ml, 2.3 ml yields maximum concentration of 6 mg/ml).
Rate of administration • Infuse over 15–60 min.
Storage • Store unreconstituted vials at room temperature. • Do not refrigerate reconstituted and/or diluted solution. Must administer within 10 hrs of preparation. • Do not use if precipitate forms or solution is discolored.

PO

• Give after meals with fluid. • Instruct pt to drink at least 2,500–3,000 ml of fluid/day (prevents risk of renal stone formation). • Dosages greater than 300 mg/day to be administered in divided doses.

IV INCOMPATIBILITIES

Amikacin (Amikin), carmustine (BiCNU), cefotaxime (Claforan), chlorpromazine (Thorazine), cimetidine (Tagamet), clindamycin (Cleocin), cytarabine (Ara-C), dacarbazine (DTIC), diphenhydramine (Benadryl), doxorubicin (Adriamycin), doxycycline (Vibramycin), droperidol (Inapsine), fludarabine (Fludara), gentamicin (Garamycin), haloperidol (Haldol), hydroxyzine (Vistaril), idarubicin (Idamycin), imipenem-cilastatin (Primaxin), meperidine (Demerol), methylprednisolone (Solu-Medrol), metoclopramide (Reglan), ondansetron (Zofran), prochlorperazine (Compazine), promethazine (Phenergan), streptozocin (Zanosar), tobramycin (Nebcin), vinorelbine (Navelbine).

IV COMPATIBILITIES

Bumetanide (Bumex), calcium gluconate, furosemide (Lasix), heparin, hydromorphone (Dilaudid), lorazepam (Ativan), morphine, potassium chloride.

INDICATIONS/ROUTES/DOSAGE

◀ALERT▶ Doses greater than 300 mg given in divided doses.

Gouty Arthritis
PO: ADULTS, CHILDREN OLDER THAN 10 YRS (Mild): 200–300 mg/day. **(Moderate to severe):** 400–600 mg/day in 2–3 divided doses. **Maximum:** 800 mg/day.

Secondary Hyperuricemia Associated with Chemotherapy
PO: ADULTS, CHILDREN OLDER THAN 10 YRS: 600–800 mg/day in 2–3 divided doses for 2–3 days starting 1–2 days before chemotherapy. **CHILDREN 6–10 YRS:** 300 mg/day 2–3 divided doses. **CHILDREN YOUNGER THAN 6 YRS:** 150 mg/day in 3 divided doses.
◀ALERT▶ IV daily dose given as single infusion or at 6-, 8-, or 12-hr intervals.
IV: ADULTS, ELDERLY, CHILDREN 10 YRS OR OLDER: 200–400 mg/m²/day beginning 24–48 hrs before initiation of chemotherapy. **CHILDREN YOUNGER THAN 10 YRS:** 200 mg/m²/day. **Maximum:** 600 mg/day.

Recurrent Calcium Oxalate Calculi
PO: ADULTS: 200–300 mg/day.

Usual Elderly Dosage
PO: Initially, 100 mg/day, gradually increase until optimal uric acid level is reached.

Dosage in Renal Impairment
Dosage is modified based on creatinine clearance. **PO:** Removed by hemodialysis, adult maintenance doses based on creatinine clearance. Administer dose posthemodialysis or administer 50% supplemental dose.

PO

Creatinine Clearance (ml/min)	Dosage (mg/day)
140	400
120	350
100	300
80	250
60	200
40	150
20	100
10	100 every 2 days
0	100 every 3 days

IV

Creatinine Clearance	Dosage
10–20 ml/min	200 mg/day
3–9 ml/min	100 mg/day
Less than 3 ml/min	100 mg at extended intervals

SIDE EFFECTS

Occasional: PO: Drowsiness, unusual hair loss. **IV:** Rash, nausea, vomiting. **Rare:** Diarrhea, headache.

ADVERSE EFFECTS/TOXIC REACTIONS

Pruritic maculopapular rash possibly accompanied by malaise, fever, chills, joint pain, nausea, vomiting should be considered a toxic reaction. Severe hypersensitivity (hypotension, wheezing, dyspnea) may follow appearance of rash. Bone marrow depression, hepatotoxicity, peripheral neuritis, acute renal failure occur rarely.

NURSING CONSIDERATIONS

BASELINE ASSESSMENT

Instruct pt to drink minimum of 2,500–3,000 ml of fluid daily while taking medication.

INTERVENTION/EVALUATION

Discontinue medication immediately if rash or other evidence of allergic reaction appears. Monitor I&O (output should be at least 2,000 ml/day). Assess CBC, uric acid, hepatic function serum levels. Assess urine for cloudiness, unusual color, odor. **Gout:** Assess for therapeutic response: relief of pain, stiffness, swelling, increased joint mobility, reduced joint tenderness, improved grip strength.

PATIENT/FAMILY TEACHING

• May take 1 wk or longer for full therapeutic effect. • Drink 2,500–3,000 ml of fluid daily while taking medication. • Avoid tasks that require alertness, motor skills until response to drug is established. • Maintain adequate hydration. • Avoid alcohol (may increase uric acid).

almotriptan

al-moe-**trip**-tan
(Axert)
Do not confuse almotriptan with alvimopan, or Axert with Antivert.

◆CLASSIFICATION

PHARMACOTHERAPEUTIC: Serotonin receptor agonist. **CLINICAL:** Antimigraine (see p. 63C).

ACTION

Binds selectively to vascular receptors, producing a vasoconstrictive effect on cranial blood vessels. **Therapeutic Effect:** Produces relief of migraine headache.

PHARMACOKINETICS

Well absorbed after PO administration. Protein binding: 35%. Metabolized by liver to inactive metabolite, primarily excreted in urine. **Half-life:** 3–4 hrs.

USES

Acute treatment of migraine headache with or without aura. Acute treatment of migraine headache in adolescents 12–17 yrs with history of migraine with or without aura, and having attacks usually lasting 4 or more hrs.

PRECAUTIONS

Contraindications: Arrhythmias associated with conduction disorders, Wolff-Parkinson-White syndrome, hemiplegic or basilar migraine, ischemic heart disease (including angina pectoris, history of MI, silent ischemia, and Prinzmetal's angina), uncontrolled hypertension, use within 24 hrs of ergotamine-containing preparation or another serotonin receptor antagonist, use within 14 days of MAOIs. **Cautions:** Mild to moderate renal or hepatic impairment, pt profile suggesting cardiovascular risks, controlled hypertension, history of CVA.

LIFESPAN CONSIDERATIONS

Pregnancy/Lactation: Unknown if distributed in breast milk. **Pregnancy Category C. Children:** Safety and efficacy not established in those younger than 12 yrs. **Elderly:** No age-related precautions noted.

INTERACTIONS

DRUG: **Ergotamine-containing drugs** may produce vasospastic reaction. **MAOIs** may increase concentration. Combined use of **fluoxetine, fluvoxamine, paroxetine, sertraline** may produce weakness, hyperreflexia, incoordination. **Erythromycin, itraconazole, ketoconazole, ritonavir** may increase plasma concentration of almotriptan. **HERBAL:** None significant. **FOOD:** None known. **LAB VALUES:** None significant.

AVAILABILITY (Rx)

Tablets: 6.5 mg, 12.5 mg.

ADMINISTRATION/HANDLING

PO

• Swallow tablets whole. • Take with full glass of water. • May give without regard to food.

INDICATIONS/ROUTES/DOSAGE

Migraine Headache

PO: ADULTS, ELDERLY, ADOLESCENTS 12–17 YRS: Initially, 6.25–12.5 mg as a single dose. If headache improves but then returns, dose may be repeated after 2 hrs. **Maximum:** 2 doses/24 hrs.

Dosage in Renal/Hepatic Impairment

For adult and elderly pts, recommended initial dose is 6.25 mg, maximum daily dose is 12.5 mg.

SIDE EFFECTS

Frequent: Nausea, dry mouth, paresthesia, flushing. **Occasional:** Changes in temperature sensation, asthenia, dizziness.

ADVERSE EFFECTS/ TOXIC REACTIONS

Excessive dosage may produce tremor, redness of extremities, decreased respirations, cyanosis, seizures, chest pain. Serious arrhythmias occur rarely but particularly in pts with hypertension, diabetes, obesity, smokers, and those with strong family history of coronary artery disease.

NURSING CONSIDERATIONS

BASELINE ASSESSMENT

Question for history of peripheral vascular disease, cardiac conduction disorders. Question pt regarding onset, location, duration of migraine, and possible precipitating symptoms.

INTERVENTION/EVALUATION

Evaluate for relief of migraine headache and resulting photophobia, phonophobia (sound sensitivity), nausea, vomiting.

PATIENT/FAMILY TEACHING

• Take a single dose as soon as symptoms of an actual migraine attack appear. • Medication is intended to relieve migraine, not to prevent or reduce number of attacks. • Lie down in quiet, dark room for additional benefit after taking medication. • Avoid tasks that require alertness, motor skills until response to drug is established. • If palpitations, pain or tightness in chest or throat, or pain or weakness of extremities occurs, contact physician immediately.

Aloxi, *see palonosetron*

alprazolam

al-**praz**-oh-lam
(Alprazolam Intensol, Apo-Alpraz ✱, Niravam, Novo-Alprazol ✱, Xanax, Xanax XR)
Do not confuse alprazolam with lorazepam, or Xanax with Tenex, Xopenex, Zantac, or Zyrtec.

CLASSIFICATION

PHARMACOTHERAPEUTIC: Benzodiazepine (**Schedule IV**). **CLINICAL:** Antianxiety (see p. 13C).

ACTION

Enhances the action of the neurotransmitter gamma-aminobutyric acid in the brain. **Therapeutic Effect:** Produces anxiolytic effect due to CNS depressant action.

PHARMACOKINETICS

Well absorbed from GI tract. Protein binding: 80%. Metabolized in liver. Primarily excreted in urine. Minimal removal by hemodialysis. **Half-life:** 6–27 hrs.

USES

Management of anxiety disorders, anxiety associated with depression, panic disorder. **OFF-LABEL:** Management of premenstrual syndrome symptoms (mood disturbances, insomnia, cramps), irritable bowel syndrome, treatment of agoraphobia, post-traumatic stress disorder, tremors, ethanol withdrawal, anxiety in children, depression.

PRECAUTIONS

Contraindications: Acute alcohol intoxication with depressed vital signs, acute angle-closure glaucoma, concurrent use of itraconazole or ketoconazole, myasthenia gravis, severe COPD. **Cautions:** Renal/hepatic impairment.

LIFESPAN CONSIDERATIONS

Pregnancy/Lactation: Crosses placenta; distributed in breast milk. Chronic ingestion during pregnancy may produce withdrawal symptoms, CNS depression in neonates. **Pregnancy Category D. Children:** Safety and efficacy not established. **Elderly:** Use small initial doses with gradual increase to avoid ataxia (muscular incoordination) or excessive sedation.

INTERACTIONS

DRUG: Potentiated effects when used with **other CNS depressants (including alcohol). Fluvoxamine, ketoconazole, nefazodone** may inhibit hepatic metabolism, increase serum concentrations. **HERBAL: Gotu kola, kava kava, St. John's wort, valerian** may increase CNS depressant effect. **St. John's wort** may decrease effectiveness. **FOOD:** None known. **LAB VALUES:** None significant.

AVAILABILITY (Rx)

Solution, Oral (Alprazolam Intensol): 1 mg/ml. **Tablets (Orally-Disintegrating [Niravam]):** 0.25 mg, 0.5 mg, 1 mg, 2 mg. **Tablets (Immediate-Release [Xanax]):** 0.25 mg, 0.5 mg, 1 mg, 2 mg.

Tablets (Extended-Release [Xanax XR]): 0.5 mg, 1 mg, 2 mg, 3 mg.

ADMINISTRATION/HANDLING

PO, Immediate-Release
• May give without regard to meals.
• Tablets may be crushed.

PO, Extended-Release
• Administer once daily. • Do not crush, chew, break extended-release tablets. Swallow whole.

PO, Orally-Disintegrating
• Place tablet on tongue, allow to dissolve. • Swallow with saliva. • Administration with water not necessary.

INDICATIONS/ROUTES/DOSAGE

Anxiety Disorders

PO (IMMEDIATE-RELEASE): ADULTS: Initially, 0.25–0.5 mg 3 times a day. May titrate q3–4 days. **Maximum:** 4 mg/day in divided doses.

PO (ORALLY-DISINTEGRATING): ADULTS: 0.25–0.5 mg 3 times a day. **Maximum:** 4 mg/day in divided doses. **ELDERLY, DEBILITATED PTS, PTS WITH HEPATIC DISEASE OR LOW SERUM ALBUMIN:** Initially, 0.25 mg 2–3 times a day. Gradually increase to optimum therapeutic response.

Anxiety with Depression

PO: ADULTS: (average dose required) 2.5–3 mg/day in divided doses.

Panic Disorder

PO (IMMEDIATE-RELEASE): ADULTS: Initially, 0.5 mg 3 times a day. May increase at 3- to 4-day intervals. Range: 5–6 mg/day. **Maximum:** 10 mg/day. **ELDERLY:** Initially, 0.125–0.25 mg twice a day. May increase in 0.125-mg increments until desired effect attained.

PO (EXTENDED-RELEASE):
◀ALERT▶ To switch from immediate-release to extended-release form, give total daily dose (immediate-release) as a single daily dose of extended-release form.
ADULTS: Initially, 0.5–1 mg once a day. May titrate at 3- to 4-day intervals. Range: 3–6 mg/day. **Maximum:** 10 mg/day. **ELDERLY:** Initially, 0.5 mg once a day.

PO (ORALLY-DISINTEGRATING): ADULTS: Initially, 0.5 mg 3 times a day. May increase at 3- to 4-day intervals. Range: 5–6 mg/day. **Maximum:** 10 mg/day.

Premenstrual Syndrome

PO: ADULTS: 0.25 mg 3 times a day.

SIDE EFFECTS

Frequent: Ataxia; light-headedness; transient, mild drowsiness; slurred speech (particularly in elderly or debilitated pts). **Occasional:** Confusion, depression, blurred vision, constipation, diarrhea, dry mouth, headache, nausea. **Rare:** Behavioral problems such as anger, impaired memory; paradoxical reactions (insomnia, nervousness, irritability).

ADVERSE EFFECTS/ TOXIC REACTIONS

Abrupt or too-rapid withdrawal may result in pronounced restlessness, irritability, insomnia, hand tremors, abdominal/muscle cramps, diaphoresis, vomiting, seizures. Overdose results in drowsiness, confusion, diminished reflexes, coma. Blood dyscrasias noted rarely. **Antidote:** Flumazenil (see Appendix M for dosage).

NURSING CONSIDERATIONS

BASELINE ASSESSMENT

Assess degree of anxiety; assess for drowsiness, dizziness, light-headedness. Assess motor responses (agitation, trembling, tension), autonomic responses (cold/clammy hands, diaphoresis).

INTERVENTION/EVALUATION

For those on long-term therapy, perform hepatic/renal function tests, blood counts periodically. Assess for paradoxical reaction, particularly during early therapy. Evaluate for therapeutic response: calm facial expression, decreased restlessness, insomnia. Monitor respiratory and cardiovascular status.

PATIENT/FAMILY TEACHING

• Drowsiness usually disappears during continued therapy. • If dizziness occurs, change positions slowly from recumbent to sitting position before standing. • Avoid tasks that require alertness, motor skills until response to drug is established. • Smoking reduces drug effectiveness. • Sour hard candy, gum, sips of tepid water may relieve dry mouth. • Do not abruptly withdraw medication after long-term therapy. • Avoid alcohol. • Do not take other medications without consulting physician.

alprostadil (prostaglandin E_1; PGE_1)

ale-**pros**-tah-dill
(Caverject, Caverject Impulse, Edex, Edex Refill, Muse, Prostin VR Pediatric)

BLACK BOX ALERT Apnea may occur in 10%–12% of neonates with congenital heart defects, esp. in those weighing less than 4.4 lb.

CLASSIFICATION

PHARMACOTHERAPEUTIC: Prostaglandin. **CLINICAL:** Patent ductus arteriosus agent, anti-impotence.

ACTION

Direct effect on vascular and ductus arteriosus smooth muscle; relaxes trabecular smooth muscle. **Therapeutic Effect:** Causes vasodilation; dilates cavernosal arteries, allowing blood flow to and entrapment in the lacunar spaces of the penis.

USES

Prostin VR Pediatric: Temporarily maintains patency of ductus arteriosus until surgery is performed in those with congenital heart defects and dependent on patent ductus for survival (e.g., pulmonary atresia or stenosis). **Caverject, Edex, Muse:** Treatment of erectile dysfunction due to neurogenic, vasculogenic, psychogenic causes. **Caverject:** Adjunct in diagnosis of erectile dysfunction. **OFF-LABEL:** Treatment of atherosclerosis, gangrene, pain due to severe peripheral arterial occlusive disease, treatment of pulmonary hypertension in infants, children.

PRECAUTIONS

Contraindications: Conditions predisposing to anatomic deformation of penis, hyaline membrane disease, penile implants, priapism, respiratory distress syndrome. **Cautions:** Severe hepatic disease, coagulation defects, leukemia, multiple myeloma, polycythemia, sickle cell disease, thrombocythemia. **Pregnancy Category X (Muse: C).**

INTERACTIONS

DRUG: **Sympathomimetics** may decrease effect. **Antihypertensives** may increase risk of hypotension. **HERBAL:** None significant. **FOOD:** None known. **LAB VALUES:** May increase serum bilirubin. May decrease serum glucose, potassium.

AVAILABILITY (Rx)

Injection, Powder for Reconstitution (Edex): 10 mcg, 20 mcg, 40 mcg. **(Caverject):** 20 mcg, 40 mcg. **(Caverject Impulse):** 10 mcg, 20 mcg. **Injection, Solution (Prostin VR Pediatric):** 500 mcg/ml. **Urethral Pellet (Muse):** 125 mcg, 250 mcg, 500 mcg, 1,000 mcg.

ADMINISTRATION/HANDLING

Urethral Pellet

Storage: Refrigerate pellet unless used within 14 days.

IV (Prostin VR Pediatric)

Reconstitution • Dilute 500-mcg ampule with D_5W or 0.9% NaCl to volume depending on infusion pump capabilities. • **Maximum concentration:** 20 mcg/ml.

Rate of administration • Infuse into a large vein or through an umbilical artery catheter placed at ductal opening. • Infuse for shortest time, lowest dose possible. • If significant decrease in arterial pressure is noted via umbilical artery catheter, auscultation, or Doppler transducer, decrease infusion rate immediately. • Discontinue infusion immediately if apnea or bradycardia occurs (overdosage).

Storage • Store parenteral form in refrigerator. • Must dilute before use. • Prepare fresh q24h. • Discard unused portions.

IV INCOMPATIBILITIES

No information available.

INDICATIONS/ROUTES/DOSAGE

Maintain Patency of Ductus Arteriosus

IV INFUSION: NEONATES: Initially, 0.05–0.1 mcg/kg/min. Maintenance: 0.01–0.4 mcg/kg/min. **Maximum:** 0.4 mcg/kg/min. Therapeutic response is indicated by increased pH in pts with acidosis or increase in oxygenation (usually seen within 30 min).

Impotence

PELLET, INTRACAVERNOSAL: ADULTS: Dosage is individualized.

SIDE EFFECTS

Frequent: **Intracavernosal (4%–1%):** Penile pain (37%), prolonged erection, hypertension, localized pain, penile fibrosis, injection site hematoma or ecchymosis, headache, respiratory infection, flu-like symptoms. **Intraurethral (3%):** Penile pain (36%), urethral pain or burning, testicular pain, urethral bleeding, headache, dizziness, respiratory infection, flu-like symptoms. **Systemic (greater than 1%):** Fever, flushing, bradycardia, hypotension, tachycardia, diarrhea. Occasional: **Intracavernosal (less than 1%):** Hypotension, pelvic pain, back pain, dizziness, cough, nasal congestion. **Intraurethral (less than 3%):** Fainting, sinusitis, back and pelvic pain. **Systemic (less than 1%):** Anxiety, lethargy, myalgia, arrhythmias, respiratory depression, anemia, bleeding, hematuria.

ADVERSE EFFECTS/ TOXIC REACTIONS

◀ALERT▶ Apnea experienced by 10%–12% of neonates with congenital heart defects.

Overdose manifested as apnea, flushing of the face/arms, bradycardia. Cardiac arrest, sepsis, seizures, thrombocytopenia occur rarely.

NURSING CONSIDERATIONS

INTERVENTION/EVALUATION

Patent Ductus Arteriosus: Monitor arterial pressure by umbilical artery catheter, auscultation, doppler transducer. If significant decrease in arterial pressure occurs, decrease infusion rate immediately. Maintain continuous cardiac monitoring. Assess heart sounds, femoral pulse (circulation to lower extremities), respiratory status frequently. Monitor for symptoms of hypotension. Assess B/P, arterial blood gases, temperature. If apnea or bradycardia occurs, discontinue infusion and notify physician. In infants with restricted systemic blood flow, efficacy should be measured by monitoring improvement of systemic B/P and blood pH.

PATIENT/FAMILY TEACHING

• **Patent Ductus Arteriosus:** Therapy maintains patency of ductus arteriousus until surgery is performed. • **Impotence:** Erection will occur within 2–5 min. • Do not use if female is pregnant (unless using condom barrier). • Inform physician if erection lasts longer than 4 hrs or becomes painful.

Altace, *see ramipril*

alteplase HIGH ALERT

all-teh-place
(Activase, Cathflo Activase)
Do not confuse alteplase or Activase with Altace, or Activase with Cathflo Activase.

◆CLASSIFICATION

PHARMACOTHERAPEUTIC: Tissue plasminogen activator (tPA). **CLINICAL:** Thrombolytic (see p. 33C).

ACTION

Binds to fibrin in a thrombus and converts entrapped plasminogen to plasmin, initiating fibrinolysis. **Therapeutic Effect:** Degrades fibrin clots, fibrinogen, other plasma proteins.

PHARMACOKINETICS

Rapidly metabolized in liver. Primarily excreted in urine. **Half-life:** 35 min.

USES

Treatment of acute MI, acute ischemic stroke, acute massive pulmonary embolism. Treatment of occluded central venous catheters. **OFF-LABEL:** Acute peripheral occlusive disease, basilar artery occlusion, cerebral infarction, deep vein thrombosis, femoropopliteal artery occlusion, mesenteric or subclavian vein occlusion, pleural effusion (parapneumonic).

PRECAUTIONS

Contraindications: Active internal bleeding, AV malformation or aneurysm, bleeding diathesis, intracranial neoplasm, intracranial or intraspinal surgery or trauma, recent (within past 2 mos) CVA, severe uncontrolled hypertension. **Cautions:** Recent (within 10 days) major surgery or GI bleeding, OB delivery, organ biopsy, recent trauma or CPR, left heart thrombus, endocarditis, severe hepatic/renal disease, pregnancy, elderly, cerebrovascular disease, diabetic retinopathy, thrombophlebitis, occluded AV cannula at infected site.

LIFESPAN CONSIDERATIONS

Pregnancy/Lactation: Use only when benefit outweighs potential risk to fetus. Unknown if drug crosses placenta or is distributed in breast milk. **Pregnancy Category C. Children:** Safety and efficacy not established. **Elderly:** Risk of bleeding with thrombolytic therapy increases; careful pt selection, monitoring recommended.

INTERACTIONS

DRUG: **Heparin, low molecular weight heparins, medications altering platelet function (e.g., clopidogrel, NSAIDs, thrombolytics), oral anticoagulants** increase risk of hemorrhage. **HERBAL:** **Cat's claw, dong quai, evening primrose, feverfew, garlic, ginkgo, ginseng, green tea, horse chestnut, red clover** may increase risk of bleeding due to antiplatelet activity. **FOOD:** None known. **LAB VALUES:** Decreases plasminogen, fibrinogen levels during infusion, decreases clotting time (confirms the presence of lysis). Decreases Hgb, Hct.

AVAILABILITY (Rx)

Injection, Powder for Reconstitution: 2 mg (Cathflo Activase), 50 mg (Activase), 100 mg (Activase).

ADMINISTRATION/HANDLING

IV

Reconstitution • Reconstitute immediately before use with Sterile Water for Injection. • Reconstitute 100-mg vial with 100 ml Sterile Water for Injection (50-mg vial with 50 ml sterile water) without preservative to provide a concentration of 1 mg/ml. **Activase Cathflo:** Add 2.2 ml Sterile Water for Injection to provide concentration of 1 mg/ml. • Avoid excessive agitation; gently swirl or slowly invert vial to reconstitute.

Rate of administration • Give by IV infusion via infusion pump (see Indications/Routes/Dosage). • If minor bleeding occurs at puncture sites, apply pressure for 30 sec; if unrelieved, apply pressure dressing. • If uncontrolled hemorrhage occurs, discontinue infusion immediately (slowing rate of infusion may produce worsening hemorrhage). • Avoid undue pressure when drug is injected into catheter (can rupture catheter or expel clot into circulation). **Activase Cathflo:** Instill dose into occluded catheter. • After 30 min assess catheter function by attempting to aspirate blood. • If still occluded, let dose dwell an additional 90 min. • If function not restored, a second dose may be instilled.

Storage • Store vials at room temperature. • After reconstitution, solution appears colorless to pale yellow. • Solution is stable for 8 hrs after reconstitution. Discard unused portions.

IV INCOMPATIBILITIES

Dobutamine (Dobutrex), dopamine (Intropin), heparin, nitroglycerin.

IV COMPATIBILITIES

Lidocaine, metoprolol (Lopressor), morphine, propranolol (Inderal).

INDICATIONS/ROUTES/DOSAGE

Acute MI

IV INFUSION: ADULTS WEIGHING MORE THAN 67 KG: Total dose: 100 mg over 90 min, starting with 15-mg bolus over 1–2 min, then 50 mg over 30 min, then 35 mg over 60 min. **ADULTS WEIGHING 67 KG OR LESS: Total dose:** Start with 15-mg bolus over 1–2 min, then 0.75 mg/kg over 30 min (**maximum:** 50 mg), then 0.5 mg/kg over 60 min (**maximum:** 35 mg).

Acute Pulmonary Emboli

IV INFUSION: ADULTS: 100 mg over 2 hrs. Institute or reinstitute heparin near end or immediately after infusion when activated partial thromboplastin time (aPTT) or thrombin time (TT) returns to twice normal or less.

Acute Ischemic Stroke

◀ALERT▶ Dose should be given within the first 3 hrs of the onset of symptoms. Recommended total dose: 0.9 mg/kg (**Maximum:** 90 mg).

IV INFUSION: ADULTS WEIGHING 100 KG OR LESS: 0.09 mg/kg as IV bolus over 1 min, then 0.81 mg/kg as continuous infusion over 60 min. **WEIGHING GREATER THAN 100 KG:** 9 mg bolus over 1 min, then 81 mg as continuous infusion over 60 min.

Central Venous Catheter Clearance

IV: ADULTS, ELDERLY: Up to 2 mg; may repeat after 2 hrs. If catheter functional, withdraw 4–5 ml blood to remove drug and residual clot.

SIDE EFFECTS

Frequent: Superficial bleeding at puncture sites, decreased B/P. **Occasional:** Allergic reaction (rash, wheezing, bruising).

ADVERSE EFFECTS/ TOXIC REACTIONS

Severe internal hemorrhage may occur. Lysis of coronary thrombi may produce atrial or ventricular arrhythmias or stroke.

NURSING CONSIDERATIONS

BASELINE ASSESSMENT

Obtain baseline B/P, apical pulse. Record weight. Evaluate 12-lead EKG, cardiac enzymes, electrolytes. Assess Hct, platelet count, thrombin time (TT), prothrombin time (PT), activated partial thromboplastin time (aPTT), fibrinogen level before therapy is instituted. Type and crossmatch, hold blood.

INTERVENTION/EVALUATION

Perform continuous cardiac monitoring for arrhythmias. Check B/P, pulse, respirations q15min until stable, then hourly. Check peripheral pulses, heart and lung sounds. Monitor for chest pain relief and notify physician of continuation or recurrence (note location, type, intensity). Assess for bleeding: overt blood, blood in any body substance. Monitor aPTT per protocol. Maintain B/P; avoid any trauma that might increase risk of bleeding (e.g., injections, shaving). Assess neurologic status frequently.

alvimopan

ale-vih-**moe**-pan
(Entereg)

BLACK BOX ALERT Available only for short-term (15 doses) use in hospitalized pts. Only hospitals that have registered in and met all requirements for Entereg Access Support and Education (E.A.S.E.) program may use this medication.

Do not confuse alvimopan with almotriptan.

◆CLASSIFICATION

PHARMACOTHERAPEUTIC: Peripherally acting mu-opioid receptor antagonist. **CLINICAL:** Anti-ileus agent.

ACTION

Binds to opioid receptors in GI tract. **Therapeutic Effect:** Accelerates GI recovery period as defined by time to first bowel movement or flatus.

PHARMACOKINETICS

Protein binding: 80%–90%. Undergoes no significant hepatic metabolism but is metabolized by intestinal flora. Excreted 50% by biliary route. Unabsorbed drug and unchanged alvimopan resulting from biliary excretion is hydrolyzed to its metabolite by gut microflora. Metabolite eliminated in feces and urine as unchanged. **Half-life:** 10–17 hrs.

USES

Accelerates time to upper and lower GI recovery following partial large or small bowel resection surgery with primary anastomosis.

PRECAUTIONS

Contraindications: Pts who have taken therapeutic doses of opioids for more than 7 consecutive days prior to initiation of alvimopan (recent exposure to opioids heightens pt's sensitivity to drug's effects, increasing susceptibility to abdominal pain, nausea, vomiting, diarrhea); severe hepatic impairment, bowel obstruction. **Cautions:** Active hepatic disease, Crohn's disease, bowel disorders associated with diarrhea, electrolyte imbalance, obstructive bowel disease for more than 7 consecutive days immediately prior to taking alvimopan, pts receiving more than 3 doses of an opioid during the wk prior to surgery.

LIFESPAN CONSIDERATIONS:

Pregnancy/Lactation: Unknown if drug crosses placenta or is distributed in breast milk. **Pregnancy Category B. Children:** Safety and efficacy not established. **Elderly:** No age-related precautions noted.

INTERACTIONS

DRUG: None significant. **HERBAL:** None significant. **FOOD:** None known. **LAB VALUES:** May reduce Hgb, Hct, serum potassium.

AVAILABILITY (Rx)

Capsules: 12 mg.

ADMINISTRATION/HANDLING

PO

• First dose given preop (NPO); remaining dosage given without regard to meals.

INDICATIONS/ROUTES/DOSAGE

PO: ADULTS, ELDERLY: 12 mg given 30 min to 5 hrs prior to surgery followed by 12 mg twice daily beginning the day after surgery for a maximum of 7 days or until discharge. Pts should receive no more than 15 doses.

SIDE EFFECTS

Occasional (9%–6%): Hypokalemia, constipation, flatulence, dyspepsia (epigastric distress, heartburn, indigestion). **Rare (3%):** Back pain, urinary retention.

ADVERSE EFFECTS/ TOXIC REACTIONS

None known.

NURSING CONSIDERATIONS

BASELINE ASSESSMENT

Inform pts that they must disclose long-term or intermittent opioid pain therapy, including any use of opioids in the wk prior to receiving alvimopan. Treatment should not be instituted unless pt is opioid-free for 7 days.

INTERVENTION/EVALUATION

Monitor closely for evidence of hepatotoxicity (abdominal pain lasting more than a few days, white bowel movements, dark urine, jaundice), increased AST, ALT, serum bilirubin.

PATIENT/FAMILY TEACHING

• Recent use of opioids may increase susceptibility to adverse reactions, primarily those limited to GI tract (e.g., abdominal pain, nausea, vomiting, diarrhea). • Inform pts that the most common side effects in those undergoing bowel resection are constipation, dyspepsia, flatulence. • Report abdominal pain, nausea, vomiting, diarrhea.

amantadine

ah-**man**-tih-deen
(Endantadine ✦, PMS-Amantadine ✦, Symmetrel)

Do not confuse amantadine with ranitidine or rimantadine, or Symmetrel with Synthroid.

◆CLASSIFICATION

PHARMACOTHERAPEUTIC: Dopaminergic agonist. **CLINICAL:** Antiviral, antiparkinson agent (see p. 67C).

ACTION

Blocks uncoating of influenza A virus, preventing penetration into the host and inhibiting M2 protein in the assembly of progeny virions. Blocks reuptake of dopamine into presynaptic neurons and causes direct stimulation of postsynaptic receptors. **Therapeutic Effect:** Antiviral, antiparkinsonian activity.

PHARMACOKINETICS

Rapidly and completely absorbed from GI tract. Protein binding: 67%. Widely distributed. Primarily excreted in urine. Minimally removed by hemodialysis. **Half-life:** 11–15 hrs (increased in elderly, decreased in renal impairment).

USES

Prevention, treatment of respiratory tract infections due to influenza virus, Parkinson's disease, drug-induced extrapyramidal reactions. **OFF-LABEL:** Treatment of ADHD, fatigue associated with multiple sclerosis, post-polio syndrome related fatigue.

PRECAUTIONS

Contraindications: None known. **Cautions:** History of seizures, orthostatic hypotension, CHF, peripheral edema, hepatic disease, recurrent eczematoid dermatitis, cerebrovascular disease, renal dysfunction, those receiving CNS stimulants.

⌛ LIFESPAN CONSIDERATIONS

Pregnancy/Lactation: Unknown if drug crosses placenta or is distributed in breast milk. **Pregnancy Category C. Children:** No age-related precautions noted in those older than 1 yr. **Elderly:** May exhibit increased sensitivity to anticholinergic effects. Age-related renal impairment may require dosage adjustment.

INTERACTIONS

DRUG: Alcohol may increase CNS effects. **Quinidine, quinine, trimethoprim/sulfamethoxazole (Bactrim, Septra)** may increase concentration. **Anticholinergics, antihistamines, phenothiazines, tricyclic antidepressants** may increase anticholinergic effects. **Hydrochlorothiazide, triamterene** may increase concentration, toxicity. **HERBAL:** None significant. **FOOD:** None known. **LAB VALUES:** None significant.

AVAILABILITY (Rx)

Capsules: 100 mg. **Solution, Oral:** 50 mg/5 ml. **Syrup:** 50 mg/5 ml. **Tablets:** 100 mg.

ADMINISTRATION/HANDLING

PO

• May give without regard to food. • Administer nighttime dose several hrs before bedtime (prevents insomnia).

INDICATIONS/ROUTES/DOSAGE

Treatment of Influenza A

PO: ADULTS: 100 mg twice a day. Initiate within 24–48 hrs after onset of symptoms; discontinue as soon as possible based on clinical response. **ELDERLY:** 100 mg once daily. **CHILDREN 10 YRS AND OLDER, WEIGHING 40 KG OR MORE:** 100 mg twice a day. **WEIGHING LESS THAN 40 KG:** 5 mg/kg/day. **Maximum:** 150 mg/day. **CHILDREN 1–9 YRS:** 5 mg/kg/day. **Maximum:** 150 mg/day.

Prevention of Influenza A

PO: ADULTS: 100 mg twice a day. **CHILDREN:** Refer to treatment dosing above.

Parkinson's Disease, Extrapyramidal Symptoms

PO: ADULTS, ELDERLY: 100 mg twice a day. May increase up to 400 mg/day in divided doses.

Dosage in Renal Impairment

Dosage and frequency are modified based on creatinine clearance.

Creatinine Clearance	Dosage
30–50 ml/min	200 mg first day; 100 mg/day thereafter
15–29 ml/min	200 mg first day; 100 mg on alternate days
Less than 15 ml/min	200 mg every 7 days

SIDE EFFECTS

Frequent (10%–5%): Nausea, dizziness, poor concentration, insomnia, nervousness. **Occasional (5%–1%):** Orthostatic hypotension, anorexia, headache, livedo reticularis (reddish-blue, netlike blotching of skin), blurred vision, urinary retention, dry mouth or nose, agitation, confusion, hallucinations. **Rare:** Vomiting, depression, irritation or swelling of eyes, rash.

ADVERSE EFFECTS/ TOXIC REACTIONS

CHF, leukopenia, neutropenia occur rarely. Hyperexcitability, seizures, ventricular arrhythmias may occur. Neuroleptic malignant syndrome (NMS) occurs rarely.

NURSING CONSIDERATIONS

BASELINE ASSESSMENT

When treating infections caused by influenza A virus, obtain specimens for viral diagnostic tests before giving first dose (therapy may begin before results are known).

INTERVENTION/EVALUATION

Monitor I&O, renal function tests if ordered; check for peripheral edema. Evaluate food tolerance, vomiting. Assess skin for mottling or rash. Assess for dizziness. **Parkinson's Disease:** Assess for clinical reversal of symptoms (improvement of tremor of head/hands at rest, mask-like facial expression, shuffling gait, muscular rigidity).

PATIENT/FAMILY TEACHING

• Do not take any other medications without consulting physician. • Avoid alcoholic beverages. • Do not drive, use machinery, or engage in other activities that require mental acuity if experiencing dizziness, blurred vision. • Get up slowly from a sitting or lying position. • Inform physician of new symptoms, esp. blotching, rash, dizziness, blurred vision, nausea/vomiting, muscle rigidity. • Take nighttime dose several hours before bedtime to prevent insomnia.

Amaryl, *see glimepiride*

Ambien, *see zolpidem*

Ambien CR, *see zolpidem*

AmBisome, *see amphotericin B*

ambrisentan

am-**bris**-en-tan
(Letairis, Volibris)

BLACK BOX ALERT Can increase hepatic enzymes AST, ALT to at least 3 times upper limit of normal. Likely to produce serious birth defects if used by pregnant women.

◆CLASSIFICATION

PHARMACOTHERAPEUTIC: Endothelin receptor antagonist. **CLINICAL:** Vasodilator.

ACTION

Blocks endothelin receptor subtypes ET_A and ET_B on vascular endothilium and smooth muscle, leading to vasodilation. **Therapeutic Effect:** Improves symptoms of pulmonary arterial hypertension (e.g., improves exercise ability), decreases rate of clinical deterioration.

PHARMACOKINETICS

Rapidly absorbed. Protein binding: high (99%). Not eliminated by renal pathways. **Half-life:** 9 hrs.

USES

Treatment of pulmonary arterial hypertension (PAH) in those with Class II or III symptoms (World Health Organization).

PRECAUTIONS

Contraindications: Pregnancy, women who may become pregnant. **Extreme Caution:** Moderate to severe hepatic impairment. **Cautions:** Mild hepatic impairment.

LIFESPAN CONSIDERATIONS

Pregnancy/Lactation: May cause serious birth defects, including malformation of heart and great vessels, facial abnormalities. Breast-feeding not recommended. **Pregnancy Category X. Children:** Safety and efficacy not established. **Elderly:** Age-related hepatic impairment requires strict monitoring.

INTERACTIONS

DRUG: **Cyclosporine, ketoconazole, omeprazole, indinavir, ritonavir** may increase plasma concentration of ambrisentan. **FOOD:** **Grapefruit/grapefruit juice** may increase levels/effect. **HERBAL:** **St. John's wort** may decrease levels/effect. **LAB VALUES:** May increase AST, ALT to at least 3 times upper limit of normal levels (ULN). May increase aminotransferase more than 3 times ULN. May increase bilirubin more than 2 times ULN. May cause marked decrease in Hgb, Hct.

AVAILABILITY (Rx)

Tablets, Film-Coated: 5 mg, 10 mg.

ADMINISTRATION/HANDLING

PO

• Swallow whole. Do not crush/break tablets. • Give without regard to food.

INDICATIONS/ROUTES/DOSAGE

Pulmonary Arterial Hypertension (PAH)

PO: ADULTS, ELDERLY: Initially, 5 mg once a day. Dose may be increased to 10 mg once a day if 5 mg is tolerated. Dosage modification based on transaminase elevation.

SIDE EFFECTS

Frequent (17%–15%): Peripheral edema, headache. **Occasional (6%–3%):** Nasal congestion, palpitations, constipation, flushing, nasopharyngitis, dyspnea, abdominal pain, sinusitis.

ADVERSE EFFECTS/ TOXIC REACTIONS

Potential for serious hepatic injury.

NURSING CONSIDERATIONS

BASELINE ASSESSMENT

Pregnancy must be excluded before the start of treatment and prevented thereafter. Obtain a negative pregnancy test prior to initiation of treatment and monthly during treatment. Measure Hgb prior to therapy, 1 mo and periodically thereafter. Assess hepatic function tests (including aminotransferase, bilirubin) prior to initiating therapy and then monthly thereafter.

INTERVENTION/EVALUATION

If elevation in hepatic enzymes is noted, changes in monitoring and treatment must be initiated, or if bilirubin level increases, stop treatment. Monitor Hgb, Hct levels at 1 and 3 mos of treatment, then every 3 mos. Monitor Hgb, Hct levels for decrease. Monitor for signs/symptoms of hepatic/injury (abdominal pain, fever, jaundice).

PATIENT/FAMILY TEACHING

• Female pts should take measures to avoid pregnancy during treatment. • Hepatic function tests, pregnancy test must be run every mo during treatment. • Report clinical symptoms of hepatic injury (nausea, vomiting, fever, abdominal pain, fatigue, jaundice) immediately.

amikacin

am-eh-**kay**-sin
(Amikin 🍁)

BLACK BOX ALERT May cause ototoxicity, nephrotoxicity, and/or neuromuscular blockade and respiratory paralysis. Ototoxicity usually is irreversible; nephrotoxicity usually is reversible.

Do not confuse amikacin or Amikin with Amicar, or amikacin with anakinra.

◆CLASSIFICATION

PHARMACOTHERAPEUTIC: Aminoglycoside. **CLINICAL:** Antibiotic (see p. 21C).

ACTION

Irreversibly binds to protein on bacterial ribosomes. **Therapeutic Effect:** Interferes with protein synthesis of susceptible microorganisms.

PHARMACOKINETICS

Rapid, complete absorption after IM administration. Protein binding: 0%–10%. Widely distributed (penetrates blood-brain barrier when meninges are inflamed). Excreted unchanged in urine. Removed by hemodialysis. **Half-life:** 2–4 hrs (increased in renal impairment, neonates; decreased in cystic fibrosis, burn pts, febrile pts).

USES

Treatment of susceptible infections due to *Pseudomonas,* other gram-negative organisms (*Proteus, Serratia,* other gram-negative bacilli) including biliary tract, bone and joint, CNS, intra-abdominal, skin and soft tissue, urinary tract. Treatment of bacterial pneumonia, septicemia.

PRECAUTIONS

Contraindications: Hypersensitivity to amikacin, other aminoglycosides (cross-sensitivity), or their components. **Cautions:** Myasthenia gravis, parkinsonism, renal impairment, 8th cranial nerve impairment (vestibulocochlear nerve).

⌛ LIFESPAN CONSIDERATIONS

Pregnancy/Lactation: Readily crosses placenta; small amounts distributed in breast milk. May produce fetal nephrotoxicity. **Pregnancy Category D. Children:** Neonates, premature infants may be more susceptible to toxicity due to immature renal function. **Elderly:** Higher risk of toxicity due to age-related renal impairment, increased risk of hearing loss.

INTERACTIONS

DRUG: **Nephrotoxic- and ototoxic-medications** may increase toxicity. May increase effects of **neuromuscular blocking agents.** **HERBAL:** None significant. **FOOD:** None known. **LAB VALUES:** May increase serum creatinine BUN, AST, ALT, bilirubin, LDH; may decrease serum calcium, magnesium, potassium, sodium concentrations. **Therapeutic levels:** Peak: life threatening infections: 25–40 mcg/ml; serious infections: 20–25 mcg/ml; urinary tract infections: 15–20 mcg/ml. **Trough:** less than 8 mcg/ml. **Toxic levels:** Peak: greater than 40 mcg/ml; **trough:** greater than 10 mcg/ml.

AVAILABILITY (Rx)

Injection Solution: 50 mg/ml, 250 mg/ml (Amikin).

ADMINISTRATION/HANDLING

IV

Reconstitution • Dilute to concentration of 0.25–5 mg/ml in 0.9% NaCl or D_5W.

Rate of administration • Infuse over 30–60 min.

Storage • Store vials at room temperature. • Solution appears clear but may become pale yellow (does not affect potency). • Intermittent IV infusion (piggyback) is stable for 24 hrs at room temperature, 2 days if refrigerated. • Discard if precipitate forms or dark discoloration occurs.

IM

• To minimize discomfort, give deep IM slowly. • Less painful if injected into gluteus maximus rather than in lateral aspect of thigh.

IV INCOMPATIBILITIES

Amphotericin, ampicillin, cefazolin (Ancef), heparin, propofol (Diprivan).

IV COMPATIBILITIES

Amiodarone (Cordarone), aztreonam (Azactam), calcium gluconate, cefepime (Maxipime), cimetidine (Tagamet), ciprofloxacin (Cipro), clindamycin (Cleocin), diltiazem (Cardizem), diphenhydramine (Benadryl), enalapril (Vasotec), esmolol (BreviBloc), fluconazole (Diflucan), furosemide (Lasix), levofloxacin (Levaquin), lorazepam (Ativan), lipids, magnesium sulfate, meperidine (Demerol), midazolam (Versed), morphine, ondansetron (Zofran), potassium chloride, ranitidine (Zantac), total parenteral nutrition (TPN), vancomycin.

INDICATIONS/ROUTES/DOSAGE

Usual Parenteral Dosage

IV, IM: ADULTS, ELDERLY, CHILDREN, INFANTS: 15–22.5 mg/kg/day in divided doses q8h. **NEONATES:** 7.5–10 mg/kg/dose q8–24h.

Dosage in Renal Impairment

Dosage and frequency are modified based on degree of renal impairment and serum drug concentration. After a loading dose of 5–7.5 mg/kg, maintenance dose and frequency are based on serum creatinine levels and creatinine clearance.

Creatinine Clearance	Dosing Interval
60 ml/min or greater	q8h
40–59 ml/min	q12h
20–39 ml/min	q24h
Less than 20 ml/min	Loading dose, monitor levels

SIDE EFFECTS

Frequent: Phlebitis, thrombophlebitis. **Occasional:** Hypersensitivity reactions (rash, fever, urticaria, pruritus). **Rare:** Neuromuscular blockade (difficulty breathing, drowsiness, weakness).

ADVERSE EFFECTS/ TOXIC REACTIONS

Serious reactions include nephrotoxicity (as evidenced by increased thirst, decreased appetite, nausea, vomiting, increased BUN and serum creatinine levels, decreased creatinine clearance); neurotoxicity (manifested as muscle twitching, visual disturbances, seizures, paresthesias); ototoxicity (as evidenced by tinnitus, dizziness, loss of hearing).

NURSING CONSIDERATIONS

BASELINE ASSESSMENT

Dehydration must be treated prior to aminoglycoside therapy. Establish pt's baseline hearing acuity before beginning therapy. Question for history of allergies, esp. to aminoglycosides and sulfite. Obtain specimen for culture, sensitivity before giving first dose (therapy may begin before results are known).

INTERVENTION/EVALUATION

Monitor I&O (maintain hydration), urinalysis (casts, RBC, WBC, decrease in specific gravity). Monitor results of serum peak/trough levels. Be alert to ototoxic, neurotoxic, nephrotoxic symptoms (see Adverse Effects/Toxic Reactions). Check IM injection site for pain, induration. Evaluate IV site for phlebitis (heat, pain, red streaking over vein). Assess for skin rash, superinfection (particularly genital/anal pruritus), changes of oral mucosa, diarrhea. When treating pts with neuromuscular disorders, assess respiratory response carefully. **Therapeutic levels:** Peak: life threatening infections: 25–40 mcg/ml; serious infections: 20–25 mcg/ml; urinary tract infections: 15–20 mcg/ml. **Trough:** less than 8 mcg/ml. **Toxic levels:** Peak: greater than 40 mcg/ml; **trough:** greater than 10 mcg/ml.

PATIENT/FAMILY TEACHING

• Continue antibiotic for full length of treatment. • Space doses evenly. • IM injection may cause discomfort. • Notify physician of any hearing, visual, balance, urinary problems even after therapy is completed. • Do not take other medications without consulting physician. • Lab tests are essential part of therapy.

aminocaproic acid

a-mee-noe-ka-**proe**-ik **ah**-sid
(Amicar)
Do not confuse Amicar with amikacin, Amikin, or Omacor.

◆CLASSIFICATION

PHARMACOTHERAPEUTIC: Systemic hemostatic. **CLINICAL:** Antifibrinolytic, antihemorrhagic.

ACTION

Inhibits activation of plasminogen, thereby reducing fibrinolysin, without inhibiting lysis of clot. **Therapeutic Effect:** Enhances hemostasis when fibrinolysis contributes to bleeding.

USES

Treatment of excessive bleeding from hyperfibrinolysis or urinary fibrinolysis as noted in anemia, abruptio placentae, cirrhosis, carcinoma of prostate, lung, stomach, cervix. **OFF-LABEL:** Control of bleeding in thrombocytopenia, control of oral bleeding in congenital and acquired coagulation disorders, prevention of recurrence of subarachnoid hemorrhage, prevention of hemorrhage in hemophiliacs following dental surgery, treatment of traumatic hyphema.

PRECAUTIONS

Contraindications: Any active intravascular clotting process, disseminated intravascular coagulation without concurrent heparin therapy, hematuria of upper urinary tract origin (unless benefit outweighs risk); newborns (parenteral form). **Cautions:** Cardiac, hepatic, renal impairment; those with hyperfibrinolysis, premature neonates. **Pregnancy Category C.**

INTERACTIONS

DRUG: **Estrogens, oral contraceptives** increase risk of hypercoagulability. **HERBAL:** None significant. **FOOD:** None known. **LAB VALUES:** May elevate serum potassium level.

AVAILABILITY (Rx)

Injection, Solution: 250 mg/ml. **Solution, Oral:** 250 mg/ml. **Syrup:** 250 mg/ml. **Tablets:** 500 mg, 1,000 mg.

ADMINISTRATION/HANDLING

IV

Reconstitution • Dilute each 1 g in up to 50 ml 0.9% NaCl, D_5W, Ringer's, or Sterile Water for Injection (do not use Sterile Water for Injection in pts with subarachnoid hemorrhage). **Maximum concentration:** 20 mg/ml.

Rate of administration • Give only by IV infusion. • Infuse 5 g or less over first hr in 250 ml of solution followed by infusion of 1–1.25 g/hr in adults or 33.3 mg/kg/hr in children.

Administration precaution • Monitor for hypotension during infusion. • Rapid infusion may produce bradycardia, arrhythmias.

IV INCOMPATIBILITY

Sodium lactate.

INDICATIONS/ROUTES/DOSAGE

Acute Bleeding

PO, IV INFUSION: ADULTS, ELDERLY: 4–5 g over first hr, then 1–1.25 g/hr. Continue for 8 hrs or until bleeding is controlled. **Maximum:** 30 g/24 hr. **CHILDREN:** 100–200 mg/kg over first hr, then 33.3 mg/kg/hr or 100 mg/kg q6h. **Maximum:** 30 g/24 hrs.

SIDE EFFECTS

Occasional: Nausea, diarrhea, cramps, decreased urination, decreased B/P, dizziness, headache, muscle fatigue and weakness, myopathy, bloodshot eyes.

ADVERSE EFFECTS/ TOXIC REACTIONS

Too-rapid IV administration produces tinnitus, rash, arrhythmias, unusual fatigue, weakness. Rarely, grand mal seizure occurs, generally preceded by weakness, dizziness, headache.

NURSING CONSIDERATIONS

INTERVENTION/EVALUATION

Question for any change in muscle strength as noted by pt. Monitor for increased serum creatine kinase (CK), AST levels (skeletal myopathy), serum potassium. Monitor heart rhythm. Assess for decrease in B/P, increase in pulse rate, abdominal/back pain, severe headache (may be evidence of hemorrhage). Assess peripheral pulses for quality, skin for ecchymoses, petechiae. Question for increased discharge during menses. Check for excessive bleeding from minor cuts, scratches. Assess gums for erythema, gingival bleeding. Observe urine for hematuria.

PATIENT/FAMILY TEACHING

• Report any sign of red/dark urine, black/red stool, coffee-ground vomitus, blood-tinged mucus from cough.

amiodarone HIGH ALERT

ah-me-**oh**-dah-roan
(Apo-Amiodarone ✱, Cordarone, Novo-Amiodarone ✱, Pacerone)

BLACK BOX ALERT Pts should be hospitalized when amiodarone is initiated. Alternative therapies to be tried first before using amiodarone. Only indicated for pts with life-threatening arrhythmias due to risk of toxicity. Lung damage may occur without symptoms. Hepatotoxicity is common, usually mild (rarely possible). Can exacerbate arrhythmias.

Do not confuse amiodarone with amiloride, or Cordarone with Cardura.

◆CLASSIFICATION

PHARMACOTHERAPEUTIC: Cardiac agent. **CLINICAL:** Antiarrhythmic (see p. 17C).

ACTION

Prolongs duration of myocardial cell action potential and refractory period by acting directly on all cardiac tissue. Decreases AV and sinus node function. **Therapeutic Effect:** Suppresses arrhythmias.

PHARMACOKINETICS

Route	Onset	Peak	Duration
PO	3 days–3 wks	1 wk–5 mos	7–50 days after discontinuation

Slowly, variably absorbed from GI tract. Protein binding: 96%. Extensively metabolized in liver to active metabolite. Excreted via bile; not removed by hemodialysis. **Half-life:** 26–107 days; metabolite, 61 days.

A

USES

PO: Management of life-threatening recurrent ventricular fibrillation, hemodynamically unstable ventricular tachycardia (VT). **IV:** Management/prophylaxis of frequently occurring ventricular fibrillation, unstable VT unresponsive to other therapy. OFF-LABEL: Control of hemodynamically stable VT, control of rapid ventricular rate due to accessory pathway conduction in pre-excited atrial arrhythmias, conversion of atrial fibrillation to normal sinus rhythm, in cardiac arrest with persistent VT or ventricular fibrillation, paroxysmal supraventricular tachycardia (PSVT), polymorphic VT or wide complex tachycardia of uncertain origin, prevention of postop atrial fibrillation.

PRECAUTIONS

Contraindications: Bradycardia-induced syncope (except in the presence of a pacemaker), second- and third-degree AV block, severe hepatic disease, severe sinus node dysfunction. Hypersensitivity to iodine. **Cautions:** Thyroid disease, electrolyte imbalance, hepatic disease, hypotension, left ventricular dysfunction, photosensitivity, pulmonary disease. May prolong QT interval.

LIFESPAN CONSIDERATIONS

Pregnancy/Lactation: Crosses placenta; distributed in breast milk. May adversely affect fetal development. **Pregnancy Category D. Children:** Safety and efficacy not established. **Elderly:** May be more sensitive to effects on thyroid function. May experience increased incidence of ataxia, other neurotoxic effects.

INTERACTIONS

DRUG: May increase cardiac effects with **other antiarrhythmics.** May increase effect of **beta-blockers, oral anticoagulants.** May increase concentration, toxicity of **digoxin, phenytoin. Simvastatin** may increase risk for myopathy, rhabdomyolysis. HERBAL: **St. John's wort** may decrease effect. FOOD: **Grapefruit, grapefruit juice** may decrease effect. LAB VALUES: May increase serum AST, ALT, alkaline phosphatase, ANA titer. May cause changes in EKG, thyroid function test results. **Therapeutic serum level:** 0.5–2.5 mcg/ml; toxic serum level not established.

AVAILABILITY (Rx)

Injection, Solution (Cordarone I.V.): 50 mg/ml. **Tablets:** 100 mg (Pacerone), 200 mg (Cordarone, Pacerone), 400 mg (Pacerone).

ADMINISTRATION/HANDLING

IV

Reconstitution • Infusions longer than 2 hrs must be administered/diluted in glass or polyolefin bottles. • Dilute loading dose (150 mg) in 100 ml D_5W (1.5 mg/ml). • Dilute maintenance dose (900 mg) in 500 ml D_5W (1.8 mg/ml). Concentrations greater than 3 mg/ml cause peripheral vein phlebitis.

Rate of administration • Does not need protection from light during administration. • Administer through central venous catheter (CVC) if possible, using in-line filter. • Bolus over 10 min (15 mg/min) not to exceed 30 mg/min; then 1 mg/min over 6 hrs; then 0.5 mg/min over 18 hrs. • Infusions longer than 1 hr, concentration not to exceed 2 mg/ml unless CVC used.

Storage • Store at room temperature. • Stable for 24 hrs when diluted in glass or polyolefin containers; stable for 2 hrs when diluted in PVC containers.

PO

• Give consistently with regard to meals to reduce GI distress. • Tablets may be crushed • Do not give with grapefruit juice, grapefruit.

IV INCOMPATIBILITIES

Aminophylline (theophylline), cefazolin (Ancef), heparin, sodium bicarbonate.

IV COMPATIBILITIES

Dobutamine (Dobutrex), dopamine (Intropin), furosemide (Lasix), insulin (regular), labetalol (Normodyne), lidocaine, lorazepam (Ativan), midazolam (Versed), morphine, nitroglycerin, norepinephrine (Levophed), phenylephrine (Neo-Synephrine), potassium chloride, vancomycin.

INDICATIONS/ROUTES/DOSAGE

Ventricular Arrhythmias

PO: ADULTS, ELDERLY: Initially, 800–1,600 mg/day in 2–4 divided doses for 1–3 wks. After arrhythmia is controlled or side effects occur, reduce to 600–800 mg/day for 4 wks. Maintenance: 200–600 mg/day. **CHILDREN:** Initially, 10–20 mg/kg/day for 4–14 days, then 5 mg/kg/day for several wks. Maintenance: 2.5 mg/kg/day or lowest effective maintenance dose for 5–7 days/wk.

IV INFUSION: ADULTS: Initially, 1,050 mg over 24 hrs; 150 mg over 10 min, then 360 mg over 6 hrs; then 540 mg over 18 hrs. May continue at 0.5 mg/min. After first 24 hrs, infuse 720 mg/24 hrs with a concentration of 1–6 mg/ml.

SIDE EFFECTS

Expected: Corneal microdeposits noted in almost all pts treated for more than 6 mos (can lead to blurry vision). **Frequent (greater than 3%): PO:** Constipation, headache, decreased appetite, nausea, vomiting, paresthesias, photosensitivity, muscular incoordination. **Parenteral:** Hypotension, nausea, fever, bradycardia. **Occasional (less than 3%): PO:** Bitter or metallic taste; decreased libido; dizziness; facial flushing; blue-gray coloring of skin (face, arms, and neck); blurred vision; bradycardia; asymptomatic corneal deposits. **Rare (less than 1%): PO:** Rash, vision loss, blindness.

ADVERSE EFFECTS/ TOXIC REACTIONS

Serious, potentially fatal pulmonary toxicity (alveolitis, pulmonary fibrosis, pneumonitis, acute respiratory distress syndrome) may begin with progressive dyspnea and cough with crackles, decreased breath sounds, pleurisy, CHF, or hepatotoxicity. May worsen existing arrhythmias or produce new arrhythmias.

NURSING CONSIDERATIONS

BASELINE ASSESSMENT

Obtain baseline pulmonary function tests, chest X-ray, hepatic enzyme tests, serum AST, ALT, alkaline phosphatase, EKG. Assess B/P, apical pulse immediately before drug is administered (if pulse is 60/min or less or systolic B/P is less than 90 mm Hg, withhold medication, contact physician).

INTERVENTION/EVALUATION

Monitor for symptoms of pulmonary toxicity (progressively worsening dyspnea, cough). Dosage should be discontinued or reduced if toxicity occurs. Assess pulse for quality, rhythm, bradycardia. Monitor EKG for cardiac changes (e.g., widening of QRS, prolongation of PR and QT intervals). Notify physician of any significant interval changes. Assess for nausea, fatigue, paresthesia, tremor. Monitor for signs of hypothyroidism (periorbital edema, lethargy, pudgy hands/feet, cool/pale skin, vertigo, night cramps) and hyperthyroidism (hot/dry skin, bulging eyes [exophthalmos], frequent urination, eyelid edema, weight loss, difficulty breathing). Monitor serum AST, ALT, alkaline phosphatase for evidence of hepatic toxicity. Assess skin, cornea for bluish discoloration in those who have been on drug therapy longer than 2 mos. Monitor hepatic function tests, thyroid test results. If elevated hepatic enzymes occur, dosage reduction or discontinuation is necessary. Monitor for therapeutic serum level (0.5–2.5 mcg/ml). Toxic serum level not established.

PATIENT/FAMILY TEACHING

• Protect against photosensitivity reaction on skin exposed to sunlight. • Bluish skin discoloration gradually disappears when drug is discontinued. • Report shortness of breath, cough. • Outpatients should monitor pulse before taking medication.

• Do not abruptly discontinue medication. • Compliance with therapy regimen is essential to control arrhythmias. • Restrict salt, alcohol intake. • Avoid grapefruit, grapefruit juice. • Recommend ophthalmic exams q6mo. • Report any vision changes, signs/symptoms of cardiac arrhythmias.

amitriptyline

a-me-**trip**-tih-leen
(Apo-Amitriptyline ✱, Elavil, Levate ✱, Novo-Tryptyn ✱)

BLACK BOX ALERT Increased risk of suicidal thinking and behavior in children, adolescents, young adults 18–24 yrs with major depressive disorder, other psychiatric disorders.

Do not confuse amitriptyline with aminophylline, imipramine, or nortriptyline, or Elavil with enalapril, Eldepryl, Equanil, or Mellaril.

FIXED-COMBINATION(S)

Etrafon, Triavil: amitriptyline/perphenazine (an antipsychotic): 10 mg/2 mg, 25 mg/2 mg, 10 mg/4 mg, 25 mg/4 mg. **Limbitrol:** amitriptyline/chlordiazepoxide (an antianxiety): 12.5 mg/5 mg, 25 mg/10 mg.

◆CLASSIFICATION

PHARMACOTHERAPEUTIC: Tricyclic. **CLINICAL:** Antidepressant, antineuralgic, antibulimic (see p. 37C).

ACTION

Blocks reuptake of neurotransmitters (norepinephrine, serotonin) at presynaptic membranes, increasing availability at postsynaptic receptor sites. Strong anticholinergic activity. **Therapeutic Effect:** Antidepressant effect.

PHARMACOKINETICS

Rapidly and well absorbed from GI tract. Protein binding: 90%. Undergoes first-pass metabolism in liver. Primarily excreted in urine. Minimal removal by hemodialysis. **Half-life:** 10–26 hrs.

USES

Treatment of various forms of depression, exhibited as persistent, prominent dysphoria (occurring nearly every day for at least 2 wks) manifested by 4 of 8 symptoms: appetite change, sleep pattern change, increased fatigue, impaired concentration, feelings of guilt or worthlessness, loss of interest in usual activities, psychomotor agitation or retardation, suicidal tendencies. **OFF-LABEL:** Relief of neuropathic pain, such as that experienced by pts with diabetic neuropathy or postherpetic neuralgia; treatment of anxiety, bulimia nervosa, migraine, nocturnal enuresis, panic disorder, peptic ulcer. Treatment of depression in children, post-traumatic stress disorder (PTSD).

PRECAUTIONS

Contraindications: Acute recovery period after MI, use within 14 days of MAOIs. **Cautions:** Prostatic hypertrophy, history of urinary retention or obstruction, glaucoma, diabetes mellitus, history of seizures, hyperthyroidism, cardiac/hepatic/renal disease, schizophrenia, increased intraocular pressure (IOP), hiatal hernia.

⌛ LIFESPAN CONSIDERATIONS

Pregnancy/Lactation: Crosses placenta; minimally distributed in breast milk. **Pregnancy Category C. Children:** More sensitive to increased dosage, toxicity, increased risk of suicidal ideation, worsening of depression. **Elderly:** Increased risk of toxicity. Increased sensitivity to anticholinergic effects. Cautions in those with cardiovascular disease.

INTERACTIONS

DRUG: CNS depressants (including alcohol, anticonvulsants, barbiturates, phenothiazines, sedative-hypnotics) may increase sedation, respiratory depression, hypotensive effects. **Antithyroid agents** may increase risk of agranulocytosis. **Phenothiazines** may increase sedative, anticholinergic effects. **Cimetidine, valproic acid** may increase concentration, toxicity. May decrease effects of **clonidine.** May increase cardiac effects with **sympathomimetics.** May increase risk of hypertensive crisis, hyperpyresis, seizures with **MAOIs.** HERBAL: **St. John's wort** may decrease levels. **Gotu kola, kava kava, St. John's wort, valerian** may increase CNS depression. FOOD: None known. LAB VALUES: May alter EKG readings (flattened T wave), serum glucose (increase or decrease). **Therapeutic serum level:** Peak: 120–250 ng/ml; **toxic serum level:** greater than 500 ng/ml.

AVAILABILITY (Rx)

Tablets (Elavil): 10 mg, 25 mg, 50 mg, 75 mg, 100 mg, 150 mg.

ADMINISTRATION/HANDLING

PO

- Give with food or milk if GI distress occurs.

INDICATIONS/ROUTES/DOSAGE

Depression

PO: ADULTS: 25–150 mg/day as a single dose at bedtime or in divided doses. May gradually increase up to 300 mg/day. Titrate to lowest effective dosage. ELDERLY: Initially, 10–25 mg at bedtime. May increase by 10–25 mg at weekly intervals. Range: 25–150 mg/day. CHILDREN 6–12 YRS: 1–5 mg/kg/day in divided doses.

Pain Management

PO: ADULTS, ELDERLY: 25–100 mg at bedtime.

SIDE EFFECTS

Frequent: Dizziness, drowsiness, dry mouth, orthostatic hypotension, headache, increased appetite, weight gain, nausea, unusual fatigue, unpleasant taste. Occasional: Blurred vision, confusion, constipation, hallucinations, delayed micturition, eye pain, arrhythmias, fine muscle tremors, parkinsonian syndrome, anxiety, diarrhea, diaphoresis, heartburn, insomnia. Rare: Hypersensitivity, alopecia, tinnitus, breast enlargement, photosensitivity.

ADVERSE EFFECTS/ TOXIC REACTIONS

Overdose may produce confusion, seizures, severe drowsiness, fast/slow/irregular heart rate, fever, hallucinations, agitation, dyspnea, vomiting, unusual fatigue, weakness. Abrupt withdrawal after prolonged therapy may produce headache, malaise, nausea, vomiting, vivid dreams. Blood dyscrasias, cholestatic jaundice occur rarely.

NURSING CONSIDERATIONS

BASELINE ASSESSMENT

Observe and record behavior. Assess psychological status, thought content, suicidal tendencies, sleep patterns, appearance, interest in environment. For those on long-term therapy, hepatic/renal function tests, blood counts should be performed periodically.

INTERVENTION/EVALUATION

Supervise suicidal-risk pt closely during early therapy (as depression lessens, energy level improves, increasing suicide potential). Assess appearance, behavior, speech pattern, level of interest, mood. Monitor B/P, pulse for hypotension, arrhythmias. **Therapeutic serum level:** Peak: 120–250 ng/ml; **toxic serum level:** greater than 500 ng/ml.

PATIENT/FAMILY TEACHING

• Change positions slowly to avoid hypotensive effect. Tolerance to postural hypotension, sedative and anticholinergic effects usually develop during early therapy. • Maximum therapeutic effect may be noted in 2–4 wks. • Sensitivity to sun may occur. • Report visual disturbances. • Do not abruptly discontinue medication. • Avoid tasks that require alertness, motor skills until response to drug is established. • Avoid alcohol. • Sips of tepid water may relieve dry mouth.

amlodipine

am-**low**-dih-peen
(Apo-Amlodipine ✦, Norvasc, Novo-Amlodipine ✦)

Do not confuse amlodipine with amiloride, or Norvasc with Navane or Vascor.

FIXED-COMBINATION(S)

Anturnide: amlodipine/aliskiren (a renin inhibitor)/hydrochlorothiazide (a diuretic): 5 mg/150 mg/12.5 mg, 5 mg/300 mg/12.5 mg, 5 mg/300 mg/25 mg, 10 mg/300 mg/12.5 mg, 10 mg/300 mg/25 mg. **Azor:** amlodipine/olmesartan (an angiotensin II receptor antagonist): 5 mg/20 mg, 10 mg/20 mg, 5 mg/40 mg, 10 mg/40 mg. **Caduet:** amlodipine/atorvastatin (hydroxamethylglutaryl-CoA [HMG-CoA] reductase inhibitor): 2.5 mg/10 mg, 2.5 mg/20 mg, 2.5 mg/40 mg, 5 mg/10 mg, 10 mg/10 mg, 5 mg/20 mg, 10 mg/20 mg, 5 mg/40 mg, 10 mg/40 mg, 5 mg/80 mg, 10 mg/80 mg. **Exforge:** amlodipine/valsartan (an angiotensin II receptor antagonist): 5 mg/160 mg, 10 mg/160 mg, 5 mg/320 mg, 10 mg/320 mg. **Exforge HCT:** amlodipine/valsartan/hydrochlorothiazide (a diuretic): 5 mg/160 mg/12.5 mg, 5 mg/160 mg/25 mg, 10 mg/160 mg/12.5 mg, 10 mg/160 mg/25 mg, 10 mg/320 mg/25 mg. **Lotrel:** amlodipine/benazepril (an angiotensin-converting enzyme [ACE] inhibitor): 2.5 mg/10 mg, 5 mg/10 mg, 5 mg/20 mg, 5 mg/40 mg, 10 mg/20 mg, 10 mg/40 mg. **Tekamlo:** amlodipine/aliskiren (a renin inhibitor): 5 mg/150 mg, 5 mg/300 mg, 10 mg/150 mg, 10 mg/300 mg. **Tribenzor:** amlodipine/olmesartan/hydrochlorothiazide: 5 mg/20 mg/12.5 mg, 5 mg/40 mg/12.5 mg, 5 mg/40 mg/25 mg, 10 mg/40 mg/12.5 mg, 10 mg/40 mg/25 mg. **Twynsta:** amlodipine/telmisartan (an angiotensin II receptor antagonist): 5 mg/40 mg, 5 mg/80 mg, 10 mg/40 mg, 10 mg/80 mg.

◆CLASSIFICATION

PHARMACOTHERAPEUTIC: Calcium channel blocker. **CLINICAL:** Antihypertensive, antianginal (see p. 77C).

ACTION

Inhibits calcium movement across cardiac and vascular smooth muscle cell membranes. **Therapeutic Effect:** Dilates coronary arteries, peripheral arteries/arterioles. Decreases total peripheral vascular resistance and B/P by vasodilation.

PHARMACOKINETICS

Route	Onset	Peak	Duration
PO	0.5–1 hr	N/A	24 hrs

Slowly absorbed from GI tract. Protein binding: 95%–98%. Undergoes first-pass metabolism in liver. Excreted primarily in urine. Not removed by hemodialysis. **Half-life:** 30–50 hrs (increased in elderly, those with hepatic cirrhosis).

USES

Management of hypertension, chronic stable angina, vasospastic (Prinzmetal's or variant) angina. May be used alone or with other antihypertensives or antianginals.

PRECAUTIONS

Contraindications: Severe hypotension. **Cautions:** Hepatic impairment, aortic stenosis, CHF.

⌛ LIFESPAN CONSIDERATIONS

Pregnancy/Lactation: Unknown if drug crosses placenta or is distributed in breast milk. **Pregnancy Category C. Children:** Safety and efficacy not established. **Elderly:** Half-life may be increased, more sensitive to hypotensive effects.

INTERACTIONS

DRUG: None significant. **HERBAL: St. John's wort** may decrease concentration. **Ephedra, yohimbe** may worsen hypertension. **Garlic** may increase antihypertensive effect. **FOOD: Grapefruit, grapefruit juice** may increase concentration, hypotensive effects. **LAB VALUES:** May increase hepatic enzymes.

AVAILABILITY (Rx)

Tablets: 2.5 mg, 5 mg, 10 mg.

ADMINISTRATION/HANDLING

PO

• May give without regard to food.

INDICATIONS/ROUTES/DOSAGE

Hypertension

PO: ADULTS: Initially, 5 mg/day as a single dose. May increase by 2.5 mg/day every 7–14 days. **Maximum:** 10 mg/day. **SMALL-FRAME, FRAGILE, ELDERLY:** Initially, 2.5 mg/day as a single dose. **CHILDREN 6–17 YRS:** 2.5–5 mg/day.

Angina (Chronic Stable or Vasospastic)

PO: ADULTS: 5–10 mg/day as a single dose. **ELDERLY, PTS WITH HEPATIC INSUFFICIENCY:** 5 mg/day as a single dose.

Dosage in Hepatic Impairment

ADULTS, ELDERLY: (Hypertension) 2.5 mg/day. (Angina) 5 mg/day.

SIDE EFFECTS

Frequent (greater than 5%): Peripheral edema, headache, flushing. **Occasional (5%–1%):** Dizziness, palpitations, nausea, unusual fatigue or weakness (asthenia). **Rare (less than 1%):** Chest pain, bradycardia, orthostatic hypotension.

ADVERSE EFFECTS/ TOXIC REACTIONS

Overdose may produce excessive peripheral vasodilation, marked hypotension with reflex tachycardia.

NURSING CONSIDERATIONS

BASELINE ASSESSMENT

Assess baseline renal/hepatic function tests, B/P, apical pulse.

INTERVENTION/EVALUATION

Assess B/P (if systolic B/P is less than 90 mm Hg, withhold medication, contact physician). Assess for peripheral edema behind medial malleolus (sacral area in bedridden pts). Assess skin for flushing. Question for headache, asthenia.

PATIENT/FAMILY TEACHING

• Do not abruptly discontinue medication. • Compliance with therapy regimen is essential to control hypertension. • Avoid tasks that require alertness, motor skills until response to drug is established. • Avoid concomitant ingestion of grapefruit juice.

amoxicillin

ah-mocks-ih-**sill**-in
(Amoxil, Apo-Amoxi ✱, Moxatag, Novamoxin ✱)

Do not confuse amoxicillin with amoxapine or Atarax.

◆ CLASSIFICATION

PHARMACOTHERAPEUTIC: Penicillin. **CLINICAL:** Antibiotic (see p. 29C).

ACTION

Inhibits bacterial cell wall synthesis. **Therapeutic Effect:** Bactericidal in susceptible microorganisms.

PHARMACOKINETICS

Well absorbed from GI tract. Protein binding: 20%. Partially metabolized in liver. Primarily excreted in urine. Removed by hemodialysis. **Half-life:** 1–1.3 hrs (increased in renal impairment).

USES

Treatment of susceptible infections due to *streptococci, E. coli, E. faecalis, P. mirabilis, H. influenzae, N. gonorrhoeae* including ear, nose and throat, lower respiratory tract, skin and skin structure, UTIs, acute uncomplicated gonorrhea, *H. pylori*. **OFF-LABEL:** Treatment of Lyme disease and typhoid fever. Postexposure prophylaxis for anthrax exposure.

PRECAUTIONS

Contraindications: Hypersensitivity to any penicillin, infectious mononucleosis. **Cautions:** History of allergies (esp. cephalosporins), antibiotic-associated colitis.

LIFESPAN CONSIDERATIONS

Pregnancy/Lactation: Crosses placenta, appears in cord blood, amniotic fluid. Distributed in breast milk in low concentrations. May lead to allergic sensitization, diarrhea, candidiasis, skin rash in infant. **Pregnancy Category B. Children:** Immature renal function in neonate/young infant may delay renal excretion. **Elderly:** Age-related renal impairment may require dosage adjustment.

INTERACTIONS

DRUG: **Allopurinol** may increase incidence of rash. **Probenecid** may increase concentration, toxicity risk. May decrease effects of **oral contraceptives. HERBAL:** None significant. **FOOD:** None known. **LAB VALUES:** May increase serum AST, ALT, LDH, bilirubin, creatinine, BUN. May cause positive Coombs' test.

AVAILABILITY (Rx)

Capsules: 250 mg, 500 mg. **Powder for Oral Suspension:** 50 mg/ml, 125 mg/5 ml, 200 mg/5 ml, 250 mg/5 ml, 400 mg/5ml. **Tablets:** 500 mg, 875 mg. **Tablets (Chewable):** 125 mg, 200 mg, 250 mg, 400 mg. **Tablets (For Oral Suspension):** 200 mg, 400 mg. **Tablets, Extended-Release (Moxatag):** 775 mg.

ADMINISTRATION/HANDLING

PO

• Store capsules, tablets at room temperature. • After reconstitution, oral solution is stable for 14 days at either room temperature or refrigerated. • Give without regard to meals. **Moxatag:** Take within 1 hr of finishing a meal. • Instruct pt to chew/crush chewable tablets thoroughly before swallowing.

INDICATIONS/ROUTES/DOSAGE

Susceptible Infections

PO: ADULTS, ELDERLY, CHILDREN 12 YRS AND OLDER: 250–500 mg q8h or 500–875 mg q12h or 775 mg (Moxatag) once daily. **CHILDREN OLDER THAN 3 MOS:** 20–50 mg/kg/day in 3 divided doses. **CHILDREN 3 MOS AND YOUNGER:** 20–30 mg/kg/day in 2 divided doses.

Lower Respiratory Tract Infection

PO: ADULTS, ELDERLY: 500 mg q8h or 875 mg q12h. **CHILDREN:** 45 mg/kg/day in divided doses q12h or 40 mg/kg/day in divided doses q8h.

***H. Pylori* Infection**

PO: ADULTS, ELDERLY: 1 g twice a day in combination with at least 1 other antibiotic and an acid-suppressing agent (proton pump inhibitor or H_2 antagonist).

Otitis Media

PO: CHILDREN: 80–90 mg/kg/day in 2 divided doses.

Pharyngitis/Tonsillitis

PO: ADULTS, CHILDREN 12 YRS AND OLDER: (MOXATAG) 775 mg once daily.

Gonorrhea

PO: ADULTS, ELDERLY: 3 g as a single dose.

Endocarditis Prophylaxis

PO: ADULTS, ELDERLY: 2 g 1 hr before procedure. **CHILDREN:** 50 mg/kg 1 hr before procedure. **Maximum:** 2 g.

Dosage in Renal Impairment

ALERT 875-mg tablet should not be used in pts with creatinine clearance less than 30 ml/min. Dosage interval is modified based on creatinine clearance. **Creatinine clearance 10–30 ml/min:** 250–500 mg q12h. **Creatinine clearance less than 10 ml/min:** 250–500 mg q24h.

SIDE EFFECTS

Frequent: GI disturbances (mild diarrhea, nausea, vomiting), headache, oral/

vaginal candidiasis. **Occasional:** Generalized rash, urticaria.

ADVERSE EFFECTS/ TOXIC REACTIONS

Antibiotic-associated colitis, other superinfections (abdominal cramps, severe watery diarrhea, fever) may result from altered bacterial balance. Severe hypersensitivity reactions, including anaphylaxis, acute interstitial nephritis, occur rarely.

NURSING CONSIDERATIONS

BASELINE ASSESSMENT

Question for history of allergies, esp. penicillins, cephalosporins.

INTERVENTION/EVALUATION

Hold medication and promptly report rash, diarrhea (fever, abdominal pain, mucus and blood in stool may indicate antibiotic-associated colitis). Be alert for superinfection: fever, vomiting, diarrhea, anal/genital pruritus, oral mucosal changes (ulceration pain, erythema). Monitor renal/hepatic function tests.

PATIENT/FAMILY TEACHING

• Continue antibiotic for full length of treatment. • Space doses evenly. • Take with meals if GI upset occurs. • Thoroughly chew the chewable tablets before swallowing. • Notify physician if rash, diarrhea, other new symptoms occur.

amoxicillin/ clavulanate

a-mocks-ih-**sill**-in/klah-view-**lan**-ate (Amoclan, Augmentin, Augmentin ES 600, Augmentin XR, Clavulin ✤)
Do not confuse Augmentin with Azulfidine.

◆ CLASSIFICATION

PHARMACOTHERAPEUTIC: Penicillin. **CLINICAL:** Antibiotic (see p. 29C).

ACTION

Amoxicillin inhibits bacterial cell wall synthesis. Clavulanate inhibits bacterial beta-lactamase. **Therapeutic Effect:** Amoxicillin is bactericidal in susceptible microorganisms. Clavulanate protects amoxicillin from enzymatic degradation.

PHARMACOKINETICS

Well absorbed from GI tract. Protein binding: 20%. Partially metabolized in liver. Primarily excreted in urine. Removed by hemodialysis. **Half-life:** 1–1.3 hrs (increased in renal impairment).

USES

Treatment of susceptible infections due to *streptococci, E. coli, E. faecalis, P. mirabilis,* beta-lactamase producing *H. influenzae, Klebsiella* spp., *M. catarrhalis*, and *S. aureus* (not methicillin-resistant *Staphylococcus aureus* [MRSA]) including lower respiratory, skin and skin structure, UTIs, otitis media, sinusitis. **OFF-LABEL:** Treatment of bronchitis, chancroid.

PRECAUTIONS

Contraindications: Hypersensitivity to any penicillins, infectious mononucleosis. **Cautions:** History of allergies, esp. cephalosporins; antibiotic-associated colitis.

⌛ LIFESPAN CONSIDERATIONS

Pregnancy/Lactation: Crosses placenta, appears in cord blood, amniotic fluid. Distributed in breast milk in low concentrations. May lead to allergic sensitization, diarrhea, candidiasis, skin rash in infant. **Pregnancy Category B. Children:** Immature renal function in neonate/young infant may delay renal excretion. **Elderly:** Age-related renal impairment may require dosage adjustment.

INTERACTIONS

DRUG: **Allopurinol** may increase incidence of rash. **Probenecid** may increase concentration, toxicity risk. May decrease effects of **oral contraceptives. HERBAL:** None significant. **FOOD:** None known. **LAB**

VALUES: May increase serum AST, ALT. May cause positive Coombs' test.

AVAILABILITY (Rx)

Powder for Oral Suspension (Amoclan, Augmentin): 125 mg–31.25 mg/5 ml, 200 mg–28.5 mg/5 ml, 250 mg–62.5 mg/5 ml, 400 mg–57 mg/5 ml, 600 mg–42.9 mg/5 ml. **Tablets (Augmentin):** 250 mg–125 mg, 500 mg–125 mg, 875 mg–125 mg. **Tablets (Chewable [Augmentin]):** 125 mg–31.25 mg, 200 mg–28.5 mg, 250 mg–62.5 mg, 400 mg–57 mg.

Tablets (Extended-Release [Augmentin XR]): 1,000 mg–62.5 mg.

ADMINISTRATION/HANDLING

PO

• Store tablets at room temperature. • After reconstitution, oral solution is stable for 10 days but should be refrigerated. • Give without regard to meals. • Instruct pt to chew/crush chewable tablets thoroughly before swallowing. • Do not crush extended-release tablets.

INDICATIONS/ROUTES/DOSAGE

Mild to Moderate Infections

PO: ADULTS, ELDERLY: 500 mg q12h or 250 mg q8h.

Severe Infections, Respiratory Tract Infections

PO: ADULTS, ELDERLY: 875 mg q12h or 500 mg q8h.

Community-Acquired Pneumonia, Sinusitis

PO: ADULTS, ELDERLY: 2 g (extended-release tablets) q12h for 7–10 days.

Usual Pediatric Dosage

PO: CHILDREN OLDER THAN 3 MOS, WEIGHING 40 KG OR LESS: 20–90 mg/kg/day divided q8–12h.

Otitis Media

PO: CHILDREN: 90 mg/kg/day (600 mg/5 ml suspension) in divided doses q12h for 10 days.

Usual Neonate Dosage

PO: NEONATES, CHILDREN YOUNGER THAN 3 MOS: 30 mg/kg/day (125 mg/5 ml suspension) in divided doses q12h.

Dosage in Renal Impairment

ALERT Do not use 875-mg tablet or extended-release tablets for creatinine clearance less than 30 ml/min.

Dosage and frequency are modified based on creatinine clearance. **Creatinine clearance 10–30 ml/min:** 250–500 mg q12h. **Creatinine clearance less than 10 ml/min:** 250–500 mg q24h.

SIDE EFFECTS

Frequent: GI disturbances (mild diarrhea, nausea, vomiting), headache, oral/vaginal candidiasis. **Occasional:** Generalized rash, urticaria.

ADVERSE EFFECTS/ TOXIC REACTIONS

Antibiotic-associated colitis, other superinfections (abdominal cramps, severe watery diarrhea, fever) may result from altered bacterial balance. Severe hypersensitivity reactions, including anaphylaxis, acute interstitial nephritis occur rarely.

NURSING CONSIDERATIONS

BASELINE ASSESSMENT

Question for history of allergies, esp. penicillins, cephalosporins.

INTERVENTION/EVALUATION

Hold medication and promptly report rash, diarrhea (fever, abdominal pain, mucus and blood in stool may indicate antibiotic-associated colitis). Be alert for signs of superinfection including fever, vomiting, diarrhea, black/hairy tongue, ulceration or changes of oral mucosa, anal/genital pruritus. Monitor renal/hepatic tests with prolonged therapy.

PATIENT/FAMILY TEACHING

• Continue antibiotic for full length of treatment. • Space doses evenly. • Take with meals if GI upset occurs. • Thoroughly chew the chewable tablets before swallowing. • Notify physician if rash, diarrhea, other new symptoms occur.

amphotericin B

HIGH ALERT

am-foe-**tear**-ih-sin
(Abelcet, AmBisome, Amphotec, Fungizone ✱)

BLACK BOX ALERT To be used primarily for pts with progressive, potentially fatal fungal infection. Not to be used for noninvasive forms of fungal disease (oral thrush, vaginal candidiasis).

◆CLASSIFICATION

CLINICAL: Antifungal, antiprotozoal.

ACTION

Generally fungistatic but may become fungicidal with high dosages or very susceptible microorganisms. Binds to sterols in fungal cell membrane. **Therapeutic Effect:** Increases fungal cell-membrane permeability, allowing loss of potassium, other cellular components, resulting in cell death.

PHARMACOKINETICS

Protein binding: 90%. Widely distributed. Metabolic fate unknown. Cleared by nonrenal pathways. Minimal removal by hemodialysis. Amphotec and Abelcet are not dialyzable. **Half-life:** Fungizone, 24 hrs (increased in neonates and children); Abelcet, 7.2 days; AmBisome, 100–153 hrs; Amphotec, 26–28 hrs.

USES

Abelcet: Treatment of aspergillosis or any type of invasive fungal infections refractory or intolerant to Fungizone. **AmBisome:** Empiric treatment of fungal infection in febrile neutropenic pts. *Aspergillus,* candida, *cryptococcus* infections refractory to Fungizone or pt with renal impairment or toxicity with Fungizone. Treatment of cryptococcal meningitis in HIV-infected pts. Treatment of visceral leishmaniasis. **Amphotec:** Treatment of invasive aspergillosis in pts with renal impairment or toxicity or prior treatment failure with Fungizone. **Fungizone:** Treatment of severe systemic and CNS infections caused by susceptible fungi including *Candida* spp., *Histoplasma, Cryptococcus, Aspergillus, Blastomyces.* Treatment of fungal peritonitis. **OFF-LABEL:** Febrile neutropenia, meningoencephalitis, paracoccidioidomycosis.

PRECAUTIONS

Contraindications: Hypersensitivity to amphotericin B or sulfites. **Cautions:** Renal impairment, in combination with antineoplastic therapy. Give only for progressive, potentially fatal fungal infection.

LIFESPAN CONSIDERATIONS

Pregnancy/Lactation: Crosses placenta; unknown if distributed in breast milk. **Pregnancy Category B. Children:** Safety and efficacy not established, but use the least amount for therapeutic regimen. **Elderly:** No age-related precautions noted.

INTERACTIONS

DRUG: Antineoplastic agents may increase potential for bronchospasm, renal toxicity, hypotension. **Steroids** may cause severe hypokalemia. **Bone marrow depressants** may worsen anemia. May increase **digoxin** toxity (due to hypokalemia). **Nephrotoxic medications** may increase nephrotoxicity. **HERBAL:** None significant. **FOOD:** None known. **LAB VALUES:** May increase serum AST, ALT, alkaline phosphatase, BUN, serum creatinine. May decrease serum calcium, magnesium, potassium.

AVAILABILITY (Rx)

Injection, Powder for Reconstitution: 50 mg (AmBisome, Amphotec, Fungizone), 100 mg (Amphotec). **Injection, Suspension (Abelcet):** 5 mg/ml.

ADMINISTRATION/HANDLING

IV

• Observe strict aseptic technique because no bacteriostatic agent or preservative is present in diluent.

Reconstitution

ABELCET

• Shake 20-ml (100-mg) vial gently until contents are dissolved. Withdraw required dose using 5-micron filter needle (supplied by manufacturer). • Dilute with D_5W to 1–2 mg/ml.

AMBISOME

• Reconstitute each 50-mg vial with 12 ml Sterile Water for Injection to provide concentration of 4 mg/ml. • Shake vial vigorously for 30 sec. Withdraw required dose and empty syringe contents through a 5-micron filter into an infusion of D_5W to provide final concentration of 1–2 mg/ml (0.2–0.5 mg/ml for infants and small children).

AMPHOTEC

• Add 10 ml Sterile Water for Injection to each 50-mg vial to provide concentration of 5 mg/ml. Shake gently. • Further dilute **only** with D_5W to a concentration of 0.1–2 mg/ml.

FUNGIZONE

• Add 10 ml Sterile Water for Injection to each 50-mg vial. • Further dilute with 250–500 ml D_5W. • Final concentration should not exceed 0.1 mg/ml (0.25 mg/ml for central infusion).

Rate of administration

• Give by slow IV infusion. Infuse conventional amphotericin over 4–6 hrs; Abelcet over 2 hrs (shake contents if infusion longer than 2 hrs); Amphotec over 2–4 hrs (avoid rate faster than 1 mg/kg/hr); AmBisome over 1–2 hrs.

Storage

ABELCET

• Refrigerate unreconstituted solution. Reconstituted solution is stable for 48 hrs if refrigerated, 6 hrs at room temperature.

AMBISOME

• Refrigerate unreconstituted solution. Reconstituted solution of 4 mg/ml is stable for 24 hrs. Concentration of 1–2 mg/ml is stable for 6 hrs.

AMPHOTEC

• Refrigerate intact vials. • Reconstituted solution is stable for 24 hrs if refrigerated.

FUNGIZONE

• Refrigerate intact vials. • Once reconstituted, vials stable for 24 hrs at room temperature, 7 days if refrigerated. • Diluted solutions stable for 24 hrs at room temperature, 2 days if refrigerated.

IV INCOMPATIBILITIES

Abelcet, AmBisome, Amphotec: Do not mix with any other drug, diluent, or solution. Fungizone: Allopurinol (Aloprim), amifostine (Ethyol), aztreonam (Azactam), calcium gluconate, cefepime (Maxipime), cimetidine (Tagamet), ciprofloxacin (Cipro), diphenhydramine (Benadryl), docetaxel (Taxotere), dopamine (Intropin), doxorubicin (Adriamycin), enalapril (Vasotec), etoposide (VP-16), filgrastim (Neupogen), fluconazole (Diflucan), fludarabine (Fludara), foscarnet (Foscavir), gemcitabine (Gemzar), lipids, magnesium sulfate, meperidine (Demerol), meropenem (Merrem IV), ondansetron (Zofran), paclitaxel (Taxol), piperacillin and tazobactam (Zosyn), potassium chloride, propofol (Diprivan), total parenteral nutrition (TPN), vinorelbine (Navelbine).

IV COMPATIBILITY

Lorazepam (Ativan).

INDICATIONS/ROUTES/DOSAGE

Usual Abelcet Dose

IV INFUSION (ABELCET): ADULTS, CHILDREN: 2.5–5 mg/kg/day at rate of 2.5 mg/kg/hr.

Usual AmBisome Dose

IV INFUSION (AMBISOME): ADULTS, CHILDREN: 3–6 mg/kg/day over 2 hrs.

Usual Amphotec Dose

IV INFUSION (AMPHOTEC): ADULTS, CHILDREN: 3–4 mg/kg/day at rate no faster than 1 mg/kg/hr. **Maximum:** 7.5 mg/kg/day.

Fungizone, Usual Dose

IV INFUSION: ADULTS, ELDERLY: Dosage based on pt tolerance and severity of infection. Initially, 1-mg test dose is given over 20–30 min. If test dose is tolerated, 0.25 mg/kg is given on same day and 0.5 mg/kg on second day; then dosage is increased until desired daily dose reached. Total daily dose: 1 mg/kg/day up to 1.5 mg/kg every other day. **Maximum:** 1.5 mg/kg/day. **CHILDREN:** Test dose of 0.1 mg/kg/dose (**Maximum:** 1 mg) is infused over 20–60 min. If test dose is tolerated, initial dose of 0.4 mg/kg may be given on same day; dosage is then increased in 0.25-mg/kg increments as needed. Maintenance dose: 0.25–1 mg/kg/day.

SIDE EFFECTS

Frequent (greater than 10%): **Abelcet:** Chills, fever, increased serum creatinine, multiple organ failure. **AmBisome:** Hypokalemia, hypomagnesemia, hyperglycemia, hypocalcemia, edema, abdominal pain, back pain, chills, chest pain, hypotension, diarrhea, nausea, vomiting, headache, fever, rigors, insomnia, dyspnea, epistaxis, increased hepatic/renal function test results. **Amphotec:** Chills, fever, hypotension, tachycardia, increased serum creatinine, hypokalemia, bilirubinemia. **Amphocin:** Fever, chills, headache, anemia, hypokalemia, hypomagnesemia, anorexia, malaise, generalized pain, nephrotoxicity.

ADVERSE EFFECTS/ TOXIC REACTIONS

Cardiovascular toxicity (hypotension, ventricular fibrillation), anaphylaxis occurs rarely. Altered vision/hearing, seizures, hepatic failure, coagulation defects, multiple organ failure, sepsis may be noted. Each alternative formulation is less nephrotoxic than conventional amphotericin (Amphocin).

NURSING CONSIDERATIONS

BASELINE ASSESSMENT

Question for history of allergies, esp. to amphotericin B, sulfite. Avoid, if possible, other nephrotoxic medications. Obtain premedication orders to reduce adverse reactions during IV therapy (antipyretics, antihistamines, antiemetics, corticosteroids).

INTERVENTION/EVALUATION

Monitor B/P, temperature, pulse, respirations; assess for adverse reactions (fever, tremors, chills, anorexia, nausea, vomiting, abdominal pain) q15min twice, then q30min for 4 hrs of initial infusion. If symptoms occur, slow infusion, administer medication for symptomatic relief. For severe reaction, stop infusion and notify physician. Evaluate IV site for phlebitis (heat, pain, red streaking over vein). Monitor I&O, renal function tests for nephrotoxicity. Check serum potassium and magnesium levels, hematologic and hepatic function test results.

PATIENT/FAMILY TEACHING

• Prolonged therapy (wks or mos) is usually necessary. • Fever reaction may decrease with continued therapy. • Muscle weakness may be noted during therapy (due to hypokalemia).

ampicillin

am-pi-**sill**-in
(Apo-Ampi ✱, Novo-Ampicillin ✱, Nu-Ampi ✱)
Do not confuse ampicillin with aminophylline.

◆ CLASSIFICATION

PHARMACOTHERAPEUTIC: Penicillin. **CLINICAL:** Antibiotic (see p. 29C).

ACTION

Inhibits cell wall synthesis in susceptible microorganisms. **Therapeutic Effect:** Bactericidal in susceptible microorganisms.

PHARMACOKINETICS

Moderately absorbed from GI tract. Protein binding: 15%–25%. Widely distributed. Partially metabolized in liver. Primarily excreted in urine. Removed by hemodialysis. **Half-life:** 1–1.5 hrs (increased in renal impairment).

USES

Treatment of susceptible infections due to *streptococci, S. pneumoniae, staphylococci* (non-penicillinase producing), *meningococci*, *Listeria*, some *Klebsiella*, *E. coli*, *H. influenzae*, *Salmonella*, *Shigella* including GI, GU, respiratory infections, meningitis, endocarditis prophylaxis.

PRECAUTIONS

Contraindications: Hypersensitivity to any penicillin, infectious mononucleosis. **Cautions:** History of allergies, esp. cephalosporins; antibiotic-associated colitis.

LIFESPAN CONSIDERATIONS

Pregnancy/Lactation: Crosses placenta; appears in cord blood, amniotic fluid. Distributed in breast milk in low concentrations. May lead to allergic sensitization, diarrhea, candidiasis, skin rash in infant. **Pregnancy Category B. Children:** Immature renal function in neonates/young infants may delay renal excretion. **Elderly:** Age-related renal impairment may require dosage adjustment.

INTERACTIONS

DRUG: Allopurinol may increase incidence of rash. **Probenecid** may increase concentration, toxicity risk. May decrease effects of **oral contraceptives. HERBAL:** None significant. **FOOD:** None known. **LAB VALUES:** May increase serum AST, ALT. May cause positive Coomb's test.

AVAILABILITY (Rx)

Capsules: 250 mg, 500 mg. **Injection, Powder for Reconsitution:** 125 mg, 250 mg, 500 mg, 1 g, 2 g. **Powder for Oral Suspension:** 125 mg/5 ml, 250 mg/5 ml.

ADMINISTRATION/HANDLING

IV

Reconstitution • For IV injection, dilute each vial with 5 ml Sterile Water for Injection or 0.9% NaCl (10 ml for 1- and 2-g vials). **Maximum concentration:** 100 mg/ml. • For intermittent IV infusion (piggyback), further dilute with 50–100 ml 0.9% NaCl. **Maximum concentration:** 30 mg/ml.

Rate of administration • For IV injection, give over 3–5 min (10–15 min for 1- to 2-g dose). • For intermittent IV infusion (piggyback), infuse over 15–30 min. • Due to potential for hypersensitivity/anaphylaxis, start initial dose at few drops per min, increase slowly to ordered rate; stay with pt first 10–15 min, then check q10min.

Storage • IV solution, diluted with 0.9% NaCl, is stable for 2–8 hrs at room temperature or 3 days if refrigerated. • If diluted with D_5W, is stable for 2 hrs at room temperature or 3 hrs if refrigerated. • Discard if precipitate forms.

IM

• Reconstitute each vial with Sterile Water for Injection or Bacteriostatic Water for Injection (consult individual vial for specific volume of diluent). • Stable for 1 hr. • Give deeply in large muscle mass.

PO

• Store capsules at room temperature. • Oral suspension, after reconstitution, is stable for 7 days at room temperature, 14 days if refrigerated. • Give orally 1 hr before or 2 hrs after meals for maximum absorption.

IV INCOMPATIBILITIES

Amikacin (Amikin), diltiazem (Cardizem), gentamicin, midazolam (Versed), ondansetron (Zofran).

IV COMPATIBILITIES

Calcium gluconate, cefepime (Maxipime), dopamine (Intropin), famotidine (Pepcid), furosemide (Lasix), heparin, hydromorphone (Dilaudid), insulin (regular), levofloxacin (Levaquin), lipids, magnesium sulfate, meperidine (Demerol), morphine, multivitamins, potassium chloride, propofol (Diprivan), total parenteral nutrition (TPN) (if ampicillin sodium concentration is less than 40 mg/ml).

INDICATIONS/ROUTES/DOSAGE

Usual Dosage

PO: ADULTS, ELDERLY: 250–500 mg q6h. **CHILDREN:** 50–100 mg/kg/day in divided doses q6h. **Maximum:** 2–3 g/day.
IV, IM: ADULTS, ELDERLY: 500 mg–3 g q4–6h. **Maximum:** 12 g/day. **CHILDREN:** 100–400 mg/kg/day in divided doses q6h. **Maximum:** 12 g/day. **NEONATES:** 50–100 mg/kg/day in divided doses q6–12h.

Dosage in Renal Impairment

Creatinine Clearance	Dosage
10–50 ml/min	Administer q6–12h
Less than 10 ml/min	Administer q12–24h

SIDE EFFECTS

Frequent: Pain at IM injection site, GI disturbances (mild diarrhea, nausea, vomiting), oral or vaginal candidiasis. **Occasional:** Generalized rash, urticaria, phlebitis or thrombophlebitis (with IV administration), headache. **Rare:** Dizziness, seizures (esp. with IV therapy).

ADVERSE EFFECTS/ TOXIC REACTIONS

Antibiotic-associated colitis, other superinfections (abdominal cramps, severe watery diarrhea, fever) may result from altered bacterial balance. Severe hypersensitivity reactions, including anaphylaxis, acute interstitial nephritis occur rarely.

NURSING CONSIDERATIONS

BASELINE ASSESSMENT

Question for history of allergies, esp. penicillins, cephalosporins.

INTERVENTION/EVALUATION

Hold medication and promptly report rash (although common with ampicillin, may indicate hypersensitivity) or diarrhea (fever, abdominal pain, mucus and blood in stool may indicate antibiotic-associated colitis). Evaluate IV site for phlebitis (heat, pain, red streaking over vein). Check IM injection site for pain, induration. Monitor I&O, urinalysis, renal function tests. Be alert for superinfection: fever, vomiting, diarrhea, anal/genital pruritus, oral mucosal changes (ulceration, pain, erythema).

PATIENT/FAMILY TEACHING

• Continue antibiotic for full length of treatment. • Space doses evenly. • More effective if taken 1 hr before or 2 hrs after food/beverages. • Discomfort may occur with IM injection. • Notify physician if rash, diarrhea, or other new symptoms occur.

ampicillin/ sulbactam

amp-ih-**sill**-in/sull-**bak**-tam
(Unasyn)

◆ CLASSIFICATION

PHARMACOTHERAPEUTIC: Penicillin.
CLINICAL: Antibiotic (see p. 29C).

ACTION

Ampicillin inhibits bacterial cell wall synthesis. Sulbactam inhibits bacterial beta-lactamase. **Therapeutic Effect:** Ampicillin is bactericidal in susceptible microorganisms. Sulbactam protects ampicillin from enzymatic degradation.

PHARMACOKINETICS

Protein binding: 28%–38%. Widely distributed. Partially metabolized in liver. Primarily excreted in urine. Removed by hemodialysis. **Half-life:** 1–1.3 hrs (increased in renal impairment).

USES

Treatment of susceptible infections, including intra-abdominal, skin/skin structure, gynecologic infections, due to beta-lactamase producing organisms including *H. influenzae, E. coli, Klebsiella, Acinetobacter, Enterobacter, S. aureus,* and *Bacteroides* spp.

PRECAUTIONS

Contraindications: Hypersensitivity to any penicillins or sulbactam, infectious mononucleosis. **Cautions:** History of allergies, esp. cephalosporins, antibiotic-associated colitis.

LIFESPAN CONSIDERATIONS

Pregnancy/Lactation: Crosses placenta; appears in cord blood, amniotic fluid. Distributed in breast milk in low concentrations. May lead to allergic sensitization, diarrhea, candidiasis, skin rash in infant. **Pregnancy Category B. Children:** Safety and efficacy not established in those younger than 1 yr. **Elderly:** Age-related renal impairment may require dosage adjustment.

INTERACTIONS

DRUG: Allopurinol may increase incidence of rash. **Probenecid** may increase concentration, toxicity risk. May decrease effects of oral contraceptives. **HERBAL:** None significant. **FOOD:** None known. **LAB VALUES:** May increase serum AST, ALT, alkaline phosphatase, LDH, creatinine. May cause positive Coomb's test.

AVAILABILITY (Rx)

Injection, Powder for Reconsitution: 1.5 g (ampicillin 1 g/sulbactam 500 g), 3 g (ampicillin 2 g/sulbactam 1 g).

ADMINISTRATION/HANDLING

IV

Reconstitution • For IV injection, dilute 1.5-g vial with 3.2 ml and 3-g vial with 6.4 ml Sterile Water for Injection to provide concentration of 375 mg/ml. • For intermittent IV infusion (piggyback), further dilute with 50–100 ml D_5W or 0.9% NaCl.

Rate of administration • For IV injection, give slowly over minimum of 10–15 min. • For intermittent IV infusion (piggyback), infuse over 15–30 min. • Due to potential for hypersensitivity/anaphylaxis, start initial dose at few drops per min, increase slowly to ordered rate; stay with pt first 10–15 min, then check q10min.

Storage • IV solution, diluted with 0.9% NaCl, is stable for 8 hrs at room temperature, 72 hrs if refrigerated. • Discard if precipitate forms.

IM

• Reconstitute each 1.5-g vial with 3.2 ml Sterile Water for Injection or lidocaine to provide concentration of 250 mg ampicillin/125 mg sulbactam/ml. • Give deeply into large muscle mass within 1 hr after preparation.

IV INCOMPATIBILITIES

Diltiazem (Cardizem), idarubicin (Idamycin), ondansetron (Zofran), sargramostim (Leukine), total parenteral nutrition (TPN).

IV COMPATIBILITIES

Famotidine (Pepcid), heparin, insulin (regular), lipids, meperidine (Demerol), morphine.

INDICATIONS/ROUTES/DOSAGE

Usual Dosage Range

IV, IM: ADULTS, ELDERLY, CHILDREN 13 YRS AND OLDER: 1.5 g (1 g ampicillin/500 mg sulbactam) to 3 g (2 g ampicillin/1 g sulbactam) q6h. **Maximum:** 12 g/day (Unasyn). **IV: CHILDREN 12 YRS AND YOUNGER:** 100–400 mg ampicillin/kg/day in divided doses q6h. **Maximum:** 12 g/day (Unasyn).

Dosage in Renal Impairment
Dosage and frequency are modified based on creatinine clearance and severity of infection.

Creatinine Clearance	Dosage
Greater than 30 ml/min	1.5–3 g q6–8h
15–30 ml/min	1.5–3 g q12h
5–14 ml/min	1.5–3 g q24h

SIDE EFFECTS

Frequent: Diarrhea, rash (most common), urticaria, pain at IM injection site, thrombophlebitis with IV administration, oral or vaginal candidiasis. **Occasional:** Nausea, vomiting, headache, malaise, urinary retention.

ADVERSE EFFECTS/ TOXIC REACTIONS

Antibiotic-associated colitis, other superinfections (abdominal cramps; severe, watery diarrhea; fever) may result from altered bacterial balance. Severe hypersensitivity reactions, including anaphylaxis, acute interstitial nephritis, blood dyscrasias, may occur. High dosage may produce seizures.

NURSING CONSIDERATIONS

BASELINE ASSESSMENT

Question for history of allergies, esp. penicillins, cephalosporins.

INTERVENTION/EVALUATION

Hold medication and promptly report rash (although common with ampicillin, may indicate hypersensitivity) or diarrhea (fever, abdominal pain, mucus and blood in stool may indicate antibiotic-associated colitis). Evaluate IV site for phlebitis (heat, pain, red streaking over vein). Check IM injection site for pain, induration. Monitor I&O, urinalysis, renal function tests. Be alert for superinfection: fever, vomiting, diarrhea, anal/genital pruritus, oral mucosal changes (ulceration, pain, erythema).

PATIENT/FAMILY TEACHING

• Take antibiotic for full length of treatment. • Space doses evenly. • Discomfort may occur with IM injection. • Notify physician if rash, diarrhea, or other new symptoms occur.

anakinra

an-a-**kin**-ra
(Kineret)
Do not confuse anakinra with amikacin.

◆ CLASSIFICATION

PHARMACOTHERAPEUTIC: Interleukin-1 receptor antagonist. **CLINICAL:** Anti-inflammatory.

ACTION

Blocks the binding of interleukin-1 (IL-1), a protein that is a major mediator of joint pathology and is present in excess amounts in pts with rheumatoid arthritis. **Therapeutic Effect:** Inhibits inflammatory response.

PHARMACOKINETICS

No accumulation of anakinra in tissues or organs was observed after daily subcutaneous doses. Excreted in urine. **Half-life:** 4–6 hrs.

USES

Treatment of signs and symptoms or to slow progression of structural damage of moderate to severely active rheumatoid arthritis (RA) in pts who have failed treatment with one or more disease-modifying antirheumatic drugs. May use alone or with other disease-modifying antirheumatic drugs.

PRECAUTIONS

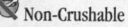

Contraindications: Known hypersensitivity to *Escherichia coli*-derived proteins, serious infection. **Cautions:** Renal impairment (risk of toxic reaction is increased), asthma (higher incidence of serious infection).

LIFESPAN CONSIDERATIONS

Pregnancy/Lactation: Unknown if distributed in breast milk. **Pregnancy Category B. Children:** Safety and efficacy not established. **Elderly:** Age-related renal impairment may require caution.

INTERACTIONS

DRUG: Live/inactive virus vaccines may be ineffective. Increased risk of infection with **etanercept. HERBAL:** None significant. **FOOD:** None known. **LAB VALUES:** May decrease WBC count, platelet count, absolute neutrophil count (ANC). May increase eosinophil count.

AVAILABILITY (Rx)

Injection Solution: 100-mg syringe.

ADMINISTRATION/HANDLING

Subcutaneous

• Store in refrigerator; do not freeze or shake. • Do not use if particulate or discoloration is noted. • Give by subcutaneous route.

INDICATIONS/ROUTES/DOSAGE

Rheumatoid Arthritis (RA)

SUBCUTANEOUS: ADULTS, ELDERLY: 100 mg/day, given at same time each day.

Dosage in Renal Impairment

Creatinine clearance less than 30 ml/min and/or end-stage renal disease: 100 mg every other day.

SIDE EFFECTS

Occasional: Injection site ecchymosis, erythema, inflammation. **Rare:** Headache, nausea, diarrhea, abdominal pain.

ADVERSE EFFECTS/ TOXIC REACTIONS

Infections, including upper respiratory tract infection, sinusitis, flu-like symptoms, and cellulitis, have been noted. Neutropenia may occur, particularly when anakinra is used in combination with tumor necrosis factor-blocking agents.

NURSING CONSIDERATIONS

BASELINE ASSESSMENT

Assess pt's range of motion, pain, swelling in joints.

INTERVENTION/EVALUATION

Monitor neutrophil count before therapy begins, monthly for 3 mos while receiving therapy, then quarterly for up to 1 yr. Assess for hypersensitivity reaction, esp. during first 4 wks of therapy (uncommon after first mo of therapy).

PATIENT/FAMILY TEACHING

• Follow dosage and administration procedures carefully. • Dispose of syringes and needles properly. • Avoid live virus vaccines during therapy.

anastrozole

HIGH ALERT

ah-**nas**-trow-zole

(Arimidex)

Do not confuse Arimidex with Imitrex, or anastrozole with letrozole.

CLASSIFICATION

PHARMACOTHERAPEUTIC: Aromatase inhibitor. **CLINICAL:** Antineoplastic hormone (see p. 80C).

ACTION

Decreases circulating estrogen level by inhibiting aromatase, the enzyme that catalyzes the final step in estrogen production. **Therapeutic Effect:** Inhibits growth of breast cancers that are stimulated by estrogens by lowering serum estradiol concentration.

PHARMACOKINETICS

Well absorbed into systemic circulation (absorption not affected by food). Protein binding: 40%. Extensively metabolized in liver. Eliminated by biliary system and, to a lesser extent, kidneys. **Mean half-life:** 50 hrs in postmenopausal women. Steady-state plasma levels reached in about 7 days.

USES

Treatment of advanced breast cancer in postmenopausal women who have developed progressive disease while receiving tamoxifen therapy. First-line therapy in advanced or metastatic breast cancer in postmenopausal women. Adjuvant treatment in early breast cancer in postmenopausal women.

PRECAUTIONS

Contraindications: Pregnancy. Cautions: None known.

LIFESPAN CONSIDERATIONS

Pregnancy/Lactation: Crosses placenta; may cause fetal harm. Unknown if distributed in breast milk. **Pregnancy Category D. Children:** Safety and efficacy not established. **Elderly:** No age-related precautions noted.

INTERACTIONS

DRUG: **Estrogen therapies** may reduce efficacy. **Tamoxifen** may reduce plasma concentration. HERBAL: Avoid **black cohosh, dong quai, licorice, red clover.** FOOD: None known. LAB VALUES: May elevate serum GGT level in pts with liver metastases. May increase serum AST, ALT, alkaline phosphate, total cholesterol, LDL.

AVAILABILITY (Rx)

Tablets: 1 mg.

ADMINISTRATION/HANDLING

PO

- Give without regard to food.

INDICATIONS/ROUTES/DOSAGE

Breast Cancer

PO: ADULTS, ELDERLY: 1 mg once a day.

SIDE EFFECTS

Frequent (16%–8%): Asthenia, nausea, headache, hot flashes, back pain, vomiting, cough, diarrhea. Occasional (6%–4%): Constipation, abdominal pain, anorexia, bone pain, pharyngitis, dizziness, rash, dry mouth, peripheral edema, pelvic pain, depression, chest pain, paresthesia. Rare (2%–1%): Weight gain, diaphoresis.

ADVERSE EFFECTS/ TOXIC REACTIONS

Thrombophlebitis, anemia, leukopenia occur rarely. Vaginal hemorrhage occurs rarely (2%).

NURSING CONSIDERATIONS

INTERVENTION/EVALUATION

Monitor for asthenia (loss of strength, energy) and dizziness and assist with ambulation if needed. Assess for headache, pain. Offer antiemetic for nausea, vomiting. Monitor for onset of diarrhea; offer antidiarrheal medication.

PATIENT/FAMILY TEACHING

- Notify physician if nausea, asthenia, hot flashes become unmanageable.

Ancef, *see cefazolin*

AndroGel, *see testosterone*

Angiomax, *see bivalirudin*

anidulafungin

a-nid-you-lah-**fun**-gin
(Eraxis)

CLASSIFICATION

PHARMACOTHERAPEUTIC: Echinocandin. **CLINICAL:** Antifungal.

ACTION

Inhibits synthesis of the enzyme glucan, (vital component of fungal cell formation), preventing fungal cell wall formation. **Therapeutic Effect:** Fungistatic.

PHARMACOKINETICS

Distributed in tissue. Moderately bound to albumin. Protein binding: 84%–99%. Slow chemical degradation; 30% excreted in feces over 9 days. Not removed by hemodialysis. **Half-life:** 40–50 hrs.

USES

Treatment of candidemia, other forms of *Candida* infections (intra-abdominal abscess, peritonitis), esophageal candidiasis. **OFF-LABEL:** Treatment of infections due to *Aspergillus*.

PRECAUTIONS

Contraindications: Hypersensitivity to anidulafungin, other echinocandins. **Cautions:** Hepatic impairment, myelosuppression, renal insufficiency.

LIFESPAN CONSIDERATIONS

Pregnancy/Lactation: May be embryotoxic. Crosses placental barrier. Unknown if distributed in breast milk. **Pregnancy Category C. Children:** Safety and efficacy not established. **Elderly:** No age-related precautions noted.

INTERACTIONS

DRUG: None significant. **HERBAL:** None significant. **FOOD:** None known. **LAB VALUES:** May increase serum ALT, AST, bilirubin, alkaline phosphatase, LDH, transferase, amylase, lipase, CPK, creatinine, calcium. May decrease serum albumin, bicarbonate, magnesium, protein, potassium, Hgb, Hct, WBCs, neutrophils, platelet count. May prolong prothrombin time (PT).

AVAILABILITY (Rx)

Injection, Powder for Reconsitution: 50-mg vial, 100-mg vial.

ADMINISTRATION/HANDLING

IV

Reconstitution • Reconstitute each 50-mg vial with 15 ml of companion diluent (20% dehydrated alcohol in Sterile Water for Injection) (100 mg with 30 ml). • Further dilute 50 mg with 100 ml D_5W or 0.9% NaCl (100 mg with 250 ml, 200 mg with 500 ml).

Rate of administration • Do not exceed infusion rate of 1.1 mg/min. Not for IV bolus injection.

Storage • May store unreconstituted vials or reconstituted vials with companion diluent at room temperature. • Final reconstituted infusion solution must be used within 24 hrs.

IV INCOMPATIBILITIES

Amphotericin B (Abelcet, AmBisome), ertapenem (Invanz), sodium bicarbonate.

IV COMPATIBILITIES

Dexamethasone (Decadron), famotidine (Pepcid), furosemide (Lasix), hydromorphone (Dilaudid), lorazepam (Ativan), meperidine (Demerol), methylprednisolone (Solu-Medrol), morphine.

INDICATIONS/ROUTES/DOSAGE

ALERT Duration of treatment based on pt's clinical response. In general, treatment is continued for at least 14 days after last positive culture.

Candidemia, Other Candida Infections

IV: ADULTS, ELDERLY: Give single 200-mg loading dose on day 1, followed by 100 mg/day thereafter for at least 14 days after last positive culture.

Esophageal Candidiasis

IV: ADULTS, ELDERLY: Give single 100-mg loading dose on day 1, followed by 50 mg/day thereafter for a minimum of 14 days and for at least 7 days following resolution of symptoms.

SIDE EFFECTS

Rare (3%–1%): Diarrhea, nausea, headache, rigors, peripheral edema.

ADVERSE EFFECTS/ TOXIC REACTIONS

Hypokalemia occurs in 4% of pts. Hypersensitivity reaction characterized by facial flushing, hypotension, pruritus, urticaria, rash occurs rarely.

NURSING CONSIDERATIONS

BASELINE ASSESSMENT

Obtain specimens for fungal culture prior to therapy. Treatment may be instituted before results are known. Obtain baseline hepatic enzyme levels.

INTERVENTION/EVALUATION

Monitor serum chemistry results for evidence of hepatic dysfunction, hypokalemia. Monitor daily pattern of bowel activity and stool consistency. Assess for rash, urticaria.

PATIENT/FAMILY TEACHING

- For esophageal candidiasis, maintain diligent oral hygiene.

antihemophilic factor (factor VIII, AHF)

an-tee-hee-moe-**fill**-ick **fak**-tor
(**Antihemophilic Factor/von Willebrand Factor Complex:** Alphanate, Humate-P. **Human:** Hemofil M, Koate-DVI, Monarc M, Monoclate-P. **Recombinant:** Advate, Hexilate FS, Kogenate FS, Recombinate, Refacto, Xyntha)

◆CLASSIFICATION

PHARMACOTHERAPEUTIC: Antihemophilic agent. **CLINICAL:** Hemostatic.

ACTION

Assists in conversion of prothrombin to thrombin, essential for blood coagulation. Replaces missing clotting factor VIII. **Therapeutic Effect:** Produces hemostasis; corrects or prevents bleeding episodes.

PHARMACOKINETICS

Half-life: 8–27 hrs.

USES

Human: Prevention/treatment of hemorrhagic episodes, perioperative management of hemophilia A. **Alphanate, Humate-P:** Prevention/treatment of hemorrhagic episodes in pts with hemophilia A. Prophylaxis with surgical/invasive procedures, treatment of bleeding in pts with von Willebrand disease (vWD) when desmopressin is known or suspected to be inadequate. **Recombinant:** Management of hemophilia A, prevention and control of bleeding episodes, perioperative management of hemophilia A, prophylaxis of joint bleeding and reduce risk of joint damage in children with hemophilia A. OFF-LABEL: Treatment of disseminated intravascular coagulation.

PRECAUTIONS

Contraindications: None known. **Cautions:** Hepatic disease, those with blood types A, B, AB.

⌛ LIFESPAN CONSIDERATIONS

Pregnancy/Lactation: Unknown if drug crosses placenta or is distributed in breast milk. **Pregnancy Category C. Children:** Safety and efficacy not established. **Elderly:** No age-related precautions noted.

INTERACTIONS

DRUG: None significant. **HERBAL:** None significant. **FOOD:** None known. **LAB VALUES:** None significant.

AVAILABILITY (Rx)

Human: Injection, Powder for Reconsitution (Hemofil M, Koate-DVI, Monarc-M, Mono-

clate-P): Actual number of units listed on each vial. Alphanate: 250 units, 500 units, 1,000 units, 1,500 units. Humate-P: 250 units, 500 units, 1,000 units. Recombinant: Injection, Powder for Reconsitution: Advate: 250 units, 500 units, 1,000 units, 1,500 units, 2,000 units, 3,000 units. Hexilate, Kogenate, Recombinate: 250 units, 500 units, 1,000 units. Refacto, Xyntha: 250 units, 500 units, 1,000 units, 2,000 units.

ADMINISTRATION/HANDLING

IV

Reconstitution • Warm concentrate and diluent to room temperature. • Using needle supplied by the manufacturer, add diluent to powder to dissolve, gently agitate or rotate. Do not shake vigorously. Complete dissolution may take 5–10 min. • Use second filtered needle supplied by the manufacturer, and add to infusion bag.
Rate of administration • **Advate:** Over 5 min or less. **Maximum:** 10 ml/min. • **Hexilate FS, Kogenate FS:** Over 1–15 min based on pt tolerance. • **Xyntha:** Over several min. • **Hemafil M, Koate-DVI, Monarc M:** Over 5–10 min. **Maximum:** 10 ml/min. • **Monoclate-P:** Infuse at 2 ml/min. • **Alphanate:** 10 ml/min. **Humate-P:** 4 ml/min.
Administration precautions • Check pulse rate prior to and following administration. If pulse rate increases, reduce or stop administration. • After administration, apply prolonged pressure on venipuncture site. • Monitor IV site for oozing q5–15min for 1–2 hrs following administration.
Storage • May refrigerate or store at room temperature. • Use within 3 hrs following reconstitution.

IV INCOMPATIBILITIES

Do not mix with other IV solutions or medications.

INDICATIONS/ROUTES/DOSAGE

Hemophilia A, Von Willebrand Disease
IV: ADULTS, ELDERLY, CHILDREN: Dosage is highly individualized and is based on pt's weight, severity of bleeding, coagulation studies.

SIDE EFFECTS

Occasional: Allergic reaction, including fever, chills, urticaria, wheezing, hypotension, nausea, feeling of chest tightness; stinging at injection site; dizziness; dry mouth; headache; altered taste.

ADVERSE EFFECTS/ TOXIC REACTIONS

Risk of transmitting viral hepatitis. Intravascular hemolysis may occur if large or frequent doses are used with blood group A, B, or AB.

NURSING CONSIDERATIONS

BASELINE ASSESSMENT

When monitoring B/P, avoid overinflation of cuff. Remove adhesive tape from any pressure dressing very carefully and slowly.

INTERVENTION/EVALUATION

Following IV administration, apply prolonged pressure on venipuncture site. Monitor IV site for oozing q5–15 min for 1–2 hrs following administration. Assess for allergic reaction. Report immediately any evidence of hematuria or change in vital signs. Assess for decreases in B/P, increased pulse rate, complaint of abdominal or back pain, severe headache (may be evidence of hemorrhage). Question for increased discharge during menses. Assess skin for bruises, petechiae. Check for excessive bleeding from minor cuts, scratches. Assess gums for erythema, gingival bleeding. Assess urine for hematuria. Evaluate for therapeutic relief of pain, reduction of swelling, restricted joint movement.

PATIENT/FAMILY TEACHING

• Use electric razor, soft toothbrush to prevent bleeding. • Report any sign of bleeding, including red or dark urine, black/red stool, coffee-ground vomitus, blood-tinged mucus from cough. • Wear identification indicating a hemolytic condition. • Bring adequate supply of agent when traveling.

Antivert, *see meclizine*

aprepitant/ fosaprepitant

ah-**prep**-ih-tant
(Emend, Emend for Injection)

◆CLASSIFICATION

PHARMACOTHERAPEUTIC: Selective receptor antagonist. **CLINICAL:** Antinausea, antiemetic.

ACTION

Inhibits chemotherapy-induced nausea, vomiting centrally in the chemoreceptor trigger zone. **Therapeutic Effect:** Prevents acute and delayed phases of chemotherapy-induced emesis, including vomiting caused by high-dose cisplatin.

PHARMACOKINETICS

Moderately absorbed from GI tract. Crosses blood-brain barrier. Extensively metabolized in liver. Protein binding: greater than 95%. Eliminated primarily by liver metabolism (not excreted renally). **Half-life:** 9–13 hrs.

USES

PO/IV: Prevention of nausea, vomiting associated with repeat courses of moderate to high emetogenic cancer chemotherapy, including high-dose cisplatin. **PO:** Prevention of postop nausea, vomiting.

PRECAUTIONS

Contraindications: Breast-feeding, concurrent use of astemizole, cisapride, pimozide, terfenadine. **Cautions:** None known.

LIFESPAN CONSIDERATIONS

Pregnancy/Lactation: Unknown if drug crosses placenta or is distributed in breast milk. **Pregnancy Category B. Children:** Safety and efficacy not established. **Elderly:** No age-related precautions noted.

INTERACTIONS

DRUG: May elevate plasma concentrations of **alprazolam, docetaxel, etoposide, ifosfamide, imatinib, irinotecan, midazolam, paclitaxol, triazolam, vinblastine, vincristine, vinorelbine.** May decrease effectiveness of **contraceptives.** Increases effects of **corticosteroids** (IV steroid dose should be reduced by 25%, PO dose by 50%). **Paroxetine** may decrease effectiveness of either drug. May decrease effectiveness of **warfarin. HERBAL: St. John's wort** may decrease plasma concentration. **FOOD: Grapefruit, grapefruit juice** may increase plasma concentration. **LAB VALUES:** May increase BUN, serum creatinine, glucose, alkaline phosphatase, AST, ALT. May produce proteinuria.

AVAILABILITY (Rx)

Capsules (Emend): 40 mg, 80 mg, 125 mg. **Emend (Combination):** 80 mg (2), 125 mg (1). **Injection, Powder for Reconstitution (Fosaprepitant):** 115-mg single-dose vial.

ADMINISTRATION/HANDLING

PO

• Give without regard to food.

IV

Reconstitution • Reconstitute each vial with 5 ml 0.9% NaCl. • Add to 110 ml 0.9% NaCl to provide a final concentration of 1 mg/ml.

Rate of administration • Infuse over 15 min 30 min prior to chemotherapy.

Storage • Store vials at room temperature. • After reconstitution, solution is stable at room temperature for 24 hrs.

IV INCOMPATIBILITIES

Do not infuse with any solutions containing calcium or magnesium.

INDICATIONS/ROUTES/DOSAGE

Prevention of Chemotherapy-Induced Nausea, Vomiting

PO: ADULTS, ELDERLY: 125 mg 1 hr before chemotherapy on day 1 and 80 mg once a day in the morning on days 2 and 3. **Note:** Emend for Injection 115 mg may be substituted for Emend 125 mg on day 1 only.

Prevention of Postop Nausea, Vomiting

PO: ADULTS, ELDERLY: 40 mg once within 3 hrs prior to induction of anesthesia.

SIDE EFFECTS

Frequent (17%–10%): Fatigue, nausea, hiccups, diarrhea, constipation, anorexia. **Occasional (8%–4%):** Headache, vomiting, dizziness, dehydration, heartburn. **Rare (3% or less):** Abdominal pain, epigastric discomfort, gastritis, tinnitus, insomnia.

ADVERSE EFFECTS/ TOXIC REACTIONS

Neutropenia, mucous membrane disorders occur rarely.

NURSING CONSIDERATIONS

BASELINE ASSESSMENT

Assess for dehydration if excessive vomiting occurs (poor skin turgor, dry mucous membranes, longitudinal furrows in tongue).

INTERVENTION/EVALUATION

Monitor hydration, nutritional status, I&O. Assess bowel sounds for peristalsis. Assist with ambulation if dizziness occurs. Provide supportive measures. Monitor daily pattern of bowel activity and stool consistency. Record time of evacuation.

PATIENT/FAMILY TEACHING

- Relief from nausea/vomiting generally occurs shortly after drug administration.
- Report persistent vomiting, headache.
- May decrease effectiveness of oral contraceptives.

Aptivus, *see tipranavir*

Aranesp, *see darbepoetin alfa*

Arava, *see leflunomide*

Aredia, *see pamidronate*

argatroban

HIGH ALERT

our-ga-**trow**-ban

Do not confuse argatroban with Aggrestat.

◆ CLASSIFICATION

PHARMACOTHERAPEUTIC: Thrombin inhibitor. **CLINICAL:** Anticoagulant.

ACTION

Direct thrombin inhibitor that reversibly binds to thrombin-active sites. Inhibits thrombin-catalyzed or thrombin-induced reactions, including fibrin formation, activation of coagulant factors V, VIII, and XIII; inhibits protein C formation, platelet aggregation. **Therapeutic Effect:** Produces anticoagulation.

PHARMACOKINETICS

Following IV administration, distributed primarily in extracellular fluid. Protein binding: 54%. Metabolized in liver. Primarily excreted in the feces, presumably through biliary secretion. **Half-life:** 39–51 min.

USES

Prophylaxis or treatment of thrombosis in heparin-induced thrombocytopenia (HIT). Prevention of HIT during percutaneous coronary procedures. OFF-LABEL: Cerebral thrombosis, MI. Maintain extrocorporeal circuit patency of continuous renal replacement therapy (CRRT) in pts with HIT.

PRECAUTIONS

Contraindications: Overt major bleeding. Cautions: Severe hypertension, immediately following lumbar puncture, spinal anesthesia, major surgery, pts with congenital or acquired bleeding disorders, ulcerations, hepatic impairment.

LIFESPAN CONSIDERATIONS

Pregnancy/Lactation: Unknown if excreted in breast milk. **Pregnancy Category C.** **Children:** Safety and efficacy not established in those younger than 18 yrs. **Elderly:** No age-related precautions noted.

INTERACTIONS

DRUG: **Antiplatelet agents, other anticoagulants, thrombolytics** may increase the risk of bleeding. HERBAL: **Dong quai, evening primrose oil, ginkgo, policosanol, willow bark** may increase risk of bleeding. FOOD: None known. LAB VALUES: Increases prothrombin time (PT), activated partial thromboplastin time (aPTT), international normalized ratio (INR). May increase Hgb, Hct.

AVAILABILITY (Rx)

Injection Solution: 100 mg/ml (2.5 ml).

ADMINISTRATION/HANDLING

IV

Reconstitution • Dilute each 250-mg vial with 250 ml 0.9% NaCl, D_5W, or lactated Ringer's solution to provide a final concentration of 1 mg/ml. • The solution must be mixed by repeated inversion of the diluent bag for 1 min. • After reconstitution, solution may show a brief haziness due to formation of microprecipitates that rapidly dissolve upon mixing.

Rate of administration • Rate of administration is based on body weight at 2 mcg/kg/min (e.g., 50-kg pt infuse at 6 ml/hr).

Storage • Discard if solution appears cloudy or an insoluble precipitate is noted. • Following reconstitution, stable for 96 hrs at room temperature or refrigerated. • Avoid direct sunlight.

IV INCOMPATIBILITY

Amiodarone (Cardarone).

IV COMPATIBILITIES

Diphenhydramine (Benadryl), dobutamine (Dobutrex), dopamine (Intropin), furosemide (Lasix), midazolam (Versed), morphine, vasopressin (Pitressin).

INDICATIONS/ROUTES/DOSAGE

Heparin-Induced Thrombocytopenia (HIT)

IV INFUSION: ADULTS, ELDERLY: Initially, 2 mcg/kg/min administered as a continuous infusion. After initial infusion, dose may be adjusted until steady-state aPTT is 1.5–3 times initial baseline value, not to exceed 100 sec. Dosage should not exceed 10 mcg/kg/min.

Percutaneous Coronary Intervention

IV INFUSION: ADULTS, ELDERLY: Initially, administer bolus of 350 mcg/kg over 3–5 min, then infuse at 25 mcg/kg/min. Check ACT (activated clotting time) 5–10 min following bolus. If ACT is less than 300 sec, give additional bolus 150 mcg/kg, increase infusion to 30 mcg/kg/min. If ACT is greater than 450 sec, decrease infusion to 15 mcg/kg/min. Once ACT of 300–450 sec achieved, proceed with procedure.

Dosage in Hepatic Impairment

ADULTS, ELDERLY: Initially, 0.5 mcg/kg/min. **CHILDREN:** Initially, 0.2 mcg/kg/min.

SIDE EFFECTS

Frequent (8%–3%): Dyspnea, hypotension, fever, diarrhea, nausea, pain, vomiting, infection, cough.

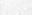

ADVERSE EFFECTS/ TOXIC REACTIONS

Ventricular tachycardia, atrial fibrillation occur occasionally. Major bleeding, sepsis occur rarely.

NURSING CONSIDERATIONS

BASELINE ASSESSMENT

Check CBC, including platelet count, PT, PTT. Determine initial B/P. Minimize need for numerous injection sites, blood draws, catheters.

INTERVENTION/EVALUATION

Assess for any sign of bleeding: bleeding at surgical site, hematuria, blood in stool, bleeding from gums, petechiae, ecchymoses, bleeding from injection sites. Handle pt carefully and infrequently to prevent bleeding. Do not obtain B/P in lower extremities (possible deep vein thrombi). Assess for decreased B/P, increased pulse rate, complaint of abdominal/back pain, severe headache (indicates evidence of hemorrhage). Monitor ACT, PT, aPTT, platelet count, Hgb, Hct. Question for increase in discharge during menses. Assess urinary output for hematuria. Observe skin for any occurring ecchymoses, petechiae, hematoma. Use care in removing any dressing, tape.

PATIENT/FAMILY TEACHING

• Use electric razor, soft toothbrush to prevent bleeding. • Report any sign of bleeding, including red/dark urine, black/red stool, coffee-ground vomitus, blood-tinged mucus from cough.

Aricept, *see donepezil*

Arimidex, *see anastrozole*

aripiprazole

air-ee-**pip**-rah-zole
(Abilify, Abilify Discmelt)

BLACK BOX ALERT Increased risk of mortality in elderly pts with dementia-related psychosis, mainly due to pneumonia, heart failure. Risk may be increased by dehydration. Increased risk of suicidal thinking and behavior in children, adolescents, young adults 18–24 yrs with major depressive disorder, other psychiatric disorders.

Do not confuse aripiprazole with esomeprazole, omeprazole, or pantoprazole (proton pump inhibitors).

◆CLASSIFICATION

PHARMACOTHERAPEUTIC: Dopamine agonist. **CLINICAL:** Antipsychotic agent.

ACTION

Provides partial agonist activity at dopamine and serotonin ($5\text{-}HT_{1A}$) receptors and antagonist activity at serotonin ($5\text{-}HT_{2A}$) receptors. **Therapeutic Effect:** Diminishes schizophrenic behavior.

PHARMACOKINETICS

Well absorbed through GI tract. Protein binding: 99% (primarily albumin). Reaches steady levels in 2 wks. Metabolized in liver. Eliminated primarily in feces and, to a lesser extent, in urine. Not removed by hemodialysis. **Half-life:** 75 hrs.

USES

Treatment of schizophrenia. Maintains stability in pts with schizophrenia. Treatment of bipolar disorder. Adjunct treatment in major depressive disorder. Treatment of irritability associated with autistic disorder in children 6–17 yrs of age. **IM:** Agitation associated with schizophrenia/bipolar disorder. **OFF-LABEL:** Schizoaffective disorder, depression with psychotic features, aggression, bipolar disorder (children), conduct disorder (children), Tourette syndrome (children), psychosis/agitation related to Alzheimer's dementia.

PRECAUTIONS

Contraindications: None known. **Cautions:** Concurrent use of CNS depressants (including alcohol), cardiovascular or cerebrovascular diseases (may induce hypotension), Parkinson's disease (potential for exacerbation), history of seizures or conditions that may lower seizure threshold (Alzheimer's disease), renal/hepatic impairment. May prolong QT interval.

LIFESPAN CONSIDERATIONS

Pregnancy/Lactation: Unknown if drug crosses placenta. May be distributed in breast milk. Breast-feeding not recommended. **Pregnancy Category C. Children:** Safety and efficacy not established. **Elderly:** No age-related precautions noted.

INTERACTIONS

DRUG: **Alcohol** may potentiate cognitive and motor effects. **Carbamazepine** may decrease concentration. **Fluoxetine, itraconazole, ketoconazole, paroxetine, quinidine** may increase concentrations. **HERBAL:** **St. John's wort** may decrease levels. **Gotu kola, kava kava, St. John's wort, valerian** may increase CNS depression. **FOOD:** None known. **LAB VALUES:** None significant.

AVAILABILITY (Rx)

Injection, Solution: 9.75 mg/1.3 ml (7.5 mg/ml). **Solution, PO:** 1 mg/ml. **Tablets:** 2 mg, 5 mg, 10 mg, 15 mg, 20 mg, 30 mg. **Tablets, Orally-Disintegrating:** 10 mg, 15 mg.

ADMINISTRATION/HANDLING

IM

• For IM use only (inject slowly into muscle mass). Do not administer IV or subcutaneous.

PO

• Give without regard to food.

Orally-Disintegrating Tablet

• Remove tablet, place entire tablet on tongue. • Do not break, split tablet. • May give without liquid.

INDICATIONS/ROUTES/DOSAGE

Schizophrenia

PO: ADULTS, ELDERLY: Initially, 10–15 mg once a day. May increase up to 30 mg/day. Titrate dose at minimum of 2-wk intervals. **CHILDREN 13–17 YRS:** Initially, 2 mg/day for 2 days, then 5 mg/day for 2 days. May further increase to target dose of 10 mg/day. May then increase in increments of 5 mg up to maximum of 30 mg/day.

Bipolar Disorder

PO: ADULTS, ELDERLY: 15 mg once a day. May increase to 30 mg/day based on pt tolerance. **CHILDREN 10–17 YRS:** Initially, 2 mg/day for 2 days, then 5 mg/day for 2 days. Give subsequent dose increases in 5-mg increments. **Maximum:** 30 mg/day.

Major Depressive Disorder

PO: ADULTS, ELDERLY: Initially, 2–5 mg/day. May increase up to 15 mg/day. Titrate dose in 5-mg increments of at least 1-wk intervals.

Agitation with Schizophrenia/Bipolar Disorder

IM: ADULTS, ELDERLY: 5.25–15 mg as a single dose. May repeat after 2 hrs. **Maximum:** 30 mg/day.

Irritability with Autistic Disorder

PO: CHILDREN 6–17 YRS: Initially, 2 mg/day. May increase up to 5–10 mg/day. **Maximum:** 15 mg/day.

SIDE EFFECTS

Frequent (11%–5%): Weight gain, headache, insomnia, vomiting. **Occasional (4%–3%):** Light-headedness, nausea, akathisia, drowsiness. **Rare (2% or less):** Blurred vision, constipation, asthenia (loss of energy/strength), anxiety, fever, rash, cough, rhinitis, orthostatic hypotension.

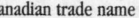

ADVERSE EFFECTS/ TOXIC REACTIONS

Extrapyramidal symptoms, neuroleptic malignant syndrome occur rarely. Prolonged QT interval occurs rarely. May cause leukopenia, neutropenia, agranulocytosis.

NURSING CONSIDERATIONS

BASELINE ASSESSMENT

Assess behavior, appearance, emotional status, response to environment, speech pattern, thought content. Correct dehydration, hypovolemia. Assess for suicidal tendencies.

INTERVENTION/EVALUATION

Periodically monitor weight. Monitor for extrapyramidal symptoms (abnormal movement), tardive dyskinesia (protrusion of tongue, puffing of cheeks, chewing/puckering of the mouth). Periodically monitor B/P, pulse (particularly in those with preexisting cardiovascular disease). Assess for therapeutic response (greater interest in surroundings, improved self-care, increased ability to concentrate, relaxed facial expression).

PATIENT/FAMILY TEACHING

• Avoid alcohol. • Avoid tasks that require alertness, motor skills until response to drug is established. • Report worsening depression, suicidal ideation, unusual changes in behavior, extrapyramidal effects.

Arixtra, *see fondaparinux*

armodafinil

HIGH ALERT

are-mode-ah-**feen**-ill
(Nuvigil)

◆CLASSIFICATION

PHARMACOTHERAPEUTIC: Alpha$_1$ agonist. **CLINICAL:** Antinarcoleptic.

ACTION

Binds to dopamine reuptake carrier sites in the brain, increasing alpha activity, decreasing delta, theta, and beta activity. **Therapeutic Effect:** Reduces number of sleep episodes, total daytime sleep.

PHARMACOKINETICS

Well absorbed. Widely distributed. Mainly eliminated by hepatic metabolism with less than 10% excreted by kidneys. Unknown if removed by hemodialysis. **Half-life:** 15 hrs.

USES

Treatment of excessive daytime sleepiness associated with obstructive sleep apnea-hypopnea syndrome, narcolepsy, shift-work sleep disorder.

PRECAUTIONS

Contraindications: History of sensitivity to modafinil. **Cautions:** History of mitral valve prolapse, left ventricular hypertrophy, hepatic impairment, recent history of MI, unstable angina. History of psychosis, renal or hepatic impairment.

LIFESPAN CONSIDERATIONS

Pregnancy/Lactation: Unknown if distributed in breast milk. Use caution if given to pregnant women. **Pregnancy Category C. Children:** Safety and efficacy not established in those younger than 17 yrs. **Elderly:** Age-related renal/hepatic impairment may require decreased dosage.

INTERACTIONS

DRUG: **Carbamazine, erythromycin, ketoconazole, phenobarbital, rifampin** can alter plasma levels of armodafinil. May reduce effects of **cyclosporine, midazolam, oral contraceptives, triazolam.** May increase concentrations of **diazepam, omeprazole, phenytoin, propanolol, tricyclic antidepressants, warfarin. Other CNS stimulants** may increase CNS stimulation. **HERBAL:** None significant. **FOOD:** **Food** slows peak concentration by 2–4 hrs; may affect time of onset, length of drug action. **LAB VALUES:**

May increase alkaline phosphatase, GGT. May decrease serum uric acid.

AVAILABILITY (Rx)

Tablets: 50 mg, 150 mg, 250 mg.

ADMINISTRATION/HANDLING

PO

• May give without regard to food. • Food slows peak concentration by 2–4 hrs, may affect time of onset, length of action. • Tablets may be crushed.

INDICATIONS/ROUTES/DOSAGE

Narcolepsy, Obstructive Sleep Apnea-Hypopnea Syndrome

PO: ADULTS, ELDERLY: 150 or 250 mg/day given as a single dose in the morning.

Shift-Work Sleep Disorder

PO: ADULTS, ELDERLY: 150 mg given daily approximately 1 hr prior to the start of work shift.

SIDE EFFECTS

Frequent (17%–7%): Headache, nausea. Occasional (5%–4%): Dizziness, insomnia, dry mouth, diarrhea, anxiety. Rare (2%): Depression, fatigue, palpitations, dyspepsia, rash, upper abdominal pain.

ADVERSE EFFECTS/ TOXIC REACTIONS

Small risk of serious rash, including Stevens-Johnson syndrome.

NURSING CONSIDERATIONS

BASELINE ASSESSMENT

Obtain baseline evidence of narcolepsy or other sleep disorders, including pattern, environmental situations, lengths of time of sleep episodes. Question for sudden loss of muscle tone (cataplexy) precipitated by strong emotional responses before sleep episode. Assess frequency/severity of sleep episodes prior to drug therapy.

INTERVENTION/EVALUATION

Monitor sleep pattern, evidence of restlessness during sleep, length of insomnia episodes at night. Assess for dizziness, anxiety; initiate fall precautions. Sips of tepid water may relieve dry mouth.

PATIENT/FAMILY TEACHING

• Avoid tasks that require alertness, motor skills until response to drug is established. • Avoid or limit alcohol. • Use alternative contraceptives during therapy and 1 mo after discontinuing drug (reduces effectiveness of oral contraceptives). Report rash, depression, diarrhea, insomnia.

Aromasin, *see exemestane*

Arranon, *see nelarbine*

arsenic trioxide HIGH ALERT

arc-sih-nic try-**ox**-idc
(Trisenox)

BLACK BOX ALERT May prolong QT interval. May lead to multiform ventricular tachycardia (torsade de pointes) or complete AV block. May cause retinoic acid–acute promyelocytic leukemia (RA-APL) syndrome or acute promyelocytic leukemia.

Do not confuse Trisenox with Trimox.

◆CLASSIFICATION

CLINICAL: Antineoplastic (see p. 79C).

ACTION

Produces morphologic changes and DNA fragmentation in promyelocytic leukemia cells. Therapeutic Effect: Produces cell death.

PHARMACOKINETICS

Distributed in liver, kidneys, heart, lungs, hair, and nails. Metabolized in liver. Eliminated by kidneys. Half-life: Not available.

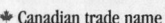

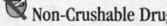

USES

Induction of remission and consolidations in pts with acute promyelocytic leukemia (APL) who are refractory to or have relapsed from retinoid and anthracycline chemotherapy. OFF-LABEL: Treatment of myelodysplastic syndrome; multiple myeloma.

PRECAUTIONS

Contraindications: None known. Cautions: Renal impairment, cardiac abnormalities.

LIFESPAN CONSIDERATIONS

Pregnancy/Lactation: Distributed in breast milk. May cause fetal harm. **Pregnancy Category D. Children:** Safety and efficacy not established in those younger than 5 yrs. **Elderly:** Age-related renal impairment may require dosage adjustment.

INTERACTIONS

DRUG: May prolong QT interval in those taking **antiarrhythmics, moxifloxacin, thioridazine. Amphotericin B, cyclosporine, diuretics** may produce electrolyte abnormalities. HERBAL: **Bilberry, fenugreek, garlic, ginger, ginseng** may worsen hypoglycemia. FOOD: None known. LAB VALUES: May decrease WBC count, Hgb, platelet count, serum magnesium, calcium. May increase serum AST, ALT. Higher risk of hypokalemia than hyperkalemia, hyperglycemia than hypoglycemia.

AVAILABILITY (Rx)

Injection Solution: 1 mg/ml.

ADMINISTRATION/HANDLING

IV

◄ALERT► Central venous line is not required for drug administration.

Reconstitution • After withdrawing drug from ampule, dilute with 100–250 ml D_5W or 0.9% NaCl.

Rate of administration • Infuse over 1–2 hrs. Duration of infusion may be extended up to 4 hrs.

Storage • Store at room temperature. • Diluted solution is stable for 24 hrs at room temperature, 48 hrs if refrigerated.

IV INCOMPATIBILITIES

Do not mix with any other medications.

INDICATIONS/ROUTES/DOSAGE

Acute Promyelocytic Leukemia

IV: ADULTS, ELDERLY, CHILDREN 5 YRS AND OLDER: Induction: 0.15 mg/kg/day until myelosuppression occurs. Do not exceed 60 induction doses. **Consolidation:** Beginning 3–6 wks after completion of induction therapy, 0.15 mg/kg/day for maximum 25 doses over a period of up to 5 wks.

SIDE EFFECTS

Expected (75%–50%): Nausea, cough, fatigue, fever, headache, vomiting, abdominal pain, tachycardia, diarrhea, dyspnea. Frequent (43%–30%): Dermatitis, insomnia, edema, rigors, prolonged QT interval, sore throat, pruritus, arthralgia, paresthesia, anxiety. Occasional (28%–20%): Constipation, myalgia, hypotension, epistaxis, anorexia, dizziness, sinusitis. (15%–8%): Ecchymosis, nonspecific pain, weight gain, herpes simplex infections, wheezing, flushing, diaphoresis, tremor, hypertension, palpitations, dyspepsia, eye irritation, blurred vision, asthenia, adventitious or diminished breath sounds (crackles). Rare: Confusion, petechiae, dry mouth, oral candidiasis, incontinence, pulmonary rhonchi.

ADVERSE EFFECTS/ TOXIC REACTIONS

Seizures, GI hemorrhage, renal impairment or failure, pleural or pericardial effusion, hemoptysis, sepsis occur rarely. Prolonged QT interval, complete AV block, unexplained fever, dyspnea, weight gain, effusion are evidence of arsenic toxicity. Treatment should be halted, steroid therapy instituted.

NURSING CONSIDERATIONS

BASELINE ASSESSMENT

Assess platelet count, Hgb, Hct, WBC, serum electrolytes, coagulation profiles before and frequently during treatment. Ask if pt is breast-feeding, pregnant, or planning to become pregnant (may cause fetal harm).

INTERVENTION/EVALUATION

Monitor hepatic function test results, CBC, serum values. Monitor for arsenic toxicity syndrome (fever, dyspnea, weight gain, confusion, muscle weakness, seizures).

PATIENT/FAMILY TEACHING

• Avoid crowds, those with known infection. • Avoid tasks that require alertness, motor skills, until response to drug is established. • Contact physician if high fever, vomiting, difficulty breathing, or rapid heart rate occur.

Arthrotec, *see diclofenac and misoprostol*

Asacol, *see mesalamine*

ascorbic acid (vitamin C)

a-**skor**-bic a-sid
(C-Gram, Proflavanol C ✦, Revitalose C-1000 ✦, Vita-C)

◆CLASSIFICATION

CLINICAL: Vitamin (see p. 162C).

ACTION

Assists in collagen formation, tissue repair and is involved in oxidation reduction reactions, other metabolic reactions. **Therapeutic Effect:** Involved in carbohydrate utilization and metabolism, as well as synthesis of carnitine, lipids, proteins. Preserves blood vessel integrity.

PHARMACOKINETICS

Readily absorbed from GI tract. Protein binding: 25%. Metabolized in liver. Excreted in urine. Removed by hemodialysis.

USES

Prevention and treatment of scurvy, acidification of urine, dietary supplement. **OFF-LABEL:** Chronic iron toxicity, control of idiopathic methemoglobinemia, macular degeneration, prevention of common cold, urinary acidifier.

PRECAUTIONS

Contraindications: None known. **Cautions:** Sodium-restricted diet, daily salicylate treatment, warfarin therapy, diabetes mellitus, history of renal stones.

⌛ LIFESPAN CONSIDERATIONS

Pregnancy/Lactation: Crosses placenta; excreted in breast milk. Large doses during pregnancy may produce scurvy in neonates. **Pregnancy Category A (C if used in doses above recommended daily allowance). Children/Elderly:** No age-related precautions noted.

INTERACTIONS

DRUG: Enhances **iron** absorption. May increase or decrease effect of **oral contraceptives. HERBAL:** None significant. **FOOD:** None known. **LAB VALUES:** May decrease serum bilirubin, urinary pH. May increase serum uric acid, urinary oxalate.

AVAILABILITY

Capsules: 500 mg, 1,000 mg. **Crystals:** 4 g/tsp. **Injection, Solution:** 500 mg/ml. **Solution, Oral:** 90 mg/ml. **Tablets:** 100 mg, 250 mg, 500 mg, 1,000 mg. **Tablets (Chewable):** 250 mg, 500 mg.

Capsules (Timed-Release): 500 mg. Tablets (Timed-Release): 500 mg, 1,000 mg.

ADMINISTRATION/HANDLING

IV

Rate of administration • May give undiluted or dilute in D_5W, 0.9% NaCl, lactated Ringer's solution. • For IV push, dilute with equal volume D_5W or 0.9% NaCl and infuse over 10 min.
Storage • Refrigerate. • Protect from freezing and light.

PO

• Give without regard to food but best given with meals. • Do not crush time-release formulations.

IV INCOMPATIBILITIES

Nafcillin, sodium bicarbonate, theophylline.

IV COMPATIBILITIES

Calcium gluconate, heparin, lipids.

INDICATIONS/ROUTES/DOSAGE

Dietary Supplement

PO: ADULTS, ELDERLY: 50–200 mg/day. **CHILDREN:** 35–100 mg/day.

Acidification of Urine

PO: ADULTS, ELDERLY: 4–12 g/day in 3–4 divided doses. **CHILDREN:** 500 mg q6–8h.

Scurvy

PO: ADULTS, ELDERLY: 100–250 mg 1–2 times a day for at least 2 wks. **CHILDREN:** 100–300 mg/day in divided doses for at least 2 wks.

Prevention, Reduction of Severity of Colds

PO: ADULTS, ELDERLY: 1–3 g/day in divided doses.

SIDE EFFECTS

Rare: Abdominal cramps, nausea, vomiting, diarrhea, increased urination with doses exceeding 1 g. **Parenteral:** Flushing, headache, dizziness, sleepiness or insomnia, soreness at injection site.

ADVERSE EFFECTS/ TOXIC REACTIONS

May acidify urine, leading to crystalluria. Large doses of IV ascorbic acid may lead to deep vein thrombosis. Prolonged use of large doses may produce rebound ascorbic acid deficiency when dosage is reduced to normal range.

NURSING CONSIDERATIONS

INTERVENTION/EVALUATION

Assess for clinical improvement (improved sense of well-being and sleep patterns). Observe for reversal of deficiency symptoms (improving gingivitis, bleeding gums, poor wound healing, digestive difficulties, joint pain).

PATIENT/FAMILY TEACHING

• Larger doses may cause diarrhea, nausea, abdominal cramping. • Foods rich in vitamin C include rose hips, guava, black currant jelly, Brussels sprouts, green peppers, spinach, watercress, strawberries, citrus fruits.

asenapine

ah-**sen**-ah-peen
(Saphris)

BLACK BOX ALERT Elderly pts with dementia-related psychosis are at increased risk for mortality due to cerebrovascular events.

Do not confuse asenapine with inapsine.

CLASSIFICATION

PHARMACOTHERAPEUTIC: Antipsychotic. **CLINICAL:** Antischizophrenia, bipolar agent.

ACTION

Exact mechanism unknown. May be mediated through antagonistic activity at D_2 and 5-HT_{2A} receptors. **Therapeutic Effect:** Assists in preventing relapse in those with schizophrenia, manic-depressive disease.

PHARMACOKINETICS

Rapidly absorbed following sublingual administration. Rapidly distributed, indicating extensive extravascular distribution. Protein binding: 95%. Primarily excreted in urine (50%), with smaller amount eliminated in feces (40%). Steady-state levels attained within 3 days. **Half-life:** 24 hrs.

USES

Acute treatment and maintenance of schizophrenia in adults, manic or mixed episodes associated with bipolar disorder in adults as monotherapy or as an adjunct to lithium or valproic acid medication.

PRECAUTIONS

Contraindications: Not recommended in pts with severe hepatic impairment, dementia-related psychosis. **Cautions:** History of cardiovascular or cerebrovascular disease, seizures, tardive dyskinesia, diabetes mellitus, leukopenia/neutropenia, concurrent use with other medications that prolong QT interval (e.g., amiodarone, quinidine). May increase risk of stroke, transient ischemic attack in pts with dementia-related psychosis.

LIFESPAN CONSIDERATIONS

Pregnancy/Lactation: Unknown if crosses placenta or is distributed in breast milk. Breast-feeding not recommended. **Pregnancy Category C. Children:** Safety and efficacy not established. **Elderly:** Potential for orthostatic hypotension.

INTERACTIONS

DRUG: Alcohol, CNS depressants may increase CNS depression. **Fluvoxamine** may increase **asenapine** plasma concentration. May decrease **cimetidine, paroxetine** concentrations. **HERBAL:** None significant. **FOOD: Food, liquids** reduce absorption of asenapine if given within 10 min of administration. **LAB VALUES:** May decrease WBC count. May increase serum glucose.

AVAILABILITY (Rx)

Tablets, Sublingual: 5 mg, 10 mg.

ADMINISTRATION/HANDLING

Sublingual

• Avoid eating/drinking for at least 10 min following sublingual dosing (reduces absorption). • Do not crush, chew, swallow tablet; place under tongue and allow tablet to dissolve completely (tablet will dissolve within seconds). • Press and hold thumb button, then pull out tablet pack. Do not push tablet through tablet pack. Do not cut or tear tablet pack. Peel back colored tab. Gently remove tablet. Slide tablet pack back into case until it clicks.

INDICATIONS/ROUTES/DOSAGE

Schizophrenia

SUBLINGUAL: ADULTS, ELDERLY: (Acute): 5 mg twice daily. **(Maintenance):** 5 mg twice daily for 1 wk, then 10 mg twice daily. **Maximum:** 10 mg twice daily.

Bipolar Disorder

SUBLINGUAL: ADULTS, ELDERLY: (Monotherapy): 10 mg twice daily. Dosage can be decreased to 5 mg twice daily if adverse effects occur. **(Adjunct):** 5 mg twice daily. May increase to 10 mg twice daily.

SIDE EFFECTS

Frequent (15%–13%): Insomnia, drowsiness. **Occasional** (6%–5%): Akathisia, constipation, decreased oral sensitivity, vomiting, dizziness, weight gain. **Rare** (3%–2%): Fatigue, dry mouth, salivary hypersecretion, abdominal discomfort, irritability, increased appetite, hypertension.

ADVERSE EFFECTS/ TOXIC REACTIONS

Extrapyramidal symptoms occur in 10% of pts (dystonia, oculogyration, dyskinesia, muscle rigidity, parkinsonism, tremors). Neuroleptic malignant syndrome (hyperpyrexia, muscle rigidity, altered mental status, irregular pulse or B/P, tachycardia, diaphoresis, cardiac arrhythmias, tardive dyskinesia [protrusion of tongue, puffing of cheeks, chewing/puckering of mouth]) may occur. Leukopenia, neutropenia, agranulocytosis have been reported.

NURSING CONSIDERATIONS

BASELINE ASSESSMENT

Assess behavior, appearance, emotional and mental status, response to environment, speech pattern, thought content, suicidal ideation, baseline weight. Pts with preexisting low WBC count or history of leukopenia/neutropenia should have CBC monitored frequently during first few months of therapy; drug should be discontinued at first sign of decline in WBC count in the absence of other causative factors.

INTERVENTION/EVALUATION

Monitor B/P, heart rate, weight, EKG. Monitor for fine tongue movement (may be first sign of tardive dyskinesia). Supervise suicidal risk pt closely during early therapy. Assess for therapeutic response (greater interest in surroundings, improved self care, increased ability to concentrate, relaxed facial expression). Monitor for potential neuroleptic malignant syndrome (fever, muscle rigidity, irregular B/P or pulse, altered mental status).

PATIENT/FAMILY TEACHING

• Avoid tasks that may require alertness, motor skills until response to drug is established (may cause drowsiness, dizziness). • Avoid alcohol. • Use caution when changing position from lying or sitting to standing. • Inform physician of trembling in fingers, altered gait, unusual muscle/skeletal movements, palpitations, severe dizziness, fainting.

asparaginase

HIGH ALERT

ah-spa-**raj**-in-ace
(Elspar, Kidrolase ✱)

Do not confuse asparaginase with pegaspargase.

◆CLASSIFICATION

PHARMACOTHERAPEUTIC: Enzyme. **CLINICAL:** Antineoplastic (see p. 80C).

ACTION

Inhibits DNA, RNA, protein synthesis by breaking down asparagine, depriving tumor cells of this essential amino acid. Cell cycle–specific for G_1 phase of cell division. **Therapeutic Effect:** Toxic to leukemic cells.

PHARMACOKINETICS

Metabolized by reticuloendothelial system through slow sequestration. **Half-life: IM:** 39–49 hrs; **IV:** 8–30 hrs.

USES

Treatment of acute lymphocytic leukemia (ALL), lymphoma in combination with other therapy. **OFF-LABEL:** Treatment of acute myelocytic leukemia, acute myelomonocytic leukemia, chronic lymphocytic leukemia, Hodgkin's disease, lymphosarcoma, melanosarcoma, reticulum cell sarcoma.

PRECAUTIONS

Contraindications: History of hypersensitivity to asparaginase, pancreatitis. **Cautions:** Existing or recent chickenpox, herpes zoster, diabetes mellitus, gout, infection, hepatic/renal impairment, recent cytotoxic/radiation therapy.

⌛ LIFESPAN CONSIDERATIONS

Pregnancy/Lactation: If possible, avoid use during pregnancy, esp. first trimester. Breast-feeding not recommended. **Pregnancy Category C. Chil-**

dren/Elderly: No age-related precautions noted.

INTERACTIONS

DRUG: **Steroids, vincristine** may increase hyperglycemia, risk of neuropathy, disturbances of erythropoiesis. May decrease effect of **antigout medications.** May block effects of **methotrexate. Live virus vaccines** may potentiate virus replication, increase vaccine side effects, decrease pt's antibody response to vaccine. HERBAL: None significant. FOOD: None known. LAB VALUES: May increase serum ammonia, BUN, uric acid, glucose, partial thromboplastin time (PTT), platelet count, prothrombin time (PT), thrombin time (TT), AST, ALT, alkaline phosphatase, bilirubin. May decrease blood clotting factors (plasma fibrinogen, antithrombin, plasminogen), serum albumin, calcium, cholesterol.

AVAILABILITY (Rx)

Injection, Powder for Reconstitution: 10,000 international units.

ADMINISTRATION/HANDLING

◀ALERT▶ May be carcinogenic, mutagenic, teratogenic. Handle with extreme care during preparation/administration. Handle voided urine as infectious waste. Powder, solution may irritate skin on contact. Wash area for 15 min if contact occurs.

IV

◀ALERT▶ Administer intradermal test dose (2 international units) before initiating therapy or when longer than 1 wk has elapsed between doses.
• Observe pt for 1 hr for appearance of wheal or erythema.

Test solution • Reconstitute 10,000 international units vial with 5 ml Sterile Water for Injection or 0.9% NaCl. • Shake to dissolve.

Reconstitution • **Test Dose:** Withdraw 0.1 ml, inject into vial containing 9.9 ml same diluent for concentration of 20 international units/ml. • **Regular Dose:** Reconstitute 10,000 international units vial with 5 ml Sterile Water for Injection or 0.9% NaCl to provide a concentration of 2,000 international units/ml. • Shake gently to ensure complete dissolution (vigorous shaking produces foam, some loss of potency). Further dilute in 50–250 ml D_5W or 0.9% NaCl.

Rate of administration • Infuse over at least 30–60 min.

Storage • Refrigerate powder for reconstitution. • Reconstituted solution stable for 8 hrs if refrigerated. • Gelatinous fiber-like particles may develop (remove via 5-micron filter during administration).

IM

• Add 2 ml 0.9% NaCl injection to 10,000 international units vial to provide a concentration of 5,000 international units/ml. • Administer no more than 2 ml at any one site.

IV INCOMPATIBILITIES

None known.

INDICATIONS/ROUTES/DOSAGE

Usual Dosage

IV: ADULTS, ELDERLY, CHILDREN: 6,000 units/m²/dose 3 times/wk for 6–9 doses or 1,000 units/kg/day for 10 days.

IM: ADULTS, ELDERLY, CHILDREN: 6,000 units/m²/dose 3 times/wk for 6–9 doses.

SIDE EFFECTS

Frequent: Allergic reaction (rash, urticaria, arthralgia, facial edema, hypotension, respiratory distress), pancreatitis (severe abdominal pain, nausea and vomiting). Occasional: CNS effects (confusion, drowsiness, depression, anxiety, fatigue), stomatitis, hypoalbuminemia or uric acid nephropathy (manifested as pedal or lower extremity edema), hyperglycemia. Rare: Hyperthermia (including fever or chills), thrombosis, seizures.

ADVERSE EFFECTS/ TOXIC REACTIONS

Hepatotoxicity usually occurs within 2 wks of initial treatment. Risk of allergic reaction, including anaphylaxis, increases after repeated therapy. Myelosuppression may be severe.

NURSING CONSIDERATIONS

BASELINE ASSESSMENT

Before giving medication, agents for adequate airway and allergic reaction, (antihistamine, epinephrine, O_2, IV corticosteroid) should be readily available. Assess baseline CNS functions. CBC, comprehensive serum chemistry should be performed before therapy begins and when 1 or more wks have elapsed between doses.

INTERVENTION/EVALUATION

Monitor vital signs, CBC, urinalysis, amylase hepatic enzymes, coagulation profile, glucose, uric acid. Discontinue medication at first sign of renal failure (oliguria, anuria), pancreatitis (abdominal pain, nausea, vomiting). Monitor for hematologic toxicity (fever, sore throat, signs of local infection, unusual bruising/bleeding), symptoms of anemia (excessive fatigue, weakness), hypersensitivity reaction.

PATIENT/FAMILY TEACHING

• Increase fluid intake (protects against renal impairment). • Nausea may decrease during therapy. • Do not have immunizations without physician's approval (drug lowers body's resistance). • Avoid contact with those who have recently taken a live virus vaccine. • Notify physician if abdominal pain, rash, nausea, vomiting occurs.

aspirin (acetylsalicylic acid, ASA)

HIGH ALERT

ass-purr-in
(Asaphen E.C. ✦, Ascriptin, Bayer, Bufferin, Ecotrin, Entrophen ✦, Halfprin, Novasen ✦, ZORprin)
Do not confuse aspirin or Ascriptin with Afrin, Aricept, or Asendin, Ecotrin with Epogen, or ZORprin with Zyloprim.

FIXED-COMBINATION(S)

Aggrenox: aspirin/dipyridamole (an antiplatelet agent): 25 mg/200 mg. **Fiorinal:** aspirin/butalbital/caffeine (a barbiturate): 325 mg/50 mg/40 mg. **Lortab/ASA:** aspirin/hydrocodone (an analgesic): 325 mg/5 mg. **Percodan:** aspirin/oxycodone (an analgesic): 325 mg/2.25 mg, 325 mg/4.5 mg. **Pravigard:** aspirin/pravastatin (a cholesterol lowering agent): 81 mg/20 mg, 81 mg/40 mg, 81 mg/80 mg, 325 mg/20 mg, 325 mg/40 mg, 325 mg/80 mg.

◆CLASSIFICATION

PHARMACOTHERAPEUTIC: Nonsteroidal salicylate. **CLINICAL:** Anti-inflammatory, antipyretic, anticoagulant (see pp. 32C, 127C).

ACTION

Inhibits prostaglandin synthesis, acts on the hypothalamus heat-regulating center, interferes with production of thromboxane A, a substance that stimulates platelet aggregation. **Therapeutic Effect:** Reduces inflammatory response, intensity of pain; decreases fever; inhibits platelet aggregation.

PHARMACOKINETICS

Route	Onset	Peak	Duration
PO	1 hr	2–4 hrs	4–6 hrs

Rapidly and completely absorbed from GI tract; enteric-coated absorption delayed; rectal absorption delayed and incomplete. Protein binding: High. Widely distributed. Rapidly hydrolyzed to salicylate. **Half-life:** 15–20 min (aspirin); 2–3 hrs (salicylate at low dose); more than 20 hrs (salicylate at high dose).

USES

Treatment of mild to moderate pain, fever. Reduces inflammation including rheumatoid arthritis (RA), juvenile arthritis, osteoarthritis, rheumatic fever. As platelet aggregation inhibitor in the prevention of transient ischemic attacks (TIAs), cerebral thromboembolism, MI or reinfarction. **OFF-LABEL:** Acute ischemic stroke, complications of pregnancy (prophylaxis), MI (prophylaxis), prevention of thromboembolism, rheumatic fever, treatment of Kawasaki's disease.

PRECAUTIONS

Contraindications: Allergy to tartrazine dye, bleeding disorders, chickenpox or flu in children and teenagers, GI bleeding or ulceration, hepatic impairment, history of hypersensitivity to aspirin or NSAIDs. **Cautions:** Vitamin K deficiency, chronic renal insufficiency, those with "aspirin triad" (rhinitis, nasal polyps, asthma).

LIFESPAN CONSIDERATIONS

Pregnancy/Lactation: Readily crosses placenta; distributed in breast milk. May prolong gestation and labor; decrease fetal birth weight; increase incidence of stillbirths, neonatal mortality, hemorrhage. Avoid use during last trimester (may adversely affect fetal cardiovascular system: premature closure of ductus arteriosus). **Pregnancy Category C (D if full dose used in third trimester of pregnancy). Children:** Caution in those with acute febrile illness (Reye's syndrome). **Elderly:** May be more susceptible to toxicity; lower dosages recommended.

INTERACTIONS

DRUG: **Alcohol, NSAIDs** may increase risk of GI effects (e.g., ulceration). **Antacids, urinary alkalinizers** increase excretion. **Anticoagulants, heparin, thrombolytics** increase risk of bleeding. **Platelet aggregation inhibitors, valproic acid** may increase risk of bleeding. May increase toxicity of **methotrexate, zidovudine. Ototoxic medications, vancomycin** may increase ototoxicity. May decrease effect of **probenecid, sulfinpyrazone.** **HERBAL:** Avoid **cat's claw, dong quai, evening primrose, feverfew, garlic, ginger, ginkgo, ginseng, green tea, horse chestnut, red clover** (possess antiplatelet activity). **FOOD:** None known. **LAB VALUES:** May alter serum AST, ALT, alkaline phosphatase, uric acid; prolongs prothrombin time (PT), bleeding time. May decrease serum cholesterol, potassium, T_3, T_4.

AVAILABILITY (OTC)

Caplets (Bayer): 81 mg, 325 mg, 500 mg. **Suppositories:** 300 mg, 600 mg. **Tablets:** 162 mg (Halfprin), 325 mg (Bayer), 500 mg (Bayer). **Tablets (Chewable [Bayer, St. Joseph]):** 81 mg.

Tablets (Enteric-Coated [Bayer, Ecotrin, St. Joseph]): 81 mg, 325 mg, 500 mg, 650 mg.

ADMINISTRATION/HANDLING

PO

- Do not crush or break enteric-coated tablets. • May give with water, milk, meals if GI distress occurs.

Rectal

- Refrigerate suppositories; do not freeze. • If suppository is too soft, chill for 30 min in refrigerator or run cold water over foil wrapper. • Moisten suppository with cold water before inserting well into rectum.

INDICATIONS/ROUTES/DOSAGE

Analgesia, Fever

PO, RECTAL: ADULTS, ELDERLY: 325–650 mg q4–6h. **CHILDREN:** 10–15 mg/kg/dose q4–6h. **Maximum:** 4 g/day.

Anti-Inflammatory

PO: ADULTS, ELDERLY: Initially, 2.4–3.6 g/day in divided doses, then 3.6–5.4 g/day. **CHILDREN:** Initially, 60–90 mg/kg/day in divided doses, then 80–100 mg/kg/day.

Platelet Aggregation Inhibitor

PO: ADULTS, ELDERLY: 80–325 mg/day.

Kawasaki's Disease

PO: CHILDREN: 80–100 mg/kg/day in divided doses q6h. After fever resolves, 3–5 mg/kg once a day.

SIDE EFFECTS

Occasional: GI distress (including abdominal distention, cramping, heartburn, mild nausea); allergic reaction (including bronchospasm, pruritus, urticaria).

ADVERSE EFFECTS/ TOXIC REACTIONS

High doses of aspirin may produce GI bleeding and/or gastric mucosal lesions. Dehydrated, febrile children may experience aspirin toxicity quickly. Reye's syndrome may occur in children with chickenpox or flu. Low-grade toxicity characterized by tinnitus, generalized pruritus (may be severe), headache, dizziness, flushing, tachycardia, hyperventilation, diaphoresis, thirst. Marked toxicity characterized by hyperthermia, restlessness, seizures, abnormal breathing patterns, respiratory failure, coma.

NURSING CONSIDERATIONS

BASELINE ASSESSMENT

Do not give to children or teenagers who have flu or chickenpox (increases risk of Reye's syndrome). Do not use if vinegar-like odor is noted (indicates chemical breakdown). Assess type, location, duration of pain, inflammation. Inspect appearance of affected joints for immobility, deformities, skin condition. **Therapeutic serum level for antiarthritic effect:** 20–30 mg/dl (toxicity occurs if level is greater than 30 mg/dl).

INTERVENTION/EVALUATION

Monitor urinary pH (sudden acidification, pH from 6.5 to 5.5, may result in toxicity). Assess skin for evidence of ecchymosis. If given as antipyretic, assess temperature directly before and 1 hr after giving medication. Evaluate for therapeutic response: relief of pain, stiffness, swelling; increased joint mobility; reduced joint tenderness; improved grip strength.

PATIENT/FAMILY TEACHING

• Do not crush or chew enteric-coated tablets. • Avoid alcohol. • Report tinnitus or persistent abdominal GI pain, bleeding. • Therapeutic anti-inflammatory effect noted in 1–3 wks. • Behavioral changes, vomiting may be early signs of Reye's syndrome. Contact physician.

Astelin, *see azelastine*

Atacand, *see candesartan*

atazanavir

ah-tah-**zan**-ah-veer
(Reyataz)
Do not confuse Reyataz with Retavase.

◆CLASSIFICATION

PHARMACOTHERAPEUTIC: Antiretroviral. **CLINICAL:** Protease inhibitor.

ACTION

Acts as an HIV-1 protease inhibitor, selectively preventing the processing of viral precursors found in cells infected with HIV-1. **Therapeutic Effect:** Prevents formation of mature HIV viral cells.

PHARMACOKINETICS

Rapidly absorbed after PO administration. Protein binding: 86%. Extensively metabolized in liver. Excreted primarily in urine and, to a lesser extent, in feces. **Half-life:** 5–8 hrs.

USES

Treatment of HIV-1 infection in combination with other antiretroviral agents.

PRECAUTIONS

Contraindications: Concurrent use with ergot derivatives, midazolam, pimozide, triazolam; severe hepatic insufficiency. **Extreme Caution:** Hepatic impairment. **Cautions:** Preexisting conduction system defects (first-, second-, or third-degree AV block), diabetes mellitus, elderly, renal impairment.

⌛ LIFESPAN CONSIDERATIONS

Pregnancy/Lactation: Unknown if drug crosses placenta or distributed in breast milk. Lactic acidosis syndrome, hyperbilirubinemia, kernicterus have been reported. **Pregnancy Category B.** **Children:** Safety and efficacy not established in those younger than 3 mos. **Elderly:** Age-related hepatic impairment may require dose reduction.

INTERACTIONS

DRUG: May increase concentration, toxicity of **amiodarone, atorvastatin, bepridil, clarithromycin, cyclosporine, diltiazem, felodipine, lidocaine, lovastatin, nicardipine, nifedipine, sildenafil, simvastatin, sirolimus, tacrolimus, tadalafil, tricyclic antidepressants, vardenafil, verapamil, warfarin.** **H_2-receptor antagonists, proton pump inhibitors, rifampin** decrease atazanavir concentration, effect. **Ritonavir, voriconazole** increase concentration. **HERBAL:** **St. John's wort** may decrease concentration, effect. **FOOD:** **High-fat meals** may decrease absorption. **LAB VALUES:** May increase serum bilirubin, AST, ALT, amylase, lipase. May decrease Hgb, neutrophil count, platelets. May alter LDL, triglycerides.

AVAILABILITY (Rx)

Capsules: 100 mg, 150 mg, 200 mg, 300 mg.

ADMINISTRATION/HANDLING

PO

• Give with food. • Swallow whole; do not open. • Administer at least 2 hrs before or 10 hrs after H_2 antagonist, 12 hrs after proton pump inhibitor.

INDICATIONS/ROUTES/DOSAGE

HIV-1 Infection

PO: ADULTS, ELDERLY (ANTIRETROVIRAL-NAIVE): 300 mg and ritonavir 100 mg, once a day, or 400 mg (2 capsules) once a day with food. **CHILDREN 6–17 YRS WEIGHING 39 KG OR MORE:** 300 mg and ritonavir 100 mg once daily. **WEIGHING 32–38 KG:** 250 mg and ritonavir 100 mg once daily. **WEIGHING 25–31 KG:** 200 mg and ritonavir 100 mg once daily. **WEIGHING 15–24 KG:** 150 mg and ritonavir 80 mg once daily. **ADULTS, ELDERLY (ANTIRETROVIRAL-EXPERIENCED):** 300 mg and ritonavir (Norvir) 100 mg once a day.

HIV-1 Infection (Concurrent Therapy with Efavirenz)

PO: ADULTS, ELDERLY: 300 mg atazanavir, 100 mg ritonavir, and 600 mg efavirenz as a single daily dose on an empty stomach.

HIV-1 Infection (Concurrent Therapy with Didanosine)

PO: ADULTS, ELDERLY: Give atazanavir with food 2 hrs before or 1 hr after didanosine.

HIV-1 Infection (Concurrent Therapy with Tenofovir)

PO: ADULTS, ELDERLY: 300 mg atazanavir, 100 mg ritonavir, and 300 mg tenofovir given as a single daily dose with food.

HIV-1 Infection in Pts with Mild to Moderate Hepatic Impairment

◀ALERT▶ Avoid use in pts with severe hepatic impairment.

PO: ADULTS, ELDERLY: 300 mg once a day with food.

SIDE EFFECTS

Frequent (16%–14%): Nausea, headache. **Occasional (9%–4%):** Rash, vomiting, depression, diarrhea, abdominal pain, fever. **Rare (3% or less):** Dizziness, insomnia, cough, fatigue, back pain.

ADVERSE EFFECTS/ TOXIC REACTIONS

Severe hypersensitivity reaction (angioedema, chest pain), jaundice may occur.

NURSING CONSIDERATIONS

BASELINE ASSESSMENT

Obtain baseline chemistries, CBC, hepatic function tests, before beginning therapy and at periodic intervals during therapy. Offer emotional support.

INTERVENTION/EVALUATION

Check lab results. Assess for nausea, vomiting; assess eating pattern. Monitor daily pattern of bowel activity and stool consistency. Assess skin for rash. Question for evidence of headache. Monitor for onset of depression.

PATIENT/FAMILY TEACHING

• Take with food. • Small, frequent meals may offset nausea, vomiting. • Pt must continue practices to prevent HIV transmission. • Report dizziness, light-headedness, yellowing of skin or whites of eyes, pain in side or when urinating, blood in urine, skin rash.

atenolol

HIGH ALERT

ay-**ten**-oh-lol
(Apo-Atenol ✱, Novo-Atenol ✱, Tenolin ✱, Tenormin)

BLACK BOX ALERT Do not abruptly discontinue; taper gradually to avoid acute tachycardia, hypertension, ischemia.

Do not confuse atenolol with albuterol, timolol, or Tylenol, or Tenormin with Imuran, Norpramin, or thiamine.

FIXED-COMBINATION(S)

Tenoretic: atenolol/chlorthalidone (a diuretic): 50 mg/25 mg, 100 mg/25 mg.

◆CLASSIFICATION

PHARMACOTHERAPEUTIC: Beta$_1$-adrenergic blocker. **CLINICAL:** Antihypertensive, antianginal, antiarrhythmic (see pp. 61C, 71C).

ACTION

Blocks beta$_1$-adrenergic receptors in cardiac tissue. **Therapeutic Effect:** Slows sinus node heart rate, decreasing cardiac output, B/P. Decreases myocardial oxygen demand.

PHARMACOKINETICS

Route	Onset	Peak	Duration
PO	1 hr	2–4 hrs	24 hrs

Incompletely absorbed from GI tract. Protein binding: 6%–16%. Minimal liver metabolism. Primarily excreted unchanged in urine. Removed by hemodialysis. **Half-life:** 6–9 hrs (increased in renal impairment).

USES

Treatment of hypertension, alone or in combination with other agents; management of angina; secondary prevention of postmyocardial infarction (MI). **OFF-LABEL:** Acute alcohol withdrawal, arrhythmia (esp. supraventricular and ventricular tachycardia), improved survival in diabetics with heart disease, mild to moderately severe CHF (adjunct); prevention of migraine, thyrotoxicosis, tremors; treatment of hypertrophic cardiomyopathy, pheochromocytoma, syndrome of mitral valve prolapse.

PRECAUTIONS

Contraindications: Cardiogenic shock, overt heart failure, second- or third-degree heart block, severe bradycardia. **Cautions:** Renal/hepatic impairment, peripheral vascular disease, hyperthyroidism, diabetes, inadequate cardiac function, bronchospastic disease.

LIFESPAN CONSIDERATIONS

Pregnancy/Lactation: Readily crosses placenta; distributed in breast milk. Avoid use during first trimester. May produce bradycardia, apnea, hypoglycemia, hypothermia during delivery; low birth-weight infants. **Pregnancy Category D. Children:** No age-related precautions noted. **Elderly:** Age-related peripheral vascular disease, renal impairment require caution.

INTERACTIONS

DRUG: **Diuretics, other hypotensives** may increase hypotensive effects. **Sympathomimetics, xanthines** may mutually inhibit effects. May mask symptoms of hypoglycemia, prolong hypoglycemic effect of **insulin, oral hypoglycemics. NSAIDs** may decrease antihypertensive effect. **Cimetidine** may increase concentration. **HERBAL:** **Ephedra, yohimbe, ginseng** may worsen hypertension. **Garlic** may increase antihypertensive effect. **FOOD:** None known. **LAB VALUES:** May increase serum ANA titer and BUN, serum creatinine, potassium, uric acid, lipoprotein, triglycerides.

AVAILABILITY (Rx)

Tablets: 25 mg, 50 mg, 100 mg.

ADMINISTRATION/HANDLING

PO

• Give without regard to food. • Tablets may be crushed.

INDICATIONS/ROUTES/DOSAGE

Hypertension

PO: ADULTS: Initially, 25–50 mg once a day. May increase dose up to 100 mg once a day. **ELDERLY:** Usual initial dose, 25 mg/day. **CHILDREN:** Initially, 0.5–1 mg/kg/dose given once a day. Range: 0.5–1.5 mg/kg/day. **Maximum:** 2 mg/kg/day or 100 mg/day.

Angina Pectoris

PO: ADULTS: Initially, 50 mg once a day. May increase dose up to 200 mg once a day. **ELDERLY:** Usual initial dose, 25 mg/day.

Post-MI

PO: ADULTS: 100 mg once a day or 50 mg twice a day for 6–9 days post-MI.

Dosage in Renal Impairment

Dosage interval is modified based on creatinine clearance.

Creatinine Clearance	Maximum Dosage
15–35 ml/min	50 mg/day
Less than 15 ml/min	50 mg every other day

SIDE EFFECTS

Atenolol is generally well tolerated, with mild and transient side effects. **Frequent:** Hypotension manifested as cold extremities, constipation or diarrhea, diaphoresis, dizziness, fatigue, headache, nausea. **Occasional:** Insomnia, flatulence, urinary frequency, impotence or decreased libido, depression. **Rare:** Rash, arthralgia, myalgia, confusion (esp. in the elderly), altered taste.

ADVERSE EFFECTS/ TOXIC REACTIONS

Overdose may produce profound bradycardia, hypotension. Abrupt withdrawal may result in diaphoresis, palpitations, headache, tremors. May precipitate CHF, MI in pts with cardiac disease; thyroid storm in those with thyrotoxicosis; peripheral ischemia in those with existing peripheral vascular disease. Hypoglycemia may occur in previously controlled diabetes. Thrombocytopenia (unusual bruising, bleeding) occurs rarely. **Antidote:** Glucagon (see Appendix M for dosage).

NURSING CONSIDERATIONS

BASELINE ASSESSMENT

Assess B/P, apical pulse immediately before drug is administered (if pulse is 60/min or less, or systolic B/P is less than 90 mm Hg, withhold medication, contact physician). **Antianginal:** Record onset, quality (sharp, dull, squeezing), radiation, location, intensity, duration of anginal pain, precipitating factors (exertion, emotional stress). Assess baseline renal/hepatic function tests.

INTERVENTION/EVALUATION

Monitor B/P for hypotension, pulse for bradycardia, respiration for difficulty in breathing, EKG. Monitor daily pattern of bowel activity and stool consistency. Assess for evidence of CHF: dyspnea (particularly on exertion or lying down), night cough, peripheral edema, distended neck veins. Monitor I&O (increased weight, decreased urinary output may indicate CHF). Assess extremities for coldness. Assist with ambulation if dizziness occurs.

PATIENT/FAMILY TEACHING

• Do not abruptly discontinue medication. • Compliance with therapy essential to control hypertension, angina. • To reduce hypotensive effect, rise slowly from lying to sitting position and permit legs to dangle from bed momentarily before standing. • Avoid tasks that require alertness, motor skills until drug reaction is established. • Advise diabetic pts to monitor blood glucose carefully (may mask signs of hypoglycemia). • Report dizziness, depression, confusion, rash, unusual bruising/bleeding. • Outpatients should monitor B/P, pulse before taking medication following correct technique. • Restrict salt, alcohol intake. • Therapeutic antihypertensive effect noted in 1–2 wks.

Ativan, *see lorazepam*

atomoxetine

ah-toe-**mocks**-eh-teen
(Strattera)

BLACK BOX ALERT Increased risk of suicidal thinking and behavior in children and adolescents with attention-deficit hyperactivity disorder (ADHD).

Do not confuse atomoxetine with atorvastatin.

◆CLASSIFICATION

PHARMACOTHERAPEUTIC: Norepinephrine reuptake inhibitor. **CLINICAL:** Psychotherapeutic agent.

ACTION

Enhances noradrenergic function by selective inhibition of the presynaptic norepinephrine transporter. **Therapeutic Effect:** Improves symptoms of ADHD.

PHARMACOKINETICS

Rapidly absorbed after PO administration. Protein binding: 98% (primarily to albumin). Eliminated primarily in urine and, to a lesser extent, in feces. Not removed by hemodialysis. **Half-life:** 4–5 hrs (increased in moderate to severe hepatic insufficiency).

USES

Treatment of ADHD. **OFF-LABEL:** Treatment of depression.

PRECAUTIONS

Contraindications: Angle-closure glaucoma, use within 14 days of MAOIs. **Cautions:** Hypertension; tachycardia; cardiovascular disease; pts at risk for urinary retention, moderate or severe hepatic impairment. May prolong QT interval.

⌛ LIFESPAN CONSIDERATIONS

Pregnancy/Lactation: Unknown if distributed in breast milk. **Pregnancy Cate-**

gory C. **Children:** Safety and efficacy not established in those younger than 6 yrs. May produce suicidal thoughts in children and adolescents. **Elderly:** Age-related hepatic/renal impairment, cardiovascular or cerebrovascular disease may increase risk of effects.

INTERACTIONS

DRUG: **MAOIs** may increase toxic effects. **Fluoxetine, paroxetine, quinidine** may increase concentrations. Avoid concurrent use of **medications that can increase heart rate or B/P.** HERBAL: None significant. FOOD: None known. LAB VALUES: May increase hepatic enzymes, serum bilirubin.

AVAILABILITY (Rx)

Capsules: 10 mg, 18 mg, 25 mg, 40 mg, 60 mg, 80 mg, 100 mg.

ADMINISTRATION/HANDLING

PO

• Give without regard to food. • Swallow capsules whole, do not open (powder in capsule is ocular irritant).

INDICATIONS/ROUTES/DOSAGE

Attention-Deficit Hyperactivity Disorder (ADHD)

PO: ADULTS, CHILDREN 6 YRS AND OLDER WEIGHING 70 KG OR MORE: 40 mg once a day. May increase after at least 3 days to 80 mg as a single daily dose or in divided doses. **Maximum:** 100 mg. **CHILDREN 6 YRS AND OLDER WEIGHING LESS THAN 70 KG:** Initially, 0.5 mg/kg/day. May increase after at least 3 days to 1.2 mg/kg/day. **Maximum:** 1.4 mg/kg/day or 100 mg, whichever is less.

Dosage in Hepatic Impairment

Expect to administer 50% of normal atomoxetine dosage to pts with moderate hepatic impairment and 25% of normal dosage to those with severe hepatic impairment.

SIDE EFFECTS

Frequent: Headache, dyspepsia, nausea, vomiting, fatigue, decreased appetite, dizziness, altered mood. Occasional: Tachycardia, hypertension, weight loss, delayed growth in children, irritability. Rare: Insomnia, sexual dysfunction in adults, fever.

ADVERSE EFFECTS/ TOXIC REACTIONS

Urinary retention, urinary hesitancy may occur. In overdose, gastric lavage, activated charcoal may prevent systemic absorption. Severe hepatic injury occurs rarely.

NURSING CONSIDERATIONS

BASELINE ASSESSMENT

Assess pulse, B/P before therapy, following dose increases, and periodically during therapy. Assess attention span, interactions with others.

INTERVENTION/EVALUATION

Monitor urinary output; complaints of urinary retention/hesitancy may be a related adverse reaction. Monitor B/P, pulse periodically and following dose increases. Monitor growth, attention, hyperactivity, unusual changes in behavior, suicidal ideation. Assist with ambulation if dizziness occurs. Be alert to mood changes. Monitor fluid and electrolyte status in those with significant vomiting.

PATIENT/FAMILY TEACHING

• Avoid tasks that require alertness, motor skills until response to drug is established. • Take last dose early in evening to avoid insomnia. • Report palpitations, fever, vomiting, irritability. • Monitor growth rate, weight. • Report new or worsened psychiatric problems (e.g., behavior, suicidal ideation), chest pain, palpitations, dyspnea.

atorvastatin

ah-**tore**-vah-stah-tin

(Lipitor)

Do not confuse atorvastatin with atomoxetine, lovastatin,

nystatin, pitavastatin, pravastatin, or simvastatin, or Lipitor with labetalol, Levatol, lisinopril, or Zocor.

FIXED-COMBINATION(S)

Caduet: atorvastatin/amlodipine (calcium channel blocker): 10 mg/2.5 mg, 10 mg/5 mg, 10 mg/10 mg, 20 mg/2.5 mg, 20 mg/5 mg, 20 mg/10 mg, 40 mg/2.5 mg, 40 mg/5 mg, 40 mg/10 mg, 80 mg/5 mg, 80 mg/10 mg.

◆CLASSIFICATION

PHARMACOTHERAPEUTIC: Hydroxymethylglutaryl CoA (HMG-CoA) reductase inhibitor. **CLINICAL:** Antihyperlipidemic (see p. 57C).

ACTION

Inhibits HMG-CoA reductase, the enzyme that catalyzes the early step in cholesterol synthesis. **Therapeutic Effect:** Decreases LDL and VLDL, plasma triglyceride levels; increases HDL concentration.

PHARMACOKINETICS

Poorly absorbed from GI tract. Protein binding: greater than 98%. Metabolized in liver. Minimally eliminated in urine, primarily eliminated in feces (biliary). **Half-life:** 14 hrs.

USES

Primary prevention of cardiovascular disease in high-risk pts. Reduces risk of stroke and heart attack in pts with type 2 diabetes with or without evidence of heart disease. Reduces risk of stroke in pts with or without evidence of heart disease with multiple risk factors other than diabetes. Adjunct to diet therapy in management of hyperlipidemias (reduces elevations in total cholesterol, LDL-C, apolipoprotein B triglycerides in pts with primary hypercholesterolemia), homozygous familial hypercholesterolemia, heterozygous familial hypercholesterolemia in pts 10–17 yrs of age, females more than 1 yr postmenarche. **OFF-LABEL:** Secondary prevention of ischemia in pts with CHF.

PRECAUTIONS

Contraindications: Active hepatic disease, lactation, pregnancy, unexplained elevated hepatic function test results. **Cautions:** Anticoagulant therapy, history of hepatic disease, substantial alcohol consumption, major surgery, severe acute infection, trauma, hypotension, severe metabolic, endocrine, electrolyte disorders, uncontrolled seizures.

⌛ LIFESPAN CONSIDERATIONS

Pregnancy/Lactation: Distributed in breast milk. Contraindicated during pregnancy. May produce skeletal malformation. **Pregnancy Category X. Children:** Safety and efficacy not established. **Elderly:** No age-related precautions noted.

INTERACTIONS

DRUG: May increase concentration/toxicity of **digoxin.** Increased risk of rhabdomyolysis, acute renal failure with **cyclosporine, erythromycin, gemfibrozil, nicotinic acid. HERBAL: St. John's wort** may decrease levels. **FOOD: Grapefruit juice in large quantities (greater than 1 quart/day)** may increase serum concentrations. **Red yeast rice** contains 2.4 mg lovastatin per 600 mg rice. **LAB VALUES:** May increase creatinine kinase, serum transaminase concentrations.

AVAILABILITY (Rx)

Tablets: 10 mg, 20 mg, 40 mg, 80 mg.

ADMINISTRATION/HANDLING

PO

• Give without regard to food or time of day. • Do not break film-coated tablets.

INDICATIONS/ROUTES/DOSAGE

Do not use in active hepatic disease.

Hyperlipidemias

PO: ADULTS, ELDERLY: Initially, 10–20 mg/day (40 mg in pts requiring greater than 45% reduction in LDL-C). Range: 10–80 mg/day.

Heterozygous Hypercholesterolemia
PO: CHILDREN 10–17 YRS: Initially, 10 mg/day. **Maximum:** 20 mg/day.

SIDE EFFECTS

Common: Atorvastatin is generally well tolerated. Side effects are usually mild and transient. **Frequent (16%):** Headache. **Occasional (5%–2%):** Myalgia, rash, pruritus, allergy. **Rare (less than 2%–1%):** Flatulence, dyspepsia, depression.

ADVERSE EFFECTS/ TOXIC REACTIONS

Potential for cataracts, photosensitivity, myalgia, rhabdomyolysis.

NURSING CONSIDERATIONS

BASELINE ASSESSMENT

Question for possibility of pregnancy before initiating therapy (Pregnancy Category X). Assess baseline lab results: cholesterol, triglycerides, hepatic function tests. Obtain dietary history.

INTERVENTION/EVALUATION

Monitor for headache. Assess for rash, pruritus, malaise. Monitor cholesterol, triglyceride lab values for therapeutic response. Monitor hepatic function tests, CPK.

PATIENT/FAMILY TEACHING

• Follow special diet (important part of treatment). • Periodic lab tests are essential part of therapy. • Do not take other medications without consulting physician. • Report dark urine, muscle fatigue, bone pain. • Avoid excessive alcohol intake, large quantities of grapefruit juice.

atovaquone

a-**toe**-va-kwone
(Mepron)

◆ CLASSIFICATION

PHARMACOTHERAPEUTIC: Systemic anti-infective. **CLINICAL:** Antiprotozoal.

ACTION

Inhibits mitochondrial electron transport system at the cytochrome bc1 complex (Complex III) interrupting nucleic acid, adenosine triphosphate synthesis. **Therapeutic Effect:** Antiprotozoal, antipneumocystic activity.

USES

Treatment or prevention of mild to moderate *Pneumocystis jiroveci* pneumonia (PCP) in those intolerant to trimethoprim-sulfamethoxazole (TMP-SMZ).

PRECAUTIONS

Contraindications: Development or history of potentially life-threatening allergic reaction to the drug. **Cautions:** Elderly, pts with severe PCP, chronic diarrhea, malabsorption syndromes. **Pregnancy Category C.**

INTERACTIONS

DRUG: **Rifabutin, rifampin, tetracycline** may decrease concentration. Atovaquone may increase **rifampin** concentration. **Metoclopramide** decreases bioavailability. **HERBAL:** None significant. **FOOD:** **High-fat meals** increase absorption. **LAB VALUES:** May elevate serum AST, ALT, alkaline phosphatase, amylase. May decrease serum sodium.

AVAILABILITY (Rx)

Suspension, Oral: 750 mg/5 ml.

ADMINISTRATION/HANDLING

PO

• Must give with meals.

INDICATIONS/ROUTES/DOSAGE

Pneumocystis Jiroveci Pneumonia (PCP)
PO: ADULTS, CHILDREN OLDER THAN 12 YRS: 750 mg twice a day with food for 21 days. **CHILDREN 4–24 MOS:** 45 mg/kg/day in 2 divided doses with food. **Maximum:** 1,500 mg/day. **CHILDREN 1–3 MOS OR OLDER THAN 24 MOS:** 30–40 mg/kg/day in 2 divided doses with food. **Maximum:** 1,500 mg/day.

A

Prevention of PCP

PO: ADULTS: 1,500 mg once a day with food. **CHILDREN 4–24 MOS:** 45 mg/kg/day as single dose. **Maximum:** 1,500 mg/day. **CHILDREN 1–3 MOS OR OLDER THAN 24 MOS:** 30 mg/kg/day as single dose. **Maximum:** 1,500 mg/day.

SIDE EFFECTS

Frequent (greater than 10%): Rash, nausea, diarrhea, headache, vomiting, fever, insomnia, cough. **Occasional (less than 10%):** Abdominal discomfort, thrush, asthenia, anemia, neutropenia.

ADVERSE EFFECTS/ TOXIC REACTIONS

None known.

NURSING CONSIDERATIONS

INTERVENTION/EVALUATION

Assess for GI discomfort, nausea, vomiting. Monitor daily pattern of bowel activity and stool consistency. Assess skin for rash. Monitor I&O, renal function tests, CBC, hepatic enzymes, serum chemistries, amylase. Monitor elderly closely for decreased hepatic, renal, cardiac function.

PATIENT/FAMILY TEACHING

• Continue therapy for full length of treatment. • Do not take any other medications unless approved by physician. • Notify physician of rash, diarrhea, or other new symptoms.

atropine

at-roe-peen
(AtroPen Auto Injector, Atropine-Care, Isopto Atropine, Sal-Tropine)

FIXED-COMBINATION(S)

Donnatal: atropine/hyoscyamine (anticholinergic)/phenobarbital (sedative)/scopolamine (anticholinergic): 0.0194 mg/0.1037 mg/16.2 mg/0.0065 mg. **Lomotil:** atropine/diphenoxylate (peristaltic inhibitor): 0.025 mg/2.5 mg.

◆CLASSIFICATION

PHARMACOTHERAPEUTIC: Acetylcholine antagonist. **CLINICAL:** Antiarrhythmic, antispasmodic, antidote, cycloplegic, antisecretory, anticholinergic.

ACTION

Competes with acetylcholine for common binding sites on muscarinic receptors located on exocrine glands, cardiac and smooth muscle ganglia, intramural neurons. **Therapeutic Effect:** Decreases GI motility, secretory activity, GU muscle tone (ureter, bladder); produces ophthalmic cycloplegia, mydriasis; abolishes various types of reflex vagal cardiac slowing or asystole.

PHARMACOKINETICS

Rapidly and well absorbed after IM administration. Widely distributed. Metabolized in liver. Excreted in urine (30%–50% as unchanged drug). **Half-life:** 2–3 hrs.

USES

Injection: Preop to inhibit salivation/secretions; treatment of symptomatic sinus bradycardia; AV block; ventricular asystole; antidote for organophosphate pesticide poisoning. **Ophthalmic:** Produce mydriasis and cycloplegia for examination of retina and optic disc; uveitis. **OFF-LABEL:** Malignant glaucoma, pulseless electric activity, asystole, neuromuscular blockage reversal.

PRECAUTIONS

Contraindications: Bladder neck obstruction due to prostatic hypertrophy, cardiospasm, intestinal atony, myasthenia gravis in those not treated with neostigmine, narrow-angle glaucoma, obstructive disease of GI tract, paralytic ileus, severe ulcerative colitis, tachycardia secondary to cardiac insufficiency or thyrotoxicosis, toxic megacolon, unstable cardiovascular status in acute hemorrhage. **Extreme Caution:** Autonomic neuropathy, known or suspected GI infections, diarrhea, mild to moderate ulcerative colitis. **Cautions:** Hyperthyroidism, hepatic/renal disease, hypertension, tachyarrhythmias, CHF, coronary artery disease, gastric ulcer, esophageal reflux or hiatal hernia associated with reflux esophagitis, infants, elderly, systemic administration in those with chronic obstructive pulmonary disease (COPD). **Ophthalmic:** Spastic paralysis, brain injury, Down syndrome.

LIFESPAN CONSIDERATIONS

Pregnancy/Lactation: Crosses placenta; distributed in breast milk. **Pregnancy Category C. Children/Elderly:** Increased susceptibility to atropine effects.

INTERACTIONS

DRUG: **Anticholinergics** may increase effects. **HERBAL:** None significant. **FOOD:** None known. **LAB VALUES:** None significant.

AVAILABILITY (Rx)

Injection (AtroPen): 0.25 mg/0.3 ml, 0.5 mg/0.7 ml, 1 mg/0.7 ml, 2 mg/0.7 ml. **Injection, Solution:** 0.05 mg/ml, 0.1 mg/ml, 0.4 mg/ml, 1 mg/ml. **Ophthalmic Ointment:** 1%. **Ophthalmic Solution:** 1%.

ADMINISTRATION/HANDLING

IV

• Must be given rapidly (prevents paradoxical slowing of heart rate).

IM

• May be given subcutaneously or IM.

IM, AtroPen

• Store at room temperature. • Give as soon as symptoms of organophosphorous or carbamate poisoning appear. • Do not use more than three AtroPen auto injectors for each person at risk for carbamate or organophosphate poisoning.

Ophthalmic

• Place gloved finger on lower eyelid and pull out until a pocket is formed between eye and lower lid. • Hold dropper above pocket and place prescribed number of drops or ¼–½ inch of ointment into pocket. • Instruct pt to close eye gently (so medication will not be squeezed out of the sac). • For solution, apply digital pressure to lacrimal sac at inner canthus for 1 min to minimize systemic absorption. • For ointment, instruct pt to roll eyeball to increase contact area of drug to eye.

IV INCOMPATIBILITY

Pentothal (Thiopental).

IV COMPATIBILITIES

Diphenhydramine (Benadryl), droperidol (Inapsine), fentanyl (Sublimaze), glycopyrrolate (Robinul), heparin, hydromorphone (Dilaudid), midazolam (Versed), morphine, potassium chloride, propofol (Diprivan).

INDICATIONS/ROUTES/DOSAGE

Asystole, Slow Pulseless Electrical Activity

IV: ADULTS, ELDERLY: 1 mg; may repeat q3–5min up to total dose of 0.04 mg/kg.

Preanesthetic

IV, IM, SUBCUTANEOUS: ADULTS, ELDERLY: 0.4–0.6 mg 30–60 min preop. **CHILDREN WEIGHING 5 KG OR MORE:** 0.01–0.02 mg/kg/dose to maximum of 0.4 mg/dose. Minimum Dose: 0.1 mg. **CHILDREN WEIGHING LESS THAN 5 KG:** 0.02 mg/kg/dose 30–60 min preop.

Bradycardia

IV: ADULTS, ELDERLY: 0.5–1 mg q5min not to exceed total of 3 mg or 0.04 mg/kg. **CHILDREN:** 0.02 mg/kg with a minimum of 0.1 mg to a maximum of 0.5 mg in children and 1 mg in adolescents. May repeat in 5 min. **Maximum total dose:** 1 mg in children, 2 mg in adolescents.

Cycloplegic Refraction, Postop Mydriasis, Uveitis
OPHTHALMIC SOLUTION: ADULTS, ELDERLY: Instill 1 drop in affected eye(s) up to 4 times a day.
OPHTHALMIC OINTMENT: ADULTS, ELDERLY: Apply ointment several hours prior to examination when used for refraction.

Antidote for Organophosphate or Carbamate Poisoning
IM: ADULTS, CHILDREN WEIGHING MORE THAN 90 LB: AtroPen 2 mg (green). **CHILDREN WEIGHING 40–90 LB:** AtroPen 1 mg (dark red). **CHILDREN WEIGHING 15–39 LB:** AtroPen 0.5 mg (blue). **INFANTS WEIGHING LESS THAN 15 LB:** 0.05 mg/kg. Do not use AtroPen.

SIDE EFFECTS

Frequent: Dry mouth, nose, throat (may be severe); decreased diaphoresis; constipation; irritation at subcutaneous or IM injection site. **Occasional:** Dyphagia, blurred vision, bloated feeling, impotence, urinary hesitancy. **Ophthalmic:** Mydriasis, blurred vision, photophobia, decreased visual acuity, tearing, dry eyes or dry conjunctiva, eye irritation, crusting of eyelid. **Rare:** Allergic reaction, including rash, urticaria; mental confusion or excitement, particularly in children; fatigue.

ADVERSE EFFECTS/ TOXIC REACTIONS

Overdose may produce tachycardia, palpitations, hot/dry/flushed skin, absence of bowel sounds, increased respiratory rate, nausea, vomiting, confusion, drowsiness, slurred speech, dizziness, CNS stimulation. Overdose may also produce psychosis as evidenced by agitation, restlessness, rambling speech, visual hallucinations, paranoid behavior, delusions, followed by depression. Opthalmic form may rarely produce increased IOP.

NURSING CONSIDERATIONS

BASELINE ASSESSMENT

Determine if pt is sensitive to atropine, homatropine, scopolamine. Treatment with AtroPen auto injector may be instituted without waiting for lab results.

INTERVENTION/EVALUATION

Monitor changes in B/P, pulse, temperature. Observe for tachycardia if pt has cardiac abnormalities. Assess skin turgor, mucous membranes to evaluate hydration status (encourage adequate fluid intake unless NPO for surgery), bowel sounds for peristalsis. Be alert for fever (increased risk of hyperthermia). Monitor I&O, palpate bladder for urinary retention. Monitor daily pattern of bowel activity and stool consistency.

PATIENT/ FAMILY TEACHING

• For preop use, explain that warm, dry, flushing feeling may occur.

Atrovent, *see ipratropium*

Augmentin, *see amoxicillin/clavulanate*

Augmentin XR, *see amoxicillin/clavulanate*

Avalide, *see hydrochlorothiazide and irbesartan*

Avandamet, *see metformin and rosiglitazone*

Avandia, *see rosiglitazone*

Avapro, *see irbesartan*

Avastin, *see bevacizumab*

Avelox, *see moxifloxacin*

Avelox IV, *see moxifloxacin*

Avinza, *see morphine*

Avodart, *see dutasteride*

Avonex, *see interferon beta-1a*

azacitidine

HIGH ALERT

ay-zah-**sigh**-tih-deen
(Vidaza)
Do not confuse azacitidine with azathioprine.

CLASSIFICATION

PHARMACOTHERAPEUTIC: Antineoplastic. **CLINICAL:** DNA demethylation agent.

ACTION

Exerts cytotoxic effect on rapidly dividing cells by causing demethylation of DNA in abnormal hematopoietic cells in bone marrow. **Therapeutic Effect:** Restores normal function to tumor-suppressor genes regulating cellular differentiation, proliferation.

PHARMACOKINETICS

Rapidly absorbed after subcutaneous administration. Metabolized by liver. Eliminated in urine. **Half-life:** 4 hrs.

USES

Treatment of myelodysplastic syndromes (MDS), specifically refractory anemia, myelomonocytic leukemia. **OFF-LABEL:** Treatment of refractory acute lymophocytic and myelogenous leukemia.

PRECAUTIONS

Contraindications: Advanced malignant hepatic tumors, hypersensitivity to mannitol. **Cautions:** Hepatic disease, renal impairment.

LIFESPAN CONSIDERATIONS

Pregnancy/Lactation: May be embryotoxic; may cause developmental abnormalities of the fetus. Mothers should avoid breast-feeding. **Pregnancy Category D. Children:** Safety and efficacy not established. **Elderly:** Age-related renal impairment may increase risk of renal toxicity.

INTERACTIONS

DRUG: Bone marrow suppressants may increase myelosuppression. **HERBAL:** None significant. **FOOD:** None known. **LAB VALUES:** May decrease Hgb, Hct, WBC, RBC, platelet counts. May increase serum creatinine, potassium, AST, ALT, alkaline phosphatase.

AVAILABILITY (Rx)

Injection, Powder for Reconstitution: 100 mg.

ADMINISTRATION/HANDLING

IV

Reconstitution • Reconstitute each vial with 10 ml Sterile Water for Injection to provide a concentration of 10 mg/ml. • Vigorously shake/roll vial until all solids are dissolved. Solution should be clear. • Further dilute desired dose with 50–100 ml 0.9% NaCl.
Rate of administration • Administer total dose over 10–40 min. • Administration should be completed within 1 hr of reconstitution of vial.
Stability • Store unreconstituted vial at room temperature. • Solution is stable for 1 hr following reconstitution.

SUBCUTANEOUS

Reconstitution • Reconstitute with 4 ml Sterile Water for Injection. • Reconstituted solution will appear cloudy.
Rate of administration • Doses greater than 4 ml should be divided equally into 2 syringes. • Contents of syringe must be resuspended by inverting the syringe 2–3 times and rolling the syringe between the palms for 30 sec immediately before administration. • Rotate site for each injection (thigh, upper arm, abdomen). New injections should be administered at least 1 inch from the old site.
Storage • Store vials at room temperature. • Reconstituted solution may be stored for up to 1 hr at room temperature or up to 8 hrs if refrigerated. • Solution may be allowed to return to room temperature and used within 30 min.

IV INCOMPATIBILITIES

Dextrose, hespan, solutions containing sodium bicarbonate.

IV COMPATIBILITIES

Lactated Ringer's, sodium chloride.

INDICATIONS/ROUTES/DOSAGE

MDS

◀ALERT▶ Dosage adjustment based on hematology testing.

IV/SUBCUTANEOUS: ADULTS, ELDERLY: 75 mg/m^2/day for 7 days every 4 wks. Dosage may be increased to 100 mg/m^2 if initial dose is insufficient and toxicity is manageable. Treatment recommended for at least 4 cycles.

SIDE EFFECTS

Frequent (71%–29%): **IV/Subcutaneous:** Nausea, vomiting, fever, diarrhea, fatigue, injection site erythema, constipation, ecchymosis, cough, dyspnea, weakness. **IV:** Petechiae, weakness, rigors, hypokalemia. Occasional (26%–16%): **IV/Subcutaneous:** Rigors, petechiae, injection site pain, pharyngitis, arthralgia, headache, limb pain, dizziness, peripheral edema, back pain, erythema, epistaxis, weight loss, myalgia. Rare (13%–8%): **IV/Subcutaneous:** Anxiety, abdominal pain, rash, depression, tachycardia, insomnia, night sweats, stomatitis.

ADVERSE EFFECTS/ TOXIC REACTIONS

Hematologic toxicity, manifested as anemia, leukopenia, neutropenia, thrombocytopenia, occurs commonly.

NURSING CONSIDERATIONS

BASELINE ASSESSMENT

Give emotional support to pt and family. Use strict aseptic technique and protect pt from infection. Obtain blood counts, electrolytes, BUN, serum creatinine, hepatic enzyme levels routinely to monitor response and toxicity but particularly before each dosing cycle.

INTERVENTION/EVALUATION

Monitor for hematologic toxicity (fever, sore throat, signs of local infections, unusual bruising/bleeding), symptoms of anemia (excessive fatigue, weakness). Assess response to medication; monitor and report nausea, vomiting, diarrhea. Avoid rectal temperatures, other traumas that may induce bleeding.

PATIENT/FAMILY TEACHING

• Do not have immunizations without physician's approval (drug lowers body's resistance). • Avoid crowds, persons with known infections. • Report signs of infection (fever, flu-like symptoms) immediately. • Contact physician if nausea/vomiting continues at home. • Men should use barrier contraception while receiving treatment.

Azactam, *see aztreonam*

azathioprine

ay-za-**thye**-oh-preen
(Apo-Azathioprine ✦, Azasan, Imuran, Novo-Azathioprine ✦)

BLACK BOX ALERT Chronic immunosuppression increases risk of neoplastic syndrome, serious infections.

Do not confuse azathioprine with Azulfidine, azacitidine, or azithromycin, or Imuran with Elmiron, Imdur, or Inderal.

CLASSIFICATION

PHARMACOTHERAPEUTIC: Immunologic agent. **CLINICAL:** Immunosuppressant.

ACTION

Antagonizes purine metabolism, inhibits DNA, protein, and RNA synthesis. **Therapeutic Effect:** Suppresses cell-mediated hypersensitivities; alters antibody production, immune response in transplant recipients. Reduces symptoms of arthritis severity.

USES

Adjunct in prevention of rejection in kidney transplantation; treatment of rheumatoid arthritis (RA) in those unresponsive to conventional therapy. **OFF-LABEL:** Treatment of biliary cirrhosis, chronic active hepatitis, glomerulonephritis, inflammatory bowel disease, inflammatory myopathy, multiple sclerosis, myasthenia gravis, nephrotic syndrome, pemphigoid, pemphigus, polymyositis, systemic lupus erythematosus. Adjunct in preventing rejection of solid organ (nonrenal) transplants. Maintenance, remission in Crohn's disease.

PRECAUTIONS

Contraindications: Pregnant pts with rheumatoid arthritis (RA). **Cautions:** Immunosuppressed pts, those previously treated for RA with alkylating agents (cyclophosphamide, chlorambucil, melphalan), chickenpox (current or recent), herpes zoster, gout, hepatic/renal impairment, active infection.

LIFESPAN CONSIDERATIONS

Pregnancy/Lactation: May depress spermatogenesis, reduction of sperm viability, count. May cause fetal harm. Do not breast-feed. **Pregnancy Category D. Children:** Safety and efficacy not established. **Elderly:** No age-related precautions noted.

INTERACTIONS

DRUG: **Allopurinol** may increase activity, toxicity. **Bone marrow depressants** may increase myelosuppression. **Other immunosuppressants** may increase risk of infection or development of neoplasms. **Live virus vaccines** may potentiate virus replication, increase vaccine side effects, decrease pt's antibody response to vaccine. **HERBAL:** Avoid **cat's claw, echinacea** (immunostimulant properties). **FOOD:** None known. **LAB VALUES:** May decrease Hgb, serum albumin, uric acid. May increase AST, ALT, alkaline phosphatase, amylase, bilirubin.

AVAILABILITY (Rx)

Injection, Powder for Reconstitution (Imuran): 100-mg vial. **Tablets:** 50 mg (Imuran), 75 mg (Azasan), 100 mg (Azasan).

ADMINISTRATION/HANDLING

IV

Reconstitution • Reconstitute 100-mg vial with 10 ml Sterile Water for Injection to provide concentration of 10 mg/ml. • Swirl vial gently to mix and dissolve solution. • May further dilute in 50 ml D_5W or 0.9% NaCl.

Rate of administration • Give IVP over 5 min at concentration not to exceed 10 mg/ml or as intermittent infusion over 15–60 min.

Storage • Store parenteral form at room temperature. • After reconstitution, IV solution stable for 24 hrs.

PO

• Give with food or in divided doses to reduce potential for GI disturbances. • Store oral form at room temperature.

IV INCOMPATIBILITIES

Methyl and propyl parabens, phenol.

INDICATIONS/ROUTES/DOSAGE

Prevention of Renal Allograft Rejection

PO, IV: ADULTS, ELDERLY, CHILDREN: 3–5 mg/kg/day on day of transplant, then 1–3 mg/kg/day as maintenance dose.

Rheumatoid Arthritis (RA)

PO: ADULTS: Initially, 1 mg/kg/day as a single dose or in 2 divided doses for 6–8 wks. May increase by 0.5 mg/kg/day after 6–8 wks at 4-wk intervals. **Maximum:** 2.5 mg/kg/day. Maintenance: Lowest effective dosage. May decrease dose by 0.5 mg/kg or 25 mg/day q4wk (while other therapies, such as rest, physiotherapy, and salicylates, are maintained). **ELDERLY:** Initially, 1 mg/kg/day (50–100 mg); may increase by 25 mg/day until response or toxicity.

Dosage in Renal Impairment

Dosage is modified based on creatinine clearance.

Creatinine Clearance	Dosage
10–50 ml/min	75% of normal
Less than 10 ml/min	50% of normal

SIDE EFFECTS

Frequent: Nausea, vomiting, anorexia (particularly during early treatment and with large doses). **Occasional:** Rash. **Rare:** Severe nausea/vomiting with diarrhea, abdominal pain, hypersensitivity reaction.

ADVERSE EFFECTS/ TOXIC REACTIONS

Increases risk of neoplasia (new abnormal-growth tumors). Significant leukopenia and thrombocytopenia may occur, particularly in those undergoing renal transplant rejection. Hepatotoxicity occurs rarely.

NURSING CONSIDERATIONS

BASELINE ASSESSMENT

Arthritis: Assess onset, type, location, and duration of pain, fever, inflammation. Inspect appearance of affected joints for immobility, deformities, skin condition.

INTERVENTION/EVALUATION

CBC, platelet count, hepatic function studies should be performed weekly during first mo of therapy, twice monthly during second and third mos of treatment, then monthly thereafter. If WBC falls rapidly, dosage should be reduced or discontinued. Assess particularly for delayed myelosuppression. Routinely watch for any change from baseline. **Arthritis:** Assess for therapeutic response: relief of pain, stiffness, swelling; increased joint mobility; reduced joint tenderness; improved grip strength.

PATIENT/FAMILY TEACHING

• Contact physician if unusual bleeding/bruising, sore throat, mouth sores, abdominal pain, fever occurs. • Therapeutic response in rheumatoid arthritis may take up to 12 wks. • Women of childbearing age must avoid pregnancy.

azelastine

aye-zeh-**las**-teen
(Astelin, Astepro, Optivar)

Do not confuse Astelin with Astepro or Optivar with Optiray.

◆CLASSIFICATION

PHARMACOTHERAPEUTIC: Antihistamine. **CLINICAL:** Antiallergy.

ACTION

Competes with histamine for histamine receptor sites on cells in blood vessels, GI tract, respiratory tract. **Therapeutic Effect:** Relieves symptoms associated with seasonal allergic rhinitis (increased mucus production, sneezing) and symptoms associated with allergic conjunctivitis (redness, itching, excessive tearing).

PHARMACOKINETICS

Route	Onset	Peak	Duration
Nasal spray	0.5–1 hr	2–3 hrs	12 hrs
Ophthalmic	N/A	3 min	8 hrs

Well absorbed through nasal mucosa. Primarily excreted in feces. Protein binding: 88%. Metabolized in liver. **Half-life:** 22 hrs.

USES

Nasal: Treatment of symptoms of seasonal and perennial allergic rhinitis. **Ophthalmic:** Treatment of itching associated with allergic conjunctivitis.

PRECAUTIONS

Contraindications: Breast-feeding women; history of hypersensitivity to antihistamines; neonates or premature infants; third trimester of pregnancy. **Cautions:** Renal impairment.

⌛ LIFESPAN CONSIDERATIONS

Pregnancy/Lactation: Unknown if drug crosses placenta or is distributed in breast milk. Do not use during third trimester. **Pregnancy Category C. Children:** Safety and efficacy not established in those younger than 12 yrs. **Elderly:** No age-related precautions noted.

INTERACTIONS

DRUG: Alcohol, CNS depressants may increase CNS depression. **Cimetidine** may increase plasma concentration. **HERBAL:** None significant. **FOOD:** None known. **LAB VALUES:** May suppress wheal and flare reaction to antigen skin testing unless drug is discontinued 4 days before testing. May increase serum ALT.

AVAILABILITY (Rx)

Nasal Spray (Astelin, Astepro): (0.1%) 137 mcg/spray. **(Astepro):** (0.15%) 205.5 mcg/spray. **Ophthalmic Solution (Optivar):** 0.05%.

ADMINISTRATION/HANDLING

Nasal

• Instruct pt to clear nasal passages as much as possible before use. • Tilt pt's head slightly forward. • Insert spray tip into nostril, pointing toward nasal passage, away from nasal septum. • Spray into nostril while pt holds the other nostril closed and concurrently inhales through nose to permit medication as high into nasal passage as possible.

Ophthalmic

• Place gloved finger on lower eyelid and pull out until a pocket is formed between eye and lower lid. • Place prescribed number of drops into pocket. • Instruct pt to close eye gently for 1–2 min (so medication will not be squeezed out of the sac) and to apply digital pressure to lacrimal sac at inner canthus for 1 min to minimize systemic absorption.

INDICATIONS/ROUTES/DOSAGE

Allergic Rhinitis

NASAL: ADULTS, ELDERLY, CHILDREN 12 YRS AND OLDER: (Astelin, Astepro): 1–2 sprays in each nostril twice a day. **(Astepro 0.15%):** 2 sprays once daily (twice daily for perennial allergic rhinitis). **CHILDREN 5–11 YRS: (Astelin):** 1 spray in each nostril twice a day.

Allergic Conjunctivitis
OPHTHALMIC: ADULTS, ELDERLY, CHILDREN 3 YRS AND OLDER: 1 drop into affected eye twice a day.

SIDE EFFECTS

Nasal: Frequent (20%–15%): Headache, bitter taste. **Rare:** Nasal burning, paroxysmal sneezing, drowsiness. **Ophthalmic:** Transient eye burning or stinging, bitter taste, headache.

ADVERSE EFFECTS/ TOXIC REACTIONS

Epistaxis occurs rarely.

NURSING CONSIDERATIONS

BASELINE ASSESSMENT

Question for hypersensitivity to antihistamines.

INTERVENTION/EVALUATION

Assess therapeutic response to medication.

PATIENT/FAMILY TEACHING

• May cause drowsiness, impair ability to perform tasks requiring mental alertness or physical coordination. • Avoid alcohol.

azithromycin

aye-zith-row-**my**-sin
(Apo-Azithromycin, AzaSite, Novo-Azithromycin, Zithromax, Zithromax TRI-PAK, Zithromax Z-PAK, Zmax)
Do not confuse azithromycin with azathioprine or erythromycin, or Zithromax with Fosamax or Zovirax.

◆CLASSIFICATION

PHARMACOTHERAPEUTIC: Macrolide. **CLINICAL:** Antibiotic (see p. 26C).

ACTION

Binds to ribosomal receptor sites of susceptible organisms, inhibiting RNA-dependent protein synthesis. **Therapeutic Effect:** Bacteriostatic or bactericidal, depending on drug dosage.

PHARMACOKINETICS

Rapidly absorbed from GI tract. Protein binding: 7%–50%. Widely distributed. Metabolized in liver. Eliminated primarily by biliary excretion. **Half-life:** 68 hrs.

USES

IV/PO: Treatment of susceptible infections due to *Chlamydia pneumoniae, C. trachomatis, H. influenzae, Legionella, M. catarrhalis, Mycoplasma pneumoniae, N. gonorrhoeae, S. aureus. S. pneumoniae, S. pyogenes* including mild to moderate infections of upper respiratory tract (pharyngitis, tonsillitis), lower respiratory tract (acute bacterial exacerbations, COPD, pneumonia), uncomplicated skin and skin-structure infections, sexually transmitted diseases (nongonococcal urethritis, cervicitis due to *Chlamydia trachomatis*), chancroid. Prevents disseminated *Mycobacterium avium* complex (MAC). Treatment of mycoplasma pneumonia, community-acquired pneumonia, pelvic inflammatory disease (PID). **Ophthalmic:** Treatment of bacterial conjunctivitis caused by susceptible infections due to *H. influenzae, S. aureus, S. mitis, S. pneumoniae.* **OFF-LABEL:** Treatment of chlamydial infections, gonococcal pharyngitis, uncomplicated gonococcal infections of cervix, urethra, rectum. Prevention/treatment of MAC in pts with advanced HIV infection; prophylaxis of endocarditis, pertussis.

PRECAUTIONS

Contraindications: Hypersensitivity to other macrolide antibiotics. **Cautions:** Hepatic/renal dysfunction. May prolong QT interval (rare).

LIFESPAN CONSIDERATIONS

Pregnancy/Lactation: Unknown if distributed in breast milk. **Pregnancy Category B. Children:** Safety and efficacy not established in those younger than 16 yrs for IV use and younger than 6 mos for oral use. **Elderly:** No age-related precautions in those with normal renal function.

INTERACTIONS

DRUG: **Aluminum/magnesium-containing antacids** may decrease concentration (give 1 hr before or 2 hrs after antacid). HERBAL: None significant. FOOD: None known. LAB VALUES: May increase serum creatine phosphokinase (CPK), AST, ALT, bilirubin, LDH, potassium.

AVAILABILITY (Rx)

Injection, Powder for Reconstitution (Zithromax): 500 mg. Ophthalmic Solution (Azasite): 1%. Suspension, Oral (Zithromax): 100 mg/5 ml, 200 mg/5 ml, 1-g single dose packet. Suspension, Oral (Extended-Release [ZMAX]): 2-g single-dose packet. Tablets: 250 mg, 500 mg, 600 mg (Zithromax). Tri-Pak: 3 × 500 mg (Zithromax TRI-PAK). Z-Pak: 6 × 250 mg (Zithromax Z-PAK).

ADMINISTRATION/HANDLING

IV

Reconstitution • Reconstitute each 500-mg vial with 4.8 ml Sterile Water for Injection to provide concentration of 100 mg/ml. • Shake well to ensure dissolution. • Further dilute with 250 or 500 ml 0.9% NaCl or D_5W to provide final concentration of 2 mg with 250 ml diluent or 1 mg/ml with 500 ml diluent.

Rate of administration • Infuse over 60 min.

Storage • Store vials at room temperature. • Following reconstitution, diluted solution is stable for 24 hrs at room temperature or 7 days if refrigerated.

PO (Immediate-release suspension)

• Give tablets without regard to food. • May store suspension at room temperature. Stable for 10 days after reconstitution.

PO (Extended-release suspension)

• Do not administer oral suspension with food. Give at least 1 hr before or 2 hrs after meals. • Give Zmax within 12 hrs of reconstitution.

Ophthalmic

• Place gloved finger on lower eyelid and pull out until a pocket is formed between eye and lower lid. • Place prescribed number of drops into pocket. • Instruct pt to close eye gently for 1 to 2 min (so medication will not be squeezed out of sac) and to apply digital pressure to lacrimal sac at inner canthus for 1 min to minimize systemic absorption.

IV INCOMPATIBILITIES

Ceftriaxone (Rocephin), ciprofloxacin (Cipro), famotidine (Pepcid), furosemide (Lasix), ketorolac (Toradol), levofloxacin (Levaquin), morphine, piperacillin/tazobactam (Zosyn), potassium chloride.

IV COMPATIBILITY

Diphenhydramine (Benadryl).

INDICATIONS/ROUTES/DOSAGE

Usual Dosage Range

PO: ADULTS, ELDERLY: 250–600 mg once daily or 1–2 g as single dose. **CHILDREN 6 MOS AND OLDER:** 5–12 mg/kg once daily or 30 mg/kg as single dose.
IV: ADULTS, ELDERLY: 250–500 mg once daily (not currently approved in children).

Acute Exacerbations of COPD

PO: ADULTS, ELDERLY, CHILDREN 16 YRS AND OLDER: 500 mg/day for 3 days or 500 mg on day 1, then 250 mg/day on days 2–5.

Acute Bacterial Sinusitis

PO (ZMAX): ADULTS, ELDERLY: 2 g as a single dose.

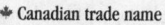

PO: ADULTS, ELDERLY: 500 mg/day for 3 days. **CHILDREN 6 MOS AND OLDER:** 10 mg/kg for 3 days. **Maximum:** 500 mg/day.

Cervicitis

PO: ADULTS, ELDERLY: 1–2 g as single dose.

Chancroid

PO: ADULTS, ELDERLY: 1 g as single dose.

MAC Prevention

PO: ADULTS, ELDERLY: 1,200 mg once weekly. **CHILDREN:** 20 mg/kg once weekly. **Maximum:** 1,200 mg/dose.

MAC Treatment

PO: ADULTS, ELDERLY: 600 mg/day with ethambutol 15 mg/kg/day. **CHILDREN:** 5–20 mg/kg/day for 1 mo or longer.

Otitis Media

PO: CHILDREN 6 MOS AND OLDER: 30 mg/kg as single dose or 10 mg/kg/day for 3 days or 10 mg/kg on day 1, then 5 mg/kg on days 2–5.

Pharyngitis, Tonsillitis

PO: ADULTS, ELDERLY, CHILDREN 16 YRS AND OLDER: 500 mg on day 1, then 250 mg on days 2–5. **CHILDREN 2–15 YRS:** 12 mg/kg daily for 5 days.

Pneumonia, Community-Acquired

PO (ZMAX): ADULTS, ELDERLY: 2 g as a single dose.

PO: ADULTS, ELDERLY, CHILDREN 16 YRS AND OLDER: 500 mg on day 1, then 250 mg on days 2–5 or 500 mg/day IV for 2 days, then 500 mg/day PO to complete course of therapy. **CHILDREN 6 MOS–15 YRS:** 10 mg/kg on day 1, then 5 mg/kg on days 2–5.

Skin and Skin-Structure Infections

PO: ADULTS, ELDERLY, CHILDREN 16 YRS AND OLDER: 500 mg on day 1, then 250 mg on days 2–5.

Pelvic Inflammatory Disease (PID)

IV: ADULTS, ELDERLY: 500 mg/day for at least 2 days, then 250 mg/day to complete a 7-day course of therapy.

Bacterial Conjunctivitis

OPHTHALMIC: ADULTS, ELDERLY: 1 drop in affected eye twice a day for 2 days, then 1 drop once a day for 5 days.

SIDE EFFECTS

Occasional: Systemic: Nausea, vomiting, diarrhea, abdominal pain. **Ophthalmic:** Eye irritation. **Rare: Systemic:** Headache, dizziness, allergic reaction.

ADVERSE EFFECTS/ TOXIC REACTIONS

Antibiotic-associated colitis, other superinfections (abdominal cramps, severe watery diarrhea, fever) may result from altered bacterial balance. Acute interstitial nephritis, hepatotoxicity occur rarely.

NURSING CONSIDERATIONS

BASELINE ASSESSMENT

Question for history of hepatitis, allergies to azithromycin, erythromycins. Assess for infection (WBC count, appearance of wound, evidence of fever).

INTERVENTION/EVALUATION

Check for GI discomfort, nausea, vomiting. Monitor daily pattern of bowel activity and stool consistency. Monitor hepatic function tests, CBC. Assess for hepatotoxicity: malaise, fever, abdominal pain, GI disturbances. Be alert for superinfection: fever, vomiting, diarrhea, anal/genital pruritus, oral mucosal changes (ulceration, pain, erythema).

PATIENT/FAMILY TEACHING

• Continue therapy for full length of treatment. • Avoid concurrent administration of aluminum- or magnesium-containing antacids. • Bacterial conjunctivitis: Do not wear contact lenses.

aztreonam

az-**tree**-oo-nam
(Azactam, Cayston)

◆CLASSIFICATION

PHARMACOTHERAPEUTIC: Monobactam. **CLINICAL:** Antibiotic.

ACTION

Inhibits bacterial cell wall synthesis. **Therapeutic Effect:** Bactericidal.

PHARMACOKINETICS

Completely absorbed after IM administration. Protein binding: 56%–60%. Partially metabolized by hydrolysis. Primarily excreted unchanged in urine. Removed by hemodialysis. **Half-life:** 1.4–2.2 hrs (increased in renal/hepatic impairment).

USES

Treatment of infections caused by susceptible gram-negative micro-organisms *P. aeruginosa, E. coli, S. marcescens, K. pneumoniae, P. mirabilis, H. influenzae, Enterobacter, Citrobacter* spp. including lower respiratory tract, skin/skin structure, intra-abdominal, gynecologic, complicated/uncomplicated UTIs; septicemia, cystic fibrosis. **Clayston:** Improve respiratory symptoms in cystic fibrosis pts with *Pseudomonas aeruginosa.* **OFF-LABEL:** Treatment of bone and joint infections.

PRECAUTIONS

Contraindications: None known. **Cautions:** History of allergy, esp. antibiotics, hepatic/renal impairment.

LIFESPAN CONSIDERATIONS

Pregnancy/Lactation: Crosses placenta, distributed in amniotic fluid; low concentration in breast milk. **Pregnancy Category B. Children:** Safety and efficacy not established in those younger than 9 mos. **Elderly:** Age-related renal impairment may require dosage adjustment.

INTERACTIONS

DRUG: None significant. **HERBAL:** None significant. **FOOD:** None known. **LAB VALUES:** May increase serum alkaline phosphatase, creatinine, LDH, AST, ALT levels. Produces a positive Coombs' test. May prolong partial thromboplastin time (PTT), prothrombin time (PT).

AVAILABILITY (Rx)

Injection, Infusion Solution (Azactam): Premix 1 g/50 ml, 2 g/50 ml. **Injection, Powder for Reconstitution (Azactam):** 500 mg, 1 g, 2 g. **Oral Inhalation, Powder for Reconstitution (Cayston):** 75 mg.

ADMINISTRATION/HANDLING

IV

Reconstitution • For IV push, dilute each gram with 6–10 ml Sterile Water for Injection. • For intermittent IV infusion, further dilute with 50–100 ml D_5W or 0.9% NaCl.

Rate of administration • For IV push, give over 3–5 min. • For IV infusion, administer over 20–60 min.

Storage • Store vials at room temperature. • Solution appears colorless to light yellow. • Following reconstitution, solution is stable for 48 hrs at room temperature or 7 days if refrigerated. • Discard if precipitate forms. Discard unused portions.

IM

• Shake immediately, vigorously after adding diluent. • Inject deeply into large muscle mass. • Following reconstitution, solution is stable for 48 hrs at room temperature or 7 days if refrigerated.

Inhalation

• Administer only with an Altera nebulizer system. • Nebulize over 2–3 min. • Give bronchodilator 15 min–4 hr (short-acting) or 30 min–12 hrs (long-acting) before administration. • Reconstituted solution must be used immediately.

IV INCOMPATIBILITIES

Acyclovir (Zovirax), amphotericin (Fungizone), daunorubicin (Cerubidine), ganciclovir (Cytovene), lorazepam (Ativan), metronidazole (Flagyl), vancomycin (Vancocin).

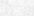

B

IV COMPATIBILITIES

Aminophylline, bumetanide (Bumex), calcium gluconate, cimetidine (Tagamet), diltiazem (Cardizem), diphenhydramine (Benadryl), dobutamine (Dobutrex), dopamine (Intropin), famotidine (Pepcid), furosemide (Lasix), heparin, hydromorphone (Dilaudid), insulin (regular), lipids, magnesium sulfate, meperidine (Demerol), morphine, potassium chloride, propofol (Diprivan), total parenteral nutrition (TPN).

INDICATIONS/ROUTES/DOSAGE

UTIs

IV, IM: ADULTS, ELDERLY: 500 mg–1 g q8–12h.

Moderate to Severe Systemic Infections

IV, IM: ADULTS, ELDERLY: 1–2 g q8–12h.

Severe or Life-Threatening Infections

IV: ADULTS, ELDERLY: 2 g q6–8h.

Cystic Fibrosis

IV: CHILDREN: 50 mg/kg/dose q6–8h up to 200 mg/kg/day. **Maximum:** 8 g/day.

INHALATION: ADULTS, CHILDREN 7 YRS OR OLDER: 75 mg 3 times/day (at least 4 hrs apart) for 28 days, then off for 28-day cycle.

Mild to Severe Infections in Children

IV: CHILDREN: 30 mg/kg q6–8h. **Maximum:** 120 mg/kg/day. **NEONATES:** 60–120 mg/kg/day divided q6–12h (dosage based on age and weight).

Dosage in Renal Impairment

Dosage and frequency are modified based on creatinine clearance and severity of infection:

Creatinine Clearance	Dosage
10–30 ml/min	½ usual dose at usual intervals
Less than 10 ml/min	¼ usual dose at usual intervals

SIDE EFFECTS

Frequent (greater than 5%): **Clayston:** Cough, nasal congestion, wheezing, pharyngolaryngeal pain, pyrexia, chest discomfort, abdominal pain, vomiting.

Occasional (less than 3%): Discomfort and swelling at IM injection site, nausea, vomiting, diarrhea, rash. Rare (less than 1%): Phlebitis or thrombophlebitis at IV injection site, abdominal cramps, headache, hypotension.

ADVERSE EFFECTS/ TOXIC REACTIONS

Antibiotic-associated colitis, other superinfections (abdominal cramps, severe watery diarrhea, fever) may result from altered bacterial balance. Severe hypersensitivity reactions, including anaphylaxis, occur rarely.

NURSING CONSIDERATIONS

BASELINE ASSESSMENT

Question for history of allergies, esp. to aztreonam, other antibiotics.

INTERVENTION/EVALUATION

Evaluate for phlebitis (heat, pain, red streaking over vein), pain at IM injection site. Assess for GI discomfort, nausea, vomiting. Monitor daily pattern of bowel activity and stool consistency. Assess skin for rash. Be alert for superinfection: fever, vomiting, diarrhea, anal/genital pruritus, oral mucosal changes (ulceration, pain, erythema). Monitor renal/hepatic function.

PATIENT/FAMILY TEACHING

- Report nausea, vomiting, diarrhea, rash.

bacitracin

bah-cih-tray-sin
(Baciguent, Baci-Rx, Bacitracin)
Do not confuse bacitracin with Bactrim or Bactroban.

FIXED-COMBINATION(S)

With polymyxin B, an antibiotic **(Polysporin);** with polymyxin B and neomycin, antibiotics **(Neosporin).**

◆CLASSIFICATION

PHARMACOTHERAPEUTIC: Anti-infective. **CLINICAL:** Antibiotic.

ACTION

Interferes with plasma membrane permeability, inhibits bacterial cell wall synthesis in susceptible microorganisms. **Therapeutic Effect:** Bacteriostatic.

USES

Ophthalmic: Superficial ocular infections (conjunctivitis, keratitis, corneal ulcers, blepharitis). **Topical:** Minor skin abrasions, superficial infections. **Irrigation:** Treatment, prophylaxis of surgical procedures.

PRECAUTIONS

Contraindications: None known. **Cautions:** None known. **Pregnancy Category C.**

INTERACTIONS

DRUG: None significant. **HERBAL:** None significant. **FOOD:** None known. **LAB VALUES:** None significant.

AVAILABILITY (Rx)

Ophthalmic Ointment: 500 units/g. **Powder for Irrigation:** 50,000 units. **Topical Ointment (Baciguent [OTC]):** 500 units/g.

ADMINISTRATION/HANDLING

Ophthalmic

• Place gloved finger on lower eyelid and pull out until a pocket is formed between eye and lower lid. Place ¼–½ inch ointment into pocket. • Instruct pt to close eye gently for 1–2 min, and roll eyeball (increases contact area of drug to eye).

Topical

• Gently cleanse area prior to application. • Without touching application tip to skin, apply on area thoroughly.

INDICATIONS/ROUTES/DOSAGE

Superficial Ocular Infections

OPHTHALMIC: ADULTS: ¼- to ½-inch ribbon in conjunctival sac q3–4h.

Skin Abrasions, Superficial Skin Infections

TOPICAL: ADULTS, CHILDREN: Apply to affected area 1–5 times a day.

Surgical Treatment, Prophylaxis

IRRIGATION: ADULTS, ELDERLY: 50,000–150,000 units, as needed.

SIDE EFFECTS

Rare: **Ophthalmic:** Burning, itching, redness, swelling, pain. **Topical:** Hypersensitivity reaction (allergic contact dermatitis, burning, inflammation, pruritus).

ADVERSE EFFECTS/ TOXIC REACTIONS

Severe hypersensitivity reaction (apnea, hypotension) occur rarely.

NURSING CONSIDERATIONS

INTERVENTION/EVALUATION

Topical: Evaluate for hypersensitivity reaction: itching, burning, inflammation. With preparations containing corticosteroids, consider masking effect on clinical signs. **Ophthalmic:** Assess eye for therapeutic response or increased redness, swelling, burning, itching (hypersensitivity reaction).

PATIENT/FAMILY TEACHING

• Continue therapy for full length of treatment. • Doses should be evenly spaced. • Report burning, itching, rash, increased irritation.

baclofen

bak-loe-fen

(Apo-Baclofen ✱, Lioresal, Liotec ✱, Nu-Baclo ✱)

BLACK BOX ALERT Abrupt withdrawal of intrathecal form has resulted in severe

B

hyperpyrexia, obtundation, rebound or exaggerated spasticity, muscle rigidity, leading to organ failure, death.

Do not confuse baclofen with Bactroban or Beclovent, or Lioresal with lisinopril or Lotensin.

◆CLASSIFICATION

PHARMACOTHERAPEUTIC: Skeletal muscle relaxant. **CLINICAL:** Antispastic, analgesic in trigeminal neuralgia (see p. 151C).

ACTION

Inhibits transmission of reflexes at spinal cord level. **Therapeutic Effect:** Relieves muscle spasticity.

PHARMACOKINETICS

Well absorbed from GI tract. Protein binding: 30%. Partially metabolized in liver. Primarily excreted in urine. **Half-life:** 2.5–4 hrs.

USES

Treatment of cerebral spasticity, reversible spasticity associated with multiple sclerosis, spinal cord lesions. **Intrathecal:** For those unresponsive to oral therapy or exhibiting intolerable side effects. **OFF-LABEL:** Treatment of bladder spasms, cerebral palsy, intractable hiccups or pain, Huntington's chorea, trigeminal neuralgia.

PRECAUTIONS

Contraindications: Skeletal muscle spasm due to cerebral palsy, Parkinson's disease, rheumatic disorders, CVA, cough, intractable hiccups, neuropathic pain. **Cautions:** Renal impairment, CVA, diabetes mellitus, epilepsy, preexisting psychiatric disorders.

⌛ LIFESPAN CONSIDERATIONS

Pregnancy/Lactation: Unknown if drug crosses placenta or is distributed in breast milk. **Pregnancy Category C.** **Children:** Safety and efficacy not established in those younger than 12 yrs. Limited published data in children. **Elderly:** Increased risk of CNS toxicity (hallucinations, sedation, confusion, mental depression); age-related renal impairment may require decreased dosage.

INTERACTIONS

DRUG: Potentiated effects when used with other **CNS depressants (including alcohol). MAOIs** may increase CNS depression, hypotensive effect. **HERBAL:** **Gotu kola, kava kava, St. John's wort, valerian** may increase CNS sedation. **FOOD:** None known. **LAB VALUES:** May increase serum AST, ALT, alkaline phosphatase, blood glucose.

AVAILABILITY (Rx)

Intrathecal Injection Solution: 50 mcg/ml, 500 mcg/ml, 2,000 mcg/ml. **Tablets:** 10 mg, 20 mg.

ADMINISTRATION/HANDLING

PO

• Give without regard to food. • Tablets may be crushed.

Intrathecal

• For screening, a 50 mcg/ml concentration should be used for injection. • For maintenance therapy, solution should be diluted for pts who require concentrations other than 500 mcg/ml or 2,000 mcg/ml.

INDICATIONS/ROUTES/DOSAGE

◀ALERT▶ Avoid abrupt withdrawal.

Spasticity

PO: ADULTS: Initially, 5 mg 3 times a day. May increase by 15 mg/day at 3-day intervals. Range: 40–80 mg/day. **Maximum:** 80 mg/day. **ELDERLY:** Initially, 5 mg 2–3 times a day. May gradually increase dosage. **CHILDREN 8 YRS AND OLDER:** 30–40 mg/day in divided doses q8h. May increase dose by 5–15 mg/day q3days. **Maximum:** 120 mg/day. **CHILDREN 2–7 YRS:** 20–30 mg/day in divided doses q8h. May increase dose by 5–15 mg/day q3days. **Maximum:** 60 mg/day. **CHILDREN YOUNGER THAN 2 YRS:** 10–20 mg/day in divided doses q8h. May increase dose by 5–15 mg/day. **Maximum:** 40 mg/day.

Intrathecal Dose

ADULTS, ELDERLY, CHILDREN: Test dose: 50–100 mcg. Dose greater than 50 mcg given in 25-mcg increments, separated by 24 hrs. Following positive response to test dose, maintenance infusion can be given via implanted intrathecal pump. Initial dose is twice the test dose.

SIDE EFFECTS

Frequent (greater than 10%): Transient drowsiness, asthenia (loss of strength, energy), dizziness, light-headedness, nausea, vomiting. **Occasional (10%–2%):** Headache, paresthesia, constipation, anorexia, hypotension, confusion, nasal congestion. **Rare (less than 1%):** Paradoxical CNS excitement or restlessness, slurred speech, tremor, dry mouth, diarrhea, nocturia, impotence.

ADVERSE EFFECTS/ TOXIC REACTIONS

Abrupt discontinuation may produce hallucinations, seizures. Overdose results in blurred vision, seizures, myosis, mydriasis, severe muscle weakness, strabismus, respiratory depression, vomiting.

NURSING CONSIDERATIONS

BASELINE ASSESSMENT

Record onset, type, location, duration of muscular spasm. Check for immobility, stiffness, swelling.

INTERVENTION/EVALUATION

Assess for paradoxical reaction. Observe pt for drowsiness, dizziness, ataxia. Assist with ambulation at all times. For those on long-term therapy, hepatic/renal function tests, blood counts should be performed periodically. Evaluate for therapeutic response: decreased intensity of skeletal muscle pain.

PATIENT/FAMILY TEACHING

• Drowsiness usually diminishes with continued therapy. • Avoid tasks that require alertness, motor skills until response to drug is established. • Do not abruptly withdraw medication after long-term therapy (may result in muscle rigidity, rebound spasticity, high fever, altered mental status). • Avoid alcohol, CNS depressants.

Bactrim, *see co-trimoxazole*

Bactroban, *see mupirocin*

Baraclude, *see entecavir*

basiliximab

bay-zul-**ix**-ah-mab
(Simulect)

BLACK BOX ALERT Must be administered by certified chemotherapy personnel under supervision of a physician experienced in immunosuppression therapy.

Do not confuse basiliximab with daclizumab.

◆CLASSIFICATION

PHARMACOTHERAPEUTIC: Monoclonal antibody. **CLINICAL:** Immunosuppressive (see p. 119C).

ACTION

Binds to and blocks receptor of interleukin-2, a protein that stimulates proliferation of T-lymphocytes, which play a major role in organ transplant rejection. **Therapeutic Effect:** Prevents lymphocytic activity, impairs response of immune system to antigens, preventing acute renal transplant rejection.

PHARMACOKINETICS

Half-life: 4–10 days (adults); 5–17 days (children).

B

USES

Adjunct with cyclosporine, corticosteroids in prevention of acute organ rejection in pts receiving renal transplant.

PRECAUTIONS

Contraindications: None known. **Cautions:** Infection, history of malignancy.

LIFESPAN CONSIDERATIONS

Pregnancy/Lactation: Unknown if drug crosses placenta or is distributed in breast milk. Breast-feeding not recommended. **Pregnancy Category B. Children/Elderly:** No age-related precautions noted.

INTERACTIONS

DRUG: May increase risk of vaccinal infection with **live vaccine** administration. **HERBAL: Echinacea** may decrease therapeutic effect. **Bilberry, garlic, ginger, ginseng** may increase hypoglycemic effect. **FOOD:** None known. **LAB VALUES:** Alters serum calcium, glucose, potassium, Hgb, Hct. Increases serum cholesterol, BUN, creatinine, uric acid. Decreases serum magnesium, phosphate, platelet count.

AVAILABILITY (Rx)

Injection, Powder for Reconstitution: 10 mg, 20 mg.

ADMINISTRATION/HANDLING

IV

Reconstitution • Reconstitute with 5 ml Sterile Water for Injection. • Shake gently to dissolve. • May further dilute with 25–50 ml 0.9% NaCl or D_5W to a final concentration of 0.4 mg/ml. • Gently invert to avoid foaming.

Rate of administration • IV bolus over 10 min. • IV infusion over 20–30 min.

Storage • Refrigerate. • After reconstitution, use within 4 hrs (24 hrs if refrigerated). • Discard if precipitate forms.

IV INCOMPATIBILITIES

Specific information not available. Do not add other medications simultaneously through same IV line.

INDICATIONS/ROUTES/DOSAGE

Prophylaxis of Organ Rejection

IV: ADULTS, ELDERLY, CHILDREN WEIGHING 35 KG OR MORE: 20 mg within 2 hrs before transplant surgery and 20 mg 4 days after transplant. **CHILDREN WEIGHING LESS THAN 35 KG:** 10 mg within 2 hrs before transplant surgery and 10 mg 4 days after transplant.

SIDE EFFECTS

Frequent (greater than 10%): GI disturbances (constipation, diarrhea, dyspepsia), CNS effects (dizziness, headache, insomnia, tremor), respiratory tract infection, dysuria, acne, leg or back pain, peripheral edema, hypertension. **Occasional (10%–3%):** Angina, neuropathy, abdominal distention, tachycardia, rash, hypotension, urinary disturbances (urinary frequency, genital edema, hematuria), arthralgia, hirsutism, myalgia.

ADVERSE EFFECTS/ TOXIC REACTIONS

Severe acute hypersensitivity reactions including anaphylaxis characterized by hypotension, tachycardia, cardiac failure, dyspnea, wheezing, bronchospasm, pulmonary edema, respiratory failure, urticaria, rash, pruritus, sneezing, as well as capillary leak syndrome and cytokine release syndrome, have been reported.

NURSING CONSIDERATIONS

BASELINE ASSESSMENT

Obtain baseline BUN, serum creatinine, potassium, uric acid, glucose, calcium, phosphatase levels and vital signs, particularly B/P, pulse rate. Breast-feeding not recommended.

INTERVENTION/EVALUATION

Diligently monitor CBC, all serum levels. Assess B/P for hypertension/hypotension; pulse for evidence of tachycardia. Question for GI disturbances, CNS effects, urinary changes. Monitor for presence of wound infection, signs of infection (fever, sore throat, unusual bleeding/bruising), hypersensitivity reaction.

B

PATIENT/FAMILY TEACHING

• Report difficulty in breathing or swallowing, palpitations, bruising/bleeding, rash, itching, swelling of lower extremities, weakness. • Female pts should take measures to avoid pregnancy.

beclomethasone

be-kloe-**meth**-a-sone
(Apo-Beclomethasone ✱, Beconase AQ, Propaderm ✱, Qvar, Rivanase AQ ✱)

Do not confuse Beconase with baclofen.

◆CLASSIFICATION

PHARMACOTHERAPEUTIC: Adrenocorticosteroid. **CLINICAL:** Anti-inflammatory, immunosuppressant (see pp. 2C, 75C, 97C).

ACTION

Controls or prevents inflammation by altering rate of protein synthesis; migration of polymorphonuclear leukocytes, fibroblasts; reverses capillary permeability. **Therapeutic Effect: Inhalation:** Inhibits bronchoconstriction, produces smooth muscle relaxation, decreases mucus secretion. **Intranasal:** Decreases response to seasonal, perennial rhinitis.

PHARMACOKINETICS

Rapidly absorbed from pulmonary, nasal, GI tissue. Hydrolyzed by pulmonary esterase prior to absorption. Metabolized in liver. Protein binding: 87%. Primarily eliminated in feces. **Half-life:** 15 hrs.

USES

Inhalation: Long-term control of bronchial asthma. Reduces need for oral corticosteroid therapy for asthma. **Intranasal:** Relief of seasonal/perennial rhinitis; prevention of nasal polyp recurrence after surgical removal; treatment of nonallergic rhinitis. **OFF-LABEL:** Prevention of seasonal rhinitis (nasal form).

PRECAUTIONS

Contraindications: Hypersensitivity to beclomethasone, acute exacerbation of asthma, status asthmaticus. **Cautions:** Cirrhosis, glaucoma, hypothyroidism, untreated systemic infections, osteoporosis, tuberculosis.

⌛ LIFESPAN CONSIDERATIONS

Pregnancy/Lactation: Unknown if drug crosses placenta or is distributed in breast milk. **Pregnancy Category C. Children:** Prolonged treatment/high dosages may decrease short-term growth rate, cortisol secretion. **Elderly:** No age-related precautions noted.

INTERACTIONS

DRUG: None significant. **HERBAL:** None significant. **FOOD:** None known. **LAB VALUES:** None significant.

AVAILABILITY (Rx)

Inhalation, Oral (Qvar): 40 mcg/inhalation, 80 mcg/inhalation. **Nasal Inhalation (Beconase AQ):** 42 mcg/inhalation.

ADMINISTRATION/HANDLING

Inhalation

• Shake container well. Instruct pt to exhale completely, place mouthpiece between lips, inhale, hold breath as long as possible before exhaling. • Allow at least 1 min between inhalations. • Rinsing mouth after each use decreases dry mouth, hoarseness.

Intranasal

• Instruct pt to clear nasal passages as much as possible before use. • Tilt pt's head slightly forward. Insert spray tip into nostril, pointing toward nasal passages, away from nasal septum. • Spray into one nostril while pt holds the other nostril closed, concurrently inhaling through nose to permit medication as high into nasal passages as possible.

INDICATIONS/ROUTES/DOSAGE

Long-Term Control of Bronchial Asthma

ORAL INHALATION: ADULTS, ELDERLY, CHILDREN 12 YRS AND OLDER: 40–160

B

mcg twice a day. **Maximum:** 320 mcg twice a day. CHILDREN 5–11 YRS: 40 mcg twice a day. **Maximum:** 80 mcg twice a day.

Rhinitis, Prevention of Recurrence of Nasal Polyps

NASAL INHALATION: ADULTS, ELDERLY, CHILDREN 6 YRS AND OLDER: 1–2 sprays in each nostril twice a day.

SIDE EFFECTS

Frequent: **Inhalation (14%–4%):** Throat irritation, dry mouth, hoarseness, cough. **Intranasal:** Nasal burning, mucosal dryness. Occasional: **Inhalation (3%–2%):** Localized fungal infection (thrush). **Intranasal:** Nasal-crusting epistaxis, sore throat, ulceration of nasal mucosa. Rare: **Inhalation:** Transient bronchospasm, esophageal candidiasis. **Intranasal:** Nasal and pharyngeal candidiasis, eye pain.

ADVERSE EFFECTS/ TOXIC REACTIONS

Acute hypersensitivity reaction (urticaria, angioedema, severe bronchospasm) occurs rarely. Change from systemic to local steroid therapy may unmask previously suppressed bronchial asthma condition.

NURSING CONSIDERATIONS

BASELINE ASSESSMENT

Establish baseline history for asthma, rhinitis. Question for hypersensitivity to any corticosteroids.

INTERVENTION/EVALUATION

Monitor respiratory status, lung sounds; observe for signs of oral candidiasis. In those receiving bronchodilators by inhalation concomitantly with inhalation of steroid therapy, advise to use bronchodilator several minutes before corticosteroid aerosol (enhances penetration of steroid into bronchial tree).

PATIENT/FAMILY TEACHING

• Do not change dose schedule or stop taking drug; must taper off gradually under medical supervision. • **Inhalation:** Maintain diligent oral hygiene. • Rinse mouth with water immediately after inhalation (prevents mouth/throat dryness, fungal infection of mouth). • Contact physician if sore throat or mouth occurs. • **Intranasal:** Contact physician if symptoms do not improve or sneezing, nasal irritation occurs. • Clear nasal passages prior to use. • Improvement noted after several days.

Benadryl, *see diphenhydramine*

benazepril

ben-**ayz**-ah-prill
(Apo-Benazepril, Lotensin)

BLACK BOX ALERT May cause fetal injury, mortality if used during second or third trimester of pregnancy.

Do not confuse benazepril with Benadryl, or Lotensin with Lioresal or lovastatin.

FIXED-COMBINATION(S)

Lotensin HCT: benazepril/hydrochlorothiazide (a diuretic): 5 mg/625 mg, 10 mg/12.5 mg, 20 mg/12.5 mg, 20 mg/25 mg. **Lotrel:** benazepril/amlodipine (a calcium blocker): 2.5 mg/10 mg, 5 mg/10 mg, 5 mg/20 mg, 5 mg/40 mg, 10 mg/20 mg, 10 mg/40 mg.

CLASSIFICATION

PHARMACOTHERAPEUTIC: Angiotensin-converting enzyme (ACE) inhibitor. CLINICAL: Antihypertensive (see p. 9C).

ACTION

Decreases rate of conversion of angiotensin I to angiotensin II, a potent vasoconstrictor. Reduces peripheral arterial resistance. Therapeutic Effect: Lowers B/P.

B

PHARMACOKINETICS

Route	Onset	Peak	Duration
PO	1 hr	2–4 hrs	24 hrs

Partially absorbed from GI tract. Protein binding: 97%. Metabolized in liver to active metabolite. Primarily excreted in urine. Minimal removal by hemodialysis. **Half-life:** 35 min; metabolite, 10–11 hrs.

USES

Treatment of hypertension. Used alone or in combination with other antihypertensives. **OFF-LABEL:** Treatment of CHF.

PRECAUTIONS

Contraindications: History of angioedema from previous treatment with ACE inhibitors, pregnancy. **Cautions:** Renal impairment, sodium depletion, diuretic therapy, dialysis, hypovolemia, coronary or cerebrovascular insufficiency, hepatic impairment, diabetes mellitus.

LIFESPAN CONSIDERATIONS

Pregnancy/Lactation: Crosses placenta. Unknown if distributed in breast milk. May cause fetal, neonatal mortality or morbidity. **Pregnancy Category D. Children:** Safety and efficacy not established. **Elderly:** May be more sensitive to hypotensive effects.

INTERACTIONS

DRUG: **Alcohol, diuretics, hypotensive agents** may increase effects. **NSAIDs, sympathomimetics** may decrease effect. **Potassium-sparing diuretics, potassium supplements** may cause hyperkalemia. May increase **lithium** concentration, toxicity. **HERBAL:** **Ephedra, ginseng, yohimbe** may worsen hypertension. **Garlic** may have increased antihypertensive effect. **FOOD:** None known. **LAB VALUES:** May increase serum potassium, AST, ALT, alkaline phosphatase, bilirubin, BUN, creatinine, glucose. May decrease serum sodium, Hgb, Hct. May cause positive ANA titer.

AVAILABILITY (Rx)

Tablets: 5 mg, 10 mg, 20 mg, 40 mg.

ADMINISTRATION/HANDLING

- Give without regard to food.

INDICATIONS/ROUTES/DOSAGE

Hypertension (Monotherapy)

PO: ADULTS: Initially, 10 mg/day. Maintenance: 20–40 mg/day as single dose or in 2 divided doses. **Maximum:** 80 mg/day. **ELDERLY:** Initially, 5–10 mg/day. Range: 20–40 mg/day.

Hypertension (Combination Therapy)

PO: ADULTS: Discontinue diuretic 2–3 days prior to initiating benazepril, then dose as noted above. If unable to discontinue diuretic, begin benazepril at 5 mg/day.

Usual Pediatric Dosage

PO: CHILDREN 6 YRS AND OLDER: Initially, 0.2 mg/kg/day (up to 10 mg/day). Range: 0.1–0.6 mg/kg/day. **Maximum:** 40 mg/day.

Dosage in Renal Impairment

For adult pts with creatinine clearance less than 30 ml/min, initially, 5 mg/day titrated up to maximum of 40 mg/day.

SIDE EFFECTS

Frequent (6%–3%): Cough, headache, dizziness. **Occasional (2%):** Fatigue, drowsiness, nausea. **Rare (less than 1%):** Rash, fever, myalgia, diarrhea, loss of taste.

ADVERSE EFFECTS/ TOXIC REACTIONS

Excessive hypotension ("first-dose syncope") may occur in those with CHF, severe salt or volume depletion. Angioedema (swelling of face, lips), hyperkalemia occur rarely. Agranulocytosis, neutropenia may be noted in those with renal impairment, collagen vascular disease (scleroderma, systemic lupus erythematosus). Nephrotic syndrome may be noted in pts with history of renal disease.

B

NURSING CONSIDERATIONS

BASELINE ASSESSMENT

Obtain B/P immediately before each dose, in addition to regular monitoring (be alert to fluctuations). If excessive reduction in B/P occurs, place pt in supine position with legs elevated. In pts with renal impairment, autoimmune disease, or taking drugs that affect leukocytes or immune response, CBC should be performed before therapy begins and q2wk for 3 mos, then periodically thereafter.

INTERVENTION/EVALUATION

Assist with ambulation if dizziness occurs. Monitor B/P, renal function, urinary protein, potassium. CBC with differential if pt has collagen vascular disease or renal impairment.

PATIENT/FAMILY TEACHING

• To reduce hypotensive effect, rise slowly from lying to sitting position, permit legs to dangle from bed momentarily before standing. • Full therapeutic effect may take 2–4 wks. • Skipping doses or noncompliance with drug therapy may produce severe, rebound hypertension. • Report light-headedness, dizziness, persistent cough.

bendamustine

ben-dah-**mus**-teen
(Treanda)
Do not confuse bendamustine with carmustine or lomustine.

◆CLASSIFICATION

PHARMACOTHERAPEUTIC: Alkylating agent. **CLINICAL:** Antineoplastic.

ACTION

Alkylates and crosslinks macromolecules, resulting in DNA, RNA, and protein synthesis inhibition. **Therapeutic Effect:** Inhibits tumor cell growth, causes cell death.

PHARMACOKINETICS

Metabolized via hydrolysis to metabolites. Protein binding: 64%–95%. Eliminated primarily in feces. **Half-life:** 40 min.

USES

Treatment of chronic lymphocytic leukemia (CLL). Treatment of indolent B-cell non-Hodgkin's lymphoma (NHL) that has progressed during or within 6 mos of treatment with rituximab or a rituximab-containing regimen. **OFF-LABEL:** Treatment of mantle cell lymphoma, relapsed multiple myeloma.

PRECAUTIONS

Contraindications: None known. **Cautions:** Preexisting immunosuppression, renal/hepatic impairment.

LIFESPAN CONSIDERATIONS:

Pregnancy/Lactation: May cause fetal harm. Unknown if distributed in breast milk. **Pregnancy Category D.** Impaired spermatogenesis, azoospermia have been reported in male pts. **Children:** Safety and efficacy not established. **Elderly:** No age-related precautions noted.

INTERACTIONS

Ciprofloxacin, fluvoxamine may increase bendamustine concentration, decrease plasma concentrations of active metabolites. **Omeprazole, smoking** may decrease concentration. **FOOD:** None known. **HERBAL: Ginkgo biloba, green tea, St. John's wort** may decrease plasma concentration. **LAB VALUES:** May increase serum AST, bilirubin, creatinine, uric acid. May decrease WBCs, neutrophils, Hgb, platelets, serum potassium.

AVAILABILITY (Rx)

Injection, Powder for Reconstitution: 100 mg.

ADMINISTRATION/HANDLING

IV

Reconstitution • Reconstitute each 100-mg vial with 20 ml Sterile Water for

Injection for a concentration of 5 mg/ml. • Powder should completely dissolve in 5 min. • Discard if particulate matter is observed. • Withdraw volume needed for required dose (based on 5 mg/ml concentration) and immediately transfer to 500-ml infusion bag of 0.9% NaCl to final concentration of 0.2–0.6 mg/ml. • Reconstituted solution must be transferred to infusion bag within 30 min of reconstitution. • After transferring, thoroughly mix contents of infusion bag.

Storage • Reconstituted solution appears clear, colorless to pale yellow solution, free from visual particulates. • Final solution is stable for 24 hrs if refrigerated or 3 hrs at room temperature. • Administration must be completed within these stability time frames.

INDICATIONS/ROUTES/DOSAGE

◀ALERT▶ During first few wks of treatment, allopurinol should be given as a preventative measure in those at risk for tumor lysis syndrome.

Chronic Lymphocytic Leukemia

IV INFUSION: ADULTS/ELDERLY: 100 mg/m² given over 30 min daily on days 1 and 2 of a 28-day cycle, up to 6 cycles.

Non-Hodgkin's Lymphoma

IV INFUSION: ADULTS/ELDERLY: 120 mg/m² on days 1 and 2 of a 21-day cycle, up to 8 cycles.

SIDE EFFECTS

Frequent (24%–16%): Fever, nausea, vomiting. **Occasional** (9%–8%): Diarrhea, fatigue, asthenia, rash, decreased weight, nasopharyngitis. **Rare** (6%–3%): Chills, pruritus, cough, herpes simplex infections.

ADVERSE EFFECTS/ TOXIC REACTIONS

Myelosuppression characterized as neutropenia (28%), thrombocytopenia (23%), anemia (19%), leukopenia (18%). Infection, including pneumonia, sepsis may occur. Tumor lysis syndrome may lead to acute renal failure. Worsening hypertension occurs rarely.

NURSING CONSIDERATIONS

BASELINE ASSESSMENT

Question for possibility of pregnancy. Offer emotional support. Obtain baseline CBC, serum chemistries including hepatic function tests (bilirubin, ALT, AST, alkaline phosphatase) before treatment begins and routinely thereafter.

INTERVENTION/EVALUATION

Offer antiemetics to control nausea, vomiting. Monitor daily pattern of bowel activity and stool consistency. Assess skin for evidence of rash. Monitor for signs of infection (fever, chills, cough, flu-like symptoms). Monitor for hypertension. Hematologic nadirs occur in 3rd week of therapy and may require dose delays if recovery to recommended values has not occurred by day 28.

PATIENT/FAMILY TEACHING

• Avoid crowds, those with known infection. • Avoid contact with anyone who recently received live virus vaccine. • Do not have immunizations without physician's approval (drug lowers body resistance). • Promptly report fever, chills, flu-like symptoms, sore throat, unusual bruising/bleeding from any site. • Male pts should be warned of potential risk to their reproductive capacities.

Benicar, *see olmesartan*

Benicar HCT, *see hydrochlorthiazide and olmesartan*

B

benzonatate

ben-**zoe**-nah-tate
(Tessalon Perles)
Do not confuse benzonatate with benazepril, benzocaine, or benztropine, or Tessalon with Tussionex.

◆CLASSIFICATION

PHARMACOTHERAPEUTIC: Non-narcotic antitussive. **CLINICAL:** Cough suppressant.

ACTION

Anesthetizes stretch or cough receptors in alveoli of lungs, bronchi, and pleura suppressing the cough reflex. **Therapeutic Effect:** Reduces cough production.

PHARMACOKINETICS

Route	Onset	Peak	Duration
PO	15–20 min	—	3–8 hrs

Metabolized in liver. Primarily excreted in urine. **Half-life:** Unknown.

USES

Relief of nonproductive cough, including acute cough of minor throat/bronchial irritation.

PRECAUTIONS

Contraindications: Allergy to topical numbing medicines (tetracaine, procaine) found in some insect bite and sunburn creams. **Cautions:** Productive cough.

LIFESPAN CONSIDERATIONS

Pregnancy/Lactation: Unknown if drug crosses placenta or is distributed in breast milk. **Pregnancy Category C. Children:** Safety and efficacy not established in those younger than 10 yrs. **Elderly:** No age-related precautions noted.

INTERACTIONS

DRUG: CNS depressants may increase effect. **HERBAL:** None significant. **FOOD:** None known. **LAB VALUES:** None significant.

AVAILABILITY (Rx)

Capsules (Liquid Filled): 100 mg, 200 mg.

ADMINISTRATION/HANDLING

PO

• Give without regard to meals. • Swallow whole; do not chew or dissolve in mouth (may produce temporary local anesthesia of oral mucosa). • Take with full glass of water.

INDICATIONS/ROUTES/DOSAGE

Antitussive

PO: ADULTS, ELDERLY, CHILDREN OLDER THAN 10 YRS: 100 mg, 200 mg 3 times a day, or every 4 hrs up to 600 mg/day.

SIDE EFFECTS

Occasional (10%–5%): Mild drowsiness, mild dizziness, constipation, nausea, skin eruptions, nasal congestion.

ADVERSE EFFECTS/ TOXIC REACTIONS

Paradoxical reaction (restlessness, insomnia, euphoria, nervousness, tremors) has been noted. Chest pain or numbness, choking feeling, sense of faintness, confusion, hallucinations may result from chewing or sucking on capsule.

NURSING CONSIDERATIONS

BASELINE ASSESSMENT

Assess type, severity, frequency of cough. Monitor amount, color, consistency of sputum.

INTERVENTION/EVALUATION

Initiate deep breathing and coughing exercises, particularly in pts with impaired pulmonary function. Monitor for paradoxical reaction. Increase fluid intake and environmental humidity to lower viscosity of lung secretions. Assess for clinical improvement and record onset of cough relief.

B

PATIENT/FAMILY TEACHING

• Avoid tasks that require alertness, motor skills until response to drug is established. • Dry mouth, drowsiness, dizziness may be expected responses to drug. • Sucking or chewing on capsule may cause numbness of mouth or throat.

benztropine

benz-**trow**-peen
(Apo-Benthropine ✤, Cogentin)
Do not confuse benztropine with bromocriptine.

◆ CLASSIFICATION

PHARMACOTHERAPEUTIC: Anticholinergic. **CLINICAL:** Antiparkinson agent.

ACTION

Selectively blocks central cholinergic receptors, assists in balancing cholinergic/dopaminergic activity. **Therapeutic Effect:** Reduces incidence/severity of akinesia, rigidity, tremor.

PHARMACOKINETICS

Well absorbed following PO and IM administration. Metabolized in liver. PO onset of action: 1–2 hrs, IM onset of action: minutes. Pharmacologic effects may not be apparent until 2–3 days after initiation of therapy and may persist for up to 24 hrs after discontinuation of drug. **Half-life:** Extended.

USES

Treatment of Parkinson's disease, drug-induced extrapyramidal reactions (except tardive dyskinesia).

PRECAUTIONS

Contraindications: Angle-closure glaucoma, benign prostatic hyperplasia, children younger than 3 yrs, GI obstruction, intestinal atony, megacolon, myasthenia gravis, paralytic ileus, severe ulcerative colitis. **Cautions:** Treated open-angle glaucoma, heart disease, hypertension; pts with tachycardia, arrhythmias, prostatic hypertrophy, hepatic/renal impairment, obstructive diseases of GI/GU tract, urinary retention.

⌛ LIFESPAN CONSIDERATIONS

Pregnancy/Lactation: Unknown if drug crosses placenta or is distributed in breast milk. **Pregnancy Category C. Children:** Safety and efficacy not established. **Elderly:** No age-related precautions noted, but there is a higher risk for adverse effects.

INTERACTIONS

DRUG: Alcohol, CNS depressants may increase sedation. **Amantadine, anticholinergics, MAOIs** may increase effects. **Antacids, antidiarrheals** may decrease absorption, effects. **HERBAL:** None significant. **FOOD:** None known. **LAB VALUES:** None significant.

AVAILABILITY (Rx)

Injection, Solution: 1 mg/ml. **Tablets:** 0.5 mg, 1 mg, 2 mg.

ADMINISTRATION/HANDLING

IM

• Inject slow, deep IM.

PO

• Give without regard to food. • Give with food if GI upset occurs.

INDICATIONS/ROUTES/DOSAGE

Parkinsonism

PO: ADULTS: 0.5–6 mg/day as a single dose or in 2 divided doses. Titrate by 0.5 mg at 5–6 day intervals. **ELDERLY:** Initially, 0.5 mg once or twice a day. Titrate by 0.5 mg at 5–6 day intervals. **Maximum:** 4 mg/day.

Drug-Induced Extrapyramidal Symptoms

PO, IM, IV: ADULTS: 1–4 mg once or twice a day. **CHILDREN OLDER THAN 3 YRS:** 0.02–0.05 mg/kg/dose once or twice a day.

Acute Dystonic Reactions

IV, IM: ADULTS: Initially, 1–2 mg; then 1–2 mg PO twice a day to prevent recurrence.

B

SIDE EFFECTS

Frequent: Drowsiness, dry mouth, blurred vision, constipation, decreased diaphoresis or urination, GI upset, photosensitivity. **Occasional:** Headache, memory loss, muscle cramps, anxiety, peripheral paresthesia, orthostatic hypotension, abdominal cramps. **Rare:** Rash, confusion, eye pain.

ADVERSE EFFECTS/ TOXIC REACTIONS

Overdose may produce severe anticholinergic effects (unsteadiness, drowsiness, tachycardia, dyspnea, skin flushing, dryness of mouth/nose/throat). Severe paradoxical reactions (hallucinations, tremor, seizures, toxic psychosis) may occur.

NURSING CONSIDERATIONS

BASELINE ASSESSMENT

Assess mental status for confusion, disorientation, agitation, psychotic-like symptoms (medication frequently produces such side effects in those older than 60 yrs).

INTERVENTION/EVALUATION

Be alert to neurologic effects: headache, drowsiness, mental confusion, agitation. Assess for clinical reversal of symptoms (improvement of tremor of head and hands at rest, mask-like facial expression, shuffling gait, muscular rigidity). Monitor for constipation, abdominal pain, bowel sounds. Monitor I/O. Assess for urinary retention.

PATIENT/FAMILY TEACHING

• Avoid tasks that require alertness, motor skills until response to drug is established. • Dry mouth, drowsiness, dizziness may be an expected response to drug. • Avoid alcoholic beverages during therapy. • Drowsiness tends to diminish or disappear with continued therapy. • Report sudden muscle weakness or stiffness.

beractant

ber-ak-tant
(Survanta Intratracheal)
Do not confuse Survanta with Sufenta.

◆CLASSIFICATION

PHARMACOTHERAPEUTIC: Natural bovine lung extract. **CLINICAL:** Pulmonary surfactant.

ACTION

Lowers alveolar surface tension during respiration, stabilizing alveoli. **Therapeutic Effect:** Improves lung compliance, respiratory gas exchange.

PHARMACOKINETICS

Not absorbed systemically.

USES

Prevention and treatment (rescue therapy) of respiratory distress syndrome (RDS—hyaline membrane disease) in premature infants. **Prevention:** Body weight less than 1,250 g in infants at risk for developing or with evidence of surfactant deficiency (give within 15 min of birth). **Rescue Therapy:** Treatment of infants with RDS confirmed by X-ray, requiring mechanical ventilation (give within 8 hrs of birth).

PRECAUTIONS

Contraindications: None known. **Cautions:** Those at risk for circulatory overload. This drug is for use only in neonates. **Pregnancy Category:** Not indicated for use in pregnant women.

INTERACTIONS

DRUG: None significant. **HERBAL:** None significant. **FOOD:** None known. **LAB VALUES:** None significant.

AVAILABILITY (Rx)

Suspension, Intratracheal: 25 mg/ml (4 ml, 8 ml).

ADMINISTRATION/HANDLING

Intratracheal

Administration • Instill through catheter inserted into infant's endotracheal tube. Do not instill into main stem bronchus. • Monitor for bradycardia, decreased O_2 saturation during administration. Stop dosing procedure if these effects occur; begin appropriate measures before reinstituting therapy.

Storage • Refrigerate vials. • Warm by standing vial at room temperature for 20 min or warm in hand 8 min. • If settling occurs, gently swirl vial (do not shake) to redisperse. • After warming, may return to refrigerator within 8 hrs one time only. • Each vial should be injected via needle only one time; discard unused portions. • Color appears off-white to light brown.

INDICATIONS/ROUTES/DOSAGE

Prevention and Treatment (Rescue Therapy) of RDS or Hyaline Membrane Disease in Premature Infants

INTRATRACHEAL: INFANTS: 100 mg of phospholipids/kg birth weight (4 ml/kg). Give within 15 min of birth if infant weighs less than 1,250 g and has evidence of surfactant deficiency; give within 8 hrs when RDS is confirmed by X-ray and pt requires mechanical ventilation. May repeat in 6 hrs or longer after preceding dose. **Maximum:** 4 doses in the first 48 hrs of life.

SIDE EFFECTS

Frequent: Transient bradycardia, oxygen (O_2) desaturation, increased carbon dioxide (CO_2) retention. **Occasional:** Endotracheal tube reflux. **Rare:** Apnea, endotracheal tube blockage, hypotension or hypertension, pallor, vasoconstriction.

ADVERSE EFFECTS/TOXIC REACTIONS

Life-threatening nosocomial sepsis may occur.

NURSING CONSIDERATIONS

BASELINE ASSESSMENT

Drug must be administered in highly supervised setting. Clinicians caring for neonate must be experienced with intubation, ventilator management. Offer emotional support to parents.

INTERVENTION/EVALUATION

Monitor infant with arterial or transcutaneous measurement of systemic O_2, CO_2. Assess for adventitious breath sounds (rales, rhonchi).

betamethasone

bay-ta-**meth**-a-sone
(Beta-Val, Betaderm ✤, Betaject ✤, Betnesol ✤, Betnovate ✤, Celestone, Celestone Soluspan, Diprolene, Diprolene AF, Ectosone ✤, Luxiq)

Do not confuse Luxiq with Lasix.

FIXED-COMBINATION(S)

Lotrisone: betamethasone/clotrimazole (an antifungal): 0.05%/1%. **Taclonex:** betamethasone/calcipotriene (an antipsoriatic): 0.064%/0.005%.

◆CLASSIFICATION

PHARMACOTHERAPEUTIC: Adrenocorticosteroid. **CLINICAL:** Anti-inflammatory, immunosuppressant (see pp. 97C, 99C, 100C).

ACTION

Controls rate of protein synthesis, depresses migration of polymorphonuclear leukocytes/fibroblasts, reverses capillary permeability, prevents or controls inflammation. **Therapeutic Effect:** Decreases tissue response to inflammatory process.

B

PHARMACOKINETICS

Rapidly and almost completely absorbed following PO administration. Protein binding: 64%. After topical application, limited absorption systemically. Metabolized in liver. Excreted in urine. **Half-life:** 6.5 hrs.

USES

Systemic: Anti-inflammatory, immunosuppressant, corticosteroid replacement therapy. **Topical:** Relief of inflammatory and pruritic dermatoses. **Foam:** Relief of inflammation, itching associated with dermatosis.

PRECAUTIONS

Contraindications: Hypersensitivity to systemic fungal infections. **Cautions:** Hypothyroidism, cirrhosis, nonspecific ulcerative colitis, pts at increased risk for peptic ulcer.

LIFESPAN CONSIDERATIONS

Pregnancy/Lactation: Crosses placenta, distributed in breast milk. **Pregnancy Category C (D if used in first trimester). Children:** Prolonged treatment, high-dose therapy may decrease short-term growth rate, cortisol secretion. **Elderly:** Higher risk for developing hypertension, osteoporosis.

INTERACTIONS

DRUG: **Amphotericin** may increase hypokalemia. May decrease effect of **diuretics, insulin, oral hypoglycemics, potassium supplements.** May increase **digoxin** toxicity (due to hypokalemia). **Hepatic enzyme inducers** may decrease effect. **Live virus vaccines** may potentiate virus replication, increase vaccine side effects, decrease pt's antibody response to vaccine. **HERBAL:** **Cat's claw, echinacea** possess immunostimulant effects. **FOOD:** None known. **LAB VALUES:** May decrease serum calcium, potassium, thyroxine. May increase serum cholesterol, lipids, glucose, sodium, amylase.

AVAILABILITY (Rx)

Cream: 0.05% **(Diprolene AF),** 0.1% **(Beta-Val). Foam: (Luxiq):** 0.12%. **Gel:** 0.05%. **Injection, Suspension (Celestone Soluspan):** 3 mg/ml. **Lotion:** 0.05% **(Diprolene),** 0.1% **(Beta-Val). Ointment:** 0.05%, 0.1%. **Syrup (Celestone):** 0.6 mg/5 ml.

ADMINISTRATION/HANDLING

IM

• Inject slowly, deep IM into large muscle mass.

PO

• Protect syrup from light and tablets from excessive moisture. • Give with milk or food (decreases GI upset). • Give single doses before 9 AM; give multiple doses at evenly spaced intervals.

Topical

• Gently cleanse area before application. • Apply sparingly and rub into area thoroughly. • When using aerosol, spray area 3 sec from 15-cm (approximately 12 in) distance; avoid inhalation.

Storage • Store all forms at room temperature. • Protect parenteral form from light.

INDICATIONS/ROUTES/DOSAGE

Anti-Inflammation, Immunosuppression, Corticosteroid Replacement Therapy

PO: ADULTS, ELDERLY: 0.6–7.2 mg/day. **CHILDREN:** 0.0175–0.25 mg/kg/day in 3–4 divided doses.

IM: ADULTS, ELDERLY: 0.6–9 mg/day in 2 divided doses. **CHILDREN:** 0.0175–0.125 mg/kg/day in 3–4 divided doses.

Relief of Inflamed and Pruritic Dermatoses

TOPICAL: ADULTS, ELDERLY: 1–3 times a day. **Foam:** Apply twice a day (morning and night).

SIDE EFFECTS

Frequent: Systemic: Increased appetite, abdominal distention, nervousness, insomnia, false sense of well-being. **Topi-**

cal: Burning, stinging, pruritus. Occasional: **Systemic:** Dizziness, facial flushing, diaphoresis, decreased or blurred vision, mood swings. **Topical:** Allergic contact dermatitis, purpura or blood-containing blisters, thinning of skin with easy bruising, telangiectases, raised dark red spots on skin, angiomas.

ADVERSE EFFECTS/ TOXIC REACTIONS

Overdose may cause systemic hypercorticism, adrenal suppression.

NURSING CONSIDERATIONS

BASELINE ASSESSMENT

Question for hypersensitivity to any corticosteroid, sulfite. Obtain baseline values for height, weight, B/P, serum glucose, electrolytes. Obtain baseline results of initial tests (tuberculosis [TB] skin test, X-rays, EKG).

INTERVENTION/EVALUATION

Monitor B/P, blood glucose, electrolytes. Apply topical preparation sparingly. Do not use on broken skin or in areas of infection. Do not apply to wet skin, face, inguinal areas.

PATIENT/FAMILY TEACHING

• Take with food, milk. • Take single daily dose in the morning. • Do not stop abruptly. • Apply topical preparations in a thin layer. • Do not receive smallpox vaccination during or immediately after therapy.

Betaseron, *see interferon beta-1b*

bethanechol

be-**than**-e-kole
(Duvoid ✦, Urecholine)
Do not confuse bethanechol with betaxolol.

◆ CLASSIFICATION

PHARMACOTHERAPEUTIC: Cholinergic (see p. 90C).

ACTION

Acts directly at cholinergic receptors in smooth muscle of urinary bladder, GI tract. Increases detrusor muscle tone. **Therapeutic Effect:** May initiate micturition, bladder emptying. Stimulates gastric, intestinal motility.

PHARMACOKINETICS

Route	Onset	Peak	Duration
PO	30–90 min	60 min	6 hrs

Poorly absorbed following PO administration. Does not cross blood-brain barrier. **Half-life:** Unknown.

USES

Treatment of nonobstructive urinary retention, retention due to neurogenic bladder. OFF-LABEL: Treatment of congenital megacolon, gastroesophageal reflux, postop gastric atony.

PRECAUTIONS

Contraindications: Active or latent bronchial asthma, acute inflammatory GI tract conditions, anastomosis, bladder wall instability, coronary artery disease, epilepsy, hypertension, hyperthyroidism, hypotension, mechanical GI or urinary tract obstruction or recent GI resection, parkinsonism, peptic ulcer, pronounced bradycardia, vasomotor instability. **Cautions:** Presence of bacteremia, urinary retention.

⌛ LIFESPAN CONSIDERATIONS

Pregnancy/Lactation: Unknown if drug crosses placenta or is distributed in breast milk. **Pregnancy Category C. Children/Elderly:** No age-related precautions noted.

INTERACTIONS

DRUG: **Cholinesterase inhibitors** may increase effects/toxicity. **Procainamide,**

B

quinidine may decrease effect. HERBAL: None significant. FOOD: None known. LAB VALUES: May increase serum amylase, lipase, AST, ALT.

AVAILABILITY (Rx)

Tablets: 5 mg, 10 mg, 25 mg, 50 mg.

ADMINISTRATION/HANDLING

PO

- Administer 1 hr before or 2 hrs after meals.

INDICATIONS/ROUTES/DOSAGE

Nonobstructive Urinary Retention, Atony of Bladder

PO: ADULTS, ELDERLY: 10–50 mg 3–4 times a day. Minimum effective dose determined by giving 5–10 mg initially, repeating same amount at 1-hr intervals until desired response is achieved. CHILDREN: 0.3–0.6 mg/kg/day in 3–4 divided doses.

SIDE EFFECTS

Occasional: Belching, changes in vision, blurred vision, diarrhea, frequent urinary urgency. Rare: Shortness of breath, chest tightness, bronchospasm.

ADVERSE EFFECTS/ TOXIC REACTIONS

Overdose produces CNS stimulation (insomnia, anxiety, orthostatic hypotension), cholinergic stimulation (headache, increased salivation/diaphoresis, nausea, vomiting, flushed skin, abdominal pain, seizures).

NURSING CONSIDERATIONS

BASELINE ASSESSMENT

Assure pt has emptied bladder prior to procedure.

INTERVENTION/EVALUATION

Monitor urine output. Palpate bladder for evidence of urinary retention.

PATIENT/FAMILY TEACHING

- Report nausea, vomiting, diarrhea, diaphoresis, increased salivary secretions, irregular heartbeat, muscle weakness, severe abdominal pain, difficulty breathing.

bevacizumab HIGH ALERT

be-vah-**ciz**-you-mab
(Avastin)

BLACK BOX ALERT May result in development of GI perforation, presented as intra-abdominal abscess, fistula, wound dehiscence, wound healing complications. Pulmonary hemorrhage, manifested as severe or fatal hemoptysis has occurred.

Do not confuse bevacizumab with cetuximab or rituximab.

◆CLASSIFICATION

PHARMACOTHERAPEUTIC: Monoclonal antibody. CLINICAL: Antineoplastic.

ACTION

Binds to and inhibits vascular endothelial growth factor, a protein that plays a major role in formation of new blood vessels to tumors. **Therapeutic Effect:** Inhibits metastatic disease progression.

PHARMACOKINETICS

Clearance varies by body weight, gender, tumor burden. **Half-life:** 20 days (range: 11–50 days).

USES

Combination chemotherapy with 5-fluorouracil (5-FU) for first-line treatment of pts with colorectal cancer. First-line treatment with carboplatin and paclitaxel for nonsquamous, non–small-cell lung cancer (NSCLC). Treatment of renal cell carcinoma (metastatic) with interferon alfa, brain cancer that has progressed following prior therapy. OFF-LABEL: Adjunctive therapy in malignant mesothelioma, ovarian cancer, prostate cancer, age-related macular degeneration.

PRECAUTIONS

Contraindications: GI perforation, hypertensive crisis, nephrotic syndrome, recent hemoptysis, serious bleeding, wound dehiscence requiring medical intervention. **Cautions:** Hypertension, proteinuria, CHF, epistaxis, renal insufficiency.

LIFESPAN CONSIDERATIONS

Pregnancy/Lactation: Teratogenic. Potential for fertility impairment. May decrease maternal and fetal body weight; increase risk of skeletal fetal abnormalities. Breast-feeding not recommended. **Pregnancy Category C. Children:** Safety and efficacy not established. **Elderly:** Higher incidence of severe adverse reactions in those older than 65 yrs.

INTERACTIONS

DRUG: **Sunitinib** may increase level/effects. **HERBAL:** None significant. **FOOD:** None known. **LAB VALUES:** May decrease serum potassium, sodium, WBC count, Hgb, Hct, platelet count.

AVAILABILITY (Rx)

Injection, Solution: 25-mg/ml vial.

ADMINISTRATION/HANDLING

IV

ALERT Do not give by IV push or bolus.

Reconstitution • Dilute prescribed dose in 100 ml 0.9% NaCl. • Avoid dextrose-containing solutions. • Discard any unused portion.

Rate of administration • Infuse IV over 90 min following chemotherapy. • If first infusion is well tolerated, second infusion may be administered over 60 min. • If 60-min infusion is well tolerated, all subsequent infusions may be administered over 30 min.

Storage • Refrigerate vials. • Diluted solution may be stored for up to 8 hrs if refrigerated.

IV INCOMPATIBILITIES

Do not mix with dextrose solutions.

INDICATIONS/ROUTES/DOSAGE

Colorectal Cancer

IV: ADULTS, ELDERLY: 5–10 mg/kg once every 14 days (with fluorouracil-based chemotherapy).

Non–Small-Cell Lung Cancer (NSCLC)

IV: ADULTS, ELDERLY: 15 mg/kg every 3 wks (in combination with carboplatin and paclitaxel).

Metastatic Renal Cell Carcinoma

IV: ADULTS, ELDERLY: 10 mg/kg once every 2 wks (with interferon alfa).

Brain Cancer

IV: ADULTS, ELDERLY: 10 mg/kg every 2 wks.

Dose Adjustment for Toxicity

Temporary Suspension: Mild to moderate proteinuria, severe hypertension not controlled with medical management. **Permanent Discontinuation:** Wound dehiscence requiring intervention, GI perforation, hypertensive crises, serious bleeding, nephrotic syndrome.

SIDE EFFECTS

Frequent (73%–25%): Asthenia, vomiting, anorexia, hypertension, epistaxis, stomatitis, constipation, headache, dyspnea. **Occasional (21%–15%):** Altered taste, dry skin, exfoliative dermatitis, dizziness, flatulence, excessive lacrimation, skin discoloration, weight loss, myalgia. **Rare (8%–6%):** Nail disorder, skin ulcer, alopecia, confusion, abnormal gait, dry mouth.

ADVERSE EFFECTS/ TOXIC REACTIONS

UTI, manifested as urinary frequency/urgency, proteinuria, occurs frequently. Most serious adverse effects include CHF, deep vein thrombosis, GI perforation, wound dehiscence, hypertensive crisis, nephrotic syndrome, severe hemorrhage. Anemia, neutropenia, thrombocytopenia occur occasionally. Hypersensitivity reactions occur rarely. May increase risk of tracheoesophageal fistula development.

B

NURSING CONSIDERATIONS

BASELINE ASSESSMENT

Monitor B/P regularly during treatment. Assess for proteinuria with urinalysis. For those with 2+ or greater urine dipstick reading, a 24-hr urine collection is advisable. Monitor CBC, serum potassium, sodium levels at regular intervals during therapy.

INTERVENTION/EVALUATION

Monitor B/P for hypertension. Assess for asthenia (loss of strength, energy). Assist with ambulation if asthenia occurs. Monitor for fever, chills, abdominal pain, epistaxis. Offer antiemetic if nausea, vomiting occur. Monitor daily pattern of bowel activity and stool consistency.

PATIENT/FAMILY TEACHING

• Report abdominal pain, vomiting, constipation, headache. • Do not have immunizations without physician's approval (lowers body's resistance). • Avoid contact with anyone who recently received a live virus vaccine. • Avoid crowds, those with infection. • Female pts should take measures to avoid pregnancy during treatment.

bexarotene

HIGH ALERT

beks-**air**-oh-teen
(Targretin)

BLACK BOX ALERT Do not administer to pregnant women (high risk of birth defects).

CLASSIFICATION

PHARMACOTHERAPEUTIC: Retinoid.
CLINICAL: Antineoplastic (see p. 80C).

ACTION

Binds to and activates retinoid X receptor subtypes that regulate the genes controlling cellular differentiation and proliferation. **Therapeutic Effect:** Inhibits growth of tumor cell lines of hematopoietic and squamous cell origin, induces tumor regression.

PHARMACOKINETICS

Moderately absorbed from GI tract. Protein binding: greater than 99%. Metabolized in liver. Primarily eliminated through the hepatobiliary system. **Half-life:** 7 hrs.

USES

PO: Treatment of cutaneous T-cell lymphoma (CTCL) in those refractory to at least one prior systemic therapy. **Topical:** Treatment of cutaneous lesions in those with refractory CTCL (stage 1A and 1B) or not tolerant of other therapies. **OFF-LABEL:** Treatment of diabetes mellitus; head, neck, lung, renal cell carcinomas; Kaposi's sarcoma.

PRECAUTIONS

Contraindications: None known. **Cautions:** Hepatic impairment, diabetes mellitus, lipid abnormalities.

LIFESPAN CONSIDERATIONS

Pregnancy/Lactation: May cause fetal harm. Unknown if distributed in breast milk. **Pregnancy Category X. Children:** Safety and efficacy not established. **Elderly:** No age-related precautions noted.

INTERACTIONS

DRUG: Bone marrow depressants, medications causing blood dyscrasias may have adverse additive effects. **Phenobarbital, phenytoin, rifampin** may decrease plasma concentration. **Erythromycin, gemfibrozil, itraconazole, ketoconazole** may increase plasma concentration. Bexarotene may reduce **tamoxifen** concentration, may enhance hypoglycemic effect of **insulin, oral hypoglycemics. Live virus vaccines** may potentiate virus replication, increase vaccine side effects, decrease pt's antibody response to vaccine. **Vitamin A** (doses greater than 15,000 units/day) may increase toxicity. **HERBAL: Dong quai, St. John's wort** may cause photosensitization. **St. John's wort** may decrease plasma concentration. **FOOD: Grapefruit, grapefruit juice** may increase concentration/toxicity. LAB VALUES: May produce abnormal hepatic function tests; increase serum cholesterol, glucose, potassium, triglycerides, total cholesterol, LDL; decrease HDL. CA-125 in ovarian cancer may be increased.

AVAILABILITY (Rx)

Capsules (Soft Gelatin [Targretin]): 75 mg. **Topical Gel (Targretin):** 1%.

ADMINISTRATION/HANDLING

PO

• Give following a high-fat meal.

Topical

• Generously coat lesions with gel. • Allow to dry before covering. • Avoid applying gel to normal skin surrounding lesions or near mucosal surfaces. • Use of occlusive dressings not recommended.

INDICATIONS/ROUTES/DOSAGE

Cutaneous T-Cell Lymphoma Refractory to at Least One Prior Systemic Therapy

PO: ADULTS: 300 mg/m^2/day. If no tumor response after 8 wks and initial dose is well tolerated, may be increased to 400 mg/m^2/day. If not tolerated, may be decreased to 200 mg/m^2/day, then to 100 mg/m^2/day, or temporarily suspended to manage toxicity. **TOPICAL: ADULTS:** Initially, apply once every other day for first wk. May increase at weekly intervals to once a day, then twice a day, then 3 times a day up to 4 times a day based on tolerance.

SIDE EFFECTS

Frequent: Hyperlipidemia (79%), headache (30%), hypothyroidism (29%), asthenia (20%). **Occasional:** Rash (17%); nausea (15%); peripheral edema (13%); dry skin, abdominal pain (11%); chills, exfoliative dermatitis (10%); diarrhea (7%).

ADVERSE EFFECTS/ TOXIC REACTIONS

Pancreatitis, hepatic failure, pneumonia occur rarely.

NURSING CONSIDERATIONS

BASELINE ASSESSMENT

Assess baseline lipid profile, WBC, hepatic function, thyroid function. Question about possibility of pregnancy (Pregnancy Category X). Warn women of childbearing age about potential fetal risk if pregnancy occurs.

INTERVENTION/EVALUATION

Monitor serum cholesterol, triglycerides, CBC, hepatic, thyroid function tests.

PATIENT/FAMILY TEACHING

• Do not use medicated, drying, abrasive soaps; wash with gentle, bland soap. • Inform physician if pregnant or planning to become pregnant (Pregnancy Category X). • Instruct on need for use of 2 reliable forms of contraceptives concurrently during therapy and for 1 mo after discontinuation of therapy, even in infertile, premenopausal woman.

Biaxin, *see clarithromycin*

Biaxin XL, *see clarithromycin*

bicalutamide HIGH ALERT

bye-ka-**loo**-ta-mide
(Apo-Bicalutamide ✦, Casodex, Novo-Bicalutamide ✦)
Do not confuse Casodex with Kapidex.

◆CLASSIFICATION

PHARMACOTHERAPEUTIC: Antiandrogen hormone. **CLINICAL:** Antineoplastic (see p. 81C).

B

ACTION

Competitively inhibits androgen action by binding to androgen receptors in target tissue. **Therapeutic Effect:** Decreases growth of prostatic carcinoma.

PHARMACOKINETICS

Well absorbed from GI tract. Protein binding: 96%. Metabolized in liver to inactive metabolite. Excreted in urine and feces. Not removed by hemodialysis. **Half-life:** 5.8–7 days.

USES

Treatment of advanced metastatic prostatic carcinoma (in combination with luteinizing hormone-releasing hormone [LHRH] agonist analogues, e.g., leuprolide). Treatment with both drugs must be started at same time. **OFF-LABEL:** Monotherapy for locally advanced prostate cancer.

PRECAUTIONS

Contraindications: Women, esp. those who may become pregnant. **Cautions:** Moderate to severe hepatic impairment.

LIFESPAN CONSIDERATIONS

Pregnancy/Lactation: May inhibit spermatogenesis, not used in women. **Pregnancy Category X. Children:** Safety and efficacy not established. **Elderly:** No age-related precautions noted.

INTERACTIONS

DRUG: May increase **warfarin** effect. **HERBAL:** None significant. **FOOD:** None known. **LAB VALUES:** May increase serum AST, ALT, alkaline phosphatase, creatinine, bilirubin, BUN, glucose. May decrease WBC, Hgb.

AVAILABILITY (Rx)

Tablets: 50 mg.

ADMINISTRATION/HANDLING

PO

• Give without regard to food. • Give at same time each day.

INDICATIONS/ROUTES/DOSAGE

Prostatic Carcinoma

PO: ADULTS, ELDERLY: 50 mg once a day in morning or evening, given concurrently with an LHRH analogue or after surgical castration.

SIDE EFFECTS

Frequent: Hot flashes (49%), breast pain (38%), muscle pain (27%), constipation (17%), asthenia (15%), diarrhea (10%), nausea (11%). **Occasional (9%–8%):** Nocturia, abdominal pain, peripheral edema. **Rare (7%–3%):** Vomiting, weight loss, dizziness, insomnia, rash, impotence, gynecomastia.

ADVERSE EFFECTS/ TOXIC REACTIONS

Sepsis, CHF, hypertension, iron deficiency anemia, interstitial pneumonitis, pulmonary fibrosis may occur. Severe hepatotoxicity occurs rarely within the first 3–4 mos after treatment initiation.

NURSING CONSIDERATIONS

BASELINE ASSESSMENT

Obtain baseline lab tests including CBC, hepatic function, PSA, serum testosterone, leutinizing hormone (LH) levels.

INTERVENTION/EVALUATION

Monitor lab studies for changes from baseline. Perform periodic hepatic function tests. If transaminases increase over 2 times the upper limit of normal (ULN) or jaundice is noted, discontinue treatment. Monitor for diarrhea, nausea, vomiting.

PATIENT/FAMILY TEACHING

• Do not stop taking medication (both drugs must be continued). • Take medications at same time each day. • Explain possible expectancy of frequent side effects. • Contact physician if persistent nausea, vomiting, diarrhea occur.

bisacodyl

bye-**sak**-oh-dil
(Alophen, Apo-Bisacodyl ✱, Dulcolax, Dulcolax Balance, Fleet Bisacodyl Enema, Veracolate)

◆CLASSIFICATION

PHARMACOTHERAPEUTIC: GI stimulant. **CLINICAL:** Laxative (see p. 122C).

ACTION

Direct effect on colonic smooth musculature by stimulating intramural nerve plexi. **Therapeutic Effect:** Promotes fluid and ion accumulation in colon increasing peristalsis, producing laxative effect.

PHARMACOKINETICS

Route	Onset	Peak	Duration
PO	6–12 hrs	N/A	N/A
Rectal	15–60 min	N/A	N/A

Minimal absorption following PO and rectal administration. Absorbed drug is excreted in urine; remainder is eliminated in feces.

USES

Treatment of constipation, colonic evacuation before examinations or procedures.

PRECAUTIONS

Contraindications: Abdominal pain, appendicitis, intestinal obstruction, nausea, undiagnosed rectal bleeding, vomiting. **Cautions:** Excessive use may lead to fluid, electrolyte imbalance.

⌛ LIFESPAN CONSIDERATIONS

Pregnancy/Lactation: Unknown if drug crosses placenta or is distributed in breast milk. **Pregnancy Category C. Children:** Use with caution in those younger than 6 yrs (usually unable to describe symptoms or more severe side effects). **Elderly:** Repeated use may cause weakness, orthostatic hypotension due to electrolyte loss.

INTERACTIONS

DRUG: Antacids, cimetidine, famotidine, ranitidine may cause rapid dissolution of bisacodyl, producing abdominal cramping, vomiting. May decrease transit time of concurrently administered **oral medications,** decreasing absorption. **HERBAL:** None significant. **FOOD: Milk** may cause rapid dissolution of bisacodyl. **LAB VALUES:** May increase blood glucose concentration. May decrease serum potassium.

AVAILABILITY (OTC)

Powder (Dulcolax Balance). Rectal Enema (Fleet Bisacodyl Enema): 10 mg/30 ml. **Suppositories (Dulcolax):** 10 mg.

Tablets (Enteric-Coated [Dulcolax]): 5 mg.

ADMINISTRATION/HANDLING

PO

• Give on empty stomach (faster action). • Offer 6–8 glasses of water a day (aids stool softening). • Administer tablets whole; do not crush or chew. • Avoid giving within 1 hr of antacids, milk, other oral medication. • Powder: Mix a capful with 4–8 oz water or favorite beverage.

Rectal, Enema

• Shake bottle, and remove orange protective shield from tip. • Position pt on left side with left knee slightly bent and right leg drawn up, or in knee-chest position. • Insert tip into rectum, aiming at pt's umbilicus.

Rectal, Suppository

• If suppository is too soft, chill for 30 min in refrigerator or run cold water over foil wrapper. • Moisten suppository with cold water before inserting well into rectum.
Storage • Store rectal enema, suppositories at room temperature.

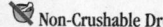

B

INDICATIONS/ROUTES/DOSAGE

Treatment of Constipation

PO: ADULTS, CHILDREN OLDER THAN 12 YRS: 5–15 mg as needed. **Maximum:** 30 mg. **Powder:** Mix a capful with 4–8 oz water or favorite beverage. **CHILDREN 3–12 YRS:** 5–10 mg or 0.3 mg/kg at bedtime or after breakfast. **ELDERLY:** Initially, 5 mg/day.

RECTAL, ENEMA: ADULTS, CHILDREN OLDER THAN 12 YRS: One 1.25-oz bottle in a single daily dose.

RECTAL, SUPPOSITORY: ADULTS, CHILDREN OLDER THAN 12 YRS: 10 mg to induce bowel movement. **CHILDREN 2–12 YRS:** 5–10 mg as a single dose. **CHILDREN YOUNGER THAN 2 YRS:** 5 mg. **ELDERLY:** 5–10 mg/day.

SIDE EFFECTS

Frequent: Some degree of abdominal discomfort, nausea, mild cramps, faintness. **Occasional:** Rectal administration: burning of rectal mucosa, mild proctitis.

ADVERSE EFFECTS/ TOXIC REACTIONS

Long-term use may result in laxative dependence, chronic constipation, loss of normal bowel function. Chronic use or overdose may result in electrolyte or metabolic disturbances (hypokalemia, hypocalcemia, metabolic acidosis, alkalosis), persistent diarrhea, vomiting, muscle weakness, malabsorption, weight loss.

NURSING CONSIDERATIONS

INTERVENTION/EVALUATION

Encourage adequate fluid intake. Assess bowel sounds for peristalsis. Monitor daily pattern of bowel activity and stool consistency; record time of evacuation. Assess for abdominal disturbances. Monitor serum electrolytes in those exposed to prolonged, frequent, or excessive use of medication.

PATIENT/FAMILY TEACHING

• Institute measures to promote defecation: increase fluid intake, exercise, high-fiber diet. • Do not take antacids, milk, or other medication within 1 hr of taking medication (decreased effectiveness). • Report unrelieved constipation, rectal bleeding, muscle pain or cramps, dizziness, weakness. • Do not crush or chew tablets.

bismuth

bis-muth

(Diotame, Kaopectate, Maalox Total Stomach Relief, Pepto-Bismol)

Do not confuse Kaopectate with Kayexalate.

FIXED-COMBINATION(S)

Helidac: bismuth/metronidazole/tetracycline: 262 mg/250 mg/500 mg.

◆CLASSIFICATION

PHARMACOTHERAPEUTIC: Antisecretory, antimicrobial. **CLINICAL:** Antidiarrheal, antinausea, antiulcer (see p. 45C).

ACTION

Absorbs water, toxins in large intestine, forms a protective coating in intestinal mucosa. Possesses antisecretory and antimicrobial effects. **Therapeutic Effect:** Prevents diarrhea.

USES

Treatment of diarrhea, indigestion, nausea. Adjunct in treatment of *H. pylori*–associated peptic ulcer disease. **OFF-LABEL:** Prevention of traveler's diarrhea.

PRECAUTIONS

Contraindications: Bleeding ulcers, gout, hemophilia, hemorrhagic states, renal impairment. **Cautions:** Elderly, diabetic pts. **Pregnancy Category C (D if used in third trimester).**

INTERACTIONS

DRUG: **Anticoagulants, heparin, thrombolytics** may increase risk of bleeding. **Aspirin, other salicylates**

may increase risk of salicylate toxicity. Large doses may increase effects of **insulin, oral antidiabetics.** May decrease absorption of **tetracyclines.** HERBAL: None significant. FOOD: None known. LAB VALUES: May alter serum alkaline phosphatase, AST, ALT, uric acid levels. May decrease serum potassium. May prolong prothrombin time (PT).

AVAILABILITY (OTC)

Caplets: (Pepto-Bismol): 262 mg. Liquid: 262 mg/15 ml (Diotame, Kaopectate, Pepto-Bismol), 525 mg/15 ml (Kaopectate Extra Strength, Maalox Total Stomach Relief, Pepto-Bismol Maximum Strength). Suspension: 262 mg/15 ml. Tablets, Chewable: (Diotame, Pepto-Bismol): 262 mg.

ADMINISTRATION/HANDLING

• Shake suspension well. • Instruct pt to chew or dissolve chewable tablet before swallowing.

INDICATIONS/ROUTES/DOSAGE

Diarrhea, Gastric Distress

PO: ADULTS, ELDERLY: 2 tablets (30 ml) q30–60min. **Maximum:** 8 doses in 24 hrs. **CHILDREN 9–12 YRS:** 1 tablet or 15 ml q30–60min. **Maximum:** 8 doses in 24 hrs. **CHILDREN 6–8 YRS:** ⅔ tablet or 10 ml q30–60min. **Maximum:** 8 doses in 24 hrs. **CHILDREN 3–5 YRS:** ⅓ tablet or 5 ml q30–60min. **Maximum:** 8 doses in 24 hrs.

H. Pylori–Associated Duodenal Ulcer, Gastritis

PO: ADULTS, ELDERLY: 525 mg 4 times a day, with 500 mg amoxicillin and 500 mg metronidazole, 3 times a day after meals, for 7–14 days.

Chronic Infant Diarrhea

PO: CHILDREN 2–24 MOS: 2.5 ml q4h; **25–48 MOS:** 5 ml q4h; **49–70 MOS:** 10 ml q4h.

SIDE EFFECTS

Frequent: Grayish black stools. Rare: Constipation.

ADVERSE EFFECTS/ TOXIC REACTIONS

Debilitated pts and infants may develop impaction.

NURSING CONSIDERATIONS

INTERVENTION/EVALUATION

Encourage adequate fluid intake. Assess bowel sounds for peristaltic activity. Monitor daily pattern of bowel activity and stool consistency.

PATIENT/FAMILY TEACHING

• Stool may appear gray/black. • Chew chewable tablets thoroughly before swallowing. • Report diarrhea lasting more than 2 days.

bisoprolol

HIGH ALERT

bye-**sew**-pro-lol
(Apo-Bisoprolol ✦, Monocor ✦, Novo-Bisoprolol ✦, Zebeta)
Do not confuse Zebeta with DiaBeta or Zetia.

FIXED-COMBINATION(S)

Ziac: bisoprolol/hydrochlorothiazide (a diuretic): 2.5 mg/6.25 mg, 5 mg/6.25 mg, 10 mg/6.25 mg.

◆ CLASSIFICATION

PHARMACOTHERAPEUTIC: Beta-adrenergic blocker. **CLINICAL:** Antihypertensive (see p. 71C).

ACTION

Blocks $beta_1$-adrenergic receptors in cardiac tissue. **Therapeutic Effect:** Slows sinus heart rate, decreases B/P.

PHARMACOKINETICS

Well absorbed from GI tract. Protein binding: 26%–33%. Metabolized in liver. Primarily excreted in urine. Not removed by hemodialysis. **Half-life:** 9–12 hrs (increased in renal impairment).

B

USES

Management of hypertension, alone or in combination with diuretics, other medications. OFF-LABEL: Angina pectoris, premature ventricular contractions, supraventricular arrhythmias, CHF.

PRECAUTIONS

Contraindications: Cardiogenic shock, marked sinus bradycardia, overt cardiac failure, second- or third-degree heart block. Cautions: Renal/hepatic impairment, peripheral vascular disease, hyperthyroidism, diabetes, inadequate cardiac function, bronchospastic disease.

LIFESPAN CONSIDERATIONS

Pregnancy/Lactation: Readily crosses placenta; distributed in breast milk. Avoid use during first trimester. May produce bradycardia, apnea, hypoglycemia, hypothermia during delivery, low birth-weight infants. **Pregnancy Category C (D if used in second or third trimester).** **Children:** Safety and efficacy not established. **Elderly:** Age-related peripheral vascular disease may increase risk of decreased peripheral circulation.

INTERACTIONS

DRUG: **Diuretics, other antihypertensives** may increase hypotensive effect. **Sympathomimetics, xanthines** may mutually inhibit effects. May mask symptoms of hypoglycemia, prolong hypoglycemic effect of **insulin, oral hypoglycemics. NSAIDs** may decrease antihypertensive effect. **Cimetidine** may increase concentration. HERBAL: **Ephedra, ginseng, yohimbe** may worsen hypertension. **Garlic** may have increased antihypertensive effect. FOOD: None known. LAB VALUES: May increase ANA titer, BUN, serum creatinine, potassium, uric acid, lipoproteins, triglycerides.

AVAILABILITY (Rx)

Tablets: 5 mg, 10 mg.

ADMINISTRATION/HANDLING

PO

• Give without regard to food. • Scored tablet may be crushed.

INDICATIONS/ROUTES/DOSAGE

Hypertension

PO: ADULTS: Initially, 2.5–5 mg/day. May increase up to 20 mg/day. **ELDERLY:** Initially, 2.5 mg/day. May increase by 2.5–5 mg/day. **Maximum:** 20 mg/day.

Dosage in Hepatic/Renal Impairment

For adults and elderly pts with cirrhosis or hepatitis whose creatinine clearance is less than 40 ml/min, initially give 2.5 mg.

SIDE EFFECTS

Frequent: Hypotension manifested as dizziness, nausea, diaphoresis, headache, cold extremities, fatigue, constipation, diarrhea. Occasional: Insomnia, flatulence, urinary frequency, impotence or decreased libido. Rare: Rash, arthralgia, myalgia, confusion (esp. in the elderly), altered taste.

ADVERSE EFFECTS/ TOXIC REACTIONS

Overdose may produce profound bradycardia, hypotension. Abrupt withdrawal may result in diaphoresis, palpitations, headache, tremors. May precipitate CHF, MI in pts with cardiac disease, thyroid storm in those with thyrotoxicosis, peripheral ischemia in those with existing peripheral vascular disease. Hypoglycemia may occur in previously controlled diabetes. Thrombocytopenia, unusual bruising/bleeding, occur rarely.

NURSING CONSIDERATIONS

BASELINE ASSESSMENT

Assess baseline renal/hepatic function tests. Assess B/P, apical pulse immediately before drug is administered (if pulse is 60/min or less or systolic B/P is less than 90 mm Hg, withhold medications, contact physician).

B

INTERVENTION/EVALUATION

Assess B/P, pulse for quality, irregular rate, bradycardia. Assist with ambulation if dizziness occurs. Assess for peripheral edema (usually, first area of lower extremity swelling is behind medial malleolus in ambulatory, sacral area in bedridden). Monitor daily pattern of bowel activity and stool consistency. Assess neurologic status.

PATIENT/FAMILY TEACHING

• Do not abruptly discontinue medication. • Compliance with therapy regimen is essential to control hypertension. • If dizziness occurs, sit or lie down immediately. • Avoid tasks that require alertness, motor skills until response to drug is established. • Teach pts how to take pulse properly before each dose and to report excessively slow pulse rate (less than 60 beats/min), peripheral numbness, dizziness. • Do not use nasal decongestants, OTC cold preparations (stimulants) without physician's approval. • Restrict salt, alcohol intake.

bivalirudin HIGH ALERT

bye-**val**-ih-rhu-din
(Angiomax)

◆CLASSIFICATION

PHARMACOTHERAPEUTIC: Thrombin inhibitor. **CLINICAL:** Anticoagulant.

ACTION

Specifically and reversibly inhibits thrombin by binding to its receptor sites. **Therapeutic Effect:** Decreases acute ischemic complications in pts with unstable angina pectoris.

PHARMACOKINETICS

Route	Onset	Peak	Duration
IV	Immediate	N/A	1 hr

Primarily eliminated by kidneys. Twenty-five percent removed by hemodialysis. **Half-life:** 25 min (increased in moderate to severe renal impairment).

USES

Anticoagulant in pts with unstable angina undergoing percutaneous transluminal coronary angioplasty (PTCA) in conjunction with aspirin. Pts with heparin-induced thrombocytopenia (HIT) and thrombosis syndrome (HITTS) while undergoing percutaneous coronary intervention.

PRECAUTIONS

Contraindications: Active major bleeding. **Cautions:** Conditions associated with increased risk of bleeding (e.g., bacterial endocarditis, recent major bleeding, CVA, stroke, intracerebral surgery, hemorrhagic diathesis, severe hypertension, severe renal/hepatic impairment, recent major surgery).

LIFESPAN CONSIDERATIONS

Pregnancy/Lactation: Unknown if drug crosses placenta or is distributed in breast milk. **Pregnancy Category B. Children:** Safety and efficacy not established. **Elderly:** Age-related renal impairment may require dosage adjustment.

INTERACTIONS

DRUG: Platelet aggregation inhibitors (except for aspirin, thrombolytics, warfarin) may increase risk of bleeding complications. **HERBAL: Ginkgo biloba** may increase risk of bleeding. **FOOD:** None known. **LAB VALUES:** Prolongs activated partial thromboplastin time (aPTT), prothrombin time (PT).

AVAILABILITY (Rx)

Injection, Powder for Reconstitution: 250 mg.

ADMINISTRATION/HANDLING

IV

Reconstitution • To each 250-mg vial add 5 ml Sterile Water for Injection.

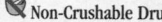

B

• Gently swirl until all material is dissolved. • Further dilute each vial in 50 ml D_5W or 0.9% NaCl to yield final concentration of 5 mg/ml (1 vial in 50 ml, 2 vials in 100 ml, 5 vials in 250 ml). • If low-rate infusion is used after initial infusion, reconstitute the 250-mg vial with added 5 ml Sterile Water for Injection. • Gently swirl until all material is dissolved. • Further dilute each vial in 500 ml D_5W or 0.9% NaCl to yield final concentration of 0.5 mg/ml. • Produces a clear, colorless solution (do not use if cloudy or contains a precipitate).

Rate of administration • Adjust IV infusion based on aPTT or pt's body weight.

Storage • Store unreconstituted vials at room temperature. • Reconstituted solution may be refrigerated for 24 hrs or less. • Diluted drug with a concentration of 0.5–5 mg/ml is stable at room temperature for up to 24 hrs.

IV INCOMPATIBILITIES

Alteplase (Activase), amiodarone (Cordarone), amphotericin B (AmBisome, Abelcet), chlorpromazine (Thorazine), diazepam (Valium), dobutamine (incompatible at 12.5 mg/ml, compatible at 4 mg/ml) (Dobutrex), prochlorperazine (Compazine), reteplase (Retavase), streptokinase (Streptase), vancomycin (Vancocin).

INDICATIONS/ROUTES/DOSAGE

Anticoagulant in Pts with Unstable Angina, HIT, or HITTS Undergoing PTCA

IV: ADULTS, ELDERLY: 0.75 mg/kg as IV bolus, followed by IV infusion at rate of 1.75 mg/kg/hr for duration of procedure and up to 4 hrs postprocedure. IV infusion may be continued beyond initial 4 hrs at rate of 0.2 mg/kg/hr for up to 20 hrs.

Dosage in Renal Impairment

ALERT Initial bolus dose remains unchanged.

Creatinine Clearance	Dosage
30 ml/min or greater	1.75 mg/kg/hr
10–29 ml/min	1 mg/kg/hr
Dialysis	0.25 mg/kg/hr

SIDE EFFECTS

Frequent (42%): Back pain. **Occasional (15%–12%):** Nausea, headache, hypotension, generalized pain. **Rare (8%–4%):** Injection site pain, insomnia, hypertension, anxiety, vomiting, pelvic or abdominal pain, bradycardia, nervousness, dyspepsia, fever, urinary retention.

ADVERSE EFFECTS/ TOXIC REACTIONS

Hemorrhagic events occur rarely, characterized by significant fall in B/P or Hct.

NURSING CONSIDERATIONS

BASELINE ASSESSMENT

Assess CBC, bleeding time, renal function. Determine initial B/P.

INTERVENTION/EVALUATION

Monitor aPTT, Hct, urine and stool specimen for occult blood, renal function studies. Monitor for evidence of bleeding. Assess for decrease in B/P, increase in pulse rate. Question for increase in amount of discharge during menses. Assess urine for hematuria.

black cohosh

(Black Cohosh Softgel, Remifemin)
Also known as baneberry, bugbane, bugwort, fairy candles.

CLASSIFICATION

HERBAL: See Appendix G.

ACTION

May target serotonin receptors to help regulate body temperature. **Effect:** Reduces symptoms of menopause (e.g., hot flashes).

USES

Treatment of symptoms of menopause, induction of labor in pregnant women. May reduce serum lipids, decrease B/P (esp. when combined with prescription medications). Mild sedative action.

PRECAUTIONS

Contraindications: Preterm pregnancy (has menstrual and uterine stimulant effects that may increase risk of miscarriage). Not to be taken for longer than 6 mos. **Cautions:** Pts with breast, uterine, ovarian cancer; endometriosis; uterine fibroids.

LIFESPAN CONSIDERATIONS

Pregnancy/Lactation: Contraindicated. **Children:** Safety and efficacy not established. **Elderly:** No age-related precautions noted.

INTERACTIONS

DRUG: May have additive antiproliferative effect with **tamoxifen.** May increase action of **antihypertensives. HERBAL:** None significant. **FOOD:** None known. **LAB VALUES:** May decrease serum luteinizing hormone (LH) concentration.

AVAILABILITY

Capsules (Soft Gelatin): 40 mg. **Tablets:** 20 mg.

INDICATIONS/ROUTES/DOSAGE

Menopause, Labor Induction, Reduce Lipids and/or B/P, Sedative

PO: ADULTS, ELDERLY: 20–80 mg twice a day.

SIDE EFFECTS

Nausea, headache, dizziness, weight gain, visual changes, migraines.

ADVERSE EFFECTS/ TOXIC REACTIONS

Overdose may cause nausea/vomiting, bradycardia, diaphoresis. May produce hepatotoxicity.

NURSING CONSIDERATIONS

BASELINE ASSESSMENT

Assess if pt is pregnant or breast-feeding (contraindicated).

INTERVENTION/EVALUATION

Monitor B/P, lipid levels.

PATIENT/FAMILY TEACHING

• Inform physician if pregnancy occurs or planning to become pregnant, breastfeeding. • Do not take for longer than 6 mos.

bleomycin HIGH ALERT

blee-oh-**my**-sin
(Blenoxane)

BLACK BOX ALERT Pulmonary fibrosis (commonly presenting as pneumonitis) occurs more often in elderly, pts receiving more than 400 units total lifetime dose or single dose more than 30 units, smokers, prior radiation treatment, or receiving concurrent oxygen. A severe reaction (hypotension, mental confusion, fever, chills, wheezing) is reported rarely.

◆CLASSIFICATION

PHARMACOTHERAPEUTIC: Glycopeptide antibiotic. **CLINICAL:** Antineoplastic, sclerosing agent (see p. 81C).

ACTION

Binds to portions of DNA, producing DNA single-strand breaks. Most effective in G_2 phase of cell division. **Therapeutic Effect:** Inhibits cell replication.

PHARMACOKINETICS

Protein binding: Low (1%). Metabolism varies. Excreted in urine as unchanged drug. **Half-life:** 115 min.

USES

Treatment of Hodgkin's and non-Hodgkin's lymphoma, malignant pleural effusions, squamous cell carcinoma (e.g., head, neck, penis, cervix, vulva), testicular carcinoma. **OFF-LABEL:** Sclerosing agent for malignant pleural effusion, treatment of mycosis fungoides, osteosarcoma, ovarian tumors, renal carcinoma, soft tissue sarcoma.

B

PRECAUTIONS

Contraindications: Previous allergic reaction. Cautions: Severe renal or pulmonary impairment.

LIFESPAN CONSIDERATIONS

Pregnancy/Lactation: May cause fetal harm. Breast-feeding not recommended. **Pregnancy Category D. Children:** Safety and efficacy not established. **Elderly:** Increased risk of pulmonary toxicity.

INTERACTIONS

DRUG: **Cisplatin** may decrease bleomycin clearance and increase risk of bleomycin toxicity (from cisplatin-induced renal impairment). **Other antineoplastics** may increase risk of toxicity. HERBAL: None significant. FOOD: None known. LAB VALUES: None significant.

AVAILABILITY (Rx)

Injection, Powder for Reconstitution, (Blenoxane): 15 units, 30 units.

ADMINISTRATION/HANDLING

◀ALERT▶ May be carcinogenic, mutagenic, teratogenic. Handle with extreme care during preparation/administration.

IV

Reconstitution • Reconstitute 15-unit vial with at least 5 ml (30-unit vial with at least 10 ml) 0.9% NaCl to provide a concentration not greater than 3 units/ml.
Rate of administration • Administer over at least 10 min for IV injection.
Storage • Refrigerate powder. • After reconstitution with 0.9% NaCl, solution is stable for 24 hrs at room temperature.

IM, Subcutaneous

Rate of administration • Reconstitute 15-unit vial with 1–5 ml (30-unit vial with 2–10 ml) Sterile Water for Injection, 0.9% NaCl, or Bacteriostatic Water for Injection to provide concentration of 3–15 units/ml. Do not use D_5W.
Storage • Refrigerate powder • After reconstitution, solution is stable for 24 hrs at room temperature.

IV INCOMPATIBILITIES

Diazepam (Valium), furosemide (Lasix), hydrocortisone sodium succinate (Solu-Cortef).

IV COMPATIBILITIES

Cefepime (Maxipime), dacarbazine (DTIC), dexamethasone (Decadron), diphenhydramine (Benadryl), fludarabine (Fludara), gemcitabine (Gemzar), ondansetron (Zofran), paclitaxel (Taxol), piperacillin/tazobactam (Zosyn), vinblastine (Velban), vinorelbine (Navelbine).

INDICATIONS/ROUTES/DOSAGE

◀ALERT▶ Maximum lifetime dose = 400 units.

Usual Dosage
(Refer to individual protocols)
IV, IM, SUBCUTANEOUS: ADULTS, ELDERLY: 10–20 units/m² (0.25–0.5 units/kg) 1–2 times a wk.
IV (CONTINUOUS): ADULTS, ELDERLY: 15 units/m² over 24 hrs for 4 days.

Sclerosing Agent
ADULTS, ELDERLY: 60 units as a single infusion. May repeat at intervals of several days if fluid continues to accumulate (may add lidocaine 100–200 mg to reduce local discomfort).

Dosage in Renal Impairment

Creatinine Clearance	Dosage
40–50 ml/min	70% of normal
30–39 ml/min	60% of normal
20–29 ml/min	55% of normal
10–19 ml/min	45% of normal
5–9 ml/min	40% of normal

SIDE EFFECTS

Frequent: Anorexia, weight loss, erythematous skin swelling, urticaria, rash, striae, vesiculation, hyperpigmentation (particularly at areas of pressure, skin folds, cuticles, IM injection sites, scars), stomatitis (usually evident 1–3 wks after initial therapy); may be accompanied by decreased skin sensitivity followed by skin hypersensitivity, nausea, vomiting, alopecia. With parenteral form, fever, chills typically occurring a few hrs after large single dose, lasting 4–12 hrs occur frequently.

ADVERSE EFFECTS/ TOXIC REACTIONS

Interstitial pneumonitis occurs in 10% of pts, occasionally progresses to pulmonary fibrosis. Appears to be dose-, age-related (older than 70 yrs, those receiving total dose greater than 400 units). Nephrotoxicity, hepatotoxicity occur infrequently.

NURSING CONSIDERATIONS

BASELINE ASSESSMENT

Obtain baseline chest X-ray.

INTERVENTION/EVALUATION

Adventitious breath sounds may indicate pulmonary toxicity (rales, rhonchi). Observe for dyspnea. Monitor hematologic, pulmonary, hepatic, renal function tests. Assess skin daily for cutaneous toxicity (erythema, rash, vesiculation). Monitor for stomatitis (burning, erythema of oral mucosa at inner margin of lips), hematologic toxicity (fever, sore throat, signs of local infection, unusual bruising/bleeding), symptoms of anemia (excessive fatigue, weakness).

PATIENT/FAMILY TEACHING

• Report fever, chills, wheezing, difficulty breathing, prolonged nausea, vomiting, oral pain or lesions. • Fever or chills reaction occurs less frequently with continued therapy. • Improvement of Hodgkin's disease, testicular tumors noted within 2 wks, squamous cell carcinoma within 3 wks. • Do not have immunizations without physician's approval (drug lowers body's resistance). • Avoid contact with those who have recently taken live virus vaccine or had a viral infection (e.g., cold virus, herpetic infection).

Boniva, *see ibandronate*

bortezomib HIGH ALERT

bor-**teh**-zoe-mib
(Velcade)

◆CLASSIFICATION

PHARMACOTHERAPEUTIC: Proteasome inhibitor. **CLINICAL:** Antineoplastic.

ACTION

Degrades conjugated proteins required for cell-cycle progression and mitosis, disrupting cell proliferation. **Therapeutic Effect:** Produces antitumor and chemosensitizing activity, cell death.

PHARMACOKINETICS

Widely distributed. Protein binding: 83%. Primarily metabolized by enzymatic action. Significant biliary excretion, with lesser amount excreted in urine. **Half-life:** 9–15 hrs.

USES

Treatment of relapsed or refractory multiple myeloma, mantle cell lymphoma. Initial treatment of multiple myeloma. **OFF-LABEL:** Treatment of non-Hodgkin's lymphoma.

PRECAUTIONS

Contraindications: Hypersensitivity to boron or mannitol. **Cautions:** History of syncope, pts receiving medication known to be associated with hypotension, dehydrated pts, renal/hepatic impairment, preexisting cardiac disease.

⌛ LIFESPAN CONSIDERATIONS

Pregnancy/Lactation: May induce degenerative effects in ovary, degenerative changes in testes. May affect male/female fertility. Breast-feeding not recommended. **Pregnancy Category D. Children:** Safety and efficacy not established. **Elderly:** Increased incidence of grades 3 or 4 thrombocytopenia.

INTERACTIONS

DRUG: **Amiodarone, antivirals, isoniazid, nitrofurantoin, statins** may increase risk of peripheral neuropathy. May alter effects of **antihypertensives, medications associated with hypotension.** May alter **oral hypoglycemic** response. HERBAL: **Green tea, green tea extracts** may diminish effect. **St. John's wort** may decrease level/effect. FOOD: **Grapefruit juice** may increase drug level. LAB VALUES: May significantly decrease WBC, Hgb, Hct, platelet count, neutrophils.

AVAILABILITY (Rx)

Injection, Powder for Reconstitution: 3.5 mg.

ADMINISTRATION/HANDLING

IV

Reconstitution • Reconstitute vial with 3.5 ml 0.9% NaCl.
Rate of administration • Give as bolus IV injection over 3–5 sec.
Storage • Store unopened vials at room temperature. • Once reconstituted, solution may be stored at room temperature for up to 3 days or for 5 days if refrigerated.

INDICATIONS/ROUTES/DOSAGE

Relapsed or Refractory Multiple Myeloma, Mantle Cell Lymphoma

IV: ADULTS, ELDERLY: Treatment cycle consists of 1.3 mg/m^2 twice weekly on days 1, 4, 8, and 11 for 2 wks followed by a 10-day rest period on days 12 to 21. Consecutive doses separated by at least 72 hrs.

Multiple Myeloma (Initial Treatment)

IV: ADULTS, ELDERLY: 1.3 mg/m^2 (with melphalan and prednisone) for a total of nine 6-wk treatment cycles (cycles 1–4 administer twice weekly; cycles 5–9 administer once weekly).

Dosage Adjustment Guidelines

Therapy is withheld at onset of grade 3 nonhematologic or grade 4 hematologic toxicities, excluding neuropathy. When symptoms resolve, therapy is restarted at a 25% reduced dosage.

Dosage Adjustment Guidelines with Neuropathic Pain, Peripheral Sensory Neuropathy

For grade 1 toxicity with pain or grade 2 (interfering with function but not activities of daily living [ADL]), 1 mg/m^2. For grade 2 toxicity with pain or grade 3 (interfering with ADL), withhold drug until toxicity is resolved, then reinitiate with 0.7 mg/m^2. For grade 4 toxicity (permanent sensory loss that interferes with function), discontinue bortezomib.

SIDE EFFECTS

Expected (65%–36%): Fatigue, malaise, asthenia, nausea, diarrhea, anorexia, constipation, fever, vomiting. Frequent (28%–21%): Headache, insomnia, arthralgia, limb pain, edema, paresthesia, dizziness, rash. Occasional (18%–11%): Dehydration, cough, anxiety, bone pain, muscle cramps, myalgia, back pain, abdominal pain, taste alteration, dyspepsia, pruritus, hypotension (including orthostatic hypotension), rigors, blurred vision.

ADVERSE EFFECTS/ TOXIC REACTIONS

Thrombocytopenia occurs in 40% of pts. Platelet count peaks at day 11, returns to baseline by day 21. GI, intracerebral hemorrhage are associated with drug-induced thrombocytopenia. Anemia occurs in 32% of pts. New onset or worsening of existing neuropathy occurs in 37% of pts. Symptoms may improve in some pts upon drug discontinuation. Pneumonia occurs occasionally.

NURSING CONSIDERATIONS

BASELINE ASSESSMENT

Obtain baseline CBC. Assure adequate hydration prior to initiation of therapy.

Antiemetics, antidiarrheals may be effective in preventing, treating nausea, vomiting, diarrhea.

INTERVENTION/EVALUATION

Routinely assess B/P; monitor pt for orthostatic hypotension. Maintain strict I&O. Monitor CBC, esp. platelet count, throughout treatment. Monitor renal, hepatic, pulmonary function throughout therapy. Encourage adequate fluid intake to prevent dehydration. Monitor temperature and be alert to high potential for fever. Monitor for peripheral neuropathy (burning sensation, neuropathic pain, paresthesia, hyperesthesia). Avoid IM injections, rectal temperatures, other traumas that may induce bleeding.

PATIENT/FAMILY TEACHING

• Report new/worsening vomiting, bruising/bleeding, breathing difficulties. • Discuss importance of pregnancy testing, avoidance of pregnancy, measures to prevent pregnancy. • Increase fluid intake. • Avoid tasks that require mental alertness, motor skills until response to drug is established.

bosentan

bo-sen-tan
(Tracleer)

BLACK BOX ALERT Do not use in pregnancy or in moderate to severe hepatic impairment.

Do not confuse Tracleer with Tricor.

◆CLASSIFICATION

PHARMACOTHERAPEUTIC: Endothelin receptor antagonist. **CLINICAL:** Vasodilator, neurohormonal blocker.

ACTION

Blocks the neurohormone that constricts pulmonary arteries. **Therapeutic Effect:** Improves exercise ability, slows clinical worsening of pulmonary arterial hypertension (PAH).

PHARMACOKINETICS

Protein binding: greater than 98%. Metabolized in liver. Eliminated by biliary excretion. **Half-life:** Approximately 5 hrs (increased in cardiac failure).

USES

Treatment of PAH in those with class III or IV symptoms (World Health Organization). **OFF-LABEL:** CHF, pulmonary hypertension secondary to scleroderma.

PRECAUTIONS

Contraindications: Administration with cyclosporine or glyburide, pregnancy. **Extreme Caution:** Moderate to severe hepatic impairment. **Cautions:** Mild hepatic impairment.

⌛ LIFESPAN CONSIDERATIONS

Pregnancy/Lactation: May induce male infertility, atrophy of seminiferous tubules of testes; reduce sperm count. Expected to cause fetal harm, teratogenic effects, including malformations of head, mouth, face, large vessels. Breast-feeding not recommended. **Pregnancy Category X. Children:** Safety and efficacy not established. **Elderly:** Use caution in dosage due to higher frequency of decreased hepatic, renal, cardiac function.

INTERACTIONS

DRUG: May decrease concentration of **atorvastatin, glyburide, hormonal contraceptives (oral, injectable, implantable), lovastatin, simvastatin, warfarin. Cyclosporine, ketoconazole** may increase plasma concentration of bosentan. **HERBAL:** None significant. **FOOD:** None known. **LAB VALUES:** May increase serum bilirubin, AST, ALT levels. May decrease Hgb, Hct levels.

B

AVAILABILITY (Rx)

Tablets: 62.5 mg, 125 mg.

ADMINISTRATION/HANDLING

• Give in morning and evening, with or without food. • Instruct pt to not chew film-coated tablets.

INDICATIONS/ROUTES/DOSAGE

Pulmonary Arterial Hypertension

PO: ADULTS, ELDERLY, CHILDREN OLDER THAN 12 YRS AND WEIGHING 40 KG OR GREATER: 62.5 mg twice a day for 4 wks; then increase to maintenance dosage of 125 mg twice a day. **ADULTS, ELDERLY, CHILDREN WEIGHING LESS THAN 40 KG:** 62.5 mg twice a day.

◀ALERT▶ When discontinuing adult/elderly dosage, reduce dosage to 62.5 mg twice a day for 3–7 days to avoid clinical deterioration.

Dosage Based on Hepatic Enzyme Elevations

Any elevation accompanied by symptoms of hepatic injury or serum bilirubin 2 or more times upper limit of normal (ULN), stop treatment. AST/ALT greater than 3 or less than 6 times ULN, reduce dose or interrupt treatment. AST/ALT greater than 5 and up to 8 times ULN, confirm with additional test and, if confirmed, stop treatment. AST/ALT greater than 8 times ULN, stop treatment.

SIDE EFFECTS

Occasional: Headache, nasopharyngitis, flushing. **Rare:** Dyspepsia (heartburn, epigastric distress), fatigue, pruritus, hypotension.

ADVERSE EFFECTS/ TOXIC REACTIONS

Abnormal hepatic function, lower extremity edema, palpitations occur rarely.

NURSING CONSIDERATIONS

BASELINE ASSESSMENT

Pregnancy must be excluded before starting treatment and prevented thereafter. A negative pregnancy test performed during the first 5 days of a normal menstrual period and at least 11 days after the last act of sexual intercourse must be obtained. Monthly follow-up pregnancy tests must be maintained. Obtain, assess baseline lab tests, esp. hepatic function.

INTERVENTION/EVALUATION

Assess hepatic enzyme levels before initiating therapy then monthly thereafter. If elevation in hepatic enzymes is noted, changes in monitoring and treatment must be initiated. If clinical symptoms of hepatic injury (nausea, vomiting, fever, abdominal pain, fatigue, jaundice) occur or if serum bilirubin level increases to 2 or more times ULN, stop treatment. Assess for peripheral edema. Monitor Hgb levels at 1 mo and 3 mos of treatment, then q3mo for decrease.

PATIENT/FAMILY TEACHING

• Discuss importance of pregnancy testing, avoidance of pregnancy, measures to prevent pregnancy. • Report palpitations, extremity swelling, unusual weight gain, fatigue, yellowing of skin or eyes, change in color of stool, urine.

Botox, *see botulinum toxin type A*

botulinum toxin type A

bot-ue-lye-num **tox**-in
(Botox, Botox Cosmetic)

BLACK BOX ALERT Effects may spread beyond treatment area; may occur hours to weeks after injection. Dysphagia, breathing difficulties, including fatalities, asthenia, diplopia, blurred vision, ptosis, have been reported. Risk greatest in children treated for spasticity.

B

◆CLASSIFICATION

PHARMACOTHERAPEUTIC: Neurotoxin. **CLINICAL:** Neuromuscular conduction blocker.

ACTION

Blocks neuromuscular conduction by binding to receptor sites on motor nerve endings, inhibiting release of acetylcholine, resulting in muscle denervation. **Therapeutic Effect:** Reduces muscle activity.

PHARMACOKINETICS

In treatment of blepharospasm, each treatment lasts approximately 3 mos. In treatment of strabismus, paralysis lasts for 2–6 wks and gradually resolves over an additional 2–6 wks. In treatment of hemifacial spasm, treatment may last 6 mos.

USES

Treatment of strabismus, blepharospasm associated with dystonia, cervical dystonia. Temporary improvement of brow furrow lines in those 65 yrs and younger. **OFF-LABEL:** Treatment of dynamic muscle contracture in children with cerebral palsy, focal task-specific dystonia, head and neck tremor unresponsive to drug therapy, hemifacial spasms, laryngeal dystonia, oromandibular dystonia, spasmoditic torticollis, mogigraphia (writer's cramp), migraine treatment, prophylaxis.

PRECAUTIONS

Contraindications: Infection at proposed injection sites. **Cautions:** Pts with neuromuscular junctional disorders (amyotrophic lateral sclerosis, motor neuropathy, myasthenia gravis, Lambert-Eaton syndrome) may experience significant systemic effects (severe dysphagia, respiratory compromise).

⌛ LIFESPAN CONSIDERATIONS

Pregnancy/Lactation: Unknown if drug crosses placenta or is distributed is breast milk. **Pregnancy Category C. Children:** Safety and efficacy not established. **Elderly:** No age-related precautions noted.

INTERACTIONS

DRUG: **Aminoglycoside antibiotics, neuromuscular blocking agents** may potentiate effects. **HERBAL:** None significant. **FOOD:** None known. **LAB VALUES:** None significant.

AVAILABILITY (Rx)

Injection, Powder for Reconstitution: 100 units/vial.

ADMINISTRATION/HANDLING

IM

Reconstitution • 0.9% NaCl is recommended diluent. • For resulting dose of units/0.1 ml, draw up 1 ml diluent to provide 10 units, 2 ml to provide 5 units, 4 ml to provide 2.5 units, 8 ml to provide 1.25 units. • Slowly, gently inject diluent into the vial, avoid bubbles, rotate vial gently to mix.

Rate of administration • Administer within 4 hrs after reconstitution. • Inject into affected muscle using 25-, 27-, or 30-gauge needle for superficial muscles and 22-gauge needle for deeper musculature.

Storage • Store in freezer. • Administer within 4 hrs after removal from freezer and reconstitution. • Store reconstituted solution in refrigerator for up to 4 hrs. • Appears as a clear, colorless solution (discard if particulates form).

INDICATIONS/ROUTES/DOSAGE

◀ALERT▶ Administer at lower dosage for pts who have not received previous treatment with this drug until tolerance is established.

Cervical Dystonia

IM: ADULTS, ELDERLY: Mean dose of 236 units (range: 198–300 units) divided among the affected muscles, based on pt's head and neck position, localization of pain, muscle hypertrophy, pt response, adverse reaction history.

B

Strabismus

IM: ADULTS, CHILDREN OLDER THAN 12 YRS: 1.25–2.5 units into any one muscle. **CHILDREN 2 MOS–12 YRS:** 1–2.5 units into any one muscle.

Blepharospasm

IM: ADULTS, CHILDREN 12 YRS AND OLDER: Initially, 1.25–2.5 units. May increase up to 2.5–5 units at repeat treatments. **Maximum:** 5 units per injection or cumulative dose of 200 units over a 30-day period.

Cerebral Palsy Spasticity

IM: CHILDREN OLDER THAN 18 MOS: 1–6 units/kg. **Maximum:** 50 units per injection site. No more than 400 units per visit or during a 3-mo period.

Improvement of Brow Furrow

IM: ADULTS 65 YRS AND YOUNGER: Individualized.

SIDE EFFECTS

ALERT Side effects usually occur within the first wk after injection. **Frequent (15%–11%):** Localized pain, tenderness, bruising at injection site; localized weakness in injected muscle; upper respiratory tract infection; neck pain; headache. **Occasional (10%–2%):** Increased cough, flu-like symptoms, back pain, rhinitis, dizziness, hypertonia, soreness at injection site, asthenia, dry mouth, nausea, drowsiness. **Rare:** Stiffness, numbness, diplopia, ptosis.

ADVERSE EFFECTS/ TOXIC REACTIONS

Mild to moderate dysphagia occurs in approximately 20% of pts. Arrhythmias and severe dysphagia (manifested as aspiration, pneumonia, dyspnea) occur rarely. Overdose produces systemic weakness, muscle paralysis.

NURSING CONSIDERATIONS

BASELINE ASSESSMENT

Assess onset, type, location, duration of dystonia.

INTERVENTION/EVALUATION

Clinical improvement begins within first 2 wks after injection. Maximum benefit appears at approximately 6 wks after injection.

PATIENT/FAMILY TEACHING

- Resume activity slowly and carefully.
- Seek medical attention immediately if swallowing, speech, respiratory difficulties occur.

botulinum toxin type B

bot-ue-lye-num **tox**-in
(Myobloc)

BLACK BOX ALERT Effects may spread beyond treatment area; may occur hours to weeks after injection. Dysphagia, breathing difficulties, including fatalities, asthenia, diplopia, blurred vision, ptosis, have been reported. Risk greatest in children treated for spasticity.

CLASSIFICATION

PHARMACOTHERAPEUTIC: Neurotoxin. **CLINICAL:** Neuromuscular conduction blocker.

ACTION

Inhibits acetylcholine release at neuromuscular junction by binding to the protein complex responsible for fusion to the presynaptic membrane, a necessary step to neurotransmitter release. **Therapeutic Effect:** Produces flaccid paralysis.

PHARMACOKINETICS

Duration of effect is 12–16 wks at doses of 5,000 or 10,000 units.

USES

Treatment of cervical dystonia to reduce severity of abnormal head position, neck pain associated with cervical dystonia. **OFF-LABEL:** Treatment of cervical dystonia in pts resistant to botulinum toxin type A.

PRECAUTIONS

Contraindications: None known. **Cautions:** Pts with neuromuscular junctional disorders (amyotrophic lateral sclerosis, motor neuropathy, myasthenia gravis, Lambert-Eaton syndrome) may experience significant systemic effects (severe dysphagia, respiratory compromise).

LIFESPAN CONSIDERATIONS

Pregnancy/Lactation: Unknown if drug crosses placenta or is distributed in breast milk. **Pregnancy Category C. Children:** Safety and efficacy not established. **Elderly:** No age-related precautions noted.

INTERACTIONS

DRUG: Aminoglycoside antibiotics, neuromuscular blocking agents may potentiate effects. **HERBAL:** None significant. **FOOD:** None known. **LAB VALUES:** None significant.

AVAILABILITY (Rx)

Injection Solution: 5,000 units/ml.

ADMINISTRATION/HANDLING

IM

Reconstitution • 0.9% NaCl is recommended diluent. • Slowly, gently inject diluent into the vial; avoid bubbles, rotate vial gently to mix.

Rate of administration • Administer within 4 hrs after reconstitution. • Inject into affected muscle using 25-, 27-, or 30-gauge needle for superficial muscles and 22-gauge needle for deeper musculature.

Storage • May be refrigerated for up to 21 mos. Do not freeze. • Administer within 4 hrs after removal from refrigerator and reconstitution. • Store reconstituted solution in refrigerator for up to 4 hrs. • Appears as a clear, colorless solution (discard if particulate forms).

INDICATIONS/ROUTES/DOSAGE

◄ALERT► Administer at lower dosage for pts who have not received previous treatment with this drug until tolerance is established.

IM: ADULTS, ELDERLY: 2,500–5,000 units divided among the affected muscles.

SIDE EFFECTS

◄ALERT► Side effects usually occur within the first wk after the injection. **Frequent (19%–12%):** Infection, neck pain, headache, injection site pain, dry mouth. **Occasional (10%–4%):** Flu-like symptoms, generalized pain, increased cough, back pain, myasthenia. **Rare:** Dizziness, nausea, rhinitis, headache, vomiting, edema, allergic reaction.

ADVERSE EFFECTS/ TOXIC REACTIONS

Mild to moderate dysphagia occurs in approximately 10% of pts. Arrhythmias and severe dysphagia (manifested as aspiration, pneumonia, dyspnea) occur rarely. Overdose produces systemic weakness, muscle paralysis.

NURSING CONSIDERATIONS

BASELINE ASSESSMENT

Assess onset, type, location, duration of dystonia.

INTERVENTION/EVALUATION

Duration of effect lasts between 12–16 wks at doses of 5,000 units or 10,000 units.

PATIENT/FAMILY TEACHING

• Resume activity slowly and carefully. • Seek medical attention immediately if swallowing, speech, respiratory difficulties occur.

Brethine, *see terbutaline*

Brevibloc, *see esmolol*

B

bromocriptine

broe-moe-**krip**-teen
(Apo-Bromocriptine, Cycloset, Parlodel)
Do not confuse bromocriptine with benztropine, or Parlodel with pindolol or Provera.

CLASSIFICATION

PHARMACOTHERAPEUTIC: Dopamine agonist. **CLINICAL:** Infertility therapy adjunct, antihyperprolactinemic, lactation inhibitor, antidyskinetic, growth hormone suppressant.

ACTION

Directly stimulates dopamine receptors in corpus striatum, inhibits prolactin secretion. Suppresses secretion of growth hormone. **Therapeutic Effect:** Improves symptoms of parkinsonism, suppresses galactorrhea, reduces serum growth hormone concentrations in acromegaly.

PHARMACOKINETICS

Indication	Onset	Peak	Duration
Prolactin lowering	1–2 hrs	5–10 hrs	8–12 hrs

Minimally absorbed from GI tract. Protein binding: 90%–96%. Metabolized in liver. Excreted in feces by biliary secretion. **Half-life:** 15 hrs.

USES

Treatment of pituitary prolactinomas, conditions associated with hyperprolactinemia (amenorrhea, galactorrhea, hypogonadism, infertility), parkinsonism, acromegaly. **Cycloset:** Control blood glucose in type 2 diabetes. **OFF-LABEL:** Treatment of cocaine addiction, hyperprolactinemia associated with pituitary adenomas, neuroleptic malignant syndrome.

PRECAUTIONS

Contraindications: Hypersensitivity to ergot alkaloids, peripheral vascular disease, pregnancy, severe ischemic heart disease, uncontrolled hypertension. **Cautions:** Impaired hepatic or cardiac function, hypertension, psychiatric disorders.

LIFESPAN CONSIDERATIONS

Pregnancy/Lactation: Not recommended during pregnancy or breastfeeding. **Pregnancy Category B. Children:** Safety and efficacy not established. **Elderly:** CNS effects may occur more frequently.

INTERACTIONS

DRUG: Disulfram-like reactions (chest pain, confusion, flushed face, nausea, vomiting) may occur with **alcohol. Estrogens, progestins** may decrease effects. **Haloperidol, MAOIs, phenothiazines** may decrease prolactin effect. **Antihypertensive agents** may increase hypotension. **Levodopa** may increase effects. **Erythromycin, ritonavir** may increase concentration, toxicity. **Risperidone** may increase serum prolactin concentration, interfere with bromocriptine effects. **HERBAL: St. John's wort** may decrease concentration. **FOOD:** None known. **LAB VALUES:** May increase plasma concentration of growth hormone.

AVAILABILITY (Rx)

Capsules: 5 mg. **Tablets:** 2.5 mg. **(Cycloset):** 0.8 mg.

ADMINISTRATION/HANDLING

PO

• Pt should be lying down before administering first dose. • Give after food intake (decreases incidence of nausea).

INDICATIONS/ROUTES/DOSAGE

Hyperprolactinemia

PO: ADULTS, ELDERLY: Initially, 1.25–2.5 mg at bedtime. May increase by 2.5 mg q3–7days up to 5–7.5 mg/day in divided doses. Maintenance: 2.5 mg 2–3 times a day. Range: 2.5–15 mg/day.

Pituitary Prolactinomas

PO: ADULTS, ELDERLY: Initially, 1.25 mg 2–3 times a day. May gradually increase over several wks to 10–20 mg/day in divided doses. Maintenance: 2.5–20 mg/day in divided doses.

Parkinsonism

PO: ADULTS, ELDERLY: Initially, 1.25 mg 1–2 times a day. May take single doses at bedtime. May increase by 2.5 mg/day at 14- to 28-day intervals. Maintenance: 2.5–40 mg/day in divided doses. Range: 30–90 mg/day in 3 divided doses. **Maximum:** 100 mg/day.

Acromegaly

PO: ADULTS, ELDERLY: Initially, 1.25–2.5 mg at bedtime. May increase by 1.25–2.5 mg q3–7days up to 30 mg/day in divided doses. Maintenance: 20–30 mg/day in divided doses. **Maximum:** 100 mg/day.

Type 2 Diabetes

PO: ADULTS, ELDERLY: Initially, 0.8 mg once daily. Increase by 0.8 mg/day weekly up to maximum of 4.8 mg/day.

SIDE EFFECTS

Frequent: Nausea (49%), headache (19%), dizziness (17%). **Occasional (7%–3%):** Fatigue, light-headedness, vomiting, abdominal cramps, diarrhea, constipation, nasal congestion, drowsiness, dry mouth. **Rare:** Muscle cramps, urinary hesitancy.

ADVERSE EFFECTS/ TOXIC REACTIONS

Visual or auditory hallucinations noted in pts with Parkinson's disease. Long-term, high-dose therapy may produce continuing rhinorrhea, syncope, GI hemorrhage, peptic ulcer, severe abdominal pain.

NURSING CONSIDERATIONS

BASELINE ASSESSMENT

Evaluation of pituitary gland (rule out tumor) should be done before treatment for hyperprolactinemia with amenorrhea or galactorrhea, infertility. Obtain baseline lab tests including CBC, hepatic function, prolactin level, pregnancy test.

INTERVENTION/EVALUATION

Assist with ambulation if dizziness is noted after administration. Assess for therapeutic response (decrease in engorgement, parkinsonism symptoms). Monitor for changes in daily bowel habits, stool consistency. Monitor cardiac function.

PATIENT/FAMILY TEACHING

• To reduce light-headedness, rise slowly from lying to sitting position, permit legs to dangle momentarily before standing. • Avoid sudden posture changes. Avoid tasks that require alertness, motor skills until response to drug is established. • Use contraceptive measures (other than oral) during treatment. • Report any watery nasal discharge to physician. • Avoid alcohol intake.

Budeprion, *see bupropion*

budesonide

byoo-**des**-oh-nide
(Entocort EC, Pulmicort Flexhaler, Pulmicort Respules, Rhinocort Aqua)

FIXED-COMBINATION(S)

Symbicort: budesonide/formoterol (bronchodilator): 80 mcg/4.5 mcg, 160 mcg/4.5 mcg.

B

◆CLASSIFICATION

PHARMACOTHERAPEUTIC: Glucocorticosteroid. **CLINICAL:** Anti-inflammatory, antiallergy (see pp. 2C, 75C, 97C).

ACTION

Inhibits accumulation of inflammatory cells, decreases and prevents tissues from responding to inflammatory process. **Therapeutic Effect:** Relieves symptoms of allergic rhinitis, Crohn's disease.

PHARMACOKINETICS

Form	Onset	Peak	Duration
Pulmicort Respules	2–8 days	4–6 wks	–
Rhinocort Aqua	10 hrs	2 wks	–

Minimally absorbed from nasal tissue; moderately absorbed from inhalation. Protein binding: 88%. Primarily metabolized in liver. **Half-life:** 2–3 hrs.

USES

Nasal: Management of seasonal or perennial allergic rhinitis, nonallergic rhinitis. **Inhalation:** Maintenance or prophylaxis therapy for bronchial asthma. **PO:** Treatment of mild to moderate active Crohn's disease. Maintenance of clinical remission of mild to moderate Crohn's disease. **OFF-LABEL:** Treatment of vasomotor rhinitis.

PRECAUTIONS

Contraindications: Hypersensitivity to any corticosteroid or its components, persistently positive sputum cultures for *Candida albicans,* primary treatment of status asthmaticus, systemic fungal infections, untreated localized infection involving nasal mucosa. **Cautions:** Adrenal insufficiency, cirrhosis, glaucoma, hypothyroidism, untreated infection, osteoporosis, tuberculosis.

⌛ LIFESPAN CONSIDERATIONS

Pregnancy/Lactation: Unknown if drug crosses placenta or is distributed in breast milk. **Pregnancy Category B (Inhalation); C (PO). Children:** Prolonged treatment or high dosages may decrease short-term growth rate, cortisol secretion. **Elderly:** No age-related precautions noted.

INTERACTIONS

DRUG: Itraconazole, ketoconazole may increase plasma concentration. **HERBAL:** None significant. **FOOD: Grapefruit, grapefruit juice** may increase systemic exposure of budesonide. **LAB VALUES:** None significant.

AVAILABILITY (Rx)

Oral Inhalation Powder (Pulmicort Flexhaler): 90 mcg per inhalation; 180 mcg per inhalation. **Inhalation Suspension for Nebulization (Pulmicort Respules):** 0.25 mg/2 ml; 0.5 mg/ 2 mg. **Nasal Spray (Rhinocort Aqua):** 32 mcg/spray.

Capsules, Enteric Coated (Entocort EC): 3 mg.

ADMINISTRATION/HANDLING

Inhalation

• Shake container well. Instruct pt to exhale completely, place mouthpiece between lips, inhale, hold breath as long as possible before exhaling. • Allow at least 1 min between inhalations. • Rinsing mouth after each use decreases dry mouth, hoarseness.

Intranasal

• Instruct pt to clear nasal passages before use. • Tilt pt's head slightly forward. • Insert spray tip into nostril, pointing toward nasal passages, away from nasal septum. • Spray into one nostril while pt holds other nostril closed and concurrently inspires through nostril to allow medication as high into nasal passages as possible.

PO

• Swallow whole. Do not crush or chew capsule.

INDICATIONS/ROUTES/DOSAGE

Rhinitis

INTRANASAL: ADULTS, ELDERLY, CHILDREN 6 YRS AND OLDER: 1 spray (32 mcg) in each nostril once a day. **Maximum:** 8 sprays (256 mcg)/day for adults and children 12 yrs and older; 4 sprays (128 mcg)/day for children younger than 12 yrs.

Bronchial Asthma

NEBULIZATION: CHILDREN 12 MOS–8 YRS: ***(Previous therapy with bronchodilators alone):*** 0.5 mg/day as a single dose or 2 divided doses. **Maximum:** 0.5 mg/day. ***(Previous therapy with inhaled corticosteroids):*** 0.5 mg/day as a single dose or 2 divided doses. **Maximum:** 1 mg/day. ***(Previous therapy of oral corticosteroids):*** 1 mg/day as a single dose in 2 divided doses. **Maximum:** 1 mg/day.

ORAL INHALATION: (PULMICORT FLEXHALER): ADULTS, ELDERLY: Initially, 360 mcg 2 times/day. **Maximum:** 720 mcg 2 times/day. **CHILDREN, 6 YRS AND OLDER:** 180 mcg 2 times/day. **Maximum:** 360 mcg 2 times/day.

Crohn's Disease

PO: ADULTS, ELDERLY: 9 mg once a day for up to 8 wks. Recurring episodes may be treated with a repeat 8-wk course of treatment.

SIDE EFFECTS

Frequent (greater than 3%): Nasal: Mild nasopharyngeal irritation, burning, stinging, dryness; headache, cough. **Inhalation:** Flu-like symptoms, headache, pharyngitis. **Occasional (3%–1%): Nasal:** Dry mouth, dyspepsia, rebound congestion, rhinorrhea, loss of taste. **Inhalation:** Back pain, vomiting, altered taste, voice changes, abdominal pain, nausea, dyspepsia.

ADVERSE EFFECTS/ TOXIC REACTIONS

Acute hypersensitivity reaction (urticaria, angioedema, severe bronchospasm) occurs rarely.

NURSING CONSIDERATIONS

BASELINE ASSESSMENT

Question for hypersensitivity to any corticosteroids, components.

INTERVENTION/EVALUATION

Monitor for relief of symptoms.

PATIENT/FAMILY TEACHING

• Improvement noted in 24 hrs, but full effect may take 3–7 days. • Contact physician if no improvement in symptoms, sneezing, nasal irritation occurs.

bumetanide

byoo-**met**-ah-nide
(Bumex, Burinex ✱)

BLACK BOX ALERT Excess dosage can lead to profound diuresis with fluid and electrolyte loss.

Do not confuse bumetanide with Buminate, or Bumex with Buprenex.

◆CLASSIFICATION

PHARMACOTHERAPEUTIC: Loop diuretic. **CLINICAL:** Diuretic (see p. 102C).

ACTION

Enhances excretion of sodium, chloride, and, to lesser degree, potassium, by direct action at ascending limb of loop of Henle and in proximal tubule. **Therapeutic Effect:** Produces diuresis.

PHARMACOKINETICS

Route	Onset	Peak	Duration
PO	30–60 min	60–120 min	4–6 hrs
IV	Rapid	15–30 min	2–3 hrs

Completely absorbed from GI tract (absorption decreased in CHF, nephrotic syndrome). Protein binding: 94%–96%. Partially metabolized in liver. Pri-

B

marily excreted in urine. Not removed by hemodialysis. **Half-life:** 1–1.5 hrs.

USES

Treatment of edema associated with CHF, chronic renal failure (including nephrotic syndrome), hepatic cirrhosis with ascites, acute pulmonary edema. OFF-LABEL: Treatment of hypercalcemia, hypertension.

PRECAUTIONS

Contraindications: Anuria, hepatic coma, severe electrolyte depletion. Cautions: Hypersensitivity to sulfonamides, renal/hepatic impairment, diabetes mellitus, elderly/debilitated pts.

LIFESPAN CONSIDERATIONS

Pregnancy/Lactation: Unknown if drug is distributed in breast milk. **Pregnancy Category C (D if used in pregnancy-induced hypertension). Children:** Safety and efficacy not established. **Elderly:** May be more sensitive to hypotension/electrolyte effects. Increased risk for circulatory collapse or thrombolytic episode. Age-related renal impairment may require reduced or extended dosage interval.

INTERACTIONS

DRUG: **Amphotericin B, nephrotoxic, ototoxic agents** may increase risk of toxicity. May decrease effect of **anticoagulants, heparin. Agents inducing hypokalemia** may have increased hypokalemic effect. May increase risk of **lithium** toxicity. HERBAL: **Ephedra, ginseng, yohimbe** may worsen hypertension. **Garlic** may have increased antihypertensive effect. FOOD: None known. LAB VALUES: May increase serum glucose, BUN, uric acid, urinary phosphate. May decrease serum calcium, chloride, magnesium, potassium, sodium.

AVAILABILITY (Rx)

Injection Solution: 0.25 mg/ml. Tablets: 0.5 mg, 1 mg, 2 mg.

ADMINISTRATION/HANDLING

IV

Rate of administration • May give undiluted but is compatible with D_5W, 0.9% NaCl, or lactated Ringer's solution. • Administer IV push over 1–2 min. • May give through Y tube or 3-way stopcock. • May give as continuous infusion.

Storage • Store at room temperature. • Stable for 24 hrs if diluted.

PO

• Give with food to avoid GI upset, preferably with breakfast (may prevent nocturia).

IV INCOMPATIBILITY

Midazolam (Versed).

IV COMPATIBILITIES

Aztreonam (Azactam), cefepime (Maxipime), diltiazem (Cardizem), dobutamine (Dobutrex), furosemide (Lasix), lipids, lorazepam (Ativan), milrinone (Primacor), morphine, piperacillin and tazobactam (Zosyn), propofol (Diprivan).

INDICATIONS/ROUTES/DOSAGE

Edema

PO: ADULTS: 0.5–2 mg as a single dose in the morning. May repeat q4–5h. **Maximum:** 10 mg/day. **ELDERLY:** 0.5 mg/day, increased as needed.

IV, IM: ADULTS, ELDERLY: 0.5–2 mg/dose; may repeat in 2–3 hrs (maximum 10 mg/day) or 0.5–2 mg/hr by continuous IV infusion.

Hypertension

PO: ADULTS, ELDERLY: Initially, 0.5 mg/day. Range: 1–4 mg/day. **Maximum:** 5 mg/day. Larger doses may be given 2–3 doses/day.

Usual Pediatric Dosage

IV, IM, PO: CHILDREN: 0.015–0.1 mg/kg/dose q6–24h. **Maximum:** 10 mg/day. **NEONATES:** 0.01–0.05 mg/kg/dose q24–48h.

SIDE EFFECTS

Expected: Increased urinary frequency and urine volume. **Frequent:** Orthostatic hypotension, dizziness. **Occasional:** Blurred vision, diarrhea, headache, anorexia, premature ejaculation, impotence, dyspepsia. **Rare:** Rash, urticaria, pruritus, asthenia (loss of strength, energy), muscle cramps, nipple tenderness.

ADVERSE EFFECTS/ TOXIC REACTIONS

Vigorous diuresis may lead to profound water and electrolyte depletion, resulting in hypokalemia, hyponatremia, dehydration, coma, circulatory collapse. Ototoxicity manifested as deafness, vertigo, tinnitus may occur, esp. in pts with severe renal impairment or those taking other ototoxic drugs. Blood dyscrasias, acute hypotensive episodes have been reported.

NURSING CONSIDERATIONS

BASELINE ASSESSMENT

Check vital signs, esp. B/P for hypotension, before administration. Assess baseline electrolytes; particularly check for low serum potassium. Assess for edema. Observe skin turgor, mucous membranes for hydration status. Initiate I&O.

INTERVENTION/EVALUATION

Continue to monitor B/P, vital signs, electrolytes, I&O, weight. Note extent of diuresis. Watch for changes from initial assessment (hypokalemia may result in muscle strength changes, tremor, muscle cramps, altered mental status, cardiac arrhythmias; hyponatremia may result in confusion, thirst, cold/clammy skin).

PATIENT/FAMILY TEACHING

• Expect increased urinary frequency/volume. • Report auditory abnormalities (e.g., sense of fullness in ears, tinnitus) to physician. • Eat foods high in potassium such as whole grains (cereals), legumes, meat, bananas, apricots, orange juice, potatoes (white, sweet), raisins. • Rise slowly from sitting/lying position.

Bumex, *see bumetanide*

Buminate, *see albumin*

buprenorphine

byew-**pren**-or-phen
(Buprenex, Butrans, Suboxone, Subutex)
Do not confuse buprenorphine with bupropion, or Buprenex with Bumex.

FIXED-COMBINATION(S)

Suboxone: buprenorphine/naloxone (narcotic antagonist): 2 mg/0.5 mg, 8 mg/2 mg.

◆CLASSIFICATION

PHARMACOTHERAPEUTIC: Opioid agonist, antagonist injection **(Schedule V)**; tablet **(Schedule III)**. **CLINICAL:** Opioid dependence adjunct, analgesic.

ACTION

Binds to opioid receptors within CNS. **Therapeutic Effect:** Suppresses opioid withdrawal symptoms, cravings. Alters pain perception, emotional response to pain.

PHARMACOKINETICS

Route	Onset	Peak	Duration
Sublingual	15 min	1 hr	6 hrs
IV	Less than 15 min	Less than 1 hr	6 hrs
IM	15 min	1 hr	6 hrs

Excreted primarily in feces with lesser amount eliminated in urine. Protein binding: High. **Half-life: Parenteral:**

B

2–3 hrs; **Sublingual:** 37 hrs (increased in hepatic impairment).

USES

Tablet: Treatment of opioid dependence. **Injection**: Relief of moderate to severe pain. **Transdermal:** Moderate to severe chronic pain requiring continuous around-the-clock opioid analgesic for extended period of time. OFF-LABEL: Heroin/opioid withdrawal.

PRECAUTIONS

Contraindications: Hypersensitivity to naloxone, significant respiratory depression, bronchial asthma, paralytic ileus. Cautions: Hepatic/renal impairment, elderly, debilitated, head injury/increased intracranial pressure, pts at risk for respiratory depression, hypothyroidism, myxedema, adrenal cortical insufficiency (e.g., Addison's disease), urethral stricture, CNS depression, toxic psychosis, prostatic hypertrophy, delirium tremens, kyphoscoliosis, biliary tract dysfunction, acute pancreatitis, acute abdominal conditions, acute alcoholism, pts with long QT syndrome, concurrent use of antiarrhythmics.

LIFESPAN CONSIDERATIONS

Pregnancy/Lactation: Crosses placenta. Distributed in breast milk. Breastfeeding not recommended. Neonatal withdrawal noted in infant if mother was treated with buprenorphine during pregnancy with onset of withdrawal symptoms generally noted on day 1, manifested as hypertonia, tremor, agitation, myoclonus. Apnea, bradycardia, seizures occur rarely. **Pregnancy Category C. Children:** Safety and efficacy of injection form not established in those 2–12 yrs. Safety and efficacy of tablet, fixed-combination form not established in those 16 yrs or younger. **Elderly:** Age-related hepatic impairment may require dosage adjustment.

INTERACTIONS

DRUG: **CNS depressants, MAOIs** may increase CNS or respiratory depression, hypotension. **Azole antifungals, macrolide antibiotics, protease inhibitors** may increase plasma concentration. **Carbamazepine, phenobarbital, phenytoin, rifampin** may cause increased clearance of buprenorphine. May decrease effects of **other opioid analgesics.** HERBAL: None significant. FOOD: None known. LAB VALUES: May increase serum amylase, lipase.

AVAILABILITY (Rx)

Injection Solution (Buprenex): 0.3 mg/1 ml. Tablets, Sublingual (Subutex): 2 mg, 8 mg. Tablets, Sublingual (Fixed-Combination [Suboxone]): 2 mg/0.5 mg, 8 mg/2 mg. Transdermal (Butrans): 5 mcg/hr, 10 mcg/hr, 20 mcg/hr.

ADMINISTRATION/HANDLING

IV

Reconstitution • May be diluted with isotonic saline, lactated Ringer's solution, D_5W, 0.9% NaCl.
Rate of administration • If given as IV push, administer over at least 2 min.

IM

• Give deep IM into large muscle mass.

Sublingual

• Instruct pt to dissolve tablet(s) under tongue; avoid swallowing (reduces drug bioavailability). • For doses greater than 2 tablets, either place all tablets at once or 2 tablets at a time under the tongue.
Storage • Store parenteral form at room temperature. • Protect from prolonged exposure to light. • Store tablets at room temperature.

Transdermal

• Apply to clean, dry, intact skin of upper outer arm, upper chest, upper back, or side of chest. • Wear for 7 days. • Wait minimum of 21 days before reapplying to same site.

IV INCOMPATIBILITIES

Amphotericin B (Abelcet, AmBisome), diazepam (Valium), furosemide (Lasix), lansoprazole (Prevacid), lorazepam (Ativan).

IV COMPATIBILITIES

Allopurinol (Aloprim, Zyloprim), aztreonam (Azactam), cefepime (Maxipime), diphenhydramine (Benadryl), granisetron (Kytril), haloperidol (Haldol), heparin, linezolid (Zyvox), lipids, midazolam (Versed), piperacillin/tazobactam (Zosyn), promethazine (Phenergan), propofol (Diprivan).

INDICATIONS/ROUTES/DOSAGE

Opioid Dependence

SUBLINGUAL: ADULTS, CHILDREN 13 YRS AND OLDER: 12–16 mg/day of Subutex used as induction with switch to Suboxone for maintenance.

Moderate to Severe Pain

IM/IV: ADULTS, CHILDREN 13 YRS AND OLDER: 0.3 mg (1 ml) q6h prn; may repeat 30–60 min after initial dose. May increase to 0.6 mg and/or reduce dosing interval to q4h if necessary. **CHILDREN 2–12 YRS:** 2–6 mcg/kg q4–6h prn.

Usual Elderly Dosage

IM/IV: 0.15 mg q6h prn.

SUBLINGUAL: ADULTS, ELDERLY: INDUCTION: 12–16 mg/day. For pts taking heroin/other short-acting opioids, give at least 4 hrs after pt last used opioids or when early signs of withdrawal appear. Maintenance: 16 mg/day. Range: 4–24 mg/day.

TRANSDERMAL: ADULTS, ELDERLY: (OPIOID NAIVE): Initial dose always 5 mcg/hr. **THOSE ALREADY RECEIVING OPIOIDS:** Refer to conversion chart in package insert. Do not increase dose until pt exposed to previous dose for 72 hrs.

SIDE EFFECTS

Frequent: Sedation (67%), dizziness, nausea (10%). **Butrans (5% or greater):** Nausea, headache, pruritus at application site, dizziness, rash, vomiting, constipation, dry mouth. **Occasional (5%–1%):** Headache, hypotension, vomiting, miosis, diaphoresis. **Rare (Less than 1%):** Dry mouth, pallor, visual abnormalities, injection site reaction.

ADVERSE EFFECTS/ TOXIC REACTIONS

Overdosage results in cold, clammy skin, weakness, confusion, severe respiratory depression, cyanosis, pinpoint pupils, extreme drowsiness progressing to seizures, stupor, coma.

NURSING CONSIDERATIONS

BASELINE ASSESSMENT

Obtain baseline B/P, pulse rate. Assess mental status, alertness. Assess type, location, intensity of pain. Obtain history of pt's last opioid use. Assess for early signs of withdrawal symptoms before initiating therapy.

INTERVENTION/EVALUATION

Monitor for change in respirations, B/P, rate/quality of pulse, mental status. Assess lab results. Initiate deep breathing, coughing exercises, particularly in those with pulmonary impairment. Assess for clinical improvement, record onset of relief of pain.

PATIENT/FAMILY TEACHING

Change positions slowly to avoid dizziness, orthostatic hypotension. Avoid tasks that require alertness, motor skills until response to drug is established. Avoid alcohol, sedatives, antidepressants, tranquilizers.

*buPROPion

byew-**pro**-peon
(Aplenzin, Budeprion SR, Budeprion XL, Buproban, Wellbutrin, Wellbutrin SR, Wellbutrin XL, Zyban)

BLACK BOX ALERT Increased risk of suicidal thinking and behavior in children, adolescents, young adults 18–24 yrs with major depressive disorder, other psychiatric disorders. Agitation, hostility, depressed mood also reported. Use in

B

smoking cessation may cause serious neuropsychiatic events.

Do not confuse Aplenzin with Relenza, bupropion with buspirone, Wellbutrin SR with Wellbutrin XL, or Zyban with Zagam or Diovan.

◆CLASSIFICATION

PHARMACOTHERAPEUTIC: Aminoketone. **CLINICAL:** Antidepressant, smoking cessation aid (see pp. 40C, 152C).

ACTION

Blocks reuptake of neurotransmitters, (serotonin, norepinephrine) at CNS presynaptic membranes, increasing availability at postsynaptic receptor sites. Reduces firing rate of noradrenergic neurons. **Therapeutic Effect:** Relieves depression. Eliminates nicotine withdrawal symptoms.

PHARMACOKINETICS

Rapidly absorbed from GI tract. Protein binding: 84%. Crosses the blood-brain barrier. Undergoes extensive first-pass metabolism in liver to active metabolite. Primarily excreted in urine. **Half-life:** 14 hrs.

USES

Treatment of depression, particularly endogenous depression, exhibited as persistent and prominent dysphoria (occurring nearly every day for at least 2 wks) manifested by 4 of 8 symptoms: appetite change, sleep pattern change, increased fatigue, impaired concentration, feelings of guilt or worthlessness, loss of interest in usual activities, psychomotor agitation or retardation, suicidal tendencies. Assists in smoking cessation. Prevents depression in pts with seasonal affective disorder (SAD). **OFF-LABEL:** Treatment of ADHD in adults, children. Depression associated with bipolar disorder.

PRECAUTIONS

Contraindications: Current or prior diagnosis of anorexia nervosa or bulimia, seizure disorder, use within 14 days of MAOIs, concomitant use of other bupropion products. **Cautions:** History of seizure, cranial trauma; those currently taking antipsychotics, antidepressants; renal/hepatic impairment.

⌛ LIFESPAN CONSIDERATIONS

Pregnancy/Lactation: Unknown if drug crosses placenta or is distributed in breast milk. **Pregnancy Category B. Children:** More sensitive to increased dosage, toxicity, increased risk of suicidal ideation, worsening of depression. Safety and efficacy not established in those younger than 18 yrs. **Elderly:** More sensitive to anticholinergic, sedative, cardiovascular effects. Age-related renal impairment may require dosage adjustment.

INTERACTIONS

DRUG: **Alcohol, lithium, ritonavir, steroids, trazodone, tricyclic antidepressants** may increase risk of seizures. **Fosphenytoin, phenobarbital, phenytoin** may decrease the effectiveness of bupropion. May increase plasma levels of **haloperidol. Levodopa** may increase risk of adverse effects (nausea, vomiting, excitation, restlessness, postural tremor). **MAOIs** may increase risk of neuroleptic malignant syndrome, acute bupropion toxicity. **HERBAL:** **Gotu kola, kava kava, St. John's wort, valerian** may increase CNS depression. **FOOD:** None known. **LAB VALUES:** May decrease WBC.

AVAILABILITY (Rx)

Tablets (Sustained-Release): 100 mg, 150 mg, 200 mg (**Wellbutrin SR**), 150 mg (**Zyban**). **Tablets (Wellbutrin):** 75 mg, 100 mg.

Tablets (Extended-Release): 174 mg, 348 mg, 522 mg (**Aplenzin**), 100 mg, 150 mg (**Budeprion XL**), 150 mg (**Buproban**), 150 mg, 300 mg (**Wellbutrin XL**).

ADMINISTRATION/HANDLING

PO

• Give without regard to food (give with food if GI irritation occurs). • Give at least 4-hr interval for immediate onset and 8-hr interval for sustained-release tablet to avoid seizures. • Give Aplenzin once daily in the morning. • Avoid bedtime dosage (decreases risk of insomnia). • Do not crush, chew, or divide extended-release preparations.

INDICATIONS/ROUTES/DOSAGE

Depression

PO (Immediate-Release): ADULTS: Initially, 100 mg twice a day. May increase to 100 mg 3 times a day no sooner than 3 days after beginning therapy. **Maximum:** 450 mg/day. **ELDERLY:** 37.5 mg twice a day. May increase by 37.5 mg q3–4 days. Maintenance: Lowest effective dosage.

PO (Sustained-Release): ADULTS: Initially, 150 mg/day as a single dose in the morning. May increase to 150 mg twice a day as early as day 4 after beginning therapy. **Maximum:** 400 mg/day in 2 divided doses. **ELDERLY:** Initially, 50–100 mg/day. May increase by 50–100 mg/day q3–4 days. Maintenance: Lowest effective dosage.

PO (Extended-Release): ADULTS: 150 mg once a day. May increase to 300 mg once a day. **Maximum:** 450 mg/day. **(Aplenzin):** Initially, 174 mg once daily in morning; may increase as soon as 4 days to 348 mg/day. **Maximum:** 522 mg/day.

Smoking Cessation

PO: ADULTS: (ZYBAN): Initially, 150 mg a day for 3 days, then 150 mg twice a day for 7–12 wks.

Prevention of Seasonal Affective Disorder

PO: ADULTS, ELDERLY: (Wellbutrin XL): 150 mg/day for 1 wk, then 300 mg/day. Begin in autumn (Sept–Nov). End of treatment begins in spring (Mar–Apr) by decreasing dose to 150 mg/day for 2 wks before discontinuation.

Dosage in Hepatic Impairment

Mild to moderate: Use caution, reduce dosage. **Severe:** Use extreme caution. Maximum dose: Aplenzin: 174 mg every other day. Wellbutrin: 75 mg/day. Wellbutrin SR: 100 mg/day or 150 mg every other day. Wellbutrin XL: 150 mg every other day. Zyban: 150 mg every other day.

SIDE EFFECTS

Frequent (32%–18%): Constipation, weight gain or loss, nausea, vomiting, anorexia, dry mouth, headache, diaphoresis, tremor, sedation, insomnia, dizziness, agitation. **Occasional (10%–5%):** Diarrhea, akinesia, blurred vision, tachycardia, confusion, hostility, fatigue.

ADVERSE EFFECTS/ TOXIC REACTIONS

Risk of seizures increases in pts taking more than 150 mg/dose, history of bulimia, seizure disorders, discontinuing drugs that may lower seizure threshold.

NURSING CONSIDERATIONS

BASELINE ASSESSMENT

Assess psychological status, thought content, suicidal tendencies, appearance. For those on long-term therapy, hepatic/renal function tests should be performed periodically.

INTERVENTION/EVALUATION

Supervise suicidal-risk pt closely during early therapy and dose changes (as depression lessens, energy level improves, increasing suicide potential). Assess appearance, behavior, speech pattern, level of interest, mood changes.

PATIENT/FAMILY TEACHING

• Full therapeutic effect may be noted in 4 wks. • Avoid tasks that require alertness, motor skills until response to drug is established. • Report signs/symptoms of seizure, worsening depression, suicidal ideation, unusual behavioral changes. • Avoid alcohol.

B

*busPIRone

byew-spear-own
(Apo-Buspirone, BuSpar, Buspirex, Bustab, Novo-Buspirone)
Do not confuse buspirone with bupropion.

◆CLASSIFICATION

PHARMACOTHERAPEUTIC: Nonbarbiturate. **CLINICAL:** Antianxiety (see p. 14C).

ACTION

Binds to serotonin, dopamine at presynaptic neurotransmitter receptors in CNS. **Therapeutic Effect:** Produces anxiolytic effect.

PHARMACOKINETICS

Rapidly and completely absorbed from GI tract. Protein binding: 95%. Undergoes extensive first-pass metabolism. Metabolized in liver to active metabolite. Primarily excreted in urine. Not removed by hemodialysis. **Half-life:** 2–3 hrs.

USES

Short-term management (up to 4 wks) of generalized anxiety disorder (GAD). **OFF-LABEL:** Augmenting medication for antidepressants; management of aggression in mental retardation, secondary mental disorders, major depression, panic attack; premenstrual syndrome (aches, pain, fatigue, irritability).

PRECAUTIONS

Contraindications: Concurrent use of MAOIs, severe hepatic/renal impairment. **Cautions:** Renal/hepatic impairment.

LIFESPAN CONSIDERATIONS

Pregnancy/Lactation: Unknown if drug crosses placenta or is distributed in breast milk. **Pregnancy Category B. Children:** Safety and efficacy not established. **Elderly:** No age-related precautions noted.

INTERACTIONS

DRUG: Alcohol, other CNS depressants potentiate effects, may increase sedation. **Erythromycin, itraconazole** may increase concentration, risk of toxicity. **MAOIs** may increase B/P. **HERBAL: Gotu kola, kava kava, St. John's wort, valerian** may increase CNS depression. **FOOD: Grapefruit, grapefruit juice** may increase concentration, risk of toxicity. **LAB VALUES:** None significant.

AVAILABILITY (Rx)

Tablets: 5 mg, 7.5 mg, 10 mg, 15 mg, 30 mg.

ADMINISTRATION/HANDLING

PO

• Give without regard to food. • Tablets may be crushed.

INDICATIONS/ROUTES/DOSAGE

Short-Term Management (up to 4 wks) of Anxiety Disorders

PO: ADULTS: 5 mg 2–3 times a day or 7.5 mg twice a day. May increase by 5 mg/day every 2–4 days. Maintenance: 15–30 mg/day in 2–3 divided doses. **Maximum:** 60 mg/day. **ELDERLY:** Initially, 5 mg twice a day. May increase by 5 mg/day every 2–3 days. **Maximum:** 60 mg/day. **CHILDREN 6 YRS AND OLDER:** Initially, 5 mg/day. May increase by 5 mg/day at weekly intervals. **Maximum:** 60 mg/day in 2–3 divided doses.

SIDE EFFECTS

Frequent (12%–6%): Dizziness, drowsiness, nausea, headache. **Occasional (5%–2%):** Nervousness, fatigue, insomnia, dry mouth, light-headedness, mood swings, blurred vision, poor concentration, diarrhea, paresthesia. **Rare:** Muscle pain/stiffness, nightmares, chest pain, involuntary movements.

ADVERSE EFFECTS/ TOXIC REACTIONS

No evidence of drug tolerance, psychological or physical dependence, withdrawal syndrome. Overdose may produce severe nausea, vomiting, dizziness, drowsiness, abdominal distention, excessive pupil contraction.

NURSING CONSIDERATIONS

BASELINE ASSESSMENT

Assess degree/manifestations of anxiety. Offer emotional support to anxious pt. Assess motor responses (agitation, trembling, tension), autonomic responses (cold, clammy hands; diaphoresis).

INTERVENTION/EVALUATION

For those on long-term therapy, hepatic/renal function tests, blood counts should be performed periodically. Assist with ambulation if drowsiness, light-headedness occur. Evaluate for therapeutic response: calm facial expression, decreased restlessness, insomnia, mental status.

PATIENT/FAMILY TEACHING

• Improvement may be noted in 7–10 days, but optimum therapeutic effect generally takes 3–4 wks. • Drowsiness usually disappears during continued therapy. • If dizziness occurs, change position slowly from recumbent to sitting position before standing. • Avoid tasks that require alertness, motor skills until response to drug is established. • Avoid alcohol, large quantities of grapefruit juice.

busulfan HIGH ALERT

bew-**sull**-fan
(Busulfex, Myleran)

BLACK BOX ALERT Must be administered by certified chemotherapy personnel. Major effect characterized by severe bone marrow suppression.

Do not confuse Myleran with Alkeran, Leukeran, or Mylicon.

CLASSIFICATION

PHARMACOTHERAPEUTIC: Alkylating agent. **CLINICAL:** Antineoplastic (see p. 81C).

ACTION

Interferes with DNA replication, RNA synthesis. Cell cycle-phase nonspecific. **Therapeutic Effect:** Disrupts nucleic acid function. Myelosuppressant.

PHARMACOKINETICS

Completely absorbed from GI tract. Protein binding: 33%. Metabolized in liver. Primarily excreted in urine. Minimally removed by hemodialysis. **Half-life:** 2.5 hrs.

USES

PO: Treatment of chronic myelogenous leukemia (CML), conditioning regimen for bone marrow transplant. **IV:** Conditioning regimen prior to allogeneic hematopoietic progenitor cell transplantation for chronic myelogenous leukemia. **OFF-LABEL:** Treatment of acute myelocytic leukemia. **PO:** Bone marrow disorders (e.g., polycythemia vera).

PRECAUTIONS

Contraindications: Disease resistance to previous therapy with this drug. **Extreme Caution:** Compromised bone marrow reserve. **Cautions:** Chickenpox, herpes zoster, infection, history of gout.

LIFESPAN CONSIDERATIONS

Pregnancy/Lactation: If possible, avoid use during pregnancy, esp. first trimester. May cause fetal harm. Unknown if distributed in breast milk. Breast-feeding not recommended. **Pregnancy Category D. Children/Elderly:** No age-related precautions noted.

INTERACTIONS

DRUG: May decrease effect of **antigout medications. Cytotoxic agents** may increase cytotoxicity. **Bone marrow depressants** may increase risk of myelosuppression. **Live virus vaccines** may potentiate virus replication, increase vaccine side effects, decrease antibody response to vaccine. **HERBAL: St. John's wort** may decrease concentration. **FOOD:** None known. **LAB VALUES:** May decrease serum magnesium, potassium, phos-

B

phate, sodium. May increase serum glucose, calcium, bilirubin, AST, ALT, creatinine, alkaline phosphatase, BUN.

AVAILABILITY (Rx)

Injection Solution (Busulfex): 6 mg/ml. Tablets (Myleran): 2 mg.

ADMINISTRATION/HANDLING

◀ALERT▶ May be carcinogenic, mutagenic, teratogenic. Handle with extreme care during administration. Use of gloves recommended. If contact occurs with skin/mucosa, wash thoroughly with water.

IV

Reconstitution • Dilute with 0.9% NaCl or D_5W only. Diluent quantity must be 10 times the volume of busulfan (e.g., 9.3 ml busulfan must be diluted with 93 ml diluent). • Use filter to withdraw busulfan from ampule. • Add busulfan to calculated diluent. • Use infusion pump to administer busulfan.

Rate of administration • Infuse over 2 hrs. • Before and after infusion, flush catheter line with 5 ml 0.9% NaCl or D_5W.

Storage • Refrigerate ampules. • Following dilution, stable for 8 hrs at room temperature, 12 hrs if refrigerated when diluted with 0.9% NaCl. • Infusion must be completed within 8- or 12-hr time frame.

PO

• May give without regard to meals.

IV INCOMPATIBILITIES

Do not mix busulfan with any other medications.

INDICATIONS/ROUTES/DOSAGE

Remission Induction in CML

PO: ADULTS, ELDERLY: 4–8 mg/day up to 12 mg/day. Maintenance: 1–4 mg/day to 2 mg/wk. Continue until WBC count is 10,000–20,000/mm³, resume when WBC count reaches 50,000/mm³. **CHILDREN:** 0.06–0.12 mg/kg/day. Maintenance: Titrate to maintain leukocyte count above 40,000/mm³, reduce dose by 50% if count is 30,000–40,000/mm³, and discontinue if the count is 20,000/mm³ or less.

Marrow Ablative Conditioning and Bone Marrow Transplantation

IV: ADULTS, ELDERLY, CHILDREN WEIGHING MORE THAN 12 KG: 0.8 mg/kg/dose q6h for total of 16 doses. (Use ideal body weight [IBW] or actual body weight [ABW], whichever is lower.) **CHILDREN WEIGHING 12 KG OR LESS:** 1.1 mg/kg/dose (IBW) q6h for 16 doses.

PO: ADULTS, ELDERLY, CHILDREN: 1 mg/kg/dose (IBW) q6h for 16 doses.

SIDE EFFECTS

Expected (98%–72%): Nausea, stomatitis, vomiting, anorexia, insomnia, diarrhea, fever, abdominal pain, anxiety. Frequent (69%–44%): Headache, rash, asthenia (loss of strength, energy), infection, chills, tachycardia, dyspepsia. Occasional (38%–16%): Constipation, dizziness, edema, pruritus, cough, dry mouth, depression, abdominal enlargement, pharyngitis, hiccups, back pain, alopecia, myalgia. Rare (13%–5%): Injection site pain, arthralgia, confusion, hypotension, lethargy.

ADVERSE EFFECTS/ TOXIC REACTIONS

Major adverse effect is myelosuppression resulting in hematologic toxicity (anemia, severe leukopenia, severe thrombocytopenia). Very high dosages may produce blurred vision, muscle twitching, tonic-clonic seizures. Long-term therapy (more than 4 yrs) may produce pulmonary syndrome ("busulfan lung"), characterized by persistent cough, congestion, adventitious breath sounds (rales, crackles), dyspnea. Hyperuricemia may produce uric acid nephropathy, renal calculi, acute renal failure.

NURSING CONSIDERATIONS

BASELINE ASSESSMENT

CBC with differential, hepatic/renal function studies should be performed weekly (dosage based on hematologic values).

INTERVENTION/EVALUATION

Monitor lab values diligently for evidence of bone marrow depression. Assess mouth for onset of stomatitis (redness/ulceration of oral mucous membranes, gum inflammation, difficulty swallowing). Initiate antiemetics to prevent nausea/vomiting. Monitor daily pattern of bowel activity and stool consistency.

PATIENT/FAMILY TEACHING

Educate pt/family regarding expected effects of therapy. • Maintain adequate daily fluid intake (may protect against renal impairment). • Report consistent cough, congestion, difficulty breathing. • Promptly report fever, sore throat, signs of local infection, unusual bruising/bleeding from any site. • Report signs of abrupt weakness, fatigue, weight loss, nausea, vomiting. • Do not have immunizations without physician's approval (drug lowers body's resistance). • Avoid contact with those who have recently taken live virus vaccine. • Take at same time each day. • Contraception is recommended during therapy.

butorphanol HIGH ALERT

byew-**tore**-phen-awl
(Apo-Butorphanol ✦, Stadol, Stadol NS)
Do not confuse butorphanol with butabarbital, or Stadol with Haldol or sotalol.

◆ CLASSIFICATION

PHARMACOTHERAPEUTIC: Opioid **(Schedule IV). CLINICAL:** Analgesic, anesthesia adjunct (see p. 141C).

ACTION

Binds to opiate receptor sites in CNS. Reduces intensity of pain stimuli incoming from sensory nerve endings. **Therapeutic Effect:** Alters pain perception, emotional response to pain.

PHARMACOKINETICS

Route	Onset	Peak	Duration
IM	15 min	30–60 min	3–4 hrs
IV	Less than 5 min	30–60 min	2–4 hrs
Nasal	15 min	1–2 hrs	4–5 hrs

Rapidly absorbed after IM injection. Protein binding: 80%. Extensively metabolized in liver. Primarily excreted in urine. **Half-life:** 2.5–4 hrs.

USES

Management of pain (including postop pain). **Nasal:** Management of moderate to severe pain, including migraine headache pain. **Parenteral:** Preop, preanesthetic medication, supplement balanced anesthesia, relief of pain during labor.

PRECAUTIONS

Contraindications: CNS disease that affects respirations, hypersensitivity to the preservative benzethonium chloride, physical dependence on other opioid analgesics, preexisting respiratory depression, pulmonary disease. **Cautions:** Hepatic/renal impairment, elderly, debilitated, head injury, hypertension, use before biliary tract surgery (produces spasm of sphincter of Oddi), MI, narcotic dependence.

⌛ LIFESPAN CONSIDERATIONS

Pregnancy/Lactation: Readily crosses placenta. Distributed in breast milk. Breast-feeding not recommended. **Pregnancy Category C (D if used for prolonged time, high dose at term). Children:** Safety and efficacy not known in those younger than 18 yrs. **Elderly:** May be more sensitive to effects; adjust dose and interval.

INTERACTIONS

DRUG: Alcohol, CNS depressants, MAOIs, muscle relaxants may increase CNS or respiratory depression, hypotension. **HERBAL: Gotu kola, kava kava, St. John's wort, valerian** may increase CNS depression. **FOOD:** None known. **LAB VALUES:** None significant.

B

AVAILABILITY (Rx)

Injection Solution (Stadol): 1 mg/ml, 2 mg/ml. **Nasal Spray (Stadol NS):** 10 mg/ml.

ADMINISTRATION/HANDLING

Intranasal

• Instruct pt to blow nose to clear nasal passages as much as possible before use. • Tilt pt's head slightly forward before use. Insert spray tip into nostril, pointing toward nasal passages, away from nasal septum. • Spray into one nostril while pt holds other nostril closed, concurrently inhaling through nose to permit medication as high into nasal passages as possible.

IV INCOMPATIBILITY

Amphotericin B complex (Abelcet, AmBisome, Amphotec).

IV COMPATIBILITIES

Atropine, diphenhydramine (Benadryl), droperidol (Inapsine), hydroxyzine (Vistaril), lipids, morphine, promethazine (Phenergan), propofol (Diprivan).

INDICATIONS/ROUTES/DOSAGE

Analgesia

IV: ADULTS: Initially 1 mg, then 0.5–2 mg q3–4h as needed. **ELDERLY:** 1 mg q4–6h as needed.

IM: ADULTS: Initially 2 mg, then 1–4 mg q3–4h as needed. **ELDERLY:** 1 mg q4–6h as needed.

NASAL: ADULTS: 1 mg or 1 spray in one nostril. May repeat in 60–90 min. May repeat 2-dose sequence q3–4h as needed. Alternatively, 2 mg (1 spray in each nostril if pt remains recumbent.) May repeat in 3–4 hrs.

SIDE EFFECTS

Frequent: Parenteral: Drowsiness (43%), dizziness (19%). **Nasal:** Nasal congestion (13%), insomnia (11%). **Occasional: Parenteral (9%–3%):** Confusion, diaphoresis, clammy skin, lethargy, headache, nausea, vomiting, dry mouth. **Nasal (9%–3%):** Vasodilation, constipation, unpleasant taste, dyspnea, epistaxis, nasal irritation, upper respiratory tract infection, tinnitus. **Rare: Parenteral:** Hypotension, pruritus, blurred vision, sensation of heat, CNS stimulation, insomnia. **Nasal:** Hypertension, tremor, ear pain, paresthesia, depression, sinusitis.

ADVERSE EFFECTS/ TOXIC REACTIONS

Abrupt withdrawal after prolonged use may produce symptoms of narcotic withdrawal (abdominal cramping, rhinorrhea, lacrimation, anxiety, increased temperature, piloerection [goose bumps]). Overdose results in severe respiratory depression, skeletal muscle flaccidity, cyanosis, extreme drowsiness progressing to seizures, stupor, coma. Tolerance to analgesic effect, physical dependence may occur with chronic use.

NURSING CONSIDERATIONS

BASELINE ASSESSMENT

Obtain vital signs before giving medication. If respirations are 12/min or less (20/min or less in children), withhold medication, contact physician. Assess onset, type, location, duration of pain. Effect of medication is reduced if full pain recurs before next dose. Protect from falls. During labor, assess fetal heart tones, uterine contractions.

INTERVENTION/EVALUATION

Monitor for change in respirations, B/P, rate/quality of pulse. Initiate deep breathing, coughing exercises, particularly in those with pulmonary impairment. Change pt's position q2–4h. Assess for clinical improvement, record onset of relief of pain.

PATIENT/FAMILY TEACHING

• Change positions slowly to avoid dizziness. • Avoid tasks that require alertness, motor skills until response to drug is established. • Instruct pt on proper use of nasal spray. • Avoid use of alcohol, CNS depressants.

Byetta, *see exenatide*

C

cabazitaxel

kah-bah-zih-**tax**-all
(Jevtana)

BLACK BOX ALERT All pts should be premedicated with a corticosteroid, an antihistamine, and an H_2 antagonist prior to infusion. Severe hypersensitivity reaction has occurred. Immediately discontinue infusion and give appropriate treatment if hypersensitivity reaction occurs. Neutropenic deaths reported. CBC, particularly ANC, should be obtained prior to and during treatment.

Do not confuse Jevtana with Januvia, Levitra, or Sentra, or cabazitaxel with paclitaxel or Paxil.

◆CLASSIFICATION

PHARMACOTHERAPEUTIC: Microtubule inhibitor. **CLINICAL:** Antineoplastic.

ACTION

Disrupts microtubular cell network, essential for cellular function. Results in inhibition of mitotic and interphase cellular functions. **Therapeutic Effect:** Blocks cells in mitotic phase of cell cycle, leading to cell death.

PHARMACOKINETICS

Demonstrates activity in tumor models insensitive to chemotherapy, including docetaxel. Subcutaneously distributed throughout total body water. Protein binding: 89%–92%. Extensively metabolized in liver. Primarily excreted in feces (76%), with lesser amount eliminated in urine (3.7%). **Half-life:** 95 hrs.

USES

Used in combination with prednisone for treatment of hormone-refractory metastatic prostate cancer previously treated with docetaxel-containing regimen.

PRECAUTIONS

Contraindications: Those with neutrophil count of 1,500/mm^3 or less, severe hepatic impairment (bilirubin equal to or greater than ULN or AST and/or ALT over 1.5 times ULN), history of hypersensitivity to polysorbate 80. Avoid concurrent use of strong CYPA3A inhibitors (atazanavir, clarithromycin, indinavir, itraconazole, ketoconazole, nefazodone, nelfinavir, ritonavir, saquinavir, voriconazole). **Extreme Caution:** Hepatic impairment. **Cautions:** Elderly, pregnancy, renal impairment (creatinine clearance less than 50 ml/min), concurrent use of moderate CYP3A inhibitors (diltiazem, erythromycin, fluconazole, fosamprenavir, verapamil).

⌛ LIFESPAN CONSIDERATIONS

Pregnancy/Lactation: May cause fetal harm. Crosses placental barrier. Do not breast-feed. **Pregnancy Category D. Children:** Safety and effectiveness not established. **Elderly:** Those 65 yrs and older have 5% greater risk of developing neutropenia, fatigue, dizziness, fever, urinary tract infection, dehydration.

INTERACTIONS

DRUG: Concurrent administration of **strong CYP3A inhibitors (atazanavir, clarithromycin, indinavir, itraconazole, ketoconazole, nefazodone, nelfinavir, ritonavir, saquinavir, voriconazole)** may increase concentration of cabazitaxel and is not recommended. **Strong CYP3A inducers (carbamazepine, phenobarbital, phenytoin, rifabutin, rifampin, rifapentine)** are expected to decrease cabazitaxel concentration. **Live virus vaccine** may potentiate virus replication, increase vaccine's side effects, decrease response to vaccine. **HERBAL: St. John's wort, valerian** may increase CNS depression. **FOOD: Grapefruit, grapefruit juice** may decrease concentration/effect. **LAB VALUES:** May increase AST, ALT, bilirubin. May decrease Hgb, Hct, neutrophils, platelets.

AVAILABILITY (Rx)

Injection, Single-Use Vials, 2 Per Kit: 60 mg/1.5 ml polysorbate 80 vial and one vial ethanol in water for injection.

ADMINISTRATION/HANDLING

◀ALERT▶ Wear gloves during preparation, handling. Two-step dilution process must be performed under aseptic conditions to prepare second (final) infusion solution. Medication undergoes two dilutions. After first dilution, administration should be initiated within 30 min.

Reconstitution

Step 1, First Dilution: • Each vial of cabazitaxel contains 60 mg/1.5 ml; must first be mixed with entire contents of supplied diluent. • Once reconstituted, resultant solution contains 10 mg/ml of cabazitaxel. • When transferring diluent, direct needle onto inside vial wall and inject slowly to limit foaming. • Remove syringe and needle, then gently mix initial diluted solution by repeated inversions for at least 45 sec to ensure full mixing of drug and diluent. • Do not shake. • Allow any foam to dissipate.

Step 2, Final Dilution: • Withdrawn recommended dose and further dilute with 250 ml 0.9% NaCl or D_5W. • If dose greater than 65 mg is required, use larger volume of 0.9% NaCl or D_5W so that concentration of 0.26 mg/ml is not exceeded. • Concentration of final infusion should be between 0.10 and 0.26 mg/ml.

Rate of administration • Use in-line 0.22-micron filter during administration. • Infuse over 1 hr.

Storage • Store vials at room temperature. • First dilution solution stable for 30 min. • Final dilution solution stable for 8 hrs at room temperature or 24 hr if refrigerated.

INDICATIONS/ROUTES/DOSAGE

◀ALERT▶ Antihistamine (dexchlorpheniramine 5 mg, diphenhydramine 25 mg, or equivalent antihistamine), corticosteroid (dexamethasone 8 mg or equivalent steroid), and H_2 antagonist (ranitidine 50 mg or equivalent H_2 antagonist) should be given 30 min before initiation of treatment and least 30 min prior to each dose to reduce risk/severity of hypersensitivity.

Hormone-Refractory Metastatic Prostate Cancer

◀ALERT▶ Monitoring of CBC is essential on weekly basis during cycle 1 and before each treatment cycle thereafter so that the dose can be adjusted.

IV INFUSION: ADULTS, ELDERLY: 25 mg/m^2 given as 1-hr infusion every 3 wks in combination with 10 mg prednisone daily throughout treatment. Dose modifications: grade 3 neutropenia, febrile neutropenia, severe or persistent diarrhea. **ADULTS, ELDERLY:** Reduce dosage to 20 mg/m^2.

SIDE EFFECTS

Frequent (47%–16%): Diarrhea, fatigue, nausea, vomiting, constipation, esthesia (decreased sensitivity to touch), abdominal pain, anorexia, back pain. **Occasional (13%–5%):** Peripheral neuropathy, fever, dyspnea, cough, arthralgia, dysgeusia, dyspepsia, alopecia, peripheral edema, weight decrease, urinary tract infection, dizziness, headache, muscle spasm, dysuria, hematuria, mucosal inflammation, dehydration.

ADVERSE EFFECTS/ TOXIC REACTIONS

Hypersensitivity reaction may include generalized rash, erythema, hypotension, bronchospasm. 94% of pts develop grade 1–4 neutropenia and associated complications, including anemia, thrombocytopenia, sepsis. GI abnormalities and its effects, hypertension, arrhythmias, renal failure may occur.

NURSING CONSIDERATIONS

BASELINE ASSESSMENT

Offer emotional support to pt/family. Monitoring of CBC, ANC is essential on weekly basis during cycle 1 and before each treatment cycle thereafter; do not administer if ANC is 1,500 cells/mm^3 or less. Obtain baseline EKG, electrolyte parameters, ALT, AST, bilirubin, alkaline phosphatase, testosterone levels prior to initiation of therapy.

INTERVENTION/EVALUATION

Assess CBC, ANC prior to each infusion; do not administer if ANC less than 1,500 cells/mm^3. Monitor ALT, AST. Monitor for hypersensitivity reaction (rash, erythema, dyspnea). Encourage adequate fluid intake. Monitor daily pattern of bowel activity and stool consistency. Offer antiemetics if nausea, vomiting occur. Maintain due diligence to signs/symptoms of neutropenia.

PATIENT/FAMILY TEACHING

• Report fever, chills, persistent sore throat, unusual bruising/bleeding, pale skin, fatigue. • Avoid tasks that require alertness, motor skills until response to drug is established. • Maintain fastidious oral hygiene. • Do not have immunizations without physician approval (drug lowers body's resistance). • Avoid those who have recently taken live virus vaccine. • Avoid crowds, those with cough, sneezing.

Caduet, *see amlodipine and atorvastatin*

caffeine citrate

(Cafcit)

ACTION

Stimulates medullary respiratory center. Appears to increase sensitivity of respiratory center to stimulatory effects of CO_2. **Therapeutic Effect:** Increases alveolar ventilation, reducing severity, frequency of apneic episodes.

USES

Short-term treatment of apnea in premature infants from 28 wks to younger than 33 wks gestational age.

PRECAUTIONS

Pregnancy Category C.

INTERACTIONS

DRUG: **CNS stimulants** may cause excessive CNS stimulation (e.g., nervousness, insomnia, seizures, arrhythmias). **HERBAL:** None signifcant. **FOOD:** None known. **LAB VALUES:** None significant.

AVAILABILITY (Rx)

Injection Solution: 20 mg/ml. **Oral Solution:** 20 mg/ml.

ADMINISTRATION/HANDLING

PO

• May give without regard to meals. • May administer injectable solution orally.

IV

• Infuse loading dose over at least 30 min; maintenance dose over at least 10 min. • May give without further dilution.

INDICATIONS/ROUTES/DOSAGE

Apnea

PO, IV: Loading dose: 10–20 mg/kg as caffeine citrate (5–10 mg/kg as caffeine base). If theophylline given within previous 72 hrs, a modified dose (50%–75%) may be given. Maintenance: 5 mg/kg/day as caffeine citrate (2.5 mg/kg/day as caffeine base). Dosage adjusted based on pt response.

SIDE EFFECTS

Frequent (10%–5%): Feeding intolerance, rash.

ADVERSE EFFECTS/ TOXIC REACTIONS

Sepsis, necrotizing enterocolitis may occur.

NURSING CONSIDERATIONS

BASELINE ASSESSMENT

Baseline serum caffeine levels should be measured in infants previously treated with theophylline (preterm infants metabolize theophylline to caffeine).

INTERVENTION/EVALUATION

Monitor respirations diligently. Assess skin for rash. Monitor heart rate, number/ severity of apnea spells, serum caffeine levels.

C

calcitonin

kal-sih-**toe**-nin
(Apo-Calcitonin ✦, Calcimar ✦, Caltine ✦, Fortical, Miacalcin, Miacalcin Nasal)

Do not confuse calcitonin with calcitriol, or Miacalcin with Micatin.

◆CLASSIFICATION

PHARMACOTHERAPEUTIC: Synthetic hormone. **CLINICAL:** Calcium regulator, bone resorption inhibitor.

ACTION

Decreases osteoclast activity in bones, decreases tubular reabsorption of sodium and calcium in kidneys, increases absorption of calcium in GI tract. **Therapeutic Effect:** Regulates serum calcium concentrations.

PHARMACOKINETICS

Nasal form rapidly absorbed. Injection form rapidly metabolized primarily in kidneys; primarily excreted in urine. **Half-life: Nasal:** 43 min; **Injection:** 70–90 min.

USES

Parenteral: Treatment of Paget's disease, hypercalcemia, postmenopausal osteoporosis. **Intranasal**: Postmenopausal osteoporosis. **OFF-LABEL:** Treatment of secondary osteoporosis due to drug therapy or hormone disturbance.

PRECAUTIONS

Contraindications: Hypersensitivity to gelatin desserts or salmon protein. **Cautions:** Renal dysfunction.

⌛ LIFESPAN CONSIDERATIONS

Pregnancy/Lactation: Does not cross placenta; unknown if distributed in breast milk. Safe usage during lactation not established (inhibits lactation in animals). **Pregnancy Category C. Children:** Safety and efficacy not established. **Elderly:** No age-related precautions noted.

INTERACTIONS

DRUG: Preparations containing calcium, vitamin D may antagonize effects. **HERBAL:** None significant. **FOOD:** None known. **LAB VALUES:** None significant.

AVAILABILITY (Rx)

Injection Solution (Miacalcin): 200 international units/ml (calcitonin-salmon). **Nasal Spray (Fortical, Miacalcin Nasal):** 200 international units/activation (calcitonin-salmon).

ADMINISTRATION/HANDLING

IM, Subcutaneous

No more than 2-ml dose should be given IM. • Skin test should be performed before therapy in pts suspected of sensitivity to calcitonin. • Bedtime administration may reduce nausea, flushing.

Intranasal

• Refrigerate unopened nasal spray. Store at room temperature after initial use. • Instruct pt to clear nasal passages as much as possible. • Tilt head slightly forward. • Insert spray tip into nostril, pointing toward nasal passages, away from nasal septum. • Spray into one nostril while pt holds other nostril closed and concurrently inspires through nose to permit medication as high into nasal passage as possible.

INDICATIONS/ROUTES/DOSAGE

Skin Testing Before Treatment in Pts with Suspected Sensitivity to Calcitonin-Salmon

INTRACUTANEOUS: ADULTS, ELDERLY: Prepare a 10-international units/ml dilution; withdraw 0.05 ml from a 200-international units/ml vial in a tuberculin syringe; fill up to 1 ml with 0.9% NaCl. Give 0.1 ml intracutaneously on inner aspect of forearm. Observe after 15 min; a positive response is the appearance of more than mild erythema or wheal.

Paget's Disease

IM, SUBCUTANEOUS: ADULTS, ELDERLY: Initially, 100 international units/day. Maintenance: 50 international units/day or 50–100 international units every 1–3 days.

Postmenopausal Osteoporosis

IM, SUBCUTANEOUS: ADULTS, ELDERLY: 100 international units every other day with adequate calcium and vitamin D intake.

INTRANASAL: ADULTS, ELDERLY: 200 international units/day as a single spray, alternating nostrils daily.

Hypercalcemia

IM, SUBCUTANEOUS: ADULTS, ELDERLY: Initially, 4 international units/kg q12h; may increase to 8 international units/kg q12h if no response in 2 days; may further increase to 8 international units/kg q6h if no response in another 2 days.

SIDE EFFECTS

Frequent: **IM, Subcutaneous (10%):** Nausea (may occur soon after injection, usually diminishes with continued therapy), inflammation at injection site. **Nasal (12%–10%):** Rhinitis, nasal irritation, redness, lesions. Occasional: **IM, Subcutaneous (5%–2%):** Flushing of face, hands. **Nasal (5%–3%):** Back pain, arthralgia, epistaxis, headache. Rare: **IM, Subcutaneous:** Epigastric discomfort, dry mouth, diarrhea, flatulence. **Nasal:** Itching of earlobes, pedal edema, rash, diaphoresis.

ADVERSE EFFECTS/ TOXIC REACTIONS

Pts with a protein allergy may develop a hypersensitivity reaction (rash, dyspnea, hypotension, tachycardia).

NURSING CONSIDERATIONS

BASELINE ASSESSMENT

Establish baseline electrolyte levels.

INTERVENTION/EVALUATION

Ensure rotation of injection sites; check for inflammation. Assess vertebral bone mass (document stabilization/improvement). Assess for allergic response: rash, urticaria, swelling, shortness of breath, tachycardia, hypotension. Monitor serum electrolytes, calcium, alkaline phosphatase.

PATIENT/FAMILY TEACHING

• Instruct pt/family on aseptic technique, proper injection of medication, including rotation of sites, proper administration of nasal medication. • Nausea is transient and usually decreases with continued therapy. • Notify physician immediately if rash, itching, shortness of breath, significant nasal irritation occur. • Explain to pt/family that improvement in biochemical abnormalities and bone pain usually occurs in the first few months of treatment. • Explain improvement may take more than a year with neurologic lesions.

calcium acetate

(PhosLo)

calcium carbonate

(Apo-Cal ✤, Caltrate, Caltrate 600 ✤, OsCal ✤, Os-Cal 500, Titralac, Tums)

calcium chloride

calcium citrate

(Cal-Citrate, Citracal, Osteocit ✤)

calcium glubionate

calcium gluconate

kal-see-um

Do not confuse OsCal with Asacol, Citracal with Citrucel, or PhosLo with ProSom.

C

◆CLASSIFICATION

PHARMACOTHERAPEUTIC: Electrolyte replenisher. **CLINICAL:** Antacid, antihypocalcemic, antihyperkalemic, antihypermagnesemic, antihyperphosphatemic (see p. 12C).

ACTION

Essential for function, integrity of nervous, muscular, skeletal systems. Plays an important role in normal cardiac/renal function, respiration, blood coagulation, cell membrane and capillary permeability. Assists in regulating release/storage of neurotransmitters/hormones. Neutralizes/reduces gastric acid (increases pH). **Calcium acetate**: Combines with dietary phosphate, forming insoluble calcium phosphate. **Therapeutic Effect:** Replaces calcium in deficiency states; controls hyperphosphatemia in end-stage renal disease, relieves heartburn, indigestion.

PHARMACOKINETICS

Moderately absorbed from small intestine (absorption depends on presence of vitamin D metabolites, pH). Primarily eliminated in feces.

USES

Parenteral: Acute hypocalcemia (e.g., neonatal hypocalcemic tetany, alkalosis), electrolyte depletion, cardiac arrest (strengthens myocardial contractions), hyperkalemia (reverses cardiac depression), hypermagnesemia (aids in reversing CNS depression). **Calcium carbonate**: Antacid, treatment/prevention of calcium deficiency, hyperphosphatemia. **Calcium citrate**: Antacid, treatment/prevention of calcium deficiency, hyperphosphatemia. **Calcium acetate**: Controls hyperphosphatemia in end-stage renal disease.

PRECAUTIONS

Contraindications: Calcium-based renal calculi, digoxin toxicity, hypercalcemia, hypercalciuria, sarcoidosis, ventricular fibrillation. **Calcium acetate**: Renal impairment, hypoparathyroidism. **Cautions:** Dehydration, history of renal calculi, chronic renal impairment, decreased cardiac function, ventricular fibrillation during cardiac resuscitation.

⌛ LIFESPAN CONSIDERATIONS

Pregnancy/Lactation: Distributed in breast milk. Unknown whether calcium chloride or gluconate is distributed in breast milk. **Pregnancy Category C. Children:** Extreme irritation, possible tissue necrosis or sloughing with IV. Restrict IV use due to small vasculature. **Elderly:** Oral absorption may be decreased.

INTERACTIONS

DRUG: Hypercalcemia may increase **digoxin** toxicity. May decrease absorption of **etidronate, fluoroquinolones, ketoconazole, phenytoin, risedronate, tetracyclines. HERBAL:** None significant. **FOOD:** Food may increase calcium absorption. **LAB VALUES:** May increase serum pH, calcium, gastrin. May decrease serum phosphate, potassium.

AVAILABILITY

CALCIUM ACETATE

Gelcap (PhosLo): 667 mg (equivalent to 169 mg elemental calcium). **Tablets (PhosLo):** 667 mg (equivalent to 169 mg elemental calcium).

CALCIUM CARBONATE

Tablets: 1,250 mg (equivalent to 500 mg elemental calcium) (Os-Cal 500); 1,500 mg (equivalent to 600 mg elemental calcium) (Caltrate 600). **Tablets (Chewable):** 500 mg (equivalent to 200 mg elemental calcium) (Tums); 1,250 mg (equivalent to 500 mg elemental calcium) (Os-Cal 500).

CALCIUM CHLORIDE

Injection Solution: 10% (100 mg/ml) equivalent to 27.2 mg elemental calcium per ml.

CALCIUM CITRATE

Tablets: 125 mg; 250 mg (equivalent to 53 mg elemental calcium) (Cal-Citrate); 950

mg (equivalent to 200 mg elemental calcium) (Citracal).
CALCIUM GLUBIONATE
Syrup: 1.8 g/5 ml (equivalent to 115 mg elemental calcium per 5 ml).
CALCIUM GLUCONATE
Injection Solution: 10% (equivalent to 9 mg elemental calcium per ml).

ADMINISTRATION/HANDLING

IV

Dilution

Calcium chloride • May give undiluted or may dilute with 0.9% NaCl or Sterile Water for Injection.
Calcium gluconate • May give undiluted or may dilute with 100 ml 0.9% NaCl or D_5W.

Rate of administration

Calcium chloride • **Note:** Rapid administration may produce bradycardia, metallic/chalky taste, drop in B/P, sensation of heart, peripheral vasodilation. • **IV push:** Infuse slowly at maximum rate of 50–100 mg/min (in cardiac arrest, may administer over 10–20 sec). • **IV infusion:** Dilute to final concentration of 20 mg/ml and infuse over 1 hr or no faster than 45–90 mg/kg/hr. Give via a central line. Do **NOT** use scalp, small hand or foot veins. Stop infusion if pt complains of pain or discomfort.
Calcium gluconate • **Note:** Rapid administration may produce vasodilation, drop in B/P, arrhythmias, syncope, cardiac arrest. • **IV push:** Infuse slowly over 3–5 min or at maximum rate of 50–100 mg/min (in cardiac arrest, may administer over 10–20 sec). • **IV infusion:** Dilute 1–2 g in 100 ml 0.9% NaCl or D_5W and infuse over 1 hr.

PO

Calcium acetate • Administer with plenty of fluids with meals to optimize effectiveness.
Calcium carbonate • Administer with or immediately following meals with plenty of water (give with meals if used for phosphate binding). Thoroughly chew chewable tablets before swallowing.
Calcium citrate • Give without regard to food (give with food when used to treat hyperphosphatemia).
Calcium glucobionate • Give with or following meals (give on empty stomach before meals when used to treat hyperphosphatemia).
Storage • Store at room temperature. • Once diluted, stable for 24 hrs at room temperature.

IV INCOMPATIBILITIES

Calcium chloride: Amphotericin B complex (Abelcet, AmBisome, Amphotec), phosphate-containing solutions, propofol (Diprivan), sodium bicarbonate. **Calcium gluconate**: Amphotericin B complex (Abelcet, AmBisome, Amphotec), fluconazole (Diflucan).

IV COMPATIBILITIES

Calcium chloride: Amikacin (Amikin), dobutamine (Dobutrex), lidocaine, milrinone (Primacor), morphine, norepinephrine (Levophed). **Calcium gluconate**: Ampicillin, aztreonam (Azactam), cefazolin (Ancef), cefepime (Maxipime), ciprofloxacin (Cipro), dobutamine (Dobutrex), enalapril (Vasotec), famotidine (Pepcid), furosemide (Lasix), heparin, lidocaine, lipids, magnesium sulfate, meropenem (Merrem IV), midazolam (Versed), milrinone (Primacor), norepinephrine (Levophed), piperacillin and tazobactam (Zosyn), potassium chloride, propofol (Diprivan).

INDICATIONS/ROUTES/DOSAGE

Hyperphosphatemia

PO (CALCIUM ACETATE): ADULTS, ELDERLY: 2 tablets 3 times a day with meals. May increase gradually to bring serum phosphate level to less than 6 mg/dl as long as hypercalcemia does not develop.

Hypocalcemia

PO (CALCIUM CARBONATE): ADULTS, ELDERLY: 1–2 g/day in 3–4 divided doses. **CHILDREN:** 45–65 mg/kg/day in 3–4 divided doses.

C

PO (CALCIUM GLUBIONATE): ADULTS, ELDERLY: 6–18 g/day in 4–6 divided doses. **CHILDREN, INFANTS:** 0.6–2 g/kg/day in 4 divided doses. **NEONATES:** 1.2 g/kg/day in 4–6 divided doses.
IV (CALCIUM CHLORIDE): ADULTS, ELDERLY: 0.5–1 g repeated q4–6h as needed. **CHILDREN:** 2.5–5 mg/kg/dose q4–6h.
IV (CALCIUM GLUCONATE): ADULTS, ELDERLY: 2–15 g/24 hr. **CHILDREN:** 200–500 mg/kg/day.

Antacid
PO (CALCIUM CARBONATE): ADULTS, ELDERLY: 1–2 tabs (5–10 ml) q2h as needed.

Osteoporosis
PO (CALCIUM CARBONATE): ADULTS, ELDERLY: 1,200 mg/day.

Cardiac Arrest
IV (CALCIUM CHLORIDE): ADULTS, ELDERLY: 500–1,000 mg. May repeat as necessary. **CHILDREN:** 20 mg/kg. May repeat as necessary.

Hypocalcemia Tetany
IV (CALCIUM CHLORIDE): ADULTS, ELDERLY: 1 g. May repeat in 6 hrs. **CHILDREN:** 10 mg/kg over 5–10 min. May repeat q6–8h.
IV (CALCIUM GLUCONATE): ADULTS, ELDERLY: 1–3 g until therapeutic response achieved. **CHILDREN:** 100–200 mg/kg/dose in 6–8 hrs.

Supplement
PO (CALCIUM CITRATE): ADULTS, ELDERLY: 0.5–2 g 2–4 times a day.

SIDE EFFECTS

Frequent: PO: Chalky taste. **Parenteral:** Pain, rash, redness, burning at injection site, flushing, feeling of warmth, nausea, vomiting, diaphoresis, hypotension. **Occasional: PO:** Mild constipation, fecal impaction, peripheral edema, metabolic alkalosis (muscle pain, restlessness, slow respirations, altered taste). **Calcium carbonate:** Milk-alkali syndrome (headache, decreased appetite, nausea, vomiting, unusual fatigue). **Rare:** Urinary urgency, painful urination.

ADVERSE EFFECTS/ TOXIC REACTIONS

Hypercalcemia: Early signs: Constipation, headache, dry mouth, increased thirst, irritability, decreased appetite, metallic taste, fatigue, weakness, depression. **Later signs:** Confusion, drowsiness, hypertension, photosensitivity, arrhythmias, nausea, vomiting, painful urination.

NURSING CONSIDERATIONS

BASELINE ASSESSMENT

Assess B/P, EKG and cardiac rhythm, renal function, serum magnesium, phosphate, potassium concentrations.

INTERVENTION/EVALUATION

Monitor B/P, EKG, cardiac rhythm, serum magnesium, phosphate, potassium, renal function. Monitor serum, urine calcium concentrations. Monitor for signs of hypercalcemia.

PATIENT/FAMILY TEACHING

- Do not take within 1–2 hrs of other oral medications, fiber-containing foods.
- Avoid excessive alcohol, tobacco, caffeine.

calfactant

cal-**fac**-tant
(Infasurf)

◆CLASSIFICATION

PHARMACOTHERAPEUTIC: Natural lung extract. **CLINICAL:** Pulmonary surfactant.

ACTION

Reduces alveolar surface tension, stabilizing the alveoli. **Therapeutic Effect:** Restores surface activity to infant lungs, improves lung compliance, respiratory gas exchange.

PHARMACOKINETICS

No studies have been performed.

USES

Prevention of respiratory distress syndrome (RDS) in premature infants younger than 29 wks of gestational age; treatment of premature infants younger than 72 hrs of age who develop RDS and require endotracheal intubation.

PRECAUTIONS

Contraindications: None known. **Cautions:** None known.

LIFESPAN CONSIDERATIONS

Pregnancy/Lactation: Not indicated in this pt population. **Pregnancy Category:** Not indicated for use in pregnant women. **Children:** Used only in neonates. No age-related precautions noted. **Elderly:** Not indicated in this pt population.

INTERACTIONS

DRUG: None significant. **HERBAL:** None significant. **FOOD:** None known. **LAB VALUES:** None significant.

AVAILABILITY (Rx)

Intratracheal Suspension: 35-mg/ml vials.

ADMINISTRATION/HANDLING

Intratracheal

• Refrigerate. • Unopened, unused vials may be returned to refrigerator within 24 hrs for future use. Avoid repeated warming to room temperature. • Do not shake. • Enter vial only once, discard unused suspension.

INDICATIONS/ROUTES/DOSAGE

Respiratory Distress Syndrome (RDS)

INTRATRACHEAL: NEONATES: 3 ml/kg of birth weight administered as soon as possible after birth in 2 doses of 1.5 ml/kg. Repeat 3-ml/kg doses, up to a total of 3 doses given 12 hrs apart.

SIDE EFFECTS

Frequent: Cyanosis (65%), airway obstruction (39%), bradycardia (34%), reflux of surfactant into endotracheal tube (21%), need for manual ventilation (16%). **Occasional:** Need for reintubation (3%).

ADVERSE EFFECTS/TOXIC REACTIONS

None known.

NURSING CONSIDERATIONS

BASELINE ASSESSMENT

Drug must be administered in highly supervised setting. Clinicians in charge of care of neonate must be experienced with intubation, ventilator management. Offer emotional support to parents.

INTERVENTION/EVALUATION

Monitor infant with arterial or transcutaneous measurement of systemic O_2, CO_2. Auscultate lungs for adventitious breath sounds (rales, crackles, rhonchi). Frequent ABG sampling necessary to prevent post-dosing hyperoxia and hypocarbia.

Camptosar, *see irinotecan*

canakinumab

can-ah-**kin**-oo-mab
(Ilaris)

◆CLASSIFICATION

PHARMACOTHERAPEUTIC: Monoclonal antibody. **CLINICAL:** Interleukin-1B blocker.

ACTION

Provides potent blockade of interleukin-1 beta (IL-1β); binds specifically to tumor

C

necrosis factor alpha (TNF-α) cell, a protein found in the immune system that causes inflammation. **Therapeutic Effect:** Relieves symptoms of cryopyrin-associated periodic syndrome (CAPS) (e.g., fever, arthralgia, myalgia, fatigue).

PHARMACOKINETICS

Peak serum concentration occurs in 2–7 days. Markers of inflammation (C-reactive protein, serum amyloid A) normalized within 8 days of treatment in majority of pts. **Half-life:** 26 days.

USES

Treatment of CAPS, including familial cold autoinflammatory syndrome and Muckle-Wells syndrome, in adults and children 4 years and older.

PRECAUTIONS

Contraindications: None known. **Cautions:** Pts with active infections, history of recurring infections, or underlying conditions that may predispose to infections. Administration of Ilaris should be discontinued if pt develops serious infection.

⧖ LIFESPAN CONSIDERATIONS

Pregnancy/Lactation: Unknown if distributed in breast milk. **Pregnancy Category C. Children:** Safety and efficacy not established in those younger than 4 yrs. **Elderly:** No age-related precautions noted.

INTERACTIONS

DRUG: **Anakinra, other TNF antagonists (adalimumab, etanercept, infliximab)** may increase risk of infection, neutropenia. May alter effects of **warfarin. Live virus vaccines** may decrease immune response. **HERBAL:** None significant. **FOOD:** None known. **LAB VALUES:** Expected to decrease serum C-reactive protein, serum amyloid A. May decrease WBC count.

AVAILABILITY (Rx)

Injection, Powder for Reconstitution: 180 mg.

ADMINISTRATION/HANDLING

Subcutaneous

Reconstitution • Reconstitute each vial by slowly injecting 1 ml Sterile Water for Injection. • Swirl vial slowly at 45° angle for approximately 1 min and allow to stand for 5 min, then gently turn vial upside down and back again 10 times. Allow to stand for approximately 15 min at room temperature to obtain a clear solution. Slight foaming of product upon reconstitution is not unusual.

Administration • Using a sterile syringe and needle, carefully withdraw required volume depending on dose to be administered (0.2–1 ml) and inject subcutaneously using 27-gauge, 0.5-inch needle. Avoid injection into scar tissue or area where skin is tender, bruised, red, hard.

Storage • Store unopened vial in refrigerator. • Reconstituted solution should be free from particulates and appear clear to opalescent. Solution should be colorless or may have a slight brownish-yellow tint. Discard if solution has a distinctly brown discoloration or contains precipitate. • Reconstituted solution is stable for up to 60 min at room temperature or 4 hrs if refrigerated.

INDICATIONS/ROUTES/DOSAGE

Cryopyrin-Associated Periodic Syndrome

SUBCUTANEOUS: ADULTS, ELDERLY, CHILDREN 4–17 YRS: Weight greater than 40 kg: 150 mg every 8 weeks. Weight 15–40 kg: Recommended dose is 2 mg/kg, given every 8 wks as a single dose. **CHILDREN WEIGHING 15–40 KG:** For pts with inadequate response, dose can be increased to 3 mg/kg, given every 8 wks as a single dose.

SIDE EFFECTS

◀ALERT▶ All effects resolved with continued treatment. **Common (34%–20%):** Nasopharyngitis, diarrhea. **Occasional (17%–9%):** Rhinitis, headache, nausea, increased weight, musculoskeletal pain, injection site reactions. Vertigo (11%) noted exclusively in Muckle-Wells syndrome.

ADVERSE EFFECTS/ TOXIC REACTIONS

Influenza occurs in 17% of pts. Gastroenteritis, bronchitis occur in 11% of pts.

NURSING CONSIDERATIONS

BASELINE ASSESSMENT

Do not initiate treatment in pts with active infections, including chronic or localized infection. Obtain baseline WBC count, C-reactive protein. Assess onset, type, location, duration of pain, inflammation.

INTERVENTION/EVALUATION

Monitor pt for signs/symptoms of infection during and after treatment and discontinue treatment if pt develops an infection. Monitor laboratory results, especially WBC count, C-reactive protein, for evidence of infection. Monitor temperature. Assess daily pattern of bowel activity and stool consistency.

PATIENT/FAMILY TEACHING

- Consult physician if cough, fever, flulike symptoms occur. Do not receive live virus vaccine during treatment. Inform physician if persistent fever, vomiting occur or diarrhea persists.

Cancidas, *see caspofungin*

candesartan

kan-de-**sar**-tan
(Atacand)

BLACK BOX ALERT May cause fetal injury, mortality if used during second or third trimester of pregnancy.

FIXED-COMBINATION(S)

Atacand HCT: candesartan/hydrochlorothiazide (a diuretic): 16 mg/12.5 mg, 32 mg/12.5 mg.

◆CLASSIFICATION

PHARMACOTHERAPEUTIC: Angiotensin II receptor antagonist. **CLINICAL:** Antihypertensive (see p. 10C).

ACTION

Blocks vasoconstrictor, aldosterone-secreting effects of angiotensin II, inhibiting binding of angiotensin II to AT_1 receptors. **Therapeutic Effect:** Produces vasodilation, decreases peripheral resistance, B/P.

PHARMACOKINETICS

Route	Onset	Peak	Duration
PO	2–3 hrs	6–8 hrs	Greater than 24 hrs

Rapidly, completely absorbed. During absorption, undergoes rapid/complete hydrolysis to form active drug. Protein binding: greater than 99%. Undergoes minor hepatic metabolism to inactive metabolite. Excreted unchanged in urine and in feces through biliary system. Not removed by hemodialysis. **Half-life:** 9 hrs.

USES

Treatment of hypertension alone or in combination with other antihypertensives, heart failure (reduces risk of death from cardiovascular causes, reduces hospitalization for heart failure).

PRECAUTIONS

Contraindications: None known. **Cautions:** Severe CHF, dehydration (increased risk for hypotension), renal/hepatic impairment, renal artery stenosis.

LIFESPAN CONSIDERATIONS

Pregnancy/Lactation: Unknown if distributed in breast milk. May cause fetal/neonatal morbidity/mortality. **Pregnancy Category C (D if used in second or third trimester). Children:** Safety and efficacy not established. **Elderly:** No age-related precautions noted.

INTERACTIONS

DRUG: May increase risk of **lithium** toxicity. **HERBAL:** **Ephedra, ginseng, yohimbe** may worsen hypertension. **Garlic** may increase antihypertensive effect. **FOOD:** None known. **LAB VALUES:** May increase BUN, serum alkaline phosphatase, bilirubin, creatinine, AST, ALT. May decrease Hgb, Hct.

AVAILABILITY (Rx)

Tablets: 4 mg, 8 mg, 16 mg, 32 mg.

ADMINISTRATION/HANDLING

PO

- Give without regard to food.

INDICATIONS/ROUTES/DOSAGE

Hypertension

PO: ADULTS, ELDERLY, PTS WITH MILD HEPATIC OR RENAL IMPAIRMENT: Initially, 16 mg once a day in those who are not volume depleted. Can be given once or twice a day with total daily doses of 8–32 mg. Give lower dosage in those treated with diuretics or with severe renal impairment.

Heart Failure

PO: ADULTS, ELDERLY: Initially, 4 mg once daily. May double dose at approximately 2-wk intervals up to a target dose of 32 mg/day.

SIDE EFFECTS

Occasional (6%–3%): Upper respiratory tract infection, dizziness, back/leg pain. **Rare (2%–1%):** Pharyngitis, rhinitis, headache, fatigue, diarrhea, nausea, dry cough, peripheral edema.

ADVERSE EFFECTS/ TOXIC REACTIONS

Overdosage may manifest as hypotension, tachycardia. Bradycardia occurs less often. Institute supportive measures.

NURSING CONSIDERATIONS

BASELINE ASSESSMENT

Obtain B/P, apical pulse immediately before each dose, in addition to regular monitoring (be alert to fluctuations). Question for possibility of pregnancy (see Black Box Alert). Assess medication history (esp. diuretic). Question for history of hepatic/renal impairment, renal artery stenosis. Obtain BUN, serum creatinine, AST, ALT, alkaline phosphatase, bilirubin, Hgb, Hct.

INTERVENTION/EVALUATION

Maintain hydration (offer fluids frequently). Assess for evidence of upper respiratory infection. Assist with ambulation if dizziness occurs. Monitor electrolytes, serum creatinine, BUN, urinalysis, (CHF): serum potassium. Assess B/P for hypertension/hypotension. If excessive reduction in B/P occurs, place pt in supine position, feet slightly elevated.

PATIENT/FAMILY TEACHING

• Inform female pt regarding potential for fetal injury, mortality with second- and third-trimester exposure to candesartan. • Report pregnancy to physician as soon as possible. • Avoid tasks that require alertness, motor skills until response to drug is established. • Report any sign of infection (sore throat, fever). • Do not stop taking medication. • Explain need for lifelong control. • Caution against exercising during hot weather (risk of dehydration, hypotension).

capecitabine

HIGH ALERT

cap-eh-**sit**-ah-bean
(<u>Xeloda</u>)

BLACK BOX ALERT May increase anticoagulant effect of warfarin.

Do not confuse Xeloda with Xenical.

◆CLASSIFICATION

PHARMACOTHERAPEUTIC: Antimetabolite. **CLINICAL:** Antineoplastic (see p. 81C).

ACTION

Enzymatically converted to 5-fluorouracil (5-FU). Inhibits enzymes necessary for synthesis of essential cellular components. **Therapeutic Effect:** Interferes with DNA synthesis, RNA processing, protein synthesis.

PHARMACOKINETICS

Readily absorbed from GI tract. Protein binding: less than 60%. Metabolized in liver. Primarily excreted in urine. **Half-life:** 45 min.

USES

Treatment of metastatic breast cancer resistant to other therapy, colorectal cancer. Adjuvant (postsurgical) treatment of Dukes C colon cancer. **OFF-LABEL:** Gastric cancer, pancreatic cancer, esophageal cancer, ovarian cancer, metastatic renal cell cancer, metastatic CNS lesions.

PRECAUTIONS

Contraindications: Severe renal impairment, dihydropyrimidine dehydrogenase (DPD) deficiency, hypersensitivity to 5-fluorouracil (5-FU). **Cautions:** Existing bone marrow depression, chickenpox, herpes zoster, hepatic impairment, moderate renal impairment, previous cytotoxic therapy/radiation therapy.

LIFESPAN CONSIDERATIONS

Pregnancy/Lactation: May be harmful to fetus. Unknown if distributed in breast milk. **Pregnancy Category D. Children:** Safety and efficacy not established in those younger than 18 yrs. **Elderly:** May be more sensitive to GI side effects.

INTERACTIONS

DRUG: **Warfarin** may increase risk of bleeding. Myelosuppression may be enhanced when given concurrently with **bone marrow depressants. Live virus vaccines** may potentiate virus replication, increase vaccine side effects, decrease pt's antibody response to vaccine. **HERBAL:** **Echinacea** may decrease levels/effect. **FOOD:** None known. **LAB VALUES:** May increase serum alkaline phosphatase, bilirubin, AST, ALT. May decrease Hgb, Hct, WBC count. May increase PT, INR.

AVAILABILITY (Rx)

Tablets: 150 mg, 500 mg.

ADMINISTRATION/HANDLING

- Give within 30 min after meals with water.

INDICATIONS/ROUTES/DOSAGE

Metastatic Breast Cancer, Colorectal Cancer, Adjuvant (Postsurgery) Treatment of Dukes C Colon Cancer

PO: ADULTS, ELDERLY: Initially, 2,500 mg/m^2/day in 2 equally divided doses approximately q12h for 2 wks. Follow with a 1-wk rest period; given in 3-wk cycles.

Dosage in Renal Impairment

Creatinine clearance 50–80 ml/min: No adjustment. **Creatinine clearance 30–49 ml/min:** 75% of normal dose. **Creatinine clearance less than 30 ml/min:** Not recommended.

SIDE EFFECTS

Frequent (greater than 5%): Diarrhea (sometimes severe), nausea, vomiting, stomatitis, hand-and-foot syndrome (painful palmar-plantar swelling with paresthesia, erythema, blistering), fatigue, anorexia, dermatitis. **Occasional (less than 5%):** Constipation, dyspepsia, nail disorder, headache, dizziness, insomnia, edema, myalgia.

ADVERSE EFFECTS/ TOXIC REACTIONS

Serious reactions include myelosuppression (neutropenia, thrombocytopenia, anemia), cardiovascular toxicity (angina, cardiomyopathy, deep vein thrombosis), respiratory toxicity (dyspnea, epistaxis, pneumonia), lymphedema.

NURSING CONSIDERATIONS

BASELINE ASSESSMENT

Assess sensitivity to capecitabine or 5-fluorouracil. Obtain baseline Hgb, Hct, serum chemistries, renal function.

INTERVENTION/EVALUATION

Monitor for severe diarrhea; if dehydration occurs, fluid and electrolyte replacement therapy should be initiated. Assess hands/feet for erythema (chemotherapy induced). Monitor CBC for evidence of bone marrow depression. Monitor renal/hepatic function. Monitor for blood dyscrasias (fever, sore throat, signs of local infection, unusual bruising/bleeding from any site), symptoms of anemia (excessive fatigue, weakness).

PATIENT/FAMILY TEACHING

• Notify physician if nausea, vomiting, diarrhea, hand-and-foot syndrome, stomatitis occur. • Do not have immunizations without physician's approval (drug lowers body's resistance). • Avoid contact with those who have recently received live virus vaccine. • Promptly report fever higher than 100.5°F, sore throat, signs of local infection, unusual bruising/bleeding from any site.

Capoten, *see captopril*

captopril

cap-toe-pril
(Apo-Capto 🍁, Capoten,
Novo-Captoril 🍁)

BLACK BOX ALERT May cause fetal injury, mortality if used during second or third trimester of pregnancy.

Do not confuse captopril with calcitriol, Capitrol, or carvedilol.

FIXED-COMBINATION(S)

Capozide: captopril/hydrochlorothiazide (a diuretic): 25 mg/15 mg, 25 mg/25 mg, 50 mg/15 mg, 50 mg/25 mg.

◆CLASSIFICATION

PHARMACOTHERAPEUTIC: Angiotensin-converting enzyme (ACE) inhibitor. **CLINICAL:** Antihypertensive, vasodilator (see p. 9C).

ACTION

Suppresses renin-angiotensin-aldosterone system (prevents conversion of angiotensin I to angiotensin II, a potent vasoconstrictor; may inhibit angiotensin II at local vascular and renal sites). Decreases plasma angiotensin II, increases plasma renin activity, decreases aldosterone secretion. **Therapeutic Effect:** Reduces peripheral arterial resistance, pulmonary capillary wedge pressure; improves cardiac output, exercise tolerance.

PHARMACOKINETICS

Route	Onset	Peak	Duration
PO	0.25 hr	0.5–1.5 hrs	Dose-related

Rapidly, well absorbed from GI tract (absorption decreased in presence of food). Protein binding: 25%–30%. Metabolized in liver. Primarily excreted in urine. Removed by hemodialysis. **Half-life:** less than 3 hrs (increased in renal impairment).

USES

Treatment of hypertension, CHF, diabetic nephropathy, post-MI for prevention of ventricular failure. **OFF-LABEL:** Treatment of hypertensive crisis, rheumatoid arthritis, diagnosis of renal artery stenosis, hypertension secondary to sclerodema renal crisis, diagnosis of aldosteronism, idiopathic edema, Bartter's syndrome to increase circulation in Raynaud's syndrome.

PRECAUTIONS

Contraindications: History of angioedema from previous treatment with ACE inhibitors. **Cautions:** Renal impairment, those with sodium depletion or on diuretic therapy, dialysis, hypovolemia, coronary/cerebrovascular insufficiency.

C

LIFESPAN CONSIDERATIONS

Pregnancy/Lactation: Crosses placenta; distributed in breast milk. May cause fetal/neonatal mortality/morbidity. **Pregnancy Category C (D if used in second or third trimester). Children:** Safety and efficacy not established. **Elderly:** May be more sensitive to hypotensive effects; caution recommended.

INTERACTIONS

DRUG: **Alcohol, antihypertensives, diuretics** may increase effects. May increase **lithium** concentration, toxicity. **NSAIDs** may decrease effect. **Potassium-sparing diuretics, potassium supplements** may cause hyperkalemia. HERBAL: **Ephedra, ginseng, yohimbe** may worsen hypertension. **Garlic** may increase antihypertensive effect. FOOD: **All foods** significantly reduce absorption. LAB VALUES: May increase BUN, serum alkaline phosphatase, bilirubin, creatinine, potassium, AST, ALT. May decrease serum sodium. May cause positive ANA titer.

AVAILABILITY (Rx)

Tablets: 12.5 mg, 25 mg, 50 mg, 100 mg.

ADMINISTRATION/HANDLING

PO

- Best taken 1 hr before or 2 hrs after meals for maximum absorption (food significantly decreases drug absorption).
- Tablets may be crushed.

INDICATIONS/ROUTES/DOSAGE

Hypertension

PO: ADULTS, ELDERLY: Initially, 12.5–25 mg 2–3 times a day. After 1–2 wks, may increase to 50 mg 2–3 times a day. Diuretic may be added if no response in additional 1–2 wks. If taken in combination with diuretic, may increase to 100–150 mg 2–3 times a day after 1–2 wks. Maintenance: 25–150 mg 2–3 times a day. **Maximum:** 450 mg/day. **CHILDREN:** 0.05–0.5 mg 3 times a day. **Maximum:** 2 mg/kg/dose 2–3 times a day. **INFANTS:** 0.15–0.3 mg/kg q12h. **Maximum:** 2 mg/kg/dose 2–3 times a day.

CHF

PO: ADULTS, ELDERLY: Initially, 6.25–25 mg 3 times a day. Increase to 50 mg 3 times a day. After at least 2 wks, may increase to 50–100 mg 3 times a day. **Maximum:** 450 mg/day.

Post-MI

PO: ADULTS, ELDERLY: Initially, 6.25 mg, then 12.5 mg 3 times a day. Increase to 25 mg 3 times a day over several days, up to 50 mg 3 times a day over several wks.

Diabetic Nephropathy, Prevention of Renal Failure

PO: ADULTS, ELDERLY: 25 mg 3 times a day.

Dosage in Renal Impairment

Creatinine clearance 10–50 ml/min: 75% of normal dosage. **Creatinine clearance less than 10 ml/min:** 50% of normal dosage.

SIDE EFFECTS

Frequent (7%–4%): Rash. Occasional (4%–2%): Pruritus, dysgeusia (altered taste). Rare (less than 2%–0.5%): Headache, cough, insomnia, dizziness, fatigue, paresthesia, malaise, nausea, diarrhea or constipation, dry mouth, tachycardia.

ADVERSE EFFECTS/ TOXIC REACTIONS

Excessive hypotension ("first-dose syncope") may occur in pts with CHF and in those who are severely sodium/volume depleted. Angioedema (swelling of face/tongue/lips), hyperkalemia occur rarely. Agranulocytosis, neutropenia may be noted in those with collagen vascular disease (scleroderma, systemic lupus erythematosus), renal impairment. Nephrotic syndrome may be noted in those with history of renal disease.

NURSING CONSIDERATIONS

BASELINE ASSESSMENT

Obtain B/P immediately before each dose, in addition to regular monitoring (be alert to fluctuations). If excessive reduction in B/P occurs, place pt in supine position with legs elevated. In pts with prior renal disease or receiving dosages greater than 150 mg/day, urine test for protein by dipstick method should be made with first urine of day before therapy begins and periodically thereafter. In pts with renal impairment, autoimmune disease, or taking drugs that affect leukocytes or immune response, CBC should be performed before beginning therapy, q2wk for 3 mos, then periodically thereafter.

INTERVENTION/EVALUATION

Assess skin for rash, pruritus. Assist with ambulation if dizziness occurs. Monitor urinalysis for proteinuria. Assess for anorexia secondary to altered taste perception. Monitor serum potassium levels in those on concurrent diuretic therapy. Monitor B/P, BUN, serum creatinine, CBC. Discontinue medication, contact physician if angioedema occurs.

PATIENT/FAMILY TEACHING

• Full therapeutic effect of B/P reduction may take several wks. • Skipping doses or voluntarily discontinuing drug may produce severe rebound hypertension. • Limit alcohol. • Notify physician if swelling of face, lips, or tongue, difficulty breathing, vomiting, diarrhea, excessive perspiration, dehydration, persistent cough, sore throat, fever occur. • Inform physician if pregnant or planning to become pregnant. • Rise slowly from sitting/lying position.

carbamazepine

car-bah-**maz**-zeh-peen
(Apo-Carbamazepine 🍁, Carbatrol, Epitol, Equetro, Novo-Carbamaz 🍁, Tegretol, Tegretol XR)

BLACK BOX ALERT Potentially fatal aplastic anemia, agranulocytosis reported. Potentially fatal, severe dermatologic reactions (e.g., Stevens-Johnson syndrome, toxic epidermal necrolysis) may occur.

Do not confuse carbamazepine with oxcarbazepine, or Tegretol with Mebaral, Toprol XL, Toradol, or Trental.

◆ CLASSIFICATION

PHARMACOTHERAPEUTIC: Iminostilbene derivative. **CLINICAL:** Anticonvulsant, antineuralgic, antimanic, antipsychotic (see p. 34C).

ACTION

Decreases sodium, calcium ion influx into neuronal membranes, reducing post-tetanic potentiation at synapses. **Therapeutic Effect:** Produces anticonvulsant effect; decreases pain response.

PHARMACOKINETICS

Slowly, completely absorbed from GI tract. Protein binding: 75%–90%. Metabolized in liver to active metabolite. Primarily excreted in urine. Not removed by hemodialysis. **Half-life:** 25–65 hrs (decreased with chronic use).

USES

Carbatrol, Epitol, Tegretol, Tegretol XR: Treatment of partial seizures with complex symptomatology, generalized tonic-clonic seizures, mixed seizure patterns, pain relief of trigeminal neuralgia, diabetic neuropathy. **Equetro:** Acute manic and mixed episodes associated with bipolar disorder. **OFF-LABEL:** Treatment of alcohol withdrawal, diabetes insipidus, neurogenic pain, psychotic disorders, post-traumatic stress disorder, resistant schizophrenia, restless legs syndrome.

PRECAUTIONS

Contraindications: Concomitant use of MAOIs, history of myelosuppression, hypersensitivity to tricyclic antidepressants.

Cautions: Mental illness, increased IOP, history of atypical absence seizures, cardiac, hepatic, renal impairment.

LIFESPAN CONSIDERATIONS

Pregnancy/Lactation: Crosses placenta; distributed in breast milk. Accumulates in fetal tissue. **Pregnancy Category D. Children:** Behavioral changes more likely to occur. **Elderly:** More susceptible to confusion, agitation, AV block, bradycardia, syndrome of inappropriate antidiuretic hormone (SIADH).

INTERACTIONS

DRUG: May decrease effects of **anticoagulants, clarithromycin, diltiazem, erythromycin, estrogens, propoxyphene, quinidine, steroids.** May increase CNS depressant effects of **antipsychotic medications, haloperidol, tricyclic antidepressants.** May increase metabolism of **other anticonvulsant medications, barbiturates, benzodiazepines, valproic acid. Cimetidine, isoniazid, itraconazole, ketoconazole** may increase concentration, toxicity. May increase metabolism of **isoniazid. MAOIs** may cause seizures, hypertensive crisis. **HERBAL: Evening primrose** may decrease seizure threshold. **Gotu kola, kava kava, St. John's wort, valerian** may increase CNS depression. **FOOD: Grapefruit, grapefruit juice** may increase absorption, concentration. **LAB VALUES:** May increase BUN, serum glucose, alkaline phosphatase, bilirubin, AST, ALT, protein, cholesterol, HDL, triglycerides. May decrease serum calcium, thyroid hormone (T_3, T_4 index) levels. **Therapeutic serum level:** 4–12 mcg/ml; **toxic serum level:** greater than 12 mcg/ml.

AVAILABILITY (Rx)

Suspension (Tegretol): 100 mg/5 ml. **Tablets (Epitol, Tegretol):** 200 mg. **Tablets (Chewable [Tegretol]):** 100 mg.

Capsules (Extended-Release [Carbatrol, Equetro]): 100 mg, 200 mg, 300 mg. **Tablets (Extended-Release [Tegretol XR]):** 100 mg, 200 mg, 400 mg.

ADMINISTRATION/HANDLING

PO

• Store oral suspension, tablets at room temperature. • Give with meals to reduce risk of GI distress. • Shake oral suspension well. Do not administer simultaneously with other liquid medicine. • Do not crush or chew extended-release capsules or tablets. • Extended-release capsules may be opened and sprinkled over food (e.g., applesauce).

INDICATIONS/ROUTES/DOSAGE

ALERT Suspension must be given on a 3–4 times/day schedule; tablets on a 2–4 times/day schedule; extended-release capsules 2 times/day.

Seizure Control

PO: ADULTS, CHILDREN OLDER THAN 12 YRS: Initially, 200 mg twice a day. May increase dosage by 200 mg/day at weekly intervals. Range: 400–1,200 mg/day in 2–4 divided doses. **Maximum: ADULTS:** 1.6–2.4 g/day; **CHILDREN OLDER THAN 15 YRS:** 1,200 mg/day; **CHILDREN 13–15 YRS:** 1,000 mg/day. **CHILDREN 6–12 YRS:** Initially, 100 mg twice a day. May increase by 100 mg/day at weekly intervals. Range: 400–800 mg/day. **Maximum:** 1,000 mg/day. **CHILDREN YOUNGER THAN 6 YRS:** Initially 10–20 mg/kg/day in 2–3 divided doses. May increase at weekly intervals until optimal response and therapeutic levels are achieved. **Maximum:** 35 mg/kg/day. **ELDERLY:** Initially 100 mg 1–2 times a day. May increase by 100 mg/day at weekly intervals. Usual dose 400–1,000 mg/day.

Trigeminal Neuralgia, Diabetic Neuropathy

PO: ADULTS: Initially, 100 mg twice a day. May increase by 100 mg twice a day up to 400–800 mg/day. **Maximum:** 1,200 mg/day. **ELDERLY:** Initially 100 mg 1–2 times a day. May increase by 100 mg/day at weekly intervals. Usual dose 400–1,000 mg/day.

C

Bipolar Disorder

PO: ADULTS, ELDERLY (Equetro): Initially, 400 mg/day in 2 divided doses. May adjust dose in 200 mg increments. **Maximum:** 1,600 mg/day in divided doses.

SIDE EFFECTS

Frequent: Drowsiness, dizziness, nausea, vomiting. Occasional: Visual abnormalities (spots before eyes, difficulty focusing, blurred vision), dry mouth/pharynx, tongue irritation, headache, fluid retention, diaphoresis, constipation, diarrhea, behavioral changes in children.

ADVERSE EFFECTS/ TOXIC REACTIONS

Toxic reactions appear as blood dyscrasias (aplastic anemia, agranulocytosis, thrombocytopenia, leukopenia, leukocytosis, eosinophilia), cardiovascular disturbances (CHF, hypotension/hypertension, thrombophlebitis, arrhythmias), dermatologic effects (rash, urticaria, pruritus, photosensitivity). Abrupt withdrawal may precipitate status epilepticus.

NURSING CONSIDERATIONS

BASELINE ASSESSMENT

Seizures: Review history of seizure disorder (intensity, frequency, duration, level of consciousness [LOC]). Provide safety precautions, quiet/dark environment. **Neuralgia:** Assess facial pain, stimuli that may cause facial pain. **Bipolar:** Assess mental status, cognitive abilities. CBC, serum iron determination, urinalysis, BUN should be performed before therapy begins and periodically during therapy.

INTERVENTION/EVALUATION

Seizures: Observe frequently for recurrence of seizure activity. Monitor for therapeutic serum levels. Assess for clinical improvement (decrease in intensity, frequency of seizures). Assess for clinical evidence of early toxic signs (fever, sore throat, mouth ulcerations, unusual bruising/bleeding, joint pain). **Neuralgia:** Avoid triggering tic douloureux (draft, talking, washing face, jarring bed, hot/warm/cold food or liquids). **Bipolar:** Monitor for suicidal ideation, behavioral changes. Observe for excessive sedation. **Therapeutic serum level:** 4–12 mcg/ml; **toxic serum level:** greater than 12 mcg/ml.

PATIENT/FAMILY TEACHING

• Do not abruptly discontinue medication after long-term use (may precipitate seizures). • Strict maintenance of drug therapy is essential for seizure control. • Avoid tasks that require alertness, motor skills until response to drug is established. • Report visual disturbances. • Blood tests should be repeated frequently during first 3 mos of therapy and at monthly intervals thereafter for 2–3 yrs. • Do not take oral suspension simultaneously with other liquid medicine. • Do not take with grapefruit juice. • Report serious skin reactions.

carbidopa/levodopa

car-bih-dope-ah/**lev**-oh-dope-ah (Apo-Levocarb 🍁, Novo-Levocarbidopa 🍁, Parcopa, Sinemet, Sinemet CR)

FIXED-COMBINATION(S)

Stalevo: carbidopa/levodopa/entacapone (antiparkinson agent): 12.5 mg/50 mg/200 mg, 18.75 mg/75 mg/200 mg, 25 mg/100 mg/200 mg, 31.25 mg/125 mg/200 mg, 37.5 mg/150 mg/200 mg, 50 mg/200 mg/200 mg.

◆CLASSIFICATION

PHARMACOTHERAPEUTIC: Dopamine precursor. **CLINICAL:** Antiparkinson agent.

ACTION

Converted to dopamine in basal ganglia, increasing dopamine concentration in brain, inhibiting hyperactive cholinergic activity. Carbidopa prevents peripheral breakdown of levodopa, making more levodopa available for transport into brain. Therapeutic Effect: Reduces tremor.

PHARMACOKINETICS

Carbidopa is rapidly and completely absorbed from GI tract. Widely distributed. Excreted primarily in urine. Levodopa is converted to dopamine. Excreted primarily in urine. Half-life: 1–2 hrs (carbidopa); 1–3 hrs (levodopa).

USES

Treatment of idiopathic Parkinson's disease (paralysis agitans), postencephalitic parkinsonism, symptomatic parkinsonism following CNS injury by CO_2 poisoning, manganese intoxication. OFF-LABEL: Restless legs syndrome.

PRECAUTIONS

Contraindications: Angle-closure glaucoma, use within 14 days of MAOIs, skin lesions (Sinemet CR), history of melanoma (Sinemet CR). Cautions: History of MI, bronchial asthma (tartrazine sensitivity), emphysema; severe cardiac, pulmonary, renal, hepatic, endocrine disease; active peptic ulcer; treated open-angle glaucoma.

LIFESPAN CONSIDERATIONS

Pregnancy/Lactation: Unknown if drug crosses placenta or is distributed in breast milk. May inhibit lactation. Breast-feeding not recommended. **Pregnancy Category C.** **Children:** Safety and efficacy not established in those younger than 18 yrs. **Elderly:** More sensitive to effects of levodopa. Anxiety, confusion, nervousness more common when receiving anticholinergics.

INTERACTIONS

DRUG: **Anticonvulsants, benzodiazepines, haloperidol, phenothiazines** may decrease effects of carbidopa and levodopa. **MAOIs** may increase risk of hypertensive crisis. **Selegiline** may increase levodopa-induced dyskinesias, nausea, orthostatic hypotension, confusion, hallucinations. HERBAL: **Kava kava** may decrease effect. FOOD: **High-protein** diets may cause decreased or erratic response to levodopa. LAB VALUES: May increase BUN, LDH, alkaline phosphatase, bilirubin, AST, ALT. May decrease Hgb, Hct, WBC count.

AVAILABILITY (Rx)

Tablets (Immediate-Release [Sinemet]): 10 mg carbidopa/100 mg levodopa, 25 mg carbidopa/100 mg levodopa, 25 mg carbidopa/250 mg levodopa. Tablets (Orally-Disintegrating [Parcopa], Immediate-Release): 10 mg carbidopa/100 mg levodopa, 25 mg carbidopa/100 mg levodopa, 25 mg carbidopa/250 mg levodopa.

Tablets (Extended-Release [Sinemet CR]): 25 mg carbidopa/100 mg levodopa, 50 mg carbidopa/200 mg levodopa.

ADMINISTRATION/HANDLING

Note: Space doses evenly over waking hours.

PO

• Scored tablets may be crushed. • Give without regard to food. • Do not crush extended-release tablets; may cut in half.

PO (Parcopa)

• Place orally-disintegrating tablet on top of tongue. Tablet will dissolve in seconds, pt to swallow with saliva. Not necessary to administer with liquid.

INDICATIONS/ROUTES/DOSAGE

Parkinsonism

PO: ADULTS (IMMEDIATE-RELEASE): Initially, 25/100 mg 3 times a day. May increase every other day by 1 tablet up to 200/2,000 mg daily. **ELDERLY:** Initially, 25/100 mg twice a day. May increase as necessary. When converting a pt from Sinemet to Sinemet CR (50 mg/200 mg), dosage is based on total daily dose of levodopa, as follows:

Sinemet or Parcopa	Sinemet CR (50/200)
300–400 mg	1 tablet twice a day
500–600 mg	1.5 tablet twice a day or 1 tablet 3 times a day
700–800 mg	4 tablets in 3 or more divided doses
900–1,000 mg	5 tablets in 3 or more divided doses

Intervals between doses of Sinemet CR should be 4–8 hrs while awake, with smaller doses at end of day if doses are not equal.

SIDE EFFECTS

Frequent: Uncontrolled movements of face, tongue, arms, upper body; nausea/vomiting (80%); anorexia (50%). **Occasional:** Depression, anxiety, confusion, nervousness, urinary retention, palpitations, dizziness, light-headedness, decreased appetite, blurred vision, constipation, dry mouth, flushed skin, headache, insomnia, diarrhea, unusual fatigue, darkening of urine and sweat. **Rare:** Hypertension, ulcer, hemolytic anemia (marked by fatigue).

ADVERSE EFFECTS/ TOXIC REACTIONS

High incidence of involuntary choreiform, dystonic, dyskinetic movements in those on long-term therapy. Numerous mild to severe CNS and psychiatric disturbances may occur (reduced attention span, anxiety, nightmares, daytime drowsiness, euphoria, fatigue, paranoia, psychotic episodes, depression, hallucinations).

NURSING CONSIDERATIONS

BASELINE ASSESSMENT

Assess symptoms of Parkinson's disease (e.g., rigidity, pill rolling, gait).

INTERVENTION/EVALUATION

Be alert to neurologic effects (headache, lethargy, mental confusion, agitation). Monitor for evidence of dyskinesia (difficulty with movement). Assess for clinical reversal of symptoms (improvement of tremor of head and hands at rest, mask-like facial expression, shuffling gait, muscular rigidity). Monitor B/P (standing, sitting, supine).

PATIENT/FAMILY TEACHING

• Avoid tasks that require alertness, motor skills until response to drug is established. • Sugarless gum, sips of tepid water may relieve dry mouth. • Take with food to minimize GI upset. • Effects may be delayed from several wks to mos. • May cause darkening of urine or sweat (not harmful). • Report any uncontrolled movement of face, eyelids, mouth, tongue, arms, hands, legs; mental changes; palpitations; severe or persistent nausea/vomiting; difficulty urinating. • Report exacerbations of asthma, underlying depression, psychosis.

carboplatin

HIGH ALERT

car-bow-**play**-tin
(Paraplatin, Paraplatin-AQ 🍁)

BLACK BOX ALERT Must be administered by personnel trained in administration/handling of chemotherapeutic agents (high potential for severe reactions, including anaphylaxis [may occur within minutes of administration] and sudden death). Profound myelosuppression (anemia, thrombocytopenia) has occurred.

Do not confuse carboplatin with Cisplatin or oxaliplatin, or Paraplatin with Platinol.

◆CLASSIFICATION

PHARMACOTHERAPEUTIC: Platinum coordination complex. **CLINICAL:** Antineoplastic (see p. 81C).

ACTION

Inhibits DNA synthesis by cross-linking with DNA strands, preventing cell division. Cell cycle-phase nonspecific. **Therapeutic Effect:** Interferes with DNA function.

PHARMACOKINETICS

Protein binding: Low. Hydrolyzed in solution to active form. Primarily excreted in urine. **Half-life:** 2.6–5.9 hrs.

USES

Treatment of ovarian carcinoma. **OFF-LABEL:** Brain tumors, Hodgkin's and non-Hodgkin's lymphomas, malignant melanoma, retinoblastoma, treatment of breast, bladder, cervical, endometrial, esophageal, small-cell lung, non–small-cell lung, head and neck, testicular carcinomas, germ cell tumors, osteogenic sarcoma.

PRECAUTIONS

Contraindications: History of severe allergic reaction to cisplatin, platinum compounds, mannitol; severe bleeding, severe myelosuppression. **Cautions:** Chickenpox, herpes zoster, renal impairment.

LIFESPAN CONSIDERATIONS

Pregnancy/Lactation: If possible, avoid use during pregnancy, esp. first trimester. May cause fetal harm. Unknown if distributed in breast milk. Breast-feeding not recommended. **Pregnancy Category D. Children:** Safety and efficacy not established. **Elderly:** Peripheral neurotoxicity increased, myelotoxicity may be more severe. Age-related renal impairment may require decreased dosage, more careful monitoring of blood counts.

INTERACTIONS

DRUG: Bone marrow depressants may increase myelosuppression. **Live virus vaccines** may potentiate virus replication, increase vaccine side effects, decrease pt's antibody response to vaccine. **Nephrotoxic, ototoxic medications** may increase risk of toxicity. **HERBAL:** Avoid **black cohosh, dong quai** in estrogen-dependent tumors. **FOOD:** None known. **LAB VALUES:** May decrease serum calcium, magnesium, potassium, sodium. May increase BUN, serum alkaline phosphatase, bilirubin, creatinine, AST.

AVAILABILITY (Rx)

Injection, Powder for Reconstitution: 50 mg, 150 mg, 450 mg. **Injection Solution:** 10 mg/ml.

ADMINISTRATION/HANDLING

◀ALERT▶ May be carcinogenic, mutagenic, teratogenic. Handle with extreme care during preparation/administration.

IV

Reconstitution • Reconstitute immediately before use. • Do not use aluminum needles or administration sets that come in contact with drug (may produce black precipitate, loss of potency). • Reconstitute each 50 mg with 5 ml Sterile Water for Injection, D_5W, or 0.9% NaCl to provide concentration of 10 mg/ml. • May be further diluted with D_5W or 0.9% NaCl to a final concentration of 0.5–2 mg/ml.

Rate of administration • Infuse over 15–60 min. • Rarely, anaphylactic reaction occurs minutes after administration. Use of epinephrine, corticosteroids alleviates symptoms.

Storage • Store vials at room temperature. •After reconstitution, solution is stable for 8 hrs. 2 mg/ml solution diluted in D_5W or 0.9% NaCl is stable for 24 hrs.

IV INCOMPATIBILITY

Amphotericin B complex (Abelcet, AmBisome, Amphotec).

IV COMPATIBILITIES

Etoposide (VePesid), granisetron (Kytril), lipids, ondansetron (Zofran), paclitaxel (Taxol).

INDICATIONS/ROUTES/DOSAGE

Ovarian Carcinoma (Monotherapy)

IV: ADULTS: 360 mg/m² on day 1, every 4 wks. Do not repeat dose until neutrophil and platelet counts are within acceptable levels. Adjust dosage in previously treated pts based on lowest post-treatment platelet or neutrophil count. Increase dosage only once to no more than 125% of starting dose.

C

Ovarian Carcinoma (Combination Therapy)
IV: ADULTS: 300 mg/m² (with cyclophosphamide) on day 1, every 4 wks. Do not repeat dose until neutrophil and platelet counts are within acceptable levels.

Usual Dose for Children
300–600 mg/m² every 4 wks for solid tumor, or 175 mg/m² every 4 wks for brain tumor.

Dosage in Renal Impairment
Initial dosage is based on creatinine clearance; subsequent dosages are based on pt's tolerance, degree of myelosuppression.

Creatinine Clearance	Dosage Day 1
60 ml/min or greater	360 mg/m²
41–59 ml/min	250 mg/m²
16–40 ml/min	200 mg/m²

SIDE EFFECTS

Frequent: Nausea (80%–75%), vomiting (65%). **Occasional:** Generalized pain (17%), diarrhea/constipation (6%), peripheral neuropathy (4%). **Rare (3%–2%):** Alopecia, asthenia, hypersensitivity reaction (erythema, pruritus, rash, urticaria).

ADVERSE EFFECTS/ TOXIC REACTIONS

Myelosuppression may be severe, resulting in anemia, infection (sepsis, pneumonia), major bleeding. Prolonged treatment may result in peripheral neurotoxicity.

NURSING CONSIDERATIONS

BASELINE ASSESSMENT

Offer emotional support. Do not repeat treatment until WBC recovers from previous therapy. Transfusions may be needed in those receiving prolonged therapy (myelosuppression increased in those with previous therapy, renal impairment).

INTERVENTION/EVALUATION

Monitor hematologic status, pulmonary function studies, hepatic/renal function tests, CBC, serum electrolytes. Monitor for fever, sore throat, signs of local infection, unusual bruising/bleeding from any site, symptoms of anemia (excessive fatigue, weakness).

PATIENT/FAMILY TEACHING

• Nausea, vomiting generally abate in less than 24 hrs. • Do not have immunizations without physician's approval (drug lowers body's resistance). • Avoid contact with those who have recently received live virus vaccine.

Cardene, *see nicardipine*

Cardizem, *see diltiazem*

Cardura, *see doxazosin*

carisoprodol

car-eye-sow-**pro**-doll
(Soma)
Do not confuse carisoprodol with carbamazepine, or Soma with senna.

FIXED-COMBINATION(S)

Soma Compound: carisoprodol/aspirin (a nonsteroidal salicylate): 200 mg/325 mg.

◆ CLASSIFICATION

PHARMACOTHERAPEUTIC: Carbamic acid ester. **CLINICAL:** Skeletal muscle relaxant.

ACTION

Skeletal muscle relaxant action may be related to its sedative properties. May produce muscle relaxation by altering interneuronal activity in the descending reticular formation of the brain and spinal cord. Does not directly affect skeletal muscle. **Therapeutic Effect:** Relieves musculoskeletal pain.

PHARMACOKINETICS

Route	Onset	Peak	Duration
PO	30 min	—	4–6 hrs

Readily absorbed from GI tract. Distributed throughout CNS. Converts to its active metabolite, meprobamate. Protein binding: 60%. Metabolized in liver; excreted in urine. Removed by hemodialysis, peritoneal dialysis. **Half-life:** 2 hrs.

USES

Relief of discomfort associated with acute, painful musculoskeletal conditions. Not to be used for more than 3 wks.

PRECAUTIONS

Contraindications: Acute intermittent porphyria, hypersensitivity to meprobamate (Equanil, Miltown), felbamate. **Cautions:** Hepatic/renal impairment, history of seizures, addiction-prone pts, elderly, debilitated.

LIFESPAN CONSIDERATIONS

Pregnancy/Lactation: Distributed in breast milk; decreases milk production. Crosses placenta. **Pregnancy Category C. Children:** Safety and efficacy not established in those younger than 16 yrs. **Elderly:** No age-related precautions noted.

INTERACTIONS

DRUG: **CNS depressants,** including **alcohol, benzodiazepines, tricyclic antidepressants,** may increase CNS effects. **HERBAL:** None significant. **FOOD:** None known. **LAB VALUES:** None significant.

AVAILABILITY (Rx)

Tablets: 250 mg, 350 mg.

ADMINISTRATION/HANDLING

• Give without regard to food.

INDICATIONS/ROUTES/DOSAGE

PO: ADULTS, ELDERLY, CHILDREN OLDER THAN 16 YRS: 250–350 mg 4 times daily with last dose at bedtime.

SIDE EFFECTS

Frequent (17%–13%): Drowsiness. **Occasional (8%–3%):** Dizziness, headache.

ADVERSE EFFECTS/ TOXIC REACTIONS

Idiosyncratic reactions and/or severe allergic reactions may occur within min or hr of first dose (severe weakness, transient quadriplesia, euphoria, temporary vision loss). Prolonged use at high dosage can lead to tolerance, dependence, withdrawal symptoms. Abrupt withdrawal following long-term use results in anxiety, abdominal cramps, insomnia, nausea, vomiting, confusion, and occasionally chills, seizures, hallucinations. Onset of withdrawal occurs 12–48 hours following cessation of use and can last another 12–48 hours. Overdose may result in tachycardia, facial flushing, ataxia, tremors, agitation, irritability. Overdose has resulted in stupor, coma, shock, respiratory depression, death. Coma may last from several hours to 1 day or more.

NURSING CONSIDERATIONS

BASELINE ASSESSMENT

Record onset, type, location, duration of musculoskeletal pain, inflammation. Inspect appearance of affected joints for immobility, stiffness, swelling.

INTERVENTION/EVALUATION

Assist with ambulation at all times. Evaluate for therapeutic response: relief of pain, stiffness, swelling, improved mobility, reduced joint tenderness, improved grip strength.

PATIENT/FAMILY TEACHING

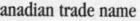

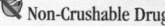

• Avoid tasks that require alertness, motor skills until response to drug is established. • Avoid alcohol. • Should only be used for short periods (2–3 wks). • Report withdrawal symptoms (syncope, tachyarrhythmia or excessive fatigue, unusual mental status changes).

C

carmustine

HIGH ALERT

car-**muss**-teen
(BiCNU, Gliadel Wafer)

BLACK BOX ALERT Profound myelosuppression (leukopenia, thrombocytopenia) is major toxicity. High risk of pulmonary toxicity. Must be administered by personnel trained in administration/handling of chemotherapeutic agents (high potential for severe reactions, including anaphylaxis, sudden death).

Do not confuse carmustine with bendamustine or lomustine.

◆CLASSIFICATION

PHARMACOTHERAPEUTIC: Alkylating agent, nitrosourea. **CLINICAL:** Antineoplastic (see p. 81C).

ACTION

Inhibits DNA, RNA synthesis by cross-linking with DNA, RNA strands, preventing cell division. Cell cycle-phase nonspecific. **Therapeutic Effect:** Interferes with DNA, RNA function.

PHARMACOKINETICS

Crosses blood-brain barrier. Metabolized in liver. Excreted in urine. **Half-life:** 15–30 min.

USES

Treatment of brain tumors, Hodgkin's lymphomas, non-Hodgkin's lymphomas, multiple myeloma. **Gliadel Wafer**: Adjunct to surgery to prolong survival in recurrent glioblastoma multiforme. **OFF-LABEL:** Treatment of colorectal, hepatic, GI carcinoma; malignant melanoma; mycosis fungoides.

PRECAUTIONS

Contraindications: None known. **Cautions:** Pts with decreased platelet, leukocyte, erythrocyte counts.

LIFESPAN CONSIDERATIONS

Pregnancy/Lactation: Avoid during pregnancy, particularly first trimester; may cause fetal harm. Unknown if distributed in breast milk. Breast-feeding not recommended. **Pregnancy Category D. Children:** Safety and efficacy not established. **Elderly:** No age-related precautions noted.

INTERACTIONS

DRUG: **Bone marrow depressants, cimetidine** may enhance myelosuppressive effect. **Hepatotoxic, nephrotoxic medications** may increase risk of hepatotoxicity, nephrotoxicity. **Live-virus vaccines** may potentiate virus replication, increase vaccine side effects, decrease pt's antibody response to vaccine. **HERBAL:** None significant. **FOOD:** None known. **LAB VALUES:** May increase BUN, serum alkaline phosphatase, bilirubin, AST, ALT.

AVAILABILITY (Rx)

Injection, Powder for Reconstitution (BiCNU): 100 mg. **Implant Device (Gliadel Wafer):** 7.7 mg.

ADMINISTRATION/HANDLING

◀ALERT▶ May be carcinogenic, mutagenic, teratogenic. Wear protective gloves during preparation of drug; may cause transient burning, brown staining of skin.

IV

Reconstitution • Reconstitute 100-mg vial with 3 ml sterile dehydrated (absolute) alcohol, followed by 27 ml Sterile Water for Injection to provide concentration of 3.3 mg/ml. • Further dilute with 50–250 ml D_5W or 0.9% NaCl to final concentration of 0.2–1 mg/ml.

Rate of administration • Infuse over 1–2 hrs (shorter duration may produce intense burning pain at injection site, intense flushing of skin, conjunctiva). • Flush IV line with 5–10 ml 0.9% NaCl or D_5W before and after administration to prevent irritation at injection site.

Storage • Refrigerate unopened vials of dry powder. • Reconstituted vials are stable for 8 hrs at room temperature or 24 hrs if refrigerated. • Solutions further diluted to 0.2 mg/ml with D_5W or 0.9% NaCl are stable for 48 hrs if refrigerated or an additional 8 hrs at room temperature. • Solutions appear clear, colorless to yellow. • Discard if precipitate forms, color change occurs, or oily film develops on bottom of vial. **Gliadel Wafers:** Store at or below −20°C (−4°F). Unopened pouches may be kept at room temperature for maximum of 6 hrs.

IV INCOMPATIBILITY

Allopurinol (Aloprim), sodium bicarbonate.

INDICATIONS/ROUTES/DOSAGE

◀ALERT▶ Refer to individual oncology protocols.

Usual Dosage

IV (BiCNU): ADULTS, ELDERLY: 150–200 mg/m^2 as a single dose q6–8wk or 75–100 mg/m^2 on 2 successive days q6–8wk. **CHILDREN:** 200–250 mg/m^2 q4–6wk as a single dose.

◀ALERT▶ Next dosage is based on clinical and hematologic response to previous dose (platelets greater than 100,000/mm^3 and leukocytes greater than 4,000/mm^3).

IMPLANTATION (GLIADEL WAFER): ADULTS, ELDERLY, CHILDREN: Up to 8 wafers (62.6 mg) may be placed in resection cavity.

SIDE EFFECTS

Frequent: Nausea/vomiting within minutes to 2 hrs after administration (may last up to 6 hrs). **Occasional:** Diarrhea, esophagitis, anorexia, dysphagia, hyperpigmentation. **Rare:** Thrombophlebitis, burning sensation, pain at injection site.

ADVERSE EFFECTS/ TOXIC REACTIONS

Hematologic toxicity due to myelosuppression occurs frequently. Thrombocytopenia occurs approximately 4 wks after carmustine treatment begins and lasts 1–2 wks. Leukopenia is evident 5–6 wks after treatment begins and lasts 1–2 wks. Anemia occurs less frequently, is less severe. Mild, reversible hepatotoxicity occurs frequently. Prolonged high-dose carmustine therapy may produce impaired renal function, pulmonary toxicity (pulmonary infiltrate/fibrosis).

NURSING CONSIDERATIONS

BASELINE ASSESSMENT

Perform CBC, renal/hepatic function studies before beginning therapy and periodically thereafter. Perform blood counts weekly during and for at least 6 wks after therapy ends.

INTERVENTION/EVALUATION

Monitor CBC, BUN, serum transaminase, alkaline phosphatase, bilirubin, pulmonary, renal/hepatic function tests. Monitor for hematologic toxicity (fever, sore throat, signs of local infection, unusual bruising/bleeding from any site), symptoms of anemia (excessive fatigue, weakness). Monitor for pulmonary toxicity: Observe for dyspnea. Monitor for adventitious breath sounds (rales, rhonchi, crackles).

PATIENT/FAMILY TEACHING

• Maintain adequate daily fluid intake (may protect against renal impairment). • Do not have immunizations without physician's approval (drug lowers body's resistance). • Avoid contact with those who have recently received live virus vaccine. • Contact physician if nausea/vomiting, fever, sore throat, chills, unusual bleeding/bruising occurs.

carvedilol HIGH ALERT

car-**veh**-dih-lol
(Apo-Carvedilol ✱, Coreg, Coreg CR, Novo-Carvedilol ✱)
Do not confuse carvedilol with atenolol, captopril, or

carteolol, or Coreg with Corgard, Cortef, or Cozaar.

◆CLASSIFICATION

PHARMACOTHERAPEUTIC: Beta-adrenergic blocker. **CLINICAL:** Antihypertensive (see p. 72C).

ACTION

Possesses nonselective beta-blocking and alpha-adrenergic blocking activity. Causes vasodilation. **Therapeutic Effect:** Reduces cardiac output, exercise-induced tachycardia, reflex orthostatic tachycardia; reduces peripheral vascular resistance.

PHARMACOKINETICS

Route	Onset	Peak	Duration
PO	30 min	1–2 hrs	24 hrs

Rapidly, extensively absorbed from GI tract. Protein binding: 98%. Metabolized in liver. Excreted primarily via bile into feces. Minimally removed by hemodialysis. **Half-life:** 7–10 hrs. Food delays rate of absorption.

USES

Treatment of mild to severe heart failure, left ventricular dysfunction following MI, hypertension. Reduces risk of recurrent MI in pts with damaged heart or heart failure. **OFF-LABEL:** Treatment of angina pectoris, idiopathic cardiomyopathy.

PRECAUTIONS

Contraindications: Bronchial asthma or related bronchospastic conditions, cardiogenic shock, pulmonary edema, second- or third-degree AV block, severe bradycardia. **Cautions:** CHF controlled with digitalis, diuretics, ACE inhibitors; peripheral vascular disease; anesthesia; diabetes mellitus; hypoglycemia; thyrotoxicosis; hepatic impairment.

⌛ LIFESPAN CONSIDERATIONS

Pregnancy/Lactation: Unknown if drug crosses placenta or is distributed in breast milk. May produce bradycardia, apnea, hypoglycemia, hypothermia during delivery; may contribute to low birth-weight infants. **Pregnancy Category C (D if used in the second or third trimester).** **Children:** Safety and efficacy not established. **Elderly:** Incidence of dizziness may be increased.

INTERACTIONS

DRUG: **Calcium channel blockers** increase risk of cardiac conduction disturbances. **Diuretics, other antihypertensives** may potentiate hypotensive effects. **Cimetidine** may increase concentration. May increase concentration of **cyclosporine, digoxin.** May decrease effect of **insulin, oral hypoglycemics. Rifampin** decreases concentration. **HERBAL:** **Ephedra, ginseng, yohimbe** may worsen hypertension. **Garlic** may increase antihypertensive effect. **FOOD:** None known. **LAB VALUE:** May increase bilirubin, transaminases, serum creatinine, PT.

AVAILABILITY (Rx)

Tablets (Immediate-Release): 3.125 mg, 6.25 mg, 12.5 mg, 25 mg.

Capsules (Extended-Release [Coreg CR]): 10 mg, 20 mg, 40 mg, 80 mg.

ADMINISTRATION/HANDLING

PO

• Give with food (slows rate of absorption, reduces risk of orthostatic effects). • Take standing systolic B/P 1 hr after dosing as guide for tolerance. • Do not crush or chew extended-release capsules.

INDICATIONS/ROUTES/DOSAGE

Hypertension

PO (IMMEDIATE-RELEASE): ADULTS, ELDERLY: Initially, 6.25 mg twice a day. May double at 7- to 14-day intervals to highest tolerated dosage. **Maximum:** 50 mg/day. **(EXTENDED-RELEASE):** Initially, 20 mg once daily. May increase to 40 mg once daily after 1–2 wks. **Maximum:** 80 mg once daily.

CHF

PO (IMMEDIATE-RELEASE): ADULTS, ELDERLY: Initially, 3.125 mg twice a day. May double at 2-wk intervals to highest tolerated dosage. **Maximum:** For pts weighing more than 85 kg, give 50 mg twice a day; for those weighing 85 kg or less, give 25 mg twice a day. **(EXTENDED-RELEASE):** Initially, 10 mg once daily for 2 wks. May increase to 20 mg, 40 mg, and 80 mg over successive intervals of at least 2 wks.

Left Ventricular Dysfunction

PO (IMMEDIATE-RELEASE): ADULTS, ELDERLY: Initially, 3.125–6.25 mg twice a day. May increase at intervals of 3–10 days up to 25 mg twice a day. **(EXTENDED-RELEASE):** Initially, 10–20 mg once daily. May increase to 40 mg and 80 mg once daily in intervals of 3–10 days.

SIDE EFFECTS

Carvedilol is generally well tolerated, with mild transient side effects. **Frequent (6%–4%):** Fatigue, dizziness. **Occasional (2%):** Diarrhea, bradycardia, rhinitis, back pain. **Rare (less than 2%):** Orthostatic hypotension, drowsiness, UTI, viral infection.

ADVERSE EFFECTS/ TOXIC REACTIONS

Overdose may produce profound bradycardia, hypotension, bronchospasm, cardiac insufficiency, cardiogenic shock, cardiac arrest. Abrupt withdrawal may result in diaphoresis, palpitations, headache, tremors. May precipitate CHF, MI in pts with cardiac disease; thyroid storm in those with thyrotoxicosis, peripheral ischemia in those with existing peripheral vascular disease. Hypoglycemia may occur in pts with previously controlled diabetes.

NURSING CONSIDERATIONS

BASELINE ASSESSMENT

Assess B/P, apical pulse immediately before drug is administered (if pulse is 60 beats/min or less or systolic B/P is less than 90 mm Hg, withhold medication, contact physician).

INTERVENTION/EVALUATION

Monitor B/P for hypotension, respiration for dyspnea. Assess pulse for quality, irregular rate, bradycardia. Monitor EKG for cardiac arrhythmias. Assist with ambulation if dizziness occurs. Assess for evidence of CHF: dyspnea (particularly on exertion or lying down), night cough, peripheral edema, distended neck veins. Monitor I&O (increase in weight, decrease in urine output may indicate CHF). Monitor renal/hepatic function tests.

PATIENT/FAMILY TEACHING

• Full antihypertensive effect noted in 1–2 wks. • Contact lens wearers may experience decreased lacrimation. • Take with food. • Do not abruptly discontinue medication. • Compliance with therapy regimen is essential to control hypertension. • Avoid tasks that require alertness, motor skills until response to drug is established. • Report excessive fatigue, prolonged dizziness. • Do not use nasal decongestants, OTC cold preparations (stimulants) without physician's approval. • Monitor B/P, pulse before taking medication. • Restrict salt, alcohol intake.

Casodex, *see bicalutamide*

caspofungin

cas-poe-**fun**-gin
(Cancidas)

◆ CLASSIFICATION

CLINICAL: Antifungal.

ACTION

Inhibits synthesis of glucan, a vital component of fungal cell wall formation, damaging fungal cell membrane. **Therapeutic Effect:** Fungistatic.

C

PHARMACOKINETICS

Distributed in tissue. Extensively bound to albumin. Protein binding: 97%. Slowly metabolized in liver to active metabolite. Excreted primarily in urine and, to a lesser extent, in feces. Not removed by hemodialysis. **Half-life:** 40–50 hrs.

USES

Treatment of invasive aspergillosis, candidemia, Candida infection in intra-abdominal abscess, peritonitis, esophageal candidiasis. Empiric therapy for presumed fungal infections in febrile neutropenia.

PRECAUTIONS

Contraindications: None known. **Cautions:** Myelosuppression, renal insufficiency, hepatic impairment.

LIFESPAN CONSIDERATIONS

Pregnancy/Lactation: May be embryotoxic. Crosses placental barrier. Distributed in breast milk. **Pregnancy Category C. Children:** Safety and efficacy not established. **Elderly:** Age-related moderate renal impairment may require dosage adjustment.

INTERACTIONS

DRUG: Cyclosporine may increase concentration. **Rifampin** may decrease concentration. May decrease concentration, effect of **tacrolimus. HERBAL:** None significant. **FOOD:** None known. **LAB VALUES:** May increase serum alkaline phosphatase, bilirubin, creatinine, AST, ALT, urine protein, RBCs. May decrease serum albumin, bicarbonate, potassium, magnesium, Hgb, Hct.

AVAILABILITY (Rx)

Injection, Powder for Reconstitution: 50-mg, 70-mg vials.

ADMINISTRATION/HANDLING

IV

Reconstitution • Reconstitute 50-mg or 70-mg vial with 10.8 ml 0.9% NaCl. Further dilute in 0.9% NaCl or D_5W to maximum concentration of 0.5 mg/ml.

Rate of administration • Infuse over 60 min.

Storage • Refrigerate but warm to room temperature before preparing with diluent. • Reconstituted solution, prior to preparation of pt infusion solution, may be stored at room temperature for 1 hr before infusion. • Final infusion solution can be stored at room temperature for 24 hrs or 48 hrs if refrigerated. • Discard if solution contains particulate or is discolored.

IV INCOMPATIBILITIES

Do not mix caspofungin with any other medication or use dextrose as a dilutent.

INDICATIONS/ROUTES/DOSAGE

Aspergillosis

IV: ADULTS, ELDERLY: Give single 70-mg loading dose on day 1, followed by 50 mg/day thereafter. For pts with moderate hepatic insufficiency, reduce daily dose to 35 mg. **CHILDREN 3 MOS–17 YRS:** 70 mg/m^2 on day 1, then 50 mg/m^2 daily. **Maximum:** 70-mg loading dose, 50-mg daily dose.

Invasive Candidiasis

IV: ADULTS, ELDERLY: Initially, 70 mg followed by 50 mg daily. **CHILDREN 3 MOS–17 YRS:** 70 mg/m^2 on day 1, then 50 mg/m^2 daily. **Maximum:** 70-mg loading dose, 50-mg daily dose.

Esophageal Candidiasis

IV: ADULTS, ELDERLY: 50 mg a day. **CHILDREN 3 MOS–17 YRS:** 50 mg/m^2 daily. **Maximum:** 50 mg.

Empiric Therapy

IV: ADULTS, ELDERLY: Initially, 70 mg then 50 mg/day. May increase to 70 mg/day. **CHILDREN 3 MOS–17 YRS:** 70 mg/m^2 on day 1, then 50 mg/m^2 daily. **Maximum:** 70 mg.

Dosage in Hepatic Impairment

Mild	No adjustment
Moderate	(Child-Pugh score 7–9): 35 mg/day
Severe	No clinical experience

C

SIDE EFFECTS

Frequent (26%): Fever. **Occasional (11%–4%):** Headache, nausea, phlebitis. **Rare (3% or less):** Paresthesia, vomiting, diarrhea, abdominal pain, myalgia, chills, tremor, insomnia.

ADVERSE EFFECTS/ TOXIC REACTIONS

Hypersensitivity reaction (rash, facial edema, pruritus, sensation of warmth) may occur.

NURSING CONSIDERATIONS

BASELINE ASSESSMENT

Determine baseline temperature, hepatic function tests. Assess for allergic or hypersensitivity reactions.

INTERVENTION/EVALUATION

Assess for signs/symptoms of hepatic dysfunction. Monitor hepatic enzyme tests in pts with preexisting hepatic dysfunction. Monitor CBC, serum potassium, Hgb. Monitor for fever, chills.

Catapres, *see clonidine*

Catapres-TTS, *see clonidine*

cefaclor

seff-uh-klor
(Apo-Cefaclor ✤, Ceclor ✤, Novo-Cefaclor ✤, Raniclor)
Do not confuse Cefaclor with cephalexin.

◆ CLASSIFICATION

PHARMACOTHERAPEUTIC: Second-generation cephalosporin. **CLINICAL:** Antibiotic (see p. 23C).

ACTION

Binds to bacterial cell membranes, inhibits cell wall synthesis. **Therapeutic Effect:** Bactericidal.

PHARMACOKINETICS

Well absorbed from GI tract. Protein binding: 25%. Widely distributed. Partially metabolized in liver. Primarily excreted in urine. Moderately removed by hemodialysis. **Half-life:** 0.6–0.9 hr (increased in renal impairment).

USES

Treatment of susceptible infections due to *S. pneumoniae, S. pyogenes, S. aureus, H. influenzae, E. coli, M. catarrhalis, Klebsiella* spp., *P. mirabilis,* including acute otitis media, bronchitis, pharyngitis/tonsillitis, respiratory tract, skin/skin structure, UTIs.

PRECAUTIONS

Contraindications: History of hypersensitivity/anaphylactic reaction to penicillins, cephalosporins. **Cautions:** Renal impairment, history of GI disease (esp. ulcerative colitis, antibiotic-associated colitis), concurrent use of nephrotoxic medications.

⧗ LIFESPAN CONSIDERATIONS

Pregnancy/Lactation: Readily crosses placenta. Distributed in breast milk. **Pregnancy Category B. Children:** No age-related precautions noted in those older than 1 mo. **Elderly:** Age-related renal impairment may require dosage adjustment.

INTERACTIONS

DRUG: **Aminoglycosides, furosemide** may increase risk of nephrotoxicity. **Probenecid** may increase concentration. Bleeding may occur with concomitant use of **warfarin. HERBAL:** None significant. **FOOD:** None known. **LAB VALUES:** May increase BUN, serum alkaline phosphatase, bilirubin, creatinine, LDH, AST, ALT. May cause positive direct/indirect Coombs' test.

C

AVAILABILITY (Rx)

Capsules: 250 mg, 500 mg. **Powder for Oral Suspension:** 125 mg/5 ml, 250 mg/5 ml, 375 mg/5 ml. **Tablets (Chewable [Raniclor]):** 250 mg, 375 mg.

ADMINISTRATION/HANDLING

PO

• After reconstitution, oral solution is stable for 14 days if refrigerated. • Shake oral suspension well before using. • Give without regard to food; if GI upset occurs, give with food, milk.

INDICATIONS/ROUTES/DOSAGE

Bronchitis

PO: ADULTS, ELDERLY, CHILDREN 16 YRS AND OLDER: 500 mg q8h for 7 days.

Lower Respiratory Tract Infections

PO: ADULTS, ELDERLY: 250–500 mg q8h. **CHILDREN:** 20–40 mg/kg/day q8h. **Maximum:** 1 g/day.

Otitis Media

PO: CHILDREN: 40 mg/kg/day divided q12h. **Maximum:** 1 g/day.

Pharyngitis

CHILDREN: 20 mg/kg/day divided q12h. **Maximum:** 1 g/day.

UTI

PO: ADULTS, ELDERLY: 250–500 mg q8h. **CHILDREN:** 20–40 mg/kg/day in 2–3 divided doses q8h. **Maximum:** 1 g/day.

Dosage in Renal Impairment

Creatinine Clearance	Dosage
10–50 ml/min	50%–100% of normal
Less than 10 ml/min	50% of normal

SIDE EFFECTS

Frequent: Oral candidiasis, mild diarrhea, mild abdominal cramping, vaginal candidiasis. **Occasional:** Nausea, serum sickness-like reaction (fever, joint pain; usually occurs after second course of therapy and resolves after drug is discontinued). **Rare:** Allergic reaction (pruritus, rash, urticaria).

ADVERSE EFFECTS/ TOXIC REACTIONS

Antibiotic-associated colitis, other superinfections (abdominal cramps, severe watery diarrhea, fever) may result from altered bacterial balance. Nephrotoxicity may occur, esp. in pts with preexisting renal disease. Pts with a history of allergies, esp. to penicillin, are at increased risk for developing a severe hypersensitivity reaction (severe pruritus, angioedema, bronchospasm, anaphylaxis).

NURSING CONSIDERATIONS

BASELINE ASSESSMENT

Question for history of allergies, particularly cephalosporins, penicillins.

INTERVENTION/EVALUATION

Assess oral cavity for white patches on mucous membranes, tongue (thrush). Monitor daily pattern of bowel activity and stool consistency. Mild GI effects may be tolerable (increasing severity may indicate onset of antibiotic-associated colitis). Monitor I&O, renal function tests for nephrotoxicity. Be alert for superinfection: fever, vomiting, diarrhea, anal/genital pruritus, oral mucosal changes (ulceration, pain, erythema).

PATIENT/FAMILY TEACHING

• Continue therapy for full length of treatment. • Doses should be evenly spaced. • May cause GI upset (may take with food, milk). • Refrigerate oral suspension. • Inform physician if persistent diarrhea occurs.

cefadroxil

sef-a-**drox**-ill
(Apo-Cefadroxil 🍁, Duricef, Novo-Cefadroxil 🍁)

✦ CLASSIFICATION

PHARMACOTHERAPEUTIC: First-generation cephalosporin. **CLINICAL:** Antibiotic (see p. 22C).

ACTION

Binds to bacterial cell membranes, inhibits cell wall synthesis. **Therapeutic Effect:** Bactericidal.

PHARMACOKINETICS

Well absorbed from GI tract. Protein binding: 15%–20%. Widely distributed. Primarily excreted unchanged in urine. Removed by hemodialysis. **Half-life:** 1.2–1.5 hrs (increased in renal impairment).

USES

Treatment of susceptible infections due to group A *streptococci, staphylococci, S. pneumoniae, H. influenzae, Klebsiella* spp., *E. coli, P. mirabilis,* including impetigo, pharyngitis/tonsillitis, skin/skin structure, UTIs.

PRECAUTIONS

Contraindications: History of hypersensitivity/anaphylactic reaction to penicillins, cephalosporins. **Cautions:** Renal impairment, history of GI disease (esp. ulcerative colitis, antibiotic-associated colitis), concurrent use of nephrotoxic medications.

⌛ LIFESPAN CONSIDERATIONS

Pregnancy/Lactation: Readily crosses placenta. Distributed in breast milk. **Pregnancy Category B. Children:** No age-related precautions noted. **Elderly:** Age-related renal impairment may require dosage adjustment.

INTERACTIONS

DRUG: **Probenecid** may increase concentration. Bleeding may occur with concomitant use of **warfarin.** **HERBAL:** None significant. **FOOD:** None known. **LAB VALUES:** May increase BUN, serum alkaline phosphatase, bilirubin, creatinine, LDH, AST, ALT. May cause positive direct/indirect Coombs' test.

AVAILABILITY (Rx)

Capsules: 500 mg. **Powder for Oral Suspension:** 250 mg/5 ml, 500 mg/5 ml. **Tablets:** 1 g.

ADMINISTRATION/HANDLING

PO

• After reconstitution, oral solution is stable for 14 days if refrigerated. • Shake oral suspension well before using. • Give without regard to meals; if GI upset occurs, give with food, milk.

INDICATIONS/ROUTES/DOSAGE

UTI

PO: ADULTS, ELDERLY: 1–2 g/day as a single dose or in 2 divided doses. **CHILDREN:** 30 mg/kg/day in 2 divided doses. **Maximum:** 2 g/day.

Skin/Skin Structure Infections, Group A Beta-Hemolytic Streptococcal Pharyngitis, Tonsillitis

PO: ADULTS, ELDERLY: 1–2 g/day in 2 divided doses. **CHILDREN:** 30 mg/kg/day in 2 divided doses. **Maximum:** 2 g/day.

Impetigo

PO: CHILDREN: 30 mg/kg/day as a single dose or in 2 divided doses. **Maximum:** 2 g/day.

Dosage in Renal Impairment

After initial 1-g dose, dosage and frequency are modified based on creatinine clearance and severity of infection.

Creatinine Clearance	Dosage
26–50 ml/min	500 mg q12h
10–25 ml/min	500 mg q24h
Less than 10 ml/min	500 mg q36h

SIDE EFFECTS

Frequent: Oral candidiasis, mild diarrhea, mild abdominal cramping, vaginal candidiasis. **Occasional:** Nausea, unusual bruising/bleeding, serum sickness-like reaction (fever, joint pain; usually occurs after second course of therapy and resolves after drug is discontinued). **Rare:**

C

Allergic reaction (rash, pruritus, urticaria), thrombophlebitis (pain, redness, swelling at injection site).

ADVERSE EFFECTS/ TOXIC REACTIONS

Antibiotic-associated colitis, other superinfections (abdominal cramps, severe watery diarrhea, fever) may result from altered bacterial balance. Nephrotoxicity may occur, esp. in pts with preexisting renal disease. Pts with a history of allergies, esp. to penicillin, are at increased risk for developing a severe hypersensitivity reaction (severe pruritus, angioedema, bronchospasm, anaphylaxis).

NURSING CONSIDERATIONS

BASELINE ASSESSMENT

Question for history of allergies, particularly cephalosporins, penicillins.

INTERVENTION/EVALUATION

Assess oral cavity for white patches on mucous membranes, tongue (thrush). Monitor daily pattern of bowel activity and stool consistency. Mild GI effects may be tolerable (increasing severity may indicate onset of antibiotic-associated colitis). Monitor I&O, renal function tests for nephrotoxicity. Be alert for superinfection: fever, vomiting, diarrhea, anal/genital pruritus, oral mucosal changes (ulceration, pain, erythema).

PATIENT/FAMILY TEACHING

• Continue therapy for full length of treatment. • Doses should be evenly spaced. • May cause GI upset (may take with food, milk). • Refrigerate oral suspension. • Report persistent diarrhea.

cefazolin

cef-ah-**zoe**-lin
(Ancef)

Do not confuse cefazolin with cefprozil, ceftriaxone, or cephalexin.

◆CLASSIFICATION

PHARMACOTHERAPEUTIC: First-generation cephalosporin. **CLINICAL:** Antibiotic (see p. 22C).

ACTION

Binds to bacterial cell membranes, inhibits cell wall synthesis. **Therapeutic Effect:** Bactericidal.

PHARMACOKINETICS

Widely distributed. Protein binding: 85%. Primarily excreted unchanged in urine. Moderately removed by hemodialysis. **Half-life:** 1.4–1.8 hrs (increased in renal impairment).

USES

Treatment of susceptible infections due to *S. aureus, S. epidermidis,* Group A *beta-hemolytic streptococci, S. pneumoniae, E. coli, P. mirabilis, Klebsiella* spp., *H. influenzae* including biliary tract, bone and joint, genital, respiratory tract, skin/skin structure, UTIs, endocarditis, perioperative prophylaxis, septicemia. **OFF-LABEL:** Prophylaxis against infective endocarditis.

PRECAUTIONS

Contraindications: History of hypersensitivity/anaphylactic reaction to penicillins, cephalosporins. **Cautions:** Renal impairment, history of GI disease (esp. ulcerative colitis, antibiotic-associated colitis), concurrent use of nephrotoxic medications.

⌛ LIFESPAN CONSIDERATIONS

Pregnancy/Lactation: Readily crosses placenta; distributed in breast milk. **Pregnancy Category B. Children:** No age-related precautions noted. **Elderly:** Age-related renal impairment may require reduced dosage.

INTERACTIONS

DRUG: Aminoglycosides, furosemide may increase risk of nephrotoxicity. **Probenecid** may increase concentration.

Bleeding may occur with concomitant use of **warfarin.** **HERBAL**: None significant. **FOOD**: None known. **LAB VALUES**: May increase BUN, serum alkaline phosphatase, bilirubin, creatinine, LDH, AST, ALT. May cause positive direct/indirect Coombs' test.

AVAILABILITY (Rx)

Injection, Powder for Reconstitution (Ancef): 500 mg, 1 g. **Ready-to-Hang Infusion (Ancef)**: 500 mg/50 ml, 1 g/50 ml, 2 g/100 ml.

ADMINISTRATION/HANDLING

IV

Reconstitution • Reconstitute each 1 g with at least 10 ml Sterile Water for Injection. • May further dilute in 50–100 ml D_5W or 0.9% NaCl (decreases incidence of thrombophlebitis).

Rate of administration • For IV push, administer over 3–5 min (**maximum concentration:** 100 mg/ml). • For intermittent IV infusion (piggyback), infuse over 10–60 min.

Storage • Solution appears light yellow to yellow. • Reconstituted solution stable for 24 hrs at room temperature or for 10 days if refrigerated. • IV infusion (piggyback) stable for 48 hrs at room temperature or for 14 days if refrigerated. • Commercially frozen solutions are stable for 48 hrs at room temperature or for 30 days if refrigerated.

IM

• To minimize discomfort, inject deep IM slowly. • Less painful if injected into gluteus maximus rather than lateral aspect of thigh.

IV INCOMPATIBILITIES

Amikacin (Amikin), amiodarone (Cordarone), hydromorphone (Dilaudid).

IV COMPATIBILITIES

Calcium gluconate, dexamethasone (Decadron), diltiazem (Cardizem), famotidine (Pepcid), heparin, insulin (regular), lidocaine, lipids, lorazepam (Ativan), magnesium sulfate, meperidine (Demerol), midazolam (Versed), morphine, multivitamins, metoclopramide (Reglan), ondansetron (Zofran), potassium chloride, propofol (Diprivan), total parenteral nutrition (TPN), vecuronium (Norcuron).

INDICATIONS/ROUTES/DOSAGE

Usual Dosage Range

IV, IM: ADULTS: 250 mg to 2g q6–12h (usually q8h). **CHILDREN OLDER THAN 1 MO**: 25–100 mg/kg/day divided q6–8h. **Maximum:** 6 g/day.

Uncomplicated UTI

IV, IM: ADULTS, ELDERLY: 1 g q12h.

Mild to Moderate Infections

IV, IM: ADULTS, ELDERLY: 500 mg–1 g q6–8h.

Severe Infections

IV, IM: ADULTS, ELDERLY: 1–2 g q6–8h.

Life-Threatening Infections

IV, IM: ADULTS, ELDERLY: 1–2 g q4–6h. **Maximum**: 12 g/day.

Perioperative Prophylaxis

IV, IM: ADULTS, ELDERLY: 1 g 30–60 min before surgery, 0.5–1 g during surgery and q6–8h for up to 24 hrs postoperatively.

Usual Pediatric Dosage

CHILDREN: 25–100 mg/kg/day in divided doses q8h. **Maximum**: 6 g/day. **NEONATES OLDER THAN 7 DAYS**: 40–60 mg/kg/day in divided doses q8–12h. **NEONATES 7 DAYS AND YOUNGER**: 40 mg/kg/day in divided doses q12h.

Dosage in Renal Impairment

Dosing frequency is modified based on creatinine clearance.

Creatinine Clearance	Dosage
11–34 ml/min	½ usual dose q12h
10 ml/min or less	½ usual dose q24h

C

SIDE EFFECTS

Frequent: Discomfort with IM administration, oral candidiasis (thrush), mild diarrhea, mild abdominal cramping, vaginal candidiasis. **Occasional:** Nausea, serum sickness-like reaction (fever, joint pain; usually occurs after second course of therapy and resolves after drug is discontinued). **Rare:** Allergic reaction (rash, pruritus, urticaria), thrombophlebitis (pain, redness, swelling at injection site).

ADVERSE EFFECTS/ TOXIC REACTIONS

Antibiotic-associated colitis, other superinfections (abdominal cramps, severe watery diarrhea, fever) may result from altered bacterial balance. Nephrotoxicity may occur, esp. in pts with preexisting renal disease. Pts with a history of allergies, esp. to penicillin, are at increased risk for developing a severe hypersensitivity reaction (severe pruritus, angioedema, bronchospasm, anaphylaxis).

NURSING CONSIDERATIONS

BASELINE ASSESSMENT

Question for history of allergies, particularly cephalosporins, penicillins.

INTERVENTION/EVALUATION

Evaluate IM site for induration and tenderness. Assess oral cavity for white patches on mucous membranes, tongue (thrush). Monitor daily pattern of bowel activity and stool consistency. Mild GI effects may be tolerable (increasing severity may indicate onset of antibiotic-associated colitis). Monitor I&O, renal function tests for nephrotoxicity. Be alert for superinfection: fever, vomiting, diarrhea, anal/genital pruritus, oral mucosal changes (ulceration, pain, erythema).

PATIENT/FAMILY TEACHING

• Discomfort may occur with IM injection.

cefdinir

sef-di-neer
(Omnicef)

◆CLASSIFICATION

PHARMACOTHERAPEUTIC: Third-generation cephalosporin. **CLINICAL:** Antibiotic (see p. 24C).

ACTION

Binds to bacterial cell membranes, inhibits cell wall synthesis. **Therapeutic Effect:** Bactericidal.

PHARMACOKINETICS

Moderately absorbed from GI tract. Protein binding: 60%–70%. Widely distributed. Not appreciably metabolized. Primarily excreted unchanged in urine. Minimally removed by hemodialysis. **Half-life:** 1–2 hrs (increased in renal impairment).

USES

Treatment of susceptible infections due to *S. pyogenes, S. pneumoniae, H. influenzae, H. parainfluenzae, M. catarrhalis* including community-acquired pneumonia, acute exacerbation of chronic bronchitis, acute maxillary sinusitis, pharyngitis, tonsillitis, uncomplicated skin/skin structure infections, otitis media.

PRECAUTIONS

Contraindications: History of anaphylactic reaction to penicillins, hypersensitivity to cephalosporins. **Cautions:** Hypersensitivity to penicillins, other drugs; history of GI disease (e.g., colitis); renal/hepatic impairment.

LIFESPAN CONSIDERATIONS

Pregnancy/Lactation: Crosses placenta. Not detected in breast milk. **Pregnancy Category B. Children:** Newborns, infants may have lower renal clearance. **Elderly:** Age-related renal impairment may require decreased dosage or increased dosing interval.

C

INTERACTIONS

DRUG: **Aminoglycosides** may increase risk of nephrotoxicity. **Antacids, iron preparations** may interfere with absorption. **Probenecid** increases concentration. HERBAL: None significant. FOOD: None known. LAB VALUES: May produce false-positive reaction for urine ketones. May increase serum alkaline phosphatase, bilirubin, LDH, AST, ALT.

AVAILABILITY (Rx)

Capsules: 300 mg. Powder for Oral Suspension: 125 mg/5 ml, 250 mg/5 ml.

ADMINISTRATION/HANDLING

PO

• Give without regard to food. • Twice daily doses should be given 12 hrs apart. • Shake oral suspension well before administering. • Store mixed suspension at room temperature. Discard unused portion after 10 days.

INDICATIONS/ROUTES/DOSAGE

Usual Dosage Range

PO: ADULTS, ELDERLY: 300 mg q12h or 600 mg once daily. **CHILDREN 6 MOS–12 YRS:** 7 mg/kg q12h or 14 mg/kg once daily. **Maximum:** 600 mg/day.

Community-Acquired Pneumonia

PO: ADULTS, ELDERLY, CHILDREN 13 YRS AND OLDER: 300 mg q12h for 10 days.

Acute Exacerbation of Chronic Bronchitis

PO: ADULTS, ELDERLY: 300 mg q12h for 5–10 days or 600 mg once daily for 10 days.

Acute Maxillary Sinusitis

PO: ADULTS, ELDERLY, CHILDREN 13 YRS AND OLDER: 300 mg q12h or 600 mg q24h for 10 days. **CHILDREN 6 MOS–12 YRS:** 7 mg/kg q12h or 14 mg/kg q24h for 10 days. **Maximum:** 600 mg/day.

Pharyngitis, Tonsillitis

PO: ADULTS, ELDERLY, CHILDREN 13 YRS AND OLDER: 300 mg q12h for 5–10 days or 600 mg q24h for 10 days. **CHILDREN 6 MOS–12 YRS:** 7 mg/kg q12h for 5–10 days or 14 mg/kg q24h for 10 days. **Maximum:** 600 mg/day.

Uncomplicated Skin/Skin Structure Infections

PO: ADULTS, ELDERLY, CHILDREN 13 YRS AND OLDER: 300 mg q12h for 10 days. **CHILDREN 6 MOS–12 YRS:** 7 mg/kg q12h for 10 days. **Maximum:** 600 mg/day.

Acute Bacterial Otitis Media

PO (CAPSULES): CHILDREN: 6 MOS–12 YRS: 7 mg/kg q12h or 14 mg/kg q24h for 10 days. **Maximum:** 600 mg/day.

Usual Pediatric Dosage for Oral Suspension

CHILDREN WEIGHING 81–95 LB (37–43 KG): 12.5 ml (2.5 tsp) q12h or 25 ml (5 tsp) q24h. **CHILDREN WEIGHING 61–80 LB (28–36 KG):** 10 ml (2 tsp) q12h or 20 ml (4 tsp) q24h. **CHILDREN WEIGHING 41–60 LB (19–27 KG):** 7.5 ml (1 tsp) q12h or 15 ml (3 tsp) q24h. **CHILDREN WEIGHING 20–40 LB (9–18 KG):** 5 ml (1 tsp) q12h or 10 ml (2 tsp) q24h. **INFANTS WEIGHING LESS THAN 20 LB (LESS THAN 9 KG):** 2.5 ml (½ tsp) q12h or 5 ml (1 tsp) q24h.

Dosage in Renal Impairment

Creatinine clearance less than 30 ml/min: 300 mg/day or 7 mg/kg as single daily dose. **Hemodialysis pts:** 300 mg or 7 mg/kg/dose every other day.

SIDE EFFECTS

Frequent: Oral candidiasis, mild diarrhea, mild abdominal cramping, vaginal candidiasis. Occasional: Nausea, serum sickness-like reaction (fever, joint pain; usually occurs after second course of therapy and resolves after drug is discontinued). Rare: Allergic reaction (rash, pruritus, urticaria).

ADVERSE EFFECTS/ TOXIC REACTIONS

Antibiotic-associated colitis, other superinfections (abdominal cramps, severe watery diarrhea, fever) may result from altered bacterial balance. Nephrotoxicity may occur, esp. in pts with preexisting renal disease. Pts with a history of allergies, esp. to penicillin, are at increased risk for developing a severe hypersensitivity reaction (severe pruritus, angioedema, bronchospasm, anaphylaxis).

NURSING CONSIDERATIONS

BASELINE ASSESSMENT

Question for hypersensitivity to cefdinir or other cephalosporins, penicillins.

INTERVENTION/EVALUATION

Observe for rash. Monitor daily pattern of bowel activity and stool consistency. Mild GI effects may be tolerable (increasing severity may indicate onset of antibiotic-associated colitis). Be alert for superinfection: fever, vomiting, diarrhea, anal/genital pruritus, oral mucosal changes (ulceration, pain, erythema). Monitor hematology reports.

PATIENT/FAMILY TEACHING

• Take antacids 2 hrs before or following medication. • Continue medication for full length of treatment; do not skip doses. • Doses should be evenly spaced. • Report persistent severe diarrhea, rash, muscle aches, fever, enlarged lymph nodes, joint pain.

cefepime

sef-eh-**peem**
(Maxipime)
Do not confuse cefepime with cefixime.

◆CLASSIFICATION

PHARMACOTHERAPEUTIC: Fourth-generation cephalosporin. **CLINICAL:** Antibiotic (see p. 24C).

ACTION

Binds to bacterial cell wall membranes, inhibits cell wall synthesis. **Therapeutic Effect:** Bactericidal.

PHARMACOKINETICS

Well absorbed after IM administration. Protein binding: 20%. Widely distributed. Primarily excreted unchanged in urine. Removed by hemodialysis. **Half-life:** 2–2.3 hrs (increased in renal impairment, elderly pts).

USES

Susceptible infections due to aerobic gram-negative organisms including *P. aeruginosa,* gram-positive organisms including *S. aureus.* Treatment of empiric febrile neutropenia, intra-abdominal, skin/skin structure, UTIs, pneumonia.

PRECAUTIONS

Contraindications: History of anaphylactic reaction to penicillins, hypersensitivity to cephalosporins. **Cautions:** Renal impairment.

⌛ LIFESPAN CONSIDERATIONS

Pregnancy/Lactation: Unknown if distributed in breast milk. **Pregnancy Category B. Children:** No age-related precautions noted in those older than 2 mos. **Elderly:** Age-related renal impairment may require reduced dosage or increased dosing interval.

INTERACTIONS

DRUG: Aminoglycosides, furosemide may increase risk of nephrotoxicity. **Probenecid** may increase concentration. **HERBAL:** None significant. **FOOD:** None known. **LAB VALUES:** May increase BUN, serum alkaline phosphatase, bilirubin, LDH, AST, ALT. May cause positive direct/indirect Coombs' test.

AVAILABILITY (Rx)

Injection, Powder for Reconstitution: 500 mg, 1 g, 2 g.

C

ADMINISTRATION/HANDLING

IV

Reconstitution • Add 5 ml to 500-mg vial (10 ml for 1-g and 2-g vials). • Further dilute with 50–100 ml 0.9% NaCl or D_5W (final concentration not to exceed 40 mg/ml).

Rate of administration • For intermittent IV infusion (piggyback), infuse over 20–30 min.

Storage • Solution is stable for 24 hrs at room temperature, 7 days if refrigerated.

IM

• Add 1.3 ml Sterile Water for Injection, 0.9% NaCl, or D_5W to 500-mg vial (2.4 ml for 1-g and 2-g vials). • Inject into a large muscle mass (e.g., upper gluteus maximus).

IV INCOMPATIBILITIES

Acyclovir (Zovirax), amphotericin (Fungizone), cimetidine (Tagamet), ciprofloxacin (Cipro), cisplatin (Platinol), dacarbazine (DTIC), daunorubicin (Cerubidine), diazepam (Valium), diphenhydramine (Benadryl), dobutamine (Dobutrex), dopamine (Intropin), doxorubicin (Adriamycin), droperidol (Inapsine), famotidine (Pepcid), ganciclovir (Cytovene), haloperidol (Haldol), magnesium, magnesium sulfate, mannitol, meperidine (Demerol), metoclopramide (Reglan), morphine, ofloxacin (Floxin), ondansetron (Zofran), vancomycin (Vancocin).

IV COMPATIBILITIES

Bumetanide (Bumex), calcium gluconate, furosemide (Lasix), hydromorphone (Dilaudid), lorazepam (Ativan), propofol (Diprivan).

INDICATIONS/ROUTES/DOSAGE

Usual Dosage Range

IV: ADULTS, ELDERLY: 1–2 g q8–12h. CHILDREN: 50 mg/kg q8–12h not to exceed adult dosing.

Pneumonia

IV: ADULTS, ELDERLY: 1–2 g q12h for 7–10 days. CHILDREN 2 MOS AND OLDER: 50 mg/kg q12h. **Maximum:** 2 g/dose.

Intra-Abdominal Infections

IV: ADULTS, ELDERLY: 2 g q12h for 7–10 days.

Skin/Skin Structure Infections

IV: ADULTS, ELDERLY: 2 g q12h for 10 days. CHILDREN 2 MOS AND OLDER: 50 mg/kg q12h. **Maximum:** 2 g/dose.

UTIs

IV: ADULTS, ELDERLY: 0.5–2 g q12h for 7–10 days. CHILDREN 2 MOS AND OLDER: 50 mg/kg q12h. **Maximum:** 2 g/dose.

Febrile Neutropenia

IV: ADULTS, ELDERLY: 2 g q8h. CHILDREN 2 MOS AND OLDER: 50 mg/kg q8h. **Maximum:** 2 g/dose.

Dosage in Renal Impairment

Dosage and frequency are modified based on creatinine clearance and severity of infection.

Creatinine Clearance	Dosage
30–60 ml/min	500 mg q24h–2 g q12h
11–29 ml/min	500 mg–2 g q24h
10 ml/min or less	250 mg–1 g q24h

SIDE EFFECTS

Frequent: Discomfort with IM administration, oral candidiasis (thrush), mild diarrhea, mild abdominal cramping, vaginal candidiasis. **Occasional:** Nausea, serum sickness-like reaction (fever, joint pain; usually occurs after second course of therapy and resolves after drug is discontinued). **Rare:** Allergic reaction (rash, pruritus, urticaria), thrombophlebitis (pain, redness, swelling at injection site).

ADVERSE EFFECTS/ TOXIC REACTIONS

Antibiotic-associated colitis, other superinfections (abdominal cramps, severe watery diarrhea, fever) may result from altered bacterial balance. Nephrotoxicity may occur, esp. in pts with preexisting renal disease. Pts with a history of allergies, esp. to penicillin, are at increased risk for developing a severe hypersensitivity reaction (severe pruritus, angioedema, bronchospasm, anaphylaxis).

NURSING CONSIDERATIONS

BASELINE ASSESSMENT

Question for history of allergies, particularly cephalosporins, penicillins.

INTERVENTION/EVALUATION

Evaluate IM site for induration and tenderness. Assess oral cavity for white patches on mucous membranes, tongue (thrush). Monitor daily pattern of bowel activity and stool consistency. Mild GI effects may be tolerable (increasing severity may indicate onset of antibiotic-associated colitis). Monitor I&O, CBC, renal function tests for nephrotoxicity. Be alert for superinfection: fever, vomiting, diarrhea, anal/genital pruritus, oral mucosal changes (ulceration, pain, erythema).

PATIENT/FAMILY TEACHING

• Discomfort may occur with IM injection. • Continue therapy for full length of treatment. • Doses should be evenly spaced. • Notify physician if persistent diarrhea occurs.

cefixime

sef-icks-zeem
(Suprax)
Do not confuse cefixime with cefepime, or Suprax with Sporanox, Surbex, or Surfak.

◆CLASSIFICATION

PHARMACOTHERAPEUTIC: Third-generation cephalosporin. **CLINICAL:** Antibiotic.

ACTION

Binds to bacterial cell membranes, inhibits cell wall synthesis. **Therapeutic Effect:** Bactericidal.

PHARMACOKINETICS

Moderately absorbed from GI tract. Protein binding: 65%–70%. Widely distributed. Primarily excreted unchanged in urine. Minimally removed by hemodialysis. **Half-life:** 3–4 hrs (increased in renal impairment).

USES

Treatment of susceptible infections due to *S. pneumoniae, S. pyogenes, M. catarrhalis, H. influenzae, N. gonorrhoeae, E. coli, P. mirabilis* including otitis media, acute bronchitis, acute exacerbations of chronic bronchitis, pharyngitis, tonsillitis, uncomplicated UTI, uncomplicated gonorrhea.

PRECAUTIONS

Contraindications: History of hypersensitivity/anaphylactic reaction to penicillins, cephalosporins. **Cautions:** History of GI disease (e.g., colitis); renal impairment.

⌛ LIFESPAN CONSIDERATIONS

Pregnancy/Lactation: Not recommended during labor and delivery. Unknown if distributed in breast milk. **Pregnancy Category B. Children:** Safety and efficacy not established in those younger than 6 mos. **Elderly:** Age-related renal impairment may require dosage adjustment.

INTERACTIONS

DRUG: Aminoglycosides, furosemide may increase risk of nephrotoxicity. **Probenecid** may increase concentration. Bleeding may occur with concomitant use of **warfarin. HERBAL:** None significant. **FOOD:** None known. **LAB VALUES:**

May increase BUN, serum alkaline phosphatase, bilirubin, creatinine, LDH, AST, ALT. May cause a positive direct/indirect Coombs' test.

AVAILABILITY (Rx)

Oral Suspension: 100 mg/5 ml, 200 mg/5 ml. Tablets: 400 mg.

ADMINISTRATION/HANDLING

PO

• Give without regard to food. • After reconstitution, oral suspension is stable for 14 days at room temperature. • Do not refrigerate. • Shake oral suspension well before administering.

INDICATIONS/ROUTES/DOSAGE

Usual Dosage

PO: ADULTS, ELDERLY, CHILDREN WEIGHING MORE THAN 50 KG: 400 mg/day as a single dose or in 2 divided doses. **CHILDREN 6 MOS–12 YRS WEIGHING LESS THAN 50 KG:** 8–20 mg/kg/day as a single dose or in 2 divided doses. **Maximum:** 400 mg.

Uncomplicated Gonorrhea

PO: ADULTS: 400 mg as a single dose.

Dosage in Renal Impairment

Dosage is modified based on creatinine clearance.

Creatinine Clearance	Dosage
21–60 ml/min	75% of usual dose
20 ml/min or less	50% of usual dose

SIDE EFFECTS

Frequent: Oral candidiasis (thrush), mild diarrhea, mild abdominal cramping, vaginal candidiasis. Occasional: Nausea, serum sickness-like reaction (arthralgia, fever; usually occurs after second course of therapy and resolves after drug is discontinued). Rare: Allergic reaction (rash, pruritus, urticaria).

ADVERSE EFFECTS/ TOXIC REACTIONS

Antibiotic-associated colitis, other superinfections (abdominal cramps, severe watery diarrhea, fever) may result from altered bacterial balance. Nephrotoxicity may occur, esp. in pts with preexisting renal disease. Pts with a history of allergies, esp. to penicillin, are at increased risk for developing a severe hypersensitivity reaction (severe pruritus, angioedema, bronchospasm, anaphylaxis).

NURSING CONSIDERATIONS

BASELINE ASSESSMENT

Question for hypersensitivity to cefixime or other cephalosporins, penicillins.

INTERVENTION/EVALUATION

Assess oral cavity for white patches on mucous membranes, tongue (thrush). Monitor daily pattern of bowel activity and stool consistency. Mild GI effects may be tolerable (increasing severity may indicate onset of antibiotic-associated colitis). Monitor renal function tests for evidence of nephrotoxicity. Be alert for superinfection: fever, vomiting, diarrhea, anal/genital pruritus, oral mucosal changes (ulceration, pain, erythema).

PATIENT/FAMILY TEACHING

• Continue medication for full length of treatment; do not skip doses. • Doses should be evenly spaced. • May cause GI upset (may take with food or milk). • Report diarrhea.

cefotaxime

sef-oh-**tax**-eem
(Claforan)

Do not confuse cefotaxime with cefoxitin, ceftizoxime, or cefuroxime, or Claforan with Claritin.

CLASSIFICATION

PHARMACOTHERAPEUTIC: Third-generation cephalosporin. **CLINICAL:** Antibiotic (see p. 24C).

C

ACTION

Binds to bacterial cell membranes, inhibits cell wall synthesis. Therapeutic Effect: Bactericidal.

PHARMACOKINETICS

Widely distributed to CSF. Protein binding: 30%–50%. Partially metabolized in liver to active metabolite. Primarily excreted in urine. Moderately removed by hemodialysis. Half-life: 1 hr (increased in renal impairment).

USES

Treatment of susceptible infections due to gram-negative organisms including bone, joint, GU, gynecologic, intra-abdominal, lower respiratory tract, skin/skin structure infections, septicemia, meningitis, preop prophylaxis. OFF-LABEL: Treatment of Lyme disease.

PRECAUTIONS

Contraindications: History of hypersensitivity/anaphylactic reaction to penicillins, cephalosporins. **Cautions:** Concurrent use of nephrotoxic medications, history of GI disease (esp. ulcerative colitis, antibiotic-associated colitis), renal impairment with creatinine clearance less than 20 ml/min.

LIFESPAN CONSIDERATIONS

Pregnancy/Lactation: Readily crosses placenta. Distributed in breast milk. **Pregnancy Category B. Children:** No age-related precautions noted. **Elderly:** Age-related renal impairment may require dosage adjustment.

INTERACTIONS

DRUG: **Aminoglycosides, furosemide** may increase risk of nephrotoxicity. **Probenecid** may increase concentration. HERBAL: None significant. FOOD: None known. LAB VALUES: May cause positive direct/indirect Coombs' test. May increase serum AST, ALT, alkaline phosphatase.

AVAILABILITY (Rx)

Injection, Powder for Reconstitution: 500 mg, 1 g, 2 g. **Intravenous Solution:** 1 g/50 ml, 2 g/50 ml.

ADMINISTRATION/HANDLING

IV

Reconstitution • Reconstitute with 10 ml Sterile Water for Injection to provide a concentration of 50 mg/ml, 95 mg/ml, or 180 mg/ml for 500-mg, 1-g, or 2-g vial, respectively. • May further dilute with 50–100 ml 0.9% NaCl or D_5W.

Rate of administration • For IV push, administer over 3–5 min. • For intermittent IV infusion (piggyback), infuse over 20–30 min.

Storage • Solution appears light yellow to amber. IV infusion (piggyback) may darken in color (does not indicate loss of potency). • IV infusion (piggyback) is stable for 24 hrs at room temperature, 5 days if refrigerated. • Discard if precipitate forms.

IM

• Reconstitute with Sterile Water for Injection or Bacteriostatic Water for Injection. • Add 2, 3, or 5 ml to 500-mg, 1-g, or 2-g vial, respectively, providing a concentration of 230 mg/ml, 300 mg/ml, or 330 mg/ml, respectively. • To minimize discomfort, inject deep IM slowly. Less painful if injected into gluteus maximus than lateral aspect of thigh. For 2-g IM dose, give at 2 separate sites.

IV INCOMPATIBILITIES

Allopurinol (Aloprim), filgrastim (Neupogen), fluconazole (Diflucan), hetastarch (Hespan), lipids, pentamidine (Pentam IV), vancomycin (Vancocin).

IV COMPATIBILITIES

Diltiazem (Cardizem), famotidine (Pepcid), hydromorphone (Dilaudid), lorazepam (Ativan), magnesium sulfate, midazolam (Versed), morphine, propofol (Diprivan), total parenteral nutrition (TPN).

C

INDICATIONS/ROUTES/DOSAGE

Usual Dosage Range

IV, IM: ADULTS, ELDERLY: 1–2 g q4–12h. **CHILDREN WEIGHING 50 KG OR MORE:** 1–2 g q4–12h. **CHILDREN 1 MOS–12 YRS WEIGHING LESS THAN 50 KG:** 100–200 mg/kg/day in divided doses q6–8h.

Uncomplicated Infections

IV, IM: ADULTS, ELDERLY: 1 g q12h.

Mild to Moderate Infections

IV, IM: ADULTS, ELDERLY: 1–2 g q8h.

Severe Infections

IV, IM: ADULTS, ELDERLY: 2 g q6–8h.

Life-Threatening Infections

IV, IM: ADULTS, ELDERLY: 2 g q4h. **CHILDREN:** 2 g q4h. **Maximum:** 12 g/day.

Gonorrhea

IM: ADULTS: (Male): 1 g as a single dose. **(Female):** 0.5 g as a single dose.

Perioperative Prophylaxis

IV, IM: ADULTS, ELDERLY: 1 g as a single dose 30–90 min before surgery.

Cesarean Section

IV: ADULTS: 1 g as soon as umbilical cord is clamped, then 1 g 6 and 12 hrs after first dose.

Dosage in Renal Impairment

Creatinine Clearance	Dosage Interval
10–50 ml/min	8–12 hrs
Less than 10 ml/min	24 hrs

SIDE EFFECTS

Frequent: Discomfort with IM administration, oral candidiasis (thrush), mild diarrhea, mild abdominal cramping, vaginal candidiasis. **Occasional:** Nausea, serum sickness-like reaction (fever, joint pain; usually occurs after second course of therapy and resolves after drug is discontinued). **Rare:** Allergic reaction (rash, pruritus, urticaria), thrombophlebitis (pain, redness, swelling at injection site).

ADVERSE EFFECTS/ TOXIC REACTIONS

Antibiotic-associated colitis, other superinfections (abdominal cramps, severe watery diarrhea, fever) may result from altered bacterial balance. Nephrotoxicity may occur, esp. in pts with preexisting renal disease. Pts with a history of allergies, esp. to penicillin, are at increased risk for developing a severe hypersensitivity reaction (severe pruritus, angioedema, bronchospasm, anaphylaxis).

NURSING CONSIDERATIONS

BASELINE ASSESSMENT

Question for history of allergies, particularly cephalosporins, penicillins.

INTERVENTION/EVALUATION

Check IM injection sites for induration, tenderness. Assess oral cavity for white patches on mucous membranes, tongue (thrush). Monitor daily pattern of bowel activity and stool consistency. Mild GI effects may be tolerable (increasing severity may indicate onset of antibiotic-associated colitis). Monitor I&O, renal function tests for nephrotoxicity. Be alert for superinfection: fever, vomiting, diarrhea, anal/genital pruritus, oral mucosal changes (ulceration, pain, erythema).

PATIENT/FAMILY TEACHING

• Discomfort may occur with IM injection. • Doses should be evenly spaced. • Continue antibiotic therapy for full length of treatment.

cefoxitin

sef-**ox**-i-tin

(Apo-Cefoxitin ✤, Mefoxin)

Do not confuse cefoxitin with cefotaxime or Cytoxan, or Mefoxin with Lanoxin.

C

◆CLASSIFICATION

PHARMACOTHERAPEUTIC: Second-generation cephalosporin. **CLINICAL:** Antibiotic (see p. 23C).

ACTION

Binds to bacterial cell membranes, inhibits cell wall synthesis. **Therapeutic Effect:** Bactericidal.

PHARMACOKINETICS

Well distributed. Protein binding: 65%–79%. Primarily excreted unchanged in urine. Removed by hemodialysis. **Half-life:** 0.8–1 hr.

USES

Treatment of susceptible infections due to *S. pneumoniae, S. aureus,* gram-negative enteric bacilli, anaerobes (e.g., bacteroides spp.) including bone, joint, gynecologic, intra-abdominal, lower respiratory, skin/skin structure, UTIs, perioperative prophylaxis.

PRECAUTIONS

Contraindications: History of hypersensitivity/anaphylactic reaction to penicillins, cephalosporins. **Cautions:** Renal impairment, history of GI disease (esp. ulcerative colitis, antibiotic-associated colitis), concurrent use of nephrotoxic medications.

⌛ LIFESPAN CONSIDERATIONS

Pregnancy/Lactation: Readily crosses placenta; distributed in breast milk. **Pregnancy Category B. Children:** No age-related precautions noted. **Elderly:** Age-related renal impairment may require dosage adjustment.

INTERACTIONS

DRUG: **Aminoglycosides, furosemide** may increase risk of nephrotoxicity. **Probenecid** may increase concentration. **HERBAL:** None significant. **FOOD:** None known. **LAB VALUES:** May increase BUN, serum alkaline phosphatase, creatinine, AST, ALT. May cause positive direct/indirect Coombs' test.

AVAILABILITY (Rx)

Injection, Powder for Reconstitution: 1 g, 2 g. **Intravenous Solution:** 1 g/50 ml, 2 g/50 ml.

ADMINISTRATION/HANDLING

◀ALERT▶ Give IM, IV push, intermittent IV infusion (piggyback).

IV

Reconstitution • Reconstitute each 1 g with 10 ml Sterile Water for Injection to provide concentration of 95 mg/ml. • May further dilute with 50–100 ml 0.9% Sterile Water for Injection, NaCl, or D_5W.

Rate of administration • For IV push, administer over 3–5 min. • For intermittent IV infusion (piggyback), infuse over 15–30 min.

Storage • Solution appears colorless to light amber but may darken (does not indicate loss of potency). • IV infusion (piggyback) is stable for 24 hrs at room temperature, 48 hrs if refrigerated. • Discard if precipitate forms.

IM

• Reconstitute each 1 g with 2 ml Sterile Water for Injection or lidocaine to provide concentration of 400 mg/ml. • To minimize discomfort, inject deep IM slowly. Less painful if injected into gluteus maximus than lateral aspect of thigh.

IV INCOMPATIBILITIES

Filgrastim (Neupogen), pentamidine (Pentam IV), vancomycin (Vancocin).

IV COMPATIBILITIES

Diltiazem (Cardizem), famotidine (Pepcid), heparin, hydromorphone (Dilaudid), lipids, magnesium sulfate, morphine, multivitamins, propofol (Diprivan).

INDICATIONS/ROUTES/DOSAGE

Mild to Moderate Infections

IV, IM: ADULTS, ELDERLY: 1–2 g q6–8h.

Severe Infections

IV, IM: ADULTS, ELDERLY: 1 g q4h or 2 g q6–8h up to 2 g q4h.

Perioperative Prophylaxis

IV, IM: ADULTS, ELDERLY: 1–2 g 30–60 min before surgery, then q6h for up to 24 hrs after surgery. **CHILDREN OLDER THAN 3 MOS:** 30–40 mg/kg 30–60 min before surgery, then q6h for up to 24 hrs after surgery.

Usual Pediatric Dosage

CHILDREN OLDER THAN 3 MOS: 80–160 mg/kg/day in 4–6 divided doses. **Maximum:** 12 g/day. **NEONATES:** 90–100 mg/kg/day in divided doses q8h.

Dosage in Renal Impairment

After a loading dose of 1–2 g, dosage and frequency are modified based on creatinine clearance and severity of infection.

Creatinine Clearance	Dosage
30–50 ml/min	1–2 g q8–12h
10–29 ml/min	1–2 g q12–24h
5–9 ml/min	500 mg–1 g q12–24h
Less than 5 ml/min	500 mg–1 g q24–48h

SIDE EFFECTS

Frequent: Discomfort with IM administration, oral candidiasis (thrush), mild diarrhea, mild abdominal cramping, vaginal candidiasis. Occasional: Nausea, serum sickness-like reaction (fever, joint pain; usually occurs after second course of therapy and resolves after drug is discontinued). Rare: Allergic reaction (pruritus, rash, urticaria), thrombophlebitis (pain, redness, swelling at injection site).

ADVERSE EFFECTS/ TOXIC REACTIONS

Antibiotic-associated colitis, other superinfections (abdominal cramps, severe watery diarrhea, fever) may result from altered bacterial balance. Nephrotoxicity may occur, esp. in pts with preexisting renal disease. Pts with a history of allergies, esp. to penicillin, are at increased risk for developing a severe hypersensitivity reaction (severe pruritus, angioedema, bronchospasm, anaphylaxis).

NURSING CONSIDERATIONS

BASELINE ASSESSMENT

Question for history of allergies, particularly cephalosporins, penicillins.

INTERVENTION/EVALUATION

Evaluate IV site for phlebitis (heat, pain, red streaking over vein). Assess IM injection sites for induration, tenderness. Assess oral cavity for white patches on mucous membranes, tongue (thrush). Monitor daily pattern of bowel activity and stool consistency. Mild GI effects may be tolerable (increasing severity may indicate onset of antibiotic-associated colitis). Monitor I&O, renal function tests for nephrotoxicity. Be alert for superinfection: fever, vomiting, diarrhea, anal/genital pruritus, oral mucosal changes (ulceration, pain, erythema).

PATIENT/FAMILY TEACHING

• Discomfort may occur with IM injection. • Doses should be evenly spaced. • Continue antibiotic therapy for full length of treatment.

cefpodoxime

seff-poh-**dox**-eem
(Vantin)
Do not confuse Vantin with Ventolin.

CLASSIFICATION

PHARMACOTHERAPEUTIC: Third-generation cephalosporin. **CLINICAL:** Antibiotic (see p. 24C).

ACTION

Binds to bacterial cell membranes, inhibits cell wall synthesis. Therapeutic Effect: Bactericidal.

PHARMACOKINETICS

Well absorbed from GI tract (food increases absorption). Protein binding: 18%–23%. Widely distributed. Primarily excreted unchanged in urine. Partially removed by hemodialysis. **Half-life:** 2.3 hrs (increased in renal impairment, elderly pts).

C

USES

Treatment of susceptible infections due to *S. pneumoniae, S. pyogenes, S. aureus, H. influenzae, M. catarrhalis, E. coli, Proteus, Klebsiella* spp., including acute maxillary sinusitis, chronic bronchitis, community-acquired pneumonia, gonorrhea, otitis media, pharyngitis, tonsillitis, skin/skin structure, UTIs.

PRECAUTIONS

Contraindications: History of hypersensitivity/anaphylactic reaction to penicillins, cephalosporins. **Cautions:** Renal impairment, history of GI disease (esp. ulcerative colitis, antibiotic-associated colitis), concurrent use of nephrotoxic medications.

LIFESPAN CONSIDERATIONS

Pregnancy/Lactation: Readily crosses placenta. Distributed in breast milk. **Pregnancy Category B. Children:** Safety and efficacy not established in those younger than 6 mos. **Elderly:** Age-related renal impairment may require dosage adjustment.

INTERACTIONS

DRUG: **Antacids containing aluminum, H_2 antagonists, magnesium** may decrease absorption. **Aminoglycosides, furosemide** may increase risk of nephrotoxicity. **Probenecid** may increase concentration. **HERBAL:** None significant. **FOOD:** **Food** enhances absorption. **LAB VALUES:** May increase BUN, serum alkaline phosphatase, bilirubin, creatinine, LDH, AST, ALT. May cause positive direct/indirect Coombs' test.

AVAILABILITY (Rx)

Oral Suspension: 50 mg/5 ml, 100 mg/5 ml. **Tablets:** 100 mg, 200 mg.

ADMINISTRATION/HANDLING

PO

• Administer tablet with food (enhances absorption). • Administer suspension without regard to food. • After reconstitution, oral suspension is stable for 14 days if refrigerated.

INDICATIONS/ROUTES/DOSAGE

Usual Dosage Range

PO: ADULTS, ELDERLY, CHILDREN OLDER THAN 12 YRS: 100–400 mg q12h. **CHILDREN 2 MOS–12 YRS:** 10 mg/kg/day in 2 divided doses. **Maximum:** 400 mg/day.

Chronic Bronchitis, Pneumonia

PO: ADULTS, ELDERLY, CHILDREN OLDER THAN 12 YRS: 200 mg q12h for 10–14 days.

Gonorrhea, Rectal Gonococcal Infection (Female Pts Only)

PO: ADULTS, CHILDREN OLDER THAN 12 YRS: 200 mg as a single dose.

Skin/Skin Structure Infections

PO: ADULTS, ELDERLY, CHILDREN OLDER THAN 13 YRS: 400 mg q12h for 7–14 days.

Pharyngitis, Tonsillitis

PO: ADULTS, ELDERLY, CHILDREN OLDER THAN 13 YRS: 100 mg q12h for 5–10 days. **CHILDREN 6 MOS–13 YRS:** 5 mg/kg q12h for 5–10 days. **Maximum:** 100 mg/dose.

Acute Maxillary Sinusitis

PO: ADULTS, CHILDREN OLDER THAN 13 YRS: 200 mg q12h for 10 days. **CHILDREN 2 MOS–13 YRS:** 5 mg/kg q12h for 10 days. **Maximum:** 200 mg/dose.

UTI

PO: ADULTS, ELDERLY, CHILDREN OLDER THAN 13 YRS: 100 mg q12h for 7 days.

Acute Otitis Media

PO: CHILDREN 6 MOS–13 YRS: 5 mg/kg q12h for 5 days. **Maximum:** 400 mg/dose.

Dosage in Renal Impairment

For pts with creatinine clearance less than 30 ml/min, usual dose is given q24h. For pts on hemodialysis, usual dose is given 3 times a wk after dialysis.

SIDE EFFECTS

Frequent: Oral candidiasis (thrush), mild diarrhea, mild abdominal cramping, vaginal candidiasis. **Occasional:** Nausea, serum sickness-like reaction (fever, joint pain; usually occurs after second course of therapy and resolves after drug is discontinued). **Rare:** Allergic reaction (pruritus, rash, urticaria).

ADVERSE EFFECTS/ TOXIC REACTIONS

Antibiotic-associated colitis, other superinfections (abdominal cramps, severe watery diarrhea, fever) may result from altered bacterial balance. Nephrotoxicity may occur, esp. in pts with preexisting renal disease. Pts with a history of allergies, esp. to penicillin, are at increased risk for developing a severe hypersensitivity reaction (severe pruritus, angioedema, bronchospasm, anaphylaxis).

NURSING CONSIDERATIONS

BASELINE ASSESSMENT

Question for history of allergies, particularly cephalosporins, penicillins.

INTERVENTION/EVALUATION

Assess oral cavity for white patches on mucous membranes, tongue (thrush). Monitor daily pattern of bowel activity and stool consistency. Mild GI effects may be tolerable (increasing severity may indicate onset of antibiotic-associated colitis). Monitor I&O, renal function tests for nephrotoxicity. Be alert for superinfection: fever, vomiting, diarrhea, anal/genital pruritus, oral mucosal changes (ulceration, pain, erythema).

PATIENT/FAMILY TEACHING

• Doses should be evenly spaced. • Shake oral suspension well before using. • Continue antibiotic therapy for full length of treatment. • Refrigerate oral suspension. • Notify physician if persistent diarrhea occurs.

cefprozil

sef-**pro**-zill

(Apo-Cefprozil ✤, Cefzil)

Do not confuse cefprozil with cefazolin, or Cefzil with Cefol, Ceftin, or Kefzol.

◆CLASSIFICATION

PHARMACOTHERAPEUTIC: Second-generation cephalosporin. **CLINICAL:** Antibiotic (see p. 23C).

ACTION

Binds to bacterial cell membranes, inhibits cell wall synthesis. **Therapeutic Effect:** Bactericidal.

PHARMACOKINETICS

Well absorbed from GI tract. Protein binding: 36%–45%. Widely distributed. Primarily excreted unchanged in urine. Moderately removed by hemodialysis. **Half-life:** 1.3 hrs (increased in renal impairment).

USES

Treatment of susceptible infections due to *S. pneumoniae, S. pyogenes, S. aureus, H. influenzae, M. catarrhalis* including pharyngitis, tonsillitis, otitis media, secondary bacterial infection of acute bronchitis, acute bacterial exacerbation of chronic bronchitis, uncomplicated skin/skin structure infections, acute sinusitis.

C

PRECAUTIONS

Contraindications: History of hypersensitivity/anaphylactic reaction to penicillins, cephalosporins. Cautions: Renal impairment, history of GI disease (esp. ulcerative colitis, antibiotic-associated colitis), concurrent use of nephrotoxic medications.

⌛ LIFESPAN CONSIDERATIONS

Pregnancy/Lactation: Readily crosses placenta. Distributed in breast milk. **Pregnancy Category B. Children:** Safety and efficacy not established in those younger than 6 mos. **Elderly:** Age-related renal impairment may require dosage adjustment.

INTERACTIONS

DRUG: **Aminoglycosides, furosemide** may increase risk of nephrotoxicity. **Probenecid** may increase concentration. HERBAL: None significant. FOOD: None known. LAB VALUES: May cause positive direct/indirect Coombs' test. May increase serum alkaline phosphatase, AST, ALT.

AVAILABILITY (Rx)

Oral Suspension: 125 mg/5 ml, 250 mg/5 ml. Tablets: 250 mg, 500 mg.

ADMINISTRATION/HANDLING

PO

• After reconstitution, oral suspension is stable for 14 days if refrigerated. • Shake oral suspension well before using. • Give without regard to food; if GI upset occurs, give with food, milk.

INDICATIONS/ROUTES/DOSAGE

Usual Dosage Range

PO: ADULTS, ELDERLY, CHILDREN OLDER THAN 12 YRS: 250–500 mg q12h or 500 mg q24h. **CHILDREN OLDER THAN 6 MOS–12 YRS:** 7.5–15 mg/kg/day in 2 divided doses.

Pharyngitis, Tonsillitis

PO: ADULTS, ELDERLY: 500 mg q24h for 10 days. **CHILDREN 2–12 YRS:** 7.5 mg/kg q12h for 10 days. **Maximum:** 1 g/day.

Acute Bacterial Exacerbation of Chronic Bronchitis, Secondary Bacterial Infection of Acute Bronchitis

PO: ADULTS, ELDERLY: 500 mg q12h for 10 days.

Skin/Skin Structure Infections

PO: ADULTS, ELDERLY, CHILDREN OLDER THAN 12 YRS: 250–500 mg q12h for 10 days. **CHILDREN 2–12 YRS:** 20 mg/kg q24h for 10 days. **Maximum:** 1 g/day.

Acute Sinusitis

PO: ADULTS, ELDERLY: 250–500 mg q12h for 10 days. **CHILDREN 6 MOS–12 YRS:** 7.5–15 mg/kg q12h for 10 days.

Otitis Media

PO: CHILDREN 6 MOS–12 YRS: 15 mg/kg q12h for 10 days. **Maximum:** 1 g/day.

Dosage in Renal Impairment

Creatinine clearance less than 30 ml/min: 50% of usual dose at usual interval.

SIDE EFFECTS

Frequent: Oral candidiasis (thrush), mild diarrhea, mild abdominal cramping, vaginal candidiasis. Occasional: Nausea, serum sickness reaction (fever, joint pain; usually occurs after second course of therapy and resolves after drug is discontinued). Rare: Allergic reaction (pruritus, rash, urticaria).

ADVERSE EFFECTS/ TOXIC REACTIONS

Antibiotic-associated colitis, other superinfections (abdominal cramps, severe watery diarrhea, fever) may result from altered bacterial balance. Nephrotoxicity may occur, esp. in pts with preexisting renal disease. Pts with a history of allergies, esp. to penicillin, are at increased risk for developing a severe hypersensitivity reaction (severe pruritus, angioedema, bronchospasm, anaphylaxis).

NURSING CONSIDERATIONS

BASELINE ASSESSMENT

Question for history of allergies, particularly cephalosporins, penicillins.

INTERVENTION/EVALUATION

Assess oral cavity for evidence of stomatitis. Monitor daily pattern of bowel activity and stool consistency. Mild GI effects may be tolerable (but increasing severity may indicate onset of antibiotic-associated colitis). Monitor I&O, renal function tests for nephrotoxicity. Be alert for superinfection: fever, vomiting, diarrhea, anal/genital pruritus, oral mucosal changes (ulceration, pain, erythema).

PATIENT/FAMILY TEACHING

• Doses should be evenly spaced. • Continue antibiotic therapy for full length of treatment. • May cause GI upset (may take with food or milk). • Notify physician if persistent diarrhea occurs.

ceftaroline

cef-**tear**-oh-leem
(Teflaro)

◆CLASSIFICATION

PHARMACOTHERAPEUTIC: Fifth-generation cephalosporin. **CLINICAL:** Antibiotic.

ACTION

Binds to bacterial cell membranes, inhibits cell wall synthesis. **Therapeutic Effect:** Bactericidal.

PHARMACOKINETICS

Protein binding: 20%. Widely distributed in plasma. Not metabolized. Primarily excreted unchanged in urine. Hemodialyzable. **Half-life:** 1.6 hrs (increased in renal impairment).

USES

Treatment of susceptible infections due to gram positive and gram negative organisms including *S. pneumoniae, S. aureus* (methicillin susceptible only), *H. influenzae, Klebsiella pneumoniae, E. coli* including acute bacterial skin and skin structure infections, community-acquired bacterial pneumonia.

PRECAUTIONS

Contraindications: History of anaphylactic reaction to penicillins, hypersensitivity to cephalosporins. **Cautions:** Concurrent use of nephrotoxic medications, history of allergies or GI disease (especially ulcerative colitis, antibiotic-associated colitis), renal impairment with creatinine clearance less than 20 ml/min.

⌛ LIFESPAN CONSIDERATIONS

Pregnancy/Lactation: Unknown if distributed in breast milk. **Pregnancy Category B. Children:** Safety and efficacy not established in those younger than 18 yrs. **Elderly:** Age-related renal impairment may require dose adjustment.

INTERACTIONS

DRUG: Aminoglycosides may increase risk of nephrotoxicity. **HERBAL:** None significant. **FOOD:** None known. **LAB VALUES:** May cause positive direct/indirect Coombs' test. May increase BUN, serum creatinine. May decrease serum potassium.

AVAILABILITY (Rx)

Injection, Powder for Reconstitution: 400-mg, 600-mg single-use vial.

ADMINISTRATION/HANDLING

◀ALERT▶ Give by intermittent IV infusion (piggyback). Do not give IV push.

Reconstitution • Reconstitute either 400-mg or 600-mg vial with 20 ml Sterile Water for Injection. • Mix gently to dissolve powder. • Further dilute with 250 ml D_5W, $D_{2.5}W$, 0.9% NaCl, or 0.45% NaCl to provide concentration of 20 mg/ml for 400-mg dose or 30 mg/ml for 600-mg dose.

Rate of administration • Infuse over 60 min.

Storage • Discard if particulate is present. • Following reconstitution, solution should appear clear, light to dark yellow. • Solution is stable for 6 hrs at room temperature or 72 hrs if refrigerated.

IV INCOMPATIBILITIES

Fluconazole (Diflucan), lipids, vancomycin (Vancomycin).

IV COMPATIBILITIES

Famotidine (Pepcid), hydromorphone (Dilaudid), lorazepam (Ativan), magnesium sulfate, midazolam (Versed), morphine, propofol (Diprivan) total parenteral nutrition (TPN).

INDICATIONS/ROUTES/DOSAGE

Acute Bacterial Skin/Skin Structure Infections

IV INFUSION: ADULTS, ELDERLY: 600 mg every 12 hrs for 5–14 days.

Community-Acquired Bacterial Pneumonia

IV INFUSION: ADULTS, ELDERLY: 600 mg every 12 hrs for 5–7 days.

Dosage in Renal Impairment

Creatinine Clearance	Dosage
30–50 ml/min	400 mg q12h
15–29 ml/min	300 mg q12h
End-stage renal disease, hemodialysis	200 mg every 12 hrs

SIDE EFFECTS

Occasional (5%–4%): Diarrhea, nausea. **Rare (3%–2%):** Allergic reaction (rash, pruritus, urticaria), phlebitis.

ADVERSE EFFECTS/ TOXIC REACTIONS

Antibiotic-associated colitis, other super infections (abdominal cramps, severe watery diarrhea, fever) may result from altered bacterial balance. Nephrotoxicity may occur, esp. with preexisting renal disease. Pts with a history of allergies, esp. to penicillin, are at increased risk for developing a severe hypersensitivity reaction (severe pruritus, angioedema, bronchospasm, anaphylaxis.

NURSING CONSIDERATIONS

BASELINE ASSESSMENT

Question for hypersensitivity to other cephalosporins, penicillins. For those on hemodialysis, administer medication after dialysis.

INTERVENTION/EVALUATION

Assess oral cavity for white patches on mucous membranes, tongue. Monitor daily pattern of bowel activity and stool consistency. Mild GI effects may be tolerable, but increasing severity may indicate onset of antibiotic-associated colitis. Monitor I&O, renal function tests for evidence of nephrotoxicity. Be alert for superinfection: fever, vomiting, severe genital/anal pruritus, moderate to severe diarrhea, oral mucosal changes (ulceration, pain, erythema).

PATIENT/FAMILY TEACHING

• Continue medication for full length of treatment. • Doses should be evenly spaced.

ceftazidime

sef-**taz**-ih-deem
(Fortaz, Tazicef)

Do not confuse ceftazidime with cefepime or ceftizoxime.

◆CLASSIFICATION

PHARMACOTHERAPEUTIC: Third-generation cephalosporin. **CLINICAL:** Antibiotic (see p. 24C).

ACTION

Binds to bacterial cell membranes, inhibits cell wall synthesis. **Therapeutic Effect:** Bactericidal.

PHARMACOKINETICS

Widely distributed including to CSF. Protein binding: 5%–17%. Primarily excreted unchanged in urine. Removed by hemodialysis. **Half-life:** 2 hrs (increased in renal impairment).

USES

Treatment of susceptible infections due to gram-negative organisms including *Pseudomonas* and *Enterobacteriaceae* including bone, joint, CNS (including meningitis), gynecologic, intra-abdominal, lower respiratory tract, skin/skin structure, UTIs, septicemia. Treatment of CNS infections due to *H. influenzae, N. meningitidis,* including meningitis.

PRECAUTIONS

Contraindications: History of hypersensitivity/anaphylactic reaction to penicillins, cephalosporins. **Cautions:** Renal impairment, history of GI disease (esp. ulcerative colitis, antibiotic-associated colitis), concurrent use of nephrotoxic medications.

LIFESPAN CONSIDERATIONS

Pregnancy/Lactation: Readily crosses placenta. Distributed in breast milk. **Pregnancy Category B. Children:** No age-related precautions noted. **Elderly:** Age-related renal impairment may require dosage adjustment.

INTERACTIONS

DRUG: Aminoglycosides, furosemide may increase risk of nephrotoxicity. **HERBAL:** None significant. **FOOD:** None known. **LAB VALUES:** May increase BUN, serum alkaline phosphatase, creatinine, LDH, AST, ALT. May cause positive direct/indirect Coombs' test.

AVAILABILITY (Rx)

Injection, Powder for Reconstitution (Fortaz, Tazicef): 500 mg, 1 g, 2 g.

ADMINISTRATION/HANDLING

ALERT Give by IM injection, direct IV injection (IV push), or intermittent IV infusion (piggyback).

IV

Reconstitution • Add 10 ml Sterile Water for Injection to each 1 g to provide concentration of 90 mg/ml. • May further dilute with 50–100 ml 0.9% NaCl, D_5W or other compatible diluent.

Rate of administration • For IV push, administer over 3–5 min (**maximum concentration:** 180 mg/ml). • For intermittent IV infusion (piggyback), infuse over 15–30 min.

Storage • Solution appears light yellow to amber, tends to darken (color change does not indicate loss of potency). • IV infusion (piggyback) stable for 12 hrs at room temperature or 3 days if refrigerated. • Discard if precipitate forms.

IM

• For reconstitution, add 1.5 ml Sterile Water for Injection or lidocaine 1% to 500-mg vial or 3 ml to 1-g vial to provide a concentration of 280 mg/ml. • To minimize discomfort, inject deep IM slowly. Less painful if injected into gluteus maximus than lateral aspect of thigh.

IV INCOMPATIBILITIES

Amphotericin B complex (Abelcet, AmBisome, Amphotec), doxorubicin liposomal (Doxil), fluconazole (Diflucan), idarubicin (Idamycin), midazolam (Versed), pentamidine (Pentam IV), total parenteral nutrition (TPN), vancomycin (Vancocin).

IV COMPATIBILITIES

Diltiazem (Cardizem), famotidine (Pepcid), heparin, hydromorphone (Dilaudid), lipids, morphine, propofol (Diprivan).

INDICATIONS/ROUTES/DOSAGE

Usual Dosage Range

ADULTS, ELDERLY: 500 mg–2 g q8–12h. **CHILDREN 1 MO–12 YRS:** 100–150 mg/kg/day in divided doses q8h. **Maximum:**

6 g/day. **NEONATES 0–4 WKS:** 100–150 mg/kg/day in divided doses q8–12h.

C

UTI

IV, IM: ADULTS: 250–500 mg q8–12h.

Mild to Moderate Infections

IV, IM: ADULTS: 1 g q8–12h.

Uncomplicated Pneumonia, Skin/Skin Structure Infections

IV, IM: ADULTS: 0.5–1 g q8h.

Bone, Joint Infections

IV, IM: ADULTS: 2 g q12h.

Meningitis, Serious Gynecologic and Intra-Abdominal Infections

IV, IM: ADULTS: 2 g q8h.

Pseudomonal Pulmonary Infections in Pts with Cystic Fibrosis

IV: ADULTS: 30–50 mg/kg q8h. **Maximum:** 6 g/day.

Usual Elderly Dosage

ELDERLY (NORMAL RENAL FUNCTION): 500 mg–1 g q12h.

Dosage in Renal Impairment

After initial 1-g dose, dosage and frequency are modified based on creatinine clearance and severity of infection.

Creatinine Clearance	Dosage
31–50 ml/min	q12h
10–30 ml/min	q24h
Less than 10 ml/min	q48–72h

SIDE EFFECTS

Frequent: Discomfort with IM administration, oral candidiasis (thrush), mild diarrhea, mild abdominal cramping, vaginal candidiasis. **Occasional:** Nausea, serum sickness-like reaction (fever, joint pain; usually occurs after second course of therapy and resolves after drug is discontinued). **Rare:** Allergic reaction (pruritus, rash, urticaria), thrombophlebitis (pain, redness, swelling at injection site).

ADVERSE EFFECTS/ TOXIC REACTIONS

Antibiotic-associated colitis, other superinfections (abdominal cramps, severe watery diarrhea, fever) may result from altered bacterial balance. Nephrotoxicity may occur, esp. in pts with preexisting renal disease. Pts with a history of allergies, esp. to penicillin, are at increased risk for developing a severe hypersensitivity reaction (severe pruritus, angioedema, bronchospasm, anaphylaxis).

NURSING CONSIDERATIONS

BASELINE ASSESSMENT

Question for history of allergies, particularly cephalosporins, penicillins.

INTERVENTION/EVALUATION

Evaluate IV site for phlebitis (heat, pain, red streaking over vein). Assess IM injection sites for induration, tenderness. Check oral cavity for white patches on mucous membranes, tongue (thrush). Monitor daily pattern of bowel activity and stool consistency. Mild GI effects may be tolerable (increasing severity may indicate onset of antibiotic-associated colitis). Monitor I&O, renal function tests for nephrotoxicity. Be alert for superinfection: fever, vomiting, diarrhea, anal/genital pruritus, oral mucosal changes (ulceration, pain, erythema).

PATIENT/FAMILY TEACHING

• Discomfort may occur with IM injection. • Doses should be evenly spaced. • Continue antibiotic therapy for full length of treatment.

ceftibuten

sef-tih-**byew**-ten

(Cedax)

◆CLASSIFICATION

PHARMACOTHERAPEUTIC: Third-generation cephalosporin. **CLINICAL:** Antibiotic (see p. 24C).

ACTION

Binds to bacterial cell membranes, inhibits cell wall synthesis. Therapeutic Effect: Bactericidal.

PHARMACOKINETICS

Rapidly absorbed from GI tract. Protein binding: 65%–77%. Excreted primarily unchanged in urine. Half-life: 2–3 hrs.

USES

Treatment of susceptible infections due to *S. pneumoniae, S. pyogenes, H. influenzae, M. catarrhalis* including chronic bronchitis, acute bacterial otitis media, pharyngitis, tonsillitis.

PRECAUTIONS

Contraindications: History of anaphylactic reaction to penicillins, hypersensitivity to cephalosporins. Cautions: Hypersensitivity to penicillins, other drugs, history of GI disease (e.g., colitis), renal impairment.

LIFESPAN CONSIDERATIONS

Pregnancy/Lactation: Unknown if drug crosses placenta or is distributed in breast milk. **Pregnancy Category B. Children:** Safety and efficacy not established in those younger than 6 mos. **Elderly:** Age-related renal impairment may require dosage adjustment.

INTERACTIONS

DRUG: **Aminoglycosides** may increase risk of nephrotoxicity. **Probenecid** may increase concentration. HERBAL: None significant. FOOD: None known. LAB VALUES: May increase BUN, serum alkaline phosphatase, bilirubin, creatinine, LDH, AST, ALT. May cause positive direct/indirect Coombs' test.

AVAILABILITY (Rx)

Capsules: 400 mg. Oral Suspension: 90 mg/5 ml.

ADMINISTRATION/HANDLING

Capsules: Administer without regard to food. Suspension: Shake well, give 2 hrs before or 1 hr after meals.

INDICATIONS/ROUTES/DOSAGE

Chronic Bronchitis

PO: ADULTS, ELDERLY: 400 mg/day once a day for 10 days.

Pharyngitis, Tonsillitis

PO: ADULTS, ELDERLY: 400 mg once a day for 10 days. **CHILDREN OLDER THAN 6 MOS:** 9 mg/kg once a day for 10 days. **Maximum:** 400 mg/day.

Otitis Media

PO: CHILDREN OLDER THAN 6 MOS: 9 mg/kg once a day for 10 days. **Maximum:** 400 mg/day.

Dosage in Renal Impairment

Dosage is modified based on creatinine clearance.

Creatinine Clearance	Dosage
50 ml/min and higher	400 mg or 9 mg/kg q24h
30–49 ml/min	200 mg or 4.5 mg/kg q24h
Less than 30 ml/min	100 mg or 2.25 mg/kg q24h

SIDE EFFECTS

Frequent: Oral candidiasis (thrush), mild diarrhea (discharge, itching). Occasional: Nausea, serum sickness-like reaction (fever, joint pain; usually occurs after second course of therapy and resolves after drug is discontinued). Rare: Allergic reaction (rash, pruritus, urticaria).

ADVERSE EFFECTS/TOXIC REACTIONS

Antibiotic-associated colitis, other superinfections (abdominal cramps, severe watery diarrhea, fever) may result from altered bacterial balance. Nephrotoxicity may occur, esp. in pts with preexisting renal disease. Pts with a history of allergies, esp. to penicillin, are at increased risk for developing a severe hypersensitivity reaction (severe pruritus, angioedema, bronchospasm, anaphylaxis).

C

NURSING CONSIDERATIONS

BASELINE ASSESSMENT

Question for history of allergies, particularly cephalosporins, penicillins.

INTERVENTION/EVALUATION

Assess oral cavity for white patches on mucous membranes, tongue (thrush). Monitor daily pattern of bowel activity and stool consistency. Mild GI effects may be tolerable (increasing severity may indicate onset of antibiotic-associated colitis). Monitor I&O, serum renal function tests for nephrotoxicity. Be alert for superinfection: fever, vomiting, diarrhea, anal/genital pruritus, oral mucosal changes (ulceration, pain, erythema).

PATIENT/FAMILY TEACHING

• Continue medication for full length of treatment; do not skip doses. • May cause GI upset (may take with food or milk). • Notify physician if persistent diarrhea occurs.

Ceftin, *see cefuroxime*

ceftriaxone

sef-try-**ax**-zone
(Rocephin)
Do not confuse ceftriaxone with cefazolin.

◆CLASSIFICATION

PHARMACOTHERAPEUTIC: Third-generation cephalosporin. **CLINICAL:** Antibiotic (see p. 24C).

ACTION

Binds to bacterial cell membranes, inhibits cell wall synthesis. **Therapeutic Effect:** Bactericidal.

PHARMACOKINETICS

Widely distributed including to CSF. Protein binding: 83%–96%. Primarily excreted unchanged in urine. Not removed by hemodialysis. **Half-life: IV:** 4.3–4.6 hrs; **IM:** 5.8–8.7 hrs (increased in renal impairment).

USES

Treatment of susceptible infections due to gram-negative aerobic organisms, some gram-positive organisms including respiratory tract, GU tract, skin, bone, intra-abdominal, biliary tract infections; septicemia; meningitis; gonorrhea; Lyme disease; acute bacterial otitis media.

PRECAUTIONS

Contraindications: History of hypersensitivity/anaphylactic reaction to penicillins, cephalosporins. Hyperbilirubinemic neonates, esp. premature infants, should not be treated with ceftriaxone (can displace bilirubin from its binding to serum albumin, causing bilirubin encephalopathy). Ceftriaxone must not be co-administered with calcium-containing IV solutions, including continuous calcium-containing infusion such as parenteral nutrition, in neonates due to the risk of precipitation of ceftriaxone-calcium salt. **Cautions:** Renal/hepatic impairment, history of GI disease (esp. ulcerative colitis, antibiotic-associated colitis), concurrent administration of nephrotoxic medications.

⌛ LIFESPAN CONSIDERATIONS

Pregnancy/Lactation: Readily crosses placenta. Distributed in breast milk. **Pregnancy Category B. Children:** May displace bilirubin from serum albumin. Caution in hyperbilirubinemic neonates. **Elderly:** Age-related renal impairment may require dosage adjustment.

INTERACTIONS

DRUG: **Probenecid** may increase excretion. **HERBAL:** None significant. **FOOD:** None known. **LAB VALUES:** May increase BUN, serum alkaline phosphatase, bilirubin, creatinine, LDH, AST,

ALT. May cause positive direct/indirect Coombs' test.

AVAILABILITY (Rx)

Injection, Powder for Reconstitution (Rocephin): 250 mg, 500 mg, 1 g, 2 g. **Intravenous Solution (Rocephin):** 1 g/50 ml, 2 g/50 ml.

ADMINISTRATION/HANDLING

IV

Reconstitution • Add 2.4 ml Sterile Water for Injection to each 250 mg to provide concentration of 100 mg/ml. • May further dilute with 50–100 ml 0.9% NaCl, D_5W.

Rate of administration • For IV push, administer over 2–4 min (**maximum concentration:** 40 mg/ml). • For intermittent IV infusion (piggyback), infuse over 15–30 min for adults, 10–30 min in children, neonates. • Alternating IV sites, use large veins to reduce potential for phlebitis.

Storage • Solution appears light yellow to amber. • IV infusion (piggyback) is stable for 3 days at room temperature, 10 days if refrigerated. • Discard if precipitate forms.

IM

• Add 0.9 ml Sterile Water for Injection, 0.9% NaCl, D_5W, or lidocaine to each 250 mg to provide concentration of 250 mg/ml. • To minimize discomfort, inject deep IM slowly. Less painful if injected into gluteus maximus than lateral aspect of thigh.

IV INCOMPATIBILITIES

Aminophylline, amphotericin B complex (Abelcet, AmBisome, Amphotec), famotidine (Pepcid), filgrastim (Neupogen), fluconazole (Diflucan), labetalol (Normodyne), pentamidine (Pentam IV), vancomycin (Vancocin).

IV COMPATIBILITIES

Diltiazem (Cardizem), heparin, lidocaine, lipids, metronidazole (Flagyl), morphine, propofol (Diprivan), total parenteral nutrition (TPN).

INDICATIONS/ROUTES/DOSAGE

Usual Dosage Range

IM/IV: ADULTS, ELDERLY: 1–2 g q12–24h. **CHILDREN:** 50–100 mg/kg/day in 1–2 divided doses.

Mild to Moderate Infections

IV, IM: ADULTS, ELDERLY: 1–2 g as a single dose or in 2 divided doses. **CHILDREN:** 50–75 mg/kg/day in 1–2 divided doses q12–24h. **Maximum:** 2 g/day.

Serious Infections

IV, IM: ADULTS, ELDERLY: Up to 4 g/day in 2 divided doses. **CHILDREN:** 80–100 mg/kg/day in divided doses q12h. **Maximum:** 4 g/day.

Meningitis

IV: CHILDREN: Initially, 75–100 mg/kg, then 100 mg/kg/day as a single dose or in divided doses q12h. **Maximum:** 4 g/day.

Lyme Disease

IV: ADULTS, ELDERLY: 2 g a day for 10–14 days.

Acute Bacterial Otitis Media

IM: CHILDREN: 50 mg/kg once. **Maximum:** 1 g/day.

Perioperative Prophylaxis

IV, IM: ADULTS, ELDERLY: 1 g 0.5–2 hrs before surgery.

Uncomplicated Gonorrhea

IM: ADULTS: 125–250 mg plus doxycycline one time.

Dosage in Renal Impairment

Dosage modification is usually unnecessary but hepatic/renal function test results should be monitored in those with renal and hepatic impairment or severe renal impairment.

SIDE EFFECTS

Frequent: Discomfort with IM administration, oral candidiasis (thrush), mild diarrhea, mild abdominal cramping, vaginal candidiasis. **Occasional:** Nausea, serum sickness-like reaction (fever, joint pain; usually occurs after second course of therapy and resolves after drug is discontinued). Rare: Allergic reaction (rash, pruritus, urticaria), thrombophlebitis (pain, redness, swelling at injection site).

ADVERSE EFFECTS/ TOXIC REACTIONS

Antibiotic-associated colitis, other superinfections (abdominal cramps, severe watery diarrhea, fever) may result from altered bacterial balance. Nephrotoxicity may occur, esp. in pts with preexisting renal disease. Pts with a history of allergies, esp. to penicillin, are at increased risk for developing a severe hypersensitivity reaction (severe pruritus, angioedema, bronchospasm, anaphylaxis).

NURSING CONSIDERATIONS

BASELINE ASSESSMENT

Question for history of allergies, particularly cephalosporins, penicillins.

INTERVENTION/EVALUATION

Assess oral cavity for white patches on mucous membranes, tongue (thrush). Monitor daily pattern of bowel activity and stool consistency. Mild GI effects may be tolerable (increasing severity may indicate onset of antibiotic-associated colitis). Monitor I&O, renal function tests for nephrotoxicity, CBC. Be alert for superinfection: fever, vomiting, diarrhea, anal/genital pruritus, oral mucosal changes (ulceration, pain, erythema).

PATIENT/FAMILY TEACHING

• Discomfort may occur with IM injection. • Doses should be evenly spaced. • Continue antibiotic therapy for full length of treatment.

cefuroxime axetil

sef-yur-ox-ime
(Apo-Cefuroxime 🍁, Ceftin)

Do not confuse Ceftin with Cefzil or Cipro, cefuroxime with cefotaxime, cefprozil, or deferoxamine, or Zinacef with Zithromax.

cefuroxime sodium

(Zinacef)

◆ CLASSIFICATION

PHARMACOTHERAPEUTIC: Second-generation cephalosporin. **CLINICAL:** Antibiotic (see p. 23C).

ACTION

Binds to bacterial cell membranes, inhibits cell wall synthesis. **Therapeutic Effect:** Bactericidal.

PHARMACOKINETICS

Rapidly absorbed from GI tract. Protein binding: 33%–50%. Widely distributed including to CSF. Primarily excreted unchanged in urine. Moderately removed by hemodialysis. **Half-life:** 1.3 hrs (increased in renal impairment).

USES

Treatment of susceptible infections due to group B streptococci, pneumococci, staphylococci, *H. influenzae, E. coli, Enterobacter, Klebsiella* including acute/chronic bronchitis, gonorrhea, impetigo, early Lyme disease, otitis media, pharyngitis/tonsillitis, sinusitis, skin/skin structure, UTIs.

PRECAUTIONS

Contraindications: History of anaphylactic reaction to penicillins, hypersensitivity to cephalosporins. **Cautions:** Renal impairment, history of GI disease (esp. ulcerative colitis, antibiotic-associated colitis), concurrent use of nephrotoxic medications.

⌛ LIFESPAN CONSIDERATIONS

Pregnancy/Lactation: Readily crosses placenta. Distributed in breast milk. **Pregnancy Category B. Children:** No age-related precautions noted. **Elderly:** Age-related renal impairment may require dosage adjustment.

INTERACTIONS

DRUG: **Aminoglycosides, furosemide** may increase risk of nephrotoxicity. **Probenecid** may increase concentration. HERBAL: None significant. FOOD: None known. LAB VALUES: May increase serum alkaline phosphatase, bilirubin, LDH, AST, ALT. May cause positive direct/indirect Coombs' test.

AVAILABILITY (Rx)

Injection, Powder for Reconstitution: 750 mg, 1.5 g. Injection, Solution: 750 mg/50 ml, 1.5 g/50 ml. Oral Suspension (Ceftin): 125 mg/5 ml, 250 mg/5 ml. Tablets (Ceftin): 250 mg, 500 mg.

ADMINISTRATION/HANDLING

IV

Reconstitution • Reconstitute 750 mg in 8 ml (1.5 g in 14 ml) Sterile Water for Injection to provide a concentration of 100 mg/ml. • For intermittent IV infusion (piggyback), further dilute with 50–100 ml 0.9% NaCl or D_5W.

Rate of administration • For IV push, administer over 3–5 min. • For intermittent IV infusion (piggyback), infuse over 15–30 min.

Storage • Solution appears light yellow to amber (may darken, but color change does not indicate loss of potency). • IV infusion (piggyback) is stable for 24 hrs at room temperature, 48 hrs if refrigerated. • Discard if precipitate forms.

IM

• To minimize discomfort, inject deep IM slowly. Less painful if injected into gluteus maximus than lateral aspect of thigh.

PO

• Give tablets without regard to food (Give 400-mg dose with food). • If GI upset occurs, give with food, milk. • Avoid crushing tablets due to bitter taste. • Suspension must be given with food. • Suspension stable at room temperature or refrigerated for 10 days.

IV INCOMPATIBILITIES

Filgrastim (Neupogen), fluconazole (Diflucan), midazolam (Versed), vancomycin (Vancocin).

IV COMPATIBILITIES

Diltiazem (Cardizem), hydromorphone (Dilaudid), lipids, morphine, propofol (Diprivan), total parenteral nutrition (TPN).

INDICATIONS/ROUTES/DOSAGE

Usual Dosage

IV, IM: ADULTS, ELDERLY: 750 mg–1.5 g q8h. **CHILDREN:** 75–150 mg/kg/day divided q8h. **Maximum:** 6 g/day. **NEONATES:** 50–100 mg/kg/day divided q12h. **PO: ADULTS, ELDERLY:** 250–500 mg twice a day, depending on the infection.

Pharyngitis, Tonsillitis

PO: CHILDREN 3 MOS–12 YRS: 125 mg (tablets) q12h or 20 mg/kg/day (suspension) in 2 divided doses for 10 days.

Acute Otitis Media, Acute Bacterial Maxillary Sinusitis, Impetigo

PO: CHILDREN 3 MOS–12 YRS: 250 mg (tablets) q12h or 30 mg/kg/day (suspension) in 2 divided doses for 10 days.

Gonorrhea

PO: ADULTS, ELDERLY: 1 g as single dose. **IM:** 1.5 g as single dose.

UTI

PO: ADULTS, ELDERLY: 125–250 mg q12h for 7–10 days.

Perioperative Prophylaxis

IV: ADULTS, ELDERLY: 1.5 g 30–60 min before surgery and 750 mg q8h after surgery.

Usual Neonatal Dosage

IV, IM: NEONATES: 20–100 mg/kg/day in divided doses q12h.

C

Dosage in Renal Impairment

Adult dosage frequency is modified based on creatinine clearance and severity of infection.

Creatinine Clearance	Dosage
Greater than 20 ml/min	q8h
10–20 ml/min	q12h
Less than 10 ml/min	q24h

SIDE EFFECTS

Frequent: Discomfort with IM administration, oral candidiasis (thrush), mild diarrhea, mild abdominal cramping, vaginal candidiasis. **Occasional:** Nausea, serum sickness-like reaction (fever, joint pain; usually occurs after second course of therapy and resolves after drug is discontinued). **Rare:** Allergic reaction (rash, pruritus, urticaria), thrombophlebitis (pain, redness, swelling at injection site).

ADVERSE EFFECTS/ TOXIC REACTIONS

Antibiotic-associated colitis, other superinfections (abdominal cramps, severe watery diarrhea, fever) may result from altered bacterial balance. Nephrotoxicity may occur, esp. in pts with preexisting renal disease. Pts with a history of allergies, esp. to penicillin, are at increased risk for developing a severe hypersensitivity reaction (severe pruritus, angioedema, bronchospasm anaphylaxis).

NURSING CONSIDERATIONS

BASELINE ASSESSMENT

Question for history of allergies, particularly cephalosporins, penicillins.

INTERVENTION/EVALUATION

Assess oral cavity for white patches on mucous membranes, tongue (thrush). Monitor daily pattern of bowel activity and stool consistency. Mild GI effects may be tolerable (increasing severity may indicate onset of antibiotic-associated colitis). Monitor I&O, renal function tests for nephrotoxicity. Be alert for superinfection: fever, vomiting, diarrhea, anal/genital pruritus, oral mucosal changes (ulceration, pain, erythema).

PATIENT/FAMILY TEACHING

• Discomfort may occur with IM injection. • Doses should be evenly spaced. • Continue antibiotic therapy for full length of treatment. • May cause GI upset (may take with food, milk).

Cefzil, *see cefprozil*

Celebrex, *see celecoxib*

celecoxib

sell-eh-**kox**-ib
(Celebrex)

BLACK BOX ALERT Increased risk of serious cardiovascular thrombotic events, including MI, CVA. Increased risk of severe GI reactions, including ulceration, bleeding, perforation of stomach, intestines.

Do not confuse Celebrex with Celexa, Cerebyx, or Clarinex.

◆CLASSIFICATION

PHARMACOTHERAPEUTIC: Nonsteroidal anti-inflammatory. **CLINICAL:** Anti-inflammatory (see p. 127C).

ACTION

Inhibits cyclooxygenase-2, the enzyme responsible for prostaglandin synthesis. **Therapeutic Effect:** Reduces inflammation, relieves pain.

PHARMACOKINETICS

Rapidly absorbed from GI tract. Widely distributed. Protein binding: 97%. Metabolized in liver. Primarily eliminated in feces. **Half-life:** 11.2 hrs.

USES

Relief of signs/symptoms of osteoarthritis, rheumatoid arthritis (RA) in adults. Treatment of acute pain, menstrual pain. Used to reduce number of adenomatous colorectal polyps in familial adenomatous polyposis (FAP). Relief of signs/symptoms associated with ankylosing spondylitis. Treatment of juvenile rheumatoid arthritis (JRA).

PRECAUTIONS

◀ALERT▶ May increase cardiovascular risk when high doses given to prevent colon cancer.

Contraindications: Hypersensitivity to aspirin, NSAIDs, sulfonamides. Treatment of perioperative pain in coronary artery bypass graft (CABG) surgery. **Cautions:** History of peptic ulcer, older than 60 yrs, those receiving anticoagulant therapy, steroids, alcohol consumption, smoking.

LIFESPAN CONSIDERATIONS

Pregnancy/Lactation: Unknown if drug crosses placenta or is distributed in breast milk. Avoid use during third trimester (may adversely affect fetal cardiovascular system: premature closure of ductus arteriosus). **Pregnancy Category C (D if used in third trimester or near delivery). Children:** Safety and efficacy not established in those younger than 18 yrs. **Elderly:** No age-related precautions noted.

INTERACTIONS

DRUG: **Fluconazole** may significantly increase concentration. May significantly increase **lithium** concentration. **Warfarin** may increase risk of bleeding. **Aspirin** may increase risk of celecoxib-induced GI ulceration, other GI complications. **HERBAL:** None significant. **FOOD:** None known. **LAB VALUES:** May increase serum AST, ALT, alkaline phosphatase, creatinine, BUN. May decrease phosphate.

AVAILABILITY (Rx)

Capsules: 50 mg, 100 mg, 200 mg, 400 mg.

ADMINISTRATION/HANDLING

PO

• Give without regard to food (may give with food to reduce GI upset). • Do not give with antacids. • Capsules may be swallowed whole or opened and mixed with applesauce.

INDICATIONS/ROUTES/DOSAGE

◀ALERT▶ Decrease dose by 50% in pts with moderate hepatic impairment.

Osteoarthritis

PO: ADULTS, ELDERLY: 200 mg/day as a single dose or 100 mg twice a day.

Rheumatoid Arthritis (RA)

PO: ADULTS, ELDERLY: 100–200 mg twice a day.

Juvenile Rheumatoid Arthritis (JRA)

PO: CHILDREN 2 YRS AND OLDER, WEIGHING MORE THAN 25 KG: 100 mg twice a day. **WEIGHING 10–25 KG:** 50 mg twice a day.

Acute Pain

PO: ADULTS, ELDERLY: Initially, 400 mg with additional 200 mg on day 1, if needed. Maintenance: 200 mg twice a day as needed.

Familial Adenomatous Polyposis (FAP)

PO: ADULTS, ELDERLY: 400 mg twice a day (with food).

Primary Dysmenorrhea

PO: ADULTS: Initially, 400 mg with additional 200 mg on day 1, then 200 mg twice a day as needed (with food).

Ankylosing Spondylitis

PO: ADULTS, ELDERLY: 200 mg/day as a single dose or in 2 divided doses. May increase to 400 mg/day if no effect is seen after 6 wks.

Dosage in Hepatic Impairment

Decrease dose by 50% in pts with moderate hepatic impairment. Not recommended in severe hepatic impairment.

SIDE EFFECTS

Frequent (greater than 5%): Diarrhea, dyspepsia, headache, upper respiratory tract infection. Occasional (5%–1%): Abdominal pain, flatulence, nausea, back pain, peripheral edema, dizziness, rash.

ADVERSE EFFECTS/ TOXIC REACTIONS

Increased risk of cardiovascular events, (MI, CVA), serious, potentially life-threatening GI bleeding.

NURSING CONSIDERATIONS

BASELINE ASSESSMENT

Assess onset, type, location, duration of pain/inflammation. Inspect appearance of affected joints for immobility, deformity, skin condition. Assess for allergy to sulfa, aspirin, or NSAIDs (contraindicated).

INTERVENTION/EVALUATION

Assess for therapeutic response: pain relief, decreased stiffness, swelling; increased joint mobility; reduced joint tenderness; improved grip strength. Observe for bleeding, bruising, weight gain.

PATIENT/FAMILY TEACHING

- If GI upset occurs, take with food.
- Avoid aspirin, alcohol (increases risk of GI bleeding).

Celexa, *see citalopram*

CellCept, *see mycophenolate*

Cenestin, *see conjugated estrogens*

cephalexin

cef-ah-lex-in
(Apo-Cephalex 🍁, Keflex, Novolexin 🍁)

Do not confuse cephalexin with ciprofloxacin.

◆CLASSIFICATION

PHARMACOTHERAPEUTIC: First-generation cephalosporin. **CLINICAL:** Antibiotic (see p. 23C).

ACTION

Binds to bacterial cell membranes, inhibits cell wall synthesis. Therapeutic Effect: Bactericidal.

PHARMACOKINETICS

Rapidly absorbed from GI tract (delayed in young children). Protein binding: 10%–15%. Widely distributed. Primarily excreted unchanged in urine. Moderately removed by hemodialysis. Half-life: 0.9–1.2 hrs (increased in renal impairment).

USES

Treatment of susceptible infections due to staphylococci, group A *streptococcus, K. pneumoniae, E. coli, P. mirabilis, H. influenzae, M. catarrhalis* including respiratory tract, genitourinary tract, skin, soft tissue, bone infections; otitis media; rheumatic fever prophylaxis; follow-up to parenteral therapy.

PRECAUTIONS

Contraindications: History of anaphylactic reaction to penicillins, hypersensitivity to cephalosporins. Cautions: Renal impairment, history of GI disease (esp. ulcerative colitis, antibiotic-associated colitis), concurrent use of nephrotoxic medications.

⌛ LIFESPAN CONSIDERATIONS

Pregnancy/Lactation: Readily crosses placenta. Distributed in breast milk. **Pregnancy Category B. Children:** No age-related precautions noted. **Elderly:** Age-related renal impairment may require dosage adjustment.

INTERACTIONS

DRUG: **Aminoglycosides, furosemide** may increase risk of nephrotoxicity. **Probenecid** increases concentration. HERBAL: None significant. FOOD: None known. LAB VALUES: May increase serum alkaline phosphatase, bilirubin, LDH, AST, ALT. May cause positive direct/indirect Coombs' test.

AVAILABILITY (Rx)

Capsules (Keflex): 250 mg, 500 mg, 750 mg. Powder for Oral Suspension (Keflex): 125 mg/5 ml, 250 mg/5 ml. Tablets: 250 mg, 500 mg.

ADMINISTRATION/HANDLING

PO

• After reconstitution, oral suspension is stable for 14 days if refrigerated. • Shake oral suspension well before using. • Give without regard to food. If GI upset occurs, give with food, milk.

INDICATIONS/ROUTES/DOSAGE

Usual Dosage Range

PO: ADULTS, ELDERLY: 250–1,000 mg q6h. **Maximum:** 4 g/day. CHILDREN: 25–100 mg/kg/day in 3–4 divided doses. **Maximum:** 4 g/day.

Streptococcal Pharyngitis, Skin/Skin Structure Infections

PO: ADULTS, ELDERLY: 500 mg q12h. CHILDREN: 25–50 mg/kg/day in 2 divided doses.

Uncomplicated Cystitis

PO: ADULTS, ELDERLY, CHILDREN OLDER THAN 15 YRS: 500 mg q12h for 7–14 days.

Otitis Media

PO: CHILDREN: 75–100 mg/kg/day in 4 divided doses.

Dosage in Renal Impairment

After usual initial dose, dosing frequency is modified based on creatinine clearance and severity of infection.

Creatinine Clearance	Dosage
10–50 ml/min	500 mg q8–12h
Less than 10 ml/min	250–500 mg q12–24h

SIDE EFFECTS

Frequent: Oral candidiasis, mild diarrhea, mild abdominal cramping, vaginal candidiasis. Occasional: Nausea, serum sickness-like reaction (fever, joint pain; usually occurs after second course of therapy and resolves after drug is discontinued). Rare: Allergic reaction (rash, pruritus, urticaria).

ADVERSE EFFECTS/ TOXIC REACTIONS

Antibiotic-associated colitis, other superinfections (abdominal cramps, severe watery diarrhea, fever) may result from altered bacterial balance. Nephrotoxicity may occur, esp. in pts with preexisting renal disease. Pts with a history of allergies, esp. to penicillin, are at increased risk for developing a severe hypersensitivity reaction (severe pruritus, angioedema, bronchospasm, anaphylaxis).

NURSING CONSIDERATIONS

BASELINE ASSESSMENT

Question for history of allergies, particularly cephalosporins, penicillins.

INTERVENTION/EVALUATION

Assess oral cavity for white patches on mucous membranes, tongue (thrush). Monitor daily pattern of bowel activity and stool consistency. Mild GI effects may be tolerable (increasing severity may indicate onset of antibiotic-associated colitis). Monitor I&O, renal function tests for nephrotoxicity. Be alert for superinfection: fever, vomiting, diarrhea, anal/genital pruritus, oral mucosal changes (ulceration, pain, erythema). With prolonged therapy, monitor renal/hepatic function tests.

PATIENT/FAMILY TEACHING

• Doses should be evenly spaced. • Continue therapy for full length of treatment.

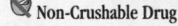

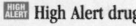

• May cause GI upset (may take with food, milk). • Refrigerate oral suspension. • Report prolonged diarrhea.

C

Cerebyx, *see fosphenytoin*

certolizumab

sir-toe-**liz**-oo-mab
(Cimzia)

BLACK BOX ALERT Tuberculosis, serious, sometimes fatal invasive fungal infections, other opportunistic infections have been reported.

CLASSIFICATION

PHARMACOTHERAPEUTIC: Tumor necrosis factor (TNF) blocker. **CLINICAL:** Crohn's disease agent.

ACTION

Binds specifically to TNF-alpha cell, a protein in the immune system that causes inflammation. **Therapeutic Effect:** Reduces signs and symptoms of Crohn's disease in those with inadequate response to conventional therapy.

PHARMACOKINETICS

Higher clearance with increasing body weight. Age, gender do not affect clearance. **Half-life:** 14 days.

USES

Reduces signs and symptoms of Crohn's disease, maintenance of clinical response in pts with moderate to severely active disease. Treatment of moderately to severely active rheumatoid arthritis.

PRECAUTIONS

Contraindications: None known. **Cautions:** Chronic, latent, or localized infection, preexisting or recent-onset CNS demyelinating disorders, heart failure, elderly. May increase risk of malignancies (e.g., lymphoma).

LIFESPAN CONSIDERATIONS:

Pregnancy/Lactation: Unknown if distributed in breast milk. **Pregnancy Category B. Children:** Safety and efficacy not established. **Elderly:** Use cautiously due to higher rate of infection.

INTERACTIONS

DRUG: Anakinra, other TNF antagonists (adalimumab, etanercept, infliximab) may increase risk of infection. **Live virus vaccines** may decrease immune response. **HERBAL: Echinacea** may decrease effect. **FOOD:** None known. **LAB VALUES:** May increase AST, ALT, alkaline phosphatase, bilirubin, aPTT.

AVAILABILITY (Rx)

Injection, Powder for Reconstitution: 200 mg. **Injection, Solution:** 200 mg/ml in a single-use prefilled syringe.

ADMINISTRATION/HANDLING

Subcutaneous

Reconstitution • Powder in each vial should be brought to room temperature before reconstitution. • Reconstitute two 200-mg vials for each dose. • Reconstitute each vial with 1 ml Sterile Water for Injection. • Gently swirl each vial without shaking, using syringe with 20-gauge needle. • Leave vials undisturbed to fully reconstitute (may take as long as 30 min). • Using a new 20-gauge needle for each vial, withdraw reconstituted solution into a separate syringe for each vial, resulting in two syringes each containing 1 ml (200 mg). • Switch each 20-gauge needle to a 23-gauge needle and inject full contents of each syringe subcutaneously into separate sites on the abdomen or thigh.

Storage • Store vial in refrigerator. • Once powder for solution is reconstituted, solution should appear as clear to opalescent, colorless to pale yellow liquid. • Discard if solution is discolored or contains precipitate. • Reconstituted solution is stable for up to 2 hrs at room temperature or 24 hrs if refrigerated.

INDICATIONS/ROUTES/DOSAGE

Crohn's Disease

SUBCUTANEOUS: Initially, 400 mg (given as 2 subcutaneous injections of 200 mg) and at weeks 2 and 4. Maintenance: In pts who obtain a therapeutic response, 400 mg every 4 wks.

Rheumatoid Arthritis

SUBCUTANEOUS: **ADULTS, ELDERLY:** Initially, 400 mg and at weeks 2 and 4. Maintenance: 200 mg q2wks or 400 mg q4wks.

SIDE EFFECTS

Occasional (6%): Arthralgia. **Rare (less than 1%):** Abdominal pain, diarrhea.

ADVERSE EFFECTS/ TOXIC REACTIONS

Upper respiratory tract infection occurs in 20% of pts. UTI occurs in 7% of pts. Serious infections manifested as pneumonia, pyelonephritis occur in 3% of pts. Hypersensitivity reaction (rash, urticaria, hypotension, dyspnea) occurs rarely.

NURSING CONSIDERATIONS

BASELINE ASSESSMENT

Do not initiate treatment in pts with active infections, including chronic or localized infection. TB test should be obtained before treatment is initiated. Obtain baseline WBC count, urinalysis, C-reactive protein.

INTERVENTION/EVALUATION

Monitor pts for signs and symptoms of infection during and after treatment. If pt develops an infection, treatment should be discontinued. Monitor lab results, especially WBC count, urinalysis, C-reactive protein for evidence of infection. Monitor temperature.

PATIENT/FAMILY TEACHING

• Consult physician/nurse if cough, fever, flu-like symptoms occur. • Do not receive live virus vaccine during treatment or within 3 months of its discontinuation.

Cervidil, *see dinoprostone*

cetirizine

sih-**tier**-eh-zeen
(Apo-Cetirizine ✱, Reactine ✱, Zyrtec)

Do not confuse cetirizine with levocetirizine, or Zyrtec with Xanax, Zantac, or Zyprexa.

FIXED-COMBINATION(S)

Zyrtec D 12 Hour Tablets: cetirizine/pseudoephedrine: 5 mg/120 mg.

◆CLASSIFICATION

PHARMACOTHERAPEUTIC: Second-generation piperazine. **CLINICAL:** Antihistamine (see p. 53C).

ACTION

Competes with histamine for H_1-receptor sites on effector cells in GI tract, blood vessels, respiratory tract. **Therapeutic Effect:** Prevents allergic response, produces mild bronchodilation, blocks histamine-induced bronchitis.

PHARMACOKINETICS

Route	Onset	Peak	Duration
PO	Less than 1 hr	4–8 hrs	Less than 24 hrs

Well absorbed from GI tract (absorption not affected by food). Protein binding: 93%. Undergoes low first-pass metabolism; not extensively metabolized. Primarily excreted in urine (more than 80% as unchanged drug). **Half-life:** 6.5–10 hrs.

USES

Relief of symptoms (sneezing, rhinorrhea, postnasal discharge, nasal pruritus, ocular pruritus, tearing) of seasonal and perennial allergic rhinitis (hay fever). Treatment of chronic urticaria (hives).

OFF-LABEL: Treatment of bronchial asthma.

PRECAUTIONS

Contraindications: Hypersensitivity to cetirizine, hydroxyzine. Cautions: Hepatic/renal impairment. May cause drowsiness at dosage greater than 10 mg/day.

LIFESPAN CONSIDERATIONS

Pregnancy/Lactation: Not recommended during first trimester of pregnancy. Distributed in breast milk. Breastfeeding not recommended. **Pregnancy Category B. Children:** Less likely to cause anticholinergic effects. **Elderly:** More sensitive to anticholinergic effects (e.g., dry mouth, urinary retention). Dizziness, sedation, confusion more likely to occur.

INTERACTIONS

DRUG: **Alcohol, other CNS depressants** may increase CNS depression. **Anticholinergics** may increase anticholinergic effects. **MAOIs** may prolong or increase anticholinergic, CNS depressant effects. HERBAL: None significant. FOOD: None known. LAB VALUES: May suppress wheal and flare reactions to antigen skin testing unless drug is discontinued 4 days before testing.

AVAILABILITY (Rx)

Syrup: 5 mg/5 ml. Tablets: 5 mg, 10 mg. Tablets (Chewable): 5 mg, 10 mg.

ADMINISTRATION/HANDLING

PO

- Give without regard to food.

INDICATIONS/ROUTES/DOSAGE

Allergic Rhinitis, Urticaria

PO: **ADULTS, ELDERLY, CHILDREN OLDER THAN 5 YRS:** Initially, 5–10 mg/day as a single or in 2 divided doses. **CHILDREN 2–5 YRS:** 2.5 mg/day. May increase up to 5 mg/day as a single or in 2 divided doses. **CHILDREN 12–23 MOS:** Initially, 2.5 mg/day. May increase up to 5 mg/day in 2 divided doses. **CHILDREN 6–11 MOS:** 2.5 mg once a day.

Dosage in Renal/Hepatic Impairment

Adult/elderly pts with renal impairment (creatinine clearance 11–31 ml/min), those receiving hemodialysis (creatinine clearance less than 7 ml/min), those with hepatic impairment: Dosage is decreased to 5 mg once a day. **CHILDREN 6–11 YRS:** Less than 2.5 mg once daily.

SIDE EFFECTS

Occasional (10%–2%): Pharyngitis; dry mucous membranes, nose, throat; nausea/vomiting; abdominal pain; headache; dizziness; fatigue; thickening of mucus; drowsiness; photosensitivity; urinary retention.

ADVERSE EFFECTS/ TOXIC REACTIONS

Children may experience paradoxical reaction (restlessness, insomnia, euphoria, nervousness, tremor). Dizziness, sedation, confusion more likely to occur in elderly.

NURSING CONSIDERATIONS

BASELINE ASSESSMENT

Assess lung sounds. Assess severity of rhinitis, urticaria, other symptoms. Obtain baseline hepatic function tests.

INTERVENTION/EVALUATION

For upper respiratory allergies, increase fluids to maintain thin secretions and offset thirst. Monitor symptoms for therapeutic response.

PATIENT/FAMILY TEACHING

- Avoid tasks that require alertness, motor skills until response to drug is established.
- Avoid alcohol during antihistamine therapy.
- Avoid prolonged exposure to sunlight.

cetuximab

HIGH ALERT

ceh-**tux**-ih-mab
(Erbitux)

C

BLACK BOX ALERT Severe infusion reactions (bronchospasm, stridor, urticaria, hypotension, cardiac arrest) have occurred, especially with first infusion. Cardiopulmonary arrest reported in pts receiving radiation in combination with cetuximab.

Do not confuse cetuximab with bevacizumab.

◆ CLASSIFICATION

PHARMACOTHERAPEUTIC: Monoclonal antibody. **CLINICAL:** Antineoplastic.

ACTION

Binds to the epidermal growth factor receptor (EGFR), a glycoprotein on normal and tumor cells. **Therapeutic Effect:** Inhibits tumor cell growth, inducing apoptosis.

PHARMACOKINETICS

Reaches steady-state levels by the third weekly infusion. Clearance decreases as dose increases. **Half-life:** 114 hrs (range: 75–188 hrs).

USES

As a single agent or in combination with irinotecan for treatment of EGFR-expressing, metastatic colorectal carcinoma in pts who are refractory or intolerant to irinotecan-based chemotherapy. Treatment of advanced squamous cell cancer of head/neck (with radiation). Treatment of recurrent or metastasized squamous cell carcinoma of head/neck progressing after platinum-based therapy. **OFF-LABEL:** Breast cancer, tumors overexpressing EGFR.

PRECAUTIONS

Contraindications: None known. **Cautions:** Hypersensitivity to murine proteins, coronary artery disease, heart failure, arrythmias, preexisting pulmonary disease.

⌛ LIFESPAN CONSIDERATIONS

Pregnancy/Lactation: Crosses placental barrier; has potential to cause fetal harm, abortifactant. Breast-feeding not recommended. **Pregnancy Category C.** **Children:** Safety and efficacy not established. **Elderly:** No age-related precautions noted.

INTERACTIONS

DRUG: None significant. **HERBAL:** None significant. **FOOD:** None known. **LAB VALUES:** May decrease WBCs, calcium, magnesium, potassium.

AVAILABILITY (Rx)

Injection Solution: 2 mg/ml (50 ml, 100 ml).

ADMINISTRATION/HANDLING

IV

◄ALERT► Do not give by IV push or bolus.

Reconstitution • Solution should appear clear, colorless; may contain a small amount of visible, white particulates. • Do not shake or dilute. • Infuse with a low protein-binding 0.22-micron in-line filter.

Rate of administration • First dose should be given as a 120-min IV infusion. • Maintenance infusion should be infused over 60 min. • Maximum infusion rate should not exceed 5 ml/min.

Storage • Refrigerate vials. • Preparations in infusion containers are stable for up to 12 hrs if refrigerated, up to 8 hrs at room temperature. • Discard any unused portion.

IV COMPATIBILITY

Irinotecan (Camptosar).

INDICATIONS/ROUTES/DOSAGE

Head/Neck Cancer, Metastatic Colorectal Carcinoma

IV: ADULTS, ELDERLY: Initially, 400 mg/m^2 as a loading dose. Maintenance: 250 mg/m^2 infused over 60 min weekly.

SIDE EFFECTS

Frequent (90%–25%): Acneiform rash, malaise, fever, nausea, diarrhea, constipation, headache, abdominal pain, anorexia, vomiting. **Occasional (16%–10%):**

Nail disorder, back pain, stomatitis, peripheral edema, pruritus, cough, insomnia. Rare (9%–5%): Weight loss, depression, dyspepsia, conjunctivitis, alopecia.

ADVERSE EFFECTS/ TOXIC REACTIONS

Anemia occurs in 10% of pts. Severe infusion reaction (rapid onset of airway obstruction, precipitous drop in B/P, severe urticaria) occurs rarely. Dermatologic toxicity, pulmonary embolus, leukopenia, renal failure occur rarely.

NURSING CONSIDERATIONS

BASELINE ASSESSMENT

Monitor Hgb, Hct, serum potassium, magnesium. Assess signs/symptoms for evidence of anemia. Question pt regarding possibility of pregnancy.

INTERVENTION/EVALUATION

Diligently monitor pt for evidence of infusion reaction (rapid onset of bronchospasm, stridor, hoarseness, urticaria, hypotension) during infusion and for at least 1 hr postinfusion. Be aware that pt may experience first severe infusion reaction during later infusions. Assess skin for evidence of dermatologic toxicity (development of inflammatory sequelae, dry skin, exfoliative dermatitis, rash).

PATIENT/FAMILY TEACHING

• Do not have immunizations without physician's approval (drug lowers resistance). • Avoid contact with anyone who recently received a live virus vaccine. • Avoid crowds, those with infection. • Wear sunscreen, limit sun exposure during therapy (sunlight can exacerbate skin reactions). • Female pts should take measures to avoid pregnancy. • Notify physician if cardiac or pulmonary symptoms, severe rash occurs.

chamomile

ka-mow-meal

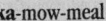

Also known as German chamomile, pinheads (Blossom 30 g/jar; 45 g/jar; 120 g/jar).

◆CLASSIFICATION

HERBAL: See Appendix G.

ACTION

Antiallergic, anti-inflammatory action due to inhibiting release of histamine. Possesses antiallergic, antiflatulent, antispasmodic, mild sedative, anti-inflammatory action. **Effect**: Reduces GI symptoms, produces mild CNS depression.

USES

Treatment of symptoms of flatulence, travel sickness, diarrhea, insomnia, GI spasms.

PRECAUTIONS

Contraindications: Pregnancy. **Cautions:** Pts with asthma (may exacerbate condition), those allergic to ragweed, aster, daisies, chrysanthemums.

LIFESPAN CONSIDERATIONS

Pregnancy/Lactation: Contraindicated. A teratogen, affects menstrual cycle, has uterine stimulant effects. **Children:** Safety and efficacy not established. **Elderly:** No age-related precautions noted.

INTERACTIONS

DRUG: May increase anticoagulation, risk of bleeding with **aspirin, clopidogrel, dalteparin, enoxaparin, heparin, warfarin.** May have additive effects with **benzodiazepines.** HERBAL: Sedative effects may increase with **ginseng, kava kava, St. John's wort, valerian.** May increase risk of bleeding with **feverfew, garlic, ginger, ginkgo, licorice.** FOOD: None known. LAB VALUES: None significant.

AVAILABILITY

Whole Flowers: 30 g/jar, 45 g/jar, 120 g/jar.

INDICATIONS/ROUTES/DOSAGE

Flatulence, Travel Sickness, Diarrhea, Insomnia, GI Spasms

PO: ADULTS, ELDERLY: 2–8 g of dried flower heads 3 times a day or 1 cup of tea 3–4 times a day.

SIDE EFFECTS

Allergic reaction (contact dermatitis, severe hypersensitivity reaction, anaphylactic reaction), eye irritation.

ADVERSE EFFECTS/ TOXIC REACTIONS

Anaphylactic reaction (bronchospasm, severe pruritus, angioedema) occurs rarely.

NURSING CONSIDERATIONS

BASELINE ASSESSMENT

Assess if pt is pregnant, breast-feeding, or asthmatic. Assess if pt is taking other medications, esp. those that increase risk of bleeding or have sedative properties. Assess for allergies to ragweed, aster, daisies, chrysanthemums.

INTERVENTION/EVALUATION

Monitor for signs of allergic reaction.

PATIENT/FAMILY TEACHING

• Inform physician if pregnancy occurs or if planning to become pregnant or breast-feed. • May cause mild sedation. • Avoid tasks that require alertness, motor skills until response to herb is established. • Avoid use with other sedatives, alcohol, anticoagulants.

chloral hydrate HIGH ALERT

klor-al **high**-drate
(Aquachloral Supprettes, PMS-Chloral Hydrate ✦, Somnote)

◆CLASSIFICATION

PHARMACOTHERAPEUTIC: Nonbarbiturate chloral derivative. **CLINICAL:** Sedative, hypnotic.

ACTION

Nonbarbiturate that produces CNS depression. **Therapeutic Effect:** Induces quiet, deep sleep, with only slight decrease in respiratory rate, B/P.

PHARMACOKINETICS

Readily absorbed from GI tract following PO administration. Well absorbed following rectal administration. Protein binding: 70%–80%. Metabolized in liver, erythrocytes to active metabolite, trichloroethanol, which may be further metabolized to inactive metabolites. Excreted in urine. **Half-life:** 7–10 hrs (trichloroethanol).

USES

Sedative/hypnotic for dental or diagnostic procedures, sedative before EEG evaluations.

PRECAUTIONS

Contraindications: Gastritis, marked hepatic/renal impairment, severe cardiac disease. **Cautions:** History of drug abuse, clinical depression.

LIFESPAN CONSIDERATIONS

Pregnancy/Lactation: Crosses placenta; distributed in breast milk. **Pregnancy Category C. Children:** Safety and efficacy not established. **Elderly:** No age-related precautions noted.

INTERACTIONS

DRUG: Alcohol, other CNS depressants may increase effects of chloral hydrate. **Furosemide (IV)** may alter B/P and cause diaphoresis, hypertension if given within 24 hrs. May increase effect of **warfarin. HERBAL:** None significant. **FOOD:** None known. **LAB VALUES:** May interfere with copper sulfate test for gly-

C

cosuria, fluorometric tests for urine catecholamines, urinary 17-hydroxycorticosteroid determinations.

AVAILABILITY (Rx)

Capsules (Somnote): 500 mg. Suppositories (Aquachloral Supprettes): 324 mg. Syrup: 500 mg/5 ml.

ADMINISTRATION/HANDLING

PO

• Give capsules with full glass of water or fruit juice. • Swallow capsules whole; do not chew. • Dilute syrup in water to minimize gastric irritation.

Rectal

• Store suppositories at room temperature.

INDICATIONS/ROUTES/DOSAGE

Premedication for Dental or Medical Procedures

PO, RECTAL: ADULTS: 0.5–1 g. **CHILDREN:** 75 mg/kg up to 1 g total.

Premedication for EEG

PO, RECTAL: ADULTS: 0.5–1.5 g. **CHILDREN:** 25–50 mg/kg/dose 30–60 min prior to EEG. May repeat in 30 min. **Maximum:** 1 g for infants, 2 g for children.

SIDE EFFECTS

Occasional: Gastric irritation (nausea, vomiting, flatulence, diarrhea), rash, sleepwalking. Rare: Headache, paradoxical CNS hyperactivity or nervousness in children, excitement or restlessness in the elderly (particularly in pts with pain).

ADVERSE EFFECTS/ TOXIC REACTIONS

Overdose may produce drowsiness, confusion, slurred speech, severe incoordination, respiratory depression, coma. Allergic-type reaction may occur in those with tartrazine sensitivity.

NURSING CONSIDERATIONS

BASELINE ASSESSMENT

Assess B/P, pulse, respirations immediately before administration. Provide safety measures, e.g., raise bedrails. Provide environment conducive to sleep (back rub, quiet environment, low lighting).

INTERVENTION/EVALUATION

Monitor mental status, vital signs. Gastric irritation decreased by diluting dose in water. Assess sleep pattern. Assess elderly and children for paradoxical reaction. Evaluate for therapeutic response to insomnia: decrease in number of nocturnal awakenings, increase in length of sleep.

PATIENT/FAMILY TEACHING

• Take capsule with full glass of water or fruit juice. • Swallow capsules whole; do not chew. • If taking at home before procedure, do not drive. • Avoid alcohol. • Do not abruptly discontinue medication after long-term use. • Tolerance, dependence may occur with prolonged use.

chlorambucil HIGH ALERT

klor-**am**-bue-sill
(Leukeran)

BLACK BOX ALERT May cause myelosuppression. Affects fertility; potential for carcinogenic, mutagenic, teratogenic effects. May cause azoospermia.

Do not confuse Leukeran with Alkeran, Leukine, or Myleran.

◆CLASSIFICATION

PHARMACOTHERAPEUTIC: Alkylating agent, nitrogen mustard. **CLINICAL:** Antineoplastic (see p. 81C).

ACTION

Inhibits DNA, RNA synthesis by cross-linking with DNA, RNA strands. Cell cycle–

phase nonspecific. Therapeutic Effect: Interferes with nucleic acid function.

PHARMACOKINETICS

Rapidly, completely absorbed from GI tract. Protein binding: 99%. Rapidly metabolized in liver to active metabolite. Not removed by hemodialysis. Half-life: 1.5 hrs; metabolite, 2.5 hrs.

USES

Treatment of chronic lymphocytic leukemia, Hodgkin's and non-Hodgkin's lymphomas. OFF-LABEL: Treatment of cutaneous T-cell lymphomas, epithelial carcinoma, hairy cell leukemia, nephrotic syndrome, ovarian or testicular carcinoma, breast cancer, polycythemia vera, trophoblastic gestational tumors.

PRECAUTIONS

Contraindications: Previous allergic reaction, disease resistance to drug. Extreme Cautions: Within 4 wks after full-course radiation therapy or myelosuppressive drug regimen. **Cautions:** Seizure disorder, head trauma, bone marrow suppression.

LIFESPAN CONSIDERATIONS

Pregnancy/Lactation: If possible, avoid use during pregnancy, esp. first trimester. Breast-feeding not recommended. **Pregnancy Category D. Children:** No age-related precautions noted. When taken for nephrotic syndrome, may increase seizures. **Elderly:** No age-related precautions noted.

INTERACTIONS

DRUG: May decrease effect of **antigout medications. Bone marrow depressants** may increase myelosuppression. **Other immunosuppressants (e.g., steroids)** may increase risk of infection or development of neoplasms. **Live virus vaccines** may potentiate virus replication, increase vaccine side effects, decrease antibody response to vaccine. HERBAL: **Echinacea** may decrease effects. FOOD: Acidic foods, hot foods, spices may delay absorption. LAB VALUES: May increase serum AST, alkaline phosphatase, uric acid.

AVAILABILITY (Rx)

Tablets: 2 mg.

ADMINISTRATION/HANDLING

PO

• Give 30–60 min before food. • Do not give with acidic foods, hot foods, spices.

INDICATIONS/ROUTES/DOSAGE

Usual Dosage

PO: ADULTS, ELDERLY, CHILDREN: For initial or short-course therapy, 0.1–0.2 mg/kg/day as a single or in divided doses for 3–6 wks (average dose, 4–10 mg/day). Alternatively, 0.4 mg/kg initially as a single daily dose every 2 wks and increased by 0.1 mg/kg every 2 wks until response and myelosuppression occur. Maintenance: 0.03–0.1 mg/kg/day (average dose, 2–4 mg/day).

SIDE EFFECTS

Expected: GI effects (nausea, vomiting, anorexia, diarrhea, abdominal distress) generally mild, last less than 24 hrs, occur only if single dose exceeds 20 mg. Occasional: Rash, dermatitis, pruritus, cold sores. Rare: Alopecia, urticaria, erythema, hyperuricemia.

ADVERSE EFFECTS/ TOXIC REACTIONS

Hematologic toxicity due to severe myelosuppression occurs frequently, manifested as neutropenia, anemia, thrombocytopenia. After discontinuation of therapy, thrombocytopenia, neutropenia usually last for 1–2 wks but may persist for 3–4 wks. Neutrophil count may continue to decrease for up to 10 days after last dose. Toxicity appears to be less severe with intermittent drug administration. Overdosage may produce seizures in children. Excessive serum uric acid level, hepatotoxicity occur rarely.

C

NURSING CONSIDERATIONS

BASELINE ASSESSMENT

CBC should be performed before therapy and each wk during therapy, WBC count performed 3–4 days following each weekly CBC during first 3–6 wks of therapy (4–6 wks if pt on intermittent dosing schedule).

INTERVENTION/EVALUATION

Monitor CBC, platelet count, serum uric acid, hepatic function tests. Monitor for hematologic toxicity (fever, sore throat, signs of local infection, unusual bruising/bleeding from any site), symptoms of anemia (excessive fatigue, weakness). Assess skin for rash, pruritus, urticaria.

PATIENT/FAMILY TEACHING

• Increase fluid intake (may protect against hyperuricemia). • Do not have immunizations without physician's approval (drug lowers resistance). • Avoid contact with those who have recently received live virus vaccine. • Promptly report fever, sore throat, signs of local infection, unusual bruising/bleeding from any site, nausea, vomiting, rash.

chlordiazepoxide

klor-dye-az-e-**pox**-ide
(Apo-Chlordiazepoxide ✱, Librium)
Do not confuse Librium with Librax.

FIXED-COMBINATION(S)

Limbitrol: amitriptyline/chlordiazepoxide: 5 mg/12.5 mg, 10 mg/25 mg. **Librax**: chlordiazepoxide-clidinium: 5 mg/2.5 mg.

◆CLASSIFICATION

PHARMACOTHERAPEUTIC: Benzodiazepine. **CLINICAL:** Antianxiety (see p. 13C).

ACTION

Enhances action of inhibitory neurotransmitter gamma-aminobutyric acid in CNS. **Therapeutic Effect:** Produces anxiolytic effect.

PHARMACOKINETICS

Widely distributed. Protein binding: 90%–98%. Metabolized in liver. Primarily excreted in urine. **Half-life:** 6.6–25 hrs.

USES

Management of anxiety disorders, acute alcohol withdrawal symptoms; short-term relief of symptoms of anxiety, pre-op anxiety, tension. **OFF-LABEL:** Treatment of panic disorder, tension headache, tremors.

PRECAUTIONS

Contraindications: Acute alcohol intoxication, acute angle-closure glaucoma. **Cautions:** Renal/hepatic impairment.

⌛ LIFESPAN CONSIDERATIONS

Pregnancy/Lactation: Crosses placenta; distributed in breast milk. **Pregnancy Category D. Children/Elderly:** Reduce initial dose, increase dosage gradually (prevents excessive sedation).

INTERACTIONS

DRUG: Alcohol, other CNS depressants may increase CNS depression. **Azole antifungals** may increase serum concentration, increase risk of toxicity. **HERBAL: Gotu kola, kava kava, St. John's wort, valerian** may increase CNS depression. **St. John's wort** may decrease effectiveness. **FOOD:** None known. **LAB VALUES: Therapeutic serum level:** 1–3 mcg/ml; **toxic serum level:** greater than 23 mcg/ml.

AVAILABILITY (Rx)

Capsules (Librium): 5 mg, 10 mg, 25 mg. **Injection, Powder for Reconstitution (Librium):** 100 mg.

ADMINISTRATION/HANDLING

◀ALERT▶ Keep pt recumbent for up to 3 hrs after parenteral administration (reduces drug's hypotensive effect).

C

Reconstitution
IM • Use diluent provided (not for IV use). **IV** • Add 5 ml 0.9% NaCl or Sterile Water for Injection.
Rate of Administration
IM • Give deep IM slowly into upper outer quadrant of gluteus muscle. **IV** • Administer slowly over at least 1 min.
Storage • Refrigerate prior to reconstitution. • Use immediately following reconstitution.

INDICATIONS/ROUTES/DOSAGE

Alcohol Withdrawal Symptoms
PO, IV: ADULTS, ELDERLY: 50–100 mg. May repeat q2–4h. **Maximum:** 300 mg/24 hrs.

Anxiety
PO: ADULTS: 15–100 mg/day in 3–4 divided doses. **ELDERLY:** 5 mg 2–4 times a day.
IV, IM: ADULTS: Initially, 50–100 mg, then 25–50 mg 3–4 times a day as needed.

Preop Anxiety
IM: ADULTS, ELDERLY: 50–100 mg once.

SIDE EFFECTS

Frequent: Pain at IM injection site; drowsiness, ataxia, dizziness, confusion with oral dose (particularly in elderly or debilitated pts). **Occasional:** Rash, peripheral edema, GI disturbances. **Rare:** Paradoxical CNS reactions (hyperactivity, nervousness in children; excitement, restlessness in the elderly, generally noted during first 2 wks of therapy, particularly in presence of uncontrolled pain).

ADVERSE EFFECTS/ TOXIC REACTIONS

IV administration may produce pain, swelling, thrombophlebitis, carpal tunnel syndrome. Abrupt or too-rapid withdrawal may result in pronounced restlessness, irritability, insomnia, hand tremors, abdominal/muscle cramps, diaphoresis, vomiting, seizures. Overdose results in drowsiness, confusion, diminished reflexes, coma.

NURSING CONSIDERATIONS

BASELINE ASSESSMENT

Assess B/P, pulse, respirations immediately before administration. Pt should remain recumbent for up to 3 hrs (individualized) after parenteral administration to reduce hypotensive effect.

INTERVENTION/EVALUATION

Monitor vital signs, esp. B/P, for changes. Assess motor responses (agitation, tremors, tension), autonomic responses (cold/clammy hands, diaphoresis). Assess children, elderly for paradoxical reaction, particularly during early therapy. Assist with ambulation if drowsiness, ataxia occur. **Therapeutic serum level:** 0.1–3 mcg/ml; **toxic serum level:** greater than 23 mcg/ml.

PATIENT/FAMILY TEACHING

• Discomfort may occur with IM injection. • Avoid tasks that require alertness, motor skills until response to drug is established or drowsiness has diminished. • Drowsiness usually disappears during continued therapy. • If dizziness occurs, change positions slowly from recumbent to sitting before standing. • Smoking reduces drug effectiveness. • Do not abruptly discontinue medication after long-term therapy. • Avoid alcohol.

*chlorproMAZINE

klor-**pro**-ma-zeen
(Largactil ✦, Novo-Chlorpromazine ✦, Thorazine)

BLACK BOX ALERT Increased risk of mortality in elderly pts with dementia-related psychosis.

Do not confuse chlorpromazine with chlorpropamide, clomipramine, or prochlorperazine, or Thorazine with thiamine or thioridazine.

C

CLASSIFICATION

PHARMACOTHERAPEUTIC: Phenothiazine. **CLINICAL:** Antipsychotic, antiemetic, antianxiety, antineuralgia adjunct (see p. 64C).

ACTION

Blocks dopamine neurotransmission at postsynaptic dopamine receptor sites. Possesses strong anticholinergic, sedative, antiemetic effects; moderate extrapyramidal effects; slight antihistamine action. Therapeutic Effect: Improves psychotic conditions; relieves nausea/vomiting; controls intractable hiccups, porphyria.

PHARMACOKINETICS

Rapidly absorbed from GI tract. Protein binding: 92%–97%. Metabolized in liver, excreted in urine. Half-life: Initial 2 hrs; **Terminal:** 30 hrs.

USES

Management of psychotic disorders, manic phase of manic-depressive illness, severe nausea/vomiting, severe behavioral disturbances in children. Relief of intractable hiccups, acute intermittent porphyria. OFF-LABEL: Treatment of choreiform movement of Huntington's disease. Management of psychotic disorders; behavioral symptoms associated with dementia; agitation related to Alzheimer's dementia.

PRECAUTIONS

Contraindications: Comatose states, myelosuppression, severe cardiovascular disease, severe CNS depression, subcortical brain damage. Cautions: Respiratory/hepatic/renal/cardiac impairment, alcohol withdrawal, history of seizures, urinary retention, glaucoma, prostatic hypertrophy, hypocalcemia (increases susceptibility to dystonias).

LIFESPAN CONSIDERATIONS

Pregnancy/Lactation: Crosses placenta; distributed in breast milk. **Pregnancy Category C. Children:** Those with acute illnesses (chickenpox, measles, gastroenteritis, CNS infection) are at risk for developing neuromuscular, extrapyramidal symptoms (EPS), particularly dystonias. **Elderly:** Susceptible to anticholinergic, neuromuscular, EPS.

INTERACTIONS

DRUG: **Alcohol, CNS depressants** may increase respiratory depression, hypotensive effects. **MAOIs, tricyclic antidepressants** may increase sedative, anticholinergic effects. **Antithyroid agents** may increase risk of agranulocytosis. Increased risk of extrapyramidal symptoms (EPS) with **EPS-producing medications. Antihypertensives** may increase hypotension. May decrease **levodopa** effects. **Lithium** may decrease absorption, produce adverse neurologic effects. HERBAL: **St. John's wort** may decrease concentration, increase photosensitization, sedative effect. **Dong quai** may increase photosensitization. **Gotu kola, kava kava, valerian** may increase sedative effect. FOOD: None known. LAB VALUES: May produce false-positive pregnancy test, phenylketonuria (PKU) test. EKG changes may occur, including Q- and T-wave disturbances. **Therapeutic serum level:** 50–300 ng/ml; **toxic serum level:** greater than 750 ng/ml.

AVAILABILITY (Rx)

Injection Solution: 25 mg/ml. Tablets: 10 mg, 25 mg, 50 mg, 100 mg, 200 mg.

ADMINISTRATION/HANDLING

IM

◀ALERT▶ Do not give chlorpromazine by subcutaneous route (risk for severe tissue necrosis).

• Dilute the injection solution as prescribed with Sodium Chloride for Injection or 2% procaine to reduce injection site irritation. • Slowly inject drug deep into large muscle, such as gluteus maximus rather than lateral aspect of the thigh, to minimize discomfort.

C

IV

• Dilute with 0.9% NaCl to maximum concentration of 1 mg/ml. • Administer slowly: 0.5 mg/min in children, 1 mg/min in adults.

PO

• Avoid skin contact with oral concentrate and syrup to prevent contact dermatitis. • Slight yellow color in oral concentrate or syrup will not affect drug's potency; discard if markedly discolored or if contains precipitate. • Dilute each dose of oral concentrate immediately before administration with 60 ml or more of water, coffee, tea, milk, carbonated beverage, tomato or fruit juice, simple syrup, orange syrup, soup, pudding. Use immediately; discard any remaining mixture.

INDICATIONS/ROUTES/DOSAGE

Severe Nausea/Vomiting

PO: ADULTS, ELDERLY: 10–25 mg q4–6h. **CHILDREN:** 0.5–1 mg/kg q4–6h.
IV, IM: ADULTS, ELDERLY: 25–50 mg q4–6h. **CHILDREN:** 0.5–1 mg/kg q6–8h.

Psychotic Disorders

PO: ADULTS, ELDERLY: 200–800 mg/day in 1–4 divided doses. **CHILDREN OLDER THAN 6 MOS:** 0.5–1 mg/kg q4–6h.
IV, IM: ADULTS, ELDERLY: Initially, 25 mg; may repeat in 1–4 hrs. May gradually increase to 400 mg q4–6h. Usual dose: 300–800 mg/day. **CHILDREN OLDER THAN 6 MOS:** 0.5–1 mg/kg q6–8h. **Maximum:** 75 mg/day for children 5–12 yrs; 40 mg/day for children younger than 5 yrs.

Intractable Hiccups

PO, IV, IM: ADULTS: 25–50 mg 3–4 times a day.

Porphyria

PO: ADULTS: 25–50 mg 3–4 times a day.
IM: ADULTS, ELDERLY: 25 mg 3–4 times a day.

SIDE EFFECTS

Frequent: Drowsiness, blurred vision, hypotension, color vision or night vision disturbances, dizziness, decreased diaphoresis, constipation, dry mouth, nasal congestion. **Occasional:** Urinary retention, photosensitivity, rash, decreased sexual function, swelling/pain in breasts, weight gain, nausea, vomiting, abdominal pain, tremors.

ADVERSE EFFECTS/ TOXIC REACTIONS

Extrapyramidal symptoms appear to be dose related (particularly high dosage) and are divided into three categories: akathisia (inability to sit still, tapping of feet), parkinsonian symptoms (mask-like face, tremors, shuffling gait, hypersalivation), acute dystonias (torticollis [neck muscle spasm], opisthotonos [rigidity of back muscles], and oculogyric crisis [rolling back of eyes]). Dystonic reaction may produce diaphoresis, pallor. Tardive dyskinesia (tongue protrusion, puffing of cheeks, puckering of the mouth) occurs rarely (may be irreversible). Abrupt discontinuation after long-term therapy may precipitate nausea, vomiting, gastritis, dizziness, tremors. Blood dyscrasias, particularly agranulocytosis mild leukopenia, may occur. May lower seizure threshold.

NURSING CONSIDERATIONS

BASELINE ASSESSMENT

Avoid skin contact with solution (contact dermatitis). **Antiemetic**: Assess for dehydration (poor skin turgor, dry mucous membranes, longitudinal furrows in tongue). **Antipsychotic**: Assess behavior, appearance, emotional status, response to environment, speech pattern, thought content.

INTERVENTION/EVALUATION

Monitor B/P for hypotension. Assess for EPS. Monitor WBC, differential count for blood dyscrasias, fine tongue movement (may be early sign of tardive dyskinesia). Supervise suicidal-risk pt closely during early therapy (as depression lessens, energy level improves, increasing suicide potential). Assess for therapeutic re-

C

sponse (interest in surroundings, improvement in self-care, increased ability to concentrate, relaxed facial expression). **Therapeutic serum level**: 50–300 ng/ml; **toxic serum level**: greater than 750 ng/ml.

PATIENT/FAMILY TEACHING

• Full therapeutic response may take up to 6 wks. • Urine may darken. • Do not abruptly withdraw from long-term drug therapy. • Report visual disturbances. • Drowsiness generally subsides with continued therapy. • Avoid tasks that require alertness, motor skills until response to drug is established. • Avoid alcohol, exposure to sunlight.

cholestyramine

coal-es-**tie**-rah-meen
(Novo-Cholamine, Prevalite, Questran, Questran Lite)

◆CLASSIFICATION

PHARMACOTHERAPEUTIC: Bile acid sequestrant. **CLINICAL:** Antihyperlipoproteinemic (see p. 56C).

ACTION

Binds with bile acids in intestine, forming insoluble complex. Binding results in partial removal of bile acid from enterohepatic circulation. **Therapeutic Effect:** Removes LDL cholesterol from plasma.

PHARMACOKINETICS

Not absorbed from GI tract. Decreases in serum LDL apparent in 5–7 days and in serum cholesterol in 1 mo. Serum cholesterol returns to baseline levels about 1 mo after drug is discontinued.

USES

Adjunct to dietary therapy to decrease elevated serum cholesterol levels in pts with primary hypercholesterolemia. Relief of pruritus associated with elevated levels of bile acids. **OFF-LABEL:** Treatment of diarrhea (due to bile acids), hyperoxaluria.

PRECAUTIONS

Contraindications: Complete biliary obstruction, hypersensitivity to cholestyramine, tartrazine (frequently seen in aspirin hypersensitivity). **Cautions:** GI dysfunction (esp. constipation), hemorrhoids, hematologic disorders, osteoporosis.

LIFESPAN CONSIDERATIONS

Pregnancy/Lactation: Not systemically absorbed. May interfere with maternal absorption of fat-soluble vitamins. **Pregnancy Category B. Children:** No age-related precautions noted. Limited experience in those younger than 10 yrs. **Elderly:** Increased risk of GI side effects, adverse nutritional effects.

INTERACTIONS

DRUG: May increase effects of **anticoagulants** by decreasing vitamin K level. May decrease **warfarin** absorption. May bind with, decrease absorption of **digoxin, folic acid, penicillins, propranolol, tetracyclines, thiazides, thyroid hormones, other medications.** May bind with, decrease effects of **oral vancomycin. HERBAL:** None significant. **FOOD:** None known. **LAB VALUES:** May increase serum alkaline phosphatase, magnesium, AST, ALT. May decrease serum calcium, potassium, sodium. May prolong PT.

AVAILABILITY (Rx)

Powder for Oral Suspension: 4 g/5.5 g powder (Questran Light), 4 g/9 g powder (Prevalite, Questran).

ADMINISTRATION/HANDLING

PO

• Give other drugs at least 1 hr before or 4–6 hrs following cholestyramine (capable of binding drugs in GI tract). • Do not give in dry form (highly irritating). Mix with 3–6 oz water, milk, fruit juice, soup. • Place powder on surface for 1–2 min (prevents lumping), then mix thoroughly. • Excessive foaming with carbonated beverages; use extra large glass, stir slowly. • Administer with meals.

INDICATIONS/ROUTES/DOSAGE

Hypercholesterolemia

PO: ADULTS, ELDERLY: Initially, 4 g 1–2 times a day. Maintenance: 8–16 g/day in divided doses. **Maximum:** 24 g/day. **CHILDREN:** 80 mg/kg 3 times a day.

Pruritis

PO: ADULTS, ELDERLY: Initially, 4 g 1–2 times a day. Maintenance: 8–16 g/day in divided doses. **Maximum:** 24 g/day.

SIDE EFFECTS

Frequent: Constipation (may lead to fecal impaction), nausea, vomiting, abdominal pain, indigestion. **Occasional:** Diarrhea, belching, bloating, headache, dizziness. **Rare:** Gallstones, peptic ulcer disease, malabsorption syndrome.

ADVERSE EFFECTS/ TOXIC REACTIONS

GI tract obstruction, hyperchloremic acidosis, osteoporosis secondary to calcium excretion may occur. High dosage may interfere with fat absorption, resulting in steatorrhea.

NURSING CONSIDERATIONS

BASELINE ASSESSMENT

Question for history of hypersensitivity to cholestyramine, tartrazine, aspirin. Obtain baseline serum cholesterol, triglycerides, electrolytes, hepatic enzyme levels.

INTERVENTION/EVALUATION

Monitor daily pattern of bowel activity and stool consistency. Evaluate food tolerance, abdominal discomfort, flatulence. Monitor cholesterol, triglycerides, PT, hepatic enzymes, CBC, serum electrolytes. Encourage several glasses of water between meals.

PATIENT/FAMILY TEACHING

• Complete full course of therapy; do not omit or change doses. • Take other drugs at least 1 hr before or 4–6 hrs after cholestyramine. • Never take in dry form; mix with 3–6 oz water, milk, fruit juice, soup (place powder on surface for 1–2 min to prevent lumping, then mix well). • Use extra large glass, stir slowly when mixing with carbonated beverages due to foaming. • Take with meals, drink several glasses of water between meals. • Eat high-fiber foods (whole grain cereals, fruits, vegetables) to reduce potential for constipation.

chorionic gonadotropin, hCG

kore-ee-**on**-ik goe-**nad**-oh-troe-pin (Novarel, Pregnyl)

◆CLASSIFICATION

PHARMACOTHERAPEUTIC: Gonadotropin. **CLINICAL:** Infertility therapy adjunct, diagnostic aid (hypogonadism).

ACTION

Stimulates production of gonadal steroid hormones by stimulating interstitial cells (Leydig cells) of testes to produce androgen and corpus luteum of the ovary to produce progesterone. **Therapeutic Effect:** Androgen stimulation in male causes production of secondary sex characteristics, may stimulate descent of testes when no anatomic impediment exists. In women of childbearing age with normally functioning ovaries, causes maturation of corpus luteum, triggers ovulation.

PHARMACOKINETICS

Excreted in urine. **Half-life:** 23–29 hrs.

USES

Treatment of hypogonadotropic hypogonadism, prepubertal cryptorchidism. Induces ovulation. **OFF-LABEL:** Diagnosis of male hypogonadism, treatment of corpus luteum dysfunction.

PRECAUTIONS

Contraindications: Precocious puberty, carcinoma of prostate, other androgen-dependent neoplasia. Undiagnosed abnormal vaginal bleeding, fibroid tumors of uterus, ovarian cyst or enlargement not associated with polycystic ovarian disease. Active thrombophlebitis. **Cautions:** Prepubertal males, conditions aggravated by fluid retention (cardiac/renal disease, epilepsy, migraine, asthma), polycystic ovarian disease. **Pregnancy Category X.**

INTERACTIONS

DRUG: None significant. **HERBAL:** None significant. **FOOD:** None known. **LAB VALUES:** May increase urine concentrations of 17-hydroxycorticosteroids, 17-ketosteroids.

AVAILABILITY (Rx)

Injection, Powder for Reconstitution: 10,000 units.

ADMINISTRATION/HANDLING

IM

• Reconstituted drug is stable for 30–90 days if refrigerated.

INDICATIONS/ROUTES/DOSAGE

Prepubertal Cryptorchidism, Hypogonadotropic Hypogonadism

IM: ADULTS, CHILDREN: Dosage is individualized based on indication, age, weight of pt, and physician preference.

Induction of Ovulation

IM: ADULTS (AFTER PRETREATMENT WITH MENOTROPINS): 5,000–10,000 international units 1 day after last dose of menotropins.

SIDE EFFECTS

Frequent: Pain at injection site. **Induction of ovulation:** Ovarian cysts, uncomplicated ovarian enlargement. **Occasional:** Gynecomastia, headache, irritability, fatigue, depression. **Induction of ovulation:** Severe ovarian hyperstimulation, peripheral edema. **Cryptorchidism:** Precocious puberty (acne, deepening voice, penile growth, pubic/axillary hair).

ADVERSE EFFECTS/ TOXIC REACTIONS

When used with menotropins: increased risk of arterial thromboembolism, ovarian hyperstimulation with high incidence (20%) of multiple births (premature deliveries and neonatal prematurity), ruptured ovarian cysts.

NURSING CONSIDERATIONS

BASELINE ASSESSMENT

Obtain baseline weight, B/P.

INTERVENTION/EVALUATION

Assess for edema: weigh every 2–3 days, report weight gain greater than 5 lb/wk; monitor B/P periodically during treatment; check for decreased urinary output, peripheral edema.

PATIENT/FAMILY TEACHING

• Promptly report abdominal pain, vaginal bleeding, signs of precocious puberty in males (deepening of voice; axillary, facial, pubic hair; acne; penile growth), signs of edema. • In anovulation treatment, begin recording daily basal temperature; initiate intercourse daily beginning the day preceding human chorionic gonadotropin (hCG) treatment. • Possibility of multiple births exists.

Cialis, *see tadalafil*

ciclesonide

sye-**kles**-oh-nide
(Alvesco HFA, Omnaris)

◆CLASSIFICATION

PHARMACOTHERAPEUTIC: Glucocorticoid. **CLINICAL:** Anti-inflammatory.

ACTION

Inhibits accumulation of inflammatory cells, decreases and prevents tissues from responding to inflammatory process. **Therapeutic Effect:** Relieves symptoms of allergic rhinitis, asthma.

PHARMACOKINETICS

Minimally absorbed from nasal tissue, moderately absorbed from inhalation. Protein binding: 99%. Primarily metabolized in liver. Excreted mainly in feces with lesser amount eliminated in urine. **Half-life:** 2–3 hrs.

USES

Intranasal: Management of symptoms of seasonal or perennial allergic rhinitis. **Oral Inhalation:** Treatment of asthma.

PRECAUTIONS

Contraindications: Hypersensitivity to any corticosteroid or components. **Caution:** Adrenal insufficiency, CHF, diabetes, GI disease, hepatic impairment, seizures, osteoporosis, glaucoma, thyroid disease, myasthenia gravis.

LIFESPAN CONSIDERATIONS

Pregnancy/Lactation: Unknown if drug crosses placenta or is distributed in breast milk. **Pregnancy Category C. Children:** Safety and efficacy not established in those younger than 12 yrs. **Elderly:** No age-related precautions noted.

INTERACTIONS

DRUG: **Ketoconazole** may increase plasma concentration. **HERBAL:** None significant. **FOOD:** None known. **LAB VALUES:** None significant.

AVAILABILITY (Rx)

Inhalation: (Alvesco HFA): 80 mcg/spray, 160 mcg/spray. **Nasal Spray: (Omnaris):** 50 mcg/spray.

ADMINISTRATION/HANDLING

Inhalation

• Shaking not necessary. • Wait 2 min before inhaling second dose (allows for deeper bronchial penetration). • Rinse mouth with water immediately after inhalation (prevents mouth/throat dryness).

Intranasal

• Instruct pt to clear nasal passages as much as possible before use. • Tilt head slightly forward. • Insert spray tip into nostril, pointing towards nasal passages, away from nasal septum. • Spray into one nostril while pt holds other nostril closed, concurrently inspires through nose to permit medication as high into nasal passages as possible.

INDICATIONS/ROUTES/DOSAGE

Perennial Allergic Rhinitis

INTRANASAL: ADULTS, ELDERLY, CHILDREN 12 YRS AND OLDER: 2 sprays in each nostril once a day.

Seasonal Allergic Rhinitis

INTRANASAL: ADULTS, ELDERLY, CHILDREN 6 YRS AND OLDER: 2 sprays in each nostril once a day.

Asthma

INHALATION: ADULTS, ELDERLY, CHILDREN 12 YRS AND OLDER: Initially, 80 mcg 2 times daily. **Maximum:** 320 mcg 2 times daily.

SIDE EFFECTS

Occasional (6%–4%): Headache, epistaxis, nasopharyngitis. **Rare (2%):** Ear pain.

ADVERSE EFFECTS/ TOXIC REACTIONS

Excessive doses over prolonged periods may result in systemic hypercortisolism.

NURSING CONSIDERATIONS

BASELINE ASSESSMENT

Question for hypersensitivity to any corticosteroids. Establish baseline history of asthma, rhinitis.

INTERVENTION/EVALUATION

Monitor for relief of symptoms. Monitor rate, depth, rhythm, type of respiration.

C

Assess lung sounds for rhonchi, wheezing, rales. Assess oral mucous membranes for candidiasis.

PATIENT/FAMILY TEACHING

• Improvement noted in 24–48 hrs, but full effect may take 1–2 wks for seasonal allergic rhinitis, 5 wks for perennial allergic rhinitis. • Improvement in asthma may take 4 wks or longer. • Oral inhalation not for acute asthma attacks. • Contact physician if no improvement in symptoms, sneezing or nasal irritation occurs.

cidofovir

ci-**doe**-fo-veer
(Vistide)

BLACK BOX ALERT Dose-dependent nephrotoxicity requires dose adjustment, discontinuation if changes in renal function occur (renal lab tests, urinalysis). May cause hypospermia. May be embryotoxic, teratogenic. Neutropenia reported: monitor neutrophil count.

◆CLASSIFICATION

PHARMACOTHERAPEUTIC: Anti-infective. **CLINICAL:** Antiviral (see p. 67C).

ACTION

Inhibits viral DNA synthesis by incorporating itself into growing viral DNA chain. **Therapeutic Effect:** Suppresses replication of cytomegalovirus (CMV).

PHARMACOKINETICS

Protein binding: less than 6%. Excreted primarily unchanged in urine. Effect of hemodialysis unknown. **Elimination Half-life:** 1.4–3.8 hrs.

USES

Treatment of CMV retinitis in those with HIV. Should be given with probenecid. **OFF-LABEL:** Treatment of acyclovir-resistant herpes simplex virus, adenovirus, foscarnet-resistant CMV, ganciclovir-resistant CMV, varicella-zoster virus.

PRECAUTIONS

Contraindications: Direct intraocular injection, history of clinically severe hypersensitivity to probenecid or other sulfa-containing drugs, renal impairment (serum creatinine level greater than 1.5 mg/dl, creatinine clearance 55 ml/min or less, or urine protein level greater than 100 mg/dl). **Caution:** Preexisting diabetes.

⌛ LIFESPAN CONSIDERATIONS

Pregnancy/Lactation: Embryotoxic (reduced fetal body weight) in animals. Unknown if distributed in breast milk. Breast-feeding not recommended. **Pregnancy Category C. Children:** Safety and efficacy not established. **Elderly:** Age-related renal impairment may require dosage adjustment.

INTERACTIONS

DRUG: **Nephrotoxic medications (e.g., aminoglycosides, amphotericin B, foscarnet, IV pentamidine)** increase risk of nephrotoxicity. **HERBAL:** None significant. **FOOD:** None known. **LAB VALUES:** May decrease neutrophil count, serum bicarbonate, phosphate, uric acid. May elevate serum creatinine.

AVAILABILITY (Rx)

Injection Solution: 75 mg/ml (5-ml ampule).

ADMINISTRATION/HANDLING

◀ALERT▶ Do not exceed recommended dosage, frequency, infusion rate.

IV

Reconstitution • Dilute in 100 ml 0.9% NaCl or D_5W not to exceed concentration of 8 mg/ml.

Rate of administration • Infuse over 1 hr. • IV hydration with 0.9% NaCl and probenecid therapy **must** be used with each cidofovir infusion (minimizes risk of nephrotoxicity). • Ingestion of food before each dose of probenecid may reduce nausea/vomiting. Antiemetic may reduce potential for nausea.

Storage • Store at controlled room temperature (68°–77°F). • Admixtures may be refrigerated for no more than 24 hrs. • Allow refrigerated admixtures to warm to room temperature before use.

IV INCOMPATIBILITIES

No information available for Y-site administration.

INDICATIONS/ROUTES/DOSAGE

Cytomegalovirus (CMV) Retinitis in Pts with AIDS (in Combination with Probenecid)

IV INFUSION: ADULTS: Induction: Usual dosage, 5 mg/kg at constant rate over 1 hr once weekly for 2 consecutive wks. Give 2 g of PO probenecid 3 hrs before cidofovir dose, then give 1 g 2 hrs and 8 hrs after completion of the 1-hr cidofovir infusion (total of 4 g). In addition, give 1 L of 0.9% NaCl over 1–2 hrs immediately before cidofovir infusion. If tolerated, a second liter may be infused over 1–3 hrs at start of infusion or immediately afterward. **CHILDREN:** 5 mg/kg one time with probenecid and hydration. Maintenance: **ADULTS, ELDERLY:** 5 mg/kg once every 2 wks. **CHILDREN:** 3 mg/kg once every wk.

Dosage in Renal Impairment

Changes During Therapy: If creatinine increases by 0.3–0.4 mg/dl, reduce dose to 3 mg/kg; if creatinine increases by 0.5 mg/dl or greater or proteinuria 3+ or greater develops, discontinue therapy.

Preexisting Renal Impairment: Do not use with serum creatinine greater than 1.5 mg/dl, creatinine clearance less than 55 ml/min, or urine protein 100 mg/dl or greater (2+ or greater proteinuria).

SIDE EFFECTS

Frequent: Nausea, vomiting (65%), fever (57%), asthenia (loss of strength, energy) (46%), rash (30%), diarrhea (27%), headache (27%), alopecia (25%), chills (24%), anorexia (22%), dyspnea (22%), abdominal pain (17%).

ADVERSE EFFECTS/ TOXIC REACTIONS

Serious adverse effects include proteinuria (80%), nephrotoxicity (53%), neutropenia (31%), elevated serum creatinine (29%), infection (24%), anemia (20%), decrease in intraocular pressure (IOP) (12%), pneumonia (9%). Concurrent use of probenecid may produce a hypersensitivity reaction characterized by rash, fever, chills, anaphylaxis. Acute renal failure occurs rarely.

NURSING CONSIDERATIONS

BASELINE ASSESSMENT

For those taking zidovudine, temporarily discontinue zidovudine administration or decrease zidovudine dose by 50% on days of infusion (probenecid reduces metabolic clearance of zidovudine). Closely monitor renal function (urinalysis, serum creatinine) during therapy.

INTERVENTION/EVALUATION

Monitor serum creatinine, BUN, WBC count, urine protein, electrolytes, hepatic function tests before each dose. Monitor for proteinuria (may be early indicator of dose-dependent nephrotoxicity). Periodically monitor visual acuity, ocular symptoms.

PATIENT/FAMILY TEACHING

• Obtain regular follow-up ophthalmologic exams. • Those of childbearing age should use effective contraception during and for 1 mo after treatment. • Men should practice barrier contraceptive methods during and for 3 mos after treatment. • Breast-feeding not recommended. • Must complete full course of probenecid with each cidofovir dose. • Report rash immediately.

cilostazol

sill-oh-**stay**-zole
(Pletal)

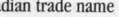

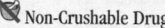

C

BLACK BOX ALERT Contraindicated in pts with CHF of any severity.

Do not confuse Pletal with Plendil.

◆CLASSIFICATION

PHARMACOTHERAPEUTIC: Phosphodiesterase enzyme inhibitor. **CLINICAL:** Antiplatelet.

ACTION

Inhibits platelet aggregation. Dilates vascular beds with greatest dilation in femoral beds. **Therapeutic Effect:** Improves walking distance in those with intermittent claudication; usually noted in 2–4 wks but may take as long as 12 wks.

PHARMACOKINETICS

Moderately absorbed from GI tract. Protein binding: 95%–98%. Extensively metabolized in liver. Excreted primarily in urine and, to a lesser extent, in feces. Not removed by hemodialysis. **Half-life:** 11–13 hrs.

USES

Management of peripheral vascular disease, primarily intermittent claudication. **OFF-LABEL:** Treatment of acute coronary syndrome, graft patency improvement in percutaneous coronary intervention with/without stenting.

PRECAUTIONS

Contraindications: CHF of any severity; hemostatic disorders or active pathologic bleeding (bleeding peptic ulcer, intracranial bleeding). **Cautions:** None known.

LIFESPAN CONSIDERATIONS

Pregnancy/Lactation: Unknown if drug crosses placenta or is distributed in breast milk. **Pregnancy Category C. Children:** Safety and efficacy not established. **Elderly:** No age-related precautions noted.

INTERACTIONS

DRUG: **Aspirin** may potentiate inhibition of platelet aggregation. **Clarithromycin, diltiazem, erythromycin, fluconazole, fluoxetine, omeprazole, sertraline** may increase concentration. **HERBAL:** None significant. **FOOD:** **Grapefruit, grapefruit juice** may increase concentration, toxicity. **LAB VALUES:** May increase BUN, serum glucose, uric acid. May decrease platelet count, WBCs.

AVAILABILITY (Rx)

Tablets: 50 mg, 100 mg.

ADMINISTRATION/HANDLING

PO

• Give at least 30 min before or 2 hrs after meals. • Do not take with grapefruit juice.

INDICATIONS/ROUTES/DOSAGE

Peripheral Vascular Disease

PO: ADULTS, ELDERLY: 100 mg twice a day at least 30 min before or 2 hrs after meals. 50 mg twice a day during concurrent therapy with CYP3A4 or CYP2C19 (e.g., clarithromycin, diltiazem, erythromycin, fluconazole, fluoxetine, omeprazole, sertraline).

SIDE EFFECTS

Frequent (34%–10%): Headache, diarrhea, palpitations, dizziness, pharyngitis. **Occasional (7%–3%):** Nausea, rhinitis, back pain, peripheral edema, dyspepsia, abdominal pain, tachycardia, cough, flatulence, myalgia. **Rare (2%–1%):** Leg cramps, paresthesia, rash, vomiting.

ADVERSE EFFECTS/ TOXIC REACTIONS

Overdose noted as severe headache, diarrhea, hypotension, cardiac arrhythmias.

NURSING CONSIDERATIONS

BASELINE ASSESSMENT

Assess platelet count, CBC before treatment and periodically during treatment.

PATIENT/FAMILY TEACHING

• Take on an empty stomach (at least 30 min before or 2 hrs after meals). • Do not take with grapefruit juice.

Ciloxan, *see ciprofloxacin*

cimetidine

sih-**met**-ih-deen
(Apo-Cimetidine ✦, Novo-Cimetidine ✦, Tagamet, Tagamet HB 200)
Do not confuse cimetidine with simethicone.

◆CLASSIFICATION

PHARMACOTHERAPEUTIC: H_2 receptor antagonist. **CLINICAL:** Antiulcer, gastric acid secretion inhibitor (see p. 107C).

ACTION

Inhibits histamine action at histamine 2 (H_2) receptor sites of parietal cells. **Therapeutic Effect:** Inhibits gastric acid secretion.

PHARMACOKINETICS

Well absorbed from GI tract. Protein binding: 15%–20%. Widely distributed. Metabolized in liver. Primarily excreted in urine. Not removed by hemodialysis. **Half-life:** 2 hrs (increased in renal impairment).

USES

Short-term treatment of active duodenal ulcer. Prevention of duodenal ulcer recurrence, upper GI bleeding in critically ill pts. Treatment of benign gastric ulcer, pathologic GI hypersecretory conditions, gastroesophageal reflux disease (GERD). **OTC use**: Heartburn, acid indigestion, sour stomach. **OFF-LABEL:** Prevention of aspiration pneumonia; treatment of acute urticaria, chronic warts, upper GI bleeding; *H. pylori* eradication.

PRECAUTIONS

Contraindications: Hypersensitivity to other H_2-antagonists. **Cautions:** Renal/hepatic impairment, elderly. Cimetidine may interfere with skin allergen testing.

⌛ LIFESPAN CONSIDERATIONS

Pregnancy/Lactation: Distributed in breast milk. Safe use in pregnancy has not been established (possible adverse effects on fetal development). **Pregnancy Category B. Children:** Long-term use may induce cerebral toxicity, affect hormonal system. **Elderly:** More likely to experience confusion, esp. in those with renal impairment.

INTERACTIONS

DRUG: May increase concentration, decrease metabolism of **metoprolol, oral anticoagulants, phenytoin, propranolol, theophylline, tricyclic antidepressants.** May decrease absorption of **itraconazole, ketoconazole. HERBAL: St. John's wort** may decrease concentration. **FOOD:** None known. **LAB VALUES:** Interferes with skin tests using allergen extracts. May increase serum prolactin, creatinine, transaminase. May decrease parathyroid hormone concentration.

AVAILABILITY (Rx)

Injection, Solution: 150 mg/ml. **Liquid, Oral:** 300 mg/5 ml. **Tablets:** 200 mg (OTC), 300 mg, 400 mg, 800 mg.

ADMINISTRATION/HANDLING

IV

Reconstitution • Dilute with 0.9% NaCl, D_5W. • For IV push, dilute to concentration not to exceed 15 mg/ml. • For intermittent IV (piggyback), dilute to concentration not to exceed 6 mg/ml.

Rate of administration • For IV push, administer over not less than 5 min (prevents arrhythmias, hypotension). • For intermittent IV (piggyback), infuse over 15–30 min. • For IV infusion, dilute with 100–1,000 ml 0.9% NaCl, D_5W, or other compatible solution (see Reconstitution) and infuse over 24 hrs.

C

Storage • Store at room temperature. • Reconstituted drug is stable for 7 days at room temperature.

IM
• Administer undiluted. • Inject deep into large muscle mass.

PO
• Give without regard to food. • Best given with meals and at bedtime. • Do not administer within 1 hr of antacids.

IV INCOMPATIBILITIES

Allopurinol (Aloprim), amphotericin B complex (Abelcet, AmBisome, Amphotec), cefepime (Maxipime).

IV COMPATIBILITIES

Aminophylline, diltiazem (Cardizem), furosemide (Lasix), heparin, hydromorphone (Dilaudid), insulin (regular), lidocaine, lipids, lorazepam (Ativan), midazolam (Versed), morphine, potassium chloride, propofol (Diprivan).

INDICATIONS/ROUTES/DOSAGE

Active Duodenal Ulcer
PO: ADULTS, ELDERLY: 300 mg 4 times a day or 400 mg twice a day or 800 mg at bedtime for up to 8 wks.
IV, IM: ADULTS, ELDERLY: 300 mg q6h or 37.5 mg/hr continuous infusion.

Prevention of Duodenal Ulcer
PO: ADULTS, ELDERLY: 400 mg at bedtime.

Gastric Hypersecretory Secretions
PO, IV, IM: ADULTS, ELDERLY: 300–600 mg q6h. **Maximum:** 2,400 mg/day.

Gastroesophageal Reflux Disease (GERD)
PO: ADULTS, ELDERLY: 800 mg twice a day or 400 mg 4 times a day for 12 wks.

OTC Use
PO: ADULTS, ELDERLY: 200 mg up to 30 min before meals. **Maximum:** 2 doses/day.

Prevention of Upper GI Bleeding
IV INFUSION: ADULTS, ELDERLY: 50 mg/hr.

Usual Pediatric Dosage
CHILDREN: 20–40 mg/kg/day in divided doses q6h. **INFANTS:** 10–20 mg/kg/day in divided doses q6–12h. **NEONATES:** 5–10 mg/kg/day in divided doses q8–12h.

Dosage in Renal Impairment
Dosage is modified based on creatinine clearance.

Creatinine Clearance	Dosage
Greater than 50 ml/min	No change
10–50 ml/min	50% of normal dose
Less than 10 ml/min	25% of normal dose

Give after hemodialysis and q12h between dialysis sessions.

SIDE EFFECTS

Occasional (4%–2%): Headache. **Elderly, pts with renal impairment, severely ill pts:** Confusion, agitation, psychosis, depression, anxiety, disorientation, hallucinations. Effects reverse 3–4 days after discontinuance. **Rare (less than 2%):** Diarrhea, dizziness, drowsiness, nausea, vomiting, gynecomastia, rash, impotence.

ADVERSE EFFECTS/ TOXIC REACTIONS

Rapid IV administration may produce cardiac arrhythmias, hypotension.

NURSING CONSIDERATIONS

BASELINE ASSESSMENT
Obtain baseline CBC, PT, aPTT, BUN, creatinine.

INTERVENTION/EVALUATION
Monitor B/P for hypotension during IV infusion. Assess for GI bleeding: hematemesis, blood in stool. Monitor for changes in mental status in elderly, severely ill, those with renal impairment.

PATIENT/FAMILY TEACHING
• May produce transient discomfort at IM injection site. • Do not take antacids within 1 hr of cimetidine administration. • Avoid tasks that require alertness, motor

skills until response to drug is established. • Avoid smoking, excessive amounts of coffee. • Report any blood in vomitus/stool, or dark, tarry stool.

cinacalcet

sin-ah-**kal**-set
(Sensipar)

◆CLASSIFICATION

PHARMACOTHERAPEUTIC: Calcium receptor agonist. **CLINICAL:** Calcimimetic.

ACTION

Increases sensitivity of calcium-sensing receptor on parathyroid gland to activation by extracellular calcium, thus lowering parathyroid hormone (PTH) levels. **Therapeutic Effect:** Decreases serum calcium, PTH levels.

PHARMACOKINETICS

Extensively distributed after PO administration. Protein binding: 93%–97%. Metabolized in liver to inactive metabolites. Primarily eliminated in urine with a lesser amount excreted in feces. **Half-life:** 30–40 hrs.

USES

Treatment of hypercalcemia in pts with parathyroid carcinoma. Treatment of secondary hyperparathyroidism in pts with chronic renal disease on dialysis. **OFF-LABEL:** Primary hyperparathyroidism.

PRECAUTIONS

Contraindications: None known. **Cautions:** Hepatic impairment.

LIFESPAN CONSIDERATIONS

Pregnancy/Lactation: May cross placental barrier; unknown if distributed in breast milk. Safe usage during lactation not established (potential adverse reaction in infants). **Pregnancy Category C.** **Children:** Safety and efficacy not established. **Elderly:** No age-related precautions noted.

INTERACTIONS

DRUG: Increases **amitriptyline** plasma concentration. **Erythromycin, itraconazole, ketoconazole** increase plasma concentration. Concurrent administration of **flecainide, thioridazine, tricyclic antidepressants, vinblastine** may require dosage adjustment. **HERBAL:** None significant. **FOOD: High-fat meals** increase plasma concentration. **LAB VALUES:** Lowers serum calcium, phosphorus level.

AVAILABILITY (Rx)

Tablets: 30 mg, 60 mg, 90 mg.

ADMINISTRATION/HANDLING

PO

• Store at room temperature. • Do not break/crush film-coated tablets. • Administer with food or shortly after a meal.

INDICATIONS/ROUTES/DOSAGE

Hypercalcemia in Parathyroid Carcinoma

PO: ADULTS, ELDERLY: Initially, 30 mg twice a day. Titrate dosage sequentially (60 mg twice a day, 90 mg twice a day, and 90 mg 3–4 times a day) every 2–4 wks as needed to normalize serum calcium level. **Maximum:** 360 mg/day.

Secondary Hyperparathyroidism in Pts on Dialysis

PO: ADULTS, ELDERLY: Initially, 30 mg once a day. Titrate dosage sequentially (60, 90, 120, and 180 mg once a day) every 2–4 wks to maintain iPTH level between 150–300 pg/ml.

SIDE EFFECTS

Frequent (31%–21%): Nausea, vomiting, diarrhea. **Occasional (15%–10%):** Myalgia, dizziness. **Rare (7%–5%):** Asthenia (loss of strength, energy), hypertension, anorexia, noncardiac chest pain.

C

ADVERSE EFFECTS/ TOXIC REACTIONS

Overdose may lead to hypocalcemia.

NURSING CONSIDERATIONS

BASELINE ASSESSMENT

Establish baseline serum electrolyte levels, serum calcium, phosphorus for hyperparathyroidism, serum calcium for parathyroid carcinoma.

INTERVENTION/EVALUATION

Monitor serum calcium, phosphorus for hyperparathyroidism. Monitor daily pattern of bowel activity and stool consistency. Obtain order for antidiarrhea, antiemetic medication to prevent serum electrolyte imbalance. Assess for evidence of dizziness, institute fall risk precautions.

PATIENT/FAMILY TEACHING

• Take cinacalcet with food or shortly after a meal. • Notify physician immediately if vomiting, diarrhea, cramping, muscle pain, numbness occurs.

Cipro, *see ciprofloxacin*

Cipro IV, *see ciprofloxacin*

ciprofloxacin

sip-row-**flocks**-ah-sin
(Apo-Ciproflox 🍁, Cetraxal, Ciloxan, Cipro, Cipro IV, Cipro XR, Novo-Ciprofloxacin 🍁, Proquin XR)

BLACK BOX ALERT May increase risk of tendonitis, tendon rupture.

Do not confuse Ciloxan with Cytoxan, or Cipro with Ceftin, or ciprofloxacin with cephalexin.

FIXED-COMBINATION(S)

Cipro HC Otic: ciprofloxacin/hydrocortisone (a steroid): 0.2%/1%. **CiproDex Otic:** ciprofloxacin/dexamethasone (a corticosteroid): 0.3%/0.1%.

◆CLASSIFICATION

PHARMACOTHERAPEUTIC: Fluoroquinolone. **CLINICAL:** Anti-infective (see p. 25C).

ACTION

Inhibits enzyme, DNA gyrase, in susceptible bacteria, interfering with bacterial cell replication. **Therapeutic Effect:** Bactericidal.

PHARMACOKINETICS

Well absorbed from GI tract. Protein binding: 20%–40%. Widely distributed including to CSF. Metabolized in liver to active metabolite (limited activity). Primarily excreted in urine. Minimal removal by hemodialysis. **Half-life:** 3–5 hrs (increased in renal impairment, elderly).

USES

Treatment of susceptible infections due to *E. coli, K. pneumoniae, E. cloacae, P. mirabilis, P. vulgaris, P. aeruginosa, H. influenzae, M. catarrhalis, S. pneumoniae, S. aureus* (methicillin susceptible), *S. epidermidis, S. pyogenes, C. jejuni,* Shigella spp., *S. typhi* including intra-abdominal, bone, joint, lower respiratory tract, skin/skin structure, UTIs, infectious diarrhea, prostatitis, sinusitis, typhoid fever, febrile neutropenia. OTIC: Treatment of acute otitis externa. **OFF-LABEL:** Treatment of chancroid. Acute pulmonary exacerbations in cystic fibrosis, disseminated gonococcal infections, prophylaxis to *Neisseria meninigitidis* following close contact with infected person.

PRECAUTIONS

Contraindications: Hypersensitivity to any fluoroquinolones, other quinolones; for ophthalmic administration: vaccinia, varicella, epithelial herpes simplex, keratitis, mycobacterial infection, fungal disease of ocular structure, use after uncomplicated removal of foreign body. Cautions: Renal impairment, CNS disorders, seizures, those taking theophylline, caffeine. Suspension not for use in NG tube. May prolong QT interval.

LIFESPAN CONSIDERATIONS

Pregnancy/Lactation: Unknown if distributed in breast milk. If possible, do not use during pregnancy/lactation (risk of arthropathy to fetus/infant). **Pregnancy Category C. Children:** Safety and efficacy not established in those younger than 18 yrs. Arthropathy may occur if given to children younger than 18 yrs. **Elderly:** Age-related renal impairment may require dosage adjustment.

INTERACTIONS

DRUG: **Antacids, iron preparations, sucralfate** may decrease absorption. May increase effects of **caffeine, oral anticoagulants.** May decrease concentration of **fosphenytoin, phenytoin.** May increase concentration, toxicity of **theophylline.** Decreases **theophylline** clearance. HERBAL: **Dong quai, St. John's wort** may increase photosensitization. FOOD: None known. LAB VALUES: May increase serum alkaline phosphatase, creatine kinase (CK), LDH, AST, ALT.

AVAILABILITY (Rx)

Infusion Solution: 200 mg/100 ml, 400 mg/200 ml. **Injection, Solution (Cipro):** 10 mg/ml. **Ophthalmic Ointment (Ciloxan):** 0.3%. **Ophthalmic Solution (Ciloxan):** 0.3%. **Otic Solution (Cetraxal):** 0.2%. **Tablets (Cipro):** 100 mg, 250 mg, 500 mg, 750 mg.

Tablets (Extended-Release) (Cipro XR, Proquin XR): 500 mg. **(Cipro XR):** 1,000 mg.

ADMINISTRATION/HANDLING

IV

Reconstitution • Available prediluted in infusion container ready for use.

Rate of administration • Infuse over 60 min (reduces risk of venous irritation).

Storage • Store at room temperature. • Solution appears clear, colorless to slightly yellow.

PO

• May be given without regard to food (preferred dosing time: 2 hrs after meals). • Do not give with dairy products. • Do not administer antacids (aluminum, magnesium) within 2 hrs of ciprofloxacin.

Ophthalmic

• Place gloved finger on lower eyelid and pull out until a pocket is formed between eye and lower lid. • Place ointment or drops into pocket. • Instruct pt to close eye gently for 1-2 min (so medication will not be squeezed out of the sac). • Instruct pt using ointment to roll eyeball to increase contact area of drug to eye. • Instruct pt using solution to apply digital pressure to lacrimal sac at inner canthus for 1 min to minimize systemic absorption. • Do not use ophthalmic solution for injection.

IV INCOMPATIBILITIES

Aminophylline, ampicillin and sulbactam (Unasyn), cefepime (Maxipime), dexamethasone (Decadron), furosemide (Lasix), heparin, hydrocortisone (Solu-Cortef), methylprednisolone (Solu-Medrol), phenytoin (Dilantin), sodium bicarbonate, total parenteral nutrition (TPN).

IV COMPATIBILITIES

Calcium gluconate, diltiazem (Cardizem), dobutamine (Dobutrex), dopamine (Intropin), lidocaine, lipids, lorazepam (Ativan), magnesium, midazolam (Versed), potassium chloride.

INDICATIONS/ROUTES/DOSAGE

Usual Dosage Range

PO: ADULTS, ELDERLY: 250–750 mg q12h.
IV: ADULTS, ELDERLY: 200–400 mg q12h.

Bone, Joint Infections

IV: ADULTS, ELDERLY: 400 mg q8–12h for 4–6 wks.

PO: ADULTS, ELDERLY: 500–750 mg q12h for 4–6 wks.

C

Conjunctivitis
OPHTHALMIC: ADULTS, ELDERLY: (Solution): 1–2 drops q2h for 2 days, then 2 drops q4h for next 5 days. **(Ointment):** ½ inch 3 times a day for 2 days, then ½ inch daily for 5 days.

Corneal Ulcer
OPHTHALMIC: ADULTS, ELDERLY: 2 drops q15min for 6 hrs, then 2 drops q30min for the remainder of first day, 2 drops q1h on second day, and 2 drops q4h on days 3–14.

Cystic Fibrosis
IV: CHILDREN: 40 mg/kg/day in 2–3 divided doses. **Maximum:** 1.2 g/day.
PO: CHILDREN: 40 mg/kg/day. **Maximum:** 2 g/day.

Febrile Neutropenia
IV: ADULTS, ELDERLY: 400 mg q8h for 7–14 days (in combination).

Gonorrhea
PO: ADULTS, ELDERLY: 250–500 mg as a single dose.

Infectious Diarrhea
PO: ADULTS, ELDERLY: 500 mg q12h for 3–7 days.

Intra-Abdominal Infections (with Metronidazole)
IV: ADULTS, ELDERLY: 400 mg q12h for 7–14 days.
PO: ADULTS, ELDERLY: 500 mg q12h for 7–14 days.

Lower Respiratory Tract Infections
IV: ADULTS, ELDERLY: 400 mg q8–12h for 7–14 days.
PO: ADULTS, ELDERLY: 500–750 mg q12h for 7–14 days.

Nosocomial Pneumonia
IV: ADULTS, ELDERLY: 400 mg q8h for 10–14 days.

Prostatitis
IV: ADULTS, ELDERLY: 400 mg q12h for 28 days.
PO: ADULTS, ELDERLY: 500 mg q12h for 28 days.

Sinusitis
IV: ADULTS, ELDERLY: 400 mg q12h for 10 days.
PO: ADULTS, ELDERLY: 500 mg q12h for 10 days.

Skin/Skin Structure Infections
IV: ADULTS, ELDERLY: 400 mg q12h for 7–14 days.
PO: ADULTS, ELDERLY: 500–750 mg q12h for 7–14 days.

Susceptible Infections
IV: ADULTS, ELDERLY: 400 mg q8–12h.
PO: ADULTS, ELDERLY: 500–750 mg q12h.

Typhoid Fever
PO: ADULTS, ELDERLY: 500 mg q12h for 10 days.

UTI
IV: ADULTS, ELDERLY: 200–400 mg q12h for 7–14 days.
PO: ADULTS, ELDERLY: Immediate-release: 250 mg q12h for 3 days for acute uncomplicated infections; 250 mg q12h for 7–14 days for mild to moderate infections; 500 mg q12h for 7–14 days for severe or complicated infections. **Extended-release: Complicated infection:** 1,000 mg q24h for 7–14 days. **Uncomplicated infection:** 500 mg q24h for 3 days.

Otitis Externa
OTIC: ADULTS, ELDERLY, CHILDREN: Contents of one single-use container 2 times a day for 7 days.

Dosage in Renal Impairment
Dosage and frequency are modified based on creatinine clearance and the severity of the infection.

Creatinine Clearance	Dosage
30–50 ml/min	PO: 250–500 mg q12h
Less than 30 ml/min	PO (extended-release): 500 mg q24h PO (immediate-release): 250–500 mg q18h IV: 200-400 q18–24h

Hemodialysis

ADULTS, ELDERLY: 250–500 mg q24h (after dialysis).

Peritoneal Dialysis

ADULTS, ELDERLY: 250–500 mg q24h (after dialysis).

SIDE EFFECTS

Frequent (5%–2%): Nausea, diarrhea, dyspepsia, vomiting, constipation, flatulence, confusion, crystalluria. **Ophthalmic:** Burning, crusting in corner of eye. **Occasional (less than 2%):** Abdominal pain/discomfort, headache, rash. **Ophthalmic:** Bad taste, sensation of foreign body in eye, eyelid redness, itching. **Rare (less than 1%):** Dizziness, confusion, tremors, hallucinations, hypersensitivity reaction, insomnia, dry mouth, paresthesia.

ADVERSE EFFECTS/ TOXIC REACTIONS

Superinfection (esp. enterococcal, fungal), nephropathy, cardiopulmonary arrest, cerebral thrombosis may occur. Hypersensitivity reaction (rash, pruritus, blisters, edema, burning skin), photosensitivity have occurred. Sensitization to ophthalmic form may contraindicate later systemic use of ciprofloxacin.

NURSING CONSIDERATIONS

BASELINE ASSESSMENT

Question for history of hypersensitivity to ciprofloxacin, quinolones.

INTERVENTION/EVALUATION

Obtain urinalysis for microscopic analysis for crystalluria prior to and during treatment. Evaluate food tolerance. Monitor daily pattern of bowel activity and stool consistency. Encourage pt to drink several glasses of water daily (reduces risk of crystalluria). Monitor for dizziness, headache, visual changes, tremors. Assess for chest, joint pain. **Ophthalmic:** Observe therapeutic response.

PATIENT/FAMILY TEACHING

• Do not skip doses; take full course of therapy. • Maintain adequate hydration to prevent crystalluria. • Do not take antacids 2 hrs before or 6 hrs after ciprofloxacin (reduces/destroys effectiveness). • Shake suspension well before using; do not chew microcapsules in suspension. • Sugarless gum, hard candy may relieve bad taste. • Avoid caffeine. • Report tendon pain or swelling. • Avoid exposure to sunlight/artificial light (may cause photosensitivity reaction). • Report persistent diarrhea. • **Ophthalmic:** Crystal precipitate may form, usual resolution in 1–7 days.

cisplatin HIGH ALERT

sis-**plah**-tin
(Platinol-AQ)

BLACK BOX ALERT Cumulative renal toxicity may be severe. Dose-related toxicities include myelosuppression, nausea, vomiting. Ototoxicity, especially pronounced in children, noted by tinnitus, loss of high-frequency hearing, deafness. Must be administered by personnel trained in administration/handling of chemotherapeutic agents. Anaphylactic reaction can occur within minutes of administration.

Do not confuse cisplatin with carboplatin or oxaliplatin.

◆CLASSIFICATION

PHARMACOTHERAPEUTIC: Platinum coordination complex. **CLINICAL:** Antineoplastic (see p. 81C).

ACTION

Inhibits DNA and, to a lesser extent, RNA protein synthesis by cross-linking with

DNA strands. Cell cycle–phase nonspecific. **Therapeutic Effect:** Prevents cellular division.

PHARMACOKINETICS

Widely distributed. Protein binding: greater than 90%. Undergoes rapid nonenzymatic conversion to inactive metabolite. Excreted in urine. Removed by hemodialysis. **Half-life:** 58–73 hrs (increased in renal impairment).

USES

Treatment of metastatic testicular tumors, metastatic ovarian tumors, advanced bladder carcinoma. **OFF-LABEL:** Adrenocortical, anal, biliary tract, breast, cervical, endometrial, esophageal, gastric, head and neck, lung (small-cell, non–small-cell), primary hepatocellular, prostatic, skin, thyroid, vulvar carcinomas; germ cell, gestational trophoblastic, ovarian germ cell tumors; Hodgkin's and non-Hodgkin's lymphomas; Kaposi's sarcoma, malignant melanoma, neuroblastoma, osteosarcoma, soft tissue sarcoma, Wilms' tumor.

PRECAUTIONS

Contraindications: Hearing impairment, myelosuppression, preexisting renal impairment. **Cautions:** Previous therapy with other antineoplastic agents, radiation.

LIFESPAN CONSIDERATIONS

Pregnancy/Lactation: If possible, avoid use during pregnancy, esp. first trimester. Breast-feeding not recommended. **Pregnancy Category D. Children:** Ototoxic effects may be more severe. **Elderly:** Age-related renal impairment may require dosage adjustment.

INTERACTIONS

DRUG: May decrease effects of **antigout medications. Bone marrow depressants** may increase myelosuppression. **Live virus vaccines** may potentiate virus replication, increase vaccine side effects, decrease pt's antibody response to vaccine. **Nephrotoxic, ototoxic agents** may increase risk of toxicity. **HERBAL:** Avoid **black cohosh, dong quai** with estrogen-dependent tumors. **FOOD:** None known. **LAB VALUES:** May increase BUN, serum creatinine, uric acid, AST. May decrease creatinine clearance, serum calcium, magnesium, phosphate, potassium, sodium. May cause positive Coombs' test.

AVAILABILITY (Rx)

Injection Solution: 1 mg/ml (50 ml, 100 ml, 200 ml).

ADMINISTRATION/HANDLING

◀ALERT▶ Wear protective gloves during handling of cisplatin. May be carcinogenic, mutagenic, teratogenic. Handle with extreme care during preparation/administration.

IV

Dilution • For IV infusion, dilute desired dose in 250–1,000 ml 0.9% NaCl, D_5/0.45% NaCl, or D_5/0.9% NaCl to concentration of 0.05–2 mg/ml. Solution should have final NaCl concentration of 0.2% or greater.

Rate of administration • Infuse over 2–24 hrs. • Avoid rapid infusion (increases risk of nephrotoxicity, ototoxicity). • Monitor for anaphylactic reaction during first few minutes of IV infusion.

Storage • Protect from sunlight; do not refrigerate (may precipitate). Discard if precipitate forms. IV infusion: Stable for 72 hrs at 39°F–77°F.

IV INCOMPATIBILITIES

Amifostine (Ethyol), amphotericin B complex (Abelcet, AmBisome, Amphotec), cefepime (Maxipime), piperacillin and tazobactam (Zosyn), sodium bicarbonate, thiotepa.

IV COMPATIBILITIES

Etoposide (VePesid), granisetron (Kytril), heparin, hydromorphone (Dilaudid), lipids, lorazepam (Ativan), magnesium sulfate, mannitol, morphine, ondansetron (Zofran).

INDICATIONS/ROUTES/DOSAGE

Note: Pretreatment hydration with 1–2 liters of fluid recommended. Adequate hydration, urine output greater than 100 ml/hr should be maintained for 24 hrs after administration.

Bladder Carcinoma

IV: ADULTS, ELDERLY: (Single agent): 50–70 mg/m² q3–4wks.

Ovarian Tumors

IV: ADULTS, ELDERLY: 75–100 mg/m² q3–4wks.

Testicular Tumors

IV: ADULTS, ELDERLY: 10–20 mg/m² daily for 5 days repeated q3–4wks.

Dosage in Renal Impairment

Dosage is modified based on creatinine clearance, BUN.

◀ALERT▶ Repeated courses of cisplatin should not be given until serum creatinine is less than 1.5 mg/100 ml and/or BUN is less than 25 mg/100 ml.

Creatinine Clearance	Dosage
10–50 ml/min	75% of normal dose
Less than 10 ml/min	50% of normal dose

SIDE EFFECTS

Frequent: Nausea, vomiting (generally beginning 1–4 hrs after administration and lasting up to 24 hrs); myelosuppression (affecting 25%–30% of pts, with recovery generally occurring in 18–23 days). **Occasional:** Peripheral neuropathy (with prolonged therapy [4–7 mos]). Pain/redness at injection site, loss of taste, appetite. **Rare:** Hemolytic anemia, blurred vision, stomatitis.

ADVERSE EFFECTS/ TOXIC REACTIONS

Anaphylactic reaction (angioedema, wheezing, tachycardia, hypotension) may occur in first few minutes of IV administration in those previously exposed to cisplatin. Nephrotoxicity occurs in 28%–36% of pts treated with single dose of cisplatin, usually during second wk of therapy. Ototoxicity (tinnitus, hearing loss) occurs in 31% of pts treated with single dose of cisplatin (more severe in children). Symptoms may become more frequent, severe with repeated doses.

NURSING CONSIDERATIONS

BASELINE ASSESSMENT

Pts should be well hydrated before and 24 hrs after medication to ensure adequate urinary output (100 ml/hr), decrease risk of nephrotoxicity.

INTERVENTION/EVALUATION

Measure all vomitus (general guideline requiring immediate notification of physician: 750 ml/8 hrs, urinary output less than 100 ml/hr). Monitor I&O q1–2h beginning with pretreatment hydration, continue for 48 hrs after cisplatin therapy. Assess vital signs q1–2h during infusion. Monitor urinalysis, electrolytes, hepatic function tests, CBC, platelet count, renal function tests for nephrotoxicity.

PATIENT/FAMILY TEACHING

• Report signs of ototoxicity (tinnitus, hearing loss). • Do not have immunizations without physician's approval (lowers body's resistance). • Avoid contact with those who have recently taken oral polio vaccine. • Contact physician if nausea/vomiting continues at home. • Report signs of peripheral neuropathy.

citalopram

sigh-**tail**-oh-pram
(Apo-Citalopram ✤, Celexa, Novo-Citalopram ✤)

BLACK BOX ALERT Increased risk of suicidal thinking and behavior in children, adolescents, young adults 18–24 yrs with major depressive disorder, other psychiatric disorders.

Do not confuse Celexa with Celebrex, Cerebyx, Ranexa, or Zyprexa.

C

◆CLASSIFICATION

PHARMACOTHERAPEUTIC: Serotonin reuptake inhibitor. **CLINICAL:** Antidepressant (see p. 39C).

ACTION

Blocks uptake of the neurotransmitter serotonin at CNS presynaptic neuronal membranes, increasing its availability at postsynaptic receptor sites. **Therapeutic Effect:** Relieves depression.

PHARMACOKINETICS

Well absorbed after PO administration. Protein binding: 80%. Extensively metabolized in liver. Excreted in urine. **Half-life:** 35 hrs.

USES

Treatment of depression. **OFF-LABEL:** Treatment of alcohol abuse, dementia, diabetic neuropathy, obsessive-compulsive disorder, panic disorder, smoking cessation.

PRECAUTIONS

Contraindications: Sensitivity to citalopram, use within 14 days of MAOIs. **Cautions:** Hepatic/renal impairment, history of seizures, mania, hypomania. May prolong QT interval.

⌛ LIFESPAN CONSIDERATIONS

Pregnancy/Lactation: Distributed in breast milk. **Pregnancy Category C. Children:** May cause increased anticholinergic effects, hyperexcitability. **Elderly:** More sensitive to anticholinergic effects (e.g., dry mouth), more likely to experience dizziness, sedation, confusion, hypotension, hyperexcitability.

INTERACTIONS

DRUG: Linezolid, MAOIs may cause serotonin syndrome (excitement, diaphoresis, rigidity, hyperthermia, autonomic hyperactivity, coma). **HERBAL: Gotu kola, kava kava, SAMe, St. John's wort, valerian** may increase CNS depression. **FOOD:** None known. **LAB VALUES:** None significant.

AVAILABILITY (Rx)

Oral Solution: 10 mg/5 ml. **Tablets:** 10 mg, 20 mg, 40 mg.

ADMINISTRATION/HANDLING

PO

• Give without regard to food. • Scored tablets may be crushed.

INDICATIONS/ROUTES/DOSAGE

Depression

PO: ADULTS: Initially, 20 mg once a day in the morning or evening. May increase in 20-mg increments at intervals of no less than 1 wk. **Maximum:** 60 mg/day. **ELDERLY, PTS WITH HEPATIC IMPAIRMENT:** 20 mg/day. May titrate to 40 mg/day only for nonresponding pts.

SIDE EFFECTS

Frequent (21%–11%): Nausea, dry mouth, drowsiness, insomnia, diaphoresis. **Occasional (8%–4%):** Tremor, diarrhea, abnormal ejaculation, dyspepsia, fatigue, anxiety, vomiting, anorexia. **Rare (3%–2%):** Sinusitis, sexual dysfunction, menstrual disorder, abdominal pain, agitation, decreased libido.

ADVERSE EFFECTS/ TOXIC REACTIONS

Overdose manifested as dizziness, drowsiness, tachycardia, confusion, seizures.

NURSING CONSIDERATIONS

BASELINE ASSESSMENT

Hepatic/renal function tests, blood counts should be performed periodically for pts on long-term therapy. Observe, record behavior. Assess psychological status, thought content, sleep pattern, appearance, interest in environment.

INTERVENTION/EVALUATION

Supervise suicidal-risk pt closely during early therapy (as depression lessens, energy level improves, increasing suicide potential). Assess appearance, behavior, speech pattern, level of interest, mood.

C

PATIENT/FAMILY TEACHING

• Do not stop taking medication or increase dosage. • Avoid alcohol. • Avoid tasks that require alertness, motor skills until response to drug is established. • Report worsening depression, suicidal ideation, unusual changes in behavior.

cladribine

HIGH ALERT

clad-rih-bean
(Leustatin)

BLACK BOX ALERT Must be administered by personnel trained in administration/handling of chemotherapeutic agents. Myelosuppression, neurologic toxicity, acute nephrotoxicity have been reported.

Do not confuse cladribine with clevidipine, clofarabine, or fludarabine, or Leustatin with lovastatin.

CLASSIFICATION

PHARMACOTHERAPEUTIC: Antimetabolite. **CLINICAL:** Antineoplastic (see p. 82C).

ACTION

Disrupts cellular metabolism by incorporating into DNA of dividing cells. Cytotoxic to both actively dividing and quiescent lymphocytes, monocytes. **Therapeutic Effect:** Prevents DNA synthesis.

PHARMACOKINETICS

Protein binding: 20%. Metabolized in liver. Primarily excreted in urine. **Half-life:** 5.4 hrs.

USES

Treatment of active hairy cell leukemia defined by clinically significant anemia, neutropenia, thrombocytopenia. **OFF-LABEL:** Treatment of chronic lymphocytic leukemia, non-Hodgkin's lymphoma, acute myeloid leukemia, autoimmune hemolytic anemia, progressive multiple sclerosis.

PRECAUTIONS

Contraindications: None known. **Cautions:** Renal/hepatic impairment, bone marrow suppression.

LIFESPAN CONSIDERATIONS

Pregnancy/Lactation: May produce fetal harm; may be embryotoxic, fetotoxic; potential for serious reactions in breast-fed infants. **Pregnancy Category D. Children:** Safety and efficacy not established. **Elderly:** No age-related precautions noted.

INTERACTIONS

DRUG: Bone marrow depressants may increase myelosuppression. Concurrent administration of **cyclophosphamide, total body irradiation** may cause severe, irreversible neurologic toxicity, acute renal dysfunction. **Nephrotoxic, neurotoxic medications** may increase toxicity. **Live virus vaccines** may potentiate virus replication, increase vaccine side effects, decrease pt's antibody response to vaccine. **HERBAL:** None significant. **FOOD:** None known. **LAB VALUES:** None significant.

AVAILABILITY (Rx)

Injection Solution: 1 mg/ml (10 ml).

ADMINISTRATION/HANDLING

IV

Reconstitution • Must dilute before administration. • Wear gloves, protective clothing during handling; if contact with skin, rinse with copious amounts of water. • Add calculated dose (0.09 mg/kg) to 500 ml 0.9% NaCl. Avoid D_5W (increases degradation of medication).

Rate of administration • Infuse over 1–2 hrs.

Storage • Refrigerate unopened vials. • May refrigerate dilution solution for no more than 8 hrs before administration. • Diluted solution is stable for at least 24 hrs at room temperature. • Discard unused portion.

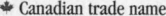

C

IV INCOMPATIBILITIES

Do not mix with other IV drugs/additives or infuse concurrently via a common IV line.

INDICATIONS/ROUTES/DOSAGE

Hairy Cell Leukemia

IV INFUSION: ADULTS, CHILDREN: 0.09–0.1 mg/kg/day as continuous infusion for 7 days. May repeat in 4–5 wks.

Chronic Lymphocytic Leukemia

IV INFUSION: ADULTS, ELDERLY: 0.1 mg/kg/day days 1–7.

Chronic Myelogenous Leukemia

IV INFUSION: ADULTS, ELDERLY: 15 mg/m^2/day days 1–5. Give as a 1-hr infusion. If no response, increase to 20 mg/m^2/day with second course.

Acute Leukemias

IV INFUSION: CHILDREN: 6.2–7.5 mg/m^2/day for days 1–5.

SIDE EFFECTS

Frequent: Fever (69%), fatigue (45%), nausea (28%), rash (27%), headache (22%), injection site reactions (19%), anorexia (17%), vomiting (13%). **Occasional (10%–5%):** Diarrhea, cough, purpura, chills, diaphoresis, constipation, dizziness, petechiae, myalgia, shortness of breath, malaise, pruritus, erythema, insomnia, edema, tachycardia, abdominal/trunk pain, epistaxis, arthralgia.

ADVERSE EFFECTS/ TOXIC REACTIONS

Myelosuppression characterized as severe neutropenia (less than 500 cells/mm^3), severe anemia (Hgb less than 8.5 g/dl), thrombocytopenia occur commonly. High-dose treatment may produce acute nephrotoxicity (increased BUN, creatinine levels), neurotoxicity (irreversible motor weakness of upper/lower extremities).

NURSING CONSIDERATIONS

BASELINE ASSESSMENT

Offer emotional support to pt, family. Perform neurologic function tests before chemotherapy. Use strict asepsis; protect pt from infection.

INTERVENTION/EVALUATION

Monitor vital signs during infusion, esp. during first hour. Observe for hypotension, bradycardia (usually both do not occur during same course). Immediately discontinue administration if severe hypersensitivity reaction occurs. Report fever promptly. Assess for signs of infection. Assess skin for evidence of rash, purpura, petechiae. Monitor Hgb, Hct, BUN, platelet count, WBC, serum creatinine, potassium, sodium.

PATIENT/FAMILY TEACHING

• Narrow margin between therapeutic and toxic response. • Avoid crowds, persons with known infections; report signs of infection at once (fever, flu-like symptoms). • Do not have immunizations without physician's approval (drug lowers resistance). • Avoid contact with those who have recently received live virus vaccine. • Discuss importance of pregnancy testing, avoidance of pregnancy measures to prevent pregnancy.

Clarinex, *see desloratadine*

clarithromycin

clair-**rith**-row-my-sin
(Apo-Clarithromycin 🍁, Biaxin, Biaxin XL, PMS-Clarithromycin 🍁)
Do not confuse clarithromycin with Claritin, clindamycin, or erythromycin.

◆CLASSIFICATION

PHARMACOTHERAPEUTIC: Macrolide. **CLINICAL:** Antibiotic (see p. 26C).

ACTION

Binds to ribosomal receptor sites of susceptible organisms, inhibiting protein synthesis of bacterial cell wall. **Therapeutic Effect:** Bacteriostatic; may be bactericidal with high dosages or very susceptible microorganisms.

PHARMACOKINETICS

Well absorbed from GI tract. Protein binding: 65%–75%. Widely distributed (except CNS). Metabolized in liver to active metabolite. Primarily excreted in urine. Not removed by hemodialysis. **Half-life:** 3–7 hrs; metabolite, 5–9 hrs (increased in renal impairment).

USES

Treatment of susceptible infections due to *C. pneumoniae, H. influenzae, H. parainfluenzae, H. pylori, M. catarrhalis, M. avium, M. pneumoniae, S. aureus, S. pneumoniae, S. pyogenes,* including bacterial exacerbation of bronchitis, otitis media, acute maxillary sinusitis, *Mycobacterium avium* complex (MAC), pharyngitis, tonsillitis, *H. pylori* duodenal ulcer, bacterial pneumonia, skin and soft tissue infections. Prevention of MAC disease. **Biaxin XL:** Treatment of community-acquired pneumonia. **OFF-LABEL:** Prophylaxis of infective endocarditis, pertussis.

PRECAUTIONS

Contraindications: Hypersensitivity to other macrolide antibiotics. **Cautions:** Hepatic/renal dysfunction, elderly with severe renal impairment. May prolong QT interval (rare).

⌛ LIFESPAN CONSIDERATIONS

Pregnancy/Lactation: Unknown if distributed in breast milk. **Pregnancy Category C. Children:** Safety and efficacy not established in those younger than 6 mos. **Elderly:** Age-related renal impairment may require dosage adjustment.

INTERACTIONS

DRUG: May increase concentration, toxicity of **carbamazepine, colchicine, digoxin, ergotamine, theophylline. Rifabutin, rifampin** may decrease plasma concentration. May increase **warfarin** effects. May decrease concentration of **zidovudine. Quinidine** may increase risk of torsade de pointes. **HERBAL: St. John's wort** may decrease plasma concentration. **FOOD:** None known. **LAB VALUES:** May increase BUN, serum AST, ALT, alkaline phosphatase, LDH, serum creatinine, PT. May decrease WBC.

AVAILABILITY (Rx)

Oral Suspension (Biaxin): 125 mg/5 ml, 250 mg/5 ml. **Tablets (Biaxin):** 250 mg, 500 mg.

Tablets (Extended-Release [Biaxin XL]): 500 mg.

ADMINISTRATION/HANDLING

PO

- Give immediate-release tablets, oral suspension without regard to food.
- Biaxin XL should be given with food.
- Do not crush/chew extended-release tablets.

INDICATIONS/ROUTES/DOSAGE

Usual Dosage Range

PO: ADULTS, ELDERLY: 250–500 mg q12h or 500–1,000 mg once daily (extended-release tablets). **CHILDREN 6 MOS AND OLDER:** 7.5 mg/kg q12h. **Maximum:** 500 mg.

Bronchitis

PO: ADULTS, ELDERLY: 250–500 mg q12h for 7–14 days.

PO (EXTENDED-RELEASE): ADULTS, ELDERLY: 1 g once daily for 7 days.

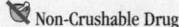

C

Skin, Soft Tissue Infections
PO: ADULTS, ELDERLY: 250 mg q12h for 7–14 days. **CHILDREN:** 7.5 mg/kg q12h for 10 days. **Maximum:** 1 g/day.

***Mycobacterium Avium* Complex (MAC) Prophylaxis**
PO: ADULTS, ELDERLY: 500 mg twice a day. **CHILDREN:** 7.5 mg/kg q12h. **Maximum:** 500 mg twice a day.

***Mycobacterium Avium* Complex (MAC) Treatment**
PO: ADULTS, ELDERLY: 500 mg twice a day in combination. **CHILDREN:** 7.5 mg/kg q12h in combination. **Maximum:** 500 mg twice a day.

Pharyngitis, Tonsillitis
PO: ADULTS, ELDERLY: 250 mg q12h for 10 days. **CHILDREN:** 7.5 mg/kg q12h for 10 days. **Maximum:** 1 g/day.

Pneumonia
PO: ADULTS, ELDERLY: 250 mg q12h for 7–14 days. **CHILDREN:** 7.5 mg/kg q12h.
PO (EXTENDED-RELEASE): ADULTS, ELDERLY: 1 g/day.

Maxillary Sinusitis
PO: ADULTS, ELDERLY: 500 mg q12h or 1,000 mg (2×500 mg extended-release) once daily for 14 days. **CHILDREN:** 7.5 mg/kg q12h. **Maximum:** 500 mg twice a day.

H. Pylori
PO: ADULTS, ELDERLY: 500 mg q8–12h for 10–14 days in combination.

Acute Otitis Media
PO: CHILDREN: 7.5 mg/kg q12h for 10 days. **Maximum:** 500 mg q12h.

Dosage in Renal Impairment
Creatinine clearance less than 30 ml/min: Reduce dose by 50% and administer once or twice a day.

SIDE EFFECTS

Occasional (6%–3%): Diarrhea, nausea, altered taste, abdominal pain. **Rare (2%–1%):** Headache, dyspepsia.

ADVERSE EFFECTS/ TOXIC REACTIONS

Antibiotic-associated colitis, other superinfections (abdominal cramps, severe watery diarrhea, fever) may result from altered bacterial balance. Hepatotoxicity, thrombocytopenia occur rarely.

NURSING CONSIDERATIONS

BASELINE ASSESSMENT

Question pt for allergies to clarithromycin, erythromycins.

INTERVENTION/EVALUATION

Monitor daily pattern of bowel activity and stool consistency. Mild GI effects may be tolerable, but increasing severity may indicate onset of antibiotic-associated colitis. Be alert for superinfection: fever, vomiting, diarrhea, anal/genital pruritus, oral mucosal changes (ulceration, pain, erythema). Monitor CBC, BUN, creatinine.

PATIENT/FAMILY TEACHING

• Continue therapy for full length of treatment. • Doses should be evenly spaced. • Take Biaxin XL with food; Biaxin may be taken without regard to food. • Report severe diarrhea.

Claritin, *see loratadine*

clemastine

klem-**as**-teen
(Dayhist Allergy, Tavist Allergy)

◆CLASSIFICATION

PHARMACOTHERAPEUTIC: Histamine H_1 antagonist. **CLINICAL:** Antihistamine (see p. 54C).

ACTION
Competes with histamine on effector cells in GI tract, blood vessels, respiratory tract. **Therapeutic Effect:** Relieves perennial, seasonal allergic rhinitis, other allergic symptoms (urticaria, rhinitis, pruritus). Anticholinergic effects cause drying of nasal mucosa.

PHARMACOKINETICS

Route	Onset	Peak	Duration
PO	15–60 min	5–7 hrs	10–12 hrs

Well absorbed from GI tract. Metabolized in liver. Excreted primarily in urine. **Half-life:** 21 hrs.

USES
Perennial and seasonal allergic rhinitis, other allergic symptoms (e.g., urticaria, pruritus).

PRECAUTIONS
Contraindications: Angle-closure glaucoma, hypersensitivity to clemastine, use within 14 days of MAOIs. **Cautions:** Peptic ulcer, GI/GU obstruction, asthma, prostatic hypertrophy.

LIFESPAN CONSIDERATIONS
Pregnancy/Lactation: Distributed in breast milk. **Pregnancy Category B. Children:** Safety and efficacy not established in those younger than 6 yrs. **Elderly:** Age-related renal impairment may require dosage adjustment.

INTERACTIONS
DRUG: **Alcohol, other CNS depressants** may increase CNS depression. **MAOIs** may increase anticholinergic, CNS depressant effects. **HERBAL:** None significant. **FOOD:** None known. **LAB VALUES:** May suppress wheal, flare reactions to antigen skin testing unless drug is discontinued 4 days before testing.

AVAILABILITY (Rx)
Syrup (Tavist): 0.67 mg/5 ml. **Tablets (Dayhist Allergy, Tavist Allergy):** 1.34 mg, 2.68 mg.

ADMINISTRATION/HANDLING
PO

• Administer with food to minimize GI disturbance. • Scored tablets may be crushed.

INDICATIONS/ROUTES/DOSAGE
Allergic Rhinitis, Allergic Symptoms

PO: ADULTS, CHILDREN OLDER THAN 11 YRS: 1.34 mg twice a day up to 2.68 mg 3 times a day. **Maximum:** 8.04 mg/day. **CHILDREN 6–11 YRS:** 0.67–1.34 mg twice a day. **Maximum:** 4.02 mg/day. **CHILDREN YOUNGER THAN 6 YRS:** 0.05 mg/kg/day or 2.5–5 ml daily divided into 2–3 doses per day. **Maximum:** 1.34 mg/day. **ELDERLY:** 1.34 mg 1–2 times a day.

SIDE EFFECTS
Frequent: Drowsiness, dizziness, urinary retention, thickening of bronchial secretions, dry mouth, nose, throat. In elderly, sedation, dizziness, hypotension. **Occasional:** Epigastric distress, flushing, blurred vision, tinnitus, paresthesia, diaphoresis, chills.

ADVERSE EFFECTS/ TOXIC REACTIONS
Children may experience paradoxical reactions (restlessness, insomnia, euphoria, anxiety, tremors). Overdose in children may result in hallucinations, seizures, death. Hypersensitivity reaction (eczema, pruritus, rash, cardiac disturbances, angioedema, photosensitivity) may occur. Overdose symptoms may vary from paradoxical reaction (hallucinations, tremors, seizure) to CNS depression (sedation, apnea, cardiovascular collapse).

NURSING CONSIDERATIONS
BASELINE ASSESSMENT
If pt is experiencing allergic reaction, obtain history of recently ingested foods, drugs, environmental exposure, recent emotional stress. Monitor rate, depth, rhythm, type of respiration; quality and rate of pulse. Assess lung sounds for rhonchi, wheezing, rales.

C

INTERVENTION/EVALUATION

Monitor B/P, esp. in elderly (increased risk of hypotension). Monitor children closely for paradoxical reaction. Monitor for therapeutic improvement.

PATIENT/FAMILY TEACHING

• Tolerance to antihistaminic effect generally does not occur; tolerance to sedative effect may occur. • Avoid tasks that require alertness, motor skills until response to drug is established. • Avoid direct exposure to sunlight. • Dry mouth, drowsiness, dizziness may be an expected response of drug. • Avoid alcoholic beverages during antihistamine therapy. • Coffee, tea may help reduce drowsiness.

clevidipine

clev-**ih**-dih-peen
(Cleviprex)
Do not confuse clevidipine with cladribine or clafarabine, or Cleviprex with Claravis.

◆CLASSIFICATION

PHARMACOTHERAPEUTIC: Short-acting calcium-channel blocker. **CLINICAL:** Antihypertensive.

ACTION

Inhibits calcium ion movement across cell membranes, depressing contraction of cardiac, vascular smooth muscle. **Therapeutic Effect:** Increases heart rate, cardiac output. Decreases systemic vascular resistance, B/P.

PHARMACOKINETICS

Route	Onset	Peak	Duration
IV	2–4 min	—	—

Full recovery to therapeutic B/P reading occurs 5–15 min following termination of infusion. Rapidly distributed and metabolized. Protein binding: 99.5%. Eliminated primarily in urine with a lesser amount excreted in feces. **Half-life:** 30 sec–1 min.

USES

Indicated for reduction in B/P when oral therapy is not feasible or desirable.

PRECAUTIONS

Contraindications: Allergy to soy or eggs, abnormal lipid metabolism, severe aortic stenosis. **Cautions:** None known.

LIFESPAN CONSIDERATIONS:

Pregnancy/Lactation: Unknown if distributed in breast milk. **Pregnancy Category C. Children:** Safety and efficacy not established in those younger than 18 yrs. **Elderly:** No age-related precautions noted.

INTERACTIONS

DRUG: Diuretics, other antihypertensives may increase hypotensive effect. **Sympathomimetics, xanthines** may mutually inhibit effect. May mask symptoms of hypoglycemia, prolong hypoglycemic effect of **insulin, oral hypoglycemics. NSAIDs** may decrease antihypertensive effect. **Cimetidine** may increase concentration. **HERBAL: Ephedra, ginseng, yohimbe** may worsen hypertension. **Garlic** may increase antihypertensive effect. **FOOD:** None known. **LAB VALUES:** May increase BUN, uric acid, potassium, triglycerides.

AVAILABILITY (Rx)

Injection, Emulsion: 0.05 mg/ml as 50-ml vial, 100-ml vial.

ADMINISTRATION/HANDLING

IV

Reconstitution • Do not dilute. • Both 50-ml and 100-ml vials supplied as concentration of 0.5 mg/ml. • Invert vial gently several times before use to ensure uniformity of emulsion.

Storage • Refrigerate vials but may be held at controlled room temperature

(77°F) for 2 mos. • Vial cannot be returned to refrigerator once warmed to room temperature. • Once stopper is punctured, use within 4 hrs; discard unused portion, including that currently being infused. • Discard if discoloration or particulate matter is present.

IV INCOMPATIBILITIES

Do not administer in same IV line as other medications.

IV COMPATIBILITIES

Sterile Water for Injection, 0.9% NaCl, D_5W, lactated Ringer's, 10% amino acid.

INDICATIONS/ROUTES/DOSAGE

◀ALERT▶ Titrate drug to achieve desired B/P reduction. Individualize dosage depending on desired B/P and pt response.

Hypertension

IV: ADULTS, ELDERLY: Initiate IV infusion at 1–2 mg/hr. Dose may be doubled at short (90-sec) intervals initially. As B/P approaches goal, increase in doses should be less than double and time between dose adjustments lengthened to every 5–10 min. Maintenance: Desired therapeutic response generally occurs at doses of 4–6 mg/hr. Pts with severe hypertension may require doses up to 32 mg/hr. **Maximum:** 16 mg/hr; no more than 21 mg/hr is recommended per 24-hr period.

Dose conversion from mg/hr to ml/hr:

mg/hr	ml/hr
1	2
2	4
4	8
6	12
8	16
10	20
12	24
14	28
16	32
18	36
20	40

SIDE EFFECTS

Generally well tolerated. **Occasional (6%–3%):** Headache, nausea, vomiting. **Rare (less than 1%):** Syncope, dyspnea.

ADVERSE EFFECTS/ TOXIC REACTIONS

Hypotension, atrial fibrillation, sinus tachycardia may occur with large doses. Can exacerbate heart failure. Acute renal failure has occurred rarely.

NURSING CONSIDERATIONS

BASELINE ASSESSMENT

Assess baseline renal/hepatic function tests. Assess B/P, apical pulse immediately before drug administration (if pulse is 60/min or less or systolic B/P is below 90 mm Hg, withhold medication, contact physician).

INTERVENTION/EVALUATION

Monitor B/P, pulse rate continually during IV infusion and then until vital signs are stable. Monitor cardiac pts diligently. Pts who receive prolonged IV infusion and are not changed to other antihypertensive therapy should be monitored for rebound hypertension for at least 8 hrs after infusion is stopped.

PATIENT/FAMILY TEACHING

• Compliance with therapy regimen is essential to control hypertension. • Do not use nasal decongestants, OTC cold preparations (stimulants) without physician approval. • Monitor B/P, pulse before beginning oral antihypertensive medication. • Restrict salt, alcohol intake.

Climara, *see estradiol*

C

clindamycin

klin-da-**mye**-sin
(Apo-Clindamycin, Cleocin, Cleocin Pediatric, Cleocin T, Cleocin Vaginal, Clindagel, Clindamax, Clindesse, Clindets Pledget, Dalacin, Novo-Clindamycin)

BLACK BOX ALERT May cause severe, potentially fatal colitis characterized by severe, persistent diarrhea, severe abdominal cramps, passage of blood and mucus.

Do not confuse Cleocin with Clinoril or Cubicin, or clindamycin with clarithromycin, Claritin, or vancomycin.

◆CLASSIFICATION

PHARMACOTHERAPEUTIC: Lincosamide. **CLINICAL:** Antibiotic.

ACTION

Inhibits protein synthesis of bacterial cell wall by binding to bacterial ribosomal receptor sites. Topically, decreases fatty acid concentration on skin. **Therapeutic Effect:** Bacteriostatic. Prevents outbreaks of acne vulgaris.

PHARMACOKINETICS

Rapidly absorbed from GI tract. Protein binding: 92%–94%. Widely distributed. Metabolized in liver to some active metabolites. Primarily excreted in urine. Not removed by hemodialysis. **Half-life:** 1.6–5.3 hrs (increased in renal impairment, premature infants).

USES

Systemic: Treatment of aerobic gram-positive staphylococci and streptococci (not enterococci), *Fusobacterium, Bacteroides* spp., and *Actinomyces* for treatment of respiratory tract infections. Skin/soft tissue infections, sepsis, intra-abdominal infections, infections of female pelvis and genital tract, bacterial endocarditis prophylaxis for dental and upper respiratory procedures in penicillin-allergic pts, perioperative prophylaxis. **Topical:** Treatment of acne vulgaris. **Intravaginal:** Treatment of bacterial vaginosis. **OFF-LABEL:** Treatment of actinomycosis, babesiosis, erysipelas, malaria, otitis media, *Pneumocystis jiroveci* pneumonia (PCP), sinusitis, toxoplasmosis. **PO:** Bacterial vaginosis.

PRECAUTIONS

Contraindications: History of antibiotic-associated colitis, regional enteritis, ulcerative colitis; hypersensitivity to clindamycin, lincomycin; known allergy to tartrazine dye. **Cautions:** Severe renal/hepatic dysfunction, concomitant use of neuromuscular blocking agents, neonates. Topical preparations should not be applied to abraded areas of skin or near eyes.

LIFESPAN CONSIDERATIONS

Pregnancy/Lactation: Readily crosses placenta. Distributed in breast milk. **Topical/vaginal:** Unknown if distributed in breast milk. **Pregnancy Category B. Children:** Caution in those younger than 1 mo. **Elderly:** No age-related precautions noted.

INTERACTIONS

DRUG: **Adsorbent antidiarrheals** may delay absorption. **Erythromycin** may antagonize effects. May increase effects of **neuromuscular blockers. HERBAL: St. John's wort** may decrease plasma concentration. **FOOD:** None known. **LAB VALUES:** May increase serum alkaline phosphatase, AST, ALT levels.

AVAILABILITY (Rx)

Capsules: 75 mg, 150 mg, 300 mg. **Cream, Vaginal (Cleocin, Clindesse):** 2%. **Gel, Topical: (Cleocin T, Clindagel, Clindamax):** 1%. **Infusion, Pre-Mix: (Cleocin):** 300 mg/50 ml, 600 mg/50 ml, 900 mg/50 ml. **Injection Solution: (Cleocin):** 150 mg/ml. **Lotion: (Cleocin T, Clindamax):** 1%. **Oral Solution: (Cleocin Pediatric):** 75 mg/5 ml. **Suppositories, Vaginal: (Cleocin):** 100 mg. **Swabs, Topical: (Clindets, Cleocin T):** 1%.

C

ADMINISTRATION/HANDLING

IV

Reconstitution • Dilute 300–600 mg with 50 ml D_5W or 0.9% NaCl (900–1,200 mg with 100 ml). • Never exceed concentration of 18 mg/ml.

Rate of administration • Infuse over at least 10–60 min at rate not exceeding 30 mg/min. Severe hypotension, cardiac arrest can occur with too-rapid administration. • No more than 1.2 g should be given in a single infusion.

Storage • Reconstituted IV infusion (piggyback) is stable for 16 days at room temperature, 32 days if refrigerated.

IM

• Do not exceed 600 mg/dose. • Administer deep IM.

PO

• Store capsules at room temperature. • After reconstitution, oral solution is stable for 2 wks at room temperature. • Do not refrigerate oral solution (avoids thickening). • Give with at least 8 oz water (minimizes esophageal ulceration). • Give without regard to food.

Topical

• Wash skin, allow to dry completely before application. • Shake topical lotion well before each use. • Apply liquid, solution, or gel in thin film to affected area. • Avoid contact with eyes or abraded areas.

Vaginal, Cream or Suppository

• Use one applicatorful or suppository at bedtime. • Fill applicator that comes with cream or suppository to indicated level. • Instruct pt to lie on back with knees drawn upward and spread apart. • Insert applicator into vagina and push plunger to release medication. • Withdraw, wash applicator with soap and warm water. • Wash hands promptly to avoid spreading infection.

IV INCOMPATIBILITIES

Allopurinol (Aloprim), filgrastim (Neupogen), fluconazole (Diflucan), idarubicin (Idamycin).

IV COMPATIBILITIES

Amiodarone (Cordarone), diltiazem (Cardizem), heparin, hydromorphone (Dilaudid), lipids, magnesium sulfate, midazolam (Versed), morphine, multivitamins, propofol (Diprivan), total parenteral nutrition (TPN).

INDICATIONS/ROUTES/DOSAGE

Susceptible Infections

IV, IM: ADULTS, ELDERLY: 1.2–2.7 g/day in 2–4 divided doses. **Maximum:** 4.8 g/day. **CHILDREN 1 MOS–16 YRS:** 20–40 mg/kg/day in 3–4 divided doses. **Maximum:** 4.8 g/day. **CHILDREN YOUNGER THAN 1 MO:** 15–20 mg/kg/day in 2–3 divided doses.

PO: ADULTS, ELDERLY: 150–450 mg q6h. **Maximum:** 1.8 g/day. **CHILDREN:** 8–25 mg/kg/day in 3–4 divided doses.

Bacterial Vaginosis

PO: ADULTS, ELDERLY: 300 mg twice a day for 7 days.

INTRAVAGINAL: ADULTS: One applicatorful at bedtime for 3–7 days or 1 suppository at bedtime for 3 days.

INTRAVAGINAL (CLINDESSE CREAM): ADULTS: One applicatorful once at any time of the day.

Acne Vulgaris

TOPICAL: ADULTS: Apply thin layer to affected area twice a day.

SIDE EFFECTS

Frequent: Systemic: Abdominal pain, nausea, vomiting, diarrhea. **Topical:** Dry, scaly skin. **Vaginal:** Vaginitis, pruritus. **Occasional: Systemic:** Phlebitis, thrombophlebitis with IV administration, pain, induration at IM injection site, allergic reaction, urticaria, pruritus. **Topical:** Contact dermatitis, abdominal pain, mild diarrhea, burning, stinging. **Vaginal:** Headache, dizziness, nausea, vomiting, abdominal pain. **Rare: Vaginal:** Hypersensitivity reaction.

C

ADVERSE EFFECTS/ TOXIC REACTIONS

Antibiotic-associated colitis, other superinfections (abdominal cramps, severe watery diarrhea, fever) may occur during and several wks after clindamycin therapy (including topical form). Blood dyscrasias (leukopenia, thrombocytopenia), nephrotoxicity (proteinuria, azotemia, oliguria) occur rarely.

NURSING CONSIDERATIONS

BASELINE ASSESSMENT

Question pt for history of allergies. Avoid, if possible, concurrent use of neuromuscular blocking agents.

INTERVENTION/EVALUATION

Monitor daily pattern of bowel activity and stool consistency. Report diarrhea promptly due to potential for serious colitis (even with topical or vaginal administration). Assess skin for rash (dryness, irritation) with topical application. With all routes of administration, be alert for superinfection: fever, vomiting, diarrhea, anal/genital pruritus, oral mucosal changes (ulceration, pain, erythema).

PATIENT/FAMILY TEACHING

• Continue therapy for full length of treatment. • Doses should be evenly spaced. • Take oral doses with at least 8 oz water. • Caution should be used when applying topical clindamycin concurrently with peeling or abrasive acne agents, soaps, alcohol-containing cosmetics to avoid cumulative effect. • Do not apply topical preparations near eyes, abraded areas. • Notify physician if severe persistent diarrhea, cramps, bloody stool occur. • **Vaginal:** In event of accidental contact with eyes, rinse with copious amounts of cool tap water. • Do not engage in sexual intercourse during treatment. • Wear sanitary napkin to protect clothes against stains. Tampons should not be used.

clofarabine

kloe-**fare**-ah-been
(Clolar)
Do not confuse clofarabine with cladribine or clevidipine.

◆CLASSIFICATION

PHARMACOTHERAPEUTIC: Antimetabolite. **CLINICAL:** Antineoplastic.

ACTION

Metabolized intracellularly to ribonucleotide reductase. Alters mitochondrial membrane necessary in DNA synthesis. **Therapeutic Effect:** Decreases cell replication, inhibits cell repair. Produces cell death.

PHARMACOKINETICS

Protein binding: 47%, primarily to albumin. Metabolized intracellularly. Primarily excreted in urine (40%–60% unchanged). **Half-life:** 5.2 hrs.

USES

Treatment of pediatric pts (1–21 yrs) with relapsed or refractory acute lymphoblastic leukemia (ALL) after at least 2 prior regimens. **OFF-LABEL:** Relapsed or refractory acute myeloid leukemia (AML), chronic myeloid leukemia (CML) in blast phase, ALL, myelodysplastic syndrome.

PRECAUTIONS

Contraindications: None known. **Cautions:** Renal/hepatic impairment, dehydration, hypotension.

LIFESPAN CONSIDERATIONS

Pregnancy/Lactation: May cause fetal harm. Breast-feeding not recommended. **Pregnancy Category D. Children:** Safety and efficacy not established. **Elderly:** No age-related precautions noted.

INTERACTIONS

DRUG: **Hepatotoxic, nephrotoxic medications** may increase risk of hepatic/renal toxicity. **HERBAL:** None significant. **FOOD:** None known. **LAB VALUES:** May increase serum creatinine, uric acid, AST, ALT, bilirubin.

AVAILABILITY (Rx)

Injection, Solution: 1 mg/ml (20-ml vial).

ADMINISTRATION/HANDLING

IV

Reconstitution • Filter clofarabine through sterile, 0.2-micrometer syringe filter prior to further dilution with D_5W or 0.9% NaCl to final concentration of 0.15–0.4 mg/ml.

Rate of administration • Administer over 2 hrs. • Continuously infuse IV fluids to decrease risk of tumor lysis syndrome, other adverse events.

Storage • Store undiluted or diluted solution at room temperature. • Use diluted solution within 24 hrs.

IV INCOMPATIBILITIES

Do not administer any other medication through same IV line.

INDICATIONS/ROUTES/DOSAGE

Acute Lymphoblastic Leukemia (ALL)

IV: CHILDREN 1–21 YRS: 52 mg/m^2 over 2 hrs once daily for 5 consecutive days; repeat q2–6wk following recovery or return to baseline organ function.

SIDE EFFECTS

Frequent: Vomiting (83%); nausea (75%); diarrhea (53%); pruritus (47%); headache (46%); fever, dermatitis (41%); rigors (38%); abdominal pain, fatigue (36%); tachycardia (34%); epistaxis (31%); anorexia (30%); petechiae, limb pain, hypotension (29%); anxiety (22%); constipation (21%); edema (20%). **Occasional:** Cough (19%); mucosal inflammation, erythema, flushing (18%); hematuria (17%); dizziness (16%); gingival bleeding (15%); injection site pain, respiratory distress, pharyngitis (14%); back pain, palmar-plantar erythrodysesthesia syndrome, myalgia, oral candidiasis (13%); hypertension, depression, irritability, arthralgia, anorexia (11%). **Rare (10%):** Tremor, weight gain, drowsiness.

ADVERSE EFFECTS/ TOXIC REACTIONS

Neutropenia occurs in 57% of pts; pericardial effusion in 35%; left ventricular systolic dysfunction in 27%; hepatomegaly, jaundice in 15%; pleural effusion, pneumonia, bacteremia in 10%; capillary leak syndrome in less than 10%.

NURSING CONSIDERATIONS

BASELINE ASSESSMENT

Monitor Hgb, Hct; assess for signs/symptoms of anemia. Question pt regarding possibility of pregnancy. Assess AST, ALT, bilirubin, creatinine clearance, BUN, creatinine levels prior to therapy.

INTERVENTION/EVALUATION

Monitor B/P, hepatic/renal function tests, cardiac function, respiratory status, CBC, platelets, uric acid. Monitor daily pattern of bowel activity and stool consistency. Assess for GI disturbances. Assess skin for pruritus, dermatitis, petechiae, erythema on palms of hands and soles of feet. Assess for fever, sore throat; obtain blood cultures to detect evidence of infection. Ensure adequate hydration throughout duration of administration.

PATIENT/FAMILY TEACHING

• Do not have immunizations without physician's approval (drug lowers resistance). • Avoid contact with anyone who recently received a live virus vaccine. • Avoid crowds, those with infection. • Avoid pregnancy due to risk of fetal harm; pts of childbearing potential should use effective contraception. • Maintain fastidious oral hygiene and frequent handwashing. • Notify physician if fever, respiratory distress, prolonged nausea, vomiting, diarrhea, easy bruising occur.

*clomiPRAMINE

kloe-**mip**-ra-meen
(Anafranil, Apo-Clomipramine 🍁)

BLACK BOX ALERT Increased risk of suicidal thinking and behavior in children, adolescents, young adults 18–24 yrs with major depressive disorder, other psychiatric disorders.

Do not confuse clomipramine with chlorpromazine, clevidipine, clomiphene, or desipramine, or Anafranil with alfentanil, enalapril, or nafarelin.

◆CLASSIFICATION

PHARMACOTHERAPEUTIC: Tricyclic. **CLINICAL:** Antidepressant (see p. 37C).

ACTION

Blocks reuptake of neurotransmitters (norepinephrine, serotonin) at CNS presynaptic membranes, increasing availability at postsynaptic receptor sites. **Therapeutic Effect:** Reduces obsessive-compulsive behavior.

PHARMACOKINETICS

Rapidly absorbed. Metabolized in liver. **Half-life:** 20–30 hrs.

USES

Treatment of obsessive-compulsive disorder manifested as repetitive tasks producing marked distress, time-consuming, or significant interference with social or occupational behavior. **OFF-LABEL:** Treatment of bulimia nervosa, cataplexy associated with narcolepsy, mental depression, neurogenic pain, chronic pain, panic disorder, ejaculatory disorders, pervasive developmental disorder.

PRECAUTIONS

Contraindications: Acute recovery period after MI, use within 14 days of MAOIs. **Cautions:** Prostatic hypertrophy, history of urinary retention/obstruction, glaucoma, diabetes mellitus, seizures, hyperthyroidism, cardiac/hepatic/renal disease, schizophrenia, increased intraocular pressure, hiatal hernia.

⌛ LIFESPAN CONSIDERATIONS

Pregnancy/Lactation: Distributed in breast milk. **Pregnancy Category D. Children:** Increased risk of suicidal thinking, behavior noted in children, adolescents. Safety and effectiveness in those younger than 10 yrs not established. **Elderly:** No age-related precautions noted.

INTERACTIONS

DRUG: Alcohol, other CNS depressants may increase CNS, respiratory depression, hypotensive effects. **Antithyroid agents** may increase the risk of agranulocytosis. **Cimetidine** may increase plasma concentration, risk of toxicity. May decrease effects of **clonidine. MAOIs** may increase risk of neuroleptic malignant syndrome, seizures, hyperpyresis, hypertensive crisis. **Phenothiazines** may increase anticholinergic, sedative effects. **Sympathomimetics** may increase the risk of cardiac effects. **HERBAL: Gota kola, kava kava, SAMe, St. John's wort, valerian** may increase CNS depression. **FOOD: Grapefruit juice** may increase serum concentration, toxicity. **LAB VALUES:** May alter serum glucose, EKG readings.

AVAILABILITY (Rx)

Capsules: 25 mg, 50 mg, 75 mg.

ADMINISTRATION/HANDLING

PO

• May give with food to decrease risk of GI disturbance.

INDICATIONS/ROUTES/DOSAGE

Obsessive-Compulsive Disorder (OCD)

PO: ADULTS, ELDERLY: Initially, 25 mg/day. May gradually increase to 100 mg/day in the first 2 wks. **Maximum:** 250 mg/day. **CHILDREN 10 YRS AND OLDER:** Initially, 25 mg/day. May gradually increase up to maximum of 3 mg/kg/day or 200 mg, whichever is smaller.

SIDE EFFECTS

Frequent: Drowsiness, fatigue, dry mouth, blurred vision, constipation, sexual dysfunction (42%), ejaculatory failure (20%), impotence, weight gain (18%), delayed micturition, orthostatic hypotension, diaphoresis, impaired concentration, increased appetite, urinary retention. **Occasional:** GI disturbances (nausea, GI distress, metallic taste), asthenia, aggressiveness, muscle weakness. **Rare:** Paradoxical reactions (agitation, restlessness, nightmares, insomnia), extrapyramidal symptoms (particularly fine hand tremor), laryngitis, seizures.

ADVERSE EFFECTS/ TOXIC REACTIONS

Overdose may produce seizures; cardiovascular effects (severe orthostatic hypotension, dizziness, tachycardia, palpitations, arrhythmias), altered temperature regulation (hyperpyrexia, hypothermia). Abrupt discontinuation after prolonged therapy may produce headache, malaise, nausea, vomiting, vivid dreams. Anemia, agranulocytosis have been noted.

NURSING CONSIDERATIONS

BASELINE ASSESSMENT

Assess psychological status, thought content, suicidal ideation or behavior.

INTERVENTION/EVALUATION

Supervise suicidal-risk pt closely during early therapy (as depression lessens, energy level improves, increasing suicide potential). Assess appearance, behavior, speech pattern, level of interest, mood.

PATIENT/FAMILY TEACHING

• May cause dry mouth, constipation, blurred vision. • Tolerance to postural hypotension, sedative, anticholinergic effects usually develop during early therapy. • Maximum therapeutic effect may be noted in 2–4 wks. • Do not abruptly discontinue medication. • Avoid tasks that require alertness, motor skills until response to drug is established. • Daily dose may be given at bedtime to minimize daytime sedation. • Avoid alcohol. • Report worsening depression, suicidal ideation, change in behavior.

clonazepam

klon-**nah**-zih-pam
(Apo-Clonazepam ✤, Clonapam ✤, Klonopin, Klonopin Wafer, Novo-Clonazepam ✤, Rivotril ✤)

Do not confuse clonazepam or Klonopin with clonidine, clozapine, or lorazepam.

◆ CLASSIFICATION

PHARMACOTHERAPEUTIC: Benzodiazepine (Schedule IV). **CLINICAL:** Anticonvulsant, antianxiety (see p. 34C).

ACTION

Depresses all levels of CNS; depresses nerve impulse transmission in motor cortex. Suppresses abnormal discharge in petit mal seizures. **Therapeutic Effect:** Produces anxiolytic, anticonvulsant effects.

PHARMACOKINETICS

Route	Onset	Peak	Duration
PO	20–60 min	–	12 hrs or less

Well absorbed from GI tract. Protein binding: 85%. Metabolized in liver. Excreted in urine. Not removed by hemodialysis. **Half-life:** 18–50 hrs.

USES

Adjunct in treatment of Lennox-Gastaut syndrome (petit mal variant epilepsy); akinetic, myoclonic seizures; absence seizures (petit mal). Treatment of panic disorder. **OFF-LABEL:** Restless legs syndrome, neuralgia, multifocal tic disorder, parkinsonian dysarthria, bipolar disorder, adjunct therapy for schizophrenia.

C

PRECAUTIONS

Contraindications: Narrow-angle glaucoma, significant hepatic disease. **Cautions:** Renal/hepatic impairment, chronic respiratory disease.

LIFESPAN CONSIDERATIONS

Pregnancy/Lactation: Crosses placenta. May be distributed in breast milk. Chronic ingestion during pregnancy may produce withdrawal symptoms, CNS depression in neonates. **Pregnancy Category D. Children:** Long-term use may adversely affect physical/mental development. **Elderly:** Usually more sensitive to CNS effects (e.g., ataxia, dizziness, oversedation). Use low dosage, increase gradually.

INTERACTIONS

DRUG: **Alcohol, other CNS depressants** may increase CNS depressant effect. **Azole antifungals** may increase serum concentration, toxicity. **HERBAL:** **Gotu kola, kava kava, SAMe, St. John's wort, valerian** may increase CNS depression. **FOOD:** None known. **LAB VALUES:** None significant.

AVAILABILITY (Rx)

Tablets (Klonopin): 0.5 mg, 1 mg, 2 mg. **Tablets (Orally-Disintegrating [Klonopin Wafer]):** 0.125 mg, 0.25 mg, 0.5 mg, 1 mg, 2 mg.

ADMINISTRATION/HANDLING

PO

• Give without regard to food. • Tablets may be crushed.

Oral-Disintegrating Tablet

• Open pouch, peel back foil; do not push tablet through foil. • Remove tablet with dry hands, place in mouth. • Swallow with or without water. • Use immediately after removing from package.

INDICATIONS/ROUTES/DOSAGE

Seizures

PO: ADULTS, ELDERLY, CHILDREN 10 YRS AND OLDER: Initial dose not to exceed 1.5 mg/day in 3 divided doses; may be increased in 0.5- to 1-mg increments every 3 days until seizures are controlled or adverse effects occur. Maintenance: 0.05–0.2 mg/kg/day. **Maximum:** 20 mg/day. **INFANTS, CHILDREN YOUNGER THAN 10 YRS OR WEIGHING LESS THAN 30 KG:** 0.01–0.03 mg/kg/day in 2–3 divided doses; may be increased by no more than 0.5 mg every 3 days until seizures are controlled or adverse effects occur. Do not exceed maintenance dosage of 0.2 mg/kg/day.

Panic Disorder

PO: ADULTS, ELDERLY: Initially, 0.25 mg twice a day; increased in increments of 0.125–0.25 mg twice a day every 3 days. **Maximum:** 4 mg/day.

SIDE EFFECTS

Frequent: Mild, transient drowsiness; ataxia; behavioral disturbances (aggression, irritability, agitation), esp. in children. **Occasional:** Rash, ankle or facial edema, nocturia, dysuria, change in appetite or weight, dry mouth, sore gums, nausea, blurred vision. **Rare:** Paradoxical CNS reactions (hyperactivity/nervousness in children; excitement, restlessness in elderly, particularly in the presence of uncontrolled pain).

ADVERSE EFFECTS/ TOXIC REACTIONS

Abrupt withdrawal may result in pronounced restlessness, irritability, insomnia, hand tremors, abdominal/muscle cramps, diaphoresis, vomiting, status epilepticus. Overdose results in drowsiness, confusion, diminished reflexes, coma.

NURSING CONSIDERATIONS

BASELINE ASSESSMENT

Review history of seizure disorder (frequency, duration, intensity, level of consciousness [LOC]). For panic attack, assess motor responses (agitation, trembling, tension), autonomic responses (cold/ clammy hands, diaphoresis).

INTERVENTION/EVALUATION

Observe for excess sedation, respiratory depression, suicidal ideation. Assess children, elderly for paradoxical reaction, particularly during early therapy. Implement safety measures, observe frequently for recurrence of seizure activity. Assist with ambulation if drowsiness, ataxia occur. For those on long-term therapy, hepatic/renal function tests, blood counts should be performed periodically. Evaluate for therapeutic response: decreased intensity and frequency of seizures or, if used in panic attack, calm facial expression, decreased restlessness.

PATIENT/FAMILY TEACHING

• Avoid tasks that require alertness, motor skills until response to drug is established. • Do not abruptly discontinue medication after long-term therapy. • Strict maintenance of drug therapy is essential for seizure control. • Avoid alcohol. • Report depression, thoughts of suicide/self harm, excessive drowsiness, GI symptoms, worsening or loss of seizure control.

clonidine

klon-ih-deen
(Apo-Clonidine ✦, Catapres, Catapres-TTS, Dixarit ✦, Duraclon, Novo-Clonidine ✦)

BLACK BOX ALERT **Epidural:** Not to be used for perioperative, obstetric, or postpartum pain.

Do not confuse Catapres with Cataflam, Cetapred, or Combipres, or clonidine with clomiphene, clorazepam, Klonopin, or quinidine.

FIXED-COMBINATION(S)

Combipres: clonidine/chlorthalidone (a diuretic): 0.1 mg/15 mg, 0.2 mg/15 mg, 0.3 mg/15 mg.

◆CLASSIFICATION

PHARMACOTHERAPEUTIC: Antiadrenergic, sympatholytic. **CLINICAL:** Antihypertensive (see pp. 60C, 154C).

ACTION

Prevents pain signal transmission to brain and produces analgesia at pre- and post-alpha-adrenergic receptors in spinal cord. **Therapeutic Effect:** Reduces peripheral resistance; decreases B/P, heart rate.

PHARMACOKINETICS

Route	Onset	Peak	Duration
PO	0.5–1 hr	2–4 hrs	6–10 hrs

Well absorbed from GI tract. Transdermal best absorbed from chest and upper arm; least absorbed from thigh. Protein binding: 20%–40%. Metabolized in liver. Primarily excreted in urine. Minimally removed by hemodialysis. **Half-life:** 6–20 hrs (increased in renal impairment).

USES

Treatment of hypertension alone or in combination with other antihypertensive agents. **Epidural:** Combined with opiates for relief of severe pain. **OFF-LABEL:** ADHD, diagnosis of pheochromocytoma, opioid withdrawal, prevention of migraine headaches, treatment of diarrhea in diabetes mellitus, treatment of dysmenorrhea, menopausal flushing, alcohol dependence, glaucoma, clozapine-induced sialorrhea.

PRECAUTIONS

Contraindications: Epidural contraindicated in pts with bleeding diathesis or infection at the injection site, those receiving anticoagulation therapy. **Cautions:** Severe coronary insufficiency, recent MI, cerebrovascular disease, chronic renal failure, Raynaud's disease, thromboangiitis obliterans.

⌛ LIFESPAN CONSIDERATIONS

Pregnancy/Lactation: Crosses placenta. Distributed in breast milk. **Preg-**

nancy Category C. **Children:** More sensitive to effects; use caution. **Elderly:** May be more sensitive to hypotensive effect. Age-related renal impairment may require dosage adjustment.

INTERACTIONS

DRUG: Discontinuation of concurrent **beta-blocker** therapy may increase risk of clonidine-withdrawal hypertensive crisis. **Tricyclic antidepressants** may decrease effect. **HERBAL: Gotu kola, kava kava, SAMe, St. John's wort, valerian** may increase CNS depression. **Ephedra, ginseng, yohimbe** may decrease antihypertensive effects. **FOOD:** None known. **LAB VALUES:** None significant.

AVAILABILITY (Rx)

Injection Solution (Duraclon): 100 mcg/ml, 500 mcg/ml. **Tablets (Catapres):** 0.1 mg, 0.2 mg, 0.3 mg. **Transdermal Patch (Catapres-TTS):** 2.5 mg (release at 0.1 mg/24 hrs), 5 mg (release at 0.2 mg/24 hrs), 7.5 mg (release at 0.3 mg/24 hrs).

ADMINISTRATION/HANDLING

PO

• Give without regard to food. • Tablets may be crushed. • Give last oral dose just before bedtime.

Transdermal

• Apply transdermal system to dry, hairless area of intact skin on upper arm or chest. • Rotate sites (prevents skin irritation). • Do not trim patch to adjust dose.

Epidural

• To be administered only by medical personnel trained in epidural management.

IV INCOMPATIBILITIES

None known.

IV COMPATIBILITIES

Bupivacaine (Marcaine, Sensorcaine), fentanyl (Sublimaze), heparin, ketamine (Ketalar), lidocaine, lorazepam (Ativan).

INDICATIONS/ROUTES/DOSAGE

Hypertension

PO: ADULTS: Initially, 0.1 mg twice a day. Increase by 0.1–0.2 mg q2–4days. Maintenance: 0.2–1.2 mg/day in 2–4 divided doses up to maximum of 2.4 mg/day. **ELDERLY:** Initially, 0.1 mg at bedtime. May increase gradually. **CHILDREN 12 YRS AND OLDER:** Initially, 0.2 mg/day in 2 divided doses. May increase gradually at 5- to 7-day intervals. **Maximum:** 2.4 mg/day.
TRANSDERMAL: ADULTS, ELDERLY: System delivering 0.1 mg/24 hrs up to 0.6 mg/24 hrs q7days. Usual dosage range: 0.1–0.3 mg once weekly.

Acute Hypertension

PO: ADULTS: Initially, 0.1–0.2 mg followed by 0.1 mg every hr if necessary, up to maximum total dose of 0.6 mg.

Attention-Deficit Hyperactivity Disorder (ADHD)

PO: CHILDREN: Initially 0.05 mg/day. May increase by 0.05 mg/day q3–7days up to 3–5 mcg/kg/day in divided doses 3–4 times a day. **Maximum:** 0.3–0.4 mg/day.

Severe Pain

EPIDURAL: ADULTS, ELDERLY: 30–40 mcg/hr. **CHILDREN:** Range: 0.5–2 mcg/kg/hr, not to exceed adult dose.

SIDE EFFECTS

Frequent: Dry mouth (40%), drowsiness (33%), dizziness (16%), sedation, constipation (10%). **Occasional (5%–1%): Tablets, Injection:** Depression, pedal edema, loss of appetite, decreased sexual function, itching eyes, dizziness, nausea, vomiting, nervousness. **Transdermal:** Pruritus, redness or darkening of skin. **Rare (less than 1%):** Nightmares, vivid dreams, feeling of coldness in distal extremities (esp. the digits).

ADVERSE EFFECTS/ TOXIC REACTIONS

Overdose produces profound hypotension, irritability, bradycardia, respiratory depression, hypothermia, miosis (pupillary constriction), arrhythmias, apnea. Abrupt withdrawal may result in rebound hypertension associated with nervousness, agitation, anxiety, insomnia, paresthesia, tremor, flushing, diaphoresis.

NURSING CONSIDERATIONS

BASELINE ASSESSMENT

Obtain B/P immediately before each dose is administered, in addition to regular monitoring (be alert to B/P fluctuations).

INTERVENTION/EVALUATION

Monitor B/P, pulse, mental status. Monitor daily pattern of bowel activity and stool consistency. If clonidine is to be withdrawn, discontinue concurrent beta-blocker therapy several days before discontinuing clonidine (prevents clonidine withdrawal hypertensive crisis). Slowly reduce clonidine dosage over 2–4 days.

PATIENT/FAMILY TEACHING

• Sugarless gum, sips of tepid water may relieve dry mouth. • Avoid tasks that require alertness, motor skills until response to drug is established. • To reduce hypotensive effect, rise slowly from lying to sitting position, permit legs to dangle momentarily before standing. • Skipping doses or voluntarily discontinuing drug may produce severe, rebound hypertension. • Avoid alcohol. If patch loosens during 7-day application period, secure with adhesive cover.

clopidogrel

HIGH ALERT

klow-**pih**-duh-grel
(Plavix)

BLACK BOX ALERT Diminished effectiveness in poor metabolizers increases risk for cardiovascular events.

Do not confuse Plavix with Elavil or Paxil.

CLASSIFICATION

PHARMACOTHERAPEUTIC: Thienopyridine derivative. **CLINICAL:** Antiplatelet (see p. 32C).

ACTION

Inhibits binding of enzyme adenosine phosphate (ADP) to its platelet receptor and subsequent ADP-mediated activation of a glycoprotein complex. **Therapeutic Effect:** Inhibits platelet aggregation.

PHARMACOKINETICS

Route	Onset	Peak	Duration
PO	2 hrs	5–7 days (with repeated doses of 75 mg/day)	5 days after last dose

Rapidly absorbed. Protein binding: 98%. Extensively metabolized by liver. Eliminated equally in the urine and feces. **Half-life:** 8 hrs.

USES

Reduction of atherosclerotic events (e.g., MI, stroke, vascular death) in pts with documented atherosclerosis. Treatment of acute coronary syndrome (reduces MI, stroke, refractory ischemia, cardiovascular death). Reduction of atherothrombotic events in pts with ST-segment elevation MI. **OFF-LABEL:** Graft patency (saphenous vein), mitral regurgitation, mitral stenosis, noncardioembolic stroke, percutaneous coronary intervention. Initial treatment of acute coronary syndrome in pts allergic to aspirin.

PRECAUTIONS

Contraindications: Active bleeding, coagulation disorders, severe hepatic disease. **Cautions:** Hypertension, hepatic/renal impairment, history of bleeding, hematologic disorders, preop pts.

LIFESPAN CONSIDERATIONS

Pregnancy/Lactation: Unknown if drug crosses placenta or is distributed in breast milk. **Pregnancy Category B.**

C

Children: Safety and efficacy not established. **Elderly:** No age-related precautions noted.

INTERACTIONS

DRUG: **Aspirin, NSAIDs** may increase risk of bleeding. May interfere with metabolism of **fluvastatin, NSAIDs, phenytoin, tamoxifen, tolbutamide, torsemide, warfarin. Proton pump inhibitors (e.g., omeprazole)** may decrease efficacy. HERBAL: **Cat's claw, dong quai, evening primrose, feverfew, garlic, ginger, ginkgo, ginseng, green tea, horse chestnut, red clover** may have additive antiplatelet effects. FOOD: None known. LAB VALUES: May increase bilirubin, hepatic enzymes, serum cholesterol, uric acid. May decrease neutrophil count, platelet count.

AVAILABILITY (Rx)

Tablets: 75 mg, 300 mg.

ADMINISTRATION/HANDLING

PO

- Give without regard to food.

INDICATIONS/ROUTES/DOSAGE

Reduction of Atherosclerotic Events

PO: ADULTS, ELDERLY: 75 mg once a day.

Acute Coronary Syndrome

PO: ADULTS, ELDERLY: Initially, 300–600 mg loading dose, then 75 mg once a day (in combination with aspirin).

ST-Segment MI

PO: ADULTS, ELDERLY: 75 mg once a day (in combination with aspirin).

SIDE EFFECTS

Frequent (15%): Skin disorders. Occasional (8%–6%): Upper respiratory tract infection, chest pain, flu-like symptoms, headache, dizziness, arthralgia. Rare (5%–3%): Fatigue, edema, hypertension, abdominal pain, dyspepsia, diarrhea, nausea, epistaxis, dyspnea, rhinitis.

ADVERSE EFFECTS/ TOXIC REACTIONS

Agranulocytosis, aplastic anemia/pancytopenia, thrombotic thrombocytopenic purpura (TTP) occur rarely. Hepatitis, hypersensitivity reaction, anaphylactoid reaction have been reported.

NURSING CONSIDERATIONS

BASELINE ASSESSMENT

Perform platelet counts before drug therapy, q2days during first wk of treatment, and weekly thereafter until therapeutic maintenance dose is reached. Abrupt discontinuation of drug therapy produces elevated platelet count within 5 days.

INTERVENTION/EVALUATION

Monitor platelet count for evidence of thrombocytopenia. Assess BUN, serum creatinine, bilirubin, AST, ALT, WBC, Hgb, Hct, signs/symptoms of hepatic insufficiency during therapy.

PATIENT/FAMILY TEACHING

• It may take longer to stop bleeding during drug therapy. • Report any unusual bleeding. • Inform physicians, dentists if clopidogrel is being taken, esp. before surgery is scheduled or before taking any new drug.

clorazepate

klor-**az**-e-pate
(Apo-Clorazepate 🍁, Novo-Clopate 🍁, Tranxene, Tranxene SD, Tranxene SD Half-Strength, Tranxene T-Tab)
Do not confuse clorazepate with clofibrate or clonazepam.

◆CLASSIFICATION

PHARMACOTHERAPEUTIC: Benzodiazepine. **CLINICAL:** Antianxiety, anticonvulsant (Schedule IV) (see p. 13C).

C

ACTION

Depresses all levels of CNS, including limbic and reticular formation, by binding to benzodiazepine receptor sites on gamma-aminobutyric acid (GABA) receptor complex. Modulates GABA, a major inhibitory neurotransmitter in the brain. **Therapeutic Effect:** Produces anxiolytic effect, suppresses seizure activity.

PHARMACOKINETICS

Readily absorbed from GI tract. Metabolized in liver to desmethyldiazepam (**Half-life:** 48–96 hrs) and oxazepam (**Half-life:** 6–8 hrs). Excreted primarily in urine.

USES

Management of anxiety disorders; short-term relief of anxiety symptoms, partial seizures, acute alcohol withdrawal symptoms.

PRECAUTIONS

Contraindications: Acute narrow-angle glaucoma. **Cautions:** Renal/hepatic impairment, acute alcohol intoxication.

LIFESPAN CONSIDERATIONS

Pregnancy/Lactation: Crosses placenta; distributed in breast milk. **Pregnancy Category D. Children:** May experience paradoxical excitement. **Elderly:** Increased risk of dizziness, sedation, confusion, hypotension, hyperexcitability.

INTERACTIONS

DRUG: **Alcohol, other CNS depressants** may increase CNS depressant effects. **Azole antifungals** may increase plasma concentration, toxicity. **HERBAL:** **Gotu kola, kava kava, SAMe, St. John's wort, valerian** may increase CNS depression. **FOOD:** None known. **LAB VALUES:** May increase BUN, serum creatinine, ALT, AST, alkaline phosphatase. May decrease Hct. **Therapeutic serum level:** 0.12–1 mcg/ml; **toxic serum level:** greater than 5 mcg/ml.

AVAILABILITY (Rx)

Tablets (Tranxene, Tranxene T-Tab): 3.75 mg, 7.5 mg, 15 mg.

Tablets (Sustained-Release): 11.25 mg (Tranxene SD Half-Strength), 22.5 mg (Tranxene SD).

ADMINISTRATION/HANDLING

ALERT If pt requires change to another anticonvulsant, decrease clorazepate dosage gradually as low-dose therapy begins with replacement drug.

PO

- May administer with food/water to decrease risk of GI disturbance.

INDICATIONS/ROUTES/DOSAGE

Anxiety

PO (REGULAR-RELEASE): ADULTS, ELDERLY: 7.5–15 mg 2–4 times a day.
PO (SUSTAINED-RELEASE): ADULTS, ELDERLY: 11.25 mg or 22.5 mg once a day at bedtime.

Partial Seizures

PO: ADULTS, ELDERLY, CHILDREN OLDER THAN 12 YRS: Initially, up to 7.5 mg 2–3 times a day. May increase by 7.5 mg at weekly intervals. **Maximum:** 90 mg/day. **CHILDREN 9–12 YRS:** Initially, 3.75–7.5 mg twice a day. May increase by 3.75 mg at weekly intervals. **Maximum:** 60 mg/day in 2–3 divided doses.

Alcohol Withdrawal

PO: ADULTS, ELDERLY: Initially, 30 mg, then 15 mg 2–4 times a day on first day. Gradually decrease dosage over subsequent days. **Maximum:** 90 mg/day.

SIDE EFFECTS

Frequent: Drowsiness. **Occasional:** Dizziness, GI disturbances, anxiety, blurred vision, dry mouth, headache, confusion,

C

ataxia, rash, irritability, slurred speech. **Rare**: Paradoxical CNS reactions (hyperactivity, nervousness in children, excitement, restlessness in elderly, debilitated, generally noted during first 2 wks of therapy, particularly in presence of uncontrolled pain).

ADVERSE EFFECTS/ TOXIC REACTIONS

Abrupt or too-rapid withdrawal may result in pronounced restlessness, irritability, insomnia, hand tremors, abdominal/muscle cramps, diaphoresis, vomiting, seizures. Overdose results in drowsiness, confusion, diminished reflexes, coma. May increase risk of suicidal ideation or behavior.

NURSING CONSIDERATIONS

BASELINE ASSESSMENT

Anxiety: Assess autonomic response (cold/clammy hands, diaphoresis), motor response (agitation, trembling, tension). Offer emotional support to anxious pt. **Seizures**: Review history of seizure disorder (intensity, frequency, duration, level of consciousness [LOC]). Observe frequently for recurrence of seizure activity. Initiate seizure precautions.

INTERVENTION/EVALUATION

Assess for paradoxical reaction, particularly during early therapy. Assist with ambulation if drowsiness, dizziness occur. Evaluate for therapeutic response: **Anxiety**: Calm facial expression; decreased restlessness. Monitor for signs/symptoms of depression, anxiety (loss of interest, mood swings, suicidal ideation or behavior). **Seizures**: Decrease in intensity/frequency of seizures. **Therapeutic serum level**: Peak: 0.12–1 mcg/ml; **toxic serum level**: greater than 5 mcg/ml.

PATIENT/FAMILY TEACHING

• Do not abruptly discontinue medication after long-term use (may precipitate seizures). • Strict maintenance of drug therapy is essential for seizure control. • Drowsiness usually disappears during continued therapy. • Avoid tasks that require alertness, motor skills until response to drug is established. • If dizziness occurs, change positions slowly from recumbent to sitting position before standing. • Smoking reduces drug effectiveness. • Avoid alcohol. • Notify physician if thoughts of suicide, worsening depression, or loss of seizure control occurs.

clotrimazole

kloe-**tri**-mah-zole
(Canesten ✦, Clotrimaderm ✦, Cruex, Gyne-Lotrimin, Lotrimin, Mycelex)
Do not confuse clotrimazole with cotrimoxazole, Lotrimin with Lotrisone, or Mycelex with Myoflex.

FIXED-COMBINATION(S)

Lotrisone: clotrimazole/betamethasone (a corticosteroid): 1%/0.05%.

◆CLASSIFICATION

PHARMACOTHERAPEUTIC: Anti-infective. **CLINICAL**: Antifungal (see p. 48C).

ACTION

Binds with phospholipids in fungal cell membrane. **Therapeutic Effect:** Alters cell membrane permeability, inhibits fungal growth.

USES

Oral Lozenges: Treatment/prophylaxis of oropharyngeal candidiasis due to *Candida* spp. **Topical**: Treatment of tinea pedis, tinea cruris, tinea corporis, tinea versicolor, cutaneous candidiasis (moniliasis) due to *Candida albicans*. **Intravaginal**: Treatment of vulvovaginal candidiasis (moniliasis) due to *Candida* spp. **OFF-LABEL**: **Topical**:

Treatment of paronychia, tinea barbae, tinea capitis.

PRECAUTIONS

Contraindications: Children younger than 3 yrs. **Cautions:** Hepatic disorder with oral therapy.

LIFESPAN CONSIDERATIONS

Pregnancy/Lactation: PO: Unknown if distributed in breast milk. **Pregnancy Category C. Topical:** Unknown if distributed in breast milk. No adverse effects noted in fetus when given in second or third trimester. **Pregnancy Category B. Vaginal:** Unknown if distributed in breast milk. **Pregnancy Category B. Children: PO:** No specific problems noted in those 3 yrs and older. Not recommended in those younger than 3 yrs. **Topical:** No age-related precautions noted. **Vaginal:** Safety and efficacy not established in those up to 12 yrs. **Elderly: PO/Topical/Vaginal:** No age-related precautions noted.

INTERACTIONS

DRUG: None significant. **HERBAL:** None significant. **FOOD:** None known. **LAB VALUES:** May increase serum AST.

AVAILABILITY (Rx)

Topical Cream (Cruex, Lotrimin): 1%. **Topical Solution (Lotrimin):** 1%. **Troche (Mycelex):** 10 mg. **Vaginal Cream (Gyne-Lotrimin):** 1%, 2%. **Vaginal Tablet (Gyne-Lotrimin):** 200 mg.

ADMINISTRATION/HANDLING

PO

• Lozenges must be dissolved in mouth longer than 15–30 min for oropharyngeal therapy. • Swallow saliva.

Topical

• Rub well into affected, surrounding areas. • Do not apply occlusive covering or other preparations to affected area.

Vaginal

• Use vaginal applicator; insert high into vagina. • Remain supine for 30 min following administration.

INDICATIONS/ROUTES/DOSAGE

Oropharyngeal

PO: ADULTS, ELDERLY, CHILDREN 3 YRS AND OLDER: 10 mg 5 times a day for 14 days.

Prophylaxis for Oropharyngeal Candidiasis

PO: ADULTS, ELDERLY: 10 mg 3 times a day.

Usual Topical Dosage

TOPICAL: ADULTS, ELDERLY, CHILDREN 3 YRS AND OLDER: Twice a day. Therapeutic effect may take up to 8 wks.

Vulvovaginal Candidiasis

VAGINAL (TABLETS): ADULTS, ELDERLY, CHILDREN 12 YRS AND OLDER: 1 tablet (100 mg) at bedtime for 7 days; 2 tablets (200 mg) at bedtime for 3 days; or 500-mg tablet one time.

VAGINAL (CREAM): ADULTS, ELDERLY, CHILDREN 12 YRS AND OLDER: (1%): One applicator at bedtime for 7 days. (2%): One applicator at bedtime for 3 days.

SIDE EFFECTS

Frequent: PO: Nausea, vomiting, diarrhea, abdominal pain. **Occasional: Topical:** Pruritis, burning, stinging, erythema, urticaria. **Vaginal:** Mild burning (tablets/cream); irritation, cystitis (cream). **Rare: Vaginal:** Pruritis, rash, lower abdominal cramping, headache.

ADVERSE EFFECTS/ TOXIC REACTIONS

None known.

NURSING CONSIDERATIONS

BASELINE ASSESSMENT

Assess pt's ability to understand, follow directions regarding use of medication.

INTERVENTION/EVALUATION

With oral therapy, assess for nausea, vomiting. With topical therapy, check skin for erythema, urticaria, blistering; inquire about pruritis, burning, stinging. With vaginal therapy, evaluate for vulvovaginal irritation, abdominal cramping, urinary frequency, discomfort.

PATIENT/FAMILY TEACHING

• Continue medication for full length of therapy. • **Topical**: • Inform physician of increased irritation. • Avoid contact with eyes. Keep areas clean, dry; wear light clothing to promote ventilation. • Separate personal items, linens. • **Vaginal**: Continue use during menses. • Refrain from sexual intercourse or advise partner to use condom during therapy. • Instruct pt to remain lying down for 30 min after insertion of medication.

clozapine

kloe-za-peen
(Apo-Clozapine, Clozaril, FazaClo)

BLACK BOX ALERT Significant risk of life-threatening agranulocytosis, increased risk of potentially fatal cardiovascular events, particularly myocarditis, in elderly pts with dementia-related psychosis. May cause severe orthostatic hypotension, dose-dependent seizures.

Do not confuse clozapine with clofazimine, clonidine, or Klonopin, or Clozaril with Clinoril or Colazal.

CLASSIFICATION

PHARMACOTHERAPEUTIC: Dibenzodiazepine derivative. CLINICAL: Antipsychotic (see p. 64C).

ACTION

Interferes with binding of dopamine at dopamine receptor sites; binds primarily at nondopamine receptor sites. **Therapeutic Effect**: Diminishes schizophrenic behavior.

PHARMACOKINETICS

Readily absorbed from GI tract. Protein binding: 97%. Metabolized in liver. Excreted in urine. **Half-life**: 12 hrs.

USES

Management of severely ill schizophrenic pts who fail to respond to other antipsychotic therapy. Treatment of recurrent suicidal behavior. OFF-LABEL: Bipolar disorder, childhood psychosis, obsessive-compulsive disorder, agitation related to Alzheimer's dementia.

PRECAUTIONS

Contraindications: Concurrent use of other drugs that may suppress bone marrow function, history of clozapine-induced agranulocytosis or severe granulocytopenia, myeloproliferative disorders, paralytic ileus, uncontrolled seizures, severe CNS depression, coma. Cautions: History of seizures, cardiovascular disease, myocarditis; respiratory, hepatic, renal impairment; alcohol withdrawal; urinary retention; glaucoma; prostatic hypertrophy. **Pregnancy Category B.**

INTERACTIONS

DRUG: **Antihypertensive medications** may increase risk of hypotension. **Alcohol, other CNS depressants** may increase CNS depressant effects. **Bone marrow depressants** may increase myelosuppression. **SSRIs (e.g., paroxetine)** may increase concentration. **Lithium** may increase risk of confusion, dyskinesia, seizures. HERBAL: None significant. FOOD: None known. LAB VALUES: May increase serum glucose, cholesterol (rare), triglycerides (rare).

AVAILABILITY (Rx)

Tablets (Clozaril): 12.5 mg, 25 mg, 100 mg, 200 mg. Tablets (Orally Disintegrating [FazaClo]): 12.5 mg, 25 mg, 100 mg.

ADMINISTRATION/HANDLING

PO

• Give without regard to food.

Orally Disintegrating Tablets

• Remove from foil blister; do not push tablet through foil. • Remove tablet with dry hands, place in mouth. • Allow to dissolve in mouth, swallow with saliva. • If dose requires splitting tablet, discard unused portion.

INDICATIONS/ROUTES/DOSAGE

Schizophrenic Disorders, Reduce Risk of Suicidal Behavior

◀ALERT▶ For initiation of therapy, must have WBC equal to or greater than 3,500 mm^3 and ANC equal to or greater than 2,000 mm^3.

PO: ADULTS: Initially, 12.5 mg once or twice a day. May increase by 25–50 mg/day over 2 wks until dosage of 300–450 mg/day is achieved. May further increase by 50–100 mg/day no more than once or twice a week. **Range:** 200–600 mg/day. **Maximum:** 900 mg/day. **ELDERLY**: Initially, 25 mg/day. May increase by 25 mg/day. **Maximum:** 450 mg/day.

SIDE EFFECTS

Frequent: Drowsiness (39%), salivation (31%), tachycardia (25%), dizziness (19%), constipation (14%). **Occasional:** Hypotension (9%); headache (7%); tremor, syncope, diaphoresis, dry mouth (6%); nausea, visual disturbances (5%); nightmares, restlessness, akinesia, agitation, hypertension, abdominal discomfort, heartburn, weight gain (4%). **Rare:** Rigidity, confusion, fatigue, insomnia, diarrhea, rash.

ADVERSE EFFECTS/ TOXIC REACTIONS

Seizures occur occasionally (3%). Overdose produces CNS depression (sedation, delirium, coma), respiratory depression, hypersalivation. Blood dyscrasias, particularly agranulocytosis, mild leukopenia, may occur.

NURSING CONSIDERATIONS

BASELINE ASSESSMENT

Obtain baseline weight, glucose, Hgb A_{1c} WBC, absolute neutrophil count (ANC) before initiating treatment. Monitor WBC, ANC count every wk for first 6 mos of continuous therapy, then biweekly for 6 mos. If CBC and ANC are normal after 12 mos, then monthly monitoring of CBC and ANC is recommended. Assess behavior, appearance, emotional status, response to environment, speech pattern, thought content.

INTERVENTION/EVALUATION

Monitor B/P for hypertension/hypotension. Assess pulse for tachycardia (common side effect). Monitor CBC for blood dyscrasias. Supervise suicidal-risk pt closely during early therapy (as depression lessens, energy level improves, increasing suicide potential). Assess for therapeutic response (interest in surroundings, improvement in self-care, increased ability to concentrate, relaxed facial expression).

PATIENT/FAMILY TEACHING

• Do not abruptly discontinue long-term drug therapy. • Drowsiness generally subsides during continued therapy. • Avoid tasks that require alertness, motor skills until response to drug is established. • Avoid alcohol, caffeine. • Report fever, sore throat, flu-like symptoms.

codeine phosphate HIGH ALERT

koe-deen
(Codeine Phosphate Injection)

codeine sulfate

(Codeine Contin ✱)
Do not confuse codeine with Cardene or Lodine.

FIXED-COMBINATION(S)

Capital with Codeine, Tylenol with Codeine: acetaminophen/codeine: 120 mg/12 mg per 5 ml. **Tylenol with Codeine**: acetaminophen/codeine: 300 mg/15 mg, 300 mg/30 mg, 300 mg/60 mg.

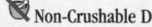

C

◆CLASSIFICATION

PHARMACOTHERAPEUTIC: Opioid agonist. **CLINICAL:** Analgesic: **Schedule II;** Fixed-combination form: **Schedule III** (see p. 141C).

ACTION

Binds to opioid receptors in CNS, particularly in medulla. Inhibits ascending pain pathways. **Therapeutic Effect:** Alters perception of, emotional response to pain; suppresses cough reflex.

PHARMACOKINETICS

Route	Onset	Peak	Duration
PO	30–60 min	1–1.5 hrs	4–6 hrs
IM	10–30 min	0.5–1 hr	4–6 hrs

Well absorbed following PO administration. Protein binding: Very low. Metabolized in liver. Excreted in urine. **Half-life:** 2.5–3.5 hrs.

USES

Relief of mild to moderate pain, nonproductive cough. **OFF-LABEL:** Treatment of diarrhea.

PRECAUTIONS

Contraindications: Premature infants. **Extreme Caution:** CNS depression, anoxia, hypercapnia, respiratory depression, seizures, acute alcoholism, shock, untreated myxedema, respiratory dysfunction. **Cautions:** Increased intracranial pressure, hepatic impairment, acute abdominal conditions, hypothyroidism, prostatic hypertrophy, Addison's disease, urethral stricture, COPD.

⌛ LIFESPAN CONSIDERATIONS

Pregnancy Category C (D if used for prolonged periods or at high dosages at term). Children: Efficacy not established in those younger than 2 years. **Elderly:** May cause confusion, oversedation; use lower dosing range.

INTERACTIONS

DRUG: Alcohol, other CNS depressants may increase CNS, respiratory depression, hypotension. **MAOIs** may produce a severe, sometimes fatal reaction (reduce dosage to ¼ usual dose). **HERBAL: St. John's wort** may decrease plasma concentration. **Gotu kola, kava kava, SAMe, St. John's wort, valerian** may increase CNS depression. **FOOD:** None known. **LAB VALUES:** May increase serum amylase, lipase.

AVAILABILITY (Rx)

Injection Solution: 15 mg/ml, 30 mg/ml. **Tablets (Phosphate):** 30 mg, 60 mg. **Tablets (Sulfate):** 15 mg, 30 mg, 60 mg.

ADMINISTRATION/HANDLING

PO

- Give with food or milk (minimizes adverse GI effects).

INDICATIONS/ROUTES/DOSAGE

◀ALERT▶ Reduce initial dosage in those with hypothyroidism, Addison's disease, renal insufficiency; those using other CNS depressants concurrently.

Analgesia

PO, IM, SUBCUTANEOUS: ADULTS, ELDERLY: 30 mg q4–6h. Range: 15–120 mg. **CHILDREN:** 0.5–1 mg/kg q4–6h. **Maximum:** 60 mg/dose.

Cough

PO: ADULTS, ELDERLY, CHILDREN 12 YRS AND OLDER: 10–20 mg q4–6yrs. **Maximum:** 120 mg/day. **CHILDREN 6–11 YRS:** 5–10 mg q4–6h. **Maximum:** 60 mg/day. **CHILDREN 2–5 YRS:** 2.5–5 mg q4–6h. **Maximum:** 30 mg/day.

Dosage in Renal Impairment

Dosage is modified based on creatinine clearance.

Creatinine Clearance	Dosage
10–50 ml/min	75% of usual dose
Less than 10 ml/min	50% of usual dose

SIDE EFFECTS

◀ALERT▶ Ambulatory pts, those not in severe pain may experience dizziness, nausea, vomiting, hypotension more frequently than those in supine position or with severe pain. **Frequent:** Constipation, drowsiness, nausea, vomiting. **Occasional:** Paradoxical excitement, confusion, palpitations, facial flushing, decreased urination, blurred vision, dizziness, dry mouth, headache, hypotension (including orthostatic hypotension), decreased appetite, injection site redness, burning, or pain. **Rare:** Hallucinations, depression, abdominal pain, insomnia.

ADVERSE EFFECTS/ TOXIC REACTIONS

Too-frequent use may result in paralytic ileus. Overdose may produce cold/clammy skin, confusion, seizures, decreased B/P, restlessness, pinpoint pupils, bradycardia, respiratory depression, decreased LOC, severe weakness. Tolerance to drug's analgesic effect, physical dependence may occur with repeated dosage.

NURSING CONSIDERATIONS

BASELINE ASSESSMENT

Analgesic: Assess onset, type, location, duration of pain. Effect of medication is reduced if full pain response recurs before next dose. **Antitussive**: Assess type, severity, frequency of cough, sputum production.

INTERVENTION/EVALUATION

Monitor daily pattern of bowel activity and stool consistency. Increase fluid intake, environmental humidity to improve viscosity of lung secretions. Initiate deep breathing, coughing exercises. Assess for clinical improvement; record onset of relief of pain, cough.

PATIENT/FAMILY TEACHING

• Change positions slowly to avoid orthostatic hypotension. • Avoid tasks that require alertness, motor skills until response to drug is established. • Tolerance, dependence may occur with prolonged use of high dosages. • Avoid alcohol.

colchicine HIGH ALERT

kol-chi-seen
(Colcrys)
Do not confuse colchicine with Cortrosyn.

◆CLASSIFICATION

PHARMACOTHERAPEUTIC: Alkaloid. **CLINICAL:** Antigout.

ACTION

Decreases leukocyte motility, phagocytosis, lactic acid production. **Therapeutic Effect:** Decreases urate crystal deposits, reduces inflammatory process.

PHARMACOKINETICS

Rapidly absorbed from GI tract. Highest concentration is in liver, spleen, kidney. Protein binding: 30%–50%. Reenters intestinal tract by biliary secretion and is reabsorbed from intestines. Partially metabolized in liver. Eliminated primarily in feces. **Half-life:** 12–30 min.

USES

Prevention and treatment of acute gouty arthritis. Used to reduce frequency of recurrence of familial Mediterranean fever (FMF). **OFF-LABEL:** Treatment of acute calcium pyrophosphate deposition, amyloidosis, biliary cirrhosis, recurrent pericarditis, sarcoid arthritis.

PRECAUTIONS

Contraindications: Blood dyscrasias; severe cardiac, GI, hepatic, renal disorders. **Cautions:** Hepatic impairment, elderly, debilitated.

⧖ LIFESPAN CONSIDERATIONS

Pregnancy/Lactation: Unknown if drug crosses placenta or is distributed in breast milk. **Pregnancy Category C. Children:** Safety and efficacy not established. **Elderly:** May be more susceptible to cumulative toxicity. Age-related renal impairment may increase risk of myopathy.

C

INTERACTIONS

DRUG: **Bone marrow depressants** may increase risk of blood dyscrasias. **Statins** increase risk of rhabdomyolysis. **Atazanavir, clarithromycin, cyclosporine, diltiazem, erythromycin, fluconazole, fosamprenavir, indinavir, itraconazole, ketoconazole, nelfinavir, ranolazine, ritonavir, saquinavir, verapamil** may increase colchicine toxicity. HERBAL: None significant. FOOD: **Grapefruit juice, grapefruit** may increase concentration/toxicity. LAB VALUES: May increase serum alkaline phosphatase, AST. May decrease platelet count.

AVAILABILITY (Rx)

Tablets: 0.6 mg.

ADMINISTRATION/HANDLING

PO

• Give without regard to food. • For FMF, give in 1 or 2 divided doses. • Give with adequate water and maintain fluid intake.

INDICATIONS/ROUTES/DOSAGE

Acute Gouty Arthritis

PO: ADULTS, ELDERLY: Initially, 1.2 mg at first sign of gout flare, then 0.6 mg 1 hr later. **Co-administration with strong CYP3A4 inhibitors:** 0.6 mg, follow in 1 hr by single 0.3 mg dose. Do not repeat for at least 3 days. **Co-administration with moderate CYP3A4 inhibitors:** 1.2 mg once. Do not repeat for at least 3 days. **Co-administration with P-glycoprotein inhibitors:** 0.6 mg once. Do not repeat for at least 3 days.

Gout Prophylaxis

PO: ADULTS, ELDERLY: 0.6 mg 1–2 times/day. **Co-administration with strong CYP3A4 inhibitors:** If dose is 0.6 mg 2 times/day, adjust dose to 0.3 mg once daily; if dose is 0.6 mg once daily, adjust dose to 0.3 mg every other day. **Co-administration with moderate CYP3A4 inhibitors:** If dose is 0.6 mg 2 times/day, adjust dose to 0.3 mg twice daily or 0.6 mg once daily; if dose is 0.6 mg once daily, adjust dose to 0.3 mg once daily. **Co-administration with P-glycoprotein inhibitors:** If dose is 0.6 mg 2 times/day, adjust dose to 0.3 mg once daily; if dose is 0.6 mg once daily, adjust dose to 0.3 mg every other day.

FMF

PO: ADULTS, ELDERLY, CHILDREN OLDER THAN 12 YRS: 1.2–2.4 mg/day. **Co-administration with strong CYP3A4 inhibitors: Maximum:** 0.6 mg once daily (or 0.3 mg twice daily). **Co-administration with moderate CYP3A4 inhibitors:** 1.2 mg/day (0.6 mg twice daily). **Co-administration with P-glycoprotein inhibitors:** 0.6 mg once daily (or 0.3 mg twice daily). **CHILDREN 6–12 YRS:** 0.9–1.8 mg/day. **CHILDREN 4–5 YRS:** 0.3–1.8 mg/day. **Note:** Increase or decrease dose by 0.3 mg/day, not to exceed maximum dose.

Dosage in Renal Impairment

Creatinine Clearance	Dosage
Less than 30 ml/min	0.3 g/day
35–49 ml/min	0.6 mg/day

No adjustment for gout flare treatment.

SIDE EFFECTS

Frequent: **PO:** Nausea, vomiting, abdominal discomfort. Occasional: **PO:** Anorexia. Rare: Hypersensitivity reaction, including angioedema. **Parenteral:** Nausea, vomiting, diarrhea, abdominal discomfort, pain/redness at injection site, neuritis in injected arm.

ADVERSE EFFECTS/ TOXIC REACTIONS

Bone marrow depression (aplastic anemia, agranulocytosis, thrombocytopenia) may occur with long-term therapy. Overdose initially causes burning feeling in skin/throat, severe diarrhea, abdominal pain. Second stage manifests as fever, seizures, delirium, renal impairment (hematuria, oliguria). Third stage causes hair loss, leukocytosis, stomatitis.

NURSING CONSIDERATIONS

BASELINE ASSESSMENT

Gout: Assess involved joints for pain, mobility, edema. **Mediterranean fever:** Assess abdominal pain, fever, chills, erythema, swollen skin lesions.

INTERVENTION/EVALUATION

Discontinue medication immediately if GI symptoms occur. Encourage high fluid intake (3,000 ml/day). Monitor I&O (output should be at least 2,000 ml/day), CBC, hepatic/renal function tests. Assess serum uric acid. Assess for therapeutic response: relief of pain, stiffness, swelling; increased joint mobility; reduced joint tenderness; improved grip strength.

PATIENT/FAMILY TEACHING

• Drink 8–10 glasses (8 oz) of fluid daily while taking medication. • Report skin rash, sore throat, fever, unusual bruising/bleeding, weakness, fatigue, numbness. • Stop medication as soon as gout pain is relieved or at first sign of nausea, vomiting, diarrhea. • Avoid grapefruit, grapefruit juice.

Combivent, *see albuterol and ipratropium*

Combivir, *see lamivudine and zidovudine*

Concerta, *see methylphenidate*

conivaptan

kon-ih-**vap**-tan
(Vaprisol)

CLASSIFICATION

PHARMACOTHERAPEUTIC: Vasopressin antagonist. **CLINICAL:** Hyponatremia adjunct.

ACTION

Promotes excretion of free water (without loss of serum electrolytes) resulting in net fluid loss, increased urine output, decreased urine osmolarlity. **Therapeutic Effect:** Restores normal serum sodium level.

PHARMACOKINETICS

Metabolized in liver to active metabolites. Protein binding: 99%. Mainly eliminated in feces with lesser amount excreted in urine. **Half-life:** 6.7–8.6 hrs.

USES

Treatment of euvolemic and hypervolemic hyponatremia (syndrome of inappropriate secretion of antidiuretic hormone, in setting of hypothyroidism, adrenal insufficiency, pulmonary disorders) in hospitalized pts.

PRECAUTIONS

Contraindications: Hypovolemic hyponatremia; concurrent use with strong CYP3A4 inhibitors (clarithromycin, ketoconazole, ritonavir). **Cautions:** Hepatic/renal impairment, underlying congestive heart failure.

LIFESPAN CONSIDERATIONS

Pregnancy/Lactation: Accumulates in placenta; systemic exposure to fetus likely. Potential for decreased neonatal viability, delayed growth/development at doses lower than those required for therapeutic efficacy. Unknown if distributed in breast milk. **Pregnancy Category C. Children:** Safety and efficacy not established. **Elderly:** No age-related precautions noted.

INTERACTIONS

DRUG: **Aminoglutethimide, carbamazepine, nafcillin, nevirapine, phenobarbital, phenytoin, rifamycins** may decrease level/effect. **Clarithromycin, itraconazole, ketoconazole, ritonavir** may increase level/effect. May increase levels/effects of **benzodiazepines, calcium channel blockers, cyclosporine, mirtazapine, nateglinide, nefazodone, sildenafil, tacrolimus, venlafaxine.** May increase level/toxicity of **digoxin.** HERBAL: None significant. FOOD: None known. LAB VALUES: May decrease Hgb, Hct, serum potassium, magnesium. May alter serum glucose.

AVAILABILITY (Rx)

Injection Solution (Vaprisol): 5 mg/ml (4-ml single-use ampule). **Premix Solution:** 20 mg/100 ml D_5W.

ADMINISTRATION/HANDLING

◀ALERT▶ Administer through large veins; change peripheral IV site every 24 hrs (minimizes risk of vascular irritation).

IV

Reconstitution • For loading dose infusion (piggyback), withdraw 4 ml (20 mg) conivaptan and dilute with 100 ml D_5W. Invert bag several times to ensure mixing solution. • For continuous infusion, withdraw 4–8 ml (20–40 mg) conivaptan and dilute with 250 ml D_5W. Invert bag several times to ensure mixing solution.
Rate of administration • For 100-ml infusion, infuse over 30 min. For 250-ml infusion, infuse over 24 hrs.
Storage • Store ampules at room temperature. • Protect from prolonged exposure to light. • Diluted solution must be used within 24 hrs of mixing.

IV INCOMPATIBILITIES

Lactated Ringer's, 0.9% NaCl.

IV COMPATIBILITIES

Do not infuse concurrently with any other medication or solution.

INDICATIONS/ROUTES/DOSAGE

Euvolemic/Hypervolemic Hyponatremia
IV: ADULTS, ELDERLY: Loading dose: 20 mg given over 30 min. Follow with 20 mg in a continuous IV infusion over 24 hrs. Administer for an additional 1–3 days as a continuous infusion of 20 mg/day. May be titrated upward to 40 mg/day as a continuous infusion if serum sodium is not rising at desired rate. Duration of infusion after loading dose should not exceed 4 days.

SIDE EFFECTS

Frequent: Peripheral injection site reactions (pain, erythema, phlebitis, swelling) (53%), headache (12%). **Occasional (10%–4%):** Thirst, vomiting, hypertension, polyuria, orthostatic hypotension, diarrhea, constipation, fever, confusion, dry mouth, nausea. **Rare (3%–2%):** Atrial fibrillation, hypotension, insomnia, dehydration, oral candidiasis.

ADVERSE EFFECTS/ TOXIC REACTIONS

Overly rapid increase in serum sodium may produce temporary neurologic symptoms. UTI, anemia, hematuria, pneumonia occur occasionally.

NURSING CONSIDERATIONS

BASELINE ASSESSMENT

Obtain baseline serum sodium, hepatic enzyme levels, BUN, creatinine, CBC. Start peripheral IV in large vein. Assess for increased pulse rate, poor skin turgor, nausea, diarrhea (signs of hyponatremia).

INTERVENTION/EVALUATION

Obtain, monitor frequent serum sodium levels. Assess peripheral IV site for pain, erythema, phlebitis, swelling; if vein irritation occurs, change IV site. New IV site should be obtained every 24 hrs (minimizes vein irritation). Monitor urine output. Observe for improvement in signs/symptoms of hyponatremia, impending signs/symptoms of hypernatremia (flushing, edema, restlessness, dry mucous membranes, fever).

PATIENT/FAMILY TEACHING

Change positions slowly to avoid orthostatic hypotension.

conjugated estrogens

ess-troe-jenz
(Cenestin, C.E.S. ✦, Enjuvia, Premarin)

BLACK BOX ALERT Risk of dementia may be increased in postmenopausal women. Do not use to prevent cardiovascular disease. May increase risk of endometrial carcinoma in postmenopausal women.

Do not confuse Enjuvia with Januvia, or Premarin with Primaxin or Remeron.

FIXED-COMBINATION(S)

Premphase, Prempro: estrogen/methyltestosterone (an androgen): 0.3 mg/1.5 mg, 0.45 mg/1.5 mg, 0.625 mg/2.5 mg, 0.625 mg/5 mg.

◆CLASSIFICATION

PHARMACOTHERAPEUTIC: Estrogen. **CLINICAL:** Hormone.

ACTION

Increases synthesis of DNA, RNA, various proteins in target tissues; reduces release of gonadotropin-releasing hormone, reduces follicle-stimulating hormone (FSH), luteinizing hormone (LH) release. **Therapeutic Effect:** Promotes normal growth, development of female sex organs, maintains GU function, vasomotor stability. Prevents accelerated bone loss by inhibiting bone resorption, restoring balance of bone resorption/formation. Inhibits LH, decreases serum concentration of testosterone.

PHARMACOKINETICS

Well absorbed from GI tract. Widely distributed. Protein binding: 50%–80%. Metabolized in liver. Primarily excreted in urine. **Half-life (total estrone):** 27 hrs.

USES

Premarin: Management of moderate to severe vasomotor symptoms associated with menopause. Treatment of atrophic vaginitis, kraurosis vulvae, female hypogonadism and castration, primary ovarian failure. Retardation of osteoporosis in postmenopausal women. Palliative treatment of inoperable, progressive cancer of the prostate in men and of the breast in postmenopausal women. Treatment of moderate to severe postmenopausal dyspareunia (painful sexual intercourse). **Cenestin**: Treatment of moderate to severe vasomotor symptoms of menopause, treatment of vulvar/vaginal atrophy. **Enjuvia**: Treatment of moderate to severe vasomotor symptoms, moderate to severe vaginal dryness and pain with intercourse, symptoms of vulvar/vaginal atrophy associated with menopause. **OFF-LABEL**: Prevention of estrogen deficiency–induced premenopausal osteoporosis. **Cream**: Prevention of nosebleeds.

PRECAUTIONS

Contraindications: Breast cancer (with some exceptions), hepatic disease, thrombophlebitis, undiagnosed vaginal bleeding. **Cautions:** Asthma, epilepsy, migraine headaches, diabetes, cardiac/renal dysfunction.

⧗ LIFESPAN CONSIDERATIONS

Pregnancy/Lactation: Distributed in breast milk. May be harmful to fetus. Not for use during lactation. **Pregnancy Category X. Children:** Safety and efficacy not established. **Elderly:** No age-related precautions noted.

INTERACTIONS

DRUG: May increase serum concentration, enhance hepatotoxic effect of **cyclosporine. Hepatotoxic medications** may increase risk of hepatotoxicity. **HERBAL**: **Black cohosh, dong quai** may increase estrogenic activity. **Ginseng, red clover, saw palmetto** may increase hormonal effects. **St. John's wort** may decrease plasma concentration. **FOOD**: **Grapefruit juice** may increase concentration/toxicity. **LAB VALUES**: May increase blood glucose, HDL, serum calcium, triglycerides. May decrease serum cholesterol, LDH. May affect serum metapyrone testing, thyroid function tests.

C

AVAILABILITY (Rx)

Cream, Vaginal: (Premarin): 0.625 mg/g.
Injection, Powder for Reconstitution: 25 mg.
Tablet (Cenestin, Enjuvia, Premarin): 0.3 mg, 0.45 mg, 0.625 mg, 0.9 mg, 1.25 mg.

ADMINISTRATION/HANDLING

IV

Reconstitution • Reconstitute with 5 ml Sterile Water for Injection containing benzyl alcohol (diluent provided). • Slowly add diluent, shaking gently. Avoid vigorous shaking.
Rate of administration • Give slowly to prevent flushing reaction.
Storage • Refrigerate vials for IV use. • Use immediately following reconstitution.

PO

- Administer at same time each day.
- Give with milk, food if nausea occurs.

IV INCOMPATIBILITIES

No information available on Y-site administration.

INDICATIONS/ROUTES/DOSAGE

Vasomotor Symptoms Associated with Menopause, Atrophic Vaginitis, Kraurosis Vulvae
PO: ADULTS, ELDERLY: 0.3–0.625 mg/day cyclically (21 days on, 7 days off) or continuously.
INTRAVAGINAL: ADULTS, ELDERLY: 0.5–2 g/day cyclically, such as 21 days on and 7 days off.

Female Hypogonadism
PO: ADULTS: 0.3–0.625 mg/day in divided doses for 20 days, then a rest period of 10 days.

Female Castration, Primary Ovarian Failure
PO: ADULTS: Initially, 1.25 mg/day cyclically. Adjust dosage, upward or downward, according to severity of symptoms and pt response. For maintenance, adjust dosage to lowest level that will provide effective control.

Osteoporosis Prevention
PO: ADULTS, ELDERLY: 0.3–0.625 mg/day, cyclically, such as 25 days on and 5 days off.

Breast Cancer
PO: ADULTS, ELDERLY: 10 mg 3 times a day for at least 3 mos.

Prostate Cancer
PO: ADULTS, ELDERLY: 1.25–2.5 mg 3 times a day.

Abnormal Uterine Bleeding
PO: ADULTS: 1.25 mg q4h for 24 hrs, then 1.25 mg/day for 7–10 days.
IV, IM: ADULTS: 25 mg; may repeat once in 6–12 hrs.

Dyspareunia
INTRAVAGINAL: ADULTS, ELDERLY: 0.5 g daily (21 days on, 7 days off).

SIDE EFFECTS

Frequent: Vaginal bleeding (spotting, breakthrough bleeding); breast pain/tenderness; gynecomastia. **Occasional:** Headache, hypertension, intolerance to contact lenses. **High-doses:** Anorexia, nausea. **Rare:** Loss of scalp hair, depression.

ADVERSE EFFECTS/ TOXIC REACTIONS

Prolonged administration may increase risk of breast, cervical, endometrial, hepatic, vaginal carcinoma; cerebrovascular disease, coronary heart disease, gallbladder disease, hypercalcemia.

NURSING CONSIDERATIONS

BASELINE ASSESSMENT

Question for hypersensitivity to estrogen, previous jaundice, thromboembolic disorders associated with pregnancy, estrogen therapy. Assess frequency/severity of vasomotor symptoms.

INTERVENTION/EVALUATION

Assess B/P periodically. Check for edema; weigh daily; Monitor for loss of vision, sudden onset of proptosis, diplopia, migraine, thromboembolic disorder.

PATIENT/FAMILY TEACHING

• Avoid smoking due to increased risk of heart attack, blood clots. • Avoid grapefruit juice. • Diet, exercise important part of therapy when used to retard osteoporosis. • Teach how to perform Homans' test, signs/symptoms of blood clots (report these to physician immediately). • Promptly report signs/symptoms of thromboembolic, thrombotic disorders: sudden severe headache, shortness of breath, vision/speech disturbance, weakness/numbness of an extremity, loss of coordination, pain in chest, groin, leg. • Notify physician of abnormal vaginal bleeding, depression. • Teach female pts to perform breast self-exam. • Report weight gain of more than 5 lbs a wk. • Stop taking medication, contact physician if pregnancy is suspected.

Copaxone, *see glatiramer*

Cordarone, *see amiodarone*

Coreg, *see carvedilol*

cortisone

kor-ti-sone
(Cortone)
Do not confuse cortisone with Cardizem.

◆ CLASSIFICATION

PHARMACOTHERAPEUTIC: Adrenocortical steroid. **CLINICAL:** Glucocorticoid (see p. 97C).

ACTION

Inhibits accumulation of inflammatory cells at inflammation sites, phagocytosis, synthesis and release of mediators of inflammation. **Therapeutic Effect:** Prevents/suppresses cell-mediated immune reactions. Decreases/prevents tissue response to inflammatory process.

PHARMACOKINETICS

Slowly absorbed from GI tract. Widely distributed. Metabolized in liver. Excreted in urine/feces. **Half-life:** 0.5–2 hrs.

USES

Treatment of adrenocortical insufficiency, conditions treated by immunosuppression, inflammatory conditions.

PRECAUTIONS

Contraindications: Hypersensitivity to corticosteroids, administration of live virus vaccine, peptic ulcers (except in life-threatening situations), systemic fungal infection. **Cautions:** Thromboembolic disorders, history of tuberculosis (may reactivate disease), hypothyroidism, cirrhosis, nonspecific ulcerative colitis, CHF, hypertension, psychosis, renal insufficiency, seizure disorders. Prolonged therapy should be discontinued slowly.

⌛ LIFESPAN CONSIDERATIONS

Pregnancy/Lactation: Crosses placenta; distributed in breast milk. **Pregnancy Category C (D if used in the first trimester). Children:** Monitor growth, development of children, infants on prolonged steroid therapy. **Elderly:** Higher risk for hypertension, osteoporosis.

INTERACTIONS

DRUG: Amphotericin may worsen hypokalemia. **Bupropion** may lower seizure threshold. May increase **digoxin**

C

toxicity caused by hypokalemia. May decrease effects of **diuretics, insulin, oral hypoglycemics, potassium supplements. Hepatic enzyme inducers** may decrease effects. **Live-virus vaccines** may decrease pt's antibody response to vaccine, increase vaccine side effects, potentiate virus replication. **HERBAL: Echinacea, ma huang** may decrease corticosteroid effectiveness. **FOOD**: None known. **LAB VALUES**: May increase blood glucose, serum cholesterol, amylase, sodium. May decrease serum calcium, potassium, thyroxine.

AVAILABILITY (Rx)

Tablets: 25 mg.

ADMINISTRATION/HANDLING

• Administer with meals, food, or milk to decrease risk of GI disturbance.

INDICATIONS/ROUTES/DOSAGE

Dosage is dependent on condition being treated and pt response.

Physiologic Replacement

PO: ADULTS, ELDERLY: 25–35 mg/day. **CHILDREN:** 0.5–0.75 mg/kg/day in 3 divided doses.

Inflammatory Conditions

PO: ADULTS, ELDERLY: 25–300 mg/day. **CHILDREN:** 2.5–10 mg/kg/day in 3–4 divided doses.

SIDE EFFECTS

Frequent: Insomnia, heartburn, anxiety, abdominal distention, increased diaphoresis, acne, mood swings, increased appetite, facial flushing, delayed wound healing, increased susceptibility to infection, diarrhea, constipation. **Occasional**: Headache, edema, change in skin color, frequent urination. **Rare:** Tachycardia, allergic reaction (rash, urticaria), psychological changes, hallucinations, depression.

ADVERSE EFFECTS/ TOXIC REACTIONS

Long-term therapy: Hypocalcemia, hypokalemia, muscle wasting (esp. arms, legs), osteoporosis, spontaneous fractures, amenorrhea, cataracts, glaucoma, peptic ulcer, CHF. **Abrupt withdrawal following long-term therapy**: Anorexia, nausea, fever, headache, joint pain, rebound inflammation, fatigue, weakness, lethargy, dizziness, orthostatic hypotension.

NURSING CONSIDERATIONS

BASELINE ASSESSMENT

Question for hypersensitivity to any of the corticosteroids. Obtain baseline values for weight, B/P, serum glucose, cholesterol, electrolytes.

INTERVENTION/EVALUATION

Be alert for infection (reduced immune response): sore throat, fever, vague symptoms. For pts on long-term therapy, monitor for hypocalcemia (muscle twitching, cramps, positive Trousseau's or Chvostek's signs), hypokalemia (weakness, muscle cramps, numbness/tingling [esp. lower extremities], nausea/vomiting, irritability, EKG changes). Assess emotional status, ability to sleep.

PATIENT/FAMILY TEACHING

• Do not change dose or schedule or stop taking drug; **must** taper off under medical supervision. • Notify physician of fever, sore throat, muscle aches, sudden weight gain/swelling. • Inform dentist, other physicians of cortisone therapy now or within past 12 mos.

Cortrosyn, *see cosyntropin*

cosyntropin

koe-sin-**troe**-pin
(Cortrosyn)
Do not confuse Cortrosyn with cortisone or Cotazym.

◆CLASSIFICATION

PHARMACOTHERAPEUTIC: Adrenocortical steroid. **CLINICAL:** Glucocorticoid.

ACTION

Stimulates initial reaction in synthesis of adrenal steroids from cholesterol. **Therapeutic Effect:** Increases endogenous corticoid synthesis.

USES

Diagnostic testing of adrenocortical function.

PRECAUTIONS

Contraindications: Hypersensitivity to cosyntropin, corticotropin. **Cautions:** None known.

LIFESPAN CONSIDERATIONS

Pregnancy/Lactation: Unknown if distributed in breast milk. **Pregnancy Category C. Children/Elderly:** No age-related precautions noted.

INTERACTIONS

DRUG: None significant. **HERBAL:** None significant. **FOOD:** None known. **LAB VALUES:** None significant.

AVAILABILITY (Rx)

Powder for Injection: 0.25 mg.

ADMINISTRATION/HANDLING

Reconstitution
• Reconstitute with 1 ml 0.9% NaCl.
IM • Give as 0.25 mg/ml concentration.
IV push: • Dilute with 2–5 ml 0.9% NaCl over 2 min.

INDICATIONS/ROUTES/DOSAGE

Adrenocortical Insufficiency
IM, IV: ADULTS, ELDERLY, CHILDREN OLDER THAN 2 YRS: 0.25–0.75 mg. **CHILDREN 2 YRS AND YOUNGER:** 0.125 mg. **NEONATES:** 0.015 mg/kg/dose.
IV INFUSION: ADULTS, ELDERLY, CHILDREN OLDER THAN 2 YRS: 0.25 mg over 4–8 hrs at 0.04 mg/hr.

SIDE EFFECTS

Occasional: Nausea, vomiting. **Rare:** Hypersensitivity reaction (fever, pruritus).

ADVERSE EFFECTS/ TOXIC REACTIONS

None known.

NURSING CONSIDERATIONS

BASELINE ASSESSMENT

Hold cortisone, hydrocortisone, spironolactone the day prior to and the day of the test. Ensure that baseline plasma cortisol concentration has been drawn before start of test or 24-hr urine for 17-KS or 17-OHCS is initiated.

INTERVENTION/EVALUATION

Adhere to time frame for blood draws; monitor urine collection if indicated.

PATIENT/FAMILY TEACHING

• Explain procedure, purpose of test.

co-trimoxazole (sulfamethoxazole-trimethoprim)

koe-try-**mox**-oh-zole
(Apo-Sulfatrim ✤, Bactrim, Bactrim DS, Novotrimel ✤, Septra, Septra DS, Sulfatrim)
Do not confuse Bactrim with bacitracin or Bactroban, co-trimoxazole with clotrimazole, or Septra with Sectral.

C

FIXED-COMBINATION(S)

Zotrim: co-trimoxazole/phenazopyridine. **Bactrim, Septra:** sulfamethoxazole/trimethoprim: 5:1 ratio remains constant in all dosage forms (e.g., 400 mg/80 mg).

◆CLASSIFICATION

PHARMACOTHERAPEUTIC: Sulfonamide/folate antagonist. **CLINICAL:** Antibiotic.

ACTION

Blocks bacterial synthesis of essential nucleic acids. **Therapeutic Effect:** Bactericidal in susceptible microorganisms.

PHARMACOKINETICS

Rapidly, well absorbed from GI tract. Protein binding: 45%–60%. Widely distributed. Metabolized in liver. Excreted in urine. Minimally removed by hemodialysis. **Half-life:** sulfamethoxazole, 6–12 hrs; trimethoprim, 6–17 hrs (increased in renal impairment).

USES

Treatment of susceptible infections due to *S. pneumoniae, H. influenzae, E. coli, Klebsiella* spp., *Enterobacter* spp., *M. morganii, P. mirabilis, P. vulgaris, S. flexneri, Pneumocystis jiroveci* including acute or complicated and recurrent or chronic UTI, *Pneumocystis jiroveci* pneumonia (PCP), shigellosis, enteritis, otitis media, chronic bronchitis, traveler's diarrhea. Prophylaxis of PCP. **OFF-LABEL:** Treatment of bacterial endocarditis; gonorrhea; meningitis; septicemia; sinusitis; biliary tract, bone, joint, chancroid, chlamydial, intra-abdominal, skin, soft-tissue infections.

PRECAUTIONS

Contraindications: Hypersensitivity to trimethoprim or any sulfonamides, infants younger than 2 mos, megaloblastic anemia due to folate deficiency. **Cautions:** Those with G6PD deficiency, renal/hepatic impairment.

⌛ LIFESPAN CONSIDERATIONS

Pregnancy/Lactation: Contraindicated during pregnancy at term and during lactation. Readily crosses placenta. Distributed in breast milk. May produce kernicterus in newborn. **Pregnancy Category C (D at term). Children:** Contraindicated in those younger than 2 mos; may increase risk of kernicterus in newborn. **Elderly:** Increased risk for severe skin reaction, myelosuppression, decreased platelet count.

INTERACTIONS

DRUG: **Hemolytics** may increase risk of toxicity. **Hepatotoxic medications** may increase risk of hepatotoxicity. May increase, prolong effects, increase toxicity of **hydantoin anticonvulsants, oral hypoglyemics, warfarin. Methenamine** may form a precipitate. May increase effects of **methotrexate.** **HERBAL:** **Dong quai, St. John's wort** may increase photosensitization reaction. **FOOD:** None known. **LAB VALUES:** May increase BUN, creatinine, AST, ALT, bilirubin.

AVAILABILITY (Rx)

◀ALERT▶ All dosage forms have same 5:1 ratio of sulfamethoxazole (SMZ) to trimethoprim (TMP).

Injection Solution: SMZ 80 mg and TMP 16 mg per ml. **Oral Suspension (Sulfatrim):** SMZ 200 mg and TMP 40 mg per 5 ml. **Tablets (Bactrim, Septra):** SMZ 400 mg and TMP 80 mg. **Tablets (Double Strength [Bactrim DS, Septra DS]):** SMZ 800 mg and TMP 160 mg.

ADMINISTRATION/HANDLING

IV

Reconstitution • For IV infusion (piggyback), dilute each 5 ml with 75–125 ml D_5W. • Do not mix with other drugs or solutions.

Rate of administration • Infuse over 60–90 min. Must avoid bolus or rapid infusion. • Do not give IM. • Ensure adequate hydration.

Storage • IV infusion (piggyback) stable for 2 hrs (5 ml/75 ml D_5W), 4 hrs (5 ml/100 ml D_5W), 6 hrs (5 ml/125 ml D_5W. • Discard if cloudy or precipitate forms.

PO

• Store tablets, suspension at room temperature. • Administer on empty stomach with 8 oz water. • Give several extra glasses of water/day.

IV INCOMPATIBILITIES

Fluconazole (Diflucan), foscarnet (Foscavir), midazolam (Versed), total parenteral nutrition (TPN), vinorelbine (Navelbine).

IV COMPATIBILITIES

Diltiazem (Cardizem), heparin, hydromorphone (Dilaudid), lorazepam (Ativan), magnesium sulfate, morphine.

INDICATIONS/ROUTES/DOSAGE

Usual Adult/Elderly Dosage Range

PO: One double-strength tablet q12–24h. **IV:** 8–20 mg/kg/day as trimethoprim in divided doses q6–12h.

Mild to Moderate Infection

PO: CHILDREN: 8–12 mg/kg/day as trimethoprim in divided doses q12h.

Severe Infections

PO: CHILDREN: 20 mg/kg/day as trimethoprim in divided doses q6h.

IV: CHILDREN: 8–12 mg/kg/day as trimethoprim in divided doses q6h.

Chronic Bronchitis

PO: ADULTS, ELDERLY: 1 double-strength or 2 single-strength tablets or 20 ml suspension q12h for 10–14 days.

***Pneumocystis Jiroveci* Pneumonia (PCP) Prophylaxis**

PO: ADULTS, ELDERLY: 1 double-strength tablet daily or 3 times a wk or 1 single-strength tablet daily. **CHILDREN 2 MOS AND OLDER:** 150 mg/m²/day as trimethoprim in 2 divided doses 3 times a wk on consecutive days.

PCP Treatment

PO, IV: ADULTS, ELDERLY, CHILDREN 2 MOS AND OLDER: 15–20 mg/kg/day as trimethoprim in 4 divided doses for 14–21 days.

Shigellosis

PO: ADULTS, ELDERLY: 1 double-strength tablet or 2 single-strength tablets or 20 ml suspension q12h for 5 days.

IV: ADULTS, CHILDREN: 8–10 mg/kg/day as trimethoprim in 2–4 divided doses for up to 5 days.

Otitis Media

PO: CHILDREN 2 MOS AND OLDER: 8 mg/kg/day trimethoprim q12h for 10 days.

UTI

PO: ADULTS, ELDERLY: 1 double-strength or 2 single-strength tablets or 20 ml suspension q12h for 3–14 days depending on severity. **CHILDREN 2 MOS AND OLDER:** 8 mg/kg/day as trimethoprim in 2 divided doses for 10 days.

Traveler's Diarrhea

PO: ADULTS, ELDERLY: 1 double-strength or 2 single-strength tablets or 20 ml suspension q12h for 5 days.

Dosage in Renal Impairment

Creatinine Clearance	Dosage
15–30 ml/min	50% of usual dosage
Less than 15 ml/min	Not recommended

SIDE EFFECTS

Frequent: Anorexia, nausea, vomiting, rash (generally 7–14 days after therapy begins), urticaria. **Occasional:** Diarrhea, abdominal pain, pain/irritation at IV infusion site. **Rare:** Headache, vertigo, insomnia, seizures, hallucinations, depression.

ADVERSE EFFECTS/ TOXIC REACTIONS

Rash, fever, sore throat, pallor, purpura, cough, shortness of breath may be early signs of serious adverse effects. Fatalities are rare but have occurred in sulfonamide therapy following Stevens-Johnson syndrome, toxic epidermal necrolysis, fulminant hepatic necrosis, agranulocytosis, aplastic anemia, other blood dyscrasias. Myelosuppression, decreased platelet count, severe dermatologic reactions may occur, esp. in the elderly.

NURSING CONSIDERATIONS

BASELINE ASSESSMENT

Obtain history for hypersensitivity to trimethoprim or any sulfonamide, sulfite sensitivity, bronchial asthma. Determine renal, hepatic, hematologic baselines.

INTERVENTION/EVALUATION

Monitor daily pattern of bowel activity and stool consistency. Assess skin for rash, pallor, purpura. Check IV site, flow rate. Monitor renal, hepatic, hematology reports. Assess I&O. Check for CNS symptoms (headache, vertigo, insomnia, hallucinations). Monitor vital signs at least twice a day. Monitor for cough, shortness of breath. Assess for overt bleeding, ecchymosis, edema.

PATIENT/FAMILY TEACHING

• Continue medication for full length of therapy. • Space doses evenly around the clock. • Take oral doses with 8 oz water and drink several extra glasses of water daily. • Notify physician immediately of new symptoms, esp. rash, other skin changes, bleeding/bruising, fever, sore throat, diarrhea. • Avoid prolonged exposure to direct sunlight.

Coumadin, *see warfarin*

Cozaar, *see losartan*

Crestor, *see rosuvastatin*

Crixivan, *see indinavir*

cromolyn

kroe-moe-lin
(Apo-Cromolyn, Crolom, Gastrocom, Intal, Nasalcrom)
Do not confuse Nasalcrom with Nasacort or Nasalide.

◆CLASSIFICATION

PHARMACOTHERAPEUTIC: Mast cell stabilizer. **CLINICAL:** Antiasthmatic, antiallergic (see pp. 3C, 139C).

ACTION

Prevents mast cell release of histamine, leukotrienes, slow-reacting substances of anaphylaxis by inhibiting degranulation after contact with antigens. **Therapeutic Effect:** Assists in preventing symptoms of asthma, allergic rhinitis, mastocytosis, exercise-induced bronchospasm.

PHARMACOKINETICS

Minimal absorption after PO, inhalation, or nasal administration. Absorbed portion excreted in urine or by biliary system. **Half-life:** 80–90 min.

USES

Oral inhalation, nebulization: Prophylactic management of allergic disorders including bronchial asthma; prevention of exercise-induced bronchospasm. **Intranasal**: Prevention/treatment of perennial or seasonal allergic rhinitis. **Systemic**: Symptomatic treatment of systemic mastocytosis. **Ophthalmic**: Conjunctivitis. **OFF-LABEL**: Food allergy, treatment of inflammatory bowel disease (IBD).

PRECAUTIONS

Contraindications: Status asthmaticus. **Cautions:** Coronary artery disease, arrhythmias; when tapering dose or discontinuing therapy (symptoms may recur).

LIFESPAN CONSIDERATIONS

Pregnancy/Lactation: Unknown if drug crosses placenta or is distributed in breast milk. **Pregnancy Category B. Children:** No age-related precautions noted. **Elderly:** Age-related renal/hepatic impairment may require dosage adjustment.

INTERACTIONS

DRUG: None significant. **HERBAL:** None significant. **FOOD:** None known. **LAB VALUES:** None significant.

AVAILABILITY (Rx)

Inhalation Aerosol (Intal): 800 mcg/inhalation. **Nasal Spray (Nasalcrom):** 40 mg/ml. **Nebulization Solution (Intal):** 10 mg/ml. **Ophthalmic Solution (Crolom):** 4%. **Oral Solution (Gastrocrom):** 100 mg/5 ml.

ADMINISTRATION/HANDLING

PO

• Give at least 30 min before meals. • Do not mix oral solution with fruit juice, milk, food.

Inhalation

• Shake container well. Instruct pt to exhale completely, place mouthpiece between lips, inhale, hold breath as long as possible before exhaling. • Wait 1–10 min before inhaling second dose (allows for deeper bronchial penetration). • Rinsing mouth after each use decreases dry mouth, hoarseness.

Nasal

• Nasal passages should be clear (may require nasal decongestant). • Inhale through nose.

Ophthalmic

• Place gloved finger on lower eyelid and pull down until pocket is formed between eye and lower lid. • Place prescribed number of drops in pocket. • Instruct pt to close eyes gently for 1–2 min (so that medication will not be squeezed out of the sac) and to apply digital pressure to lacrimal sac at inner canthus for 1 min (to minimize systemic absorption).

INDICATIONS/ROUTES/DOSAGE

Asthma

INHALATION (NEBULIZATION): ADULTS, ELDERLY, CHILDREN OLDER THAN 2 YRS: 20 mg 3–4 times a day.
AEROSOL SPRAY: ADULTS, ELDERLY, CHILDREN 12 YRS AND OLDER: Initially, 2 sprays 4 times a day. Maintenance: 2–4 sprays 3–4 times a day. **CHILDREN 5–11 YRS:** Initially, 2 sprays 4 times a day, then 1–2 sprays 3–4 times a day.

Prevention of Bronchospasm

INHALATION (NEBULIZATION): ADULTS, ELDERLY, CHILDREN OLDER THAN 2 YRS: 20 mg within 1 hr before exercise or exposure to allergens.
AEROSOL SPRAY: ADULTS, ELDERLY, CHILDREN OLDER THAN 5 YRS: 2 sprays within 1 hr before exercise or exposure to allergens.

Food Allergy, Inflammatory Bowel Disease

PO: ADULTS, ELDERLY, CHILDREN OLDER THAN 12 YRS: 200–400 mg 4 times a day. **CHILDREN 2–12 YRS:** 100–200 mg 4 times a day. **Maximum:** 40 mg/kg/day.

Allergic Rhinitis

INTRANASAL: ADULTS, ELDERLY, CHILDREN 2 YRS AND OLDER: 1 spray each nostril 3–4 times a day. May increase up to 6 times a day.

Systemic Mastocytosis

PO: ADULTS, ELDERLY, CHILDREN OLDER THAN 12 YRS: 200 mg 4 times a day. **CHILDREN 2–12 YRS:** 100 mg 4 times a day. **Maximum:** 40 mg/kg/day. **CHILDREN YOUNGER THAN 2 YRS:** 20 mg/kg/day in 4 divided doses. **Maximum:** 30 mg/kg/day (children 6 mos–2 yrs).

Conjunctivitis

OPHTHALMIC: ADULTS, ELDERLY, CHILDREN OLDER THAN 4 YRS: 1–2 drops in both eyes 4–6 times a day.

C

SIDE EFFECTS

Frequent: PO: Headache, diarrhea. **Inhalation:** Cough, dry mouth/throat, nasal congestion, throat irritation, unpleasant taste. **Nasal:** Nasal burning, stinging, irritation; increased sneezing. **Ophthalmic:** Eye burning/stinging. **Occasional: PO:** Rash, abdominal pain, arthralgia, nausea, insomnia. **Inhalation:** Bronchospasm, hoarseness, lacrimation. **Nasal:** Cough, headache, unpleasant taste, postnasal drip. **Ophthalmic:** Lacrimation, itching of eye. **Rare: Inhalation:** Dizziness, painful urination, arthralgia, myalgia, rash. **Nasal:** Epistaxis, rash. **Ophthalmic:** Chemosis or edema of conjunctiva, eye irritation.

ADVERSE EFFECTS/ TOXIC REACTIONS

Anaphylaxis occurs rarely when given by inhalation, nasal, oral route.

NURSING CONSIDERATIONS

INTERVENTION/EVALUATION

Monitor rate, depth, rhythm, type of respiration; quality/rate of pulse. Assess lung sounds for rhonchi, wheezing, rales. Observe for cyanosis (lips, fingernails for blue or dusky color in light-skinned pts; gray in dark-skinned pts).

PATIENT/FAMILY TEACHING

• Increase fluid intake (decreases lung secretion viscosity). • Rinsing mouth with water immediately after inhalation may prevent mouth/throat dryness. • Effect of therapy dependent on administration at regular intervals.

Cubicin, *see daptomycin*

cyanocobalamin (vitamin B_{12})

sye-an-oh-koe-**bal**-a-min
(CaloMist, Nascobal)

◆CLASSIFICATION

PHARMACOTHERAPEUTIC: Coenzyme. **CLINICAL:** Vitamin, antianemic (see p. 162C).

ACTION

Coenzyme for metabolic functions (fat, carbohydrate metabolism, protein synthesis). **Therapeutic Effect:** Necessary for cell growth and replication, hematopoiesis, myelin synthesis.

PHARMACOKINETICS

In presence of calcium, absorbed systemically in lower half of ileum. Initially, bound to intrinsic factor; this complex passes down intestine, binding to receptor sites on ileal mucosa. Protein binding: High. Metabolized in liver. Primarily eliminated unchanged in urine. **Half-life:** 6 days.

USES

Treatment of pernicious anemia, vitamin B_{12} deficiency due to malabsorption diseases, increased B_{12} requirement due to pregnancy, thyrotoxicosis, hemorrhage, malignancy, hepatic/renal disease.

PRECAUTIONS

Contraindications: Folic acid deficiency anemia, hereditary optic nerve atrophy, history of allergy to cobalamins. **Cautions:** None known.

LIFESPAN CONSIDERATIONS

Pregnancy/Lactation: Crosses placenta. Distributed in breast milk. **Pregnancy Category A (C if used in doses above recommended daily allowance; C for intranasal). Children/Elderly:** No age-related precautions noted.

INTERACTIONS

DRUG: None significant. **HERBAL:** None significant. **FOOD:** None known. **LAB VALUES:** None significant.

AVAILABILITY (Rx)

Injection Solution: 1,000 mcg/ml. **Nasal Gel (Nascobal):** 500 mcg/0.1 ml. **(Calo-**

Mist) 25 mcg/0.1 ml. **Tablets:** 50 mcg, 100 mcg, 250 mcg, 500 mcg, 1,000 mcg. **Tablets (Extended-Release):** 1,000 mcg, 1,500 mcg.

ADMINISTRATION/HANDLING

IM, Subcutaneous

• Avoid IV route.

PO

• Give with food (increases absorption).

Intranasal

• Clear both nostrils. • Pull clear cover off top of pump. • Press down firmly and quickly on pump's finger grips until a droplet of gel appears at top of the pump. Then press down on finger grips two more times. • Place the tip of pump halfway into nostril, pointing tip toward back of nose. • Press down firmly and quickly on finger grips to release medication into one nostril while pressing other nostril closed. • Massage medicated nostril for a few seconds. • Administer nasal preparation at least 1 hr before or 1 hr after hot foods or liquids are consumed.

INDICATIONS/ROUTES/DOSAGE

Pernicious Anemia

IM, SUBCUTANEOUS: ADULTS, ELDERLY: 100 mcg/day for 7 days, then every other day for 7 days, then every 3–4 days for 2–3 wks. Maintenance: 100 mcg/mo (PO 1,000–2,000 mcg/day). **CHILDREN:** 30–50 mcg/day for 2 or more wks. Maintenance: 100 mcg/mo. **NEONATES:** 0.2 mcg/kg for 2 days, then 1,000 mcg/day for 2–7 days. Maintenance: 100 mcg/mo.

Vitamin Deficiency

IM, SUBCUTANEOUS: ADULTS, ELDERLY: 30 mcg/day for 5–10 days, then 100–200 mcg/mo.

PO: ADULTS, ELDERLY: 250 mcg/day.

INTRANASAL: ADULTS, ELDERLY: (NASCOBAL): 500 mcg in one nostril once weekly. **(CALOMIST):** Maintenance: 25 mcg in each nostril daily.

SIDE EFFECTS

Occasional: Diarrhea, pruritus.

ADVERSE EFFECTS/ TOXIC REACTIONS

Impurities in preparation may cause rare allergic reaction. Peripheral vascular thrombosis, pulmonary edema, hypokalemia, CHF occur rarely.

NURSING CONSIDERATIONS

BASELINE ASSESSMENT

Before and during therapy, assess for signs, symptoms of vitamin B_{12} deficiency (anorexia, ataxia, fatigue, hyporeflexia, insomnia, irritability, loss of positional sense, pallor, palpitations on exertion).

INTERVENTION/EVALUATION

Assess for CHF, pulmonary edema, hypokalemia in cardiac pts receiving subcutaneous/IM therapy. Monitor serum potassium (3.5–5 mEq/L), serum B_{12} (200–800 mcg/ml), rise in reticulocyte count (peaks in 5–8 days). Assess for reversal of deficiency symptoms (hyporeflexia, loss of positional sense, ataxia, fatigue, irritability, insomnia, anorexia, pallor, palpitations on exertion). Therapeutic response to treatment usually dramatic within 48 hrs.

PATIENT/FAMILY TEACHING

• Lifetime treatment may be necessary with pernicious anemia. • Report symptoms of infection. • Foods rich in vitamin B_{12} include organ meats, clams, oysters, herring, red snapper, muscle meats, fermented cheese, dairy products, egg yolks. • Use nasal preparation at least 1 hr before or 1 hr after consuming hot foods, liquids.

cyclobenzaprine

sye-kloe-**ben**-za-preen
(Amrix, Apo-cyclobenzaprine ✱, Flexeril, Flexitec ✱, Flexmid, Novo-Cycloprine ✱)

C

Do not confuse cyclobenzaprine with cycloserine or cyproheptadine, or Flexeril with Floxin.

◆CLASSIFICATION

CLINICAL: Skeletal muscle relaxant.

ACTION

Centrally acting skeletal muscle relaxant that reduces tonic somatic muscle activity at level of brainstem. **Therapeutic Effect:** Relieves local skeletal muscle spasm.

PHARMACOKINETICS

Route	Onset	Peak	Duration
PO	1 hr	3–4 hrs	12–24 hrs

Well but slowly absorbed from GI tract. Protein binding: 93%. Metabolized in GI tract and liver. Primarily excreted in urine. **Half-life:** 8–37 hrs.

USES

Treatment of muscle spasm associated with acute, painful musculoskeletal conditions. **OFF-LABEL:** Treatment of fibromyalgia.

PRECAUTIONS

Contraindications: Acute recovery phase of MI, arrhythmias, CHF, heart block, conduction disturbances, hyperthyroidism, use within 14 days of MAOIs. **Cautions:** Renal/hepatic impairment, history of urinary retention, angle-closure glaucoma, increased intraocular pressure (IOP).

LIFESPAN CONSIDERATIONS

Pregnancy/Lactation: Unknown if drug crosses placenta or is distributed in breast milk. **Pregnancy Category B. Children:** Safety and efficacy not established. **Elderly:** Increased sensitivity to anticholinergic effects (e.g., confusion, urinary retention).

INTERACTIONS

DRUG: Alcohol, other CNS depressant medications (e.g., tricyclic antidepressants) may increase CNS depression. **MAOIs** may increase risk of hypertensive crisis, seizures. **Tramadol** may increase risk of seizures. **HERBAL: Gotu kola, kava kava, SAMe, St. John's wort, valerian** may increase CNS depression. **FOOD:** None known. **LAB VALUES:** None significant.

AVAILABILITY (Rx)

Tablets (Flexeril): 5 mg, 10 mg. **(Flexmid):** 7.5 mg.

Capsules (Extended-Release [Amrix]): 15 mg, 30 mg.

ADMINISTRATION/HANDLING

PO

• Give without regard to food. • Do not crush or chew extended-release capsule.

INDICATIONS/ROUTES/DOSAGE

◀ALERT▶ Do not use longer than 2–3 wks.

Acute, Painful Musculoskeletal Conditions

PO: ADULTS: Initially, 5 mg 3 times a day. May increase to 7.5–10 mg 3 times a day. **ELDERLY:** 5 mg 3 times a day.

PO (EXTENDED-RELEASE): ADULTS, ELDERLY: 15–30 mg once daily.

Dosage in Hepatic Impairment

MILD: 5 mg 3 times a day. **MODERATE AND SEVERE:** Not recommended.

SIDE EFFECTS

Frequent: Drowsiness (39%), dry mouth (27%), dizziness (11%). **Rare (3%–1%):** Fatigue, asthenia, blurred vision, headache, anxiety, confusion, nausea, constipation, dyspepsia, unpleasant taste.

ADVERSE EFFECTS/ TOXIC REACTIONS

Overdose may result in visual hallucinations, hyperactive reflexes, muscle rigidity, vomiting, hyperpyrexia.

NURSING CONSIDERATIONS

BASELINE ASSESSMENT

Record onset, type, location, duration of muscular spasm. Check for immobility, stiffness, swelling.

INTERVENTION/EVALUATION

Assist with ambulation at all times. Assess for therapeutic response. Assess pain relief, decreased stiffness, swelling; increased joint mobility; reduced joint tenderness; improved grip strength.

PATIENT/FAMILY TEACHING

• Drowsiness usually diminishes with continued therapy. • Avoid tasks that require alertness, motor skills until response to drug is established. • Avoid alcohol, other depressants while taking medication. • Avoid sudden changes in posture. • Sugarless gum, sips of water may relieve dry mouth.

cyclophosphamide

HIGH ALERT

sye-kloe-**foss**-fa-mide
(Cytoxan, Cytoxan Lyophilized, Procytox ✦)
Do not confuse Cytoxan with cefoxitin, Ciloxan, Cytosar, or Cytotec, or cyclophosphamide with cyclosporine or ifosfamide.

◆ CLASSIFICATION

PHARMACOTHERAPEUTIC: Alkylating agent. **CLINICAL:** Antineoplastic (see p. 82C).

ACTION

Inhibits DNA, RNA protein synthesis by cross-linking with DNA, RNA strands. Cell cycle–phase nonspecific. **Therapeutic Effect:** Prevent cell growth. Potent immunosuppressant.

PHARMACOKINETICS

Well absorbed from GI tract. Protein binding: 10%–60%. Crosses blood-brain barrier. Metabolized in liver to active metabolites. Primarily excreted in urine. Removed by hemodialysis. **Half-life:** 3–12 hrs.

USES

Treatment of acute lymphocytic, acute nonlymphocytic, chronic myelocytic, chronic lymphocytic leukemias; ovarian, breast carcinomas; neuroblastoma, retinoblastoma, Hodgkin's, non-Hodgkin's lymphomas; multiple myeloma, mycosis fungoides, nephrotic syndrome. **OFF-LABEL:** Treatment of adrenocortical, bladder, cervical, endometrial, prostatic, testicular carcinomas; Ewing's sarcoma; multiple sclerosis; non–small-cell, small-cell lung cancer; organ transplant rejection; osteosarcoma; ovarian germ cell, primary brain, trophoblastic tumors; rheumatoid arthritis; soft-tissue sarcomas; systemic dermatomyositis; systemic lupus erythematosus; Wilms' tumor.

PRECAUTIONS

Contraindications: Severe myelosuppression. **Cautions:** Severe leukopenia, thrombocytopenia, tumor infiltration of bone marrow, previous therapy with other antineoplastic agents, radiation.

⌛ LIFESPAN CONSIDERATIONS

Pregnancy/Lactation: If possible, avoid use during pregnancy. May cause fetal malformations (limb abnormalities, cardiac anomalies, hernias). Distributed in breast milk. Breast-feeding not recommended. **Pregnancy Category D. Children:** No age-related precautions noted. **Elderly:** Age-related renal impairment may require dosage adjustment.

INTERACTIONS

DRUG: Allopurinol, bone marrow depressants may increase myelosuppression. May decrease effects of **antigout medications. Cytarabine** may increase risk of cardiomyopathy. **Immunosuppressants** may increase risk of infection, development of neoplasms. **Live virus vaccines** may potentiate virus replication, increase vaccine side effects, decrease pt's antibody response to vaccine. **HERBAL:** None significant. **FOOD:** None known. **LAB VALUES:** May increase serum uric acid.

C

AVAILABILITY (Rx)

Injection, Powder for Reconstitution (Cytoxan): 500 mg, 1 g, 2 g. **Tablets (Cytoxan):** 25 mg, 50 mg.

ADMINISTRATION/HANDLING

◀ALERT▶ May be carcinogenic, mutagenic, teratogenic. Handle with extreme care during preparation/administration.

IV

Reconstitution • For IV push, reconstitute each 100 mg with 5 ml Sterile Water for Injection, 0.9% NaCl or D_5W to provide concentration of 20 mg/ml. • Shake to dissolve. Allow to stand until clear.

Rate of administration • May give by IV push or further dilute with 250 ml D_5W, 0.9% NaCl. • IV infusions may be given over 1–24 hrs. • Doses of 500 mg to 2g may be given over 20–30 min. • IV route may produce faintness, facial flushing, diaphoresis, oropharyngeal sensation.

Storage • Reconstituted solution is stable for 24 hrs at room temperature or up to 6 days if refrigerated.

PO

• Give on an empty stomach. If GI upset occurs, give with food. • Do not cut or crush. • To minimize risk of bladder irritation, do not give at bedtime.

IV INCOMPATIBILITY

Amphotericin B complex (Abelcet, AmBisome, Amphotec).

IV COMPATIBILITIES

Granisetron (Kytril), heparin, hydromorphone (Dilaudid), lipids, lorazepam (Ativan), morphine, ondansetron (Zofran), propofol (Diprivan).

INDICATIONS/ROUTES/DOSAGE

Usual Dosage (Refer to Individual Protocols)

IV: ADULTS, ELDERLY, CHILDREN: (Single Dose): 400–1,800 mg/m^2 (30–50 mg/kg) per treatment course (1–5 days), which may be repeated q2–4wk. (Continuous Daily Dose): 60–120 mg/m^2 (1–2.5 mg/kg).

PO: ADULTS, ELDERLY, CHILDREN: 50–100 mg/m^2 day as continuous therapy or 400–1,000 mg/m^2 in divided doses over 4–5 days as intermittent therapy.

Biopsy-Proven Minimal-Change Nephrotic Syndrome

PO: ADULTS, CHILDREN: 2–3 mg/kg/day for 60–90 days.

SIDE EFFECTS

Expected: Marked leukopenia 8–15 days after initial therapy. **Frequent:** Nausea, vomiting (beginning about 6 hrs after administration and lasting about 4 hrs); alopecia (33%). **Occasional:** Diarrhea, darkening of skin/fingernails, stomatitis, headache, diaphoresis. **Rare:** Pain/redness at injection site.

ADVERSE EFFECTS/ TOXIC REACTIONS

Major toxic effect is myelosuppression resulting in blood dyscrasias (leukopenia, anemia, thrombocytopenia, hypoprothrombinemia). Expect leukopenia to resolve in 17–28 days. Anemia generally occurs after large doses or prolonged therapy. Thrombocytopenia may occur 10–15 days after drug initiation. Hemorrhagic cystitis occurs commonly in long-term therapy (esp. in children). Pulmonary fibrosis, cardiotoxicity noted with high doses. Amenorrhea, azoospermia, hyperkalemia may occur.

NURSING CONSIDERATIONS

BASELINE ASSESSMENT

Obtain WBC count weekly during therapy or until maintenance dose is established, then at 2- to 3-wk intervals.

INTERVENTION/EVALUATION

Monitor CBC, platelets, serum creatinine, BUN, urine output, serum uric acid, electrolytes. Monitor WBC counts closely during initial therapy. Monitor for hematologic toxicity (fever, sore throat, signs of local infection, unusual bruising/bleeding from any site), symptoms of anemia (excessive fatigue, weakness). Recovery from marked leukopenia due to myelosuppression can be expected in 17–28 days.

PATIENT/FAMILY TEACHING

• Encourage copious fluid intake, frequent voiding (assists in preventing cystitis) at least 24 hrs before, during, after therapy. • Do not have immunizations without physician's approval (drug lowers resistance). • Avoid contact with those who have recently received live virus vaccine. • Promptly report fever, sore throat, signs of local infection, difficulty or pain with urination, unusual bruising/bleeding from any site. • Alopecia is reversible, but new hair growth may have different color, texture.

*cycloSPORINE

sye-kloe-**spor**-in
(Gengraf, Neoral, Restasis, Sandimmune)

BLACK BOX ALERT Renal impairment may occur with high dosage. Increased risk of skin cancer, particularly in transplant pts, those with history of radiation, treatment with methotrexate or other immunosuppressants, use of phototherapy. Increased risk of mortality due to infection. May cause hypertension.

Do not confuse cyclosporine with cycloserine or cyclophosphamide, Gengraf with ProGraf, Neoral with Neurontin or Nizoral, or Sandimmune with Sandostatin.

◆CLASSIFICATION

PHARMACOTHERAPEUTIC: Cyclic polypeptide. **CLINICAL:** Immunosuppressant (see p. 119C).

ACTION

Inhibits cellular, humoral immune responses by inhibiting interleukin-2, a proliferative factor needed for T-cell activity. **Therapeutic Effect:** Prevents organ rejection, relieves symptoms of psoriasis, arthritis.

PHARMACOKINETICS

Variably absorbed from GI tract. Protein binding: 90%. Widely distributed. Metabolized in liver. Eliminated primarily by biliary or fecal excretion. Not removed by hemodialysis. **Half-life:** Adults, 10–27 hrs; children, 7–19 hrs.

USES

Prevents organ rejection of kidney, liver, heart in combination with steroid therapy. Treatment of chronic allograft rejection in those previously treated with other immunosuppressives. **Capsules/Solution**: Treatment of severe, active rheumatoid arthritis, psoriasis. **Ophthalmic**: Chronic dry eyes. **OFF-LABEL:** Treatment of alopecia areata, aplastic anemia, atopic dermatitis, Behçet's disease, biliary cirrhosis, prevention of corneal transplant rejection, ulcerative colitis.

PRECAUTIONS

Contraindications: History of hypersensitivity to cyclosporine, polyoxyethylated castor oil. **Cautions:** Hepatic, renal, cardiac impairment; malabsorption syndrome; pregnancy; chickenpox; herpes zoster infection; hypokalemia. **Ophthalmic**: Active eye infection.

⌛ LIFESPAN CONSIDERATIONS

Pregnancy/Lactation: Readily crosses placenta. Distributed in breast milk. Breast-feeding not recommended. **Pregnancy Category C. Children:** No age-related precautions noted in transplant pts. **Elderly:** Increased risk of hypertension, increased serum creatinine.

C

INTERACTIONS

DRUG: **Allopurinol, bromocriptine, cimetidine, clarithromycin, danazol, diltiazem, estrogens, erythromycin, fluconazole, itraconazole, ketoconazole** may increase plasma concentration, risk of hepatic/renal toxicity. **ACE inhibitors, potassium-sparing diuretics, potassium supplements** may cause hyperkalemia. **Immunosuppressants** may increase risk of infection, lymphoproliferative disorders. **Lovastatin** may increase risk of rhabdomyolysis, acute renal failure. **Live virus vaccines** may potentiate virus replication, increase vaccine side effects, decrease pt's response to vaccine. **HERBAL:** Avoid **cat's claw, echinacea** (possess immunostimulant properties). **St. John's wort** may decrease plasma concentration. **FOOD:** **Grapefruit, grapefruit juice** may increase absorption, risk of toxicity. **LAB VALUES:** May increase BUN, serum alkaline phosphatase, amylase, bilirubin, creatinine, potassium, uric acid, AST, ALT. May decrease serum magnesium. Therapeutic peak serum level: 50–400 ng/ml; toxic serum level: greater than 400 ng/ml.

AVAILABILITY (Rx)

Capsules (Gengraf, Neoral [Modified], Sandimmune [Nonmodified]): 25 mg, 100 mg. **Injection, Solution (Sandimmune):** 50 mg/ml. **Ophthalmic Emulsion (Restasis):** 0.05%. **Oral Solution (Gengraf, Neoral [Modified], Sandimmune [Nonmodified]):** 100 mg/ml.

ADMINISTRATION/HANDLING

◀ALERT▶ Oral solution available in bottle form with calibrated liquid measuring device. Oral form should replace IV administration as soon as possible.

IV

Reconstitution • Dilute each ml (50 mg) concentrate with 20–100 ml 0.9% NaCl or D_5W (**maximum concentration:** 2.5 mg/ml).

Rate of administration • Infuse over 2–6 hrs. • Monitor pt continuously for first 30 min after instituting infusion and frequently thereafter for hypersensitivity reaction (facial flushing, dyspnea).

Storage • Store parenteral form at room temperature. • Protect IV solution from light. • After diluted, stable for 6 hrs in PVC; 24 hrs in Excel or glass.

PO

• Administer consistently with relation to time of day and meals. • Oral solution may be mixed in glass container with milk, chocolate milk, orange juice, or apple juice (preferably at room temperature). Stir well. • Drink immediately. • Add more diluent to glass container. Mix with remaining solution to ensure total amount is given. • Dry outside of calibrated liquid measuring device before replacing cover. • Do not rinse with water. • Avoid refrigeration of oral solution (solution may separate). • Discard oral solution after 2 mos once bottle is opened.

Ophthalmic

• Invert vial several times to obtain uniform suspension. • Instruct pt to remove contact lenses before administration (may reinsert 15 min after administration). • May use with artificial tears.

IV INCOMPATIBILITIES

Amphotericin B complex (Abelcet, AmBisome, Amphotec), magnesium.

IV COMPATIBILITIES

Lipids, propofol (Diprivan).

INDICATIONS/ROUTES/DOSAGE

Transplantation, Prevention of Organ Rejection

PO: ADULTS, ELDERLY, CHILDREN: NOT MODIFIED: 10–18 mg/kg/dose given 4–12 hrs prior to organ transplantation. Maintenance: 5–15 mg/kg/day in divided doses then tapered to 3–10 mg/kg/day. **MODIFIED:** (dose dependent upon type of transplant): Renal: 6–12 mg/kg/day in 2 divided doses. Hepatic: 4–12 mg/kg/day in 2 divided doses. Heart: 4–10 mg/kg/day in 2 divided doses.

IV: ADULTS, ELDERLY, CHILDREN: Initially, 5–6 mg/kg/dose given 4–12 hrs prior to organ transplantation. Maintenance: 2–10 mg/kg/day in divided doses.

Rheumatoid Arthritis

PO: ADULTS, ELDERLY: Initially, 2.5 mg/kg a day in 2 divided doses. May increase by 0.5–0.75 mg/kg/day. **Maximum:** 4 mg/kg/day.

Psoriasis

PO: ADULTS, ELDERLY: Initially, 2.5 mg/kg/day in 2 divided doses. May increase by 0.5 mg/kg/day. **Maximum:** 4 mg/kg/day.

Dry Eye

OPHTHALMIC: ADULTS, ELDERLY: Instill 1 drop in each affected eye q12h.

SIDE EFFECTS

Frequent: Mild to moderate hypertension (26%), hirsutism (21%), tremor (12%). **Occasional (4%–2%):** Acne, leg cramps, gingival hyperplasia (red, bleeding, tender gums), paresthesia, diarrhea, nausea, vomiting, headache. **Rare (less than 1%):** Hypersensitivity reaction, abdominal discomfort, gynecomastia, sinusitis.

ADVERSE EFFECTS/ TOXIC REACTIONS

Mild nephrotoxicity occurs in 25% of renal transplants, 38% of cardiac transplants, 37% of liver transplants, generally 2–3 mos after transplantation (more severe toxicity may occur soon after transplantation). Hepatotoxicity occurs in 4% of renal, 7% of cardiac, and 4% of liver transplants, generally within first mo after transplantation. Both toxicities usually respond to dosage reduction. Severe hyperkalemia, hyperuricemia occur occasionally.

NURSING CONSIDERATIONS

BASELINE ASSESSMENT

If nephrotoxicity occurs, mild toxicity is generally noted 2–3 mos after transplantation; more severe toxicity noted early after transplantation; hepatotoxicity may be noted during first mo after transplantation.

INTERVENTION/EVALUATION

Diligently monitor BUN, serum creatinine, bilirubin, AST, ALT, LDH levels for evidence of hepatotoxicity, nephrotoxicity (mild toxicity noted by slow rise in serum levels; more overt toxicity noted by rapid rise in levels; hematuria also noted in nephrotoxicity). Monitor serum potassium for evidence of hyperkalemia. Encourage diligent oral hygiene (gingival hyperplasia). Monitor B/P for evidence of hypertension. Note: Reference ranges dependent on organ transplanted, organ function, cyclosporine toxicity. Trough levels should be obtained immediately prior to next dose. **Therapeutic serum level**: 50–400 ng/ml; **toxic serum level**: greater than 400 ng/ml.

PATIENT/FAMILY TEACHING

• Essential to repeat blood testing on a routine basis while receiving medication. • Report severe headache, persistent nausea/vomiting, unusual swelling of extremities, chest pain. • Avoid grapefruit, grapefruit juice (increases concentration, side effects), St. John's wort (decreases concentration).

Cymbalta, *see duloxetine*

cytarabine

HIGH ALERT

sigh-**tar**-ah-bean
(Ara-C, Cytosar-U ✤, Depo-Cyt)

BLACK BOX ALERT Must be administered by personnel trained in administration/handling of chemotherapeutic agents. ***Conventional:*** Potent myelosuppressant. High risk of multiple toxicities (GI, CNS, pulmonary, cardiac). ***Liposomal:*** Profound nausea, vomiting, fever may be fatal if untreated.

Do not confuse cytarabine with Cytoxan or vidarabine, or Cytosar with Cytoxan or Neosar.

C

◆CLASSIFICATION

PHARMACOTHERAPEUTIC: Antimetabolite. **CLINICAL:** Antineoplastic (see p. 82C).

ACTION

Converted intracellularly to nucleotide. Cell cycle–specific for S phase of cell division. **Therapeutic Effect:** Appears to inhibit DNA synthesis. Potent immunosuppressive activity.

PHARMACOKINETICS

Widely distributed; moderate amount crosses blood-brain barrier. Protein binding: 15%. Primarily excreted in urine. **Half-life:** 1–3 hrs.

USES

Ara-C: Treatment of acute lymphocytic, acute nonlymphocytic, chronic myelocytic, meningeal leukemias. **Depo-Cyt:** Treatment of lymphomatous meningitis. **OFF-LABEL: Ara-C:** Carcinomatous meningitis, Hodgkin's and non-Hodgkin's lymphomas, myelodysplastic syndrome.

PRECAUTIONS

Contraindications: None known. **Cautions:** Hepatic impairment.

LIFESPAN CONSIDERATIONS

Pregnancy/Lactation: If possible, avoid use during pregnancy. May cause fetal malformations. Unknown if distributed in breast milk. Breast-feeding not recommended. **Pregnancy Category D. Children:** No age-related precautions noted. **Elderly:** Age-related renal impairment may require dosage adjustment.

INTERACTIONS

DRUG: May decrease effects of **antigout medications. Bone marrow depressants** may increase myelosuppression. **Immunosuppressants (e.g., cyclosporin, tacrolimus)** may increase risk of infection. **Cyclophosphamide** may increase risk of cardiomyopathy. **Live virus vaccines** may potentiate virus replication, increase vaccine side effects, decrease pt's response to vaccine. **HERBAL:** None significant. **FOOD:** None known. **LAB VALUES:** May increase serum alkaline phosphatase, bilirubin, uric acid, AST.

AVAILABILITY (Rx)

Injection, Powder for Reconstitution: (Ara-C): 100 mg, 500 mg, 1 g, 2 g. **Injection, Solution (Ara-C):** 20 mg/ml, 100 mg/ml. **Injection, Suspension (Depo-Cyt):** 10 mg/ml.

ADMINISTRATION/HANDLING

◀ALERT▶ May give by subcutaneous, IV push, IV infusion, intrathecal routes at concentration not to exceed 100 mg/ml. May be carcinogenic, mutagenic, teratogenic (embryonic deformity). Handle with extreme care during preparation/administration. Depo-Cyt for intrathecal use only.

IV, Subcutaneous, Intrathecal

IV

Reconstitution • Reconstitute with Bacteriostatic Water for Injection. • Dose may be further diluted with 250–1,000 ml D_5W or 0.9% NaCl for IV infusion. • For intrathecal use, reconstitute vial with preservative-free 0.9% NaCl or pt's spinal fluid. Dose usually administered in 5–15 ml of solution, after equivalent volume of CSF removed.

Rate of administration • For IV infusion, give over 1–3 hrs or as continuous infusion.

Storage • Store Cytosar at room temperature. • Reconstituted solution is stable for 48 hrs at room temperature. • Use diluted solution within 24 hrs. • Discard if slight haze develops. • DepoCyt: Refrigerate; use within 4 hrs.

IV INCOMPATIBILITIES

Amphotericin B complex (Abelcet, AmBisome, Amphotec), ganciclovir (Cytovene), heparin, insulin (regular).

IV COMPATIBILITIES

Dexamethasone (Decadron), diphenhydramine (Benadryl), filgrastim (Neupogen), granisetron (Kytril), hydromorphone (Dilaudid), lipids, lorazepam (Ativan), morphine, ondansetron (Zofran), potassium chloride, propofol (Diprivan), total parenteral nutrition (TPN).

INDICATIONS/ROUTES/DOSAGE

Usual Dosage for Induction

IV: ADULTS, ELDERLY, CHILDREN: (Induction): 75–200 mg/m^2/day for 5–10 days q2–4wk.

INTRATHECAL: ADULTS, ELDERLY, CHILDREN: 5–75 mg/m^2 q2–7 days.

Usual Maintenance Dosage

IV: ADULTS, ELDERLY, CHILDREN: 70–200 mg/m^2/day for 2–5 days q mo.

IM, SUBCUTANEOUS: ADULTS, ELDERLY, CHILDREN: 1–1.5 mg/m^2 as single dose q1–4wk.

Usual Dosage for Depo-Cyt

INTRATHECAL: ADULTS, ELDERLY: (Induction): 50 mg q14days for 2 doses (wks 1, 3). **(Consolidation):** 50 mg q14days for 3 doses (wks 5, 7, 9) followed by additional dose at wk 13. **(Maintenance):** 50 mg q28days for 4 doses (wks 17, 21, 25, 29).

SIDE EFFECTS

Frequent: **IV, Subcutaneous (33%–16%):** Asthenia, fever, pain, altered taste/smell, nausea, vomiting (risk greater with IV push than with continuous IV infusion). **Intrathecal (28%–11%):** Headache, asthenia, altered taste/smell, confusion, drowsiness, nausea, vomiting. Occasional: **IV, Subcutaneous (11%–7%):** Abnormal gait, drowsiness, constipation, back pain, urinary incontinence, peripheral edema, headache, confusion. **Intrathecal (7%–3%):** Peripheral edema, back pain, constipation, abnormal gait, urinary incontinence.

ADVERSE EFFECTS/ TOXIC REACTIONS

Major toxic reaction is myelosuppression resulting in blood dyscrasias (leukopenia, anemia, thrombocytopenia, megaloblastosis, reticulocytopenia) occurring minimally after single IV dose. Leukopenia, anemia, thrombocytopenia should be expected with daily or continuous IV therapy. Cytarabine syndrome (fever, myalgia, rash, conjunctivitis, malaise, chest pain), hyperuricemia may occur. High-dose therapy may produce severe CNS, GI, pulmonary toxicity.

NURSING CONSIDERATIONS

BASELINE ASSESSMENT

Obtain baseline CBC, platelet count, renal/hepatic function tests. Leukocyte count decreases within 24 hrs after initial dose, continues to decrease for 7–9 days followed by brief rise at 12 days, decreases again at 15–24 days, then rises rapidly for next 10 days. Platelet count decreases 5 days after drug initiation to its lowest count at 12–15 days, then rises rapidly for next 10 days.

INTERVENTION/EVALUATION

Monitor BUN, creatinine, uric acid, AST, ALT, bilirubin, alkaline phosphatase. Monitor CBC for evidence of myelosuppression. Monitor for blood dyscrasias (fever, sore throat, signs of local infection, unusual bruising/bleeding from any site), symptoms of anemia (excessive fatigue, weakness). Monitor for signs of neuropathy (gait disturbances, handwriting difficulties, paresthesias).

PATIENT/FAMILY TEACHING

• Increase fluid intake (may protect against hyperuricemia). • Do not have immunizations without physician's approval (drug lowers resistance). • Avoid contact with those who have recently received live virus vaccine. • Promptly report fever, sore throat, signs of local infection, unusual bruising/bleeding from any site.

dabigatran

dab-ih-**gah**-tran
(Pradaxa)

◆CLASSIFICATION

PHARMACOTHERAPEUTIC: Thrombin inhibitor. **CLINICAL:** Anticoagulant.

ACTION

Direct thrombin inhibitor, preventing the conversion of fibrinogen into fibrin during coagulation cascade. **Therapeutic Effect:** Produces anticoagulation, preventing development of thrombus.

PHARMACOKINETICS

Metabolized in liver. Protein binding: 35%. Eliminated primarily in urine. **Half-life:** 12–17 hrs.

USES

Indicated to reduce risk of stroke, systemic embolism in pts with nonvalvular atrial fibrillation.

PRECAUTIONS

Contraindications: Overt major bleeding. **Cautions:** Severe hypertension, invasive procedures, spinal anesthesia, major surgery, those with congenital or acquired bleeding disorders, ulcerations.

⌛ LIFESPAN CONSIDERATIONS:

Pregnancy/Lactation: Unknown if distributed in breast milk. **Pregnancy Category C. Children:** Safety and efficacy not established in those younger than 18 yrs. **Elderly:** Severe renal impairment may require dosage adjustment.

INTERACTIONS

DRUG: Rifampin may decrease dabigatran levels. **Antiplatelet agents, NSAIDs, other anticoagulants, thrombolytics** may increase risk of bleeding. **HERBAL: Chamomile, feverfew, ginkgo biloba, green tea, red clover** may increase risk of bleeding. **FOOD: High-fat meal** delays absorption approximately 2 hrs. **LAB VALUES:** May increase aPTT, PT, INR.

AVAILABILITY (Rx)

Capsules: 75 mg, 150 mg.

ADMINISTRATION/HANDLING

PO

- May be given without regard to food.
- Do not break, chew, open capsules.

INDICATIONS/ROUTES/DOSAGE

◀ALERT▶ Medication should be discontinued prior to invasive or surgical procedures.

Anticoagulant

PO: ADULTS, ELDERLY: 150 mg twice daily.

Moderate Renal Impairment

Creatinine Clearance 15–30 ml/min: 75 mg twice daily.

SIDE EFFECTS

Frequent (15% and less): Dyspepsia (heartburn, nausea, indigestion), diarrhea, upper abdominal pain.

ADVERSE EFFECTS/ TOXIC REACTIONS

Gastrointestinal bleeding occurs rarely.

NURSING CONSIDERATIONS

BASELINE ASSESSMENT

Assess CBC, including platelet count. Check PT, PTT. Determine initial B/P.

INTERVENTION/EVALUATION

Assess for any sign of bleeding (hematuria, stool for occult blood, bleeding from gums, petechiae, bruising). Handle pt carefully and as infrequently as possible to prevent bleeding. Do not obtain B/P in lower extremities (possible deep vein thrombosis). Assess for decrease in B/P, increase in pulse rate, complaint of abdominal pain, diarrhea, aPTT, PT platelet count. Question for increase in discharge during menses. Monitor for any occurring hematoma. Use care in removing any dressing, tape.

PATIENT/FAMILY TEACHING

• Do not break, open, chew capsules. • Use electric razor, soft toothbrush to prevent bleeding. • Report any sign of red or dark urine, black or red stool, coffee-ground vomitus, red-speckled mucus from cough. • Keep in original container. Do not transfer to pill box/organizer. Use within 30 days after opening bottle.

dacarbazine

HIGH ALERT

da-**car**-bah-zeen
(DTIC ✤)

BLACK BOX ALERT Myelosuppression is most common toxicity. May cause hepatic necrosis, hepatic vein thrombosis.

Do not confuse dacarbazine with Dicarbosil or procarbazine.

CLASSIFICATION

PHARMACOTHERAPEUTIC: Alkylating agent. **CLINICAL:** Antineoplastic (see p. 82C).

ACTION

Forms methyldiazonium ions, which attack nucleophilic groups in DNA. Cross-links DNA strands. **Therapeutic Effect:** Inhibits DNA, RNA, protein synthesis.

PHARMACOKINETICS

Minimally crosses blood-brain barrier. Protein binding: 5%. Metabolized in liver. Excreted in urine. **Half-life:** 5 hrs (increased in renal impairment).

USES

Treatment of metastatic malignant melanoma, second-line therapy of Hodgkin's disease. **OFF-LABEL:** Treatment of islet cell carcinoma, neuroblastoma, soft-tissue sarcoma, fibrosarcomas, medullary carcinoma of thyroid.

PRECAUTIONS

Contraindications: Demonstrated hypersensitivity to dacarbazine. **Cautions:** Hepatic impairment.

LIFESPAN CONSIDERATIONS

Pregnancy/Lactation: If possible, avoid use during pregnancy, esp. first trimester. Breast-feeding not recommended. **Pregnancy Category C. Children:** Safety and efficacy not established. **Elderly:** Age-related renal impairment may require dosage adjustment.

INTERACTIONS

DRUG: **Bone marrow depressants** may enhance myelosuppression. **Live virus vaccines** may potentiate virus replication, increase vaccine side effects, decrease pt's antibody response to the vaccine. **HERBAL:** **Dong quai, St. John's wort** may increase photosensitization. **FOOD:** None known. **LAB VALUES:** May increase BUN, serum alkaline phosphatase, AST, ALT.

AVAILABILITY (Rx)

Injection, Powder for Reconstitution: 100-mg vial, 200-mg vial.

ADMINISTRATION/HANDLING

◀ALERT▶ Give by IV push or IV infusion. May be carcinogenic, mutagenic, teratogenic. Handle with extreme care during preparation/administration.

IV

Reconstitution • Reconstitute 100-mg vial with 9.9 ml Sterile Water for Injection (19.7 ml for 200-mg vial) to provide concentration of 10 mg/ml.

Rate of administration • Give IV push over 2–3 min. • For IV infusion, further dilute with up to 250 ml D_5W or 0.9% NaCl at a concentration not to exceed 10 mg/ml. Infuse over 30–60 min. • Apply hot packs if local pain, burning sensation, irritation at injection site occur. • Avoid extravasation (stinging, swelling, coolness, slight or no blood return at injection site).

Storage • Protect from light; refrigerate vials. • Color change from ivory to pink indicates decomposition; discard. • Solution containing 10 mg/ml is stable for 8 hrs at room temperature or 72 hrs if refrigerated. • Solution diluted with up to 500 ml D_5W or 0.9% NaCl is stable for at least 8 hrs at room temperature or 24 hrs if refrigerated.

D

IV INCOMPATIBILITIES

Allopurinol (Aloprim), cefepime (Maxipime), heparin, piperacillin and tazobactam (Zosyn).

IV COMPATIBILITIES

Etoposide (VePesid), granisetron (Kytril), ondansetron (Zofran), paclitaxel (Taxol).

INDICATIONS/ROUTES/DOSAGE

Refer to individual protocols.

Malignant Melanoma

IV: ADULTS, ELDERLY: 150–250 mg/m²/day for 5 days, repeat q3–4wk.

Hodgkin's Disease

IV: ADULTS, ELDERLY: 100 mg/m²/day for 5 days, repeat q4wk; or 375 mg/m² once, repeat q15 days (as combination therapy). **CHILDREN:** 375 mg/m² on days 1 and 15; repeat q28 days (as combination therapy).

Solid Tumors

IV: CHILDREN: 200–470 mg/m²/day over 5 days q21–28 days.

Neuroblastoma

IV: CHILDREN: 800–900 mg/m² as single dose on day 1 of therapy, repeat q3–4wk (as combination therapy).

SIDE EFFECTS

Frequent (90%): Nausea, vomiting, anorexia (occurs within 1 hr of initial dose, may last up to 12 hrs). **Occasional:** Facial flushing, paresthesia, alopecia, flu-like symptoms (fever, myalgia, malaise), dermatologic reactions, confusion, blurred vision, headache, lethargy. **Rare:** Diarrhea, stomatitis, photosensitivity.

ADVERSE EFFECTS/ TOXIC REACTIONS

Myelosuppression resulting in blood dyscrasias (leukopenia, thrombocytopenia) generally appears 2–4 wks after last dacarbazine dose. Hepatotoxicity occurs rarely.

NURSING CONSIDERATIONS

BASELINE ASSESSMENT

Some clinicians recommend food, fluid restriction 4–6 hrs before treatment; other clinicians believe good hydration to within 1 hr of treatment will prevent dehydration due to vomiting. Conflicting reports of effectiveness of administering antiemetics for nausea, vomiting.

INTERVENTION/EVALUATION

Monitor leukocyte, erythrocyte, platelet counts for evidence of myelosuppression. Monitor for hematologic toxicity (fever, sore throat, signs of local infection, unusual bleeding/bruising from any site).

PATIENT/FAMILY TEACHING

• Tolerance to GI effects occurs rapidly (generally after 1–2 days of treatment). • Do not have immunizations without physician's approval (drug lowers resistance). • Avoid contact with those who have recently received live virus vaccine. • Promptly report fever, sore throat, signs of local infection, unusual bleeding/bruising from any site. • Notify physician of persistent nausea, vomiting.

daclizumab

da-**cly**-zu-mab
(Zenapax)

BLACK BOX ALERT Must be administered by personnel trained in administration/handling of immunosuppressive therapy/organ transplant management.

CLASSIFICATION

PHARMACOTHERAPEUTIC: Monoclonal antibody. **CLINICAL:** Immunosuppressive (see p. 119C).

ACTION

Binds to interleukin-2 (IL-2) receptor complex, inhibiting IL-2–mediated activation of T lymphocytes, a critical pathway in cellular immune response involved in allograft rejection. **Therapeutic Effect:** Prevents organ rejection.

PHARMACOKINETICS

Half-life: Adults, 20 days; children, 13 days.

USES

Prophylaxis of acute organ rejection in pts receiving renal transplants (in combination with an immunosuppressive regimen). **OFF-LABEL:** Treatment of aplastic anemia, graft-vs-host disease. Prevention of organ rejection following heart transplant.

PRECAUTIONS

Contraindications: None known. **Cautions:** Infection, history of malignancy.

LIFESPAN CONSIDERATIONS

Pregnancy/Lactation: Unknown if drug crosses placenta or is distributed in breast milk. **Pregnancy Category C. Children/Elderly:** No age-related precautions noted.

INTERACTIONS

DRUG: None significant. **HERBAL:** **Echinacea** may decrease effects. **FOOD:** None known. **LAB VALUES:** May increase blood glucose.

AVAILABILITY (Rx)

Injection Solution: 5 mg/ml (5 ml).

ADMINISTRATION/HANDLING

IV

Reconstitution • Dilute in 50 ml 0.9% NaCl. • Invert gently. • Avoid shaking.

Rate of administration • Infuse over 15 min.

Storage • Protect from light; refrigerate vials. • Once reconstituted, stable for 4 hrs at room temperature, 24 hrs if refrigerated.

IV INCOMPATIBILITIES

Do not mix daclizumab with any other drugs.

INDICATIONS/ROUTES/DOSAGE

Prophylaxis of Acute Renal Transplant Rejection (in Combination with an Immunosuppressive)

IV: ADULTS, CHILDREN: 1 mg/kg over 15 min q14days for 5 doses, with initial dose beginning no more than 24 hrs before transplantation. **Maximum:** 100 mg.

SIDE EFFECTS

Occasional (greater than 2%): Constipation, nausea, diarrhea, vomiting, abdominal pain, edema, headache, dizziness, fever, pain, fatigue, insomnia, weakness, arthralgia, myalgia, diaphoresis.

ADVERSE EFFECTS/ TOXIC REACTIONS

Hypersensitivity reaction (dyspnea, tachycardia, dysphagia, peripheral edema, rash, pruritus) occurs rarely.

NURSING CONSIDERATIONS

BASELINE ASSESSMENT

Obtain baseline laboratory studies, vital signs, particularly B/P, pulse.

INTERVENTION/EVALUATION

Diligently monitor all serum levels, renal function, tests, glucose levels, CBC. Assess B/P for hypertension/hypotension; pulse for evidence of tachycardia. Question for GI disturbances, urinary changes. Monitor for presence of wound infection, signs of systemic infection (fever, sore throat), unusual bleeding/bruising.

PATIENT/FAMILY TEACHING

- Report difficulty in breathing or swallowing, tachycardia, rash, pruritus, swelling of lower extremities, weakness.
- Avoid pregnancy.

dalfampridine

dale-**fam**-prih-deen
(Ampyra)

◆CLASSIFICATION

PHARMACOTHERAPEUTIC: Potassium channel blocker. **CLINICAL:** Multiple sclerosis agent.

ACTION

Increases conduction of action potentials in demyelinated axons, inhibiting potassium channels. **Therapeutic Effect:** Improves walking in those with multiple sclerosis (MS).

PHARMACOKINETICS

Rapidly, completing absorbed from GI tract. Minimally metabolized in liver. Primarily unbound to plasma proteins. Primarily excreted in urine. **Half-life:** 5.2–6.5 hrs.

USES

Indicated to improve walking in pts with MS, as demonstrated by increase in walking speed.

PRECAUTIONS

Contraindications: History of seizures, moderate to severe renal impairment (creatinine clearance [CrCl] equal to or less than 50 ml/min). **Cautions:** Mild renal impairment (CrCl equal to 51–80 ml/min).

LIFESPAN CONSIDERATIONS:

Pregnancy/Lactation: Unknown if drug crosses placenta or is distributed in breast milk. **Pregnancy Category C. Children:** Safety and efficacy not established in those younger than 18 years. **Elderly:** Age-related renal impairment may require dosage adjustment.

INTERACTIONS

DRUG: None significant. **HERBAL:** None significant. **FOOD:** None known. **LAB VALUES:** May increase creatinine clearance.

AVAILABILITY (Rx)

Tablet, Film-Coated, Extended-Release: 10 mg.

ADMINISTRATION/HANDLING

PO

• May give without regard to food. • Do not crush, chew, split tablets.

INDICATIONS/ROUTES/DOSAGE

Multiple Sclerosis

PO: ADULTS 18 YEARS AND OLDER, ELDERLY: 10 mg twice daily, approximately 12 hrs apart.

SIDE EFFECTS

Frequent (9%–5%): Insomnia, dizziness, headache, nausea, asthenia (loss of strength, energy), back pain.
Rare (4%–2%): Paresthesia, nasopharyngitis, constipation, dyspepsia (heartburn, GI upset), pharyngolaryngeal pain.

ADVERSE EFFECTS/ TOXIC REACTIONS

Urinary tract infection occurs in 12% of pts.

NURSING CONSIDERATIONS

BASELINE ASSESSMENT

Creatinine clearance, BUN, CBC, serum chemistries should be obtained prior to treatment and routinely thereafter. Offer emotional support to pt, family.

INTERVENTION/EVALUATION

Periodically monitor CBC, serum chemistries, renal function tests, particularly creatinine clearance. Monitor for signs/symptoms of urinary, respiratory infection. Assess for therapeutic response (improvement in walking as demonstrated by increase in walking speed).

PATIENT/FAMILY TEACHING

• Avoid tasks that require alertness, motor skills until response to drug is established.

• Report difficulty in sleeping, dizziness, headache, nausea, back pain, loss of strength or energy.

Dalmane, *see flurazepam*

see flurazepam

dalteparin HIGH ALERT

dawl-teh-pear-in
(Fragmin)

BLACK BOX ALERT Epidural or spinal anesthesia greatly increases potential for spinal or epidural hematoma, subsequent long-term or permanent paralysis.

◆CLASSIFICATION

PHARMACOTHERAPEUTIC: Low-molecular-weight-heparin. **CLINICAL:** Anticoagulant (see p. 31C).

ACTION

Antithrombin in presence of low-molecular-weight heparin inhibits factor Xa, thrombin. Only slightly influences platelet aggregation, PT, aPTT. **Therapeutic Effect:** Produces anticoagulation.

PHARMACOKINETICS

Route	Onset	Peak	Duration
Subcutaneous	N/A	4 hrs	N/A

Protein binding: less than 10%. **Half-life:** 3–5 hrs.

USES

Treatment of unstable angina, non–Q-wave MI to prevent ischemic events. Prevention of deep vein thrombosis (DVT) in pts undergoing hip replacement or abdominal surgery who are at risk for thromboembolic complications. Those at risk are 40 yrs and older, obese, undergoing surgery under general anesthesia lasting longer than 30 min, malignancy, history of DVT, pulmonary embolism. Extended treatment of symptomatic venous thromboembolism (VTE) to reduce recurrence of VTE in cancer pts. Prevention of DVT or pulmonary embolism in acutely ill pts with severely restricted mobility. **OFF-LABEL:** Treatment of DVT.

PRECAUTIONS

Contraindications: Active major bleeding; concurrent heparin therapy; hypersensitivity to dalteparin, heparin, pork products; thrombocytopenia associated with positive in vitro test for antiplatelet antibody. **Cautions:** Conditions with increased risk for hemorrhage, bacterial endocarditis, history of heparin-induced thrombocytopenia, renal/hepatic impairment, uncontrolled hypertension, history of recent GI ulceration/hemorrhage, hypertensive/diabetic retinopathy.

LIFESPAN CONSIDERATIONS

Pregnancy/Lactation: Use with caution, particularly during last trimester, immediate postpartum period (increased risk of maternal hemorrhage). Unknown if distributed in breast milk. **Pregnancy Category B. Children:** Safety and efficacy not established. **Elderly:** No age-related precautions noted.

INTERACTIONS

DRUG: **Anticoagulants, NSAIDs, platelet inhibitors** may increase risk of bleeding. **HERBAL:** **Cat's claw, dong quai, evening primrose, garlic, ginseng** may increase antiplatelet activity. **FOOD:** None known. **LAB VALUES:** May increase AST, ALT. May decrease serum triglycerides.

AVAILABILITY (Rx)

Injection, Solution: 2,500 international units/0.2 ml, 5,000 international units/0.2 ml, 7,500 international units/0.3 ml, 10,000 international units/ml, 25,000 international units/ml, 12,500 international units/0.5 ml, 15,000 international units/0.6 ml, 18,000 international units/0.72 ml.

D

ADMINISTRATION/HANDLING

Subcutaneous

• Store at room temperature. • Instruct pt to sit/lie down before administering by deep subcutaneous injection. • Inject in U-shaped area around the navel, upper outer side of thigh, upper outer quadrangle of buttock. • Use fine needle (25–26 gauge) to minimize tissue trauma. • Introduce entire length of needle (½ inch) into skin fold held between thumb and forefinger, holding needle during injection at 45°–90° angle. • Do not rub injection site after administration (prevents bruising). • Alternate administration site with each injection. • New injections should be administered at least 1 inch from the old site. Never inject into an area where skin is tender, bruised, red, or hard.

INDICATIONS/ROUTES/DOSAGE

Low to Moderate DVT Risk

SUBCUTANEOUS: ADULTS, ELDERLY: 2,500 international units 1–2 hrs before surgery, then daily for 5–10 days.

High DVT Risk

SUBCUTANEOUS: ADULTS, ELDERLY: 5,000 international units 1–2 hrs before surgery, then daily for 5–10 days.

Total Hip Surgery

SUBCUTANEOUS: ADULTS, ELDERLY: 2,500 international units 1–2 hrs before surgery, then 2,500 units 6 hrs after surgery, then 5,000 units/day for 7–10 days.

Unstable Angina, Non–Q-Wave MI

SUBCUTANEOUS: ADULTS, ELDERLY: 120 international units/kg q12h (**Maximum:** 10,000 international units/dose) given with aspirin until clinically stable.

Venous Thromboembolism (Cancer Pts)

SUBCUTANEOUS: ADULTS, ELDERLY: Initially (1 mo), 200 international units/kg (**Maximum:** 18,000 international units) daily for 30 days. Maintenance (2–6 mos): 150 international units/kg once daily (**Maximum:** 18,000 international units).

Prevention of Deep Vein Thrombosis (DVT), Acutely Ill Pt, Immobile Pt

SUBCUTANEOUS: ADULTS, ELDERLY: 5,000 international units once a day.

Dosage in Renal Impairment

For creatinine clearance less than 30 ml/min, monitor anti-Xa levels to determine appropriate dose.

SIDE EFFECTS

Occasional (7%–3%): Hematoma at injection site. **Rare (less than 1%):** Hypersensitivity reaction (chills, fever, pruritus, urticaria, asthma, rhinitis, lacrimation, headache); mild, local skin irritation.

ADVERSE EFFECTS/ TOXIC REACTIONS

Overdose may lead to bleeding complications ranging from local ecchymoses to major hemorrhage. Thrombocytopenia occurs rarely.

NURSING CONSIDERATIONS

BASELINE ASSESSMENT

Assess CBC, esp. platelet count. Determine baseline B/P.

INTERVENTION/EVALUATION

Periodically monitor CBC, platelet count, stool for occult blood (no need for daily monitoring in pts with normal presurgical coagulation parameters). Assess for any sign of bleeding (bleeding at surgical site, hematuria, blood in stool, bleeding from gums, petechiae, bruising/bleeding at injection sites).

PATIENT/FAMILY TEACHING

• Usual length of therapy is 5–10 days. • Do not take any OTC medication (esp. aspirin) without consulting physician. • Report bleeding, bruising, dizziness, light-headedness, rash, itching, fever, swelling, breathing difficulty. • Rotate injection sites daily. • Teach proper injection technique. • Excessive bruising at injection site may be lessened by ice massage before injection.

danazol

dan-ah-zole
(Cyclomen ✤, Danocrine)

BLACK BOX ALERT Do not use during pregnancy (Pregnancy Category X). Thromboembolism, thrombotic events, including fatal strokes, reported. Long-term use may cause hepatitis, hepatic adenoma. May cause intracranial hypertension.

Do not confuse Danocrine with Dantrium.

◆CLASSIFICATION

PHARMACOTHERAPEUTIC: Testosterone derivative. **CLINICAL:** Androgen, hormone.

ACTION

Suppresses pituitary-ovarian axis by inhibiting output of pituitary gonadotropins. In endometriosis, causes atrophy of both normal and ectopic endometrial tissue. For fibrocystic breast disease, follicle-stimulating hormone (FSH), luteinizing hormone (LH) are depressed. Inhibits steroid synthesis, binding of steroids to their receptors in breast tissue. Increases serum esterase inhibitor. **Therapeutic Effect:** Produces anovulation, amenorrhea. Reduces estrogen production. Corrects biochemical deficiency as seen in hereditary angioedema.

PHARMACOKINETICS

Metabolized in liver. Excreted in urine. **Half-life:** 4.5 hrs.

USES

Palliative treatment of endometriosis, fibrocystic breast disease; prophylactic treatment of hereditary angioedema. **OFF-LABEL:** Treatment of gynecomastia, menorrhagia, precocious puberty.

PRECAUTIONS

Contraindications: Severe cardiac/hepatic/renal impairment. Active or history of thromboembolic disease, androgen tumor, abnormal vaginal bleeding. **Cautions:** Renal impairment, cardiac impairment, epilepsy, migraine headaches, diabetes. **Pregnancy Category X.**

INTERACTIONS

DRUG: May enhance effects of **anticoagulants.** May increase nephrotoxicity with **cyclosporine, tacrolimus. HERBAL:** None significant. **FOOD: High-fat meals** increase concentration. **LAB VALUES:** May increase hepatic function values.

AVAILABILITY (Rx)

Capsules: 50 mg, 100 mg, 200 mg.

ADMINISTRATION/HANDLING

PO

• Avoid administration with fatty meals.

INDICATIONS/ROUTES/DOSAGE

◀ALERT▶ Initiate therapy during menstruation or when pt is not pregnant.

Endometriosis

PO: ADULTS: 200–800 mg a day in 2 divided doses for 3–9 mos.

Fibrocystic Breast Disease

PO: ADULTS: 100–400 mg a day in 2 divided doses.

Hereditary Angioedema

PO: ADULTS: Initially, 200 mg 2–3 times a day. Decrease dosage by 50% or less at 1- to 3-mo intervals. If attack occurs, increase dosage by up to 200 mg a day.

SIDE EFFECTS

Frequent: Females: Amenorrhea, breakthrough bleeding/spotting, decreased breast size, weight gain, irregular menstrual period. **Occasional: Males/Females:** Edema, rhabdomyolysis (abnormal urine color [dark, red, cola colored], muscle cramps, unusual fatigue), virilism (acne, oily skin), flushed skin, altered moods. **Rare: Males/Females:** Hematuria, gingivitis, carpal tunnel syndrome, cataracts, severe headache, vomiting, rash, photosensitivity. **Females:** Enlarged clitoris, hoarseness, deepening voice, hair growth, monilial vaginitis. **Males:** Decreased testicle size.

D

ADVERSE EFFECTS/ TOXIC REACTIONS

Jaundice may occur in those receiving 400 mg or more per day. Hepatic dysfunction, eosinophilia, thrombocytopenia, pancreatitis occur rarely.

NURSING CONSIDERATIONS

BASELINE ASSESSMENT

Inquire about menstrual cycle. Determine pregnancy status prior to beginning therapy. Therapy should begin during menstruation. Establish baseline weight, B/P.

INTERVENTION/EVALUATION

Weigh pt 2–3 times a wk; report 5 lb or more/wk gain or swelling of fingers/feet. Periodically monitor B/P, hepatic function tests. Check for jaundice (yellow sclera/skin, dark urine, clay-colored stools).

PATIENT/FAMILY TEACHING

• Use nonhormonal contraceptive during therapy. • Do not take drug, notify physician if pregnancy suspected (risk to fetus). • Complete full length of therapy. • Regular visits to physician's office are needed for hepatic function tests, CBC, serum amylase, lipase. • Notify physician promptly of masculinizing effects (may not be reversible), weight gain, muscle cramps, fatigue, dark urine, yellowing of whites of eyes. • Spotting/bleeding may occur in first mos of therapy for endometriosis (does not mean lack of efficacy). • In fibrocystic breast disease, irregular menstrual periods, amenorrhea may occur with or without ovulation.

dantrolene

dan-troe-leen
(Dantrium, Dantrium Intravenous)

BLACK BOX ALERT Potential for hepatotoxicity.

Do not confuse Dantrium with danazol or Daraprim.

◆ CLASSIFICATION

CLINICAL: Skeletal muscle relaxant.

ACTION

Reduces muscle contraction by interfering with release of calcium ion. Reduces calcium ion concentration. **Therapeutic Effect:** Dissociates excitation-contraction coupling. Interferes with catabolic process associated with malignant hyperthermic crisis.

PHARMACOKINETICS

Poorly absorbed from GI tract. Protein binding: High. Metabolized in liver. Primarily excreted in urine. **Half-life: IV:** 4–8 hrs; **PO:** 8.7 hrs.

USES

PO: Relief of symptoms of spasticity due to spinal cord injuries, stroke, cerebral palsy, multiple sclerosis, esp. flexor spasms, concomitant pain, clonus, muscular rigidity. **Parenteral:** Management of fulminant hypermetabolism of skeletal muscle due to malignant hyperthermia crisis. Prevention of malignant hyperthermia (pre- or postoperative administration). **OFF-LABEL:** Relief of exercise-induced pain in pts with muscular dystrophy; treatment of flexor spasms, neuroleptic malignant syndrome.

PRECAUTIONS

Contraindications: Active hepatic disease. **Cautions:** Cardiac/pulmonary impairment, history of previous hepatic disease.

LIFESPAN CONSIDERATIONS

Pregnancy/Lactation: Readily crosses placenta. Breast-feeding not recommended. **Pregnancy Category C. Children:** No age-related precautions noted in those 5 yrs and older. **Elderly:** No information available.

INTERACTIONS

DRUG: CNS depressants may increase CNS depression with short-term use. **Hepatotoxic medications** may increase risk of hepatic toxicity with chronic use. **HERBAL: Gotu kola, kava kava, St. John's wort, valerian** may increase CNS depression. **FOOD:** None known. **LAB VALUES:** May alter hepatic function test results.

AVAILABILITY (Rx)

Capsules (Dantrium): 25 mg, 50 mg, 100 mg. **Injection, Powder for Reconstitution (Dantrium Intravenous):** 20-mg vial.

ADMINISTRATION/HANDLING

IV

Reconstitution • Reconstitute 20-mg vial with 60 ml Sterile Water for Injection to provide concentration of 0.33 mg/ml.
Rate of administration • For therapeutic emergency dose, give IV over 2–3 min. • For IV infusion, administer over 1 hr. • Diligently monitor for extravasation (high pH of IV preparation). May produce severe complications.
Storage • Store at room temperature. • Use within 6 hrs after reconstitution. • Solution is clear, colorless. Discard if cloudy, precipitate forms.

PO

• Give without regard to food.

IV INCOMPATIBILITY

None known.

INDICATIONS/ROUTES/DOSAGE

Spasticity

PO: ADULTS, ELDERLY: Initially, 25 mg/day. Increase to 25 mg 2–4 times a day, then by 25-mg increments up to 100 mg 2–4 times a day. **CHILDREN:** Initially, 0.5 mg/kg twice a day. Increase to 0.5 mg/kg 3–4 times a day, then in increments of 0.5 mg/kg/day up to 3 mg/kg 2–4 times a day. **Maximum:** 400 mg/day.

Prevention of Malignant Hyperthermic Crisis

PO: ADULTS, ELDERLY, CHILDREN: 4–8 mg/kg/day in 3–4 divided doses 1–2 days before surgery; give last dose 3–4 hrs before surgery.
IV: ADULTS, ELDERLY, CHILDREN: 2.5 mg/kg about 1.25 hrs before surgery.

Management of Malignant Hyperthermic Crisis

IV: ADULTS, ELDERLY, CHILDREN: Initially a minimum of 2.5 mg/kg rapid IV; may repeat up to total cumulative dose of 10 mg/kg. May follow with 4–8 mg/kg/day PO in 4 divided doses up to 3 days after crisis.

SIDE EFFECTS

Frequent: Drowsiness, dizziness, weakness, general malaise, diarrhea (mild). **Occasional:** Confusion, diarrhea (severe), headache, insomnia, constipation, urinary frequency. **Rare:** Paradoxical CNS excitement or restlessness, paresthesia, tinnitus, slurred speech, tremor, blurred vision, dry mouth, nocturia, impotence, rash, pruritus.

ADVERSE EFFECTS/ TOXIC REACTIONS

Risk of hepatotoxicity, most notably in females, those 35 yrs and older, those taking other hepatotoxic medications concurrently. Overt hepatitis noted most frequently between 3rd and 12th mo of therapy. Overdosage results in vomiting, muscular hypotonia, muscle twitching, respiratory depression, seizures.

NURSING CONSIDERATIONS

BASELINE ASSESSMENT

Obtain baseline hepatic function tests (AST, ALT, alkaline phosphatase, total bilirubin). Record onset, type, location, duration of muscular spasm. Check for immobility, stiffness, swelling.

INTERVENTION/EVALUATION

Assist with ambulation. For those on long-term therapy, hepatic/renal function tests, CBC should be performed periodically. Assesss for therapeutic response: relief of pain, stiffness, spasm.

PATIENT/FAMILY TEACHING

• Drowsiness usually diminishes with continued therapy. • Avoid tasks that require alertness, motor skills until response to drug is established. • Avoid alcohol/other depressants while taking medication. • Report continued weakness, fatigue, nausea, diarrhea, skin rash, itching, bloody/tarry stools.

daptomycin

dap-toe-my-sin
(Cubicin)
Do not confuse daptomycin with dactinomycin, or Cubicin with Cleocin.

◆CLASSIFICATION

PHARMACOTHERAPEUTIC: Lipopeptide antibacterial agent. **CLINICAL:** Antibiotic.

ACTION

Binds to bacterial membranes and causes rapid depolarization of membrane potential. Inhibits protein, DNA, RNA synthesis. **Therapeutic Effect:** Bactericidal.

PHARMACOKINETICS

Widely distributed. Protein binding: 90%. Primarily excreted unchanged in urine. Moderately removed by hemodialysis. **Half-life:** 7–8 hrs (increased in renal impairment).

USES

Treatment of complicated skin/skin structure infections caused by susceptible strains of gram-positive pathogens, including penicillin-resistant *Streptococcus pneumoniae,* methicillin-resistant *Staphyloccus aureus* (MRSA), vancomycin-resistant enterococci (VRE). Treatment of *S. aureus* systemic infections caused by methicillin susceptible and resistant *S. aureus.*

PRECAUTIONS

Contraindications: None known. **Cautions:** Renal impairment, history of or current musculoskeletal disorders (risk of exacerbation), pregnancy.

⌛ LIFESPAN CONSIDERATIONS

Pregnancy/Lactation: Unknown if drug is distributed in breast milk. **Pregnancy Category B. Children:** Safety and efficacy not established in those younger than 18 yrs. **Elderly:** No age-related precautions noted.

INTERACTIONS

DRUG: Concurrent use with **HMG-CoA reductase inhibitors (statins)** may cause myopathy (discontinue use). **HERBAL:** None significant. **FOOD:** None known. **LAB VALUES:** May increase serum CPK levels. May alter hepatic function test results.

AVAILABILITY (Rx)

Injection, Powder for Reconstitution: 500 mg/vial.

ADMINISTRATION/HANDLING

IV

Reconstitution • Reconstitute 500-mg vial with 10 ml 0.9% NaCl to provide a concentration of 50 mg/ml. May further dilute in 0.9% NaCl at a concentration not to exceed 20 mg/ml.

Rate of administration • For IV injection, give over 2 min (concentration: 50 mg/ml). • For intermittent IV infusion (piggyback), infuse over 30 min.

Storage • Refrigerate. • Appears as pale yellow to light brown lyophilized cake. • Reconstituted solution is stable for 12 hrs at room temperature or up to 48 hrs if refrigerated. • Discard if particulate forms.

IV INCOMPATIBILITIES

Diluents containing dextrose. If same IV line is used to administer different drugs, flush line with 0.9% NaCl.

IV COMPATIBILITIES

0.9% NaCl, lactated Ringer's.

INDICATIONS/ROUTES/DOSAGE

Complicated Skin/Skin Structure Infections

IV: ADULTS, ELDERLY: 4 mg/kg every 24 hrs for 7–14 days.

Systemic Infections

IV: ADULTS, ELDERLY: 6 mg/kg once daily.

Dosage in Renal Impairment

Creatinine clearance less than 30 ml/min: Dosage is 4 mg/kg q48h for skin and soft tissue infections, 6 mg/kg q48h for staphylococcal bacteremia.

SIDE EFFECTS

Frequent (6%–5%): Constipation, nausea, peripheral injection site reactions, headache, diarrhea. **Occasional (4%–3%):** Insomnia, rash, vomiting. **Rare (less than 3%):** Pruritus, dizziness, hypotension.

ADVERSE EFFECTS/ TOXIC REACTIONS

Skeletal muscle myopathy (muscle pain/weakness, particularly of distal extremities) occurs rarely. Antibiotic-associated colitis, other superinfections (abdominal cramps, severe watery diarrhea, fever) may result from altered bacterial balance.

NURSING CONSIDERATIONS

BASELINE ASSESSMENT

Obtain blood culture, sensitivity test before first dose (therapy may begin before results are known).

INTERVENTION/EVALUATION

Assess oral cavity for white patches on mucous membranes, tongue (thrush). Monitor for myopathy (muscle pain, weakness), CPK levels, renal function tests. Monitor daily pattern of bowel activity and stool consistency. Mild GI effects may be tolerable, but increasing severity may indicate onset of antibiotic-associated colitis. Be alert for superinfection: fever, vomiting, diarrhea, anal/genital pruritus, oral mucosal changes (ulceration, pain, erythema). Monitor for dizziness, institute appropriate measures.

PATIENT/FAMILY TEACHING

- Report rash, headache, nausea, dizziness, constipation, diarrhea, muscle pain, or any new symptom.

darbepoetin alfa

dar-bee-eh-poe-**ee**-tin
(Aranesp)

BLACK BOX ALERT Increased risk of serious cardiovascular events, thromboembolic events, mortality, time-to-tumor progression when administered to a target hemoglobin greater than 12 g/dl.

Do not confuse Aranesp with Aricept, or darbepoetin with dalteparin or epoetin.

CLASSIFICATION

PHARMACOTHERAPEUTIC: Glycoprotein. **CLINICAL:** Hematopoietic.

ACTION

Stimulates formation of RBCs in bone marrow; increases serum half-life of epoetin. **Therapeutic Effect:** Induces erythropoiesis, release of reticulocytes from bone marrow.

PHARMACOKINETICS

Well absorbed after subcutaneous administration. **Half-life:** 48.5 hrs.

USES

Treatment of anemia associated with chronic renal failure (including pts on dialysis and pts not on dialysis), chemotherapy-induced anemia (nonmyeloid malignancies).

PRECAUTIONS

Contraindications: History of sensitivity to mammalian cell-derived products or human albumin, uncontrolled hypertension. **Cautions:** Pts with known porphyria (impairment of erythrocyte formation in bone marrow or responsible for hepatic impairment), hemolytic anemia, sickle cell anemia, thalassemia, history of seizures. **Cancer pts:** Tumor growth, shortened survival may occur when Hgb levels of 12 g/dl or greater are achieved with darbepoetin alfa. **Chronic renal failure pts:** Increased risk for serious cardiovascular reactions (e.g., stroke, MI) when Hgb levels greater than 12 g/dl are achieved with darbepoetin alfa.

LIFESPAN CONSIDERATIONS

Pregnancy/Lactation: Unknown if drug crosses placenta or is distributed in breast milk. **Pregnancy Category C. Children:** Safety and efficacy not established. **Elderly:** Age-related renal impairment may require dosage adjustment.

INTERACTIONS

DRUG: None significant. **HERBAL:** None significant. **FOOD:** None known. **LAB VALUES:** May decrease serum ferritin, serum transferrin saturation.

AVAILABILITY (Rx)

Injection Solution: 25 mcg/ml, 40 mcg/ml, 60 mcg/ml, 100 mcg/ml, 150 mcg/ml, 200 mcg/ml, 300 mcg/ml. **Prefilled Syringe:** 25 mcg/0.42 ml, 40 mcg/0.4 ml, 60 mcg/0.3 ml, 100 mcg/0.5 ml, 150 mcg/0.3 ml, 200 mcg/0.4 ml, 300 mcg/0.6 ml, 500 mcg/ml.

ADMINISTRATION/HANDLING

◀ALERT▶ Avoid excessive agitation of vial; do not shake (will cause foaming).

IV

Reconstitution • No reconstitution necessary.

Rate of administration • May be given as IV bolus.

Storage • Refrigerate vials. • Vigorous shaking may denature medication, rendering it inactive.

Subcutaneous

• Use 1 dose per vial; do not reenter vial. Discard unused portion. • May be mixed in a syringe with Bacteriostatic 0.9% NaCl with Benzyl Alcohol 0.9% (Bacteriostatic Saline) at a 1:1 ratio (benzyl alcohol acts as a local anesthetic; may reduce injection site discomfort).

IV INCOMPATIBILITIES

Do not mix with other medications.

INDICATIONS/ROUTES/DOSAGE

Anemia in Chronic Renal Failure

◀ALERT▶ Individualize dosing to achieve/maintain hemoglobin between 10–12 g/dl. Do not exceed 12 g/dl or increase by greater than 1g/dl in any 2-wk period.

IV, SUBCUTANEOUS: ADULTS, ELDERLY: Initially, 0.45 mcg/kg once weekly. Alternate for nondialysis pts: 0.75 mcg/kg once q2wks. Titrate to response.

Decrease dose by 25%: If hemoglobin approaches 12 g/dl or increases greater than 1 g/dl in any 2-wk period.

Increase dose by 25%: If hemoglobin does not increase by 1 g/dl after 4 wks of therapy and Hgb is below target range (with adequate iron stores), do not increase dose more frequently than every 4 wks.

Note: If pt does not attain hemoglobin range of 10–12 g/dl after appropriate dosing over 12 wks, do not continue to increase dose and use minimum effective dose to maintain hemoglobin level that will avoid red blood cell transfusions.

Anemia Associated with Chemotherapy

◀ALERT▶ Use minimum effective dose to maintain hemoglobin level that will avoid red blood cell transfusions. Do not exceed hemoglobin level of 12 g/dl or increase by greater than 1g/dl in any 2-wk period.

SUBCUTANEOUS: ADULTS, ELDERLY: 2.25 mcg/kg once weekly or 500 mcg every 3 wks.

Increase dose: If hemoglobin does not increase by 1 g/dl after 6 wks and Hgb is below target range, increase dose to 4.5 mcg/kg once weekly.

Decrease dose: Decrease dose by 40% if hemoglobin increases greater than 1 g/dl in any 2-wk period or hemoglobin reaches level that will avoid red blood cell transfusions. Note: Withhold dose when Hgb exceeds 12 g/dl, resume at dose 40% lower when Hgb approaches a concentration where transfusions may be required.

SIDE EFFECTS

Frequent: Myalgia, hypertension/hypotension, headache, diarrhea. **Occasional:** Fatigue, edema, vomiting, reaction at injection site, asthenia (loss of strength, energy), dizziness.

ADVERSE EFFECTS/ TOXIC REACTIONS

Vascular access thrombosis, CHF, sepsis, arrhythmias, anaphylactic reaction occur rarely.

NURSING CONSIDERATIONS

BASELINE ASSESSMENT

Assess B/P before drug administration (80% of pts with chronic renal failure have history of hypertension). B/P often rises during early therapy in those with history of hypertension. Assess serum iron (transferrin saturation should be greater than 20%), serum ferritin (greater than 100 ng/ml) before and during therapy. Consider that all pts will eventually need supplemental iron therapy. Establish baseline CBC (esp. note Hct).

INTERVENTION/EVALUATION

Monitor Hgb, Hct, serum ferritin, CBC with differential, serum creatinine, BUN, potassium, phosphorus, reticulocyte count. Monitor B/P aggressively for increase (25% of pts taking medication require antihypertension therapy, dietary restrictions).

PATIENT/FAMILY TEACHING

• Frequent blood tests needed to determine correct dose. • Inform physician of swollen extremities, breathing difficulty, extreme fatigue, or severe headache. • Avoid tasks requiring alertness, motor skills until response to drug is established.

D

darifenacin

dare-ih-**fen**-ah-sin
(Enablex)

◆CLASSIFICATION

PHARMACOTHERAPEUTIC: Muscarinic receptor antagonist. **CLINICAL:** Urinary antispasmodic.

ACTION

Acts as a direct antagonist at muscarinic receptor sites in cholinergically innervated organs. Blockade of the receptor limits bladder contractions. **Therapeutic Effect:** Reduces symptoms of bladder irritability/overactivity (urge incontinence, urinary urgency/ frequency), improves bladder capacity.

PHARMACOKINETICS

Well absorbed following PO administration. Protein binding: 98%. Extensively metabolized in liver. Primarily excreted in urine with a lesser amount eliminated in feces. **Half-life:** 13–19 hrs.

USES

Management of symptoms of bladder overactivity (urge incontinence, urinary urgency/frequency).

PRECAUTIONS

Contraindications: Uncontrolled narrow-angle glaucoma, paralytic ileus, GI/GU obstruction, urine retention, severe hepatic impairment. **Cautions:** Bladder outflow obstruction, nonobstructive prostatic hyperplasia, GI obstructive disorders, decreased GI motility, constipation, hiatal hernia, reflux esophagitis, ulcerative colitis, controlled narrow-angle glaucoma, myasthenia gravis.

LIFESPAN CONSIDERATIONS

Pregnancy/Lactation: Unknown if drug crosses placenta or is distributed in breast milk. **Pregnancy Category C. Children:** Safety and efficacy not established. **Elderly:** No age-related precautions noted.

INTERACTIONS

DRUG: **CYP3A4 inhibitors (clarithromycin, erythromycin, isoniazid, protease inhibitors)** may increase effects. **HERBAL:** **St. John's wort** may decrease effect. **FOOD:** None known. **LAB VALUES:** None known.

AVAILABILITY (Rx)

Tablets (Extended-Release): 7.5 mg, 15 mg.

ADMINISTRATION/HANDLING

PO

• Give without regard to food. • Swallow extended-release tablets whole; do not crush, chew, or split tablet.

INDICATIONS/ROUTES/DOSAGE

Overactive Bladder

PO: ADULTS, ELDERLY: Initially, 7.5 mg once daily. If response is not adequate after at least 2 wks, may increase to 15 mg once daily. Do not exceed 7.5 mg once daily in moderate hepatic impairment or concurrent use with CYP3A4 inhibitors (clarithromycin, fluconazole, protease inhibitors, isoniazid).

SIDE EFFECTS

Frequent (35%–21%): Dry mouth, constipation. **Occasional (8%–4%):** Dyspepsia, headache, nausea, abdominal pain. **Rare (3%–2%):** Asthenia (loss of strength, energy), diarrhea, dizziness, ocular dryness.

ADVERSE EFFECTS/ TOXIC REACTIONS

UTI occurs occasionally.

NURSING CONSIDERATIONS

BASELINE ASSESSMENT

Monitor voiding pattern, assess signs/symptoms of overactive bladder prior to therapy as baseline.

INTERVENTION/EVALUATION

Monitor I&O. Palpate bladder for urine retention. Monitor daily pattern of bowel activity and stool consistency for evidence of constipation. Dry mouth may be relieved with sips of tepid water. Assess for relief of symptoms of overactive bladder (urge incontinence, urinary frequency/urgency).

PATIENT/FAMILY TEACHING

• Swallow tablet whole; do not crush, divide, chew. • Increase fluid intake to reduce risk of constipation. • Avoid tasks that require alertness, motor skills until response to drug is established.

darunavir

dah-**run**-ah-vir
(Prezista)

CLASSIFICATION

PHARMACOTHERAPEUTIC: Antiretroviral. **CLINICAL:** Protease inhibitor.

ACTION

Prevents virus-specific processing of polyproteins, HIV-1 protease infected cells. **Therapeutic Effect:** Prevents formation of mature viral cells.

PHARMACOKINETICS

Readily absorbed following PO administration. Protein binding: 95%. Metabolized in liver. Eliminated mainly in feces with a lesser amount eliminated in urine. Not significantly removed by hemodialysis. **Half-life:** 15 hrs.

USES

Treatment of HIV infection in combination with ritonavir and other antiretroviral agents in adults and children 6 yrs and older.

PRECAUTIONS

Contraindications: Concurrent therapy with alfuzosin, dihydroergotamine, ergonovine, ergotamine, lovastatin, methylergonovine, oral midazolam, pimozide, rifampin, sildenafil (for treatment PAH), simvastatin, St. John's wort, triamzolam. **Cautions:** Diabetes mellitus, hemophilia, known sulfonamide allergy, hepatic impairment.

LIFESPAN CONSIDERATIONS

Pregnancy/Lactation: Unknown if drug crosses placenta or is distributed in breast milk. Breast-feeding not recommended. **Pregnancy Category B. Children:** Safety and efficacy not established. **Elderly:** No age-related precautions noted.

INTERACTIONS

DRUG: May interfere with metabolism of **amiodarone, bepredil, lidocaine, midazolam, oral contraceptives, paroxetine, quinidine, sertraline, triazolam. Dexamethasone, lopinavir, rifabutin, rifampin** may decrease darunavir concentration. May increase concentration of **atorvastatin, clarithromycin, cyclosporine, felodipine, inhaled fluticasone, lovastatin, nicardipine, nifedipine, pravastatin, simvastatin, sirolimus, tacrolimus, trazodone.** May alter **methadone, sildenafil, tadalafil, vardenafil, warfarin** concentration. **Efavirenz, itraconazole, ketoconazole, voriconazole** may increase darunavir concentration. **Ergot derivatives** may cause peripheral vasospasm/ischemia. **HERBAL: St. John's wort** may lead to loss of virologic response, potential resistance to darunavir. **FOOD: Food** increases plasma concentration of darunavir. **LAB VALUES:** May increase aPTT, PT, serum alkaline phosphatase, bilirubin, amylase, lipase, cholesterol, triglycerides, uric acid. May decrease lymphocytes/neutrophil count, platelets, WBC count, serum bicarbonate, albumin, calcium. May alter glucose, sodium.

AVAILABILITY (Rx)

Tablets (Prezista): 75 mg, 150 mg, 300 mg, 400 mg, 600 mg.

ADMINISTRATION/HANDLING

PO

• Give with food (increases plasma concentration). • Do not crush, chew film-coated tablets.

INDICATIONS/ROUTES/DOSAGE

HIV Infection, Treatment Experienced

PO: ADULTS, ELDERLY: 600 mg administered with 100 mg ritonavir and with food twice daily or 800 mg (two 400 mg tablets) with 100 mg ritonavir and with food once daily.

HIV Infection, Treatment Naive

PO: ADULTS, ELDERLY: 800 mg (two 400-mg tablets) administered with 100 mg ritonavir and with food once daily.

Usual Pediatric Dose

ALERT Do not use once-daily dosing in pediaric pts.

PO: CHILDREN WEIGHING 40 KG OR MORE: 600 mg twice daily. **WEIGHING 30–39 KG:** 450 mg twice daily. **WEIGHING 20–29 KG:** 375 mg twice daily.

SIDE EFFECTS

Frequent (19%–13%): Diarrhea, nausea, headache, nasopharyngitis. **Occasional (3%–2%):** Constipation, abdominal pain, vomiting. **Rare (less than 2%):** Allergic dermatitis, dyspepsia, flatulence, abdominal distention, anorexia, arthralgia, myalgia, paresthesia, memory impairment.

ADVERSE EFFECTS/ TOXIC REACTIONS

Hypertension, MI, transient ischemic attack occur in less than 2% of pts. Acute renal failure, diabetes mellitus, dyspnea, worsening of hepatic impairment, skin reactions including Stevens-Johnson syndrome, toxic epidermal necrolysis occur rarely.

D

NURSING CONSIDERATIONS

BASELINE ASSESSMENT

Obtain baseline laboratory testing, esp. hepatic function tests, before beginning therapy and at periodic intervals during therapy. Offer emotional support. Obtain medication history.

INTERVENTION/EVALUATION

Closely monitor for evidence of GI discomfort. Monitor daily pattern of bowel activity and stool consistency. Assess skin for evidence of rash, other skin reactions. Monitor serum chemistry tests for marked laboratory abnormalities, particularly hepatic profile, glucose, cholesterol, triglycerides. Assess for opportunistic infections (onset of fever, oral mucosa changes, cough, other respiratory symptoms).

PATIENT/FAMILY TEACHING

• Take medication with food. • Continue therapy for full length of treatment. • Doses should be evenly spaced. • Darunavir is not a cure for HIV infection, nor does it reduce risk of transmission to others. • Pt may continue to experience illnesses, including opportunistic infections. • Diarrhea can be controlled with OTC medication. • Notify physician if skin reactions occur.

dasatinib

HIGH ALERT

dah-**sah**-tin-ib
(Sprycel)
Do not confuse dasatinib with erlotinib, imatinib, or lapatinib.

◆CLASSIFICATION

PHARMACOTHERAPEUTIC: Protein-tyrosine kinase inhibitor. **CLINICAL:** Antineoplastic.

ACTION

Reduces activity of proteins responsible for uncontrolled growth of leukemia cells by binding to most imatinib-resistant BCR-ABL mutations of pts with chronic myelogenous leukemia (CML) or acute lymphoblastic leukemia (ALL). **Therapeutic Effect:** Inhibits proliferation, tumor growth of CML and ALL cancer cell lines.

PHARMACOKINETICS

Extensively distributed in extravascular space. Protein binding: 96%. Metabolized in liver. Eliminated primarily in feces. **Half-life:** 3–5 hrs.

USES

Treatment of adults with chronic, accelerated, myeloid or lymphoid blast phase of chronic myelogenous leukemia (CML) with resistance, intolerance to prior therapy, including imatinib. Treatment of adults with Philadelphia chromosome-positive (Ph+) acute lymphoblastic leukemia (ALL) with resistance or intolerance to prior therapy. Treatment of Philadelphia chromosome-positive (Ph+) chronic myeloid leukemia (CML) in chronic phase of newly diagnosed pts. **OFF-LABEL:** Post stem cell transplant follow-up treatment of CML.

PRECAUTIONS

Contraindications: None known. **Cautions:** Hepatic/renal impairment, myelosuppression, particularly thrombocytopenia, pts prone to fluid retention, those with prolonged QT interval.

⌛ LIFESPAN CONSIDERATIONS

Pregnancy/Lactation: Has potential for severe teratogenic effects, fertility impairment. Breast-feeding not recommended. **Pregnancy Category D. Children:** Safety and efficacy not established in those younger than 18 yrs. **Elderly:** No age-related precautions noted.

INTERACTIONS

DRUG: **Atazanavir, clarithromycin, erythromycin, indinavir, itracon-**

azole, ketoconazole, nefazodone, nelfinavir, ritonavir, saquinavir may increase dasatinib concentrations. **Carbamazepine, phenobarbital, phenytoin, rifampicin** may decrease dasatinib concentrations. **Antacids** alter pH-dependent solubility of dasatinib. **Famotidine, omeprazole** reduce dasatinib exposure. HERBAL: **St. John's wort** may decrease dasatinib concentration. FOOD: **Grapefruit juice** may increase concentration. LAB VALUES: May decrease WBC, platelets, Hgb, Hct, RBC, serum calcium, phosphates. May increase serum bilirubin, ALT, AST, creatinine.

AVAILABILITY (Rx)

Tablets (Film-Coated): 20 mg, 50 mg, 70 mg, 100 mg.

ADMINISTRATION/HANDLING

PO

• Give without regard to food. • Do not chew/crush/cut film-coated tablets. • Store at room temperature. • Do not give antacids either 2 hrs prior to or within 2 hrs after dasatinib administration.

INDICATIONS/ROUTES/DOSAGE

Chronic Myelogenous Leukemia (CML)

PO: ADULTS, ELDERLY: (Chronic phase): 100 mg once daily. **(Accelerated or blast phase):** 70 mg 2 times/day.

PH+ ALL

PO: ADULTS, ELDERLY: 70 mg 2 times/day. Dose increase or reduction in 20-mg increments per dose is recommended based on pt safety, tolerance, ANC, platelet count, concomitant CYP3A4 inhibitors or inducers.

SIDE EFFECTS

Frequent (50%–32%): Fluid retention, diarrhea, headache, fatigue, musculoskeletal pain, fever, rash, nausea, dyspnea. Occasional (28%–12%): Cough, abdominal pain, vomiting, anorexia, asthenia (loss of strength, energy), arthralgia, stomatitis, dizziness, constipation, peripheral neuropathy, myalgia. Rare (less than 12%): Abdominal distention, chills, weight increase, pruritus.

ADVERSE EFFECTS/ TOXIC REACTIONS

Pleural effusion occurs in 8% of pts, febrile neutropenia in 7%, GI bleeding, pneumonia in 6%, thrombocytopenia in 5%, dyspnea in 4%, anemia, cardiac failure in 3%.

NURSING CONSIDERATIONS

BASELINE ASSESSMENT

Obtain CBC weekly for first mo, biweekly for second mo, and periodically thereafter. Monitor hepatic function tests (bilirubin, alkaline phosphatase, AST, ALT) before treatment begins and monthly thereafter.

INTERVENTION/EVALUATION

Assess lower extremities for pedal edema for early evidence of fluid retention. Weigh, monitor for unexpected rapid weight gain. Offer antiemetics to control nausea, vomiting. Monitor daily pattern of bowel activity and stool consistency. Assess oral mucous membranes for evidence of stomatitis. Monitor CBC for neutropenia, thrombocytopenia; monitor hepatic function tests for hepatotoxicity.

PATIENT/FAMILY TEACHING

• Avoid crowds, those with known infection. • Avoid contact with anyone who recently received live virus vaccine; do not receive vaccinations. • Antacids may be taken up to 2 hrs before or 2 hrs after taking dasatinib. • Avoid grapefruit juice.

*DAUNOrubicin

HIGH ALERT

dawn-oh-**rue**-bih-sin
(Cerubidine, DaunoXome)

BLACK BOX ALERT Irreversible cardiotoxicity may occur. Myelosuppresant. Lipid component may cause infusion-related effects (back pain, flushing, chest tightness) within first 5 min of infusion. Must be administered by personnel trained in administration/handling of chemotherapeutic agents.

Do not confuse daunorubicin with dactinomycin, doxorubicin, epirubicin, idarubicin, or valrubicin.

CLASSIFICATION

PHARMACOTHERAPEUTIC: Anthracycline antibiotic. **CLINICAL:** Antineoplastic (see p. 82C).

ACTION

Inhibits DNA, DNA-dependent RNA synthesis by binding with DNA strands. Liposomal encapsulation increases uptake by tumors, prolongs drug action, may decrease toxicity. Cell cycle-phase nonspecific. **Therapeutic Effect:** Prevents cell division.

PHARMACOKINETICS

Widely distributed. Protein binding: High. Does not cross blood-brain barrier. Metabolized in liver to active metabolite. Excreted in urine; eliminated by biliary excretion. **Half-life:** 18.5 hrs; metabolite: 26.7 hrs.

USES

Cerubidine: Treatment of leukemias (acute lymphocytic [ALL], acute nonlymphocytic [ANLL]) in combination with other agents. **DaunoXome:** Advanced HIV-related Kaposi's sarcoma. **OFF-LABEL: Cerubidine:** Treatment of chronic myelocytic leukemia, Ewing's sarcoma, neuroblastoma, non-Hodgkin's lymphoma, Wilms tumor.

PRECAUTIONS

Contraindications: Arrhythmias, CHF, left ventricular ejection fraction less than 40%, preexisting myelosuppression. **Cautions:** Hepatic, biliary, renal impairment.

LIFESPAN CONSIDERATIONS

Pregnancy/Lactation: If possible, avoid use during pregnancy, esp. first trimester. May cause fetal harm. Breastfeeding not recommended. **Pregnancy Category D. Children:** Safety and efficacy not established. **Elderly:** Cardiotoxicity may be more frequent; reduced bone marrow reserves require caution. Age-related renal impairment may require dosage adjustment.

INTERACTIONS

DRUG: May decrease effects of **antigout medications. Bone marrow depressants** may enhance myelosuppression. **Live virus vaccines** may potentiate virus replication, increase vaccine side effects, decrease pt's antibody response to vaccine. **HERBAL:** None significant. **FOOD:** None known. **LAB VALUES:** May increase serum alkaline phosphatase, bilirubin, uric acid, AST.

AVAILABILITY (Rx)

Injection, Powder for Reconstitution (Cerubidine): 20 mg. **Injection Solution (Cerubidine):** 5 mg/ml. **Injection Solution (DaunoXome):** 2 mg/ml.

ADMINISTRATION/HANDLING

IV

◀ALERT▶ Give by IV push or IV infusion. Peripheral IV infusion not recommended due to vein irritation, risk of thrombophlebitis. Avoid small veins, swollen/edematous extremities, areas overlying joints/tendons. May be carcinogenic, mutagenic, teratogenic. Handle with extreme care during preparation/administration.

Reconstitution

Cerubidine • Reconstitute each 20-mg vial with 4 ml Sterile Water for Injection to provide concentration of 5 mg/ml. • Gently agitate vial until completely dissolved.
DaunoXome • Must dilute with equal part D_5W to provide concentration of 1 mg/ml. • Do not use any other diluent.

Rate of administration

Cerubidine • For IV push, withdraw desired dose into syringe containing 10–15 ml 0.9% NaCl. Inject over 2–3 min into tubing of running IV solution of D_5W or

0.9% NaCl. • For IV infusion, further dilute with 100 ml D_5W or 0.9% NaCl. Infuse over 30–45 min. • Extravasation produces immediate pain, severe local tissue damage. Aspirate as much infiltrated drug as possible, then infiltrate area with hydrocortisone sodium succinate injection (50–100 mg hydrocortisone) and/or isotonic sodium thiosulfate injection or ascorbic acid injection (1 ml of 5% injection). Apply cold compresses.
DaunoXome • Infuse over 60 min.

Storage

Cerubidine • Reconstituted solution is stable for 4 days at room temperature. Diluted solution in D_5W or 0.9% NaCl is stable for 4 wks at room temperature if protected from light. • Color change from red to blue-purple indicates decomposition; discard.
DaunoXome • Refrigerate unopened vials • Reconstituted solution is stable for 6 hrs if refrigerated. • Do not use if opaque.

IV INCOMPATIBILITIES

Allopurinol (Aloprim), aztreonam (Azactam), cefepime (Maxipime), dexamethasone (Decadron), fludarabine (Fludara), heparin, piperacillin and tazobactam (Zosyn). **DaunoXome:** Do not mix with any other solution, esp. NaCl or bacteriostatic agents (e.g., benzyl alcohol).

IV COMPATIBILITIES

Cytarabine (Cytosar), etoposide (VePesid), filgrastim (Neupogen), granisetron (Kytril), ondansetron (Zofran).

INDICATIONS/ROUTES/DOSAGE

ALERT Refer to individual protocols. **Cerubidine:** Cumulative dose should not exceed 550 mg/m^2 in adult (increased risk of cardiotoxicity) or 400 mg/m^2 in those receiving chest irradiation.

Acute Lymphoblastic Leukemia (ALL)

IV (CERUBIDINE): ADULTS, ELDERLY: 45 mg/m^2 on days 1, 2, and 3 of induction course. **CHILDREN 2 YRS AND OLDER, BODY SURFACE AREA 0.5 OR GREATER:** 25 mg/m^2 on day 1 of every wk for up to 4–6 cycles. **CHILDREN YOUNGER THAN 2 YRS, BODY SURFACE AREA LESS THAN 0.5:** 1 mg/kg/dose per protocol.

Acute Non-lymphocytic Leukemia (ANLL)

IV (CERUBIDINE): ADULTS YOUNGER THAN 60 YRS: 45 mg/m^2 on days 1, 2, and 3 of induction course then on days 1 and 2 of subsequent courses. **ADULTS 60 YRS AND OLDER:** 30 mg/m^2 on days 1, 2, and 3 of induction course, then on days 1 and 2 of subsequent courses.

Kaposi's Sarcoma

IV (DAUNOXOME): ADULTS: 40 mg/m^2 over 1 hr repeated q2wk.

Dosage in Renal Impairment

CERUBIDINE: SERUM CREATININE GREATER THAN 3 MG/DL: 50% of normal dose.
DAUNOXOME: SERUM CREATININE GREATER THAN 3 MG/DL: 50% of normal dose.

Dosage in Hepatic Impairment

CERUBIDINE: BILIRUBIN 1.2–3 MG/DL: 75% of normal dose. **BILIRUBIN 3.1–5 MG/DL:** 50% of normal dose. **BILIRUBIN GREATER THAN 5 MG/DL:** Daunorubicin is not recommended for use in this pt population.
DAUNOXOME: BILIRUBIN 1.2–3 MG/DL: 75% of normal dose. **BILIRUBIN GREATER THAN 3 MG/DL:** 50% of normal dose.

SIDE EFFECTS

Frequent: Complete alopecia (scalp, axillary, pubic), nausea, vomiting (beginning a few hrs after administration and lasting 24–48 hrs). **DAUNOXOME:** Mild to moderate nausea, fatigue, fever. **Occasional:** Diarrhea, abdominal pain, esophagitis, stomatitis, transverse pigmentation of fingernails, toenails. **Rare:** Transient fever, chills.

ADVERSE EFFECTS/ TOXIC REACTIONS

Myelosuppression manifested as hematologic toxicity (severe leukopenia, anemia, thrombocytopenia). Decrease in platelet count, WBC count occurs in 10–14 days, returns to normal level by third week. Cardiotoxicity noted as either acute, transient, abnormal. EKG findings and/or cardiomyopathy manifested as CHF (risk increases when cumulative dose exceeds 550 mg/m^2 in adults, 300 mg/m^2 in children 2 yrs and older, or total dosage greater than 10 mg/kg in children younger than 2 yrs).

NURSING CONSIDERATIONS

BASELINE ASSESSMENT

Obtain WBC, platelet, erythrocyte counts before and at frequent intervals during therapy. EKG should be obtained before therapy. Antiemetics may be effective in preventing, treating nausea.

INTERVENTION/EVALUATION

Monitor for stomatitis (burning, erythema of oral mucosa). May lead to ulceration within 2–3 days. Assess skin, nailbeds for hyperpigmentation. Monitor hematologic status, renal/hepatic function studies, serum uric acid. Monitor daily pattern of bowel activity and stool consistency. Monitor for hematologic toxicity (fever, sore throat, signs of local infection, unusual bruising/bleeding from any site), symptoms of anemia (excessive fatigue, weakness).

PATIENT/FAMILY TEACHING

• Urine may turn reddish color for 1–2 days after beginning therapy. • Alopecia is reversible, but new hair growth may have different color, texture. • New hair growth resumes about 5 wks after last therapy dose. • Maintain fastidious oral hygiene. • Do not have immunizations without physician's approval (drug lowers resistance). • Avoid contact with those who have recently received live virus vaccine. • Promptly report fever, sore throat, signs of local infection, unusual bruising/bleeding from any site, yellowing of whites of eyes/skin, difficulty breathing. • Increase fluid intake (may protect against hyperuricemia). • Contact physician for persistent nausea, vomiting.

DDAVP, *see desmopressin*

Decadron, *see dexamethasone*

decitabine HIGH ALERT

deh-**sit**-tah-bean
(Dacogen)

◆CLASSIFICATION

PHARMACOTHERAPEUTIC: Antineoplastic. **CLINICAL:** DNA demethylation agent.

ACTION

Exerts cytotoxic effect on rapidly dividing cells by causing demethylation of DNA in abnormal hematopoietic cells in bone marrow. **Therapeutic Effect:** Restores normal function to tumor suppressor genes regulating cellular differentiation, proliferation.

PHARMACOKINETICS

Protein binding: Less than 1%. Elimination appears to occur by removal of an amino group from the enzyme cytidine deaminase, found principally in liver, but also in granulocytes, intestinal epithelium, whole blood. **Half-life:** 30 min.

USES

Treatment of myelodysplastic syndromes, specifically refractory anemia, myelomonocytic leukemia. **OFF-LABEL:** Treatment of acute and chronic myelogenous leukemia, sickle cell anemia.

PRECAUTIONS

Contraindications: None known. **Cautions:** Hepatic/renal impairment.

LIFESPAN CONSIDERATIONS

Pregnancy/Lactation: May be embryotoxic; may cause developmental abnormalities of fetus. Breast-feeding not recommended. Men should not father a child while receiving treatment and for 2 mos after treatment. **Pregnancy Category D. Children:** Safety and efficacy not established. **Elderly:** No age-related precautions noted.

INTERACTIONS

DRUG: None significant. **HERBAL:** None significant. **FOOD:** None known. **LAB VALUES:** May decrease Hgb, Hct, WBC, RBC, platelets. May increase serum creatinine, AST, alkaline phosphatase, bicarbonate, lactate dehydrogenase, BUN, bilirubin, glucose, albumin, magnesium, sodium.

AVAILABILITY (Rx)

Injection, Powder for Reconstitution: 50 mg.

ADMINISTRATION/HANDLING

IV

Reconstitution • Reconstitute with 10 ml Sterile Water for Injection. • Further dilute with 50–250 ml 0.9% NaCl, D_5W, or lactated Ringer's.

Rate of administration • Give by continuous IV infusion over 1–6 hrs.

Storage • Store vials at room temperature. • Unless used within 15 min of reconstitution, diluted solution must be prepared using cold infusion fluids and stored in refrigerator up to maximum of 7 hrs until administration.

INDICATIONS/ROUTES/DOSAGE

ALERT Premedicate with antiemetics prior to therapy.

Myelodysplastic Syndrome

IV INFUSION: ADULTS, ELDERLY: (Option 1): 15 mg/m^2 given over 3 hrs q8h (45 mg/m^2/day) for 3 days. Subsequent treatment cycles should be repeated every 6 wks for a minimum of 4 cycles. **(Option 2):** 20 mg/m^2 given over 1 hr daily for 5 days. Repeat cycle q4wks. Adjust dose for delayed hematologic recovery. Hold treatment until resolution of serum creatinine 2 mg/dl or greater; ALT or bilirubin 2 times upper limit of normal; active or controlled infection.

SIDE EFFECTS

Frequent (53%–20%): Fever, nausea, cough, petechiae, constipation, diarrhea, insomnia, headache, vomiting, peripheral edema, pallor, ecchymosis, rigors, arthralgia. **Occasional (19%–11%):** Rash, limb pain, dizziness, back pain, anorexia, pharyngitis, abdominal pain, erythema, oral mucosal petechiae, stomatitis, confusion, lethargy, dyspepsia, anxiety, pruritus, hypoesthesia. **Rare (10%–5%):** Candidiasis, ascites, alopecia, chest wall pain, rales, catheter site infection, facial edema, hypotension, urticaria, dehydration, blurred vision, musculoskeletal discomfort, malaise, sinusitis, gastroesophageal reflux.

ADVERSE EFFECTS/ TOXIC REACTIONS

Pneumonia occurs in 22% of pts, cellulitus in 12%. Hematologic toxicity manifested most commonly as neutropenia (90%; recovery 28–50 days), thrombocytopenia (89%), anemia (82%), febrile neutropenia (29%), leukopenia (28%), lymphadenopathy (12%). UTI occurs in 7%.

NURSING CONSIDERATIONS

BASELINE ASSESSMENT

Give emotional support to pt, family. Use strict asepsis, protect pt from infection. Perform blood counts as needed to monitor response, toxicity but esp. prior to each dosing cycle.

INTERVENTION/EVALUATION

Monitor for hematologic toxicity (fever, sore throat, signs of local infections, unusual bleeding/bruising), symptoms of anemia (excessive fatigue, weakness). Assess response to medication; monitor, report nausea, vomiting, diarrhea. Avoid rectal temperatures, other traumas that may induce bleeding. Monitor CBC, platelets, serum creatinine, hepatic enzyme tests. If serum creatinine increases to 2 mg/dl, ALT, total bilirubin at least 2 times upper limit of normal, and pt has active or uncontrolled infection, treatment should be stopped and not restarted until toxicity is resolved.

D

PATIENT/FAMILY TEACHING

• Do not have immunizations without physician's approval (drug lowers resistance). • Avoid crowds, persons with known infections. • Report signs of infection (fever, flu-like symptoms) immediately. • Contact physician if nausea/vomiting continues at home. • Men should use barrier contraception while receiving treatment.

deferasirox

daeh-fur-**ah**-sir-ox
(Exjade)

BLACK BOX ALERT May cause renal/hepatic failure, gastrointestinal hemorrhage.

Do not confuse deferasirox with deferoxamine.

◆CLASSIFICATION

PHARMACOTHERAPEUTIC: Iron-chelating agent. **CLINICAL:** Iron reduction.

ACTION

Selective for iron. Binds iron with high affinity in a 2:1 ratio. **Therapeutic Effect:** Induces iron excretion.

PHARMACOKINETICS

Well absorbed following PO administration. Protein binding: 99%. Metabolized in liver. Primarily excreted in feces with a lesser amount eliminated in urine. **Half-life:** 8–16 hrs.

USES

Treatment of chronic iron overload due to blood transfusions (transfusional hemosiderosis).

PRECAUTIONS

Contraindications: None known. **Cautions:** Renal/hepatic impairment, preexisting hearing loss, vision disturbances.

⌛ LIFESPAN CONSIDERATIONS

Pregnancy/Lactation: Unknown if drug crosses placenta or is distributed in breast milk. **Pregnancy Category B. Children:** Not recommended for those younger than 2 yrs. **Elderly:** No age-related precautions noted.

INTERACTIONS

DRUG: **Antacids containing aluminium, cholestyramine** decrease effects. **Iron-chelating agents** may increase risk of toxic effects. **HERBAL:** None significant. **FOOD:** Bioavailability is variably increased when given with **food. LAB VALUES:** Decreases serum ferritin. May increase serum creatinine, transaminase, AST, ALT, urine protein.

AVAILABILITY (Rx)

Tablets for Oral Suspension (Exjade): 125 mg, 250 mg, 500 mg.

ADMINISTRATION/HANDLING

PO

• Give on empty stomach 30 min before food. • Do not give simultaneously with aluminum-containing antacids, cholestyramine. • Tablets should not be chewed or swallowed whole. • Disperse tablet by stirring in water, apple juice, orange juice until fine suspension is achieved. • Dosage less than 1 g should be dispersed in 3.5 oz of liquid, dosage more than 1 g should be dispersed in 7 oz of liquid. If any residue remains in glass, re-suspend with a small amount of liquid.

INDICATIONS/ROUTES/DOSAGE

Iron Overload

PO: ADULTS, ELDERLY, CHILDREN 2 YRS AND OLDER: Initially, 20 mg/kg once daily. Adjust dosage of 5 or 10 mg/kg every 3–6 mos based on serum ferritin levels. Hold dose for serum ferritin less than 500 mcg/L. **Maximum:** 30 mg/kg once daily.

Dosage in Renal Impairment

For increase in serum creatinine greater than 33% on 2 consecutive measures, reduce daily dose by 10 mg/kg.

Dosage in Liver Impairment

For severe or persistent elevations in hepatic function tests, consider dose reduction or discontinuation.

SIDE EFFECTS

Frequent (19%–10%): Fever, headache, abdominal pain, cough, nasopharyngitis, diarrhea, nausea, vomiting. **Occasional (9%–4%):** Rash, arthralgia, fatigue, back pain, urticaria. **Rare (1%):** Edema, sleep disorder, dizziness, anxiety.

ADVERSE EFFECTS/ TOXIC REACTIONS

Bronchitis, pharyngitis, acute tonsillitis, ear infection occur occasionally. Hepatitis, auditory disturbances, ocular abnormalities occur rarely. Acute renal failure, cytopenias (e.g., agranulocytosis, neutropenia, thrombocytopenia) may occur.

NURSING CONSIDERATIONS

BASELINE ASSESSMENT

Obtain baseline serum creatinine, ALT, AST, transaminase, then monthly thereafter. Auditory, ophthalmic testing should be obtained before therapy and annually therafter. Monitor CBC, urine protein, serum ferritin monthly.

INTERVENTION/EVALUATION

Treatment should be interrupted if serum ferritin levels are consistently less than 500 mcg/L. Suspend treatment if severe rash occurs.

PATIENT/FAMILY TEACHING

• Take on empty stomach 30 min before food. • Do not chew or swallow tablet whole; disperse tablet completely in water, apple juice, orange juice; drink resulting suspension immediately. • Do not take aluminum-containing antacids concurrently. • Inform physician if severe skin rash, changes in vision/hearing, or yellowing of skin/eyes occur.

D

deferoxamine

deaf-er-**ox**-ah-meen
(Desferal)
Do not confuse deferoxamine with cefuroxime or deferasirox, or Desferal with Desyrel or Disophrol.

◆ CLASSIFICATION

CLINICAL: Antidote.

ACTION

Binds with iron to form complex. **Therapeutic Effect:** Promotes urinary excretion of iron.

PHARMACOKINETICS

Erratic absorption following IM administration. Widely distributed. Rapidly metabolized in tissues, plasma. Excreted in urine, eliminated in feces via biliary excretion. Removed by hemodialysis. **Half-life:** 6 hrs.

USES

Treatment of acute iron toxicity, chronic iron toxicity secondary to multiple transfusions associated with some chronic anemias (e.g., thalassemia). **OFF-LABEL:** Treatment/diagnosis of aluminum toxicity associated with chronic kidney disease.

PRECAUTIONS

Contraindications: Severe renal disease, anuria, primary hemochromatosis. **Cautions:** Renal impairment. **Pregnancy Category C.**

INTERACTIONS

DRUG: **Vitamin C** may increase effect. **HERBAL:** None significant. **FOOD:** None known. **LAB VALUES:** May cause falsely elevated total iron-binding capacity (TIBC).

AVAILABILITY (Rx)

Injection, Powder for Reconstitution: 500 mg, 2 g.

ADMINISTRATION/HANDLING

◀ALERT▶ Reconstitute each 500-mg vial with 2 ml Sterile Water for Injection or 8 ml to each 2-g vial to provide a concentration of 213 mg/ml.

IV

• For IV infusion, further dilute with 0.9% NaCl, D_5W, and administer at no more than 15 mg/kg/hr for first 1,000 mg, followed by 500 mg over 4 hrs. • Too-rapid IV administration may produce skin flushing, urticaria, hypotension, shock.

IM

• Inject deeply into upper outer quadrant of buttock. No further dilution necessary.

Subcutaneous

• Administer subcutaneous very slowly. No further dilution necessary. Following reconstitution, stable for 7 days at room temperature.

IV INCOMPATIBILITY

Do not mix with any other IV medications.

INDICATIONS/ROUTES/DOSAGE

Acute Iron Intoxication

IV, IM: ADULTS: Initially, 1 g, then 0.5 g q4h for 2 doses; may give additional doses of 0.5 g q4–12h. **IM: CHILDREN 3 YRS AND OLDER:** 90 mg/kg/dose q8h. **Maximum:** 6 g/day.

IV: CHILDREN: 15 mg/kg/hr. **Maximum:** 6 g/day.

Chronic Iron Overload

SUBCUTANEOUS: ADULTS: 1–2 g/day over 8–24 hrs. **CHILDREN 3 YRS AND OLDER:** 20–40 mg/kg/day over 8–12 hrs. **Maximum:** 2 g/day.

IM: ADULTS: 0.5–1 g/day. Also, 2 g with each unit blood.

IV: CHILDREN: 15 mg/kg/hr. **Maximum:** 12 g/day.

SIDE EFFECTS

Frequent: Pain, induration at injection site, urine color change (to orange-rose). **Occasional:** Abdominal discomfort, diarrhea, leg cramps, impaired vision.

ADVERSE EFFECTS/ TOXIC REACTIONS

High-frequency hearing loss, tinnitus have been noted.

NURSING CONSIDERATIONS

BASELINE ASSESSMENT

Assess serum iron levels, total iron-binding capacity (TIBC) before and during therapy.

INTERVENTION/EVALUATION

Question for evidence of hearing loss (neurotoxicity). Periodic slit-lamp ophthalmic exams should be obtained in those treated for chronic iron overload. For IV administration, monitor serum ferritin, iron, TIBC, body weight, growth, B/P. If using subcutaneous technique, monitor for pruritus, erythema, skin irritation, edema.

PATIENT/FAMILY TEACHING

• Medication may produce discomfort at IM or subcutaneous injection site. • Urine will appear reddish. • Notify physician if hearing or vision changes occur.

degarelix

deg-ah-**rel**-ix
(Firmagon)
Do not confuse degarelix with cetrorelix or ganirelix.

◆CLASSIFICATION

PHARMACOTHERAPEUTIC: Gonadotropin-releasing hormone antagonist. **CLINICAL:** Antineoplastic.

ACTION

Antagonizes pituitary gonadotropin-releasing hormone (GnRH) receptors (binds immediately and reversibly), suppressing release of luteinizing hormone (LH) from pituitary gland, leading to rapid and sustained suppression of testosterone release from testes. **Therapeutic Effect:** Reduces size and growth of prostate cancer.

PHARMACOKINETICS

Subcutaneously distributed throughout total body water. Protein binding: 90%. Metabolized due to peptide hydrolysis during hepatobiliary system passage. Primarily excreted as peptide fragments in feces, with a lesser amount eliminated in urine. **Half-life:** 53 days.

USES

Treatment of advanced prostate cancer.

PRECAUTIONS

Contraindications: Pregnancy (Pregnancy Category X). **Cautions:** Those with QT prolongation, hypokalemia, CHF, severe hepatic impairment, renal impairment (creatinine clearance less than 50 ml/min).

LIFESPAN CONSIDERATIONS

Pregnancy/Lactation: Not indicated for use in this pt population. **Pregnancy Category X. Children:** Not indicated for use in this pt population. **Elderly:** No age-related precautions noted.

INTERACTIONS

DRUG: Dronedarone, phenothiazines increase risk of QT prolongation. **HERBAL:** None significant. **FOOD:** None known. **LAB VALUES:** Expected to decrease testosterone levels. May increase transaminase levels.

AVAILABILITY (Rx)

Injection, Powder for Solution: 80 mg, 120 mg.

ADMINISTRATION/HANDLING

Subcutaneous

• Reconstitute 80-mg vial with 4.2 ml Sterile Water for Injection (SWI) to provide 20 mg/ml concentration (120 mg with 3 ml SWI to provide 40 mg/ml concentration). • Administer within 1 hr following reconstitution. • Wear gloves during preparation and administration. • Vial must be kept vertical at all times; do not shake. • Give in abdominal region in areas that will not be exposed to pressure (on or close to waistband area).

INDICATIONS/ROUTES/DOSAGE

Prostate Cancer

SUBCUTANEOUS: ADULTS, ELDERLY: 240 mg given as 2 injections of 120 mg (40 mg/ml). Administer maintenance dose every 28 days after initial treatment begins. Maintenance: 80 mg.

SIDE EFFECTS

Frequent: (27%–11%): Hot flashes, injection site pain, erythema, increased weight. **Occasional (7%–5%):** Hypertension, local edema, fatigue, back pain, constipation, urinary tract infection, asthenia (lack of strength, energy), arthralgia, chills. **Rare: (1%):** Insomnia, headache, nausea, dizziness, erectile dysfunction, gynecomastia, testicular atrophy, night sweats.

ADVERSE EFFECTS/ TOXIC REACTIONS

Long-term androgen deprivation therapy may prolong QT interval. Loss of bone density may occur.

NURSING CONSIDERATIONS

BASELINE ASSESSMENT

Obtain baseline EKG, electrolyte parameters, ALT, AST, bilirubin, alkaline phosphatase, testosterone levels prior to initiation of therapy.

INTERVENTION/EVALUATION

Monitor serum electrolytes, prostate-specific antigen (PSA) periodically. If PSA increases, measure testosterone serum concentrations. Monitor routine EKG for QT prolongation. Assess for decrease in testosterone levels throughout therapy.

Monitor daily pattern of bowel activity and stool consistency.

PATIENT/FAMILY TEACHING

• Advise pt that swelling, itching, redness may occur at injection site. • Avoid tasks that require alertness, motor skills until response to drug is established.

D

delavirdine

deh-la-**ver**-deen
(Rescriptor)
Do not confuse Rescriptor with Ritonavir.

◆CLASSIFICATION

PHARMACOTHERAPEUTIC: Nonnucleoside reverse transcriptase inhibitor. **CLINICAL:** Antiretroviral (see pp. 66C, 116C).

ACTION

Binds directly to HIV-1 reverse transcriptase, blocks RNA- and DNA-dependent DNA polymerase activities. **Therapeutic Effect:** Interrupts HIV replication, slowing progression of HIV infection.

PHARMACOKINETICS

Rapidly absorbed after PO administration. Protein binding: 98%. Primarily distributed in plasma. Metabolized in liver. Eliminated in feces and urine. **Half-life:** 2–11 hrs.

USES

Treatment of HIV infection (in combination with other antiretrovirals).

PRECAUTIONS

Contraindications: None known. **Cautions:** Hepatic impairment.

⌛ LIFESPAN CONSIDERATIONS

Pregnancy/Lactation: Unknown if drug crosses placenta or is distributed in breast milk. **Pregnancy Category C. Children:** Safety and efficacy not established in those younger than 16 yrs. **Elderly:** Safety and efficacy not established.

INTERACTIONS

DRUG: Concurrent administration of **alprazolam, carbamazepine, ergotamine, lovastatin, midazolam, phenobarbital, phenytoin, rifabutin, rifampin, simvastatin** may cause serious adverse effects. **H_2 blockers, proton pump inhibitors** may decrease absorption. May increase concentration/effect of **amprenavir, antiarrhythmic agents (e.g., amiodarone, lidocaine), atorvastatin, bepridil, calcium channel blockers (e.g., amlodipine, diltiazem), clarithromycin, fluvastatin, immunosuppressants (e.g., cyclosporine, tacrolimus), indinavir, methadone, ritonavir, saquinavir, warfarin. HERBAL: St. John's wort** may increase concentration. **FOOD:** None known. **LAB VALUES:** May increase serum AST, ALT. May decrease neutrophil count.

AVAILABILITY (Rx)

Tablets: 100 mg, 200 mg.

ADMINISTRATION/HANDLING

PO

• May disperse 100-mg tablets in water before consumption. 200-mg tablets should remain intact. • Give without regard to food. • Pts with achlorhydria should take with orange juice, cranberry juice.

INDICATIONS/ROUTES/DOSAGE

HIV Infection (in Combination with Other Antiretrovirals)

PO: ADULTS: 400 mg 3 times a day.

SIDE EFFECTS

Frequent (18%): Rash, pruritus. **Occasional (greater than 2%):** Headache, nausea, diarrhea, fatigue, anorexia.

ADVERSE EFFECTS/ TOXIC REACTIONS

Hepatic failure, severe rash, hemolytic anemia, rhabdomyolysis, erythema multiforme, Stevens-Johnson syndrome, acute renal failure have been reported.

NURSING CONSIDERATIONS

BASELINE ASSESSMENT

Obtain baseline lab tests, esp. hepatic function tests, before initiation of therapy and at periodic intervals during therapy. Offer emotional support.

INTERVENTION/EVALUATION

Assess skin for rash. Question if nausea is noted. Monitor daily pattern of bowel activity and stool consistency. Assess eating pattern; monitor for weight loss. Monitor lab values carefully, particularly hepatic function, especially if taken with saquinavir.

PATIENT/FAMILY TEACHING

• Do not take any medications, including OTC drugs, without consulting physician. • Small, frequent meals may offset anorexia, nausea. • Delavirdine is not a cure for HIV infection, nor does it reduce risk of transmission to others.

Demadex, *see torsemide*

demeclocycline

deh-meh-clo-**sigh**-clean
(Declomycin)

◆CLASSIFICATION

PHARMACOTHERAPEUTIC: Tetracycline. **CLINICAL:** Antibiotic.

ACTION

Inhibits bacterial protein synthesis by binding to ribosomal receptor sites; inhibits antidiuretic hormone (ADH)-induced water reabsorption. **Therapeutic Effect:** Bacteriostatic. Produces water diuresis.

PHARMACOKINETICS

Food, dairy products interfere with absorption. Protein binding: 41%–91%. Metabolized in liver. Excreted in urine. Removed by hemodialysis. **Half-life:** 10–15 hrs.

USES

Treatment of acne, gonorrhea, pertussis, chronic bronchitis, UTI caused by both gram-negative and gram-positive organisms, syndrome of inappropriate antidiuretic hormone secretion (SIADH).

PRECAUTIONS

Contraindications: Children 8 yrs and younger, last half of pregnancy. **Cautions:** Renal/hepatic impairment, sun/ultraviolet exposure (severe photosensitivity reaction).

⌛ LIFESPAN CONSIDERATIONS

Pregnancy/Lactation: Crosses placenta; distributed in breast milk. May inhibit skeletal growth of fetus; avoid use in last half of pregnancy. **Pregnancy Category D. Children:** Not recommended in those 8 yrs and younger; may cause permanent discoloration of teeth, enamel hypoplasia; may inhibit skeletal growth. **Elderly:** No age-related precautions noted.

INTERACTIONS

DRUG: **Antacids** containing aluminum, calcium, or magnesium, **laxatives** containing magnesium, **oral iron preparations** impair absorption. **Cholestyramine, colestipol** may decrease absorption. May decrease effects of **oral contraceptives. HERBAL: Dong quai, St. John's wort** may increase photosensitization. **FOOD: Dairy products** may decrease absorption. **LAB VALUES:** May increase BUN, serum alkaline phosphatase, amylase, bilirubin, AST, ALT.

AVAILABILITY (Rx)

Tablets: 150 mg, 300 mg.

ADMINISTRATION/HANDLING

PO

• Give 1 hr before or 2 hrs after meals. • Give antacids containing aluminum, calcium, magnesium, laxatives containing magnesium, oral iron preparations

1–2 hrs before or after demeclocycline (impair drug's absorption).

INDICATIONS/ROUTES/DOSAGE

Mild to Moderate Infection, Including Acne, Pertussis, Chronic Bronchitis, UTI

PO: ADULTS, ELDERLY: 150 mg 4 times a day or 300 mg 2 times a day. **CHILDREN OLDER THAN 8 YRS:** 8–12 mg/kg/day in 2–4 divided doses.

SIADH

PO: ADULTS, ELDERLY: Initially, 900–1,200 mg/day in 3–4 divided doses, then decrease dose to 600–900 mg/day in divided doses.

SIDE EFFECTS

Frequent: Anorexia, nausea, vomiting, diarrhea, dysphagia, possibly severe photosensitivity (with moderate to high demeclocycline dosage). **Occasional:** Urticaria, rash. Long-term therapy may result in diabetes insipidus syndrome (polydipsia, polyuria, weakness).

ADVERSE EFFECTS/ TOXIC REACTIONS

Superinfection (esp. fungal), anaphylaxis, benign intracranial hypertension occur rarely. Bulging fontanelles occur rarely in infants.

NURSING CONSIDERATIONS

BASELINE ASSESSMENT

Question for history of allergies, esp. to tetracyclines.

INTERVENTION/EVALUATION

Monitor daily pattern of bowel activity and stool consistency. Assess food intake, tolerance. Monitor I&O, renal/hepatic function test results. Assess for rash. Be alert for superinfection: fever, vomiting, diarrhea, anal/genital pruritus, oral mucosal changes (ulceration, pain, erythema). Monitor B/P, LOC (potential for increased ICP).

PATIENT/FAMILY TEACHING

• Continue antibiotic for full length of treatment. • Space doses evenly. • Take oral doses on empty stomach with full glass of water. • Avoid sun/ultraviolet light exposure.

Demerol, *see meperidine*

denileukin

HIGH ALERT

den-ee-**lew**-kin
(Ontak)

BLACK BOX ALERT Must be administered by personnel trained in administration/handling of chemotherapeutic agents. Has been associated with severe capillary leak syndrome; severe and fatal infusion reactions; loss of visual acuity, usually with loss of color vision.

◆CLASSIFICATION

PHARMACOTHERAPEUTIC: Biologic response modifier. **CLINICAL:** Antineoplastic (see p. 82C).

ACTION

Cytotoxic fusion protein that targets cells expressing interleukin-2 (IL-2) receptors. After binding to IL-2 receptor, directs cytocidal action to malignant cutaneous T-cell lymphoma (CTCL) cells. **Therapeutic Effect:** Causes inhibition of protein synthesis, cell death.

PHARMACOKINETICS

Metabolized in liver. **Half-life:** 70–80 min.

USES

Treatment of persistent/recurrent cutaneous T-cell lymphoma (CTCL) whose malignant cells express CD25 component of IL-2 receptor. **OFF-LABEL:** Treatment of CTCL types mycosis fungoides and sezary syndrome.

PRECAUTIONS

Contraindications: None known. **Cautions:** Preexisting cardiovascular disease, hypoalbuminemia. **Pregnancy Category C.**

INTERACTIONS

DRUG: None significant. **HERBAL:** None significant. **FOOD:** None known. **LAB VALUES:** May decrease serum albumin, calcium, potassium, WBC, Hgb, Hct. Increases serum transaminase.

AVAILABILITY (Rx)

Injection Solution: 150 mcg/ml.

ADMINISTRATION/HANDLING

IV

Reconstitution • Thaw in refrigerator for up to 24 hrs or at room temperature for 1–2 hrs. • Inject calculated dose into empty infusion bag. Add no more than 9 ml 0.9% NaCl to each ml denileukin.

Rate of administration • Infuse over 30–60 min.

Storage • Store frozen. • Solutions for IV infusion stable for 6 hrs.

IV INCOMPATIBILITIES

Do not mix with any other IV medications.

INDICATIONS/ROUTES/DOSAGE

Cutaneous T-Cell Lymphoma (CTCL)

IV INFUSION: ADULTS: 9 or 18 mcg/kg/day for 5 consecutive days q21days. Infuse over at least 30 min. Hold if serum albumin less than 3 g/dl.

SIDE EFFECTS

Frequent: Two distinct syndromes occur commonly: a hypersensitivity reaction (69%), consisting of 2 or more of the following: hypotension, back pain, dyspnea, vasodilation, vascular leak syndrome characterized by hypotension, edema, hypoalbuminemia, rash, chest tightness, tachycardia, dysphagia, syncope; and a flu-like symptom complex (91%), consisting of 2 or more of the following: fever, chills, nausea, vomiting, diarrhea, myalgia, arthralgia. **Occasional (25%–10%):** Dizziness, peripheral edema, chest pain, weight loss, rhinitis, pruritus.

ADVERSE EFFECTS/ TOXIC REACTIONS

Pancreatitis, acute renal insufficiency, hematuria, hypothyroidism/hyperthyroidism occur rarely.

D

NURSING CONSIDERATIONS

BASELINE ASSESSMENT

CBC, blood chemistries (including renal/hepatic function tests), chest X-ray should be performed before therapy and weekly thereafter. Assess serum albumin level before initiation of each treatment (should be equal to or greater than 3 g/dl).

INTERVENTION/EVALUATION

Monitor serum albumin for hypoalbuminemia (generally occurs 1–2 wks after administration). Monitor for evidence of infection (lowered immune response: sore throat, fever, other vague symptoms). Monitor weight, B/P, hypersensitivity reaction. Assess for peripheral edema.

PATIENT/FAMILY TEACHING

• At home, increase fluid intake (protects against renal impairment). • Do not have immunizations without physician's approval (drug lowers resistance); avoid contact with those who have recently taken live virus vaccine.

denosumab

deh-**new**-sue-mab
(Prolia)

Do not confuse denosumab with daclizumab or Prolia with Avandia or Zebeta.

◆CLASSIFICATION

PHARMACOTHERAPEUTIC: Monoclonal antibody. **CLINICAL:** Bone resorption inhibitor.

ACTION

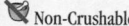

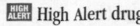

Binds to RANK ligand (transmembrane protein). Essential for formation, function, survival of osteoclasts. **Therapeutic Effect:** Decreases bone resorption; increases bone mass, strength.

PHARMACOKINETICS

Serum level detected 1 hr after administration. **Half-life:** 32 days.

USES

Treatment of postmenopausal women with osteoporosis at high risk for fracture.

PRECAUTIONS

Contraindications: Preexisting hypocalcemia (must be corrected prior to surgery). **Cautions:** History of hypoparathyroidism, thyroid/parathyroid surgery, malabsorption syndromes, excision of small intestine, immunocompromised. Those with severe renal impairment (creatinine clearance less than 30 ml/min) or receiving dialysis are at greater risk for developing hypocalcemia.

LIFESPAN CONSIDERATIONS

Pregnancy/Lactation: Approved for use only in postmenopausal women. **Pregnancy Category C. Children:** Approved for use only in postmenopausal women. **Elderly:** No age-related precautions noted.

INTERACTIONS

DRUG: None significant. **HERBAL:** None significant. **FOOD:** None known. **LAB VALUES:** May decrease calcium, may increase cholesterol.

AVAILABILITY (Rx)

Injection, Solution (Prefilled Syringe): 60 mg/ml.

ADMINISTRATION/HANDLING

Subcutaneous

• Administer in upper arm, upper thigh, or abdomen.

Storage • Refrigerate vials. • Solution appears as clear, colorless to pale yellow.

INDICATIONS/ROUTES/DOSAGE

Osteoporosis

SUBCUTANEOUS: ADULTS, ELDERLY: 60 mg every 6 wks.

SIDE EFFECTS

Frequent (35%–12%): Back pain, extremity pain. **Occasional (8%–5%):** Musculoskeletal pain, vertigo, peripheral edema, sciatica. **Rare (4%–2%):** Bone pain, upper abdominal pain, rash, insomnia, flatulence, pruritus, myalgia, asthenia (loss of strength, energy), GI reflux.

ADVERSE EFFECTS/ TOXIC REACTIONS

Increases risk of infection, specifically cystitis, upper respiratory tract infection, pneumonia, pharyngitis, herpes zoster (shingles) occur in 2%–6% of pts. Osteonecrosis of the jaw (OJN). Suppression of bone turnover, pancreatitis has been reported.

NURSING CONSIDERATIONS

BASELINE ASSESSMENT

Hypocalcemia must be corrected prior to treatment. Calcium 1,000 mg/day and vitamin D at least 400 international units/day should be given. Dental exam should be provided prior to treatment.

INTERVENTION/EVALUATION

Monitor magnesium, calcium, phosphorus. In pts predisposed with hypocalcemia and disturbances of mineral metabolism, clinical monitoring of calcium, mineral levels is highly recommended. Adequately supplement all pts with calcium and vitamin D. Monitor for delayed fracture healing.

PATIENT/FAMILY TEACHING

• Report rash, new-onset eczema. • Seek prompt medical attention if signs, symptoms of severe infection (rash, itching, reddened skin, cellulitis) occur. • Report muscle stiffness, numbness, cramps, spasms (signs of hypocalcemia); swelling or drainage from jaw, mouth, or teeth.

Depacon, *see valproic acid*

D

Depakene, *see valproic acid*

Depakote, *see valproic acid*

Depakote ER, *see valproic acid*

DepoMedrol, *see methylprednisolone acetate*

Depo-Provera, *see medroxyprogesterone*

desipramine

deh-**sip**-rah-meen
(Apo-Desipramine ✱, Norpramin)

BLACK BOX ALERT Increased risk of suicidal thinking and behavior in children, adolescents, young adults 18–24 yrs with major depressive disorder, other psychiatric disorders.

Do not confuse desipramine with clomipramine, dalfampridine, diphenhydramine, disopyramide, or imipramine, or Norpramin with nortriptyline.

◆CLASSIFICATION

PHARMACOTHERAPEUTIC: Tricyclic. **CLINICAL:** Antidepressant (see p. 37C).

ACTION

Blocks reuptake of neurotransmitters, (norepinephrine, serotonin) at presynaptic membranes, increasing their availability at postsynaptic receptor sites. Strong anticholinergic activity. **Therapeutic Effect:** Relieves depression.

PHARMACOKINETICS

Rapidly, well absorbed from GI tract. Protein binding: 90%. Metabolized in liver. Primarily excreted in urine. Minimally removed by hemodialysis. **Half-life:** 7–60 hrs.

USES

Treatment of depression, often in conjunction with psychotherapy. **OFF-LABEL:** Treatment of ADHD, bulimia nervosa, cataplexy associated with narcolepsy, cocaine withdrawal, neurogenic pain, panic disorder, depression in children 6–12 yrs.

PRECAUTIONS

Contraindications: Angle-closure glaucoma, within 14 days of MAOIs. **Cautions:** Cardiovascular disease, cardiac conduction disturbances, urinary retention, seizure disorders, hyperthyroidism, those taking thyroid replacement therapy.

⌛ LIFESPAN CONSIDERATIONS

Pregnancy/Lactation: Crosses placenta. Minimally distributed in breast milk. **Pregnancy Category C. Children:** Not recommended in those 6 yrs and younger. Children and adolescents with major depressive disorder (MDD), other psychiatric disorders are at increased risk for suicidal thinking, behavior while taking desipramine, esp. during first few mos of treatment. **Elderly:** Use lower dosages (higher dosages not tolerated, increases risk of toxicity).

INTERACTIONS

DRUG: Alcohol, other CNS depressants may increase CNS, respiratory depression; hypotensive effects. **Antithyroid agents** may increase risk of agranulocytosis. **Cimetidine** may increase desipramine blood concentration, risk of toxicity.

D

Clonidine may decrease effects. **MAOIs** may increase risk of neuroleptic malignant syndrome, hyperpyrexia, hypertensive crisis, seizures. **Phenothiazines** may increase anticholinergic, sedative effects. **Phenytoin** may decrease concentration. **Sympathomimetics** may increase risk of cardiac effects. HERBAL: **Kava kava, SAMe, St. John's wort, valerian** may increase sedation, risk of serotonin syndrome. FOOD: **Grapefruit, grapefruit juice** may increase concentration/toxicity. LAB VALUES: May alter serum glucose, EKG readings. **Therapeutic serum level:** 115–300 ng/ml; **toxic serum level:** greater than 400 ng/ml.

AVAILABILITY (Rx)

Tablets: 10 mg, 25 mg, 50 mg, 75 mg, 100 mg, 150 mg.

ADMINISTRATION/HANDLING

PO

◀ALERT▶ Fourteen days must elapse between use of MAOIs and despiramine. • Give with food, milk if GI distress occurs.

INDICATIONS/ROUTES/DOSAGE

Depression

PO: ADULTS: 75 mg/day. May gradually increase to 150–200 mg/day. **Maximum:** 300 mg/day. ELDERLY: Initially, 10–25 mg/day. May gradually increase to 75–100 mg/day. **Maximum:** 150 mg/day. CHILDREN OLDER THAN 12 YRS: Initially, 25–50 mg/day. May gradually increase to 100 mg/day. **Maximum:** 150 mg/day. CHILDREN 6–12 YRS (OFF-LABEL): 1–3 mg/kg/day. **Maximum:** 5 mg/kg/day.

SIDE EFFECTS

Frequent: Drowsiness, fatigue, dry mouth, blurred vision, constipation, delayed micturition, orthostatic hypotension, diaphoresis, impaired concentration, increased appetite, urinary retention. Occasional: GI disturbances (nausea, GI distress, metallic taste). Rare: Paradoxical reactions (agitation, restlessness, nightmares, insomnia), extrapyramidal symptoms (particularly fine hand tremor).

ADVERSE EFFECTS/ TOXIC REACTIONS

Overdose may produce confusion, seizures, drowsiness, arrhythmias, fever, hallucinations, dyspnea, vomiting, unusual fatigue, weakness. Abrupt discontinuation after prolonged therapy may produce severe headache, malaise, nausea, vomiting, vivid dreams.

NURSING CONSIDERATIONS

BASELINE ASSESSMENT

For those on long-term therapy, hepatic/renal function tests, blood counts should be performed periodically. For those at risk for arrhythmias, perform baseline EKG.

INTERVENTION/EVALUATION

Monitor for worsening of depression, suicidal ideation. Assess appearance, behavior, speech pattern, level of interest, mood. **Therapeutic serum level:** 115–300 ng/ml; **toxic serum level:** greater than 400 ng/ml. Monitor EKG if pt has history of arrhythmias.

PATIENT/FAMILY TEACHING

• Change positions slowly to avoid hypotensive effect. • Tolerance to postural hypotension, sedative, anticholinergic effects usually develops during early therapy. • Maximum therapeutic effect may be noted in 2–4 wks. • Do not abruptly discontinue medication. • Avoid alcohol. • Report worsening depression, suicidal ideation, unusual changes in behavior (esp. at initiation of therapy or with changes in dosage).

desloratadine

des-low-**rah**-tah-deen
(Aerius 🍁, Clarinex, Clarinex Redi-Tabs)

Do not confuse Clarinex with Celebrex or Claritin.

FIXED-COMBINATION(S)

Clarinex-D 24 Hour: desloratadine/pseudoephedrine (a sympathomimetic): 5 mg/240 mg. **Clarinex-D 12 Hour:** desloratadine/pseudoephedrine: 2.5 mg/120 mg.

◆CLASSIFICATION

PHARMACOTHERAPEUTIC: H_1 antagonist. **CLINICAL:** Nonsedating antihistamine.

ACTION

Exhibits selective peripheral histamine H_1 receptor blocking action. Competes with histamine at receptor sites. **Therapeutic Effect:** Prevents allergic response mediated by histamine (rhinitis, urticaria).

PHARMACOKINETICS

Rapidly, almost completely absorbed from GI tract. Distributed mainly in liver, lungs, GI tract, bile. Protein binding: 82%. Metabolized in liver to active metabolite and undergoes extensive first-pass metabolism. Eliminated in urine, feces. **Half-life:** 27 hrs (increased in elderly, renal/hepatic impairment).

USES

Relief of nasal/non-nasal symptoms of seasonal and perennial rhinitis (sneezing, rhinorrhea, itching/tearing of eyes, stuffiness), chronic idiopathic urticaria (hives).

PRECAUTIONS

Contraindications: None known. **Cautions:** Renal/hepatic impairment. Safety in children younger than 6 yrs unknown.

LIFESPAN CONSIDERATIONS

Pregnancy/Lactation: Excreted in breast milk. **Pregnancy Category C. Children/Elderly:** More sensitive to anticholinergic effects (e.g., dry mouth, nose, throat).

INTERACTIONS

DRUG: **Erythromycin, ketoconazole** may increase concentration. **HERBAL:** None significant. **FOOD:** None known. **LAB VALUES:** May suppress wheal, flare reactions to antigen skin testing unless antihistamines are discontinued 4 days before testing.

AVAILABILITY (Rx)

Syrup (Clarinex): 2.5 mg/5 ml. **Tablets (Clarinex):** 5 mg. **Tablets (Orally Disintegrating [Clarinex RediTabs]):** 2.5 mg, 5 mg.

ADMINISTRATION/HANDLING

PO

- May give with or without food.

Orally Disintegrating Tablet

- Use immediately after removing from blister pack. • Place on tongue. • May give with or without water.

INDICATIONS/ROUTES/DOSAGE

Allergic Rhinitis, Urticaria

PO: ADULTS, ELDERLY, CHILDREN OLDER THAN 12 YRS: 5 mg once a day. **CHILDREN 6–12 YRS:** 2.5 mg once a day. **CHILDREN 1–5 YRS:** 1.25 mg once a day. **CHILDREN 6–11 MOS:** 1 mg once a day.

Dosage in Hepatic/Renal Impairment

Dosage is decreased to 5 mg every other day.

SIDE EFFECTS

Frequent (12%): Headache. **Occasional (3%):** Dry mouth, drowsiness. **Rare (less than 3%):** Fatigue, dizziness, diarrhea, nausea.

ADVERSE EFFECTS/ TOXIC REACTIONS

None known.

NURSING CONSIDERATIONS

BASELINE ASSESSMENT

Assess lung sounds for wheezing; skin for urticaria, hives.

INTERVENTION/EVALUATION

For upper respiratory allergies, increase fluids to decrease viscosity of secretions, offset thirst, replace loss of fluids from diaphoresis. Monitor symptoms for therapeutic response.

PATIENT/FAMILY TEACHING

• Drink plenty of water (may cause dry mouth). • Avoid tasks that require alertness, motor skills until response to drug is established (may cause drowsiness). • Avoid alcohol.

desmopressin

des-moe-**press**-in
(Apo-Desmopressin ✱, DDAVP, DDAVP Nasal, DDAVP Rhinal Tube, Minirin ✱, Novo-Desmopressin ✱, Octostim ✱, Stimate)

◆CLASSIFICATION

PHARMACOTHERAPEUTIC: Synthetic pituitary hormone. **CLINICAL:** Antidiuretic.

ACTION

Increases reabsorption of water by increasing permeability of collecting ducts of kidneys. Plasminogen activator. **Therapeutic Effect:** Increases plasma factor VIII (antihemophilic factor). Decreases urinary output.

PHARMACOKINETICS

Route	Onset	Peak	Duration
PO	1 hr	2–7 hrs	8–12 hrs
IV	15–30 min	1.5–3 hrs	8–12 hrs
Intranasal	15 min–1 hr	1–5 hrs	8–12 hrs

Poorly absorbed after PO, nasal administration. Metabolism: Unknown. **Half-life: PO:** 1.5–2.5 hrs. **Intranasal:** 3.3–3.5 hrs. **IV:** 0.4–4 hrs.

USES

DDAVP Nasal: Central cranial diabetes insipidus. **Parenteral:** Central cranial diabetes insipidus. Maintain hemostasis and control bleeding in hemophilia A, von Willebrand's disease (type I). **Stimate intranasal:** Maintain hemostasis and control bleeding in hemophilia A, von Willebrand's disease (type I). **PO:** Central cranial diabetes insipidus, primary nocturnal enuresis. **OFF-LABEL:** Prophylaxis, treatment of central diabetes insipidus, treatment of hemophilia A, primary nocturnal enuresis.

PRECAUTIONS

Contraindications: Hemophilia A with factor VIII levels less than 5%; hemophilia B; severe type I, type IIB, platelet-type von Willebrand's disease. **Cautions:** Predisposition to thrombus formation, conditions with fluid, electrolyte imbalance, coronary artery disease, hypertensive cardiovascular disease.

LIFESPAN CONSIDERATIONS

Pregnancy/Lactation: Pregnancy Category B. Children: Caution in neonates, those younger than 3 mos (increased risk of fluid balance problems). Careful fluid restrictions recommended in infants. **Elderly:** Increased risk of hyponatremia, water intoxication.

INTERACTIONS

DRUG: Carbamazepine, chlorpropamide, clofibrate may increase effects. **Demeclocycline, lithium, norepinephrine** may decrease effects. **HERBAL:** None significant. **FOOD:** None known. **LAB VALUES:** None significant.

AVAILABILITY (Rx)

Injection Solution (DDAVP): 4 mcg/ml. **Nasal Solution (DDAVP):** 100 mcg/ml. **Nasal Spray:** 1.5 mg/ml (150 mcg/spray) (Stimate), 100 mcg/ml (10 mcg/spray) (DDAVP). **Tablets (DDAVP):** 0.1 mg, 0.2 mg.

ADMINISTRATION/HANDLING

IV

Reconstitution • For IV infusion, dilute in 10–50 ml 0.9% NaCl to a maximum concentration of 0.5 mcg/ml.

Rate of administration • Infuse over 15–30 min. • For preop use, administer 30 min before procedure. • Monitor B/P, pulse during IV infusion.
Storage • Refrigerate. • Stable for 2 wks at room temperature.

Subcutaneous
• Withdraw dose from vial. Further dilution not required.

Intranasal
• Refrigerate DDAVP nasal solution, Stimate nasal spray. • Nasal solution, Stimate nasal spray are stable for 3 wks at room temperature if unopened. • DDAVP nasal spray is stable at room temperature. • Calibrated catheter (rhinyle) is used to draw up measured quantity of desmopressin; with one end inserted in nose, pt blows on other end to deposit solution deep in nasal cavity. • For infants, young children, obtunded pts, air-filled syringe may be attached to catheter to deposit solution.

INDICATIONS/ROUTES/DOSAGE

Primary Nocturnal Enuresis
PO: CHILDREN 6 YRS AND OLDER: 0.2–0.6 mg once before bedtime. Limit fluid intake 1 hr prior and at least 8 hrs after dose.

Central Cranial Diabetes Insipidus
◀ALERT▶ Fluid restriction should be observed.
PO: ADULTS, ELDERLY, CHILDREN 12 YRS AND OLDER: Initially, 0.05 mg twice a day. Range: 0.1–1.2 mg/day in 2–3 divided doses. **CHILDREN YOUNGER THAN 12 YRS:** Initially, 0.05 mg, then twice a day. Range: 0.1–0.8 mg daily.
IV, SUBCUTANEOUS: ADULTS, ELDERLY, CHILDREN 12 YRS AND OLDER: 2–4 mcg/day in 2 divided doses or 1/10 of maintenance intranasal dose.
INTRANASAL (USE 100 MCG/ML CONCENTRATION): ADULTS, ELDERLY, CHILDREN OLDER THAN 12 YRS: 10–40 mcg (0.1–0.4 ml) in 1–3 doses/day. **CHILDREN 3 MOS–12 YRS:** Initially, 5 mcg (0.05 ml)/day. Range: 5–30 mcg (0.05–0.3 ml)/day.

Hemophilia A, von Willebrand's Disease (Type I)
IV INFUSION: ADULTS, ELDERLY, CHILDREN WEIGHING MORE THAN 10 KG: 0.3 mcg/kg diluted in 50 ml 0.9% NaCl. **CHILDREN WEIGHING 10 KG AND LESS:** 0.3 mcg/kg diluted in 10 ml 0.9% NaCl.
INTRANASAL (USE 1.5 MG/ML CONCENTRATION PROVIDING 150 MCG/SPRAY): ADULTS, ELDERLY, CHILDREN 12 YRS AND OLDER WEIGHING MORE THAN 50 KG: 300 mcg; use 1 spray in each nostril. **ADULTS, ELDERLY, CHILDREN 12 YRS AND OLDER WEIGHING 50 KG OR LESS:** 150 mcg as a single spray.

Dosage in Renal Impairment
Creatinine clearance less than 50: Not recommended.

SIDE EFFECTS

Occasional: IV: Pain, redness, swelling at injection site; headache; abdominal cramps; vulvular pain; flushed skin; mild B/P elevation; nausea with high dosages. **Nasal:** Rhinorrhea, nasal congestion, slight B/P elevation.

ADVERSE EFFECTS/ TOXIC REACTIONS

Water intoxication, hyponatremia (headache, drowsiness, confusion, decreased urination, rapid weight gain, seizures, coma) may occur in overhydration. Children, elderly pts, infants are esp. at risk.

NURSING CONSIDERATIONS

BASELINE ASSESSMENT

Establish baselines for B/P, pulse, weight, serum electrolytes, urine specific gravity. Check lab values for factor VIII coagulant concentration for hemophilia A, von Willebrand's disease; bleeding times.

INTERVENTION/EVALUATION

Check B/P, pulse with IV infusion. Monitor pt weight, fluid intake, urine volume, urine specific gravity, osmolality, serum electrolytes for diabetes insipidus. Assess factor VIII antigen levels, aPTT, factor VIII activity level for hemophilia.

PATIENT/FAMILY TEACHING

• Avoid overhydration. • Follow guidelines for proper intranasal administration. • Inform physician if headache, shortness of breath, heartburn, nausea, abdominal cramps occur.

desvenlafaxine

des-ven-lah-**facks**-een
(Pristiq)

BLACK BOX ALERT Increased risk of suicidal thinking and behavior in children, adolescents, young adults 18–24 yrs with major depressive disorder, other psychiatric disorders.

◆CLASSIFICATION

PHARMACOTHERAPEUTIC: Phenethylamine derivative. **CLINICAL:** Antidepressant (see p. 40C).

ACTION

Appears to inhibit serotonin and norepinephrine reuptake at CNS neuronal presynaptic membranes (weakly inhibits dopamine reuptake). **Therapeutic Effect:** Produces antidepressant effect.

PHARMACOKINETICS

Well absorbed from GI tract. Protein binding: 30%. Extensively metabolized to active metabolites. Excreted primarily in urine. Steady-state plasma levels occurs in 4–5 days. **Half-life:** 9–11 hrs.

USES

Treatment of major depression exhibited as persistent, prominent dysphoria (occurring nearly every day for at least 2 wks) manifested by 4 of 8 symptoms: change in appetite, change in sleep pattern, increased fatigue, impaired concentration, feelings of guilt or worthlessness, loss of interest in usual activities, psychomotor agitation or retardation, or suicidal tendencies.

PRECAUTIONS

Contraindications: Use of MAO inhibitors within 14 days or in those currently taking MAOIs (may cause neuroleptic malignant syndrome). Allow at least 7 days after discontinuing desvenlafaxine before starting an MAOI. **Cautions:** Renal/hepatic impairment, history of seizures, mania, conditions that may slow gastric emptying, those with suicidal ideation and behavior.

⌛ LIFESPAN CONSIDERATIONS:

Pregnancy/Lactation: Distributed in breast milk. **Pregnancy Category C. Children:** Safety and efficacy not established. **Elderly:** No age-related precautions noted.

INTERACTIONS

DRUG: Concurrent use of **MAOIs** may cause hyperthermia, rigidity, myoclonus, autonomic instability (including rapid fluctuations of vital signs), mental status changes, coma, extreme agitation. **Alcohol** increases CNS depressant effects. Decreases **midazolam** concentration. Increases **desipramine** concentration. **Aspirin, NSAIDs, warfarin** increase risk of bleeding. **Ketoconazole** may increase desvenlafaxine concentration. **HERBAL: Gotu kola, kava kava, St. John's wort, valerian** may increase CNS depressant effects. **FOOD:** None known. **LAB VALUES:** May increase total cholesterol, LDL cholesterol, triglycerides, hepatic function tests, prolactin level.

AVAILABILITY (Rx)

Tablets: 50 mg, 100 mg.

ADMINISTRATION/HANDLING

PO

• Give without regard to food. • Give with food or milk if GI distress occurs. • Do not divide, crush, dissolve tablets. • Must be swallowed whole, with fluid. • Give at same time each day.

INDICATIONS/ROUTES/DOSAGE

Major Depressive Disorder

PO: ADULTS: 50 mg once daily.

Dosage in Renal Impairment

Creatinine clearance less than 30 ml/min: 50 mg every other day.

SIDE EFFECTS

Frequent (22%–20%): Nausea, headache. **Occasional** (13%–7%): Dizziness, dry mouth, diarrhea, sweating, constipation, insomnia, fatigue. **Rare** (5%–2%): Anorexia, drowsiness, decreased libido, erectile dysfunction in men, anxiety, blurred vision, vomiting, decreased weight, tremor, paresthesia, irritability, abnormal dreams, blurred vision, tinnitus.

ADVERSE EFFECTS/ TOXIC REACTIONS

Seizures, syncope, extrapyramidal disorder, depersonalization, hypomania, epistaxis occur rarely. Ischemic cardiac events, including myocardial ischemia, myocardial infarction, and coronary occlusion requiring revascularization, may occur. Sustained increase in diastolic B/P (10–15 mm Hg) occurs occasionally.

NURSING CONSIDERATIONS

BASELINE ASSESSMENT

Obtain initial weight, B/P. Assess appearance, behavior, speech pattern, level of interest, mood, sleep pattern. For those on long-term therapy, blood serum chemistry profile to assess hepatic function should be performed periodically.

INTERVENTION/EVALUATION

Assess sleep pattern for evidence of insomnia. Monitor for suicidal ideation (esp. at initiation of therapy or changes in dosage). Assess appearance, behavior, speech pattern, level of interest, mood for therapeutic response.

PATIENT/FAMILY TEACHING

• Take with food to minimize GI distress. • Do not increase, decrease, or suddenly discontinue medication. • For those on long-term therapy, obtain periodic blood serum chemistry profile to assess hepatic function. • Therapeutic effect may be noted within 1–4 wks. • Avoid tasks that require alertness, motor skills until response to drug is established. • Avoid alcohol. • Report worsening depression, suicidal ideation, unusual changes in behavior.

D

Desyrel, *see trazodone*

Detrol, *see tolterodine*

Detrol LA, *see tolterodine*

dexamethasone

dex-a-**meth**-a-sone
(Apo-Dexamethasone ✱, Decadron, Dexamethasone Intensol, DexPak TaperPak, Diodex ✱, Maxidex)

Do not confuse dexamethasone with dextroamphetamine, Decadron with Percodan, or Maxidex with Maxzide.

FIXED-COMBINATION(S)

Ciprodex Otic: dexamethasone/ciprofloxacin (antibiotic): 0.1%/0.3%. **Dexacidin, Maxitrol:** dexamethasone/neomycin/polymyxin (anti-infectives): 0.1%/3.5 mg/10,000 units per g or ml.

◆CLASSIFICATION

PHARMACOTHERAPEUTIC: Long-acting glucocorticoid. **CLINICAL:** Corticosteroid (see pp. 97C, 100C).

ACTION

Inhibits accumulation of inflammatory cells at inflammation sites, phagocytosis, lysosomal enzyme release and synthesis, and/or release of mediators of inflammation. **Therapeutic Effect:** Prevents/suppresses cell/tissue immune reactions, inflammatory process.

PHARMACOKINETICS

Rapidly, completely absorbed from GI tract after PO administration. Widely distributed. Protein binding: High. Metabolized in liver. Primarily excreted in urine. Minimally removed by hemodialysis. **Half-life:** 3–4.5 hrs.

USES

Acute exacerbations of chronic allergic disorders, cerebral edema, conditions treated by immunosuppression, inflammatory conditions, otitis externa, ophthalmic conditions (corneal injury, inflammatory conditions, infective conjunctivitis). **OFF-LABEL:** Antiemetic, treatment of croup, dexamethasone suppression test (indicator consistent with suicide and/or depression), accelerate fetal lung maturation.

PRECAUTIONS

Contraindications: Active untreated infections, fungal, tuberculosis, viral diseases of the eye. **Cautions:** Respiratory tuberculosis, untreated systemic infections, ocular herpes simplex, hyperthyroidism, cirrhosis, ulcerative colitis, hypertension, osteoporosis pts at high thromboembolic risk, CHF, seizure disorders, peptic ulcer, diabetes. Prolonged use may result in cataracts, glaucoma.

LIFESPAN CONSIDERATIONS

Pregnancy/Lactation: Crosses placenta. Distributed in breast milk. **Pregnancy Category C (D if used in the first trimester). Children:** Prolonged treatment with high-dose therapy may decrease short-term growth rate, cortisol secretion. **Elderly:** Higher risk for developing hypertension, osteoporosis.

INTERACTIONS

DRUG: **Amphotericin** may increase hypokalemia. May increase **digoxin** toxicity caused by hypokalemia. May decrease effects of **diuretics, insulin, oral hypoglycemics, potassium supplements. Hepatic enzyme inducers** may decrease effects. **Live virus vaccines** may decrease pt's antibody response to vaccine, increase vaccine side effects, potentiate virus replication. **HERBAL:** **Cat's claw, echinacea** may increase immunosuppressant effect. **FOOD:** Interferes with **calcium** absorption. **LAB VALUES:** May increase serum glucose, lipids, sodium levels. May decrease serum calcium, potassium, thyroxine, WBC.

AVAILABILITY (Rx)

Elixir: 0.5 mg/5 ml. **Injection, Solution:** 4 mg/ml, 10 mg/ml. **Ophthalmic Solution:** 0.1%. **Ophthalmic Suspension (Maxidex):** 0.1%. **Solution, Oral:** 0.5 mg/5 ml. **Solution, Oral Concentrate (Dexamethasone Intensol):** 1 mg/ml. **Tablets:** 0.5 mg, 0.75 mg, 1 mg, 1.5 mg, 2 mg, 4 mg, 6 mg. **Tablets (TaperPak [DexPak]):** 1.5 mg (35 or 51 tablets on taper dose card).

ADMINISTRATION/HANDLING

IV

◀ALERT▶ Dexamethasone sodium phosphate may be given by IV push or IV infusion.

• For IV push, give over 1–4 min if dose is less than 10 mg. • For IV infusion, mix with 50–100 ml 0.9% NaCl or D_5W and infuse over 15–30 min. • For neonates, solution must be preservative free. • IV solution must be used within 24 hrs.

IM

• Give deep IM, preferably in gluteus maximus.

PO

• Give with milk, food (to decrease GI effect).

Ophthalmic Solution, Suspension

• Place gloved finger on lower eyelid and pull out until a pocket is formed between eye and lower lid. • Place prescribed number of drops or ¼–½ inch ointment into pocket. • Instruct pt to close eye gently for 1–2 min (so medication will not be squeezed out of the sac). • Instruct pt to apply digital pressure to lacrimal sac at inner canthus for 1–2 min to minimize systemic absorption.

IV INCOMPATIBILITIES

Ciprofloxacin (Cipro), daunorubicin (Cerubidine), idarubicin (Idamycin), midazolam (Versed).

IV COMPATIBILITIES

Aminophylline, cimetidine (Tagamet), cisplatin (Platinol), cyclophosphamide (Cytoxan), cytarabine (Cytosar), docetaxel (Taxotere), doxorubicin (Adriamycin), etoposide (VePesid), furosemide (Lasix), granisetron (Kytril), heparin, hydromorphone (Dilaudid), lipids, lorazepam (Ativan), morphine, ondansetron (Zofran), paclitaxel (Taxol), potassium chloride, propofol (Diprivan), total parenteral nutrition (TPN).

INDICATIONS/ROUTES/DOSAGE

Anti-Inflammatory

PO, IV, IM: ADULTS, ELDERLY: 0.75–9 mg/day in divided doses q6–12h. **CHILDREN:** 0.08–0.3 mg/kg/day in divided doses q6–12h.

Cerebral Edema

IV: ADULTS, ELDERLY: Initially, 10 mg, then 4 mg (IV or IM) q6h.
PO, IV, IM: CHILDREN: Loading dose of 1–2 mg/kg, then 1–1.5 mg/kg/day in divided doses q4–6h.

Nausea/Vomiting in Chemotherapy Pts

IV: ADULTS, ELDERLY: 8–20 mg once, then 4 mg (PO, IM, IV) q4–6h. **CHILDREN:** 10 mg/m^2/dose (**Maximum:** 20 mg), then 5 mg/m^2/dose q6h.

Usual Topical Dosage

TOPICAL: ADULTS, ELDERLY, CHILDREN: Apply to affected area 3–4 times a day.

Physiologic Replacement

PO, IV, IM: ADULTS, ELDERLY, CHILDREN: 0.03–0.15 mg/kg/day in divided doses q6–12h.

Usual Ophthalmic Dosage, Ocular Inflammatory Conditions

SUSPENSION: ADULTS, ELDERLY, CHILDREN: Initially, 2 drops q1h while awake and q2h at night for 1 day, then reduce to 3–4 times a day.

SIDE EFFECTS

Frequent: **Inhalation:** Cough, dry mouth, hoarseness, throat irritation. **Intranasal:** Burning, mucosal dryness. **Ophthalmic:** Blurred vision. **Systemic:** Insomnia, facial edema (cushingoid appearance ["moon face"]), moderate abdominal distention, indigestion, increased appetite, nervousness, facial flushing, diaphoresis. Occasional: **Inhalation:** Localized fungal infection (thrush). **Intranasal:** Crusting inside nose, epistaxis, sore throat, ulceration of nasal mucosa. **Ophthalmic:** Decreased vision; watering of eyes; eye pain; burning, stinging, redness of eyes; nausea; vomiting. **Systemic:** Dizziness, decreased/blurred vision. Rare: **Inhalation:** Increased bronchospasm, esophageal candidiasis. **Intranasal:** Nasal/pharyngeal candidiasis, eye pain. **Systemic:** Generalized allergic reaction (rash, urticaria); pain, redness, swelling at injection site; psychological changes; false sense of well-being; hallucinations; depression.

ADVERSE EFFECTS/ TOXIC REACTIONS

Long-term therapy: Muscle wasting (esp. arms, legs), osteoporosis, spontaneous fractures, amenorrhea, cataracts, glaucoma, peptic ulcer disease, CHF. **Ophthalmic:** Glaucoma, ocular hypertension, cataracts. **Abrupt withdrawal following long-term therapy:** Severe joint pain, severe headache, anorexia, nausea, fever, rebound inflammation, fatigue, weakness, lethargy, dizziness, orthostatic hypotension.

D

NURSING CONSIDERATIONS

BASELINE ASSESSMENT

Question for hypersensitivity to any corticosteroids. Obtain baselines for height, weight, B/P, serum glucose, electrolytes.

INTERVENTION/EVALUATION

Monitor I&O, daily weight. Assess for edema. Evaluate food tolerance. Monitor daily pattern of bowel activity and stool consistency. Report hyperacidity promptly. Check vital signs at least twice a day. Be alert to infection (sore throat, fever, vague symptoms). Monitor serum electrolytes, esp. for hypercalcemia (muscle twitching, cramps), hypokalemia (weakness, muscle cramps, paresthesia [esp. lower extremities], nausea/vomiting, irritability), Hgb, occult blood loss. Assess emotional status, ability to sleep.

PATIENT/FAMILY TEACHING

• Do not change dose/schedule or stop taking drug. • **Must** taper off gradually under medical supervision. • Notify physician if fever, sore throat, muscle aches, sudden weight gain, edema, exposure to measles/chicken pox occur. • Severe stress (serious infection, surgery, trauma) may require increased dosage. • Inform dentist, other physicians of dexamethasone therapy now or within past 12 mos. • Avoid alcohol, limit caffeine.

dexlansoprazole

dex-lan-sew-**prah**-zoll
(Dexilant)
Do not confuse dexlansoprazole with aripiprazole, lansoprazole, omeprazole, pantoprazole, or rabeprazole, or Kapidex with Atarax, Casodex, or Xanax.

◆ CLASSIFICATION

CLINICAL: Proton pump inhibitor.

ACTION

Binds to and inhibits hydrogen-potassium adenosine triphosphatase, an enzyme on surface of gastric parietal cells, blocking the final step of acid production. **Therapeutic Effect:** Reduces gastric acid production.

PHARMACOKINETICS

Extensively metabolized in liver. Mainly excreted in urine, with slightly lesser amount eliminated in feces. Protein binding: 97%. **Half-life:** 1–2 hrs.

USES

Healing of all grades of erosive esophagitis; maintenance healing of erosive esophagitis. Treatment of heartburn associated with nonerosive gastroesophageal reflux disease (GERD).

PRECAUTIONS

Contraindications: None known. **Cautions:** Hepatic impairment.

LIFESPAN CONSIDERATIONS

Pregnancy/Lactation: Unknown if distributed in breast milk. **Pregnancy Category B. Children:** Safety and efficacy not established. **Elderly:** No age-related precautions noted.

INTERACTIONS

Drug: May decrease **atazanavir** concentration. May interfere with **ampicillin, digoxin, iron salts, ketoconazole** absorption. May increase effect of **warfarin. Sucralfate** may delay dexlansoprazole absorption (give dexlansoprazole 30 min before sucralfate). **HERBAL:** None significant. **FOOD:** None known. **LAB VALUES:** None known.

AVAILABILITY (Rx)

Capsules (Delayed-Release): 30 mg, 60 mg.

ADMINISTRATION/HANDLING

PO

• Do not chew/crush delayed-release capsules. • Swallow whole. May take with or without regard to food. • If pt has difficulty swallowing capsules, open capsules, sprinkle granules on 1 tbsp of applesauce, and have pt swallow immediately.

INDICATIONS/ROUTES/DOSAGE

Erosive Esophagitis

PO: ADULTS, ELDERLY: 60 mg once daily for up to 8 wks. Maintenance of healed erosive esophagitis: 30 mg once daily for up to 6 mos.

GERD

PO: ADULTS, ELDERLY: 30 mg once daily for 4 wks.

Moderate Hepatic Impairment

PO: ADULTS, ELDERLY: Consider 30 mg maximum daily dose.

SIDE EFFECTS

Occasional (5%–4%): Diarrhea, abdominal pain. **Rare (3%–1%):** Nausea, vomiting, flatulence.

ADVERSE EFFECTS/ TOXIC REACTIONS

Upper respiratory tract infection occurs rarely.

NURSING CONSIDERATIONS

BASELINE ASSESSMENT

Obtain baseline lab values. Assess for epigastric or abdominal pain, occult blood.

INTERVENTION/EVALUATION

Assess for therapeutic response (relief of GI symptoms). Question for occurrence of diarrhea, GI discomfort, nausea. Monitor CBC, renal/hepatic function tests.

PATIENT/FAMILY TEACHING

• Do not chew/crush delayed-release capsules. • For pts who have difficulty swallowing capsules, open capsules, sprinkle granules on 1 tbsp of applesauce, and have pt swallow immediately.

dexmedetomidine

decks-meh-deh-**tome**-ih-deen
(Precedex)
Do not confuse Precedex with Percocet or Peridex.

◆CLASSIFICATION

PHARMACOTHERAPEUTIC: Alpha$_2$-agonist. **CLINICAL:** Nonbarbiturate sedative, hypnotic.

ACTION

Selective alpha$_2$-adrenergic agonist. **Therapeutic Effect:** Produces analgesic, hypnotic, sedative effects.

PHARMACOKINETICS

Protein binding: 94%. Metabolized in liver. Excreted in urine. **Half-life:** 2 hrs.

USES

Sedation of initially intubated, mechanically ventilated adults during treatment in intensive care setting. Use in nonintubated pts requiring sedation before and/ or during surgical and other procedures. **OFF-LABEL:** Pain relief, treatment of shivering.

PRECAUTIONS

Contraindications: None known. **Cautions:** Advanced heart block, severe CHF, hepatic/renal impairment, hypovolemia. **Pregnancy Category C.**

INTERACTIONS

DRUG: **Isoniazid, miconazole** may increase concentration/effects. May increase concentration/effects of **beta-blockers, fluoxetine, lidocaine, mirtazapine, paroxetine, risperidone, ritonavir, thioridazine, tricyclic antidepressants, venlafaxine. Vasodilators** may increase hypotensive effect. May decrease concentration of **codeine, hydrocodone, oxycodone, tramadol.** **HERBAL:**

None significant. **FOOD:** None known. **LAB VALUES:** May increase serum alkaline phosphatase, potassium, AST, ALT.

AVAILABILITY (Rx)

Injection Solution: 100 mcg/ml.

ADMINISTRATION/HANDLING

IV

Reconstitution • Dilute 2 ml of dexmedetomidine with 48 ml 0.9% NaCl.
Rate of administration • Individualized, titrated to desired effect.
Storage • Store at room temperature.

IV INCOMPATIBILITIES

Do not mix dexmedetomidine with any other medications.

INDICATIONS/ROUTES/DOSAGE

Sedation
IV: ADULTS: Loading dose of 1 mcg/kg over 10 min followed by maintenance infusion of 0.2–0.7 mcg/kg/hr. **ELDERLY:** May require decreased dosage. No guidelines available.

SIDE EFFECTS

Frequent: Hypotension (30%), nausea (11%). **Occasional (3%–2%):** Pain, fever, oliguria, thirst.

ADVERSE EFFECTS/ TOXIC REACTIONS

Bradycardia, atrial fibrillation, hypoxia, anemia, pain, pleural effusion may occur with too-rapid IV infusion.

NURSING CONSIDERATIONS

INTERVENTION/EVALUATION

Monitor EKG for atrial fibrillation, pulse for bradycardia, B/P for hypotension, level of sedation. Assess respiratory rate, rhythm. Monitor ventilator settings. Do not discontinue abruptly.

dexmethylphenidate

dex-meth-ill-**fen**-i-date
(Focalin, Focalin XR)

BLACK BOX ALERT Chronic use can lead to marked tolerance, psychological dependence. Frank psychosis may occur, especially with IV use. Severe depression may occur during drug withdrawal.

◆CLASSIFICATION

CLINICAL: CNS stimulant **(Schedule II).**

ACTION

Blocks reuptake of norepinephrine, dopamine into presynaptic neurons, increasing release of these neurotransmitters into synaptic cleft. **Therapeutic Effect:** Decreases motor restlessness, fatigue; increases motor activity, mental alertness, attention span; elevates mood.

PHARMACOKINETICS

Readily absorbed from GI tract. Plasma concentrations increase rapidly. Metabolized in liver. Excreted in urine. **Half-life:** 2.2 hrs.

USES

Adjunct in treatment of ADHD with moderate to severe distractability, short attention spans, hyperactivity, emotional impulsivity in children 6 yrs and older. Focalin XR extended-release capsule approved for 30-minute onset of action for treatment of ADHD.

PRECAUTIONS

Contraindications: Diagnosis or family history of Tourette syndrome; glaucoma; history of marked agitation, anxiety, tension; motor tics; use of MAOIs within 14 days. **Cautions:** Cardiovascular disease, seizure disorder, psychosis. Avoid use in those with history of substance abuse.

LIFESPAN CONSIDERATIONS

Pregnancy/Lactation: Unknown if excreted in breast milk. **Pregnancy Cate-**

gory C. **Children:** May be more susceptible to developing anorexia, insomnia, abdominal pain, weight loss. Chronic use may inhibit growth. In psychotic children, may exacerbate symptoms of behavior disturbance, thought disorder. **Elderly:** No age-related precautions noted.

INTERACTIONS

DRUG: **Acid suppressants, antacids** may alter absorption. Other **CNS stimulants** may have additive effects. **MAOIs** may increase effects. Decreased dosages for **phenobarbital, phenytoin, primidone, tricyclic antidepressants** may be necessary. May inhibit effects of **warfarin.** HERBAL: **Ephedra** may cause hypertension, arrhythmias. **Yohimbe** may increase CNS stimulation. FOOD: None known. LAB VALUES: None significant.

AVAILABILITY (Rx)

Tablets (Focalin): 2.5 mg, 5 mg, 10 mg.

Capsules (Extended-Release [Focalin XR]): 5 mg, 10 mg, 15 mg, 20 mg.

ADMINISTRATION/HANDLING

PO

- Do not give drug in afternoon or evening (causes insomnia).
- Tablets may be crushed.
- Give without regard to food.
- Swallow extended-release capsules whole; do not chew, crush, divide.
- May sprinkle contents of extended-release capsules on small amount of applesauce.
- Give extended-release capsules once each day in the morning, before breakfast.

INDICATIONS/ROUTES/DOSAGE

ADHD

Pts not currently taking methylphenidate:

Capsules

PO: ADULTS, ELDERLY: Initially, 10 mg/day. May increase in increments of 10 mg/day at weekly intervals. **Maximum:** 20 mg/day. CHILDREN 6 YRS AND OLDER: Initially, 5 mg/day. May increase in increments of 5 mg/day at weekly intervals. **Maximum:** 20 mg/day.

Tablets

PO: ADULTS, ELDERLY, CHILDREN 6 YRS AND OLDER: Initially, 2.5 mg 2 times a day. Doses should be given at least 4 hrs apart. May increase in increments of 2.5–5 mg at weekly intervals. **Maximum:** 20 mg/day. **Conversion from methylphenidate:** Initially, half the dose of methylphenidate. **Maximum:** 20 mg/day. **Conversion from dexmethylphenidate immediate-release to extended-release:** Switch to same dose using extended-release formulation. **Maximum:** 20 mg/day.

SIDE EFFECTS

Frequent: Abdominal pain, nausea, anorexia, fever. Occasional: Tachycardia, arrhythmias, palpitations, insomnia, twitching. Rare: Blurred vision, rash, arthralgia.

ADVERSE EFFECTS/ TOXIC REACTIONS

Withdrawal after prolonged therapy may unmask symptoms of underlying disorder. May lower seizure threshold in those with history of seizures. Overdose produces excessive sympathomimetic effects (vomiting, tremor, hyperreflexia, seizures, confusion, hallucinations, diaphoresis). Prolonged administration to children may delay growth. Neuroleptic malignant syndrome occurs rarely.

NURSING CONSIDERATIONS

BASELINE ASSESSMENT

Evaluate pt for cardiac disease, psychiatric conditions.

INTERVENTION/EVALUATION

CBC, differential, platelet count, B/P, heart rate should be performed routinely during therapy. If paradoxical return of attention deficit occurs, dosage should be reduced or discontinued. Weigh pediatric pt regularly to detect delayed growth.

PATIENT/FAMILY TEACHING

• Avoid tasks that require alertness, motor skills until response to drug is established. • Report any increase in seizures, chest pain, unexplained syncope. • Avoid caffeine. • Last dose should be given several hours before bedtime to prevent insomnia. • Report anxiety, fever.

D

dexrazoxane

dex-ray-**zoks**-ane
(Tolect, Zinecard)
Do not confuse Zinecard with Gemzar.

CLASSIFICATION

PHARMACOTHERAPEUTIC: Antineoplastic. **CLINICAL:** Cytoprotective agent.

ACTION

Rapidly penetrates myocardial cell membrane. Binds intracellular iron, prevents generation of free radicals by anthracyclines. **Therapeutic Effect:** Protects against anthracycline-induced cardiomyopathy.

PHARMACOKINETICS

Rapidly distributed after IV administration. Not bound to plasma proteins. Primarily excreted in urine. Removed by peritoneal dialysis. **Half-life:** 2.1–2.5 hrs.

USES

Tolect: Treatment of anthracycline-induced extravasation. **Zinecard:** Reduction of incidence, severity of cardiomyopathy associated with doxorubicin therapy in women with metastatic breast cancer having received a cumulative dose of 300 mg/m^2 and would benefit from continued doxorubicin therapy. Not recommended with initiation of doxorubicin therapy.

PRECAUTIONS

Contraindications: Hypersensitivity to nonanthracycline chemotherapy regimens. **Cautions:** Chemotherapeutic agents that are additive to myelosuppression, concurrent fluorouracil, adriamycin, cyclophosphamide (FAC) therapy.

LIFESPAN CONSIDERATIONS

Pregnancy/Lactation: May be embryotoxic, teratogenic. Unknown if distributed in breast milk. Breast-feeding not recommended. **Pregnancy Category C. Children:** Safety and efficacy not established. **Elderly:** Information not available.

INTERACTIONS

DRUG: Bone marrow depressants may increase myelosuppression. **HERBAL:** None significant. **FOOD:** None known. **LAB VALUES:** None significant.

AVAILABILITY (Rx)

Injection, Powder for Reconstitution: (Zinecard): 250 mg (10 mg/ml reconstituted in 25-ml single-use vial). **(Tolect, Zinecard):** 500 mg (10 mg/ml reconstituted in 50-ml single-use vial).

ADMINISTRATION/HANDLING

◀ALERT▶ Do not mix with other drugs. Use caution in handling/preparation of reconstituted solution (glove use recommended).

IV

Reconstitution • Reconstitute with 0.167 molar (M/6) sodium lactate injection to give concentration of 10 mg dexrazoxane for each ml of sodium lactate. • May further dilute with 0.9% NaCl or D_5W. Concentration should range from 1.3–5 mg/ml. Treatment of extravasation: Further dilute reconstituted vial in 1,000 ml 0.9% NaCl.

Rate of administration • Give reconstituted solution by slow IV push or IV infusion over 15–30 min. • After infusion is complete and before total elapsed time of 30 min from beginning of dexrazoxane infusion, give IV injection of doxorubicin. Treatment of extravasation:

Infuse over 1–2 hrs in large vein other than in area of extravasation.

Storage • Store vials at room temperature. • **Zinecard:** Reconstituted solution is stable for 6 hrs at room temperature or if refrigerated. Discard unused solution. **Tolect:** Stable for 4 hrs in 0.9% NaCl.

IV INCOMPATIBILITIES

Do not mix dexrazoxane with other medications.

INDICATIONS/ROUTES/DOSAGE

Cardioprotective

IV: ADULTS, CHILDREN: (ZINECARD): Recommended dosage ratio is 10 parts dexrazoxane to 1 part doxorubicin (e.g., 500 mg/m^2 dexrazoxane for every 50 mg/m^2 doxorubicin).

Anthracycline Extravasation

IV: ADULTS, ELDERLY: (TOLECT): 1,000 mg/m^2 on days 1 and 2 (**Maximum:** 2,000 mg), then 500 mg/m^2 on day 3 (**Maximum:** 1,000 mg). Begin treatment within 6 hrs of extravasation.

Dosage in Renal Impairment

IV: ADULTS, ELDERLY: Moderate to severe (creatinine clearance less than 40 ml/min): Reduce dose by 50%.

SIDE EFFECTS

Frequent: Alopecia, nausea, vomiting, fatigue, malaise, anorexia, stomatitis, fever, infection, diarrhea. **Occasional:** Pain at injection site, neurotoxicity, phlebitis, dysphagia, streaking/erythema at injection site. **Rare:** Urticaria, skin reaction.

ADVERSE EFFECTS/ TOXIC REACTIONS

Fluorouracil, adriamycin, cyclophosphamide (FAC) therapy with dexrazoxane increases risk for severe leukopenia, granulocytopenia, thrombocytopenia compared with those receiving FAC without dextrazoxane. Overdose can be removed with peritoneal dialysis or hemodialysis.

NURSING CONSIDERATIONS

BASELINE ASSESSMENT

Use gloves when preparing solution. If powder/solution comes in contact with skin, wash immediately with soap and water. Antiemetics may be effective in preventing, treating nausea.

INTERVENTION/EVALUATION

Frequently monitor platelets, CBC with differential for evidence of blood dyscrasias. Assess for stomatitis (burning/erythema of oral mucosa at inner margin of lips, sore throat, difficulty swallowing). Monitor hematologic status, renal/hepatic function studies, cardiac function. Monitor daily pattern of bowel activity and stool consistency. Monitor for hematologic toxicity (fever, signs of local infection, unusual bruising/bleeding from any site).

PATIENT/FAMILY TEACHING

• Alopecia is reversible, but new hair growth may have different color/texture. • New hair growth resumes 2–3 mos after last therapy dose. • Maintain fastidious oral hygiene. • Promptly report fever, sore throat, signs of local infection, bleeding, bruising. • Contact physician if persistent nausea/vomiting continues at home.

dextroamphetamine and amphetamine

dex-troe-am-**fet**-ah-meen/am-**fet**-ah-meen

(Adderall, Adderall-XR)

BLACK BOX ALERT High potential for abuse. Prolonged administration may lead to drug dependence.

Do not confuse Adderall with Inderal.

CLASSIFICATION

PHARMACOTHERAPEUTIC: Amphetamine **(Schedule II). CLINICAL:** CNS stimulant.

D

ACTION

Enhances action of dopamine, norepinephrine by blocking reuptake from synapses. Inhibits monoamine oxidase, facilitates release of catecholamines. **Therapeutic Effect:** Increases motor activity, mental alertness; decreases drowsiness, fatigue; suppresses appetite.

PHARMACOKINETICS

Well absorbed following PO administration. Widely distributed including CNS. Metabolized in liver. Excreted in urine. Removed by hemodialysis. **Half-life:** 10–13 hrs.

USES

Treatment of narcolepsy; treatment of ADHD in hyperactive children.

PRECAUTIONS

Contraindications: Advanced arteriosclerosis, agitated mental states, glaucoma, history of drug abuse, hypersensitivity to sympathomimetic amines, hyperthyroidism, moderate to severe hypertension, symptomatic cardiovascular disease, use of MAOIs within 14 days. **Cautions:** Elderly, debilitated pts; tartrazine-sensitive pts. May prolong QT interval.

LIFESPAN CONSIDERATIONS

Pregnancy/Lactation: Distributed in breast milk. **Pregnancy Category C. Children:** Safety and efficacy not established in those younger than 3 yrs. **Elderly:** Age-related cardiovascular, cerebrovascular disease, hepatic/renal impairment may increase risk of side effects.

INTERACTIONS

DRUG: **Beta-blockers** may increase risk of bradycardia, heart block, hypertension. **Digoxin** may increase risk of arrhythmias. **MAOIs** may prolong, intensify effects. **Meperidine** may increase risk of hypotension, respiratory depression, seizures, vascular collapse. **Other CNS stimulants** may increase effects. **Thyroid hormones** may increase effects. **Tricyclic antidepressants** may increase cardiovascular effects. **HERBAL:** None significant. **FOOD:** None known. **LAB VALUES:** May increase plasma corticosteroid.

AVAILABILITY (Rx)

Tablets (Adderall): 5 mg, 7.5 mg, 10 mg, 12.5 mg, 15 mg, 20 mg, 30 mg.

Capsules (Extended-Release [Adderall-XR]): 5 mg, 10 mg, 15 mg, 20 mg, 25 mg, 30 mg.

ADMINISTRATION/HANDLING

PO

- Give at least 6 hrs before bedtime.
- Extended-release capsules should be swallowed whole; do not break, crush, or chew.

INDICATIONS/ROUTES/DOSAGE

Narcolepsy

PO: ADULTS, CHILDREN OLDER THAN 12 YRS: Initially, 10 mg/day. Increase by 10 mg/day at weekly intervals until therapeutic response is achieved. **Maximum:** 60 mg/day given in 1–3 divided doses with interval of 4–6 hrs between doses. **CHILDREN 6–12 YRS:** Initially, 5 mg/day. Increase by 5 mg/day at weekly intervals until therapeutic response is achieved. **Maximum:** 60 mg/day given in 1–3 divided doses with interval of 4–6 hrs between doses.

ADHD

ADULTS, ELDERLY: (ADDERALL-XR): Initially, 20 mg once daily in the morning. May increase up to 60 mg/day. **CHILDREN 13–17 YRS: (ADDERALL-XR):** Initially, 10 mg once daily in the morning. May increase to 20 mg/day after 1 wk if symptoms are not controlled. May increase up to 60 mg/day. **CHILDREN 6–12 YRS: (ADDERALL):** Initially, 5 mg 1–2 times a day. May increase in 5-mg increments at weekly intervals until optimal response is obtained. **Maximum:** 40 mg/day given in 1–3 divided doses (use intervals of 4–6 hrs between additional doses). **(ADDERALL-XR):** Initially, 5-10 mg once daily in the morning. May increase daily dose in 5- to 10-mg increments at weekly intervals. **Maximum:** 30 mg/day. **CHILDREN 3–5 YRS: (AD-**

DERALL): Initially, 2.5 mg/day given every morning. May increase daily dose in 2.5-mg increments at weekly intervals until optimal response is obtained. **Maximum:** 40 mg/day given in 1–3 divided doses (use intervals of 4–6 hrs between additional doses). Not recommended in children younger than 3 yrs.

SIDE EFFECTS

Frequent: Increased motor activity, talkativeness, nervousness, mild euphoria, insomnia. **Occasional:** Headache, chills, dry mouth, GI distress, worsening depression in pts who are clinically depressed, tachycardia, palpitations, chest pain, dizziness, decreased appetite.

ADVERSE EFFECTS/ TOXIC REACTIONS

Overdose may produce skin pallor/flushing, arrhythmias, psychosis. Abrupt withdrawal after prolonged use of high doses may produce lethargy (may last for wks). Prolonged administration to children with ADHD may temporarily suppress normal weight/height pattern.

NURSING CONSIDERATIONS

BASELINE ASSESSMENT

Assess child's attention span, impulse control, interaction with others.

INTERVENTION/EVALUATION

Monitor for CNS overstimulation, increase in B/P, growth rate, change in pulse rate, respirations, weight loss. **Narolepsy:** Observe/document frequency of narcoleptic episodes. **ADHD:** Observe for improved attention span.

PATIENT/FAMILY TEACHING

• Normal dosage levels may produce tolerance to drug's anorexic mood-elevating effects within a few wks. • Avoid tasks that require alertness, motor skills until response to drug is established. • Dry mouth may be relieved with sugarless gum, sips of tepid water. • Take early in day. • May mask extreme fatigue. • Report pronounced anxiety, dizziness, decreased appetite, dry mouth, new or worsening behavior, chest pain, palpitations. • Avoid large amounts of caffeine.

DHEA

Also known as prasterone.

◆CLASSIFICATION

HERBAL: See Appendix G.

ACTION

Produced in adrenal glands, liver; metabolized to androstenedione, major precursor to androgens and estrogens. Also produced in CNS, concentrated in limbic regions; may function as excitatory neuroregulator. **Effect:** Androgen, estrogen-like hormonal effects may be responsible for DHEA benefits.

USES

Increases strength, energy, muscle mass; stimulates immune system; improves cognitive function and memory; improves depressed mood/fatigue in HIV pts. Treatment of atherosclerosis, hyperglycemia, cancer; prevention of osteoporosis; increases bone mineral density.

PRECAUTIONS

Contraindications: None known. **Cautions:** May increase risk of prostate, breast, hormone-sensitive cancers. Avoid use in those with breast, uterine, ovarian cancer; endometriosis; uterine fibroids; diabetes (can increase insulin resistance/sensitivity); depression (may increase risk of adverse psychiatric effects).

LIFESPAN CONSIDERATIONS

Pregnancy/Lactation: May adversely affect pregnancy by increasing androgen levels; avoid use. **Children:** Safety and efficacy not established. **Elderly:** Age-related hepatic impairment may require dosage adjustment.

INTERACTIONS

DRUG: May interfere with **estrogen/androgen therapy.** May increase **triazolam** concentration. **HERBAL:** None significant. **FOOD:** None known. **LAB VALUES:** None significant.

AVAILABILITY (OTC)

Capsules: 25 mg. **Tablets:** 25 mg.

INDICATIONS/ROUTES/DOSAGE

Depression

PO: ADULTS, ELDERLY: 30–90 mg/day.

Usual Adult Dosage

PO: ADULTS, ELDERLY: 25–50 mg/day.

SIDE EFFECTS

Acne, hair loss, hirsutism, voice deepening, insulin resistance, altered menstrual cycle, hypertension, abdominal pain, fatigue, headache, nasal congestion.

ADVERSE EFFECTS/ TOXIC REACTIONS

None known.

NURSING CONSIDERATIONS

BASELINE ASSESSMENT

Assess for hormone-sensitive tumors (may stimulate growth). Avoid use of hormone replacement therapy.

INTERVENTION/EVALUATION

Assess changes in mood, sleep pattern. Monitor changes in aggressiveness, irritability, restlessness.

PATIENT/FAMILY TEACHING

- Avoid use in pregnancy/lactation; concurrent hormone replacement therapy.
- Lower dosage if acne develops.

Diabeta, *see glyburide*

diazepam

dye-**az**-e-pam

(Apo-Diazepam ✱, Diastat, Diazemuls ✱, Diazepam Intensol, Novo-Dipam ✱, Valium)

Do not confuse diazepam with diazoxide, diltiazem, Ditropan, or lorazepam, or Valium with Valcyte.

◆CLASSIFICATION

PHARMACOTHERAPEUTIC: Benzodiazepine **(Schedule IV). CLINICAL:** Anti-anxiety, skeletal muscle relaxant, anti-convulsant (see pp. 13C, 153C).

ACTION

Depresses all levels of CNS by enhancing action of gamma-aminobutyric acid, a major inhibitory neurotransmitter in the brain. **Therapeutic Effect:** Produces anxiolytic effect, elevates seizure threshold, produces skeletal muscle relaxation.

PHARMACOKINETICS

Well absorbed from GI tract. Widely distributed. Protein binding: 98%. Metabolized in liver to active metabolite. Excreted in urine. Minimally removed by hemodialysis. **Half-life:** 20–70 hrs (increased in hepatic dysfunction, elderly).

USES

Short-term relief of anxiety symptoms, relief of acute alcohol withdrawal. Adjunct for relief of acute musculoskeletal conditions, treatment of seizures (IV route used for termination of status epilepticus). **Gel:** Control of increased seizure activity in refractory epilepsy in those on stable regimens. **OFF-LABEL:** Treatment of panic disorder, tension headache, tremors.

PRECAUTIONS

Contraindications: Angle-closure glaucoma, coma, preexisting CNS depression, respiratory depression, severe, uncontrolled pain. **Cautions:** Those receiving other CNS depressants, renal/hepatic impairment, hypoalbuminemia.

LIFESPAN CONSIDERATIONS

Pregnancy/Lactation: Crosses placenta. Distributed in breast milk. May increase risk of fetal abnormalities if administered during first trimester of pregnancy. Chronic ingestion during pregnancy may produce withdrawal symptoms, CNS depression in neonates. **Pregnancy Category D. Children/Elderly:** Use small initial doses with gradual increases to avoid ataxia, excessive sedation.

INTERACTIONS

DRUG: Alcohol, CNS depressants may increase CNS depression. **Fluvoxamine, itraconazole, ketoconazole** may increase concentration/toxicity. **HERBAL: Gotu kola, kava kava, St. John's wort, valerian** may increase CNS depression. **FOOD:** None known. **LAB VALUES:** None significant. **Therapeutic serum level:** 0.5–2 mcg/ml; **toxic serum level:** greater than 3 mcg/ml.

AVAILABILITY (Rx)

Injection, Solution: 5 mg/ml. **Oral Concentrate (Diazepam Intensol):** 5 mg/ml. **Oral Solution:** 5 mg/5 ml. **Rectal Gel (Diastat):** 5 mg/ml. **Tablet (Valium):** 2 mg, 5 mg, 10 mg.

ADMINISTRATION/HANDLING

IV

Rate of administration • Give by IV push into tubing of flowing IV solution as close as possible to vein insertion point. • Administer directly into large vein (reduces risk of thrombosis/phlebitis). Do not use small veins (e.g., wrist/dorsum of hand). • Administer IV at rate not exceeding 5 mg/min. For children, give over a 3-min period (too-rapid IV may result in hypotension, respiratory depression). • Monitor respirations q5–15min for 2 hrs.
Storage • Store at room temperature.

IM

• Injection may be painful. Inject deeply into deltoid muscle.

PO

• Give without regard to meals. • Dilute oral concentrate with water, juice, carbonated beverages; may be mixed in semisolid food (applesauce, pudding). • Tablets may be crushed.

IV INCOMPATIBILITIES

Amphotericin B complex (Abelcet, AmBisome, Amphotec), cefepime (Maxipime), diltiazem (Cardizem), fluconazole (Diflucan), foscarnet (Foscavir), furosemide (Lasix), heparin, hydrocortisone (Solu-Cortef), hydromorphone (Dilaudid), meropenem (Merrem IV), potassium chloride, propofol (Diprivan), vitamins.

IV COMPATIBILITIES

Dobutamine (Dobutrex), fentanyl, morphine.

INDICATIONS/ROUTES/DOSAGE

Anxiety

PO: ADULTS: 2–10 mg 2–4 times a day. **ELDERLY:** Initially, 1–2 mg 1–2 times a day.
IV, IM: ADULTS: 2–10 mg, may repeat in 3–4 hrs if needed.

Skeletal Muscle Relaxation

PO: ADULTS: 2–10 mg 2–4 times a day. **ELDERLY:** Initially, 1–2 mg 1–2 times a day. **CHILDREN:** 0.12–0.8 mg/kg/day in divided doses q6–8h.
IV, IM: ADULTS: 2–10 mg repeated in 3–4 hrs. **CHILDREN:** 0.04–0.3 mg/kg/dose q2–4h. **Maximum:** 0.6 mg/kg in an 8-hr period.

Alcohol Withdrawal

PO: ADULTS, ELDERLY: 10 mg 3–4 times during first 24 hrs, then reduced to 5 mg 3–4 times a day as needed.
IV, IM: ADULTS, ELDERLY: Initially, 10 mg, followed by 5–10 mg q3–4h.

Status Epilepticus

IV: ADULTS, ELDERLY: 5–10 mg q5–10min. **Maximum:** 30 mg. **CHILDREN 5 YRS AND OLDER:** 1 mg q2–5min up to maximum total dose of 10 mg; may be repeated in 2–4 hrs if needed. **CHILDREN 1 MO TO 5 YRS:**

0.2–0.5 mg q2–5min up to maximum total dose of 5 mg; may be repeated in 2–4 hrs if needed.

Control of Increased Seizure Activity (Breakthrough Seizures) in Pts with Refractory Epilepsy Who Are on Stable Regimens of Anticonvulsants

RECTAL GEL: ADULTS, CHILDREN 12 YRS AND OLDER: 0.2 mg/kg; may be repeated in 4–12 hrs. **CHILDREN 6–11 YRS:** 0.3 mg/kg; may be repeated in 4–12 hrs. **CHILDREN 2–5 YRS:** 0.5 mg/kg; may be repeated in 4–12 hrs.

SIDE EFFECTS

Frequent: Pain with IM injection, drowsiness, fatigue, ataxia. **Occasional:** Slurred speech, orthostatic hypotension, headache, hypoactivity, constipation, nausea, blurred vision. **Rare:** Paradoxical CNS reactions (hyperactivity/nervousness in children, excitement/restlessness in elderly/debilitated) generally noted during first 2 wks of therapy, particularly in presence of uncontrolled pain.

ADVERSE EFFECTS/ TOXIC REACTIONS

IV route may produce pain, swelling, thrombophlebitis, carpal tunnel syndrome. Abrupt or too-rapid withdrawal may result in pronounced restlessness, irritability, insomnia, hand tremor, abdominal/muscle cramps, diaphoresis, vomiting, seizures. Abrupt withdrawal in pts with epilepsy may produce increase in frequency/severity of seizures. Overdose results in drowsiness, confusion, diminished reflexes, CNS depression, coma. **Antidote:** Flumazenil (see Appendix M for dosage).

NURSING CONSIDERATIONS

BASELINE ASSESSMENT

Assess B/P, pulse, respirations immediately before administration. **Anxiety:** Assess autonomic response (cold, clammy hands, diaphoresis), motor response (agitation, trembling, tension). **Musculoskeletal spasm:** Record onset, type, location, duration of pain. Check for immobility, stiffness, swelling. **Seizures:** Review history of seizure disorder (length, intensity, frequency, duration, LOC). Observe frequently for recurrence of seizure activity. Initiate seizure precautions.

INTERVENTION/EVALUATION

Monitor heart rate, respiratory rate, B/P, mental status. Assess children, elderly for paradoxical reaction, particularly during early therapy. Evaluate for therapeutic response (decrease in intensity/frequency of seizures; calm, facial expression, decreased restlessness; decreased intensity of skeletal muscle pain). **Therapeutic serum level:** 0.5–2 mcg/ml; **toxic serum level:** greater than 3 mcg/ml.

PATIENT/FAMILY TEACHING

• Avoid alcohol. • Limit caffeine. • May cause drowsiness. • Avoid tasks that require alertness, motor skills until response to drug is established. • May be habit forming. • Avoid abrupt discontinuation after prolonged use.

diclofenac

dye-**klo**-feh-nak
(Apo-Diclo ✦, Cambia, Cataflam, Flector, Novo-Difenac ✦, Pennsaid, Solaraze, Voltaren, Voltaren Gel, Voltaren Ophthalmic, Voltaren XR, Zipsor)

BLACK BOX ALERT Increased risk of serious cardiovascular thrombotic events, including myocardial infarction, CVA. Increased risk of severe GI reactions, including ulceration, bleeding, perforation of stomach, intestines.

Do not confuse Cataflam with Catapres, diclofenac with Diflucan or Duphalac, or Voltaren with tramadol, Ultram, or Verelan.

FIXED-COMBINATION(S)

Arthrotec: diclofenac/misoprostol (an antisecretory gastric protectant): 50 mg/200 mcg, 75 mg/200 mcg.

CLASSIFICATION

PHARMACOTHERAPEUTIC: Nonsteroidal anti-inflammatory. **CLINICAL:** Analgesic, anti-inflammatory (see p. 127C).

ACTION

Inhibits prostaglandin synthesis, intensity of pain stimulus reaching sensory nerve endings. Constricts iris sphincter. **Therapeutic Effect:** Produces analgesic, anti-inflammatory effects. Prevents miosis during cataract surgery.

PHARMACOKINETICS

Route	Onset	Peak	Duration
PO	30 min	2–3 hrs	Up to 8 hrs

Completely absorbed from GI tract; penetrates cornea after ophthalmic administration (may be systemically absorbed). Protein binding: greater than 99%. Widely distributed. Metabolized in liver. Primarily excreted in urine. Minimally removed by hemodialysis. **Half-life:** 1.2–2 hrs.

USES

PO: (Immediate-release): Treatment of rheumatoid arthritis, osteoarthritis, ankylosing spondylitis, primary dysmenorrhea. **(Zipsor):** Mild to moderate pain. **(Delayed-release):** Treatment of rheumatoid arthritis, osteoarthritis, ankylosing spondylitis. **(Extended-release):** Treatment of rheumatoid arthritis, osteoarthritis. **Oral Solution (Cambia):** Treatment of migraine. **Topical Patch:** Treatment of acute pain due to minor strains, sprains, contusions. **Ophthalmic:** Treatment of photophobia, pain in pts undergoing corneal refractive surgery. **Topical Gel (3%):** Treatment of actinic keratoses. **(1%):** Treatment of osteoarthritis, joint pain (e.g., ankle, elbow, wrist). **Topical Solution:** Treatment of pain associated with osteoarthritis of knee. **OFF-LABEL:** Treatment of vascular headaches (PO); reduce occurrence/severity of cystoid macular edema after cataract surgery (ophthalmic form); treatment of juvenile rheumatoid arthritis.

PRECAUTIONS

Contraindications: Hypersensitivity to aspirin, diclofenac, other NSAIDs; porphyria. **Cautions:** CHF, hypertension, renal/hepatic impairment, history of GI disease. Avoid topical gel in open skin wounds, infections, exfoliative dermatitis, eyes, neonates, infants, children.

LIFESPAN CONSIDERATIONS

Pregnancy/Lactation: Crosses placenta. Unknown if distributed in breast milk. Avoid use during third trimester (may adversely affect fetal cardiovascular system: premature closure of ductus arteriosus). **Pregnancy Category B (D if used in third trimester or near delivery; C for ophthalmic solution). Children:** Safety and efficacy not established. **Elderly:** GI bleeding, ulceration more likely to cause serious adverse effects. Age-related renal impairment may increase risk of hepatic/renal toxicity; reduced dosage recommended.

INTERACTIONS

DRUG: May decrease effects of **antihypertensives, diuretics. Aspirin, other salicylates** may increase risk of GI side effects/bleeding. **Bone marrow depressants** may increase risk of hematologic reactions. May increase effects of **heparin, oral anticoagulants, thrombolytics.** May increase serum **lithium** concentration/toxicity. May increase risk of **methotrexate** toxicity. **Probenecid** may increase concentration. **Ophthalmic:** May decrease antiglaucoma effects of **antiglaucoma agents, epinephrine.** May decrease effects of **acetylcholine, carbachol.** **HERBAL:** **Cat's claw, dong quai, evening primrose, garlic, ginseng** may increase antiplatelet activity. **FOOD:** None known. **LAB VALUES:** May increase urine protein, BUN, serum alkaline phosphatase, creatinine, LDH, potassium, AST, ALT. May decrease serum uric acid.

AVAILABILITY (Rx)

Adhesive Patch (Flector): 10×14 cm patch containing 180 mg diclofenac.

Capsules (Zipsor): 25 mg. **Ophthalmic Solution (Voltaren Ophthalmic):** 0.1%. **Oral Solution (Cambia):** 50-mg packets. **Tablets (Cataflam):** 50 mg. **Topical Gel (Solaraze):** 3%. **(Voltaren Gel):** 1%. **Topical Solution (Pennsaid):** 1.5%.

Tablets (Delayed-Release [Voltaren]): 25 mg, 50 mg, 75 mg. **Tablets (Extended-Release [Voltaren XR]):** 100 mg.

ADMINISTRATION/HANDLING

PO

• Do not crush, break enteric-coated tablets. • May give with food, milk, antacids if GI distress occurs. • Cambia: Mix one packet in 1–2 oz water, stir well, and instruct pt to drink immediately.

Ophthalmic

• Place finger on lower eyelid and pull out until pocket is formed between eye and lower lid. • Place prescribed number of drops in pocket. • Instruct pt to close eye gently for 1–2 min (so medication will not be squeezed out of the sac) and to apply digital pressure to lacrimal sac for 1 min to minimize system absorption. • Remove excess solution with tissue.

Topical Solution

• Apply only to clean, dry skin. • Squeeze 10 drops into hand or directly onto knee. • Spread evenly onto knee (front, back, sides). • Repeat until 40 drops applied and knee completely covered.

Topical Gel

• Do not apply to eyes, mucous membranes, open wounds. • Avoid sunlight exposure to treated areas.

Transdermal Patch

• Apply to intact skin; avoid contact with eyes. • Do not wear when bathing/showering. • Wash hands after handling.

INDICATIONS/ROUTES/DOSAGE

Osteoarthritis

PO (CATAFLAM, VOLTAREN): ADULTS, ELDERLY: 50 mg 2–3 times a day.

PO (VOLTAREN XR): ADULTS, ELDERLY: 100–200 mg/day as a single dose.

TOPICAL (VOLTAREN GEL): 2–4 g 4 times a day. **Maximum:** (upper extremities): 8g per joint per day. (lower extremities): 16 g per joint per day.

TOPICAL (PENNSAID): 40 drops to knee 4 times/day.

Rheumatoid Arthritis (RA)

PO (CATAFLAM, VOLTAREN): ADULTS, ELDERLY: 50 mg 2–4 times a day. **Maximum:** 225 mg/day.

PO (VOLTAREN XR): ADULTS, ELDERLY: 100 mg once a day. **Maximum:** 100 mg twice a day.

Ankylosing Spondylitis

PO (VOLTAREN): ADULTS, ELDERLY: 100–125 mg/day in 4–5 divided doses.

Analgesia, Primary Dysmenorrhea

PO (CATAFLAM): ADULTS, ELDERLY: 50 mg 3 times a day.

Acute Pain

TOPICAL PATCH (FLECTOR): ADULTS, ELDERLY: Apply 2 times a day.

Mild–Moderate Pain

PO: ADULTS, ELDERLY: 25 mg 4 times a day.

Migraine

PO: ADULTS, ELDERLY: 50 mg once.

Usual Pediatric Dosage

CHILDREN: 2–3 mg/kg/day in 2–4 divided doses.

Actinic Keratoses

TOPICAL (SOLARAZE): ADULTS, ADOLESCENTS: Apply twice a day to lesion for 60–90 days.

Cataract Surgery

OPHTHALMIC: ADULTS, ELDERLY: Apply 1 drop to eye 4 times a day commencing 24 hrs after cataract surgery. Continue for 2 wks afterward.

Pain, Relief of Photophobia in Pts Undergoing Corneal Refractive Surgery
OPHTHALMIC: ADULTS, ELDERLY: Apply 1–2 drops to affected eye 1 hr before surgery, within 15 min after surgery, then 4 times a day for up to 3 days.

SIDE EFFECTS

Frequent (9%–4%): PO: Headache, abdominal cramps, constipation, diarrhea, nausea, dyspepsia. **Ophthalmic:** Burning, stinging on instillation, ocular discomfort. **Occasional (3%–1%): PO:** Flatulence, dizziness, epigastric pain. **Ophthalmic:** Ocular itching, tearing. **Rare (less than 1%): PO:** Rash, peripheral edema, fluid retention, visual disturbances, vomiting, drowsiness.

ADVERSE EFFECTS/ TOXIC REACTIONS

Overdose may result in acute renal failure. In those treated chronically, peptic ulcer, GI bleeding, gastritis, severe hepatic reaction (jaundice), nephrotoxicity (hematuria, dysuria, proteinuria), severe hypersensitivity reaction (bronchospasm, angioedema) occur rarely.

NURSING CONSIDERATIONS

BASELINE ASSESSMENT

Anti-inflammatory: Assess onset, type, location, duration of pain, inflammation. Inspect appearance of affected joints for immobility, deformities, skin condition.

INTERVENTION/EVALUATION

Monitor CBC, hepatic/renal function tests, urine output, occult blood test. Monitor for headache, dyspepsia. Monitor daily pattern of bowel activity and stool consistency. Assess for therapeutic response: relief of pain, stiffness, swelling; increased joint mobility; reduced joint tenderness; improved grip strength.

PATIENT/FAMILY TEACHING

• Swallow tablet whole; do not crush, chew. • Avoid aspirin, alcohol during therapy (increases risk of GI bleeding). • If GI upset occurs, take with food, milk. • Report skin rash, itching, weight gain, changes in vision, black stools, bleeding, jaundice, upper quadrant pain, persistent headache. • **Ophthalmic:** Do not use hydrogel soft contact lenses. • **Topical:** Avoid exposure to sunlight, sun lamps. • Inform physician if rash occurs.

dicyclomine

dye-**sye**-kloe-meen
(Bentyl, Bentylol ✱, Formulex ✱, Lomine ✱)
Do not confuse Bentyl with Aventyl, Benadryl, Proventil, or Trental, or dicyclomine with diphenhydramine or doxycycline.

◆ CLASSIFICATION

CLINICAL: GI antispasmodic, anticholinergic.

ACTION

Directly acts as smooth muscle relaxant. **Therapeutic Effect:** Reduces tone, motility of GI tract.

PHARMACOKINETICS

Readily absorbed from GI tract. Widely distributed. Metabolized in liver. **Half-life:** 9–10 hrs.

USES

Treatment of functional disturbances of GI motility (e.g., irritable bowel syndrome). **OFF-LABEL:** Urinary incontinence.

PRECAUTIONS

Contraindications: Bladder neck obstruction due to prostatic hyperplasia, coronary vasospasm, intestinal atony, myasthenia gravis in pts not treated with neostigmine, narrow-angle glaucoma, obstructive disease of GI tract, paralytic ileus, severe ulcerative colitis, tachycardia secondary to cardiac insufficiency/ thyrotoxicosis, toxic megacolon, unstable cardiovascular status in acute hemorrhage. **Extreme Caution:** Autonomic neuropathy, known/suspected GI infections, diarrhea, mild to moderate ulcerative colitis. **Cautions:** Hyperthyroidism, hepatic/renal disease, hypertension, tachyarrhythmias, CHF, coronary artery disease, gastric ulcer, esophageal reflux/hiatal hernia associated with reflux esophagitis, infants, elderly, COPD.

D

⌛ LIFESPAN CONSIDERATIONS

Pregnancy/Lactation: Unknown if drug crosses placenta or is distributed in breast milk. **Pregnancy Category B. Children:** Infants, young children more susceptible to toxic effects. **Elderly:** May cause excitement, agitation, drowsiness, confusion.

INTERACTIONS

DRUG: **Antacids, antidiarrheals** may decrease absorption. May decrease absorption of **ketoconazole. Other anticholinergics** may increase effects. **Potassium chloride** may increase severity of GI lesions with wax matrix formulation. **HERBAL:** None significant. **FOOD:** None known. **LAB VALUES:** None significant.

AVAILABILITY (Rx)

Capsules (Bentyl): 10 mg. **Injection Solution (Bentyl):** 10 mg/ml. **Syrup (Bentyl):** 10 mg/5 ml. **Tablets (Bentyl):** 20 mg.

ADMINISTRATION/HANDLING

• Store capsules, tablets, syrup, parenteral form at room temperature • Administer 30 mins before food.

IM

• Injection should appear colorless.
• Do not administer IV or subcutaneous.
• Inject deep into large muscle mass.
• Do not give for longer than 2 days.

PO

• Dilute oral solution with equal volume of water just before administration.
• May give without regard to meals (food may slightly decrease absorption).

INDICATIONS/ROUTES/DOSAGE

Functional Disturbances of GI Motility

PO: ADULTS: 10–20 mg 3–4 times a day up to 40 mg 4 times a day. **ELDERLY:** 10–20 mg 4 times a day. May increase up to 160 mg/day. **CHILDREN OLDER THAN 2 YRS:** 10 mg 3–4 times a day. **CHILDREN 6 MOS–2 YRS:** 5 mg 3–4 times a day.
IM: ADULTS: 20 mg q4–6h.

SIDE EFFECTS

Frequent: Dry mouth (sometimes severe), constipation, diminished sweating ability. **Occasional:** Blurred vision; photophobia; urinary hesitancy; drowsiness (with high dosage); agitation, excitement, confusion, drowsiness noted in elderly (even with low dosages); transient light-headedness (with IM route), irritation at injection site (with IM route). **Rare:** Confusion, hypersensitivity reaction, increased intraocular pressure, nausea, vomiting, unusual fatigue.

ADVERSE EFFECTS/ TOXIC REACTIONS

Overdose may produce temporary paralysis of ciliary muscle; pupillary dilation; tachycardia; palpitations; hot/dry/flushed skin; absence of bowel sounds; hyperthermia; increased respiratory rate; EKG abnormalities; nausea; vomiting; rash over face/upper trunk; CNS stimulation, psychosis (agitation, restlessness, rambling speech, visual hallucinations, paranoid behavior, delusions) followed by depression.

NURSING CONSIDERATIONS

BASELINE ASSESSMENT

Assess symptoms of irritable bowel syndrome (abdominal cramping, bloating, excessive flatus).

INTERVENTION/EVALUATION

Monitor daily pattern of bowel activity and stool consistency. Monitor I/O. Assess for urinary retention. Monitor changes in B/P, temperature. Be alert for fever (increased risk of hyperthermia). Assess skin turgor, mucous membranes to evaluate hydration status (encourage adequate fluid intake), bowel sounds for peristalsis.

PATIENT/FAMILY TEACHING

• Do not become overheated during exercise in hot weather (may result in heat stroke). • Avoid hot baths, saunas. • Avoid tasks that require alertness, motor skills until response to drug is established. • Do not take antacids or antidiarrheals within 1 hr of taking dicyclomine (decreased effectiveness).

didanosine

dye-**dan**-o-seen
(Videx, Videx-EC)

BLACK BOX ALERT Pancreatitis, sometimes fatal, has been reported. Serious, sometimes fatal, hypersensitivity reactions, lactic acidosis, severe hepatomegaly with steatosis (fatty liver) have occurred.

Do not confuse Videx with Lidex.

◆ CLASSIFICATION

PHARMACOTHERAPEUTIC: Purine nucleoside analogue. **CLINICAL:** Antiviral (see pp. 68C, 114C).

ACTION

Intracellularly converted into triphosphate, which interferes with RNA-directed DNA polymerase (reverse transcriptase). **Therapeutic Effect:** Inhibits replication of retroviruses, including HIV.

PHARMACOKINETICS

Variably absorbed from GI tract. Protein binding: less than 5%. Rapidly metabolized intracellularly to active form. Primarily excreted in urine. Partially (20%) removed by hemodialysis. **Half-life:** 1.5 hrs; metabolite, 8–24 hrs.

USES

Treatment of HIV infection in combination with other antiretroviral agents.

PRECAUTIONS

Contraindications: Hypersensitivity to didanosine or any of its components. **Cautions:** Renal/hepatic impairment, alcoholism, elevated triglycerides, T-cell counts less than 100 cells/mm^3; extreme caution with history of pancreatitis. Phenylketonuria, sodium-restricted diets due to phenylalanine, sodium content of preparations.

LIFESPAN CONSIDERATIONS

Pregnancy/Lactation: Use during pregnancy only if clearly needed. Breast-feeding not recommended. **Pregnancy Category B.** **Children:** Well tolerated in those older than 3 mos. **Elderly:** Age-related renal impairment may require dosage adjustment.

INTERACTIONS

DRUG: May decrease absorption of **dapsone, fluoroquinolones, itraconazole, ketoconazole, tetracyclines. Medications producing pancreatitis or peripheral neuropathy** may increase risk of pancreatitis, peripheral neuropathy. **Stavudine** may increase risk of fatal lactic acidosis in pregnancy. **HERBAL:** None significant. **FOOD: All foods** decrease absorption. **LAB VALUES:** May increase serum alkaline phosphatase, amylase, bilirubin, lipase, triglycerides, AST, ALT, uric acid. May decrease serum potassium, WBC, CBC.

AVAILABILITY (Rx)

◀ALERT▶ Chewable/dispersible buffered tablets not available in United States. **Pediatric Powder for Oral Solution (Videx):** 2 g, 4 g (makes 10 mg/ml after final mixing).

Capsules (Delayed-Release): (Videx EC): 125 mg, 200 mg, 250 mg, 400 mg.

ADMINISTRATION/HANDLING

PO

• Store at room temperature. • Administer oral solution or tablets 30 min before or 2 hrs after a meal. • Pediatric powder for oral solution, following reconstitution as directed, is stable for 30 days if refrig-

D

erated. • **Powder for oral solution:** Add 100–200 ml water to 2 or 4 g, respectively, to provide concentration of 20 mg/ml. Immediately mix with equal amount of antacid to provide concentration of 10 mg/ml. Shake thoroughly before removing each dose. • **Enteric-coated capsules:** Swallow whole; do not break, open, chew, capsules.

INDICATIONS/ROUTES/DOSAGE

HIV Infection

PO (DELAYED-RELEASE CAPSULES): ADULTS, CHILDREN 13 YRS AND OLDER, WEIGHING 60 KG OR MORE: 400 mg once a day. **ADULTS, CHILDREN 13 YRS AND OLDER, WEIGHING 25 KG TO LESS THAN 60 KG:** 250 mg once a day. **WEIGHING 20 KG TO LESS THAN 25 KG:** 200 mg once a day.

PO (ORAL SOLUTION): ADULTS, CHILDREN 13 YRS AND OLDER WEIGHING 60 KG OR MORE: 200 mg q12h or 400 mg once a day. **ADULTS, CHILDREN 13 YRS AND OLDER, WEIGHING LESS THAN 60 KG:** 125 mg q12h or 250 mg once a day. **CHILDREN 8 MOS–12 YRS:** 90–150 mg/m^2 2 times a day. **CHILDREN YOUNGER THAN 8 MOS:** 100 mg/m^2 2 times a day.

Dosage in Renal Impairment

Pts weighing less than 60 kg:

Creatinine Clearance	Oral Solution	Delayed-Release Capsules
30–59 ml/min	75 mg twice a day (or 150 mg once a day)	125 mg once a day
10–29 ml/min	100 mg once a day	125 mg once a day
Less than 10 ml/min	75 mg once a day	N/A

Pts weighing 60 kg or more:

Creatinine Clearance	Oral Solution	Delayed-Release Capsules
30–59 ml/min	100 mg twice a day (or 200 mg once a day)	200 mg once a day
10–29 ml/min	150 mg once a day	125 mg once a day
Less than 10 ml/min	100 mg once a day	125 mg once a day

SIDE EFFECTS

Frequent: **Adults (greater than 10%):** Diarrhea, neuropathy, chills, fever. **Children (greater than 25%):** Chills, fever, decreased appetite, pain, malaise, nausea, vomiting, diarrhea, abdominal pain, headache, nervousness, cough, rhinitis, dyspnea, asthenia (loss of strength, energy), rash, pruritus. Occasional: **Adults (9%–2%):** Rash, pruritus, headache, abdominal pain, nausea, vomiting, pneumonia, myopathy, decreased appetite, dry mouth, dyspnea. **Children (25%–10%):** Failure to thrive, weight loss, stomatitis, oral thrush, ecchymosis, arthritis, myalgia, insomnia, epistaxis, pharyngitis.

ADVERSE EFFECTS/ TOXIC REACTIONS

Pneumonia, opportunistic infections occur occasionally. Peripheral neuropathy, potentially fatal pancreatitis are major toxic effects.

NURSING CONSIDERATIONS

BASELINE ASSESSMENT

Obtain baseline values for CBC, serum renal/hepatic function tests, vital signs, weight.

INTERVENTION/EVALUATION

In event of abdominal pain, nausea, vomiting, elevated serum amylase, triglycerides, contact physician before administering medication (potential for pancreatitis). Be alert to sensation of burning feet, "restless leg syndrome" (unable to find comfortable position for legs or feet), lack of coordination, other signs of peripheral neuropathy. Monitor daily pattern of bowel activity and stool consistency. Check skin for rash, eruptions. Monitor serum electrolytes, CBC, glucose, renal/hepatic function tests, Hgb, platelet count. Assess for opportunistic infections (onset of fever, oral mucosa changes, cough, other respiratory symptoms). Check weight at least twice per wk. Assess for visual, auditory difficulty; provide protection from light if photophobia develops.

PATIENT/FAMILY TEACHING

• Avoid alcohol. • Inform physician if numbness, tingling, persistent severe abdominal pain, nausea, vomiting, change in vision occur. • Shake oral suspension well before use, keep refrigerated. • Discard solution after 30 days, obtain new supply.

Diflucan, *see fluconazole*

Digitek, *see digoxin*

digoxin HIGH ALERT

di-**jox**-in
(Apo-Digoxin ✤, Digitek, Lanoxin)
Do not confuse digoxin with Desoxyn or doxepin, or Lanoxin with Lasix, Levoxyl, Levsinex, Lonox, or Mefoxin.

◆CLASSIFICATION

PHARMACOTHERAPEUTIC: Cardiac glycoside. **CLINICAL:** Antiarrhythmic, cardiotonic.

ACTION

Increases influx of calcium from extracellular to intracellular cytoplasm. **Therapeutic Effect:** Potentiates activity of contractile cardiac muscle fibers, increases force of myocardial contraction. Slows the heart rate by decreasing conduction through SA, AV nodes.

PHARMACOKINETICS

Route	Onset	Peak	Duration
PO	0.5–2 hrs	2–8 hrs	3–4 days
IV	5–30 min	1–4 hrs	3–4 days

Readily absorbed from GI tract. Widely distributed. Protein binding: 30%. Partially metabolized in liver. Primarily excreted in urine. Minimally removed by hemodialysis. **Half-life:** 36–48 hrs (increased in renal impairment, elderly).

USES

Prophylactic management/treatment of CHF, control of ventricular rate in pts with atrial fibrillation/atrial flutter. Treatment/prevention of recurrent paroxysmal atrial tachycardia.

PRECAUTIONS

Contraindications: Ventricular fibrillation, ventricular tachycardia unrelated to CHF. **Cautions:** Renal/hepatic impairment, hypokalemia, advanced cardiac disease, acute MI, incomplete AV block, cor pulmonale, hyperthyroidism, hypothyroidism, pulmonary disease, severe bradycardia, sick sinus syndrome, Wolff-Parkinson-White syndrome.

⌛ LIFESPAN CONSIDERATIONS

Pregnancy/Lactation: Crosses placenta. Distributed in breast milk. **Pregnancy Category C. Children:** Premature infants more susceptible to toxicity. **Elderly:** Age-related hepatic/renal impairment may require dosage adjustment. Increased risk of loss of appetite.

INTERACTIONS

DRUG: **Amiodarone** may increase concentration/toxicity. **Beta-blockers, calcium channel blockers** may have additive effect on slowing AV nodal conduction. **Potassium-depleting diuretics** may increase toxicity due to hypokalemia. **Sympathomimetics** may increase risk of arrhythmias. **HERBAL:** **Ephedra** may increase risk of arrhythmias. **Licorice** may cause sodium and water retention, loss of potassium. **FOOD:** **Meals with increased fiber**

(bran) or high in pectin may decrease absorption. LAB VALUES: None significant.

AVAILABILITY (Rx)

Elixir (Lanoxin): 50 mcg/ml. Injection Solution (Lanoxin): 100 mcg/ml, 250 mcg/ml. Tablets (Digitek, Lanoxin): 125 mcg, 250 mcg.

ADMINISTRATION/HANDLING

ALERT IM rarely used (produces severe local irritation, erratic absorption). If no other route possible, give deep into muscle followed by massage. Give no more than 2 ml at any one site.

IV

- May give undiluted or dilute with at least a 4-fold volume of Sterile Water for Injection or D_5W (less may cause precipitate). • Use immediately. • Give IV slowly over at least 5 min.

PO

- May give without regard to meals.
- Tablets may be crushed.

IV INCOMPATIBILITIES

Amphotericin B complex (Abelcet, AmBisome, Amphotec), fluconazole (Diflucan), foscarnet (Foscavir), propofol (Diprivan).

IV COMPATIBILITIES

Cimetidine (Tagamet), diltiazem (Cardizem), furosemide (Lasix), heparin, insulin regular (physically compatible for 3 hrs in 0.9% NaCl. In D_5W, a slight haze develops within 1 hr), lidocaine, lipids, midazolam (Versed), milrinone (Primacor), morphine, potassium chloride.

INDICATIONS/ROUTES/DOSAGE

Loading Dose

PO: ADULTS, ELDERLY: Initially, 0.5–0.75 mg, additional doses of 0.125–0.375 mg at 6- to 8-hr intervals. Range: 0.75–1.5 mg. CHILDREN 10 YRS AND OLDER: 10–15 mcg/kg. CHILDREN 5–9 YRS: 20–35 mcg/kg. CHILDREN 2–4 YRS: 30–40 mcg/kg. CHILDREN 1–23 MOS: 35–60 mcg/kg. NEONATE, FULL-TERM: 25–35 mcg/kg. NEONATE, PREMATURE: 20–30 mcg/kg.

IV: ADULTS, ELDERLY: 0.5–1 mg. CHILDREN 10 YRS AND OLDER: 8–12 mcg/kg. CHILDREN 5–9 YRS: 15–30 mcg/kg. CHILDREN 2–4 YRS: 25–35 mcg/kg. CHILDREN 1–23 MOS: 30–50 mcg/kg. NEONATES, FULL-TERM: 20–30 mcg/kg. NEONATES, PREMATURE: 15–25 mcg/kg.

Maintenance Dosage

	PO	IV/IM
Preterm infant	5–7.5 mcg/kg	4–6 mcg/kg
Full-term infant	6–10 mcg/kg	5–8 mcg/kg
1 mos–2 yrs	10–15 mcg/kg	7.5–12 mcg/kg
2–5 yrs	7.5–10 mcg/kg	6–9 mcg/kg
5–10 yrs	5–10 mcg/kg	4–8 mcg/kg
11–18 yrs	2.5–5 mcg/kg	2–3 mcg/kg
Adults	0.125–0.5 mg	0.1–0.4 mg

Dosage in Renal Impairment

Dosage adjustment is based on creatinine clearance. Total digitalizing dose: decrease by 50% in end-stage renal disease.

Creatinine Clearance	Dosage
10–50 ml/min	25%–75% of usual dose or q36h
Less than 10 ml/min	10%–25% of usual dose or q48h

SIDE EFFECTS

Dizziness, headache, diarrhea, rash, visual disturbances.

ADVERSE EFFECTS/ TOXIC REACTIONS

Most common early manifestations of digoxin toxicity are GI disturbances (anorexia, nausea, vomiting), neurologic abnormalities (fatigue, headache, depression, weakness, drowsiness, confusion, nightmares). Facial pain, personality change, ocular disturbances (photophobia, light flashes, halos around bright objects, yellow or green color perception) may occur. Sinus bradycardia, AV block, ventricular arrhythmias noted. **Antidote:** Digoxin immune FAB (see Appendix M for dosage).

NURSING CONSIDERATIONS

BASELINE ASSESSMENT

Assess apical pulse for 60 sec (30 sec if on maintenance therapy). If pulse is 60 or less/min (70 or less/min for children), withhold drug, contact physician. Blood samples are best taken 6–8 hrs after dose or just before next dose.

INTERVENTION/EVALUATION

Monitor pulse for bradycardia, EKG for arrhythmias for 1–2 hrs after administration (excessive slowing of pulse may be first clinical sign of toxicity). Assess for GI disturbances, neurologic abnormalities (signs of toxicity) q2–4h during loading dose (daily during maintenance). Monitor serum potassium, magnesium, calcium. **Therapeutic serum level:** 0.8–2 ng/ml; **toxic serum level:** greater than 2 ng/ml.

PATIENT/FAMILY TEACHING

• Follow-up visits, blood tests are an important part of therapy. • Follow guidelines to take apical pulse and report pulse 60 or less/min (or as indicated by physician). • Notify physician if any signs of toxicity occur. • Wear/carry identification of digoxin therapy and inform dentist, other physician of taking digoxin. • Do not increase or skip doses. • Do not take OTC medications without consulting physician. • Inform physician of decreased appetite, nausea/vomiting, diarrhea, visual changes.

digoxin immune FAB

di-**jox**-in
(Digibind, DigiFab)
Do not confuse digoxin immune FAB with Desoxyn or doxepin.

◆CLASSIFICATION

CLINICAL: Antidote.

ACTION

Binds molecularly to digoxin in extracellular space. **Therapeutic Effect:** Makes digoxin unavailable for binding at its site of action on cells in the body.

PHARMACOKINETICS

Route	Onset	Peak	Duration
IV	2–30 min	N/A	3–4 days

Widely distributed into extracellular space. Excreted in urine. **Half-life:** 15–20 hrs.

USES

Treatment of potentially life-threatening digoxin toxicity.

PRECAUTIONS

Contraindications: None known. **Cautions:** Cardiac, renal impairment.

LIFESPAN CONSIDERATIONS

Pregnancy/Lactation: Unknown if drug crosses placenta or is distributed in breast milk. **Pregnancy Category C. Children:** No age-related precautions noted. **Elderly:** Age-related renal impairment may require dosage adjustment.

INTERACTIONS

DRUG: None significant. **HERBAL:** None significant. **FOOD:** None known. **LAB VALUES:** May alter serum potassium. Serum digoxin may increase precipitously and persist for up to 1 wk until FAB/digoxin complex is eliminated from body.

AVAILABILITY (Rx)

Injection, Powder for Reconstitution: 38-mg vial (Digibind), 40-mg vial (DigiFab).

ADMINISTRATION/HANDLING

IV

Reconstitution • Reconstitute each 38-mg vial with 4 ml Sterile Water for Injection to provide concentration of 9.5 mg/ml. • Further dilute with 50 ml 0.9% NaCl. **Rate of administration** • Infuse over 30 min (recommended that solution be infused

through a 0.22-micron filter). • If cardiac arrest is imminent, may give IV push.
Storage • Refrigerate vials. • After reconstitution, stable for 4 hrs if refrigerated. • Use immediately after reconstitution.

D

IV INCOMPATIBILITY

None known.

INDICATIONS/ROUTES/DOSAGE

Potentially Life-Threatening Digoxin Overdose

IV: ADULTS, ELDERLY, CHILDREN: Dosage varies according to amount of digoxin to be neutralized. Refer to manufacturer's dosing guidelines.

SIDE EFFECTS

Rare: Allergic reaction.

ADVERSE EFFECTS/ TOXIC REACTIONS

Digoxin toxicity may result in hyperkalemia (diarrhea, paresthesias, heaviness of legs, decreased B/P, cold skin, grayish pallor, hypotension, mental confusion, irritability, flaccid paralysis, tented T waves, widening QRS, ST depression). When effect of digitalis is reversed, hypokalemia may develop rapidly (muscle cramping, nausea, vomiting, hypoactive bowel sounds, abdominal distention, difficulty breathing, postural hypotension). Low cardiac output conditions, CHF occur rarely.

NURSING CONSIDERATIONS

BASELINE ASSESSMENT

Obtain serum digoxin level before administering drug. If drawn less than 6 hrs before last digoxin dose, test result may be unreliable. Those with renal impairment may require more than 1 wk before serum digoxin assay is reliable. Assess muscle strength, mental status.

INTERVENTION/EVALUATION

Closely monitor temperature, B/P, EKG, serum potassium during and after drug is administered. Watch for changes from initial assessment (hypokalemia may result in muscle strength changes, tremor, muscle cramps, altered mental status, cardiac arrhythmias; hyponatremia may result in confusion, thirst, cold/clammy skin).

dihydroergotamine,

See ergotamine

dihydrotachysterol,

See vitamin D

Dilacor XR, *see diltiazem*

Dilantin, *see phenytoin*

Dilaudid, *see hydromorphone*

diltiazem

dil-**tye**-a-zem
(Apo-Diltiaz 🍁, Cardizem, Cardizem CD, Cardizem LA, Cartia XT, Dilacor XR, Dilt-CD, Dilt-XR, Diltia XT, Novo-Diltiazem 🍁, Taztia XT, Tiazac)
Do not confuse Cardizem with Cardene or Cardene SR, Cartia XT with Procardia XL, diltiazem with Calan, diazepam, or Dilantin, or Tiazac with Ziac.

FIXED-COMBINATION(S)

Teczem: diltiazem/enalapril (ACE inhibitor): 180 mg/5 mg.

◆CLASSIFICATION

PHARMACOTHERAPEUTIC: Calcium channel blocker. **CLINICAL:** Antianginal, antihypertensive, antiarrhythmic (see pp. 18C, 77C).

ACTION

Inhibits calcium movement across cardiac, vascular smooth-muscle cell membranes (causes dilation of coronary arteries, peripheral arteries, arterioles). **Therapeutic Effect:** Decreases heart rate, myocardial contractility; slows SA, AV conduction; decreases total peripheral vascular resistance by vasodilation.

PHARMACOKINETICS

Route	Onset	Peak	Duration
PO	0.5–1 hr	N/A	N/A
PO (extended-release)	2–3 hrs	N/A	N/A
IV	3 min	N/A	N/A

Well absorbed from GI tract. Protein binding: 70%–80%. Undergoes first-pass metabolism in liver to active metabolite. Primarily excreted in urine. Not removed by hemodialysis. **Half-life:** 3–8 hrs.

USES

PO: Treatment of angina due to coronary artery spasm (Prinzmetal's variant angina), chronic stable angina (effort-associated angina). **Extended-release:** Treatment of essential hypertension, angina. **Cardizem LA:** Treatment of chronic stable angina. **Parenteral:** Temporary control of rapid ventricular rate in atrial fibrillation/flutter. Rapid conversion of paroxysmal supraventricular tachycardia (PSVT) to normal sinus rhythm. **OFF-LABEL:** Therapy for Duchenne muscular dystrophy, pediatric hypertension.

PRECAUTIONS

Contraindications: Acute MI, pulmonary congestion, hypersensitivity to diltiazem or other calcium channel blockers, second- or third-degree AV block (except in presence of pacemaker), severe hypotension (less than 90 mm Hg, systolic), sick sinus syndrome. **Cautions:** Renal/hepatic impairment, CHF.

LIFESPAN CONSIDERATIONS

Pregnancy/Lactation: Distributed in breast milk. **Pregnancy Category C. Children:** No age-related precautions noted. **Elderly:** Age-related renal impairment may require dosage adjustment.

INTERACTIONS

DRUG: **Beta-blockers** may have additive effect. **Carbamazepine, quinidine, theophylline** may increase concentration, risk of toxicity. May increase serum **digoxin** concentration. **Procainamide, quinidine** may increase risk of QT-interval prolongation. **HERBAL:** **Ephedra** may worsen arrhythmias, hypertension. **Garlic** may increase antihypertensive effect. **Ginseng, yohimbe** may worsen hypertension. **St. John's wort** may decrease concentration. **FOOD:** None known. **LAB VALUES:** May increase PR interval.

AVAILABILITY (Rx)

Injection, Infusion (Ready to Hang): 1 mg/ml. **Injection, Solution:** 5 mg/ml (5 ml, 10 ml, 25 ml). **Tablets, Immediate-Release:** 30 mg, 60 mg, 90 mg, 120 mg.

Capsules, Extended-Release: (Cardizem CD): 120 mg, 180 mg, 240 mg, 300 mg, 360 mg. **(Cartia XT):** 120 mg, 180 mg, 240 mg, 300 mg. **(Dilacor XR, Dilt-XR, Diltia XT):** 120 mg, 180 mg, 240 mg. **(Taztia XT):** 120 mg, 180 mg, 240 mg, 300 mg, 360 mg. **(Tiazac):** 120 mg, 180 mg, 240 mg, 300 mg, 360 mg, 420 mg. **Capsules, Sustained-Release:** 60 mg, 90 mg, 120 mg. **Tablets, Extended-Release: (Cardizem LA):** 120 mg, 180 mg, 240 mg, 300 mg, 360 mg, 420 mg.

ADMINISTRATION/HANDLING

IV

Reconstitution • Add 125 mg to 100 ml D_5W, 0.9% NaCl to provide concentration of 1 mg/ml. Add 250 mg to 250 or 500 ml diluent to provide concentration of 0.83 mg/ml or 0.45 mg/ml, respectively. Maximum concentration: 1.25 g/250 ml (5 mg/ml).

Rate of administration • Infuse per dilution/rate chart provided by manufacturer.

D

Storage • Refrigerate vials. • After dilution, stable for 24 hrs.

PO

• Give immediate-release tablets before meals and at bedtime. • Tablets may be crushed. • Do not open, chew, or crush sustained-release capsules or extended-release capsules or tablets. Swallow whole. • Taztia XT capsules may be opened and mixed with applesauce; follow with glass of water. • Cardizem CD, Cardizem LA, Cartia XT, Dilt-CD may be given without regard to meals. • Dilacor XR, Dilt-XR, Diltia XT to be given on empty stomach.

IV INCOMPATIBILITIES

Acetazolamide (Diamox), acyclovir (Zovirax), aminophylline, ampicillin, ampicillin/sulbactam (Unasyn), cefoperazone (Cefobid), diazepam (Valium), furosemide (Lasix), heparin, insulin, nafcillin, phenytoin (Dilantin), rifampin (Rifadin), sodium bicarbonate.

IV COMPATIBILITIES

Albumin, aztreonam (Azactam), bumetanide (Bumex), cefazolin (Ancef), cefotaxime (Claforan), ceftazidime (Fortaz), ceftriaxone (Rocephin), cefuroxime (Zinacef), cimetidine (Tagamet), ciprofloxacin (Cipro), clindamycin (Cleocin), digoxin (Lanoxin), dobutamine (Dobutrex), dopamine (Intropin), gentamicin (Garamycin), hydromorphone (Dilaudid), lidocaine, lorazepam (Ativan), metoclopramide (Reglan), metronidazole (Flagyl), midazolam (Versed), morphine, multivitamins, nitroglycerin, norepinephrine (Levophed), potassium chloride, potassium phosphate, tobramycin (Nebcin), vancomycin (Vancocin).

INDICATIONS/ROUTES/DOSAGE

Angina

PO (IMMEDIATE-RELEASE) (CARDIZEM): ADULTS, ELDERLY: Initially, 30 mg 4 times a day. Range: 180–360 mg/day.

PO (EXTENDED-RELEASE) (CARDIZEM CD, CARTIA XT, DILACOR XR, DILTIA XT, TIAZAC): ADULTS, ELDERLY: Initially, 120–180 mg/day. **Maximum:** 480 mg/day.

PO (EXTENDED-RELEASE) (CARDIZEM LA): ADULTS, ELDERLY: Initially, 180 mg/day. May increase at 7- to 14-day intervals. **Maximum:** 360 mg/day.

Hypertenison

PO (CARDIZEM CD, CARTIA XT, DILACOR XR, DILTIA XT, TIAZAC): ADULTS, ELDERLY: Initially, 180–240 mg/day. Range: 180–420 mg/day, **Tiazac:** 120–540 mg/day.

PO (SUSTAINED-RELEASE): ADULTS, ELDERLY: Initially, 60–120 mg twice a day. May increase at 14-day intervals. Maintenance: 240–360 mg/day.

PO (CARDIZEM LA): ADULTS, ELDERLY: Initially, 180–240 mg/day. May increase at 14-day intervals. Range: 120–540 mg/day.

Temporary Control of Rapid Ventricular Rate in Atrial Fibrillation/Flutter; Rapid Conversion of Paroxysmal Supraventricular Tachycardia to Normal Sinus Rhythm

IV PUSH: ADULTS, ELDERLY: Initially, 0.25 mg/kg (average dose: 20 mg) actual body weight over 2 min. May repeat in 15 min at dose of 0.35 mg/kg (average dose: 25 mg) actual body weight. Subsequent doses individualized.

IV INFUSION: ADULTS, ELDERLY: After initial bolus injection, may begin infusion at 5–10 mg/hr; may increase by 5 mg/hr up to a maximum of 15 mg/hr. Infusion duration should not exceed 24 hrs.

SIDE EFFECTS

Frequent (10%–5%): Peripheral edema, dizziness, light-headedness, headache, bradycardia, asthenia (loss of strength, energy). **Occasional (5%–2%):** Nausea, constipation, flushing, EKG changes. **Rare (less than 2%):** Rash, micturition disorder (polyuria, nocturia, dysuria, frequency of urination), abdominal discomfort, drowsiness.

ADVERSE EFFECTS/ TOXIC REACTIONS

Abrupt withdrawal may increase frequency, duration of angina, CHF, second-

and third-degree AV block occur rarely. Overdose produces nausea, drowsiness, confusion, slurred speech, profound bradycardia. **Antidote:** Glucagon (see Appendix M for dosage).

NURSING CONSIDERATIONS

BASELINE ASSESSMENT

Record onset, type (sharp, dull, squeezing), radiation, location, intensity, duration of anginal pain, precipitating factors (exertion, emotional stress). Assess baseline renal/hepatic function tests. Assess B/P, apical pulse immediately before drug is administered.

INTERVENTION/EVALUATION

Assist with ambulation if dizziness occurs. Assess for peripheral edema behind medial malleolus (sacral area in bedridden pts). Monitor pulse rate for bradycardia. Assess B/P, renal/hepatic function tests, EKG with IV therapy. Question for asthenia, headache.

PATIENT/FAMILY TEACHING

• Do not abruptly discontinue medication. • Compliance with therapy regimen is essential to control anginal pain. • To avoid hypotensive effect, rise slowly from lying to sitting position, wait momentarily before standing. • Avoid tasks that require alertness, motor skills until response to drug is established. • Contact physician if palpitations, shortness of breath, pronounced dizziness, nausea, constipation occurs. • Avoid alcohol (may increase risk of hypotension or vasodilation).

dimenhydrinate

dye-men-**high**-dra-nate
(Dramamine)
Do not confuse dimenhydrinate with diphenhydramine.

◆CLASSIFICATION

PHARMACOTHERAPEUTIC: Anticholinergic, antihistamine. **CLINICAL:** Antiemetic, antivertigo.

ACTION

Depressant action on labyrinthine function. **Therapeutic Effect:** Prevents, treats nausea, vomiting, vertigo associated with motion sickness.

PHARMACOKINETICS

	Onset	Peak	Duration
PO	15-60 min	1–2 hrs	4–6 hrs

Well absorbed following PO administration. Metabolized in liver. Primarily excreted in urine. **Half-life:** 1.5 hrs.

USES

Prevention and treatment of nausea, vomiting, dizziness, vertigo of motion sickness. **OFF-LABEL:** Treatment of Meniere's disease.

PRECAUTIONS

Contraindications: Neonates. **Cautions:** Narrow-angle glaucoma, peptic ulcer, prostatic hyperplasia, pyloro-duodenal or bladder neck obstruction, asthma, COPD, increased IOP, cardiovascular disease, hyperthyroidism, hypertension, seizure disorders.

LIFESPAN CONSIDERATIONS

Pregnancy/Lactation: Small amount detected in breast milk. **Pregnancy Category B. Children/Elderly:** Paradoxical excitement may occur. **Elderly:** Increased risk for dizziness, sedation, confusion, hyperexcitability.

INTERACTIONS

DRUG: **Alcohol, other CNS depressants** may increase CNS depressant effects. **Anticholinergics** may increase anticholinergic, CNS depressant effects. **HERBAL:** **Gotu kola, kava kava, St. John's wort, valerian** may increase CNS depression. **FOOD:** None known. **LAB**

VALUES: May suppress wheal/flare reactions to antigen skin testing unless antihistamines are discontinued 4 days before testing.

AVAILABILITY (OTC)

Tablets: 50 mg. **Tablets, Chewable:** 50 mg.

ADMINISTRATION/HANDLING

PO

• Give without regard to meals. • Scored tablets may be crushed.

INDICATIONS/ROUTES/DOSAGE

Nausea, Vomiting, Motion Sickness

PO: ADULTS, ELDERLY: 50–100 mg q4–6h. **Maximum:** 400 mg in 24 hrs. **CHILDREN 6–12 YRS:** 25–50 mg q6–8h. **Maximum:** 150 mg in 24 hrs. **CHILDREN 2–5 YRS:** 12.5–25 mg q6–8h. **Maximum:** 75 mg in 24 hrs.

SIDE EFFECTS

Occasional: Drowsiness, restlessness, dry mouth, hypotension, insomnia (esp. in children), excitation, lassitude. Sedation, dizziness, hypotension more likely noted in elderly. **Rare:** Visual disturbances, hearing disturbances, paresthesia.

ADVERSE EFFECTS/ TOXIC REACTIONS

Children may experience dominant paradoxical reactions (restlessness, insomnia). Overdosage may result in seizures, respiratory depression.

NURSING CONSIDERATIONS

BASELINE ASSESSMENT

Assess for dehydration if excessive vomiting occurs (poor skin turgor, dry mucous membranes, longitudinal furrows in tongue).

INTERVENTION/EVALUATION

Monitor B/P, esp. in elderly (increased risk of hypotension). Monitor children closely for paradoxical reaction. Monitor serum electrolytes in those with severe vomiting. Assess hydration status.

PATIENT/FAMILY TEACHING

• Avoid tasks that require alertness, motor skills until response to drug is established. • Avoid alcoholic beverages during therapy. • Sugarless gum, sips of tepid water may relieve dry mouth. • Coffee, tea may help reduce drowsiness.

dinoprostone

dye-noe-**pros**-tone
(Cervidil, Prepidil, Prostin E_2)

BLACK BOX ALERT To be used only by personnel medically trained in dinoprostone-specific drug effects in a hospital setting.

Do not confuse Cervidil or Prepidil with bepridil.

◆ CLASSIFICATION

PHARMACOTHERAPEUTIC: Prostaglandin. **CLINICAL:** Oxytocic, abortifacient.

ACTION

Directly acts on myometrium, causing softening, dilation effect of cervix. **Therapeutic Effect:** Stimulates myometrial contractions in gravid uterus.

PHARMACOKINETICS

	Onset	Peak	Duration
Uterine stimulation	10 min (contractions begin)	1–2 hrs (abortion time)	2–6 hrs (contractions persist)

Undergoes rapid enzymatic deactivation primarily in maternal lungs. Protein binding: 73%. Primarily excreted in urine. **Half-life:** Less than 5 min.

USES

Vaginal suppository: To induce abortion from wk 12 of pregnancy through the second trimester, to evacuate uterine contents in missed abortion or intrauterine fetal death up to 28 wks gestational age (as calculated from first day of last normal menstrual period), benign hydatidiform mole. **Gel:** Ripening unfavorable cervix in pregnant women at or near term with medical/obstetric need for labor induction. Induction of labor at or near term. **Vaginal insert:** Initiation and/or cervical ripening in pts with medical indication for induction of labor.

PRECAUTIONS

Contraindications: Gel: Active cardiac, hepatic, pulmonary, renal disease; acute pelvic inflammatory disease (PID); fetal malpresentation; grand multiparae with 6 or more previous term pregnancy cases with nonvertex presentation; history of cesarean section, major uterine surgery; history of difficult labor, traumatic delivery; hypersensitivity to other prostaglandins; placenta previa, unexplained vaginal bleeding during this pregnancy; pts for whom vaginal delivery is not indicated (vasa previa, active herpes genitalia); significant cephalopelvic disproportion. **Vaginal suppository:** Active cardiac, hepatic, pulmonary, renal disease; acute PID. **Cautions:** Cervicitis, infected endocervical lesions, acute vaginitis, history of asthma, hypotension/hypertension, anemia, jaundice, diabetes, epilepsy, uterine fibroids, compromised (scarred) uterus, history of cardiovascular, renal/hepatic disease.

LIFESPAN CONSIDERATIONS

Pregnancy/Lactation: Suppository: Teratogenic, therefore abortion must be complete. **Gel:** Sustained uterine hyperstimulation may affect fetus (e.g., abnormal heart rate). **Pregnancy Category C. Children/Elderly:** Not used in these pt populations.

INTERACTIONS

DRUG: Oxytocics may cause uterine hypertonus, possibly resulting in uterine rupture, cervical laceration. **HERBAL:** None significant. **FOOD:** None known. **LAB VALUES:** May alter B/P, heart rate. May increase body temperature.

AVAILABILITY (Rx)

Endocervical Gel (Prepidil): 0.5 mg/3 g syringe. **Vaginal Inserts (Cervidil):** 10 mg. **Vaginal Suppositories (Prostin E_2):** 20 mg.

ADMINISTRATION/HANDLING

Gel

• Refrigerate. • Use caution in handling; prevent skin contact. Wash hands thoroughly with soap and water following administration. • Bring to room temperature just before use (avoid forcing the warming process). • Assemble dosing apparatus as described in manufacturer's insert. • Place pt in dorsal position with cervix visualized using a speculum. • Introduce gel into cervical canal just below level of internal os. • Have pt remain in supine position at least 15–30 min (minimizes leakage from cervical canal).

Suppository, Vaginal Inserts

• Keep frozen (−4°F); bring to room temperature just before use. • Administer only in hospital setting with emergency equipment available. • Warm suppository to room temperature before removing foil wrapper. • Avoid skin contact (risk of absorption). • Insert high into vagina. • Pt should remain supine for 10 min after administration of suppository, 2 hrs after vaginal insert.

INDICATIONS/ROUTES/DOSAGE

Abortifacient

INTRAVAGINAL: ADULTS (VAGINAL SUPPOSITORY): 20 mg (or one suppository) high into vagina. May repeat at 3- to 5-hr intervals until abortion occurs. Do not administer for longer than 2 days.

Ripening of Unfavorable Cervix

INTRACERVICAL (PREPIDIL): ADULTS (ENDOCERVICAL GEL): Initially, 0.5 mg (2.5 ml); if no cervical or uterine response, may repeat 0.5-mg dose in 6 hrs. **Maximum:** 1.5 mg (7.5 ml) for a 24-hr period.

INTRACERVICAL (CERVIDIL): ADULTS (VAGINAL INSERT): 10 mg over 12-hr period; remove upon onset of active labor or 12 hrs after insertion.

SIDE EFFECTS

D

Frequent: Vomiting (66%), diarrhea (40%), nausea (33%). Occasional: Headache (10%), chills/shivering (10%), urticaria, bradycardia, increased uterine pain accompanying abortion, peripheral vasoconstriction. Rare: Flushing of skin, vulvar edema.

ADVERSE EFFECTS/ TOXIC REACTIONS

Overdose may cause uterine hypertonicity with spasm and tetanic contraction, leading to cervical laceration/perforation, uterine rupture/hemorrhage.

NURSING CONSIDERATIONS

BASELINE ASSESSMENT

Offer emotional support. **Suppository:** Obtain orders for antiemetics, antidiarrheals, meperidine, other pain medication for abdominal cramps. Assess any uterine activity, vaginal bleeding. **Gel:** Assess Bishop score. Assess degree of effacement (determines size of shielded endocervical catheter).

INTERVENTION/EVALUATION

Suppository: Check strength, duration, frequency of contractions. Monitor vital signs q15min until stable, then hourly until abortion complete. Check resting uterine tone. Administer medications for relief of GI effects if indicated or for abdominal cramps. **Gel:** Monitor uterine activity (onset of uterine contractions), fetal status (heart rate), character of cervix (dilation, effacement). Have pt remain recumbent 12 hrs after application with continuous electronic monitoring of fetal heart rate, uterine activity. Record maternal vital signs at least hourly in presence of uterine activity. Reassess Bishop score.

PATIENT/FAMILY TEACHING

- **Suppository:** Report promptly fever, chills, foul-smelling/increased vaginal discharge, uterine cramps, pain.

Diovan, *see valsartan*

Diovan HCT, *see hydrochlorothiazide and valsartan*

*diphenhydrAMINE

dye-fen-**hye**-dra-meen
(Allerdryl 🍁, Banophen, Benadryl, Benadryl Children's Allergy, Diphen, Diphenhist, Dytan, Genahist, Nytol 🍁)

Do not confuse diphenhydramine with desipramine, dicyclomine, or dimenhydrinate, or Benadryl with benazepril, Bentyl, or Benylin.

FIXED-COMBINATION(S)

Advil PM: diphenhydramine/ibuprofen (NSAID): 38 mg/200 mg. With calamine, an astringent, and camphor, a counterirritant **(Caladryl).**

◆CLASSIFICATION

PHARMACOTHERAPEUTIC: Ethanolamine. CLINICAL: Antihistamine, anticholinergic, antipruritic, antitussive, antiemetic, antidyskinetic (see p. 54C).

ACTION

Competitively blocks effects of histamine at peripheral H_1 receptor sites. Therapeutic Effect: Produces anticholinergic, antipruritic, antitussive, antiemetic, antidyskinetic, sedative effects.

PHARMACOKINETICS

Route	Onset	Peak	Duration
PO	15–30 min	1–4 hrs	4–6 hrs
IV, IM	Less than 15 min	1–4 hrs	4–6 hrs

Well absorbed after PO, parenteral administration. Protein binding: 98%–99%.

Widely distributed. Metabolized in liver. Primarily excreted in urine. **Half-life:** 1–4 hrs.

USES

Treatment of allergic reactions, parkinsonism; prevention/treatment of nausea, vomiting, vertigo due to motion sickness; antitussive; short-term management of insomnia. Topical form used for relief of pruritus, insect bites, skin irritations.

PRECAUTIONS

Contraindications: Acute exacerbation of asthma, use of MAOIs within 14 days. **Cautions:** Narrow-angle glaucoma, peptic ulcer, prostatic hypertrophy, pyloroduodenal/bladder neck obstruction, asthma, COPD, increased IOP, cardiovascular disease, hyperthyroidism, hypertension, seizure disorders.

LIFESPAN CONSIDERATIONS

Pregnancy/Lactation: Crosses placenta. Detected in breast milk (may produce irritability in breast-fed infants). Increased risk of seizures in neonates, premature infants if used during third trimester of pregnancy. May prohibit lactation. **Pregnancy Category B. Children:** Not recommended in newborns, premature infants (increased risk of paradoxical reaction, seizures). **Elderly:** Increased risk for dizziness, sedation, confusion, hypotension, hyperexcitability.

INTERACTIONS

DRUG: **Alcohol, other CNS depressants** may increase CNS depressant effects. **Anticholinergics** may increase anticholinergic effects. **MAOIs** may increase anticholinergic, CNS depressant effects. **HERBAL:** **Gotu kola, kava kava, St. John's wort, valerian** may increase CNS depression. **FOOD:** None known. **LAB VALUES:** May suppress wheal/flare reactions to antigen skin testing unless drug is discontinued 4 days before testing.

AVAILABILITY (OTC)

Capsules: 25 mg (Banophen, Diphen, Genahist), 50 mg. **Cream (Benadryl):** 1%, 2%. **Injection Solution (Benadryl):** 50 mg/ml. **Syrup (Diphen, Diphenhist):** 12.5 mg/5 ml. **Tablets (Banophen, Benadryl, Genahist):** 25 mg, 50 mg. **Tablets, Chewable: Benadryl Children's Allergy, Dytan:** 12.5 mg, 25 mg. **Tablets, Orally Disintegrating: Benadryl Children's Allergy:** 12.5 mg, 25 mg.

ADMINISTRATION/HANDLING

IV

• May be given undiluted. • Give IV injection over at least 1 min. **Maximum rate:** 25 mg/min.

IM

• Give deep IM into large muscle mass.

PO

• Give with food to decrease GI distress.
• Scored tablets may be crushed.

IV INCOMPATIBILITIES

Allopurinol (Aloprim), amphotericin B complex (Abelcet, AmBisome, Amphotec), cefepime (Maxipime), dexamethasone (Decadron), foscarnet (Foscavir).

IV COMPATIBILITIES

Atropine, cisplatin (Platinol), cyclophosphamide (Cytoxan), cytarabine (Ara-C), droperidol (Inapsine), fentanyl, glycopyrrolate (Robinul), heparin, hydrocortisone (Solu-Cortef), hydromorphone (Dilaudid), hydroxyzine (Vistaril), lidocaine, lipids, metoclopramide (Reglan), ondansetron (Zofran), potassium chloride, promethazine (Phenergan), propofol (Diprivan).

INDICATIONS/ROUTES/DOSAGE

Moderate to Severe Allergic Reaction

PO, IV, IM: ADULTS, ELDERLY: 25–50 mg q6–8h. **Maximum:** 400 mg/day. **CHILDREN:** 5 mg/kg/day in divided doses q6–8h. **Maximum:** 300 mg/day.

Motion Sickness

PO: ADULTS, ELDERLY, CHILDREN 12 YRS AND OLDER: 25–50 mg q4–6h. **Maximum:** 300 mg/day. **CHILDREN 6–11 YRS:**

12.5–25 mg q4–6h. **Maximum:** 150 mg/day. **CHILDREN 2–5 YRS:** 6.25 mg q4–6h. **Maximum:** 37.5 mg/day.

Parkinson's Disease

PO: ADULTS, ELDERLY: 25–50 mg 3–4 times a day.

Antitussive

PO: ADULTS, ELDERLY, CHILDREN 12 YRS AND OLDER: 25 mg q4h. **Maximum:** 150 mg/day. **CHILDREN 6–11 YRS:** 12.5 mg q4h. **Maximum:** 75 mg/day. **CHILDREN 2–5 YRS:** 6.25 mg q4h. **Maximum:** 37.5 mg/day.

Nighttime Sleep Aid

PO: ADULTS, ELDERLY, CHILDREN 12 YRS AND OLDER: 50 mg at bedtime. **CHILDREN 2–11 YRS:** 1 mg/kg/dose. **Maximum:** 50 mg.

Pruritus

TOPICAL: ADULTS, ELDERLY, CHILDREN 12 YRS AND OLDER: Apply 1% or 2% cream or spray 3–4 times a day. **CHILDREN 2–11 YRS:** Apply 1% cream or spray 3–4 times a day.

SIDE EFFECTS

Frequent: Drowsiness, dizziness, muscle weakness, hypotension, urinary retention, thickening of bronchial secretions, dry mouth, nose, throat, lips; in elderly: sedation, dizziness, hypotension. **Occasional:** Epigastric distress, flushing, visual/hearing disturbances, paresthesia, diaphoresis, chills.

ADVERSE EFFECTS/ TOXIC REACTIONS

Hypersensitivity reactions (eczema, pruritus, rash, cardiac disturbances, photosensitivity) may occur. Overdose symptoms may vary from CNS depression (sedation, apnea, hypotension, cardiovascular collapse, death) to severe paradoxical reactions (hallucinations, tremor, seizures). Children, infants, neonates may experience paradoxical reactions (restlessness, insomnia, euphoria, nervousness, tremors). Overdosage in children may result in hallucinations, seizures, death.

NURSING CONSIDERATIONS

BASELINE ASSESSMENT

If pt is having acute allergic reaction, obtain history of recently ingested foods, drugs, environmental exposure, emotional stress. Monitor B/P rate, depth, rhythm, type of respiration; quality, rate of pulse. Assess lung sounds for rhonchi, wheezing, rales.

INTERVENTION/EVALUATION

Monitor B/P, esp. in elderly (increased risk of hypotension). Monitor children closely for paradoxical reaction.

PATIENT/FAMILY TEACHING

• Tolerance to antihistaminic effect generally does not occur; tolerance to sedative effect may occur. • Avoid tasks that require alertness, motor skills until response to drug is established. • Dry mouth, drowsiness, dizziness may be an expected response of drug. • Avoid alcohol.

diphenoxylate with atropine

dye-fen-**ox**-i-late
(Lomotil, Lonox)
Do not confuse Lomotil with Lamictal, Lamisil, or Lasix, or Lonox with Lanoxin, Loprox, or Lovenox.

FIXED-COMBINATION(S)

Lomotil: diphenoxylate/atropine (anticholinergic, antispasmodic): 2.5 mg/0.025 mg.

◆CLASSIFICATION

PHARMACOTHERAPEUTIC: Meperidine derivative. **CLINICAL:** Antidiarrheal (see p. 45C).

ACTION

Acts locally and centrally on gastric mucosa. **Therapeutic Effect:** Reduces intestinal motility.

PHARMACOKINETICS

	Onset	Peak	Duration
Antidiarrheal	45–60 min	—	3–4 hrs

Well absorbed from GI tract. Metabolized in liver to active metabolite. Primarily eliminated in feces. **Half-life:** 2.5 hrs; metabolite, 12–24 hrs.

USES

Adjunctive treatment of acute, chronic diarrhea.

PRECAUTIONS

Contraindications: Children younger than 2 yrs, dehydration, jaundice, narrow-angle glaucoma, severe hepatic disease. **Cautions:** Cirrhosis, renal/hepatic disease, renal impairment, acute ulcerative colitis.

LIFESPAN CONSIDERATIONS

Pregnancy/Lactation: Unknown if drug crosses placenta or is distributed in breast milk. **Pregnancy Category C. Children:** Not recommended (increased susceptibility to toxicity, including respiratory depression). **Elderly:** More susceptible to anticholinergic effects, confusion, respiratory depression.

INTERACTIONS

DRUG: **Alcohol, other CNS depressants** may increase CNS depressant effects. **Anticholinergics** may increase the effects of atropine. May increase serum **digoxin** levels. **MAOIs** may precipitate hypertensive crisis. **HERBAL:** None significant. **FOOD:** None known. **LAB VALUES:** May increase serum amylase.

AVAILABILITY (Rx)

Liquid (Lomotil): 2.5 mg/5 ml. **Tablets (Lomotil, Lonox):** 2.5 mg diphenoxylate/0.025 mg atropine.

ADMINISTRATION/HANDLING

PO

• Give without regard to meals. If GI irritation occurs, give with food. • Use liquid for children 2–12 yrs (use graduated dropper for administration of liquid medication).

INDICATIONS/ROUTES/DOSAGE

Diarrhea

PO: ADULTS, ELDERLY: Initially, 15–20 mg/day in 3–4 divided doses; then 5–15 mg/day in 2–3 divided doses. **CHILDREN 9–12 YRS:** 2 mg 5 times a day. **CHILDREN 6–8 YRS:** 2 mg 4 times a day. **CHILDREN 2–5 YRS:** 2 mg 3 times a day.

SIDE EFFECTS

Frequent: Drowsiness, light-headedness, dizziness, nausea. **Occasional:** Headache, dry mouth. **Rare:** Flushing, tachycardia, urinary retention, constipation, paradoxical reaction (marked by restlessness, agitation), blurred vision.

ADVERSE EFFECTS/ TOXIC REACTIONS

Dehydration may predispose pt to diphenoxylate toxicity. Paralytic ileus, toxic megacolon (constipation, decreased appetite, abdominal pain with nausea/vomiting) occur rarely. Severe anticholinergic reaction (severe lethargy, hypotonic reflexes, hyperthermia) may result in severe respiratory depression, coma.

NURSING CONSIDERATIONS

BASELINE ASSESSMENT

Check baseline hydration status: skin turgor, mucous membranes for dryness, urinary status.

INTERVENTION/EVALUATION

Encourage adequate fluid intake. Assess bowel sounds for peristalsis. Monitor daily pattern of bowel activity and stool consistency. Record time of evacuation. Assess for abdominal disturbances. Discontinue medication if abdominal distention occurs.

PATIENT/FAMILY TEACHING

• Avoid tasks that require alertness, motor skills until response to drug is established. • Avoid alcohol. • Contact physician if fever, palpitations occur or diarrhea persists. • Report abdominal distention.

Diprivan, *see propofol*

D

dipyridamole

HIGH ALERT

dye-pie-**rid**-ah-mole
(Apo-Dipyridamole FC, Persantine)

Do not confuse Aggrenox with Aggrastat, dipyridamole with disopyramide, or Persantine with Periactin.

FIXED-COMBINATION(S)

Aggrenox: dipyridamole/aspirin (antiplatelet): 200 mg/25 mg.

CLASSIFICATION

PHARMACOTHERAPEUTIC: Blood modifier, platelet aggregation inhibitor. **CLINICAL:** Antiplatelet, antianginal, diagnostic agent (see p. 32C).

ACTION

Inhibits activity of adenosine deaminase and phosphodiesterase, enzymes causing accumulation of adenosine, cyclic adenosine monophosphate (AMP). Therapeutic Effect: Inhibits platelet aggregation; may cause coronary vasodilation.

PHARMACOKINETICS

Slowly, variably absorbed from the GI tract. Widely distributed. Protein binding: 91%–99%. Metabolized in liver. Primarily eliminated via biliary excretion. Half-life: 10–15 hrs.

USES

Adjunct to warfarin (Coumadin) anticoagulant therapy in prevention of postop thromboembolic complications of cardiac valve replacement. **IV:** Alternative to exercise in thallium myocardial perfusion imaging for evaluation of coronary artery disease. **OFF-LABEL:** Reduces risk of reinfarction in pts recovering from MI, treatment of transient ischemic attacks (TIAs).

PRECAUTIONS

Contraindications: None known. **Cautions:** Hypotension.

LIFESPAN CONSIDERATIONS

Pregnancy/Lactation: Distributed in breast milk. **Pregnancy Category B. Children:** Safety and efficacy not established. **Elderly:** No age-related precautions noted.

INTERACTIONS

DRUG: **Anticoagulants, aspirin, heparin, salicylates, thrombolytics** may increase risk of bleeding. **HERBAL:** **Cat's claw, dong quai, evening primrose, garlic, ginseng** may increase antiplatelet activity. **FOOD:** None known. **LAB VALUES:** None significant.

AVAILABILITY (Rx)

Injection Solution: 5 mg/ml. **Tablets:** 25 mg, 50 mg, 75 mg.

ADMINISTRATION/HANDLING

IV

- Dilute to at least 1:2 ratio with 0.9% NaCl or D_5W for total volume of 20–50 ml (undiluted may cause irritation).
- Infuse over 4 min.
- Inject thallium within 5 min after dipyridamole infusion.

PO

- Best taken on empty stomach with full glass of water.

IV INCOMPATIBILITIES

No information available on Y-site administration.

INDICATIONS/ROUTES/DOSAGE

Prevention of Thromboembolic Disorders

PO: ADULTS, ELDERLY: 75–100 mg 4 times a day in combination with other medications. **CHILDREN:** 3–6 mg/kg/day in 3 divided doses.

Diagnostic Aid

IV: ADULTS, ELDERLY (BASED ON WEIGHT): 0.142 mg/kg/min infused over 4 min;

doses greater than 60 mg have been determined to be unnecessary for any pt.

SIDE EFFECTS

Frequent (14%): Dizziness. **Occasional (6%–2%):** Abdominal distress, headache, rash. **Rare (less than 2%):** Diarrhea, vomiting, flushing, pruritus.

ADVERSE EFFECTS/ TOXIC REACTIONS

Overdose produces peripheral vasodilation, resulting in hypotension.

NURSING CONSIDERATIONS

BASELINE ASSESSMENT

Assess for presence of chest pain. Obtain baseline B/P, pulse. When used as antiplatelet, check hematologic status.

INTERVENTION/EVALUATION

Assist with ambulation if dizziness occurs. Assess B/P for hypotension. Monitor for change in heart rate. Assess skin for flushing, rash.

PATIENT/FAMILY TEACHING

• Avoid alcohol. • If nausea occurs, cola, unsalted crackers, dry toast may relieve effect. • Therapeutic response may not be achieved before 2–3 mos of continuous therapy. • Use caution when rising suddenly from lying or sitting position.

disopyramide

dye-soe-**peer**-a-mide
(Norpace, Norpace CR, Rythmodan ✤, Rythmodan LA ✤)

BLACK BOX ALERT Increase in mortality or nonfatal myocardial arrest has occurred.

Do not confuse disopyramide with desipramine or dipyridamole, or Norpace with Norpramin.

◆CLASSIFICATION

CLINICAL: Antiarrhythmic (see p. 16C).

ACTION

Prolongs refractory period of cardiac cell by direct effect, decreasing myocardial excitability, conduction velocity. **Therapeutic Effect:** Depresses myocardial contractility. Has anticholinergic, negative inotropic effects.

PHARMACOKINETICS

Route	Onset	Peak	Duration
PO	0.5–3.5 hrs	–	1.5–8.5 hrs

Rapidly, almost completely absorbed from GI tract. Protein binding: 20%–65%. Metabolized in liver. Excreted in urine. Removed by hemodialysis. **Half-life:** 4–10 hrs.

USES

Suppression/prevention of ventricular ectopy (premature ventricular contractions, ventricular tachycardia). **OFF-LABEL:** Prophylaxis/treatment of supraventricular tachycardia, hypertrophic obstructive cardiomyopathy.

PRECAUTIONS

Contraindications: Cardiogenic shock, congenital QT-interval prolongation, narrow-angle glaucoma (unless pt is undergoing cholinergic therapy), preexisting second- or third-degree AV block, preexisting urinary retention. **Cautions:** CHF, myasthenia gravis, prostatic hypertrophy, sick sinus syndrome (bradycardia/tachycardia), Wolff-Parkinson-White syndrome, bundle-branch block, renal/hepatic impairment.

LIFESPAN CONSIDERATIONS

Pregnancy/Lactation: Distributed in breast milk. **Pregnancy Category C. Children:** Safety and efficacy not established. **Elderly:** Increased sensitivity to anticholinergic effects.

INTERACTIONS

DRUG: Other antiarrhythmics (e.g., diltiazem, propranolol, verapamil) may prolong cardiac conduction, decrease cardiac output. **Erythromycin**

may increase concentration. **Medications prolonging QT-interval (e.g., clarithromycin, tricyclic antidepressants)** may have additive effects. HERBAL: **Ephedra** may worsen arrhythmias. **St. John's wort** may decrease concentration. FOOD: None known. LAB VALUES: May decrease serum glucose. **Therapeutic serum level:** 2–8 mcg/ml; **toxic serum level:** greater than 8 mcg/ml.

AVAILABILITY (Rx)

Capsules (Norpace): 100 mg, 150 mg.

Capsules (Extended-Release [Norpace CR]): 100 mg, 150 mg.

ADMINISTRATION/HANDLING

PO

• Administer on empty stomach. • Administer immediate-release capsules in divided doses. • Extended-release capsules should be swallowed whole. • Do not crush, break, chew extended-release capsules.

INDICATIONS/ROUTES/DOSAGE

Suppression/Prevention of Ventricular Ectopy

PO: ADULTS, ELDERLY WEIGHING 50 KG OR MORE: 150 mg q6h (300 mg q12h with extended-release). **ADULTS, ELDERLY WEIGHING LESS THAN 50 KG:** 100 mg q6h (200 mg q12h with extended-release).

Usual Pediatric Dosage

PO (IMMEDIATE-RELEASE CAPSULES): CHILDREN 12–18 YRS: 6–15 mg/kg/day in divided doses q6h. **CHILDREN 5–11 YRS:** 10–15 mg/kg/day in divided doses q6h. **CHILDREN 1–4 YRS:** 10–20 mg/kg/day in divided doses q6h. **CHILDREN YOUNGER THAN 1 YR:** 10–30 mg/kg/day in divided doses q6h.

Dosage in Renal Impairment

With or without loading dose of 150 mg:

Creatinine Clearance	Dosage
40 ml/min and higher	100 mg q6h (extended-release 200 mg q12h)
30–39 ml/min	100 mg q8h
15–29 ml/min	100 mg q12h
Less than 15 ml/min	100 mg q24h

Dosage in Hepatic Impairment

ADULTS, ELDERLY WEIGHING 50 KG OR MORE: 100 mg q6h (200 mg q12h with extended-release).

Dosage in Cardiomyopathy, Cardiac Decompensation

ADULTS, ELDERLY WEIGHING 50 KG OR MORE: No loading dose; 100 mg q6–8h with gradual dosage adjustments.

SIDE EFFECTS

Frequent (greater than 9%): Dry mouth (32%), urinary hesitancy, constipation. **Occasional (9%–3%):** Blurred vision; dry eyes, nose, throat; urinary retention; headache; dizziness; fatigue; nausea. **Rare (less than 1%):** Impotence, hypotension, edema, weight gain, shortness of breath, syncope, chest pain, nervousness, diarrhea, vomiting, decreased appetite, rash, pruritus.

ADVERSE EFFECTS/ TOXIC REACTIONS

May produce/aggravate CHF. May produce severe hypotension, shortness of breath, chest pain, syncope (esp. in pts with primary cardiomyopathy, CHF). Hepatotoxicity occurs rarely.

NURSING CONSIDERATIONS

BASELINE ASSESSMENT

Before giving medication, instruct pt to void (reduces risk of urinary retention).

INTERVENTION/EVALUATION

Monitor EKG for cardiac changes, particularly widening of QRS complex, prolongation of PR, QT intervals. Monitor B/P, EKG, serum potassium, glucose, hepatic enzymes. Monitor I&O (be alert to urinary retention). Assess for evidence of CHF (cough, dyspnea [particularly on exertion], rales at base of lungs, fatigue). Assist with ambulation if dizziness occurs. **Therapeutic serum level:** 2–8 mcg/ml; **toxic serum level:** greater than 8 mcg/ml.

PATIENT/FAMILY TEACHING

• Report shortness of breath, productive cough. • Do not use nasal decongestants, OTC cold preparations (stimulants) without physician approval. • Restrict salt, alcohol intake.

Ditropan, *see oxybutynin*

Ditropan XL, *see oxybutynin*

*DOBUTamine HIGH ALERT

doe-**byoo**-ta-meen
(Dobutrex)
Do not confuse dobutamine with dopamine.

◆CLASSIFICATION

PHARMACOTHERAPEUTIC: Sympathomimetic. **CLINICAL:** Cardiac stimulant (see p. 158C).

ACTION

Direct-action inotropic agent acting primarily on $beta_1$-adrenergic receptors, decreasing preload, afterload. **Therapeutic Effect:** Enhances myocardial contractility, stroke volume, cardiac output. Improves renal blood flow, urinary output.

PHARMACOKINETICS

Route	Onset	Peak	Duration
IV	1–2 min	10 min	Length of infusion

Metabolized in liver. Primarily excreted in urine. Not removed by hemodialysis. **Half-life:** 2 min.

USES

Short-term management of cardiac decompensation. **OFF-LABEL:** Positive inotropic agent in myocardial dysfunction or sepsis, stress echocardiography.

PRECAUTIONS

Contraindications: Hypovolemia, idiopathic hypertrophic subaortic stenosis, sulfite sensitivity. **Cautions:** Atrial fibrillation, hypertension, severe coronary artery disease, MI.

⌛ LIFESPAN CONSIDERATIONS

Pregnancy/Lactation: Unknown if drug crosses placenta or is distributed in breast milk. Has not been administered to pregnant women. **Pregnancy Category B. Children/Elderly:** No age-related precautions noted.

INTERACTIONS

DRUG: **Beta-blockers** may increase risk of severe hypotension effects. **MAOIs, oxytocics, tricyclic antidepressants** may increase adverse effects (e.g., arrhythmias, hypertension). **HERBAL:** None significant. **FOOD:** None known. **LAB VALUES:** Slightly decreases serum potassium.

AVAILABILITY (Rx)

Infusion (Ready-to-Use): 1 mg/ml, 2 mg/ml, 4 mg/ml. **Injection Solution:** 12.5-mg/ml vial.

ADMINISTRATION/HANDLING

◀ALERT▶ Correct hypovolemia with volume expanders before dobutamine infusion. Those with atrial fibrillation should be digitalized before infusion. Administer by IV infusion only.

IV

Reconstitution • Dilute vial in 0.9% NaCl or D_5W to maximum concentration of 5,000 mcg/ml (5 mg/ml).

Rate of administration • Use infusion pump to control flow rate. • Titrate dosage to individual response. • Infiltration causes local inflammatory changes. • Extravasation may cause dermal necrosis.

D

Storage • Store at room temperature (freezing produces crystallization). • Pink discoloration of solution (due to oxidation) does not indicate loss of potency if used within recommended time period. • Further diluted solution for infusion is stable for 48 hrs at room temperature, 7 days if refrigerated.

IV INCOMPATIBILITIES

Acyclovir (Zovirax), alteplase (Activase), amphotericin B complex (Abelcet, AmBisome, Amphotec), bumetanide (Bumex), cefepime (Maxipime), foscarnet (Foscavir), furosemide (Lasix), heparin, piperacillin/tazobactam (Zosyn), sodium bicarbonate.

IV COMPATIBILITIES

Amiodarone (Cordarone), calcium chloride, calcium gluconate, diltiazem (Cardizem), dopamine (Intropin), enalapril (Vasotec), epinephrine, famotidine (Pepcid), hydromorphone (Dilaudid), insulin (regular), lidocaine, lipids, lorazepam (Ativan), magnesium sulfate, midazolam (Versed), milrinone (Primacor), morphine, nitroglycerin, nitroprusside (Nipride), norepinephrine (Levophed), potassium chloride, propofol (Diprivan), total parenteral nutrition (TPN).

INDICATIONS/ROUTES/DOSAGE

◀ALERT▶ Dosage determined by pt response to drug.

Management of Cardiac Decompensation

IV INFUSION: ADULTS, ELDERLY, CHILDREN: 2.5–20 mcg/kg/min titrated to desired response. May be infused at a rate of up to 40 mcg/kg/min to increase cardiac output. **NEONATES:** 2–15 mcg/kg/min titrated to desired response.

SIDE EFFECTS

Frequent (greater than 5%): Increased heart rate, B/P. **Occasional (5%–3%):** Pain at injection site. **Rare (3%–1%):** Nausea, headache, anginal pain, shortness of breath, fever.

ADVERSE EFFECTS/ TOXIC REACTIONS

Overdose may produce marked increase in heart rate (30 beats/min or higher), marked increase in B/P (50 mm Hg or higher), anginal pain, premature ventricular contractions (PVCs).

NURSING CONSIDERATIONS

BASELINE ASSESSMENT

Pt must be on continuous cardiac monitoring. Determine weight (for dosage calculation). Obtain initial B/P, heart rate, respirations. Correct hypovolemia before drug therapy.

INTERVENTION/EVALUATION

Continuously monitor for cardiac rate, arrhythmias. With physician, establish parameters for adjusting rate, stopping infusion. Maintain accurate I&O; measure urinary output frequently. Assess serum potassium, plasma dobutamine (therapeutic range: 40–190 ng/ml). Monitor B/P continuously (hypertension risk greater in pts with preexisting hypertension). Check cardiac output, pulmonary wedge pressure/central venous pressure (CVP) frequently. Immediately notify physician of decreased urinary output, cardiac arrhythmias, significant increase in B/P, heart rate, or less commonly hypotension.

Dobutrex, *see dobutamine*

docetaxel

HIGH ALERT

dox-eh-**tax**-el
(Taxotere)

BLACK BOX ALERT Pts with hepatic impairment are at increased risk for grade 4 neutropenia, infections, severe thrombocytopenia, severe stomatitis, skin toxicity, death. Severe hypersensitivity reaction (rash, hypotension, bronchospasm, anaphylaxis) may occur. Fluid retention syndrome (pleural effusions, ascites, edema, dyspnea at rest) has been reported.

Do not confuse docetaxel or Taxotere with Taxol.

◆CLASSIFICATION

PHARMACOTHERAPEUTIC: Antimitotic agent, taxoid. **CLINICAL:** Antineoplastic (see p. 81C).

ACTION

Disrupts microtubular cell network, essential for cellular function. **Therapeutic Effect:** Inhibits cellular mitosis.

PHARMACOKINETICS

Widely distributed. Protein binding: 94%. Extensively metabolized in liver. Excreted primarily in feces, with lesser amount in urine. **Half-life:** 11.1 hrs.

USES

Treatment of locally advanced or metastatic breast carcinoma after failure of prior chemotherapy. Treatment of metastatic non–small-cell lung cancer. Treatment of metastatic prostate cancer, head and neck cancer (with prednisone). Treatment of stomach cancer. **OFF-LABEL:** Bladder, esophageal, gastric, ovarian, small-cell lung carcinoma, soft tissue carcinoma.

PRECAUTIONS

Contraindications: History of severe hypersensitivity to drugs formulated with polysorbate 80, neutrophil count less than 1,500 cells/mm^3. **Cautions:** Hepatic impairment; myelosuppression; herpes zoster (shingles); varicella–zoster (chickenpox); preexisting pleural effusion, infection, chemotherapy, radiation.

LIFESPAN CONSIDERATIONS

Pregnancy/Lactation: May cause fetal harm. Unknown if distributed in breast milk. Breast-feeding not recommended. **Pregnancy Category D. Children:** Safety and efficacy not established in those younger than 16 yrs. **Elderly:** No age-related precautions noted.

INTERACTIONS

DRUG: **Hepatic enzyme inhibitors (e.g., erythromycin, ketoconazole)** may increase concentration/toxicity. **Immunosuppressants (e.g., cyclophosphamide, cyclosporine)** may increase risk of infection. **Live virus vaccines** may potentiate replication, increase vaccine side effects, decrease pt's antibody response to vaccine. **HERBAL:** **St. John's wort** may decrease concentration. **FOOD:** None known. **LAB VALUES:** May increase serum alkaline phosphatase, bilirubin, AST, ALT. Reduces neutrophil, platelet counts, Hgb, Hct.

AVAILABILITY (Rx)

Injection Solution: 20 mg/0.5 ml, 80 mg/2 ml.

ADMINISTRATION/HANDLING

◄ALERT► Pt should be premedicated with oral corticosteroids (e.g., dexamethasone 16 mg/day for 5 days beginning day 1 before docetaxel therapy); reduces severity of fluid retention, hypersensitivity reaction.

IV

Reconstitution • Withdraw dose and add to 250–1,000 ml 0.9% NaCl or D_5W in glass or polyolefin container to provide a final concentration of 0.3–0.9 mg/ml.

Rate of administration • Administer as a 1-hr infusion. • Monitor closely for hypersensitivity reaction (flushing, localized skin reaction, bronchospasm [may occur within a few min after beginning infusion]).

Storage • Store vials between 36–77°F. • Protect from bright light. • If refrigerated, stand vial at room temperature for 5 min before administering (do not store in PVC bags). • Diluted solution should be used within 4 hrs.

D

IV INCOMPATIBILITIES

Amphotericin B (Fungizone), doxorubicin liposomal (DaunoXome), methylprednisolone (Solu-Medrol), nalbuphine (Nubain).

IV COMPATIBILITIES

Bumetanide (Bumex), calcium gluconate, dexamethasone (Decadron), diphenhydramine (Benadryl), dobutamine (Dobutrex), dopamine (Intropin), furosemide (Lasix), granisetron (Kytril), heparin, hydromorphone (Dilaudid), lorazepam (Ativan), magnesium sulfate, mannitol, morphine, ondansetron (Zofran), potassium chloride.

INDICATIONS/ROUTES/DOSAGE

Breast Carcinoma

IV: ADULTS: 60–100 mg/m^2 given over 1 hr q3wk. If pt develops febrile neutropenia, neutrophil count less than 500 cells/mm^3 for longer than 1 wk, severe or cumulative cutaneous reactions, severe peripheral neuropathy with initial dose of 100 mg/m^2, dosage should be decreased to 75 mg/m^2. If reaction continues, dosage should be further reduced to 55 mg/m^2 or therapy should be discontinued. Pts who do not experience these symptoms at a dose of 60 mg/m^2 may tolerate an increased docetaxel dose.

Non–Small-Cell Lung Carcinoma (NSCLC)

IV: ADULTS: 75 mg/m^2 q3wk. Adjust dosage if toxicity occurs.

Prostate Cancer

IV: ADULTS, ELDERLY: 75 mg/m^2 q3wk with concurrent administration of prednisone 5 mg twice a day.

Stomach Cancer, Head/Neck Cancer

IV: ADULTS, ELDERLY: 75 mg/m^2 followed by cisplatin 75 mg/m^2 on day 1 only, then followed by 5-fluorouracil 750 mg/m^2 as 24-hr infusion for 5 days. Repeat q3wk.

SIDE EFFECTS

Frequent: Alopecia (80%), asthenia (62%), hypersensitivity reaction (e.g., dermatitis) (59%), which decreases to 16% in those pretreated with oral corticosteroids, fluid retention (49%), stomatitis (43%), nausea, diarrhea (40%), fever (30%), nail changes (28%), vomiting (24%), myalgia (19%). **Occasional:** Hypotension, edema, anorexia, headache, weight gain, infection (urinary tract, injection site, indwelling catheter tip), dizziness. **Rare:** Dry skin, sensory disorders (vision, speech, taste), arthralgia, weight loss, conjunctivitis, hematuria, proteinuria.

ADVERSE EFFECTS/ TOXIC REACTIONS

In pts with normal hepatic function tests, neutropenia (neutrophil count less than 2,000 cells/mm^3), leukopenia (WBC count less than 4,000 cells/mm^3) occur in 96% of pts; anemia (hemoglobin level less than 11 g/dl) occurs in 90% of pts; thrombocytopenia (platelet count less than 100,000 cells/mm^3) occurs in 8% of pts; infection occurs in 28% of pts. Neurosensory, neuromotor disturbances (distal paresthesias, weakness) occur in 54% and 13% of pts, respectively.

NURSING CONSIDERATIONS

BASELINE ASSESSMENT

Offer emotional support to pt, family. Antiemetics may be effective in preventing, treating nausea/vomiting. Pt should be pretreated with corticosteroids before therapy to reduce fluid retention, hypersensitivity reaction.

INTERVENTION/EVALUATION

Frequent monitoring of blood counts is essential, particularly neutrophil count (less than 1,500 cells/mm^3 requires discontinuation of therapy). Monitor renal/hepatic function tests; serum uric acid levels. Observe for cutaneous reactions (rash with eruptions, mainly on hands, feet). Assess for extravascular fluid accumulation: rales in lungs, dependent edema, dyspnea at rest, pronounced abdominal distention (due to ascites).

PATIENT/FAMILY TEACHING

• Alopecia is reversible, but new hair growth may have different color or texture. • New hair growth resumes 2–3 mos after last therapy dose. • Maintain fastidious oral hygiene. • Do not have immunizations without physician's approval (drug lowers resistance). • Avoid those who have recently taken any live virus vaccine. • Notify physician if persistent nausea, diarrhea, respiratory difficulty, chest pain, fever, chills, unusual bleeding, bruising occurs.

docusate

dok-yoo-sate
(Apo-Docusate ✤, Colace, Diocto, Docusoft-S, Novo-Docusate ✤, PMS-Docusate ✤, Regulex ✤, Selax ✤, Soflax ✤, Surfak)
Do not confuse Colace with Calan or Cozaar, or Surfak with Surbex.

FIXED COMBINATION(S)

Peri-Colace, Senokot-S: colace/senna (a laxative): 50 mg/8.6 mg.

◆CLASSIFICATION

PHARMACOTHERAPEUTIC: Bulk-producing laxative. **CLINICAL:** Stool softener (see p. 121C).

ACTION

Decreases surface film tension by mixing liquid with bowel contents. **Therapeutic Effect:** Increases infiltration of liquid to form a softer stool.

PHARMACOKINETICS

Minimal absorption from GI tract. Acts in small and large intestines. Results usually occur 1–2 days after first dose but may take 3–5 days.

USES

Stool softener for those who need to avoid straining during defecation; constipation associated with hard, dry stools.

PRECAUTIONS

Contraindications: Acute abdominal pain, concomitant use of mineral oil, intestinal obstruction, nausea, vomiting. **Cautions:** Do not use for longer than 1 wk.

⌛ LIFESPAN CONSIDERATIONS

Pregnancy/Lactation: Unknown if drug is distributed in breast milk. **Pregnancy Category C. Children:** Not recommended in those younger than 6 yrs. **Elderly:** No age-related precautions noted.

INTERACTIONS

DRUG: None significant. **HERBAL:** None significant. **FOOD:** None known. **LAB VALUES:** None significant.

AVAILABILITY (OTC)

Capsules: 50 mg (Colace), 100 mg (Colace, Docusoft-S), 240 mg (Surfak). **Liquid (Colace, Diocto):** 50 mg/5 ml. **Syrup (Colace, Diocto):** 60 mg/15 ml.

ADMINISTRATION/HANDLING

• Drink 6–8 glasses of water a day (aids stool softening). • Give each dose with full glass of water, fruit juice. • Administer docusate liquid with milk, fruit juice, infant formula (masks bitter taste).

INDICATIONS/ROUTES/DOSAGE

Stool Softener

PO: ADULTS, ELDERLY, CHILDREN 12 YRS AND OLDER: 50–500 mg/day in 1–4 divided doses. **CHILDREN 6–11 YRS:** 40–150 mg/day in 1–4 divided doses. **CHILDREN 3–5 YRS:** 20–60 mg/day in 1–4 divided doses. **CHILDREN YOUNGER THAN 3 YRS:** 10–40 mg in 1–4 divided doses.

SIDE EFFECTS

Occasional: Mild GI cramping, throat irritation (with liquid preparation). **Rare:** Rash.

ADVERSE EFFECTS/ TOXIC REACTIONS

None known.

D

NURSING CONSIDERATIONS

INTERVENTION/EVALUATION

Encourage adequate fluid intake. Assess bowel sounds for peristalsis. Monitor daily pattern of bowel activity and stool consistency. Record time of evacuation.

PATIENT/FAMILY TEACHING

• Institute measures to promote defecation: increase fluid intake, exercise, high-fiber diet. • Do not use for longer than 1 wk.

dofetilide

doe-**fet**-ill-ide
(Tikosyn)

BLACK BOX ALERT Pt must be placed in a setting with continuous EKG monitoring for minimum of 3 days and monitored by staff familiar with treatment of life-threatening arrhythmias.

◆ CLASSIFICATION

PHARMACOTHERAPEUTIC: Potassium channel blocker. **CLINICAL:** Antiarrhythmic: Class III.

ACTION

Prolongs repolarization without affecting conduction velocity by blocking one or more time-dependent potassium currents. No effect on sodium channels, alpha-adrenergic, beta-adrenergic receptors. **Therapeutic Effect:** Terminates reentrant tachyarrhythmias, preventing reinduction.

PHARMACOKINETICS

Well absorbed following PO administration. 80% eliminated in urine as unchanged drug, 20% excreted as minimally active metabolites. Protein binding: 60%–70%. **Half-life:** 2–3 hrs.

USES

Maintenance of normal sinus rhythm (NSR) in pts with chronic atrial fibrillation/atrial flutter of longer than 1-wk duration who have been converted to NSR. Conversion of atrial fibrillation/flutter to NSR.

PRECAUTIONS

Contraindications: Paroxysmal atrial fibrillation, congenital or acquired QT syndrome, severe renal impairment, concurrent use of drugs that may prolong QT interval, hypokalemia, hypomagnesemia, concurrent use with verapamil, prochlorperazine, megestrol, amiodarone. **Cautions:** Severe hepatic impairment, renal impairment.

⌛ LIFESPAN CONSIDERATIONS

Pregnancy/Lactation: Unknown if drug is distributed in breast milk. **Pregnancy Category C. Children:** No age-related precautions noted. **Elderly:** Age-related renal impairment may require dosage adjustment.

INTERACTIONS

DRUG: Amiloride, megestrol, metformin, prochlorperazine, triamterine increases dofetilide serum levels. **Bepredil, phenothiazines, tricyclic antidepressants** may increase QT interval. **Cimetidine, verapamil** increases dofetilide serum plasma levels. **Ketoconazole, trimethoprim** increases maximum plasma concentration. **HERBAL: St. John's wort** may decrease concentration. **FOOD:** None known. **LAB VALUES:** None significant.

AVAILABILITY (Rx)

Capsules: 125 mcg, 250 mcg, 500 mcg.

ADMINISTRATION/HANDLING

PO

• Give without regard to meals. • Do not open capsules.

INDICATIONS/ROUTES/DOSAGE

Antiarrhythmias

PO: ADULTS, ELDERLY: Individualized using a 7-step dosing algorithm dependent upon calculated creatinine clearance and QT measurements.

SIDE EFFECTS

Rare (less than 2%): Headache, chest pain, dizziness, dyspnea, nausea, insomnia, back/abdominal pain, diarrhea, rash.

ADVERSE EFFECTS/ TOXIC REACTIONS

Angioedema, bradycardia, cerebral ischemia, facial paralysis, serious arrhythmias (ventricular, various forms of block) may be noted.

NURSING CONSIDERATIONS

BASELINE ASSESSMENT

Prior to initiating treatment, QTc must be determined using an average of 5 to 10 beats. Do not use if heart rate is less than 50 beats/min. Provide continuous EKG monitoring, calculation of creatinine clearance, equipment for resuscitation available for minimum of 3 days. Anticipate proarrhythmic events.

INTERVENTION/EVALUATION

Assess for conversion of ventricular arrhythmias and absence of new arrhythmias. Constantly monitor EKG. Provide emotional support to pt and family. Monitor serum creatinine for electrolyte imbalance (prolonged or excessive diarrhea, sweating, vomiting, thirst).

PATIENT/FAMILY TEACHING

- Instruct pt on need for compliance and requirement for periodic monitoring of QTc and renal function.

dolasetron

dole-**ah**-seh-tron
(Anzemet)

Do not confuse Anzemet with Aldomet, Antivert, or Avandamet, or dolasetron with granisetron, ondansetron, or palonosetron.

◆CLASSIFICATION

PHARMACOTHERAPEUTIC: Selective receptor antagonist. **CLINICAL:** Antiemetic.

ACTION

Acts centrally in chemoreceptor trigger zone, peripherally at the vagal nerve terminals to antagonize 5-HT_3 receptors. **Therapeutic Effect:** Prevents nausea/vomiting.

PHARMACOKINETICS

Readily absorbed from GI tract after PO administration. Protein binding: 69%–77%. Metabolized in liver. Primarily excreted in urine. Unknown if removed by hemodialysis. **Half-life:** 5–10 hrs.

USES

PO: Prevention of nausea/vomiting associated with cancer chemotherapy, including high-dose cisplatin; prevention of postop nausea/vomiting. **Injection:** Treatment of postop nausea/vomiting. **OFF-LABEL:** Radiation therapy-induced nausea/vomiting.

PRECAUTIONS

Contraindications: None known. **Cautions:** Those who have or may have prolongation of cardiac conduction intervals, hypokalemia, hypomagnesemia, those taking diuretics with potential for inducing electrolyte disturbances, congenital prolonged QT interval syndrome, those taking antiarrhythmics that may lead to QT prolongation, cumulative high-dose anthracycline therapy.

⌛ LIFESPAN CONSIDERATIONS

Pregnancy/Lactation: Unknown if drug is distributed in breast milk. **Pregnancy Category B. Children:** Safety and efficacy not established in those younger than 2 yrs. **Elderly:** No age-related precautions noted.

INTERACTIONS

DRUG: **Medications prolonging QT interval (e.g., clarithromycin, tricy-**

clic antidepressants) may have additive effects. **HERBAL:** **St. John's wort** may decrease concentration. **FOOD:** None known. **LAB VALUES:** May transiently increase AST, ALT.

D

AVAILABILITY (Rx)

Injection, Solution: 20 mg/ml in single-use 0.625-ml ampules, 0.625 ml fill in 2-ml Carpuject and 5-ml vials.

Tablets: 50 mg, 100 mg.

ADMINISTRATION/HANDLING

IV

Reconstitution • May dilute in 0.9% NaCl, D_5W, D_5W with 0.45% NaCl, D_5W with lactated Ringer's, lactated Ringer's, or 10% mannitol injection to 50 ml.
Rate of administration • Can be given as IV push as rapidly as 100 mg/30 sec. • Intermittent IV infusion (piggyback) may be infused over 15 min.
Storage • Store vials at room temperature. • After dilution, solution is stable for 24 hrs at room temperature or 48 hrs if refrigerated.

PO

• May give with or without food. • Do not cut, break, chew film-coated tablets. • For children 2–16 yrs, injection form may be mixed in juice for oral dosing at 1.8 mg/kg up to a maximum of 100 mg.

IV INCOMPATIBILITIES

No information available on Y-site administration.

INDICATIONS/ROUTES/DOSAGE

Treatment/Prevention of Chemotherapy-Induced Nausea/Vomiting

PO: ADULTS: 100 mg within 1 hr of chemotherapy. **CHILDREN 2–16 YRS:** 1.8 mg/kg within 1 hr of chemotherapy. **Maximum:** 100 mg.

IV: ADULTS, CHILDREN 1–16 YRS: 1.8 mg/kg as a single dose 30 min before chemotherapy. **Maximum:** 100 mg.

Treatment/Prevention of Postop Nausea/Vomiting

PO: ADULTS: 100 mg within 2 hrs of surgery. **CHILDREN 2–16 YRS:** 1.2 mg/kg within 2 hrs of surgery. **Maximum:** 100 mg.

IV: ADULTS: 12.5 mg 15 min before cessation of anesthesia or as soon as nausea occurs. **CHILDREN 2–16 YRS:** 0.35 mg/kg 15 min before cessation of anesthesia or as soon as nausea occurs. **Maximum:** 12.5 mg.

SIDE EFFECTS

Frequent (10%–5%): Headache, diarrhea, fatigue. **Occasional (5%–1%):** Fever, dizziness, tachycardia, dyspepsia.

ADVERSE EFFECTS/ TOXIC REACTIONS

Overdose may produce a combination of CNS stimulant, depressant effects.

NURSING CONSIDERATIONS

BASELINE ASSESSMENT

Assess for dehydration if excessive vomiting occurs (poor skin turgor, dry mucous membranes, longitudinal furrows in tongue). Provide emotional support.

INTERVENTION/EVALUATION

Monitor for therapeutic relief from nausea/vomiting, electrolytes, EKG in high-risk pts. Maintain quiet, supportive atmosphere.

Dolobid, *see diflunisal*

Dolophine, *see methadone*

donepezil

doh-**neh**-peh-zil
(Aricept, Aricept ODT)

Do not confuse Aricept with Aciphex, Ascriptin, or Azilect.

◆CLASSIFICATION

PHARMACOTHERAPEUTIC: Cholinesterase inhibitor. **CLINICAL:** Cholinergic.

ACTION

Inhibits enzyme acetylcholinesterase, increasing concentration of acetylcholine at cholinergic synapses, enhancing cholinergic function in CNS. **Therapeutic Effect:** Slows progression of Alzheimer's disease.

PHARMACOKINETICS

Well absorbed after PO administration. Protein binding: 96%. Extensively metabolized. Eliminated in urine, feces. **Half-life:** 70 hrs.

USES

Treatment of dementia of Alzheimer's disease. **OFF-LABEL:** Treatment of attention deficit hyperactivity disorder, autism, behavioral syndromes in dementia, dementia associated with Parkinson's disease, Lewy body dementia.

PRECAUTIONS

Contraindications: History of hypersensitivity to piperidine derivatives. **Cautions:** Asthma, COPD, bladder outflow obstruction, history of ulcer disease, those taking concurrent NSAIDs, supraventricular cardiac conduction disturbances (e.g., "sick sinus syndrome," Wolff-Parkinson-White syndrome), seizures.

LIFESPAN CONSIDERATIONS

Pregnancy/Lactation: Unknown if drug is distributed in breast milk. **Pregnancy Category C. Children:** Safety and efficacy not established. **Elderly:** No age-related precautions noted.

INTERACTIONS

DRUG: May decrease effect of **anticholinergic medications.** May increase synergistic effects of **cholinergic agonists, neuromuscular blockers, succinylcholine. Ketoconazole, quinidine** may inhibit metabolism of donepezil. May increase gastric acid secretion with **NSAIDs. Paroxetine** may decrease metabolism, increase concentration of donepezil. **HERBAL: St. John's wort** may decrease concentration. **FOOD:** None known. **LAB VALUES:** None significant.

AVAILABILITY (Rx)

Tablets (Aricept): 5 mg, 10 mg, 23 mg. **Tablets (Orally-Disintegrating [Aricept ODT]):** 5 mg, 10 mg.

ADMINISTRATION/HANDLING

PO

• May be given at bedtime without regard to meals. • **ODT:** Allow to dissolve completely on tongue. • Follow dose with water.

INDICATIONS/ROUTES/DOSAGE

Alzheimer's Disease

PO: ADULTS, ELDERLY: Initially 5 mg/day at bedtime. May increase at 4- to 6-wk intervals to 10 mg/day at bedtime. A dose of 23 mg once daily can be administered once pt has been taking 10 mg once daily for at least 3 mos.

SIDE EFFECTS

Frequent (11%–8%): Nausea, diarrhea, headache, insomnia, nonspecific pain, dizziness. **Occasional (6%–3%):** Mild muscle cramps, fatigue, vomiting, anorexia, ecchymosis. **Rare (3%–2%):** Depression, abnormal dreams, weight loss, arthritis, drowsiness, syncope, frequent urination.

ADVERSE EFFECTS/ TOXIC REACTIONS

Overdose may result in cholinergic crisis (severe nausea, increased salivation, diaphoresis, bradycardia, hypotension, flushed skin, abdominal pain, respiratory depression, seizures, cardiorespiratory collapse). Increasing muscle weakness may occur, resulting in death if muscles of respiration become involved. **Antidote:** Atropine sulfate 1–2 mg IV with subsequent doses based on therapeutic response.

NURSING CONSIDERATIONS

BASELINE ASSESSMENT

Assess cognitive function (e.g., memory, attention, reasoning). Obtain baseline vital signs. Assess history for peptic ulcer, urinary obstruction, asthma, COPD, seizure disorder, cardiac conduction disturbances.

INTERVENTION/EVALUATION

Monitor behavior, mood/cognitive function, activities of daily living. Monitor for cholinergic reaction (GI discomfort/cramping, feeling of facial warmth, excessive salivation/diaphoresis), lacrimation, pallor, urinary urgency, dizziness. Monitor for nausea, diarrhea, headache, insomnia.

PATIENT/FAMILY TEACHING

• Report nausea, vomiting, diarrhea, diaphoresis, increased salivary secretions, severe abdominal pain, dizziness. • May take without regard to food (best taken at bedtime). • Not a cure for Alzheimer's disease but may slow progression of symptoms.

dong quai

Also known as Chinese angelica, dang gui, tang kuei, toki.

◆CLASSIFICATION

HERBAL: See Appendix G.

ACTION

Competitively inhibits estradiol binding to estrogen receptors. Has vasodilatory, antispasmodic, CNS stimulant. **Effect:** Reduces symptoms of menopause.

USES

Gynecologic ailments, including menstrual cramps, menopause symptoms; uterine stimulant. Used as antihypertensive, anti-inflammatory, vasodilator, immunosuppressant, analgesic, antipyretic.

PRECAUTIONS

Contraindications: Pregnancy (due to uterine stimulant effect), bleeding disorders, excessive menstrual flow. Cautions: Lactation; breast, ovarian, uterine cancer.

⌛ LIFESPAN CONSIDERATIONS

Pregnancy/Lactation: Contraindicated. **Children:** Safety and efficacy not established. **Elderly:** No age-related precautions noted.

INTERACTIONS

DRUG: Anticoagulant effect, risk of bleeding increased with **warfarin.** HERBAL: **Feverfew, garlic, ginger, ginkgo, ginseng** may increase risk of bleeding. FOOD: None known. LAB VALUES: May increase PT, INR.

AVAILABILITY (Rx)

Dong Quai Softgel: 200 mg, 530 mg, 565 mg.

INDICATIONS/ROUTES/DOSAGE

Gynecologic Ailments, Other Uses

PO: ADULTS, ELDERLY: 3–4 g a day in divided doses with meals.

SIDE EFFECTS

Diarrhea, photosensitivity, nausea, vomiting, anorexia, increased menstrual flow.

ADVERSE EFFECTS/ TOXIC REACTIONS

None known.

NURSING CONSIDERATIONS

BASELINE ASSESSMENT

Assess if pt is pregnant or breast-feeding, taking other medications, esp. those that increase risk of bleeding.

INTERVENTION/EVALUATION

Assess for hypersensitivity reaction.

PATIENT/FAMILY TEACHING

• Inform physician if pregnant or planning to become pregnant. • Do not breast-feed.

• May cause photosensitivity reaction; sunscreen, protective clothing should be worn.

*DOPamine

HIGH ALERT

dope-a-meen
(Intropin)

BLACK BOX ALERT If extravasation occurs, infiltrate area with phentolamine (5–10 ml 0.9% NaCl) as soon as possible, no later than 12 hrs after extravasation.

Do not confuse dopamine with dobutamine or Dopram, or Intropin with Isoptin.

CLASSIFICATION

PHARMACOTHERAPEUTIC: Sympathomimetic (adrenergic agonist). **CLINICAL:** Cardiac stimulant, vasopressor (see p. 158C).

ACTION

Stimulates adrenergic receptors. Effects are dose dependent. Lower dosage stimulates dopaminergic receptors, causing renal vasodilation. Higher doses stimulate both dopaminergic and beta$_1$-adrenergic receptors, causing cardiac stimulation and renal vasodilation. Therapeutic Effect: **Low dosage (1–3 mcg/kg/min):** Increases renal blood flow, urinary flow, sodium excretion. **Low to moderate dosage (4–10 mcg/kg/min):** Increase myocardial contractility, stroke volume, cardiac output. **High dosage (greater than 10 mcg/kg/min):** Increases peripheral resistance, renal vasoconstriction, B/P.

PHARMACOKINETICS

Route	Onset	Peak	Duration
IV	1–2 min	N/A	Less than 10 min

Widely distributed. Does not cross blood-brain barrier. Metabolized in liver, kidney, plasma. Primarily excreted in urine. Not removed by hemodialysis. Half-life: 2 min.

USES

Prophylaxis/treatment of acute hypotension, shock (associated with MI, trauma, renal failure, cardiac decompensation, open heart surgery), treatment of low cardiac output, congestive heart failure (CHF). OFF-LABEL: Symptomatic bradycardia or heart block unresponsive to atropine or cardiac pacing.

PRECAUTIONS

Contraindications: Pheochromocytoma, sulfite sensitivity, uncorrected tachyarrhythmias, ventricular fibrillation. Cautions: Ischemic heart disease, occlusive vascular disease, hypovolemia, recent use of MAOIs, ventricular arrhythmias.

LIFESPAN CONSIDERATIONS

Pregnancy/Lactation: Unknown if drug crosses placenta or is distributed in breast milk. **Pregnancy Category C. Children:** Recommended close hemodynamic monitoring (gangrene due to extravasation reported). **Elderly:** No age-related precautions noted.

INTERACTIONS

DRUG: May increase effects of **sympathomimetics. COMT inhibitors** may increase levels/effects. HERBAL: None significant. FOOD: None known. LAB VALUES: None significant.

AVAILABILITY (Rx)

Injection Solution: 40 mg/ml, 80 mg/ml, 160 mg/ml. Injection (Premix with Dextrose): 0.8 mg/ml (250 ml, 500 ml), 1.6 mg/ml (250 ml, 500 ml), 3.2 mg/ml (250 ml).

ADMINISTRATION/HANDLING

ALERT Blood volume depletion must be corrected before administering dopamine (may be used concurrently with fluid replacement).

IV

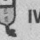

Reconstitution • Available prediluted in 250 or 500 ml D_5W or dilute in 250–500 ml 0.9% NaCl, D_5W, or lactated Ringer's to

D

maximum concentration of 3,200 mcg/ml (3.2 mg/ml).

Rate of administration • Administer into large vein (antecubital fossa, central line preferred) to prevent extravasation. • Use infusion pump to control flow rate. • Titrate drug to desired hemodynamic, renal response (optimum urinary flow determines dosage).

Storage • Do not use solutions darker than slightly yellow or discolored to yellow, brown, pink to purple (indicates decomposition of drug). • Stable for 24 hrs after dilution.

IV INCOMPATIBILITIES

Acyclovir (Zovirax), amphotericin B complex (Abelcet, AmBisome, Amphotec), cefepime (Maxipime), furosemide (Lasix), insulin, sodium bicarbonate.

IV COMPATIBILITIES

Amiodarone (Cordarone), calcium chloride, diltiazem (Cardizem), dobutamine (Dobutrex), enalapril (Vasotec), epinephrine, heparin, hydromorphone (Dilaudid), labetalol (Trandate), levofloxacin (Levaquin), lidocaine, lipids, lorazepam (Ativan), methylprednisolone (Solu-Medrol), midazolam (Versed), milrinone (Primacor), morphine, nicardipine (Cardene), nitroglycerin, norepinephrine (Levophed), piperacillin/tazobactam (Zosyn), potassium chloride, propofol (Diprivan), total parenteral nutrition (TPN).

INDICATIONS/ROUTES/DOSAGE

◀ALERT▶ Effects of dopamine are dose dependent. Titrate to desired response.

Acute Hypotension, Shock

IV INFUSION: ADULTS, ELDERLY: Initially, 1–5 mcg/kg/min. Increase in 5–10 mcg/kg/min increments. **Maximum:** 50 mcg/kg/min. **CHILDREN:** Initially, 1–5 mcg/kg/min. Increase in 5–10 mcg/kg/min increments. **Maximum:** 50 mcg/kg/min.

CHF

IV INFUSION: ADULTS, ELDERLY: Initially, 1–5 mcg/kg/min. Increase in 5–10 mcg/kg/min increments. **Maximum:** 50 mcg/kg/min. **CHILDREN:** Initially, 1–5 mcg/kg/min. Increase in 5–10 mcg/kg/min increments. **Maximum:** 50 mcg/kg/min.

SIDE EFFECTS

Frequent: Headache, arrhythmias, tachycardia, anginal pain, palpitations, vasoconstriction, hypotension, nausea, vomiting, dyspnea. **Occasional:** Piloerection (goose bumps), bradycardia, widening of QRS complex.

ADVERSE EFFECTS/ TOXIC REACTIONS

High doses may produce ventricular arrhythmias. Pts with occlusive vascular disease are at high risk for further compromise of circulation to extremities, which may result in gangrene. Tissue necrosis with sloughing may occur with extravasation of IV solution.

NURSING CONSIDERATIONS

BASELINE ASSESSMENT

Pt must be on continuous cardiac monitoring. Determine weight (for dosage calculation). Obtain initial B/P, heart rate, respirations.

INTERVENTION/EVALUATION

Continuously monitor for cardiac arrhythmias. Measure urinary output frequently. If extravasation occurs, immediately infiltrate affected tissue with 10–15 ml 0.9% NaCl solution containing 5–10 mg phentolamine mesylate. Monitor B/P, heart rate, respirations q15min during administration (more often if indicated). Assess cardiac output, pulmonary wedge pressure, or central venous pressure (CVP) frequently. Assess peripheral circulation (palpate pulses, note color/temperature of extremities). Immediately notify physician of decreased urinary output, cardiac arrhythmias, significant changes in B/P, heart rate, or failure to respond to increase or decrease in infusion rate, decreased peripheral circulation (cold, pale, mottled extremities). Taper dosage before discontinuing (abrupt cessation of therapy may result in marked hypotension). Be alert to excessive vasoconstriction (decreased urine output, increased heart rate, arrhythmias, disproportionate increase in diastolic B/P, decrease in pulse pressure); slow or temporarily stop infusion, notify physician.

doripenem

door-ih-**pen**-em
(Doribax)
Do not confuse doripenem with ertapenem, imipenem, or meropenem.

◆CLASSIFICATION

PHARMACOTHERAPEUTIC: Carbapenem. **CLINICAL:** Antibiotic.

ACTION

Inactivates penicillin-binding proteins, resulting in inhibition of cell wall synthesis. **Therapeutic Effect:** Produces bacterial cell death.

PHARMACOKINETICS

Penetrates into body fluids, tissues. Widely distributed. Protein binding: 8%. Primarily excreted in urine. Removed by dialysis. **Half-life:** 1 hr.

USES

Treatment of complicated intra-abdominal infections, complicated UTIs due to susceptible gram-positive, gram-negative (including *Pseudomonas aeruginosa)* and anaerobic bacteria. **OFF-LABEL:** Treatment of nosocomial pneumonia.

PRECAUTIONS

Contraindications: History of serious hypersensitivity to carbapenems (meropenem, imipenem-cilastin, ertapenem). Anaphylactic reactions to beta-lactam antibiotics. **Cautions:** Hypersensitivity to penicillins, cephalosporins, other allergens; impaired renal function, CNS disorders, particularly with brain lesions or history of seizures.

⌛ LIFESPAN CONSIDERATIONS

Pregnancy/Lactation: Distributed in breast milk. **Pregnancy Category B. Children:** Safety and efficacy not established in those younger than 18 yrs. **Elderly:** Advanced renal insufficiency, end-stage renal insufficiency may require dosage adjustment.

INTERACTIONS

DRUG: Probenecid reduces renal excretion of doripenem. May decrease valproic acid concentrations (do not use concurrently). **HERBAL:** None known. **FOOD:** None known. **LAB VALUES:** May increase AST, ALT, alkaline phosphatase. May decrease Hgb, Hct, platelet count, potassium.

AVAILABILITY (Rx)

Injection, Powder for Reconstitution: 250 mg, 500 mg.

ADMINISTRATION/HANDLING

IV

Reconstitution • Reconstitute 250-mg or 500-mg vial with 10 ml Sterile Water for Injection or 0.9% NaCl. • Shake well to dissolve. • Further dilute with 100 ml 0.9% NaCl or D_5W.

Rate of administration • Give by intermittent IV infusion (piggyback). • Do not give IV push. • Infuse over 60 min.

Storage • Stable for 12 hrs at room temperature, 72 hrs if refrigerated when diluted in 0.9% NaCl; 4 hrs at room temperature, 24 hrs if refrigerated when diluted in D_5W.

D

IV INCOMPATIBILITIES

Diazepam (Valium), potassium phosphate, propofol (Diprivan).

IV COMPATIBILITIES

Amiodarone, bumetanide (Bumex), calcium gluconate, dexamethasone, diltiazem (Cardizem), diphenhydramine (Benadryl), furosemide (Lasix), heparin, hydrocortisone (Solu-Cortef), hydromorphone (Dilaudid), insulin, labetalol (Trandate), lorazepam (Ativan), magnesium sulfate, methylprednisolone (Solu-Medrol), metoclopramide (Reglan), milrinone, morphine, ondansetron (Zofran), pantoprazole (Protonix), potassium chloride.

INDICATIONS/ROUTES/DOSAGE

Intra-Abdominal Infections

IV: ADULTS, ELDERLY: 500 mg q8h for 5–14 days.

Urinary Tract Infections

IV: ADULTS, ELDERLY: 500 mg q8h for 10–14 days.

Dosage in Renal Impairment

Creatinine Clearance	Dosage
30–50 ml/min	250 mg q8h
11–29 ml/min	250 mg q12h

SIDE EFFECTS

Frequent (10%–6%): Diarrhea, nausea, headache. **Occasional (5%–2%):** Altered mental status, insomnia, rash, abdominal pain, constipation, vomiting, edema, fever. **Rare (less than 2%):** Dizziness, cough, oral candidiasis, anxiety, tachycardia, phlebitis at IV site.

ADVERSE REACTIONS/ TOXIC EFFECTS

Antibiotic-associated colitis, other superinfections (abdominal cramps, severe watery diarrhea, fever) may occur. Anaphylactic reactions in those receiving beta lactams have occurred. Seizures may occur in those with CNS disorders (brain lesions, history of seizures) or with bacterial meningitis or severe impaired renal function.

NURSING CONSIDERATIONS

BASELINE ASSESSMENT

Question pt for history of allergies, particularly to beta lactams, penicillins, cephalosporins. Inquire about history of seizures.

INTERVENTION/EVALUATION

Monitor for signs of hypersensitivity reaction during first dose. Monitor daily pattern of bowel activity and stool consistency. Monitor for nausea, vomiting. Evaluate hydration status. Evaluate for inflammation at IV injection site. Assess skin for rash. Check mental status; be alert to tremors, possible seizures. Assess sleep pattern for evidence of insomnia.

PATIENT/FAMILY TEACHING

- Notify physician in event of tremors, seizures, rash, diarrhea, or other new symptom.

doxazosin

dox-ay-**zoe**-sin
(Apo-Doxazosin ♣, Cardura, Cardura XL, Novo-Doxazosin ♣)
Do not confuse Cardura with Cardene, Cordarone, Coumadin, K-Dur, or Ridaura, or doxazosin with doxapram, doxepin, or doxorubicin.

CLASSIFICATION

PHARMACOTHERAPEUTIC: Alpha-adrenergic blocker. **CLINICAL:** Antihypertensive (see p. 60C).

ACTION

Selectively blocks $alpha_1$-adrenergic receptors, decreasing peripheral vascular resistance. **Therapeutic Effect:** Causes peripheral vasodilation, lowering B/P. Relaxes smooth muscle of bladder, prostate.

D

PHARMACOKINETICS

Route	Onset	Peak	Duration
PO (antihypertensive)	1–2 hrs	2–6 hrs	24 hrs

Well absorbed from GI tract. Protein binding: 98%–99%. Metabolized in liver. Primarily eliminated in feces. Not removed by hemodialysis. **Half-life:** 19–22 hrs.

USES

CARDURA: Treatment of mild to moderate hypertension. Used alone or in combination with other antihypertensives. Treatment of benign prostatic hyperplasia. **CARDURA XL:** Treatment of benign prostatic hyperplasia. **OFF-LABEL:** Pediatric hypertension.

PRECAUTIONS

Contraindications: Hypersensitivity to other quinazolines. **Cautions:** Carcinoma of the prostate, chronic renal failure, hepatic impairment, recent CVA.

LIFESPAN CONSIDERATIONS

Pregnancy/Lactation: Unknown if drug crosses placenta or is distributed in breast milk. **Pregnancy Category C. Children:** Safety and efficacy not established. **Elderly:** May be more sensitive to hypotensive effects.

INTERACTIONS

DRUG: **NSAIDs** may decrease effect. **Hypotension-producing medications (e.g., antihypertensives, diuretics)** may increase effect. **Sympathomimetics** may decrease antihypertensive effect. **HERBAL:** **Ephedra, ginseng, yohimbe** may worsen hypertension. **Garlic** may increase antihypertensive effect. Avoid **saw palmetto** (limited experience with this combination). **FOOD:** None known. **LAB VALUES:** None significant.

AVAILABILITY (Rx)

Tablets: 1 mg, 2 mg, 4 mg, 8 mg.

Tablets, Extended-Release: 4 mg, 8 mg.

ADMINISTRATION/HANDLING

PO

• Give without regard to food. • Do not crush, chew, divide extended-release tablet. • Immediate-release tablets given morning or evening; extended-release tablets given with morning meal.

INDICATIONS/ROUTES/DOSAGE

Hypertension

PO: ADULTS: Initially, 1 mg once a day. May increase upward over several weeks to a maximum of 16 mg/day. **ELDERLY:** Initially, 0.5 mg once a day. May increase upward over several weeks.

BENIGN PROSTATIC HYPERPLASIA

PO: ADULTS, ELDERLY: Initially, 1 mg/day. May increase q1–2wk. **Maximum:** 8 mg/day. **EXTENDED-RELEASE:** Initially, 4 mg/day. May increase to 8 mg in 3–4 wks. Note: When switching to extended-release, omit evening dose prior to starting morning dose.

SIDE EFFECTS

Frequent (20%–10%): Dizziness, asthenia (loss of strength, energy), headache, edema. **Occasional (9%–3%):** Nausea, pharyngitis, rhinitis, pain in extremities, drowsiness. **Rare (2%–1%):** Palpitations, diarrhea, constipation, dyspnea, myalgia, altered vision, anxiety.

ADVERSE EFFECTS/ TOXIC REACTIONS

First-dose syncope (hypotension with sudden loss of consciousness) may occur 30–90 min following initial dose of 2 mg or greater, too-rapid increase in dosage, addition of another antihypertensive agent to therapy. First-dose syncope may be preceded by tachycardia (pulse rate 120–160 beats/min).

NURSING CONSIDERATIONS

BASELINE ASSESSMENT

Give first dose at bedtime. If initial dose is given during daytime, pt must remain recumbent for 3–4 hrs. Assess B/P, pulse immediately before each dose, and q15–30 min until B/P is stabilized (be alert to fluctuations).

INTERVENTION/EVALUATION

Monitor B/P, I/O. Monitor pulse diligently (first-dose syncope may be preceded by tachycardia). Assess for edema, headache. Assist with ambulation if dizziness, light-headedness occurs.

PATIENT/FAMILY TEACHING

• Full therapeutic effect may not occur for 3–4 wks. • May cause syncope (fainting); Rise slowly from sitting/lying position. • Avoid tasks that require alertness, motor skills until response to drug is established.

doxepin

dox-eh-pin
(Apo-Doxepin ✦, Novo-Doxepin ✦, Prudoxin, Silenor, Sinequan, Zonalon)

BLACK BOX ALERT Increased risk of suicidal thinking and behavior in children, adolescents, young adults 18–24 yrs with major depressive disorder, other psychiatric disorders.

Do not confuse doxepin with digoxin, doxapram, doxazosin, Doxidan, or doxycycline, or Sinequan with saquinavir, Seroquel, or Singulair.

◆CLASSIFICATION

PHARMACOTHERAPEUTIC: Tricyclic. **CLINICAL:** Antidepressant, antianxiety, antineuralgic, antiulcer, antipruritic (see p. 38C).

ACTION

Increases synaptic concentrations of norepinephrine, serotonin. **Therapeutic Effect:** Produces antidepressant, anxiolytic effects.

PHARMACOKINETICS

PO: Rapidly, well absorbed from GI tract. Protein binding: 80%–85%. Metabolized in liver to active metabolite. Primarily excreted in urine. Not removed by hemodialysis. **Half-life:** 6–8 hrs. **Topical:** Absorbed through skin. Distributed to body tissues. Metabolized to active metabolite. Excreted in urine.

USES

Treatment of depression, often in conjunction with psychotherapy. Treatment of anxiety. **Silenor:** Treatment of insomnia in pts with difficulty staying asleep. **Topical:** Treatment of pruritus associated with atopic dermatitis. **OFF-LABEL:** Treatment of neurogenic pain, panic disorder; prophylaxis for vascular headache, pruritus in idiopathic urticaria.

PRECAUTIONS

Contraindications: Angle-closure glaucoma, hypersensitivity to other tricyclic antidepressants, urinary retention. **Cautions:** Schizophrenia, cardiac/hepatic/renal disease, diabetes mellitus, increased IOP, glaucoma, history of seizures, history of urinary retention/obstruction, hyperthyroidism, prostatic hypertrophy, hiatal hernia.

LIFESPAN CONSIDERATIONS

Pregnancy/Lactation: Crosses placenta. Distributed in breast milk. **Pregnancy Category C (B for topical form). Children:** Safety and efficacy not established in those younger than 12 yrs. **Elderly:** Increased risk of toxicity (lower dosages recommended).

INTERACTIONS

DRUG: Alcohol, other CNS depressants may increase CNS, respiratory depression, hypotensive effects. **Antithyroid agents** may increase risk of agranulocytosis. **Cimetidine** may increase concentration, risk of toxicity. May decrease effects of **clonidine. MAOIs** may increase risk of seizures, hyperpyrexia, hypertensive crisis. **Phenothiazines** may increase anticholinergic, sedative effects. **Sympathomimetics** may increase cardiac effects. **HERBAL: Kava kava, SAMe, St. John's wort, va-**

lerian may increase sedation, risk of serotonin syndrome. FOOD: **Grapefruit, grapefruit juice** may increase concentration/toxicity. LAB VALUES: May alter serum glucose, EKG readings. **Therapeutic serum level:** 110–250 ng/ml; **toxic serum level:** greater than 300 ng/ml.

AVAILABILITY (Rx)

Capsules (Sinequan): 10 mg, 25 mg, 50 mg, 75 mg, 100 mg, 150 mg. Cream (Prudoxin, Zonalon): 5%. Oral Concentrate (Sinequan): 10 mg/ml. Tablets (Silenor): 3 mg, 6 mg.

ADMINISTRATION/HANDLING

PO

• Give with food, milk if GI distress occurs. • Dilute concentrate in 4-oz glass of water, milk, orange, tomato, prune, pineapple juice. Incompatible with carbonated drinks. • Give larger portion of daily dose at bedtime. • **Silenor:** Give within 30 min of bedtime but not within 3 hrs of a meal.

Topical

• Apply thin film of cream on affected areas of skin. • Do not use for more than 8 days. • Do not use occlusive dressing.

INDICATIONS/ROUTES/DOSAGE

Depression, Anxiety

PO: ADULTS: 25–150 mg/day at bedtime or in 2–3 divided doses. May increase gradually to 300 mg/day (single dose should not exceed 150 mg). ELDERLY: Initially, 10–25 mg at bedtime. May increase by 10–25 mg/day every 3–7 days. **Maximum:** 75 mg/day. ADOLESCENTS: Initially, 25–50 mg/day as a single dose or in divided doses. May increase to 100 mg/day. CHILDREN 12 YRS AND YOUNGER: 1–3 mg/kg/day.

Insomnia

PO: ADULTS: 6 mg. ELDERLY: 3 mg (give within 30 min of bedtime).

Pruritus Associated with Atopic Dermatitis

TOPICAL: ADULTS, ELDERLY: Apply thin film 4 times a day at 3- to 4-hr intervals. Not recommended for more than 8 days.

SIDE EFFECTS

Frequent: **PO:** Orthostatic hypotension, drowsiness, dry mouth, headache, increased appetite, weight gain, nausea, unusual fatigue, unpleasant taste. **Topical:** Edema; increased pruritus, eczema; burning, tingling, stinging at application site; altered taste; dizziness; drowsiness; dry skin; dry mouth; fatigue; headache; thirst. Occasional: **PO:** Blurred vision, confusion, constipation, hallucinations, difficult urination, eye pain, irregular heartbeat, fine muscle tremors, nervousness, impaired sexual function, diarrhea, diaphoresis, heartburn, insomnia. **Silenor:** Nausea, upper respiratory infection. **Topical:** Anxiety, skin irritation/cracking, nausea. Rare: **PO:** Allergic reaction, alopecia, tinnitus, breast enlargement. **Topical:** Fever, photosensitivity.

ADVERSE EFFECTS/ TOXIC REACTIONS

Abrupt or too-rapid withdrawal may result in headache, malaise, nausea, vomiting, vivid dreams. Overdose may produce confusion, severe drowsiness, agitation, tachycardia, arrhythmias, shortness of breath, vomiting.

NURSING CONSIDERATIONS

BASELINE ASSESSMENT

Assess B/P, pulse, EKG (those with history of cardiovascular disease). Perform CBC, serum electrolyte tests before long-term therapy. Assess pt's appearance, behavior, level of interest, mood, suicidal ideation, sleep pattern.

INTERVENTION/EVALUATION

Monitor B/P, pulse, weight. Perform CBC, serum electrolyte tests periodically to assess renal/hepatic function. Monitor mental status, suicidal ideation. Supervise suicidal-risk pt closely during early therapy (as depression lessens, energy level improves, increasing suicide potential). Assess appearance, behavior, speech pattern, level of interest, mood. **Therapeutic serum level:** 110–250 ng/ml; **toxic serum level:** greater than 300 ng/ml.

PATIENT/FAMILY TEACHING

• Do not discontinue abruptly. • Change positions slowly to avoid dizziness. • Avoid tasks that require alertness, motor skills until response to drug is established. • Do not cover affected area with occlusive dressing after applying cream. • May cause dry mouth. • Avoid alcohol, limit caffeine. • May increase appetite. • Avoid exposure to sunlight/artificial light source. • Therapeutic effect may be noted within 2–5 days, maximum effect within 2–3 wks. • Notify physician of worsening depression, suicidal ideation, unusual changes in behavior (esp. at initiation of therapy or with changes in dosage).

doxercalciferol

(Hectorol)
See vitamin D

Doxil, *see doxorubicin*

*DOXOrubicin

HIGH ALERT

dox-o-**roo**-bi-sin
(Adriamycin, Caelyx, Doxil, Rubex)

BLACK BOX ALERT May cause concurrent or cumulative myocardial toxicity. Acute allergic or anaphylaxis-like infusion reaction may be life-threatening. Severe myelosuppresion may occur. Must be administered by personnel trained in administration/handling of chemotherapeutic agents. Secondary acute myelogenous leukemia and myelodysplastic syndrome have been reported.

Do not confuse doxorubicin with dactinoycin, daunorubicin, doxazosin, epirubicin, idarubicin, or valrubicin, or Adriamycin with Aredia or idamycin.

CLASSIFICATION

PHARMACOTHERAPEUTIC: Anthracycline antibiotic. **CLINICAL:** Antineoplastic (see p. 82C).

ACTION

Inhibits DNA, DNA-dependent RNA synthesis by binding with DNA strands. Liposomal encapsulation increases uptake by tumors, prolongs drug action, may decrease toxicity. **Therapeutic Effect:** Prevents cell division.

PHARMACOKINETICS

Widely distributed. Protein binding: 74%–76%. Does not cross blood-brain barrier. Metabolized rapidly in liver to active metabolite. Primarily eliminated by biliary system. Not removed by hemodialysis. **Half-life:** 20–48 hrs.

USES

Adriamycin, Rubex: Treatment of acute lymphocytic, nonlymphocytic leukemia, breast, gastric, small-cell lung, ovarian, epithelial, thyroid, bladder carcinomas, neuroblastoma, Wilms tumor, Hodgkin's/non-Hodgkin's lymphoma, osteosarcoma, soft tissue sarcoma. **Doxil:** Treatment of AIDS-related Kaposi's sarcoma, metastatic ovarian cancer. Used with bortezomib to treat multiple myeloma in pts who have not previously received bortezomib and have received at least one previous treatment. OFF-LABEL: **Adriamycin, Rubex:** Ewing's sarcoma; germ cell, gestational trophoblastic, prostatic tumors; retinoblastoma; treatment of cervical, endometrial, esophageal, head/neck, non–small-cell lung, pancreatic carcinoma. **Doxil:** Metastatic breast cancer, Hodgkin's lymphoma, cutaneous T-cell lymphomas, advanced soft tissue sarcomas.

PRECAUTIONS

Contraindications: Cardiomyopathy; preexisting myelosuppression; previous or concomitant treatment with cyclophosphamide, idarubicin, mitoxantrone, or irradiation of cardiac region; severe CHF. Cautions: Hepatic impairment.

LIFESPAN CONSIDERATIONS

Pregnancy/Lactation: If possible, avoid use during pregnancy, esp. first trimester. Breast-feeding not recommended. **Pregnancy Category D. Children/Elderly:** Cardiotoxicity may be more frequent in those younger than 2 yrs or older than 70 yrs.

INTERACTIONS

DRUG: May decrease effects of **antigout medications. Bone marrow depressants** may increase myelosuppression. **Daunorubicin** may increase risk of cardiotoxicity. **Live virus vaccines** may potentiate virus replication, increase vaccine side effects, decrease pt's antibody response to vaccine. HERBAL: **St. John's wort** may decrease concentration. Avoid **black cohosh, dong quai** in estrogen-dependent tumors. FOOD: None known. LAB VALUES: May cause EKG changes, increase serum uric acid. May reduce neutrophil, RBC counts.

AVAILABILITY (Rx)

Injection, Powder for Reconstitution: 10 mg (Adriamycin), 20 mg (Adriamycin), 50 mg (Adriamycin RDF, Rubex). Injection Solution (Adriamycin): 2 mg/ml (5-ml, 10-ml, 25-ml, 100-ml vial). Lipid Complex (Doxil): 2 mg/ml.

ADMINISTRATION/HANDLING

◀ALERT▶ Wear gloves. If powder or solution comes in contact with skin, wash thoroughly. Avoid small veins; swollen/edematous extremities; areas overlying joints, tendons. **Doxil:** Do not use with in-line filter or mix with any diluent except D_5W. May be carcinogenic, mutagenic, teratogenic. Handle with extreme care during preparation/administration.

IV

Reconstitution • Reconstitute vials of powder with 0.9% NaCl to provide concentration of 2 mg/ml. • Shake vial; allow contents to dissolve. • Withdraw appropriate volume of air from vial during reconstitution (avoids excessive pressure buildup). • May be further diluted with 50–1,000 ml D_5W or 0.9% NaCl and given as continuous infusion. **Doxil:** Dilute each dose in 250 ml D_5W (doses greater than 90 mg in 500 ml D_5W).

Rate of administration • For IV push, administer into tubing of freely running IV infusion of D_5W or 0.9% NaCl, preferably via butterfly needle over 3–5 min (avoids local erythematous streaking along vein and facial flushing). • Must test for flashback q30sec to be certain needle remains in vein during injection. For IV infusion, administer over 1–4 hrs at concentration not to exceed 2 mg/ml. • Extravasation produces immediate pain, severe local tissue damage. Terminate administration immediately; withdraw as much medication as possible, obtain extravasation kit, follow protocol. **Doxil:** Give as infusion over 60 min. Do not use in-line filter.

Storage • Store at room temperature. • Reconstituted vials stable for 7 days at room temperature, 15 days if refrigerated. Infusions stable for 48 hrs at room temperature. • Protect from prolonged exposure to sunlight; discard unused solution. **Doxil:** Refrigerate unopened vials. After solution is diluted, use within 24 hrs.

IV INCOMPATIBILITIES

Doxorubicin: Allopurinol (Aloprim), amphotericin B complex (Abelcet, AmBisome, Amphotec), cefepime (Maxipime), furosemide (Lasix), ganciclovir (Cytovene), heparin, lipids, piperacillin/tazobactam (Zosyn), propofol (Diprivan). **Doxil:** Do not mix with any other medications.

IV COMPATIBILITIES

Dexamethasone (Decadron), diphenhydramine (Benadryl), etoposide (VePesid), granisetron (Kytril), hydromorphone (Dilaudid), lorazepam (Ativan), morphine, ondansetron (Zofran), paclitaxel (Taxol).

D

INDICATIONS/ROUTES/DOSAGE

ALERT Refer to individual protocols.

Usual Dosage

IV: ADULTS (ADRIAMYCIN, RUBEX): 60–75 mg/m^2 as a single dose every 21 days, 20 mg/m^2 once weekly, or 20–30 mg/m^2/day on 2–3 successive days q4wk. Because of risk of cardiotoxicity, do not exceed cumulative dose of 550 mg/m^2 (400–450 mg/m^2 for those previously treated with related compounds or irradiation of cardiac region). **CHILDREN:** 35–75 mg/m^2 as a single dose q3wk or 20–30 mg/m^2 weekly, or 60–90 mg/m^2 as continuous infusion over 96 hrs q3–4wk.

Kaposi's Sarcoma

IV (DOXIL): ADULTS: 20 mg/m^2 q3wk infused over 30 min.

Ovarian Cancer

IV (DOXIL): ADULTS: 50 mg/m^2 q4wk.

Multiple Myeloma

IV (DOXIL): ADULTS: 30 mg/m^2/dose every 3 wks (with bortezomib).

Dosage in Renal Impairment

Creatinine Clearance	Dosage
Less than 10 ml/min	75% of normal dose

Dosage in Hepatic Impairment

Hepatic Function	Dosage
ALT/AST 2–3 times ULN	75% of normal dose
ALT/AST greater than 3 times ULN or bilirubin 1.2–3 mg/dl	50% of normal dose
Bilirubin 3.1–5 mg/dl	25% of normal dose
Bilirubin greater than 5 mg/dl	Not recommended

ULN = upper limit of normal.

SIDE EFFECTS

Frequent: Complete alopecia (scalp, axillary, pubic hair), nausea, vomiting, stomatitis, esophagitis (esp. if drug is given on several successive days), reddish urine. **Doxil:** Nausea. **Occasional:** Anorexia, diarrhea; hyperpigmentation of nailbeds, phalangeal, dermal creases. **Rare:** Fever, chills, conjunctivitis, lacrimation.

ADVERSE EFFECTS/ TOXIC REACTIONS

Myelosuppression manifested as hematologic toxicity (principally leukopenia and, to lesser extent, anemia, thrombocytopenia) generally occurs within 10–15 days, returns to normal levels by third wk. Cardiotoxicity (either acute, manifested as transient EKG abnormalities, or chronic, manifested as CHF) may occur.

NURSING CONSIDERATIONS

BASELINE ASSESSMENT

Obtain WBC, platelet, erythrocyte counts before and at frequent intervals during therapy. Obtain EKG before therapy, hepatic function studies before each dose. Antiemetics may be effective in preventing, treating nausea.

INTERVENTION/EVALUATION

Monitor for stomatitis (burning or erythema of oral mucosa at inner margin of lips, difficulty swallowing). Observe IV injection site for infiltration, vein irritation. May lead to ulceration of mucous membranes within 2–3 days. Assess dermal creases, nailbeds for hyperpigmentation. Monitor hematologic status, renal/hepatic function studies, serum uric acid levels. Monitor daily pattern of bowel activity and stool consistency. Monitor for hematologic toxicity (fever, sore throat, signs of local infection, unusual bruising/bleeding from any site), symptoms of anemia (excessive fatigue, weakness).

PATIENT/FAMILY TEACHING

• Alopecia is reversible, but new hair growth may have different color, texture. New hair growth resumes 2–3 mos after last therapy dose. • Maintain fastidious oral hygiene. • Do not have immunizations without physician's approval (drug lowers resistance). • Avoid contact with those who have recently received live virus vaccine. • Promptly report fever, sore throat, signs of local infection, unusual bruising/bleeding from any site. • Contact physician for persistent nausea/vomiting. • Avoid alcohol (may cause GI irritation, a common side effect with liposomal doxorubicin).

doxycycline

dox-i-**sye**-kleen
(Adoxa, Apo-Doxy ✤, Doryx, Doxy-100, Doxycin ✤, Monodox, Novo-Doxylin ✤, Oracea, Periostat, Vibramycin, Vibra-Tabs).
Do not confuse doxycycline with dicyclomine or doxepin, Monodox with Maalox, Oracea with Orencia, Vibramycin with Vancomycin or Vibativ, or Vibra-Tabs with Vibativ.

◆ CLASSIFICATION

PHARMACOTHERAPEUTIC: Tetracycline. **CLINICAL:** Antibiotic.

ACTION

Inhibits bacterial protein synthesis by binding to ribosomes. **Therapeutic Effect:** Bacteriostatic.

PHARMACOKINETICS

Rapidly, almost completely absorbed after PO administration. Protein binding: 90%. Partially inactivated in GI tract by chelate formation. Partially excreted in urine; partially eliminated in bile. **Half-life:** 15–24 hrs.

USES

Treatment of susceptible infections due to *H. ducreyi, Pasteurella pestis, P. tularensis,* Bacteroides spp., *V. cholerae,* Brucella spp., *Rickettsiae, Y. pestis, Francisella tularensis, M. pneumoniae* including brucellosis, chlamydia, cholera, granuloma inguinale, lymphogranuloma venereum, malaria prophylaxis, nongonococcal urethritis, pelvic inflammatory disease (PID), plague, psittacosis, relapsing fever, rickettsia infections, primary and secondary syphilis, tularemia. Treatment of inflammatory lesions in adults with rosacea. **OFF-LABEL:** Treatment of atypical mycobacterial infections, gonorrhea, malaria, rheumatoid arthritis, prevention of Lyme disease; prevention, treatment of traveler's diarrhea.

PRECAUTIONS

Contraindications: Children 8 yrs and younger, hypersensitivity to tetracyclines or sulfites, last half of pregnancy, severe hepatic dysfunction. **Cautions:** Sun, ultraviolet light exposure (severe photosensitivity reaction).

⌛ LIFESPAN CONSIDERATIONS

Pregnancy/Lactation: Crosses placenta; distributed in breast milk. **Pregnancy Category D. Children:** May cause permanent discoloration of teeth, enamel hypoplasia. **Elderly:** No age-related precautions noted.

INTERACTIONS

DRUG: **Antacids containing aluminum, calcium, magnesium; laxatives containing magnesium** decrease absorption. **Barbiturates, carbamazepine, phenytoin** may decrease concentration. **Cholestyramine, colestipol** may decrease absorption. May decrease effects of **oral contraceptives. Oral iron preparations** impair absorption. **HERBAL:** **Dong quai, St. John's wort** may increase photosensitization. **FOOD:** None known. **LAB VALUES:** May increase serum alkaline phosphatase, amylase, bilirubin, AST, ALT. May alter CBC.

AVAILABILITY (Rx)

Capsules: 40 mg (Oracea), 50 mg (Monodox), 100 mg (Doryx, Monodox, Vibramycin). **Injection, Powder for Reconstitution (Doxy-100):** 100 mg. **Oral Suspension (Vibramycin):** 25 mg/5 ml. **Syrup (Vibramycin):** 50 mg/5 ml. **Tablets:** 20 mg (Periostat), 50 mg (Adoxa), 75 mg (Adoxa), 100 mg (Adoxa, Vibra-Tabs), 150 mg (Adoxa).

ADMINISTRATION/HANDLING

◀ALERT▶ Do not administer IM or subcutaneous. Space doses evenly around clock.

IV

Reconstitution • Reconstitute each 100-mg vial with 10 ml Sterile Water for Injection for concentration of 10 mg/ml. • Further dilute each 100 mg with at least 100 ml D_5W, 0.9% NaCl, lactated Ringer's.
Rate of administration • Give by intermittent IV infusion (piggyback). • Infuse over 1–4 hrs.
Storage • After reconstitution, IV infusion (piggyback) is stable for 12 hrs at room temperature or 72 hrs if refrigerated. • Protect from direct sunlight. Discard if precipitate forms.

PO

• Store capsules, tablets at room temperature. • Oral suspension is stable for 2 wks at room temperature. • Give with full glass of fluid. • Instruct pt to sit up for 30 min after taking to reduce risk of esophageal irritation and ulceration. • Give without regard to food. Oracea should be given 1 hr before or 2 hrs after meals. • Avoid concurrent use of antacids, milk; separate by 2 hrs.

IV INCOMPATIBILITIES

Allopurinol (Aloprim), heparin, lipids, piperacillin/tazobactam (Zosyn).

IV COMPATIBILITIES

Acyclovir (Zovirax), amiodarone (Cordarone), diltiazem (Cardizem), granisetron (Kytril), hydromorphone (Dilaudid), magnesium sulfate, meperidine (Demerol), morphine, ondansetron (Zofran), propofol (Diprivan), total parenteral nutrition (TPN).

INDICATIONS/ROUTES/DOSAGE

Usual Dosage

IV/PO: ADULTS, ELDERLY: 100–200 mg/day in 1–2 divided doses. **CHILDREN 8 YRS AND OLDER:** 2–5 mg/kg/day (maximum: 200 mg/day) in 1–2 divided doses or 100–200 mg/day in 1–2 divided doses.

Acute Gonococcal Infections

PO: ADULTS: Initially, 200 mg, then 100 mg at bedtime on first day; then 100 mg twice a day for 14 days.

Syphilis

PO, IV: ADULTS: 200 mg/day in divided doses for 14–28 days.

Traveler's Diarrhea

PO: ADULTS, ELDERLY: 100 mg/day during a period of risk (up to 14 days) and for 2 days after returning home.

Rosacea

PO: ADULTS, ELDERLY: 40 mg (Oracea) once daily.

Periodontitis

PO: ADULTS: 20 mg twice a day.

SIDE EFFECTS

Frequent: Anorexia, nausea, vomiting, diarrhea, dysphagia, photosensitivity (may be severe). **Occasional:** Rash, urticaria.

ADVERSE EFFECTS/ TOXIC REACTIONS

Superinfection (esp. fungal), benign intracranial hypertension (headache, visual changes) may occur. Hepatotoxicity, fatty degeneration of liver, pancreatitis occur rarely.

NURSING CONSIDERATIONS

BASELINE ASSESSMENT

Question for history of allergies, esp. to tetracyclines, sulfites.

INTERVENTION/EVALUATION

Monitor daily pattern of bowel activity and stool consistency. Assess skin for rash. Monitor LOC due to potential for increased intracranial pressure (ICP). Be alert for superinfection: fever, vomiting, diarrhea, anal/genital pruritus, oral mucosal changes (ulceration, pain, erythema). Monitor CBC, renal/hepatic function tests.

PATIENT/FAMILY TEACHING

• Avoid unnecessary exposure to sunlight. • Do not take with antacids, iron products. • Complete full course of therapy. • After application of dental gel, avoid brushing teeth, flossing the treated areas for 7 days. • Report severe diarrhea.

Dramamine, *see dimenhydrinate*

dronabinol

droe-**nab**-i-nol
(Marinol)
Do not confuse dronabinol with droperidol.

CLASSIFICATION

PHARMACOTHERAPEUTIC: Controlled substance **(Schedule III).** **CLINICAL:** Antinausea, antiemetic, appetite stimulant.

ACTION

Inhibits vomiting control mechanisms in medulla oblongata. **Therapeutic Effect:** Inhibits nausea/vomiting, stimulates appetite.

PHARMACOKINETICS

Well absorbed after PO administration, only 10%–20% reaches systemic circulation. Protein binding: 97%. Undergoes first-pass metabolism. Highly lipid soluble. Primarily excreted in feces. **Half-life:** 25–36 hrs.

USES

Prevention, treatment of nausea/vomiting due to cancer chemotherapy; appetite stimulant in AIDS, cancer pts. **OFF-LABEL:** Postop nausea/vomiting, cancer-related anorexia.

PRECAUTIONS

Contraindications: Treatment of nausea/vomiting not caused by chemotherapy, hypersensitivity to sesame oil, tetrahydrocannabinol products. **Cautions:** Cardiac disorders, history of psychiatric illness, history of substance abuse, hypertension.

LIFESPAN CONSIDERATIONS

Pregnancy/Lactation: Unknown if drug crosses placenta. Distributed in breast milk. **Pregnancy Category C. Children:** Not recommended. **Elderly:** Monitor carefully during therapy.

INTERACTIONS

DRUG: Alcohol, other CNS suppressants may increase CNS depression. **HERBAL: St. John's wort** may decrease concentration. **FOOD:** None known. **LAB VALUES:** None significant.

AVAILABILITY (Rx)

Capsules (Gelatin [Marinol]): 2.5 mg, 5 mg, 10 mg.

ADMINISTRATION/HANDLING

PO

• Store in cool environment. May refrigerate capsules. • May administer without regard to meals. Give before meals if used for appetite stimulant.

INDICATIONS/ROUTES/DOSAGE

Prevention of Chemotherapy-Induced Nausea and Vomiting

PO: ADULTS, CHILDREN: Initially, 5 mg/m^2 1–3 hrs before chemotherapy, then q2–4h after chemotherapy for total of 4–6 doses a day. May increase by 2.5 mg/m^2 up to 15 mg/m^2 per dose.

Appetite Stimulant

PO: ADULTS: Initially, 2.5 mg twice a day (before lunch and dinner). Range: 2.5–20 mg/day.

D

SIDE EFFECTS

Frequent (24%–3%): Euphoria, dizziness, paranoid reaction, drowsiness. **Occasional (less than 3%–1%):** Asthenia (loss of strength, energy), ataxia, confusion, abnormal thinking, depersonalization. **Rare (less than 1%):** Diarrhea, depression, nightmares, speech difficulties, headache, anxiety, tinnitus, flushed skin.

ADVERSE EFFECTS/ TOXIC REACTIONS

Mild intoxication may produce increased sensory awareness (taste, smell, sound), altered time perception, reddened conjunctiva, dry mouth, tachycardia. Moderate intoxication may produce memory impairment, urine retention. Severe intoxication may produce lethargy, decreased motor coordination, slurred speech, orthostatic hypotension.

NURSING CONSIDERATIONS

BASELINE ASSESSMENT

Assess dehydration status if excessive vomiting occurs (skin turgor, mucous membranes, urinary output).

INTERVENTION/EVALUATION

Supervise closely for serious mood, behavior responses, esp. in pts with history of psychiatric illness. Monitor B/P, heart rate.

PATIENT/FAMILY TEACHING

• Change positions slowly to avoid dizziness. • Relief from nausea/vomiting generally occurs within 15 min of drug administration. • Do not take any other medications, including OTC, without physician approval. • Avoid alcohol, barbiturates. • Avoid tasks that require alertness, motor skills until response to drug is established. • For appetite stimulation, take before lunch and dinner.

dronedarone

dro-**ned**-dah-roan
(Multaq)

BLACK BOX ALERT Contraindicated in those with Class II–III congestive heart failure (CHF) with recent decompensation requiring hospitalization or referral to specialized CHF clinic or with Class IV CHF (over 2-fold increased mortality risk).

Do not confuse dronedarone with amiodarone, dexamethasone, methyltrexone, milrinone, prednisone, or risperidone, or Multaq with Adalat, Atarax, Betaloc, Carac, or Titralac.

◆CLASSIFICATION

PHARMACOTHERAPEUTIC: Cardiac agent. **CLINICAL:** Antiarrhythmic.

ACTION

Exact mechanism unknown. Has antiarrhythmic properties of all 4 Vaughan-Williams classes, but contribution of each of these to clinical effect unknown. **Therapeutic Effect:** Suppresses arrhythmias.

PHARMACOKINETICS

Derivative of amiodarone. Protein binding: 98%. Metabolized extensively in liver via isoenzyme system. Eliminated mainly in feces, with smaller amount excreted in urine. **Half-life:** 13–19 hrs.

USES

Outpatient management to reduce cardiovascular hospitalization in those with persistent or paroxysmal atrial fibrillation, atrial flutter in those in sinus rhythm.

PRECAUTIONS

Contraindications: Class II–III CHF with recent decompensation requiring hospitalization or referral to specialized CHF clinic, Class IV CHF, sick sinus syndrome without pacemaker, bradycardia less than 50 beats/min, concurrent use of drugs that prolong QT interval (QTc Bazett interval equal to or greater than 500 ms or PR interval greater than 280 ms), pregnancy, breast-feeding, severe hepatic impairment, hypomagnesemia, hypokalemia. Concomitant use of strong CYP3A4 inhibitors (e.g., ketoconazole, cyclosporine, clarithromycin). **Cautions:** Thyroid disease, mild to moderate hepatic impairment, hypotension, photosensitivity.

LIFESPAN CONSIDERATIONS

Pregnancy/Lactation: May be distributed in breast milk. May cause fetal harm; teratogenic. **Pregnancy Category X. CHILDREN:** Safety and efficacy not established in those younger than 18 yrs. **ELDERLY:** No age-related precautions noted.

INTERACTIONS

DRUG: May increase cardiac effects with other **antiarrhythmics.** May increase effect of **beta-blockers (bradycardia), oral anticoagulants.** May increase concentration, toxicity of **digoxin, phenytoin. Simvastatin** may increase risk of myopathy, rhabdomyolysis. **Digoxin** can potentiate effects of dronedarone. **Rifampin** may decrease effect. May increase concentration of **tacrolimus, sirolimus. HERBAL: St. John's wort** may decrease effect. **FOOD: Grapefruit, grapefruit juice** may decrease effect. **LAB VALUES:** May increase AST, ALT, alkaline phosphatase, ANA titer. May cause changes in EKG, thyroid function tests. Expected to increase serum creatinine by about 0.1 mg/dl; elevation has rapid onset, reaches plateau after 7 days, and is reversible after discontinuation.

AVAILABILITY (Rx)

Tablets (Film-Coated): 400 mg.

ADMINISTRATION/HANDLING

PO

• Give with meals to reduce risk of GI distress. • Do not crush/chew/break film-coated tablets.

INDICATIONS/ROUTES/DOSAGE

Atrial Fibrillation/Atrial Flutter

PO: ADULTS, ELDERLY: 400 mg twice daily: 1 tablet with morning meal, 1 tablet with evening meal.

SIDE EFFECTS

Frequent (9%–5%): Diarrhea, asthenia (lack of strength, weakness), nausea, rash (including pruritus, dermatitis, eczema). **Occasional (4%–3%):** Abdominal pain, bradycardia. **Rare (2%–1%):** Vomiting, dyspepsia, photosensitivity reaction, dysgeusia (distortion or loss of taste).

ADVERSE EFFECTS/ TOXIC REACTIONS

Overdose manifested as arrhythmias, B/P changes.

NURSING CONSIDERATIONS

BASELINE ASSESSMENT

Premenopausal women who have not undergone a hysterectomy or oophorectomy must use effective contraception (Pregnancy Category X). Obtain baseline pulmonary function tests, chest X-ray, AST, ALT, alkaline phosphatase, serum potassium, magnesium, creatinine. Potassium levels should be within normal range prior to administration and maintained in normal range during administration.

INTERVENTION/EVALUATION

If serum creatinine increases and plateaus, use increased value as pt's new baseline. Stop medication if QTc Bazett interval is equal to or greater than 500 ms. Assess pulse for strength/weakness, irregular rate, bradycardia. Monitor EKG for cardiac changes, particularly widening of QRS, prolongation of PR and QT intervals. Notify physician of any significant interval changes. Assess for diarrhea, nausea, rash, weakness.

PATIENT/FAMILY TEACHING

• Protect against photosensitivity reaction on skin exposed to sunlight. Wear protective clothing; avoid suntanning booths. • Report increased shortness of breath, cough, sudden weight gain, dependent edema. • Pt should monitor pulse before taking medication. • Compliance with therapy regimen is essential to control arrhythmias. • Use appropriate contraception to avoid pregnancy (Pregnancy Category X).

D

droperidol

droe-**pear**-ih-dall
(Inapsine)

BLACK BOX ALERT May alter cardiac conduction by prolonging QT interval, torsade de pointes (dose-dependent).

Do not confuse droperidol with dronabinol.

CLASSIFICATION

PHARMACOTHERAPEUTIC: General anesthetic. **CLINICAL:** Anesthesia adjunct, antiemetic.

ACTION

Antagonizes dopamine neurotransmission at synapses by blocking postsynaptic dopamine receptor sites; partially blocks adrenergic receptor binding sites. **Therapeutic Effect:** Produces tranquilization, antiemetic effect.

PHARMACOKINETICS

Onset	Peak	Duration
IM		
3–10 min	30 min	2–4 hrs
IV		
3–10 min	30 min	2–4 hrs

Well absorbed after IM administration. Protein binding: extensive. Crosses blood-brain barrier. Metabolized in liver. Primarily excreted in urine. **Half-life:** 2.3 hrs.

USES

Treatment of nausea/vomiting associated with surgical and diagnostic procedures. **OFF-LABEL:** Adjunct in induction and maintenance of general and regional anesthesia, produces sedation for diagnostic procedures, treatment of acute psychotic episodes.

PRECAUTIONS

Contraindications: Known or suspected QT interval prolongation, congenital long QT syndrome. **Cautions:** Hepatic/renal/cardiac impairment (may cause cardiac arrhythmias during administration).

LIFESPAN CONSIDERATIONS

Pregnancy/Lactation: Crosses placenta. Unknown if drug is distributed in breast milk. **Pregnancy Category C. Children:** Dystonias more likely. **Elderly:** May be more sensitive to sedative, hypotensive effects.

INTERACTIONS

DRUG: **Antihypertensives** may increase hypotension. **CNS depressants** may increase CNS depressant effect. **Benzodiazepines, diuretics, IV opioids, volatile anesthetics** may have additive effect on prolongation of QT interval. **HERBAL:** None significant. **FOOD:** None known. **LAB VALUES:** None significant.

AVAILABILITY (Rx)

Injection Solution: 2.5 mg/ml.

ADMINISTRATION/HANDLING

◀ALERT▶ Pt must remain recumbent for 30–60 min in head-low position with legs raised to minimize hypotensive effect. **Storage** • Store parenteral form at room temperature.

IV

• May give undiluted as IV push over 2–5 min. • Dose for high-risk pts should be added to 0.9% NaCl, D_5W, or lactated Ringer's injection to a concentration of 1 mg/50 ml and given as an IV infusion.

IM

• Inject slowly, deep IM into upper outer quadrant of gluteus maximus.

IV INCOMPATIBILITIES

Allopurinol (Aloprim), amphotericin B complex (Abelcet, AmBisome, Amphotic), cefepime (Maxipime), foscarnet (Foscavir), heparin, lipids, methotrexate, piperacillin/tazobactam (Zosyn).

IV COMPATIBILITIES

Atropine, diphenhydramine (Benadryl), glycopyrrolate (Robinul), metoclopramide (Reglan), midazolam (Versed), morphine, potassium chloride, promethazine (Phenergan).

INDICATIONS/ROUTES/DOSAGE

Nausea, Vomiting

IM, IV: ADULTS, ELDERLY: Initially, 0.625–2.5 mg. Additional doses of 1.25 mg may be given to achieve desired effect. **CHILDREN 2–12 YRS:** 0.05–0.06 mg/kg. **Maximum initial dose:** 0.1 mg/kg. Additional dose may be given to achieve desired effect.

SIDE EFFECTS

Frequent: Mild to moderate hypotension. **Occasional:** Tachycardia, postop drowsiness, dizziness, chills, shivering. **Rare:** Postop nightmares, facial diaphoresis, bronchospasm.

ADVERSE EFFECTS/ TOXIC REACTIONS

May produce cardiac arrhythmias. Extrapyramidal symptoms (EPS) may appear as akathisia (motor restlessness), dystonias: torticollis (neck muscle spasm), opisthotonos (rigidity of back muscles), oculogyric crisis (rolling back of eyes).

NURSING CONSIDERATIONS

BASELINE ASSESSMENT

Assess vital signs. Have pt void. Raise side rails. Instruct pt to remain recumbent.

INTERVENTION/EVALUATION

Monitor B/P, pulse diligently for hypotensive reaction during and after procedure. Monitor respiratory rate. Assess pulse for tachycardia. Monitor for extrapyramidal symptoms (EPS). Evaluate for therapeutic response from anxiety (calm facial expression, decreased restlessness). Monitor for decreased nausea, vomiting.

drotrecogin alfa

dro-trae-**coe**-gin **al**-fa
(Xigris)

CLASSIFICATION

PHARMACOTHERAPEUTIC: Activated protein C. **CLINICAL:** Antisepsis agent.

ACTION

Recombinant form of human-activated protein C that exerts antithrombotic effect. Also exerts anti-inflammatory effect by inhibiting tumor necrosis factor (TNF) production. **Therapeutic Effect:** Produces anti-inflammatory, antithrombotic, profibrinolytic effects.

PHARMACOKINETICS

Inactivated by endogenous plasma protease inhibitors. Clearance occurs within 2 hrs of initiating infusion. **Half-life:** 1.6 hrs.

USES

Treatment of severe sepsis, septic shock with evidence of organ dysfunction in pts at high risk for death. **OFF-LABEL:** Purpura fulminans.

PRECAUTIONS

Contraindications: Active internal bleeding, evidence of cerebral herniation, intracranial neoplasm/mass lesion, presence of epidural catheter, recent (within the past 3 mos) hemorrhagic stroke, recent (within the past 2 mos) intracranial or intraspinal surgery or severe head trauma, trauma with increased risk of life-threatening bleeding. **Cautions:** Concurrent use of heparin, platelet count less than 30,000/mm^3, prolonged PT, recent (6 wks or less) GI bleeding, recent (3 days or less) thrombolytic therapy, recent (7 days or less) anticoagulant or aspirin therapy, intracranial aneurysm, chronic severe hepatic disease.

LIFESPAN CONSIDERATIONS

Pregnancy/Lactation: Unknown if drug can cause fetal harm. Unknown if distributed in breast milk. **Pregnancy Category C.** **Children/Elderly:** Safety and efficacy not established.

INTERACTIONS

DRUG: **Aspirin, heparin, platelet inhibitors, thrombolytic agents, warfarin** may increase risk of bleeding. HERBAL: **Cat's claw, dong quai, evening primrose, garlic, ginseng** may increase antiplatelet activity. FOOD: None known. LAB VALUES: May prolong aPTT.

AVAILABILITY (Rx)

Injection, Powder for Reconstitution: 5 mg, 20 mg.

ADMINISTRATION/HANDLING

IV

Reconstitution • Reconstitute 5-mg vials with 2.5 ml Sterile Water for Injection and 20-mg vials with 10 ml Sterile Water for Injection. Resulting concentration is 2 mg/ml. • Slowly add Sterile Water for Injection by swirling; do not shake, invert vial. • Further dilute with 0.9% NaCl. Must be further diluted within 3 hrs of reconstitution. • Withdraw amount from vial and add to infusion bag containing 0.9% NaCl for final concentration between 100 and 200 mcg/ml; direct stream to side of bag (minimizes agitation). • Invert infusion bag to mix solution.

Rate of administration • Administer via dedicated IV line or dedicated lumen of multilumen central venous line (CVL). • Administer infusion rate of 24 mcg/kg/hr for 96 hrs. • If infusion is interrupted, restart drug at 24 mcg/kg/hr.

Storage • Refrigerate vials. • Once reconstituted and further diluted, infusion must be completed wtihin 12 hrs.

IV INCOMPATIBILITIES

Amiodarone (Cordarone), ciprofloxacin (Ciloxan), cyclosporine (Sandimmune), furosemide (Lasix), levofloxacin (Levoquin).

IV COMPATIBILITIES

Lactated Ringer's, 0.9% NaCl, dextrose are only solutions that can be administered through same line.

INDICATIONS/ROUTES/DOSAGE

Severe Sepsis

IV INFUSION: ADULTS, ELDERLY: 24 mcg/kg/hr for 96 hrs. Immediately stop infusion if clinically significant bleeding is identified.

SIDE EFFECTS

None known.

ADVERSE EFFECTS/ TOXIC REACTIONS

Bleeding (intrathoracic, retroperitoneal, GI, GU, intra-abdominal, intracranial) occurs in 2% of pts.

NURSING CONSIDERATIONS

BASELINE ASSESSMENT

Criteria that must be met before initiating drug therapy: age older than 18 yrs, no pregnancy or breast-feeding, actual body weight less than 135 kg, 3 or more systemic inflammatory response criteria (fever, heart rate over 90 beats/min, respiratory rate over 20 breaths/min, increased WBC count), and at least one sepsis-induced organ or system failure (cardiovascular, renal, respiratory, hematologic, unexplained metabolic acidosis).

INTERVENTION/EVALUATION

Monitor closely for hemorrhagic complication.

Dulcolax, *see bisacodyl*

duloxetine

dew-**lox**-ah-teen

(Cymbalta)

BLACK BOX ALERT Increased risk of suicidal thinking and behavior in children, adolescents, young adults 18–24 yrs with major depressive disorder, other psychiatric disorders.

Do not confuse duloxetine with fluoxetine.

CLASSIFICATION

CLINICAL: Antidepressant.

ACTION

Appears to inhibit serotonin and norepinephrine reuptake at CNS neuronal presynaptic membranes; is a less potent inhibitor of dopamine reuptake. **Therapeutic Effect:** Produces antidepressant effect.

PHARMACOKINETICS

Well absorbed from GI tract. Protein binding: greater than 90%. Extensively metabolized to active metabolites. Excreted primarily in urine and, to a lesser extent, in feces. **Half-life:** 8–17 hrs.

USES

Treatment of major depression exhibited as persistent, prominent dysphoria (occurring nearly every day for at least 2 wks) manifested by 4 of 8 symptoms: appetite change, sleep pattern change, increased fatigue, impaired concentration, feelings of guilt or worthlessness, loss of interest in usual activities, psychomotor agitation or retardation, suicidal tendencies. Treatment of pain associated with diabetic neuropathy, fibromyalgia. Treatment of generalized anxiety disorder. **OFF-LABEL:** Treatment of chronic pain syndromes, stress incontinence, urinary incontinence.

PRECAUTIONS

Contraindications: End-stage renal disease (creatinine clearance less than 30 ml/min), severe hepatic impairment, uncontrolled angle-closure glaucoma, use within 14 days of MAOIs. **Cautions:** Renal impairment, history of alcoholism, chronic hepatic disease, hepatic insufficiency, history of seizures, history of mania, conditions that may slow gastric emptying, those with suicidal ideation and behavior.

LIFESPAN CONSIDERATIONS

Pregnancy/Lactation: May produce neonatal adverse reactions (constant crying, feeding difficulty, hyperreflexia, irritability). Unknown if distributed in breast milk. Breast-feeding not recommended. **Pregnancy Category C. Children:** Safety and efficacy not established. **Elderly:** Caution required when increasing dosage.

INTERACTIONS

DRUG: **Alcohol** increases risk of hepatic injury. **Fluoxetine, fluvoxamine, paroxetine, quinidine, quinolone antimicrobials** may increase plasma concentration. **MAOIs** may cause serotonin syndrome (autonomic hyperactivity, coma, diaphoresis, excitement, hyperthermia, rigidity). May increase concentration, potential toxicity of **phenothiazines, propafenone, tricyclic antidepressants. Thioridazine** may produce ventricular arrhythmias. **HERBAL:** **Gotu kola, kava kava, St. John's wort, valerian** may increase CNS depression. **FOOD:** None known. **LAB VALUES:** May increase serum bilirubin, AST, ALT, alkaline phosphatase.

AVAILABILITY (Rx)

Capsules: 20 mg, 30 mg, 60 mg.

ADMINISTRATION/HANDLING

◀ALERT▶ Allow at least 14 days to elapse between use of MAOIs and duloxetine.

PO

- Give without regard to meals. Give with food, milk if GI distress occurs.
- Do not crush, chew enteric-coated capsules.
- Do not sprinkle capsule contents on food or mix with liquids.

INDICATIONS/ROUTES/DOSAGE

Fibromyalgia

PO: ADULTS: Initially, 30 mg/day for 1 wk. Increase to 60 mg/day. **Maximum:** 120 mg/day.

D

Major Depressive Disorder

PO: ADULTS: 20 mg twice a day, increased up to 60 mg/day as a single dose or in 2 divided doses. For doses greater than 60 mg/day, titrate in increments of 30 mg/day over 1 wk. **Maximum:** 120 mg/day. **ELDERLY:** Initially, 20 mg 1–2 times day. May increase to 40–60 mg/day as single or divided doses.

Diabetic Neuropathy Pain

PO: ADULTS, ELDERLY: 60 mg once a day. **Maximum:** 120 mg/day.

Generalized Anxiety Disorder

PO: ADULTS, ELDERLY: Initially, 30–60 mg once daily. May increase up to 120 mg/day in 30-mg increments weekly.

SIDE EFFECTS

Frequent (20%–11%): Nausea, dry mouth, constipation, insomnia. **Occasional (9%–5%):** Dizziness, fatigue, diarrhea, drowsiness, anorexia, diaphoresis, vomiting. **Rare (4%–2%):** Blurred vision, erectile dysfunction, delayed or failed ejaculation, anorgasmia, anxiety, decreased libido, hot flashes.

ADVERSE EFFECTS/ TOXIC REACTIONS

May slightly increase heart rate. Colitis, dysphagia, gastritis, irritable bowel syndrome occur rarely.

NURSING CONSIDERATIONS

BASELINE ASSESSMENT

Assess appearance, behavior, speech pattern, level of interest, mood, sleep pattern, suicidal tendencies. Question pain level, intensity, location of pain.

INTERVENTION/EVALUATION

For those on long-term therapy, serum chemistry profile to assess hepatic/renal function should be performed periodically. Supervise suicidal risk pt closely during early therapy (as depression lessens, energy level improves, increasing suicide potential). Monitor B/P, mental status, anxiety, social functioning, glucose levels.

PATIENT/FAMILY TEACHING

• Therapeutic effect may be noted within 1–4 wks. • Do not abruptly discontinue medication. • Avoid tasks that require alertness, motor skills until response to drug is established. • Inform physician of intention of pregnancy or if pregnancy occurs. • Inform physician of anxiety, agitation, panic attacks, worsening of depression occurs. • Avoid heavy alcohol intake (associated with severe hepatic injury).

DuoNeb, *see albuterol and ipratropium*

Duragesic, *see fentanyl*

Duramorph, *see morphine*

dutasteride

do-tah-**stir**-eyed
(Avodart)

FIXED-COMBINATION(S)

Jalyn: dutasteride/tamsulosin (alpha-adrenergic blocker): 0.5 mg/0.4 mg.

◆CLASSIFICATION

PHARMACOTHERAPEUTIC: Androgen hormone inhibitor. **CLINICAL:** Benign prostatic hyperplasia agent.

ACTION

Inhibits 5-alpha reductase, an intracellular enzyme that converts testosterone into dihydrotestosterone (DHT) in the prostate gland, reducing serum DHT level. **Therapeutic Effect:** Reduces enlarged prostate gland.

PHARMACOKINETICS

Route	Onset	Peak	Duration
PO	24 hrs	N/A	3–8 wks

Moderately absorbed after PO administration. Widely distributed. Protein binding: 99%. Metabolized in liver. Primarily excreted in feces. Half-life: Up to 5 wks.

USES

Treatment of benign prostatic hyperplasia (BPH), alone or in combination with tamsulosin (Flomax). OFF-LABEL: Treatment of hair loss. Prostate cancer prevention.

PRECAUTIONS

Contraindications: Females, physical handling of tablets by those who are or may be pregnant. Cautions: Hepatic disease/impairment, obstructive uropathy, preexisting sexual dysfunction (reduced male libido, impotence). **Pregnancy Category X.**

INTERACTIONS

DRUG: **Cimetidine, ciprofloxacin, diltiazem, ketoconazole, ritonavir, verapamil** may increase concentration. HERBAL: Avoid **saw palmetto** (limited experience with this combination). **St. John's wort** may decrease concentration. FOOD: None known. LAB VALUES: Decreases serum prostate-specific antigen (PSA) level.

AVAILABILITY (Rx)

Capsules: 0.5 mg.

ADMINISTRATION/HANDLING

PO

• Do not open/break capsules. • Give without regard to meals.

INDICATIONS/ROUTES/DOSAGE

Benign Prostatic Hyperplasia (BPH)

PO: ADULTS, ELDERLY (MEN ONLY): 0.5 mg once a day.

SIDE EFFECTS

Occasional: Gynecomastia, sexual dysfunction (decreased libido, impotence, decreased volume of ejaculate).

ADVERSE EFFECTS/ TOXIC REACTIONS

Toxicity manifested as rash, diarrhea, abdominal pain.

NURSING CONSIDERATIONS

BASELINE ASSESSMENT

Serum prostate-specific antigen (PSA) determination should be performed in pts with benign prostatic hyperplasia (BPH) before beginning therapy and periodically thereafter. Question possibility of sexual dysfunction.

INTERVENTION/EVALUATION

Diligently monitor I&O. Assess for signs/symptoms of BPH (hesitancy, reduced force of urinary stream, postvoid dribbling, sensation of incomplete bladder emptying).

PATIENT/FAMILY TEACHING

• Discuss potential for impotence; volume of ejaculate may be decreased during treatment. • May not notice improved urinary flow for up to 6 mos after treatment. • Women who are or may be pregnant should not handle capsules (risk of fetal anomaly to male fetus). • Do not donate blood for at least 6 mos after last dose.

Dyazide, *see hydrochlorothiazide and triamterene*

DynaCirc, *see isradipine*

ecallantide

ee-**cal**-an-tide
(Kalbitor)

BLACK BOX ALERT Risk of anaphylactic reaction. Must be administered by healthcare personnel with appropriate support to manage anaphylaxis, hereditary angioedema and an understanding of the similarity of symptoms.

◆CLASSIFICATION

PHARMACOTHERAPEUTIC: Plasma kallikrein inhibitor. **CLINICAL:** Proteolytic complex.

ACTION

Blocks inflammatory and coagulation pathways; converts kininogen to bradykinin by inactivating enzymatic active components. **Therapeutic Effect:** Reduces conversion of kininogen to bradykinin, thereby treating symptoms of hereditary angioedema.

PHARMACOKINETICS

Half-life: 1.5–2.5 hrs.

USES

Treatment of acute attacks of hereditary angioedema in pts 16 yrs and older.

PRECAUTIONS

Contraindications: History of life-threatening immediate hypersensitivity reactions. **Cautions:** Known hypersensitivity to other medications.

⌛ LIFESPAN CONSIDERATIONS

Pregnancy/Lactation: Unknown if distributed in breast milk. **Pregnancy Category C. Children:** Safety and efficacy not established in those younger than 16 yrs. **Elderly:** Age-related renal, hepatic, cardiac impairment may require dosage adjustment. Initiate treatment at low end of dosage range.

INTERACTIONS

DRUG: None significant. **HERBAL:** None significant. **FOOD:** None known. **LAB VALUES:** May prolong aPTT.

AVAILABILITY (Rx)

Single-Use Vial: 10 mg/ml. Dose supplied as three single-use vials in one carton.

ADMINISTRATION/HANDLING

Subcutaneous

Reconstitution • Withdraw 1 ml (10 mg) from each vial.

Rate of administration • Administer as 3 subcutaneous injections. • Injection site for each injection may be in same or different anatomic locations (abdomen, thigh, upper arm). There is no need for site rotation. Injection sites should be located at least 2 inches away from anatomic site of attack.

Storage • Refrigerate unused vials. • Liquid appears as clear, colorless. Discard if solution contains particulate or is discolored. • Vials kept at room temperature must be used within 14 days or returned to refrigeration.

INDICATIONS/ROUTES/DOSAGE

Hereditary Angioedema

SUBCUTANEOUS: ADULTS, ELDERLY, ADOLESCENTS 16 YRS AND OLDER: 30 mg (3 ml) administered as three injections of 10 mg (1 ml) each. If attack persists, an additional 30-mg dose may be administered within 24 hrs.

SIDE EFFECTS

Occasional (8%–3%): Headache, nausea, diarrhea, fever, injection site reactions, nasopharyngitis.

ADVERSE EFFECTS/ TOXIC REACTIONS

Symptoms associated with anaphylactic reactions may include chest discomfort, flushing, pharyngeal edema, pruritus, rhinorrhea, sneezing, urticaria, rash, wheezing, hypotension. Reactions occur within first hr after dosing.

NURSING CONSIDERATIONS

BASELINE ASSESSMENT

Assess for history of immediate hypersensitivity reactions, including anaphylaxis.

INTERVENTION/EVALUATION

Observe pt following drug administration. Given the similarity between hypersensitivity reactions and acute hereditary angioedema symptoms, pt should be monitored closely in the event of a hypersensitivity reaction.

PATIENT/FAMILY TEACHING

• Immediately report signs, symptoms of allergic reactions. Pt should be advised that medication may cause anaphylaxis, other hypersensitivity reactions. • A second 30-mg subcutaneous dose administered within 24 hrs following initial dose may be given if symptoms persist or relapse occurs.

echinacea

Also known as black susan, comb flower, red sunflower, scurvy root.

◆CLASSIFICATION

HERBAL: See Appendix G.

ACTION

Stimulates immune system. Possesses antiviral/immune stimulatory effects. Increases phagocytosis, lymphocyte activity (possibly by releasing tumor necrosis factor [TNF], interleukin-1, interferon). **Effect:** Prevents/reduces symptoms associated with upper respiratory infection.

USES

Immune system stimulant used for treatment/prevention of the common cold, other upper respiratory infections. Also used for UTI, vaginal candidiasis.

PRECAUTIONS

Contraindications: Pregnancy/lactation, children 2 yrs and younger, those with autoimmune disease (e.g., multiple sclerosis, systemic lupus erythematosus [SLE], HIV/AIDS), tuberculosis, history of allergic conditions. **Cautions:** Diabetes (may alter control of blood sugar). Do not use for more than 8 wks (may decrease effectiveness).

⌛ LIFESPAN CONSIDERATIONS

Pregnancy/Lactation: Contraindicated. **Pregnancy Category C. Children:** Safety and efficacy not established in those younger than 2 yrs. **Elderly:** No age-related precautions noted.

INTERACTIONS

DRUG: May interfere with **immunosuppressant therapy (corticosteroids, cyclosporine, mycophenolate). Topical econazole** may reduce recurring vaginal candida infections. **HERBAL:** None significant. **FOOD:** None known. **LAB VALUES:** None significant.

AVAILABILITY (OTC)

Capsules: 200 mg, 380 mg, 400 mg, 500 mg. **Powder:** 25 g, 100 g, 500 g. **Tincture:** 475 mg/ml.

INDICATIONS/ROUTES/DOSAGE

Usual Adult Dosage

PO: ADULTS, ELDERLY: 6–9 ml herbal juice for maximum of 8 wks.

◀ALERT▶ A variety of doses have been used depending on the preparation.

SIDE EFFECTS

Well tolerated. May cause allergic reaction (urticaria, acute asthma/dyspnea, angioedema), fever, nausea, vomiting, diarrhea, unpleasant taste, abdominal pain, dizziness.

ADVERSE EFFECTS/ TOXIC REACTIONS

None known.

NURSING CONSIDERATIONS

BASELINE ASSESSMENT

Assess if pt is pregnant or breast-feeding, has history of autoimmune disease, is receiving immunosuppressant therapy.

INTERVENTION/EVALUATION

Assess for hypersensitivity reaction, improvement in infection.

PATIENT/FAMILY TEACHING

• Do not use during pregnancy or lactation, children younger than 2 yrs. • Do not use for more than 8 wks without at least 1-wk break in therapy.

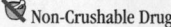

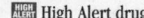

Ecotrin, *see aspirin*

E

eculizumab

ek-you-**liz**-zoo-mab
(Soliris)

BLACK BOX ALERT Increased risk for septicemia, meningitis in those with paroxysmal nocturnal hemoglobinemia. Meningoccal vaccination to be given 2 wks before initiation of treatment.

Do not confuse Soliris with Synagis, or eculizumab with efalizumab or palivizumab.

◆CLASSIFICATION

PHARMACOTHERAPEUTIC: Monoclonal antibody. **CLINICAL:** Hemostatic agent.

ACTION

Binds to complement protein C5, preventing terminal intravascular hemolysis. **Therapeutic Effect:** Prevents intravascular hemolysis in paroxysmal nocturnal hemoglobinuria.

PHARMACOKINETICS

Route	Onset	Peak	Duration
IV	Rapid	End of infusion	1–2 wks

Complete bioavailablity. Unknown metabolism. **Half-life:** 11.3 days.

USES

Reduces hemolysis in pts with paroxysmal nocturnal hemoglobinuria.

PRECAUTIONS

Contraindications: Unresolved serious *Neisseria meningitides* infection, pts not currently vaccinated against *N. meningitides*. **Cautions:** Systemic infection.

⌛ LIFESPAN CONSIDERATIONS

Pregnancy/Lactation: Crosses placenta. Distributed in breast milk. **Pregnancy Category C. Children:** Safety and efficacy not established in those younger than 18 yrs. **Elderly:** No age-related precautions noted.

INTERACTIONS

DRUG: May increase levels/effect of **leflunomide, natalizumab. Trastuzumab** may increase eculizumab concentration. **HERBAL: Echinacea** may decrease effects. **FOOD:** None known. **LAB VALUES:** Reduces serum LDH levels.

AVAILABILITY (Rx)

Injection, Solution: 10 mg/ml (30-ml vial).

ADMINISTRATION/HANDLING

◀ALERT▶ Vaccination with a meningococcal vaccine must be given at least 2 wks prior to receiving first dose of eculizumab. Must be given by IV infusion; do not give by bolus or IV push.

IV

Reconstitution • Withdraw required amount of eculizumab from vial and dilute with equal volume of 0.9% NaCl, D_5W, or lactated Ringer's to provide final concentration of 5 mg/ml. • Final admixture is 120 ml for 600 mg dose or 180 ml for 900 mg dose. • Gently invert bag to ensure thorough mixing. • Prior to administration, allow admixture to adjust to room temperature.

Rate of administration • Administer as IV infusion over 35 min. • Total infusion time should not exceed 2 hrs.

Storage • Refrigerate vials. • Discard solution that is discolored or contains particulate matter. • Solution is stable for 24 hrs at room temperature or if refrigerated.

INDICATIONS/ROUTES/DOSAGE

Paroxysmal Nocturnal Hemoglobinuria

IV INFUSION: ADULTS, ELDERLY: 600 mg every 7 days for 4 doses, followed by 900 mg 7 days later, then 900 mg every 14 days thereafter.

SIDE EFFECTS

Frequent (44%–23%): Headache, pharyngitis. **Occasional (19%–12%):** Back pain, nausea, cough, fatigue. **Rare (7%):** Constipation, myalgia, sinusitis, herpes simplex infection, extremity pain, influenza-like symptoms.

ADVERSE EFFECTS/ TOXIC REACTIONS

Eculizumab increases susceptibility to serious meningococcal infections (septicemia, meningitis), encapsulated bacteria. Pts who discontinue treatment may be at increased risk for serious hemolysis.

NURSING CONSIDERATIONS

BASELINE ASSESSMENT

Vaccinate pts with meningococcal vaccine at least 2 wks prior to receiving first dose of eculizumab.

INTERVENTION/EVALUATION

Observe for infusion site reaction. Monitor CBC, LDH, AST, urinalysis results. Monitor for early signs of meningococcal infection (moderate to severe headache with nausea or vomiting; moderate to severe headache and fever; moderate to severe headache with stiff neck or stiff back; fever 103°F or higher; fever with rash, confusion, severe myalgia with flu-like symptoms, photosensitivity).

PATIENT/ FAMILY TEACHING

- Vaccination may not prevent meningococcal infection.

EES, *see erythromycin*

efavirenz

eh-fah-**vir**-enz
(Sustiva)

FIXED COMBINATION(S)

Atripla: efavirenz/emtricitabine (an antiretroviral)/tenofovir (an antiretroviral): 600 mg/200 mg/300 mg.

◆CLASSIFICATION

PHARMACOTHERAPEUTIC: Nonnucleoside reverse transcriptase inhibitor. **CLINICAL:** Antiretroviral (see pp. 68C, 116C).

ACTION

Inhibits activity of HIV-1 reverse transcriptase. **Therapeutic Effect:** Interrupts HIV replication, slowing progression of HIV infection.

PHARMACOKINETICS

Rapidly absorbed after PO administration. Protein binding: 99%. Metabolized in liver. Eliminated in urine, feces. **Half-life:** 40–55 hrs.

USES

Treatment of HIV infection in combination with other appropriate antiretroviral agents.

PRECAUTIONS

Contraindications: Concurrent use with ergot derivatives, midazolam, triazolam; efavirenz as monotherapy. **Cautions:** History of mental illness, substance abuse, hepatic impairment.

LIFESPAN CONSIDERATIONS

Pregnancy/Lactation: Breast-feeding not recommended. **Pregnancy Category C. Children:** Safety and efficacy not established in those younger than 3 yrs; may have increased incidence of rash. **Elderly:** No age-related precautions noted.

INTERACTIONS

DRUG: Ergot derivatives, midazolam, triazolam may cause serious or life-threatening reactions (cardiac arrhythmias, prolonged sedation, respiratory depression). Decreases plasma concentrations of **amprenavir, indinavir, saquinavir.** Increases plasma concentrations of **ritonavir. Phenobarbital, rifabutin, rifampin** decrease concentration. Alters **warfarin** plasma concentration. HERBAL: **St. John's wort** may decrease concentration. FOOD: **High-fat meals** may increase drug absorption. LAB VALUES: May produce false-positive urine test results for cannabinoid; increases AST, ALT. May decrease neutrophils.

AVAILABILITY (Rx)

Capsules: 50 mg, 100 mg, 200 mg. Tablets: 600 mg.

ADMINISTRATION/HANDLING

PO

• Give with water at bedtime (decreases CNS adverse effects). • Avoid high-fat meals (may increase absorption) • Capsules may be opened and added to small amount of food/liquid. • Do not break tablets.

INDICATIONS/ROUTES/DOSAGE

HIV Infection (in Combination with Other Antiretrovirals)

PO: ADULTS, ELDERLY, CHILDREN 3 YRS AND OLDER WEIGHING 40 KG OR MORE: 600 mg once a day at bedtime. **CHILDREN 3 YRS AND OLDER WEIGHING 32.5 KG–LESS THAN 40 KG:** 400 mg once a day. **CHILDREN 3 YRS AND OLDER WEIGHING 25 KG–LESS THAN 32.5 KG:** 350 mg once a day. **CHILDREN 3 YRS AND OLDER WEIGHING 20 KG–LESS THAN 25 KG:** 300 mg once a day. **CHILDREN 3 YRS AND OLDER WEIGHING 15 KG–LESS THAN 20 KG:** 250 mg once a day. **CHILDREN 3 YRS AND OLDER WEIGHING 10 KG–LESS THAN 15 KG:** 200 mg once a day.

SIDE EFFECTS

Frequent (52%): **Mild to severe:** Dizziness, vivid dreams, insomnia, confusion, impaired concentration, amnesia, agitation, depersonalization, hallucinations, euphoria. Occasional: **Mild to moderate:** Maculopapular rash (27%); nausea, fatigue, headache, diarrhea, fever, cough (less than 26%).

ADVERSE EFFECTS/ TOXIC REACTIONS

Serious psychiatric adverse experiences (aggressive reactions, agitation, delusions, emotional lability, mania, neurosis, paranoia, psychosis, suicide) have been reported.

NURSING CONSIDERATIONS

BASELINE ASSESSMENT

Offer emotional support to pt and family. Obtain baseline AST, ALT in pts with history of hepatitis B or C; serum cholesterol or triglycerides before initiating therapy and at intervals during therapy. Obtain history of all prescription and OTC medications (high level of drug interaction).

INTERVENTION/EVALUATION

Monitor for CNS, psychological symptoms: severe acute depression, including suicidal ideation or attempts, dizziness, impaired concentration, drowsiness, abnormal dreams, insomnia (begins during first or second day of therapy, generally resolves in 2–4 wks). Assess for evidence of rash (common side effect). Monitor hepatic enzyme studies for abnormalities. Assess for headache, nausea, diarrhea.

PATIENT/FAMILY TEACHING

• Avoid high-fat meals during therapy. • If rash appears, contact physician immediately. • CNS, psychological symptoms occur in more than half of pts (dizziness, impaired concentration, delusions, depression). • Take medication every day as prescribed. • Do not alter dose or discontinue medication without informing physician. • Avoid tasks that require alertness, motor skills until response to drug is established. • Avoid alcohol. • Efavirenz is not a cure for HIV infection, nor does it reduce risk of transmission to others.

Effexor, *see venlafaxine*

Effexor XR, *see venlafaxine*

Efudex, *see fluorouracil, 5-FU*

Elavil, *see amitriptyline*

eletriptan

el-eh-**trip**-tan
(Relpax)

CLASSIFICATION

PHARMACOTHERAPEUTIC: Serotonin receptor agonist. **CLINICAL:** Antimigraine.

ACTION

Binds selectively to vascular receptors, producing vasoconstrictive effect on cranial blood vessels. **Therapeutic Effect:** Relieves migraine headache.

PHARMACOKINETICS

Well absorbed after PO administration. Metabolized by liver to inactive metabolite. Eliminated in urine. **Half-life:** 4.4 hrs (increased in hepatic impairment, elderly [older than 65 yrs]).

USES

Treatment of acute migraine headache with or without aura.

PRECAUTIONS

Contraindications: Arrhythmias associated with conduction disorders, cerebrovascular syndrome including strokes and transient ischemic attacks (TIAs), coronary artery disease, hemiplegic or basilar migraine, ischemic heart disease, peripheral vascular disease including ischemic bowel disease, severe hepatic impairment, uncontrolled hypertension; use within 24 hrs of treatment with another 5-HT1 agonist, an ergotamine-containing or ergot-type medication such as dihydroergotamine (DHE) or methysergide. **Cautions:** Mild to moderate renal/hepatic impairment, controlled hypertension, history of CVA.

LIFESPAN CONSIDERATIONS

Pregnancy/Lactation: May decrease possibility of ovulation. Distributed in breast milk. **Pregnancy Category C. Children:** Safety and efficacy not established in those younger than 18 yrs. **Elderly:** Increased risk of hypertension in those older than 65 yrs.

INTERACTIONS

DRUG: **Clarithromycin, itraconazole, ketoconazole, nefazodone, nelfinavir, ritonavir** may decrease metabolism. **Ergotamine-containing medications** may produce vasospastic reaction. **HERBAL:** None significant. **FOOD:** None known. **LAB VALUES:** None significant.

AVAILABILITY (Rx)

Tablets: 20 mg, 40 mg.

ADMINISTRATION/HANDLING

PO

• Do not crush, break film-coated tablets.

INDICATIONS/ROUTES/DOSAGE

Acute Migraine Headache

PO: ADULTS, ELDERLY: 20–40 mg. If headache improves but then returns, dose may be repeated after 2 hrs. **Maximum:** 80 mg/day.

SIDE EFFECTS

Occasional (6%–5%): Dizziness, drowsiness, asthenia (loss of strength, energy), nausea. **Rare (3%–2%):** Paresthesia, headache, dry mouth, warm or hot sensation, dyspepsia, dysphagia.

ADVERSE EFFECTS/ TOXIC REACTIONS

Cardiac reactions (ischemia, coronary artery vasospasm, MI), noncardiac vasospasm-related reactions (hemorrhage, CVA) occur rarely, particularly in pts with hypertension, obesity, diabetes, strong family history of coronary artery disease; smokers; males older than 40 yrs; postmenopausal women.

E

NURSING CONSIDERATIONS

BASELINE ASSESSMENT

Question pt regarding onset, location, duration of migraine, possible precipitating symptoms. Obtain baseline B/P for evidence of uncontrolled hypertension (contraindication).

INTERVENTION/EVALUATION

Assess for relief of migraine headache, potential for photophobia, phonophobia (sound sensitivity), nausea, vomiting.

PATIENT/FAMILY TEACHING

• Take a single dose as soon as symptoms of an actual migraine attack appear. • Medication is intended to relieve migraine headaches, not to prevent or reduce number of attacks. • Avoid tasks that require alertness, motor skills until response to drug is established. • Contact physician immediately if palpitations, pain/tightness in chest/throat, sudden or severe abdominal pain, pain/weakness of extremities occur.

Ellence, *see epirubicin*

Eloxatin, *see oxaliplatin*

eltrombopag

ell-**trom**-bow-pag
(Promacta)

BLACK BOX ALERT May cause hepatotoxicity. Measure ALT, AST, and bilirubin prior to initiation of eltrombopag, every 2 wks during dose adjustment phase, and monthly following establishment of a stable dose. If bilirubin is elevated, perform fractionation. Discontinue eltrombopag if ALT levels increase to 3 times or greater upper limit of normal and are progressive, persistent for 4 or more wks, accompanied by increased direct bilirubin, clinical symptoms of hepatic injury, or evidence of hepatic decompensation.

◆CLASSIFICATION

PHARMACOTHERAPEUTIC: Thrombopoietin receptor agonist. **CLINICAL:** Prevents thrombocytopenia.

ACTION

Interacts with the human thrombopoietin receptor and initiates signaling cascades. **Therapeutic Effect:** Induces proliferation and differentiation of megakaryocytes from bone marrow progenitor cells.

PHARMACOKINETICS

Readily absorbed from gastrointestinal tract. Primarily distributed in blood cells. Protein binding: 99%. Extensively metabolized including oxidation, conjugation with glucoronic acid or cysteine. Excreted primarily in feces. **Half-life:** 26–35 hrs.

USES

Treatment of thrombocytopenia in pts with chronic immune (idiopathic) thrombocytopenic purpura with insufficient response with corticosteroids, immunoglobulins, or splenectomy. Use only in pts who are at increased risk for bleeding; should not be used to normalize platelet counts.

PRECAUTIONS

Contraindications: None significant. **Cautions:** Hepatic impairment, myelodysplastic syndrome (may increase risk for hematologic malignancies).

⌛ LIFESPAN CONSIDERATIONS:

Pregnancy/lactation: Unknown if distributed in breast milk. **Pregnancy Cate-**

gory C. **Children:** Safety and efficacy not established. **Elderly:** Use caution due to increased frequency of hepatic, renal, cardiac function.

INTERACTIONS

DRUG: May increase concentration/toxicity of **atorvastatin, fluvastatin, methotrexate, nateglinide, pravastatin, repaglinide, rifampin, rosuvastatin. Aluminum, antacids, calcium, iron, magnesium** may decrease concentration/effect. HERBAL: None significant. FOOD: **Dairy products** may decrease concentration/effect. LAB VALUES: May increase ALT, AST.

AVAILABILITY (Rx)

Tablets: 25 mg, 50 mg.

ADMINISTRATION/HANDLING

PO

• Give on an empty stomach, either 1 hr before or 2 hrs after eating food. • Give at least 4 hrs before or 4 hrs after ingestion of dairy products or calcium fortified juices.

INDICATIONS/ROUTES/DOSAGE

Thrombocytopenia

PO: ADULTS, ELDERLY: Initially, 50 mg once daily (25 mg for pts of East Asian ancestry or moderate to severe hepatic insufficiency). After initiating eltrombopag, adjust dose (25 mg to 75 mg once daily) to achieve and maintain platelet count of 50×10^9/L or greater as necessary to reduce risk of bleeding. **Maximum:** 75 mg once daily.

SIDE EFFECTS

Frequent (6%–4%): Nausea, vomiting, menorrhagia. Occasional (3%–2%): Myalgia, paresthesia, dyspepsia, ecchymosis, cataract, conjunctival hemorrhage.

ADVERSE REACTIONS/ TOXIC EFFECTS

May cause hepatotoxicity. Increases risk of reticulin fiber deposits within bone marrow (may lead to bone marrow fibrosis). May produce hematologic malignancies. May cause excessive increase in platelets, leading to thrombotic complications.

NURSING CONSIDERATIONS

BASELINE ASSESSMENT

Assess CBCs, including platelet counts and peripheral blood smears; hepatic function tests (ALT, AST, bilirubin) prior to initiating therapy. Examine peripheral blood smear to establish extent of RBC and WBC abnormalities. Obtain baseline ocular examination.

INTERVENTION/EVALUATION

Monitor CBC, platelet counts, peripheral blood smears, hepatic function tests (ALT, AST, bilirubin) throughout and following discontinuation of eltrombopag. Monitor for signs of cataracts during therapy.

PATIENT/FAMILY TEACHING

• Inform pt of need to monitor hepatic function, CBC, platelet counts, peripheral blood smears throughout therapy and for at least 4 wks following discontinuation of therapy. • Report any of the following signs and symptoms of hepatotoxicity: yellowing of the skin or whites of eyes, unusual darkening of the urine, unusual tiredness, right upper stomach area pain.

emtricitabine

em-trih-**sit**-ah-bean
(Emtriva)

BLACK BOX ALERT Serious, sometimes fatal, hypersensitivity reaction, lactic acidosis, severe hepatomegaly with steatosis (fatty liver) have occurred. May exacerbate hepatitis B following completion of emtricitabine therapy.

FIXED-COMBINATION(S)

Atripla: emtricitabine/efavirenz (an antiretroviral)/tenofovir (an antiretroviral): 200 mg/600 mg/300 mg.

Truvada: emtricitabine/tenofovir (an antiretroviral): 200 mg/300 mg.

◆CLASSIFICATION

PHARMACOTHERAPEUTIC: Nucleoside reverse transcriptase inhibitor. **CLINICAL:** Antiretroviral agent.

E

ACTION

Inhibits HIV-1 reverse transcriptase by incorporating itself into viral DNA, resulting in chain termination. **Therapeutic Effect:** Impairs HIV replication, slowing progression of HIV infection.

PHARMACOKINETICS

Rapidly, extensively absorbed from GI tract. Protein binding: Less than 4%. Excreted primarily in urine. **Half-life:** 10 hrs.

USES

Used in combination with at least two other antiretroviral agents for treatment of HIV-1 infection in adults.

PRECAUTIONS

Contraindications: None known. **Cautions:** Hepatic/renal impairment.

⌛ LIFESPAN CONSIDERATIONS

Pregnancy/Lactation: Breast-feeding not recommended. **Pregnancy Category B.** **Children:** Safety and efficacy not established. **Elderly:** Age-related renal impairment may require dosage adjustment.

INTERACTIONS

DRUG: None significant. **HERBAL:** None significant. **FOOD:** None known. **LAB VALUES:** May increase serum amylase, lipase, ALT, AST, triglycerides. May alter serum glucose.

AVAILABILITY (Rx)

Capsules: 200 mg. **Oral Solution:** 10 mg/ml.

ADMINISTRATION/HANDLING

PO

- Give without regard to food.

INDICATIONS/ROUTES/DOSAGE

HIV

Capsules

PO: ADULTS, ELDERLY, CHILDREN 3 MOS–17 YRS, WEIGHING MORE THAN 33 KG: 200 mg once daily.

Oral Solution

PO: ADULTS, ELDERLY: 240 mg once daily. **CHILDREN 3 MOS–17 YRS:** 6 mg/kg once daily. **Maximum:** 240 mg once daily. **CHILDREN 0–3 MOS:** 3 mg/kg/day.

Dosage in Renal Impairment

Creatinine Clearance	Capsule	Oral Solution
30–49 ml/min	200 mg q48h	120 mg q24h
15–29 ml/min	200 mg q72h	80 mg q24h
Less than 15 ml/min; hemodialysis pts	200 mg q96h	60 mg q24h

Administer after dialysis on dialysis days.

SIDE EFFECTS

Frequent (23%–13%): Headache, rhinitis, rash, diarrhea, nausea. **Occasional (14%–4%):** Cough, vomiting, abdominal pain, insomnia, depression, paresthesia, dizziness, peripheral neuropathy, dyspepsia, myalgia. **Rare (3%–2%):** Arthralgia, abnormal dreams.

ADVERSE EFFECTS/ TOXIC REACTIONS

Lactic acidosis, hepatomegaly with steatosis (excess fat in liver) occur rarely; may be severe.

NURSING CONSIDERATIONS

BASELINE ASSESSMENT

Obtain baseline laboratory tests, esp. serum hepatic function, triglycerides before beginning and at periodic intervals during emtricitabine therapy. Offer emotional support.

INTERVENTION/EVALUATION

Monitor daily pattern of bowel activity and stool consistency. Question for evidence of nausea, pruritus. Assess skin for rash, urticaria. Monitor serum chemistry tests, hepatic function tests for marked abnormalities, signs/symptoms of lactic acidosis.

PATIENT/FAMILY TEACHING

• May cause redistribution of body fat. • Continue therapy for full length of treatment. • Emtricitabine is not a cure for HIV infection, nor does it reduce risk of transmission to others. • Pts may continue to acquire illnesses associated with advanced HIV infection. • Avoid tasks that require alertness, motor skills until response to drug is established. • Notify physician if persistent severe abdominal pain, nausea, vomiting, numbness occur.

enalapril

en-**al**-ah-pril
(Apo-Enalapril ✤, Novo-Enalapril ✤, Vasotec)

BLACK BOX ALERT May cause fetal injury, mortality if used during second or third trimester of pregnancy.

Do not confuse enalapril with Anafranil, Elavil, Eldepryl, or ramipril.

FIXED-COMBINATION(S)

Lexxel: enalapril/felodipine (calcium channel blocker): 5 mg/2.5 mg, 5 mg/5 mg. **Teczem:** enalapril/diltiazem (calcium channel blocker): 5 mg/180 mg. **Vaseretic:** enalapril/hydrochlorothiazide (diuretic): 5 mg/12.5 mg, 10 mg/25 mg.

◆ CLASSIFICATION

PHARMACOTHERAPEUTIC: Angiotensin-converting enzyme (ACE) inhibitor. **CLINICAL:** Antihypertensive, vasodilator (see p. 9C).

ACTION

Suppresses renin-angiotensin-aldosterone system (prevents conversion of angiotensin I to angiotensin II, a potent vasoconstrictor; may inhibit angiotensin II at local vascular, renal sites). Decreases plasma angiotensin II, increases plasma renin activity, decreases aldosterone secretion. **Therapeutic Effect:** In hypertension, reduces peripheral arterial resistance. In CHF, increases cardiac output; decreases peripheral vascular resistance, B/P, pulmonary capillary wedge pressure, heart size.

PHARMACOKINETICS

Route	Onset	Peak	Duration
PO	1 hr	4–6 hrs	24 hrs
IV	15 min	1–4 hrs	6 hrs

Readily absorbed from GI tract. Protein binding: 50%–60%. Converted to active metabolite. Primarily excreted in urine. Removed by hemodialysis. **Half-life:** 11 hrs (increased in renal impairment).

USES

Treatment of hypertension alone or in combination with other antihypertensives. Adjunctive therapy for CHF. **OFF-LABEL:** Diabetic nephropathy, hypertension due to scleroderma, renal crisis, hypertensive crisis, idiopathic edema, renal artery stenosis, rheumatoid arthritis, post MI for prevention of ventricular failure.

PRECAUTIONS

Contraindications: History of angioedema from previous treatment with ACE inhibitors. **Cautions:** Renal impairment, those with sodium depletion or on diuretic therapy, dialysis, hypovolemia, coronary/cerebrovascular insufficiency.

⌛ LIFESPAN CONSIDERATIONS

Pregnancy/Lactation: Crosses placenta. Distributed in breast milk. May cause fetal/neonatal mortality, morbidity. **Pregnancy Category D (C if used in first trimester). Children:** Safety and efficacy not established. **Elderly:** May be more susceptible to hypotensive effects.

INTERACTIONS

DRUG: Alcohol, antihypertensive agents, diuretics may increase effect.

NSAIDs may decrease effect. **Potassium-sparing diuretics, potassium supplements** may cause hyperkalemia. May increase **lithium** concentration, toxicity. HERBAL: **Ephedra, ginseng, yohimbe** may worsen hypertension. **Garlic** may increase antihypertensive effect. **Licorice** may cause sodium/water retention, loss of potassium. FOOD: None known. LAB VALUES: May increase BUN, serum alkaline phosphatase, bilirubin, creatinine, potassium, AST, ALT. May decrease serum sodium. May cause positive ANA titer.

AVAILABILITY (Rx)

Injection Solution: 1.25 mg/ml. **Tablets:** 2.5 mg, 5 mg, 10 mg, 20 mg.

ADMINISTRATION/HANDLING

IV

Reconstitution • May give undiluted or dilute with D_5W or 0.9% NaCl.
Rate of administration • For IV push, give undiluted over 5 min. • For IV piggyback, infuse over 10–15 min.
Storage • Store parenteral form at room temperature. • Use only clear, colorless solution. • Diluted IV solution is stable for 24 hrs at room temperature.

PO

• Give without regard to food. • Tablets may be crushed.

IV INCOMPATIBILITIES

Amphotericin B (Fungizone), amphotericin B complex (Abelcet, AmBisome, Amphotec), cefepime (Maxipime), phenytoin (Dilantin).

IV COMPATIBILITIES

Calcium gluconate, dobutamine (Dobutrex), dopamine (Intropin), fentanyl (Sublimaze), heparin, lidocaine, lipids, magnesium sulfate, morphine, nitroglycerin, potassium chloride, potassium phosphate, propofol (Diprivan).

INDICATIONS/ROUTES/DOSAGE

Hypertension

PO: ADULTS, ELDERLY: Initially, 2.5–5 mg/day. May increase at 1- to 2-wk intervals. Range: 2.5–40 mg/day in 1–2 divided doses. **CHILDREN 1 MO–16 YRS:** 0.1 mg/kg/day in 1–2 divided doses. **Maximum:** 0.5 mg/kg/day. **NEONATES:** 0.1 mg/kg/day q24h.
IV: ADULTS, ELDERLY: 0.625–1.25 mg q6h up to 5 mg q6h. **CHILDREN, NEONATES:** 5–10 mcg/kg/dose q8–24h.

Adjunctive Therapy for CHF

PO: ADULTS, ELDERLY: Initially, 2.5–5 mg/day. Range: 5–40 mg/day in 2 divided doses.

Dosage in Renal Impairment

Creatinine Clearance	PO	IV
30 ml/min or greater	5 mg/day; titrate to maximum 40 mg/day	1.25 mg q6h; titrate to desired response
Less than 30 ml/min	2.5 mg/day; titrate to control B/P	0.626 mg q6h; titrate to desired response

SIDE EFFECTS

Frequent (7%–5%): Headache, dizziness. **Occasional (3%–2%):** Orthostatic hypotension, fatigue, diarrhea, cough, syncope. **Rare (less than 2%):** Angina, abdominal pain, vomiting, nausea, rash, asthenia (loss of strength, energy).

ADVERSE EFFECTS/ TOXIC REACTIONS

Excessive hypotension ("first-dose syncope") may occur in pts with CHF, severe salt or volume depletion. Angioedema (facial, lip swelling), hyperkalemia occur rarely. Agranulocytosis, neutropenia may be noted in pts with renal impairment, collagen vascular diseases (scleroderma, systemic lupus erythematosus). Nephrotic syndrome may be noted in those with history of renal disease.

NURSING CONSIDERATIONS

BASELINE ASSESSMENT

Obtain B/P immediately before each dose (be alert to fluctuations). In pts with renal impairment, autoimmune disease, or taking drugs that affect leukocytes/immune response, CBC should be performed before beginning therapy, q2wks for 3 mos, then periodically thereafter.

INTERVENTION/EVALUATION

Assist with ambulation if dizziness occurs. Monitor serum potassium, BUN, serum creatinine, CBC, B/P. Monitor daily pattern of bowel activity and stool consistency.

PATIENT/FAMILY TEACHING

• To reduce hypotensive effect, rise slowly from lying to sitting position, permit legs to dangle from bed momentarily before standing. • Several wks may be needed for full therapeutic effect of B/P reduction. • Skipping doses or voluntarily discontinuing drug may produce severe, rebound hypertension. • Limit alcohol intake. • Inform physician if vomiting, diarrhea, diaphoresis, persistent cough, swelling of face, lips, tongue, difficulty in breathing occurs.

Enbrel, *see etanercept*

enfuvirtide

en-few-vir-tide
(Fuzeon)

◆CLASSIFICATION

PHARMACOTHERAPEUTIC: Fusion inhibitor. **CLINICAL:** Antiretroviral agent.

ACTION

Interferes with entry of HIV-1 into $CD4^+$ cells by inhibiting fusion of viral, cellular membranes. **Therapeutic Effect:** Impairs HIV replication, slowing progression of HIV infection.

PHARMACOKINETICS

Comparable absorption when injected into subcutaneous tissue of abdomen, arm, thigh. Protein binding: 92%. Undergoes catabolism to amino acids. **Half-life:** 3.8 hrs.

USES

Used in combination with other antiretroviral agents for treatment of HIV-1 infection in treatment-experienced pts with evidence of HIV-1 replication.

PRECAUTIONS

Contraindications: None known. **Cautions:** None known.

LIFESPAN CONSIDERATIONS

Pregnancy/Lactation: Breast-feeding not recommended. **Pregnancy Category B. Children:** Safety and effectiveness not established in those 6 yrs and younger. **Elderly:** No age-related precautions noted.

INTERACTIONS

DRUG: None significant. **HERBAL:** None significant. **FOOD:** None known. **LAB VALUES:** May elevate serum glucose, amylase, creatine kinase (CK), lipase, triglycerides, AST, ALT. May decrease Hgb.

AVAILABILITY (Rx)

Injection, Powder for Reconstitution: 108 mg (approximately 90 mg/ml when reconstituted) vials.

ADMINISTRATION/HANDLING

Subcutaneous

Reconstitution • Reconstitute with 1.1 ml Sterile Water for Injection. • Visually inspect vial for particulate matter. Solution should appear clear, colorless (may take up to 45 min to form clear, colorless solution). • Discard unused portion.

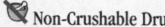

Rate of administration • Administer into upper arm, anterior thigh, abdomen. Rotate injection sites.

Storage • Store at room temperature. • Refrigerate reconstituted solution; use within 24 hrs. • Bring reconstituted solution to room temperature before injection.

INDICATIONS/ROUTES/DOSAGE

HIV Infection

SUBCUTANEOUS: ADULTS, ELDERLY: 90 mg (1 ml) twice a day. **CHILDREN 6–16 YRS:** 2 mg/kg twice a day. **Maximum:** 90 mg twice a day.

Pediatric Dosing Guidelines

Weight: kg (lb)	Dose: mg (ml)
11–15.5 (24–34)	27 (0.3)
15.6–20 (35–44)	36 (0.4)
20.1–24.5 (45–54)	45 (0.5)
24.6–29 (55–64)	54 (0.6)
29.1–33.5 (65–74)	63 (0.7)
33.6–38 (75–84)	72 (0.8)
38.1–42.5 (85–94)	81 (0.9)
Greater than 42.5 (greater than 94)	90 (1)

SIDE EFFECTS

Expected (98%): Local injection site reactions (pain, discomfort, induration, erythema, nodules, cysts, pruritus, ecchymosis). **Frequent (26%–16%):** Diarrhea, nausea, fatigue. **Occasional (11%–4%):** Insomnia, peripheral neuropathy, depression, cough, decreased appetite or weight loss, sinusitis, anxiety, asthenia (loss of strength, energy), myalgia, cold sores. **Rare (3%–2%):** Constipation, influenza, upper abdominal pain, anorexia, conjunctivitis.

ADVERSE EFFECTS/ TOXIC REACTIONS

May potentiate bacterial pneumonia. Hypersensitivity (rash, fever, chills, rigors, hypotension), thrombocytopenia, neutropenia, renal insufficiency/failure occur rarely.

NURSING CONSIDERATIONS

BASELINE ASSESSMENT

Obtain baseline laboratory tests, esp. serum hepatic function, triglycerides before beginning enfuvirtide therapy and at periodic intervals during therapy. Offer emotional support.

INTERVENTION/EVALUATION

Assess skin for local injection site hypersensitivity reaction. Question for evidence of nausea, fatigue. Assess sleep pattern. Monitor for insomnia, signs/symptoms of depression, pneumonia. Monitor serum chemistry tests for marked abnormalities.

PATIENT/FAMILY TEACHING

• Increased rate of bacterial pneumonia has occurred with enfuvirtide therapy; seek medical attention if cough with fever, difficult breathing occurs. • Continue therapy for full length of treatment. • Enfuvirtide is not a cure for HIV infection, nor does it reduce risk of transmission to others. • Pt must continue practices to prevent HIV transmission. • Notify physician if injection site reaction is severe.

enoxaparin

HIGH ALERT

en-**ox**-ah-pear-in
(Lovenox)

BLACK BOX ALERT Epidural or spinal anesthesia greatly increases potential for spinal or epidural hematoma, subsequent long-term or permanent paralysis.

Do not confuse Lovenox with Lasix, Levaquin, Lotronex, or Protonix.

◆CLASSIFICATION

PHARMACOTHERAPEUTIC: Low-molecular-weight heparin. **CLINICAL:** Anticoagulant (see p. 31C).

ACTION

Potentiates action of antithrombin III, inactivates coagulation factor Xa. **Therapeutic Effect:** Produces anticoagulation. Does not significantly influence bleeding time, PT, aPTT.

PHARMACOKINETICS

Route	Onset	Peak	Duration
Subcutaneous	N/A	3–5 hrs	12 hrs

Well absorbed after subcutaneous administration. Eliminated primarily in urine. Not removed by hemodialysis. **Half-life:** 4.5 hrs.

USES

Prevention of postop deep vein thrombosis (DVT) following hip or knee replacement surgery, abdominal surgery. Long-term DVT prevention following hip replacement surgery, nonsurgical acute illness. Treatment of unstable angina, non–Q-wave MI, acute ST-segment elevation MI (STEMI), acute DVT (with warfarin). **OFF-LABEL:** Prevention of DVT following general surgical procedures.

PRECAUTIONS

Contraindications: Active major bleeding, concurrent heparin therapy, hypersensitivity to heparin, pork products, thrombocytopenia associated with positive in vitro test for antiplatelet antibodies. **Cautions:** Conditions with increased risk of hemorrhage, history of heparin-induced thrombocytopenia, renal impairment, elderly, uncontrolled arterial hypertension, history of recent GI ulceration or hemorrhage. When neuraxial anesthesia (epidural or spinal anesthesia) or spinal puncture is used, pts anticoagulated or scheduled to be anticoagulated with enoxaparin for prevention of thromboembolic complications are at risk for developing an epidural or spinal hematoma that can result in long-term or permanent paralysis.

LIFESPAN CONSIDERATIONS

Pregnancy/Lactation: Use with caution, particularly during third trimester, immediate postpartum period (increased risk of maternal hemorrhage). Unknown if distributed in breast milk. **Pregnancy Category B. Children:** Safety and efficacy not established. **Elderly:** May be more susceptible to bleeding.

INTERACTIONS

DRUG: **Antiplatelet agents, aspirin, NSAIDs, thrombolytics** may increase risk of bleeding. **HERBAL:** **Cat's claw, dong quai, evening primrose, feverfew, garlic, ginger, ginkgo, ginseng** may increase antiplatelet action. **FOOD:** None known. **LAB VALUES:** Increases serum alkaline phosphatase, AST, ALT. May decrease Hgb, Hct, RBCs.

AVAILABILITY (Rx)

Injection Solution: 30 mg/0.3 ml, 40 mg/0.4 ml, 60 mg/0.6 ml, 80 mg/0.8 ml, 100 mg/ml, 120 mg/0.8 ml, 150 mg/ml in prefilled syringes.

ADMINISTRATION/HANDLING

◀ALERT▶ Do not mix with other injections, infusions. Do not give IM.

Subcutaneous

• Parenteral form appears clear, colorless to pale yellow. • Store at room temperature. • Instruct pt to lie down before administering by deep subcutaneous injection. • Inject between left and right anterolateral and left and right posterolateral abdominal wall. • Introduce entire length of needle (½ inch) into skin fold held between thumb and forefinger, holding skin fold during injection.

INDICATIONS/ROUTES/DOSAGE

Prevention of Deep Vein Thrombosis (DVT) After Hip and Knee Surgery

SUBCUTANEOUS: ADULTS, ELDERLY: 30 mg twice a day, generally for 7–10 days, with initial dose given within 12–24 hrs

E

following surgery. Once-daily dosing following hip surgery: 40 mg with initial dose within 9–15 hrs before surgery.

Prevention of DVT After Abdominal Surgery
SUBCUTANEOUS: ADULTS, ELDERLY: 40 mg a day for 7–10 days, with initial dose given 2h prior to surgery.

Prevention of Long-Term DVT in Nonsurgical Acute Illness
SUBCUTANEOUS: ADULTS, ELDERLY: 40 mg once a day for 3 wks.

Prevention of Ischemic Complications of Unstable Angina, Non–Q-Wave MI (with Oral Aspirin Therapy), Acute ST-Segment Elevation MI (STEMI)
SUBCUTANEOUS: ADULTS, ELDERLY: 1 mg/kg q12h.

Acute DVT
SUBCUTANEOUS: ADULTS, ELDERLY: 1 mg/kg q12h or 1.5 mg/kg once daily.

Usual Pediatric Dosage
SUBCUTANEOUS: CHILDREN: 0.5 mg/kg q12h (prophylaxis); 1 mg/kg q12h (treatment).

Dosage in Renal Impairment
Clearance is decreased when creatinine clearance is less than 30 ml/min. Monitor and adjust dosage as necessary.

Use	Dosage
Abdominal surgery, pts with acute illness	30 mg once/day
Hip, knee surgery	30 mg once/day
DVT, angina, MI	1 mg/kg once/day

SIDE EFFECTS

Occasional (4%–1%): Injection site hematoma, nausea, peripheral edema.

ADVERSE EFFECTS/ TOXIC REACTIONS

Overdose may lead to bleeding complications ranging from local ecchymoses to major hemorrhage. **Antidote:** IV injection of protamine sulfate (1% solution) equal to dose of enoxaparin injected. One mg protamine sulfate neutralizes 1 mg enoxaparin. A second dose of 0.5 mg protamine sulfate per 1 mg enoxaparin may be given if aPTT tested 2–4 hrs after first injection remains prolonged.

NURSING CONSIDERATIONS

BASELINE ASSESSMENT

Assess CBC, including platelet count.

INTERVENTION/EVALUATION

Periodically monitor CBC, platelet count, stool for occult blood (no need for daily monitoring in pts with normal presurgical coagulation parameters). Assess for any sign of bleeding (bleeding at surgical site, hematuria, blood in stool, bleeding from gums, petechiae, bruising, bleeding from injection sites).

PATIENT/FAMILY TEACHING

• Usual length of therapy is 7–10 days. • Do not take any OTC medication (esp. aspirin) without consulting physician. • Notify physician if unusual bleeding or bruising occurs.

entacapone

en-**tah**-cah-pone
(Comtan)

FIXED-COMBINATION(S)

Stalevo: entacapone/carbidopa/levodopa (an antiparkinson agent): 200 mg/12.5 mg/50 mg, 200 mg/25 mg/100 mg, 200 mg/37.5 mg/150 mg.

◆CLASSIFICATION

PHARMACOTHERAPEUTIC: Enzyme inhibitor. **CLINICAL:** Antiparkinson agent.

ACTION

Inhibits the enzyme, catechol-*O*-methyltransferase (COMT), potentiating dopamine activity, increasing duration of action of levodopa. Therapeutic Effect: Decreases signs, symptoms of Parkinson's disease.

PHARMACOKINETICS

Rapidly absorbed after PO administration. Protein binding: 98%. Metabolized in liver. Primarily eliminated by biliary excretion. Not removed by hemodialysis. Half-life: 2.4 hrs.

USES

In conjunction with levodopa/carbidopa, improves quality of life in pts with Parkinson's disease.

PRECAUTIONS

Contraindications: Hypersensitivity, use within 14 days of MAOIs. Cautions: Renal/hepatic impairment. May increase risk of orthostatic hypotension and syncope, exacerbate dyskinesias.

LIFESPAN CONSIDERATIONS

Pregnancy/Lactation: Unknown if distributed in breast milk. **Pregnancy Category C.** **Children:** Not used in this pt population. **Elderly:** No age-related precautions noted.

INTERACTIONS

DRUG: **Bitolterol, dobutamine, dopamine, epinephrine, isoetharine, isoproterenol, methyldopa, norepinephrine** may increase risk of arrhythmias, alter B/P. **Nonselective MAOIs (including phenelzine)** may inhibit catecholamine metabolism. HERBAL: None significant. FOOD: None known. LAB VALUES: Serum iron may decrease.

AVAILABILITY (Rx)

Tablets: 200 mg.

ADMINISTRATION/HANDLING

PO

- Give without regard to food.

INDICATIONS/ROUTES/DOSAGE

◀ALERT▶ Always administer with levodopa/carbidopa.

Adjunctive Treatment of Parkinson's Disease

PO: ADULTS, ELDERLY: 200 mg concomitantly with each dose of carbidopa and levodopa up to a maximum of 8 times a day (1,600 mg).

SIDE EFFECTS

Frequent (greater than 10%): Dyskinesia (uncontrolled body movements), nausea, dark yellow or orange urine and sweat, diarrhea. Occasional (9%–3%): Abdominal pain, vomiting, constipation, dry mouth, fatigue, back pain. Rare (less than 2%): Anxiety, drowsiness, agitation, dyspepsia, flatulence, diaphoresis, asthenia (loss of strength, energy), dyspnea.

ADVERSE EFFECTS/ TOXIC REACTIONS

Hallucinations may be noted.

NURSING CONSIDERATIONS

INTERVENTION/EVALUATION

Monitor for evidence of dyskinesia (difficulty with movement). Assess for clinical reversal of symptoms (improvement of tremor of head and hands at rest, masklike facial expression, shuffling gait, muscular rigidity). Monitor B/P, hepatic function tests. Assess for orthostatic hypotension, diarrhea.

PATIENT/FAMILY TEACHING

• Avoid tasks that require alertness, motor skills until response to drug is established. • May cause color change in urine or sweat (dark yellow, orange). • Report any uncontrolled movement of face, eyelids, mouth, tongue, arms, hands, legs.

entecavir

en-**tech**-ah-veer
(Baraclude)

BLACK BOX ALERT Serious, sometimes fatal, hypersensitivity reaction, lactic acidosis, severe hepatomegaly with steatosis (fatty liver) have occurred. May cause HIV resistance in chronic hepatitis B pts.

◆CLASSIFICATION

PHARMACOTHERAPEUTIC: Reverse transcriptase inhibitor. **CLINICAL:** Antiretroviral.

E

ACTION

Inhibits hepatitis B viral polymerase, an enzyme blocking reverse transcriptase activity. **Therapeutic Effect:** Interferes with viral DNA synthesis.

PHARMACOKINETICS

Poorly absorbed from GI tract. Protein binding: 13%. Extensively distributed into tissues. Partially metabolized in liver. Eliminated mainly in urine. **Half-life:** 5–6 days (increased in renal impairment).

USES

Treatment of chronic hepatitis B infection with evidence of active viral replication and evidence of either persistent transaminase elevations or histologically active disease or evidence of decompensated hepatic disease.

PRECAUTIONS

Contraindications: None known. **Cautions:** Renal impairment, pts receiving concurrent therapy that may reduce renal function, hepatic transplant pts receiving concurrent therapy of cyclosporine or tacrolimus.

⌛ LIFESPAN CONSIDERATIONS

Pregnancy/Lactation: Unknown if drug crosses placenta or is distributed in breast milk. **Pregnancy Category C. Children:** Safety and efficacy not established in those younger than 16 yrs. **Elderly:** Age-related renal impairment may require dosage adjustment.

INTERACTIONS

DRUG: **Ganciclovir, ribavirin, valganciclovir** may increase concentration. **HERBAL:** None significant. **FOOD:** **Food** delays absorption, decreases concentration. **LAB VALUES:** May increase serum amylase, lipase, bilirubin, ALT, AST, creatinine, glucose. May decrease serum albumin, platelets.

AVAILABILITY (Rx)

Oral Solution: 0.05 mg/ml. **Tablets:** 0.5 mg, 1 mg.

ADMINISTRATION/HANDLING

PO

• Administer tablets on an empty stomach (at least 2 hrs after a meal and 2 hrs before the next meal). • Do not dilute, mix oral solution with water or any other liquid. • Each bottle of oral solution is accompanied by a dosing spoon. Before administering, hold spoon in vertical position, fill it gradually to mark corresponding to prescribed dose.

Storage • Store tablets, oral solution at room temperature.

INDICATIONS/ROUTES/DOSAGE

Chronic Hepatitis B (No Previous Nucleoside Treatment)

PO: ADULTS, ELDERLY, CHILDREN 16 YRS AND OLDER: 0.5 mg once daily.

Chronic Hepatitis B (Receiving Lamivudine, Known Lamivudine Resistance)

PO: ADULTS, ELDERLY, CHILDREN 16 YRS AND OLDER: 1 mg once daily.

Dosage in Renal Impairment

Creatinine Clearance	Dosage
50 ml/min and greater	0.5 mg once daily
30–49 ml/min	0.25 mg once daily
10–29 ml/min	0.15 mg once daily
9 ml/min and less	0.05 mg once daily

SIDE EFFECTS

Occasional (4%–3%): Headache, fatigue. **Rare (less than 1%):** Diarrhea, dyspepsia, nausea, vomiting, dizziness, insomnia.

ADVERSE EFFECTS/ TOXIC REACTIONS

Lactic acidosis, severe hepatomegaly with steatosis have been reported. Severe, acute exacerbations of hepatitis B have been reported in pts who have discontinued therapy; reinitiation of antihepatitis B therapy may be required. Hematuria occurs occasionally. May cause development of HIV resistance if HIV untreated.

NURSING CONSIDERATIONS

BASELINE ASSESSMENT

Obtain baseline laboratory tests, esp. hepatic function, before beginning therapy and at periodic intervals during therapy. Offer emotional support. Obtain medication history.

INTERVENTION/EVALUATION

Hepatic function should be monitored closely with both clinical and laboratory follow-up for at least several mos in pts who discontinue antihepatitis B therapy. For pts on therapy, closely monitor amylase, lipase, bilirubin, ALT, AST, creatinine, glucose, albumin, platelet count. Assess for evidence of GI discomfort.

PATIENT/FAMILY TEACHING

• Take medication at least 2 hrs after a meal and 2 hrs before the next meal. • Avoid transmission of hepatitis B infection to others through sexual contact, blood contamination. • Notify physician immediately if unusual muscle pain, abdominal pain with nausea/vomiting, cold feeling in extremities, dizziness occur (signs and symptoms signaling onset of lactic acidosis).

epinephrine

HIGH ALERT

eh-pih-**nef**-rin
(Adrenalin, EpiPen, EpiPen Jr., Primatene Mist, Twinject)
Do not confuse epinephrine with ephedrine.

FIXED-COMBINATION(S)

LidoSite: epinephrine/lidocaine (anesthetic): 0.1%/10%.

◆CLASSIFICATION

PHARMACOTHERAPEUTIC: Sympathomimetic (adrenergic agonist). **CLINICAL:** Antiglaucoma, bronchodilator, cardiac stimulant, antiallergic, antihemorrhagic, priapism reversal agent (see p. 158C).

ACTION

Stimulates alpha-adrenergic receptors (vasoconstriction, pressor effects), $beta_1$-adrenergic receptors (cardiac stimulation), $beta_2$-adrenergic receptors (bronchial dilation, vasodilation). **Ophthalmic:** Increases outflow of aqueous humor from anterior eye chamber. **Therapeutic Effect:** Relaxes smooth muscle of bronchial tree, produces cardiac stimulation, dilates skeletal muscle vasculature. **Ophthalmic:** Dilates pupils, constricts conjunctival blood vessels.

PHARMACOKINETICS

Route	Onset	Peak	Duration
IM	5–10 min	20 min	1–4 hrs
Subcutaneous	5–10 min	20 min	1–4 hrs
Inhalation	3–5 min	20 min	1–3 hrs
Ophthalmic	1 hr	4–8 hrs	12–24 hrs

Well absorbed after parenteral administration; minimally absorbed after inhalation. Metabolized in liver, other tissues, sympathetic nerve endings. Excreted in urine. Ophthalmic form may be systemically absorbed as a result of drainage into nasal pharyngeal passages. Mydriasis occurs within several min and persists several hrs; vasoconstriction occurs within 5 min and lasts less than 1 hr.

USES

Systemic: Treatment of asthma (acute exacerbation, reversible bronchospasm), anaphylaxis, hypersensitivity reaction, cardiac arrest. Added to local anesthetics to decrease systemic absorption and increase duration of activity of local anesthetic. **Ophthalmic:** Management of chronic open-angle glaucoma. OFF-LABEL: **Systemic:** Treatment of gingival, pulpal hemorrhage; priapism. Ventricular fibrillation or pulseless ventricular tachycardia unresponsive to initial defibrillatory shocks; pulseless electrical activity, asystole, hypotension unresponsive to volume resuscitation; bradycardia/hypotension unresponsive to atropine or pacing; inotropic support. **Ophthalmic:** Treatment of conjunctival congestion during surgery, secondary glaucoma.

PRECAUTIONS

Contraindications: Cardiac arrhythmias, cerebrovascular insufficiency, hypertension, hyperthyroidism, ischemic heart disease, narrow-angle glaucoma, shock-type states. Cautions: Elderly, diabetes mellitus, angina pectoris, tachycardia, MI, severe renal/hepatic impairment, psychoneurotic disorders, hypoxia.

LIFESPAN CONSIDERATIONS

Pregnancy/Lactation: Crosses placenta. Distributed in breast milk. **Pregnancy Category C.** **Children/Elderly:** No age-related precautions noted.

INTERACTIONS

DRUG: May decrease effects of **beta-blockers. Digoxin, sympathomimetics** may increase risk of arrhythmias. **Ergonovine, methergine, oxytocin** may increase vasoconstriction. **MAOIs, tricyclic antidepressants** may increase cardiovascular effects. HERBAL: **Ephedra, yohimbe** may increase CNS stimulation. FOOD: None known. LAB VALUES: May decrease serum potassium.

AVAILABILITY (Rx)

Aerosol for Oral Inhalation:
(Primatene Mist): 0.22 mg/inhalation.

Injection, Solution (Prefilled Syringes):
(EpiPen): 0.3 mg/0.3 ml, **(EpiPen Jr.):** 0.15 mg/0.3 ml, **(Twinject):** 0.15 mg/0.15 ml. Injection, Solution: 0.1 mg/ml (1:10,000), 1 mg/ml (1:1,000).

Solution for Oral Inhalation:
(Adrenalin): 2.25% (0.5 ml).

ADMINISTRATION/HANDLING

IV

Reconstitution • For injection, dilute each 1 mg of 1:1,000 solution with 10 ml 0.9% NaCl to provide 1:10,000 solution and inject each 1 mg or fraction thereof over 1 min or more (except in cardiac arrest). • For infusion, further dilute with 250–500 ml D_5W. Maximum concentration 64 mcg/ml.
Rate of administration • For IV infusion, give at 1–10 mcg/min (titrate to desired response).
Storage • Store parenteral forms at room temperature. • Do not use if solution appears discolored or contains a precipitate.

Subcutaneous

• Shake ampule thoroughly. • Use tuberculin syringe for injection into lateral deltoid region. • Massage injection site (minimizes vasoconstriction effect).

Inhalation

• Shake container well. • Instruct pt to exhale completely, place mouthpiece between lips, inhale deeply and slowly while pressing top of canister, hold breath as long as possible, then exhale slowly. • Allow at least 1 min between inhalations when multiple inhalations are ordered (allows for deeper bronchial penetration). • Rinsing mouth after each use decreases dry mouth, hoarseness.

Nebulizer

• No more than 10 drops Adrenalin Chloride solution 1:100 should be placed in reservoir of nebulizer. • Place nozzle just inside pt's partially opened mouth. • As bulb is squeezed once or twice, instruct pt to inhale deeply, drawing vaporized solution into lungs. • Rinse mouth with water immediately after inhalation (prevents mouth/throat dryness). • When nebulizer is not in use, replace stopper, keep in upright position.

IV INCOMPATIBILITIES

Aminophylline, ampicillin (Omnipen, Polycillin), sodium bicarbonate.

IV COMPATIBILITIES

Calcium chloride, calcium gluconate, diltiazem (Cardizem), dobutamine (Dobutrex), dopamine (Intropin), fentanyl (Sublimaze), heparin, hydromorphone (Dilaudid), lorazepam (Ativan), midazolam (Versed), milrinone (Primacor), morphine, nitroglycerin, norepinephrine (Levophed), potassium chloride, propofol (Diprivan).

INDICATIONS/ROUTES/DOSAGE

Anaphylaxis

IM: ADULTS, ELDERLY: 0.3–0.5 mg (0.3–0.5 ml of 1:1,000 solution). May repeat if anaphylaxis persists. **CHILDREN WEIGHING 30 KG OR MORE:** 0.15–0.3 mg. **WEIGHING LESS THAN 30 KG:** 0.01 mg/kg. May repeat if anaphylaxis persists.

Asthma

SUBCUTANEOUS: ADULTS, ELDERLY: 0.3–0.5 mg (0.3–0.5 ml of 1:1,000 solution) q2h as needed. In severe attacks, may repeat q20min times 3 doses. **CHILDREN:** 0.01 ml/kg/dose (1:1,000 solution). **Maximum:** 0.4–0.5 ml/dose. May repeat q15–20min for 3–4 doses or q4h as needed.

INHALATION: ADULTS, ELDERLY, CHILDREN 4 YRS AND OLDER: 1 inhalation, wait at least 1 min. May repeat once. Do not use again for at least 3 hrs.

Cardiac Arrest

IV: ADULTS, ELDERLY: Initially, 1 mg. May repeat q3–5min as needed. **CHILDREN:** Initially, 0.01 mg/kg (0.1 ml/kg of a 1:10,000 solution). May repeat q3–5min as needed.

ENDOTRACHEAL: CHILDREN: 0.1 mg/kg (0.1 ml/kg of a 1:1,000 solution). May repeat q3–5min as needed.

Hypersensitivity Reaction

IM, SUBCUTANEOUS: ADULTS, ELDERLY: 0.3–0.5 mg (1:1,000) q15–20min.

IV: 0.1 mg (1:10,000) over 5 min.

SUBCUTANEOUS: CHILDREN: 0.01 mg/kg every 20 min. **Maximum single dose:** 0.5 mg.

SIDE EFFECTS

Frequent: **Systemic:** Tachycardia, palpitations, anxiety. **Ophthalmic:** Headache, eye irritation, watering of eyes. Occasional: **Systemic:** Dizziness, lightheadedness, facial flushing, headache, diaphoresis, increased B/P, nausea, trembling, insomnia, vomiting, fatigue. **Ophthalmic:** Blurred/decreased vision, eye pain. Rare: **Systemic:** Chest discomfort/pain, arrhythmias, bronchospasm, dry mouth/throat.

ADVERSE EFFECTS/ TOXIC REACTIONS

Excessive doses may cause acute hypertension, arrhythmias. Prolonged/excessive use may result in metabolic acidosis due to increased serum lactic acid. Metabolic acidosis may cause disorientation, fatigue, hyperventilation, headache, nausea, vomiting, diarrhea.

NURSING CONSIDERATIONS

INTERVENTION/EVALUATION

Monitor for vital sign changes. Assess lung sounds for rhonchi, wheezing, rales. Monitor ABGs. In cardiac arrest, monitor EKG, pt condition.

PATIENT/FAMILY TEACHING

• Avoid excessive use of caffeine derivatives (chocolate, coffee, tea, cola, cocoa). • Report any new symptoms (tachycardia, shortness of breath, dizziness) immediately: may be systemic effects.

E

epirubicin

HIGH ALERT

eh-pea-**rew**-bih-sin
(Ellence, Pharmorubicin 🍁)

BLACK BOX ALERT Potential for cardiotoxicity, severe myelosuppresion. May increase risk of secondary leukemias. With IV, severe local tissue damage, necrosis may occur. Must be administered by personnel trained in administration/handling of chemotherapeutic agents.

Do not confuse epirubicin with daunorubicin, doxorubicin, or idarubicin, or Ellence with Elase.

CLASSIFICATION

PHARMACOTHERAPEUTIC: Anthracycline antibiotic. **CLINICAL:** Antineoplastic (see p. 83C).

ACTION

May include formation of complex with DNA, subsequent inhibition of DNA, RNA, protein synthesis. Inhibits DNA helicase activity, preventing enzymatic separation of double-stranded DNA, interfering with replication, transcription. **Therapeutic Effect:** Produces antiproliferative, cytotoxic activity.

PHARMACOKINETICS

Widely distributed into tissues. Protein binding: 77%. Metabolized in liver and RBCs. Primarily eliminated through biliary excretion. Not removed by hemodialysis. **Half-life:** 33 hrs.

USES

Component of adjuvant therapy in pts with evidence of axillary node tumor involvement following resection of primary breast cancer. **OFF-LABEL:** Esophageal, gastric, small-cell lung, non–small-cell lung, ovarian carcinomas; Hodgkin's, non-Hodgkin's lymphomas; soft tissue sarcoma; neoplasms of bladder.

PRECAUTIONS

Contraindications: Baseline neutrophil count less than 1,500/mm^3, hypersensitivity to epirubicin, previous treatment with anthracyclines up to maximum cumulative dose, recent MI, severe hepatic impairment, severe myocardial insufficiency. **Cautions:** Renal/hepatic impairment.

⌛ LIFESPAN CONSIDERATIONS

Pregnancy/Lactation: May cause fetal harm. Unknown if distributed in breast milk. **Pregnancy Category D. Children:** Safety and efficacy not established. **Elderly:** No age-related precautions noted but monitor for toxicity.

INTERACTIONS

DRUG: **Medications causing blood dyscrasias** may increase risk of developing leukopenia, thrombocytopenia. **Bone marrow depressants** may cause additive myelosuppression. **Calcium channel blockers** may increase risk of developing heart failure. **Cimetidine** may increase serum concentration, toxicity. **Daunorubicin, doxorubicin, idarubicin, mitoxantrone** may increase risk of GI, hematologic, hepatic effects; cardiotoxicity. **Hepatotoxic medications** may increase risk of hepatotoxicity. **Live virus vaccines** may potentiate virus replication, increase vaccine side effects, decrease pt's antibody response to vaccine. **HERBAL:** **St. John's wort** may decrease concentration. Avoid **black cohosh, dong quai** in estrogen-dependent tumors. **FOOD:** None known. **LAB VALUES:** May increase uric acid.

AVAILABILITY (Rx)

Injection Solution: 2-mg/ml single-use vials (25 ml, 100 ml). **Injection, Powder for Reconstitution:** 50 mg, 200 mg.

ADMINISTRATION/HANDLING

◀ALERT▶ Exclude pregnant staff from working with epirubicin; wear protective clothing. If accidental contact with skin or eyes occurs, flush area immediately with copious amounts of water.

IV

Reconstitution • Ready-to-use vials require no reconstitution. **Powder:** Reconstitute with Sterile Water for Injection to final concentration of 2 mg/ml.
Rate of administration • **IV Push:** Infuse medication into tubing of free-flowing IV of 0.9% NaCl or D_5W over 3–10 min. **IV Infusion:** Further dilute with 50–250 ml 0.9% NaCl or D_5W and infuse over 15–20 min.
Storage • Refrigerate vial of solution; store vials of powder at room temperature. • Protect from light. • Use within 24 hrs of first penetration of rubber stopper. • Discard unused portion.

IV INCOMPATIBILITIES

Fluorouracil (5-FU), heparin. Do not mix epirubicin in same syringe with other medications.

INDICATIONS/ROUTES/DOSAGE

Breast Cancer

IV: ADULTS: Initially, 100–120 mg/m^2 in repeated cycles of 3–4 wks, in combination with 5-fluorouracil (5-FU) and Cytoxan. Total dose may be given on day 1 of each cycle or in equally divided doses on days 1 and 8 of each cycle.

SIDE EFFECTS

Frequent (83%–70%): Nausea, vomiting, alopecia, amenorrhea. **Occasional (9%–5%):** Stomatitis, diarrhea, hot flashes. **Rare (2%–1%):** Rash, pruritus, fever, lethargy, conjunctivitis.

ADVERSE EFFECTS/ TOXIC REACTIONS

Risk of cardiotoxicity (either acute, manifested as transient EKG abnormalities, or chronic, manifested as CHF) increases when total cumulative dose exceeds 900 mg/m^2. Extravasation during administration may result in severe local tissue necrosis. Myelosuppression may produce hematologic toxicity, manifested principally as leukopenia and, to lesser extent, anemia, thrombocytopenia.

NURSING CONSIDERATIONS

BASELINE ASSESSMENT

Obtain WBC, platelet, erythrocyte counts before and at frequent intervals during therapy. Obtain EKG before therapy, serum hepatic function studies before each dose. Antiemetics may be effective in preventing, treating nausea.

INTERVENTION/EVALUATION

Monitor for stomatitis (may lead to ulceration of mucous membranes within 2–3 days). Monitor blood counts for evidence of myelosuppression, renal/hepatic function studies, cardiac function. Monitor daily pattern of bowel activity and stool consistency. Monitor for hematologic toxicity (fever, sore throat, signs of local infection, unusual bruising/bleeding from any site), symptoms of anemia (excessive fatigue, weakness). Monitor EKG changes. Assess injection site for extravasation, local skin reactions.

PATIENT/FAMILY TEACHING

• Alopecia is reversible, but new hair growth may have different color, texture. New hair growth resumes 2–3 mos after last therapy dose. • Maintain fastidious oral hygiene. • Do not have immunizations without physician's approval (drug lowers resistance). • Avoid contact with those who have recently received live virus vaccine. • Promptly report fever, sore throat, signs of local infection, unusual bruising/bleeding from any site.

Epivir, *see lamivudine*

eplerenone

eh-**pleh**-reh-known
(Inspra)
Do not confuse Inspra with Spiriva.

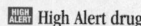

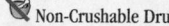

◆**CLASSIFICATION**

PHARMACOTHERAPEUTIC: Aldosterone receptor antagonist. **CLINICAL:** Antihypertensive.

E

ACTION

Binds to mineralocorticoid receptors in kidney, heart, blood vessels, brain, blocking binding of aldosterone. **Therapeutic Effect:** Reduces B/P.

PHARMACOKINETICS

Absorption unaffected by food. Protein binding: 50%. Metabolized in liver. Excreted in urine, with lesser amount eliminated in feces. Not removed by hemodialysis. **Half-life:** 4–6 hrs.

USES

Treatment of hypertension alone or in combination with other antihypertensive agents. Treatment of CHF following acute myocardial infarction (AMI).

PRECAUTIONS

Contraindications: Concurrent use of potassium supplements, potassium-sparing diuretics (e.g., amiloride, spironolactone, triamterene), strong inhibitors of cytochrome P450 3A4 enzyme system (e.g., ketoconazole, itraconazole), creatinine clearance less than 50 ml/min (30 ml/min or less in pts with hypertension), serum creatinine level greater than 2 mg/dl in males or 1.8 mg/dl in females, serum potassium level greater than 5.5 mEq/L, type 2 diabetes mellitus with microalbuminuria. **Cautions:** Hepatic insufficiency, hyperkalemia.

LIFESPAN CONSIDERATIONS

Pregnancy/Lactation: Unknown if drug crosses placenta or is distributed in breast milk. **Pregnancy Category B. Children:** Safety and efficacy not established. **Elderly:** No age-related precautions noted.

INTERACTIONS

DRUG: **ACE inhibitors, angiotensin II antagonists, erythromycin, fluconazole, saquinavir, verapamil** increase risk of hyperkalemia. **Potassium-sparing diuretics (e.g., spironolactone), potassium supplements** increase risk of hyperkalemia. **Itraconazole, ketoconazole** increase concentration fivefold (use is contraindicated). **HERBAL:** **St. John's wort** decreases effectiveness. **FOOD:** **Grapefruit, grapefruit juice** produces slight increase in serum potassium. **LAB VALUES:** May increase serum potassium, ALT, AST, cholesterol, triglycerides, serum creatinine, uric acid. May decrease serum sodium.

AVAILABILITY (Rx)

Tablets: 25 mg, 50 mg.

ADMINISTRATION/HANDLING

• Do not break, crush, chew film-coated tablets. • May give without regard to food.

INDICATIONS/ROUTES/DOSAGE

Hypertension

PO: ADULTS, ELDERLY: 50 mg once a day. If 50 mg once a day produces an inadequate B/P response, may increase dosage to 50 mg twice a day. If pt is concurrently receiving CYP3A4 inhibitors (e.g., erythromycin, saquinavir, verapamil, or fluconazole), reduce initial dose to 25 mg once a day.

CHF Following MI

PO: ADULTS, ELDERLY: Initially, 25 mg once a day. If tolerated, titrate up to 50 mg once a day within 4 wks.

Dosage Adjustment for Serum Potassium Concentrations in CHF

Less than 5 mEq/L: Increase from 25 mg daily to 50 mg daily. Increase from 25 mg every other day to 25 mg daily.
5–5.4 mEq/L: No adjustment needed.
5.5–5.9 mEq/L: Decrease dose from 50 mg daily to 25 mg daily. Decrease dose from 25 mg daily to 25 mg every other day. Decrease dose from 25 mg every other day to withhold medication.
6 mEq/L or greater: Withhold medication until potassium is less than 5.5 mEq/L.

Dosage in Renal Impairment

Use is contraindicated in pts with hypertension with creatinine clearance less than 50 ml/min or serum creatinine greater than 2 mg/dl in males or greater than 1.8 mg/dl in females. All other indications, creatinine clearance less than 30 ml/min, use is contraindicated.

SIDE EFFECTS

Rare (3%–1%): Dizziness, diarrhea, cough, fatigue, flu-like symptoms, abdominal pain.

ADVERSE EFFECTS/ TOXIC REACTIONS

Hyperkalemia may occur, particularly in pts with type 2 diabetes mellitus and microalbuminuria.

NURSING CONSIDERATIONS

BASELINE ASSESSMENT

Obtain B/P, apical pulse immediately before each dose, in addition to regular monitoring (be alert to fluctuations). If excessive reduction in B/P occurs, place pt in supine position, feet slightly elevated.

INTERVENTION/EVALUATION

Assist with ambulation if dizziness occurs. Monitor serum potassium levels. Assess B/P for hypertension and hypotension. Monitor daily pattern of bowel activity and stool consistency. Assess for evidence of flu-like symptoms.

PATIENT/FAMILY TEACHING

• Avoid tasks that require alertness, motor skills until response to drug is established (possible dizziness effect). • Hypertension requires lifelong control. • Avoid exercising during hot weather (risk of dehydration, hypotension).

epoetin alfa

eh-po-**ee**-tin **al**-fa
(Epogen, Eprex ✱, Procrit)

BLACK BOX ALERT Increased risk of serious cardiovascular events, thromboembolic events, mortality, time-to-tumor progression in pts with head and neck cancer, metastatic breast cancer, non–small-cell lung cancer when administered to a target hemoglobin of more than 12 g/dl. Increases rate of deep vein thrombosis in perioperative pts not receiving anticoagulant therapy.

Do not confuse Epogen with Neupogen, or epoetin with darbepoetin.

◆CLASSIFICATION

PHARMACOTHERAPEUTIC: Glycoprotein. **CLINICAL:** Erythropoietin.

ACTION

Stimulates division, differentiation of erythroid progenitor cells in bone marrow. **Therapeutic Effect:** Induces erythropoiesis, releases reticulocytes from bone marrow.

PHARMACOKINETICS

Well absorbed after subcutaneous administration. Following administration, an increase in reticulocyte count occurs within 10 days, and increases in Hgb, Hct, and RBC count are seen within 2–6 wks. **Half-life:** 4–13 hrs.

USES

Treatment of anemia in pts receiving or who have received chemotherapy, those with chronic renal failure, HIV-infected pts on zidovudine (AZT) therapy, those scheduled for elective noncardiac, nonvascular surgery, reducing need for allogenic blood transfusions. **OFF-LABEL:** Anemia associated with frequent blood donations, anemia in critically ill pts, malignancy, management of hepatitis C, myelodysplastic syndromes.

PRECAUTIONS

Contraindications: History of sensitivity to mammalian cell-derived products or human albumin, uncontrolled hypertension. **Cautions:** Pts with known porphyria (impairment of erythrocyte formation in bone marrow); history of seizures. **Cancer pts:**

Tumor growth, shortened survival may occur when Hgb levels of 12 g/dl or greater are achieved with epoetin alfa. **Chronic kidney failure pts:** Increased risk for serious cardiovascular reactions (e.g., stroke, MI) when Hgb levels greater than 12 g/dl are achieved with epoetin alfa.

E

LIFESPAN CONSIDERATIONS

Pregnancy/Lactation: Unknown if drug crosses placenta or is distributed in breast milk. **Pregnancy Category C. Children:** Safety and efficacy not established in those 12 yrs and younger. **Elderly:** No age-related precautions noted.

INTERACTIONS

DRUG: None significant. **HERBAL:** None significant. **FOOD:** None known. **LAB VALUES:** May increase BUN, serum phosphorus, potassium, creatinine, uric acid, sodium. May decrease bleeding time, iron concentration, serum ferritin.

AVAILABILITY (Rx)

Injection Solution (Epogen, Procrit): 2,000 units/ml, 3,000 units/ml, 4,000 units/ml, 10,000 units/ml, 20,000 units/ml, 40,000 units/ml.

ADMINISTRATION/HANDLING

◀ALERT▶ Avoid excessive agitation of vial; do not shake (foaming).

IV

Reconstitution • No reconstitution necessary.
Rate of administration • May be given as an IV bolus.
Storage • Refrigerate. • Vigorous shaking may denature medication, rendering it inactive.

Subcutaneous

• Mix in syringe with bacteriostatic 0.9% NaCl with benzyl alcohol 0.9% (bacteriostatic saline) at a 1:1 ratio (benzyl alcohol acts as local anesthetic; may reduce injection site discomfort). • Use 1 dose per vial; do not reenter vial. Discard unused portion.

IV INCOMPATIBILITIES

Do not mix injection form with other medications.

INDICATIONS/ROUTES/DOSAGE

Anemia Associated with Chemotherapy

◀ALERT▶ Use minimum effective dose to maintain hemoglobin level that will avoid red blood cell transfusions. Hemoglobin level should not exceed 12 g/dl and should not rise greater than 1 g/dl per 2-wk time period in any pt. Treatment of pts with erythropoietin levels greater than 200 mU/ml not recommended.

SUBCUTANEOUS: ADULTS, ELDERLY: Initially, 150 units/kg 3 times/wk (commonly used dose of 10,000 units 3 times/wk) or 40,000 units once weekly. **CHILDREN:** 600 units/kg once weekly. **Maximum:** 40,000 units.

Increase dose: (Adults, elderly): If response is not satisfactory (no reduction in transfusion requirements or increase in Hgb) after 8 wks of 3 times/wk dosing, 4 wks after once weekly dosing, dose may be increased q4wks to 300 units/kg 3 times/wk or 60,000 units once weekly. ***(Children):*** If hemoglobin does not increase by 1 g/dl after 4 wks of once weekly dosing, may increase dose to 900 units/kg/wk. **Maximum:** 60,000 units once weekly.

Decrease dose: Decrease dose by 25% if hemoglobin increases greater than 1 g/dl in any 2-wk period or hemoglobin levels reaches level that will avoid red blood cell transfusions.

Reduction of Allogenic Blood Transfusions in Elective Surgery

SUBCUTANEOUS: ADULTS, ELDERLY: 300 units/kg/day for 10 days before and 4 days after surgery.

Anemia in Chronic Renal Failure

◀ALERT▶ Individualize dosing to achieve/maintain hemoglobin between 10–12 g/dl. Hemoglobin level should not exceed 12 g/dl and should not rise greater than 1 g/dl per 2-wk time period in any pt.

IV, SUBCUTANEOUS: ADULTS, ELDERLY: 50–100 units/kg 3 times/wk. **CHIL-**

DREN: 50 units/kg 3 times/wk. Maintenance: Individualize to maintain hemoglobin range of 10–12 g/dl.
Decrease dose by 25%: If hemoglobin approaches 12 g/dl or increases greater than 1 g/dl in any 2-wk period. If hemoglobin continues to increase, temporarily discontinue until hemoglobin begins to decrease. Resume therapy at 25% reduction from previous dose.
Increase dose by 25%: If hemoglobin is less than 10 g/dl and does not increase by 1 g/dl after 4 wks of therapy (with adequate iron stores) or hemoglobin decreases below 10 g/dl. If transferrin saturation is greater than 20%, may increase dose. Do not increase dose more frequently than every 4 wks.
Note: If pt does not attain hemoglobin range of 10–12 g/dl after appropriate dosing over 12 wks, do not continue to increase dose and use minimum effective dose to maintain hemoglobin level that will avoid red blood cell transfusions.

HIV Infection in Pts Treated with Zidovudine (AZT)

IV, SUBCUTANEOUS: ADULTS: Initially, 100 units/kg 3 times a wk for 8 wks; may increase by 50–100 units/kg 3 times a wk. Evaluate response q4–8wk thereafter. Adjust dosage by 50–100 units/kg 3 times a wk. If dosages larger than 300 units/kg 3 times a wk are not eliciting response, it is unlikely pt will respond. Maintenance: Titrate to maintain desired hemoglobin level. Hemoglobin levels should not exceed 12 g/dl.

SIDE EFFECTS

Pts Receiving Chemotherapy

Frequent (20%–17%): Fever, diarrhea, nausea, vomiting, edema. **Occasional (13%–11%):** Asthenia (loss of strength, energy), shortness of breath, paresthesia. **Rare (5%–3%):** Dizziness, trunk pain.

Pts with Chronic Renal Failure

Frequent (24%–11%): Hypertension, headache, nausea, arthralgia. **Occasional (9%–7%):** Fatigue, edema, diarrhea, vomiting, chest pain, skin reactions at administration site, asthenia (loss of strength, energy), dizziness.

Pts with HIV Infection Treated with AZT

Frequent (38%–15%): Fever, fatigue, headache, cough, diarrhea, rash, nausea. **Occasional (14%–9%):** Shortness of breath, asthenia (loss of strength, energy), skin reaction at injection site, dizziness.

ADVERSE EFFECTS/ TOXIC REACTIONS

Hypertensive encephalopathy, thrombosis, cerebrovascular accident, MI, seizures occur rarely. Hyperkalemia occurs occasionally in pts with chronic renal failure, usually in those who do not comply with medication regimen, dietary guidelines, frequency of dialysis regimen.

NURSING CONSIDERATIONS

BASELINE ASSESSMENT

Assess B/P before drug initiation (80% of pts with chronic renal failure have history of hypertension). B/P often rises during early therapy in pts with history of hypertension. Consider that all pts eventually need supplemental iron therapy. Assess serum iron (should be greater than 20%), serum ferritin (should be greater than 100 ng/ml) before and during therapy. Establish baseline CBC (esp. note Hct). Monitor aggressively for increased B/P (25% of pts on medication require antihypertensive therapy, dietary restrictions).

INTERVENTION/EVALUATION

Assess CBC routinely. Monitor Hgb, Hct, B/P. Monitor temperature, esp. in cancer pts on chemotherapy and zidovudine-treated HIV pts. Monitor BUN, serum uric acid, creatinine, phosphorus, potassium, esp. in chronic renal failure pts.

PATIENT/FAMILY TEACHING

• Frequent blood tests needed to determine correct dosage. • Inform physician if severe headache develops. • Avoid potentially hazardous activity during first 90 days of therapy (increased risk of seizures in pts with chronic renal failure during first 90 days).

Epogen, *see epoetin alfa*

E

eprosartan

eh-pro-**sar**-tan
(Teveten)

BLACK BOX ALERT May cause fetal injury, mortality if used during second or third trimester of pregnancy.

FIXED COMBINATION(S)

Teveten HCT: eprosartan/hydrochlorothiazide (a diuretic): 400 mg/12.5 mg.

◆CLASSIFICATION

PHARMACOTHERAPEUTIC: Angiotensin II receptor antagonist. **CLINICAL:** Antihypertensive (see p. 10C).

ACTION

Potent vasodilator. Blocks vasoconstrictor, aldosterone-secreting effects of angiotensin II, inhibiting binding of angiotensin II to AT_1 receptors. **Therapeutic Effect:** Causes vasodilation, decreases peripheral resistance, decreases B/P.

PHARMACOKINETICS

Rapidly absorbed after PO administration. Protein binding: 98%. Minimally metabolized in liver. Primarily excreted via urine, biliary system. Minimally removed by hemodialysis. **Half-life:** 5–9 hrs.

USES

Treatment of hypertension (alone or in combination with other medications).

PRECAUTIONS

Contraindications: Bilateral renal artery stenosis, hyperaldosteronism. **Cautions:** Unilateral renal artery stenosis, preexisting renal insufficiency, significant aortic/mitral stenosis.

LIFESPAN CONSIDERATIONS

Pregnancy/Lactation: Has caused fetal and neonatal morbidity and mortality. Potential for adverse effects on breast-feeding infant. Breast-feeding not recommended. **Pregnancy Category C (D if used in second or third trimester). Children:** Safety and efficacy not established. **Elderly:** No age-related precautions noted.

INTERACTIONS

DRUG: Potassium-sparing diuretics, potassium supplements may increase risk of hyperkalemia. May produce additive effect with **antihypertensive agents. HERBAL: Ephedra, ginseng, yohimbe** may worsen hypertension. **Garlic** may increase antihypertensive effect. **FOOD:** None known. **LAB VALUES:** May increase BUN, serum alkaline phosphatase, bilirubin, creatinine, AST, ALT. May decrease Hgb, Hct.

AVAILABILITY (Rx)

Tablets: 400 mg, 600 mg.

ADMINISTRATION/HANDLING

PO

• Give without regard to food. • Do not crush tablets.

INDICATIONS/ROUTES/DOSAGE

Hypertension

PO: ADULTS, ELDERLY: Initially, 600 mg/day. Range: 400–800 mg/day as single dose or 2 divided doses.

SIDE EFFECTS

Occasional (5%–2%): Headache, cough, dizziness. **Rare (less than 2%):** Muscle pain, fatigue, diarrhea, upper respiratory tract infection, dyspepsia.

ADVERSE EFFECTS/ TOXIC REACTIONS

Overdosage may manifest as hypotension, tachycardia. Bradycardia occurs less often.

E

NURSING CONSIDERATIONS

BASELINE ASSESSMENT

Obtain B/P, apical pulse immediately before each dose, in addition to regular monitoring (be alert to fluctuations). Question for possibility of pregnancy (see Pregnancy Category), history of hepatic/renal impairment, renal artery stenosis. Assess medication history (esp. diuretics).

INTERVENTION/EVALUATION

Monitor B/P, electrolytes, serum creatinine, BUN, urinalysis, pulse for tachycardia.

PATIENT/FAMILY TEACHING

• Inform female pt regarding consequences of second- and third-trimester exposure to medication. • Avoid tasks that require alertness, motor skills until response to drug is established. • Restrict sodium, alcohol intake. • Follow diet, control weight. • Do not stop taking medication. • Hypertension requires lifelong control. • Avoid exercising during hot weather (risk of dehydration, hypotension). • Check B/P regularly.

eptifibatide HIGH ALERT

ep-tih-**fye**-bah-tide
(Integrilin)

◆CLASSIFICATION

PHARMACOTHERAPEUTIC: Glycoprotein IIb/IIIa inhibitor. **CLINICAL:** Antiplatelet, antithrombotic (see p. 33C).

ACTION

Produces rapid inhibition of platelet aggregation by preventing binding of fibrinogen to receptor sites on platelets. **Therapeutic Effect:** Prevents thrombus formation within coronary arteries. Prevents acute cardiac ischemic complications.

PHARMACOKINETICS

Protein binding: 25%. Excreted in urine. **Half-life:** 2.5 hrs.

USES

Treatment of pts with acute coronary syndrome (ACS), including those managed medically and those undergoing percutaneous coronary intervention (PCI).

PRECAUTIONS

Contraindications: Active internal bleeding, AV malformation or aneurysm, history of CVA within 2 yrs or CVA with residual neurologic defect, history of vasculitis, intracranial neoplasm, oral anticoagulant use within last 7 days unless PT is less than 1.22 times the control, recent (6 wks or less) GI/GU bleeding, recent (6 wks or less) surgery or trauma, prior IV dextran use prior to or during PTCA, severe uncontrolled hypertension, thrombocytopenia (less than 100,000 cells/mcl). **Cautions:** Pts who weigh less than 75 kg; those 65 yrs and older; history of GI disease; pts receiving thrombolytics, heparin, aspirin; PTCA less than 12 hrs of onset of symptoms for acute MI; prolonged PTCA (greater than 70 min); failed PTCA. **Pregnancy Category B.**

INTERACTIONS

DRUG: **Anticoagulants, heparin** may increase risk of hemorrhage. **Dextran, other platelet aggregation inhibitors (e.g., aspirin, thrombolytics), thrombolytic agents** may increase risk of bleeding. **HERBAL:** **Cat's claw, dong quai, evening primrose, feverfew, garlic, ginger, ginkgo, ginseng** may increase antiplatelet effects. **FOOD:** None known. **LAB VALUES:** Increases PT, aPTT, clotting time. Decreases platelet count.

AVAILABILITY (Rx)

Injection Solution: 0.75 mg/ml, 2 mg/ml.

ADMINISTRATION/HANDLING

IV

Reconstitution • Withdraw bolus dose from 10-ml vial (2 mg/ml); for IV infusion, withdraw from 100-ml vial (0.75 mg/ml). • IV push and infusion administration may be given undiluted.

Rate of administration • Give bolus dose IV push over 1–2 min.
Storage • Store vials in refrigerator. • Solution appears clear, colorless. • Do not shake. • Discard any unused portion left in vial or if preparation contains *any* opaque particles.

IV INCOMPATIBILITIES

Administer in separate line; do not add other medications to infusion solution.

INDICATIONS/ROUTES/DOSAGE

Adjunct to Percutaneous Coronary Intervention (PCI)

IV BOLUS, IV INFUSION: ADULTS, ELDERLY: 180 mcg/kg (**Maximum:** 22.6 mg) before PCI initiation; then continuous drip of 2 mcg/kg/min and a second 180 mcg/kg (**Maximum:** 22.6 mg) bolus 10 min after the first. **Maximum:** 15 mg/hr. Continue until hospital discharge or for up to 18–24 hrs. Minimum 12 hrs is recommended. Concurrent aspirin and heparin therapy is recommended.

Acute Coronary Syndrome (ACS)

IV BOLUS, IV INFUSION: ADULTS, ELDERLY: 180 mcg/kg (**Maximum:** 22.6 mg) bolus then 2 mcg/kg/min until discharge or coronary artery bypass graft, up to 72 hrs. **Maximum:** 15 mg/hr. Concurrent aspirin and heparin therapy is recommended.

Dosage in Renal Impairment

Creatinine clearance less than 50 ml/min: Use 180 mcg/kg bolus (**Maximum:** 22.6 mg) and 1 mcg/kg/min infusion (**Maximum:** 7.5 mg/hr).

SIDE EFFECTS

Occasional (7%): Hypotension.

ADVERSE EFFECTS/ TOXIC REACTIONS

Minor to major bleeding complications may occur, most commonly at arterial access site for cardiac catheterization.

NURSING CONSIDERATIONS

BASELINE ASSESSMENT

Assess platelet count, Hgb, Hct before treatment and during therapy. If platelet count less than 90,000/mm^3, additional platelet counts should be obtained routinely to avoid thrombocytopenia.

INTERVENTION/EVALUATION

Diligently monitor for potential bleeding, particularly at other arterial, venous puncture sites. If possible, urinary catheters, nasogastric tubes should be avoided.

Epzicom, *see abacavir and lamivudine*

Erbitux, *see cetuximab*

ergotamine

er-**got**-a-meen
(Ergomar)

dihydroergotamine

(D.H.E. 45, Migranal)

BLACK BOX ALERT Concurrent use with macrolide antibiotics, azole antifungals, protease inhibitors increases risk of vasospasm, producing ischemia of brain and peripheral extremities.

FIXED-COMBINATION(S)

Bellergal-S: ergotamine/belladonna (anticholinergic)/phenobarbital (sedative-hypnotic): 0.6 mg/0.2 mg/40 mg. **Cafergot, Wigraine:** ergotamine/caffeine (stimulant): 1 mg/100 mg, 2 mg/100 mg.
Do not confuse Cafergot with Carafate.

◆ **CLASSIFICATION**

PHARMACOTHERAPEUTIC: Ergotamine derivative. **CLINICAL:** Antimigraine.

ACTION

Directly stimulates vascular smooth muscle, resulting in peripheral and cerebral vasoconstriction. May have antagonist effects on serotonin. **Therapeutic Effect:** Suppresses vascular headaches, migraine headaches.

PHARMACOKINETICS

Slowly, incompletely absorbed from GI tract; rapidly and extensively absorbed after rectal administration. Protein binding: greater than 90%. Undergoes extensive first-pass metabolism in liver to active metabolite. Eliminated in feces by the biliary system. **Half-life:** 21 hrs.

USES

Ergotamine: Prevents or aborts vascular headaches (e.g., migraine, cluster headaches). **Dihydroergotamine:** Treatment of migraine headache with or without aura. Injection used to treat cluster headache. **OFF-LABEL:** Prevention of deep venous thrombosis (DVT), prevention and treatment of orthostatic hypotension, pulmonary thromboembolism.

PRECAUTIONS

Contraindications: Coronary artery disease, hypertension, hepatic/renal impairment, malnutrition, peripheral vascular diseases (e.g., thromboangitis obliterans, syphilitic arteritis, severe arteriosclerosis, thrombophlebitis, Raynaud's disease), sepsis, severe pruritus. **Cautions:** None known.

⌛ LIFESPAN CONSIDERATIONS

Pregnancy/Lactation: Contraindicated in pregnancy (produces uterine stimulant action, resulting in possible fetal death or retarded fetal growth); increases vasoconstriction of placental vascular bed. Drug distributed in breast milk. May produce diarrhea, vomiting in neonate. May prohibit lactation. **Pregnancy Category X. Children:** No precautions in those 6 yrs and older, but use only when unresponsive to other medication. **Elderly:** Age-related occlusive peripheral vascular disease increases risk of peripheral vasoconstriction. Age-related renal impairment may require dosage adjustment.

INTERACTIONS

DRUG: **Beta-blockers, erythromycin** may increase risk of vasospasm. **Ergot alkaloids, 5-hydroxytryptamine agonists (e.g., sumatriptan), systemic vasoconstrictors** may increase pressor effect. May decrease effects of **nitroglycerin.** **HERBAL:** None significant. **FOOD:** **Coffee, cola, tea** may increase absorption. **Grapefruit, grapefruit juice** may increase concentration/toxicity. **LAB VALUES:** None significant.

AVAILABILITY (Rx)

Ergotamine Tablets, Sublingual (Ergomar): 2 mg. **Dihydroergotamine Injection, Solution:** 1 mg/ml. **Intranasal Spray, Solution (Migranal):** 4 mg/ml (0.5 mg/spray).

ADMINISTRATION/HANDLING

Sublingual

- Place under tongue; do not swallow.

INDICATIONS/ROUTES/DOSAGE

Vascular Headaches

Ergotamine

PO: ADULTS, ELDERLY: *(Cafergot):* 2 mg at onset of headache, then 1–2 mg q30min. **Maximum:** 6 mg/episode; 10 mg/wk.

Sublingual: ADULTS, ELDERLY: *(Ergomar):* 1 tablet at onset of headache, then 1 tablet q30min. **Maximum:** 3 tablets/24 hrs; 5 tabs/wk.

Dihydroergotamine

IM/SUBCUTANEOUS: ADULTS, ELDERLY: 1 mg at onset of headache; repeat hourly. **Maximum:** 3 mg/day; 6 mg/wk.

IV: ADULTS, ELDERLY: 1 mg at onset of headache; repeat hourly. **Maximum:** 2 mg/day; 6 mg/wk.
Intranasal: ADULTS, ELDERLY: 1 spray (0.5 mg) into each nostril; repeat in 15 min. **Maximum:** 4 sprays/day; 8 sprays/wk.

E

SIDE EFFECTS

Occasional (5%–2%): Cough, dizziness. **Rare (less than 2%):** Myalgia, fatigue, diarrhea, upper respiratory tract infection, dyspepsia.

ADVERSE EFFECTS/ TOXIC REACTIONS

Prolonged administration, excessive dosage may produce ergotamine poisoning, manifested as nausea, vomiting; paresthesia of fingers/toes, muscle pain/weakness; precordial pain; tachycardia/bradycardia; hypertension/hypotension. Vasoconstriction of peripheral arteries/arterioles may result in localized edema, pruritus. Feet, hands will become cold, pale. Muscle pain will occur when walking and later, even at rest. Other rare effects include confusion, depression, drowsiness, seizures, gangrene.

NURSING CONSIDERATIONS

BASELINE ASSESSMENT

Question for history of peripheral vascular disease, renal/hepatic impairment, possibility of pregnancy. Question regarding onset, location, duration of migraine, possible precipitating symptoms.

INTERVENTION/EVALUATION

Monitor closely for evidence of ergotamine overdosage as result of prolonged administration or excessive dosage.

PATIENT/FAMILY TEACHING

• Initiate therapy at first sign of migraine headache. • Report if there is need to progressively increase dose to relieve vascular headaches or if palpitations, nausea, vomiting, paresthesias, pain or weakness of extremities, chest pain are noted. • Female pts should take measures to avoid pregnancy. • Report suspected pregnancy immediately (Pregnancy Category X).

eribulin

air-ih-**buh**-lin
(Halaven)

◆CLASSIFICATION

PHARMACOTHERAPEUTIC: Microtubule inhibitor. **CLINICAL:** Antineoplastic.

ACTION

Binds directly on microtubules during active stage of G_2 and M phases of cell cycle, preventing formation of microtubules, an essential part of process of separation of chromosomes. **Therapeutic Effect:** Blocks cells in mitotic phase of cell division, leading to cell death.

PHARMACOKINETICS

Extensively metabolized in liver. Protein binding: 49%–65%. Excreted unchanged mainly in feces, with lesser amount eliminated in urine. **Half-life:** 40 hrs.

USES

Treatment of metastatic breast cancer in those who previously received at least 2 chemotherapeutic regimens for treatment, including an anthracycline and a taxane agent.

PRECAUTIONS

Contraindications: None significant. **Cautions:** Prolonged QTc, hepatic/renal impairment, moderate to severe neuropathy.

⌛ LIFESPAN CONSIDERATIONS

Pregnancy/Lactation: May cause embryo-fetal toxicity. Unknown if distributed in breast milk. **Pregnancy Category D. Children:** Safety and efficacy not established in those younger than

18 yrs. **Elderly:** No age-related precautions noted.

INTERACTIONS

DRUG: None significant. **FOOD:** None known. **HERBAL:** None significant. **LAB VALUES:** May decrease WBC, Hgb, Hct, platelet count.

AVAILABILITY (Rx)

Injection, Solution: 1 mg/2 ml (0.5-mg/ml single-use vial).

ADMINISTRATION/HANDLING

IV

Reconstitution • May administer undiluted or dilute in 100 ml 0.9% NaCl.
Rate of administration • Administer over 2–5 min.
Storage • Store at room temperature. • Once diluted, syringe or diluted solution may be stored for up to 4 hrs at room temperature or up to 24 hrs if refrigerated.

IV INCOMPATIBILITIES

Do not dilute with D_5W or administer through IV line containing solutions with dextrose or in same IV line with other medications.

INDICATIONS/ROUTES/DOSAGE

Metastatic Breast Cancer
IV: ADULTS, ELDERLY: 1.4 mg/m² over 2–5 min on days 1 and 8 of 21-day cycle.

Mild Hepatic/Renal Impairment (Creatinine Clearance 30–50 ml/min)
IV: ADULTS, ELDERLY: 1.1 mg/m² over 2–5 min on days 1 and 8 of 21-day cycle.

Moderate Hepatic Impairment
IV: ADULTS, ELDERLY: 0.7 mg/m² over 2–5 min on days 1 and 8 of 21-day cycle.

Recommended Dose Delays
Do not administer day 1 or day 8 of treatment for any of the following: ANC less than 1,000/mm³, platelets less than 75,000/mm³, grade 3 or 4 nonhematologic toxicities. Day 8 dose may be delayed for maximum of 1 wk. If toxicities do not resolve or improve to grade 2 severity by day 15, omit dose. If toxicities resolve or improve to grade 2 severity by day 15, continue treatment at reduced dose and initiate next cycle no sooner than 2 wks later. Do not re-escalate dose after it has been reduced.

SIDE EFFECTS

Common (54%–35%): Fatigue, asthenia (loss of strength, energy), alopecia, peripheral sensory neuropathy, nausea. **Frequent (25%–18%):** Constipation, arthralgia/myalgia, decreased weight, anorexia, pyrexia, headache, diarrhea, vomiting. **Occasional (16%–9%):** Back pain, dyspnea, cough, bone pain, extremity pain, urinary tract infection, oral mucosal inflammation.

ADVERSE EFFECTS/ TOXIC REACTIONS

Neutropenia occurs in 82% of pts, with 57% developing grade 3 neutropenia. Severe neutropenia (ANC less than 500/mm³) lasting more than 1 wk occurred in 12%. Anemia occurs in 58% of pts. Peripheral neuropathy occurs in 8% of pts but is the most common adverse reaction requiring discontinuation of therapy. Prolonged QTc may be noted on day 8 of treatment.

NURSING CONSIDERATIONS

BASELINE ASSESSMENT

Question for possibility of pregnancy. Obtain baseline CBC, serum chemistries before treatment begins and diligently monitor for neutropenia, peripheral neuropathy (most frequent cause of drug discontinuation). Obtain CBC prior to each dose.

INTERVENTION/EVALUATION

Monitor for symptoms of neuropathy (burning sensation, hyperesthesia, hypoesthesia, paresthesia, discomfort, neuropathic pain). Assess hands, feet for erythema. Monitor CBC for evidence of neutropenia, thrombocytopenia. Assess mouth for stomatitis (erythema, ulceration, mucosal burning).

PATIENT/FAMILY TEACHING

• Avoid crowds, those with known infection. • Avoid contact with anyone who recently received live virus vaccine. • Do not have immunizations without physician's approval (drug lowers body resistance). • Promptly report fever over 100.5°F, chills, cough, burning or pain urinating, numbness, tingling, burning sensation, erythema of hands/feet.

erlotinib

HIGH ALERT

er-**low**-tih-nib
(Tarceva)
Do not confuse erlotinib with dasatinib, geftinib, imatinib, or lapatinib.

◆CLASSIFICATION

PHARMACOTHERAPEUTIC: Human epidermal growth factor. **CLINICAL:** Antineoplastic.

ACTION

Inhibits tyrosine kinases (TK) associated with transmembrane cell surface receptors found on both normal and cancer cells. One such receptor is epidermal growth factor receptor (EGFR). **Therapeutic Effect:** TK activity appears to be vitally important to cell proliferation and survival.

PHARMACOKINETICS

About 60% is absorbed after PO administration; bioavailability is increased by food to almost 100%. Protein binding: 93%. Extensively metabolized in liver. Primarily eliminated in feces; minimal excretion in urine. **Half-life:** 24–36 hrs.

USES

Treatment of locally advanced or metastatic non–small-cell lung cancer after failure of at least one prior chemotherapy regimen. Treatment of locally advanced, unresectable, or metastatic pancreatic cancer (in combination with gemcitabine). **OFF-LABEL:** Salvage therapy of advanced or metastatic breast, colorectal, and head and neck tumors.

PRECAUTIONS

Contraindications: Pregnancy. **Cautions:** Severe hepatic/renal impairment.

LIFESPAN CONSIDERATIONS

Pregnancy/Lactation: Unknown if drug crosses placenta or is distributed in breast milk. **Pregnancy Category D. Children:** Safety and efficacy not established. **Elderly:** No age-related precautions noted.

INTERACTIONS

DRUG: **Atanzavir, clarithromycin, indinavir, itraconazole, ketoconazole, nefazodone, nelfinavir, ritonavir, saquinavir, telithromycin** may increase concentration, effects. **Carbamazepine, phenobarbital, phenytoin, rifampin** may decrease concentration, effects. **Warfarin** may increase risk of bleeding. **HERBAL:** **St. John's wort** may decrease concentration, effects. **FOOD:** **Grapefruit, grapefruit juice** may reduce absorption. **LAB VALUES:** May increase ALT, AST, serum bilirubin.

AVAILABILITY (Rx)

Tablets: 25 mg, 100 mg, 150 mg.

ADMINISTRATION/HANDLING

PO

• Give at least 1 hr before or 2 hrs after ingestion of food. • Avoid grapefruit, grapefruit juice. • May dissolve in 3–4 oz water and give orally or via feeding tube.

INDICATIONS/ROUTES/DOSAGE

◀ALERT▶ Dosage adjustment for toxicity: Reduce dose in 50-mg increments.

Lung Cancer

PO: ADULTS, ELDERLY: 150 mg/day until disease progression or unacceptable toxicity occurs.

Pancreatic Cancer

PO: ADULTS, ELDERLY: 100 mg/day in combination with gemcitabine until disease progression or unacceptable toxicity occurs.

Dosage in Renal Impairment

Interrupt dosing for renal disease due to dehydration.

Dosage in Hepatic Impairment

Reduce starting dose to 75 mg and individualize dose escalation if tolerated.

SIDE EFFECTS

Frequent (greater than 10%): Fatigue, anxiety, headache, depression, insomnia, rash, pruritus, dry skin, erythema, diarrhea, anorexia, nausea, vomiting, mucositis, constipation, dyspepsia, weight loss, dysphagia, abdominal pain, arthralgia, dyspnea, cough. **Occasional (10%–1%):** Keratitis. **Rare (less than 1%):** Corneal ulceration.

ADVERSE EFFECTS/ TOXIC REACTIONS

UTI occurs occasionally. Pneumonitis, GI bleeding occur rarely.

NURSING CONSIDERATIONS

BASELINE ASSESSMENT

Obtain hepatic enzyme levels, CBC before beginning therapy.

INTERVENTION/EVALUATION

Assess hepatic enzyme levels, CBC, renal function, serum electrolytes, hydration status periodically.

PATIENT/FAMILY TEACHING

• Take drug on empty stomach. • Notify physician if rash, blood in stool, diarrhea, irritated eyes, fever occur. • Avoid grapefruit, grapefruit juice.

ertapenem

er-tah-**pen**-em

(Invanz)

Do not confuse ertapenem with doripenem, imipenem, or meropenem, or Invanz with Avinza.

◆CLASSIFICATION

PHARMACOTHERAPEUTIC: Carbapenem. **CLINICAL:** Antibiotic.

ACTION

Penetrates bacterial cell wall of microorganisms, binds to penicillin-binding proteins, inhibiting cell wall synthesis. **Therapeutic Effect:** Produces bacterial cell death.

PHARMACOKINETICS

Almost completely absorbed after IM administration. Protein binding: 85%–95%. Widely distributed. Primarily excreted in urine with smaller amount eliminated in feces. Removed by hemodialysis. **Half-life:** 4 hrs.

USES

Treatment of susceptible infections due to *S. aureus* (methicillin-susceptible only), *S. agalactiae, S. pneumoniae* (penicillin-susceptible only), *S. pyogenes, E. coli, H. influenzae* (beta-lactamase negative strains only), *K. pneumoniae, M. catarrhalis, Bacteroides* spp., *C. clostridioforme, Peptostreptococcus* spp., including moderate to severe intra-abdominal, skin/skin-structure infections; community-acquired pneumonia; complicated UTI; acute pelvic infection; adult diabetic foot infections without osteomyelitis. Prevention of surgical site infection.

PRECAUTIONS

Contraindications: History of hypersensitivity to beta-lactams (imipenem and cilastin, meropenem), hypersensitivity to amide-type local anesthetics (IM). **Cautions:** Hypersensitivity to penicillins, cephalosporins, other allergens; renal impairment; CNS disorders, esp. brain lesions or history of seizures.

LIFESPAN CONSIDERATIONS

Pregnancy/Lactation: Distributed in breast milk. **Pregnancy Category B.** **Children:** Safety and efficacy not established in those younger than 18 yrs. **Elderly:** Advanced or end-stage renal insufficiency may require dosage adjustment.

INTERACTIONS

DRUG: **Probenecid** reduces renal excretion of ertapenem (do not use concurrently). **HERBAL:** None significant. **FOOD:** None known. **LAB VALUES:** May increase serum alkaline phosphatase, AST, ALT, bilirubin, BUN, creatinine, glucose, PT, aPTT, sodium. May decrease platelet count, Hgb, Hct, WBC.

AVAILABILITY (Rx)

Injection, Powder for Reconstitution: 1 g.

ADMINISTRATION/HANDLING

IV

Reconstitution • Dilute 1-g vial with 10 ml 0.9% NaCl or Bacteriostatic Water for Injection. • Shake well to dissolve. • Further dilute with 50 ml 0.9% NaCl (**maximum concentration:** 20 mg/ml).
Rate of administration • Give by intermittent IV infusion (piggyback). Do not give IV push. • Infuse over 30 min.
Storage • Solution appears colorless to yellow (variation in color does not affect potency). • Discard if solution contains precipitate. • Reconstituted solution is stable for 6 hrs at room temperature or 24 hrs if refrigerated.

IM

• Reconstitute with 3.2 ml 1% lidocaine HCl injection (without epinephrine). • Shake vial thoroughly. • Inject deep in large muscle mass (gluteal or lateral part of thigh). • Administer suspension within 1 hr after preparation.

IV INCOMPATIBILITIES

Do not mix or infuse with any other medications. Do not use diluents or IV solutions containing dextrose.

IV COMPATIBILITIES

Heparin, potassium chloride, Sterile Water for Injection, 0.9% NaCl.

INDICATIONS/ROUTES/DOSAGE

Usual Dosage Range
IM, IV: ADULTS, ELDERLY: 1 g/day. **CHILDREN 3 MOS–12 YRS:** 15 mg/kg 2 times/day. **Maximum:** 1 g/day.

Intra-Abdominal Infection
IV, IM: ADULTS, ELDERLY: 1 g/day for 5–14 days. **CHILDREN 3 MOS–12 YRS:** 15 mg/kg 2 times/day. **Maximum:** 1 g/day.

Skin/Skin Structure Infection
IV, IM: ADULTS, ELDERLY: 1 g/day for 7–14 days. **CHILDREN 3 MOS–12 YRS:** 15 mg/kg 2 times/day. **Maximum:** 1 g/day.

Pneumonia, UTI
IV, IM: ADULTS, ELDERLY: 1 g/day for 10–14 days. **CHILDREN 3 MOS–12 YRS:** 15 mg/kg 2 times/day. **Maximum:** 1 g/day.

Pelvic Infection
IV, IM: ADULTS, ELDERLY: 1 g/day for 3–10 days. **CHILDREN 3 MOS–12 YRS:** 15 mg/kg 2 times/day. **Maximum:** 1 g/day.

Diabetic Foot Infection
IV, IM: ADULTS, ELDERLY: 1 g/day for 7–14 days.

Prevention of Surgical Site Infection
IV: ADULTS, ELDERLY: 1 g given 1 hr preoperatively.

Dosage in Renal Impairment
Adults and elderly pts with creatinine clearance less than 30 ml/min: 500 mg once a day.

SIDE EFFECTS

Frequent (10%–6%): Diarrhea, nausea, headache. **Occasional (5%–2%):** Altered mental status, insomnia, rash, abdominal pain, constipation, chest pain, vomiting, edema, fever. **Rare (less than 2%):** Dizziness, cough, oral candidiasis, anxiety, tachycardia, phlebitis at IV site.

ADVERSE EFFECTS/ TOXIC REACTIONS

Antibiotic-associated colitis, other superinfections (abdominal cramps, severe watery diarrhea, fever) may result from altered bacterial balance. Anaphylactic reactions have been reported. Seizures may occur in those with CNS disorders (brain lesions, history of seizures), bacterial meningitis, severe renal impairment.

NURSING CONSIDERATIONS

BASELINE ASSESSMENT

Question for history of allergies, particularly to beta-lactams, penicillins, cephalosporins. Inquire about history of seizures.

INTERVENTION/EVALUATION

Monitor renal/hepatic function. Monitor daily pattern of bowel activity and stool consistency. Monitor for nausea, vomiting. Evaluate hydration status. Evaluate for inflammation at IV injection site. Assess skin for rash. Observe mental status; be alert to tremors, possible seizures. Assess sleep pattern for evidence of insomnia.

PATIENT/FAMILY TEACHING

• Notify physician in event of tremors, seizures, rash, prolonged diarrhea, chest pain, other new symptoms.

Eryc, *see erythromycin*

Erythrocin, *see erythromycin*

erythromycin

er-rith-row-**my**-sin
(Akne-Mycin, Apo-Erythro Base ✤, EES, Erybid ✤, Eryc, EryDerm, Erygel, EryPed, Ery-Tab, Erythrocin, PCE Dispertab, Romycin)
Do not confuse erythromycin with azithromycin or clarithromycin, or Eryc with Emcyt.

FIXED-COMBINATION(S)

Eryzole, Pediazole: erythromycin/sulfisoxazole (sulfonamide): 200 mg/600 mg per 5 ml.

◆ CLASSIFICATION

PHARMACOTHERAPEUTIC: Macrolide. **CLINICAL:** Antibiotic, antiacne (see p. 26C).

ACTION

Penetrates bacterial cell membranes, reversibly binds to bacterial ribosomes, inhibiting protein synthesis. **Therapeutic Effect:** Bacteriostatic.

PHARMACOKINETICS

Variably absorbed from GI tract (depending on dosage form used). Protein binding: 70%–90%. Widely distributed. Metabolized in liver. Primarily eliminated in feces by bile. Not removed by hemodialysis. **Half-life:** 1.4–2 hrs (increased in renal impairment).

USES

Treatment of susceptible infections due to *S. pyogenes, S. pneumoniae, S. aureus, M. pneumoniae, Legionella,* diphtheria, pertussis, chancroid, *Chlamydia, N. gonorrheae, E. histolytica,* syphilis, nongonococcal urethritis, *Campylobacter* gastroenteritis. **Topical:** Treatment of acne vulgaris. **Ophthalmic:** Prevention of gonococcal ophthalmia neonatorum, superficial ocular infections. **OFF-LABEL: Systemic:** Treatment of acne vulgaris, chancroid, *Campylobacter* enteritis, gastroparesis, Lyme disease, preoperative gut sterilization. **Topical:** Treatment of minor bacterial skin infections. **Ophthalmic:** Treatment of blepharitis, conjunctivitis, keratitis, chlamydial trachoma.

PRECAUTIONS

Contraindications: Administration of fixed-combination product, Pediazole, to infants younger than 2 mos; history of hepatitis due to macrolides; hypersensitivity to macrolides; preexisting hepatic disease. **Cautions:** Hepatic dysfunction. If combination therapy is used (Pediazole), consider precautions of sulfonamides. IV route may cause tachycardia, prolonged QT interval.

LIFESPAN CONSIDERATIONS

Pregnancy/Lactation: Crosses placenta. Distributed in breast milk. Erythromycin estolate may increase hepatic enzymes in pregnant women. **Pregnancy Category B. Children/Elderly:** No age-related precautions noted. High dosage in those with decreased hepatic/renal function increases risk of hearing loss.

INTERACTIONS

DRUG: May increase concentration, toxicity of **buspirone, cyclosporine, felodipine, lovastatin, simvastatin, valproic acid.** May inhibit metabolism of **carbamazepine, valproic acid.** May decrease effects of **clindamycin. Hepatotoxic medications** may increase risk of hepatotoxicity. **Theophylline** may increase risk of theophylline toxicity. May increase effects of **warfarin. HERBAL: St. John's wort** may decrease concentration. **FOOD:** None known. **LAB VALUES:** May increase serum alkaline phosphatase, bilirubin, AST, ALT.

AVAILABILITY (Rx)

Gel, Topical: (Erygel): 2%. **Ointment, Ophthalmic: (Romycin):** 0.5%. **Ointment, Topical: (Akne-Mycin):** 2%. **Oral Suspension: (EES, EryPed):** 100 mg/2.5 ml, 200 mg/5 ml, 400 mg/5ml. **Tablet as Base:** 250 mg, 333 mg, 500 mg. **Tablet as Ethylsuccinate (EES):** 400 mg. **Tablet as Stearate (Erythrocin):** 250 mg, 500 mg. **Tablets, Chewable (EryPed):** 200 mg.

Capsules, Delayed-Release (Eryc): 250 mg. **Tablets, Delayed-Release (Ery-Tab):** 250 mg, 333 mg, 500 mg.

ADMINISTRATION/HANDLING

IV

Reconstitution • Reconstitute each 500 mg with 10 ml Sterile Water for Injection without preservative to provide a concentration of 50 mg/ml. • Further dilute with 100–250 ml D_5W or 0.9% NaCl to maximum concentration of 5 mg/ml.

Rate of administration • For intermittent IV infusion (piggyback), infuse over 20–60 min.

Storage • Store parenteral form at room temperature. • Initial reconstituted solution in vial is stable for 2 wks refrigerated or 24 hrs at room temperature. • Diluted IV solution stable for 8 hrs at room temperature or 24 hrs if refrigerated. • Discard if precipitate forms.

PO

• Store capsules, tablets at room temperature. • Oral suspension is stable for 14 days at room temperature. • Administer erythromycin base, stearate 1 hr before or 2 hrs following ingestion of food. Erythromycin estolate, ethylsuccinate may be given without regard to meals, but optimal absorption occurs when given on empty stomach. • Give with 8 oz water. • If swallowing difficulties occur, sprinkle capsule contents on teaspoon of applesauce, follow with water. • Do not swallow chewable tablets whole. • Do not crush delayed-release capsules, tablets.

Ophthalmic

• Place gloved finger on lower eyelid and pull out until a pocket is formed between eye and lower lid. • Place ¼–½ inch of ointment into pocket. • Instruct pt to close eye gently for 1–2 min (so medication will not be squeezed out of the sac) and to roll eyeball to increase contact area of drug to eye.

IV INCOMPATIBILITIES

Fluconazole (Diflucan), furosemide (Lasix), metoclopramide (Reglan).

IV COMPATIBILITIES

Aminophylline, amiodarone (Cordarone), diltiazem (Cardizem), heparin, hydromorphone (Dilaudid), lidocaine, lipids, lorazepam (Ativan), magnesium sulfate, midazolam (Versed), morphine, multivitamins, potassium chloride, total parenteral nutrition (TPN).

INDICATIONS/ROUTES/DOSAGE

Mild to Moderate Infections of Upper and Lower Respiratory Tract, Pharyngitis, Skin Infections

PO: ADULTS, ELDERLY: BASE: 250–500 mg q6–12h. **ETHYLSUCCINATE:** 400–800 mg q6–12h. **Maximum:** 4 g/day. **CHILDREN:** 30–50 mg/kg/day in divided doses. **NEONATES:** 20–40 mg/kg/day in divided doses q6–12h.
IV: ADULTS, ELDERLY: 15–20 mg/kg/day divided q6h. **Maximum:** 4 g/day. **CHILDREN, INFANTS:** 15–50 mg/kg/day divided q6h.

Preop Intestinal Antisepsis

PO: ADULTS, ELDERLY: 1 g at 1 PM, 2 PM, and 11 PM on day before surgery (with neomycin). **CHILDREN:** 20 mg/kg at 1 PM, 2 PM, and 11 PM on day before surgery (with neomycin).

Acne Vulgaris

TOPICAL: ADULTS: Apply thin layer to affected area twice a day.

Gonococcal Ophthalmia Neonatorum

OPHTHALMIC: NEONATES: 0.5–2 cm no later than 1 hr after delivery.

SIDE EFFECTS

Frequent: IV: Abdominal cramping/discomfort, phlebitis/thrombophlebitis. **Topical:** Dry skin (50%). **Occasional:** Nausea, vomiting, diarrhea, rash, urticaria. **Rare: Ophthalmic:** Sensitivity reaction with increased irritation, burning, itching, inflammation. **Topical:** Urticaria.

ADVERSE EFFECTS/ TOXIC REACTIONS

Antibiotic-associated colitis, other super infections (abdominal cramps, severe watery diarrhea, fever), reversible cholestatic hepatitis may occur. High dosage in pts with renal impairment may lead to reversible hearing loss. Anaphylaxis occurs rarely. Ventricular arrhythmias, prolonged QT interval occur rarely with IV form.

NURSING CONSIDERATIONS

BASELINE ASSESSMENT

Question for history of allergies (particularly erythromycins), hepatitis.

INTERVENTION/EVALUATION

Monitor daily pattern of bowel activity and stool consistency. Assess skin for rash. Assess for hepatotoxicity (malaise, fever, abdominal pain, GI disturbances). Be alert for superinfection: fever, vomiting, diarrhea, anal/genital pruritus, oral mucosal changes (ulceration, pain, erythema). Check for phlebitis (heat, pain, red streaking over vein). Monitor for high-dose hearing loss.

PATIENT/FAMILY TEACHING

• Continue therapy for full length of treatment. • Doses should be evenly spaced. • Do *not* swallow chewable tablets whole. • Take medication with 8 oz water 1 hr before or 2 hrs following food or beverage. • **Ophthalmic:** Report burning, itching, inflammation. • **Topical:** Report excessive skin dryness, itching, burning. • Improvement of acne may not occur for 1–2 mos; maximum benefit may take 3 mos; therapy may last mos or yrs. • Use caution if using other topical acne preparations containing peeling or abrasive agents, medicated or abrasive soaps, cosmetics containing alcohol (e.g., astringents, aftershave lotion).

escitalopram

es-sih-**tail**-oh-pram
(Cipralex, Lexapro)

BLACK BOX ALERT Increased risk of suicidal thinking and behavior in children, adolescents, young adults 18–24 yrs with major depressive disorder, other psychiatric disorders.

CLASSIFICATION

PHARMACOTHERAPEUTIC: Serotonin reuptake inhibitor. **CLINICAL:** Antidepressant (see p. 39C).

ACTION

Blocks uptake of neurotransmitter serotonin at neuronal presynaptic membranes, increasing its availability at postsynaptic receptor sites. **Therapeutic Effect:** Antidepressant effect.

PHARMACOKINETICS

Well absorbed after PO administration. Protein bindings: 56%. Primarily metabolized in liver. Primarily excreted in feces, with a lesser amount eliminated in urine. **Half-life:** 35 hrs.

USES

Treatment of major depressive disorder exhibited as persistent, prominent dysphoria (occurring nearly every day for at least 2 wks) manifested by 4 of 8 symptoms: appetite change, sleep pattern change, increased fatigue, impaired concentration, feelings of guilt or worthlessness, loss of interest in usual activities, psychomotor agitation or retardation, suicidal tendencies. Treatment of generalized anxiety disorder (GAD). **OFF-LABEL:** Mixed anxiety and depressive disorder. Treatment of mild dementia-associated agitation in nonpsychotic pt.

PRECAUTIONS

Contraindications: Breast-feeding, use within 14 days of MAOIs. **Cautions:** Hepatic/renal impairment; history of seizures, mania, hypomania; concurrent use of CNS depressants. May prolong QT interval.

LIFESPAN CONSIDERATIONS

Pregnancy/Lactation: Distributed in breast milk. **Pregnancy Category C. Children:** May cause increased anticholinergic effects or hyperexcitability. **Elderly:** More sensitive to anticholinergic effects (e.g., dry mouth), more likely to experience dizziness, sedation, confusion, hypotension, hyperexcitability.

INTERACTIONS

DRUG: **Alcohol, other CNS suppressants** may increase CNS depression. **Linezolid, MAOIs** may cause serotonin syndrome (autonomic hyperactivity, diaphoresis, excitement, hyperthermia, rigidity, neuroleptic malignant syndrome, coma). **Sumatriptan** may cause weakness, hyperreflexia, poor coordination. **HERBAL:** **Gotu kola, kava kava, SAMe, St. John's wort, valerian** may increase CNS depression. **Ginkgo biloba, St. John's wort** may increase risk of serotonin syndrome. **FOOD:** None known. **LAB VALUES:** None significant.

AVAILABILITY (Rx)

Oral Solution: 5 mg/5 ml.

Tablets: 5 mg, 10 mg, 20 mg.

ADMINISTRATION/HANDLING

PO

• Give without regard to food. • Do not crush, chew tablets.

INDICATIONS/ROUTES/DOSAGE

Depression

PO: ADULTS: Initially, 10 mg once a day in the morning or evening. May increase to 20 mg after a minimum of 1 wk. **ELDERLY:** 10 mg/day. **CHILDREN 12–17 YRS:** Initially, 10 mg once daily. **Maximum:** 20 mg once daily. Recommended: 10 mg once daily.

Generalized Anxiety Disorder

PO: ADULTS: Initially, 10 mg once a day in morning or evening. May increase to 20 mg after minimum of 1 wk. **ELDERLY:** 10 mg/day.

Dosage in Renal Impairment
Use caution in pts with creatinine clearance less than 20 ml/min.

Dosage in Hepatic Impairment
10 mg/day.

SIDE EFFECTS

Frequent (21%–11%): Nausea, dry mouth, drowsiness, insomnia, diaphoresis. **Occasional (8%–4%):** Tremor, diarrhea, abnormal ejaculation, dyspepsia, fatigue, anxiety, vomiting, anorexia. **Rare (3%–2%):** Sinusitis, sexual dysfunction, menstrual disorder, abdominal pain, agitation, decreased libido.

ADVERSE EFFECTS/ TOXIC REACTIONS

Overdose manifested as dizziness, drowsiness, tachycardia, confusion, seizures.

NURSING CONSIDERATIONS

BASELINE ASSESSMENT

For pts on long-term therapy, hepatic/renal function tests, blood counts should be performed periodically. Observe, record behavior. Assess psychological status, thought content, sleep pattern, appearance, interest in environment.

INTERVENTION/EVALUATION

Supervise suicidal-risk pt closely during early therapy (as depression lessens, energy level improves, suicide potential increases). Assess appearance, behavior, speech pattern, level of interest, mood, suicidal ideation (esp. at beginning of therapy or when doses are increased or decreased), social functioning, mania, panic attacks.

PATIENT/FAMILY TEACHING

• Do not stop taking medication or increase dosage. • Avoid use of alcohol. • Avoid tasks that require alertness, motor skills until response to drug is established. • Report worsening depression, suicidal ideation, unusual changes in behavior.

Eskalith, *see lithium carbonate*

esmolol HIGH ALERT

ess-moe-lol
(Brevibloc)
Do not confuse esmolol with Osmitrol, or Brevibloc with Bumex or Buprenex.

◆CLASSIFICATION

PHARMACOTHERAPEUTIC: Beta$_1$-adrenergic blocker. **CLINICAL:** Antiarrhythmic (see pp. 17C, 72C).

ACTION

Selectively blocks beta$_1$-adrenergic receptors. **Therapeutic Effect:** Slows sinus heart rate, decreases cardiac output, reducing B/P.

PHARMACOKINETICS

Rapidly metabolized primarily by esterase in cytosol of red blood cells. Protein binding: 55%. Less than 1%–2% excreted in urine. **Half-life:** 9 min.

USES

Rapid, short-term control of ventricular rate in supraventricular tachycardia, atrial fibrillation or flutter; treatment of tachycardia and/or hypertension (esp. intraop or postop).

PRECAUTIONS

Contraindications: Cardiogenic shock, overt cardiac failure, second- or third-degree heart block, sinus bradycardia. **Cautions:** History of allergy, bronchial asthma, emphysema, bronchitis, CHF, diabetes, renal impairment.

E

LIFESPAN CONSIDERATIONS

Pregnancy/Lactation: Crosses placenta; distributed in breast milk. **Pregnancy Category C. Children:** Safety and efficacy not established. **Elderly:** No age-related precautions noted.

INTERACTIONS

DRUG: May mask symptoms of hypoglycemia, prolong hypoglycemic effect of **insulin, oral hypoglycemics. MAOIs** may cause significant hypertension. **Sympathomimetics, xanthines** may mutually inhibit effects. HERBAL: None significant. FOOD: None known. LAB VALUES: None significant.

AVAILABILITY (Rx)

Injection Solution: 10 mg/ml (250 ml), 20 mg/ml (100 ml).

ADMINISTRATION/HANDLING

◀ALERT▶ Give by IV infusion. Avoid butterfly needles, very small veins.

IV

Rate of administration • Administer by controlled infusion device; titrate to tolerance and response. • Infuse IV loading dose over 1–2 min. • Hypotension (systolic B/P less than 90 mm Hg) is greatest during first 30 min of IV infusion.

Storage • Use only clear and colorless to light yellow solution. • Discard solution if discolored or precipitate forms.

IV INCOMPATIBILITIES

Amphotericin B complex (Abelcet, AmBisome, Amphotec), furosemide (Lasix).

IV COMPATIBILITIES

Amiodarone (Cordarone), diltiazem (Cardizem), dopamine (Intropin), heparin, magnesium, midazolam (Versed), potassium chloride, propofol (Diprivan).

INDICATIONS/ROUTES/DOSAGE

Rate Control in Supraventricular Arrhythmias

IV: ADULTS, ELDERLY: Initially, loading dose of 500 mcg/kg/min for 1 min, followed by 50 mcg/kg/min for 4 min. If optimum response is not attained in 5 min, give second loading dose of 500 mcg/kg/min for 1 min, followed by infusion of 100 mcg/kg/min for 4 min. A third (and final) loading dose can be given and infusion increased by 50 mcg/kg/min, up to 200 mcg/kg/min, for 4 min. Once desired response is attained, increase infusion by no more than 25 mcg/kg/min. Infusion usually administered over 24–48 hrs in most pts. Range: 50–200 mcg/kg/min (average dose 100 mcg/kg/min).

Intraop/Postop Tachycardia Hypertension (Immediate Control)

IV: ADULTS, ELDERLY: Initially, 80 mg over 30 sec, then 150 mcg/kg/min infusion up to 300 mcg/kg/min.

SIDE EFFECTS

Generally well tolerated, with transient, mild side effects. Frequent: Hypotension (systolic B/P less than 90 mm Hg) manifested as dizziness, nausea, diaphoresis, headache, cold extremities, fatigue. Occasional: Anxiety, drowsiness, flushed skin, vomiting, confusion, inflammation at injection site, fever.

ADVERSE EFFECTS/ TOXIC REACTIONS

Overdose may produce profound hypotension, bradycardia, dizziness, syncope, drowsiness, breathing difficulty, bluish fingernails or palms of hands, seizures. May potentiate insulin-induced hypoglycemia in diabetic pts.

NURSING CONSIDERATIONS

BASELINE ASSESSMENT

Assess B/P, apical pulse immediately before drug is administered (if pulse is 60 or less/min or systolic B/P is 90 mm Hg or less, withhold medication, contact physician).

INTERVENTION/EVALUATION

Monitor B/P for hypotension, EKG, heart rate, respiratory rate, development of diaphoresis, dizziness (usually first sign of impending hypotension). Assess pulse for quality, irregular rate, bradycardia, extremities for coldness. Assist with ambulation if dizziness occurs. Assess for nausea, diaphoresis, headache, fatigue.

esomeprazole

es-oh-**mep**-rah-zole
(Nexium)
Do not confuse esomeprazole with aripiprazole or omeprazole, or Nexium with Nexavar.

FIXED-COMBINATION(S)

Vimovo: esomeprazole/naproxen (nonsteroidal anti-inflammatory): 20 mg/375 mg, 20 mg/500 mg.

◆ CLASSIFICATION

PHARMACOTHERAPEUTIC: Proton pump inhibitor. **CLINICAL:** Gastric acid inhibitor (see p. 148C).

ACTION

Converted to active metabolites that irreversibly bind to, inhibit hydrogen-potassium adenosine triphosphates, enzymes on surface of gastric parietal cells. Inhibits hydrogen ion transport into gastric lumen. **Therapeutic Effect:** Increases gastric pH, reducing gastric acid production.

PHARMACOKINETICS

Well absorbed after PO administration. Protein binding: 97%. Extensively metabolized in liver. Primarily excreted in urine. **Half-life:** 1–1.5 hrs.

USES

PO: Short-term treatment (4–8 wks) of erosive esophagitis (diagnosed by endoscopy); symptomatic gastroesophageal reflux disease (GERD). Treatment of Zollinger-Ellison syndrome. Used in triple therapy with amoxicillin and clarithromycin for treatment of *H. pylori* infection in pts with duodenal ulcer. Reduce risk of NSAID gastric ulcer. **IV:** Short-term treatment of GERD when oral therapy is not appropriate.

PRECAUTIONS

Contraindications: Hypersensitivity to benzimidazoles. **Cautions:** May increase risk of hip, wrist, spine fractures.

LIFESPAN CONSIDERATIONS

Pregnancy/Lactation: Unknown if drug crosses placenta or is distributed in breast milk. **Pregnancy Category B. Children:** Safety and efficacy not established. **Elderly:** No age-related precautions noted.

INTERACTIONS

DRUG: May decrease concentration of **digoxin, iron, ketoconazole.** May increase effect of **warfarin.** May decrease effect of **clopidogrel. HERBAL:** None significant. **FOOD:** None known. **LAB VALUES:** None significant.

AVAILABILITY (Rx)

Injection, Powder for Reconstitution (Sodium): 20 mg, 40 mg. **Oral Suspension, Delayed-Release:** 10 mg, 20 mg, 40 mg.

Capsules (Delayed-Release [Nexium]): 20 mg, 40 mg.

ADMINISTRATION/HANDLING

IV

Reconstitution • For IV push, add 5 ml of 0.9% NaCl to esomeprazole vial.
Infusion • For IV infusion, dissolve content of one vial in 50 ml 0.9% NaCl, D_5W, or lactated Ringer's.
Rate of administration • For IV push, administer over not less than 3 min. For intermittent infusion (piggyback) infuse over 10–30 min. • Flush line with 0.9% NaCl, lactated Ringer's, or D_5W, both before and after administration.
Storage • Use only clear and colorless to very slightly yellow solution. • Discard solution if particulate forms. • IV infusion stable for 12 hrs in 0.9% NaCl or lactated Ringer's; 6 hrs in D_5W.

PO (Capsules)
• Give 1 hr or more before eating (best before breakfast). • Do not crush, chew capsule; swallow whole. • For those with difficulty swallowing capsules, open capsule and mix pellets with 1 tbsp applesauce. Swallow spoonful without chewing.

PO (Oral Suspension)
• Empty contents into 15 ml water and stir. • Let stand 2–3 min to thicken. • Stir and drink within 30 min.

IV INCOMPATIBILITIES

Do not mix esomeprazole with any other medications through the same IV line or tubing.

INDICATIONS/ROUTES/DOSAGE

Erosive Esophagitis
PO: ADULTS, ELDERLY, CHILDREN 12 YRS AND OLDER: 20–40 mg once daily for 4–8 wks. May continue for additional 4–8 wks. **CHILDREN 1–11 YRS:** 10–20 mg/day for up to 8 wks.

Maintenance Therapy for Erosive Esophagitis
PO: ADULTS, ELDERLY: 20 mg/day.

Treatment of NSAID-Induced Gastric Ulcers
PO: ADULTS, ELDERLY: 20 mg/day for 4–8 wks.

Prevention of NSAID-Induced Gastric Ulcer
PO: ADULTS, ELDERLY: 20–40 mg once a day for up to 6 mos.

Gastroesophageal Reflux Disease (GERD)
IV: ADULTS, ELDERLY: 20 or 40 mg once daily.
PO: ADULTS, ELDERLY, CHILDREN, 12–17 YRS: 20–40 mg once daily. **CHILDREN 1–11 YRS:** 10 mg/day for up to 8 wks.

Zollinger-Ellison Syndrome
PO: ADULTS, ELDERLY: 40 mg 2 times a day. Doses up to 240 mg/day have been used.

Duodenal Ulcer Caused by *Helicobacter Pylori*
PO: ADULTS, ELDERLY: 40 mg (esomeprazole) once a day, with amoxicillin 1,000 mg and clarithromycin 500 mg twice a day for 10 days.

SIDE EFFECTS

Frequent (7%): Headache. **Occasional (3%–2%):** Diarrhea, abdominal pain, nausea. **Rare (less than 2%):** Dizziness, asthenia (loss of strength, energy), vomiting, constipation, rash, cough.

ADVERSE EFFECTS/ TOXIC REACTIONS

Pancreatitis, hepatotoxicity, interstitial nephritis occur rarely.

NURSING CONSIDERATIONS

BASELINE ASSESSMENT

Assess epigastric/abdominal pain.

INTERVENTION/EVALUATION

Evaluate for therapeutic response (relief of GI symptoms). Question if GI discomfort, nausea, diarrhea occur. Monitor for rebleeding in pts with peptic ulcer bleed.

PATIENT/FAMILY TEACHING

• Report headache. • Take more than 1 hr before eating. • If swallowing capsules is difficult, open capsule and mix pellets with 1 tbsp applesauce. Swallow spoonful without chewing.

Estrace, *see estradiol*

Estraderm, *see estradiol*

estradiol

ess-tra-**dye**-ole
(Alora, Climara, Delestrogen, Depo-Estradiol, Divigel, Elestrin,

Estrace, Estraderm, Estrasorb, Estring, Estrogel, Evamist, Femring, Femtrace, Menostar, Vagifem, Vivelle, Vivelle Dot)

BLACK BOX ALERT Increased risk of dementia when given to women 65 yrs and older. Use of estrogen without progestin increases risk of endometrial cancer in postmenopausal women with intact uterus. Do not use to prevent cardiovascular disease.

Do not confuse Alora with Aldara, or Estraderm with Testoderm.

FIXED-COMBINATION(S)

Activella: estradiol/norethindrone (hormone): 1 mg/0.5 mg. **Climara PRO:** estradiol/levonorgestrel (progestin): 0.045 mg/24 hr, 0.015 mg/24 hr. **Combi-patch:** estradiol/norethindrone (hormone): 0.05 mg/0.14 mg, 0.05 mg/0.25 mg. **Femhrt:** estradiol/norethindrone (hormone): 5 mcg/1 mg. **Lunelle:** estradiol/medroxy-progesterone (progestin): 5 mg/25 mg per 0.5 ml.

◆ CLASSIFICATION

PHARMACOTHERAPEUTIC: Estrogen. **CLINICAL:** Estrogen, antineoplastic.

ACTION

Increases synthesis of DNA, RNA, proteins in target tissues; reduces release of gonadotropin-releasing hormone from hypothalamus; reduces follicle-stimulating hormone (FSH), luteinizing hormone (LH) release from pituitary. **Therapeutic Effect:** Promotes normal growth/development of female sex organs, maintains GU function, vasomotor stability. Prevents accelerated bone loss by inhibiting bone resorption, restoring balance of bone resorption, formation. Inhibits LH, decreases serum testosterone concentration.

PHARMACOKINETICS

Well absorbed from GI tract. Widely distributed. Protein binding: 50%–80%. Metabolized in liver. Primarily excreted in urine. **Half-life:** Unknown.

USES

Treatment of moderate to severe vasomotor symptoms associated with menopause, hypoestrogenism (due to hypogonadism, primary ovarian failure), breast cancer, prostate cancer, prevention of osteoporosis, vaginal atrophy, atrophic vaginitis, abnormal uterine bleeding due to hormone imbalance, postmenopausal urogenital symptoms of lower urinary tract. **OFF-LABEL:** Treatment of Turner's syndrome.

PRECAUTIONS

Contraindications: Undiagnosed abnormal vaginal bleeding, active arterial thrombosis, blood dyscrasias, estrogen-dependent cancer, known or suspected breast cancer, pregnancy, thrombophlebitis or thromboembolic disorders, thyroid dysfunction. **Cautions:** Renal/hepatic insufficiency, diseases that may be exacerbated by fluid retention, diabetes mellitus, endometriosis, hypercalcemia, hyperlipidemias, hypertension, hypocalcemia, hypothyroidism, history of jaundice during pregnancy, vaginal infection, children in whom bone growth is not complete.

⌛ LIFESPAN CONSIDERATIONS

Pregnancy/Lactation: Distributed in breast milk. May be harmful to infant. Breast-feeding not recommended. **Pregnancy Category X. Children:** Caution in those for whom bone growth is not complete (may accelerate epiphyseal closure). **Elderly:** No age-related precautions noted.

INTERACTIONS

DRUG: May increase **cyclosporine** concentration, risk of hepatotoxicity, nephrotoxicity. **Hepatotoxic medications** may increase risk of hepatotoxicity. **HERBAL:** Avoid **black cohosh, dong quai, saw palmetto. St. John's wort** may decrease plasma concentration, effectiveness of estrogens. **FOOD:** None known. **LAB VALUES:** May increase serum glucose, calcium, HDL, triglycerides. May decrease serum cholesterol, LDL. May affect metapyrone testing, thyroid function tests.

AVAILABILITY (Rx)

Emulsion, topical (Estrasorb): 4.35 mg estradiol/1.74 g pouch (contents of 2 pouches deliver estradiol 0.05 mg/day). **Gel, topical (Divigel):** 0.1% (0.25-g packet delivers estradiol 0.25 mg, 0.5 g-packet delivers estradiol 0.5 mg, 1-g packet delivers 1 mg). **(Elestrin):** 0.06% delivers 0.52 mg estradiol/actuation. **(Estrogel):** 0.06% delivers 0.75 mg/actuation. **Injection (Cypionate): Depo-Estradiol:** 5 mg/ml. **(Valerate): Delestrogen:** 10 mg/ml, 20 mg/ml, 40 mg/ml. **Tablets (Estrace):** 0.5 mg, 1 mg, 2 mg. **Femtrace:** 0.45 mg, 0.9 mg, 1.8 mg. **Topical Spray (Evamist):** 1.53 mg/spray. **Transdermal System (Alora):** twice weekly: 0.025 mg/24 hrs, 0.05 mg/24 hrs, 0.075 mg/24 hrs, 0.1 mg/24 hrs. **Transdermal System (Climara):** once weekly: 0.025 mg/24 hrs, 0.0375 mg/24 hrs, 0.05 mg/24 hrs, 0.06 mg/24 hrs, 0.075 mg/24 hrs, 0.1 mg/24 hrs. **Transdermal System (Estraderm):** twice weekly: 0.05 mg/24 hrs, 0.1 mg/24 hrs. **Transdermal System (Menostar):** once weekly: 0.014 mg/24 hrs. **Transdermal System (Vivelle):** twice weekly: 0.05 mg/24 hrs, 0.1 mg/24 hrs. **Transdermal System (Vivelle Dot):** twice weekly: 0.025 mg/24 hrs, 0.0375 mg/24 hrs, 0.05 mg/24 hrs, 0.075 mg/24 hrs, 0.1 mg/24 hrs. **Vaginal Cream (Estrace):** 0.1 mg/g. **Vaginal Ring (Estring):** 2 mg (releases 7.5 mcg/day over 90 days). **Vaginal Ring (Femring):** 0.05 mg/day (total estradiol 12.4 mg-release 0.05 mg/day over 3 mos); 0.1 mg/day (total estradiol 24.8 mg-release 0.1 mg/day over 3 mos). **Vaginal Tablet (Vagifem):** 25 mcg.

ADMINISTRATION/HANDLING

IM

- Rotate vial to disperse drug in solution.
- Inject deep IM in large muscle mass.

PO

- Administer at same time each day.
- Administer with food.

Transdermal

- Remove old patch; select new site (buttocks are alternative application site). • Peel off protective strip to expose adhesive surface. • Apply to clean, dry, intact skin on trunk of body (area with as little hair as possible). • Press in place for at least 10 sec (do not apply to breasts or waistline).

Vaginal

- Apply at bedtime for best absorption.
- Insert end of filled applicator into vagina, directed slightly toward sacrum; push plunger down completely. • Avoid skin contact with cream (prevents skin absorption).

INDICATIONS/ROUTES/DOSAGE

Prostate Cancer

IM (DELESTROGEN): ADULTS, ELDERLY: 30 mg or more q1–2wk.
PO: ADULTS, ELDERLY: 1–2 mg tid for at least 3 mos.

Breast Cancer

PO: ADULTS, ELDERLY: 10 mg 3 times a day for at least 3 mos.

Osteoporosis Prophylaxis in Postmenopausal Females

PO: ADULTS, ELDERLY: 0.45–0.5 mg/day cyclically (3 wks on, 1 wk off).
TRANSDERMAL (CLIMARA): ADULTS, ELDERLY: Initially, 0.025 mg/24 hrs weekly, adjust dose as needed.
TRANSDERMAL (ALORA, VIVELLE, VIVELLE DOT): ADULTS, ELDERLY: Initially, 0.025 mg/24 hrs patch twice weekly, adjust dose as needed.
TRANSDERMAL (ESTRADERM): ADULTS, ELDERLY: 0.05 mg/24 hrs twice weekly.
TRANSDERMAL (MENOSTAR): ADULTS, ELDERLY: 0.014 mg/24 hrs patch weekly.

Female Hypoestrogenism

PO: ADULTS, ELDERLY: 0.9–2 mg/day, adjust dose as needed.

IM (DEPO-ESTRADIOL): ADULTS, ELDERLY: 1.5–2 mg monthly.
IM (DELESTROGEN): ADULTS, ELDERLY: 10–20 mg q4wk.

Vasomotor Symptoms Associated with Menopause
PO: ADULTS, ELDERLY: 0.9–2 mg/day cyclically (3 wks on, 1 wk off), adjust dose as needed.
IM (DEPO-ESTRADIOL): ADULTS, ELDERLY: 1–5 mg q3–4wk.
IM (DELESTROGEN): ADULTS, ELDERLY: 10–20 mg q4wk.
TOPICAL EMULSION (ESTRASORB): ADULTS, ELDERLY: 3.48 g (contents of 2 pouches) once a day in the morning.
TOPICAL GEL (ESTROGEL): ADULTS, ELDERLY: 1.25 g/day.
TRANSDERMAL SPRAY (EVAMIST): Initially, 1 spray daily. May increase to 2–3 sprays daily.
TRANSDERMAL (CLIMARA): ADULTS, ELDERLY: 0.025 mg/24 hrs weekly. Adjust dose as needed.
TRANSDERMAL (ALORA, ESTRADERM, VIVELLE DOT): ADULTS, ELDERLY: 0.05 mg/24 hrs twice a wk.
TRANSDERMAL (VIVELLE): ADULTS, ELDERLY: 0.0375 mg/24 hrs twice a wk.
VAGINAL RING (FEMRING): ADULTS, ELDERLY: 0.05 mg. May increase to 0.1 mg if needed.

Vaginal Atrophy
VAGINAL RING (ESTRING): ADULTS, ELDERLY: 2 mg.
VAGINAL CREAM (ESTRACE): Insert 2–4 g/day intravaginally for 2 wks, then reduce dose by ½ initial dose for 2 wks, then maintenance dose of 1 g 1–3 times a wk.

Atrophic Vaginitis
VAGINAL TABLET (VAGIFEM): ADULTS, ELDERLY: Initially, 1 tablet/day for 2 wks. Maintenance: 1 tablet twice a wk.

SIDE EFFECTS

Frequent: Anorexia, nausea, swelling of breasts, peripheral edema marked by swollen ankles and feet. **Transdermal:** Skin irritation, redness. **Occasional:** Vomiting (esp. with high doses), headache (may be severe), intolerance to contact lenses, hypertension, glucose intolerance, brown spots on exposed skin. **Vaginal:** Local irritation, vaginal discharge, changes in vaginal bleeding (spotting, breakthrough, prolonged bleeding). **Rare:** Chorea (involuntary movements), hirsutism (abnormal hairiness), loss of scalp hair, depression.

ADVERSE EFFECTS/ TOXIC REACTIONS

Prolonged administration increases risk of gallbladder disease, thromboembolic disease, breast, cervical, vaginal, endometrial, hepatic carcinoma. Cholestatic jaundice occurs rarely.

NURSING CONSIDERATIONS

BASELINE ASSESSMENT

Assess frequency/severity of vasomotor symptoms. Question for hypersensitivity to estrogen, previous jaundice, thromboembolic disorders associated with pregnancy, estrogen therapy. Question for possibility of pregnancy (Pregnancy Category X).

INTERVENTION/EVALUATION

Monitor B/P, weight, serum calcium, glucose, hepatic enzymes. Monitor for loss of vision, sudden onset of proptosis, diplopia, migraine, thromoembolic disorders.

PATIENT/FAMILY TEACHING

• Limit alcohol, caffeine. • Avoid grapefruit, grapefruit juice. • Inform physician if sudden headache, vomiting, disturbance of vision/speech, numbness/weakness of extremities, chest pain, calf pain, shortness of breath, severe abdominal pain, mental depression, unusual bleeding occurs. • Avoid smoking. • Report abnormal vaginal bleeding. • Never place patch on breast or waistline.

estramustine

HIGH ALERT

es-trah-**mew**-steen
(Emcyt)
Do not confuse Emcyt with Eryc, or estramustine with exemestane.

E

◆CLASSIFICATION

PHARMACOTHERAPEUTIC: Alkylating agent, estrogen/nitrogen mustard. **CLINICAL:** Antineoplastic (see p. 82C).

ACTION

Binds to microtubule-associated proteins, causing their disassembly. **Therapeutic Effect:** Reduces serum testosterone concentration.

PHARMACOKINETICS

Well absorbed from GI tract. Highly localized in prostatic tissue. Rapidly dephosphorylated during absorption into peripheral circulation. Metabolized in liver. Primarily eliminated in feces by biliary system. **Half-life:** 20 hrs.

USES

Treatment of metastatic or progressive carcinoma of prostate gland.

PRECAUTIONS

Contraindications: Active thrombophlebitis or thromboembolic disorders (unless tumor is cause of thromboembolic disorder and benefits outweigh risk), hypersensitivity to estradiol nitrogen mustard. **Cautions:** History of thrombophlebitis, thrombosis, thromboembolic disorders; cerebrovascular, coronary artery disease; hepatic impairment; metabolic bone disease in those with hypercalcemia, renal insufficiency.

⌛ LIFESPAN CONSIDERATIONS

Pregnancy/Lactation: Not indicated for use in women. **Children:** Not used in this pt population. **Elderly:** Age-related renal impairment and/or peripheral vascular disease may require dosage adjustment.

INTERACTIONS

DRUG: Hepatotoxic medications may increase risk of hepatotoxicity. **HERBAL:** None significant. **FOOD: Milk, dairy products, other calcium-rich foods** may impair absorption. **LAB VALUES:** May increase serum glucose, bilirubin, cortisol, LDH, phospholipid, prolactin, AST, sodium, triglyceride. May decrease phosphate. May alter thyroid function test results.

AVAILABILITY (Rx)

Capsules: 140 mg.

ADMINISTRATION/HANDLING

PO

• Refrigerate capsules (may remain at room temperature for 24–48 hrs without loss of potency). • Give with water 1 hr before or 2 hrs after meals.

INDICATIONS/ROUTES/DOSAGE

Prostatic Carcinoma

PO: ADULTS, ELDERLY: 10–16 mg/kg/day (most common: 14 mg/kg/day) or 140 mg 4 times a day.

SIDE EFFECTS

Frequent: Peripheral edema (esp. lower extremities), breast tenderness/enlargement, diarrhea, flatulence, nausea. **Occasional:** Increase in B/P, thirst, dry skin, ecchymosis, flushing, alopecia, night sweats. **Rare:** Headache, rash, fatigue, insomnia, vomiting.

ADVERSE EFFECTS/ TOXIC REACTIONS

May exacerbate CHF; increased risk of pulmonary emboli, thrombophlebitis, CVA.

NURSING CONSIDERATIONS

INTERVENTION/EVALUATION

Monitor serum calcium, hepatic function tests, B/P periodically.

PATIENT/FAMILY TEACHING

• Do not take with milk, milk products, calcium-rich food, calcium-containing antacids. • Use contraceptive measures during therapy. • If headache (migraine or severe), vomiting, disturbed speech/vision, dizziness, numbness, shortness of breath, calf pain, chest pain/pressure, unexplained cough occurs, contact physician.

Estrasorb, *see estradiol*

Estring, *see estradiol*

Estrogel, *see estradiol*

estropipate

ess-troe-**pie**-pate
(Ogen, Ortho-Est)

CLASSIFICATION

PHARMACOTHERAPEUTIC: Estrogen.
CLINICAL: Hormone.

ACTION

Increases synthesis of DNA, RNA, proteins in target tissues; reduces release of gonadotropin-releasing hormone from hypothalamus; reduces follicle-stimulating hormone (FSH), luteinizing hormone (LH) from pituitary. **Therapeutic Effect:** Promotes normal growth, development of female sex organs, maintains GU function, vasomotor stability. Prevents accelerated bone loss by inhibiting bone resorption, restoring balance of bone resorption, formation. Inhibits LH, decreases serum testosterone.

PHARMACOKINETICS

Well absorbed from GI tract. Metabolized in liver. **Half-life:** Not available.

USES

Treatment of vasomotor symptoms associated with menopause, vulvar/vaginal atrophy, hypoestrogenism, osteoporosis prophylaxis.

PRECAUTIONS

Contraindications: Abnormal vaginal bleeding, active arterial thrombosis, blood dyscrasias, estrogen-dependent cancer, known or suspected breast cancer, pregnancy, thrombophlebitis, thromboembolic disorders, thyroid dysfunction. **Cautions:** Renal/hepatic insufficiency, diseases that may be exacerbated by fluid retention. **Pregnancy Category X.**

INTERACTIONS

DRUG: May increase **cyclosporine** concentration, risk of hepatotoxicity, nephrotoxicity. **Hepatotoxic medications** may increase risk of hepatotoxicity. **HERBAL:** **St. John's wort** may decrease concentration. Avoid **black cohosh, dong quai, saw palmetto.** **FOOD:** None known. **LAB VALUES:** May increase serum glucose, calcium, HDL, triglycerides. May decrease serum cholesterol, LDL. May affect metapyrone testing, thyroid function tests.

AVAILABILITY (Rx)

Tablets (Ogen, Ortho-EST): 0.625 mg (0.75 mg estropipate), 1.25 mg (1.5 mg estropipate), 2.5 mg (3 mg estropipate).

ADMINISTRATION/HANDLING

• Administer at same time each day.

INDICATIONS/ROUTES/DOSAGE

Vasomotor Symptoms, Atrophic Vaginitis, Kraurosis Vulvae

PO: ADULTS, ELDERLY: 0.75–6 mg estropiate/day cyclically.

Female Hypogonadism, Castration, Primary Ovarian Failure

PO: ADULTS, ELDERLY: 1.25–9 mg estropiate/day for 21 days, then off for 8–10 days. Repeat if bleeding does not occur by end of off cycle.

Prevention of Osteoporosis
PO: ADULTS, ELDERLY: 0.75 mg estropiate/day (25 days of 31-day cycle/mo).

SIDE EFFECTS

Frequent: Anorexia, nausea, swelling of breasts, peripheral edema marked by swollen ankles and feet. **Occasional:** Vomiting (esp. with high doses), headache (may be severe), intolerance to contact lenses, hypertension, glucose intolerance, brown spots on exposed skin. **Vaginal:** Local irritation, vaginal discharge, changes in vaginal bleeding (spotting, breakthrough, prolonged bleeding). **Rare:** Chorea (involuntary movements), hirsutism (abnormal hairiness), loss of scalp hair, depression.

ADVERSE EFFECTS/ TOXIC REACTIONS

Prolonged administration increases risk of cerebrovascular disease, coronary artery disease, gallbladder disease, hypercalcemia; breast, cervical, vaginal, endometrial, hepatic carcinoma. Cholestatic jaundice occurs rarely.

NURSING CONSIDERATIONS

BASELINE ASSESSMENT

Question for hypersensitivity to estrogen, previous jaundice, thromboembolic disorders associated with pregnancy, estrogen therapy. Question for possibility of pregnancy (Pregnancy Category X).

INTERVENTION/EVALUATION

Promptly report signs/symptoms of thromboembolic/thrombotic disorders (sudden severe headache, shortness of breath, vision/speech disturbance, numbness of an extremity).

PATIENT/FAMILY TEACHING

• Avoid smoking due to increased risk of heart attack and blood clots. • Notify physician of abnormal vaginal bleeding, depression. • With vaginal application, remain recumbent at least 30 min after application; do not use tampons. • Stop taking medication and contact physician at once if pregnancy is suspected.

eszopiclone

es-zoe-**pick**-lone
(Lunesta)
Do not confuse Lunesta with Neulasta.

◆CLASSIFICATION

PHARMACOTHERAPEUTIC: Non-benzodiazepine. **CLINICAL:** Hypnotic **(Schedule IV).**

ACTION

May interact with GABA-receptor complexes at binding domains located close to or allosterically coupled to benzodiazepine receptors. **Therapeutic Effect:** Prevents insomnia, difficulty maintaining normal sleep.

PHARMACOKINETICS

Rapidly absorbed following PO administration. Protein binding: 52%–59%. Metabolized in liver. Excreted in urine. **Half-life:** 5–6 hrs.

USES

Long-term treatment of insomnia in pts who experience difficulty falling asleep or are unable to sleep through the night (sleep maintenance difficulty).

PRECAUTIONS

Contraindications: None known. **Cautions:** Hepatic impairment, compromised respiratory function, clinical depression.

⌛ LIFESPAN CONSIDERATIONS

Pregnancy/Lactation: Unknown if drug crosses placenta or is distributed in breast milk. **Pregnancy Category C. Children:** Safety and efficacy not established. **Elderly:** Those with impaired motor or cognitive performance may require dosage adjustment.

INTERACTIONS

DRUG: **Alcohol, anticonvulsants, antihistamines, other CNS depressants** may increase CNS depression. **Clarithromycin, itraconazole, ketoconazole, nelfinavir, ritonavir** may increase concentration/toxicity. HERBAL: **Gotu kola, kava kava, St. John's wort, valerian** may increase CNS depression. FOOD: Onset of action may be reduced if taken with or immediately after a **high-fat meal.** LAB VALUES: None significant.

AVAILABILITY (Rx)

Tablets, Film-Coated: 1 mg, 2 mg, 3 mg.

ADMINISTRATION/HANDLING

PO

• Should be administered immediately before bedtime. • Do not give with or immediately following a high-fat or heavy meal. • Do not crush, break, or chew tablet.

INDICATIONS/ROUTES/DOSAGE

Insomnia

PO: ADULTS: 2 mg before bedtime. **Maximum:** 3 mg. **Concurrent use with CYP3A4 inhibitors** (e.g., clarithromycin, erythromycin, azole antifungals): 1 mg before bedtime; if needed, dose may be increased to 2 mg. ELDERLY: Initially, 1 mg before bedtime. **Maximum:** 2 mg.

Sleep Maintenance Difficulty

PO: ADULTS: 2 mg before bedtime.

SIDE EFFECTS

Frequent (34%–21%): Unpleasant taste, headache. **Occasional** (10%–4%): Drowsiness, dry mouth, dyspepsia, dizziness, nervousness, nausea, rash, pruritus, depression, diarrhea. **Rare** (3%–2%): Hallucinations, anxiety, confusion, abnormal dreams, decreased libido, neuralgia.

ADVERSE EFFECTS/ TOXIC REACTIONS

Chest pain, peripheral edema occur occasionally.

NURSING CONSIDERATIONS

BASELINE ASSESSMENT

Assess B/P, pulse, respirations. Raise bed rails, provide call light. Provide environment conducive to sleep (quiet environment, low or no lighting, TV off).

INTERVENTION/EVALUATION

Assess sleep pattern of pt. Evaluate for therapeutic response (decrease in number of nocturnal awakenings, increase in length of sleep).

PATIENT/FAMILY TEACHING

• Take only when experiencing insomnia. Do not take when insomnia is not present. • Avoid alcohol. • At least 8 hrs must be devoted for sleep time before daily activity begins. • Take eszopiclone immediately before bedtime. • Report insomnia that worsens or persists longer than 7–10 days; abnormal thoughts or behavior, memory loss, anxiety.

etanercept

ee-**tan**-er-cept
(Enbrel)

BLACK BOX ALERT Serious, potentially fatal, infection, including bacterial sepsis, tuberculosis have occurred.

Do not confuse Enbrel with Levbid.

◆ CLASSIFICATION

PHARMACOTHERAPEUTIC: Protein. CLINICAL: Antiarthritic.

ACTION

Binds to tumor necrosis factor (TNF), blocking its interaction with cell surface receptors. Elevated levels of TNF, involved in inflammatory and immune responses, are found in synovial fluid of rheumatoid arthritis pts. **Therapeutic Effect:** Relieves symptoms of rheumatoid arthritis.

PHARMACOKINETICS

Well absorbed after subcutaneous administration. Half-life: 72–132 hrs.

USES

Reduces signs/symptoms of moderate to severely active rheumatoid arthritis (RA). Treatment of active juvenile rheumatoid arthritis, ankylosing spondylitis, psoriatic arthritis. Treatment of chronic, moderate to severe plaque psoriasis. Improvement of physical function in pts with psoriatic arthritis. **OFF-LABEL:** Treatment of Crohn's disease, reactive arthritis.

PRECAUTIONS

Contraindications: Serious active infection or sepsis. **Cautions:** History of recurrent infections, illnesses that predispose to infection (e.g., diabetes).

LIFESPAN CONSIDERATIONS

Pregnancy/Lactation: Unknown if distributed in breast milk. **Pregnancy Category B. Children:** No age-related precautions noted in those 4 yrs and older. **Elderly:** No age-related precautions noted.

INTERACTIONS

DRUG: **Anakinra** may increase risk of infection. Use of **live virus vaccines** may potentiate virus replication, increase vaccine side effects, decrease pt's antibody response to vaccine. **HERBAL:** None significant. **FOOD:** None known. **LAB VALUES:** May increase AST, ALT, bilirubin, alkaline phosphatase.

AVAILABILITY (Rx)

Injection, Powder for Reconstitution: 25 mg. **Injection, Solution Prefilled Syringe:** 25 mg/0.5 ml, 50 mg/ml. **Injection, Solution (Auto Injector):** 50 mg/ml.

ADMINISTRATION/HANDLING

◀ALERT▶ Do not add other medications to solution. Do not use filter during reconstitution or administration.

Subcutaneous

• Refrigerate prefilled syringes, powder for reconstitution. • Reconstitute with 1 ml Bacteriostatic Water for Injection (0.9% benzyl alcohol). Do not reconstitute with other diluents. • Slowly inject diluent into vial. Some foaming will occur. To avoid excessive foaming, slowly swirl contents until powder is dissolved (less than 5 min). • Visually inspect solution for particles, discoloration. Reconstituted solution should appear clear, colorless. If discolored, cloudy, or particles remain, discard solution; do not use. • Withdraw all of the solution into syringe. Final volume should be approximately 1 ml. • Inject into thigh, abdomen, upper arm. Rotate injection sites. • Give new injection at least 1 inch from an old site and never into area where skin is tender, bruised, red, hard. • Once reconstituted, may be stored in vial for up to 14 days.

INDICATIONS/ROUTES/DOSAGE

Rheumatoid Arthritis (RA), Psoriatic Arthritis, Ankylosing Spondylitis

SUBCUTANEOUS: ADULTS, ELDERLY: 25 mg twice weekly given 72–96 hrs apart or 50 mg once weekly. **Maximum:** 50 mg/wk.

Juvenile Rheumatoid Arthritis

SUBCUTANEOUS: CHILDREN 2–17 YRS: 0.4 mg/kg. **Maximum:** 25-mg dose: twice weekly given 72–96 hrs apart or 0.8 mg/kg. **Maximum:** 50 mg/dose: once weekly.

Plaque Psoriasis

SUBCUTANEOUS: ADULTS, ELDERLY: 50 mg twice a wk (give 3–4 days apart) for 3 mos. Maintenance: 50 mg once a wk.

SIDE EFFECTS

Frequent (37%): Injection site erythema, pruritus, pain, swelling; abdominal pain, vomiting (more common in children than adults). **Occasional (16%–4%):** Headache, rhinitis, dizziness, pharyngitis, cough, asthenia (loss of strength, energy), abdominal pain, dyspepsia. Rare (less than 3%): Sinusitis, allergic reaction.

ADVERSE EFFECTS/ TOXIC REACTIONS

Infection (pyelonephritis, cellulitis, osteomyelitis, wound infection, leg ulcer, septic arthritis, diarrhea, bronchitis, pneumonia) occur in 29%–38% of pts. Rare adverse effects include heart failure, hypertension, hypotension, pancreatitis, GI hemorrhage.

NURSING CONSIDERATIONS

BASELINE ASSESSMENT

Assess onset, type, location, duration of pain, inflammation. If significant exposure to varicella virus has occurred during treatment, therapy should be temporarily discontinued and treatment with varicella-zoster immune globulin considered.

INTERVENTION/EVALUATION

Assess for joint swelling, pain, tenderness. Monitor erythrocyte sedimentation rate (ESR), C-reactive protein level, CBC with differential, platelet count, signs of infection.

PATIENT/FAMILY TEACHING

• Instruct pt in subcutaneous injection technique, including areas of body acceptable as injection sites. • Injection site reaction generally occurs in first mo of treatment and decreases in frequency during continued therapy. • Do not receive live vaccines during treatment. • Inform physician if persistent fever, bruising, bleeding, pallor occurs.

ethambutol

eth-**am**-bew-tol
(Etibi ✤, Myambutol)

◆CLASSIFICATION

PHARMACOTHERAPEUTIC: Isonicotinic acid derivative. **CLINICAL:** Antitubercular.

ACTION

Interferes with RNA synthesis. **Therapeutic Effect:** Suppresses multiplication of mycobacteria.

PHARMACOKINETICS

Rapidly, well absorbed from GI tract. Protein binding: 20%–30%. Widely distributed. Metabolized in liver. Primarily excreted in urine. Removed by hemodialysis. **Half-life:** 3–4 hrs (increased in renal impairment).

USES

In conjunction with at least one other antitubercular agent for initial treatment and retreatment of clinical tuberculosis. OFF-LABEL: Treatment of atypical mycobacterial infections (e.g., *Mycobacterium avium* complex [MAC]).

PRECAUTIONS

Contraindications: Optic neuritis. **Cautions:** Renal dysfunction, gout, ocular defects: diabetic retinopathy, cataracts, recurrent ocular inflammatory conditions. Not recommended for children 13 yrs and younger.

LIFESPAN CONSIDERATIONS

Pregnancy/Lactation: Crosses placenta. Distributed in breast milk. **Pregnancy Category B. Children:** Safety and efficacy not established in those younger than 13 yrs. **Elderly:** Age-related renal impairment may require dosage adjustment.

INTERACTIONS

DRUG: **Neurotoxic medications** may increase risk of neurotoxicity. **Aluminum hydroxide** may decrease concentration/effects. HERBAL: None significant. FOOD: None known. LAB VALUES: May increase serum uric acid.

AVAILABILITY (Rx)

Tablets: 100 mg, 400 mg.

ADMINISTRATION/HANDLING

PO

• May be crushed and mixed with apple juice or applesauce. • Administer at least 4 hrs before giving aluminum hydroxide. • Give with food (decreases GI upset).

INDICATIONS/ROUTES/DOSAGE

Tuberculosis, Other Mycobacterial Diseases

PO: ADULTS, ELDERLY: 15–25 mg/kg/day. **Maximum:** 1.6 g/dose **or** 50 mg/kg/dose twice weekly. **Maximum:** 4 g regardless of weight. **CHILDREN:** 15–20 mg/kg/day. **Maximum:** 1 g/day **or** 50 mg/kg/dose twice weekly. **Maximum:** 4 g regardless of weight.

Dosage in Renal Impairment

Dosage interval is modified based on creatinine clearance.

Creatinine Clearance	Dosage
10–50 ml/min	q24–36h
Less than 10 ml/min	q48h

SIDE EFFECTS

Occasional: Acute gouty arthritis (chills, pain, swelling of joints with hot skin), confusion, abdominal pain, nausea, vomiting, anorexia, headache. **Rare:** Rash, fever, blurred vision, red-green color blindness.

ADVERSE EFFECTS/ TOXIC REACTIONS

Optic neuritis (more common with high-dosage, long-term therapy), peripheral neuritis, thrombocytopenia, anaphylactoid reaction occur rarely.

NURSING CONSIDERATIONS

BASELINE ASSESSMENT

Evaluate initial CBC, renal/hepatic function test results, and monitor periodically.

INTERVENTION/EVALUATION

Assess for vision changes (altered color perception, decreased visual acuity may be first signs): discontinue drug and notify physician immediately. Give with food if GI distress occurs. Monitor serum uric acid. Assess for hot, painful, swollen joints, esp. great toe, ankle, knee (gout). Report numbness, tingling, burning of extremities (peripheral neuritis).

PATIENT/FAMILY TEACHING

• Do not skip doses; take for full length of therapy (may take mos or yrs). • Notify physician immediately of any visual problem (visual effects generally reversible with discontinuation of ethambutol but in rare cases may take up to 1 yr to disappear or may be permanent). • Promptly report swelling or pain of joints, numbness or tingling/burning of extremities, fever, chills.

etodolac

eh-**toe**-doe-lack
(Apo-Etodolac, Lodine,
Lodine XL, Ultradol)

BLACK BOX ALERT Increased risk of serious cardiovascular thrombotic events, including myocardial infarction, CVA. Increased risk of severe GI reactions, including ulceration, bleeding, perforation of stomach, intestines.

Do not confuse Lodine with codeine, iodine, or Lopid.

CLASSIFICATION

PHARMACOTHERAPEUTIC: NSAID. **CLINICAL:** Nonsteroidal anti-inflammatory, analgesic (see p. 127C).

ACTION

Produces analgesic, anti-inflammatory effects by inhibiting prostaglandin synthesis. **Therapeutic Effect:** Reduces inflammatory response, intensity of pain.

PHARMACOKINETICS

Route	Onset	Peak	Duration
PO (analgesic)	2–4 hrs	N/A	4–12 hrs

Completely absorbed from GI tract. Protein binding: greater than 99%. Widely distributed. Metabolized in liver. Primarily excreted in urine. Not removed by hemodialysis. **Half-life:** 6–7 hrs. **Extended-release:** 12 hrs.

USES

Acute and long-term treatment of osteoarthritis, management of pain, treatment of rheumatoid arthritis (RA), juvenile rheumatoid arthritis (JRA). OFF-LABEL: Treatment of acute gouty arthritis, vascular headache.

PRECAUTIONS

Contraindications: Active peptic ulcer disease, chronic inflammation of GI tract, GI bleeding/ulceration, history of hypersensitivity to aspirin, NSAIDs. **Cautions:** Renal/hepatic impairment, history of GI tract disease, predisposition to fluid retention.

⌛ LIFESPAN CONSIDERATIONS

Pregnancy/Lactation: Unknown if drug crosses placenta or is distributed in breast milk. Avoid use during third trimester (may adversely affect fetal cardiovascular system: premature closure of ductus arteriosus). **Pregnancy Category C (D if used in third trimester or near delivery). Children:** Safety and efficacy not established. **Elderly:** GI bleeding, ulceration more likely to cause serious adverse effects. Age-related renal impairment may increase risk of hepatic/renal toxicity; decreased dosage recommended.

INTERACTIONS

DRUG: May decrease effects of **antihypertensives, diuretics. Aspirin, other salicylates** may increase risk of GI side effects, bleeding. May increase concentration/toxicity of **cyclosporine. Bone marrow depressants** may increase risk of hematologic reactions. May increase effects of **heparin, oral anticoagulants, thrombolytics.** May increase concentration, risk of toxicity of **lithium.** May increase risk of **methotrexate** toxicity. **Probenecid** may increase concentration. HERBAL: **Cat's claw, dong quai, evening primrose, feverfew, garlic, ginger, ginkgo, ginseng** may increase antiplatelet action, risk of bleeding. FOOD: None known. LAB VALUES: May increase bleeding time, hepatic function test results, serum creatinine. May decrease serum uric acid.

AVAILABILITY (Rx)

Tablets (Lodine): 400 mg, 500 mg.

Capsules (Lodine): 200 mg, 300 mg.
Tablets (Extended-Release [Lodine XL]): 400 mg, 500 mg, 600 mg.

ADMINISTRATION/HANDLING

PO

• Do not crush, break, or chew capsules, extended-release tablets. • May give with food, milk, antacids if GI distress occurs.

INDICATIONS/ROUTES/DOSAGE

Osteoarthritis, Rheumatoid Arthritis (RA)

PO (IMMEDIATE-RELEASE): ADULTS, ELDERLY: Initially, 300 mg 2–3 times a day or 400 mg twice a day. Maintenance: 600–1,000 mg/day in 2–4 divided doses.
PO (EXTENDED-RELEASE): ADULTS, ELDERLY: 400–1,000 mg once daily.

Juvenile Rheumatoid Arthritis (JRA)

PO (EXTENDED-RELEASE): CHILDREN 6–16 YRS: 1,000 mg in children weighing more than 60 kg, 800 mg once daily in children weighing 46–60 kg, 600 mg once daily in children weighing 31–45 kg, 400 mg once daily in children weighing 20–30 kg.

Analgesia

PO: ADULTS, ELDERLY: 200–400 mg q6–8h as needed. **Maximum:** 1,000 mg/day.

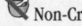

SIDE EFFECTS

Occasional (9%–4%): Dizziness, headache, abdominal pain/cramping, bloated feeling, diarrhea, nausea, indigestion. **Rare** (3%–1%): Constipation, rash, pruritus, visual disturbances, tinnitus.

E

ADVERSE EFFECTS/ TOXIC REACTIONS

Overdose may result in acute renal failure. Increased risk of cardiovascular events (MI, CVA) and serious, potentially life-threatening GI bleeding. Rare reactions with long-term use include peptic ulcer, gastritis, jaundice, nephrotoxicity (hematuria, dysuria, proteinuria), severe hypersensitivity reaction (bronchospasm, angioedema).

NURSING CONSIDERATIONS

BASELINE ASSESSMENT

Assess onset, type, location, duration of pain/inflammation. Inspect appearance of affected joints for immobility, deformities, skin condition.

INTERVENTION/EVALUATION

Monitor CBC, hepatic/renal function tests. Observe for bleeding/ecchymosis. Evaluate for therapeutic response: relief of pain, stiffness, swelling; increased joint mobility; reduced joint tenderness; improved grip strength.

PATIENT/FAMILY TEACHING

• Swallow capsule whole; do not crush, break, or chew. • Avoid aspirin, alcohol during therapy (increases risk of GI bleeding). • Report GI distress, visual disturbances, rash, edema, headache. • Report any signs of bleeding. • Take with food, milk, antacid if GI distress occurs. • Avoid tasks that require alertness, motor skills until response to drug is established.

etoposide, VP-16 HIGH ALERT

eh-**toe**-poe-side
(Etopophos, Toposar, VePesid)

BLACK BOX ALERT Severe myelosuppression with resulting infection, bleeding may occur. Must be administered by personnel trained in administration/handling of chemotherapeutic agents.

Do not confuse VePesid with Pepcid or Versed, or etoposide with teniposide.

◆CLASSIFICATION

PHARMACOTHERAPEUTIC: Epipodophyllotoxin. **CLINICAL:** Antineoplastic (see p. 82C).

ACTION

Induces single- and double-stranded breaks in DNA. Cell cycle-dependent and phase-specific; most effective in S and G_2 phases of cell division. **Therapeutic Effect:** Inhibits, alters DNA synthesis.

PHARMACOKINETICS

Variably absorbed from GI tract. Rapidly distributed, low concentrations in CSF. Protein binding: 97%. Metabolized in liver. Primarily excreted in urine. Not removed by hemodialysis. **Half-life:** 3–12 hrs.

USES

Treatment of refractory testicular tumors, small-cell lung carcinoma. **OFF-LABEL:** Acute lymphocytic, acute nonlymphocytic leukemias; Ewing's and Kaposi's sarcoma; Hodgkin's and non-Hodgkin's lymphomas; endometrial, gastric, non–small-cell lung carcinomas; multiple myeloma; myelodysplastic syndromes; neuroblastoma; osteosarcoma; ovarian germ cell tumors; primary brain, gestational trophoblastic tumors; soft tissue sarcomas; Wilms tumor.

PRECAUTIONS

Contraindications: Pregnancy. **Cautions:** Hepatic/renal impairment, myelosuppression.

⌛ LIFESPAN CONSIDERATIONS

Pregnancy/Lactation: If possible, avoid use during pregnancy, esp. first trimester. May cause fetal harm. Breast-feeding not recommended. **Pregnancy Category D. Children:** Safety and efficacy not established. **Elderly:** Age-related renal impairment may require dosage adjustment.

INTERACTIONS

DRUG: **Bone marrow depressants** may increase myelosuppression. **Live-virus vaccines** may potentiate virus replication, increase vaccine side effects, decrease pt's antibody response to vaccine. HERBAL: **St. John's wort** may decrease concentration. FOOD: None known. LAB VALUES: None significant.

AVAILABILITY (Rx)

Capsules (VePesid): 50 mg. Injection, Powder for Renconstitution (Water-Soluble [Etopophos]): 100 mg. Injection Solution (Toposar): 20 mg/ml (5 ml, 25 ml, 50 ml).

ADMINISTRATION/HANDLING

◀ALERT▶ Administer by slow IV infusion. Wear gloves when preparing solution. If powder or solution comes in contact with skin, wash immediately and thoroughly with soap, water. May be carcinogenic, mutagenic, teratogenic. Handle with extreme care during preparation, administration.

IV

Reconstitution

VEPESID • Dilute each 100 mg (5 ml) with at least 250 ml D_5W or 0.9% NaCl to provide concentration of 0.4 mg/ml (500 ml for concentration of 0.2 mg/ml).

ETOPOPHOS • Reconstitute each 100 mg with 5–10 ml Sterile Water for Injection, D_5W, or 0.9% NaCl to provide concentration of 20 mg/ml or 10 mg/ml, respectively. • May give without further dilution or further dilute to concentration as low as 0.1 mg/ml with 0.9% NaCl or D_5W.

Rate of administration

VEPESID • Infuse slowly, at least 60 min (rapid IV may produce marked hypotension) at a rate not to exceed 100 mg/m^2/hr. • Monitor for anaphylactic reaction during infusion (chills, fever, dyspnea, diaphoresis, lacrimation, sneezing, throat, back, chest pain).

ETOPOPHOS • May give over as little as 5 min up to 210 min.

Storage

VEPESID • Store injection at room temperature before dilution. • Concentrate for injection is clear, yellow. • Diluted solution is stable at room temperature for 96 hrs at 0.2 mg/ml, 24 hrs at 0.4 mg/ml. • Discard if crystallization occurs.

ETOPOPHOS • Refrigerate vials. • Stable for 24 hrs after reconstitution.

PO

Storage • Refrigerate gelatin capsules.

IV INCOMPATIBILITIES

VePesid: Cefepime (Maxipime), filgrastim (Neupogen), idarubicin (Idamycin). **Etopophos:** Amphotericin B (Fungizone), cefepime (Maxipime), chlorpromazine (Thorazine), methylprednisolone (Solu-Medrol), prochlorperazine (Compazine).

IV COMPATIBILITIES

VePesid: Carboplatin (Paraplatin), cisplatin (Platinol), cytarabine (Cytosar), daunorubicin (Cerubidine), doxorubicin (Adriamycin), granisetron (Kytril), mitoxantrone (Novantrone), ondansetron (Zofran). **Etopophos:** Carboplatin (Paraplatin), cisplatin (Platinol), cytarabine (Cytosar), dacarbazine (DTIC-Dome), daunorubicin (Cerubidine), dexamethasone (Decadron), diphenhydramine (Benadryl), doxorubicin (Adriamycin), granisetron (Kytril), magnesium sulfate, mannitol, mitoxantrone (Novantrone), ondansetron (Zofran), potassium chloride.

INDICATIONS/ROUTES/DOSAGE

◀ALERT▶ Dosage individualized based on clinical response, tolerance to adverse effects. Treatment repeated at 3- to 4-wk intervals. Refer to individual protocols.

Refractory Testicular Tumors

IV: ADULTS: 50–100 mg/m^2/day on days 1–5, or 100 mg/m^2/day on days 1, 3, 5 (as combination therapy). Give q3–4wk for 3–4 courses.

Acute Myelocytic Leukemia
IV: CHILDREN: 150 mg/m²/day for 2–3 days and 2–3 cycles.

E

Brain Tumor
IV: CHILDREN: 150 mg/m²/day on days 2 and 3 of treatment course.

Neuroblastoma
IV: CHILDREN: 100 mg/m²/day on days 1–5 of treatment course; repeated q4wk.

Small-Cell Lung Carcinoma
PO: ADULTS: Twice the IV dose rounded to nearest 50 mg. Give once a day for doses 400 mg or less, in divided doses for dosages greater than 400 mg.
IV: ADULTS: 35 mg/m²/day for 4 consecutive days up to 50 mg/m²/day for 5 consecutive days (as combination therapy).

Usual Pediatric Dosage
IV: CHILDREN: 60–120 mg/m²/day for 3–5 days q3–6wk.

Dosage in Renal Impairment

Creatinine Clearance	Dosage
10–50 ml/min	75% of normal dose
Less than 10 ml/min	50% of normal dose

SIDE EFFECTS

Frequent (66%–43%): Mild to moderate nausea/vomiting, alopecia. **Occasional (13%–6%):** Diarrhea, anorexia, stomatitis. **Rare (2% or less):** Hypotension, peripheral neuropathy.

ADVERSE EFFECTS/ TOXIC REACTIONS

Myelosuppression manifested as hematologic toxicity, principally anemia, leukopenia (occurring 7–14 days after drug administration), thrombocytopenia (occurring 9–16 days after administration) and, to lesser extent, pancytopenia. Bone marrow recovery occurs by day 20. Hepatotoxicity occurs occasionally.

NURSING CONSIDERATIONS

BASELINE ASSESSMENT

Obtain hematologic tests before and at frequent intervals during therapy. Antiemetics readily control nausea, vomiting.

INTERVENTION/EVALUATION

Monitor Hgb, Hct, WBC, platelet count, B/P, hepatic/renal function tests. Monitor daily pattern of bowel activity and stool consistency. Monitor for hematologic toxicity (fever, sore throat, signs of local infection, unusual bruising/bleeding from any site), symptoms of anemia (excessive fatigue, weakness). Assess for paresthesias (peripheral neuropathy). Monitor for stomatitis.

PATIENT/FAMILY TEACHING

• Alopecia is reversible, but new hair growth may have different color, texture. • Do not have immunizations without physician's approval (drug lowers resistance). • Avoid contact with those who have recently received live virus vaccine. • Promptly report fever, sore throat, signs of local infection, unusual bruising or bleeding from any site, burning or pain with urination, numbness in extremities, yellowing of skin, whites of eyes.

etravirine

et-ra-**vir**-een
(Intelence)

◆CLASSIFICATION

PHARMACOTHERAPEUTIC: Nonnucleoside reverse transcriptase inhibitor. **CLINICAL:** Antiretroviral.

ACTION

Binds directly to human immunodeficiency virus type 1 (HIV-1) reverse transcriptase, changing shape of enzyme, blocking RNA-, DNA-dependent DNA polymerase activity. **Therapeutic Effect:** Interferes with HIV replication, slowing progression of HIV infection.

PHARMACOKINETICS

Well absorbed following PO administration if given following a meal. Protein binding: 99.6%. Metabolized in liver. Eliminated in feces and urine. **Half-life:** 41 hrs.

USES

Used in combination with other antiretroviral agents for treatment of HIV-1 infection in antiretroviral treatment-experienced adult pts who have evidence of viral replication and HIV-1 strains resistant to other antiretroviral drugs. Traditional approval for treatment of HIV-1 in combination with other antiretrovirals.

PRECAUTIONS

Contraindications: None known. **Cautions:** Severe hepatic impairment, renal impairment, elderly.

LIFESPAN CONSIDERATIONS

Pregnancy/Lactation: Unknown if distributed in breast milk. **Pregnancy Category B. Children:** Safety and efficacy not established. **Elderly:** Age-related hepatic, renal, cardiac impairment may require dosage adjustment.

INTERACTIONS

DRUG: May decrease concentration of **antiarrhythmics, clarithromycin, indinavir, ketoconazole, oral contraceptives, protease inhibitors, saquinavir.** Increases **diazepam, nelfinavir, ritonavir, warfarin** concentration. **Rifabutin, rifampin** may decrease etravirine concentration. Alters **warfarin** plasma concentrations. **HERBAL:** **Gotu kola, kava kava, St. John's wort, valerian** may increase CNS depressant effects. **FOOD:** None known. **LAB VALUES:** May increase amylase, cholesterol, lipase, creatinine, triglycerides, glucose, ALT, AST. May decrease Hgb, neutrophil, platelet count.

AVAILABILITY (Rx)

Tablets: 100 mg, 200 mg.

ADMINISTRATION/HANDLING

PO

• Give following a meal. • Tablets may be dissolved in water. • Stir dispersion well and instruct pt to swallow immediately after dispersion. • Glass should be rinsed several times with water and each rinse swallowed to ensure entire dose is consumed.

INDICATIONS/ROUTES/DOSAGE

HIV-1 Infection

PO: ADULTS: 200 mg (one 200 mg or two 100-mg tablets) twice daily following a meal.

SIDE EFFECTS

Occasional (17%–16%): Rash (mild to moderate, occurring primarily during wk 2 of therapy and infrequently after wk 4), nausea. **Rare (6%–3%):** Diarrhea, fatigue, abdominal pain, hypertension, peripheral neuropathy, headache.

ADVERSE EFFECTS/ TOXIC REACTIONS

Severe/life-threatening rash presenting as Stevens-Johnson syndrome, hypersensitivity reaction, erythema multiforme occurs rarely.

NURSING CONSIDERATIONS

BASELINE ASSESSMENT

Obtain baseline lab tests before beginning therapy and at periodic intervals thereafter. Offer emotional support to pt and family.

INTERVENTION/EVALUATION

Closely monitor for evidence of rash (usually appears on trunk, face, extremities during second wk of drug initiation). Rash generally resolves within 1–2 wks on continued therapy.

PATIENT/FAMILY TEACHING

• Do not take any medications, including OTC drugs, without consulting physician.

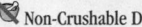

• Small, frequent meals may offset anorexia, nausea. • Etravirine is not a cure for HIV infection, nor does it reduce risk of transmission to others. • If rash appears, contact physician before continuing therapy.

E

everolimus

eh-**vear**-oh-lee-mus
(Afinitor, Zortress)
Do not confuse everolimus with sirolimus, tacrolimus, or temsirolimus, or Afinitor with Lipitor.

◆CLASSIFICATION

PHARMACOTHERAPEUTIC: Enzyme inhibitor. **CLINICAL:** Antineoplastic, immunosuppressant.

ACTION

Prevents activation of rapamycin (MTOR) kinase activity. **Therapeutic Effect:** Reduces cell proliferation, produces cell death.

PHARMACOKINETICS

Peak concentration occurs in 1–2 hrs following administration, with steady-state levels achieved in 2 wks. Undergoes extensive hepatic metabolism. Protein binding: 74%. Eliminated primarily in feces, with lesser amount excreted in urine. **Half-life:** 30 hrs.

USES

Afinitor: Treatment of advanced renal cell carcinoma after failure of treatment with sunitinib or sorafenib. Treatment of subependymal giant cell astrocytoma (SEGA) associated with tuberous sclerosis. **Zortress:** Prophylaxis of organ rejection after kidney transplant.

PRECAUTIONS

Contraindications: None significant. **Cautions:** Noninfectious pneumonitis; viral, fungal or bacterial infection; oral ulceration, mucositis, current immunosuppression.

LIFESPAN CONSIDERATIONS

Pregnancy/Lactation: May cause fetal harm. Unknown if distributed in breast milk. **Pregnancy Category D. Children:** Safety and efficacy not established. **Elderly:** No age-related precautions noted.

INTERACTIONS

DRUG: CYP3A4 inhibitors: Atazanavir, clarithromycin, indinavir, itraconazole, ketoconazole, nefazodone, nelfinavir, ritonavir, saquinavir, voriconazole may increase everolimus concentration. **CYP3A4 inducers: Carbamazepine, dexamethasone, phenobarbital, phenytoin, rifabutin, rifampin, rifapentine** may decrease everolimus concentration. **P-gp inhibitors: cyclosporine** may increase everolimus concentrations. **FOOD: High-fat meal** reduces plasma concentration. **Grapefruit juice, grapefruit** may increase concentration. **HERBAL: St. John's wort** may decrease plasma concentration. **LAB VALUES:** May increase BUN, serum creatinine, glucose, triglycerides, lipids. May decrease WBCs, neutrophils, Hgb, platelets.

AVAILABILITY (Rx)

Tablets (Zortress): 0.25 mg, 0.5 mg, 0.75 mg. **Tablets (Afinitor):** 2.5 mg, 5 mg, 10 mg.

ADMINISTRATION/HANDLING

• Give without regard to food. • Do not crush/chew Afinitor or Zortress. • Avoid direct contact of crushed tablets with skin or mucous membranes.

INDICATIONS/ROUTES/DOSAGE

◀ALERT▶ If pt requires co-administration of a strong CYP3A4 inducer (carbamazepine, dexamethasone, phenobarbital, phenytoin, rifabutin, rifampin), consider doubling the dose. If strong inducer is discontinued, reduce everolimus to dose used prior to initiation. If moderate CYP3A4 inhibitors are required, reduce dose by 50%.

Renal Carcinoma

PO: ADULTS, ELDERLY: (Afinitor): 10 mg once daily at same time every day. Co-administration with CYP3A4 inhibitors or P-gp inhibitors: 2.5 mg once daily. May increase to 5 mg/day. Co-administration with CYP3A4 inducers: Increase by 5-mg increments up to 20 mg/day.

Transplant Prophylaxis

PO: ADULTS, ELDERLY: (Zortress): Initially, 0.75 mg 2 times/day. Give in combination with basiliximab and concurrent with reduced doses of cyclosporine and corticosteroids.

Astrocytoma

PO: ADULTS, ELDERLY: Initial dose based on body surface area, titrated to attain trough concentration of 5–10 ng/ml.

Moderate Hepatic Impairment

50% normal dose at same time every day.

SIDE EFFECTS

Common (44%–26%): Stomatitis, asthenia (weakness, fatigue), diarrhea, cough, rash, nausea. **Frequent (25%–20%):** Peripheral edema, anorexia, dyspnea, vomiting, pyrexia. **Occasional (19%–10%):** Mucosal inflammation, headache, epistaxis, pruritus, dry skin, epigastric distress, extremity pain. **Rare (less than 10%):** Abdominal pain, insomnia, dry mouth, dizziness, paresthesia, eyelid edema, hypertension, nail disorder, chills.

ADVERSE EFFECTS/ TOXIC REACTIONS

Noninfectious pneumonitis characterized as hypoxia, pleural effusion, cough, or dyspnea was reported in 14% of pts; grade 3 noninfectious pneumonitis reported in 4%. Localized and systemic infections, including pneumonia, other bacterial infections, and invasive fungal infections, have occurred due to everolimus immunosuppressive properties. Renal failure occurs in 3% of pts.

NURSING CONSIDERATIONS

BASELINE ASSESSMENT

Assess medical history, esp. renal function, use of other immunosuppressants. Obtain baseline CBC, serum chemistries including hepatic function tests (bilirubin, AST, alkaline phosphatase), BUN, creatinine before treatment begins and routinely thereafter.

INTERVENTION/EVALUATION

Offer antiemetics to control nausea, vomiting. Monitor daily pattern of bowel activity and stool consistency. Assess skin for evidence of rash, edema. Monitor CBC, particularly Hgb, platelet, neutrophil count, BUN, creatinine, hepatic function tests (AST, ALT, total bilirubin). Monitor for shortness of breath, fatigue, hypertension. Assess mouth for stomatitis, mucositis.

PATIENT/FAMILY TEACHING

• Take dose at same time each day. • Avoid crowds, those with known infection. • Avoid contact with anyone who recently received live virus vaccine. • Do not have immunizations without physician's approval (drug lowers body resistance). • Promptly report fever, unusual bruising/bleeding from any site. • Swallow tablet whole. Do not crush, avoid direct contact of crushed tablets with skin or mucus membrane (wash thoroughly if contact occurs). • Do not drink grapefruit juice or eat grapefruit.

Evista, *see raloxifene*

Exelon, *see rivastigmine*

exemestane HIGH ALERT

x-eh-**mess**-tane
(Aromasin)

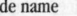

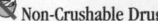

Do not confuse Aromasin with Arimidex, or exemestane with estramustine.

◆CLASSIFICATION

PHARMACOTHERAPEUTIC: Hormone. **CLINICAL:** Antineoplastic (see p. 83C).

E

ACTION

Inactivates aromatase, the principal enzyme that converts androgens to estrogens in both premenopausal and postmenopausal women, lowering circulating estrogen level. **Therapeutic Effect:** Inhibits growth of breast cancers stimulated by estrogens.

PHARMACOKINETICS

Rapidly absorbed after PO administration. Protein binding: 90%. Distributed extensively into tissues. Metabolized in liver; eliminated in urine and feces. **Half-life:** 24 hrs.

USES

Treatment of advanced breast cancer in postmenopausal women whose disease has progressed following tamoxifen therapy. Adjuvant treatment of postmenopausal women with estrogen-receptor positive early breast cancer after 2–3 yrs of tamoxifen therapy for completion of 5 consecutive yrs of adjuvant hormonal therapy. **OFF-LABEL:** Prevention of prostate cancer.

PRECAUTIONS

Contraindications: Pregnancy. **Cautions:** Do not give to premenopausal women.

⌛ LIFESPAN CONSIDERATIONS

Pregnancy/Lactation: Indicated for postmenopausal women. **Pregnancy Category D. Children:** Not indicated for use in this pt population. **Elderly:** No age-related precautions noted.

INTERACTIONS

DRUG: **Estrogens** may interfere with action. **HERBAL:** **St. John's wort** may decrease concentration. Avoid **black cohosh, dong quai** in estrogen-dependent tumors. **FOOD:** None known. **LAB VALUES:** May increase serum alkaline phosphatase, AST, ALT.

AVAILABILITY (Rx)

Tablets: 25 mg.

ADMINISTRATION/HANDLING

PO

- Give after meals.

INDICATIONS/ROUTES/DOSAGE

Breast Cancer

PO: ADULTS, ELDERLY: 25 mg once a day after a meal. 50 mg/day when used concurrently with potent CYP3A4 inducers (e.g., rifampin, phenytoin).

SIDE EFFECTS

Frequent (22%–10%): Fatigue, nausea, depression, hot flashes, pain, insomnia, anxiety, dyspnea. **Occasional (8%–5%):** Headache, dizziness, vomiting, peripheral edema, abdominal pain, anorexia, flu-like symptoms, diaphoresis, constipation, hypertension. **Rare (4%):** Diarrhea.

ADVERSE EFFECTS/ TOXIC REACTIONS

MI has been noted.

NURSING CONSIDERATIONS

INTERVENTION/EVALUATION

Monitor for onset of depression. Assess sleep pattern. Monitor for and assist with ambulation if dizziness occurs. Assess for headache. Offer antiemetic for nausea/vomiting.

PATIENT/FAMILY TEACHING

• Notify physician if nausea, hot flashes become unmanageable. • Avoid tasks that require alertness, motor skills until response to drug is established. • Best taken after meals and at same time each day.

exenatide

HIGH ALERT

ex-**en**-ah-tide
(Byetta)

◆CLASSIFICATION

PHARMACOTHERAPEUTIC: Incretin mimetic. **CLINICAL:** Antidiabetic.

ACTION

Stimulates release of insulin from beta cells of pancreas, mimics enhancement of glucose-dependent insulin secretion, suppresses elevated glucagon secretion, slows gastric emptying (central action increases satiety). **Therapeutic Effect:** Improves glycemic control by increasing postmeal insulin secretion, decreasing postmeal glucagon levels, delaying gastric emptying, and increasing satiety.

PHARMACOKINETICS

Minimal systemic metabolism. Eliminated by glomerular filtration with subsequent proteolytic degradation. **Half-life:** 2.4 hrs.

USES

Adjunct to diet, exercise to improve glycemic control in pts with type 2 diabetes mellitus who are taking metformin (Glucophage) and a sulfonylurea (e.g., glyburide) or metformin and a thiazolidinedione (e.g., pioglitazone).

PRECAUTIONS

Contraindications: Diabetic ketoacidosis, type 1 diabetes mellitus. Not recommended in severe renal impairment, severe GI disease. **Cautions:** Mild-to-moderate renal impairment.

LIFESPAN CONSIDERATIONS

Pregnancy/Lactation: Unknown if distributed in breast milk. **Pregnancy Category C. Children:** Safety and efficacy not established. **Elderly:** No age-related precautions noted.

INTERACTIONS

DRUG: None significant. **HERBAL:** None significant. **FOOD:** None known. **LAB VALUES:** None significant.

AVAILABILITY (Rx)

Injection, Solution: (Prefilled Pen): 250 mcg/ml (1.2 ml provides 5 mcg/dose; 2.4 ml provides 10 mcg/dose).

ADMINISTRATION/HANDLING

Subcutaneous

• May be given in thigh, abdomen, upper arm. • Rotation of injection sites is essential; maintain careful injection site record. • Give within 60 min before morning and evening meals.

Storage • Refrigerate prefilled pens. • Discard if freezing occurs. • May be stored at room temperature after first use. • Discard pen 30 days after initial use.

INDICATIONS/ROUTE/DOSAGE

Diabetes Mellitus

SUBCUTANEOUS: ADULTS, ELDERLY: 5 mcg per dose given twice a day at any time within the 60-min period before the morning and evening meals. Dose may be increased to 10 mcg twice a day after 1 mo of therapy.

◀ALERT▶ Not recommended in pts with creatinine clearance less than 30 ml/min.

SIDE EFFECTS

Frequent (44%): Nausea. **Occasional (13%–6%):** Diarrhea, vomiting, dizziness, anxiety, dyspepsia. **Rare (less than 6%):** Weakness.

ADVERSE EFFECTS/ TOXIC REACTIONS

With concurrent sulfonylurea, hypoglycemia occurs in 36% when given a 10-mcg dose of exenatide, 16% when given a 5-mcg dose. May cause acute pancreatitis.

NURSING CONSIDERATIONS

BASELINE ASSESSMENT

Check serum glucose before administration. Discuss lifestyle to determine extent of learning, emotional needs. Assure follow-up instruction if pt or family does not thoroughly understand diabetes management, glucose-testing technique. At least 1 mo should elapse to assess response to drug before new dose adjustment is made.

E

INTERVENTION/EVALUATION

Monitor serum glucose, food intake, renal function. Assess for hypoglycemia (cool wet skin, tremors, dizziness, anxiety, headache, tachycardia, numbness in mouth, hunger, diplopia), hyperglycemia (polyuria, polyphagia, polydipsia, nausea, vomiting, dim vision, fatigue, deep rapid breathing). Be alert to conditions that alter glucose requirements (fever, increased activity or stress, surgical procedure).

PATIENT/FAMILY TEACHING

• Diabetes mellitus requires lifelong control. • Prescribed diet and exercise are principal parts of treatment. Do not skip, delay meals. • Continue to adhere to dietary instructions, regular exercise program, regular testing of serum glucose. • When taking combination therapy with a sulfonylurea, have source of glucose available to treat symptoms of hypoglycemia. • Report any unexplained severe abdominal pain with or without nausea and vomiting.

Exforge, *see amlodipine and valsartan*

ezetimibe

eh-**zeh**-tih-myb
(Ezetrol ✦, Zetia)
Do not confuse Zetia with Zebeta or Zestril.

FIXED-COMBINATION(S)

Vytorin: ezetimibe/simvastatin (hydroxymethylglutaryl-CoA [HMG-CoA] reductase inhibitor): 10 mg/10 mg, 10 mg/20 mg, 10 mg/40 mg, 10 mg/80 mg.

◆ CLASSIFICATION

PHARMACOTHERAPEUTIC: Antihyperlipidemic. **CLINICAL:** Anticholesterol agent.

ACTION

Inhibits cholesterol absorption in small intestine, leading to decrease in delivery of intestinal cholesterol to liver. **Therapeutic Effect:** Reduces total serum cholesterol, LDL, triglyceride; increases HDL.

PHARMACOKINETICS

Well absorbed following PO administration. Protein binding: greater than 90%. Metabolized in small intestine and liver. Excreted by kidneys and bile. **Half-life:** 22 hrs.

USES

Adjunct to diet for treatment of primary hypercholesterolemia (monotherapy or in combination with HMG-CoA reductase inhibitors [statins] or fenofibrate), homozygous sitosterolemia, homozygous familial hypercholesterolemia (combined with atrovastatin or simvastatin).

PRECAUTIONS

Contraindications: Concurrent use of an HMG-CoA reductase inhibitor (atorvastatin, fluvastatin, lovastatin, pravastatin, simvastatin) in pts with active hepatic disease or unexplained persistent elevations in serum transaminase; moderate or severe hepatic insufficiency. **Cautions:** Diabetes, hypothyroidism, obstructive hepatic disease, chronic renal failure, hepatic impairment.

⌛ LIFESPAN CONSIDERATIONS

Pregnancy/Lactation: Unknown if drug crosses placenta or is distributed in breast milk. **Pregnancy Category C. Children:** Safety and efficacy not established in those 10 yrs or younger. **Elderly:** Age-related mild hepatic impairment may require dosage adjustment. Not recommended in those with moderate or severe hepatic impairment.

INTERACTIONS

DRUG: **Antacids containing aluminum or magnesium, cyclosporine, fenofibrate, gemfibrozil** increase plasma concentration. **Cholestyramine resin** decreases drug effectiveness. **HERBAL:** None significant. **FOOD:** None known. **LAB VALUES:** May increase serum alkaline phosphatase, bilirubin, AST, ALT.

AVAILABILITY (Rx)

Tablets: 10 mg.

ADMINISTRATION/HANDLING

• Give without regard to food. • May give at same time as statins. Give at least 2 hrs before or 4 hrs after cholestyramine, colestipol, colesevelam.

INDICATIONS/ROUTES/DOSAGE

Hypercholesterolemia

PO: ADULTS, ELDERLY, CHILDREN, 10 YRS AND OLDER: Initially, 10 mg once a day, given with or without food. If pt is also receiving a bile acid sequestrant, give ezetimibe at least 2 hrs before or at least 4 hrs after bile acid sequestrant.

Sitosterolemia

PO: ADULTS, ELDERLY: 10 mg/day.

SIDE EFFECTS

Occasional (4%–3%): Back pain, diarrhea, arthralgia, sinusitis, abdominal pain. **Rare (2%):** Cough, pharyngitis, fatigue, depression.

ADVERSE EFFECTS/ TOXIC REACTIONS

Hepatitis, hypersensitivity reaction, myopathy, rhabdomyolysis occur rarely.

NURSING CONSIDERATIONS

BASELINE ASSESSMENT

Obtain diet history, esp. fat consumption. Obtain serum cholesterol, triglycerides, hepatic function tests, blood counts during initial therapy and periodically during treatment. Treatment should be discontinued if hepatic enzyme levels persist more than 3 times normal limit.

INTERVENTION/EVALUATION

Monitor daily pattern of bowel activity and stool consistency. Question pt for signs/symptoms of back pain, abdominal disturbances. Monitor serum cholesterol, triglycerides for therapeutic response.

PATIENT/FAMILY TEACHING

• Periodic laboratory tests are essential part of therapy. • Do not stop medication without consulting physician. • Report muscular or bone pain. • May give at same time as statins. Give at least 2 hrs before or 4 hrs after cholestyramine, colestipol, colesevelam.

famciclovir

fam-**sih**-klo-veer
(Apo-Famciclovir ✤, Famvir)
Do not confuse Famvir with Femara.

CLASSIFICATION

PHARMACOTHERAPEUTIC: Synthetic nucleoside. **CLINICAL:** Antiviral (see p. 68C).

ACTION

Inhibits viral DNA synthesis. **Therapeutic Effect:** Suppresses replication of herpes simplex virus, varicella-zoster virus.

PHARMACOKINETICS

Rapidly, extensively absorbed after PO administration. Protein binding: 20%–25%. Rapidly metabolized to penciclovir by enzymes in GI tract, liver, plasma. Eliminated unchanged in urine. Removed by hemodialysis. **Half-life:** 2–3 hrs (increased in severe renal failure).

USES

Management of acute herpes zoster (shingles), treatment and suppression of recurrent genital herpes in immunocompetent pts, treatment of recurrent mucocutaneous herpes simplex in HIV-infected pts. Treatment of recurrent herpes labialis (cold sores).

F

PRECAUTIONS

Contraindications: Hypersensitivity to penciclovir cream. **Cautions:** Renal/hepatic impairment.

LIFESPAN CONSIDERATIONS

Pregnancy/Lactation: Increased mammary adenocarcinoma in animals. Unknown if excreted in breast milk. **Pregnancy Category B. Children:** Safety and efficacy not established. **Elderly:** Age-related renal impairment may require dosage adjustment.

INTERACTIONS

DRUG: **Probenecid** may increase concentration. **HERBAL:** None significant. **FOOD:** None known. **LAB VALUES:** May increase hepatic enzymes, bilirubin.

AVAILABILITY (Rx)

Tablets: 125 mg, 250 mg, 500 mg.

ADMINISTRATION/HANDLING

PO

• Give without regard to meals. • Give with food to decrease GI distress.

INDICATIONS/ROUTES/DOSAGE

Acute Herpes Zoster (Shingles)

PO: ADULTS: 500 mg q8h for 7 days. Begin within 72 hrs of rash onset.

Recurrent Genital Herpes

PO: ADULTS: 1,000 mg twice a day for 1 day.

Suppression of Recurrent Genital Herpes

PO: ADULTS: 250 mg twice a day for up to 1 yr.

Recurrent Herpes Simplex in HIV Pts

PO: ADULTS: 500 mg twice a day for 7 days.

Herpes Labialis (Cold Sores)

PO: ADULTS, ELDERLY: 1,500 mg as a single dose. Initiate at first sign or symptom.

Dosage in Renal Impairment

Dosage and frequency are modified based on creatinine clearance.

Dosage in Hemodialysis Pts

For adults with herpes zoster, give 250 mg after each dialysis treatment; for adults with genital herpes, give 125 mg after each dialysis treatment.

SIDE EFFECTS

Frequent: Headache (23%), nausea (12%). **Occasional (10%–2%):** Dizziness, drowsiness, paresthesia (esp. feet), diarrhea, vomiting, constipation, decreased appetite, fatigue, fever, pharyngitis, sinusitis, pruritus. **Rare (less than 2%):** Insomnia, abdominal pain, dyspepsia, flatulence, back pain, arthralgia.

ADVERSE EFFECTS/ TOXIC REACTIONS

Urticaria, hallucinations, confusion (delirium, disorientation occurs predominantly in elderly) have been reported.

Creatinine Clearance	Herpes Zoster	Recurrent Genital Herpes (single-day regimen)	Recurrent Genital Herpes (suppression)	Recurrent Herpes Labialis Treatment (single-day regimen)	Recurrent Orolabial or Genital Herpes in HIV Pts
40–59 ml/min	500 mg q12h	500 mg q12h	—	750 mg	—
20–39 ml/min	500 mg q24h	500 mg	125 mg q12h	500 mg	500 mg q24h
Less than 20 ml/min	250 mg q24h	250 mg	125 mg q24h	250 mg	250 mg q24h

NURSING CONSIDERATIONS

INTERVENTION/EVALUATION

Evaluate cutaneous lesions. Be alert to neurologic effects: headache, dizziness. Provide analgesics, comfort measures; esp. exhausting in elderly. Monitor renal function, hepatic enzymes, CBC.

PATIENT/FAMILY TEACHING

• Drink adequate fluids. • Fingernails should be kept short, hands clean. • Do not touch lesions with fingers to avoid spreading infection to new site. • **Genital herpes:** Continue therapy for full length of treatment. • Space doses evenly. • Avoid contact with lesions during duration of outbreak to prevent cross-contamination. • Notify physician if lesions recur or do not improve. • Change position slowly from sitting/lying to standing. • Avoid tasks that require alertness, motor skills until response to drug is established.

famotidine

fah-**mow**-tih-deen
(Apo-Famotidine ✱, Novo-Famotidine ✱, Pepcid, Pepcid AC, Pepcid AC Maximum Strength, Ulcidine ✱)

Do not confuse famotidine with fluoxetine or furosemide.

FIXED-COMBINATION(S)

Pepcid Complete: famotidine/calcium chloride/magnesium hydroxide (antacids): 10 mg/800 mg/165 mg.

◆CLASSIFICATION

PHARMACOTHERAPEUTIC: H_2 receptor antagonist. **CLINICAL:** Antiulcer, gastric acid secretion inhibitor (see p. 108C).

ACTION

Inhibits histamine action H_2 receptors of parietal cells. **Therapeutic Effect:** Inhibits gastric acid secretion (fasting, nocturnal, or stimulated by food, caffeine, insulin).

PHARMACOKINETICS

Route	Onset	Peak	Duration
PO	1 hr	1–4 hrs	10–12 hrs
IV	0.5 hr	0.5–3 hrs	10–12 hrs

Rapidly, incompletely absorbed from GI tract. Protein binding: 15%–20%. Partially metabolized in liver. Primarily excreted in urine. Not removed by hemodialysis. **Half-life:** 2.5–3.5 hrs (increased in renal impairment).

USES

Short-term treatment of active duodenal ulcer. Prevention, maintenance of duodenal ulcer recurrence. Treatment of active benign gastric ulcer, pathologic GI hypersecretory conditions. Short-term treatment of gastroesophageal reflux disease (GERD), including erosive esophagitis. OTC formulation for relief of heartburn, acid indigestion, sour stomach. **OFF-LABEL:** Autism, prophylaxis of aspiration pneumonitis, *H. pylori* eradication, stress ulcer prophylaxis in critically ill pts, relief of gastritis.

PRECAUTIONS

Contraindications: None known. **Cautions:** Renal/hepatic impairment.

⌛ LIFESPAN CONSIDERATIONS

Pregnancy/Lactation: Unknown if drug crosses placenta or is distributed in breast milk. **Pregnancy Category B. Children:** No age-related precautions noted. **Elderly:** Confusion more likely to occur, esp. in those with renal/hepatic impairment.

INTERACTIONS

DRUG: May decrease absorption of **itraconazole, ketoconazole. HERBAL:** None significant. **FOOD:** None known. **LAB VALUES:** Interferes with skin tests using allergen extracts. May increase serum alkaline phosphatase, AST, ALT.

AVAILABILITY (Rx)

Infusion, premix: 20 mg in 50 ml 0.9% NaCl. **Injection, Solution: (Pepcid):** 10 mg/ml. **Powder for Oral Suspension: (Pepcid):** 40 mg/5 ml. **Tablets: (Pepcid AC):** 10 mg. **(Pepcid):** 20 mg, 40 mg. **Tablets, Chewable: (Pepcid AC Maximum Strength):** 20 mg.

F

ADMINISTRATION/HANDLING

IV

Reconstitution • For IV push, dilute 20 mg with 5–10 ml 0.9% NaCl. • For intermittent IV infusion (piggyback), dilute with 50–100 ml D_5W, or 0.9% NaCl.
Rate of administration • Give IV push over at least 2 min. • Infuse piggyback over 15–30 min.
Storage • Refrigerate unreconstituted vials. • IV solution appears clear, colorless. • After dilution, IV solution is stable for 48 hrs if refrigerated.

PO

• Store tablets, suspension at room temperature. • Following reconstitution, oral suspension is stable for 30 days at room temperature. • Give without regard to meals. • Shake suspension well before use.

IV INCOMPATIBILITIES

Amphotericin B complex (Abelcet, AmBisome, Amphotec), cefepime (Maxipime), ceftriaxone (Rocephin), furosemide (Lasix), piperacillin/tazobactam (Zosyn).

IV COMPATIBILITIES

Calcium gluconate, dexamethasone (Decadron), dobutamine (Dobutrex), dopamine (Intropin), doxorubicin (Adriamycin), furosemide (Lasix), haloperidol (Haldol), heparin, hydromorphone (Dilaudid), insulin (regular), lidocaine, lipids, lorazepam (Ativan), magnesium sulfate, meperidine (Demerol), midazolam (Versed), morphine, nitroglycerin, norepinephrine (Levophed), ondansetron (Zofran), potassium chloride, potassium phosphate, propofol (Diprivan), total parenteral nutrition (TPN).

INDICATIONS/ROUTES/DOSAGE

Duodenal, Gastric Ulcers

PO: ADULTS, ELDERLY, CHILDREN 12 YRS AND OLDER: 40 mg/day at bedtime for 4–8 wks. **CHILDREN 1–11 YRS:** 0.5 mg/kg/day at bedtime. **Maximum:** 40 mg/day.

Duodenal Ulcer, Prevention and Maintenance

PO: ADULTS, ELDERLY: 20 mg/day at bedtime.

Gastroesophageal Reflux Disease (GERD)

PO: ADULTS, ELDERLY, CHILDREN 12 YRS AND OLDER: 20 mg twice a day for 6 wks. **CHILDREN 1–11 YRS:** 1 mg/kg/day in 2 divided doses. **CHILDREN 3 MOS–11 MOS:** 0.5 mg/kg/dose twice a day. **CHILDREN YOUNGER THAN 3 MOS:** 0.5 mg/kg/dose once a day.

Esophagitis

PO: ADULTS, ELDERLY, CHILDREN 12 YRS AND OLDER: 20–40 mg twice a day for up to 12 wks.

Hypersecretory Conditions

PO: ADULTS, ELDERLY, CHILDREN 12 YRS AND OLDER: Initially, 20 mg q6h. May increase up to 160 mg q6h.

Acid Indigestion, Heartburn (OTC Use)

PO: ADULTS, ELDERLY, CHILDREN 12 YRS AND OLDER: 10–20 mg 15–60 min before eating. **Maximum:** 2 doses per day.

Usual Parenteral Dosage

IV: ADULTS, ELDERLY, CHILDREN OLDER THAN 12 YRS: 20 mg q12h. **CHILDREN 1–12 YRS:** 0.25–0.5 mg/kg q12h. **Maximum:** 40 mg/day.

Dosage in Renal Impairment

Creatinine Clearance	Dosage
10–50 ml/min	Normal dose q24h or 50% of dose at normal dosing interval
Less than 10 ml/min	Normal dose q36–48h

SIDE EFFECTS

Occasional (5%): Headache. **Rare (2% or less):** Confusion, constipation, diarrhea, dizziness.

ADVERSE EFFECTS/ TOXIC REACTIONS

Agranulocytosis, pancytopenia, thrombocytopenia occur rarely.

NURSING CONSIDERATIONS

BASELINE ASSESSMENT

Assess epigastric/abdominal pain.

INTERVENTION/EVALUATION

Monitor daily pattern of bowel activity and stool consistency. Monitor for diarrhea, constipation, headache. Assess confusion in elderly.

PATIENT/FAMILY TEACHING

• May take without regard to meals, antacids. • Report headache. • Avoid excessive amounts of coffee, aspirin. • If symptoms of heartburn, acid indigestion, sour stomach persist with medication, consult physician.

Famvir, *see famciclovir*

Faslodex, *see fulvestrant*

febuxostat

feb-**ux**-oh-stat

(Uloric)

Do not confuse febuxostat with Femstat.

◆CLASSIFICATION

PHARMACOTHERAPEUTIC: Xanthine oxidase inhibitor. **CLINICAL:** Antigout.

ACTION

Decreases uric acid production by inhibiting the enzyme xanthine oxidase. **Therapeutic Effect:** Reduces uric acid concentrations in serum and urine.

PHARMACOKINETICS

Well absorbed from GI tract. Widely distributed. Protein binding: 99%. Metabolized in liver to active metabolite. Eliminated primarily in urine, with lesser amount excreted in feces. Removed by hemodialysis. **Half-life:** 5–8 hrs.

USES

Management of hyperuricemia in pts with gout. Not recommended for treatment of asymptomatic hyperuricemia.

PRECAUTIONS

Contraindications: Pts being treated with azathioprine, mercaptopurine, or theophylline. **Cautions:** Severe renal/hepatic impairment, history of heart disease or stroke.

LIFESPAN CONSIDERATIONS

Pregnancy/Lactation: Unknown if drug crosses placenta or is distributed in breast milk. **Pregnancy Category C. Children:** Safety and efficacy not established. **Elderly:** No age-related precautions noted.

INTERACTIONS

DRUG: May increase concentration, toxicity of **azathioprine, mercaptopurine, theophylline. HERBAL:** None significant. **FOOD:** None known. **LAB VALUES:** May increase AST, ALT, serum alkaline phosphatase, LDH, amylase, sodium, potassium, cholesterol, triglycerides, BUN, creatinine. May decrease platelet count, Hgb, Hct, neutrophil count. May prolong prothrombin time.

AVAILABILITY (Rx)

Tablets: 40 mg, 80 mg.

ADMINISTRATION/HANDLING

PO

• May give without regard to meals or antacids.

INDICATIONS/ROUTES/DOSAGE

Hyperuricemia

PO: ADULTS, ELDERLY: 40 mg once daily. If pt does not achieve serum uric acid level less than 6 mg/dl after 2 wks with 40 mg, may give 80 mg once daily.

SIDE EFFECTS

Rare (1%): Nausea, arthralgia, rash, dizziness.

F

ADVERSE EFFECTS/ TOXIC REACTIONS

Hepatic function abnormalities occur in 6% of pts.

NURSING CONSIDERATIONS

BASELINE ASSESSMENT

Assess baseline renal/hepatic function; concomitant medication (azathioprine, mercaptopurine, theophylline) contraindicated.

INTERVENTION/EVALUATION

Discontinue medication immediately if rash appears. Encourage high fluid intake (3,000 ml/day). Monitor I&O (output should be at least 2,000 ml/day). Monitor CBC, uric acid, serum hepatic function levels. Assess urine for cloudiness, unusual color, odor. Assess for therapeutic response (reduced joint tenderness, swelling, redness, limitation of motion).

PATIENT/FAMILY TEACHING

• Encourage drinking 8–10 glasses (8 oz) of fluid daily while taking medication. • Report rash, chest pain, shortness of breath, symptoms suggestive of stroke. • Gout attacks may occur for several months after starting treatment (medication is not a pain reliever). • Continue taking even if gout attack occurs.

felodipine

feh-**low**-dih-peen
(Plendil, Renedil)

Do not confuse Plendil with Isordil, Pletal, Prilosec, or Prinivil, or Renedil with Prinivil.

FIXED-COMBINATION(S)

Lexxel: felodipine/enalapril (ACE inhibitor): 2.5 mg/5 mg, 5 mg/5 mg.

CLASSIFICATION

PHARMACOTHERAPEUTIC: Calcium channel blocker. **CLINICAL:** Antihypertensive, antianginal (see p. 77C).

ACTION

Inhibits calcium movement across cardiac, vascular smooth muscle cell membranes (does not depress SA, AV nodes). Potent peripheral vasodilator. **Therapeutic Effect:** Increases myocardial contractility, heart rate, cardiac output; decreases peripheral vascular resistance, B/P.

PHARMACOKINETICS

Route	Onset	Peak	Duration
PO	2–5 hrs	N/A	24 hrs

Rapidly, completely absorbed from GI tract. Protein binding: greater than 99%. Undergoes first-pass metabolism in liver. Primarily excreted in urine. Not removed by hemodialysis. **Half-life:** 11–16 hrs.

USES

Management of hypertension. May be used alone or with other antihypertensives. **OFF-LABEL:** Pediatric hypertension.

PRECAUTIONS

Contraindications: None known. **Cautions:** Severe left ventricular dysfunction, CHF, hepatic/renal impairment, hypertrophic cardiomyopathy, edema, concomitant administration with beta-blockers/digoxin.

LIFESPAN CONSIDERATIONS

Pregnancy/Lactation: Unknown if drug crosses placenta or is distributed in breast milk. **Pregnancy Category C. Children:** Safety and efficacy not established.

Elderly: May experience greater hypotension response. Constipation may be more problematic.

INTERACTIONS

DRUG: **Beta-blockers** may have additive effect. May increase **digoxin** concentration. **Erythromycin** may increase concentration, risk of toxicity. **Agents producing hypokalemia (e.g., furosemide)** may increase risk of arrhythmias. **Procainamide, quinidine** may increase risk of QT-interval prolongation. **HERBAL:** **DHEA** may increase concentration. **St. John's wort** may decrease concentration. **Ephedra, ginseng, yohimbe** may worsen hypertension. **Garlic** may increase antihypertensive effect. **FOOD:** **Grapefruit, grapefruit juice** may increase absorption, concentration. **LAB VALUES:** None significant.

AVAILABILITY (Rx)

Tablets (Extended-Release): 2.5 mg, 5 mg, 10 mg.

ADMINISTRATION/HANDLING

PO

• Give without food. • Do not chew, crush, break extended-release tablets. Swallow whole.

INDICATIONS/ROUTES/DOSAGE

Hypertension

PO: ADULTS: Initially, 5 mg/day as single dose. **ELDERLY, PTS WITH HEPATIC IMPAIRMENT:** Initially, 2.5 mg/day. Adjust dosage at no less than 2-wk intervals. Maintenance: 2.5–10 mg/day. Range: 2.5–20 mg/day.

SIDE EFFECTS

Frequent (22%–18%): Headache, peripheral edema. **Occasional (6%–4%):** Flushing, respiratory infection, dizziness, light-headedness, asthenia (loss of strength, energy). **Rare (less than 3%):** Angina, gingival hyperplasia, paresthesia, abdominal discomfort, anxiety, muscle cramping, cough, diarrhea, constipation.

ADVERSE EFFECTS/ TOXIC REACTIONS

Overdose produces nausea, drowsiness, confusion, slurred speech, hypotension, bradycardia.

NURSING CONSIDERATIONS

BASELINE ASSESSMENT

Assess B/P, apical pulse immediately before drug administration (if pulse is 60 or less/min or systolic B/P is less than 90 mm Hg, withhold medication, contact physician).

INTERVENTION/EVALUATION

Assist with ambulation if light-headedness, dizziness occur. Assess for peripheral edema behind media malleolus (sacral area in bedridden pts). Monitor pulse rate for bradycardia. Assess skin for flushing. Monitor hepatic enzyme tests. Question for headache, asthenia.

PATIENT/FAMILY TEACHING

• Do not abruptly discontinue medication. • Compliance with therapy regimen is essential to control hypertension. • To avoid hypotensive effect, rise slowly from lying to sitting position. Wait momentarily before standing. • Avoid tasks that require alertness, motor skills until response to drug is established. • Contact physician if palpitations, shortness of breath, pronounced dizziness, nausea occur. • Swallow tablet whole; do not crush, chew. • Avoid grapefruit, grapefruit juice, alcohol. • Report exacerbation of angina.

fenofibrate

fen-oh-**fye**-brate
(Antara, Apo-Fenofibrate ✤, Fenoglide, Lipofen, Lofibra, Novo-Fenofibrate ✤, Tricor, Triglide)
Do not confuse Tricor with Tracleer.

◆CLASSIFICATION

CLINICAL: Antihyperlipidemic (see p. 56C).

F

ACTION

Enhances synthesis of lipoprotein lipase (VLDL). **Therapeutic Effect:** Increases VLDL catabolism, reduces total plasma triglycerides.

PHARMACOKINETICS

Well absorbed from GI tract. Absorption increased when given with food. Protein binding: 99%. Rapidly metabolized in liver to active metabolite. Excreted primarily in urine, with lesser amount in feces. Not removed by hemodialysis. **Half-life:** 10–35 hrs.

USES

Adjunct to diet for reduction of low-density lipoprotein cholesterol (LDL-C), total cholesterol, triglycerides, apo-lipoprotein B in pts with primary hypercholesterolemia, mixed dyslipidemia. Treatment of hyperlipidemia in combination with ezetimibe.

PRECAUTIONS

Contraindications: Gallbladder disease, severe renal/hepatic dysfunction (including primary biliary cirrhosis, unexplained persistent hepatic function abnormality). **Cautions:** Anticoagulant therapy, history of hepatic disease, substantial alcohol consumption.

⌛ LIFESPAN CONSIDERATIONS

Pregnancy/Lactation: Safety in pregnancy not established. Breast-feeding not recommended. **Pregnancy Category C.** **Children:** Safety and efficacy not established. **Elderly:** No age-related precautions noted.

INTERACTIONS

DRUG: Potentiates effects of **anticoagulants. Bile acid sequestrants** may impede absorption. **Cyclosporine** may increase risk of nephrotoxicity. **HMG-CoA reductase inhibitors** may increase risk of severe myopathy, rhabdomyolysis, acute renal failure. **HERBAL:** None significant. **FOOD: All foods** increase absorption. **LAB VALUES:** May increase serum creatine kinase (CK), AST, ALT. May decrease Hgb, Hct, serum uric acid, WBC count.

AVAILABILITY (Rx)

Capsules: 43 mg (Antara), 50 mg (Lipofen), 67 mg (Lofibra), 100 mg (Lipofen), 130 mg (Antara), 134 mg (Lofibra), 150 mg (Lipofen), 200 mg (Lofibra). **Tablets:** 40 mg (Fenoglide), 48 mg (Tricor), 50 mg (Triglide), 54 mg (Lofibra), 120 mg (Fenoglide), 145 mg (Tricor), 160 mg (Lofibra, Triglide).

ADMINISTRATION/HANDLING

PO

• Give Fenoglide, Lipofen, Lofibra with meals. • Antara, Tricor, and Triglide may be given without regard to food.

INDICATIONS/ROUTES/DOSAGE

Hypertriglyceridemia

PO (ANTARA): ADULTS, ELDERLY: 43–130 mg/day.

PO (FENOGLIDE): ADULTS, ELDERLY: 40–120 mg/day with meals.

PO (LIPOFEN): ADULTS, ELDERLY: 50–150 mg/day with meals.

PO (LOFIBRA): ADULTS, ELDERLY: 67–200 mg/day with meals.

PO (TRICOR): ADULTS, ELDERLY: 48–145 mg/day.

PO (TRIGLIDE): ADULTS, ELDERLY: 50–160 mg/day.

Hypercholesterolemia

PO (ANTARA): ADULTS, ELDERLY: 130 mg/day.

PO (FENOGLIDE): ADULTS, ELDERLY: 120 mg/day with meals.

PO (LIPOFEN): ADULTS, ELDERLY: 150 mg/day with meals.

PO (LOFIBRA): ADULTS, ELDERLY: 200 mg/day with meals.

PO (TRICOR): ADULTS, ELDERLY: 145 mg/day.

PO (TRIGLIDE): ADULTS, ELDERLY: 160 mg/day.

Dosage in Renal Impairment

Monitor renal function/lipid profile before adjusting dose. Decrease dose or increase dosing interval for pts with renal failure.

Initial doses:	Antara: 43 mg/day	Lofibra: 67 mg/day
	Fenoglide: 40 mg/day	Tricor: 48 mg/day
	Lipofen: 50 mg/day	Triglide: 50 mg/day

SIDE EFFECTS

Frequent (8%–4%): Pain, rash, headache, asthenia (loss of strength, energy), fatigue, flu-like symptoms, dyspepsia, nausea/vomiting, rhinitis. **Occasional (3%–2%):** Diarrhea, abdominal pain, constipation, flatulence, arthralgia, decreased libido, dizziness, pruritus. **Rare (less than 2%):** Increased appetite, insomnia, polyuria, cough, blurred vision, eye floaters, earache.

ADVERSE EFFECTS/ TOXIC REACTIONS

May increase cholestrol excretion into bile, leading to cholelithiasis. Pancreatitis, hepatitis, thrombocytopenia, agranulocytosis occur rarely.

NURSING CONSIDERATIONS

BASELINE ASSESSMENT

Obtain diet history, esp. fat consumption. Obtain serum cholesterol, triglycerides, hepatic function tests (including ALT), blood counts during initial therapy and periodically during treatment. Treatment should be discontinued if hepatic enzyme levels persist greater than 3 times normal limit.

INTERVENTION/EVALUATION

For pts on concurrent therapy with HMG-CoA reductase inhibitors, monitor for complaints of myopathy (muscle pain, weakness). Monitor serum creatine kinase (CK). Monitor serum cholesterol, triglyceride for therapeutic response.

PATIENT/FAMILY TEACHING

• Inform physician if diarrhea, constipation, nausea becomes severe. • Report skin rash/irritation, insomnia, muscle pain, tremors, dizziness.

fenofibric acid

fen-oh-**fye**-brick ah-sid
(Fibricor, Trilipix)
Do not confuse Fibricor with Tricor or Trilipix with Trileptal.

CLASSIFICATION

PHARMACOTHERAPEUTIC: Fibric acid derivative. **CLINICAL:** Antihyperlipoproteinemic.

ACTION

Increases lipolysis and elimination of triglyceride-rich particles from plasma by activating lipoprotein lipase, reducing production of lipase activity. **Therapeutic Effect:** Produces alteration in size, composition of LDL allowing for greater affinity for catabolism, decreasing plasma triglycerides, cholesterol.

PHARMACOKINETICS

Well absorbed from GI tract. Protein binding: 99%. Does not undergo oxidative metabolism. Excreted primarily in urine. **Half-life:** 20 hrs.

USES

Adjunct to diet in combination with a statin for treatment of mixed dyslipidemia. Monotherapy to treat severe hypertriglyceridemia, primary hyperlipidemia, mixed dyslipidemia.

PRECAUTIONS

Contraindications: Severe renal impairment, primary biliary cirrhosis, active hepatic disease, gallbladder disease, nursing mothers. **Cautions:** Anticoagulant therapy, history of hepatic disease, substantial alcohol consumption.

LIFESPAN CONSIDERATIONS:

Pregnancy/Lactation: Safety in pregnancy not established. Avoid use in nursing mothers. **Pregnancy Category C. Children:** Safety and efficacy not established.

Elderly: Age-related renal impairment may require monitoring.

INTERACTIONS

DRUG: Potentiates effects of **anticoagulants**. **Bile acid sequestrants (cholestyramine, colestipol)** may impede absorption; give Trilipix 1 hr before or 4–6 hrs after dosing. **Cyclosporine** may increase risk of nephrotoxicity. **HMG-CoA reductase inhibitors** may increase risk of severe myopathy, rhabdomyolysis, acute renal failure. HERBAL: None significant. FOOD: **All foods** increase absorption. LAB VALUES: May increase serum creatine kinase (CK), AST, ALT. May decrease Hgb, Hct, serum uric acid, WBC count.

AVAILABILITY (Rx)

Delayed-Release Capsules (Trilipix): 45 mg, 135 mg. **Tablets (Fibricor):** 35 mg, 105 mg.

ADMINISTRATION/HANDLING

PO

• Give without regard to meals. • Do not break, crush, or half capsule. • May be given at the same time as a statin.

INDICATIONS/ROUTE/DOSAGE

Mixed Dyslipidemia

PO: ADULTS, ELDERLY: **(Trilipix):** 135 mg once daily. **(Fibricor):** 105 mg once daily.

Hypertriglyceridemia

PO: ADULTS, ELDERLY: **(Trilipix):** 45–135 mg once daily. **(Fibricor):** 35–105 mg once daily.

Renal Impairment

PO: ADULTS, ELDERLY: **(Trilipix):** 45 mg once daily. **(Fibricor):** 35 mg once daily. (Contraindicated with creatinine clearance less than 30 ml/min).

SIDE EFFECTS

Frequent (13%): Headache. **Occasional (6%–4%):** Back pain, upper respiratory tract infection, extremity pain, nausea, dizziness, diarrhea, arthralgia, dyspepsia, nasopharyngitis. **Rare (3%–2%):** Constipation, sinusitis, myalgia, fatigue, muscle spasm.

ADVERSE EFFECTS/ TOXIC REACTIONS

Increased risk for myopathy, rhabdomyolysis, particularly in elderly, those with diabetes, renal failure, hypothyroidism. May increase cholesterol excretion into the bile, leading to cholelithiasis. Pancreatitis, hepatitis, thrombocytopenia, agranulocytosis occur rarely.

NURSING CONSIDERATIONS

BASELINE ASSESSMENT

Assess baseline cholesterol, triglycerides, hepatic function tests, blood counts during initial therapy and periodically during treatment.

INTERVENTION/EVALUATION

For those on concurrent therapy with HMG-CoA reductase inhibitors, monitor for complaints of myopathy (muscle pain, weakness), including serum creatinine kinase levels. Monitor cholesterol, triglyceride concentrations for therapeutic response.

PATIENT/FAMILY TEACHING

• Periodic lab tests are essential part of therapy. • Follow special diet (important part of treatment). • Inform physician if diarrhea, constipation, nausea become severe. • Report muscle pain, back/extremity pain, dizziness.

fenoldopam

fen-**nahl**-doe-pam
(Corlopam)

◆CLASSIFICATION

PHARMACOTHERAPEUTIC: Vasodilator (dopamine receptor agonist). CLINICAL: Antihypertensive.

ACTION

Rapid-acting vasodilator. Agonist for D_1-like dopamine receptors, produces vasodilation in coronary, renal, mesenteric, peripheral arteries. **Therapeutic Ef-**

fect: Reduces systolic, diastolic B/P, increases heart rate.

PHARMACOKINETICS

Route	Onset	Peak	Duration
IV	10 min	–	1 hr

After IV administration, metabolized in liver. Primarily excreted in urine. Unknown if removed by hemodialysis. **Half-life:** Approximately 5 min.

USES

Short-term (48 hrs or less) management of severe hypertension when rapid, but quickly reversible; emergency reduction of B/P is clinically indicated, including malignant hypertension with deteriorating end-organ function; short-term (up to 4 hrs) B/P reduction in pediatric pts. **OFF-LABEL:** Prevention of contrast media-induced nephrotoxicity.

PRECAUTIONS

Contraindications: None known. **Cautions:** Glaucoma, intraocular hypertension, angina, tachycardia, hypotension, hypokalemia, sulfite sensitivity.

LIFESPAN CONSIDERATIONS

Pregnancy/Lactation: Unknown if distributed in breast milk. **Pregnancy Category B. Children:** Safety and efficacy not established. **Elderly:** No age-related precautions noted.

INTERACTIONS

DRUG: Beta-blockers may produce excessive hypotension. **HERBAL:** None significant. **FOOD:** None known. **LAB VALUES:** May elevate BUN, serum glucose, LDH, transaminase. May decrease serum potassium.

AVAILABILITY (Rx)

Injection, Solution: 10 mg/ml.

ADMINISTRATION/HANDLING

ALERT Must give by continuous IV infusion, not as bolus injection. B/P must be monitored diligently during infusion.

IV

Reconstitution • Each 10 mg (1 ml) must be diluted with 0.9% NaCl or D_5W to provide a concentration of 40 mcg/ml.

Rate of administration • Administer as IV infusion at initial rate of 0.1–0.3 mcg/kg/min. • Use infusion pump.

Storage • Store ampules at room temperature. • Diluted solution is stable for 24 hrs. Discard any solution not used within 24 hrs.

IV INCOMPATIBILITIES

Bumetanide (Bumex), dexamethasone (Decadron), diazepam, fosphenytoin (Cerebyx), furosemide (Lasix), ketorolac (Toradol), methylprednisolone (Solu-Medrol), phenytoin (Dilantin), prochlorperazine (Compazine).

IV COMPATIBILITIES

Amiodarone (Cordarone), calcium gluconate, diltiazem (Cardizem), dobutamine, dopamine, epinephrine, heparin, hydromorphone (Dilaudid), lidocaine, lorazepam (Ativan), magnesium, midazolam (Versed), milrinone (Primacor), morphine, nitroglycerin, norepinephrine, potassium chloride, propofol (Diprivan).

INDICATIONS/ROUTES/DOSAGE

Short-Term Management of Severe Hypertension

IV INFUSION (CONTINUOUS): ADULTS, ELDERLY: Initially, 0.1–0.3 mcg/kg/min. May increase in increments of 0.05–0.1 mcg/kg/min until target B/P is achieved. Usual length of treatment is 1–6 hrs with tapering of dose q15–30min. Average rate: 0.25–0.5 mcg/kg/min. **Maximum rate:** 1.6 mcg/kg/min. **CHILDREN:** Initially, 0.2 mcg/kg/min. May increase in increments of 0.3–0.5 mcg/kg/min q20–30min. Dosage greater than 0.8 mcg/kg/min has resulted in tachycardia with no additional benefit.

SIDE EFFECTS

ALERT Avoid concurrent use of beta-blockers (may cause significant hypotension). **Occasional:** Headache (7%),

F

flushing (3%), nausea (4%), hypotension (2%). **Rare (2% or less):** Anxiety, vomiting, constipation, nasal congestion, diaphoresis, back pain.

ADVERSE EFFECTS/ TOXIC REACTIONS

Excessive hypotension occurs occasionally. Substantial tachycardia may lead to ischemic cardiac events, worsened heart failure. Allergic-type reactions, including anaphylaxis, life-threatening asthmatic exacerbation, may occur in pts with sulfite sensitivity.

NURSING CONSIDERATIONS

BASELINE ASSESSMENT

Determine initial B/P, apical pulse. It is essential to diligently monitor B/P, EKG during infusion to avoid hypotension and too-rapid decrease of B/P. Assess medication history (esp. for beta-blockers). Obtain baseline serum electrolytes, particularly potassium, and monitor periodically thereafter during infusion. Question asthmatic pts for history of sulfite sensitivity. Check with physician for desired B/P parameters.

INTERVENTION/EVALUATION

Monitor renal/hepatic function tests. Monitor rate of infusion frequently. Monitor EKG for tachycardia (may lead to ischemic heart disease, MI, angina, arrhythmias, worsening heart failure). Monitor closely for symptomatic hypotension.

fentanyl HIGH ALERT

fen-ta-nill
(Abstral, Actiq, Duragesic, Fentora, Novo-Fentanyl 🍁, Onsolis, Sublimaze)

BLACK BOX ALERT Physical and psychological dependence may occur with prolonged use. Use with strong agonist/antagonist analgesics may result in potentially fatal respiratory depression. **Buccal:** Tablet and lozenge contains enough medication that may be fatal to children. **Transdermal patch:** Serious or life-threatening hypoventilation has occurred. Exposure to direct heat source increases drug release, resulting in overdose/death.

Do not confuse fentanyl with alfentanil or sufentanil.

◆CLASSIFICATION

PHARMACOTHERAPEUTIC: Opioid, narcotic agonist **(Schedule II).** **CLINICAL:** Analgesic (see p. 141C).

ACTION

Binds to opioid receptors in CNS, reducing stimuli from sensory nerve endings, inhibits ascending pain pathways. **Therapeutic Effect:** Alters pain reception, increases pain threshold.

PHARMACOKINETICS

Route	Onset	Peak	Duration
IV	1–2 min	3–5 min	0.5–1 hr
IM	7–15 min	20–30 min	1–2 hrs
Transdermal	6–8 hrs	24 hrs	72 hrs
Transmucosal	5–15 min	20–30 min	1–2 hrs

Well absorbed after IM or topical administration. Transmucosal form absorbed through buccal mucosa and GI tract. Protein binding: 80%–85%. Metabolized in liver. Primarily eliminated by biliary system. **Half-life:** 2–4 hrs IV; 17 hrs transdermal; 6.6 hrs transmucosal.

USES

For sedation, pain relief, preop medication; adjunct to general or regional anesthesia. **Duragesic:** Management of chronic pain *(transdermal)*. **Actiq:** Treatment of breakthrough pain in chronic cancer or AIDS-related pain. **Fentora:** Breakthrough pain in pts on chronic opioids. **Onsolis:** Breakthrough pain in pts with cancer currently receiving opioids and tolerant to opioid therapy.

PRECAUTIONS

Contraindications: Increased intracranial pressure (ICP), severe hepatic/renal impairment; severe respiratory depression. Cautions: Bradycardia; renal, hepatic, respiratory disease; head injuries; altered LOC; use of MAOIs within 14 days; transdermal not recommended in those younger than 12 yrs or younger than 18 yrs and weighing less than 50 kg.

LIFESPAN CONSIDERATIONS

Pregnancy/Lactation: Readily crosses placenta. Unknown if distributed in breast milk. May prolong labor if administered in latent phase of first stage of labor or before cervical dilation of 4–5 cm has occurred. Respiratory depression may occur in neonate if mother received opiates during labor. **Pregnancy Category C (D if used for prolonged periods or at high dosages at term). Children:** PATCH: Safety and efficacy not established in those younger than 12 yrs. Neonates more susceptible to respiratory depressant effects. **Elderly:** May be more susceptible to respiratory depressant effects. Age-related renal impairment may require dosage adjustment.

INTERACTIONS

DRUG: **Benzodiazepines** may increase risk of hypotension, respiratory depression. **Buprenorphine** may decrease effects of fentanyl. **Alcohol, CNS depressant medications** may increase CNS depression. **Erythromycin, itraconazole, ketoconazole, protease inhibitors (e.g., ritonavir)** may increase effects of transmucosal fentanyl. **MAOIs** may potentiate effects. HERBAL: **Gotu kola, kava kava, St. John's wort, valerian** may increase CNS depression. FOOD: None known. LAB VALUES: May increase serum amylase, lipase.

AVAILABILITY (Rx)

Buccal Tablet (Fentora): 100 mcg, 200 mcg, 400 mcg, 600 mcg, 800 mcg. Buccal Soluble Film (Onsolis): 200 mcg, 400 mcg, 600 mcg, 800 mcg, 1,200 mcg. Injection Solution (Sublimaze): 50 mcg/ml. Sublingual Tablets (Abstral): 50 mcg, 100 mcg, 200 mcg, 300 mcg, 400 mcg, 600 mcg, 800 mcg. Transdermal Patch (Duragesic): 12 mcg/hr, 25 mcg/hr, 50 mcg/hr, 75 mcg/hr, 100 mcg/hr. Transmucosal Lozenges (Actiq): 200 mcg, 400 mcg, 600 mcg, 800 mcg, 1,200 mcg, 1,600 mcg.

ADMINISTRATION/HANDLING

IV

Rate of administration • Give by slow IV injection (over 1–2 min). • Too-rapid IV increases risk of severe adverse reactions (skeletal, thoracic muscle rigidity resulting in apnea, laryngospasm, bronchospasm, peripheral circulatory collapse, anaphylactoid effects, cardiac arrest).

Storage • Store parenteral form at room temperature. • Opiate antagonist (naloxone) should be readily available.

Transdermal

• Apply to hairless area of intact skin of upper torso. • Use flat, nonirritated site. • Firmly press evenly for 10–20 sec, ensuring adhesion is in full contact with skin and edges are completely sealed. • Use only water to cleanse site before application (soaps, oils may irritate skin). • Rotate sites of application. • Carefully fold used patches so that system adheres to itself; discard in toilet.

Buccal Film

• Wet inside of cheek. • Place film inside mouth with pink side of unit against cheek. • Press film against cheek and hold for 5 sec. • Leave in place until dissolved (15–30 min). • Do not chew, swallow, cut film. • Liquids may be given after 5 min of application; food after film dissolves.

Buccal Tablets

• Place tablet above a rear molar between upper cheek and gum. • Dissolve over 30 min. • Swallow remaining pieces with water. • Do not split tablet.

Sublingual Tablets

• Place under tongue. • Dissolves rapidly. • Do not suck, chew, or swallow tablet.

F

Transmucosal

• Suck lozenge vigorously. • Allow to dissolve over 15 min. • Do not chew.

IV INCOMPATIBILITIES

Azithromycin (Zithromax), pantoprazole (Protonix), phenytoin (Dilantin).

IV COMPATIBILITIES

Atropine, bupivacaine (Marcaine, Sensorcaine), clonidine (Duraclon), diltiazem (Cardizem), diphenhydramine (Benadryl), dobutamine (Dobutrex), dopamine (Intropin), droperidol (Inapsine), heparin, hydromorphone (Dilaudid), ketorolac (Toradol), lipids, lorazepam (Ativan), metoclopramide (Reglan), midazolam (Versed), milrinone (Primacor), morphine, nitroglycerin, norepinephrine (Levophed), ondansetron (Zofran), potassium chloride, propofol (Diprivan).

INDICATIONS/ROUTES/DOSAGE

Note: Doses titrated to desired effect dependent upon degree of analgesia, pt status.

Acute Pain Management

IM/IV: ADULTS, ELDERLY: 50–100 mcg/dose q1–2h as needed. **CHILDREN:** 0.5–2 mcg/kg/dose q1–2h as needed.

Premedication

IV, IM: ADULTS, ELDERLY, CHILDREN 12 YRS AND OLDER: 50–100 mcg/dose 30–60 min prior to surgery.

Adjunct to Regional Anesthesia

IV: ADULTS, ELDERLY, CHILDREN 12 YRS AND OLDER: 25–100 mcg/dose over 1–2 min.

Adjunct to General Anesthesia

IV: ADULTS, ELDERLY, CHILDREN 12 YRS AND OLDER: 2–50 mcg/kg.

Usual Buccal Dose

ADULTS, ELDERLY: Initially, 100 mcg. Titrate dose providing adequate analgesia with tolerable side effects.

Usual Buccal Soluble Film

Note: All pts must initiate with 200 mcg. **ADULTS, ELDERLY:** Initially, 200 mcg up to 1,200 mcg. **Maximum:** No more than 4 doses per day, separate by at least 2 hrs.

Usual Sublingual Dose

ADULTS, ELDERLY: Titrate to desired dose/effect.

Usual Transdermal Dose

ADULTS, ELDERLY, CHILDREN 12 YRS AND OLDER: Initially, 25 mcg/hr. May increase after 3 days.

Usual Transmucosal Dose

ADULTS, CHILDREN: 200–400 mcg for breakthrough pain.

Dosage in Renal Impairment

Dosage is modified based on creatinine clearance.

Creatinine Clearance	Dosage
10–50 ml/min	75% of usual dose
Less than 10 ml/min	50% of usual dose

SIDE EFFECTS

Frequent: IV: Postop drowsiness, nausea, vomiting. **Transdermal (10%–3%):** Headache, pruritus, nausea, vomiting, diaphoresis, dyspnea, confusion, dizziness, drowsiness, diarrhea, constipation, decreased appetite. **Occasional: IV:** Postop confusion, blurred vision, chills, orthostatic hypotension, constipation, difficulty urinating. **Transdermal (3%–1%):** Chest pain, arrhythmias, erythema, pruritus, syncope, agitation, skin irritations.

ADVERSE EFFECTS/ TOXIC REACTIONS

Overdose or too-rapid IV administration may produce severe respiratory depression, skeletal/thoracic muscle rigidity (may lead to apnea, laryngospasm, bronchospasm, cold/clammy skin, cyanosis, coma). Tolerance to analgesic effect may occur with repeated use. **Antidote:** Naloxone (see Appendix M for dosage).

NURSING CONSIDERATIONS

BASELINE ASSESSMENT

Resuscitative equipment, opiate antagonist (naloxone 0.5 mcg/kg) must be available. Establish baseline B/P, respirations. Assess type, location, intensity, duration of pain.

INTERVENTION/EVALUATION

Assist with ambulation. Encourage postop pt to turn, cough, deep breathe q2h. Monitor respiratory rate, B/P, heart rate, oxygen saturation. Assess for relief of pain.

PATIENT/FAMILY TEACHING

• Avoid alcohol; do not take other medications without consulting physician. • Avoid tasks that require alertness, motor skills until response to drug is established. • Teach pt proper transdermal, buccal, lozenge administration. **Transdermal:** Avoid saunas (increases drug release time). • Use as directed to avoid overdosage; potential for physical dependence with prolonged use. • Report absence of pain relief, constipation. • After long-term use, must be discontinued slowly.

Feosol, *see ferrous sulfate*

Fergon, *see ferrous gluconate*

Fer-In-Sol, *see ferrous sulfate*

Ferrlecit, *see sodium ferric gluconate complex*

ferrous fumarate

fair-us **fume**-ah-rate
(Femiron, Ferro-Sequels, Nephro-Fer, Palafer ✤)

ferrous gluconate

fair-us **glue**-kuh-nate
(Apo-Ferrous Gluconate ✤, Fergon)

ferrous sulfate

fair-us **sul**-fate
(Apo-Ferrous Sulfate ✤, Fer-In-Sol, Fer-Iron, Slow-Fe)

FIXED-COMBINATION(S)

Ferro-Sequels: ferrous fumarate/docusate (stool softener): 150 mg/100 mg.

◆CLASSIFICATION

PHARMACOTHERAPEUTIC: Enzymatic mineral. **CLINICAL:** Iron preparation (see p. 109C).

ACTION

Essential component in formation of Hgb, myoglobin, enzymes. Promotes effective erythropoiesis and transport, utilization of oxygen. **Therapeutic Effect:** Prevents iron deficiency.

PHARMACOKINETICS

Absorbed in duodenum and upper jejunum. Ten percent absorbed in pts with normal iron stores; increased to 20%–30% in those with inadequate iron stores. Primarily bound to serum transferrin. Excreted in urine, sweat, sloughing of intestinal mucosa, by menses. **Half-life:** 6 hrs.

USES

Prevention, treatment of iron deficiency anemia due to inadequate diet, malabsorption, pregnancy, blood loss.

PRECAUTIONS

Contraindications: Hemochromatosis, hemosiderosis, hemolytic anemias, peptic ulcer disease, regional enteritis, ulcerative colitis. **Cautions:** Bronchial asthma, iron hypersensitivity, GI tract inflammation.

LIFESPAN CONSIDERATIONS

Pregnancy/Lactation: Crosses placenta; distributed in breast milk. **Pregnancy Category A. Children/Elderly:** No age-related precautions noted.

INTERACTIONS

DRUG: **Antacids, calcium supplements, pancreatin, pancrelipase** may decrease absorption of ferrous compounds. May decrease absorption of **etidronate, quinolones, tetracyclines.** HERBAL: None significant. FOOD: **Cereal, coffee, dietary fiber, eggs, milk, tea** decrease absorption. LAB VALUES: May increase serum bilirubin, iron. May decrease serum calcium. May obscure occult blood in stools.

AVAILABILITY (OTC)

Ferrous Fumarate

Tablets: 63 mg (20 mg elemental iron) (Femiron), 350 mg (115 mg elemental iron) (Nephro-Fer).

Tablets (Timed-Release [Ferro-Sequels]): 150 mg (50 mg elemental iron).

Ferrous Gluconate

Tablets: 240 mg (27 mg elemental iron) (Fergon), 325 mg (36 mg elemental iron).

Ferrous Sulfate

Oral Drops (Fer-In-Sol, Fer-Iron): 75 mg/0.6 ml (15 mg/0.6 ml elemental iron). **Tablets:** 325 mg (65 mg elemental iron). **Elixir:** 220 mg/5 ml (44 mg elemental iron per 5 ml).

Tablets (Timed-Release [Slow-Fe]): 160 mg (50 mg elemental iron).

ADMINISTRATION/HANDLING

PO

• Store all forms (tablets, capsules, suspension, drops) at room temperature. • Ideally, give between meals with water or juice but may give with meals if GI discomfort occurs. • Transient staining of mucous membranes, teeth occurs with liquid iron preparation. To avoid staining, place liquid on back of tongue with dropper or straw. • Do not give with milk or milk products. • Do not crush timed-release preparations.

INDICATIONS/ROUTES/DOSAGE

Iron Deficiency Anemia

Dosage is expressed in terms of milligrams of elemental iron, degree of anemia, pt weight, presence of any bleeding. Expect to use periodic hematologic determinations as guide to therapy.

PO (FERROUS FUMARATE): ADULTS, ELDERLY: 60–100 mg twice a day. **CHILDREN:** 3–6 mg/kg/day in 2–3 divided doses.

PO (FERROUS GLUCONATE): ADULTS, ELDERLY: 60 mg 2–4 times a day. **CHILDREN:** 3–6 mg/kg/day in 2–3 divided doses.

PO (FERROUS SULFATE): ADULTS, ELDERLY: 65 mg 2–4 times a day. **CHILDREN:** 3–6 mg/kg/day in 2–3 divided doses.

Prevention of Iron Deficiency

PO (FERROUS FUMARATE): ADULTS, ELDERLY: 60–100 mg/day. **CHILDREN:** 1–2 mg/kg/day.

PO (FERROUS GLUCONATE): ADULTS, ELDERLY: 60 mg/day. **CHILDREN:** 1–2 mg/kg/day.

PO (FERROUS SULFATE): ADULTS, ELDERLY: 65 mg/day. **CHILDREN:** 1–2 mg/kg/day.

SIDE EFFECTS

Occasional: Mild, transient nausea. **Rare:** Heartburn, anorexia, constipation, diarrhea.

ADVERSE EFFECTS/ TOXIC REACTIONS

Large doses may aggravate existing GI tract disease (peptic ulcer, regional enteritis, ulcerative colitis). Severe iron poisoning occurs most often in children, manifested as vomiting, severe abdominal pain, diarrhea, dehydration, followed by hyperventilation, pallor, cyanosis, cardiovascular collapse.

NURSING CONSIDERATIONS

BASELINE ASSESSMENT

Assess nutritional status, dietary history. To prevent mucous membrane and teeth staining with liquid preparation, use dropper or straw and allow solution to drop on back of tongue. Eggs, milk inhibit absorption.

INTERVENTION/EVALUATION

Monitor serum iron, total iron-binding capacity, reticulocyte count, Hgb, ferritin. Monitor daily pattern of bowel activity and stool consistency. Assess for clinical improvement, record relief of iron deficiency symptoms (fatigue, irritability, pallor, paresthesia of extremities, headache).

PATIENT/FAMILY TEACHING

• Expect stool color to darken. • Oral liquid may stain teeth. • If GI discomfort occurs, take after meals or with food. • Do not take within 2 hrs of other medication or eggs, milk, tea, coffee, cereal.

ferumoxytol

fer-you-**mox**-eh-toll
(Feraheme)
Do not confuse ferumoxytol with metoprolol or Oxytrol.

◆CLASSIFICATION

PHARMACOTHERAPEUTIC: Iron oxide. **CLINICAL:** Iron hemostasis agent.

ACTION

An iron-carbohydrate complex that enters the reticuloendothelial system macrophages of liver, spleen, bone marrow. Iron is then released from the iron-carbohydrate complex within vesicles in macrophages and either enters the intracellular storage iron pool (e.g., ferritin) or is transferred to plasma transferrin for transport to erythroid precursor cells for incorporation into Hgb. **Therapeutic Effect:** Increases RBC counts, Hgb, serum iron; prevents iron deficiency.

PHARMACOKINETICS

Highest tissue concentrations in liver, spleen, lymph node pool. Renal excretion of iron is insignificant; carbohydrate coating significantly excreted in urine and feces. Not removed by hemodialysis. **Half-life:** 15 hrs (increases with higher doses).

USES

Treatment of iron deficiency anemia in adult pts with chronic kidney disease. **OFF-LABEL:** Diagnostic agent for vascular-enhanced MRI to assess peripheral arterial disease.

PRECAUTIONS

Contraindications: Evidence of iron overload, anemia not caused by iron deficiency (pernicious, aplastic, normocytic, refractory). **Cautions:** History of allergies, hypotensive pts, elderly.

LIFESPAN CONSIDERATIONS

Pregnancy/Lactation: Unknown if distributed in breast milk. **Pregnancy Category C. Children:** Safety and efficacy not established. **Elderly:** Cautious use due to greater frequency of decreased hepatic, renal, cardiac function, concurrent disease, or other drug therapy.

INTERACTIONS

DRUG: May reduce absorption of concurrently administered **oral iron preparations. HERBAL:** None significant. **FOOD:** None known. **LAB VALUES:** Expected to increase RBC count, Hgb, serum iron. May alter MRI studies for up to 3 mos following last dose.

AVAILABILITY (Rx)

Injection: 510 mg/17 ml (30 mg elemental iron/ml) single-use vial.

ADMINISTRATION/HANDLING

IV

Reconstitution • Give as undiluted IV injection.
Rate of administration • May deliver at rate up to 1 ml/sec (30 mg/sec).
Storage • Store vials at room temperature. • Discard if solution contains precipitate or is discolored.

F

INDICATIONS/ROUTES/DOSAGE

◀ALERT▶ Dosage expressed in terms of mg of elemental iron, with each ml ferumoxytol containing 30 mg elemental iron. Use periodic hematologic determinations as guide to therapy.

Iron Deficiency Anemia
IV: ADULTS, ELDERLY: Initially, 510-mg IV injection, followed by second 510-mg IV injection 3–8 days later. Recommended dose may be readministered to pts with persistent or recurrent iron deficiency anemia.

Hemodialysis Pts
IV: ADULTS, ELDERLY: Administer medication once B/P is stable and pt has completed at least 1 hr of hemodialysis.

SIDE EFFECTS

Occasional (4%–2%): Hypersensitivity reaction (pruritus, rash, urticaria, wheezing), nausea, dizziness, hypotension, peripheral edema, headache. **Rare (1%):** Edema, vomiting, abdominal pain, chest pain, cough, pyrexia, muscle spasm, back pain.

ADVERSE EFFECTS/ TOXIC REACTIONS

May cause serious hypersensitivity reactions, including anaphylaxis, anaphylactoid reactions.

NURSING CONSIDERATIONS

BASELINE ASSESSMENT

Do not give concurrently with oral iron form (may produce excessive iron storage [hemosiderosis]). Anticipated MRI studies should be conducted prior to administration of ferumoxytol. Alteration of MRI studies may persist for up to 3 mos following last dose.

INTERVENTION/EVALUATION

Monitor for signs, symptoms of hypotension following each injection. Evaluate hematologic response (Hgb, ferritin, iron and transferrin saturation) at least 1 mo following second injection. Observe for signs, symptoms of hypersensitivity for at least 30 min following injection, and administer drug only when therapy for hypersensitivity is readily available. In the 24 hrs following administration, laboratory assays may overestimate serum iron and transferrin bound iron by also measuring the iron in the iron-carbohydrate complex.

PATIENT/FAMILY TEACHING

• Oral iron should not be taken when receiving iron injections. • Report any signs, symptoms of hypersensitivity (rash, pruritus, urticaria, wheezing) that develop during and following administration.

fesoterodine

fess-oh-**tare**-oh-deen
(Toviaz)
Do not confuse fesoterodine with fexofenadine or tolteradine.

◆CLASSIFICATION

PHARMACOTHERAPEUTIC: Muscarinic receptor antagonist. **CLINICAL:** Antispasmodic.

ACTION

Exhibits antimuscarinic activity by interceding via cholinergic muscarinic receptors, thereby inhibiting urinary bladder contraction. **Therapeutic Effect:** Decreases urinary frequency, urgency.

PHARMACOKINETICS

Well absorbed following PO administration. Protein binding: 50%. Rapidly and extensively hydrolyzed to its active metabolite. Primarily excreted in urine. **Half-life:** 7 hours.

USES

Treatment of overactive bladder with symptoms including urinary incontinence, urgency, frequency.

PRECAUTIONS

Contraindications: Gastric retention, uncontrolled angle-closure glaucoma, urinary retention, severe hepatic impairment. **Cautions:** Renal impairment, clinically significant bladder outflow obstruction (risk of urinary retention), GI obstructive disorders (e.g., pyloric stenosis [risk of gastric retention], treated narrow-angle glaucoma, myasthenia gravis.

LIFESPAN CONSIDERATIONS

Pregnancy/lactation: Unknown if distributed in breast milk. **Pregnancy Category C. Children:** Safety and efficacy not established. **Elderly:** Increased incidence of antimuscarinic adverse events including dry mouth, constipation, dyspepsia, increase in residual urine, dizziness, urinary tract infections higher in pts 75 yrs of age and older.

INTERACTIONS

DRUG: Clarithromycin, erythromycin, itraconazole, ketoconazole, miconazole may increase concentration. **HERBAL:** None significant. **FOOD:** None known. **LAB VALUES:** May increase ALT, GGT.

AVAILABILITY (Rx)

Tablets, Extended-Release: 4 mg, 8 mg.

ADMINISTRATION/HANDLING

PO

- Take with liquid and swallow whole.
- May be administered with or without food. • Do not chew, divide, or crush.

INDICATIONS/ROUTES/DOSAGE

Overactive Bladder

PO: ADULTS, ELDERLY: Initially, 4 mg once daily. May increase to 8 mg once daily. Maximum dose for pts with creatinine clearance less than 30 ml/min or concurrent use of clarithromycin, erythromycin, itraconazole, ketoconazole, or miconazole is 4 mg once daily. Not recommended for use in severe hepatic impairment.

F

SIDE EFFECTS

Frequent: Dry mouth (34%–18%), constipation (6%–4%), urinary tract infection (4.2%–3.2%), dry eyes (3.7%–1.4%). **Occasional: (2% or less):** Nausea, dysuria, back pain, rash, insomnia, peripheral edema.

ADVERSE EFFECTS/ TOXIC REACTIONS

Severe anticholinergic effects including abdominal cramps, facial warmth, excessive salivation/lacrimation, diaphoresis, pallor, urinary urgency, blurred vision.

NURSING CONSIDERATIONS

INTERVENTION/EVALUATION

Assist with ambulation if dizziness occurs. Question for visual changes. Monitor incontinence, post-void residuals.

PATIENT/FAMILY TEACHING

• May produce constipation and urinary retention. • Blurred vision may occur, use caution until drug effects have been determined. • Heat prostration (due to decreased sweating) can occur if used in a hot environment.

feverfew

Also known as bachelor's button, featherfew, midsummer daisy, santa maria.

CLASSIFICATION

HERBAL: See Appendix G.

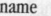

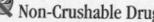

ACTION

May inhibit platelet aggregation, serotonin release from platelets, leukocytes. Inhibits/blocks prostaglandin synthesis. **Effect:** Reduces pain intensity, vomiting, noise sensitivity with severe migraine headaches.

USES

Fever, headache, prevention of migraine and menstrual irregularities, arthritis, psoriasis, allergies, asthma, vertigo.

PRECAUTIONS

Contraindications: Pregnancy/lactation (may cause uterine contraction/abortion). Allergies to ragweed, chrysanthemums, marigolds, daisies. **Cautions:** None known.

LIFESPAN CONSIDERATIONS

Pregnancy/Lactation: Contraindicated. **Children:** Safety and efficacy not established; avoid use. **Elderly:** No age-related precautions noted.

INTERACTIONS

DRUG: **Anticoagulants, antiplatelet agents** may increase risk of bleeding. **NSAIDs** may decrease effectiveness. **HERBAL:** **Garlic, ginger, ginkgo** may increase risk of bleeding. **FOOD:** None known. **LAB VALUES:** None significant.

AVAILABILITY (Rx)

Capsules: 100 mg. **Feverfew leaf:** 380 mg.

INDICATIONS/ROUTES/DOSAGE

Migraine Headache

PO: ADULTS, ELDERLY: 50–100 mg extract a day. **Leaf:** 50–125 mg a day.

SIDE EFFECTS

PO: Abdominal pain, muscle stiffness, pain, indigestion, diarrhea, flatulence, nausea, vomiting. **Chewing Leaf:** Mouth ulceration, inflammation of oral mucosa and tongue, swelling of lips, loss of taste.

ADVERSE EFFECTS/ TOXIC REACTIONS

Hypersensitivity reaction occurs rarely.

NURSING CONSIDERATIONS

BASELINE ASSESSMENT

Assess if pt is pregnant or breast-feeding (contraindicated).

INTERVENTION/EVALUATION

Assess for hypersensitivity reaction, mouth ulcers, muscle/joint pain.

PATIENT/FAMILY TEACHING

• Do not use during pregnancy or lactation. • Avoid use in children.

fexofenadine

fex-**oh**-fen-eh-deen
(Allegra)
Do not confuse Allegra with Viagra, or fexofenadine with fesoterodine.

FIXED-COMBINATION(S)

Allegra-D 12 Hour: fexofenadine/pseudoephedrine (sympathomimetic): 60 mg/120 mg. **Allegra-D 24 Hour:** fexofenadine/pseudoephedrine (sympathomimetic): 180 mg/240 mg.

CLASSIFICATION

PHARMACOTHERAPEUTIC: Piperidine. **CLINICAL:** Antihistamine (see p. 54C).

ACTION

Prevents, antagonizes most histamine effects (urticaria, pruritus). **Therapeutic Effect:** Relieves allergic rhinitis symptoms.

PHARMACOKINETICS

	Onset	Peak	Duration
PO	60 min	–	12 hrs or greater

Rapidly absorbed after PO administration. Protein binding: 60%–70%. Does not cross blood-brain barrier. Minimally metabolized. Eliminated in feces, urine. Not removed by hemodialysis.

Half-life: 14.4 hrs (increased in renal impairment).

USES

Relief of seasonal allergic rhinitis, chronic idiopathic urticaria.

PRECAUTIONS

Contraindications: None known. **Cautions:** Severe renal impairment.

LIFESPAN CONSIDERATIONS

Pregnancy/Lactation: Unknown if drug crosses placenta or is distributed in breast milk. **Pregnancy Category C. Children:** Safety and efficacy not established in those younger than 12 yrs. **Elderly:** No age-related precautions noted.

INTERACTIONS

DRUG: Antacids may decrease absorption if given within 15 min of fexofenadine. **HERBAL: St. John's wort** may decrease concentration. **FOOD: Fruit juices** may decrease bioavailability. **LAB VALUES:** May suppress wheal, flare reactions to antigen skin testing unless drug is discontinued at least 4 days before testing.

AVAILABILITY (Rx)

Oral Suspension: 6 mg/ml. **Tablets:** 30 mg, 60 mg, 180 mg. **Tablets (Orally-Disintegrating):** 30 mg.

ADMINISTRATION/HANDLING

PO

• Give without regard to food. • Avoid giving with fruit juices (apple, grapefruit, orange).

INDICATIONS/ROUTES/DOSAGE

Allergic Rhinitis

PO: ADULTS, ELDERLY, CHILDREN 12 YRS AND OLDER: 60 mg twice a day or 180 mg once a day. **CHILDREN 2–11 YRS:** 30 mg twice a day.

Urticaria

PO: ADULTS, ELDERLY, CHILDREN 12 YRS AND OLDER: 60 mg twice a day or 180 mg once a day. **CHILDREN 2–11 YRS:** 30 mg twice a day. **CHILDREN 6 MOS–LESS THAN 2 YRS:** 15 mg twice a day.

Dosage in Renal Impairment (Creatinine Clearance Less Than 80 ml/min)

PO: ADULTS, ELDERLY, CHILDREN 12 YRS AND OLDER: 60 mg once daily. **CHILDREN 2–11 YRS:** 30 mg once daily. **CHILDREN 6 MOS–LESS THAN 2 YRS:** 15 mg once daily.

SIDE EFFECTS

Rare (less than 2%): Drowsiness, headache, fatigue, nausea, vomiting, abdominal distress, dysmenorrhea.

ADVERSE EFFECTS/ TOXIC REACTIONS

Hypersensitivity reaction occurs rarely.

NURSING CONSIDERATIONS

BASELINE ASSESSMENT

If pt is having an allergic reaction, obtain history of recently ingested foods, drugs, environmental exposure, emotional stress. Monitor rate, depth, rhythm, type of respiration; quality, rate of pulse. Assess lung sounds for rhonchi, wheezing, rales.

INTERVENTION/EVALUATION

Assess for therapeutic response; relief from allergy: itching, red, watery eyes, rhinorrhea, sneezing.

PATIENT/FAMILY TEACHING

• Avoid tasks that require alertness, motor skills until response to drug is established. • Avoid alcohol during antihistamine therapy. • Coffee, tea may help reduce drowsiness. • Do not take with fruit juices.

filgrastim

fill-**gra**-stim

(GCSF, Neupogen)

Do not confuse Neupogen with Epogen, Neulasta, Neumega, or Nutramigen.

CLASSIFICATION

PHARMACOTHERAPEUTIC: Biologic modifier. **CLINICAL:** Granulocyte colony-stimulating factor (G-CSF).

ACTION

Stimulates production, maturation, activation of neutrophils. **Therapeutic Effect:** Increases migration, activation of neutrophils.

F

PHARMACOKINETICS

Readily absorbed after subcutaneous administration. Onset of action: 24 hrs (plateaus in 3–5 days). White counts return to normal in 4–7 days. Not removed by hemodialysis. **Half-life:** 3.5 hrs.

USES

Decreases infection incidence in pts with malignancies receiving chemotherapy associated with severe neutropenia, fever. Reduces neutropenia duration, sequelae, in pts with nonmyeloid malignancies having myeloablative therapy followed by bone marrow transplant (BMT). Mobilization of hematopoietic progenitor cells into peripheral blood for collection by leukapheresis. Treatment of chronic, severe neutropenia. **OFF-LABEL:** Treatment of AIDS-related neutropenia, drug-induced neutropenia, treatment of anemia in myelodysplastic syndrome. Treatment of drug-induced agranulocytosis in the elderly.

PRECAUTIONS

Contraindications: Hypersensitivity to *Escherichia coli*–derived proteins, 24 hrs before or after cytotoxic chemotherapy, concurrent use of other drugs that may result in lowered platelet count. **Cautions:** Malignancy with myeloid characteristics (due to G-CSF's potential to act as growth factor), gout, psoriasis, preexisting cardiac conditions, those taking lithium.

LIFESPAN CONSIDERATIONS

Pregnancy/Lactation: Unknown if drug crosses placenta or is distributed in breast milk. **Pregnancy Category C. Children/Elderly:** No age-related precautions noted.

INTERACTIONS

DRUG: None significant. **HERBAL:** None significant. **FOOD:** None known. **LAB VALUES:** May increase LDH, leukocyte alkaline phosphatase (LAP) scores, serum alkaline phosphatase, uric acid.

AVAILABILITY (Rx)

Injection Solution: 300 mcg/ml (1 ml, 1.6 ml) vial, 600 mcg/ml (0.5 ml, 0.8 ml) prefilled syringe.

ADMINISTRATION/HANDLING

ALERT May be given by subcutaneous injection, short IV infusion (15–30 min), or continuous IV infusion.

IV

Reconstitution • Use single-dose vial; do not reenter vial. • Do not shake. • Dilute with 10–50 ml D_5W to concentration of 15 mcg/ml or greater. For concentration from 5–14 mcg/ml, add 2 ml of 5% albumin to each 50 ml D_5W to provide a final concentration of 2 mg/ml. Do not dilute to final concentration less than 5 mcg/ml.

Rate of administration • For intermittent infusion (piggyback), infuse over 15–30 min. • For continuous infusion, give single dose over 4–24 hrs. • In all situations, flush IV line with D_5W before and after administration.

Storage • Refrigerate vials. • Stable for up to 24 hrs at room temperature (provided vial contents are clear and contain no particulate matter). Remains stable if accidentally exposed to freezing temperature.

Subcutaneous

• Aspirate syringe before injection (avoid intra-arterial administration).

Storage • Store in refrigerator, but remove before use and allow to warm to room temperature.

IV INCOMPATIBILITIES

Amphotericin (Fungizone), cefepime (Maxipime), cefotaxime (Claforan), cefoxitin (Mefoxin), ceftizoxime (Cefizox), ceftriaxone (Rocephin), cefuroxime (Zinacef), clindamycin (Cleocin), dactinomycin (Cosmegen), etoposide (VePesid), fluorouracil, furosemide (Lasix), heparin, mannitol, methylprednisolone (Solu-Medrol), mitomycin (Mutamycin), prochlorperazine (Compazine), total parenteral nutrition (TPN).

IV COMPATIBILITIES

Bumetanide (Bumex), calcium gluconate, hydromorphone (Dilaudid), lorazepam (Ativan), morphine, potassium chloride.

INDICATIONS/ROUTES/DOSAGE

◀ALERT▶ Begin therapy at least 24 hrs after last dose of chemotherapy and at least 24 hrs after bone marrow infusion. Dosing based on actual body weight.

Chemotherapy-Induced Neutropenia

IV OR SUBCUTANEOUS INFUSION, SUBCUTANEOUS INJECTION: ADULTS, ELDERLY, CHILDREN: Initially, 5 mcg/kg/day. May increase by 5 mcg/kg for each chemotherapy cycle based on duration/severity of neutropenia; continue for up to 14 days or until absolute neutrophil count (ANC) reaches 10,000/mm^3.

Bone Marrow Transplant

IV OR SUBCUTANEOUS INFUSION: ADULTS, ELDERLY, CHILDREN: 5–10 mcg/kg/day. Adjust dosage daily during period of neutrophil recovery based on neutrophil response.

Mobilization of Progenitor Cells

IV OR SUBCUTANEOUS INFUSION: ADULTS: 10 mcg/kg/day beginning at least 4 days before first leukapheresis and continuing until last leukapheresis.

Chronic Neutropenia, Congenital Neutropenia

SUBCUTANEOUS: ADULTS, CHILDREN: 6 mcg/kg/dose twice a day.

Idiopathic or Cyclic Neutropenia

SUBCUTANEOUS: ADULTS, CHILDREN: 5 mcg/kg/dose once a day.

SIDE EFFECTS

Frequent: Nausea/vomiting (57%), mild to severe bone pain (22%) (more frequent with high-dose IV form, less frequent with low-dose subcutaneous form), alopecia (18%), diarrhea (14%), fever (12%), fatigue (11%). **Occasional (9%–5%):** Anorexia, dyspnea, headache, cough, rash. **Rare (less than 5%):** Psoriasis, hematuria, proteinuria, osteoporosis.

ADVERSE EFFECTS/ TOXIC REACTIONS

Long-term administration occasionally produces chronic neutropenia, splenomegaly. Thrombocytopenia, MI, arrhythmias occur rarely. Adult respiratory distress syndrome may occur in septic pts.

NURSING CONSIDERATIONS

BASELINE ASSESSMENT

CBC, platelet count (differential) should be obtained before therapy initiation and twice weekly thereafter.

INTERVENTION/EVALUATION

In septic pts, be alert for adult respiratory distress syndrome. Closely monitor those with preexisting cardiac conditions. Monitor B/P (transient decrease in B/P may occur), temperature, CBC with differential, platelet count, Hct, serum uric acid, hepatic function tests.

PATIENT/FAMILY TEACHING

- Inform physician of fever, chills, severe bone pain, chest pain, palpitations.

finasteride

fin-**as**-ter-ide
(Propecia, Proscar)
Do not confuse finasteride with furosemide, or Proscar with ProSom, Provera, or Prozac.

◆CLASSIFICATION

PHARMACOTHERAPEUTIC: Androgen hormone inhibitor. **CLINICAL:** Benign prostatic hyperplasia agent.

ACTION

Inhibits 5-alpha reductase, an intracellular enzyme that converts testosterone into dihydrotestosterone (DHT) in prostate gland, resulting in decreased serum DHT. **Therapeutic Effect:** Reduces size of prostate gland.

F

PHARMACOKINETICS

Route	Onset	Peak	Duration
PO (reduction of DHT)	8 hrs	–	24 hrs

Rapidly absorbed from GI tract. Protein binding: 90%. Widely distributed. Metabolized in liver. **Half-life:** 6–8 hrs. Onset of clinical effect: 3–6 mos of continued therapy.

USES

Proscar: Reduces risk of acute urinary retention, need for surgery in symptomatic benign prostatic hyperplasia (BPH) alone or in combination with doxazosin (Carura). Most improvement noted in urinary hesitancy, feeling of incomplete bladder emptying, interruption of urinary stream, difficulty initiating flow, dysuria, impaired volume, force of urinary stream. **Propecia:** Treatment of hair loss. **OFF-LABEL:** Adjuvant monotherapy after radical prostatectomy in treatment of prostate cancer, female hirsutism.

PRECAUTIONS

Contraindications: Exposure to semen of treated pt or handling of finasteride tablets by those who are or may be pregnant. **Cautions:** Hepatic function abnormalities.

⧖ LIFESPAN CONSIDERATIONS

Pregnancy/Lactation: Physical handling of tablet by those who are or may become pregnant may produce abnormalities of external genitalia of male fetus. **Pregnancy Category X. Children:** Not indicated for use in children. **Elderly:** Efficacy not established.

INTERACTIONS

DRUG: None significant. **HERBAL: St. John's wort** may decrease concentration. Avoid concurrent use with **saw palmetto** (not adequately studied). **FOOD:** None known. **LAB VALUES:** Decreases serum prostate-specific antigen (PSA) level, even in presence of prostate cancer. Decreases dihydrotestosterone (DHT). Increases follicle-stimulating hormone (FSH), luteinizing hormone (LH), testosterone.

AVAILABILITY (Rx)

Tablets: 1 mg (Propecia), 5 mg (Proscar).

ADMINISTRATION/HANDLING

PO

• Do not break, crush film-coated tablets. • Give without regard to meals.

INDICATIONS/ROUTES/DOSAGE

Benign Prostatic Hyperplasia (BPH)

PO: ADULTS, ELDERLY: (Proscar): 5 mg once a day (for minimum of 6 mos).

Hair Loss

PO: ADULTS: (Propecia): 1 mg/day.

SIDE EFFECTS

Rare (4%–2%): Gynecomastia, sexual dysfunction (impotence, decreased libido, decreased volume of ejaculate).

ADVERSE EFFECTS/ TOXIC REACTIONS

Hypersensitivity reaction, circumoral swelling, testicular pain occur rarely.

NURSING CONSIDERATIONS

BASELINE ASSESSMENT

Digital rectal exam, serum prostate-specific antigen (PSA) determination should be performed in those with benign prostatic hyperplasia (BPH) before initiating therapy and periodically thereafter.

INTERVENTION/EVALUATION

Diligent monitoring of I&O, esp. in those with large residual urinary volume, severely diminished urinary flow for obstructive uropathy.

PATIENT/FAMILY TEACHING

• Pt should be aware of potential for impotence. • May not notice improved urinary flow even if prostate gland shrinks. • Need to take medication longer than 6 mos, and it is unknown if medication decreases need for surgery. • Because of potential risk to male fetus, women who are or may become pregnant should not handle tablets or be exposed to pt's semen. • Volume of ejaculate may be decreased during treatment.

fingolimod

fin-**go**-lih-mode
(Gilenya)

CLASSIFICATION

PHARMACOTHERAPEUTIC: Immunomodulator. **CLINICAL:** Multiple sclerosis agent.

ACTION

Blocks capacity of lymphocytes to move out from lymph nodes, reducing number of lymphocytes in peripheral blood. **Therapeutic Effect:** May involve reduction of lymphocyte migration into central nervous system.

PHARMACOKINETICS

Metabolized by the enzyme sphingosine kinase to active metabolite. Highly distributed in red blood cells (85%). Minimally metabolized in liver. Protein binding: 99.7%. Primarily excreted in urine. **Half-life:** 6–9 days.

USES

Treatment of pts with relapsing forms of multiple sclerosis (MS) to reduce frequency of clinical exacerbations, delay accumulation of physical disability.

PRECAUTIONS

Contraindications: None significant. **Cautions:** Antiarrhythmic drugs, beta-blockers, calcium channel blockers, those with low heart rate, history of syncope, sick sinus syndrome, second-degree or higher conduction block, ischemic heart disease, congestive heart failure are at increased risk for developing bradycardia, heart blocks. Severe hepatic impairment.

LIFESPAN CONSIDERATIONS:

Pregnancy/Lactation: May cause fetal harm. Unknown if distributed in breast milk. **Pregnancy Category C. Children:** Safety and efficacy not established in those younger than 18 yrs. **Elderly:** Age-related severe hepatic impairment may increase risk of adverse reactions.

INTERACTIONS

DRUG: **Antineoplastics, immunosuppressives, immunomodulators** increase risk of immunosuppression. **Ketoconazole** increases concentration/adverse effects. **HERBAL:** None significant. **FOOD:** None known. **LAB VALUES:** Expect decrease in neutrophil count. May increase AST, ALT, alkaline phosphatase, bilirubin, triglycerides.

AVAILABILITY (Rx)

Capsules: 0.5 mg.

ADMINISTRATION/HANDLING

PO

• May give without regard to food.

INDICATIONS/ROUTES/DOSAGE

Multiple Sclerosis

PO: ADULTS 18 YRS AND OLDER, ELDERLY: 0.5 mg once daily.

SIDE EFFECTS

Frequent (25%–10%): Headache, diarrhea, back pain, cough. **Occasional (8%–5%):** Dyspnea, clinical depression, dizziness, hypertension, migraine, paresthesia, decreased weight. **Rare (4%–2%):** Blurred vision, alopecia, eye pain, asthenia (loss of energy, strength), eczema, pruritus.

ADVERSE EFFECTS/ TOXIC REACTIONS

May increase risk of infections (influenza, herpes viral infection, bronchitis, sinusitis, gastroenteritis, ear infection) in 13%–4% of pts. Pts with diabetes or history of uveitis are at increased risk for developing macular edema.

NURSING CONSIDERATIONS

BASELINE ASSESSMENT

Obtain baseline CBC, serum chemistries prior to initial treatment. At initial treatment (within first 4–6 hrs after dose), medication reduces heart rate, AV conduction, followed by progressive increase after first day of treatment. Obtain baseline vitals, with particular attention to pulse rate. Perform ophthalmologic evaluation prior to treatment and 3–4 mos after initiation of treatment.

INTERVENTION/EVALUATION

Monitor for bradycardia for 6 hrs after first dose, followed by progressive increase after first day of treatment. Periodically monitor CBC, serum chemistries, particularly lymphocyte count (expected to decrease approximately 80% from baseline with continued treatment). Monitor for signs of systemic or local infection.

PATIENT/FAMILY TEACHING

• Obtain regular eye examinations during and for 2 mos following treatment. • Use effective methods of contraception during and for 3 mos following treatment. • Report fever, chills, aches, weakness, cough, nausea, symptoms of infection, visual changes, yellowing of skin, eyes, dark urine.

Fioricet, *see acetaminophen*

Fiorinal, *see aspirin*

Flagyl, *see metronidazole*

flavoxate

fla-vox-ate
(Apo-Flavoxate ✦, Urispas)
Do not confuse flavoxate with fluvoxamine, or Urispas with Urised.

◆ CLASSIFICATION

PHARMACOTHERAPEUTIC: Anticholinergic. **CLINICAL:** Antispasmodic.

ACTION

Relaxes detrusor, other smooth muscle by cholinergic blockade, counteracting muscle spasm in urinary tract. **Therapeutic Effect:** Produces anticholinergic, local anesthetic, analgesic effects, relieving urinary symptoms.

PHARMACOKINETICS

Well absorbed from GI tract. Protein binding: 50%–80%. Excreted in urine. **Half-life:** 10–20 hrs.

USES

Urinary analgesic, anesthetic for symptomatic relief of dysuria, nocturia, urinary urgency, frequency, incontinence associated with cystitis, prostatitis, urethritis, urethrocystitis, urethrotrigonitis.

PRECAUTIONS

Contraindications: Duodenal, pyloric obstruction; GI hemorrhage, obstruction; ileus; lower urinary tract obstruction. **Cautions:** Glaucoma.

⌛ LIFESPAN CONSIDERATIONS

Pregnancy/Lactation: Unknown if drug crosses placenta or is distributed in breast milk. **Pregnancy Category B. Children:** Safety and efficacy not established in those younger than 12 yrs. **Elderly:** Higher risk of confusion.

INTERACTIONS

DRUG: None significant. **HERBAL:** None significant. **FOOD:** None known. **LAB VALUES:** None significant.

AVAILABILITY (Rx)

Tablets: 100 mg.

INDICATIONS/ROUTES/DOSAGE

Urinary Analgesic, Anesthetic

PO: ADULTS, ELDERLY, ADOLESCENTS: 100–200 mg 3–4 times a day.

SIDE EFFECTS

Frequent: Drowsiness, dry mouth/throat. **Occasional:** Constipation, difficult urination, blurred vision, dizziness, headache, photosensitivity, nausea, vomiting, abdominal pain. **Rare:** Confusion (primarily in elderly), hypersensitivity, increased IOP, leukopenia.

ADVERSE EFFECTS/ TOXIC REACTIONS

Overdose may produce anticholinergic effects (unsteadiness, severe dizziness, drowsiness, fever, facial flushing, dyspnea, anxiety, irritability).

NURSING CONSIDERATIONS

BASELINE ASSESSMENT

Assess for dysuria, urgency, frequency, incontinence, suprapubic pain.

INTERVENTION/EVALUATION

Monitor for symptomatic relief. Observe elderly, esp. for mental confusion.

PATIENT/FAMILY TEACHING

• Avoid tasks that require alertness, motor skills until response to drug is established. • Do not become overheated in hot weather or during exercise or other activities.

Flexeril, *see cyclobenzaprine*

Flomax, *see tamsulosin*

Flonase, *see fluticasone*

Flovent, *see fluticasone*

Floxin Otic, *see ofloxacin*

fluconazole

flu-con-ah-zole
(Apo-Fluconazole ✤, Diflucan, Novo-Fluconazole ✤)

Do not confuse Diflucan with diclofenac, Diprivan, or disulfiram, or fluconazole with fluoxetine, furosemide, or itraconazole.

◆CLASSIFICATION

CLINICAL: Antifungal.

ACTION

Interferes with cytochrome P-450, an enzyme necessary for ergosterol formation. **Therapeutic Effect:** Directly damages fungal membrane, altering its function. Fungistatic.

PHARMACOKINETICS

Well absorbed from GI tract. Widely distributed, including to CSF. Protein binding: 11%. Partially metabolized in liver. Excreted unchanged primarily in urine. Partially removed by hemodialysis. **Half-life:** 20–30 hrs (increased in renal impairment).

USES

Prevention of candidiasis in pts undergoing bone marrow transplant, receiving chemotherapy and/or radiation therapy; treatment of esophageal, oropharyngeal, disseminated, vulvovaginal, urinary tract candidiasis; treatment and suppression of cryptococcal meningitis. **OFF-LABEL:** Treatment of coccidioidomycosis, cryptococcosis, fungal pneumonia, onychomycosis, ringworm of the hand, septicemia.

F

PRECAUTIONS

Contraindications: None known. **Cautions:** Hepatic/renal impairment, hypersensitivity to other triazoles (e.g., itraconazole, terconazole), imidazoles (e.g., butoconazole, ketoconazole). May prolong QT interval.

LIFESPAN CONSIDERATIONS

Pregnancy/Lactation: Unknown if distributed in breast milk. **Pregnancy Category C. Children:** No age-related precautions noted. **Elderly:** Age-related renal impairment may require dosage adjustment.

INTERACTIONS

DRUG: High fluconazole dosages increase **cyclosporine, sirolimus, tacrolimus** concentrations. **Isoniazid, rifampin** may increase drug metabolism. May increase concentration, effects of **oral antidiabetic medication.** May decrease metabolism of **phenytoin, warfarin. HERBAL:** None significant. **FOOD:** None known. **LAB VALUES:** May increase serum alkaline phosphatase, bilirubin, AST, ALT.

AVAILABILITY (Rx)

Injection, Solution: 2 mg/ml (in 100- or 200-ml containers). **Powder for Oral Suspension:** 10 mg/ml, 40 mg/ml. **Tablets:** 50 mg, 100 mg, 150 mg, 200 mg.

ADMINISTRATION/HANDLING

IV

Rate of administration • Do not exceed maximum flow rate of 200 mg/hr.

Storage • Store at room temperature. • Do not remove from outer wrap until ready to use. • Squeeze inner bag to check for leaks. • Do not use parenteral form if solution is cloudy, precipitate forms, seal is not intact, or it is discolored. • Do not add supplementary medication.

PO

• Give without regard to meals. • PO and IV therapy equally effective; IV therapy for pt intolerant of drug or unable to take orally.

IV INCOMPATIBILITIES

Amphotericin B (Fungizone), amphotericin B complex (Abelcet, AmBisome, Amphotec), ampicillin (Polycillin), calcium gluconate, cefotaxime (Claforan), ceftazidime (Fortaz), ceftriaxone (Rocephin), cefuroxime (Zinacef), chloramphenicol (Chloromycetin), clindamycin (Cleocin), co-trimoxazole (Bactrim), diazepam (Valium), digoxin (Lanoxin), erythromycin (Erythrocin), furosemide (Lasix), haloperidol (Haldol), hydroxyzine (Vistaril), imipenem and cilastatin (Primaxin), total parenteral nutrition (TPN).

IV COMPATIBILITIES

Diltiazem (Cardizem), dobutamine (Dobutrex), dopamine (Intropin), heparin, lipids, lorazepam (Ativan), midazolam (Versed), propofol (Diprivan).

INDICATIONS/ROUTES/DOSAGE

Oropharyngeal Candidiasis

PO, IV: ADULTS, ELDERLY: 200 mg once, then 100 mg/day for at least 14 days. **CHILDREN:** 6 mg/kg/day once, then 3 mg/kg/day.

Esophageal Candidiasis

PO, IV: ADULTS, ELDERLY: 200 mg once, then 100 mg/day (up to 400 mg/day) for 21 days and at least 14 days following resolution of symptoms. **CHILDREN:** 6 mg/kg/day once, then 3 mg/kg/day (up to 12 mg/kg/day) for 21 days and at least 14 days following resolution of symptoms.

Urinary Candidiasis
PO, IV: ADULTS, ELDERLY: 200 mg/day for 1–2 wks.

Vaginal Candidiasis
PO: ADULTS: 150 mg once.

Prevention of Candidiasis in Pts Undergoing Bone Marrow Transplantation
PO: ADULTS: 400 mg/day. Begin 3 days before onset of neutropenia and continue for 7 days after neutrophils greater than 10,000 cells/mm^3.

Systemic Candidiasis
PO, IV: ADULTS, ELDERLY: 400–800 mg/day for at least 28 days and at least 14 days following resolution of symptoms. **CHILDREN:** 6–12 mg/kg/day for 28 days.

Cryptococcal Meningitis
PO, IV: ADULTS, ELDERLY: 400 mg once, then 200 mg/day (up to 800 mg/day) for 10–12 wks after CSF becomes negative (200 mg/day for suppression of relapse in pts with AIDS). **CHILDREN:** 12 mg/kg/day once, then 6–12 mg/kg/day (6 mg/kg/day for suppression of relapse).

Dosage in Renal Impairment
After a loading dose of 400 mg, daily dosage is based on creatinine clearance.

Creatinine Clearance	Dosage
Greater than 50 ml/min	100%
50 ml/min or less	50%
Dialysis	100% of dose after dialysis

SIDE EFFECTS

Occasional (4%–1%): Hypersensitivity reaction (chills, fever, pruritus, rash), dizziness, drowsiness, headache, constipation, diarrhea, nausea, vomiting, abdominal pain.

ADVERSE EFFECTS/ TOXIC REACTIONS

Exfoliative skin disorders, serious hepatic effects, blood dyscrasias (eosinophilia, thrombocytopenia, anemia, leukopenia) have been reported rarely.

NURSING CONSIDERATIONS

BASELINE ASSESSMENT

Assess infected area. Establish baselines for CBC, serum potassium, hepatic function studies.

INTERVENTION/EVALUATION

Assess for hypersensitivity reaction (chills, fever). Monitor serum hepatic/renal function tests, potassium, CBC, platelet count. Report rash, itching promptly. Monitor temperature at least daily. Monitor daily pattern of bowel activity and stool consistency. Assess for dizziness; provide assistance as needed.

PATIENT/FAMILY TEACHING

• Avoid tasks that require alertness, motor skills until response to drug is established. • Notify physician of dark urine, pale stool, jaundiced skin or sclcra of eyes, rash, pruritus. • Pts with oropharyngeal infections should maintain fastidious oral hyglene. • Consult physician before taking any other medication.

fludarabine

HIGH ALERT

flew-**dare**-ah-bean
(Fludara)

BLACK BOX ALERT Must be administered by certified chemotherapy personnel. Severe neurologic toxicity reported. Life-threatening hemolytic anemia, autoimmune thrombocytopenic purpura, hemophilia have occurred. Risk of severe myelosuppression (anemia, thrombocytopenia, neutropenia). Concurrent use with pentostatin may produce, severe/fatal pulmonary toxicity.

Do not confuse Fludara with FUDR, or fludarabine with cladribine or Flumadine.

◆CLASSIFICATION

PHARMACOTHERAPEUTIC: Antimetabolite. **CLINICAL:** Antineoplastic (see p. 83C).

ACTION

Inhibits DNA synthesis by interfering with DNA polymerase alpha, ribonucleotide reductase, DNA primase. **Therapeutic Effect:** Induces cell death.

PHARMACOKINETICS

Rapidly dephosphorylated in serum, then phosphorylated intracellularly to active triphosphate. Primarily excreted in urine. **Half-life:** 7–20 hrs.

USES

Treatment of chronic lymphocytic leukemia (CLL) in those who have not responded to or have not progressed with another standard alkylating agent. **Tablets:** Treatment of CLL. **OFF-LABEL:** Treatment of non-Hodgkin's lymphoma, acute leukemias in children.

PRECAUTIONS

Contraindications: Concurrent use with pentostatin. **Cautions:** Preexisting neurologic problems, renal insufficiency, myelosuppression.

LIFESPAN CONSIDERATIONS

Pregnancy/Lactation: If possible, avoid use during pregnancy, esp. first trimester. May cause fetal harm. Not known whether distributed in breast milk. Breast-feeding not recommended. **Pregnancy Category D. Children:** Safety and efficacy not established. **Elderly:** Age-related renal impairment may require dosage adjustment.

INTERACTIONS

DRUG: May decrease effects of **antigout medications. Bone marrow depressants** may increase risk of myelosuppression. **Live virus vaccines** may potentiate virus replication, increase vaccine side effects, decrease pt's antibody response to vaccine. **HERBAL:** None significant. **FOOD:** None known. **LAB VALUES:** May increase serum alkaline phosphatase, uric acid, AST.

AVAILABILITY (Rx)

Injection, Powder for Reconstitution: 50 mg. **Injection, Solution:** 25 mg/ml.

Tablets: 10 mg.

ADMINISTRATION/HANDLING

ALERT Give by IV infusion. Do not add to other IV infusions. Avoid small veins, swollen, edematous extremities; areas overlying joints, tendons.

IV

Reconstitution • Reconstitute 50-mg vial with 2 ml Sterile Water for Injection to provide concentration of 25 mg/ml. • Further dilute with 100–125 ml 0.9% NaCl or D_5W.

Rate of administration • Infuse over 30 min.

Storage • Store in refrigerator. • Handle with extreme care during preparation/administration. If contact with skin or mucous membranes occurs, wash thoroughly with soap and water; rinse eyes profusely with plain water. • Reconstituted vials stable for 16 days at room temperature or refrigerated. • Diluted solutions stable for 48 hrs at room temperature or refrigerated.

PO

• May give with or without food. • Swallow whole; do not chew, break, or crush tablets.

IV INCOMPATIBILITIES

Acyclovir (Zovirax), amphotericin B (Fungizone), daunorubicin, hydroxyzine (Vistaril), prochlorperazine (Compazine).

IV COMPATIBILITIES

Heparin, hydromorphone (Dilaudid), lorazepam (Ativan), magnesium sulfate, morphine, multivitamins, potassium chloride.

INDICATIONS/ROUTES/DOSAGE

Chronic Lymphocytic Leukemia (CLL, Non-Hodgkin's Lymphoma)

IV: ADULTS: 25 mg/m^2 daily for 5 consecutive days. Continue for up to 3 additional cycles. Begin each course of treatment every 28 days.

CLL

PO: ADULTS, ELDERLY: 40 mg/m^2 once daily for 5 days every 28 days.

Dosage in Renal Impairment

Creatinine Clearance	Dosage
30–70 ml/min	Decrease dose by 20%
Less than 30 ml/min	IV: Not recommended PO: 50% of dose

SIDE EFFECTS

Frequent: Fever (60%), nausea/vomiting (36%), chills (11%). **Occasional (20%–10%):** Fatigue, generalized pain, rash, diarrhea, cough, asthenia (loss of strength, energy), stomatitis, dyspnea, peripheral edema. **Rare (7%–3%):** Anorexia, sinusitis, dysuria, myalgia, paresthesia, headache, visual disturbances.

ADVERSE EFFECTS/ TOXIC REACTIONS

Pneumonia occurs frequently. Severe hematologic toxicity (anemia, thrombocytopenia, neutropenia), GI bleeding may occur. Tumor lysis syndrome may begin with flank pain, hematuria; may also include hypercalcemia, hyperphosphatemia, hyperuricemia, resulting in renal failure. High-dosage therapy may produce acute leukemia, blindness, coma. Neurotoxicity (progressive demyelinating encephalopathy, mental status deterioration) occurs rarely.

NURSING CONSIDERATIONS

BASELINE ASSESSMENT

Assess baseline CBC, platelet count, serum creatinine, Hgb, AST, ALT, electrolytes, uric acid and monitor during treatment. Drug should be discontinued if intractable vomiting, diarrhea, stomatitis, GI bleeding occurs.

INTERVENTION/EVALUATION

Assess for fatigue, visual disturbances, peripheral edema. Assess for onset of pneumonia. Monitor for dyspnea, cough, rapid decrease in WBC count, intractable vomiting, diarrhea, GI bleeding (bright red or tarry stool). Assess oral mucosa for erythema, ulceration at inner margin of lips, sore throat, difficulty swallowing (stomatitis). Assess skin for rash. Be alert to possible tumor lysis syndrome (onset of flank pain, hematuria), signs of neurotoxicity.

PATIENT/FAMILY TEACHING

• Avoid crowds, exposure to infection. • Maintain fastidious oral hygiene. • Promptly report fever, sore throat, signs of local infection, unusual bruising/bleeding from any site. • Contact physician if nausea/vomiting continues.

flumazenil

flew-**maz**-ah-nil
(Anexate ✤, Romazicon)

BLACK BOX ALERT Benzodiazepine reversal may produce seizures.

◆CLASSIFICATION

PHARMACOTHERAPEUTIC: Benzodiazepine receptor antagonist. **CLINICAL:** Antidote.

ACTION

Antagonizes effect of benzodiazepines on gamma-aminobutyric acid (GABA) receptor complex in CNS. **Therapeutic Effect:** Reverses sedative effect of benzodiazepines.

PHARMACOKINETICS

Route	Onset	Peak	Duration
IV	1–2 min	6–10 min	Less than 1 hr

Duration, degree of benzodiazepine reversal directly related to dosage, plasma concentration. Protein binding: 50%. Metabolized by liver; excreted in urine. **Half-life:** 41–79 min.

USES

Complete or partial reversal of sedative effects of benzodiazepines when general

F

anesthesia has been induced and/or maintained with benzodiazepines, when sedation has been produced with benzodiazepines for diagnostic and therapeutic procedures, management of benzodiazepine overdosage.

PRECAUTIONS

Contraindications: History of hypersensitivity to benzodiazepines; pts who have been administered benzodiazepines for control of a potentially life-threatening condition (increased ICP, status epilepticus); pts exhibiting signs/symptoms of tricyclic antidepressant overdose (anticholinergic signs [mydriasis, dry mucosa, hypoperistalsis], arrhythmias, motor abnormalities, cardiovascular collapse). **Cautions:** Head injury, hepatic impairment, alcoholism, drug dependency.

LIFESPAN CONSIDERATIONS

Pregnancy/Lactation: Unknown whether drug crosses placenta or is distributed in breast milk. Not recommended during labor, delivery. **Pregnancy Category C. Children:** No age-related precautions noted. **Elderly:** Benzodiazepine-induced sedation tends to be deeper, more prolonged, requiring careful monitoring.

INTERACTIONS

DRUG: Toxic effects (e.g., seizures, arrhythmias) of other drugs taken in overdosage (esp. **tricyclic antidepressants)** may emerge with reversal of sedative effects of **benzodiazepines. HERBAL:** None significant. **FOOD:** None known. **LAB VALUES:** None significant.

AVAILABILITY (Rx)

Injection Solution: 0.1 mg/ml (5 ml, 10 ml).

ADMINISTRATION/HANDLING

ALERT Compatible with D_5W, lactated Ringer's, 0.9% NaCl.

Rate of administration • **Reversal of conscious sedation or general anesthesia:** Give over 15 sec. • **Reversal of benzodiazepine overdose:** Give over 30 sec. • Administer through freely running IV infusion into large vein (local injection produces pain, inflammation at injection site). Do not exceed 0.2 mg/min in children, adults (reversal general anesthesia); 0.5 mg/min in adults (reversal benzodiazepine overdose).

Storage • Store parenteral form at room temperature. • Discard after 24 hrs once medication is drawn into syringe, is mixed with any solutions, or if particulate/discoloration is noted. • Rinse spilled medication from skin with cool water.

IV INCOMPATIBILITIES

No information available for Y-site administration.

IV COMPATIBILITIES

Aminophylline, cimetidine (Tagamet), dobutamine (Dobutrex), dopamine (Intropin), famotidine (Pepcid), heparin, lidocaine, procainamide (Pronestyl), ranitidine (Zantac).

INDICATIONS/ROUTES/DOSAGE

Reversal of Conscious Sedation or General Anesthesia

IV: ADULTS, ELDERLY: Initially, 0.2 mg (2 ml) over 15 sec; may repeat dose in 45 sec; then at 60-sec intervals. **Maximum:** 1 mg (usual 0.6–1 mg). If re-sedation occurs, repeat doses may be given at 20-min intervals with 1 mg/dose and 3 mg/hr maximum dose. **CHILDREN, NEONATES:** Initially, 0.01 mg/kg (**Maximum:** 0.2 mg); may repeat in 45 sec, then at 60-sec intervals at dose of 0.005–0.01 mg/kg. **Maximum:** 0.2 mg single dose. **Maximum total dose:** 1 mg or 0.05 mg/kg (whichever is less).

Benzodiazepine Overdose

IV: ADULTS, ELDERLY: Initially, 0.2 mg (2 ml) over 30 sec; if desired LOC is not achieved after 30 sec, 0.3 mg (3 ml) may be given over 30 sec. Additional doses of 0.5 mg (5 ml) may be administered over 30 sec at 60-sec intervals. **Maximum:** 1 mg/dose or 3 mg/hr. Pts with partial response at 3 mg may require titration to total dose of 5 mg. If no response at 5 mg, major cause of sedation not likely benzodiazepine.

SIDE EFFECTS

Frequent (11%–3%): Agitation, anxiety, dry mouth, dyspnea, insomnia, palpitations, tremors, headache, blurred vision, dizziness, ataxia, nausea, vomiting, pain at injection site, diaphoresis. **Occasional (2%–1%):** Fatigue, flushing, auditory disturbances, thrombophlebitis, rash. **Rare (less than 1%):** Urticaria, pruritus, hallucinations.

ADVERSE EFFECTS/ TOXIC REACTIONS

Toxic effects (seizures, arrhythmias) of other drugs taken in overdose (esp. tricyclic antidepressants) may emerge with reversal of sedative effect of benzodiazepines. May provoke panic attack in those with a history of panic disorder.

NURSING CONSIDERATIONS

BASELINE ASSESSMENT

ABGs should be obtained prior to and at 30-min intervals during IV administration. Prepare to intervene in reestablishing airway, assisting ventilation (drug may not fully reverse ventilatory insufficiency induced by benzodiazepines). Note that effects of flumazenil may dissipate before effects of benzodiazepines.

INTERVENTION/EVALUATION

Properly manage airway, assist breathing, maintain circulatory access and support, perform internal decontamination by lavage and charcoal as indicated, provide adequate clinical evaluation. Monitor for reversal of benzodiazepine effect. Assess for possible resedation, respiratory depression, hypoventilation. Assess closely for return of unconsciousness (narcosis) for at least 1–2 hrs after pt is fully alert.

PATIENT/FAMILY TEACHING

- Avoid ingestion of alcohol, tasks that require alertness, motor skills or taking nonprescription drugs until at least 24 hrs after discharge.

flunisolide

floo-**niss**-oh-lide
(AeroBid, AeroBid-M, Apo-Flunisolide ✤, Bronalide ✤, Nasalide ✤, Nasarel, Rhinalar ✤)
Do not confuse flunisolide with fluocinonide, or Nasarel with Nizoral.

◆CLASSIFICATION

PHARMACOTHERAPEUTIC: Adrenocorticosteroid. **CLINICAL:** Antiasthmatic, anti-inflammatory (see pp. 2C, 75C, 98C).

ACTION

Controls rate of protein synthesis, depresses migration of polymorphonuclear leukocytes, reverses capillary permeability, stabilizes lysosomal membranes. **Therapeutic Effect:** Prevents, controls inflammation.

PHARMACOKINETICS

Rapidly absorbed from lungs and GI tract following inhalation. About 50% of dose is absorbed from nasal mucosa following intranasal administration. Metabolized in liver. Partially excreted in urine and feces. **Half-life:** 1–2 hrs.

USES

Inhalation: Long-term control of persistent bronchial asthma. Assists in reducing, discontinuing oral corticosteroid therapy. **Intranasal:** Relieves symptoms of seasonal, perennial rhinitis. **OFF-LABEL:** Prevents recurrence of nasal polyps after surgery.

PRECAUTIONS

Contraindications: Hypersensitivity to any corticosteroid, persistently positive sputum cultures for *Candida albicans*, primary treatment of status asthmaticus, systemic fungal infections. **Cautions:** Adrenal insufficiency. Increased susceptibility to infections.

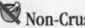

LIFESPAN CONSIDERATIONS

Pregnancy/Lactation: Unknown if distributed in breast milk. **Pregnancy Category C. Children:** Safety and efficacy not established. **Elderly:** No age-related cautions noted.

INTERACTIONS

DRUG: May decrease effects of **live vaccines. HERBAL: Echinacea** may decrease effects. **FOOD:** None known. **LAB VALUES:** None significant.

AVAILABILITY (Rx)

Aerosol with Adapter (AeroBid): 250 mcg/activation. **Aerosol (AeroBid-M):** 250 mcg/activation. **Nasal Spray (Nasarel):** 25 mcg/activation.

ADMINISTRATION/HANDLING

Inhalation

• Shake container well. Instruct pt to exhale completely, place mouthpiece fully into mouth, inhale, hold breath as long as possible before exhaling. • Allow at least 1 min between inhalations. • Rinsing mouth after each use decreases dry mouth, hoarseness.

Intranasal

• Instruct pt to clear nasal passages as much as possible before use (topical nasal decongestants may be needed 5–15 min before use). • Tilt head slightly forward. • Insert spray tip into nostril, pointing toward inflamed nasal turbinates, away from nasal septum. • Pump medication into one nostril while pt holds other nostril closed, concurrently inspires through nose. • Discard opened nasal solution after 3 mos.

INDICATIONS/ROUTES/DOSAGE

Usual Inhalation Dosage

INHALATION: ADULTS, ELDERLY, CHILDREN 16 YRS AND OLDER: 2 inhalations twice a day, morning and evening. **Maximum:** 4 inhalations twice a day. **CHILDREN 6–15 YRS:** 2 inhalations, twice a day. **Maximum:** 4 inhalations/day.

Usual Intranasal Dosage

◄ALERT► Improvement usually seen within a few days; may take up to 3 wks. Discontinue use after 3 wks if no significant improvement occurs.

INTRANASAL: ADULTS, ELDERLY, CHILDREN 15 YRS AND OLDER: Initially, 2 sprays each nostril twice a day, may increase at 4- to 7-day intervals to 2 sprays 3 times a day. **Maximum:** 8 sprays in each nostril daily. **CHILDREN 6–14 YRS:** Initially, 1 spray 3 times a day or 2 sprays twice a day. **Maximum:** 4 sprays in each nostril daily. Maintenance: 1 spray into each nostril daily.

SIDE EFFECTS

Frequent: Inhalation (25%–10%): Unpleasant taste, nausea, vomiting, sore throat, diarrhea, cold symptoms, nasal congestion. **Occasional: Inhalation (9%–3%):** Dizziness, irritability, anxiety, tremors, abdominal pain, heartburn, oropharyngeal candidiasis, edema. **Nasal:** Mild nasopharyngeal irritation/dryness, rebound congestion, bronchial asthma, rhinorrhea, altered taste.

ADVERSE EFFECTS/ TOXIC REACTIONS

Acute hypersensitivity reaction (urticaria, angioedema, severe bronchospasm) occurs rarely. Transfer from systemic to local steroid therapy may unmask previously suppressed bronchial asthma condition.

NURSING CONSIDERATIONS

BASELINE ASSESSMENT

Establish baseline assessment of asthma, rhinitis.

INTERVENTION/EVALUATION

Advise pts receiving bronchodilators by inhalation concomitantly with steroid inhalation therapy to use bronchodilator several min before corticosteroid aerosol (enhances penetration of steroid into bronchial tree). Monitor rate, depth, rhythm, type of respiration;

quality/rate of pulse. Assess lung sounds for rhonchi, wheezing, rales. Monitor ABGs.

PATIENT/FAMILY TEACHING

• Notify physician if exposed to measles, chicken pox. • Do not change dose/schedule or stop taking drug; must taper off gradually under medical supervision. • Maintain fastidious oral hygiene. • Rinse mouth with water immediately after inhalation (prevents mouth/throat dryness, oral fungal infection). • Increase fluid intake (decreases lung secretion viscosity). • **Intranasal:** • Clear nasal passages before use. • Contact physician if no improvement in symptoms, sneezing or nasal irritation occurs. • Improvement usually noted in several days.

fluorouracil, 5-FU HIGH ALERT

flur-oh-**your**-ah-sill
(Adrucil, Carac, Efudex, Fluoroplex)

BLACK BOX ALERT Must be administered by personnel trained in administration/handling of chemotherapeutic agents.

Do not confuse Efudex with Efidac.

CLASSIFICATION

PHARMACOTHERAPEUTIC: Antimetabolite. **CLINICAL:** Antineoplastic (see p. 83C).

ACTION

Blocks formation of thymidylic acid. Cell cycle-specific for S phase of cell division. **Therapeutic Effect:** Inhibits DNA, RNA synthesis. **Topical:** Destroys rapidly proliferating cells.

PHARMACOKINETICS

Widely distributed. Crosses blood-brain barrier. Metabolized in liver. Primarily excreted by lungs as carbon dioxide. Removed by hemodialysis. **Half-life:** 16 min.

USES

Parenteral: Treatment of carcinoma of colon, rectum, breast, stomach, pancreas. Used in combination with levamisole after surgical resection in pts with Dukes stage C colon cancer. **Topical:** Treatment of multiple actinic or solar keratoses, superficial basal cell carcinomas. **OFF-LABEL:** **Parenteral:** Treatment of bladder, cervical, endometrial, head/neck, liver, lung, ovarian, prostate carcinomas; treatment of pericardial, peritoneal, pleural effusions. **Topical:** Treatment of actinic cheilitis, radiodermatitis.

PRECAUTIONS

Contraindications: Major surgery (within previous 30 days), myelosuppression, poor nutritional status, potentially serious infections. **Cautions:** History of high-dose pelvic irradiation, metastatic cell infiltration of bone marrow, hepatic/renal impairment.

LIFESPAN CONSIDERATIONS

Pregnancy/Lactation: If possible, avoid use during pregnancy, esp. first trimester. May cause fetal harm. Unknown if distributed in breast milk. Breast-feeding not recommended. **Pregnancy Category D. Topical: Pregnancy Category X. Children:** No age-related precautions noted. **Elderly:** Age-related renal impairment may require dosage adjustment.

INTERACTIONS

DRUG: **Bone marrow depressants** may increase risk of myelosuppression. **Live virus vaccines** may potentiate virus replication, increase vaccine side effects, decrease pt's antibody response to vaccine. **HERBAL:** Avoid use of **black cohosh, dong quai** in pts with estrogen-dependent tumors. **FOOD:** None known. **LAB VALUES:** May decrease serum albumin. **Topical:** May cause eosinophilia, leukocytosis, thrombocytopenia, toxic granulation.

AVAILABILITY (Rx)

Cream, Topical: (Carac): 0.5%: **(Efudex):** 5%: **(Fluoroplex):** 1%. **Injection Solution:**

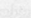

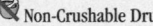

(Adrucil): 50 mg/ml. Solution, Topical: (Efudex): 2%, 5%.

ADMINISTRATION/HANDLING

◀ALERT▶ Give by IV injection or IV infusion. Do not add to other IV infusions. Avoid small veins, swollen/edematous extremities, areas overlying joints, tendons. May be carcinogenic, mutagenic, teratogenic. Handle with extreme care during preparation/administration.

IV

Reconstitution • IV push does not need to be diluted or reconstituted. • Inject through Y-tube or 3-way stopcock of free-flowing solution. • For IV infusion, further dilute with 50–1,000 ml D_5W or 0.9% NaCl.

Rate of administration • Give IV push slowly over 1–2 min. • IV infusion is administered over 30 min–24 hrs. • Extravasation produces immediate pain, severe local tissue damage. • Follow protocol.

Storage • Solution appears colorless to faint yellow. Slight discoloration does not adversely affect potency or safety. • If precipitate forms, redissolve by heating, shaking vigorously; allow to cool to body temperature. • Diluted solutions stable for 72 hrs at room temperature.

IV INCOMPATIBILITIES

Amphotericin B complex (Abelcet, AmBisome, Amphotec), droperidol (Inapsine), filgrastim (Neupogen), ondansetron (Zofran), vinorelbine (Navelbine).

IV COMPATIBILITIES

Granisetron (Kytril), heparin, hydromorphone (Dilaudid), leucovorin, morphine, potassium chloride, propofol (Diprivan), total parenteral nutrition (TPN).

INDICATIONS/ROUTES/DOSAGE

Refer to individual protocols.

Usual Therapy

IV BOLUS: ADULTS, ELDERLY: 500–600 mg/m² q3–4 wks.

IV INFUSION: ADULTS, ELDERLY: 1,000 mg/m²/day for 4–5 days every 3–4 wks.

Multiple Actinic or Solar Keratoses

TOPICAL (CARAC): ADULTS, ELDERLY: Apply once a day for up to 4 wks.

TOPICAL (EFUDEX, FLUOROPLEX): ADULTS, ELDERLY: Apply twice a day for 2–6 wks.

Basal Cell Carcinoma

TOPICAL (EFUDEX): ADULTS, ELDERLY: Apply twice a day for 3–6 wks up to 10–12 wks.

SIDE EFFECTS

Occasional: **Parenteral:** Anorexia, diarrhea, minimal alopecia, fever, dry skin, skin fissures, scaling, erythema. **Topical:** Pain, pruritus, hyperpigmentation, irritation, inflammation, burning at application site, photosensitivity. Rare: Nausea, vomiting, anemia, esophagitis, proctitis, GI ulcer, confusion, headache, lacrimation, visual disturbances, angina, allergic reaction.

ADVERSE EFFECTS/ TOXIC REACTIONS

Earliest sign of toxicity (4–8 days after beginning therapy) is stomatitis (dry mouth, burning sensation, mucosal erythema, ulceration at inner margin of lips). Most common dermatologic toxicity is pruritic rash (generally on extremities, less frequently on trunk). Leukopenia generally occurs within 9–14 days after drug administration but may occur as late as 25th day. Thrombocytopenia occasionally occurs within 7–17 days after administration. Pancytopenia, agranulocytosis occur rarely.

NURSING CONSIDERATIONS

BASELINE ASSESSMENT

Obtain baseline CBC with differential, platelet count, serum renal/hepatic function tests and monitor during therapy.

INTERVENTION/EVALUATION

Monitor for rapidly falling WBC count, intractable diarrhea, GI bleeding (bright red or tarry stool). Assess oral mucosa for stomatitis. Drug should be discontinued if intractable diarrhea, stomatitis, GI bleeding occurs. Assess skin for rash.

PATIENT/FAMILY TEACHING

• Maintain fastidious oral hygiene. • Inform physician of signs/symptoms of infection, unusual bruising/bleeding, visual changes, nausea, vomiting, diarrhea, chest pain, palpitations. • Avoid sunlight, artificial light sources; wear protective clothing, sunglasses, sunscreen. • **Topical:** Apply only to affected area. • Do not use occlusive coverings. • Be careful near eyes, nose, mouth. • Wash hands thoroughly after application. • Treated areas may be unsightly for several weeks after therapy.

fluoxetine

floo-**ox**-e-teen
(Apo-Fluoxetine ✤, Novo-Fluoxetine ✤, Prozac, Prozac Weekly, Sarafem, Selfemra)

BLACK BOX ALERT Increased risk of suicidal thinking and behavior in children, adolescents, young adults 18–24 yrs of age with major depressive disorder, other psychiatric disorders.

Do not confuse fluoxetine with duloxetine, famotidine, fluconazole, or fluvastatin, Prozac with Prilosec, Proscar, or ProSom, or Sarafem with Serophene.

FIXED-COMBINATION(S)

Symbyax: fluoxetine/olanzapine (an antipsychotic): 25 mg/6 mg, 25 mg/12 mg, 50 mg/6 mg, 50 mg/12 mg.

◆CLASSIFICATION

PHARMACOTHERAPEUTIC: Psychotherapeutic. **CLINICAL:** Antidepressant, antiobsessional agent, antibulimic (see p. 39C).

ACTION

Selectively inhibits serotonin uptake in CNS, enhancing serotonergic function. **Therapeutic Effect:** Relieves depression; reduces obsessive-compulsive, bulimic behavior.

PHARMACOKINETICS

Well absorbed from GI tract. Crosses blood-brain barrier. Protein binding: 94%. Metabolized in liver to active metabolite. Primarily excreted in urine. Not removed by hemodialysis. **Half-life:** 2–3 days; metabolite, 7–9 days.

USES

Treatment of clinical depression, obsessive-compulsive disorder (OCD), bulimia nervosa, premenstrual dysphoric disorder (PMDD), panic disorder. **OFF-LABEL:** Treatment of body dysmorphic disorder, fibromyalgia, hot flashes, post-traumatic stress disorder (PTSD), Raynaud's phenomena, premature ejaculation, selective mutism.

PRECAUTIONS

Contraindications: Use within 14 days of MAOIs. **Cautions:** Seizure disorder, cardiac dysfunction, diabetes, those at high risk for suicide. May prolong QT interval.

⌛ LIFESPAN CONSIDERATIONS

Pregnancy/Lactation: Unknown whether drug crosses placenta or is distributed in breast milk. **Pregnancy Category C. Children:** May be more sensitive to behavioral side effects (e.g., insomnia, restlessness). **Elderly:** No age-related precautions noted.

INTERACTIONS

DRUG: Aspirin, NSAIDs may increase risk of bleeding. **Alcohol, other CNS depressants** may increase CNS depression. **Highly protein-bound medications (e.g., oral anticoagulants)** may increase adverse effects. **MAOIs** may produce serotonin syndrome and neuroleptic malignant syndrome. May increase **phenytoin** concentration, risk of toxicity. May increase concentration/toxicity of **tricyclic antidepressants.** HERBAL: **Gotu kola, kava kava, St. John's wort, valerian** may increase CNS depression. **St. John's wort** may increase effects, risk of toxicity. FOOD: None known. LAB VALUES: None significant.

F

AVAILABILITY (Rx)

Capsules: 10 mg (Prozac, Sarafem, Selfemra), 20 mg (Prozac, Sarafem, Selfemra), 40 mg (Prozac). **Oral Solution (Prozac):** 20 mg/5 ml. **Tablets (Sarafem):** 10 mg, 20 mg.

Capsules (Delayed-Release [Prozac Weekly]): 90 mg.

ADMINISTRATION/HANDLING

PO

- Give without regard to food, but give with food, milk if GI distress occurs.

INDICATIONS/ROUTES/DOSAGE

◄ALERT► Use lower or less frequent doses in pts with renal/hepatic impairment, those with concurrent disease or multiple medications, the elderly.

Depression

PO: ADULTS: Initially, 20 mg each morning. If therapeutic improvement does not occur after 2 wks, gradually increase to maximum of 80 mg/day in 2 equally divided doses in morning and at noon. **ELDERLY:** Initially, 10 mg/day. May increase by 10–20 mg q2wk. **Prozac Weekly:** 90 mg/wk, begin 7 days after last dose of 20 mg. **CHILDREN 7–17 YRS:** Initially, 5–10 mg/day. Titrate upward as needed. Usual dosage: 20 mg/day.

Panic Disorder

PO: ADULTS, ELDERLY: Initially, 10 mg/day. May increase to 20 mg/day after 1 wk. **Maximum:** 60 mg/day.

Bulimia Nervosa

PO: ADULTS: 60–80 mg each morning.

Obsessive-Compulsive Disorder (OCD)

PO: ADULTS, ELDERLY: 40–80 mg/day. **CHILDREN 7–18 YRS:** Initially, 10 mg/day. May increase to 20 mg/day after 2 wks. Range: 10–60 mg/day.

Premenstrual Dysphoric Disorder (PMDD) (Sarafem)

PO: ADULTS: 20 mg/day **or** 20 mg/day beginning 14 days prior to menstruation and continuing through first full day of menses (repeated with each cycle).

SIDE EFFECTS

Frequent (greater than 10%): Headache, asthenia (loss of strength, energy), insomnia, anxiety, drowsiness, nausea, diarrhea, decreased appetite. **Occasional (9%–2%):** Dizziness, tremor, fatigue, vomiting, constipation, dry mouth, abdominal pain, nasal congestion, diaphoresis, rash. **Rare (less than 2%):** Flushed skin, light-headedness, impaired concentration.

ADVERSE EFFECTS/ TOXIC REACTIONS

Overdose may produce seizures, nausea, vomiting, excessive agitation, restlessness.

NURSING CONSIDERATIONS

BASELINE ASSESSMENT

Assess appearance, behavior, mood, suicidal tendencies. For pts on long-term therapy, baseline hepatic/renal function tests, blood counts; testing should be performed periodically thereafter.

INTERVENTION/EVALUATION

Supervise suicidal-risk pt closely during early therapy (as depression lessens, energy level improves, increasing suicide potential). Monitor mental status, anxiety, social functioning, appetite, nutritional intake. Monitor daily pattern of bowel activity and stool consistency. Assess skin for rash. Monitor serum hepatic function tests, glucose, sodium, weight.

PATIENT/FAMILY TEACHING

• Maximum therapeutic response may require 4 or more wks of therapy. • Do not abruptly discontinue medication. • Avoid tasks that require alertness, motor skills until response to drug is established. • Avoid alcohol. • To avoid insomnia, take last dose of drug before 4 PM.

fluphenazine hydrochloride (oral)

fluphenazine decanoate (injection)

floo-**fen**-a-zeen
(Apo-Fluphenazine ✤, Modecate ✤, Prolixin, Prolixin Decanoate)

BLACK BOX ALERT Increased mortality in elderly with dementia-related psychosis.

Do not confuse Prolixin with Proloprim.

◆CLASSIFICATION

PHARMACOTHERAPEUTIC: Phenothiazine. **CLINICAL:** Antipsychotic (see p. 65C).

ACTION

Antagonizes dopamine neurotransmission at synapses by blocking postsynaptic dopaminergic receptors in brain. **Therapeutic Effect:** Decreases psychotic behavior. Produces weak anticholinergic, sedative, antiemetic effects; strong extrapyramidal effects.

PHARMACOKINETICS

Erratic absorption. Protein binding: greater than 90%. Metabolized in liver. Excreted in urine. **Half-life:** 33 hrs (Decanoate: 163–232 hrs).

USES

Management of psychotic disturbances (schizophrenia, delusions, hallucinations). **OFF-LABEL:** Treatment of neurogenic pain (adjunct to tricyclic antidepressants), pervasive developmental disorder, psychosis, agitation related to Alzheimer's dementia.

PRECAUTIONS

Contraindications: Narrow-angle glaucoma, myelosuppression, severe cardiac/hepatic disease, severe hypertension/hypotension, subcortical brain damage. **Cautions:** Seizures, Parkinson's disease.

⌛ LIFESPAN CONSIDERATIONS

Pregnancy/Lactation: Crosses placenta; distributed in breast milk. **Pregnancy Category C. Children:** Those with acute illnesses (e.g., chickenpox, measles, gastroenteritis, CNS infection) are at risk for developing neuromuscular, extrapyramidal symptoms (EPS), particularly dystonias. **Elderly:** Susceptible to anticholinergic effects.

INTERACTIONS

DRUG: **Alcohol, other CNS depressants** may increase hypotensive, CNS, respiratory depressant effects. **Antithyroid agents** may increase risk of agranulocytosis. Extrapyramidal symptoms (EPS) may increase with **medications producing EPS. Antihypertensive medications, hypotensive agents** may increase hypotension. May decrease effects of **levodopa. Lithium** may decrease absorption, produce adverse neurologic effects. **MAOIs, tricyclic antidepressants** may increase anticholinergic, sedative effects. **Medications prolonging QT interval (e.g., erythromycin)** may have additive effect. **HERBAL:** **Dong quai, St. John's wort** may increase photosensitization. **Gotu kola, kava kava, St. John's wort, valerian** may increase CNS depression. **FOOD:** None known. **LAB VALUES:** May produce false-positive pregnancy, phenylketonuria test results. May cause EKG changes, including Q- and T-wave disturbances.

AVAILABILITY (Rx)

Elixir (Prolixin): 2.5 mg/5 ml. **Injection, Oil (Prolixin Decanoate):** 25 mg/ml. **Injection Solution (Prolixin):** 2.5 mg/ml. **Oral Concentrate (Prolixin):** 5 mg/ml. **Tablets (Prolixin):** 1 mg, 2.5 mg, 5 mg, 10 mg.

ADMINISTRATION/HANDLING

• Avoid skin contact with fluphenazine solution (may cause contact dermatitis). • Dilute oral liquid only with water, milk, juice. Do not dilute with caffeine-containing beverages.

INDICATIONS/ROUTES/DOSAGE

Psychosis

PO: ADULTS, ELDERLY: 0.5–10 mg/day in divided doses q6–8h. **Maximum:** 40 mg/day.
IM: ADULTS, ELDERLY: 2.5–10 mg/day in divided doses q6–8h (or 12.5–37.5 mg q2wk as decanoate).

SIDE EFFECTS

Frequent: Hypotension, dizziness, syncope (occur frequently after first injection, occasionally after subsequent injections, rarely with oral doses). **Occasional:** Drowsiness (during early therapy), dry mouth, blurred vision, lethargy, constipation or diarrhea, nasal congestion, peripheral edema, urinary retention. **Rare:** Ocular changes, altered skin pigmentation (with prolonged use of high doses).

ADVERSE EFFECTS/ TOXIC REACTIONS

Extrapyramidal symptoms (EPS) appear dose related (particularly high dosage), divided into 3 categories: akathisia (inability to sit still, tapping of feet, urge to move around), parkinsonian symptoms (hypersalivation, mask-like facial expression, shuffling gait, tremors), acute dystonias (torticollis [neck muscle spasm], opisthotonos [rigidity of back muscles], oculogyric crisis [rolling back of eyes]). Dystonic reaction may produce diaphoresis, pallor. Tardive dyskinesia (tongue protrusion, puffing of cheeks, chewing/puckering of the mouth) occurs rarely but may be irreversible. Abrupt withdrawal after long-term therapy may precipitate dizziness, gastritis, nausea, vomiting, tremors. Blood dyscrasias, particularly agranulocytosis, mild leukopenia, may occur. May lower seizure threshold.

NURSING CONSIDERATIONS

BASELINE ASSESSMENT

Avoid skin contact with solution (may cause contact dermatitis). Assess behavior, appearance, emotional status, response to environment, speech pattern, thought content.

INTERVENTION/EVALUATION

Monitor B/P for hypotension. Monitor CBC for blood dyscrasias. Monitor for fine tongue movement (may be early sign of tardive dyskinesia). Supervise suicidal-risk pt closely during early therapy (as depression lessens, energy level improves, increasing suicide potential). Assess for therapeutic response (interest in surroundings, improvement in self-care, increased ability to concentrate, relaxed facial expression).

PATIENT/FAMILY TEACHING

• Full therapeutic effect may take up to 6 wks. • Urine may darken. • Do not abruptly withdraw from long-term drug therapy. • Avoid tasks that require alertness, motor skills until response to drug is established. • Drowsiness generally subsides during continued therapy.

flurazepam

flur-**az**-e-pam
(Apo-Flurazepam ✦, Dalmane)
Do not confuse Dalmane with Dialume, or flurazepam with temazepam.

◆CLASSIFICATION

PHARMACOTHERAPEUTIC: Benzodiazepine (**Schedule IV**). **CLINICAL:** Sedative-hypnotic (see p. 149C).

ACTION

Enhances action of inhibitory neurotransmitter gamma-aminobutyric acid (GABA). **Therapeutic Effect:** Produces hypnotic effect due to CNS depression.

PHARMACOKINETICS

Route	Onset	Peak	Duration
PO	15–20 min	3–6 hrs	7–8 hrs

Well absorbed from GI tract. Protein binding: 97%. Crosses blood-brain barrier. Widely distributed. Metabolized in liver to active metabolite. Primarily excreted in urine. Not removed by hemodialysis. **Half-life:** 2.3 hrs; metabolite, 40–114 hrs.

USES

Short-term treatment of insomnia (4 wks or less). Reduces sleep-induction time, number of nocturnal awakenings; increases length of sleep.

PRECAUTIONS

Contraindications: Acute alcohol intoxication, narrow angle glaucoma, hypersensitivity to other benzodiazepines, pregnancy, breast-feeding. **Cautions:** Renal/hepatic impairment.

LIFESPAN CONSIDERATIONS

Pregnancy/Lactation: Crosses placenta; may be distributed in breast milk. Chronic ingestion during pregnancy may produce withdrawal symptoms, CNS depression in neonates. **Pregnancy Category X. Children:** Safety and efficacy not established in those younger than 15 yrs. **Elderly:** Use small initial doses with gradual dose increases to avoid ataxia, excessive sedation.

INTERACTIONS

DRUG: **Alcohol, CNS depressants** may increase CNS depression. **Azole antifungals** may increase concentration, risk of toxicity. **HERBAL:** **Gotu kola, kava kava, St. John's wort, valerian** may increase CNS depression. **FOOD:** None known. **LAB VALUES:** None significant.

AVAILABILITY (Rx)

Capsules: 15 mg, 30 mg.

ADMINISTRATION/HANDLING

PO

• Give without regard to meals. • Capsules may be emptied and mixed with food.

INDICATIONS/ROUTES/DOSAGE

Insomnia

PO: ELDERLY, DEBILITATED, HEPATIC DISEASE, LOW SERUM ALBUMIN: 15 mg at bedtime. **ADULTS:** 15–30 mg at bedtime. **CHILDREN OLDER THAN 15 YRS:** 15 mg at bedtime.

SIDE EFFECTS

Frequent: Drowsiness, dizziness, ataxia, sedation. Morning drowsiness occurs initially. **Occasional:** GI disturbances, anxiety, blurred vision, dry mouth, headache, confusion, skin rash, irritability, slurred speech. **Rare:** Paradoxical CNS excitement, restlessness (esp. in elderly, debilitated).

ADVERSE EFFECTS/ TOXIC REACTIONS

Abrupt or too-rapid withdrawal after long-term use may result in pronounced restlessness/irritability, insomnia, hand tremors, abdominal/muscle cramps, vomiting, diaphoresis, seizures. Overdose results in drowsiness, confusion, diminished reflexes, coma.

NURSING CONSIDERATIONS

BASELINE ASSESSMENT

Assess B/P, pulse, respirations immediately before administration. Provide safe environment conducive to sleep (back rub, quiet environment, low lighting, raise bed rails).

INTERVENTION/EVALUATION

Assess for paradoxical reaction, particularly during early therapy. Evaluate for therapeutic response (decrease in number of nocturnal awakenings, increase in sleep duration).

PATIENT/FAMILY TEACHING

• Smoking reduces drug effectiveness. • Do not abruptly withdraw medication after long-term use. • May have disturbed sleep pattern 1–2 nights after discontinuing. • Notify physician if pregnant or planning to become pregnant (Pregnancy Category X). • Avoid alcohol, other CNS depressants. • May be habit forming.

F

flurbiprofen

flur-bi-proe-fen
(Apo-Flurbiprofen ✱, Ansaid ✱, Froben ✱, Froben SR ✱, Ocufen)

BLACK BOX ALERT Increased risk of serious cardiovascular thrombotic events, including myocardial infarction, CVA. Increased risk of severe GI reactions, including ulceration, bleeding, perforation of stomach, intestines.

Do not confuse Ansaid with Asacol or Axid, flurbiprofen with fenoprofen, or Ocufen with Ocuflox.

◆CLASSIFICATION

PHARMACOTHERAPEUTIC: Phenylalkanoic acid. **CLINICAL:** Nonsteroidal anti-inflammatory, antidysmenorrheal (see p. 128C).

ACTION

Produces analgesic, anti-inflammatory effect by inhibiting prostaglandin synthesis. Relaxes iris sphincter. **Therapeutic Effect:** Reduces inflammatory response, intensity of pain. Prevents, decreases miosis during cataract surgery.

PHARMACOKINETICS

Well absorbed from GI tract; ophthalmic solution penetrates cornea after administration (may be systemically absorbed). Protein binding: 99%. Widely distributed. Metabolized in liver. Primarily excreted in urine. **Half-life:** 5.7 hrs.

USES

PO: Symptomatic treatment of acute and/or chronic rheumatoid arthritis, osteoarthritis, dysmenorrhea, pain. **Ophthalmic:** Inhibits intraoperative miosis. **OFF-LABEL: PO:** Ankylosing spondylitis, dental pain, postop gynecologic pain.

PRECAUTIONS

Contraindications: Active peptic ulcer; chronic inflammation of GI tract; GI bleeding, ulceration; history of hypersensitivity to aspirin, NSAIDs. **Cautions:** Renal/hepatic impairment, history of GI tract disease, predisposition to fluid retention, soft contact lens wearers, surgical pts with bleeding tendencies.

⌛ LIFESPAN CONSIDERATIONS

Pregnancy/Lactation: Crosses placenta. Unknown if distributed in breast milk. Avoid use during last trimester (may adversely affect fetal cardiovascular system, i.e., premature closure of ductus arteriosus). **Pregnancy Category C (D if used in third trimester or near delivery). Ophthalmic: Pregnancy Category C. Children:** Safety and efficacy not established. **Elderly:** GI bleeding/ulceration more likely to cause serious adverse effects. Age-related renal impairment may increase risk of hepatic/renal toxicity; decreased dosage recommended.

INTERACTIONS

DRUG: May decrease effects of **antihypertensives, diuretics. Aspirin, other salicylates** may increase risk of GI side effects, bleeding. May increase effects of **heparin, oral anticoagulants, thrombolytics.** May increase concentration, risk of toxicity of **cyclosporine, lithium.** May increase risk of **methotrexate** toxicity. **Probenecid** may increase concentration. **HERBAL: Cat's claw, dong quai, evening primrose, feverfew, garlic, ginger, ginkgo, ginseng, horse chestnut, red clover, SAMe** may increase antiplatelet activity. **FOOD:** None known. **LAB VALUES:** May increase bleeding time, serum alkaline phosphatase, LDH, AST, ALT. May decrease Hgb, Hct.

AVAILABILITY (Rx)

Ophthalmic Solution (Ocufen): 0.03%.

Tablets (Ansaid): 50 mg, 100 mg.

ADMINISTRATION/HANDLING

PO

• Do not crush, break enteric-coated tablets. • May give with food, milk, antacids if GI distress occurs.

Ophthalmic

• Place gloved finger on lower eyelid and pull out until pocket is formed between eye and lower lid. • Place prescribed number of drops into pocket. Instruct pt to close eye gently for 1–2 min (so medication will not be squeezed out of the sac) and to apply digital pressure to lacrimal sac at inner canthus for 1 min to minimize systemic absorption. • Remove excess solution with tissue.

INDICATIONS/ROUTES/DOSAGE

Rheumatoid Arthritis (RA), Osteoarthritis

PO: ADULTS, ELDERLY: 200–300 mg/day in 2–4 divided doses. **Maximum:** 100 mg/dose or 300 mg/day.

Dysmenorrhea, Pain

PO: ADULTS: 50 mg 4 times a day.

Usual Ophthalmic Dosage

ADULTS, ELDERLY, CHILDREN: Apply 1 drop q30min starting 2 hrs before surgery for total of 4 doses.

SIDE EFFECTS

Occasional: PO (9%–3%): Headache, abdominal pain, diarrhea, indigestion, nausea, fluid retention. **Ophthalmic:** Burning/stinging on instillation, keratitis, elevated intraocular pressure. **Rare (less than 3%): PO:** Blurred vision, flushed skin, dizziness, drowsiness, anxiety, insomnia, unusual fatigue, constipation, decreased appetite, vomiting, confusion.

ADVERSE EFFECTS/ TOXIC REACTIONS

Overdose may result in acute renal failure. Rare reactions with long-term use include peptic ulcer, GI bleeding, gastritis, severe hepatic reaction (jaundice), nephrotoxicity (hematuria, dysuria, proteinuria), severe hypersensitivity reaction (angioedema, bronchospasm), cardiac arrhythmias.

NURSING CONSIDERATIONS

BASELINE ASSESSMENT

Anti-inflammatory: Assess onset, type, location, duration of pain/inflammation. Inspect appearance of affected joints for immobility, deformities, skin condition.

INTERVENTION/EVALUATION

Monitor for headache, dyspepsia, dizziness. Monitor daily pattern of bowel activity and stool consistency. **Systemic Use:** Monitor CBC, platelet count, BUN, serum creatinine, hepatic function tests. Monitor stool for occult blood loss. **Ocular:** Obtain periodic eye exams. **Anti-inflammatory:** Assess for therapeutic response: relief of pain, stiffness, swelling; increased joint mobility; reduced joint tenderness; improved grip strength.

PATIENT/FAMILY TEACHING

• Swallow tablet whole; do not crush, chew. • Avoid aspirin, alcohol (increases risk of GI bleeding). • If GI upset occurs, take with food, milk. • Report GI distress, visual disturbances, rash, edema, headache. • **Ophthalmic:** Eye burning may occur with instillation.

flutamide HIGH ALERT

flew-tah-mide
(Apo-Flutamide ♣, Euflex ♣, Eulexin, Novo-Flutamide ♣)

BLACK BOX ALERT Hospitalization and, rarely, death due to flutamide-associated hepatic failure have been reported.

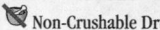

Do not confuse Eulexin with Edecrin, or flutamide with Flumadine.

◆CLASSIFICATION

PHARMACOTHERAPEUTIC: Antiandrogen, hormone. **CLINICAL:** Antineoplastic (see p. 83C).

F

ACTION

Inhibits androgen uptake and/or binding of androgen in target tissue. Used in conjunction with leuprolide to inhibit stimulant effects of flutamide on serum testosterone. **Therapeutic Effect:** Suppresses testicular androgen production, decreases growth of prostate carcinoma.

PHARMACOKINETICS

Completely absorbed from GI tract. Protein binding: 94%–96%. Metabolized in liver to active metabolite. Primarily excreted in urine. Not removed by hemodialysis. **Half-life:** 6 hrs (increased in elderly).

USES

Treatment of metastatic carcinoma of prostate (in combination with luteinizing hormone-releasing hormone [LHRH] analogues, e.g., leuprolide). Management of locally confined stages B_2-C, D_2 carcinoma. **OFF-LABEL:** Female hirsutism.

PRECAUTIONS

Contraindications: Severe hepatic impairment. **Cautions:** None known.

⌛ LIFESPAN CONSIDERATIONS

Pregnancy/Lactation: Not used in this pt population. **Pregnancy Category D. Children:** Not used in children. **Elderly:** No age-related precautions noted.

INTERACTIONS

DRUG: May increase effects of **oral anticoagulants. HERBAL: St. John's wort** may decrease concentration. **FOOD:** None known. **LAB VALUES:** May increase serum glucose, estradiol, testosterone, bilirubin, creatinine, alkaline phosphatase, BUN, AST, ALT. May decrease Hgb, WBC.

AVAILABILITY (Rx)

Capsules: 125 mg.

ADMINISTRATION/HANDLING

PO

• Give without regard to food. • May open and mix with soft food (e.g., applesauce, pudding).

INDICATIONS/ROUTES/DOSAGE

Prostatic Carcinoma

PO: ADULTS, ELDERLY: 250 mg q8h.

SIDE EFFECTS

Frequent: Hot flashes (50%); decreased libido, diarrhea (24%); generalized pain (23%); asthenia (loss of strength, energy) (17%); constipation (12%); nausea, nocturia (11%). **Occasional (8%–6%):** Dizziness, paresthesia, insomnia, impotence, peripheral edema, gynecomastia. **Rare (5%–4%):** Rash, diaphoresis, hypertension, hematuria, vomiting, urinary incontinence, headache, flu-like syndrome, photosensitivity.

ADVERSE EFFECTS/ TOXIC REACTIONS

Hepatotoxicity (including hepatic encephalopathy), hemolytic anemia may occur.

NURSING CONSIDERATIONS

INTERVENTION/EVALUATION

Obtain baseline hepatic function tests and periodically during long-term therapy.

PATIENT/FAMILY TEACHING

• Do not stop taking medication (both drugs must be continued). • Urine color may change to amber or yellow-green. • Avoid prolonged exposure to sun, tanning beds. Wear clothing to protect from ultraviolet exposure until tolerance is determined.

fluticasone

flew-**tih**-cah-sewn
(Cutivate, Flonase, Flovent Diskus, Flovent HFA, Veramyst)
Do not confuse Cutivate with Ultravate, or Flonase with Flovent.

FIXED-COMBINATION(S)

Advair, Advair Diskus, Advair HFA: fluticasone/salmeterol (bronchodilator): 100 mcg/50 mcg, 250 mcg/50 mcg, 500 mcg/50 mcg.

◆ CLASSIFICATION

PHARMACOTHERAPEUTIC: Corticosteroid. **CLINICAL:** Anti-inflammatory, antipruritic (see pp. 3C, 75C, 76C, 98C, 100C).

ACTION

Controls rate of protein synthesis, depresses migration of polymorphonuclear leukocytes, reverses capillary permeability, stabilizes lysosomal membranes. **Therapeutic Effect:** Prevents, controls inflammation.

PHARMACOKINETICS

Inhalation/intranasal: Protein binding: 91%. Undergoes extensive first-pass metabolism in liver. Excreted in urine. **Half-life:** 3–7.8 hrs. **Topical:** Amount absorbed depends on affected area and skin condition (absorption increased with fever, hydration, inflamed or denuded skin).

USES

Nasal: Relief of seasonal/perennial allergic rhinitis. **Topical:** Relief of inflammation/pruritus associated with steroid-responsive disorders (e.g., contact dermatitis, eczema). **Inhalation:** Long-term control of persistent bronchial asthma. Assists in reducing, discontinuing oral corticosteroid therapy.

PRECAUTIONS

Contraindications: Untreated localized infection of nasal mucosa. **Inhalation:** Primary treatment of status asthmaticus, acute excacerbation of asthma, other acute asthmatic conditions. **Cautions:** Untreated systemic ocular herpes simplex viral infection; untreated fungal, bacterial infection; active or quiescent tuberculosis.

⌛ LIFESPAN CONSIDERATIONS

Pregnancy/Lactation: Unknown if drug crosses placenta or is distributed in breast milk. **Pregnancy Category C. Children:** Safety and efficacy not established in those younger than 4 yrs. Children 4 yrs and older may experience growth suppression with prolonged or high doses. **Elderly:** No age-related precautions noted.

INTERACTIONS

DRUG: **Ritonavir** may increase concentration, reduce serum cortisol concentration. **HERBAL:** None significant. **FOOD:** None known. **LAB VALUES:** None significant.

AVAILABILITY (Rx)

Aerosol for Oral Inhalation (Flovent HFA): 44 mcg/inhalation, 110 mcg/inhalation, 220 mcg/inhalation. **Cream (Cutivate):** 0.05%. **Ointment (Cutivate):** 0.005%. **Powder for Oral Inhalation (Flovent Diskus):** 50 mcg, 100 mcg, 250 mcg, 500 mcg. **Suspension Intranasal Spray (Flonase):** 50 mcg/inhalation. **(Veramyst):** 27.5 mcg/spray.

ADMINISTRATION/HANDLING

Inhalation

• Shake container well. Instruct pt to exhale completely. Place mouthpiece fully into mouth, inhale, hold breath as long as possible before exhaling. • Allow at least 1 min between inhalations. • Rinsing mouth after each use decreases dry mouth, hoarseness.

Intranasal

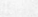

• Instruct pt to clear nasal passages as much as possible before use (topical nasal decongestants may be needed 5–15 min before use). • Tilt head slightly forward. • Insert spray tip into 1 nostril, pointing toward inflamed nasal turbinates, away from nasal septum. • Pump medication into 1 nostril while pt holds other nostril closed, concurrently inspires through nose.

INDICATIONS/ROUTES/DOSAGE

Allergic Rhinitis

INTRANASAL (FLONASE): ADULTS, ELDERLY: Initially, 200 mcg (2 sprays in each nostril once daily or 1 spray in each nostril q12h). Maintenance: 1 spray in each nostril once daily. May increase to 100 mcg (2 sprays) in each nostril. **Maximum:** 200 mcg/day. **CHILDREN 4 YRS AND OLDER:** Initially, 100 mcg (1 spray in each nostril once daily). **Maximum:** 200 mcg/day.

(VERAMYST): ADULTS, ELDERLY, CHILDREN 12 YRS AND OLDER: 110 mcg (2 sprays in each nostril) once daily. Maintenance: 55 mcg (1 spray in each nostril) once daily. **CHILDREN 2–11 YRS:** 55 mcg (1 spray in each nostril) once daily. May increase to 110 mcg (2 sprays each nostril) once daily.

Usual Topical Dosage

TOPICAL: ADULTS, ELDERLY, CHILDREN 3 MOS AND OLDER: Apply sparingly to affected area once or twice a day.

Maintenance Treatment for Asthma (Previously Treated with Bronchodilators)

INHALATION POWDER (FLOVENT DISKUS): ADULTS, ELDERLY, CHILDREN 12 YRS AND OLDER: Initially, 100 mcg q12h. **Maximum:** 500 mcg/day.

INHALATION (ORAL): ADULTS, ELDERLY, CHILDREN 12 YRS AND OLDER: 88 mcg twice a day. **Maximum:** 440 mcg twice a day.

Maintenance Treatment for Asthma (Previously Treated with Inhaled Steroids)

INHALATION POWDER (FLOVENT DISKUS): ADULTS, ELDERLY, CHILDREN 12 YRS AND OLDER: Initially, 100–250 mcg q12h. **Maximum:** 500 mcg q12h.

INHALATION (ORAL): ADULTS, ELDERLY, CHILDREN 12 YRS AND OLDER: 88–220 mcg twice a day. **Maximum:** 440 mcg twice a day.

Maintenance Treatment for Asthma (Previously Treated with Oral Steroids)

INHALATION POWDER (FLOVENT DISKUS): ADULTS, ELDERLY, CHILDREN 12 YRS AND OLDER: 500–1,000 mcg twice a day.

INHALATION (ORAL): ADULTS, ELDERLY, CHILDREN 12 YRS AND OLDER: 440–880 mcg twice a day.

Usual Pediatric Dose (4–11 yrs)

FLOVENT DISKUS: Initially, 50 mcg twice a day. May increase to 100 mcg twice a day.

SIDE EFFECTS

Frequent: **Inhalation:** Throat irritation, hoarseness, dry mouth, cough, temporary wheezing, oropharyngeal candidiasis (particularly if mouth is not rinsed with water after each administration). **Intranasal:** Mild nasopharyngeal irritation; nasal burning, stinging, dryness; rebound congestion; rhinorrhea; altered sense of taste. Occasional: **Inhalation:** Oral candidiasis. **Intranasal:** Nasal/pharyngeal candidiasis, headache. **Topical:** Stinging, burning of skin.

ADVERSE EFFECTS/ TOXIC REACTIONS

None known.

NURSING CONSIDERATIONS

BASELINE ASSESSMENT

Establish baseline history of skin disorder, asthma, rhinitis.

INTERVENTION/EVALUATION

Monitor rate, depth, rhythm, type of respiration; quality/rate of pulse. Assess lung sounds for rhonchi, wheezing, rales. Monitor ABGs. Assess oral mucous membranes for evidence of candidiasis. Monitor growth in pediatric pts. **Topical:** Assess involved area for therapeutic response to irritation.

PATIENT/FAMILY TEACHING

• Pts receiving bronchodilators by inhalation concomitantly with steroid inhalation therapy should use bronchodilator several min before corticosteroid aerosol (enhances penetration of steroid into bronchial tree). • Do not change dose/schedule or stop taking drug; must taper off gradually under medical supervision. • Maintain fastidious oral hygiene. • Rinse mouth with water immediately after inhalation (prevents mouth/throat dryness, oral fungal infection). • Increase fluid intake (decreases lung secretion viscosity). • **Intranasal:** • Clear nasal passages before use. • Contact physician if no improvement in symptoms or sneezing/nasal irritation occurs. • Improvement noted in several days. • **Topical:** Rub thin film gently into affected area. • Use only for prescribed area and no longer than ordered. • Avoid contact with eyes.

fluvastatin

flu-vah-**stah**-tin
(Lescol, Lescol XL)
Do not confuse fluvastatin with fluoxetine, nystatin, or pitavastatin.

CLASSIFICATION

PHARMACOTHERAPEUTIC: Hydroxymethylglutaryl-CoA (HMG-CoA) reductase inhibitor. **CLINICAL:** Antihyperlipidemic (see p. 58C).

ACTION

Inhibits hydroxymethylglutaryl-CoA (HMG-CoA) reductase, the enzyme that catalyzes the early step in cholesterol synthesis. **Therapeutic Effect:** Decreases LDL cholesterol, VLDL, plasma triglyceride. Slightly increases HDL.

PHARMACOKINETICS

Well absorbed from GI tract. Unaffected by food. Does not cross blood-brain barrier. Protein binding: greater than 98%. Primarily eliminated in feces. **Half-life:** 3 hrs; extended-release, 9 hrs.

USES

Adjunct to diet therapy to decrease elevated total, LDL cholesterol in those with primary hypercholesterolemia (types IIa, IIb); those with combined hypercholesterolemia and hypertriglyceridemia. Treatment of elevated triglycerides, apolipoprotein; secondary prevention of coronary events, heterozygous familial hypercholesterolemia in children 10–16 yrs.

PRECAUTIONS

Contraindications: Active hepatic disease, lactation, pregnancy, unexplained increased serum transaminase. **Cautions:** Anticoagulant therapy; history of hepatic disease; substantial alcohol consumption; major surgery; severe acute infection; trauma; hypotension; severe metabolic, endocrine, electrolyte disorders; uncontrolled seizures. Withholding/discontinuing fluvastatin may be necessary when pt is at risk for renal failure (secondary to rhabdomyolysis).

LIFESPAN CONSIDERATIONS

Pregnancy/Lactation: Contraindicated in pregnancy (suppression of cholesterol biosynthesis may cause fetal toxicity), lactation. Unknown if drug is distributed in breast milk. **Pregnancy Category X. Children:** Safety and efficacy not established. **Elderly:** No age-related precautions noted.

INTERACTIONS

DRUG: Increased risk of acute renal failure, rhabdomyolysis with **cyclosporine, erythromycin, gemfibrozil, immunosuppressants, niacin.** May increase concentration/toxicity of **digoxin. HERBAL:** None significant. **FOOD:** None known. **LAB VALUES:** May increase serum creatine kinase (CK), transaminase.

AVAILABILITY (Rx)

Capsules (Lescol): 20 mg, 40 mg.

Tablets (Extended-Release [Lescol XL]): 80 mg.

ADMINISTRATION/HANDLING

PO

• Give without regard to food. • Do not break, chew, or crush extended-release tablets. • Do not open capsules.

INDICATIONS/ROUTES/DOSAGE

Hyperlipoproteinemia

PO: ADULTS, ELDERLY: Initially, 20 mg/day (capsule) in the evening. May increase up to 40 mg/day. **Maximum:** 80 mg/day. Maintenance: 20–40 mg/day in a single dose or divided doses. **PATIENTS REQUIRING MORE THAN 25% DECREASE IN LDL:** 40 mg 1–2 times a day or 80-mg extended-release tablet once a day.

Heterozygous Familial Hypercholesterolemia

PO: CHILDREN 10–16 YRS: Initially, 20 mg/day. May increase q6wks to maximum dose of 80 mg/day, given in 2 divided doses or a single daily dose (extended-release).

SIDE EFFECTS

Frequent (8%–5%): Headache, dyspepsia, back pain, myalgia, arthralgia, diarrhea, abdominal cramping, rhinitis. **Occasional (4%–2%):** Nausea, vomiting, insomnia, constipation, flatulence, rash, pruritus, fatigue, cough, dizziness.

ADVERSE EFFECTS/ TOXIC REACTIONS

Myositis (inflammation of voluntary muscle) with or without increased creatine kinase (CK), muscle weakness, occur rarely. May progress to frank rhabdomyolysis, renal impairment, renal failure.

NURSING CONSIDERATIONS

BASELINE ASSESSMENT

Question for possibility of pregnancy before initiating therapy (Pregnancy Category X). Assess baseline lab results (serum cholesterol, triglycerides, hepatic function test, CPK).

INTERVENTION/EVALUATION

Monitor daily pattern of bowel activity, stool consistency. Assess for headache, dizziness. Assess for rash, pruritus. Monitor serum cholesterol, triglyceride lab results for therapeutic response. Be alert for malaise, muscle cramping, weakness.

PATIENT/FAMILY TEACHING

• Follow special diet (important part of treatment). • Periodic lab tests are essential part of therapy. • Report promptly vision changes, unusual bruising, yellowing of skin or eyes, any muscle pain/weakness, esp. if accompanied by fever, malaise.

fluvoxamine

floo-**vox**-a-meen

(Apo-Fluvoxumine ✱, Luvox, Luvox CR, Novo-Fluvoxamine ✱)

BLACK BOX ALERT Increased risk of suicidal thinking and behavior in children, adolescents, young adults 18–24 yrs with major depressive disorder, other psychiatric disorders.

Do not confuse fluvoxamine with flavoxate or fluoxetine, or Luvox with Lasix, Levoxyl, or Lovenox.

◆CLASSIFICATION

PHARMACOTHERAPEUTIC: Serotonin reuptake inhibitor. **CLINICAL:** Antidepressant, antiobsessive (see p. 39C).

ACTION

Selectively inhibits neuronal reuptake of serotonin. **Therapeutic Effect:** Relieves depression, symptoms of obsessive-compulsive disorder (OCD).

PHARMACOKINETICS

Well absorbed following PO administration. Protein binding: 77%. Metabolized in liver. Excreted in urine. **Half-life:** 15–20 hrs.

USES

Treatment of obsessive-compulsive disorder (OCD). **Luvox CR:** Treatment of OCD, social anxiety disorder (SAD). OFF-LABEL: Treatment of anxiety disorders in children, depression, panic disorder, mild dementia associated agitation in nonpsychotic pts.

PRECAUTIONS

Contraindications: Use within 14 days of MAOIs. **Cautions:** Renal/hepatic impairment, elderly.

LIFESPAN CONSIDERATIONS

Pregnancy/Lactation: Unknown if drug crosses the placenta; distributed in breast milk. **Children:** Safety and efficacy not established in those younger than 8 yrs. **Elderly:** Potential for reduced serum clearance; maintain caution.

INTERACTIONS

DRUG: May increase concentration, risk of toxicity of **benzodiazepines, carbamazepine, clozapine, theophylline. Lithium, tryptophan** may enhance fluvoxamine's serotonergic effects. **MAOIs** may produce serious reactions (hyperthermia, rigidity, myoclonus). **Tricyclic antidepressants** may increase concentration. May increase effects of **warfarin.** HERBAL: **St. John's wort** may increase pharmacologic effects, risk of toxicity. FOOD: None known. LAB VALUES: None significant.

AVAILABILITY (Rx)

Tablets: (Luvox): 25 mg, 50 mg, 100 mg.

Capsules (Extended-Release): (Luvox CR): 100 mg, 150 mg.

ADMINISTRATION/HANDLING

• Do not chew or crush capsules. • May give with or without food.

INDICATIONS/ROUTES/DOSAGE

Obsessive-Compulsive Disorder (OCD)

PO (IMMEDIATE-RELEASE): ADULTS: 50 mg at bedtime; may increase by 50 mg every 4–7 days. Dosages greater than 100 mg/day given in 2 divided doses. **Maximum:** 300 mg/day. **CHILDREN 8–17 YRS:** 25 mg at bedtime; may increase by 25 mg every 4–7 days. Dosages greater than 50 mg/day given in 2 divided doses. **Maximum:** 200 mg/day.

OCD, Social Anxiety Disorder

PO (EXTENDED-RELEASE): (LUVOX CR): ADULTS, ELDERLY: Initially, 100 mg once daily. May increase by 50 mg at weekly intervals. Range: 100–300 mg/day.

SIDE EFFECTS

Frequent: Nausea (40%), headache, drowsiness, insomnia (22%–21%). **Occasional (14%–8%):** Dizziness, diarrhea, dry mouth, asthenia (loss of strength, energy), dyspepsia, constipation, abnormal ejaculation. **Rare (6%–3%):** Anorexia, anxiety, tremor, vomiting, flatulence, urinary frequency, sexual dysfunction, altered taste.

ADVERSE EFFECTS/ TOXIC REACTIONS

Overdose may produce seizures, nausea, vomiting, excessive agitation, extreme restlessness.

NURSING CONSIDERATIONS

INTERVENTION/EVALUATION

Supervise suicidal-risk pt closely during early therapy (as depression lessens, energy level improves, increasing suicide potential). Assess appearance, behavior, speech pattern, level of interest, mood. Assist with ambulation if dizziness, drowsiness occurs. Monitor daily pattern of bowel activity, stool consistency.

PATIENT/FAMILY TEACHING

• Maximum therapeutic response may require 4 wks or more of therapy. • Dry mouth may be relieved by sugarless gum, sips of tepid water. • Do not abruptly discontinue medication. • Avoid tasks that require alertness, motor skills until response to drug is established.

Focalin, *see dexmethylphenidate*

F

Focalin XR, *see dexmethylphenidate*

folic acid

foe-lik
(Apo-Folic ♣, Folacin-800, Folvite)
Do not confuse folic acid with folinic acid.

◆CLASSIFICATION

PHARMACOTHERAPEUTIC: Coenzyme. **CLINICAL:** Nutritional supplement.

ACTION

Stimulates production of platelets, RBCs, WBCs. **Therapeutic Effect:** Essential for nucleoprotein synthesis, maintenance of normal erythropoiesis.

PHARMACOKINETICS

PO form almost completely absorbed from GI tract (upper duodenum). Protein binding: High. Metabolized in liver and plasma to active form. Excreted in urine. Removed by hemodialysis.

USES

Treatment of megaloblastic and macrocytic anemias due to folate deficiency (e.g., pregnancy, inadequate dietary intake). Supplement to prevent neural tube defects. **OFF-LABEL:** Adjunct therapy in methanol toxicity.

PRECAUTIONS

Contraindications: Anemias (aplastic, normocytic, pernicious, refractory). **Cautions:** None known.

⌛ LIFESPAN CONSIDERATIONS

Pregnancy/Lactation: Distributed in breast milk. **Pregnancy Category A (C if more than recommended daily allowance). Children/Elderly:** No age-related precautions noted.

INTERACTIONS

DRUG: **Analgesics, carbamazepine, estrogens** may increase folic acid requirements. **Antacids, cholestyramine** may decrease absorption. May decrease the effects of **hydantoin anticonvulsants. Methotrexate, triamterene, trimethoprim** may antagonize effects. **HERBAL:** None significant. **FOOD:** None known. **LAB VALUES:** May decrease vitamin B_{12} concentration.

AVAILABILITY (Rx)

Injection Solution: 5 mg/ml. **Tablets:** 0.4 mg (OTC), 0.8 mg (OTC), 1 mg.

ADMINISTRATION/HANDLING

PO

May give without regard to food.

◀ALERT▶ Parenteral form used in acutely ill, parenteral/enteral alimentation, those unresponsive to oral route in GI malabsorption syndrome. Dosage greater than 0.1 mg/day may conceal pernicious anemia.

INDICATIONS/ROUTES/DOSAGE

Anemia

IM/IV/SUBCUTANEOUS/PO: ADULTS, ELDERLY, CHILDREN 4 YRS AND OLDER: 0.4 mg/day. **CHILDREN YOUNGER THAN 4 YRS:** Up to 0.3 mg/day. **INFANTS:** 0.1 mg/day. **PREGNANT/LACTATING WOMEN:** 0.8 mg/day.

Prevention of Neural Tube Defects

PO: WOMEN OF CHILD-BEARING AGE: 400 mcg/day. **WOMEN AT HIGH RISK OR FAMILY HISTORY OF NEURAL TUBE DEFECTS:** 4 mg/day.

SIDE EFFECTS

None known.

ADVERSE EFFECTS/ TOXIC REACTIONS

Allergic hypersensitivity occurs rarely with parenteral form. Oral folic acid is nontoxic.

NURSING CONSIDERATIONS

BASELINE ASSESSMENT

Pernicious anemia should be ruled out with Schilling test and vitamin B_{12} blood level before initiating therapy (may produce irreversible neurologic damage). Resistance to treatment may occur if decreased hematopoiesis, alcoholism, antimetabolic drugs, deficiency of vitamin B_6, B_{12}, C, E is evident.

INTERVENTION/EVALUATION

Assess for therapeutic improvement: improved sense of well-being, relief from iron deficiency symptoms (fatigue, shortness of breath, sore tongue, headache, pallor).

PATIENT/FAMILY TEACHING

- Eat foods rich in folic acid, including fruits, vegetables, organ meats.

fondaparinux HIGH ALERT

fond-dah-**pear**-in-ux
(Arixtra)

BLACK BOX ALERT Epidural or spinal anesthesia greatly increases potential for spinal or epidural hematoma, subsequent long-term or permanent paralysis.

◆CLASSIFICATION

PHARMACOTHERAPEUTIC: Factor Xa inhibitor, pentasaccharide. **CLINICAL:** Antithrombotic.

ACTION

Factor Xa inhibitor and pentasaccharide that selectively binds to antithrombin and increases its affinity for factor Xa, inhibiting factor Xa, stopping blood coagulation cascade. **Therapeutic Effect:** Indirectly prevents formation of thrombin and subsequently fibrin clot.

PHARMACOKINETICS

Well absorbed after subcutaneous administration. Undergoes minimal, if any, metabolism. Highly bound to antithrombin III. Distributed mainly in blood and to a minor extent in extravascular fluid. Excreted unchanged in urine. Removed by hemodialysis. **Half-life:** 17–21 hrs (increased in renal impairment).

USES

Prevention of venous thromboembolism in pts undergoing total hip replacement, hip fracture surgery, knee replacement surgery. Treatment of acute deep vein thrombosis (DVT), acute pulmonary embolism. Used concurrently with warfarin therapy. Prevention of DVT in pts undergoing abdominal surgery. **OFF-LABEL:** Prophylaxis of DVT in pts with history of heparin-induced thrombocytopenia.

PRECAUTIONS

Contraindications: Active major bleeding, bacterial endocarditis, body weight less than 50 kg, severe renal impairment (creatinine clearance less than 30 ml/min), thrombocytopenia associated with antiplatelet antibody formation in presence of fondaparinux. **Cautions:** Conditions with increased risk of hemorrhage (GI ulceration, hemophilia, concurrent use of antiplatelet agents, severe uncontrolled hypertension, history of CVA), history of heparin-induced thrombocytopenia, renal impairment, elderly, neuraxial anesthesia, indwelling epidural catheter use.

LIFESPAN CONSIDERATIONS

Pregnancy/Lactation: Use with caution, particularly during third trimester, immediate postpartum period (increased risk of maternal hemorrhage). Unknown if excreted in breast milk. **Pregnancy Category B. Children:** Safety and efficacy not established. **Elderly:** Age-related renal impairment may increase risk of bleeding.

INTERACTIONS

DRUG: **Anticoagulants, antiplatelet medications, aspirin, drotrecogin**

alfa, NSAIDs, thrombolytics may increase risk of bleeding. HERBAL: **Cat's claw, dong quai, evening primrose, feverfew, garlic, ginger, ginkgo, ginseng, horse chestnut, red clover, SAMe** may increase antiplatelet activity. FOOD: None known. LAB VALUES: May cause reversible increases in serum creatinine, AST, ALT. May decrease Hgb, Hct, platelet count.

F

AVAILABILITY (Rx)

Injection, Solution: 2.5 mg/0.5 ml, 5 mg/0.4 ml, 7.5 mg/0.6 ml, 10 mg/0.8 ml.

ADMINISTRATION/HANDLING

Subcutaneous

- Parenteral form appears clear, colorless. Discard if discoloration or particulate matter is noted.
- Store at room temperature.
- Do not expel air bubble from prefilled syringe before injection.
- Pinch fold of skin at injection site between thumb and forefinger. Introduce entire length of subcutaneous needle into skin fold during injection. Inject into fatty tissue between left and right anterolateral or left and right posterolateral abdominal wall.
- Rotate injection sites.

INDICATIONS/ROUTES/DOSAGE

Prevention of Venous Thromboembolism

SUBCUTANEOUS: ADULTS: 2.5 mg once a day for 5–9 days after surgery. Initial dose should be given 6–8 hrs after surgery. Dosage should be adjusted in elderly and those with renal impairment.

Treatment of Venous Thromboembolism, Pulmonary Embolism

SUBCUTANEOUS: ADULTS, ELDERLY WEIGHING GREATER THAN 100 KG: 10 mg once daily. **ADULTS, ELDERLY WEIGHING 50–100 KG:** 7.5 mg once daily. **ADULTS, ELDERLY WEIGHING LESS THAN 50 KG:** 5 mg once daily.

Dosage in Renal Impairment

Creatinine clearance 30–50 ml/min: Use caution. **Creatinine clearance less than 30 ml/min:** Contraindicated.

SIDE EFFECTS

Occasional (14%): Fever. Rare (4%–1%): Injection site hematoma, nausea, peripheral edema.

ADVERSE EFFECTS/ TOXIC REACTIONS

Accidental overdose may lead to bleeding complications ranging from local ecchymoses to major hemorrhage. Thrombocytopenia occurs rarely.

NURSING CONSIDERATIONS

BASELINE ASSESSMENT

Assess CBC, including platelet count, baseline BUN, creatinine clearance.

INTERVENTION/EVALUATION

Periodically monitor CBC, platelet count, stool for occult blood (no need for daily monitoring in pts with normal presurgical coagulation parameters). Assess for any signs of bleeding: bleeding at surgical site, hematuria, blood in stool, bleeding from gums, petechiae, ecchymosis, bleeding from injection sites. Monitor B/P, pulse; hypotension, tachycardia may indicate bleeding, hypovolemia.

PATIENT/FAMILY TEACHING

- Usual length of therapy is 5–9 days.
- Do not take any OTC medication (esp. aspirin, NSAIDs).
- Consult physician if swelling of hands/feet, unusual back pain, unusual bleeding/bruising, weakness, sudden or severe headache occurs.

formoterol

for-**moe**-ter-ol
(Foradil Aerolizer, Oxeze ✱, Perforomist)

BLACK BOX ALERT Long-acting beta-agonists (salmeterol, formoterol) increase risk of asthma-related deaths.

Do not confuse formoterol or Foradil with toradol.

FIXED COMBINATION(S)

Dulera: formoterol/mometasone (a corticosteroid): 5 mcg/100 mcg, 5 mcg/200 mcg. **Symbicort:** formoterol/budesonide (a glucocorticoid): 4.5 mcg/80 mcg, 4.5 mcg/160 mcg.

◆CLASSIFICATION

PHARMACOTHERAPEUTIC: Sympathomimetic ($beta_2$-adrenergic agonist). **CLINICAL:** Bronchodilator (see pp. 74C, 75C).

ACTION

Stimulates $beta_2$-adrenergic receptors in lungs, resulting in relaxation of bronchial smooth muscle. Inhibits release of mediators from various cells in lungs, including mast cells, with little effect on heart rate. **Therapeutic Effect:** Relieves bronchospasm, reduces airway resistance. Improves bronchodilation, nighttime asthma control, peak flow rates.

PHARMACOKINETICS

Route	Onset	Peak	Duration
Inhalation	1–3 min	15 min	12 hrs

Absorbed from bronchi after inhalation. Protein binding: 61%–64%. Metabolized in liver. Primarily excreted in urine. Unknown if removed by hemodialysis. **Half-life:** 10–14 hrs.

USES

FORADIL: For long-term maintenance treatment of asthma, prevention of exercise-induced bronchospasm, treatment of bronchoconstriction in pts with COPD. Can be used concomitantly with short-acting beta-agonists, inhaled or systemic corticosteroids, theophylline therapy. **PERFOROMIST:** Maintenance treatment of bronchoconstriction in pts with COPD.

PRECAUTIONS

Contraindications: None known. **Cautions:** Hypertension, cardiovascular disease, seizure disorder, thyrotoxicosis. May increase risk of severe excacerbation of asthma.

⌛ LIFESPAN CONSIDERATIONS

Pregnancy/Lactation: Unknown if drug crosses placenta or is distributed in breast milk. **Pregnancy Category C. Children:** Safety and efficacy not established in those younger than 5 yrs. **Elderly:** May be more sensitive to tremor, tachycardia due to age-related increased sympathetic sensitivity.

INTERACTIONS

DRUG: **Beta-blockers** may antagonize bronchodilating effects. **Diuretics, steroids, xanthine derivatives** may increase risk of hypokalemia. **Drugs that can prolong QT interval (e.g., erythromycin, quinidine, thioridazine), MAOIs, tricyclic antidepressants** may potentiate cardiovascular effects. **HERBAL:** None significant. **FOOD:** None known. **LAB VALUES:** May decrease serum potassium. May increase serum glucose.

AVAILABILITY (Rx)

Inhalation Powder (Foradil): 12 mcg. **Inhalation Solution for Nebulization (Perforomist):** 20 mcg/2 ml.

ADMINISTRATION/HANDLING

Inhalation

• Pull off Aerolizer Inhaler cover, twisting mouthpiece in direction of arrow to open. • Place capsule in chamber. Capsule is pierced by pressing and releasing buttons on side of Aerolizer, once only. • Instruct pt to exhale completely; place mouthpiece into mouth, close lips and inhale quickly, deeply through mouth (this causes capsule to spin, dispensing the drug). Pt should hold breath as long as possible before exhaling slowly. • Check capsule to ensure all the powder is gone. If not, pt should inhale again to receive rest of the dose. Rinse mouth with water immediately after inhalation (prevents mouth/throat dryness).

Storage • Maintain capsules in individual blister pack until immediately before use. • Do not swallow capsules. • Do not use with a spacer.

Nebulization

• No diluent necessary. • Protect from heat. • Remove from foil pouch immediately before use. • Do not mix with other medications.

F

INDICATIONS/ROUTES/DOSAGE

Asthma

INHALATION POWDER: ADULTS, ELDERLY, CHILDREN 5 YRS AND OLDER: 12 mcg capsule inhaled q12h.

COPD

INHALATION POWDER: ADULTS, ELDERLY, CHILDREN 5 YRS AND OLDER: 12 mcg capsule q12h.

INHALATION SOLUTION FOR NEBULIZATION: ADULTS, ELDERLY: 20 mcg q12h.

Exercise-Induced Bronchospasm

INHALATION POWDER: ADULTS, ELDERLY, CHILDREN 5 YRS AND OLDER: 12 mcg capsule inhaled at least 15 min before exercise. Do not repeat for another 12 hrs.

SIDE EFFECTS

Occasional: Tremor, muscle cramps, tachycardia, insomnia, headache, irritability, mouth/throat irritation.

ADVERSE EFFECTS/ TOXIC REACTIONS

Excessive sympathomimetic stimulation may produce palpitations, extrasystoles, chest pain.

NURSING CONSIDERATIONS

INTERVENTION/EVALUATION

Assess rate, depth, rhythm, type of respiration; quality/rate of pulse. Monitor EKG, serum potassium, ABG determinations. Assess lung sounds for wheezing (bronchoconstriction), rales, pulmonary function tests.

PATIENT/FAMILY TEACHING

• Follow manufacturer guidelines for proper use of inhaler. • Increase fluid intake (decreases lung secretion viscosity). • Rinsing mouth with water immediately after inhalation may prevent mouth/throat irritation. • Avoid excessive use of caffeine derivatives (chocolate, coffee, tea, cola).

Fortaz, *see ceftazidime*

Fosamax, *see alendronate*

Fosamax Plus D, *see alendronate*

fosamprenavir

foss-am-**pren**-ah-vear

(Lexiva, Telzir ♣)

Do not confuse Lexiva with Levitra.

◆CLASSIFICATION

PHARMACOTHERAPEUTIC: Antiretroviral. **CLINICAL:** Protease inhibitor.

ACTION

Rapidly converted to amprenavir, inhibiting HIV-1 protease by binding to enzyme's active site, preventing processing of viral precursors, forming immature, noninfectious viral particles. **Therapeutic Effect:** Impairs HIV replication, proliferation.

PHARMACOKINETICS

Rapidly absorbed after PO administration. Protein binding: 90%. Metabolized in liver. Primarily excreted in feces. **Half-life:** 7.7 hrs.

USES

Treatment of HIV infection in combination with other antiretroviral agents.

PRECAUTIONS

Contraindications: Concurrent use of amprenavir, dihydroergotamine, ergonovine, ergotamine, methylergonovine, midazolam, pimozide, triazolam. If fosamprenavir is given concurrently with ritonavir, then flecainide and propafenone are also contraindicated. **Extreme Caution:** Hepatic impairment. **Cautions:** Diabetes mellitus, elderly, renal impairment, known sulfonamide allergy.

LIFESPAN CONSIDERATIONS

Pregnancy/Lactation: Unknown if drug crosses placenta or is distributed in breast milk. **Pregnancy Category C. Children:** Safety and efficacy not established in those younger than 4 yrs. **Elderly:** Age-related hepatic impairment may require decreased dosage.

INTERACTIONS

DRUG: May interfere with metabolism of **amiodarone, bepridil, ergotamine, lidocaine, midazolam, oral contraceptives, quinidine, triazolam, tricyclic antidepressants. Antacids, didanosine** may decrease absorption. **Carbamazepine, phenobarbital, phenytoin, rifampin** may decrease concentration. May increase concentrations of **clozapine, hydroxymethylglutaryl-CoA (HMG-CoA) reductase inhibitors (statins), warfarin. HERBAL: St. John's wort** may decrease concentration. **FOOD:** None known. **LAB VALUES:** May increase serum lipase, triglycerides, AST, ALT. May decrease neutrophil count.

AVAILABILITY (Rx)

Oral Suspension: 50 mg/ml.

Tablets: 700 mg (equivalent to 600 mg amprenavir).

ADMINISTRATION/HANDLING

PO

• Give tablets without regard to meals. • Do not crush, break film-coated tablets. • Adults should take oral suspension without food. Children should take oral suspension with food.

INDICATIONS/ROUTES/DOSAGE

HIV Infection without Previous Protease Inhibitor Therapy

PO: ADULTS, ELDERLY: (Unboosted regimen) 1,400 mg twice daily without ritonavir; or (Ritonavir boosted regimen) 1,400 mg once daily plus ritonavir 100 mg or 200 mg once daily; or 700 mg twice daily plus ritonavir 100 mg twice daily. **CHILDREN 6 YRS AND OLDER:** (Unboosted regimen) 30 mg/kg twice daily. **Maximum:** 1,400 mg twice daily. (Ritonavir boosted regimen) or 18 mg/kg plus 3 mg/kg ritonavir twice daily. **Maximum:** 700 mg fosamprenavir plus 100 mg ritonavir twice daily. **CHILDREN 2–5 YRS:** 30 mg/kg twice daily. **Maximum:** 1,400 mg twice daily.

HIV Infection with Previous Protease Inhibitor Therapy

PO: ADULTS, ELDERLY: 700 mg twice daily plus ritonavir 100 mg twice daily. **CHILDREN 6 YRS AND OLDER:** 18 mg/kg plus 3 mg/kg ritonavir twice daily. **Maximum:** 700 mg plus 100 mg ritonavir twice daily.

Concurrent Therapy with Efavirenz

PO: ADULTS, ELDERLY: In pts receiving fosamprenavir plus once-daily ritonavir in combination with efavirenz, an additional 100 mg/day ritonavir (300 mg total/day) should be given.

Dosage in Hepatic Impairment:

Mild to moderate impairment: Reduce fosamprenavir to 700 mg twice daily (without concurrent ritonavir). **Severe impairment:** Reduce fosamprenavir to 350 mg twice daily (without ritonavir).

SIDE EFFECTS

Frequent (39%–35%): Nausea, rash, diarrhea. **Occasional (19%–8%):** Headache, vomiting, fatigue, depression. Rare (7%–2%): Pruritus, abdominal pain, perioral paresthesia.

ADVERSE EFFECTS/ TOXIC REACTIONS

Severe or life-threatening dermatologic reactions, including Stevens-Johnson syndrome, occur rarely.

F

NURSING CONSIDERATIONS

BASELINE ASSESSMENT

Obtain baseline lab testing, esp. hepatic function tests, before beginning therapy and at periodic intervals during therapy. Offer emotional support. Obtain medication history.

INTERVENTION/EVALUATION

Closely monitor for evidence of GI discomfort. Monitor daily pattern of bowel activity and stool consistency. Assess skin for rash. Monitor serum chemistry tests for marked abnormalities, particularly hepatic profile, glucose, triglycerides, cholesterol. Assess for opportunistic infections (onset of fever, oral mucosa changes, cough, other respiratory symptoms).

PATIENT/FAMILY TEACHING

• Eat small, frequent meals to offset nausea, vomiting. • Continue therapy for full length of treatment. • Doses should be evenly spaced. • Fosamprenavir is not a cure for HIV infection, nor does it reduce risk of transmission to others. • Pt may continue to experience illnesses, including opportunistic infections. • Diarrhea can be controlled with OTC medication. • Notify physician if rash develops.

foscarnet

foss-**car**-net
(Foscavir)

BLACK BOX ALERT Renal toxicity occurs to some degree in majority of pts. For use only in immunocompromised pts with CMV retinitis and mucocutaneous acyclovir-resistant HSV infection. Seizures due to electrolyte/mineral imbalance may occur.

◆CLASSIFICATION

CLINICAL: Antiviral (see p. 68C).

ACTION

Selectively inhibits binding sites on virus-specific DNA polymerase, reverse transcriptase. **Therapeutic Effect:** Inhibits replication of herpes virus.

PHARMACOKINETICS

Sequestered into bone, cartilage. Protein binding: 14%–17%. Primarily excreted unchanged in urine. Removed by hemodialysis. **Half-life:** 3.3–6.8 hrs (increased in renal impairment).

USES

Treatment of herpes virus infections suspected to be caused by acyclovir-resistant or ganciclovir-resistant strains. Treatment of cytomegalovirus (CMV) retinitis. OFF-LABEL: Other CMV infections (e.g., colitis, esophagitis); CMV prophylaxis for cancer pts receiving alemtuzumab or allogenic stem cell transplant.

PRECAUTIONS

Contraindications: None known. **Cautions:** Neurologic/cardiac abnormalities, history of renal impairment, altered calcium, other electrolyte imbalances.

⌛ LIFESPAN CONSIDERATIONS

Pregnancy/Lactation: Unknown if distributed in breast milk. **Pregnancy Category C. Children:** Safety and efficacy not established. **Elderly:** Age-related renal impairment may require dosage adjustment.

INTERACTIONS

DRUG: **Nephrotoxic medications** may increase risk of renal toxicity. **Pentamidine (IV)** may cause reversible hypocalcemia, hypomagnesemia, nephrotoxicity. **Zidovudine (AZT)** may increase risk of anemia. HERBAL: None significant. FOOD:

None known. **LAB VALUES:** May increase serum alkaline phosphatase, bilirubin, creatinine, AST, ALT. May decrease serum magnesium, potassium. May alter serum calcium, phosphate concentrations.

AVAILABILITY (Rx)

Injection Solution: 24 mg/ml.

ADMINISTRATION/HANDLING

IV

Reconstitution • Standard 24 mg/ml solution may be used without dilution when central venous catheter is used for infusion; 24 mg/ml solution *must* be diluted to maximum concentration of 12 mg/ml when peripheral vein catheter is being used. • Dilute only with D_5W or 0.9% NaCl solution.

Rate of administration • Because dosage is calculated on body weight, unneeded quantity may be removed before start of infusion to avoid overdosage. Aseptic technique must be used and solution administered within 24 hrs of first entry into sealed bottle. • Do not give by IV injection or rapid infusion (increases toxicity). • Administer by IV infusion at rate not faster than 1 hr for doses up to 60 mg/kg and 2 hrs for doses greater than 60 mg/kg. • To minimize toxicity and phlebitis, use central venous lines or veins with adequate blood flow to permit rapid dilution, dissemination of foscarnet. • Use IV infusion pump to prevent accidental overdose.

Storage • Store parenteral vials at room temperature. • After dilution, stable for 24 hrs at room temperature. • Do not use if solution is discolored or particulate forms.

IV INCOMPATIBILITIES

Acyclovir (Zovirax), amphotericin B (Fungizone), calcium, co-trimoxazole (Bactrim), diazepam (Valium), digoxin (Lanoxin), diphenhydramine (Benadryl), dobutamine (Dobutrex), droperidol (Inapsine), ganciclovir (Cytovene), haloperidol (Haldol), leucovorin, magnesium, midazolam (Versed), pentamidine (Pentam IV), prochlorperazine (Compazine), total parenteral nutrition (TPN), vancomycin (Vancocin).

IV COMPATIBILITIES

Dopamine (Intropin), heparin, hydromorphone (Dilaudid), lorazepam (Ativan), morphine, potassium chloride.

INDICATIONS/ROUTES/DOSAGE

Cytomegalovirus (CMV) Retinitis

IV: ADULTS, ELDERLY: Initially, 60 mg/kg q8h or 90 mg/kg q12h for 2–3 wks. Maintenance: 90–120 mg/kg/day as a single IV infusion.

Herpes Infection

IV: ADULTS: 40 mg/kg q8–12h for 2–3 wks or until healed.

Dosage in Renal Impairment

Dosages are individualized based on creatinine clearance. Refer to dosing guide provided by manufacturer.

SIDE EFFECTS

Frequent: Fever (65%); nausea (47%); vomiting, diarrhea (30%). **Occasional (29%–5%):** Anorexia, pain/inflammation at injection site, rigors, malaise, altered B/P, headache, paresthesia, dizziness, rash, diaphoresis, abdominal pain. **Rare (4%–1%):** Back/chest pain, edema, flushing, pruritus, constipation, dry mouth.

ADVERSE EFFECTS/ TOXIC REACTIONS

Nephrotoxicity occurs to some extent in most pts. Seizures, serum mineral/ electrolyte imbalances may be life-threatening.

NURSING CONSIDERATIONS

BASELINE ASSESSMENT

Obtain baseline serum mineral and electrolyte levels, vital signs, CBC values, renal function tests. Risk of renal impairment can be reduced by sufficient fluid intake to assure diuresis prior to and during therapy.

INTERVENTION/EVALUATION

Monitor serum creatinine, calcium, phosphorus, potassium, magnesium, Hgb, Hct. Obtain periodic ophthalmologic exams. Assess for signs of serum electrolyte imbalance, esp. hypocalcemia (perioral paresthesia, paresthesia of extremities), hypokalemia (weakness, muscle cramps, paresthesia of extremities, irritability). Monitor renal function tests. Assess for tremors; provide safety measures for potential seizures. Assess for bleeding, anemia, developing superinfections.

PATIENT/FAMILY TEACHING

• Important to report perioral tingling, numbness in extremities, paresthesias during or following infusion (may indicate electrolyte abnormalities). • Tremors should be reported promptly due to potential for seizures.

fosfomycin

foss-fo-**mye**-sin
(Monurol)
Do not confuse Monurol with Monopril.

CLASSIFICATION

PHARMACOTHERAPEUTIC: Bactericidal. **CLINICAL:** Antibiotic.

ACTION

Prevents bacterial cell wall formation by inhibiting synthesis of peptidoglycan. **Therapeutic Effect:** Bactericidal.

PHARMACOKINETICS

Well absorbed following PO administration. Not bound to plasma proteins. Not metabolized. Partially excreted in urine; minimal elimination in feces. **Half-life:** 4–8 hrs.

USES

Single-dose treatment for uncomplicated UTI in women. **OFF-LABEL:** Serious UTI in men.

PRECAUTIONS

Contraindications: None known. **Cautions:** Renal impairment.

LIFESPAN CONSIDERATIONS

Pregnancy/Lactation: Unknown if drug crosses placenta or is distributed in breast milk. **Pregnancy Category B. Children:** Safety and efficacy not established in those younger than 12 yrs. **Elderly:** Age-related renal impairment may require dosage adjustment.

INTERACTIONS

DRUG: **Metoclopramide** lowers concentration, urinary excretion. **HERBAL:** None significant. **FOOD:** None known. **LAB VALUES:** May increase eosinophil count, serum alkaline phosphatase, bilirubin, AST, ALT. May alter platelet, WBC counts. May decrease serum Hct, Hgb levels.

AVAILABILITY (Rx)

Powder for Oral Solution: 3 g.

ADMINISTRATION/HANDLING

• Give without regard to food.

INDICATIONS/ROUTES/DOSAGE

UTI

PO (UNCOMPLICATED): FEMALES: 3 g mixed in 4 oz water as a single dose.
PO (COMPLICATED): MALES: 3 g q2–3days for 3 doses.

SIDE EFFECTS

Occasional (9%–3%): Diarrhea, nausea, headache, back pain. **Rare (less than 2%):** Dysmenorrhea, pharyngitis, abdominal pain, rash.

ADVERSE EFFECTS/ TOXIC REACTIONS

None known.

NURSING CONSIDERATIONS

PATIENT/FAMILY TEACHING

• Symptoms should improve in 2–3 days. • Always mix medication with water before taking.

fosinopril

fo-**sin**-o-pril
(Apo-Fosinopril ✦, Monopril, Novo-Fosinopril✦)

BLACK BOX ALERT May cause fetal injury, mortality if used during second or third trimester of pregnancy.

Do not confuse Monopril with Accupril, minoxidil, moexipril, or ramipril, or fosinopril with lisinopril.

◆CLASSIFICATION

PHARMACOTHERAPEUTIC: ACE inhibitor. **CLINICAL:** Antihypertensive (see p. 9C).

ACTION

Suppresses renin-angiotensin-aldosterone system (prevents conversion of angiotensin I to angiotensin II, a potent vasoconstrictor; may inhibit angiotensin II at local vascular, renal sites). Decreases plasma angiotensin II, increases plasma renin activity, decreases aldosterone secretion. **Therapeutic Effect:** Reduces peripheral arterial resistance, pulmonary capillary wedge pressure; improves cardiac output, exercise tolerance.

PHARMACOKINETICS

Route	Onset	Peak	Duration
PO	1 hr	2–6 hrs	24 hrs

Slowly absorbed from GI tract. Protein binding: 97%–98%. Metabolized in liver and GI mucosa to active metabolite. Primarily excreted in urine. Minimal removal by hemodialysis. **Half-life:** 11.5 hrs.

USES

Treatment of hypertension, used alone or in combination with other antihypertensives. Treatment of heart failure. **OFF-LABEL:** Treatment of diabetic, nondiabetic nephropathy; post-MI left ventricular dysfunction; renal crisis in scleroderma.

PRECAUTIONS

Contraindications: History of angioedema from previous treatment with ACE inhibitors. **Cautions:** Renal impairment, those with sodium depletion or on diuretic therapy, dialysis, hypovolemia, coronary/cerebrovascular insufficiency.

⌛ LIFESPAN CONSIDERATIONS

Pregnancy/Lactation: Crosses placenta. Distributed in breast milk. May cause fetal or neonatal mortality or morbidity. **Pregnancy Category C (D if used in second or third trimester). Children:** Safety and efficacy not established. Neonates, infants may be at increased risk for oliguria, neurologic abnormalities. **Elderly:** May be more sensitive to hypotensive effects.

INTERACTIONS

DRUG: **Alcohol, antihypertensive agents, diuretics** may increase effect. **NSAIDs** may decrease effect. **Potassium-sparing diuretics, potassium supplements** may cause hyperkalemia. May increase **lithium** concentration/toxicity. **HERBAL:** **Ephedra, ginseng, yohimbe** may worsen hypertension. **Garlic** may increase antihypertensive effect. **Licorice** may cause sodium/water retention, loss of potassium. **FOOD:** None known. **LAB VALUES:** May increase BUN, serum alkaline phosphatase, bilirubin, creatinine, potassium, AST, ALT. May decrease serum sodium. May cause positive antinuclear antibody titer (ANA).

AVAILABILITY (Rx)

Tablets: 10 mg, 20 mg, 40 mg.

ADMINISTRATION/HANDLING

PO

• Give without regard to food. • Tablets may be crushed.

INDICATIONS/ROUTES/DOSAGE

Hypertension

PO: ADULTS, ELDERLY: Initially, 10 mg/day. Maintenance: 20–40 mg/day as a single or 2 divided doses. **Maximum:** 80 mg/day. **CHILDREN 6–16 YRS WEIGHING MORE**

THAN 50 KG: Initially, 5–10 mg/day. **Maximum:** 40 mg/day.

Heart Failure

PO: ADULTS, ELDERLY: Initially, 10 mg/day. Maintenance: 20–40 mg/day. **Maximum:** 40 mg/day.

SIDE EFFECTS

Frequent (12%–9%): Dizziness, cough. **Occasional (4%–2%):** Hypotension, nausea, vomiting, upper respiratory tract infection.

ADVERSE EFFECTS/ TOXIC REACTIONS

Excessive hypotension ("first-dose syncope") may occur in pts with CHF, severely salt/volume depleted. Angioedema (swelling of face/lips), hyperkalemia occur rarely. Agranulocytosis, neutropenia may be noted in those with renal impairment, collagen vascular disease (scleroderma, systemic lupus erythematosus). Nephrotic syndrome may be noted in those with history of renal disease.

NURSING CONSIDERATIONS

BASELINE ASSESSMENT

Obtain B/P immediately before each dose, in addition to regular monitoring (be alert to fluctuations). Renal function tests should be performed before beginning therapy. In pts with renal impairment, autoimmune disease, or taking drugs that affect leukocytes or immune response, CBC, differential count should be performed before therapy begins and q2wks for 3 mos, then periodically thereafter.

INTERVENTION/EVALUATION

If excessive reduction in B/P occurs, place pt in supine position with legs elevated. Assist with ambulation if dizziness occurs. Assess for urinary frequency. Auscultate lung sounds for rales, wheezing in those with CHF. Monitor renal function tests, CBC, urinalysis for proteinuria. Observe for angioedema (circumoral swelling, edema around eyes). Monitor serum potassium in those on concurrent diuretic therapy.

PATIENT/FAMILY TEACHING

• Report any sign of infection (sore throat, fever). • Several wks may be needed for full therapeutic effect of B/P reduction. • Skipping doses or voluntarily discontinuing drug may produce severe, rebound hypertension. • To reduce hypotensive effect, rise slowly from lying to sitting position, permit legs to dangle from bed momentarily before standing. • Inform physician if swelling of face, lips, tongue, difficulty breathing, vomiting, excessive perspiration, persistent cough develops.

fosphenytoin

fos-phen-ih-**toyn**

(Cerebyx)

Do not confuse Cerebyx with Celebrex or Celexa, or fosphenytoin with fospropafol.

◆CLASSIFICATION

PHARMACOTHERAPEUTIC: Hydantoin. **CLINICAL:** Anticonvulsant (see p. 35C).

ACTION

Stabilizes neuronal membranes, limits spread of seizure activity. Decreases sodium, calcium ion influx into neurons. Decreases post-tetanic potentiation, repetitive discharge. **Therapeutic Effect:** Decreases seizure activity.

PHARMACOKINETICS

Completely absorbed after IM administration. Protein binding: 95%–99%. Rapidly and completely hydrolyzed to phenytoin after IM or IV administration. Time of complete conversion to phenytoin: 4 hrs after IM injection; 2 hrs after IV infusion. **Half-life:** 8–15 min (for conversion to phenytoin).

USES

Acute treatment, control of generalized convulsive status epilepticus; prevention, treatment of seizures occurring during neurosurgery; short-term substitution of oral phenytoin.

PRECAUTIONS

Contraindications: Adams-Stokes syndrome; hypersensitivity to ethotoin, phosphenytoin, phenytoin, mephenytoin; second- or third-degree AV block; severe bradycardia; SA block. **Cautions:** Porphyria, hypotension, severe myocardial insufficiency, renal/hepatic disease, hypoalbuminemia.

LIFESPAN CONSIDERATIONS

Pregnancy/Lactation: May increase frequency of seizures during pregnancy. Increased risk of congenital malformations. Unknown if excreted in breast milk. **Pregnancy Category D. Children:** Safety not established. **Elderly:** Lower dosage recommended.

INTERACTIONS

DRUG: **Alcohol, other CNS depressants** may increase CNS depression. **Amiodarone, anticoagulants, cimetidine, disulfiram, fluoxetine, isoniazid, sulfonamides** may increase concentration, effects, risk of toxicity. **Fluconazole, ketoconazole, miconazole** may increase concentration. May decrease effects of **glucocorticoids. Lidocaine, propranolol** may increase cardiac depressant effects. **Valproic acid** may increase concentration, decrease metabolism. May increase metabolism of **xanthines.** HERBAL: None significant. FOOD: None known. LAB VALUES: May increase serum glucose, GGT, alkaline phosphatase.

AVAILABILITY (Rx)

Injection Solution: 75 mg/ml (equivalent to 50 mg/ml phenytoin).

ADMINISTRATION/HANDLING

IV

Reconstitution • Dilute in D_5W or 0.9% NaCl to a concentration ranging from 1.5–25 mg phenytoin equivalents (PE)/ml.

Rate of administration • Administer at rate less than 150 mg PE/min (decreases risk of hypotension, arrhythmias). Children: 1–3 mg PE/kg/min.

Storage • Refrigerate. • Do not store at room temperature for longer than 48 hrs. • After dilution, solution is stable for 8 hrs at room temperature or 24 hrs if refrigerated.

IV INCOMPATIBILITY

Midazolam (Versed).

IV COMPATIBILITIES

Lorazepam (Ativan), phenobarbital, potassium chloride.

INDICATIONS/ROUTES/DOSAGE

◀ALERT▶ 150 mg fosphenytoin yields 100 mg phenytoin. Dosage, concentration solution, infusion rate of fosphenytoin are expressed in terms of phenytoin equivalents (PE).

Status Epilepticus

IV: ADULTS: Loading dose: 15–20 mg PE/kg infused at rate of 100–150 mg PE/min.

Nonemergent Seizures

IV, IM: ADULTS: Loading dose: 10–20 mg PE/kg. Maintenance: 4–6 mg PE/kg/day.

Short-Term Substitution for Oral Phenytoin

IV, IM: ADULTS: May substitute for oral phenytoin at same total daily dose.

SIDE EFFECTS

Frequent: Dizziness, paresthesia, tinnitus, pruritus, headache, drowsiness. **Occasional:** Morbilliform rash.

ADVERSE EFFECTS/ TOXIC REACTIONS

Too-high fosphenytoin blood concentration may produce ataxia (muscular incoordination), nystagmus (rhythmic oscillation of eyes), diplopia, lethargy, slurred speech, nausea, vomiting, hypotension. As drug level increases, extreme lethargy may progress to coma.

F

NURSING CONSIDERATIONS

BASELINE ASSESSMENT

Review history of seizure disorder (intensity, frequency, duration, LOC). Initiate seizure precautions. Obtain vital signs, medication history (esp. use of phenytoin, other anticonvulsants). Observe clinically.

INTERVENTION/EVALUATION

Monitor EKG, measure cardiac function, respiratory function, B/P during and immediately following infusion (10–20 min). Discontinue if skin rash appears. Interrupt or decrease rate if hypotension, arrhythmias are detected. Assess pt postinfusion (may feel dizzy, ataxic, drowsy). Assess blood levels of fosphenytoin (2 hrs post IV infusion or 4 hrs post IM injection).

PATIENT/FAMILY TEACHING

• If noncompliance is an issue in causing acute seizures, discuss and address reasons for noncompliance. • Avoid tasks that require alertness, motor skills until response to drug is established.

fospropofol

fos-pro-**poe**-foal
(Lusedra)
Do not confuse fospropofol with fosphenytoin or propofol.

CLASSIFICATION

PHARMACOTHERAPEUTIC: Rapid-acting general anesthetic. **CLINICAL:** Sedative-hypnotic **(Schedule IV).**

ACTION

Inhibits sympathetic vasoconstrictor nerve activity, decreases vascular resistance. **Therapeutic Effect:** Produces rapid hypnosis.

PHARMACOKINETICS

Route	Onset	Peak	Duration
IV	2–4 min	5–7 min	21–45 min

Rapidly, extensively distributed. Completely metabolized by alkaline phosphatase to active metabolite propofol. Primarily excreted in urine. **Half-life:** 80 min.

USES

Induction and maintenance of monitored anesthesia care (MAC) sedation in adult pts undergoing diagnostic or therapeutic procedures.

PRECAUTIONS

Contraindications: None significant. **Cautions:** Hypoxemia, hypotension, respiratory depression, hepatic impairment, severe renal impairment.

⌛ LIFESPAN CONSIDERATIONS:

Pregnancy/Lactation: Not recommended for obstetrics, breast-feeding mothers. **Pregnancy Category B. Children:** Safety and efficacy not established in those younger than 18 yrs. May be associated with neonatal respiratory, cardiovascular depression. **Elderly:** Lower doses recommended in those 65 yrs and older.

INTERACTIONS

DRUG: Alcohol, CNS depressants may increase CNS, respiratory depression, hypotensive effects. **HERBAL:** None significant. **FOOD:** None known. **LAB VALUES:** None significant.

AVAILABILITY (Rx)

Injection: 35 mg/ml.

ADMINISTRATION/HANDLING

IV

◀ALERT▶ Do not give through same IV line with blood or plasma.

Reconstitution • No reconstitution necessary.

Rate of administration • Administer as a bolus injection through a secure, freely flowing, peripheral IV line. • Flush infusion line with NaCl before and after administration.

Storage: • Store at room temperature. • Discard if precipitate is present or discoloration is noted. • For single-pt use only; discard unused portions.

IV INCOMPATIBILITIES

Meperidine (Demerol), Midazolam (Versed).

IV COMPATIBILITIES

D_5W, 0.2% NaCl, 0.45% NaCl, 0.9% NaCl, lactated Ringer's, potassium chloride.

INDICATIONS/ROUTES/DOSAGE

◀ALERT▶ Use supplemental O_2 in all pts undergoing sedation. Adults who weigh over 90 kg should be dosed as if they are 90 kg; adults who weigh less than 60 kg should be dosed as if they are 60 kg.

Standard Dosing Regimen

IV: ADULTS 18–64 YRS, THOSE WITH MILD SYSTEMIC DISEASE: Initial IV bolus dose of 6.5 mg/kg followed by supplemental doses of 1.6 mg/kg as needed. No initial dose should exceed 16.5 ml; no supplemental dose should exceed 4 ml.

Modified Dosing Regimen

IV: ELDERLY 65 YRS AND OLDER, THOSE WITH SEVERE SYSTEMIC DISEASE: 75% of standard dosing regimen. Administer supplemental doses only when pts can demonstrate purposeful movement in response to verbal or light tactile stimulation and no more frequently than every 4 min.

SIDE EFFECTS

Frequent (20%): Paresthesia manifested as genital or vaginal burning, tingling, stinging; pruritus (either generalized or in perineal region). **Occasional (4%):** Hypoxemia, hypotension. **Rare (1%):** Apnea may produce additive cardiorespiratory effects when administered with other cardiorespiratory depressants (benzodiazepines, narcotic analgesics).

ADVERSE EFFECTS/ TOXIC REACTIONS

Nonsustained irregular tachycardia has occurred. Continuous/repeated intermittent infusion may result in extreme drowsiness, respiratory/circulatory depression.

NURSING CONSIDERATIONS

BASELINE ASSESSMENT

Resuscitative equipment, endotracheal tube, suction, O_2 must be available. Obtain vital signs before administration. Use supplemental oxygen in all pts undergoing sedation.

INTERVENTION/EVALUATION

Continuously monitor with pulse oximetry, EKG, frequent B/P measurements. Monitor for hypotension, bradycardia q3–5 min during and after administration until recovery is achieved. Assess diligently for apnea during administration. Pts should be continuously monitored during sedation and through the recovery process for signs of hypotension, apnea, airway obstruction, and/or oxygen desaturation.

Fragmin, *see dalteparin*

frovatriptan

froe-va-**trip**-tan
(Frova)

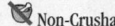

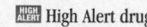

◆CLASSIFICATION

PHARMACOTHERAPEUTIC: Serotonin receptor agonist. **CLINICAL:** Antimigraine (see p. 63C).

ACTION

Binds selectively to vascular receptors, producing vasoconstrictive effect on cranial blood vessels. **Therapeutic Effect:** Relieves migraine headache.

F

PHARMACOKINETICS

Well absorbed after PO administration. Protein binding: 15%. Metabolized by liver to inactive metabolite. Primarily eliminated in feces (62%), urine (32%). **Half-life:** 26 hrs (increased in hepatic impairment).

USES

Treatment of acute migraine headache with or without aura in adults.

PRECAUTIONS

Contraindications: Basilar or hemiplegic migraine, cerebrovascular or peripheral vascular disease, coronary artery disease, ischemic heart disease (angina pectoris, history of MI, silent ischemia, Prinzmetal's angina), severe hepatic impairment (Child-Pugh grade C), uncontrolled hypertension, use within 24 hrs of ergotamine-containing preparations or another serotonin receptor agonist, use within 14 days of MAOIs. **Cautions:** Mild to moderate hepatic impairment, pt profile suggesting cardiovascular risks.

⌛ LIFESPAN CONSIDERATIONS

Pregnancy/Lactation: Unknown if drug is excreted in breast milk. **Pregnancy Category C. Children:** Safety and efficacy not established. **Elderly:** Not recommended for use in this pt population.

INTERACTIONS

DRUG: **Ergotamine-containing medications** may produce vasospastic reaction. **Fluoxetine, fluvoxamine, paroxetine, sertraline** may produce weakness, hyperreflexia, uncoordination. **Oral contraceptives** decrease frovatriptan clearance, volume of distribution. **Propranolol** may dramatically increase plasma concentration. **HERBAL:** None significant. **FOOD:** None known. **LAB VALUES:** None significant.

AVAILABILITY (Rx)

Tablets: 2.5 mg.

ADMINISTRATION/HANDLING

PO

• Give with fluids. • Do not crush, chew film-coated tablets.

INDICATIONS/ROUTES/DOSAGE

Acute Migraine Headache

PO: ADULTS, ELDERLY: Initially 2.5 mg. If headache improves but then returns, dose may be repeated after 2 hrs. **Maximum:** 7.5 mg/day.

SIDE EFFECTS

Occasional (8%–4%): Dizziness, paresthesia, fatigue, flushing. **Rare (3%–2%):** Hot/cold sensation, dry mouth, dyspepsia (heartburn, epigastric distress).

ADVERSE EFFECTS/ TOXIC REACTIONS

Cardiac reactions (ischemia, coronary artery vasospasm, MI), noncardiac vasospasm-related reactions (cerebral hemorrhage, CVA), occur rarely, particularly in pts with hypertension, obesity, smokers, diabetes, strong family history of coronary artery disease; males older than 40 yrs; postmenopausal women.

NURSING CONSIDERATIONS

BASELINE ASSESSMENT

Question for history of peripheral vascular disease, renal/hepatic impairment, possibility of pregnancy. Question regarding onset, location, duration of migraine, possible precipitating symptoms.

INTERVENTION/EVALUATION

Assess for relief of migraine headache, potential for photophobia, phonophobia (sound sensitivity), nausea, vomiting.

PATIENT/FAMILY TEACHING

• Take a single dose as soon as symptoms of an actual migraine attack appear. • Medication is intended to relieve migraine headaches, not to prevent or reduce number of attacks. • Avoid tasks that require alertness, motor skills until response to drug is established. • Contact physician immediately if palpitations, pain, tightness in chest or throat, sudden or severe abdominal pain, pain or weakness of extremities occur.

fulvestrant HIGH ALERT

full-ves-trant
(Faslodex)
Do not confuse Faslodex with Fosamax.

CLASSIFICATION

PHARMACOTHERAPEUTIC: Estrogen antagonist. **CLINICAL:** Antineoplastic (see p. 83C).

ACTION

Competes with endogenous estrogen at estrogen receptor binding sites. **Therapeutic Effect:** Inhibits tumor growth.

PHARMACOKINETICS

Extensively, rapidly distributed after IM administration. Protein binding: 99%. Metabolized in liver. Eliminated by hepatobiliary route; excreted in feces. **Half-life:** 40 days in postmenopausal women. Peak serum levels occur in 7–9 days.

USES

Treatment of hormone receptor–positive metastatic breast cancer in postmenopausal women with disease progression following antiestrogen therapy. **OFF-LABEL:** Endometriosis, uterine bleeding.

PRECAUTIONS

Contraindications: Known or suspected pregnancy. **Cautions:** Thrombocytopenia, bleeding diathesis, anticoagulant therapy, hepatic disease, reduced hepatic blood flow, estrogen receptor–negative breast cancer.

LIFESPAN CONSIDERATIONS

Pregnancy/Lactation: Do not administer to pregnant women. Unknown if excreted in breast milk. May cause fetal harm. **Pregnancy Category D. Children:** Not used in this pt population. **Elderly:** No age-related precautions noted.

INTERACTIONS

DRUG: **Anticoagulants** may increase risk of bleeding/bruising. **HERBAL:** None significant. **FOOD:** None known. **LAB VALUES:** None significant.

AVAILABILITY (Rx)

Injection, Solution: 50 mg/ml in 2.5-ml and 5-ml syringes, 500 mg (2 × 250 mg/5 ml).

ADMINISTRATION/HANDLING

IM

• Administer slowly into upper, outer quadrant or ventro-gluteal area of buttock as two injections, one in each buttock.

INDICATIONS/ROUTES/DOSAGE

Breast Cancer

IM: ADULTS, ELDERLY: Two 250-mg injections on days 1, 15, and 29, and once monthly thereafter.

SIDE EFFECTS

Frequent (26%–13%): Nausea, hot flashes, pharyngitis, asthenia (loss of strength, energy), vomiting, vasodilatation, headache. **Occasional (12%–5%):** Injection site pain, constipation, diarrhea, abdominal pain, anorexia, dizziness, insomnia, paresthesia, bone/back pain, depression, anxiety, peripheral edema, rash, diaphoresis, fever. **Rare (2%–1%):** Vertigo, weight gain.

ADVERSE EFFECTS/ TOXIC REACTIONS

UTI occurs occasionally. Vaginitis, anemia, thromboembolic phenomena, leukopenia occur rarely.

NURSING CONSIDERATIONS

BASELINE ASSESSMENT

Estrogen receptor assay should be done before beginning therapy. Baseline CT should be performed initially and periodically thereafter for evidence of tumor regression.

INTERVENTION/EVALUATION

Monitor blood chemistry, plasma lipids. Be alert to increased bone pain, ensure adequate pain relief. Check for edema, esp. of dependent areas. Monitor for and assist with ambulation if asthenia (loss of strength, energy) or dizziness occurs. Assess for headache. Offer antiemetic for nausea/vomiting.

PATIENT/FAMILY TEACHING

• Notify physician if nausea/vomiting, asthenia (loss of strength, energy), hot flashes become unmanageable.

F

furosemide

feur-**oh**-sah-mide
(Apo-Furosemide ♣, Lasix, Novo-Semide ♣)

BLACK BOX ALERT Large amounts can lead to profound diuresis with water and electrolyte depletion.

Do not confuse Lasix with Lidex, Lovenox, Luvox, or Luxiq, or furosemide with famotidine, finasteride, fluconazole, fluoxetine, loperamide, or torsemide.

◆CLASSIFICATION

PHARMACOTHERAPEUTIC: Loop. **CLINICAL:** Diuretic (see p. 102C).

ACTION

Enhances excretion of sodium, chloride, potassium by direct action at ascending limb of loop of Henle. **Therapeutic Effect:** Produces diuresis, lowers B/P.

PHARMACOKINETICS

Route	Onset	Peak	Duration
PO	30–60 min	1–2 hrs	6–8 hrs
IV	5 min	20–60 min	2 hrs
IM	30 min	N/A	N/A

Well absorbed from GI tract. Protein binding: greater than 98%. Partially metabolized in liver. Primarily excreted in urine (nonrenal clearance increases in severe renal impairment). Not removed by hemodialysis. **Half-life:** 30–90 min (increased in renal/hepatic impairment, neonates).

USES

Treatment of edema associated with CHF, chronic renal failure (including nephrotic syndrome), hepatic cirrhosis, acute pulmonary edema. Treatment of hypertension, either alone or in combination with other antihypertensives. **OFF-LABEL:** Treatment of hypercalcemia.

PRECAUTIONS

Contraindications: Anuria, hepatic coma, severe electrolyte depletion. **Cautions:** Hepatic cirrhosis.

⌛ LIFESPAN CONSIDERATIONS

Pregnancy/Lactation: Crosses placenta. Distributed in breast milk. **Pregnancy Category C. Children:** Half-life increased in neonates; may require increased dosage interval. **Elderly:** May be more sensitive to hypotensive, electrolyte effects, developing circulatory collapse, thromboembolic effect. Age-related renal impairment may require dosage adjustment.

INTERACTIONS

DRUG: Amphotericin B, nephrotoxic, ototoxic medications may increase risk of nephrotoxicity, ototoxicity. May decrease effects of **anticoagulants, heparin.** May increase risk of **lithium** toxicity. **Other medications causing hypokalemia** may increase risk of hypokalemia. **HERBAL: Ephedra, ginseng, yohimbe** may worsen hypertension. **Garlic** may increase antihypertensive effect. **FOOD:** None known. **LAB VALUES:** May increase serum glucose, BUN, uric acid. May decrease serum calcium, chloride, magnesium, potassium, sodium.

AVAILABILITY (Rx)

Injection Solution: 10 mg/ml. **Oral Solution:** 10 mg/ml, 40 mg/5 ml. **Tablets:** 20 mg, 40 mg, 80 mg.

ADMINISTRATION/HANDLING

IV

Rate of administration • May give undiluted but is compatible with D_5W or 0.9% NaCl. • Administer each 40 mg or fraction by IV push over 1–2 min. Do not exceed administration rate of 4 mg/min in those with renal impairment.
Storage • Solution appears clear, colorless. • Discard yellow solutions. • Stable for 24 hrs at room temperature when mixed with 0.9% NaCl or D_5W.

IM

• Temporary pain at injection site may be noted.

PO

• Give with food to avoid GI upset, preferably with breakfast (may prevent nocturia).

IV INCOMPATIBILITIES

Ciprofloxacin (Cipro), diltiazem (Cardizem), dobutamine (Dobutrex), dopamine (Intropin), doxorubicin (Adriamycin), droperidol (Inapsine), esmolol (Brevibloc), famotidine (Pepcid), filgrastim (Neupogen), fluconazole (Diflucan), gemcitabine (Gemzar), gentamicin (Garamycin), idarubicin (Idamycin), labetalol (Trandate), meperidine (Demerol), metoclopramide (Reglan), midazolam (Versed), milrinone (Primacor), nicardipine (Cardene), ondansetron (Zofran), quinidine, thiopental (Pentothal), vecuronium (Norcuron), vinblastine (Velban), vincristine (Oncovin), vinorelbine (Navelbine).

IV COMPATIBILITIES

Aminophylline, amiodarone (Cordarone), bumetanide (Bumex), calcium gluconate, cimetidine (Tagamet), heparin, hydromorphone (Dilaudid), lidocaine, lipids, morphine, nitroglycerin, norepinephrine (Levophed), potassium chloride, propofol (Diprivan).

INDICATIONS/ROUTES/DOSAGE

Edema, Hypertension
PO: ADULTS, ELDERLY: Initially, 20–80 mg/dose; may increase by 20–40 mg/dose q6–8h. May titrate up to 600 mg/day in severe edematous states. **CHILDREN:** 1–6 mg/kg/day in divided doses q6–12h. **NEONATES:** 1–4 mg/kg/dose 1–2 times a day.
IV, IM: ADULTS, ELDERLY: 20–40 mg/dose; may increase by 20 mg/dose q1–2h. **Maximum Single Dose:** 160–200 mg. **CHILDREN:** 1–2 mg/kg/dose q6–12h. **Maximum:** 6 mg/kg/dose. **NEONATES:** 1–2 mg/kg/dose q12–24h.
IV INFUSION: ADULTS, ELDERLY: Bolus of 20–40 mg, followed by infusion of 10–40 mg/hr; may double q2h. **Maximum:** 80–160 mg/hr. **CHILDREN:** 0.05 mg/kg/hr; titrate to desired effect.

SIDE EFFECTS

Expected: Increased urinary frequency/volume. **Frequent:** Nausea, dyspepsia, abdominal cramps, diarrhea or constipation, electrolyte disturbances. **Occasional:** Dizziness, light-headedness, headache, blurred vision, paresthesia, photosensitivity, rash, fatigue, bladder spasm, restlessness, diaphoresis. **Rare:** Flank pain.

ADVERSE EFFECTS/ TOXIC REACTIONS

Vigorous diuresis may lead to profound water loss/electrolyte depletion, resulting

F

in hypokalemia, hyponatremia, dehydration. Sudden volume depletion may result in increased risk of thrombosis, circulatory collapse, sudden death. Acute hypotensive episodes may occur, sometimes several days after beginning therapy. Ototoxicity (deafness, vertigo, tinnitus) may occur, esp. in pts with severe renal impairment. Can exacerbate diabetes mellitus, systemic lupus erythematosus, gout, pancreatitis. Blood dyscrasias have been reported.

G

NURSING CONSIDERATIONS

BASELINE ASSESSMENT

Check vital signs, esp. B/P, pulse, for hypotension before administration. Assess baseline serum electrolytes, esp. for hypokalemia. Assess skin turgor, mucous membranes for hydration status; observe for edema. Assess muscle strength, mental status. Note skin temperature, moisture. Obtain baseline weight. Initiate I&O monitoring.

INTERVENTION/EVALUATION

Monitor B/P, vital signs, serum electrolytes, I&O, weight. Note extent of diuresis. Watch for changes from initial assessment (hypokalemia may result in changes in muscle strength, tremor, muscle cramps, altered mental status, cardiac arrhythmias). Hyponatremia may result in confusion, thirst, cold/clammy skin.

PATIENT/FAMILY TEACHING

• Expect increased frequency, volume of urination. • Report palpitations, signs of electrolyte imbalances (noted previously), hearing abnormalities (sense of fullness in ears, tinnitus). • Eat foods high in potassium such as whole grains (cereals), legumes, meat, bananas, apricots, orange juice, potatoes (white, sweet), raisins. • Avoid sunlight, sunlamps.

Fuzeon, *see enfuvirtide*

gabapentin

gah-bah-**pen**-tin
(Apo-Gabapentin 🍁, Neurontin, Novo-Gabapentin 🍁)
Do not confuse Neurontin with Motrin, Neoral, nitrofurantoin, Noroxin, or Zarontin.

◆ CLASSIFICATION

CLINICAL: Anticonvulsant, antineuralgic (see p. 35C).

ACTION

May increase synthesis or accumulation of gamma-aminobutyric acid (GABA) by binding to as-yet-undefined receptor sites in brain tissue. **Therapeutic Effect:** Reduces seizure activity, neuropathic pain.

PHARMACOKINETICS

Well absorbed from GI tract (not affected by food). Protein binding: less than 5%. Widely distributed. Crosses blood-brain barrier. Primarily excreted unchanged in urine. Removed by hemodialysis. **Half-life:** 5–7 hrs (increased in renal impairment, elderly).

USES

Adjunct in treatment of partial seizures (with or without secondary generalized seizures) in children 13 yrs and older and adults. Adjunct to treatment of partial seizures in children 3–12 yrs; adjunct to treatment of neuropathic pain, postherpetic neuralgia. **OFF-LABEL:** Treatment of bipolar disorder, chronic pain, diabetic peripheral neuropathy, essential tremor, hot flashes, hyperhidrosis, migraines, psychiatric disorders (social phobia), agitation in dementia, uremic pruritus.

PRECAUTIONS

Contraindications: None known. **Cautions:** Renal impairment.

LIFESPAN CONSIDERATIONS

Pregnancy/Lactation: Unknown if distributed in breast milk. **Pregnancy Category C. Children:** Safety and efficacy not established in those 3 yrs and younger. **Elderly:** Age-related renal impairment may require dosage adjustment.

INTERACTIONS

DRUG: **Antacids** decrease absorption. **Morphine** may increase CNS depression. HERBAL: **Evening primrose** may decrease seizure threshold. **Gotu kola, kava kava, St. John's wort, valerian** may increase CNS depression. FOOD: None known. LAB VALUES: May alter serum WBC count, glucose. May increase alkaline phosphatase, ALT, AST, bilirubin.

AVAILABILITY (Rx)

Capsules (Neurontin): 100 mg, 300 mg, 400 mg. **Oral Solution (Neurontin):** 250 mg/5 ml. **Tablets (Neurontin):** 100 mg, 300 mg, 400 mg, 600 mg, 800 mg.

ADMINISTRATION/HANDLING

PO

• Give without regard to meals; may give with food to avoid, reduce GI upset. • If treatment is discontinued or anticonvulsant therapy is added, do so gradually over at least 1 wk (reduces risk of loss of seizure control).

INDICATIONS/ROUTES/DOSAGE

Note: When given 3 times/day, maximum time between doses should not exceed 12 hrs.

Adjunctive Therapy for Seizure Control

PO: ADULTS, ELDERLY, CHILDREN 13 YEARS AND OLDER: Initially, 300 mg 3 times a day. May titrate dosage. Range: 900–1,800 mg/day in 3 divided doses. **Maximum:** 3,600 mg/day. **CHILDREN 3–12 YRS:** Initially, 10–15 mg/kg/day in 3 divided doses. May titrate up to 25–35 mg/kg/day (for children 5–12 yrs) and 40 mg/kg/day (for children 3–4 yrs). **Maximum:** 50 mg/kg/day.

Adjunctive Therapy for Neuropathic Pain

PO: ADULTS, ELDERLY: Initially, 100 mg 3 times a day; may increase by 300 mg/day at weekly intervals. **Maximum:** 3,600 mg/day in 3 divided doses. **CHILDREN:** Initially, 5 mg/kg/dose at bedtime, followed by 5 mg/kg/dose for 2 doses on day 2, then 5 mg/kg/dose for 3 doses on day 3. Range: 8–35 mg/kg/day in 3 divided doses.

Postherpetic Neuralgia

PO: ADULTS, ELDERLY: 300 mg once on day 1, 300 mg twice a day on day 2, and 300 mg 3 times a day on day 3. Titrate up to 1,800 mg/day.

Dosage in Renal Impairment

Dosage and frequency are modified based on creatinine clearance:

Creatinine Clearance	Dosage
60 ml/min or higher	300–1,200 mg tid
30–59 ml/min	200–700 mg q12h
16–29 ml/min	200–700 mg/day
Less than 16 ml/min	100–300 mg/day
Hemodialysis	125–300 mg after each 4-hr hemodialysis session

SIDE EFFECTS

Frequent (19%–10%): Fatigue, drowsiness, dizziness, ataxia. **Occasional (8%–3%):** Nystagmus (rapid eye movements), tremor, diplopia (blurred vision), rhinitis, weight gain. **Rare (less than 2%):** Anxiety, dysarthria (speech difficulty), memory loss, dyspepsia, pharyngitis, myalgia.

ADVERSE EFFECTS/ TOXIC REACTIONS

Abrupt withdrawal may increase seizure frequency. Increased risk of suicidal behavior/thoughts. Overdosage may result in slurred speech, drowsiness, lethargy, diarrhea.

NURSING CONSIDERATIONS

BASELINE ASSESSMENT

Review history of seizure disorder (type, onset, intensity, frequency, duration, LOC). Assess location, intensity of neuralgia/neuropathic pain. Routine laboratory monitoring of serum levels unnecessary for safe use.

INTERVENTION/EVALUATION

Provide safety measures as needed. Monitor seizure frequency/duration, renal function, weight, behavior in children. Monitor signs/symptoms of depression, suicidal tendencies, other unusual behavior.

PATIENT/FAMILY TEACHING

• Take gabapentin only as prescribed; do not abruptly stop taking drug (may increase seizure frequency). • Avoid tasks that require alertness, motor skills until response to drug is established. • Avoid alcohol. • Carry identification card/bracelet to note seizure disorder/anticonvulsant therapy. • Report suicidal ideation, depression, unusual behavioral changes (esp. with changes in dosage), worsening of seizure activity or loss of seizure control.

galantamine

gal-**an**-tah-mean
(Razadyne, Razadyne ER, Reminyl ✤, Reminyl ER ✤)
Do not confuse Razadyne with Rozerem, or Reminyl with Amaryl.

◆CLASSIFICATION

PHARMACOTHERAPEUTIC: Cholinesterase inhibitor. **CLINICAL:** Antidementia.

ACTION

Elevates acetylcholine concentrations by slowing degeneration of acetylcholine released by still intact cholinergic neurons (Alzheimer's disease involves degeneration of cholinergic neuronal pathways). **Therapeutic Effect:** Slows progression of Alzheimer's disease.

PHARMACOKINETICS

Rapidly, completely absorbed from GI tract. Protein binding: 18%. Distributed to blood cells; binds to plasma proteins, mainly albumin. Metabolized in liver. Excreted in urine. **Half-life:** 7 hrs.

USES

Treatment of mild to moderate dementia of Alzheimer's type. **OFF-LABEL:** Severe dementia associated with Alzheimer's disease, mild to moderate dementia associated with Parkinson's disease.

PRECAUTIONS

Contraindications: Severe hepatic/renal impairment. **Cautions:** Moderate renal/hepatic impairment, history of ulcer disease, those on concurrent NSAIDs, asthma, COPD, bladder outflow obstruction, supraventricular cardiac conduction conditions.

⌛ LIFESPAN CONSIDERATIONS

Pregnancy/Lactation: Unknown if drug crosses placenta or is distributed in breast milk. **Pregnancy Category B. Children:** Not prescribed for this pt population. **Elderly:** No age-related precautions noted, but use is not recommended in those with severe hepatic/renal impairment (creatinine clearance less than 9 ml/min).

INTERACTIONS

DRUG: May interfere with the effects of **bethanechol, succinylcholine. Cimetidine, erythromycin, ketoconazole, paroxetine** may increase concentration. **HERBAL: St. John's wort** may decrease concentration. **FOOD:** None known. **LAB VALUES:** None significant.

AVAILABILITY (Rx)

Oral Solution (Razadyne): 4 mg/ml. **Tablets (Razadyne):** 4 mg, 8 mg, 12 mg.

Capsules (Extended-Release [Razadyne ER]): 8 mg, 16 mg, 24 mg.

ADMINISTRATION/HANDLING

PO

• Give tablet or solution with morning and evening meals. Capsule should be given at breakfast.

INDICATIONS/ROUTES/DOSAGE

Alzheimer's Disease

PO (IMMEDIATE-RELEASE): ADULTS, ELDERLY: Initially, 4 mg twice a day (8 mg/day). After a minimum of 4 wks (if well tolerated), may increase to 8 mg twice a day (16 mg/day). After another 4 wks, may increase to 12 mg twice daily (24 mg/day). Range: 16–24 mg/day in 2 divided doses.
PO (EXTENDED-RELEASE): ADULTS, ELDERLY: Initially, 8 mg once daily for 4 wks; then increase to 16 mg once daily for 4 wks or longer. If tolerated, may increase to 24 mg once daily. Range: 16–24 mg once daily.

Dosage in Renal/Hepatic Impairment

For moderate impairment, maximum dosage is 16 mg/day. Drug is not recommended for pts with severe impairment.

SIDE EFFECTS

Frequent (17%–7%): Nausea, vomiting, diarrhea, anorexia, weight loss. **Occcasional (5%–4%):** Abdominal pain, insomnia, depression, headache, dizziness, fatigue, rhinitis. **Rare (less than 3%):** Tremors, constipation, confusion, cough, anxiety, urinary incontinence.

ADVERSE EFFECTS/ TOXIC REACTIONS

Overdose may cause cholinergic crisis (increased salivation, lacrimation, urination, defecation, bradycardia, hypotension, muscle weakness). Treatment aimed at generally supportive measures, use of anticholinergics (e.g., atropine).

NURSING CONSIDERATIONS

BASELINE ASSESSMENT

Assess cognitive, behavioral, functional deficits of pt. Assess serum hepatic/renal function tests.

INTERVENTION/EVALUATION

Monitor cognitive, behavioral, functional status of pt. Evaluate EKG, periodic rhythm strips in pts with underlying arrhythmias. Assess for evidence of GI disturbances (nausea, vomiting, diarrhea, anorexia, weight loss).

PATIENT/FAMILY TEACHING

• Take with meals (reduces risk of nausea). • Avoid tasks that require alertness, motor skills until response to drug is established. • Report persistent GI disturbances, excessive salivation, diaphoresis, excessive tearing, excessive fatigue, insomnia, depression, dizziness, increased muscle weakness.

G

Gammagard S/D, *see immune globulin IV*

ganciclovir

gan-**sy**-clo-ver
(Cytovene, Vitrasert, Zirgan)

BLACK BOX ALERT Toxicity presents as neutropenia, thrombocytopenia, anemia. Studies suggest carcinogenic and teratogenic effects, inhibition of spermatogenesis.

Do not confuse Cytovene with Cytosar, or ganciclovir with acyclovir.

◆CLASSIFICATION

PHARMACOTHERAPEUTIC: Synthetic nucleoside. **CLINICAL:** Antiviral (see p. 68C).

ACTION

Competes with viral DNA polymerase and incorporation into growing viral DNA chains. **Therapeutic Effect:** Interferes with DNA synthesis, viral replication.

PHARMACOKINETICS

Widely distributed (including CSF and ocular tissue). Protein binding: 1%–2%.

Undergoes minimal metabolism. Excreted primarily in urine. Removed by hemodialysis. Half-life: 1.7–5.8 hrs (increased in renal impairment).

USES

Parenteral: Treatment of cytomegalovirus (CMV) retinitis in immunocompromised pts (e.g., HIV), prophylaxis of CMV infection in transplant pts. **PO:** Maintenance treatment of CMV retinitis. **Implant:** Treatment of CMV retinitis. **Ophthalmic:** Treatment of acute herpetic keratitis. OFF-LABEL: Treatment of other CMV infections (gastroenteritis, hepatitis, pneumonitis).

PRECAUTIONS

Contraindications: Absolute neutrophil count less than 500/mm³, platelet count less than 25,000/mm³, hypersensitivity to acyclovir, ganciclovir, immunocompetent pts, pts with congenital or neonatal cytomegalovirus (CMV) disease. Cautions: Pts with neutropenia, thrombocytopenia, renal impairment; children (long-term safety not determined due to potential for long-term carcinogenic, adverse reproductive effects).

LIFESPAN CONSIDERATIONS

Pregnancy/Lactation: Effective contraception should be used during therapy; ganciclovir should not be used during pregnancy. Breast-feeding should be discontinued; may be resumed no sooner than 72 hrs after the last dose of ganciclovir. **Pregnancy Category C. Children:** Safety and efficacy not established in those younger than 12 yrs. **Elderly:** Age-related renal impairment may require dosage adjustment.

INTERACTIONS

DRUG: **Bone marrow depressants** may increase myelosuppression. **Nephrotoxic medications** may increase risk of renal impairment, increase concentration/toxicity. **Zidovudine (AZT)** may increase risk of hepatotoxicity. HERBAL: None significant. FOOD: None known. LAB VALUES: May increase BUN, serum creatinine, serum alkaline phosphatase, bilirubin, AST, ALT.

AVAILABILITY (Rx)

Capsules (Cytovene): 250 mg, 500 mg. Implant (Vitrasert): 4.5 mg. Injection, Powder for Reconstitution (Cytovene): 500 mg. Ophthalmic Gel (Zirgan): 0.15%.

ADMINISTRATION/HANDLING

IV

Reconstitution • Reconstitute 500-mg vial with 10 ml Sterile Water for Injection to provide concentration of 50 mg/ml; do **not** use Bacteriostatic Water (contains parabens, which is incompatible with ganciclovir). • Further dilute with 250–1,000 ml D_5W, 0.9% NaCl, lactated Ringer's, or any combination thereof to provide a concentration of 10 mg/ml or less for infusion.

Rate of administration • Administer only by IV infusion over 1 hr. • Do not give by IV push or rapid IV infusion (increases risk of toxicity); protect from infiltration (high pH causes severe tissue irritation). • Use large veins to permit rapid dilution, dissemination of ganciclovir (minimizes phlebitis); central venous ports may reduce catheter-associated infection.

Storage • Store vials at room temperature. Do not refrigerate. • Reconstituted solution in vial is stable for 12 hrs at room temperature. • After dilution, stable for 5 days at room tempearture or if refrigerated. • Discard if precipitate forms, discoloration occurs. • Avoid exposure to skin, eyes, mucous membranes. • Use latex gloves, safety glasses during preparation/handling of solution. • Avoid inhalation. • If solution contacts skin or mucous membranes, wash thoroughly with soap and water; rinse eyes thoroughly with plain water.

PO

• Give with food. • Do not open capsules.

IV INCOMPATIBILITIES

Aldesleukin (Proleukin), amifostine (Ethyol), aztreonam (Azactam), cefepime (Maxipime), cytarabine (ARA-C), doxorubicin (Adriamycin), fludarabine (Fludara), foscarnet (Foscavir), gemcitabine (Gemzar), lipids, ondansetron (Zofran), piperacillin and tazobactam (Zosyn), sargramostim (Leukine), total parenteral nutrition (TPN), vinorelbine (Navelbine).

IV COMPATIBILITIES

Amphotericin B, enalapril (Vasotec), filgrastim (Neupogen), fluconazole (Diflucan), granisetron (Kytril), propofol (Diprivan).

INDICATIONS/ROUTES/DOSAGE

Cytomegalovirus (CMV) Retinitis

IV: ADULTS, CHILDREN 3 MOS AND OLDER: 10 mg/kg/day in divided doses q12h for 14–21 days, then 5 mg/kg/day as a single daily dose or 6 mg/kg 5 days a wk.

PO: ADULTS, ELDERLY: 1,000 mg 3 times a day or 500 mg 6 times a day. **CHILDREN:** 30 mg/kg q8h.

Prevention of CMV in Transplant Pts

IV: ADULTS, CHILDREN: 10 mg/kg/day in divided doses q12h for 7–14 days, then 5 mg/kg/day as a single daily dose.

Prevention of CMV in Pts with Advanced HIV Infection

PO: ADULTS: 1,000 mg 3 times a day.

Other CMV Infections

IV: ADULTS: Initially, 10 mg/kg/day in divided doses q12h for 14–21 days, then 5 mg/kg/day as a single daily dose. Maintenance (PO): 1,000 mg 3 times a day or 500 mg q3h (6 times a day). **CHILDREN:** Initially, 10 mg/kg/day in divided doses q12h for 14–21 days, then 5 mg/kg/day as a single daily dose. Maintenance (PO): 30 mg/kg/dose q8h.

INTRAVITREAL IMPLANT: ADULTS: 1 implant q5–8mo plus oral ganciclovir 1–1.5 g 3 times a day. **CHILDREN 9 YRS AND OLDER:** 1 implant q5–8mo plus oral ganciclovir (30 mg/dose q8h).

Acute Herpetic Keratitis

OPHTHALMIC: ADULTS, ELDERLY: 1 drop 5 times/day until ulcer heals, then 1 drop 3 times/day for 7 days.

Dosage in Renal Impairment

Dosage and frequency are modified based on creatinine clearance.

Creatinine Clearance	Dosage: IV Induction	IV Maintenance	PO
50–69 ml/min	2.5 mg/kg q12h	2.5 mg/kg q24h	1,500 mg/day
25–49 ml/min	2.5 mg/kg q24h	1.25 mg/kg q24h	1,000 mg/day
10–24 ml/min	1.25 mg/kg q24h	0.625 mg/kg q24h	500 mg/day
Less than 10 ml/min	1.25 mg/kg 3 times a wk	0.625 mg/kg 3 times a wk	500 mg 3 times a wk

SIDE EFFECTS

Frequent: Diarrhea (41%), fever (40%), nausea (25%), abdominal pain (17%), vomiting (13%). **Occasional (11%–6%):** Diaphoresis, infection, paresthesia, flatulence, pruritus. **Rare (4%–2%):** Headache, stomatitis, dyspepsia, phlebitis.

ADVERSE EFFECTS/ TOXIC REACTIONS

Hematologic toxicity occurs commonly: leukopenia (41%–29%), anemia (25%–19%). Intraocular implant occasionally results in visual acuity loss, vitreous hemorrhage, retinal detachment. GI hemorrhage occurs rarely.

NURSING CONSIDERATIONS

BASELINE ASSESSMENT

Evaluate hematologic baseline. Obtain specimens for support of differential diagnosis (urine, feces, blood, throat) because retinal infection is usually due to hematogenous dissemination.

INTERVENTION/EVALUATION

Monitor I&O, ensure adequate hydration (minimum 1,500 ml/24 hrs). Diligently evaluate hematology reports for neutropenia, thrombocytopenia, decreased platelets. Question pt regarding visual acuity, therapeutic improvement, complications. Assess for rash, pruritus.

PATIENT/FAMILY TEACHING

• Ganciclovir provides suppression, not cure, of cytomegalovirus (CMV) retinitis. • Frequent blood tests, eye exams are necessary during therapy because of toxic nature of drug. • Report any new symptom promptly. • May temporarily or permanently inhibit sperm production in men, suppress fertility in women. • Barrier contraception should be used during and for 90 days after therapy because of mutagenic potential.

garlic

Also known as ail, allium, nectar of the gods, poor man's treacle, stinking rose.

CLASSIFICATION

HERBAL: See Appendix G.

ACTION

Possesses antithrombotic properties, can increase fibrinolytic activity, decrease platelet aggregation, increase PT. Acts as HMG-CoA reductase inhibitor (statins). **Effect:** Lowers serum cholesterol. Causes smooth muscle relaxation/vasodilation, reducing B/P. Reduces oxidative stress and LDL oxidation, preventing age-related vascular changes, atherosclerosis. Prevents endothelial cell depletion, producing antioxidant effect.

USES

Treatment of hypertension, prevention of coronary artery disease, age-related vascular changes, atherosclerosis.

PRECAUTIONS

Contraindications: Pts with bleeding disorders. **Cautions:** Diabetes (may decrease blood glucose levels), inflammatory GI conditions (may irritate GI tract). Hypothyroidism (may reduce iodine uptake). May prolong bleeding time (discontinue 1–2 wks before surgery).

LIFESPAN CONSIDERATIONS

Pregnancy/Lactation: Caution: May stimulate labor and cause colic in infants. **Children:** Safety and efficacy not established (may be beneficial in those with hypercholesterolemia). **Elderly:** No age-related precautions noted.

INTERACTIONS

DRUG: May enhance effects of **anticoagulants, antiplatelets (aspirin, clopidogrel, enoxaparin, warfarin).** May decrease effects of **cyclosporine, oral contraceptives. Insulin, oral antidiabetic agents** may increase hypoglycemic effects. **Saquinavir, other antiretrovirals** may decrease concentration, effect of garlic. **HERBAL: Feverfew, ginger, ginkgo, ginseng** may increase risk of bleeding. **FOOD:** None known. **LAB VALUES:** May decrease serum glucose, cholesterol. May increase INR.

AVAILABILITY (OTC)

Capsules: 100 mg, 300 mg, 500 mg, 1,000 mg, 1.5 g. **Extract. Oil. Powder. Tablets:** 400 mg, 1,250 mg. **Tea.**

INDICATIONS/ROUTES/DOSAGE

Hyperlipidemia, Hypertension

PO (CAPSULES, POWDER, TEA): ADULTS, ELDERLY: 600–1,200 mg a day in divided doses 3 times a day.

ALERT Appropriate doses for other conditions vary depending on the preparation used.

SIDE EFFECTS

Breath/body odor, oropharyngeal/esophageal burning, heartburn, nausea, vomiting, diarrhea, allergic reactions (rhinitis, urticaria, angioedema).

ADVERSE EFFECTS/ TOXIC REACTIONS

None known.

NURSING CONSIDERATIONS

BASELINE ASSESSMENT

Assess serum lipid levels; determine whether pt is taking anticoagulants, antiplatelets. Assess if diabetic, taking insulin or oral hypoglycemic agents.

INTERVENTION/EVALUATION

Monitor CBC, coagulation studies, serum lipid, creatinine, glucose levels. Assess for hypersensitivity reaction, contact dermatitis.

PATIENT/FAMILY TEACHING

• Avoid use in pregnancy or breast-feeding. • Inform all health care providers of garlic use. • Discontinue 1–2 wks before any procedure in which excessive bleeding may occur.

gemcitabine

HIGH ALERT

gem-**cih**-tah-bean
(Gemzar)
Do not confuse Gemzar with Zinecard.

◆ CLASSIFICATION

PHARMACOTHERAPEUTIC: Antimetabolite. **CLINICAL:** Antineoplastic (see p. 84C).

ACTION

Inhibits ribonucleotide reductase, the enzyme necessary for catalyzing DNA synthesis. **Therapeutic Effect:** Produces death of cells undergoing DNA synthesis.

PHARMACOKINETICS

Not extensively distributed after IV infusion (increased with length of infusion). Protein binding: less than 10%. Metabolized intracellularly by nucleoside kinases. Excreted primarily in urine as metabolite. **Half-life:** Influenced by duration of infusion. Infusion 1 hr or less: 42–94 min; infusion 3–4 hrs: 4–10.5 hrs.

USES

Metastatic breast cancer in combination with paclitaxel. Treatment of locally advanced (stage II, III) or metastatic (stage IV) adenocarcinoma of pancreas. Indicated for pts previously treated with 5-fluorouracil. Monotherapy or in combination with cisplatin for treatment of locally advanced or metastatic non–small-cell lung cancer (NSCLC), ovarian cancer. **OFF-LABEL:** Treatment of biliary tract carcinoma, bladder carcinoma, gall bladder carcinoma, germ cell tumors (e.g., testicular), Hodgkin's lymphoma, non-Hodgkin's lymphoma, acute leukemia.

PRECAUTIONS

Contraindications: None known. **Cautions:** Renal/hepatic impairment.

LIFESPAN CONSIDERATIONS

Pregnancy/Lactation: If possible, avoid use during pregnancy, esp. first trimester. May cause fetal harm. Unknown if distributed in breast milk. Breast-feeding not recommended. **Pregnancy Category D. Children:** Safety and efficacy not established. **Elderly:** Increased risk of hematologic toxicity.

INTERACTIONS

DRUG: **Bone marrow depressants** may increase risk of myelosuppression. **Immunosuppressants (e.g., cyclosporine, tacrolimus)** may increase risk of infection. **Live virus vaccines** may potentiate virus replication, increase vaccine side effects, decrease pt's antibody response to vaccine. **HERBAL:** **Echinacea** may decrease effects. **FOOD:** None known. **LAB VALUES:** May increase BUN, serum alkaline phosphatase, bilirubin, creatinine, AST, ALT. May decrease Hgb, Hct, leukocyte count, platelet count.

AVAILABILITY (Rx)

Injection, Powder for Reconstitution: 200-mg, 1-g vials.

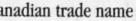

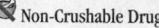

ADMINISTRATION/HANDLING

IV

Reconstitution • Use gloves when handling/preparing gemcitabine. • Reconstitute 200-mg or 1-g vial with 0.9% NaCl injection without preservative (5 ml or 25 ml, respectively) to provide concentration of 40 mg/ml. • Shake to dissolve.

Rate of administration • May give without further dilution. • May be further diluted with 50–500 ml 0.9% NaCl to a concentration as low as 0.1 mg/ml. • Infuse over 30 min. • Infusion time greater than 60 min increases toxicity.

Storage • Store at room temperature (refrigeration may cause crystallization). • Reconstituted solution is stable for 24 hrs at room temperature.

IV INCOMPATIBILITIES

Acyclovir (Zovirax), amphotericin B (Fungizone), cefotaxime (Claforan), furosemide (Lasix), ganciclovir (Cytovene), imipenem and cilastatin (Primaxin), irinotecan (Camptosar), methotrexate, methylprednisolone (Solu-Medrol), mitomycin (Mutamycin), piperacillin/tazobactam (Zosyn), prochlorperazine (Compazine).

IV COMPATIBILITIES

Bumetanide (Bumex), calcium gluconate, dexamethasone (Decadron), diphenhydramine (Benadryl), dobutamine (Dobutrex), dopamine (Intropin), granisetron (Kytril), heparin, hydrocortisone (Solu-Cortef), lorazepam (Ativan), ondansetron (Zofran), potassium.

INDICATIONS/ROUTES/DOSAGE

ALERT Dosage is individualized based on clinical response, tolerance to adverse effects. When used in combination therapy, consult specific protocols for optimum dosage, sequence of drug administration.

Breast Cancer

IV: ADULTS, ELDERLY: 1,250 mg/m² over 30 min on days 1 and 8 of each 21-day cycle.

Non–Small-Cell Lung Cancer (NSCLC)

IV: ADULTS, ELDERLY, CHILDREN: 1,000 mg/m² on days 1, 8, and 15, repeated every 28 days; or 1,250 mg/m² on days 1 and 8. Repeat every 21 days.

Ovarian Cancer

IV: ADULTS, ELDERLY: 1,000 mg/m² on days 1 and 8 of each 21-day cycle (in combination with carboplatin).

Pancreatic Cancer

IV: ADULTS: 1,000 mg/m² once weekly for up to 7 wks or until toxicity necessitates decreasing dosage or withholding the dose, followed by 1 wk of rest. Subsequent cycles should consist of once-weekly dose for 3 consecutive wks out of every 4 wks. For pts completing cycles at 1,000 mg/m², increase dose to 1,250 mg/m² as tolerated. Dose for next cycle may be increased to 1,500 mg/m².

Dosage Reduction Guidelines

Pancreatic Cancer, Non–Small-Cell Lung Cancer (NSCLC)

Dosage adjustments should be based on granulocyte count and platelet count, as follows:

Absolute Granulocyte Counts (cells/mm³)	Platelet Count (cells/mm³)	% of Full Dose
1,000 and	100,000	100
500–999 or	50,000–99,000	75
Less than 500 or	Less than 50,000	Hold

Breast Cancer

Absolute Granulocyte Counts (cells/mm³)	Platelet Count (cells/mm³)	% of Full Dose
Equal to or greater than 1,200 and	Greater than 75,000	100
1,000–1,199 or	50,000–75,000	75

Absolute Granulocyte Counts (cells/mm³)	Platelet Count (cells/mm³)	% of Full Dose
700–999 and	Equal to or greater than 50,000	50
Less than 700	Less than 50,000	Hold

Ovarian Cancer

Absolute Granulocyte Counts (cells/mm³)	Platelet Count (cells/mm³)	% of Full Dose
1,500 or greater and	100,000 or greater	100
1,000–1,499 and/or	75,000–99,999	50
Less than 1,000 and/or	Less than 75,000	Hold

SIDE EFFECTS

Frequent: Nausea, vomiting (69%); generalized pain (48%); fever (41%); mild to moderate pruritic rash (30%); mild to moderate dyspnea, constipation (23%); peripheral edema (20%). **Occasional (19%–10%):** Diarrhea, petechiae, alopecia, stomatitis, infection, drowsiness, paresthesia. **Rare:** Diaphoresis, rhinitis, insomnia, malaise.

ADVERSE EFFECTS/ TOXIC REACTIONS

Severe myelosuppression (anemia, thrombocytopenia, leukopenia) occurs commonly.

NURSING CONSIDERATIONS

BASELINE ASSESSMENT

CBC, platelets, renal/hepatic function tests should be performed before starting therapy and periodically thereafter (CBC, platelets before each dose). Drug should be suspended or dosage modified if myelosuppression is detected.

INTERVENTION/EVALUATION

Assess all lab results before giving each dose. Monitor for dyspnea, fever, pruritic rash, dehydration. Assess oral mucosa for erythema, ulceration at inner margin of lips, sore throat, difficulty swallowing (stomatitis). Assess skin for rash. Monitor for, report diarrhea. Provide antiemetics as needed.

PATIENT/FAMILY TEACHING

• Avoid crowds, exposure to infection. • Maintain fastidious oral hygiene. • Promptly report fever, sore throat, signs of local infection, easy bruising, rash, yellowing of skin or eyes. • Contact physician if nausea or vomiting continues at home.

G

gemfibrozil

gem-fi-broe-zil
(Apo-Gemfibrozil ✤, Lopid, Novo-Gemfibrozil ✤)
Do not confuse Lopid with Levbid, Lipitor, Lodine, or Slo-Bid.

◆CLASSIFICATION

PHARMACOTHERAPEUTIC: Fibric acid derivative. **CLINICAL:** Antihyperlipoproteinemic (see p. 57C).

ACTION

Inhibits lipolysis of fat in adipose tissue; decreases hepatic uptake of free fatty acids (reduces hepatic triglyceride production). Inhibits synthesis of VLDL carrier apolipoprotein B. **Therapeutic Effect:** Lowers serum cholesterol, triglycerides (decreases VLDL, LDL; increases HDL).

PHARMACOKINETICS

Well absorbed from GI tract. Protein binding: 99%. Metabolized in liver. Primarily excreted in urine. Not removed by hemodialysis. **Half-life:** 1.5 hrs.

USES

Treatment of hypertriglyceridemia in types IV and V hyperlipidemia for pts who are at greater risk for pancreatitis and those who have not responded to dietary intervention.

PRECAUTIONS

Contraindications: Hepatic dysfunction (including primary biliary cirrhosis), preexisting gallbladder disease, severe renal dysfunction. **Cautions:** Hypothyroidism, diabetes mellitus, estrogen or anticoagulant therapy.

LIFESPAN CONSIDERATIONS

Pregnancy/Lactation: Unknown if drug crosses placenta or is distributed in breast milk. Decision to discontinue nursing or drug should be based on potential for serious adverse effects. **Pregnancy Category C. Children:** Not recommended in those younger than 2 yrs (cholesterol necessary for normal development). **Elderly:** Age-related renal impairment may require dosage adjustment.

INTERACTIONS

DRUG: May increase levels of **statins** (increasing risk of rhabdomyolysis). May increase effect of **pioglitazone, repaglinide, warfarin. HERBAL:** None significant. **FOOD:** None known. **LAB VALUES:** May increase serum alkaline phosphatase, bilirubin, creatinine kinase, LDH, AST, ALT. May decrease Hgb, Hct, leukocyte counts, serum potassium.

AVAILABILITY (Rx)

Tablets: 600 mg.

ADMINISTRATION/HANDLING

PO

- Give 30 min before morning and evening meals.

INDICATIONS/ROUTES/DOSAGE

Hyperlipidemia

PO: ADULTS, ELDERLY: 600 mg twice daily 30 min before breakfast and dinner.

SIDE EFFECTS

Frequent (20%): Dyspepsia. **Occasional (10%–2%):** Abdominal pain, diarrhea, nausea, vomiting, fatigue. **Rare (less than 2%):** Constipation, acute appendicitis, vertigo, headache, rash, pruritus, altered taste.

ADVERSE EFFECTS/ TOXIC REACTIONS

Cholelithiasis, cholecystitis, acute appendicitis, pancreatitis, malignancy occur rarely.

NURSING CONSIDERATIONS

BASELINE ASSESSMENT

Obtain diet history, esp. fat/alcohol consumption. Assess baseline lab results: serum glucose, triglyceride, cholesterol, hepatic function tests; CBC.

INTERVENTION/EVALUATION

Monitor daily pattern of bowel activity and stool consistency. Monitor LDL, VLDL, serum triglyceride, cholesterol lab results for therapeutic response. Assess for rash, pruritus. Check for headache, dizziness. Monitor hepatic function, hematology tests. Assess for pain, esp. right upper quadrant or epigastric pain suggestive of adverse gallbladder effects. Monitor serum glucose in those receiving insulin, oral antihyperglycemics.

PATIENT/FAMILY TEACHING

- Follow special diet (important part of treatment). • Take before meals. • Periodic lab tests are essential part of therapy. • Notify physician if dizziness, blurred vision, abdominal pain, diarrhea, nausea, vomiting becomes pronounced. • Report signs/symptoms of rhabdomyolysis, cholelithiasis.

gemifloxacin

gem-ih-**flocks**-ah-sin
(Factive)

BLACK BOX ALERT Increased risk of tendonitis, tendon rupture.

◆CLASSIFICATION

PHARMACOTHERAPEUTIC: Fluoroquinolone. **CLINICAL:** Antibacterial.

ACTION

Inhibits the enzyme DNA gyrase in susceptible microorganisms, interfering with bacterial cell replication, repair. **Therapeutic Effect:** Bactericidal.

PHARMACOKINETICS

Rapidly, well absorbed from GI tract. Protein binding: 70%. Widely distributed. Penetrates well into lung tissue and fluid. Undergoes limited metabolism in liver. Primarily excreted in feces; lesser amount eliminated in urine. Partially removed by hemodialysis. **Half-life:** 4–12 hrs.

USES

Treatment of susceptible infections due to *S. pneumoniae, H. influenzae, H. parainfluenzae, M. catarrhalis, M. pneumoniae, C. pneumoniae, K. pneumoniae* including acute bacterial exacerbation of chronic bronchitis, community-acquired pneumonia of mild to moderate severity. **OFF-LABEL:** Acute sinusitis.

PRECAUTIONS

Contraindications: Concurrent use of amiodarone, procainamide, quinidine, sotalol; history of prolonged QT interval; hypersensitivity to fluoroquinolones; uncorrected electrolyte disorders (esp. hypokalemia, hypomagnesemia). **Cautions:** Hepatic/renal impairment, clinically significant bradycardia, acute myocardial ischemia.

⌛ LIFESPAN CONSIDERATIONS

Pregnancy/Lactation: Has potential for teratogenic effects. Substitute formula feedings for breast-feedings. **Pregnancy Category C. Children:** Safety and efficacy not established in those 18 yrs and younger. **Elderly:** Age-related renal impairment may require dosage adjustment.

INTERACTIONS

DRUG: **Aluminum-, magnesium-containing antacids, bismuth subsalicylate, didanosine, iron preparations and other metals, sucralfate, zinc preparations** may decrease absorption of gemifloxacin. **Antipsychotics, class IA and class III antiarrhythmics, erythromycin, tricyclic antidepressants** may increase risk of prolonged QT interval, life-threatening arrhythmias. **HERBAL:** **Dong quai, St. John's wort** may increase risk of photosensitization. **FOOD:** None known. **LAB VALUES:** May increase BUN, serum alkaline phosphatase, bilirubin, LDH, creatinine, AST, ALT. May alter platelets, neutrophils, Hgb, Hct, RBCs.

AVAILABILITY (Rx)

Tablets: 320 mg.

ADMINISTRATION/HANDLING

PO

• Give without regard to meals. • Do not crush, break tablets. • Take 3 hrs before or 2 hrs after supplements containing iron, zinc, or magnesium, antacids.

INDICATIONS/ROUTES/DOSAGE

Acute Bacterial Exacerbation of Chronic Bronchitis

PO: ADULTS, ELDERLY: 320 mg once a day for 5 days.

Community-Acquired Pneumonia

PO: ADULTS, ELDERLY: 320 mg once a day for 7 days.

Dosage in Renal Impairment

Dosage and frequency are modified based on creatinine clearance.

Creatinine Clearance	Dosage
Greater than 40 ml/min	320 mg once a day
40 ml/min or less	160 mg once a day

SIDE EFFECTS

Occasional (4%–2%): Diarrhea, rash, nausea. **Rare (1% or less):** Headache, abdominal pain, dizziness.

ADVERSE EFFECTS/ TOXIC REACTIONS

Antibiotic-associated colitis, other superinfections (abdominal cramps, severe watery diarrhea, fever) may result from altered bacterial balance. Hypersensitivity reaction, including photosensitivity (rash, pruritus, blisters, edema, burning skin) may occur.

G

NURSING CONSIDERATIONS

BASELINE ASSESSMENT

Question for history of hypersensitivity to fluoroquinolone antibiotics.

INTERVENTION/EVALUATION

Monitor for signs/symptoms of infection. Assess WBC count, renal/hepatic function tests. Encourage adequate fluid intake. Monitor daily pattern of bowel activity and stool consistency. Assess skin for rash. Be alert for superinfection: fever, vomiting, diarrhea, anal/genital pruritus, oral mucosal changes (ulceration, pain, erythema).

PATIENT/FAMILY TEACHING

• Take with 8 oz of water, without regard to food. • Drink several glasses of water between meals. • Complete full course of therapy. • Take 3 hrs before or 2 hrs after supplements containing iron, zinc, or magnesium, antacids.

Gemzar, *see gemcitabine*

gentamicin

jen-ta-**my**-sin
(Alcomicin ✤, Garamycin ✤, Gentak, Gentasol)

BLACK BOX ALERT Aminoglycoside antibiotics may cause neurotoxicity, nephrotoxicity. Risk of ototoxicity directly proportional to dosage, duration of treatment; ototoxicity usually is irreversible, precipitated by tinnitus, vertigo.

Do not confuse gentamicin with vancomycin.

◆CLASSIFICATION

PHARMACOTHERAPEUTIC: Aminoglycoside. **CLINICAL:** Antibiotic (see p. 21C).

ACTION

Irreversibly binds to protein of bacterial ribosomes. **Therapeutic Effect:** Interferes with protein synthesis of susceptible microorganisms. Bactericidal.

PHARMACOKINETICS

Rapid, complete absorption after IM administration. Protein binding: less than 30%. Widely distributed (does not cross blood-brain barrier, low concentrations in CSF). Excreted unchanged in urine. Removed by hemodialysis. **Half-life:** 2–4 hrs (increased in renal impairment, neonates; decreased in cystic fibrosis, burn, or febrile pts).

USES

Parenteral: Treatment of infections susceptible to *Pseudomonas* and other gram-negative organisms including skin/skin-structure, bone, joint, respiratory tract, intra-abdominal, complicated urinary tract, acute pelvic infections; burns; septicemia; meningitis. **Ophthalmic:** Ointment or solution for superficial eye infections. **Topical:** Cream or ointment for superficial skin infections. Ophthalmic or topical applications may be combined with systemic administration for serious, extensive infections. **OFF-LABEL: Topical:** Prophylaxis of minor bacterial skin infections, treatment of dermal ulcer.

PRECAUTIONS

Contraindications: Hypersensitivity to other aminoglycosides (cross-sensitivity) or their components. Sulfite sensitivity may result in anaphylaxis, esp. in asthmatic pts. **Cau-**

tions: Elderly, neonates due to renal insufficiency or immaturity; neuromuscular disorders (potential for respiratory depression), prior hearing loss, vertigo, renal impairment. Cumulative effects may occur with concurrent systemic administration and topical application to large areas.

LIFESPAN CONSIDERATIONS

Pregnancy/Lactation: Readily crosses placenta; unknown if distributed in breast milk. **Pregnancy Category C. Children:** Caution in neonates: Immature renal function increases half-life and toxicity. **Elderly:** Age-related renal impairment may require dosage adjustment.

INTERACTIONS

DRUG: **Nephrotoxic, ototoxic medications** may increase risk of nephrotoxicity, ototoxicity. May increase neuromuscular blockade with concurrent use of **neuromuscular blockers.** HERBAL: None significant. FOOD: None known. LAB VALUES: May increase serum creatinine, bilirubin, BUN, LDH, AST, ALT. May decrease serum calcium, magnesium, potassium, sodium. **Therapeutic serum level:** peak: 6–10 mcg/ml; trough: 0.5–2 mcg/ml. **Toxic serum level:** peak: greater than 10 mcg/ml; trough: greater than 2 mcg/ml.

AVAILABILITY (Rx)

Cream, Topical: 0.1%. **Injection, Infusion:** 40 mg/50 ml, 60 mg/50 ml, 60 mg/100 ml, 80 mg/50 ml, 80 mg/100 ml, 100 mg/50 ml, 100 mg/100 ml. **Injection, Solution:** 10 mg/ml, 40 mg/ml. **Ointment, Ophthalmic:** 0.3%. **Ointment, Topical:** 0.1%. **Solution, Ophthalmic: (Gentak, Gentasol)** 0.3%.

ADMINISTRATION/HANDLING

IV

Reconstitution • Dilute with 50–200 ml D_5W or 0.9% NaCl. Amount of diluent for infants, children depends on individual needs.

Rate of administration • Infuse over 30–60 min for adults, older children; over 60–120 min for infants, young children.

Storage • Store vials at room temperature. • Solution appears clear or slightly yellow. • Intermittent IV infusion (piggyback) is stable for 24 hrs at room temperature. • Discard if precipitate forms.

IM

• To minimize discomfort, give deep IM slowly. • Less painful if injected into gluteus maximus than lateral aspect of thigh.

Intrathecal

• Use only 2 mg/ml intrathecal preparation without preservative. • Mix with 10% estimated CSF volume or NaCl. • Use intrathecal forms immediately after preparation. • Discard unused portion. • Give over 3–5 min.

Ophthalmic

• Place gloved finger on lower eyelid and pull out until a pocket is formed between eye and lower lid. • Place prescribed number of drops or ¼–½ inch ointment into pocket. Instruct pt to close eye gently for 1–2 min (so medication will not be squeezed out of the sac). • **Solution:** Instruct pt to apply digital pressure to lacrimal sac at inner canthus for 1 min to minimize systemic absorption. • **Ointment:** Instruct pt to roll eyeball to increase contact area of drug to eye. • Remove excess solution or ointment around eye with tissue.

Topical

• Wash affected area with soap and water; allow to dry before applying. • Apply a small amount of gentamicin to the affected area and rub in gently.

IV INCOMPATIBILITIES

Allopurinol (Aloprim), amphotericin B complex (Abelcet, AmBisome, Amphotec), furosemide (Lasix), heparin, heta-starch (Hespan), idarubicin (Idamycin), indomethacin (Indocin), propofol (Diprivan).

IV COMPATIBILITIES

Amiodarone (Cordarone), diltiazem (Cardizem), enalapril (Vasotec), filgrastim (Neupogen), hydromorphone (Di-

G

laudid), insulin, lipids, lorazepam (Ativan), magnesium sulfate, midazolam (Versed), morphine, multivitamins, total parenteral nutrition (TPN).

INDICATIONS/ROUTES/DOSAGE

◀ALERT▶ Space parenteral doses evenly around the clock. Dosage based on ideal body weight. Peak, trough levels are determined periodically to maintain desired serum concentrations and minimize risk of toxicity.

G

Usual Parenteral Dosage

IV, IM: ADULTS, ELDERLY: 3–7.5 mg/kg/day in divided doses q8h or 4–7 mg/kg once a day. **CHILDREN 5–12 YRS:** 2–2.5 mg/kg/dose q8h. **CHILDREN YOUNGER THAN 5 YRS:** 2.5 mg/kg/dose q8h. **NEONATES:** 2.5 mg/kg/dose q8–24h.

Hemodialysis

IV, IM: ADULTS, ELDERLY: 0.5–0.7 mg/kg/dose after dialysis. **CHILDREN:** 1.25–1.75 mg/kg/dose after dialysis.

INTRATHECAL: ADULTS: 4–8 mg/day. **CHILDREN 3 MOS–12 YRS:** 1–2 mg/day. **NEONATES:** 1 mg/day.

Usual Ophthalmic Dosage

OPHTHALMIC OINTMENT: ADULTS, ELDERLY: Apply thin strip to conjunctiva 2–4 times/day.

OPHTHALMIC SOLUTION: ADULTS, ELDERLY, CHILDREN: 1–2 drops q2–4h up to 2 drops/hr.

Usual Topical Dosage

TOPICAL: ADULTS, ELDERLY: Apply 3–4 times a day.

Dosage in Renal Impairment

Creatinine Clearance	Dosage
41–60 ml/min	q12h
20–40 ml/min	q24h
Less than 20 ml/min	Monitor levels to determine dosage interval

SIDE EFFECTS

Occasional: IM: Pain, induration at injection site. **IV:** Phlebitis, thrombophlebitis, hypersensitivity reactions (fever, pruritus, rash, urticaria). **Ophthalmic:** Burning, tearing, itching, blurred vision. **Topical:** Redness, itching. **Rare:** Alopecia, hypertension, fatigue.

ADVERSE EFFECTS/ TOXIC REACTIONS

Nephrotoxicity (increased BUN, serum creatinine; decreased creatinine clearance) may be reversible if drug is stopped at first sign of symptoms. Irreversible ototoxicity (tinnitus, dizziness, diminished hearing), neurotoxicity (headache, dizziness, lethargy, tremor, visual disturbances) occur occasionally. Risk increases with higher dosages, prolonged therapy, or if solution is applied directly to mucosa. Superinfections, particularly with fungi, may result from bacterial imbalance via any route of administration. Ophthalmic application may cause paresthesia of conjunctiva, mydriasis.

NURSING CONSIDERATIONS

BASELINE ASSESSMENT

Dehydration must be treated before beginning parenteral therapy. Establish baseline hearing acuity. Question for history of allergies, esp. aminoglycosides, sulfites (parabens for topical/ophthalmic routes).

INTERVENTION/EVALUATION

Monitor I&O (maintain hydration), urinalysis (casts, RBCs, WBCs, decrease in specific gravity). Be alert to ototoxic, neurotoxic symptoms (see Adverse Effects/Toxic Reactions). Check IM injection site for induration. Evaluate IV site for phlebitis (heat, pain, red streaking over vein). Assess for rash (**Ophthalmic:** redness, burning, itching, tearing; **Topical:** redness, itching). Be alert for superinfection (genital/anal pruritus, changes in oral mucosa, diarrhea). When treating pts with neuromuscular disorders, assess respiratory response carefully. **Therapeutic serum level:** peak: 4–12 mcg/ml; peak levels are 2–3 times greater with once-daily dosing trough: 0.5–2 mcg/ml. **Toxic serum level:** peak: greater than 12 mcg/ml; trough: greater than 2 mcg/ml.

PATIENT/FAMILY TEACHING

• Discomfort may occur with IM injection. • Blurred vision, tearing may occur briefly after each ophthalmic dose. • Notify physician if hearing, visual, balance, urinary problems occur, even after therapy is completed. • **Ophthalmic:** Contact physician if tearing, redness, irritation continues. • **Topical:** Cleanse area gently before applying; notify physician if redness, itching occurs.

Geodon, *see ziprasidone*

ginger

Also known as black ginger, race ginger, zingiber.

◆CLASSIFICATION

HERBAL: See Appendix G.

ACTION

Possesses antipyretic, analgesic, antitussive, sedative properties. Increases GI motility; may act on serotonin receptors, primarily 5-HT_3. **Effect:** Reduces nausea/vomiting.

USES

Prevention of nausea/vomiting caused by motion sickness, early pregnancy, dyspepsia; treatment of rheumatoid arthritis (RA).

PRECAUTIONS

Contraindications: None known. **Cautions:** Pregnancy; pts with bleeding conditions, diabetes (may cause hypoglycemia).

LIFESPAN CONSIDERATIONS

Pregnancy/Lactation: Use during pregnancy is controversial (large amounts act as an abortifacient). **Children:** Safety and efficacy not established. **Elderly:** No age-related precautions noted.

INTERACTIONS

DRUG: Large amounts may increase risk of bleeding with **anticoagulants, antiplatelets.** **HERBAL:** **Feverfew, garlic, ginkgo, ginseng** may increase risk of bleeding. **FOOD:** None known. **LAB VALUES:** None significant.

AVAILABILITY (Rx)

Capsules: 470 mg, 550 mg. **Extract. Powder. Root:** 470 mg, 550 mg. **Tablets. Tea. Tincture.**

INDICATIONS/ROUTES/DOSAGE

Morning Sickness

PO: ADULTS: 250 mg 4 times a day. **Maximum:** 4 g a day.

Motion Sickness

PO: ADULTS: 1 g (dried powder root) 30 min before travel.

Nausea

PO: ADULTS: 550–1,100 mg 3 times a day.

Arthritis

PO: ADULTS: 170 mg 3 times a day or 255 mg twice a day.

SIDE EFFECTS

Abdominal discomfort, heartburn, diarrhea, hypersensitivity reaction, nausea.

ADVERSE EFFECTS/ TOXIC REACTIONS

CNS depression, arrhythmias.

NURSING CONSIDERATIONS

BASELINE ASSESSMENT

Assess for use of anticoagulants, antiplatelets (may increase risk of bleeding).

INTERVENTION/EVALUATION

Monitor for hypersensitivity reaction.

PATIENT/FAMILY TEACHING

- Use cautiously during pregnancy or breast-feeding.

ginkgo biloba

Also known as fossil tree, maidenhair tree, tanakan.

CLASSIFICATION

HERBAL: See Appendix G.

G

ACTION

Possesses antioxidant, free radical scavenging properties. **Effect:** Protects tissues from oxidative damage, prevents progression of tissue degeneration in pts with dementia. Inhibits platelet-activating factor bonding at numerous sites, decreasing platelet aggregation, smooth muscle contraction; may increase cardiac contractility, coronary blood flow. Decreases blood viscosity, improving circulation by relaxing vascular smooth muscle. Increases cerebral, peripheral blood flow, reduces vascular permeability. May influence neurotransmitter system (e.g., cholinergic).

USES

Treatment of dementia syndromes, including Alzheimer's. Improves cerebral, peripheral circulation. Improves conditions associated with cerebral vascular insufficiency (memory loss, difficulty concentrating, vertigo, tinnitus). Improves cognitive behavior, sleep patterns in pts with depression. Acts as antioxidant.

PRECAUTIONS

Contraindications: Pregnancy, lactation. Cautions: Pts with bleeding disorders, diabetes, epilepsy, or those prone to seizures. Avoid use in couples having difficulty conceiving.

LIFESPAN CONSIDERATIONS

Pregnancy/Lactation: Contraindicated. **Children:** Safety and efficacy not established. Avoid use. **Elderly:** No age-related precautions noted.

INTERACTIONS

DRUG: **Anticoagulants, antiplatelets (aspirin, clopidogrel, heparin, warfarin)** may increase risk of bleeding. Effects may be increased with concurrent use of **MAOIs.** HERBAL: **Feverfew, garlic, ginger, ginseng** may increase risk of bleeding. FOOD: None known. LAB VALUES: May alter glucose.

AVAILABILITY (OTC)

Capsules: 40 mg, 60 mg. Fluid Extract. Tablets: 40 mg, 60 mg. Tincture.

INDICATIONS/ROUTES/DOSAGE

Dementia

PO: ADULTS, ELDERLY: 120–240 mg a day (extract) in 2–3 doses.

Vertigo, Tinnitus

PO: ADULTS, ELDERLY: 120–160 mg a day.

Cognitive Function

PO: ADULTS, ELDERLY: 120–600 mg a day.

ALERT Appropriate doses for other conditions vary; should be started at low doses, titrated to higher doses as needed.

SIDE EFFECTS

Headache, dizziness, palpitations, constipation, allergic skin reactions. Large doses may cause nausea, vomiting, diarrhea, fatigue, diminished muscle tone.

ADVERSE EFFECTS/ TOXIC REACTIONS

None known.

NURSING CONSIDERATIONS

BASELINE ASSESSMENT

Assess for use of anticoagulants, antiplatelets, MAOIs. Assess for history of bleeding disorders, diabetes, seizures.

INTERVENTION/EVALUATION

Monitor for hypersensitivity reaction, serum glucose.

PATIENT/FAMILY TEACHING

• Avoid use with anticoagulants, antiplatelets. • May take up to 6 mos before effectiveness is noted. • Do not use during pregnancy, breast-feeding. • Avoid use in children.

ginseng

Also known as Asian ginseng, Chinese ginseng, red ginseng.

CLASSIFICATION

HERBAL: See Appendix G.

ACTION

Affects hypothalamic-pituitary-adrenal axis. Appears to stimulate lymphocytic action. **Effect:** Reduces stress. Affects immune function.

USES

Increases resistance to stress. Enhances energy level, brain activity. Increases physical endurance. Aids in serum glucose control. Improves cognitive function, concentration, memory, work efficiency. Relieves debilitating fatigue in cancer pts.

PRECAUTIONS

Contraindications: Pts with bleeding tendencies, thrombosis. Avoid use during pregnancy, lactation. **Cautions:** Pts with cardiac disorders, diabetes, hormone-sensitive cancers (breast, uterine, ovarian), endometriosis, uterine fibroids.

LIFESPAN CONSIDERATIONS

Pregnancy/Lactation: Insufficient information. Do not use. **Children:** Safety and efficacy not established. **Elderly:** No age-related precautions noted.

INTERACTIONS

DRUG: **Anticoagulants, antiplatelets (aspirin, clopidogrel, enoxaparin, heparin, warfarin)** may increase risk of bleeding. May increase effects of **insulin, oral antidiabetic agents.** Effects may be decreased with concurrent use of **furosemide.** Ginseng may interfere with effects of **immunosuppressants (e.g., cyclosporine, prednisone).** **HERBAL:** **Chamomile, feverfew, garlic, ginger, ginkgo** may increase risk of bleeding. **FOOD:** **Coffee, tea** may increase effect. **LAB VALUES:** May prolong aPTT, decrease serum glucose.

AVAILABILITY (OTC)

Capsules: 100 mg, 250 mg, 410 mg, 500 mg. **Dried Root. Extract. Powder. Tablets:** 250 mg, 1,000 mg. **Tea** (usually 1,500 mg/bag). **Tincture.**

INDICATIONS/ROUTES/DOSAGE

Usual Dosage

PO: ADULTS, ELDERLY: (Tablets/capsules): 200–600 mg a day. **(Powder, root):** 0.6–3 g 1–3 times a day. **(Tea—1,500 mg):** 1–3 times a day.

SIDE EFFECTS

Frequent: Insomnia. **Occasional:** Vaginal bleeding, amenorrhea, palpitations, hypertension, diarrhea, headache, allergic reactions.

ADVERSE EFFECTS/ TOXIC REACTIONS

None known.

NURSING CONSIDERATIONS

BASELINE ASSESSMENT

Assess if pt is pregnant, breast-feeding. Assess if pt is diabetic, taking oral hypoglycemic agents, insulin. Assess for anticoagulant, immunosuppressant use. Determine baseline serum glucose.

INTERVENTION/EVALUATION

Monitor coagulation studies, serum glucose. Assess for hypersensitivity reaction, rash.

PATIENT/FAMILY TEACHING

• Avoid use in pregnancy or breast-feeding, children. • Avoid continuous use for longer than 3 mos.

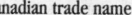

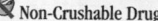

glatiramer

gla-**tir**-ah-mer
(Copaxone)
Do not confuse Copaxone with Compazine.

◆CLASSIFICATION

PHARMACOTHERAPEUTIC: Immunosuppressive. **CLINICAL:** Neurologic agent.

G

ACTION

May act by modifying immune processes thought to be responsible for pathogenesis of multiple sclerosis. **Therapeutic Effect:** Slows progression of multiple sclerosis.

PHARMACOKINETICS

Substantial fraction of glatiramer is hydrolyzed locally. Some fraction of injected material enters lymphatic circulation, reaching regional lymph nodes; some may enter systemic circulation intact.

USES

Treatment of relapsing, remitting multiple sclerosis.

PRECAUTIONS

Contraindications: Hypersensitivity to glatiramer, mannitol. **Cautions:** Pts exhibiting immediate postinjection reaction (flushing, chest pain, palpitations, anxiety, dyspnea, urticaria).

⌛ LIFESPAN CONSIDERATIONS

Pregnancy/Lactation: Unknown if distributed in breast milk. **Pregnancy Category B. Children:** Safety and efficacy not established. **Elderly:** Information not available.

INTERACTIONS

DRUG: None significant. **HERBAL:** **Echinacea** may decrease effects. **FOOD:** None known. **LAB VALUES:** None significant.

AVAILABILITY (Rx)

Injection Solution: 20 mg/ml in prefilled syringes.

ADMINISTRATION/HANDLING

Subcutaneous

• Refrigerate syringes (bring to room temperature before use). • May be stored at room temperature for up to 1 mo. • Avoid heat, intense light. • Inject into deltoid region, abdomen, gluteus maximus, or lateral aspect of thigh. • Prefilled syringe suitable for single use only; discard unused portions.

INDICATIONS/ROUTES/DOSAGE

Multiple Sclerosis

SUBCUTANEOUS: ADULTS, ELDERLY: 20 mg once a day.

SIDE EFFECTS

Expected (73%–40%): Pain, erythema, inflammation, pruritus at injection site; asthenia (loss of strength, energy). **Frequent (27%–18%):** Arthralgia, vasodilation, anxiety, hypertonia, nausea, transient chest pain, dyspnea, flu-like symptoms, rash, pruritus. **Occasional (17%–10%):** Palpitations, back pain, diaphoresis, rhinitis, diarrhea, urinary urgency. **Rare (8%–6%):** Anorexia, fever, neck pain, peripheral edema, ear pain, facial edema, vertigo, vomiting.

ADVERSE EFFECTS/ TOXIC REACTIONS

Infection occurs commonly. Lymphadenopathy occurs occasionally.

NURSING CONSIDERATIONS

BASELINE ASSESSMENT

Establish baseline neurologic function.

INTERVENTION/EVALUATION

Observe injection site for reaction. Monitor for fever, chills (evidence of infection). Observe for improvement in neurologic function.

PATIENT/FAMILY TEACHING

• Report difficulty in breathing/swallowing, rash, itching, swelling of lower extremities, fatigue. • Avoid pregnancy.

Gleevec, *see imatinib*

Gliadel, *see carmustine*

glimepiride HIGH ALERT

glim-**eh**-purr-eyd
(Amaryl, Apo-Glimepiride ✦, Novo-Glimepiride ✦)
Do not confuse Amaryl with Altace, Amerge, or Reminyl, Avandaryl with Benadryl, or glimepiride with glipizide or glyburide.

FIXED-COMBINATION(S)

Avandaryl: glimepiride/rosiglitazone (an antidiabetic): 1 mg/4 mg, 2 mg/4 mg, 4 mg/4 mg.
Duetact: glimepiride/pioglitazone (an antidiabetic): 2 mg/30 mg, 4 mg/30 mg.

CLASSIFICATION

PHARMACOTHERAPEUTIC: Second-generation sulfonylurea. **CLINICAL:** Hypoglycemic (see p. 43C).

ACTION

Promotes release of insulin from beta cells of pancreas, increases insulin sensitivity at peripheral sites. **Therapeutic Effect:** Lowers serum glucose.

PHARMACOKINETICS

Route	Onset	Peak	Duration
PO	N/A	2–3 hrs	24 hrs

Completely absorbed from GI tract. Protein binding: greater than 99%. Metabolized in liver. Excreted in urine, eliminated in feces. **Half-life:** 5–9.2 hrs.

USES

Adjunct to diet, exercise in management of non–insulin-dependent diabetes mellitus (type 2, NIDDM). Use in combination with insulin or metformin in pts whose diabetes is not controlled by diet, exercise in conjunction with a single oral hypoglycemic agent.

PRECAUTIONS

Contraindications: Diabetic complications (ketosis, acidosis, diabetic coma); monotherapy for type 1 diabetes mellitus; severe hepatic/renal impairment; stress situations (severe infection, trauma, surgery). **Cautions:** Severe diarrhea, intestinal obstruction, prolonged vomiting, hepatic disease, hyperthyroidism (uncontrolled), renal impairment, adrenal insufficiency, debilitation, malnutrition, pituitary insufficiency.

LIFESPAN CONSIDERATIONS

Pregnancy/Lactation: Not recommended for use during pregnancy. Unknown if distributed in breast milk. **Pregnancy Category C. Children:** Safety and efficacy not established. **Elderly:** Hypoglycemia may be difficult to recognize. Age-related renal impairment may increase sensitivity to glucose-lowering effect.

INTERACTIONS

DRUG: **Beta-blockers** may increase hypoglycemic effect, mask signs of hypoglycemia. **Cimetidine, ciprofloxacin, fluconazole, MAOIs, quinidine, ranitidine, large doses of salicylates** may increase effect. **Corticosteroids, lithium, thiazide diuretics** may decrease effect. May increase effects of **oral anticoagulants. HERBAL: Garlic** may worsen hypoglycemia. **FOOD:** None known. **LAB VALUES:** May increase LDH concentrations, serum alkaline phosphatase, AST, ALT, bilirubin, C-peptide.

AVAILABILITY (Rx)

Tablets: 1 mg, 2 mg, 4 mg.

ADMINISTRATION/HANDLING

PO

- Give with breakfast or first main meal.

G

INDICATIONS/ROUTES/DOSAGE

Diabetes Mellitus

PO: ADULTS, ELDERLY: Initially, 1–2 mg once a day with breakfast or first main meal. Maintenance: 1–4 mg once a day. After dose of 2 mg is reached, dosage should be increased in increments of up to 2 mg q1–2wks, based on serum glucose response. **Maximum:** 8 mg/day. **ELDERLY:** Initially, 1 mg/day. Titrate dose to avoid hypoglycemia.

Dosage in Renal Impairment

Creatinine clearance less than 22 ml/min: Initially, 1 mg/day, then titrate dose based on fasting serum glucose levels.

SIDE EFFECTS

Frequent: Altered taste, dizziness, drowsiness, weight gain, constipation, diarrhea, heartburn, nausea, vomiting, stomach fullness, headache. **Occasional:** Increased sensitivity of skin to sunlight, peeling of skin, pruritus, rash.

ADVERSE EFFECTS/ TOXIC REACTIONS

Overdose or insufficient food intake may produce hypoglycemia (esp. with increased glucose demands). GI hemorrhage, cholestatic hepatic jaundice, leukopenia, thrombocytopenia, pancytopenia, agranulocytosis, aplastic or hemolytic anemia occur rarely.

NURSING CONSIDERATIONS

BASELINE ASSESSMENT

Check serum glucose level. Discuss lifestyle to determine extent of learning, emotional needs. Ensure follow-up instruction if pt or family does not thoroughly understand diabetes management or serum glucose testing technique.

INTERVENTION/EVALUATION

Monitor serum glucose level, food intake. Assess for hypoglycemia (cool/wet skin, tremors, dizziness, anxiety, headache, tachycardia, perioral numbness, hunger, diplopia), hyperglycemia (polyuria, polyphagia, polydipsia, nausea, vomiting, dim vision, fatigue, deep or rapid breathing). Be alert to conditions that alter glucose requirements (fever, increased activity or stress, trauma, surgical procedure).

PATIENT/ FAMILY TEACHING

• Prescribed diet is principal part of treatment; do not skip or delay meals. • Avoid alcohol. • Carry candy, sugar packets, other quick-acting sugar supplements for immediate response to hypoglycemia. • Wear medical alert identification. • Check with physician when glucose demands are altered (fever, infection, trauma, stress, heavy physical activity). • Avoid direct exposure to sunlight.

*glipiZIDE

HIGH ALERT

glip-ih-zide
(Glucotrol, Glucotrol XL)
Do not confuse glipizide with glimepiride or glyburide, or Glucotrol with Glucophage or Glucotrol XL.

FIXED-COMBINATION(S)

Metaglip: glipizide/metformin (an antidiabetic): 2.5 mg/250 mg, 2.5 mg/500 mg, 5 mg/500 mg.

◆CLASSIFICATION

PHARMACOTHERAPEUTIC: Second-generation sulfonylurea. **CLINICAL:** Hypoglycemic (see p. 43C).

ACTION

Promotes release of insulin from beta cells of pancreas, increases insulin sensitivity at peripheral sites. **Therapeutic Effect:** Lowers serum glucose.

PHARMACOKINETICS

Route	Onset	Peak	Duration
PO	15–30 min	2–3 hrs	12–24 hrs
Extended-release	2–3 hrs	6–12 hrs	24 hrs

Well absorbed from GI tract. Protein binding: 92%–99%. Metabolized in liver. Excreted in urine. **Half-life:** 2–4 hrs.

USES

Adjunct to diet, exercise in management of stable, mild to moderately severe non–insulin-dependent diabetes mellitus (type 2, NIDDM). May be used to supplement insulin in those with type 1 diabetes mellitus. May be used concomitantly with insulin or metformin to improve glycemic control.

PRECAUTIONS

Contraindications: Diabetic ketoacidosis with or without coma, type 1 diabetes mellitus. **Cautions:** Adrenal/pituitary insufficiency, hypoglycemic reactions, hepatic/renal impairment.

LIFESPAN CONSIDERATIONS

Pregnancy/Lactation: Insulin is drug of choice during pregnancy; glipizide given within 1 mo of delivery may produce neonatal hypoglycemia. Drug crosses placenta. Distributed in breast milk. **Pregnancy Category C. Children:** Safety and efficacy not established. **Elderly:** Hypoglycemia may be difficult to recognize. Age-related renal impairment may increase sensitivity to glucose-lowering effect.

INTERACTIONS

DRUG: **Beta-blockers** may increase hypoglycemic effect, mask signs of hypoglycemia. **Cimetidine, ciprofloxacin, fluconazole, MAOIs, quinidine, ranitidine, large doses of salicylates** may increase effect. **Corticosteroids, lithium, thiazide diuretics** may decrease the effect. May increase effects of **oral anticoagulants. HERBAL:** **Garlic** may worsen hypoglycemia. **FOOD:** None known. **LAB VALUES:** May increase serum alkaline phosphatase, LDH, AST, ALT, bilirubin, C-peptide.

AVAILABILITY (Rx)

Tablets (Glucotrol): 5 mg, 10 mg.

Tablets (Extended-Release [Glucotrol XL]): 2.5 mg, 5 mg, 10 mg.

ADMINISTRATION/HANDLING

PO

• Give immediate-release tablets 30 min before meals. Give extended-release tablets with breakfast. • Do not crush extended-release tablets.

INDICATIONS/ROUTES/DOSAGE

Diabetes Mellitus

PO: ADULTS: Initially, 5 mg/day or 2.5 mg in elderly or those with hepatic disease. Adjust dosage in 2.5- to 5-mg increments at intervals of several days. Immediate-release tablet: **Maximum single dose:** 15 mg. **Maximum dose/day:** 40 mg. Extended-release tablet: **Maximum dose:** 20 mg/day. **ELDERLY:** Initially, 2.5–5 mg/day. May increase by 2.5–5 mg/day q1–2wks.

Dosage in Renal Impairment

Not recommended for pts with creatinine clearance less than 10 ml/min.

Dosage in Hepatic Impairment

Initial dose: 2.5 mg/day.

SIDE EFFECTS

Frequent: Altered taste, dizziness, drowsiness, weight gain, constipation, diarrhea, heartburn, nausea, vomiting, stomach fullness, headache. **Occasional:** Increased sensitivity of skin to sunlight, peeling of skin, pruritus, rash.

ADVERSE EFFECTS/ TOXIC REACTIONS

Overdose or insufficient food intake may produce hypoglycemia (esp. with increased glucose demands). GI hemorrhage, cholestatic hepatic jaundice, leukopenia, thrombocytopenia, pancytopenia, agranulocytosis, aplastic or hemolytic anemia occur rarely.

NURSING CONSIDERATIONS

BASELINE ASSESSMENT

Check serum glucose level. Discuss lifestyle to determine extent of learning, emotional needs. Ensure follow-up instruction if pt or family does not thoroughly understand diabetes management or serum glucose testing technique.

INTERVENTION/EVALUATION

Monitor serum glucose level, food intake. Assess for hypoglycemia (cool/wet skin, tremors, dizziness, anxiety, headache, tachycardia, perioral numbness, hunger, diplopia), hyperglycemia (polyuria, polyphagia, polydipsia, nausea, vomiting, dim vision, fatigue, deep or rapid breathing). Be alert to conditions that alter glucose requirements (fever, increased activity or stress, trauma, surgical procedure).

PATIENT/ FAMILY TEACHING

• Prescribed diet is principal part of treatment; do not skip or delay meals. • Avoid alcohol. • Carry candy, sugar packets, other quick-acting sugar supplements for immediate response to hypoglycemia. • Wear medical alert identification. • Check with physician when glucose demands are altered (fever, infection, trauma, stress, heavy physical activity). • Avoid direct exposure to sunlight.

glucagon

glue-ka-gon
(GlucaGen, GlucaGen Diagnostic Kit, Glucagon, Glucagon Diagnostic Kit, Glucagon Emergency Kit)
Do not confuse glucagon with Glaucon.

◆CLASSIFICATION

PHARMACOTHERAPEUTIC: Glucose elevating agent. **CLINICAL:** Antihypoglycemic, antispasmodic, antidote.

ACTION

Promotes hepatic glycogenolysis, gluconeogenesis. Stimulates cAMP, an enzyme, resulting in increased serum glucose concentration, smooth muscle relaxation, and exerts inotropic myocardial effect. **Therapeutic Effect:** Increases serum glucose level.

PHARMACOKINETICS

Route	Onset	Peak	Duration
IV	5–20 min	—	60–90 min
IM	30 min	—	60–90 min
Subcutaneous	30–45 min	—	60–90 min

Metabolized in liver. **Half-life:** 3–10 min.

USES

Treatment of severe hypoglycemia in diabetic pts. Not for use in chronic hypoglycemia or hypoglycemia due to starvation, adrenal insufficiency (hepatic glycogen unavailable). Diagnostic aid in radiographic examination of GI tract. **OFF-LABEL:** Treatment of esophageal obstruction due to foreign bodies; toxicity associated with beta-blockers, calcium channel blockers.

PRECAUTIONS

Contraindications: Hypersensitivity to glucagon, beef/pork proteins, known pheochromocytoma. **Cautions:** History of insulinoma, pheochromocytoma.

⌛ LIFESPAN CONSIDERATIONS

Pregnancy/Lactation: Unknown if drug crosses placenta or is distributed in breast milk. **Pregnancy Category B. Children/Elderly:** No age-related precautions noted.

INTERACTIONS

DRUG: May increase effects of **anticoagulants. HERBAL:** None significant. **FOOD:** None known. **LAB VALUES:** May decrease serum potassium.

AVAILABILITY (Rx)

Injection Powder (GlucaGen, GlucaGen Diagnostic Kit, Glucagon, Glucagon Diagnostic Kit, Glucagon Emergency Kit): 1 mg.

ADMINISTRATION/HANDLING

◀ALERT▶ Place pt in side-lying position to prevent aspiration (glucagon, hypoglycemia may produce nausea/vomiting).

IV, IM, Subcutaneous

Reconstitution • Reconstitute powder with manufacturer's diluent when prepar-

ing doses of 2 mg or less. For doses greater than 2 mg, dilute with Sterile Water for Injection. • To provide 1 mg glucagon/ml, use 1 ml diluent. For 1-mg vial of glucagon, use 10 ml diluent for 10-mg vial.
Rate of administration • Pt usually awakens in 5–20 min. Although 1–2 additional doses may be administered, concern for effects of continuing cerebral hypoglycemia requires consideration of parenteral glucose. • When pt awakens, give supplemental carbohydrate to restore hepatic glycogen and prevent secondary hypoglycemia. If pt fails to respond to glucagon, IV dextrose is necessary.
Storage • Store vial at room temperature. • After reconstitution, is stable for 48 hrs if refrigerated. If reconstituted with Sterile Water for Injection, use immediately. Do not use glucagon solution unless clear.

IV INCOMPATIBILITIES

Do not mix glucagon with any other medications.

INDICATIONS/ROUTES/DOSAGE

Hypoglycemia

◀ALERT▶ Administer IV dextrose if pt fails to respond to glucagon.

IV, IM, SUBCUTANEOUS: ADULTS, ELDERLY, CHILDREN WEIGHING MORE THAN 20 KG: 0.5–1 mg. May repeat in 20 min. **CHILDREN WEIGHING 20 KG OR LESS:** 0.5 mg. May repeat in 20 min.

Diagnostic Aid

IV, IM: ADULTS, ELDERLY: 0.25–2 mg 10 min prior to procedure.

SIDE EFFECTS

Occasional: Nausea, vomiting. **Rare:** Allergic reaction (urticaria, respiratory distress, hypotension).

ADVERSE EFFECTS/ TOXIC REACTIONS

Overdose may produce persistent nausea/vomiting, hypokalemia (severe fatigue, decreased appetite, palpitations, muscle cramps).

NURSING CONSIDERATIONS

BASELINE ASSESSMENT

Obtain immediate assessment, including history, clinical signs/symptoms. If presence of hypoglycemic coma is established, give glucagon promptly.

INTERVENTION/EVALUATION

Monitor blood glucose, B/P, pulse, mental status. Monitor response time carefully. Have IV dextrose readily available in event pt does not awaken within 5–20 min. Assess for possible allergic reaction (urticaria, respiratory difficulty, hypotension). When pt is conscious, give oral carbohydrate.

PATIENT/FAMILY TEACHING

• Recognize significance of identifying symptoms of hypoglycemia: pale, cool skin; anxiety, difficulty concentrating, headache, hunger, nausea, shakiness, diaphoresis, unusual fatigue, unusual weakness, unconsciousness. • If symptoms of hypoglycemia develop, give sugar form first (orange juice, honey, hard candy, sugar cubes, table sugar dissolved in water or juice) followed by cheese and crackers, half a sandwich, glass of milk.

Glucophage, *see metformin*

Glucophage XR, *see metformin*

glucosamine/ chondroitin

◆CLASSIFICATION

HERBAL: See Appendix G.

ACTION

Glucosamine: Necessary for synthesis of mucopolysaccharides, which comprise body's tendons, ligaments, cartilage, synovial fluid. May decrease glucose-induced insulin secretion. **Effect:** Relieves symptoms of osteoarthritis. **Chondroitin:** Endogenously found in cartilage tissue, substrate for forming joint matrix structure. May possess anticoagulant properties. **Effect:** Relieves symptoms of osteoarthritis.

G

USES

Treatment of osteoarthritis.

PRECAUTIONS

Contraindications: None known. **Cautions:** **Glucosamine:** Diabetes (may increase insulin resistance). **Chondroitin:** None known.

INTERACTIONS

DRUG: **Warfarin** may increase effect. **Anticoagulants** may increase risk of bleeding with chondroitin. **HERBAL:** None significant. **FOOD:** None known. **LAB VALUES:** May increase serum glucose, antifactor Xa.

AVAILABILITY (OTC)

GLUCOSAMINE
Capsules: 500 mg. **Tablets:** 500 mg.
CHONDROITIN
Capsules: 250 mg.
◀ALERT▶ Many combination products are available.

INDICATIONS/ROUTES/DOSAGE

Osteoarthritis

PO: **(Glucosamine): ADULTS, ELDERLY:** 500 mg 3 times a day or 1–2 g a day. **(Chondroitin):** 200–400 mg 2–3 times a day.

SIDE EFFECTS

GLUCOSAMINE: Mild GI symptoms (gas, bloating, cramps). **CHONDROITIN:** Well tolerated. May cause nausea, diarrhea, constipation, edema, alopecia, allergic reactions.

ADVERSE EFFECTS/ TOXIC REACTIONS

None known.

NURSING CONSIDERATIONS

BASELINE ASSESSMENT

Determine whether pt is taking anticoagulants, antiplatelets, antidiabetic drugs. Assess if pt is pregnant or breast-feeding.

INTERVENTION/EVALUATION

Monitor effectiveness of therapy in relieving osteoarthritis symptoms. Monitor serum glucose levels.

PATIENT/FAMILY TEACHING

• Avoid use in pregnancy, breast-feeding, children. • May take several mos of therapy to be effective. • Glucosamine may alter serum glucose levels.

Glucotrol, *see glipizide*

Glucovance, *see glyburide and metformin*

*glyBURIDE

HIGH ALERT

glye-byoo-ride
(Apo-Glyburide ✦, DiaBeta, Euglucon ✦, Glynase Pres-Tab, Micronase, Novo-Glyburide ✦)
Do not confuse DiaBeta with Zebeta, glyburide with glimepiride, glipizide, or Glucotrol, or Micronase with Micro-K or Micronor.

FIXED-COMBINATION(S)

Glucovance: glyburide/metformin (an antidiabetic): 1.25 mg/250 mg, 2.5 mg/500 mg, 5 mg/500 mg.

◆CLASSIFICATION

PHARMACOTHERAPEUTIC: Second-generation sulfonylurea. **CLINICAL:** Hypoglycemic (see p. 43C).

ACTION

Promotes release of insulin from beta cells of pancreas, increases insulin sensitivity at peripheral sites. **Therapeutic Effect:** Lowers serum glucose level.

PHARMACOKINETICS

Route	Onset	Peak	Duration
PO	0.25–1 hr	1–2 hrs	12–24 hrs

Well absorbed from GI tract. Protein binding: 99%. Metabolized in liver to weakly active metabolite. Primarily excreted in urine. Not removed by hemodialysis. **Half-life:** 5–16 hrs.

USES

Adjunct to diet, exercise in management of stable, mild to moderately severe non–insulin-dependent diabetes mellitus (type 2, NIDDM). May be used to supplement insulin in those with type 1 diabetes mellitus. May be used concomitantly with insulin or metformin to improve glycemic control.

PRECAUTIONS

Contraindications: Diabetic ketoacidosis with or without coma, monotherapy for type 1 diabetes mellitus. **Cautions:** Adrenal or pituitary insufficiency, hypoglycemic reactions, hepatic/renal impairment.

⌛ LIFESPAN CONSIDERATIONS

Pregnancy/Lactation: Crosses placenta. Distributed in breast milk. May produce neonatal hypoglycemia if given within 2 wks of delivery. **Pregnancy Category C. Children:** Safety and efficacy not established. **Elderly:** Hypoglycemia may be difficult to recognize. Age-related renal impairment may increase sensitivity to glucose-lowering effect.

INTERACTIONS

DRUG: **Beta-blockers** may increase hypoglycemic effect, mask signs of hypoglycemia. **Cimetidine, ciprofloxacin, fluconazole, MAOIs, quinidine, ranitidine, large doses of salicylates** may increase effect. **Corticosteroids, lithium, thiazide diuretics** may decrease effect. May increase effects of **oral anticoagulants. HERBAL:** **Garlic** may worsen hypoglycemia. **FOOD:** None known. **LAB VALUES:** May increase serum alkaline phosphatase, LDH, AST, ALT, bilirubin, C-peptide.

AVAILABILITY (Rx)

Tablets (DiaBeta, Micronase): 1.25 mg, 2.5 mg, 5 mg. **Tablets, Micronized (Glynase Pres-Tab):** 1.5 mg, 3 mg, 6 mg.

ADMINISTRATION/HANDLING

PO

- May give with food (response better if taken 15–30 min before meals).

INDICATIONS/ROUTES/DOSAGE

Diabetes Mellitus

PO: ADULTS: Initially 2.5–5 mg. May increase by 2.5 mg/day at weekly intervals. Maintenance: 1.25–20 mg/day. **Maximum:** 20 mg/day. **ELDERLY:** Initially, 1.25–2.5 mg/day. May increase by 1.25–2.5 mg/day at 1- to 3-wk intervals.

PO (MICRONIZED TABLETS): ADULTS, ELDERLY: Initially 0.75–3 mg/day. May increase by 1.5 mg/day at weekly intervals. Maintenance: 0.75–12 mg/day as a single dose or in divided doses.

Dosage in Renal Impairment

Not recommended for pts with creatinine clearance less than 50 ml/min.

SIDE EFFECTS

Frequent: Altered taste, dizziness, drowsiness, weight gain, constipation, diarrhea, heartburn, nausea, vomiting, stomach fullness, headache. **Occasional:** Increased sensitivity of skin to sunlight, peeling of skin, pruritus, rash.

G

ADVERSE EFFECTS/ TOXIC REACTIONS

Overdose or insufficient food intake may produce hypoglycemia (esp. in pts with increased glucose demands). Cholestatic jaundice, leukopenia, thrombocytopenia, pancytopenia, agranulocytosis, aplastic or hemolytic anemia occur rarely.

NURSING CONSIDERATIONS

BASELINE ASSESSMENT

Check serum glucose level. Discuss lifestyle to determine extent of learning, emotional needs. Ensure follow-up instruction if pt or family does not thoroughly understand diabetes management or glucose testing technique.

INTERVENTION/EVALUATION

Monitor serum glucose level, food intake. Assess for hypoglycemia (cool/wet skin, tremors, dizziness, anxiety, headache, tachycardia, perioral numbness, hunger, diplopia), hyperglycemia (polyuria, polyphagia, polydipsia, nausea, vomiting, dim vision, fatigue, deep or rapid breathing). Be alert to conditions that alter glucose requirements (fever, increased activity or stress, trauma, surgical procedure).

PATIENT/ FAMILY TEACHING

• Prescribed diet is principal part of treatment; do not skip or delay meals. • Avoid alcohol. • Carry candy, sugar packets, other quick-acting sugar supplements for immediate response to hypoglycemia. • Wear medical alert identification. • Check with physician when glucose demands are altered (fever, infection, trauma, stress, heavy physical activity). • Avoid direct exposure to sunlight.

glycopyrrolate

glye-koe-**pye**-roe-late
(Robinul)
Do not confuse Robinul with Reminyl.

◆ CLASSIFICATION

PHARMACOTHERAPEUTIC: Quaternary anticholinergic. **CLINICAL:** Antimuscarinic, antiarrhythmic, cholinergic adjunct.

ACTION

Inhibits action of acetylcholine at postganglionic parasympathetic sites in smooth muscle, secretory glands, CNS. **Therapeutic Effect:** Reduces salivation/excessive secretions of respiratory tract; reduces gastric secretions, acidity.

USES

Inhibits salivation/excessive secretions of respiratory tract preoperatively. Reverses neuromuscular blockade postsurgically.

PRECAUTIONS

Contraindications: Acute hemorrhage, myasthenia gravis, narrow-angle glaucoma, obstructive uropathy, paralytic ileus, tachycardia, ulcerative colitis. **Cautions:** Those with fever, hyperthyroidism, hepatic/renal disease, hypertension, CHF, GI infection, diarrhea, reflux esophagitis. **Pregnancy Category B.**

INTERACTIONS

DRUG: **Other anticholinergics** may increase effect. **HERBAL:** None significant. **FOOD:** None known. **LAB VALUES:** May decrease serum uric acid.

AVAILABILITY (Rx)

Injection Solution (Robinul): 0.2 mg/ml.

ADMINISTRATION/HANDLING

IV

• Administer undiluted as IV push through tubing of free-flowing compatible IV solution (D_5W, $D_{10}W$, 0.9% NaCl).

IM

• Administer undiluted.

IV INCOMPATIBILITY

None known.

IV COMPATIBILITIES

Diphenhydramine (Benadryl), droperidol (Inapsine), hydromorphone (Dilaudid), hydroxyzine (Vistaril), lidocaine, midazolam (Versed), morphine, promethazine (Phenergan).

INDICATIONS/ROUTES/DOSAGE

Preop Inhibition of Salivation, Excessive Respiratory Tract Secretions

IM: ADULTS, ELDERLY: 4 mcg/kg 30–60 min before procedure. **CHILDREN 2 YRS AND OLDER:** 4 mcg/kg. **CHILDREN YOUNGER THAN 2 YRS:** 4–9 mcg/kg.

Reverse Neuromuscular Blockade

IV: ADULTS, ELDERLY, CHILDREN: 0.2 mg for each 1 mg neostigmine or 5 mg pyridostigmine.

SIDE EFFECTS

Frequent: Dry mouth, decreased diaphoresis, constipation. **Occasional:** Blurred vision, gastric bloating, urinary hesitancy, drowsiness (with high dosage), headache, photosensitivity, altered taste, anxiety, flushing, insomnia, impotence, mental confusion or excitement (particularly in elderly, children), temporary lightheadedness (with parenteral form), local irritation (with parenteral form). **Rare:** Dizziness, faintness.

ADVERSE EFFECTS/ TOXIC REACTIONS

Overdose may produce temporary paralysis of ciliary muscle, pupillary dilation, tachycardia, palpitations, hot/dry/flushed skin, absence of bowel sounds, hyperthermia, increased respiratory rate, EKG abnormalities, nausea, vomiting, rash over face/upper trunk, CNS stimulation, psychosis (agitation, restlessness, rambling speech, visual hallucinations, paranoid behavior, delusions, followed by depression).

NURSING CONSIDERATIONS

INTERVENTION/EVALUATION

Monitor heart rate, changes in B/P, temperature.

PATIENT/FAMILY TEACHING

- May cause dry mouth.

golimumab

go-**lim**-you-mab
(Simponi)

BLACK BOX ALERT Tuberculosis, invasive fungal infections, other opportunistic infections have occurred; most infections occur in combination with other immunosuppressants. Test for tuberculosis prior to and during treatment.

◆CLASSIFICATION

PHARMACOTHERAPEUTIC: Monoclonal antibody. **CLINICAL:** Immune modulator, tumor necrosis factor inhibitor.

ACTION

Binds specifically to tumor necrosis factor (TNF) alpha cell, blocking its interaction with cell surface TNF receptors. **Therapeutic Effect:** Reduces inflammation, alters immune response.

PHARMACOKINETICS

Serum concentration appears to reach maximum steady state by week 12. **Half-life:** 7–20 days.

USES

Used alone or in combination with methotrexate for treatment of adult pts with active psoriatic arthritis. Used in combination with methotrexate for treatment of adult pts with moderately to severely active rheumatoid arthritis. Used alone for treatment of adult pts with active ankylosing spondylitis.

PRECAUTIONS

Contraindications: None significant. **Cautions:** History of opportunistic infections (bacterial, mycobacterial, invasive fungal, viral, protozoal), esp. tuberculosis, histoplasmosis, aspergillosis, candidiasis, coccidioidomycosis, listeriosis, pneumocystosis; preexisting or recent-onset CNS demyelinating disorders, including multiple sclerosis; those with chronic or recurrent infection or who have been exposed to tuberculosis; hematologic cytopenia; cardiovascular disease; COPD (may increase risk of malignancy); hepatitis B chronic carriers.

LIFESPAN CONSIDERATIONS

Pregnancy/Lactation: Unknown if distributed in breast milk. **Pregnancy Category B. Children:** Safety and efficacy not established. **Elderly:** Cautious use due to increased risk of serious infections, malignancy.

G

INTERACTIONS

DRUG: **Abatacept, anakinra, immunosuppressive therapy, natalizumab, rituximab** may increase risk of infections. May decrease efficacy of immune response with **live vaccines.** May alter narrow therapeutic index of **cyclosporine, theophylline, warfarin.** HERBAL: **Echinacea** may decrease effects. FOOD: None known. LAB VALUES: May increase levels of ALT, AST.

AVAILABILITY (Rx)

Injection Solution: 50 mg/0.5 ml in single-dose prefilled autoinjector or prefilled syringe.

ADMINISTRATION/HANDLING

Subcutaneous

• Remove prefilled syringe or autoinjector from refrigerator. Allow to sit at room temperature for 30 min; do not warm by any other method. • Avoid areas where skin is scarred, tender, bruised, red, scaly, hard. • Recommended injection site is front of middle thighs, but lower abdomen 2 inches below navel or outer, upper arms are acceptable. • Inject within 5 min after cap has been removed.

Autoinjector • Push open end of autoinjector firmly against skin at 90-degree angle. • Do not pull autoinjector away from skin until a first "click" sound and then a second "click" sound are heard (injection is finished and needle is pulled back). This usually takes 3–6 sec, but second click may take up to 15 sec to be heard. • If autoinjector is pulled away from skin before injection is completed, full dose may not be administered.

Prefilled syringe • Gently pinch skin and hold firmly. Use quick, dart-like motion to insert needle into pinched skin at 45-degree angle.

Storage • Refrigerate; do not freeze. • Do not shake. • Solution appears slightly opalescent, colorless to light yellow. Discard if cloudy or contains particulate.

INDICATIONS/ROUTES/DOSAGE

Active Psoriatic Arthritis

SUBCUTANEOUS: ADULTS, ELDERLY: 50 mg once monthly. Use alone or in combination with methotrexate.

Moderate to Severely Active Rheumatoid Arthritis

SUBCUTANEOUS: ADULTS, ELDERLY: 50 mg once monthly. Use in combination with methotrexate.

Active Ankylosing Spondylitis

SUBCUTANEOUS: ADULTS, ELDERLY: 50 mg once monthly.

SIDE EFFECTS

Occasional (7%–6%): Upper respiratory tract infection, nasopharyngitis. **Rare (3%–1%):** Injection site erythema, hypertension, dizziness, bronchitis, pyrexia, paresthesia.

ADVERSE EFFECTS/ TOXIC REACTIONS

New-onset psoriasis, exacerbation of preexisting psoriasis have been reported. Serious infections noted, including sepsis, pneumonia, cellulitis, abscess, tuberculosis, invasive fungal infections, hepatitis B infection. Increased risk of lymphoma, melanoma. New-onset or exacerbation of CNS demyelinating disorders, including multiple sclerosis, new-onset or worsening of CHF noted.

NURSING CONSIDERATIONS

BASELINE ASSESSMENT

Pts should be evaluated for active tuberculosis and tested for latent infection prior to initiating treatment and periodically during therapy. Induration of 5 mm or greater with tuberculin skin testing should be considered a positive test result when assessing if treatment for latent tuberculosis is necessary. Antifungal therapy should be considered for those who reside or travel to regions where mycoses are endemic. Do not initiate therapy during an active infection.

INTERVENTION/EVALUATION

Monitor hepatitis B carriers during and several months following therapy. If reactivation occurs, therapy should be discontinued and antiviral therapy begun. Pts should be closely monitored for development of signs/symptoms of tuberculosis, including those who tested negative for latent tuberculosis infection prior to initiating therapy. Treatment should be discontinued if pt develops a serious infection, opportunistic infection, or sepsis and appropriate antimicrobial therapy initiated.

PATIENT/FAMILY TEACHING

• Inform pt that therapy may lower immune system response and ask pt to report any symptoms of infection. • Counsel pt regarding risk of lymphoma, melanoma. • Advise those with latex sensitivity that needle cover on prefilled syringe and autoinjector contains dry natural rubber (latex derivative). • Avoid live vaccines during therapy. Advise on proper injection sites, rotation.

goserelin HIGH ALERT

go-**suh**-reh-lin
(Zoladex, Zoladex LA ✤)

CLASSIFICATION

PHARMACOTHERAPEUTIC: Gonadotropin-releasing hormone analogue. **CLINICAL:** Antineoplastic (see pp. 84C, 105C).

ACTION

Stimulates release of luteinizing hormone (LH) and follicle-stimulating hormone (FSH) from anterior pituitary. **Therapeutic Effect:** In females, reduces ovarian, uterine, mammary gland size, regresses hormone-responsive tumors. In males, decreases testosterone level, reduces growth of abnormal prostate tissue.

PHARMACOKINETICS

Protein binding: 27%. Metabolized in liver. Excreted in urine. **Half-life:** 4.2 hrs (male); 2.3 hrs (female).

USES

Treatment of advanced carcinoma of prostate as alternative when orchiectomy, estrogen therapy is either not indicated or unacceptable to pt. In combination with flutamide before and during radiation therapy for early stages of prostate cancer. Management of endometriosis. Treatment of advanced breast cancer in premenopausal and perimenopausal women. Endometrial thinning before ablation for dysfunctional uterine bleeding.

PRECAUTIONS

Contraindications: Pregnancy. **Cautions:** None known.

LIFESPAN CONSIDERATIONS

Pregnancy/Lactation: Crosses placenta; unknown if distributed in breast milk. **Pregnancy Category D (advanced breast cancer), X (endometriosis, endometrial thinning). Children:** Safety and efficacy not established. **Elderly:** No age-related precautions noted.

INTERACTIONS

DRUG: None significant. **HERBAL:** None significant. **FOOD:** None known. **LAB VALUES:** May increase serum prostatic acid phosphatase, testosterone.

AVAILABILITY (Rx)

Injection, Solution (Zoladex): 3.6 mg, 10.8 mg.

ADMINISTRATION/HANDLING

Injection

• Clean area of skin on upper abdominal wall with alcohol swab. • Stretch or pinch pt's skin with one hand, and insert needle into subcutaneous tissue. • Direct needle so that it parallels the abdominal wall. Push needle in until barrel hub touches pt's skin. Withdraw needle 1 cm to create a space to discharge goserelin. Fully depress plunger. • Withdraw needle, bandage site.

INDICATIONS/ROUTES/DOSAGE

Prostatic Carcinoma

IMPLANT: ADULTS OLDER THAN 18 YRS, ELDERLY: 3.6 mg every 28 days or 10.8 q12wks subcutaneously into upper abdominal wall.

Breast Carcinoma, Endometriosis

IMPLANT: ADULTS: 3.6 mg every 28 days subcutaneously into upper abdominal wall.

Endometrial Thinning

IMPLANT: ADULTS: 3.6 mg subcutaneously into upper abdominal wall as a single dose or in 2 doses 4 wks apart.

SIDE EFFECTS

Frequent: Headache (60%), hot flashes (55%), depression (54%), diaphoresis (45%), sexual dysfunction (21%), impotence (18%), lower urinary tract symptoms (13%). **Occasional (10%–5%):** Pain, lethargy, dizziness, insomnia, anorexia, nausea, rash, upper respiratory tract infection, hirsutism, abdominal pain. **Rare:** Pruritus.

ADVERSE EFFECTS/ TOXIC REACTIONS

Arrhythmias, CHF, hypertension occur rarely. Ureteral obstruction, spinal cord compression observed (immediate orchiectomy may be necessary).

NURSING CONSIDERATIONS

INTERVENTION/EVALUATION

Monitor pt closely for worsening signs/symptoms of prostatic cancer, esp. during first mo of therapy.

PATIENT/FAMILY TEACHING

• Use nonhormonal methods of contraceptive measures during therapy. • Inform physician if pt becomes pregnant or regular menstruation persists. • Breakthrough menstrual bleeding may occur if dose is missed.

granisetron

gran-**is**-eh-tron
(Granisol, Kytril, Sancuso)

Do not confuse granisetron with dolasetron, ondansetron, or palonosetron.

◆CLASSIFICATION

PHARMACOTHERAPEUTIC: Serotonin receptor antagonist. **CLINICAL:** Antiemetic.

ACTION

Selectively blocks serotonin stimulation at receptor sites at chemoreceptor trigger zone, vagal nerve terminals. **Therapeutic Effect:** Prevents nausea/vomiting.

PHARMACOKINETICS

Route	Onset	Peak	Duration
IV	1–3 min	N/A	24 hrs

Rapidly, widely distributed to tissues. Protein binding: 65%. Metabolized in liver to active metabolite. Eliminated in urine, feces. **Half-life:** 10–12 hrs (increased in elderly).

USES

Prevents nausea/vomiting associated with emetogenic cancer therapy (includes high-dose cisplatin). Prevention, treatment of postop nausea, vomiting. Prophylaxis of nausea/vomiting associated with cancer radiation therapy. **OFF-LABEL: PO:** Prophylaxis of nausea/vomiting associated with radiation therapy.

PRECAUTIONS

Contraindications: None known. **Cautions:** Safety not established in children younger than 2 yrs.

LIFESPAN CONSIDERATIONS

Pregnancy/Lactation: Unknown if distributed in breast milk. **Pregnancy Category B. Children:** Safety and efficacy not established in those younger than 2 yrs. **Elderly:** No age-related precautions noted.

INTERACTIONS

DRUG: Hepatic enzyme inducers may decrease effect. **HERBAL:** None significant. **FOOD:** None known. **LAB VALUES:** May increase AST, ALT.

AVAILABILITY (Rx)

Injection Solution (Kytril): 0.1 mg/ml, 1 mg/ml. **Oral Solution (Granisol, Kytril):** 2 mg/10 ml. **Tablets (Kytril):** 1 mg. **Transdermal Patch (Sancuso):** 52-cm^2 patch containing 34.3 mg granisetron delivering 3.1 mg/24 hrs.

ADMINISTRATION/HANDLING

IV

Reconstitution • May be given undiluted or dilute with 20–50 ml 0.9% NaCl or D_5W. Do not mix with other medications.
Rate of administration • May give undiluted as IV push over 30 sec. • For IV piggyback, infuse over 5–20 min depending on volume of diluent used.
Storage • Appears as a clear, colorless solution. • Store at room temperature. • After dilution, stable for at least 24 hrs at room temperature. • Inspect for particulates, discoloration.

PO

• Give 30 min to 1 hr prior to initiating chemotherapy.

Transdermal

• Apply to clean, dry, intact skin on upper outer arm. • Remove immediately from pouch before application. • Do not cut patch.

IV INCOMPATIBILITY

Amphotericin B (Fungizone).

IV COMPATIBILITIES

Allopurinol (Aloprim), bumetanide (Bumex), calcium gluconate, carboplatin (Paraplatin), cisplatin (Platinol), cyclophosphamide (Cytoxan), cytarabine (Ara-C), dacarbazine (DTIC-Dome), dexamethasone (Decadron), diphenhydramine (Benadryl), docetaxel (Taxotere), doxorubicin (Adriamycin), etoposide (VePesid), gemcitabine (Gemzar), lipids, magnesium, mitoxantrone (Novantrone), paclitaxel (Taxol), potassium.

INDICATIONS/ROUTES/DOSAGE

Prevention of Chemotherapy-Induced Nausea/Vomiting
PO: ADULTS, ELDERLY: 2 mg 1 hr before chemotherapy or 1 mg 1 hr before and 12 hrs after chemotherapy.
IV: ADULTS, ELDERLY, CHILDREN 2 YRS AND OLDER: 10 mcg/kg/dose (or 1 mg/dose) within 30 min of chemotherapy.
TRANSDERMAL: ADULTS, ELDERLY: Apply 24–48 hrs prior to chemotherapy. Remove minimum 24 hrs after completion of chemotherapy. May be worn up to 7 days, depending on chemotherapy duration.

Prevention of Radiation-Induced Nausea/Vomiting
PO: ADULTS, ELDERLY: 2 mg once a day, given 1 hr before radiation therapy.

Postop Nausea/Vomiting
IV: ADULTS, ELDERLY: 1 mg as a single postop dose. **CHILDREN OLDER THAN 4 YRS:** 20–40 mcg/kg. **Maximum:** 1 mg.

SIDE EFFECTS

Frequent (21%–14%): Headache, constipation, asthenia (loss of strength, energy). **Occasional (8%–6%):** Diarrhea, abdominal pain. Rare (less than 2%): Altered taste, fever.

ADVERSE EFFECTS/ TOXIC REACTIONS

Hypersensitivity reaction, hypertension, hypotension, arrhythmias (sinus bradycardia, atrial fibrillation, AV block, ventricular ectopy), EKG abnormalities occur rarely.

NURSING CONSIDERATIONS

BASELINE ASSESSMENT

Ensure that granisetron is given within 30 min of starting chemotherapy.

INTERVENTION/EVALUATION

Monitor for therapeutic effect. Assess for headache. Monitor daily pattern of bowel activity and stool consistency.

PATIENT/FAMILY TEACHING

- Granisetron is effective shortly following administration; prevents nausea/vomiting.
- Transitory taste disorder may occur.

griseofulvin

griz-ee-oh-**full**-vin
(Grifulvin V, Gris-PEG)

◆CLASSIFICATION

CLINICAL: Antifungal.

ACTION

Inhibits fungal cell mitosis by disrupting mitotic spindle structure. Therapeutic Effect: Fungistatic.

PHARMACOKINETICS

Ultramicrosize is almost completely absorbed. Absorption is significantly enhanced after a fatty meal. Extensively metabolized in liver. Minimal excretion in urine. Half-life: 9-22 hrs.

USES

Treatment of susceptible tinea (ringworm) infections of the skin, hair, and nails: *t. capitis, t. corporis, t. cruris, t. pedis, t. unguium.*

PRECAUTIONS

Contraindications: Hepatocellular failure, porphyria. Cautions: Exposure to sun/ultraviolet light (photosensitivity), hypersensitivity to penicillins.

LIFESPAN CONSIDERATIONS

Pregnancy/Lactation: Crosses placenta; unknown if distributed in breast milk. **Pregnancy Category C. Children:** Safety and efficacy not established in those younger than 2 yrs. **Elderly:** No age-related precautions noted.

INTERACTIONS

DRUG: May decrease effects of **oral contraceptives, warfarin.** HERBAL: None significant. FOOD: **High-fat foods** enhance absorption. LAB VALUES: None significant.

AVAILABILITY (Rx)

Oral Suspension (Grifulvin V): 125 mg/5 ml. Tablets (Microsize Grifulvin V): 500 mg. Tablets (Ultramicrosize, Gris-PEG): 125 mg, 250 mg.

ADMINISTRATION/HANDLING

• Administer with fatty meal, food, or milk to reduce GI irritation. • Ultramicrosize tablets may be crushed and sprinkled on applesauce.

INDICATIONS/ROUTES/DOSAGE

Usual Dosage

◄ALERT► Duration of therapy depends on site of infection.

PO (MICROSIZE TABLETS, ORAL SUSPENSION): ADULTS: 500–1,000 mg as a single dose or in divided doses. **CHILDREN 2 YRS AND OLDER:** 10–20 mg/kg/day in single or divided doses.

PO (ULTRAMICROSIZE TABLETS): ADULTS: 375–750 mg/day as a single dose or in divided doses. **CHILDREN 2 YRS AND OLDER:** 5–15 mg/kg/day in single or divided doses. **Maximum:** 750 mg/day.

SIDE EFFECTS

Occasional: Hypersensitivity reaction (pruritus, rash, urticaria), headache, nausea, diarrhea, excessive thirst, flatulence, oral thrush, dizziness, insomnia. **Rare:** Paresthesia of hands/feet, proteinuria, photosensitivity reaction.

ADVERSE EFFECTS/ TOXIC REACTIONS

Granulocytopenia occurs rarely and should necessitate discontinuation of drug.

NURSING CONSIDERATIONS

BASELINE ASSESSMENT

Question for history of allergies, esp. to griseofulvin, penicillins.

INTERVENTION/EVALUATION

Assess skin for rash, response to therapy. Monitor daily pattern of bowel activity and stool consistency. Question presence of headache: onset, location, type of discomfort. Assess for dizziness.

PATIENT/FAMILY TEACHING

• Prolonged therapy (wks or mos) is usually necessary. • Do not miss a dose; continue therapy as long as ordered. • Avoid alcohol (may produce tachycardia, flushing). • May cause photosensitivity reaction; avoid exposure to sunlight. • Maintain good hygiene (prevents superinfection). • Separate personal items in direct contact with affected areas. • Keep affected areas dry; wear light clothing for ventilation. • Take with foods high in fat such as milk, ice cream (reduces GI upset, assists absorption).

guaifenesin

gwye-**fen**-e-sin
(Guiatuss, Mucinex, Organidin, Phanasin, Robitussin)
Do not confuse guaifenesin with guanfacine, or Mucinex with Mucomyst.

FIXED-COMBINATION(S)

Mucinex D: guaifenesin/pseudoephedrine (a sympathomimetic): 600 mg/60 mg, 1,200 mg/120 mg. **Mucinex DM:** guaifenesin/dextromethorphan (a cough suppressant): 600 mg/30 mg, 1,200 mg/60 mg. **Robitussin AC:** guaifenesin/codeine (a narcotic analgesic): 100 mg/10 mg, 75 mg/2.5 mg per 5 ml. **Robitussin DM:** guaifenesin/dextromethorphan (a cough suppressant): 100 mg/10 mg per 5 ml.

CLASSIFICATION

CLINICAL: Expectorant.

ACTION

Stimulates respiratory tract secretions by decreasing adhesiveness, viscosity of phlegm. **Therapeutic Effect:** Promotes removal of viscous mucus.

PHARMACOKINETICS

Well absorbed from GI tract. Metabolized in liver. Excreted in urine. **Half-life:** 1 hr.

USES

Expectorant for symptomatic treatment of coughs.

PRECAUTIONS

Contraindications: None known. **Cautions:** None known.

LIFESPAN CONSIDERATIONS

Pregnancy/Lactation: Unknown if drug crosses placenta or is distributed in breast milk. **Pregnancy Category C. Children:** Caution advised in those younger than 2 yrs with persistent cough. **Elderly:** No age-related precautions noted.

INTERACTIONS

DRUG: None significant. **HERBAL:** None significant. **FOOD:** None known. **LAB VALUES:** None significant.

AVAILABILITY (OTC)

Liquid: 100 mg/5 ml. **Syrup:** 100 mg/5 ml. **Tablets:** 200 mg, 400 mg.

G

Tablets, Extended-Release: (Mucinex): 600 mg, 1,200 mg.

ADMINISTRATION/HANDLING

PO

• Store syrup, liquid, tablets at room temperature. • Give without regard to meals. • Do not crush, break extended-release tablet. May sprinkle contents on soft food, then swallow without crushing/chewing.

G

INDICATIONS/ROUTES/DOSAGE

Expectorant

PO: ADULTS, ELDERLY, CHILDREN OLDER THAN 12 YRS: 200–400 mg q4h. **CHILDREN 6–12 YRS:** 100–200 mg q4h. **Maximum:** 1.2 g/day. **CHILDREN 2–5 YRS:** 50–100 mg q4h. **Maximum:** 600 mg/day. **CHILDREN 6 MOS–2 YRS:** 25–50 mg of q4h. **Maximum:** 300 mg/day.

PO (EXTENDED-RELEASE): ADULTS, ELDERLY, CHILDREN OLDER THAN 12 YRS: 600–1,200 mg q12h. **Maximum:** 2.4 g/day. **CHILDREN 6–12 YRS:** 600 mg q12h. **Maximum:** 1.2 g/day.

SIDE EFFECTS

Rare: Dizziness, headache, rash, diarrhea, nausea, vomiting, abdominal pain.

ADVERSE EFFECTS/ TOXIC REACTIONS

Overdose may produce nausea, vomiting.

NURSING CONSIDERATIONS

BASELINE ASSESSMENT

Assess type, severity, frequency of cough. Increase fluid intake, environmental humidity to lower viscosity of lung secretions.

INTERVENTION/EVALUATION

Initiate deep breathing, coughing exercises, particularly in pts with pulmonary impairment. Assess for clinical improvement; record onset of relief of cough.

PATIENT/FAMILY TEACHING

• Avoid tasks that require alertness, motor skills until response to drug is established. • Do not take for chronic cough. • Inform physician if cough persists or if fever, rash, headache, sore throat is present with cough. • Maintain adequate hydration.

guanfacine

gwan-fah-seen
(Intuniv)

Do not confuse guanfacine with colchicine, guaifenesin, or guanidine.

CLASSIFICATION

PHARMACOTHERAPEUTIC: Alpha$_{2A}$-adrenergic agonist. **CLINICAL:** Psychotherapeutic agent.

ACTION

Not a CNS stimulant. Interacts with alpha$_{2A}$-adrenergic receptors in prefrontal cortex of brain. Behaviors (inattention, hyperactivity, impulsiveness) related to attention-deficit hyperactivity disorder (ADHD) may be controlled in this part of the brain. **Therapeutic Effect:** Improves symptoms of ADHD.

PHARMACOKINETICS

Readily absorbed from GI tract. Protein binding: 70%. Metabolized in liver. Excreted in urine. **Half-life:** 14–22 hrs.

USES

Treatment of ADHD.

PRECAUTIONS

Contraindications: History of hypersensitivity to other products containing guanfacine (e.g., Tenex). **Cautions:** History of hypotension, heart block, bradycardia, cardiovascular disease, syncope, those treated with antihypertensives (increases risk of hypotension, bradycardia, syncope).

LIFESPAN CONSIDERATIONS

Pregnancy/Lactation: Unknown if distributed in breast milk. **Pregnancy Category B. Children:** Safety and efficacy not established in those younger than 6 yrs.

Efficacy beyond 9 weeks and safety beyond 2 years of treatment not established for children and adolescents older than 6 yrs. **Elderly:** Safety and efficacy not established. Not used in this pt population.

INTERACTIONS

DRUG: **Atazanavir, clarithromycin, indinavir, itraconazole, ketoconazole, nefazodone, nelfinavir, ritonavir, saquinavir** increase risk of hypotension, bradycardia, sedation. **Rifampin** decreases guanfacine concentration. May increase **valproic acid** concentration. Increased risk of cardiovascular effects with **antihypertensives. Alcohol, antipsychotics, barbiturates, benzodiazepines, sedative/hypnotics** may produce additive sedative effects. HERBAL: None significant. FOOD: None known. LAB VALUES: None significant.

AVAILABILITY (Rx)

Tablets, Extended-Release: 1 mg, 2 mg, 3 mg, 4 mg.

ADMINISTRATION/HANDLING

PO

• Do not give with high-fat meal. • Do not break, crush, chew extended-release tablets.

INDICATIONS/ROUTES/DOSAGE

◀ALERT▶ Dosing should be considered on a mg/kg basis.

ADHD

PO: ADULTS, CHILDREN 6 YRS AND OLDER: Begin at dose of 1 mg/day and adjust in increments of no more than 1 mg/wk until clinical response and tolerability are observed. Improvements observed at starting doses of 0.05–0.08 mg/kg once daily. Doses up to 0.12 mg/kg once daily may provide additional benefit. Maintain dose within range of 1–4 mg once daily. If switching from immediate-release guanfacine, discontinue that treatment and titrate with extended-release guanfacine. When discontinuing, taper dose in decrements of no more than 1 mg every 3–7 days.

SIDE EFFECTS

Frequent (38%–10%): Sedation, headache, fatigue, upper abdominal pain. **Occasional (6%–3%):** Nausea, lethargy, dizziness, irritability, hypotension or decreased B/P, decreased appetite, dry mouth, constipation. **Rare (2%–1%):** Dyspepsia, asthenia, increased B/P, increased weight, orthostatic hypotension, increased urinary frequency.

ADVERSE EFFECTS/ TOXIC REACTIONS

Abrupt discontinuation may produce infrequent, transient elevations in B/P above original baseline (taper dose in decrements of no more than 1 mg every 3–7 days). Abrupt withdrawal following prolonged administration of high dosage may produce extreme fatigue (may last for wks). Prolonged administration to children may produce suppression of weight and/or height patterns. AV block, bradycardia, arrhythmias occur rarely.

NURSING CONSIDERATIONS

BASELINE ASSESSMENT

Measure pulse, B/P prior to initiation of therapy, following dose increases, and periodically during therapy.

INTERVENTION/EVALUATION

Assist with ambulation if sedation, dizziness, fatigue, lethargy occur. Be alert to mood changes. Assess for nausea, headache. Monitor B/P, blood serum chemistries, particularly renal/hepatic function studies for change from baseline. Monitor daily pattern of bowel activity and stool consistency.

PATIENT/FAMILY TEACHING

• Avoid tasks that require alertness, motor skills until response to drug is established. • Avoid alcohol. • Dry mouth may be relieved with sugarless gum, sips of tepid water. • Advise pts to avoid becoming dehydrated, overheated. • Do not substitute for immediate-release guanfacine tablets. • Swallow whole, do not break, crush, or chew. • Do not take with high-fat meal.

Haldol, *see haloperidol*

haloperidol

hal-oh-**pear**-ih-dawl
(Apo-Haloperidol 🍁, Haldol, Haldol Decanoate, Novo-Peridol 🍁, Peridol 🍁)

BLACK BOX ALERT Increased risk of mortality in elderly pts with dementia-related psychosis with use of injections.

Do not confuse Haldol with Halcion or Stadol.

◆ CLASSIFICATION

CLINICAL: Antipsychotic, antiemetic, antidyskinetic (see p. 65C).

ACTION

Competitively blocks postsynaptic dopamine receptors, interrupts nerve impulse movement, increases turnover of dopamine in brain. **Therapeutic Effect:** Produces tranquilizing effect. Strong extrapyramidal, antiemetic effects; weak anticholinergic, sedative effects.

PHARMACOKINETICS

Readily absorbed from GI tract. Protein binding: 92%. Extensively metabolized in liver. Primarily excreted in urine. Not removed by hemodialysis. **Half-life:** 20 hrs.

USES

Treatment of psychoses (including schizophrenia), Tourette's disorder, severe behavioral problems in children, emergency sedation of severely agitated/psychotic pts. OFF-LABEL: Treatment of Huntington's chorea, infantile autism, nausea/vomiting associated with cancer chemotherapy, ethanol dependence, psychosis/agitation related to Alzheimer's dementia.

PRECAUTIONS

Contraindications: Narrow-angle glaucoma, CNS depression, myelosuppression, Parkinson's disease, severe cardiac, hepatic disease. **Cautions:** Renal/hepatic impairment, cardiovascular disease, history of seizures.

⌛ LIFESPAN CONSIDERATIONS

Pregnancy/Lactation: Crosses placenta. Distributed in breast milk. **Pregnancy Category C. Children:** More susceptible to dystonias; not recommended in those younger than 3 yrs. **Elderly:** More susceptible to orthostatic hypotension, anticholinergic effects, sedation; increased risk for extrapyramidal effects. Decreased dosage recommended.

INTERACTIONS

DRUG: **Alcohol, other CNS depressants** may increase CNS depression. **Epinephrine** may block alpha-adrenergic effects. **Medications producing extrapyramidal symptoms (EPS)** may increase EPS. **Lithium** may increase neurologic toxicity. HERBAL: **Gotu kola, kava kava, St. John's wort, valerian** may increase CNS depression. FOOD: None known. LAB VALUES: None known. **Therapeutic serum level:** 0.2–1 mcg/ml; **toxic serum level:** greater than 1 mcg/ml.

AVAILABILITY (Rx)

Injection, Oil (Decanoate [Haldol Decanoate]): 50 mg/ml, 100 mg/ml. **Injection, Solution (Lactate [Haldol]):** 5 mg/ml. **Oral Concentrate:** 2 mg/ml. **Tablets (Haldol):** 0.5 mg, 1 mg, 2 mg, 5 mg, 10 mg, 20 mg.

ADMINISTRATION/HANDLING

IV

◀ALERT▶ Only haloperidol lactate is given IV.

Reconstitution • May give undiluted. • Flush with at least 2 ml 0.9% NaCl before and after administration. • May add to 30–50 ml of most solutions (D_5W preferred).

Rate of administration • Give IV push at rate of 5 mg/min. • Infuse IV piggyback over 30 min. • For IV infusion, up to 25 mg/hr has been used (titrated to pt response).

Storage • Discard if precipitate forms, discoloration occurs. • Store at room temperature; do not freeze. • Protect from light.

IM

Parental administration • Pt should remain recumbent for 30–60 min in head-low position with legs raised to minimize hypotensive effect. • Prepare Decanoate IM injection using 21-gauge needle. • Do not exceed maximum volume of 3 ml per IM injection site. • Inject slow, deep IM into upper outer quadrant of gluteus maximus.

PO

• Give without regard to meals. • Scored tablets may be crushed. • Dilute oral concentrate with water or juice.

IV INCOMPATIBILITIES

Allopurinol (Aloprim), amphotericin B complex (Abelcet, AmBisome, Amphotec), cefepime (Maxipime), fluconazole (Diflucan), foscarnet (Foscavir), heparin, lipids, nitroprusside (Nipride), piperacillin/tazobactam (Zosyn).

IV COMPATIBILITIES

Dobutamine (Dobutrex), dopamine (Intropin), fentanyl (Sublimaze), hydromorphone (Dilaudid), lidocaine, lorazepam (Ativan), midazolam (Versed), morphine, nitroglycerin, norepinephrine (Levophed), propofol (Diprivan).

INDICATIONS/ROUTES/DOSAGE

Tourette's Syndrome

PO: ADULTS, ELDERLY, CHILDERN 12 YRS AND OLDER: 0.5–2 mg (moderate symptoms) or 3–5 mg (severe symptoms) 2–3 times a day. **CHILDREN 3–11 YRS, WEIGHING 15–40 KG:** 0.05–0.075 mg/kg/day in 2–3 divided doses. May increase by 0.25–0.5 mg/day at 5- to 7-day intervals.

Psychotic Disorders

PO: ADULTS, CHILDREN 12 YRS AND OLDER: 0.5–2 mg (moderate symptoms) or 3–5 mg (severe symptoms) 2–3 times a day. **Maximum**: 30 mg/day. **CHILDREN 3–11 YRS, WEIGHING 15–40 KG:** 0.05 mg/kg/day in 2–3 divided doses. May increase by 0.25–0.5 mg/day at 5- to 7-day intervals. **Maximum**: 0.15 mg/kg/day.

Schizophrenia

IM: ADULTS, ELDERLY: 2–5 mg, may repeat q4–8h up to every hr as needed.

IM (DECANOATE): ADULTS, ELDERLY: Stabilized on low daily oral doses (up to 10 mg/day): 10–15 times previous daily oral dose IM monthly or q4wks. **Maximum initial dose**: 100 mg. Stabilized on high daily oral doses, 20 times previous daily oral dose IM for the first mo, then 10–15 times previously daily oral dose IM monthly or q4wks. **Maximum initial dose**: 100 mg.

PO: ADULTS, ELDERLY, CHILDREN 12 YRS AND OLDER: 0.5–2 mg (moderate symptoms) or 3–5 mg (severe symptoms) 2–3 times a day. **Maximum**: 30 mg/day. **CHILDREN 3–11 YRS, WEIGHING 15–40 KG:** 0.05 mg/kg/day in 2–3 divided doses. May increase by 0.25–0.5 mg/day at 5- to 7-day intervals. **Maximum**: 0.15 mg/kg/day.

Behavioral Disorders

CHILDREN 3–11 YRS, WEIGHING 15–40 KG: 0.05–0.075 mg/kg/day in 2–3 divided doses. May increase by 0.25–0.5 mg/day at 5- to 7-day intervals.

Delirium in ICU

IV: ADULTS: Monitor EKG and QT interval. Initially, 2–10 mg. May repeat q20–30 min until calm achieved then 25% of maximum dose q6h or 0.03–0.15 mg/kg q30min to q6h.

Rapid Tranquilization of Severely Agitated Pt

IM: ADULTS: 5 mg q30–60 min.

PO: ADULTS: 5–10 mg q30–60 min. Average total dose: 10–20 mg.

Usual Elderly Dosage

PO: 0.25–0.5 mg 1–2 times a day. May increase at 5- to 7-day intervals by 0.25–0.5 mg/day. May increase dosing intervals (e.g., 2 times a day to 3 times a day, etc.) as needed to control response or side effects.

SIDE EFFECTS

Frequent: Blurred vision, constipation, orthostatic hypotension, dry mouth, swelling or soreness of female breasts, peripheral edema. **Occasional:** Allergic reaction, difficulty urinating, decreased thirst, dizziness, diminished sexual function, drowsiness, nausea, vomiting, photosensitivity, lethargy.

ADVERSE EFFECTS/ TOXIC REACTIONS

Extrapyramidal symptoms (EPS) appear to be dose related and typically occur in first few days of therapy. Marked drowsiness/lethargy, excessive salivation, fixed stare may be mild to severe in intensity. Less frequently noted are severe akathisia (motor restlessness), acute dystonias: torticollis (neck muscle spasm), opisthotonos (rigidity of back muscles), oculogyric crisis (rolling back of eyes). Tardive dyskinesia (tongue protrusion, puffing of cheeks, chewing/puckering of the mouth) may occur during long-term therapy or after drug discontinuance and may be irreversible. Elderly female pts have greater risk of developing this reaction.

NURSING CONSIDERATIONS

BASELINE ASSESSMENT

Assess behavior, appearance, emotional status, response to environment, speech pattern, thought content.

INTERVENTION/EVALUATION

Monitor B/P, heart rate. Supervise suicidal-risk pt closely during early therapy (as depression lessens, energy level improves, increasing suicide potential). Monitor for rigidity, tremor, mask-like facial expression, fine tongue movement. Assess for therapeutic response (interest in surroundings, improvement in self-care, increased ability to concentrate, relaxed facial expression). Monitor EKG and QT interval. **Therapeutic serum level:** 0.2–1 mcg/ml. **Toxic serum level:** greater than 1 mcg/ml.

PATIENT/FAMILY TEACHING

• Full therapeutic effect may take up to 6 wks. • Do not abruptly withdraw from long-term drug therapy. • Sugarless gum, sips of tepid water may relieve dry mouth. • Drowsiness generally subsides during continued therapy. • Avoid tasks that require alertness, motor skills until response to drug is established. • Avoid alcohol. • Report muscle stiffness. • Avoid exposure to sunlight, overheating, dehydration (increased risk of heat stroke).

heparin

HIGH ALERT

hep-a-rin

(Hepalean ✱, Hepalean Leo ✱, Hep-Lock)

Do not confuse heparin with Hespan.

◆CLASSIFICATION

PHARMACOTHERAPEUTIC: Blood modifier. **CLINICAL:** Anticoagulant (see p. 31C).

ACTION

Interferes with blood coagulation by blocking conversion of prothrombin to thrombin and fibrinogen to fibrin. **Therapeutic Effect:** Prevents further extension of existing thrombi or new clot formation. No effect on existing clots.

PHARMACOKINETICS

Well absorbed following subcutaneous administration. Protein binding: Very high. Metabolized in liver. Removed from circulation via uptake by reticuloendothelial system. Primarily excreted in urine. Not removed by hemodialysis. **Half-life:** 1–6 hrs.

USES

Prophylaxis, treatment of thromboembolic disorders, including venous thrombosis, pulmonary embolism, peripheral arterial embolism, atrial fibrillation with embolism. Prevention of thromboembolus in cardiac and vascular surgery, dialysis procedures, blood transfusions, blood sampling for laboratory purposes. Adjunct in treatment of coronary occlusion with acute MI. Maintains patency of indwelling intravascular devices. Diagnosis, treatment of acute/chronic consumptive coagulation pathology (e.g., disseminated intravascular coagulation [DIC]). Prevents cerebral thrombosis in progressive strokes. OFF-LABEL: Acute MI.

PRECAUTIONS

Contraindications: Intracranial hemorrhage, severe hypotension, severe thrombocytopenia, subacute bacterial endocarditis, uncontrolled bleeding. **Cautions:** IM injections, peptic ulcer disease, menstruation, recent surgery or invasive procedures, severe hepatic/renal disease.

LIFESPAN CONSIDERATIONS

Pregnancy/Lactation: Use with caution, particularly during last trimester, immediate postpartum period (increased risk of maternal hemorrhage). Does not cross placenta. Not distributed in breast milk. **Pregnancy Category C. Children:** No age-related precautions noted. Benzyl alcohol preservative may cause gasping syndrome in infants. **Elderly:** More susceptible to hemorrhage. Age-related renal impairment may increase risk of bleeding.

INTERACTIONS

DRUG: **Antithyroid medications, valproic acid** may cause hypoprothrombinemia. **Other anticoagulants, platelet aggregation inhibitors, thrombolytics** may increase risk of bleeding. **Probenecid** may increase effect. HERBAL: **Cat's claw, dong quai, evening primrose, feverfew, garlic, ginkgo, ginseng, horse chestnut, red clover** may increase antiplatelet activity. FOOD: None known. LAB VALUES: May increase free fatty acids, serum AST, ALT. May decrease serum cholesterol.

AVAILABILITY (Rx)

Injection Solution: 10 units/ml (Hep-Lock), 100 units/ml, 1,000 units/ml, 5,000 units/ml, 10,000 units/ml, 20,000 units/ml, 25,000 units/250 ml infusion, 25,000 units/500 ml infusion.

ADMINISTRATION/HANDLING

◄ALERT► Do **not** give by IM injection (pain, hematoma, ulceration, erythema).

IV

◄ALERT► Used in full-dose therapy. Intermittent IV dosage produces higher incidence of bleeding abnormalities. Continuous IV route preferred.

Reconstitution • Dilute IV infusion in isotonic sterile saline, D_5W, or lactated Ringer's. • Invert container at least 6 times (ensures mixing, prevents pooling of medication).

Rate of administration • Use constant-rate IV infusion pump.

Storage • Store at room temperature.

Subcutaneous

◄ALERT► Used in low-dose therapy. • After withdrawal of heparin from vial, change needle before injection (prevents leakage along needle track). • Inject above iliac crest or in abdominal fat layer. Do not inject within 2 inches of umbilicus or any scar tissue. • Withdraw needle rapidly, apply prolonged pressure at injection site. Do not massage. • Rotate injection sites.

IV INCOMPATIBILITIES

Amiodarone (Cordarone), amphotericin B complex (Abelcet, AmBisome, Amphotec), ciprofloxacin (Cipro), dacarbazine (DTIC), diazepam (Valium), dobutamine (Dobutrex), doxorubicin (Adriamycin), droperidol (Inapsine), filgrastim (Neupogen), gentamicin (Garamycin), haloperidol (Haldol), idarubicin (Idamycin), labetalol (Trandate), lipids, nicardipine (Cardene), phenytoin (Dilantin), quinidine, tobramycin (Nebcin), vancomycin (Vancocin).

IV COMPATIBILITIES

Aminophylline, ampicillin/sulbactam (Unasyn), aztreonam (Azactam), calcium gluconate, cefazolin (Ancef), ceftazidime (Fortaz), ceftriaxone (Rocephin), digoxin (Lanoxin), diltiazem (Cardizem), dopamine (Intropin), enalapril (Vasotec), famotidine (Pepcid), fentanyl (Sublimaze), furosemide (Lasix), hydromorphone (Dilaudid), insulin, lidocaine, lorazepam (Ativan), magnesium sulfate, methylprednisolone (Solu-Medrol), midazolam (Versed), milrinone (Primacor), morphine, nitroglycerin, norepinephrine (Levophed), oxytocin (Pitocin), piperacillin/tazobactam (Zosyn), procainamide (Pronestyl), propofol (Diprivan), total parenteral nutrition (TPN).

INDICATIONS/ROUTES/DOSAGE

Line Flushing

IV: ADULTS, ELDERLY, CHILDREN: 100 units q6–8h. **INFANTS WEIGHING LESS THAN 10 KG:** 10 units q6–8h.

Treatment of Thromboembolic Disorders

INTERMITTENT IV: ADULTS, ELDERLY: Initially, 10,000 units, then 50–70 units/kg (5,000–10,000 units) q4–6h. **CHILDREN 1 YR AND OLDER:** Initially, 50–100 units/kg, then 50–100 units q4h.

IV INFUSION: Weight-based dosing per institutional nomogram is recommended.

Unstable Angina, NSTEMI, Acute Coronary Syndrome

ADULTS, ELDERLY: 60 units/kg bolus (**Maximum:** 4,000 units), then 12 units/kg/hr (**Maximum:** 1,000 units/hr).

Treatment of DVT/PE

ADULTS, ELDERLY: 80 units/kg bolus (**Maximum:** 5,000 units), then 18 units/kg/hr.

Usual Pediatric Dose

75 units/kg bolus over 10 min, then 20 units/kg/hr to maintain aPTT of 60–85 sec.

Prevention of Thromboembolic Disorders

SUBCUTANEOUS: ADULTS, ELDERLY: 5,000 units q8–12h.

SIDE EFFECTS

Occasional: Pruritus, burning (particularly on soles of feet) caused by vasospastic reaction. **Rare:** Pain, cyanosis of extremity 6–10 days after initial therapy lasting 4–6 hrs, hypersensitivity reaction (chills, fever, pruritus, urticaria, asthma, rhinitis, lacrimation, headache).

ADVERSE EFFECTS/ TOXIC REACTIONS

Bleeding complications ranging from local ecchymoses to major hemorrhage occur more frequently in high-dose therapy, intermittent IV infusion, women 60 yrs and older. **Antidote:** Protamine sulfate 1–1.5 mg IV for every 100 units heparin subcutaneous within 30 min of overdose, 0.5–0.75 mg for every 100 units heparin subcutaneous if within 30–60 min of overdose, 0.25–0.375 mg for every 100 units heparin subcutaneous if 2 hrs have elapsed since overdose, 25–50 mg if heparin was given by IV infusion.

NURSING CONSIDERATIONS

BASELINE ASSESSMENT

Cross-check dose with co-worker. Determine aPTT before administration and 24 hrs following initiation of therapy, then q24–48hrs for first wk of therapy or until maintenance dose is established. Follow with aPTT determinations 1–2 times weekly for 3–4 wks. In long-term therapy, monitor 1–2 times a mo.

INTERVENTION/EVALUATION

Monitor aPTT (therapeutic dosage at 1.5–2.5 times normal) diligently. Assess Hct, platelet count, AST, ALT, urine and stool for occult blood, regardless of route of administration. Assess for decrease in B/P, increase in pulse rate, complaint of abdominal/back pain, severe headache (may be evidence of hemorrhage). Question for increase in amount of discharge during menses. Assess peripheral pulses; skin for ecchymosis, petechiae. Check for excessive bleeding from minor cuts, scratches. Assess gums for erythema, gingival bleeding. Assess urine output for hematuria. Avoid IM injections of other medications due to potential for hematomas. When converting to warfarin (Coumadin) therapy, monitor PT results (will be 10%–20% higher while heparin is given concurrently).

PATIENT/FAMILY TEACHING

• Use electric razor, soft toothbrush to prevent bleeding. • Report any sign of red or dark urine, black or red stool, coffee-ground vomitus, blood-tinged mucus from cough. • Do not use any OTC medication without physician approval (may interfere with platelet aggregation). • Wear or carry identification that notes anticoagulant therapy. • Inform dentist, other physicians of heparin therapy. • Limit alcohol.

Hepsera, *see adefovir*

Herceptin, *see trastuzumab*

Humalog, *see insulin*

Humalog Mix 75/25, *see insulin*

Humira, *see adalimumab*

Humulin 70/30, *see insulin*

Humulin N, *see insulin*

Humulin R, *see insulin*

Hycamtin, *see topotecan*

*hydrALAZINE

hye-**dral**-a-zeen
(Apo-Hydralazine ♣, Apresoline, Novo-Hylazin ♣)
Do not confuse hydralazine with hydroxyzine.

FIXED-COMBINATION(S)

Apresazide: hydralazine/hydrochlorothiazide (a diuretic): 25 mg/25 mg, 50 mg/50 mg, 100 mg/50 mg. **BiDil:** hydralazine/isosorbide (a nitrate): 37.5 mg/20 mg.

◆ CLASSIFICATION

PHARMACOTHERAPEUTIC: Vasodilator. **CLINICAL:** Antihypertensive (see p. 62C).

ACTION

Direct vasodilating effects on arterioles. **Therapeutic Effect:** Decreases B/P, systemic resistance.

PHARMACOKINETICS

Route	Onset	Peak	Duration
PO	20–30 min	N/A	Up to 8 hrs
IV	5–20 min	N/A	1–4 hrs

Well absorbed from GI tract. Widely distributed. Protein binding: 85%–90%. Metabolized in liver to active metabolite. Primarily excreted in urine. Not removed by hemodialysis. **Half-life:** 3–7 hrs (increased in renal impairment).

USES

Management of moderate to severe hypertension. Treatment of CHF. **OFF-LABEL:** Hypertension secondary to eclampsia, preeclampsia, primary pulmonary hypertension.

PRECAUTIONS

Contraindications: Coronary artery disease, lupus erythematosus, positive ANA titer, rheumatic heart disease. **Cautions:** Renal impairment, cerebrovascular disease.

LIFESPAN CONSIDERATIONS

Pregnancy/Lactation: Drug crosses placenta. Unknown if distributed in breast milk. Thrombocytopenia, leukopenia, petechial bleeding, hematomas have occurred in newborns (resolved within 1–3 wks). **Pregnancy Category C. Children:** No age-related precautions noted. **Elderly:** More sensitive to hypotensive effects. Age-related renal impairment may require dosage adjustment.

INTERACTIONS

DRUG: Diuretics, other antihypertensives may increase hypotensive effect. **HERBAL: Ephedra, ginseng, yohimbe** may worsen hypertension. **Garlic** may increase antihypertensive effect. **FOOD:** None known. **LAB VALUES:** May produce positive direct Coombs' test.

AVAILABILITY (Rx)

Injection Solution: 20 mg/ml. **Tablets:** 10 mg, 25 mg, 50 mg, 100 mg.

ADMINISTRATION/HANDLING

IV

Rate of administration • May give undiluted. • Administer slowly: maximum rate 5 mg/min (0.2 mg/kg/min for children).
Storage • Store at room temperature.

PO

• Best given with food at regularly spaced meals. • Tablets may be crushed.

IV INCOMPATIBILITIES

Aminophylline, ampicillin (Polycillin), furosemide (Lasix).

IV COMPATIBILITIES

Dobutamine (Dobutrex), heparin, hydrocortisone (Solu-Cortef), nitroglycerin, potassium.

INDICATIONS/ROUTES/DOSAGE

Moderate to Severe Hypertension

PO: ADULTS: Initially, 10 mg 4 times a day. May increase by 10–25 mg/dose q2–5 days. **Maximum:** 300 mg/day. **ELDERLY:** Initially, 10 mg 2–3 times a day. May increase by 10–25 mg q2–5 days. **CHILDREN:** Initially, 0.75–1 mg/kg/day in 2–4 divided doses, not to exceed 25 mg/dose. May increase over 3–4 wks. **Maximum:** 7.5 mg/kg/day (5 mg/kg/day in infants). **Maximum daily dose:** 200 mg.
IV, IM: ADULTS, ELDERLY: Initially, 10–20 mg/dose q4–6h. May increase to 40 mg/dose. **CHILDREN:** Initially, 0.1–0.2 mg/kg/dose (**Maximum:** 20 mg) q4–6h, as needed, up to 1.7–3.5 mg/kg/day in divided doses q4–6h.

CHF

PO: ADULTS, ELDERLY: Initially, 10–25 mg 3–4 times/day up to 225–300 mg/day in combination with isosorbide dinitrate.

Dosage in Renal Impairment

Dosage interval is based on creatinine clearance.

Creatinine Clearance	Dosage
10–50 ml/min	q8h
Less than 10 ml/min	q8–24h

SIDE EFFECTS

Frequent: Headache, palpitations, tachycardia (generally disappears in 7–10 days). **Occasional:** GI disturbance (nausea, vomiting, diarrhea), paresthesia, fluid retention, peripheral edema, dizziness, flushed face, nasal congestion.

ADVERSE EFFECTS/ TOXIC REACTIONS

High dosage may produce lupus erythematosus–like reaction (fever, facial rash, muscle/joint aches, splenomegaly). Severe orthostatic hypotension, skin flushing, severe headache, myocardial ischemia, cardiac arrhythmias may develop. Profound shock may occur with severe overdosage.

NURSING CONSIDERATIONS

BASELINE ASSESSMENT

Obtain B/P, pulse immediately before each dose, in addition to regular monitoring (be alert to fluctuations).

INTERVENTION/EVALUATION

Monitor B/P, pulse, ANA titer. Monitor for headache, palpitations, tachycardia. Assess for peripheral edema of hands, feet. Monitor daily pattern of bowel activity and stool consistency.

PATIENT/FAMILY TEACHING

• To reduce hypotensive effect, rise slowly from lying to sitting position, permit legs to dangle from bed momentarily before standing. • Unsalted crackers, dry toast may relieve nausea. • Report muscle/joint aches, fever (lupus-like reaction), flu-like symptoms. • Limit alcohol use.

hydrochlorothiazide

high-drow-chlor-oh-**thigh**-ah-zide (Apo-Hydro ✤, HydroDIURIL, Microzide, Novo-Hydrazide ✤)

FIXED-COMBINATION(S)

Accuretic: hydrochlorothiazide/quinapril (an angiotensin-converting enzyme [ACE] inhibitor): 12.5 mg/10 mg, 12.5 mg/20 mg, 25 mg/20 mg. **Aldactazide:** hydrochlorothiazide/spironolactone (a potassium-sparing diuretic): 25 mg/25 mg, 50 mg/50 mg. **Aldoril:** hydrochlorothiazide/methyldopa (an antihypertensive): 15 mg/250 mg, 25 mg/250 mg, 30 mg/500 mg, 50 mg/500 mg. **Anturnide:** hydrochlorothiazide/aliskiren (renin inhibitor)/amlodipine (calcium channel blocker): 12.5 mg/150 mg/5 mg, 12.5 mg/300 mg/5 mg, 25 mg/300 mg/5 mg, 12.5 mg/300 mg/10 mg, 25 mg/300 mg/10 mg. **Apresazide:** hydrochlorothiazide/hydralazine (a vasodilator): 25 mg/25 mg, 50 mg/50 mg, 50 mg/100 mg. **Atacand HCT:** hydrochlorothiazide/candesartan (an angiotensin II receptor antagonist): 12.5 mg/16 mg, 12.5 mg/32 mg. **Avalide:** hydrochlorothiazide/irbesartan (an angiotensin II receptor antagonist): 12.5 mg/150 mg, 12.5 mg/300 mg, 25 mg/300 mg. **Benicar HCT:** hydrochlorothiazide/olmesartan (an angiotensin II receptor antagonist): 12.5 mg/20 mg, 12.5 mg/40 mg, 25 mg/40 mg. **Capozide:** hydrochlorothiazide/captopril (an ACE inhibitor): 15 mg/25 mg, 15 mg/50 mg, 25 mg/25 mg, 25 mg/50 mg. **Diovan HCT:** hydrochlorothiazide/valsartan (an angiotensin II receptor antagonist): 12.5 mg/80 mg, 12.5 mg/160 mg. **Dyazide/Maxide:** hydrochlorothiazide/triamterene (a potassium-sparing diuretic): 25 mg/37.5 mg, 25 mg/50 mg, 50 mg/75 mg. **Exforge HCT:** hydrochlorothiazide/amlodipine (a calcium channel blocker)/valsartan (an angiotensin II receptor blocker): 12.5 mg/5 mg/160 mg, 25 mg/5 mg/160 mg, 12.5 mg/10 mg/160 mg, 25 mg/10 mg/160 mg, 25 mg/10 mg/320 mg. **Hyzaar:** hydrochlorothiazide/losartan (an angiotensin II receptor antagonist): 12.5 mg/50 mg, 12.5 mg/100 mg, 25 mg/100 mg. **Inderide:** hydrochlorothiazide/propranolol (a beta-blocker): 25 mg/40 mg, 25 mg/80 mg, 50 mg/80 mg, 50 mg/120 mg, 50 mg/160 mg. **Lopressor HCT:** hydrochlorothiazide/metoprolol (a beta-blocker): 25 mg/50 mg, 25 mg/100 mg, 50 mg/100 mg. **Lotensin HCT:** hydrochlorothiazide/bepridil (a calcium channel blocker): 6.25 mg/5 mg, 12.5 mg/10 mg, 12.5 mg/20 mg, 25 mg/20 mg. **Micardis HCT:** hydrochlorothiazide/telmisartan (an angiotensin

H

II receptor antagonist): 12.5 mg/40 mg, 12.5 mg/80 mg. **Moduretic:** hydrochlorothiazide/amiloride (a potassium-sparing diuretic): 50 mg/5 mg. **Normozide:** hydrochlorothiazide/labetalol (a beta-blocker): 25 mg/100 mg, 25 mg/300 mg. **Prinzide/Zestoretic:** hydrochlorothiazide/lisinopril (an ACE inhibitor): 12.5 mg/10 mg, 12.5 mg/20 mg, 25 mg/20 mg. **Tekturna HCT:** hydrochlorothiazide/aliskiren (a renin inhibitor): 12.5 mg/150 mg, 25 mg/300 mg. **Teveten HCT:** hydrochlorothiazide/eprosartan (an angiotensin II receptor antagonist): 12.5 mg/600 mg, 25 mg/600 mg. **Timolide:** hydrochlorothiazide/timolol (a beta-blocker): 25 mg/10 mg. **Tribeuzor:** hydrochlorothiazide/olmesartan/amlodipine: 12.5 mg/20 mg/5 mg, 12.5 mg/40 mg/5 mg, 25 mg/40 mg/5 mg, 12.5 mg/40 mg/10 mg, 25 mg/40 mg/10 mg. **Uniretic:** hydrochlorothiazide/moexipril (an ACE inhibitor): 12.5 mg/7.5 mg, 25 mg/15 mg. **Vaseretic:** hydrochlorothiazide/enalapril (an ACE inhibitor): 12.5 mg/5 mg, 25 mg/10 mg. **Ziac:** hydrochlorothiazide/bisoprolol (a beta-blocker): 6.25 mg/5 mg, 6.25 mg/10 mg.

◆CLASSIFICATION

PHARMACOTHERAPEUTIC: Sulfonamide derivative. **CLINICAL:** Thiazide diuretic, antihypertensive (see p. 102C).

ACTION

Diuretic: Blocks reabsorption of water, sodium, potassium at cortical diluting segment of distal tubule. **Antihypertensive:** Reduces plasma, extracellular fluid volume, peripheral vascular resistance by direct effect on blood vessels. **Therapeutic Effect:** Promotes diuresis; reduces B/P.

PHARMACOKINETICS

Route	Onset	Peak	Duration
PO (diuretic)	2 hrs	4–6 hrs	6–12 hrs

Variably absorbed from GI tract. Primarily excreted unchanged in urine. Not removed by hemodialysis. **Half-life:** 5.6–14.8 hrs.

USES

Treatment of mild to moderate hypertension, edema in CHF, nephrotic syndrome. **OFF-LABEL:** Treatment of lithium-induced diabetes insipidus, prevention of calcium-containing renal calculi.

PRECAUTIONS

Contraindications: Anuria, history of hypersensitivity to sulfonamides or thiazide diuretics, renal decompensation, concurrent use with dofetilide. **Cautions:** Severe renal disease, hepatic impairment, diabetes mellitus, elderly or debilitated, thyroid disorders.

⌛ LIFESPAN CONSIDERATIONS

Pregnancy/Lactation: Crosses placenta. Small amount distributed in breast milk. Breast-feeding not recommended. **Pregnancy Category B (D if used in pregnancy-induced hypertension). Children:** No age-related precautions noted, except jaundiced infants may be at risk for hyperbilirubinemia. **Elderly:** May be more sensitive to hypotensive, electrolyte effects. Age-related renal impairment may require dosage adjustment.

INTERACTIONS

DRUG: **Cholestyramine, colestipol** may decrease absorption, effects. May increase risk of **digoxin** toxicity associated with hydrochlorothiazide-induced hypokalemia. May increase risk of **lithium** toxicity. **HERBAL:** **Ephedra, ginseng, yohimbe** may worsen hypertension. **Garlic** may increase antihypertensive effect. **FOOD:** None known. **LAB VALUES:** May increase serum glucose, cholesterol, LDL, bilirubin, calcium, creatinine, uric acid, triglycerides. May decrease urinary calcium, serum magnesium, potassium, sodium.

AVAILABILITY (Rx)

Capsules (Microzide): 12.5 mg. **Tablets:** 25 mg, 50 mg.

ADMINISTRATION/HANDLING

PO

• If GI upset occurs, give with food or milk, preferably with breakfast (may prevent nocturia). • Give last dose no later than 6 PM unless instructed otherwise.

INDICATIONS/ROUTES/DOSAGE

Edema

PO: ADULTS: 25–100 mg/day in 1–2 divided doses. **Maximum:** 200 mg/day.

Hypertension

PO: ADULTS: 12.5–50 mg/day.

Usual Elderly Dosage

PO: 12.5–25 mg once daily.

Usual Pediatric Dosage

PO: CHILDREN 2–17 YRS: Initially, 1 mg/kg/day. **Maximum:** 3 mg/kg/day (50 mg). **CHILDREN 6 MOS TO 2 YRS:** 1–3 mg/kg/day in 1–2 divided doses. **Maximum:** 37.5 mg/day. **CHILDREN YOUNGER THAN 6 MOS:** 1–3 mg/kg/day in 2 divided doses.

SIDE EFFECTS

Expected: Increased urinary frequency, urine volume. Frequent: Potassium depletion. Occasional: Orthostatic hypotension, headache, GI disturbances, photosensitivity.

ADVERSE EFFECTS/ TOXIC REACTIONS

Vigorous diuresis may lead to profound water loss/electrolyte depletion, resulting in hypokalemia, hyponatremia, dehydration. Acute hypotensive episodes may occur. Hyperglycemia may occur during prolonged therapy. Pancreatitis, blood dyscrasias, pulmonary edema, allergic pneumonitis, dermatologic reactions occur rarely. Overdose can lead to lethargy, coma without changes in electrolytes or hydration.

NURSING CONSIDERATIONS

BASELINE ASSESSMENT

Check vital signs, esp. B/P for hypotension before administration. Assess baseline electrolytes, esp. for hypokalemia. Evaluate skin turgor, mucous membranes for hydration status. Evaluate for peripheral edema. Assess muscle strength, mental status. Note skin temperature, moisture. Obtain baseline weight. Initiate I&O.

INTERVENTION/EVALUATION

Continue to monitor B/P, vital signs, electrolytes, I&O, daily weight. Note extent of diuresis. Watch for changes from initial assessment (hypokalemia may result in weakness, tremor, muscle cramps, nausea, vomiting, altered mental status, tachycardia; hyponatremia may result in confusion, thirst, cold/clammy skin). Be esp. alert for potassium depletion in pts taking digoxin (cardiac arrhythmias). Potassium supplements are frequently ordered. Check for constipation (may occur with exercise diuresis).

PATIENT/FAMILY TEACHING

• Expect increased frequency, volume of urination. • To reduce hypotensive effect, rise slowly from lying to sitting position, permit legs to dangle momentarily before standing. • Eat foods high in potassium, such as whole grains (cereals), legumes, meat, bananas, apricots, orange juice, potatoes (white, sweet), raisins. • Protect skin from sun, ultraviolet rays (photosensitivity may occur).

hydrocodone

HIGH ALERT

high-drough-**koe**-doan
(Hycodan ✦, Robidone ✦)

FIXED-COMBINATION(S)

Anexsia: hydrocodone/acetaminophen (a non-narcotic analgesic): 5 mg/500 mg, 7.5 mg/650 mg, 10 mg/650 mg. **Duocet**: hydrocodone/acetaminophen: 5 mg/500 mg. **Hycet**: hydrocodone/acetaminophen: 7.5 mg/325 mg per 15 ml. **Hycodan**: hydrocodone/homatropine (an anti-cholinergic): 5 mg/1.5 mg. **Hycotuss, Vitussin**: hydrocodone/guaifenesin (an expectorant): 5 mg/100 mg. **Lorcet**:

hydrocodone/acetaminophen: 7.5 mg/650 mg, 10 mg/650 mg. **Lortab**: hydrocodone/acetaminophen: 2.5 mg/500 mg, 5 mg/500 mg, 7.5 mg/500 mg, 10 mg/500 mg. **Lortab Elixer**: hydrocodone/acetaminophen: 2.5 mg/167 mg per 5 ml. **Lortab with ASA**: hydrocodone/aspirin: 5 mg/500 mg. **Norco**: hydrocodone/acetaminophen: 10 mg/325 mg. **Reprexain CIII**: hydrocodone/ibuprofen (an NSAID): 5 mg/200 mg. **Tussend**: hydrocodone/pseudoephedrine (a sympathomimetic)/guaifenesin (an expectorant): 2.5 mg/30 mg/100 mg per 5 ml. **Vicodin**: hydrocodone/acetaminophen: 5 mg/500 mg. **Vicodin ES**: hydrocodone/acetaminophen: 7.5 mg/750 mg. **Vicodin HP**: hydrocodone/acetaminophen: 10 mg/650 mg. **Vicoprofen**: hydrocodone/ibuprofen (an NSAID): 7.5 mg/200 mg. **Xodol**: hydrocodone/acetaminophen: 5 mg/300 mg. **Zydone**: hydrocodone/acetaminophen: 5 mg/400 mg, 7.5 mg/400 mg, 10 mg/400 mg.

CLASSIFICATION

PHARMACOTHERAPEUTIC: Opioid agonist (Schedule III). **CLINICAL:** Narcotic analgesic, antitussive.

ACTION

Binds with opioid receptors in CNS. **Therapeutic Effect:** Reduces intensity of pain stimuli incoming from sensory nerve endings, altering pain perception, emotional response to pain; suppresses cough reflex.

PHARMACOKINETICS

Route	Onset	Peak	Duration
PO (analgesic)	10–20 min	30–60 min	4–6 hrs
PO (antitussive)	N/A	N/A	4–6 hrs

Well absorbed from GI tract. Metabolized in liver. Primarily excreted in urine. **Half-life:** 3.8 hrs (increased in elderly).

USES

Relief of moderate to moderately severe pain, nonproductive cough.

PRECAUTIONS

Contraindications: None known. **Extreme Caution:** CNS depression, anoxia, hypercapnia, respiratory depression, seizures, acute alcoholism, shock, untreated myxedema, respiratory dysfunction. **Cautions:** Increased ICP, hepatic impairment, acute abdominal conditions, hypothyroidism, prostatic hypertrophy, Addison's disease, urethral stricture, COPD.

LIFESPAN CONSIDERATIONS

Pregnancy/Lactation: Readily crosses placenta. Distributed in breast milk. May prolong labor if administered in latent phase of first stage of labor or before cervical dilation of 4–5 cm has occurred. Respiratory depression may occur in neonate if mother received opiates during labor. Regular use of opiates during pregnancy may produce withdrawal symptoms (irritability, excessive crying, tremors, hyperactive reflexes, fever, vomiting, diarrhea, yawning, sneezing, seizures) in the neonate. **Pregnancy Category C (D if used for prolonged periods or at high dosages at term). Children:** Those younger than 2 yrs may be more susceptible to respiratory depression. **Elderly:** May be more susceptible to respiratory depression, may cause paradoxical excitement. Age-related renal impairment, prostatic hypertrophy or obstruction may increase risk of urinary retention; dosage adjustment recommended.

INTERACTIONS

DRUG: Alcohol, other CNS depressants may increase CNS or respiratory depression, hypotension. **MAOIs** may produce a severe, sometimes fatal reaction with hydrocodone; plan to administer ¼ of usual hydrocodone dose. **HERBAL: Gotu kola, kava kava, St. John's wort, valerian** may increase CNS depression. **FOOD:** None known. **LAB VALUES:** May increase serum amylase, lipase.

AVAILABILITY (Rx)

Combination only (see Fixed Combinations).

ADMINISTRATION/HANDLING

PO

• Give without regard to meals. • Tablets may be crushed.

INDICATIONS/ROUTES/DOSAGE

Analgesia

PO: ADULTS, CHILDREN WEIGHING 50 KG OR MORE: Initially, 10 mg q3–4h as needed. **ADULTS, CHILDREN WEIGHING LESS THAN 50 KG:** Initially, 0.2 mg/kg q3–4h as needed. **ELDERLY:** 2.5–5 mg q4–6h.

Cough

PO: ADULTS, ELDERLY: 5–10 mg q4–6h as needed. **Maximum**: 15 mg/dose. **CHILDREN:** 0.6 mg/kg/day in 3–4 divided doses at intervals of at least 4 hrs. **Maximum single dose**: 10 mg (children older than 12 yrs), 5 mg (children 2–12 yrs), 1.25 mg (children younger than 2 yrs).

SIDE EFFECTS

Frequent: Sedation, hypotension, diaphoresis, facial flushing, dizziness, drowsiness. **Occasional:** Urine retention, blurred vision, constipation, dry mouth, headache, nausea, vomiting, difficult/painful urination, euphoria, dysphoria.

ADVERSE EFFECTS/ TOXIC REACTIONS

Overdose results in respiratory depression, skeletal muscle flaccidity, cold/clammy skin, cyanosis, extreme drowsiness progressing to seizures, stupor, coma. Tolerance to analgesic effect, physical dependence may occur with repeated use. Prolonged duration of action, cumulative effect may occur in those with hepatic/renal impairment.

NURSING CONSIDERATIONS

BASELINE ASSESSMENT

Obtain vital signs before giving medication. If respirations are 12/min or less (20/min or less in children), withhold medication, contact physician. **Analgesic**: Assess onset, type, location, duration of pain. Effect of medication is reduced if full pain recurs before next dose. **Antitussive**: Assess type, severity, frequency of cough.

INTERVENTION/EVALUATION

Palpate bladder for urinary retention. Monitor daily pattern of bowel activity and stool consistency. Initiate deep breathing and coughing exercises, particularly in pts with pulmonary impairment. Assess for clinical improvement; record onset of relief of pain, cough.

PATIENT/FAMILY TEACHING

• Change positions slowly to avoid orthostatic hypotension. • Avoid tasks that require alertness, motor skills until response to drug is established. • Avoid alcohol. • Tolerance or dependence may occur with prolonged use at high dosages. • Report nausea, vomiting, constipation, shortness of breath, difficulty breathing. • May take with food.

hydrocortisone

hye-dro-**kor**-ti-sone
(Anusol HC, Caldecort, Colocort, Cortaid, Cortef, Cortenema ♣, Cortizone-10, Hytone, Nupercainal Hydrocortisone Cream, Preparation H Hydrocortisone, Proctocort, Solu-Cortef, Westcort).

Do not confuse hydrocortisone with hydrochlorothiazide, hydrocodone, or hydroxychloroquine, Cortef with Coreg, or Solu-Cortef with Solu Medrol.

FIXED-COMBINATION(S)

Cortisporin: hydrocortisone/neomycin/polymyxin (anti-infective): 5 mg/10,000 units/5 mg, 10 mg/10,000 units/5 mg. **Liposivir:** hydrocortisone/acyclovir (an antiviral): 1%/5%.

CLASSIFICATION

PHARMACOTHERAPEUTIC: Adrenal corticosteroid. **CLINICAL:** Glucocorticoid (see pp. 98C, 100C).

ACTION

Inhibits accumulation of inflammatory cells at inflammation sites, phagocytosis, lysosomal enzyme release, synthesis and/or release of mediators of inflammation. **Therapeutic Effect:** Prevents/suppresses cell-mediated immune reactions. Decreases/prevents tissue response to inflammatory process.

PHARMACOKINETICS

Route	Onset	Peak	Duration
IV	N/A	4–6 hrs	8–12 hrs

Well absorbed after IM administration. Widely distributed. Metabolized in liver. **Half-life:** Plasma, 1.5–2 hrs; biologic, 8–12 hrs.

USES

Management of adrenocortical insufficiency; relief of inflammation of corticosteroid-responsive dermatoses; adjunctive treatment of ulcerative colitis, status asthmaticus, shock. **OFF-LABEL:** Management of septic shock.

PRECAUTIONS

Contraindications: Fungal, tuberculosis, viral skin lesions; serious infections. **Cautions:** Hyperthyroidism, cirrhosis, ulcerative colitis, hypertension, osteoporosis, thromboembolic tendencies, CHF, seizure disorders, thrombophlebitis, peptic ulcer, diabetes.

LIFESPAN CONSIDERATIONS

Pregnancy/Lactation: Crosses placenta; distributed in breast milk. May produce cleft palate if used chronically during first trimester. Breast-feeding not recommended. **Pregnancy Category C (D if used in first trimester). Children:** Prolonged treatment or high dosages may decrease short-term growth rate, cortisol secretion. **Elderly:** May be more susceptible to developing hypertension or osteoporosis.

INTERACTIONS

DRUG: **Amphotericin** may worsen hypokalemia. **Bupropion** may lower seizure threshold. May increase risk of **digoxin** toxicity caused by hypokalemia. May decrease effects of **diuretics, insulin, oral hypoglycemics, potassium supplements. Hepatic enzyme inducers** may decrease effects. **Live virus vaccines** may decrease pt's antibody response to vaccine, increase vaccine side effects, potentiate virus replication. **HERBAL:** **St. John's wort** may decrease concentration. **Cat's claw, echinacea** may increase immunostimulant properties. **FOOD:** None known. **LAB VALUES:** May increase serum glucose, lipids, sodium. May decrease serum calcium, potassium, thyroxine, WBC count.

AVAILABILITY (Rx)

Cream, Rectal: (Cortizone-10, Nupercainal Hydrocortisone Cream, Preparation H Hydrocortisone): 1%. **Cream, Topical:** 0.2%, 0.5%, 1%, 2.5%. **Injection, Powder for Reconstitution: (Solu-Cortef):** 100 mg, 250 mg, 500 mg, 1 g. **Ointment, Topical:** 0.2%, 0.5%, 1%, 2.5%. **Suppository: (Anusol HC):** 25 mg. **Suspension, Rectal: (Colocort):** 100 mg/60 ml. **Tablets: (Cortef):** 5 mg, 10 mg, 20 mg.

ADMINISTRATION/HANDLING

IV

Hydrocortisone Sodium Succinate

Reconstitution • Initially, reconstitute vial per manufacturer's instructions. • May further dilute with D_5W or 0.9% NaCl. For IV push, dilute to 50 mg/ml; for intermittent infusion, dilute to 1 mg/ml. Note: 100–3,000 mg may be added to 50 ml D_5W or 0.9% NaCl.

Rate of administration • Administer IV push over 3–5 min (over 10 min for doses 500 mg or greater). Give intermittent infusion over 20–30 min.

Storage • Store at room temperature. • Once reconstituted, stable for 3 days at room temperature. Once further diluted with 0.9% NaCl or D_5W stability concentration dependent: 1 mg/ml (24 hrs) 2 mg/ml to 60 mg/ml (4 hrs).

PO
• Give with food if GI distress occurs.

Rectal
• Shake homogeneous suspension well. • Instruct pt to lie on left side with left leg extended, right leg flexed. • Gently insert applicator tip into rectum, pointed slightly toward navel (umbilicus). Slowly instill medication.

Topical
• Gently cleanse area before application. • Use occlusive dressings only as ordered. • Apply sparingly; rub into area thoroughly.

IV INCOMPATIBILITIES

Ciprofloxacin (Cipro), diazepam (Valium), idarubicin (Idamycin), midazolam (Versed), phenytoin (Dilantin).

IV COMPATIBILITIES

Aminophylline, amphotericin, calcium gluconate, cefepime (Maxipime), digoxin (Lanoxin), diltiazem (Cardizem), diphenhydramine (Benadryl), dopamine (Intropin), insulin, lidocaine, lipids, lorazepam (Ativan), magnesium sulfate, morphine, norepinephrine (Levophed), procainamide (Pronestyl), potassium chloride, propofol (Diprivan).

INDICATIONS/ROUTES/DOSAGE

Acute Adrenal Insufficiency
IV: ADULTS, ELDERLY: 100 mg IV bolus, then 300 mg/day in divided doses q8h. **CHILDREN:** 1–2 mg/kg IV bolus, then 150–250 mg/day in divided doses q––8h. **INFANTS:** 1–2 mg/kg/dose IV bolus, then 25–150 mg/day in divided doses q6–8h.

Anti-Inflammation, Immunosuppression
IV, IM: ADULTS, ELDERLY: 15–240 mg q12h. **CHILDREN:** 1–5 mg/kg/day in divided doses q12h.
PO: ADULTS, ELDERLY: 15–240 mg q12h. **CHILDREN:** 2.5–10 mg/kg/day.

Physiologic Replacement
PO: CHILDREN: 0.5–0.75 mg/kg/day in divided doses q8h.
IM: CHILDREN: 0.25–0.35 mg/kg/day as a single dose.

Status Asthmaticus
IV: ADULTS, ELDERLY: 1–2 mg/kg/dose q6h. **CHILDREN:** 1–2 mg/kg/dose q6h. Maintenance: 0.5–1 mg/kg q6h.

Shock
IV: ADULTS, ELDERLY, CHILDREN 12 YRS AND OLDER: 500 mg–2 g q2–6h. **CHILDREN YOUNGER THAN 12 YRS:** 50 mg/kg. May repeat in 4 hrs, then q24h as needed.

Adjunctive Treatment of Ulcerative Colitis
RECTAL: ADULTS, ELDERLY: 100 mg at bedtime for 21 nights or until clinical and proctologic remission occurs (may require 2–3 mos of therapy).
RECTAL: ADULTS, ELDERLY: 1 applicator 1–2 times a day for 2–3 wks, then every second day until therapy ends.
USUAL TOPICAL DOSAGE: ADULTS, ELDERLY: Apply sparingly 2–4 times a day.

SIDE EFFECTS

Frequent: Insomnia, heartburn, anxiety, abdominal distention, diaphoresis, acne, mood swings, increased appetite, facial flushing, delayed wound healing, increased susceptibility to infection, diarrhea or constipation. **Occasional:** Headache, edema, change in skin color, frequent urination. **Topical:** Pruritus, redness, irritation. **Rare:** Tachycardia, allergic reaction (rash, hives), psychological changes, hallucinations, depression. **Topical:** Allergic contact dermatitis, purpura. **Systemic:** Absorption more likely with use of occlusive dressings or extensive application in young children.

ADVERSE EFFECTS/ TOXIC REACTIONS

Long-term therapy: Hypocalcemia, hypokalemia, muscle wasting (esp. arms, legs), osteoporosis, spontaneous fractures, amenorrhea, cataracts, glaucoma, peptic ulcer, CHF. **Abrupt withdrawal after long-term therapy:** Nausea, fever, headache, sudden severe joint pain, rebound inflammation, fatigue, weakness, lethargy, dizziness, orthostatic hypotension.

NURSING CONSIDERATIONS

BASELINE ASSESSMENT

Obtain baseline values for weight, B/P, serum glucose, cholesterol, electrolytes. Check results of initial tests (tuberculosis [TB] skin test, X-rays, EKG).

INTERVENTION/EVALUATION

Assess for edema. Be alert to infection (reduced immune response): sore throat, fever, vague symptoms. Monitor daily pattern of bowel activity and stool consistency. Monitor electrolytes, B/P, weight, serum glucose. Watch for hypocalcemia (muscle twitching, cramps), hypokalemia (weakness, paresthesias [esp. lower extremities], nausea/vomiting, irritability, EKG changes). Assess emotional status, ability to sleep.

PATIENT/FAMILY TEACHING

• Notify physician of fever, sore throat, muscle aches, sudden weight gain, swelling, visual disturbances, behavioral changes. • Do not take aspirin or any other medication without consulting physician. • Limit caffeine, avoid alcohol. • Inform dentist, other physicians of cortisone therapy now or within past 12 mos. • Caution against overusing joints injected for symptomatic relief. • **Topical**: Apply after shower or bath for best absorption. • Do not cover unless physician orders; do not use tight diapers, plastic pants, coverings. • Avoid contact with eyes.

HydroDIURIL, *see hydrochlorothiazide*

hydromorphone HIGH ALERT

hye-droe-**mor**-fone
(Dilaudid, Dilaudid HP, Exalgo, Hydromorph Contin ✱)

BLACK BOX ALERT High abuse potential, respiratory depression risk. Other opioids, alcohol, CNS depressants increase risk of potentially fatal respiratory depression. Highly concentrated (Dilaudid HP, 10 mg/ml) form not to be interchanged with less concentrated (Dilaudid) form; overdose, death may result.

Do not confuse hydromorphone with hydrocodone or morphine, or Dilaudid with demerol or Dilantin.

◆CLASSIFICATION

PHARMACOTHERAPEUTIC: Opioid agonist **(Schedule II). CLINICAL:** Narcotic analgesic, antitussive (see p. 142C).

ACTION

Binds to opioid receptors in CNS, reducing intensity of pain stimuli from sensory nerve endings. **Therapeutic Effect:** Alters perception, emotional response to pain; suppresses cough reflex.

PHARMACOKINETICS

Route	Onset	Peak	Duration
PO	30 min	90–120 min	4 hrs
IV	10–15 min	15–30 min	2–3 hrs
IM	15 min	30–60 min	4–5 hrs
Subcutaneous	15 min	30–90 min	4 hrs
Rectal	15–30 min	N/A	N/A

Well absorbed from GI tract after IM administration. Widely distributed. Metabolized in liver. Excreted in urine. **Half-life:** 2.6–4 hrs.

USES

Relief of moderate to severe pain. Extended-release tablet (Exalgo): Around the clock, continuous analgesia for extended period. OFF-LABEL: Persistent nonproductive cough.

PRECAUTIONS

Contraindications: Obstetric analgesia, respiratory depression in absence of resuscitative equipment, status asthmaticus. **Extreme Caution:** CNS depression, anoxia, hypercapnia, respiratory depression, seizures, acute alcoholism, shock status, untreated myxedema, respiratory dysfunction. **Cautions:** Increased ICP, hepatic impairment, acute abdominal conditions, hypothyroidism, prostatic hypertrophy, Addison's disease, urethral stricture, COPD.

LIFESPAN CONSIDERATIONS

Pregnancy/Lactation: Readily crosses placenta. Unknown if distributed in breast milk. May prolong labor if administered in latent phase of first stage of labor or before cervical dilation of 4–5 cm has occurred. Respiratory depression may occur in neonate if mother receives opiates during labor. Regular use of opiates during pregnancy may produce withdrawal symptoms in the neonate (irritability, excessive crying, tremors, hyperactive reflexes, fever, vomiting, diarrhea, yawning, sneezing, seizures). **Pregnancy Category C (D if used for prolonged periods or at high dosages at term). Children:** Those younger than 2 yrs may be more susceptible to respiratory depression. **Elderly:** May be more susceptible to respiratory depression, may cause paradoxical excitement. Age-related renal impairment, prostatic hypertrophy or obstruction may increase risk of urinary retention; dosage adjustment recommended.

INTERACTIONS

DRUG: **Alcohol, other CNS depressants** may increase CNS, respiratory depression, hypotension. **MAOIs** may produce a severe, sometimes fatal reaction with hydromorphone; plan to administer ¼ of usual hydromorphone dose. HERBAL: **Gotu kola, kava kava, St. John's wort, valerian** may increase CNS depression. FOOD: None known. LAB VALUES: May increase serum amylase, lipase.

AVAILABILITY (Rx)

Injection, Powder for Reconstitution: (Dilaudid HP): 250 mg. **Injection, Solution: (Dilaudid):** 1 mg/ml, 2 mg/ml, 4 mg/ml, 10 mg/ml. **Liquid, Oral:** 1 mg/ml. **Suppository: (Dilaudid):** 3 mg. **Tablets: (Dilaudid):** 2 mg, 4 mg, 8 mg.

Tablets, Extended-Release (Exalgo): 8 mg, 12 mg, 16 mg.

ADMINISTRATION/HANDLING

IV

ALERT High concentration injection (10 mg/ml) should be used only in those tolerant to opiate agonists, currently receiving high doses of another opiate agonist for severe, chronic pain due to cancer.

Reconstitution • May give undiluted. • May further dilute with 5 ml Sterile Water for Injection or 0.9% NaCl.

Rate of administration • Administer IV push very slowly (over 2–3 min). • Rapid IV increases risk of severe adverse reactions (chest wall rigidity, apnea, peripheral circulatory collapse, anaphylactoid effects, cardiac arrest).

Storage • Store at room temperature; protect from light. • Slight yellow discoloration of parenteral form does not indicate loss of potency.

IM, Subcutaneous

• Use short 25- to 30-gauge needle for subcutaneous injection. • Administer slowly; rotate injection sites. • Pts with circulatory impairment experience higher risk of overdosage due to delayed absorption of repeated administration.

PO

• Give without regard to meals. • Tablets may be crushed. • Extended-release tablets must be swallowed whole; do not break, crush, dissolve, or inject.

Rectal

• Refrigerate suppositories. • Moisten suppository with cold water before inserting well up into rectum.

IV INCOMPATIBILITIES

Amphotericin B complex (Abelcet, AmBisome, Amphotec), cefazolin (Ancef, Kefzol), diazepam (Valium), lipids, phenobarbital, phenytoin (Dilantin), total parenteral nutrition (TPN).

IV COMPATIBILITIES

Diltiazem (Cardizem), diphenhydramine (Benadryl), dobutamine (Dobutrex), dopamine (Intropin), fentanyl (Sublimaze), furosemide (Lasix), heparin, lorazepam (Ativan), magnesium sulfate, metoclopramide (Reglan), midazolam (Versed), milrinone (Primacor), morphine, propofol (Diprivan).

H

INDICATIONS/ROUTES/DOSAGE

Analgesia

PO: ADULTS, ELDERLY, CHILDREN WEIGHING 50 KG AND MORE: 2–4 mg q3–4h. Range: 2–8 mg/dose. **CHILDREN OLDER THAN 6 MOS AND WEIGHING LESS THAN 50 KG:** 0.03–0.08 mg/kg/dose q3–4h.
EXTENDED-RELEASE: ADULTS, ELDERLY: Range: 8–64 mg once daily.
IV: ADULTS, ELDERLY, CHILDREN WEIGHING MORE THAN 50 KG (FOR OPIATE-NAIVE PT): 0.2–0.6 mg q2–3h. **USUAL DOSAGE:** 1–2 mg q3–4h. **CHILDREN WEIGHING 50 KG OR LESS:** 0.015 mg/kg/dose q3–6h as needed.
RECTAL: ADULTS, ELDERLY: 3 mg q4–8h.

Patient-Controlled Analgesia (PCA)

IV: ADULTS, ELDERLY: 0.05–0.5 mg at 5–15 min lockout. **Maximum (4-hr):** 4–6 mg.
EPIDURAL: ADULTS, ELDERLY: Bolus dose of 1–1.5 mg infusion (concentration: 0.05–0.075 mg/ml) at rate of 0.04–0.4 mg/hr. Demand dose of 0.15 mg at 30 min lockout.

Cough (Off-Label)

PO: ADULTS, ELDERLY, CHILDREN OLDER THAN 12 YRS: 1 mg q3–4h. **CHILDREN 6–12 YRS:** 0.5 mg q3–4h.

SIDE EFFECTS

Frequent: Drowsiness, dizziness, hypotension (including orthostatic hypotension), decreased appetite. **Occasional:** Confusion, diaphoresis, facial flushing, urinary retention, constipation, dry mouth, nausea, vomiting, headache, pain at injection site. **Rare:** Allergic reaction, depression.

ADVERSE EFFECTS/ TOXIC REACTIONS

Overdose results in respiratory depression, skeletal muscle flaccidity, cold/clammy skin, cyanosis, extreme drowsiness progressing to seizures, stupor, coma. Tolerance to analgesic effect, physical dependence may occur with repeated use. Prolonged duration of action, cumulative effect may occur in those with hepatic/renal impairment.

NURSING CONSIDERATIONS

BASELINE ASSESSMENT

Obtain vital signs before giving medication. If respirations are 12/min or less (20/min or less in children), withhold medication, contact physician. **Analgesic**: Assess onset, type, location, duration of pain. Effect of medication is reduced if full pain recurs before next dose. **Antitussive**: Assess type, severity, frequency of cough.

INTERVENTION/EVALUATION

Monitor vital signs; assess for pain relief, cough. Assess breathing sounds. Increase fluid intake, environmental humidity to decrease viscosity of lung secretions. To prevent pain cycles, instruct pt to request pain medication as soon as discomfort begins. Monitor daily pattern of bowel activity and stool consistency (esp. in long-term use). Initiate deep breathing and coughing exercises, particularly in pts with pulmonary impairment. Assess for clinical improvement; record onset of relief of pain, cough.

PATIENT/FAMILY TEACHING

• Avoid alcohol, tasks that require alertness/motor skills until response to drug is established. • Tolerance or dependence may occur with prolonged use at high dosages. • Change positions slowly to avoid orthostatic hypotension. • Do not break, crush, chew, dissolve extended-release tablets.

hydroxychloroquine

hye-drox-ee-**klor**-oh-kwin
(Apo-Hydroxyquine ✱, Plaquenil)

BLACK BOX ALERT Should be given by physicians familiar with prescribing information before use.

Do not confuse hydroxychloroquine with hydrocortisone or hydroxyzine, or Plaquenil with Platinol.

◆CLASSIFICATION

CLINICAL: Antimalarial, antirheumatic.

ACTION

Concentrates in parasite acid vesicles, interfering with parasite protein synthesis. Antirheumatic action may involve suppressing formation of antigens responsible for hypersensitivity reactions. **Therapeutic Effect:** Inhibits parasite growth.

PHARMACOKINETICS

Variable rate of absorption. Widely distributed in body tissues (eyes, kidneys, liver, lungs). Protein binding: 45%. Partially metabolized in liver. Partially excreted in urine. **Half-life:** 32 days (in plasma), 50 days (in blood).

USES

Treatment of falciparum malaria (terminates acute attacks, cures nonresistant strains); suppression of acute attacks, prolongation of interval between treatment/relapse in vivax, ovale, malariae malaria. Treatment of discoid or systematic lupus erythematosus, acute and chronic rheumatoid arthritis (RA). OFF-LABEL: Treatment of juvenile arthritis, sarcoid-associated hypercalcemia, porphyria.

PRECAUTIONS

Contraindications: Long-term therapy for children, psoriasis, retinal or visual field changes. **Cautions:** Alcoholism, hepatic disease, G6PD deficiency. Children are esp. susceptible to hydroxychloroquine fatalities.

⌛ LIFESPAN CONSIDERATIONS

Pregnancy/Lactation: Crosses placenta; distributed in breast milk. **Pregnancy Category C. Children:** Long-term therapy not recommended. **Elderly:** No age-related precautions noted.

INTERACTIONS

DRUG: May increase **penicillamine** concentration, risk of hematologic, renal, severe skin reactions. HERBAL: None significant. FOOD: None known. LAB VALUES: None significant.

AVAILABILITY (Rx)

Tablets: 200 mg (155 mg base).

ADMINISTRATION/HANDLING

PO

• Give with food or milk.

INDICATIONS/ROUTES/DOSAGE

Treatment of Acute Attack of Malaria (Dosage in mg Base)

PO:

Dose	Times	Adults	Children
Initial	Day 1	620 mg	10 mg/kg
Second	6 hrs later	310 mg	5 mg/kg
Third	Day 2	310 mg	5 mg/kg
Fourth	Day 3	310 mg	5 mg/kg

Suppression of Malaria

PO: ADULTS: 310 mg base weekly on same day each wk, beginning 2 wks before entering an endemic area and continuing for 4–6 wks after leaving the area. **CHILDREN:** 5 mg base/kg/wk, beginning 2 wks before entering an endemic area and continuing for 4–6 wks after leaving the area. If therapy is not begun before exposure, administer a loading dose of 10 mg base/kg in 2 equally divided doses 6 hrs apart, followed by the usual dosage regimen.

Rheumatoid Arthritis (RA)
PO: ADULTS: Initially, 400–600 mg (310–465 mg base) daily for 5–10 days, gradually increased to optimum response level. Maintenance (usually within 4–12 wks): Dosage decreased by 50% and then continued at maintenance dose of 200–400 mg (155–310 mg base) daily. Maximum effect may not be seen for several mos.

Lupus Erythematosus
PO: ADULTS: Initially, 400 mg (310 mg base) once or twice a day for several wks or mos. Maintenance: 200–400 mg/day (155–310 mg base).

H

SIDE EFFECTS

Frequent: Transient headache, anorexia, nausea, vomiting. **Occasional:** Visual disturbances, anxiety, fatigue, pruritus (esp. palms, soles, scalp), irritability, personality changes, diarrhea, photosensitivity. **Rare:** Stomatitis, dermatitis, impaired hearing.

ADVERSE EFFECTS/ TOXIC REACTIONS

Ocular toxicity (esp. retinopathy) may progress even after drug is discontinued. **Prolonged therapy:** Peripheral neuritis, neuromyopathy, hypotension, EKG changes, agranulocytosis, aplastic anemia, thrombocytopenia, seizures, psychosis. **Overdosage:** Headache, vomiting, visual disturbances, drowsiness, seizures, hypokalemia followed by cardiovascular collapse, death.

NURSING CONSIDERATIONS

BASELINE ASSESSMENT

Evaluate CBC, hepatic function tests, vision.

INTERVENTION/EVALUATION

Monitor CBC, muscular weakness. Evaluate for GI distress. Monitor hepatic function tests. Assess skin/buccal mucosa; inquire about pruritus. Report impaired vision/hearing immediately.

PATIENT/FAMILY TEACHING

• Avoid exposure to direct sunlight. • Avoid alcohol. • Explain need for eye exams q3 mos with prolonged therapy. • Immediately notify physician of **any** new symptom of visual difficulties, muscular weakness, impaired hearing, tinnitus, numbness, tremors, rash, persistent diarrhea, emotional change.

hydroxyurea

HIGH ALERT

high-**drox**-ee-your-ee-ah
(Apo-Hydroxyurea, Droxia, Hydrea, Mylocel)

BLACK BOX ALERT Must be administered by personnel trained in administration/handling of chemotherapeutic agents or in treatment of sickle cell anemia. Carcinogenic risk; secondary leukemias reported with long-term treatment.

Do not confuse hydroxyurea with hydroxyzine.

CLASSIFICATION

PHARMACOTHERAPEUTIC: Synthetic urea analogue. **CLINICAL:** Antineoplastic (see p. 84C).

ACTION

Inhibits DNA synthesis without interfering with RNA synthesis or protein. **Therapeutic Effect:** Interferes with normal repair process of cancer cells damaged by irradiation.

PHARMACOKINETICS

Well absorbed from GI tract. Protein binding: 75%–80%. Metabolized in liver. Excreted in urine as urea and unchanged drug. **Half-life:** 3–4 hrs.

USES

Treatment of melanoma; resistant chronic myelocytic leukemia; recurrent, metastatic, inoperable ovarian carcinoma. Used in combination with radiation therapy for local control of primary squamous cell carcinoma of head/neck, excluding lip. Treatment of sickle cell anemia. **OFF-LABEL:** Treatment of HIV, psoriasis, hematologic conditions (e.g., polycythemia vera), uterine, cervical, non–small cell lung cancer, primary brain tumors, renal cell cancer, prostate cancer.

PRECAUTIONS

Contraindications: WBC count less than 2,500/mm^3 or platelet count less than 100,000/mm^3. **Cautions:** Previous irradiation therapy, other cytoxic drugs, renal/hepatic impairment.

LIFESPAN CONSIDERATIONS

Pregnancy/Lactation: Crosses placenta; distributed in breast milk. May be harmful to fetus. **Pregnancy Category D. Children:** Safety and efficacy not established. **Elderly:** More sensitive to hydroxyurea effects; may require lower dosage.

INTERACTIONS

DRUG: May decrease effects of **antigout medications. Antiretroviral agents (e.g., didanosine, stavudine)** may cause pancreatitis, hepatotoxicity, peripheral neuropathy. **Bone marrow depressants** may increase myelosuppression. **Live virus vaccines** may potentiate virus replication, increase vaccine side effects, decrease the pt's antibody response to vaccine. **HERBAL:** None significant. **FOOD:** None known. **LAB VALUES:** May increase BUN, serum creatinine, uric acid.

AVAILABILITY (Rx)

Capsules: 200 mg (Droxia), 300 mg (Droxia), 400 mg (Droxia), 500 mg (Hydrea). **Tablets (Mylocel):** 1,000 mg.

ADMINISTRATION/HANDLING

Capsules may be opened and emptied into water (will not dissolve completely).

INDICATIONS/ROUTES/DOSAGE

◀ALERT▶ Therapy interrupted when platelet count falls below 100,000/mm^3 or WBC count falls below 2,500/mm^3. Resume when counts return to normal.

Melanoma; Recurrent, Metastatic, Inoperable Ovarian Carcinoma

PO: ADULTS, ELDERLY: 80 mg/kg every 3 days or 20–30 mg/kg/day as a single dose.

Control of Primary Squamous Cell Carcinoma of Head/Neck, Excluding Lips (in Combination with Radiation Therapy)

PO: ADULTS, ELDERLY: 80 mg/kg every 3 days, beginning at least 7 days before starting radiation therapy.

Resistant Chronic Myelocytic Leukemia

PO: ADULTS, ELDERLY: 20–30 mg/kg once a day. **CHILDREN:** 10–20 mg/kg once a day.

HIV Infection

PO: ADULTS, ELDERLY: 1,000–1,500 mg/day as single dose or in divided doses.

Sickle Cell Anemia

PO: ADULTS, ELDERLY, CHILDREN: Initially, 15 mg/kg once a day. May increase by 5 mg/kg/day every 12 weeks. **Maximum:** 35 mg/kg/day.

SIDE EFFECTS

Frequent: Nausea, vomiting, anorexia, constipation or diarrhea. **Occasional:** Mild, reversible rash; facial flushing; pruritus; fever; chills; malaise. **Rare:** Alopecia, headache, drowsiness, dizziness, disorientation.

ADVERSE EFFECTS/ TOXIC REACTIONS

Myelosuppression manifested as hematologic toxicity (leukopenia and, to a lesser extent, thrombocytopenia, anemia).

NURSING CONSIDERATIONS

BASELINE ASSESSMENT

Obtain bone marrow studies, hepatic/renal function tests before therapy begins, periodically thereafter. Obtain Hgb, WBC, platelet count, serum uric acid at baseline and weekly during therapy. Those with marked renal impairment may develop visual or auditory hallucinations, marked hematologic toxicity.

INTERVENTION/EVALUATION

Monitor daily pattern of bowel activity and stool consistency. Monitor for hematologic toxicity (fever, sore throat, signs of local infection, unusual bleeding/

H

bruising from any site), symptoms of anemia (excessive fatigue, weakness). Assess skin for rash, erythema. Monitor CBC with differential, platelet count, Hgb, renal/hepatic function, uric acid.

PATIENT/FAMILY TEACHING

• Promptly report fever, sore throat, signs of local infection, unusual bleeding/bruising from any site.

H

*hydrOXYzine

high-**drox**-ih-zeen
(Apo-Hydroxyzine, Atarax, Novo-Hydroxyzin, Vistaril)
Do not confuse hydroxyzine with hydralazine or hydroxyurea, or Vistaril with Restoril, Versed, or Zestril.

CLASSIFICATION

PHARMACOTHERAPEUTIC: Piperazine derivative. **CLINICAL:** Antihistamine, antianxiety, antispasmodic, antiemetic, antipruritic (see pp. 14C, 54C).

ACTION

Competes with histamine for receptor sites in GI tract, blood vessels, respiratory tract. Diminishes vestibular stimulation, depresses labyrinthine function. **Therapeutic Effect:** Produces anxiolytic, anticholinergic, antihistaminic, analgesic effects; relaxes skeletal muscle; controls nausea, vomiting.

PHARMACOKINETICS

Route	Onset	Peak	Duration
PO	15–30 min	N/A	4–6 hrs

Well absorbed from GI tract and after parenteral administration. Metabolized in liver. Primarily excreted in urine. Not removed by hemodialysis. **Half-life:** 3–7 hrs (increased in elderly).

USES

Treatment of anxiety, preop sedation, antipruitic. **OFF-LABEL:** Antiemetic, alcohol withdrawal symptoms.

PRECAUTIONS

Contraindications: None known. **Cautions:** Narrow-angle glaucoma, prostatic hypertrophy, bladder neck obstruction, asthma, COPD.

LIFESPAN CONSIDERATIONS

Pregnancy/Lactation: Unknown if drug crosses placenta or is distributed in breast milk. **Pregnancy Category C. Children:** Not recommended in newborns or premature infants (increased risk of anticholinergic effects). Paradoxical excitement may occur. **Elderly:** Increased risk of dizziness, sedation, confusion. Hypotension, hyperexcitability may occur.

INTERACTIONS

DRUG: Alcohol, other CNS depressants may increase CNS depressant effects. **MAOIs** may increase anticholinergic, CNS depressant effects. **HERBAL: Gotu kola, kava kava, St. John's wort, valerian** may increase CNS depression. **FOOD:** None known. **LAB VALUES:** May cause false-positive urine 17-hydroxycorticosteroid determinations.

AVAILABILITY (Rx)

Injection Solution (Vistaril): 25 mg/ml, 50 mg/ml. **Oral Suspension (Vistaril):** 25 mg/5 ml. **Syrup:** 10 mg/5 ml. **Tablets:** 10 mg, 25 mg, 50 mg.

Capsules (Vistaril): 25 mg, 50 mg, 100 mg.

ADMINISTRATION/HANDLING

IM

ALERT Significant tissue damage, thrombosis, gangrene may occur if injection is given subcutaneous, intra-arterial, or by IV.

• IM may be given undiluted. • Use Z-track technique of injection to prevent subcutaneous infiltration. • Inject deep IM into gluteus maximus or midlateral thigh in adults, midlateral thigh in children.

PO

• May give without regard to food. • Shake oral suspension well. • Scored tablets may be crushed; do not crush/break capsule.

INDICATIONS/ROUTES/DOSAGE

Anxiety

PO: ADULTS, ELDERLY: 25–100 mg 4 times a day. **Maximum:** 600 mg/day. **CHILDREN 6 YRS AND OLDER:** 50–100 mg/day in divided doses. **CHILDREN YOUNGER THAN 6 YEARS:** 50 mg/day in divided doses.

Nausea/Vomiting

IM: ADULTS, ELDERLY: 25–100 mg/dose q4–6h.

Pruritus

PO: ADULTS, ELDERLY: 25 mg 3–4 times a day. **CHILDREN 6 YRS AND OLDER:** 50–100 mg/day in divided doses. **CHILDREN YOUNGER THAN 6 YEARS:** 50 mg/day in divided doses.

Preop Sedation

PO: ADULTS, ELDERLY: 50–100 mg. **CHILDREN:** 0.6 mg/kg/dose.

IM: ADULTS, ELDERLY: 25–100 mg. **CHILDREN:** 0.5–1 mg/kg/dose.

SIDE EFFECTS

Side effects are generally mild, transient. Frequent: Drowsiness, dry mouth, marked discomfort with IM injection. Occasional: Dizziness, ataxia, asthenia (loss of strength, energy), slurred speech, headache, agitation, increased anxiety. Rare: Paradoxical reactions (hyperactivity, anxiety in children; excitement, restlessness in elderly or debilitated pts) generally noted during first 2 wks of therapy, particularly in presence of uncontrolled pain.

ADVERSE EFFECTS/ TOXIC REACTIONS

Hypersensitivity reaction (wheezing, dyspnea, chest tightness) may occur.

NURSING CONSIDERATIONS

BASELINE ASSESSMENT

Anxiety: Offer emotional support to anxious pt. Assess motor responses (agitation, trembling, tension), autonomic responses (cold/clammy hands, diaphoresis). **Antiemetic:** Assess for dehydration (poor skin turgor, dry mucous membranes, longitudinal furrows in tongue).

INTERVENTION/EVALUATION

For those on long-term therapy, hepatic/renal function tests, blood counts should be performed periodically. Monitor lung sounds for signs of hypersensitivity reaction. Monitor serum electrolytes in pts with severe vomiting. Assess for paradoxical reaction, particularly during early therapy. Assist with ambulation if drowsiness, light-headedness occur.

PATIENT/FAMILY TEACHING

• Marked discomfort may occur with IM injection. • Sugarless gum, sips of tepid water may relieve dry mouth. • Drowsiness usually diminishes with continued therapy. • Avoid tasks that require alertness, motor skills until response to drug is established.

hyoscyamine

hye-oh-**sye**-a-meen

(Anaspaz, Hyosine, Levbid, Levsin, Levsin S/L, Symax SL, Symax SR)

Do not confuse Anaspaz with Anaprox, or Levbid with Lithobid or Lopid.

FIXED COMBINATIONS

Donnatal: hyoscyamine/atropine (anticholinergic)/phenobarbital (sedative)/scopolamine (anticholinergic): 0.1037 mg/0.0194 mg/16.2 mg/0.0065 mg.

◆CLASSIFICATION

PHARMACOTHERAPEUTIC: Anticholinergic. **CLINICAL:** Antimuscarinic, antispasmodic.

ACTION

Inhibits action of acetylcholine at postganglionic (muscarinic) receptor sites. **Therapeutic Effect:** Decreases secretions (bronchial, salivary, sweat gland, gastric juices). Reduces motility of GI, urinary tracts.

PHARMACOKINETICS

Route	Onset	Peak	Duration
PO	15–30 min	–	4–6 hrs

Well absorbed following PO administration. Protein binding: 50%. Metabolized in liver. Majority excreted in urine. Removed by hemodialysis. **Half-life:** 3.5 hrs (immediate-release); 7 hrs (sustained-release).

USES

PO: Adjunctive therapy for peptic ulcer disease, irritable bowel syndrome, neurogenic bladder or bowel; treatment of infantile colic, GI tract disorders caused by spasm; reduce abdominal rigidity; reduce tremors associated with Parkinson's disease; drying agent in acute rhinitis. **Parenteral**: Preoperatively to reduce secrections, block cardiac vagal inhibitory reflexes; relief of biliary, renal colic; reduce GI motility to facilitate diagnostic procedures; reduce pain, hypersecretion in pancreatitis; reversal of neuromuscular blockade.

PRECAUTIONS

Contraindications: GI/GU obstruction, myasthenia gravis, narrow-angle glaucoma, paralytic ileus, severe ulcerative colitis. **Cautions:** Hyperthyroidism, CHF, cardiac arrhythmias, prostatic hypertrophy, neuropathy, chronic lung disease.

⌛ LIFESPAN CONSIDERATIONS

Pregnancy/Lactation: Crosses placenta; distributed in breast milk. **Pregnancy Category C. Children:** Safety and efficacy not established. **Elderly:** No age-related precautions noted.

INTERACTIONS

DRUG: Antacids, antidiarrheals may decrease absorption. May decrease absorption of **ketoconazole. Other anticholinergics** may increase effects. May increase severity of GI lesions with matrix formulation of **potassium chloride. HERBAL:** None significant. **FOOD:** None known. **LAB VALUES:** None significant.

AVAILABILITY (Rx)

Capsules, Timed-Release: 0.375 mg. **Elixir: (Hyosine, Levsin):** 0.125 mg/5 ml. **Injection, Solution: (Levsin):** 0.5 mg/ml. **Solution, Oral Drops: (Hyosine, Levsin):** 0.125 mg/ml. **Tablets: (Anaspaz, Levsin):** 0.125 mg. **Tablets, Orally-Disintegrating: (Anaspaz):** 0.125 mg. **Tablets, Sublingual: (Levsin S/L, Symax SL):** 0.125 mg.

Tablets, Extended-Release: (Levbid, Symax SR): 0.375 mg.

ADMINISTRATION/HANDLING

PO

• Give before meals. • Immediate-release tablets may be crushed, chewed. • Extended-release tablet should be swallowed whole. • Allow orally-disintegrating tablet placed on tongue to dissolve before swallowing; may give with or without water. • Sublingual: place under tongue.

Parenteral

• May give undiluted.

INDICATIONS/ROUTES/DOSAGE

GI Tract Disorders

PO, SUBLINGUAL: ADULTS, ELDERLY, CHILDREN 12 YRS AND OLDER: 0.125–0.25 mg q4h as needed. **EXTENDED-RELEASE:** 0.375–0.75 mg q12h. **Maximum:** 1.5 mg/day. **CHILDREN 2–11 YRS:** 0.0625–0.125 mg q4h as needed. **Maximum:** 0.75 mg/day.

IV, IM: ADULTS, ELDERLY, CHILDREN 12 YRS AND OLDER: 0.25–0.5 mg. May repeat as needed up to 4 times/day at 4-hr intervals.

Hypermotility of Lower Urinary Tract
PO: SUBLINGUAL: ADULTS, ELDERLY: 0.15–0.3 mg 4 times a day; **EXTENDED-RELEASE:** 0.375 mg q12h.

Infant Colic
PO: INFANTS: Drops dosed q4h as needed (based on weight): 2.3 kg: 3 drops; 3.4 kg: 4 drops; 5 kg: 5 drops; 7 kg: 6 drops; 10 kg: 8 drops; 15 kg: 11 drops.

SIDE EFFECTS

Frequent: Dry mouth (sometimes severe), decreased diaphoresis, constipation. **Occasional:** Blurred vision, bloated feeling, urinary hesitancy, drowsiness (with high dosage), headache, intolerance to light, loss of taste, anxiety, flushing, insomnia, impotence, mental confusion or excitement (particularly in elderly, children), temporary light-headedness (with parenteral form), local irritation (with parenteral form). **Rare:** Dizziness, faintness.

ADVERSE EFFECTS/ TOXIC REACTIONS

Overdose may produce temporary paralysis of ciliary muscle, pupillary dilation, tachycardia, palpitations, hot/dry/flushed skin, absence of bowel sounds, hyperthermia, increased respiratory rate, EKG abnormalities, nausea, vomiting; rash over face/upper trunk, CNS stimulation, psychosis (agitation, restlessness, rambling speech, visual hallucinations, paranoid behavior, delusions) followed by depression.

NURSING CONSIDERATIONS

BASELINE ASSESSMENT

Before giving medication, instruct pt to void (reduces risk of urinary retention).

INTERVENTION/EVALUATION

Monitor daily pattern of bowel activity and stool consistency. Palpate bladder for urinary retention. Monitor changes in B/P, temperature. Assess skin turgor, mucous membranes to evaluate hydration status (encourage adequate fluid intake), bowel sounds for peristalsis. Be alert for fever (increased risk of hyperthermia).

PATIENT/FAMILY TEACHING

• May cause dry mouth; maintain good oral hygiene habits (lack of saliva may increase risk of cavities). • Inform physician of rash, eye pain, difficulty in urinating, constipation. • Avoid tasks that require alertness, motor skills until response to drug is established. • Avoid hot baths, saunas.

I

Hyzaar, *see hydrochlorothiazide and losartan*

ibandronate

eye-**band**-droh-nate
(Bondronat ✤, Boniva)

◆CLASSIFICATION

PHARMACOTHERAPEUTIC: Bisphosphonate. **CLINICAL:** Calcium regulator.

ACTION

Binds to bone hydroxyapatite (part of mineral matrix of bone), inhibits osteoclast activity. **Therapeutic Effect:** Reduces rate of bone turnover, bone resorption, resulting in net gain in bone mass.

PHARMACOKINETICS

Absorbed in upper GI tract. Extent of absorption impaired by food, beverages (other than plain water). Protein binding: 85%–99%. Rapidly binds to bone. Unabsorbed portion eliminated in urine. **Half-life: PO:** 37–157 hrs; **IV:** 5–25 hrs.

USES

Treatment/prevention of osteoporosis in postmenopausal women. **OFF-LABEL:** Hypercalcemia of malignancy; steroid-induced osteoporosis; Paget's disease; reduces bone pain from metastatic bone disease.

PRECAUTIONS

Contraindications: Hypersensitivity to other bisphosphonates (e.g., alendronate, etidronate, pamidronate, risedronate, tiludronate), inability to stand or sit upright for at least 60 min, severe renal impairment with creatinine clearance less than 30 ml/min, uncorrected hypocalcemia. **Cautions:** GI diseases (duodenitis, dysphagia, esophagitis, gastritis, ulcers [drug may exacerbate these conditions]), mild to moderate renal impairment.

I

LIFESPAN CONSIDERATIONS

Pregnancy/Lactation: Potential for teratogenic effects. Unknown if distributed in breast milk. Breast-feeding not recommended. **Pregnancy Category C. Children:** Safety and efficacy not established. **Elderly:** No age-related precautions noted.

INTERACTIONS

DRUG: **Antacids containing aluminum, calcium, magnesium; vitamin D** decrease absorption. **Aspirin, NSAIDs** may increase GI irritation. **HERBAL:** None significant. **FOOD:** **Beverages (other than plain water), dietary supplements, food** interfere with absorption. **LAB VALUES:** May decrease serum alkaline phosphatase. May increase serum cholesterol.

AVAILABILITY (Rx)

Injection Solution: 3 mg/3 ml syringe. **Tablets:** 2.5 mg, 150 mg.

ADMINISTRATION/HANDLING

PO

- Give 60 min before first food, beverage of the day, on an empty stomach with 6–8 oz plain water (not mineral water) while pt is standing or sitting in upright position.
- Pt cannot lie down for 60 min following drug administration.
- Swallow whole; do not chew, suck tablet (potential for oropharyngeal ulceration).

IV

- Give over 15–30 sec.

INDICATIONS/ROUTES/DOSAGE

Osteoporosis

PO: ADULTS, ELDERLY: 2.5 mg daily. Alternatively, 150 mg once monthly.
IV: ADULTS, ELDERLY: 3 mg q3mo.

Dosage in Renal Impairment

Not recommended for pts with creatinine clearance less than 30 ml/min.

SIDE EFFECTS

Frequent (13%–6%): Back pain, dyspepsia (epigastric distress, heartburn), peripheral discomfort, diarrhea, headache, myalgia. **IV:** Abdominal pain, dyspepsia, constipation, nausea, diarrhea. **Occasional (4%–3%):** Dizziness, arthralgia, asthenia (loss of strength, energy). **Rare (2% or less):** Vomiting, hypersensitivity reaction.

ADVERSE EFFECTS/ TOXIC REACTIONS

Upper respiratory infection occurs occasionally. Overdose results in hypocalcemia, hypophosphatemia, significant GI disturbances.

NURSING CONSIDERATIONS

BASELINE ASSESSMENT

Hypocalcemia, vitamin D deficiency must be corrected before beginning therapy. Obtain laboratory baselines, esp. serum electrolytes, renal function. Obtain results of bone density study.

INTERVENTION/EVALUATION

Monitor electrolytes, esp. serum calcium, alkaline phosphatase. Monitor renal function tests.

PATIENT/FAMILY TEACHING

- Expected benefits occur only when medication is taken with full glass (6–8 oz) of plain water, first thing in the morning and at least 60 min before first food, beverage, medication of the day. Any other beverage (mineral water, orange juice, coffee) significantly reduces absorption of medication. • Do not lie down for at least 60 min after taking medication (potentiates delivery to stomach, reduces risk of esophageal irritation). • Consider weight-bearing exercises; modify behavioral factors (e.g., cigarette smoking, alcohol consumption).

ibritumomab HIGH ALERT

i-brit-uh-**moe**-mab
(Zevalin)

BLACK BOX ALERT Severe, potentially fatal infusion reactions (angioedema, hypoxia, marked hypotension, myocardial infarction) reported, usually within 30–130 min of rituximab infusion (co-therapy). Prolonged, severe cytopenia occurs in most pts. Severe cutaneous, mucocutaneous reactions (including fatalities) have been reported. Must be administered by personnel trained in administration/handling of radioisotopes.

◆CLASSIFICATION

PHARMACOTHERAPEUTIC: Monoclonal antibody. **CLINICAL:** Antineoplastic (see p. 84C).

ACTION

Combines targeting power of monoclonal antibodies (MAbs) with cancer-killing ability of radiation. **Therapeutic Effect:** Targets CD antigen (present in greater than 90% of pts with B-cell non-Hodgkin's lymphoma) inducing cellular damage.

PHARMACOKINETICS

Tumor uptake is greater than normal tissue in non-Hodgkin's lymphoma. Most of dose cleared by binding to tumor. Minimally excreted in urine. **Half-life:** 27–30 hrs.

USES

Treatment of non-Hodgkin's lymphoma (NHL) in combination with rituxumab in pts with relapsed or refractory low-grade, follicular, or CD20-positive transformed B-cell non-Hodgkin's lymphoma. Pts with previously untreated follicular NHL who achieve a partial or complete response to first-line chemotherapy.

PRECAUTIONS

Contraindications: Platelet count less than 100,000 cells/mm^3, neutrophil count less than 1,500 cells/mm^3, history of failed stem cell collection. **Cautions:** Mild thrombocytopenia, prior external beam radiation, cardiovascular disease, hypertension/hypotension.

LIFESPAN CONSIDERATIONS

Pregnancy/Lactation: Has potential to cause fetal harm. Those with childbearing potential should use contraceptive methods during and up to 12 mos after therapy. **Pregnancy Category D. Children:** Safety and efficacy not established. **Elderly:** No age-related precautions noted.

INTERACTIONS

DRUG: **Medications that interfere with platelet function, anticoagulants** increase potential for prolonged/severe thrombocytopenia. **Bone marrow depressants** may increase myelosuppression. **Live virus vaccines** may potentiate virus replication, increase vaccine side effects, decrease pt's antibody response to vaccine. **HERBAL:** **Cat's claw, dong quai, evening primrose, feverfew, garlic, ginkgo, ginseng, horse chestnut, red clover** may increase antiplatelet activity. **FOOD:** None known. **LAB VALUES:** May decrease platelet count, WBC count, neutrophil count, Hgb, Hct.

AVAILABILITY (Rx)

Injection Solution: 3.2-mg vial (1.6 mg/ml).

ADMINISTRATION/HANDLING

Rate of administration • Give IV push over 10 min.

IV INCOMPATIBILITIES

Do not mix with any medications.

INDICATIONS/ROUTES/DOSAGE

Non-Hodgkin's Lymphoma

IV: ADULTS, ELDERLY: Regimen consists of two steps: Step 1: Single infusion of 250 mg/m^2 rituximab preceding (4 hrs or less) a fixed dose of 5 mCi (1.6 mg total antibody dose) of indium-111 ibritumomab administered IV push over 10 min. Step 2: Follows step 1 by 7–9 days and consists of a second infusion of 250 mg/m^2 rituximab preceding (4 hrs or less) a fixed dose of 0.4 mCi/kg of Y-90 ibritumomab administered IV push over 10 min.

◀ALERT▶ Reduce dosage to 0.3 mCi/kg if platelet count is 100,000–149,000 $cells/mm^3$. Do not administer if platelet count is less than 100,000 $cells/mm^3$.

I

SIDE EFFECTS

Frequent (43%–24%): Asthenia (loss of strength, energy), nausea, chills. **Occasional (17%–10%):** Fever, abdominal pain, dyspnea, headache, vomiting, dizziness, cough, oral candidiasis. **Rare (9%–5%):** Pruritus, diarrhea, back pain, peripheral edema, anorexia, rash, flushing, arthralgia, myalgia, ecchymosis, rhinitis, constipation, insomnia.

ADVERSE EFFECTS/ TOXIC REACTIONS

Thrombocytopenia (95%), neutropenia (77%), anemia (61%) may be severe and prolonged; may be followed by infection (29%). Hypersensitivity reaction produces hypotension, bronchospasm, angioedema. Severe cutaneous or mucocutaneous reactions (erythema multiforme, Stevens-Johnson syndrome, toxic epidermal necrolysis) has been noted.

NURSING CONSIDERATIONS

BASELINE ASSESSMENT

Pretreatment with acetaminophen and diphenhydramine before each infusion may prevent infusion-related effects. Offer emotional support. Use strict asepsis. CBC, blood chemistries should be obtained as baseline before beginning therapy. Absolute neutrophil count (ANC) nadir is 62 days before recovery begins.

INTERVENTION/EVALUATION

Diligently monitor lab values for possibly severe/prolonged thrombocytopenia, neutropenia, anemia. Monitor for hematologic toxicity (fever, sore throat, signs of local infections, unusual bruising/bleeding), symptoms of anemia (excessive fatigue, weakness), infusion-related allergic reaction. Assess for GI symptoms (nausea, vomiting, abdominal pain, diarrhea).

PATIENT/FAMILY TEACHING

• Do not have immunizations without physician's approval (drug lowers resistance). • Avoid crowds, persons with known infections. • Report signs of infection at once (fever, flu-like symptoms). • Contact physician if nausea/vomiting continues at home. • Avoid pregnancy during therapy.

ibuprofen

eye-**byoo**-pro-fen
(Advil, Advil Children's, Advil Infants', Advil Junior, Advil Migraine, Apo-Ibuprofen 🍁, Caldolor, Genpril, Ibu-200, Motrin, Motrin Children's, Motrin IB, Motrin Infants', Motrin Junior Strength, NeoProfen, Novo-profen 🍁)

BLACK BOX ALERT Increased risk of serious cardiovascular thrombotic events, including myocardial infarction, CVA. Increased risk of severe GI reactions, including ulceration, bleeding, perforation. Increased risk of new onset or worsening of preexisting hypertension.

Do not confuse Motrin with Neurontin.

FIXED-COMBINATION(S)

Children's Advil Cold: ibuprofen/pseudoephedrine (a nasal decongestant): 100 mg/15 mg per 5 ml. **Combunox:** ibuprofen/oxycodone (a narcotic analgesic): 400 mg/5 mg. **Reprexain CIII:** ibuprofen/hydrocodone: 200 mg/5 mg. **Vicoprofen:** ibuprofen/hydrocodone (a narcotic analgesic): 200 mg/7.5 mg.

◆CLASSIFICATION

PHARMACOTHERAPEUTIC: Nonsteroidal anti-inflammatory. **CLINICAL:** Antirheumatic, analgesic, antipyretic, antidysmenorrheal, vascular headache suppressant (see p. 128C).

ACTION

Inhibits prostaglandin synthesis. Produces vasodilation acting on heat-regulating center of hypothalamus. **Therapeutic Effect:** Produces analgesic, anti-inflammation effects, decreases fever.

PHARMACOKINETICS

Route	Onset	Peak	Duration
PO (analgesic)	0.5 hr	N/A	4–6 hrs
PO (antirheumatic)	2 days	1–2 wks	N/A

Rapidly absorbed from GI tract. Protein binding: 90%–99%. Metabolized in liver. Primarily excreted in urine. Not removed by hemodialysis. **Half-life:** 2–4 hrs.

USES

Treatment of fever, juvenile rheumatoid arthritis (JRA), osteoarthritis, minor pain, mild to moderate pain, primary dysmenorrhea. **NeoProfen:** Closes clinically significant patent ductus arteriosus (PDA) in premature infants weighing between 500 and 1,500 g who are no more than 32 wks gestational age when usual medical management is ineffective. **OFF-LABEL:** Treatment of psoriatic arthritis, vascular headaches, cystic fibrosis, ankylosing spondylitis.

PRECAUTIONS

Contraindications: Active peptic ulcer, chronic inflammation of GI tract, GI bleeding disorders/ulceration, history of hypersensitivity to aspirin, NSAIDs. Treatment of perioperative pain in coronary artery bypass graft (CABG) surgery. **NeoProfen:** Infants with proven or suspected untreated infection, congenital heart disease in whom patency of the patent ductus arteriosus is necessary for satisfactory pulmonary or systemic blood flow (e.g., pulmonary atresia), bleeding, thrombocytopenia, coagulation defects, suspected necrotizing enterocolitis, significant renal impairment. **Cautions:** CHF, hypertension, renal/hepatic impairment, dehydration, GI disease (e.g., bleeding, ulcers), concurrent anticoagulant use. **NeoProfen:** Presence of controlled infection or infants at risk for infection.

⌛ LIFESPAN CONSIDERATIONS

Pregnancy/Lactation: Unknown if drug crosses placenta or is distributed in breast milk. Avoid use during third trimester (may adversely affect fetal cardiovascular system: premature closure of ductus arteriosus). **Pregnancy Category B (D if used in third trimester or near delivery). Children:** Safety and efficacy not established in those younger than 6 mos. **Elderly:** GI bleeding, ulceration more likely to cause serious adverse effects. Age-related renal impairment may increase risk of hepatic/renal toxicity; reduced dosage recommended.

INTERACTIONS

DRUG: May decrease effects of **antihypertensives, diuretics. Aspirin, other salicylates** may increase risk of GI side effects, bleeding. **Bone marrow depressants** may increase risk of hematologic reactions. May increase concentration/nephrotoxicity with **cyclosporine.** May increase effects of **heparin, oral anticoagulants, thrombolytics.** May increase concentration, risk of toxicity of **lithium.** May increase risk of **methotrexate** toxicity. **Probenecid** may increase concentration. **HERBAL: Cat's claw, dong quai, evening primrose, feverfew, garlic, ginkgo, ginseng, horse chestnut, red clover** may increase antiplatelet activity. **FOOD:** None known. **LAB VALUES:** May prolong bleeding time. May alter serum glucose level. May increase BUN, serum creatinine, potassium, AST, ALT. May decrease serum calcium, glucose, Hgb, Hct, platelets.

AVAILABILITY (Rx)

Caplets: (Advil, IBU-200, Motrin IB): 200 mg. **Capsules:** (Advil, Advil Migraine): 200 mg. **Gelcaps:** (Advil, Motrin IB): 200 mg. **Injection, Solution:** (NeoProfen): 10 mg/ml. (Caldolor): 100 mg/ml. **Suspension, Oral:** (Advil Children's, Motrin Children's): 100 mg/5 ml. **Suspension, Oral Drops:** (Advil Infants', Motrin Infants'): 40 mg/ml. **Tablets:** (Advil, Genpril): 200 mg. (Motrin): 400 mg, 600 mg, 800 mg. **Tablets, Chewable:** (Advil Children's, Motrin Children's): 50 mg. (Advil Junior, Motrin Junior Strength): 100 mg.

ADMINISTRATION/HANDLING

IV (Caldolor)

Reconstitution • Dilute with D_5W or 0.9% NaCl to final concentration of 4 mg/ml or less.
Rate of administration • Infuse over at least 30 min.
Storage • Store at room temperature. • Stable for 24 hrs after dilution.

IV (NeoProfen)

Reconstitution • Dilute to appropriate volume with D_5W or 0.9% NaCl. • Discard any remaining medication after first withdrawal from vial.
Rate of administration • Administer via IV port nearest the insertion site. • Infuse continuously over 15 min.
Storage • Store at room temperature. • Stable for 30 min after dilution.

PO

• Give with food, milk, antacids if GI distress occurs.

INDICATIONS/ROUTES/DOSAGE

Fever

PO: ADULTS, ELDERLY, CHILDREN 12 YRS AND OLDER: 200–400 mg q4–6h prn. **Maximum:** 1,200 mg/day. **CHILDREN 6 MOS–11 YRS:** 5–10 mg/kg q6–8h prn. **Maximum:** 40 mg/kg/day.
IV: ADULTS, ELDERLY: 400 mg q4–6h or 100–200 mg q4h as needed.

Osteoarthritis, Rheumatoid Arthritis (RA)

PO: ADULTS, ELDERLY: 1,200–3,200 mg/day in 3–4 divided doses.

Minor Pain

PO: ADULTS, ELDERLY, CHILDREN 12 YRS AND OLDER: 200–400 mg q4–6h prn. **Maximum:** 1,200 mg/day. **CHILDREN 6 MOS–11 YRS:** 4–10 mg/kg q6–8h prn. **Maximum:** 40 mg/kg/day.

Mild to Moderate Pain

PO: ADULTS, ELDERLY: 400 mg q4h prn.
IV: ADULTS, ELDERLY: 400–800 mg q6h prn.

Primary Dysmenorrhea

PO: ADULTS: 200–400 mg q4–6h prn.

Juvenile Rheumatoid Arthritis (JRA)

PO: CHILDREN: 30–50 mg/kg/day in 3–4 divided doses. **Maximum:** 2.4 g/day.

Patent Ductus Arteriosus (PDA)

IV: INFANTS: Initially, 10 mg/kg then 2 doses of 5 mg/kg, after 24 hrs and 48 hrs. All doses based on birth weight.

SIDE EFFECTS

Occasional (9%–3%): Nausea with or without vomiting, dyspepsia, dizziness, rash. **Rare (less than 3%):** Diarrhea or constipation, flatulence, abdominal cramps or pain, pruritus.

ADVERSE EFFECTS/TOXIC REACTIONS

Acute overdose may result in metabolic acidosis. Rare reactions with long-term use include peptic ulcer, GI bleeding, gastritis, severe hepatic reaction (cholestasis, jaundice), nephrotoxicity (dysuria, hematuria, proteinuria, nephrotic syndrome), severe hypersensitivity reaction (particularly in pts with systemic lupus erythematosus or other collagen diseases). **NeoProfen:** Hypoglycemia, hypocalcemia, respiratory failure, UTI, edema, atelectasis may occur.

Caldolor: Abdominal pain, anemia, cough, dizziness, dyspnea, edema, hypertension, nausea, vomiting.

NURSING CONSIDERATIONS

BASELINE ASSESSMENT

Assess onset, type, location, duration of pain, inflammation. Inspect appearance of affected joints for immobility, deformities, skin condition. Assess temperature.

INTERVENTION/EVALUATION

Monitor for evidence of nausea, dyspepsia. Monitor CBC, hepatic/renal function tests, occult blood loss. Monitor daily pattern of bowel activity and stool consistency. Assess skin for rash. Observe for bleeding, bruising. Evaluate for therapeutic response: relief of pain, stiffness, swelling; increased joint mobility; reduced joint tenderness; improved grip strength. Monitor temperature for fever.

PATIENT/FAMILY TEACHING

• Avoid aspirin, alcohol during therapy (increases risk of GI bleeding). • If GI upset occurs, take with food, milk, antacids. • May cause dizziness. • Avoid tasks that require alertness, motor skills until response to drug is established. • Report ringing in ears, persistent stomach pain, respiratory difficulty, unusual bruising/bleeding, swelling of extremities, chest pain/palpitations.

idarubicin HIGH ALERT

eye-dah-**roo**-bi-sin
(Idamycin PFS)

BLACK BOX ALERT Cardiotoxicity may occur (CHF, arrhythmias, cardiomyopathy). Severe myelosuppressant. Must be administered by personnel trained in administration/handling of chemotherapeutic agents. Severe local tissue damage, necrosis if extravasation occurs.

Do not confuse idarubicin with daunorubicin, doxorubicin, or epirubicin, or Idamycin with Adriamycin.

◆CLASSIFICATION

PHARMACOTHERAPEUTIC: Anthracycline antibiotic. **CLINICAL:** Antineoplastic (see p. 84C).

ACTION

Inhibits nucleic acid synthesis by interacting with enzyme topoisomerase II, promoting DNA strand supercoiling. **Therapeutic Effect:** Produces death of rapidly dividing cells.

PHARMACOKINETICS

Widely distributed. Protein binding: 97%. Rapidly metabolized in liver to active metabolite. Primarily eliminated by biliary excretion. Not removed by hemodialysis. **Half-life:** 12–27 hrs.

USES

Treatment of acute leukemias (acute myelogenous leukemia [AML], acute nonlymphocytic leukemia [ANLL], acute lymphocytic leukemia [ALL]), accelerated phase or blast phase of chronic myelogenous leukemia (CML), breast cancer. **OFF-LABEL:** Autologous hematopoietic stem cell transplantation (in combination with busulfan).

PRECAUTIONS

Contraindications: Arrhythmias, cardiomyopathy, preexisting myelosuppression, pregnancy, severe CHF. **Cautions:** Renal/hepatic impairment, concurrent radiation therapy.

LIFESPAN CONSIDERATIONS

Pregnancy/Lactation: If possible, avoid use during pregnancy (may be embryotoxic). Unknown if drug is distributed in breast milk (advise to discontinue breast-feeding before drug initiation). **Pregnancy Category D. Children:** Safety and efficacy not established. **Elderly:** Cardiotoxicity may be more prevalent. Caution in those with inadequate bone marrow reserves. Age-related renal impairment may require dosage adjustment.

INTERACTIONS

DRUG: May decrease effects of **antigout medications. Bone marrow depressants** may increase myelosuppression. **Live virus vaccines** may potentiate virus replication, increase vaccine side effects, decrease pt's antibody response to vaccine. **HERBAL:** None significant. **FOOD:** None known. **LAB VALUES:** May increase serum alkaline phosphatase, bilirubin, uric acid, AST, ALT. May cause EKG changes.

AVAILABILITY (Rx)

Injection Solution: 1 mg/ml in 5-ml, 10-ml, 20-ml vials.

ADMINISTRATION/HANDLING

◀ALERT▶ Give by free-flowing IV infusion (**never** subcutaneous or IM). Gloves, gowns, eye goggles recommended during preparation/administration of medication. If powder/solution comes in contact with skin, wash thoroughly. Avoid small veins, swollen/edematous extremities, areas overlying joints/tendons.

IV

Reconstitution • May give undiluted or dilute with 0.9% NaCl or D_5W.

Rate of administration • Administer IV push into tubing of freely running IV infusion of D_5W or 0.9% NaCl, preferably via butterfly needle, **slowly** over 3–5 min. • May give intermittent infusion over 10–15 min. • Extravasation produces immediate pain, severe local tissue damage. Terminate infusion immediately. Apply cold compresses for 30 min immediately, then q30min 4 times a day for 3 days. Keep extremity elevated.

Storage • Refrigerate vials. • Diluted solutions in 0.9% NaCl or D_5W are stable for 72 hrs at room temperature or 7 days if refrigerated.

IV INCOMPATIBILITIES

Acyclovir (Zovirax), allopurinol (Aloprim), ampicillin and sulbactam (Unasyn), cefazolin (Ancef, Kefzol), cefepime (Maxipime), ceftazidime (Fortaz), clindamycin (Cleocin), dexamethasone (Decadron), furosemide (Lasix), hydrocortisone (Solu-Cortef), lorazepam (Ativan), meperidine (Demerol), methotrexate, piperacillin and tazobactam (Zosyn), sodium bicarbonate, teniposide (Vumon), vancomycin (Vancocin), vincristine (Oncovin).

IV COMPATIBILITIES

Diphenhydramine (Benadryl), granisetron (Kytril), magnesium, potassium.

INDICATIONS/ROUTES/DOSAGE

◀ALERT▶ Refer to individual protocols.

Usual Dosage

IV: ADULTS: 10–12 mg/m^2/day for 3 days. **CHILDREN (SOLID TUMOR):** 5 mg/m^2 once a day for 3 days q3wks. **CHILDREN (LEUKEMIA):** 10–12 mg/m^2 once a day for 3 days q3wks.

Dosage in Renal Impairment

ADULTS: Creatinine clearance 10–50 ml/min: Give 75% of dose. Creatinine clearance less than 10 ml/min: Give 50% of dose. **CHILDREN:** Creatinine clearance less than 50 ml/min: Give 75% of dose.

Dosage in Hepatic Impairment

Bilirubin 2.6–5 mg/dl: Give 50% of dose. Bilirubin greater than 5 mg/dl: Avoid use.

SIDE EFFECTS

Frequent: Nausea, vomiting (82%), complete alopecia (scalp, axillary, pubic hair) (77%), abdominal cramping, diarrhea (73%), mucositis (50%). **Occasional:** Hyperpigmentation of nailbeds, phalangeal, dermal creases (46%), fever (36%), headache (20%). **Rare:** Conjunctivitis, neuropathy.

ADVERSE EFFECTS/ TOXIC REACTIONS

Myelosuppression manifested as hematologic toxicity (principally leukopenia and, to lesser extent, anemia, thrombocytopenia) generally occurs within 10–15 days after starting therapy, returns to normal levels by third wk. Cardiotoxicity (either acute, manifested as transient EKG abnormalities, or chronic, manifested as CHF) may occur.

NURSING CONSIDERATIONS

BASELINE ASSESSMENT

Determine baseline renal/hepatic function, CBC results. Obtain EKG before therapy. Antiemetic medication before and during therapy may prevent or relieve nausea, vomiting. Inform pt of high potential for alopecia.

INTERVENTION/EVALUATION

Monitor CBC, platelet count, serum electrolytes, EKG, renal/hepatic function tests. Monitor for hematologic toxicity (fever, sore throat, signs of local infection, unusual bruising/bleeding from any site), symptoms of anemia (excessive fatigue, weakness). Avoid IM injections, rectal temperatures, other trauma that may precipitate bleeding. Check infusion site frequently for extravasation (causes severe local necrosis). Assess for potentially fatal CHF (dyspnea, rales, pulmonary edema), life-threatening arrhythmias.

PATIENT/FAMILY TEACHING

• Total body alopecia is frequent but reversible. • New hair growth resumes 2–3 mos after last therapy dose and may have different color, texture. • Maintain fastidious oral hygiene. • Avoid crowds, those with infections. • Inform physician of fever, sore throat, bruising/bleeding. • Urine may turn pink or red. • Use contraceptive measures during therapy.

ifosfamide HIGH ALERT

eye-**fos**-fah-mide
(Ifex)

BLACK BOX ALERT Hemorrhagic cystitis may occur. Severe myelosuppressant. May cause CNS toxicity, including confusion, coma. Must be administered by personnel trained in administration/handling of chemotherapeutic agents.

Do not confuse ifosfamide with cyclophosphamide.

◆CLASSIFICATION

PHARMACOTHERAPEUTIC: Alkylating agent. **CLINICAL:** Antineoplastic (see p. 84C).

ACTION

Inhibits DNA, RNA protein synthesis by cross-linking with DNA, RNA strands, preventing cell growth. Cell cycle-phase nonspecific. **Therapeutic Effect:** Interferes with DNA, RNA function.

PHARMACOKINETICS

Metabolized in liver to active metabolite. Protein binding: Negligible. Crosses blood-brain barrier (to a limited extent). Primarily excreted in urine. Removed by hemodialysis. **Half-life:** 11–15 hrs (high dose); 4–7 hrs (low dose).

USES

Treatment of germ cell testicular carcinoma (used in combination with agents that protect against hemorrhagic cystitis). **OFF-LABEL:** Head/neck, breast, cervical, small-cell lung, non–small-cell lung, ovarian, epithelial, bladder, endometrial carcinomas, soft tissue sarcomas, Hodgkin's, non-Hodgkin's lymphomas, neuroblastoma, osteosarcoma, germ cell ovarian tumors, Wilm's tumor.

PRECAUTIONS

Contraindications: Pregnancy, severe myelosuppression. **Cautions:** Renal/hepatic impairment, compromised bone marrow function.

LIFESPAN CONSIDERATIONS

Pregnancy/Lactation: If possible, avoid use during pregnancy, esp. first trimester. May cause fetal harm. Distributed in breast milk. Breast-feeding not recommended. **Pregnancy Category D. Children:** Not intended for this pt population.

I

Elderly: Age-related renal impairment may require dosage adjustment.

INTERACTIONS

DRUG: **Bone marrow depressants** may increase myelosuppression. **Live virus vaccines** may potentiate virus replication, increase vaccine side effects, decrease pt's antibody response to vaccine. HERBAL: **St. John's wort** may decrease concentration. FOOD: None known. LAB VALUES: May increase BUN, serum bilirubin, creatinine, uric acid, AST, ALT.

AVAILABILITY (Rx)

Injection, Powder for Reconstitution (Ifex): 1 g, 3 g. Injection, Solution: 50 mg/ml.

ADMINISTRATION/HANDLING

◄ALERT► Hemorrhagic cystitis occurs if mesna is not given concurrently. Mesna should always be given with ifosfamide.

IV

Reconstitution • Reconstitute vial with Sterile Water for Injection or Bacteriostatic Water for Injection to provide concentration of 50 mg/ml. Shake to dissolve. • Further dilute with 50–1,000 ml D_5W or 0.9% NaCl to provide concentration of 0.6–20 mg/ml.

Rate of administration • Infuse over minimum of 30 min. • Give with at least 2,000 ml PO or IV fluid (prevents bladder toxicity). • Give with protectant against hemorrhagic cystitis (i.e., mesna).

Storage • Store vials of powder at room temperature. • Refrigerate vials of solution. • After reconstitution with Bacteriostatic Water for Injection, solution is stable for 3 wks if refrigerated (further diluted solution is stable for 7 days at room temperature or 6 wks if refrigerated).

IV INCOMPATIBILITIES

Cefepime (Maxipime), methotrexate.

IV COMPATIBILITIES

Granisetron (Kytril), ondansetron (Zofran).

INDICATIONS/ROUTES/DOSAGE

◄ALERT► Dosage individualized based on clinical response, tolerance to adverse effects. When used in combination therapy, consult specific protocols for optimum dosage, sequence of drug administration.

Germ Cell Testicular Carcinoma

IV: ADULTS: 1,200 mg/m²/day for 5 consecutive days. Repeat q3–4wks or after recovery from hematologic toxicity. Administer with mesna.

SIDE EFFECTS

Frequent: Alopecia (83%); nausea, vomiting (58%). Occasional (15%–5%): Confusion, drowsiness, hallucinations, infection. Rare (less than 5%): Dizziness, seizures, disorientation, fever, malaise, stomatitis (mucosal irritation, glossitis, gingivitis).

ADVERSE EFFECTS/ TOXIC REACTIONS

Hemorrhagic cystitis with hematuria, dysuria occurs frequently if protective agent (mesna) is not used. Myelosuppression, characterized by leukopenia and, to a lesser extent, thrombocytopenia, occurs frequently. Pulmonary toxicity, hepatotoxicity, nephrotoxicity, cardiotoxicity, CNS toxicity (confusion, hallucinations, drowsiness, coma) may require discontinuation of therapy.

NURSING CONSIDERATIONS

BASELINE ASSESSMENT

Obtain urinalysis before each dose. If hematuria occurs (greater than 10 RBCs per field), therapy should be withheld until resolution occurs. Obtain WBC, platelet count, Hgb before each dose.

INTERVENTION/EVALUATION

Monitor hematologic studies, urinalysis, renal/hepatic function tests diligently. Assess for fever, sore throat, signs of local infection, unusual bruising/bleeding from any site, symptoms of anemia (excessive fatigue, weakness).

PATIENT/FAMILY TEACHING

• Alopecia is reversible, but new hair growth may have a different color or texture. • Maintain copious daily fluid intake (protects against cystitis). • Do not have immunizations without physician's approval (drug lowers resistance). • Avoid contact with those who have recently received live virus vaccine. • Avoid crowds, those with infections. • Report unusual bleeding/bruising, fever, chills, sore throat, joint pain, sores in mouth or on lips, yellowing skin or eyes.

iloperidone

eye-loe-**per**-i-doan
(Fanapt)

BLACK BOX ALERT Elderly pts with dementia-related psychosis are at increased risk for mortality due to cerebrovascular events.

Do not confuse iloperidone with dronedarone or amiodarone.

◆ CLASSIFICATION

PHARMACOTHERAPEUTIC: Piperidinyl-benzisoxazole derivative. **CLINICAL:** Antipsychotic.

ACTION

Exact mechanism unknown; may be mediated through combination of dopamine type 2 (D_2) and serotonin type 2 ($5\text{-}HT_2$) antagonisms. **Therapeutic Effect:** Diminishes symptoms of schizophrenia.

PHARMACOKINETICS

Steady-state concentration occurs in 3–4 days. Well absorbed from GI tract (unaffected by food). Protein binding: 95%. Extensively metabolized in liver. Primarily excreted in urine, with a lesser amount eliminated in feces. **Half-life:** 18–33 hrs.

USES

Acute treatment of schizophrenia in adults.

PRECAUTIONS

Contraindications: None known. **Cautions:** Cardiovascular disease (heart failure, history of MI, ischemia, cardiac conduction abnormalities), cerebrovascular disease (increases risk of CVA in pts with dementia, seizure disorders). Those with bradycardia, hypokalemia, hypomagnesemia may be at greater risk for torsade de pointes. History of seizures, conditions lowering seizure threshold. High risk of suicide.

⌛ LIFESPAN CONSIDERATIONS

Pregnancy/Lactation: Unknown if drug crosses placenta or is excreted in breast milk. Breast-feeding not recommended. **Pregnancy Category C. Children:** Safety and efficacy not established. **Elderly:** More susceptible to postural hypotension. Increased risk of cerebrovascular events, mortality, including stroke in elderly pts with psychosis.

INTERACTIONS

DRUG: **Alcohol, CNS depressants** may increase CNS depression. **Carbamazepine** may decrease concentration. **Strong CYP3A4 inhibitors (e.g., clarithromycin, ketoconazole)** or **strong CYP2D6 inhibitors (e.g., fluoxetine, paroxetine)** may increase concentration. **Medications causing prolongation of QT interval (amiodarone, dofetilide, sotalol)** may increase effects on cardiac conduction, leading to malignant arrhythmias (torsade de pointes). May decrease effects of **dopamine agonists, levodopa.** May increase **dextromethorphan** concentration. **HERBAL:** **Gotu kola, kava kava, St. John's wort, valerian** may increase CNS depression. **FOOD:** None known. **LAB VALUES:** May increase serum prolactin levels.

AVAILABILITY (Rx)

Tablets: 1 mg, 2 mg, 4 mg, 6 mg, 8 mg, 10 mg, 12 mg.

ADMINISTRATION/HANDLING

PO

• Give without regard to food. • Tablets may be crushed.

I

INDICATIONS/ROUTES/DOSAGE

Antipsychotic

PO: ADULTS: To avoid orthostatic hypotension, begin with 1 mg twice daily, then adjust dosage to 2 mg twice daily, 4 mg twice daily, 6 mg twice daily, 8 mg twice daily, 10 mg twice daily, and 12 mg twice daily on days 2, 3, 4, 5, 6, and 7, respectively, to reach target daily dose of 12–24 mg, given twice daily. Note: Reduce dose by 50% when receiving strong CYP3A4 or CYP2D6 inhibitors (see Interactions).

SIDE EFFECTS

Frequent (20%–12%): Dizziness, drowsiness, tachycardia. **Occasional (10%–4%):** Nausea, dry mouth, nasal congestion, weight increase, diarrhea, fatigue, orthostatic hypotension. **Rare (3%–1%):** Arthralgia, musculoskeletal stiffness, abdominal discomfort, nasopharyngitis, tremor, hypotension, rash, ejaculatory failure, dyspnea, blurred vision, lethargy.

ADVERSE EFFECTS/ TOXIC REACTIONS

Extrapyramidal disorders, including tardive dyskinesia (protrusion of tongue, puffing of cheeks, chewing/puckering of the mouth), occurs in 4% of pts. Upper respiratory infection occurs in 3% of pts. Prolongation of QT interval (as seen on EKG) may produce torsade de pointes, a form of ventricular tachycardia. Neuroleptic malignant syndrome (e.g., hyperpyrexia, muscle rigidity, altered mental status, irregular pulse or B/P noted).

NURSING CONSIDERATIONS

BASELINE ASSESSMENT

Assess pt's behavior, appearance, emotional status, response to environment, speech pattern, thought content. EKG should be obtained to assess for QT prolongation before instituting medication.

INTERVENTION/EVALUATION

Monitor for orthostatic hypotension; assist with ambulation. Monitor for fine tongue movement (may be first sign of tardive dyskinesia, possibly irreversible). Monitor serum potassium, magnesium in pts at risk for electrolyte disturbances. Assess for therapeutic response (greater interest in surroundings, improved self-care, increased ability to concentrate, relaxed facial expression).

PATIENT/FAMILY TEACHING

• Avoid tasks that require alertness, motor skills until response to drug is established. • Be alert to symptoms of orthostatic hypotension; rise slowly from sitting or lying position. • Consult physician if feeling faint, experience heart palpitations or if fever or muscle rigidity occurs. • Report extra-pyramidal symptoms (e.g., involuntary muscle movements, tics) immediately.

iloprost

eye-loe-prost
(Ventavis)

◆CLASSIFICATION

PHARMACOTHERAPEUTIC: Prostaglandin. **CLINICAL:** Vasodilator.

ACTION

Dilates systemic, pulmonary arterial vascular beds, alters pulmonary vascular resistance, suppresses vascular smooth muscle proliferation. **Therapeutic Effect:** Improves symptoms, exercise tolerance in pts with pulmonary hypertension; delays deterioration of condition.

PHARMACOKINETICS

Protein binding: 60%. Metabolized in liver. Primarily excreted in urine; minimal elimination in feces. **Half-life:** 20–30 min.

USES

Treatment of pulmonary arterial hypertension in pts with NYHA class III, IV symptoms. May be used in combination with bosentan for treatment of pulmonary arterial hypertension.

PRECAUTIONS

Contraindications: None known. **Cautions:** Hepatic impairment, concurrent conditions or medications that may increase risk of syncope.

⌛ LIFESPAN CONSIDERATIONS

Pregnancy/Lactation: Unknown if drug crosses placenta or is distributed in breast milk. **Pregnancy Category C. Children:** Safety and efficacy not established. **Elderly:** No age-related precautions noted.

INTERACTIONS

DRUG: **Anticoagulants, antiplatelet agents** may increase risk of bleeding. **Antihypertensives, other vasodilators** may increase hypotensive effects. **HERBAL:** None significant. **FOOD:** None known. **LAB VALUES:** May increase serum alkaline phosphatase, GGT.

AVAILABILITY (Rx)

Solution for Oral Inhalation: 10 mcg/ml (1-ml, 2-ml ampules).

ADMINISTRATION/HANDLING

Oral Inhalation

• For inhalation only, using Prodose ADD system. • Transfer entire contents of ampule into the medication chamber. • After use, discard remainder of medicine.

INDICATIONS/ROUTES/DOSAGE

Pulmonary Hypertension

ORAL INHALATION: ADULTS: Initially, 2.5 mcg/dose; if tolerated, increase to 5 mcg/dose. Administer 6–9 times a day at intervals of 2 hrs or longer while pt is awake. Maintenance: 5 mcg/dose. **Maximum daily dose:** 45 mcg.

SIDE EFFECTS

Frequent (39%–27%): Increased cough, headache, flushing. **Occasional (13%–11%):** Flu-like symptoms, nausea, lockjaw, jaw pain, hypotension. **Rare (8%–2%):** Insomnia, syncope, palpitations, vomiting, back pain, muscle cramps.

ADVERSE EFFECTS/ TOXIC REACTIONS

Hemoptysis, pneumonia occur occasionally. CHF, renal failure, dyspnea, chest pain occur rarely.

NURSING CONSIDERATIONS

BASELINE ASSESSMENT

Assess B/P, pulse.

INTERVENTION/EVALUATION

Monitor pulse, B/P during therapy. Assess for signs of pulmonary venous hypertension.

PATIENT/FAMILY TEACHING

• Follow manufacturer guidelines for proper administration of medication using supplied inhalation system. • Discard any remaining solution in the medication chamber after each inhalation session.

imatinib HIGH ALERT

ih-**mah**-tin-ib
(Gleevec)

Do not confuse imatinib with dasatininb, erlotinib, lapatinib, nilotinib, sorafenib, or sunitinib.

◆ CLASSIFICATION

PHARMACOTHERAPEUTIC: Protein tyrosine kinase inhibitor. **CLINICAL:** Antineoplastic (see p. 84C).

ACTION

Inhibits Bcr-Abl tyrosine kinase, an enzyme created by Philadelphia chromosome abnormality found in pts with chronic myeloid leukemia (CML). **Therapeutic Effect:** Suppresses tumor growth during the three stages of CML: blast crisis, accelerated phase, chronic phase.

PHARMACOKINETICS

Well absorbed after PO administration. Protein binding: 95% to albumin. Metabolized in liver to active metabolite. Eliminated mainly in feces as metabolites. **Half-life:** 18 hrs; metabolite, 40 hrs.

USES

Newly diagnosed chronic-phase Philadelphia chromosome positive chronic myeloid leukemia (Ph+ CML) in children and adults. Pts in blast crisis, accelerated phase, or chronic phase Ph+ CML who have already failed interferon therapy. Adults with relapsed or refractory Ph+ acute lymphoblastic leukemia (ALL). Adults with myelodysplastic/myeloproliferative disease (MDS/MPD) associated with platelet-derived growth factor receptor (PDGFR) gene rearrangements. Adults with aggressive systemic mastocytosis (ASM) without mutation of the D816V c-Kit or unknown mutation status of the c-Kit. Adults with hypereosinophilic syndrome (HES) and/or chronic eosinophilic leukemia (CEL) with positive, negative, or unknown FIP1L1-PDGFR fusion kinase. Adults with dermatofibrosarcoma protuberans (DFSP) that is unresectable, recurrent, and/or metastatic. Pts with malignant gastrointestinal stromal tumors (GIST) that are unresectable and/or metastatic. Prevents recurrence of cancer in pts following surgical removal of GIST. **OFF-LABEL:** Treatment of desmoid tumors (soft tissue sarcoma).

PRECAUTIONS

Contraindications: Pregnancy. **Cautions:** Hepatic/renal impairment.

LIFESPAN CONSIDERATIONS

Pregnancy/Lactation: Has potential for severe teratogenic effects. Breast-feeding not recommended. **Pregnancy Category D. Children:** Safety and efficacy not established. **Elderly:** Increased frequency of fluid retention.

INTERACTIONS

DRUG: Carbamazepine, dexamethasone, phenobarbital, phenytoin, rifampicin decrease concentration. **Clarithromycin, erythromycin, itraconazole, ketoconazole** increase concentration. May alter therapeutic effects of **cyclosporine, pimozide.** May increase concentration of **benzodiazepines, calcium channel blockers, dihydropyridine, simvastatin, triazolodiazepines. Bone marrow depressants** may increase myelosuppression. **Live virus vaccines** may potentiate virus replication, increase vaccine side effects, decrease pt's antibody response to vaccine. Reduces effect of **warfarin. HERBAL: St. John's wort** decreases concentration. **FOOD: Grapefruit juice** may increase concentration. **LAB VALUES:** May increase serum bilirubin, AST, ALT. May decrease platelet count, WBC count, serum potassium.

AVAILABILITY (Rx)

Tablets: 100 mg, 400 mg.

ADMINISTRATION/HANDLING

PO

- Give with a meal and large glass of water.
- Tablets may be dispersed in water or apple juice.

INDICATIONS/ROUTES/DOSAGE

Ph+ Chronic Myeloid Leukemia (CML) (Chronic Phase)

PO: ADULTS, ELDERLY: 400 mg once daily; may increase to 600 mg/day.

Ph+ CML (Accelerated Phase)

PO: ADULTS, ELDERLY: 600 mg once daily. May increase to 800 mg/day in 2 divided doses.

Ph+ Acute Lymphoblastic Leukemia (ALL)

PO: ADULTS, ELDERLY: 600 mg once daily.

Gastrointestinal Stromal Tumors (GIST)

PO: ADULTS, ELDERLY: 400–600 mg/day.

Aggressive Systemic Mastocytosis (ASM) with Eosinophilia

PO: ADULTS, ELDERLY: Initially, 100 mg/day. May increase up to 400 mg/day.

ASM without Mutation of the D816V C-Kit or Unknown Mutation Status of C-Kit

PO: ADULTS, ELDERLY: 400 mg once daily.

Dermatofibrosarcoma Protuberans (DFSP)
PO: ADULTS, ELDERLY: 400 mg twice a day.

Hypereosinophilic Syndrome (HES)/
Chronic Eosinophilic Leukemia (CEL)
PO: ADULTS, ELDERLY: 400 mg once daily.

HES/CEL with Positive or Unknown
FIP1L1-PDGFR Fusion Kinase
PO: ADULTS, ELDERLY: Initially, 100 mg/day. May increase up to 400 mg/day.

Myelodysplastic/Myeloproliferative
Disease (MDS/MPD)
PO: ADULTS, ELDERLY: 400 mg once daily.

GI Stromal Tumors
PO: ADULTS, ELDERLY: 400 or 600 mg once daily.

Usual Dosage for Children (2 Yrs and Older)
Ph+ CML (Chronic Phase, Recurrent or Resistant): 260 mg/m^2/day. **Maximum:** 600 mg/day.
Ph+ CML (Chronic Phase, Newly Diagnosed): 340 mg/m^2/day. **Maximum:** 600 mg/day.

Dosage in Hepatic Impairment (Severe)
Reduce dosage by 25%.

SIDE EFFECTS

Frequent (68%–24%): Nausea, diarrhea, vomiting, headache, fluid retention (periorbital, lower extremities), rash, musculoskeletal pain, muscle cramps, arthralgia. Occasional (23%–10%): Abdominal pain, cough, myalgia, fatigue, fever, anorexia, dyspepsia, constipation, night sweats, pruritus. Rare (less than 10%): Nasopharyngitis, petechiae, asthenia (loss of strength, energy), epistaxis.

ADVERSE EFFECTS/ TOXIC REACTIONS

Severe fluid retention (pleural effusion, pericardial effusion, pulmonary edema, ascites), hepatotoxicity occur rarely. Neutropenia, thrombocytopenia are expected responses to the drug. Respiratory toxicity is manifested as dyspnea, pneumonia. Heart damage (left ventricular dysfunction, CHF) may occur.

NURSING CONSIDERATIONS

BASELINE ASSESSMENT

Obtain CBC weekly for first mo, biweekly for second mo, periodically thereafter. Monitor hepatic function tests (serum transaminase, bilirubin, alkaline phosphatase) before beginning treatment, monthly thereafter.

INTERVENTION/EVALUATION

Assess periorbital area, lower extremities for early evidence of fluid retention. Monitor for unexpected, rapid weight gain. Offer antiemetics to control nausea, vomiting. Monitor daily pattern of bowel activity, stool consistency. Monitor CBC for evidence of neutropenia, thrombocytopenia; assess hepatic function tests for hepatotoxicity. Monitor renal function, serum electrolytes. Duration of neutropenia or thrombocytopenia ranges from 2–4 wks.

PATIENT/FAMILY TEACHING

• Avoid crowds, those with known infection. • Avoid contact with anyone who recently received live virus vaccine; do not receive vaccinations. • Take with food and a full glass of water. • Avoid grapefruit juice. • Notify physician if chest pain, swelling of extremities, weight gain greater than 5 lb, easy bruising/bleeding occur. • Avoid tasks requiring alertness, motor skills until response to drug is established.

Imdur, *see isosorbide mononitrate*

imipenem/cilastatin

im-ih-**pen**-em/sye-la-**stat**-in
(Primaxin)

I

Do not confuse imipenem with doripenem, ertapenem, or meropenem, or Primaxin with Premarin or Primacor.

◆CLASSIFICATION

PHARMACOTHERAPEUTIC: Fixed-combination carbapenem. **CLINICAL:** Antibiotic.

ACTION

Imipenem: Penetrates bacterial cell membrane, inhibiting cell wall synthesis. **Cilastatin:** Competitively inhibits the enzyme dehydropeptidase, preventing renal metabolism of imipenem. **Therapeutic Effect:** Produces bacterial cell death.

PHARMACOKINETICS

Readily absorbed after IM administration. Protein binding: **Imipenem:** 20%; **Cilastatin:** 40%. Widely distributed. Metabolized in kidneys. Primarily excreted in urine. Removed by hemodialysis. **Half-life:** 1 hr (increased in renal impairment).

USES

Treatment of susceptible infections due to gram-negative, gram-positive, anaerobic organisms including respiratory tract, skin/skin structure, gynecologic, bone, joint, intra-abdominal, complicated or uncomplicated UTIs; endocarditis; polymicrobic infections; septicemia; serious nosocomial infections. **OFF-LABEL:** Hepatic abscess, neutropenic fever, melioidosis.

PRECAUTIONS

Contraindications: IM: Severe shock, heart block, hypersensitivity to local anesthetics of the amide type. **IV:** Pts with meningitis. **Cautions:** History of seizures, sensitivity to penicillins, renal impairment.

LIFESPAN CONSIDERATIONS

Pregnancy/Lactation: Crosses placenta. Distributed in cord blood, amniotic fluid, breast milk. **Pregnancy Category C. Children:** No precautions noted. **Elderly:** Age-related renal impairment may require dosage adjustment.

INTERACTIONS

DRUG: None significant. **HERBAL:** None significant. **FOOD:** None known. **LAB VALUES:** May increase BUN, serum alkaline phosphatase, bilirubin, creatinine, LDH, AST, ALT. May decrease Hgb, Hct.

AVAILABILITY (Rx)

IM Injection, Powder for Reconstitution (Primaxin): 500 mg. **IV Injection, Powder for Reconstitution (Primaxin):** 250 mg, 500 mg.

ADMINISTRATION/HANDLING

IV

Reconstitution • Dilute each 250 or 500 mg vial with 100 ml D_5W or 0.9% NaCl.

Rate of administration • Give by intermittent IV infusion (piggyback). • Do not give IV push. • Infuse over 15–30 min (doses greater than 500 mg over 40–60 min). • Observe pt during initial 30 min of first-time infusion for possible hypersensitivity reaction.

Storage • Solution appears colorless to yellow; discard if solution turns brown. • IV infusion (piggyback) diluted with D_5W is stable for 4 hrs at room temperature, 24 hrs if refrigerated. Stable for 10 hrs at room temperature or 48 hrs if refrigerated when diluted with 0.9% NaCl. • Discard if precipitate forms.

IM

• Prepare with 1% lidocaine without epinephrine; 500 mg vial with 2 ml, 750 mg vial with 3 ml lidocaine HCl. • Administer suspension within 1 hr of preparation. • Do not mix with any other medications. • Inject deep in large muscle mass.

IV INCOMPATIBILITIES

Allopurinol (Aloprim), amphotericin B complex (Abelcet, AmBisome, Amphotec), fluconazole (Diflucan).

IV COMPATIBILITIES

Diltiazem (Cardizem), insulin, lipids, propofol (Diprivan), total parenteral nutrition (TPN).

INDICATIONS/ROUTES/DOSAGE

Mild to Moderate Infections

IV: ADULTS, ELDERLY, WEIGHING 70 KG OR MORE: 250 mg q6h up to 1,000 mg q6h. **60–69 KG:** 250 mg q8h up to 1 g q8h. **50–59 KG:** 125 mg q6h up to 750 mg q8h. **40–49 KG:** 125 mg q6h up to 500 mg q6h. **30–39 KG:** 125 mg q8h up to 500 mg q8h. **CHILDREN OLDER THAN 3 MOS–12 YRS:** 60–100 mg/kg/day in divided doses q6h. **Maximum:** 4 g/day. **CHILDREN 1–3 MOS:** 100 mg/kg/day in divided doses q6h. **CHILDREN 1–4 WKS:** 25 mg/kg q6h. **CHILDREN YOUNGER THAN 1 WK:** 25 mg/kg q12h.

IM: ADULTS, ELDERLY: 500–750 mg q12h. **Maximum:** 1,500 mg/day.

Dosage in Renal Impairment

Dosage and frequency are modified based on creatinine clearance and severity of infection.

Creatinine Clearance (ml/min)	70 kg or greater	60–69 kg	50–59 kg	40–49 kg	30–39 kg
41–70	250 mg q8h–750 mg q8h	125 mg q6h–750 mg q8h	125 mg q6h–500 mg q6h	125 mg q6h–500 mg q8h	125 mg q8h–250 mg q6h
21–40	250 mg q12h–500 mg q6h	250 mg q12h–500 mg q8h	125 mg q8h–500 mg q8h	125 mg q12h–250 mg q6h	125 mg q12h–250 mg q8h
6–20	250 mg q12h–500 mg q12h	125 mg q12h–500 mg q12h	125 mg q12h–500 mg q12h	125 mg q12h–250 mg q12h	125 mg q12h–250 mg q12h

SIDE EFFECTS

Occasional (3%): Diarrhea, nausea, vomiting. **Rare (1%):** Rash.

ADVERSE EFFECTS/ TOXIC REACTIONS

Antibiotic-associated colitis, other superinfections (abdominal cramps, severe watery diarrhea, fever) may result from altered bacterial balance. Anaphylactic reactions have been reported.

NURSING CONSIDERATIONS

BASELINE ASSESSMENT

Question for history of allergies, particularly to beta-lactams, penicillins, cephalosporins. Inquire about history of seizures.

INTERVENTION/EVALUATION

Monitor renal, hepatic, hematologic function tests. Evaluate for phlebitis (heat, pain, red streaking over vein), pain at IV injection site. Assess for GI discomfort, nausea, vomiting. Monitor daily pattern of bowel activity, stool consistency. Assess skin for rash. Be alert to tremors, possible seizures.

imipramine

i-**mip**-ra-meen
(Apo-Imipramine ✱, Novo-Pramine ✱, Tofranil, Tofranil-PM)

BLACK BOX ALERT Increased risk of suicidal thinking and behavior in children, adolescents, young adults 18–24 yrs with major depressive disorder, other psychiatric disorders.

Do not confuse imipramine with amitriptyline, desipramine, or Norpramin.

◆ CLASSIFICATION

PHARMACOTHERAPEUTIC: Tricyclic. **CLINICAL:** Antidepressant, antineuritic, antipanic, antineuralgic, antinarcoleptic adjunct, anticataplectic, antibulimic (see p. 38C).

ACTION

Blocks reuptake of neurotransmitters (norepinephrine, serotonin) at presynaptic membranes, increasing their concentration at postsynaptic receptor sites. **Therapeutic Effect:** Relieves depression, controls nocturnal enuresis.

USES

Treatment of various forms of depression, often in conjunction with psychotherapy. Treatment of nocturnal enuresis in children older than 6 yrs. **OFF-LABEL:** Treatment of ADHD, cataplexy associated with narcolepsy, neurogenic pain, panic disorder.

I

PRECAUTIONS

Contraindications: Acute recovery period after MI, use within 14 days of MAOIs. **Cautions:** Prostatic hypertrophy; history of urinary retention, obstruction; glaucoma; diabetes mellitus; history of seizures; hyperthyroidism; cardiac, hepatic, renal disease; schizophrenia; increased intraocular pressure; hiatal hernia. **Pregnancy Category D.**

INTERACTIONS

DRUG: **Alcohol, other CNS depressants** may increase hypotensive effects, CNS, respiratory depression caused by imipramine. **Antithyroid agents** may increase risk of agranulocytosis. **Cimetidine** may increase concentration, risk of toxicity. May decrease effects of **clonidine. MAOIs** may increase risk of neuroleptic malignant syndrome, hyperpyrexia, hypertensive crisis, seizures. **Phenothiazines** may increase anticholinergic, sedative effects. **Phenytoin** may decrease concentration. **Sympathomimetics** may increase risk of cardiac effects. **HERBAL:** **Kava kava, SAMe, St. John's wort, valerian** may increase risk of serotonin syndrome, CNS depression. **FOOD:** **Grapefruit, grapefruit juice** may increase concentration/toxicity. **LAB VALUES:** May alter serum glucose, EKG readings. **Therapeutic serum level:** 225–300 ng/ml; **toxic serum level:** greater than 500 ng/ml.

AVAILABILITY (Rx)

Capsules (Tofranil-PM): 75 mg, 100 mg, 125 mg, 150 mg. **Tablets (Tofranil):** 10 mg, 25 mg, 50 mg.

ADMINISTRATION/HANDLING

PO

• Give with food, milk if GI distress occurs.

INDICATIONS/ROUTES/DOSAGE

Depression

PO: ADULTS: Initially, 75–100 mg/day in 3–4 divided doses. May gradually increase to maximum of 200 mg/day (outpatient) or 300 mg/day (inpatient). **ELDERLY:** Initially, 25–50 mg/day at bedtime. May increase by 10–25 mg every 3–7 days. **Maximum:** 100 mg/day. **CHILDREN:** 1.5 mg/kg/day. May increase by 1 mg/kg every 3–4 days. **Maximum:** 5 mg/kg/day in 1–4 divided doses.

Enuresis

PO: CHILDREN, 6 YRS AND OLDER: Initially, 25 mg 1 hr before bedtime. May increase by 25 mg if inadequate response seen after 1 wk. **Maximum:** 2.5 mg/kg/day or 50 mg at bedtime for ages 6–12 yrs; 75 mg at bedtime for ages over 12 yrs.

SIDE EFFECTS

Frequent: Drowsiness, fatigue, dry mouth, blurred vision, constipation, delayed micturition, orthostatic hypotension, diaphoresis, impaired concentration, increased appetite, urinary retention, photosensitivity. **Occasional:** GI disturbances (nausea, metallic taste). **Rare:** Paradoxical reactions (agitation, restlessness, nightmares, insomnia), extrapyramidal symptoms (EPS) (particularly fine hand tremor).

ADVERSE EFFECTS/ TOXIC REACTIONS

Overdose may produce seizures; cardiovascular effects (severe orthostatic hypotension, dizziness, tachycardia, palpitations, arrhythmias). May result in altered temperature regulation (hyperpyrexia, hypothermia). Abrupt withdrawal from prolonged therapy may produce headache, malaise, nausea, vomiting, vivid dreams.

NURSING CONSIDERATIONS

BASELINE ASSESSMENT

Assess appearance, behavior, speech pattern, level of interest, mood. Obtain baseline CBC, hepatic/renal function tests.

INTERVENTION/EVALUATION

Supervise suicidal-risk pt closely during early therapy (as depression lessens, energy level improves, increasing suicide potential). Monitor appearance, behavior, speech pattern, level of interest, mood. For pts on long-term therapy, hepatic/renal function tests, blood counts should be performed periodically. Monitor daily pattern of bowel activity, stool consistency. Monitor B/P, pulse for hypotension, arrhythmias. Assess for urinary retention by bladder palpation. **Therapeutic serum level:** 225–300 ng/ml; **toxic serum level:** greater than 500 ng/ml.

PATIENT/FAMILY TEACHING

• Notify physician if depression worsens, thoughts of suicide, agitation, irritability occur. • Change positions slowly to avoid hypotensive effect. • Tolerance to postural hypotension, sedative, anticholinergic effects usually develops during early therapy. • Avoid tasks that require alertness, motor skills until response to drug is established. • Therapeutic effect may be noted within 2–5 days, maximum effect within 2–3 wks. • Sugarless gum, sips of tepid water may relieve dry mouth. • Do not abruptly discontinue medication. • Limit caffeine; avoid alcohol.

Imitrex, *see sumatriptan*

immune globulin IV (IGIV)

im-**mune glob**-u-lin
(Carimune NF, Flebogamma, Gammagard Liquid, Gammagard S/D, Gamunex, Octagam 5%, Privigen)

BLACK BOX ALERT Acute renal impairment characterized by increased serum creatinine, oliguria, acute renal failure, osmotic nephrosis, particularly pts with any degree of renal insufficiency, diabetes mellitus, volume depletion, sepsis, and those older than age 65 yrs.

◆ CLASSIFICATION

CLINICAL: Immune serum.

ACTION

Blocks Fc receptor on macrophages in pts with idiopathic thrombocytopenia purpura (ITP). Immunomodulatory effects on T cells and macrophages, esp. cytokine synthesis, B-cell immune function. Provides antibodies that neutralize bacteria, viral toxins. **Therapeutic Effect:** Provides passive immunity against infection; induces rapid increase in platelet count; produces anti-inflammatory effect.

PHARMACOKINETICS

Evenly distributed between intravascular and extravascular space. **Half-life:** 21–23 days.

USES

Treatment of pts with primary immunodeficiency syndromes, idiopathic thrombocytopenic purpura (ITP), prevention of coronary artery aneurysms associated with Kawasaki disease, prevention of recurrent bacterial infections in pts with hypogammaglobulinemia associated with B-cell chronic lymphocytic leukemia (CLL). Treatment of chronic inflammatory demyelinating polyneuropathies. **OFF-LABEL:** Control/prevention of infections in infants, children with immunosuppression due to

AIDS or AIDS-related complex; prevention of acute infections in immunosuppressed pts; prevention, treatment of infection in high-risk, preterm, low-birth-weight neonates; treatment of multiple sclerosis.

PRECAUTIONS

Contraindications: Hypersensitivity to gamma globulin, thimerosal, anti-IgA antibodies; isolated IgA deficiency. **Cautions:** Cardiovascular disease, history of thrombosis, renal impairment, diabetes, volume depletion, sepsis, concomitant nephrotoxic drugs.

LIFESPAN CONSIDERATIONS

Pregnancy/Lactation: Unknown if drug crosses placenta or is distributed in breast milk. **Pregnancy Category C. Children/Elderly:** No age-related precautions noted.

INTERACTIONS

DRUG: **Live virus vaccines** may increase vaccine side effects, potentiate virus replication, decrease pt's antibody response to vaccine. **HERBAL:** None significant. **FOOD:** None known. **LAB VALUES:** None significant.

AVAILABILITY (Rx)

Injection, Powder for Reconstitution (Carimune NF): 3 g, 6 g, 12 g. **(Gammagard S/D):** 2.5 g, 5 g, 10 g. **Injection, Solution (Flebogamma, Gammagard Liquid 10%, Gamunex, Octagam 5%, Privigen):** 1 g, 2.5 g, 5 g, 10 g.

ADMINISTRATION/HANDLING

IV

◀ALERT▶ Monitor vital signs, B/P diligently during and immediately after IV administration (precipitous fall in B/P may indicate anaphylactic reaction). Stop infusion immediately. Epinephrine should be readily available.

Reconstitution • Reconstitute only with diluent provided by manufacturer. • Discard partially used or turbid preparations.

Rate of administration • Give by infusion only. • After reconstitution, administer via separate tubing. • Avoid mixing with other medication or IV infusion fluids. • Rate of infusion varies with product used.

Storage • Refer to individual IV preparations for storage requirements, stability after reconstitution.

IV INCOMPATIBILITIES

Do not mix with any other medications.

INDICATIONS/ROUTES/DOSAGE

Primary Immunodeficiency Syndrome
IV: ADULTS, ELDERLY, CHILDREN: 200–800 mg/kg once monthly.

Idiopathic Thrombocytopenic Purpura (ITP)
IV: ADULTS, ELDERLY, CHILDREN: 400–1,000 mg/kg/day for 2–5 days.

Kawasaki Disease
IV: ADULTS, ELDERLY, CHILDREN: 1,000 mg/kg as a single dose or 400/mg/kg daily for 4 days. Must be used in combination with aspirin.

Chronic Leukocytic Leukemia (CLL)
IV: ADULTS, ELDERLY, CHILDREN: (Acute): 400 mg/kg/day for 2–5 days. **(Chronic):** 400 mg/kg as needed to maintain platelet count at or above 30,000/mm^3 or to control significant bleeding.

Polyneuropathies
IV: ADULTS, ELDERLY, CHILDREN: 2,000 mg/kg divided over 2–4 days (consecutive). Maintenance: 1,000 mg/kg/day for 1 day q3wks or 500 mg/kg for 2 consecutive days q3wks.

SIDE EFFECTS

Frequent: Tachycardia, backache, headache, arthralgia, myalgia. **Occasional:** Fatigue, wheezing, injection site rash/pain, leg cramps, urticaria, bluish color of lips/nailbeds, light-headedness.

ADVERSE EFFECTS/ TOXIC REACTIONS

Anaphylactic reactions occur rarely but incidence increases with repeated injections. Epinephrine should be readily available. Overdose may produce chest tightness, chills, diaphoresis, dizziness, facial flushing, nausea, vomiting, fever, hypotension. Hypersensitivity reaction (anxiety, arthralgia, dizziness, flushing, myalgia, palpitations, pruritus) occurs rarely.

NURSING CONSIDERATIONS

BASELINE ASSESSMENT

Inquire about history of exposure to disease for pt/family as appropriate. Have epinephrine readily available. Pt should be well hydrated prior to administration.

INTERVENTION/EVALUATION

Control rate of IV infusion carefully; too-rapid infusion increases risk of precipitous fall in B/P, signs of anaphylaxis (facial flushing, chest tightness, chills, fever, nausea, vomiting, diaphoresis). Assess pt closely during infusion, esp. first hr; monitor vital signs continuously. Stop infusion if aforementioned signs noted. For treatment of idiopathic thrombocytopenic purpura (ITP), monitor platelet count.

PATIENT/FAMILY TEACHING

• Explain rationale for therapy. • Inform physician if sudden weight gain, fluid retention, edema, decreased urine output, shortness of breath occur.

immune globulin subcutaneous

im-**mune** **glob**-u-lin
(Hizentra, Vivaglobulin)

◆ CLASSIFICATION

CLINICAL: Immune globulin.

ACTION

Immune globulin replacement therapy for IgG antibodies against bacteria/viruses. **Therapeutic Effect:** Provides immunity against infection.

PHARMACOKINETICS

Bioavailability 73% (compared to IGIV). Time to peak plasma levels: 2.5 days.

USES

Treatment of primary immune deficiency.

PRECAUTIONS

Contraindications: History of anaphylactic or severe systemic reaction to immune globulins, selective IgA deficiency with known antibody against IgA. **Cautions:** Cardiovascular disease, renal impairment, diabetes, sepsis, concomitant nephrotoxic medications.

⌛ LIFESPAN CONSIDERATIONS

Pregnancy/Lactation: Unknown if drug crosses placenta or is distributed in breast milk. **Pregnancy Category C. Children/Elderly:** No age-related precautions noted.

INTERACTIONS

DRUG: **Live virus vaccines** may potentiate virus replication, increase vaccine side effects, decrease pt's antibody response to vaccine. **HERBAL:** None significant. **FOOD:** None known. **LAB VALUES:** None significant.

AVAILABILITY (Rx)

Injection, Solution: (Hizentra): IgG 200 mg/ml. **(Vivaglobulin):** IgG 160 mg/ml (3 ml, 10 ml, 20 ml).

ADMINISTRATION/HANDLING

• Refrigerate; do not freeze; do not shake. • Allow vial to reach room temperature prior to use. • Do not use if cloudy or precipitate forms. • Follow manufacturer's instructions for filling reservoir, preparing pump. • Inject via infusion pump into abdomen, thigh, upper arm, lateral hip.

INDICATIONS/ROUTES/DOSAGE

Primary Immune Deficiency

SUBCUTANEOUS INFUSION: ADULTS, ELDERLY, CHILDREN 2 YRS AND OLDER: (Vivaglobulin): 100–200 mg/kg/wk. Adjust dose over time to achieve desired clinical response or target IgG levels. **Maximum rate:** 20 ml/hr. Doses greater than 15 ml should be divided and injected in different sites. **(Hizentra):** Initial dose calculated to achieve serum IgG to previous IVIG treatment. For first infusion up to 15 ml/hr (may be increased to 25 ml/hr per site as tolerated). Maximum flow rate not to exceed 50 ml/hr for all sites.

SIDE EFFECTS

Frequent: Local injection site reactions (92%), headache (48%), fever (25%), nausea (18%), sore throat, rash (17%). **Occasional:** Pain, diarrhea, cough (10%), weakness (5%), tachycardia, skin disorder, urine abnormality (3%).

ADVERSE EFFECTS/ TOXIC REACTIONS

Anaphylactic reactions are rare, but epinephrine should be readily available. Overdose may produce chest tightness, chills, diaphoresis, dizziness, facial flushing, nausea, vomiting, fever, hypotension. Hypersensitivity reaction (anxiety, arthralgia, dizziness, flushing, myalgia, palpitations, pruritus) occurs rarely.

NURSING CONSIDERATIONS

BASELINE ASSESSMENT

Inquire about history of exposure to disease for pt/family. Epinephrine should be readily available.

INTERVENTION/EVALUATION

Monitor for infusion-related adverse reaction, clinical response, anaphylaxis. Monitor IgG level.

PATIENT/FAMILY TEACHING

• Explain rationale for therapy. • Report to physician any sudden weight gain, fluid retention, edema, decreased urine output, shortness of breath, unusual reactions.

Imodium A-D, *see loperamide*

Imuran, *see azathioprine*

indapamide

in-**dap**-a-mide
(Apo-Indapamide 🍁, Lozide 🍁, Lozol, Novo-Indapamide 🍁)
Do not confuse indapamide with lopidine.

CLASSIFICATION

PHARMACOTHERAPEUTIC: Thiazide. **CLINICAL:** Diuretic, antihypertensive (see p. 102C).

ACTION

Diuretic: Blocks reabsorption of water, sodium, potassium at cortical diluting segment of distal tubule. **Antihypertensive:** Reduces plasma, extracellular fluid volume and peripheral vascular resistance by direct effect on blood vessels. **Therapeutic Effect:** Promotes diuresis, reduces B/P.

PHARMACOKINETICS

Route	Onset	Peak	Duration
PO	1–2 hrs	–	up to 36 hrs

Almost completely absorbed following PO administration. Protein binding: 71%–79%. Extensively metabolized in liver. Excreted in urine. **Half-life:** 14–18 hrs.

USES

Management of hypertension. Treatment of edema associated with CHF, nephrotic syndrome.

PRECAUTIONS

Contraindications: None known. **Cautions:** History of hypersensitivity to sulfonamides or thiazide diuretics, renal decompensation, anuria. Severe renal disease, hepatic impairment, diabetes mellitus, elderly, debilitated, thyroid disorders.

LIFESPAN CONSIDERATIONS

Pregnancy/Lactation: Unknown if drug crosses placenta or is distributed in breast milk. **Pregnancy Category B (D if used in pregnancy-induced hypertension). Children:** Safety and efficacy not established. **Elderly:** May be more sensitive to hypotensive, electrolyte effects.

INTERACTIONS

DRUG: May increase risk of **digoxin** toxicity associated with indapamide-induced hypokalemia. May increase risk of **lithium** toxicity. HERBAL: **Ephedra, ginseng, yohimbe** may worsen hypertension. **Garlic** may increase antihypertensive effect. FOOD: None known. LAB VALUES: May increase plasma renin activity. May decrease protein-bound iodine, serum calcium, potassium, sodium.

AVAILABILITY (Rx)

Tablets: 1.25 mg, 2.5 mg.

ADMINISTRATION/HANDLING

PO

• Give with food, milk if GI upset occurs, preferably with breakfast (may prevent nocturia).

INDICATIONS/ROUTES/DOSAGE

Edema

PO: ADULTS: Initially, 2.5 mg/day, may increase to 5 mg/day after 1 wk.

Hypertension

PO: ADULTS, ELDERLY: Initially, 1.25 mg. May increase to 2.5 mg/day after 4 wks or 5 mg/day after additional 4 wks.

SIDE EFFECTS

Frequent (5% and greater): Fatigue, paresthesia of extremities, tension, irritability, agitation, headache, dizziness, lightheadedness, insomnia, muscle cramps. **Occasional (less than 5%):** Urinary frequency, urticaria, rhinorrhea, flushing, weight loss, orthostatic hypotension, depression, blurred vision, nausea, vomiting, diarrhea, constipation, dry mouth, impotence, rash, pruritus.

ADVERSE EFFECTS/ TOXIC REACTIONS

Vigorous diuresis may lead to profound water and electrolyte depletion, resulting in hypokalemia, hyponatremia, dehydration. Acute hypotensive episodes may occur. Hyperglycemia may be noted during prolonged therapy. Pancreatitis, blood dyscrasias, pulmonary edema, allergic pneumonitis, dermatologic reactions occur rarely. Overdose can lead to lethargy, coma without changes in electrolytes or hydration.

NURSING CONSIDERATIONS

BASELINE ASSESSMENT

Check vital signs, esp. B/P for hypotension, before administration. Assess baseline electrolytes, particularly check for hypokalemia. Observe for edema; assess skin turgor, mucous membranes for hydration status. Assess muscle strength, mental status. Note skin temperature, moisture. Obtain baseline weight. Initiate I&O.

INTERVENTION/EVALUATION

Continue to monitor B/P, vital signs, electrolytes, I&O, weight. Note extent of diuresis. Watch for electrolyte disturbances (hypokalemia may result in weakness, tremor, muscle cramps, nausea, vomiting, altered mental status, tachycardia; hyponatremia may result in confusion, thirst, cold/clammy skin).

PATIENT/FAMILY TEACHING

• Expect increased frequency, volume of urination. • To reduce hypotensive effect, rise slowly from lying to sitting position, permit legs to dangle momentarily before standing. • Eat foods high in potassium such as whole grains (cereals), legumes, meat, bananas, apricots, orange juice, potatoes (white, sweet), raisins. • Take early in the day to avoid nocturia.

Inderal, *see propranolol*

Inderal LA, *see propranolol*

indinavir

in-**din**-ah-vir
(Crixivan)
Do not confuse indinavir with Denavir.

◆CLASSIFICATION

PHARMACOTHERAPEUTIC: Protease inhibitor. **CLINICAL:** Antiviral (see pp. 68C, 117C).

ACTION

Suppresses HIV protease, an enzyme necessary for splitting viral polyprotein precursors into mature infectious viral particles. **Therapeutic Effect:** Interrupts HIV replication, slowing progression of HIV infection.

PHARMACOKINETICS

Rapidly absorbed after PO administration. Protein binding: 60%. Metabolized in liver. Primarily eliminated in feces. Unknown if removed by hemodialysis. **Half-life:** 1.4–2.2 hrs (increased in hepatic impairment).

USES

Treatment of HIV infection as part of a multidrug regimen (at least 3 antiretroviral agents). **OFF-LABEL:** Prophylaxis following occupational exposure to HIV.

PRECAUTIONS

Contraindications: Concurrent use with astemizole, cisapride, ergot derivatives, midazolam, pimozide, terfenadine, triazolam; nephrolithiasis. **Cautions:** Renal/hepatic impairment.

LIFESPAN CONSIDERATIONS

Pregnancy/Lactation: Unknown if excreted in breast milk. Breast-feeding not recommended in HIV-infected women. **Pregnancy Category C. Children:** Safety and efficacy not established. **Elderly:** Information not available.

INTERACTIONS

DRUG: May increase concentration/toxicity of **midazolam, sildenafil, triazolam. Efavirenz, rifabutin, rifampin** may decrease concentration/effect. **HMG-CoA inhibitors (e.g., lovastatin, simvastatin)** may increase risk of myopathy. **Delavirdine, itraconazole, ketoconazole** may increase concentration. **HERBAL: St. John's wort** may decrease concentration, effect. **FOOD: Grapefruit, grapefruit juice** may decrease concentration, effect. **High-fat, high-calorie, high-protein meals** may decrease concentration. **LAB VALUES:** May increase serum bilirubin, amylase, glucose, AST, ALT. May alter serum triglycerides, cholesterol.

AVAILABILITY (Rx)

Capsules: 100 mg, 200 mg, 400 mg.

ADMINISTRATION/HANDLING

PO

• Store at room temperature. • Protect from moisture (capsules sensitive to moisture; keep in original bottle). • Best given without food 1 hr before or 2 hrs following a meal but may give with water, skim milk, juice, coffee, tea, light meal (e.g., dry toast with jelly). • Do not give with meal high in fat, calories, protein. • If indinavir and didanosine are given concurrently, give at least 1 hr apart on an empty stomach.

INDICATIONS/ROUTES/DOSAGE

HIV Infection (in Combination with Other Antiretrovirals)

PO: ADULTS: 800 mg (two 400-mg capsules) q8h.

DOSAGE ADJUSTMENTS WHEN GIVEN CONCOMITANTLY: DELAVIRDINE, ITRACONAZOLE, KETOCONAZOLE: Reduce dose to 600 mg q8h. **EFAVIRENZ:** Increase dose to 1,000 mg q8h. **LOPINAVIR/RITONAVIR:** Reduce dose to 600 mg twice a day. **NEVIRAPINE:** Increase dose to 1,000 mg q8h. **RIFABUTIN:** Reduce rifabutin by ½ and increase indinavir to 1,000 mg q8h. **RITONAVIR:** 100–200 mg twice a day and indinavir 800 mg twice a day or ritonavir 400 mg twice a day and indinavir 400 mg twice a day.

HIV Infection in Pts with Hepatic Insufficiency

PO: ADULTS: 600 mg q8h.

SIDE EFFECTS

Frequent: Nausea (12%), abdominal pain (9%), headache (6%), diarrhea (5%). **Occasional:** Vomiting, asthenia (loss of strength, energy), fatigue (4%); insomnia; accumulation of fat in waist, abdomen, back of neck. **Rare:** Altered taste, heartburn, symptomatic urinary tract disease, transient renal dysfunction.

ADVERSE EFFECTS/ TOXIC REACTIONS

Nephrolithiasis (flank pain with or without hematuria) occurs in 4% of pts.

NURSING CONSIDERATIONS

BASELINE ASSESSMENT

Offer emotional support. Establish baseline lab values. Emphasize need for close monitoring of renal function (urinalysis, serum creatinine) during therapy.

INTERVENTION/EVALUATION

Encourage adequate hydration. Pt should drink 48 oz (1.5 L) of liquid for each 24 hrs during therapy. Monitor for evidence of nephrolithiasis (flank pain, hematuria); contact physician if symptoms occur (therapy should be interrupted for 1–3 days). Monitor daily pattern of bowel activity, stool consistency. Assess for abdominal discomfort, headache. Monitor serum bilirubin, glucose, cholesterol, triglycerides, amylase, lipase, hepatic function tests, CD4 cell count, CBC.

PATIENT/FAMILY TEACHING

• Indinavir is not a cure for HIV infection, nor does it reduce risk of transmission to others. Condition may progress despite treatment. • If dose is missed, take next dose at regularly scheduled time (do **not** double the dose). • Best taken without food but water only (optimal absorption) 1 hr before or 2 hrs following a meal; may take with water, skim milk, juice, coffee, tea, light carbohydrate meal. • Avoid St. John's wort, grapefruit, grapefruit juice.

indomethacin

in-doe-**meth**-a-sin

(Apo-Indomethacin ✱, Indocid ✱, Indocin, Indocin-IV, Novo-Methacin ✱)

BLACK BOX ALERT Increased risk of serious cardiovascular thrombotic events, including myocardial infarction, CVA. Increased risk of severe GI reactions, including ulceration, bleeding, perforation.

Do not confuse Indocin with Imodium, Minocin, or Vicodin.

◆ CLASSIFICATION

PHARMACOTHERAPEUTIC: Nonsteroidal anti-inflammatory. **CLINICAL:** Anti-inflammatory, analgesic (see p. 128C).

ACTION

Produces analgesic, anti-inflammatory effects by inhibiting prostaglandin synthesis. Increases sensitivity of premature ductus to dilating effects of prostaglandins. **Therapeutic Effect:** Reduces inflammatory response, intensity of pain. Closure of patent ductus arteriosus.

PHARMACOKINETICS

Route	Onset	Peak	Duration
PO	30 min	–	4–6 hrs

Well absorbed from GI tract. Protein binding: 99%. Metabolized in liver. Excreted in urine. **Half-life:** 4.5 hrs.

USES

Treatment of active stages of rheumatoid arthritis, osteoarthritis, ankylosing spondylitis, acute gouty arthritis. Relieves acute bursitis, tendonitis. For closure of hemodynamically significant patent ductus arteriosus of premature infants weighing 500–1,750 g. OFF-LABEL: Treatment of fever due to malignancy, pericarditis, psoriatic arthritis, rheumatic complications associated with Paget's disease of bone, vascular headache.

PRECAUTIONS

Contraindications: Active GI bleeding, ulcerations; hypersensitivity to aspirin, indomethacin, other NSAIDs; renal impairment; thrombocytopenia. **Cautions:** Cardiac dysfunction, hypertension, renal/hepatic impairment, epilepsy, concurrent anticoagulant therapy.

LIFESPAN CONSIDERATIONS

Pregnancy/Lactation: Crosses placenta; distributed in breast milk. **Pregnancy Category C (D if used after 34 wks gestation, close to delivery, or for longer than 48 hrs). Children:** Safety and efficacy not established in those younger than 14 yrs. **Elderly:** GI bleeding, ulceration increase risk of serious adverse effects.

INTERACTIONS

DRUG: May increase concentration of **aminoglycosides** in neonates. May decrease effects of **antihypertensives, diuretics. Aspirin, other salicylates** may increase risk of GI side effects, bleeding. **Bone marrow depressants** may increase risk of hematologic reactions. May increase effects of **heparin, oral anticoagulants, thrombolytics.** May increase concentration, risk of toxicity of **lithium.** May increase risk of **methotrexate** toxicity. **Probenecid** may increase concentration. Do not give **triamterene** concurrently as it may potentiate renal failure. HERBAL: **Cat's claw, dong quai, evening primrose, feverfew, garlic, ginkgo, ginseng, horse chestnut, red clover** may increase antiplatelet activity. FOOD: None known. LAB VALUES: May prolong bleeding time. May alter serum glucose. May increase BUN, serum creatinine, potassium, AST, ALT. May decrease serum sodium, platelet count, leukocytes.

AVAILABILITY (Rx)

Capsules (Indocin): 25 mg, 50 mg. **Injection, Powder for Reconstitution (Indocin IV):** 1 mg. **Oral Suspension (Indocin):** 25 mg/5 ml.

ADMINISTRATION/HANDLING

IV

Reconstitution • To 1-mg vial, add 1–2 ml preservative-free Sterile Water for Injection or 0.9% NaCl to provide concentration of 1 mg/ml or 0.5 mg/ml, respectively. • Do not further dilute.

Rate of administration • Administer over 20–30 min. • Restrict fluid intake.

Storage • IV solutions made without preservatives should be used immediately. • Use IV solution immediately following reconstitution. • IV solution appears clear; discard if cloudy or precipitate forms. • Discard unused portion.

PO

• Give after meals or with food, antacids.

Rectal

ALERT IV injection preferred for patent ductus arteriosus in neonate (but may give dose PO via NG tube or rectally).

IV INCOMPATIBILITIES

Amino acid injection, calcium gluconate, cimetidine (Tagamet), dobutamine (Dobutrex), dopamine (Intropin), gentamicin (Garamycin), tobramycin (Nebcin).

IV COMPATIBILITIES

Insulin, potassium.

INDICATIONS/ROUTES/DOSAGE

Moderate to Severe Rheumatoid Arthritis (RA), Osteoarthritis, Ankylosing Spondylitis

PO: ADULTS, ELDERLY: Initially, 25–50 mg 2–3 times a day; increased by 25–50 mg/wk up to 200 mg/day. **CHILDREN 2 YRS AND OLDER:** 1–2 mg/kg/day in 2–4 divided doses. **Maximum:** 4 mg/kg/day not to exceed 150–200 mg/day.

Acute Gouty Arthritis
PO: ADULTS, ELDERLY: 50 mg 3 times a day for 3–5 days.

Acute Bursitis, Tendonitis
PO: ADULTS, ELDERLY: 75–150 mg/day in 3–4 divided doses for 7–14 days.

Patent Ductus Arteriosus
IV: NEONATES: Initially, 0.2 mg/kg. Subsequent doses are based on age, as follows: **NEONATES OLDER THAN 7 DAYS:** 0.25 mg/kg for 2nd and 3rd doses. **NEONATES 2–7 DAYS:** 0.2 mg/kg for 2nd and 3rd doses. **NEONATES LESS THAN 48 HRS:** 0.1 mg/kg for 2nd and 3rd doses. In general, dosing interval is 12 hrs if urine output is greater than 1 ml/kg/hr after prior dose, 24 hrs if urine output is less than 1 ml/kg/hr but greater than 0.6 ml/kg/hr. Dose is held if urine output is less than 0.6. ml/kg/hr or if neonate is anuric.

SIDE EFFECTS

Frequent (11%–3%): Headache, nausea, vomiting, dyspepsia (heartburn, indigestion, epigastric pain), dizziness. **Occasional (less than 3%):** Depression, tinnitus, diaphoresis, drowsiness, constipation, diarrhea. **Patent ductus arteriosus:** Bleeding abnormalities. **Rare:** Hypertension, confusion, urticaria, pruritus, rash, blurred vision.

ADVERSE EFFECTS/ TOXIC REACTIONS

Paralytic ileus, ulceration of esophagus, stomach, duodenum, small intestine may occur. Pts with renal impairment may develop hyperkalemia with worsening of renal impairment. May aggravate depression or other psychiatric disturbances, epilepsy, parkinsonism. Nephrotoxicity (dysuria, hematuria, proteinuria, nephrotic syndrome) occurs rarely. Metabolic acidosis/alkalosis, bradycardia occur rarely in pts with patent ductus arteriosus.

NURSING CONSIDERATIONS

BASELINE ASSESSMENT

Assess onset, type, location, duration of pain, fever, inflammation. Inspect appearance of affected joints for immobility, deformities, skin condition.

INTERVENTION/EVALUATION

Monitor for evidence of nausea, dyspepsia. Assist with ambulation if dizziness occurs. Evaluate for therapeutic response: relief of pain, stiffness, swelling; increased joint mobility; reduced joint tenderness; improved grip strength. Monitor BUN, serum creatinine, potassium, hepatic function tests. Observe for weight gain, edema, bleeding, bruising. In neonates, also monitor heart rate, heart sounds for murmur, B/P, urine output, EKG, serum sodium, glucose, platelets.

PATIENT/FAMILY TEACHING

• Avoid aspirin, alcohol during therapy (increases risk of GI bleeding). • If GI upset occurs, take with food, milk. • Avoid tasks that require alertness, motor skills until response to drug is established. • Report ringing in ears, persistent stomach pain, unusual bruising/bleeding.

infliximab

in-**flix**-ih-mab
(Remicade)

BLACK BOX ALERT Risk of severe/fatal opportunistic infections (tuberculosis, sepsis, fungal), reactivation of latent infections. Very rare cases of very aggressive, usually fatal hepatosplenic T-cell lymphoma reported in adolescents, young adults with Crohn's disease.

Do not confuse infliximab with rituximab, or Remicade with Reminyl or Rituxan.

◆ CLASSIFICATION

PHARMACOTHERAPEUTIC: Monoclonal antibody. **CLINICAL:** GI anti-inflammatory.

ACTION

Binds to tumor necrosis factor (TNF), inhibiting functional activity of TNF. Reduces infiltration of inflammatory cells. **Therapeutic Effect:** Decreases inflamed areas of intestine.

PHARMACOKINETICS

Absorbed into GI tissue; primarily distributed in vascular compartment. **Half-life:** 8–9.5 days.

USES

In combination with methotrexate, reduces signs/symptoms, inhibits progression of structural damage, improves physical function in moderate to severe active rheumatoid arthritis (RA), psoriatic arthritis. Reduces signs/symptoms, induces and maintains remission in moderate to severe active Crohn's disease. Reduces number of draining enterocutaneous/rectovaginal fistulas, maintains fistula closure in fistulizing Crohn's disease. Reduces sign/symptoms of active ankylosing spondylitis. Treatment of chronic severe plaque psoriasis in pts who are candidates for systemic therapy. Reduces sign/symptoms, induces and maintains clinical remission and mucosal healing, eliminates corticosteroid use in moderate to severe active ulcerative colitis. **OFF-LABEL:** CHF, juvenile rheumatoid arthritis (JRA), psoriasis, reactive arthritis, sciatica, acute graft vs. host disease.

PRECAUTIONS

Contraindications: Sensitivity to murine proteins, sepsis, serious active infection. **Cautions:** History of recurrent infections.

LIFESPAN CONSIDERATIONS

Pregnancy/Lactation: Unknown if distributed in breast milk. **Pregnancy Category B. Children:** Safety and efficacy not established. **Elderly:** Use cautiously due to higher rate of infection.

INTERACTIONS

DRUG: **Anakinra** may increase risk of infection. **Immunosuppressants** may reduce frequency of infusion reactions, antibodies to infliximab. **Live virus vaccines** may decrease immune response. **HERBAL:** **Echinacea** may decrease effect. **FOOD:** None known. **LAB VALUES:** May increase AST, ALT, serum alkaline phosphatase, bilirubin.

AVAILABILITY (Rx)

Injection, Powder for Reconstitution: 100 mg.

ADMINISTRATION/HANDLING

IV

Reconstitution • Reconstitute each vial with 10 ml Sterile Water for Injection, using 21-gauge or smaller needle. Direct stream of Sterile Water for Injection to glass wall of vial. • Swirl vial gently to dissolve contents (do not shake). • Allow solution to stand for 5 min and inject into 250 ml bag 0.9% NaCl; gently mix. Concentration should range between 0.4 and 4 mg/ml. • Begin infusion within 3 hrs after reconstitution.

Rate of administration • Administer IV infusion over 2–3 hrs using a low protein-binding filter.

Storage • Refrigerate vials. • Solution should appear colorless to light yellow and opalescent; do not use if discolored or particulate forms.

IV INCOMPATIBILITIES

Do not infuse in same IV line with other agents.

INDICATIONS/ROUTES/DOSAGE

◀ALERT▶ Premedicate with antihistamines, acetaminophen, steroids to prevent/manage infusion reactions.

Rheumatoid Arthritis (RA)

IV INFUSION: ADULTS, ELDERLY: 3 mg/kg followed by additional doses at 2 and 6 wks after first infusion, then q8wk thereafter. Range: 3–10 mg/kg at 4- to 8-wk intervals.

Crohn's Disease
IV INFUSION: ADULTS, ELDERLY, CHILDREN: 5 mg/kg followed by additional doses at 2 and 6 wks after first infusion, then q8wk thereafter. For adults who respond then lose response, consideration may be given to treatment with 10 mg/kg.

Fistulizing Crohn's Disease
IV INFUSION: ADULTS, ELDERLY: 5 mg/kg followed by additional doses at 2 and 6 wks after first infusion, then q8wk thereafter. For pts who respond then lose response, consideration may be given to treatment with 10 mg/kg.

Ankylosing Spondylitis
IV INFUSION: ADULTS, ELDERLY: 5 mg/kg followed by additional doses at 2 and 6 wks after first infusion, then q6wk thereafter.

Psoriatric Arthritis
IV INFUSION: ADULTS, ELDERLY: 5 mg/kg followed by additional doses at 2 and 6 wks after first infusion, then q8wk thereafter. May be used with or without methotrexate.

Plaque Psoriasis
IV INFUSION: ADULTS, ELDERLY: 5 mg/kg followed by additional doses at 2 and 6 wks after first infusion, then q8wk thereafter.

Ulcerative Colitis
IV INFUSION: ADULTS, ELDERLY: 5 mg/kg followed by additional doses at 2 and 6 wks after first infusion, then q8wk thereafter.

SIDE EFFECTS

Frequent (22%–10%): Headache, nausea, fatigue, fever. **Occasional (9%–5%):** Fever/chills during infusion, pharyngitis, vomiting, pain, dizziness, bronchitis, rash, rhinitis, cough, pruritus, sinusitis, myalgia, back pain. **Rare (4%–1%):** Hypotension or hypertension, paresthesia, anxiety, depression, insomnia, diarrhea, UTI.

ADVERSE EFFECTS/ TOXIC REACTIONS

Serious infections, including sepsis, occur rarely. Potential for hypersensitivity reaction, lupus-like syndrome, severe hepatic reaction.

NURSING CONSIDERATIONS

BASELINE ASSESSMENT

Check baseline hydration status (skin turgor for tenting mucous membranes, urinary status).

INTERVENTION/EVALUATION

Monitor urinalysis, erythrocyte sedimentation rate (ESR), B/P. Monitor for signs of infection. Monitor daily pattern of bowel activity, stool consistency. **Crohn's Disease:** Monitor C-reactive protein, frequency of stools. Assess for abdominal pain. **Rheumatoid Arthritis (RA):** Monitor C-reactive protein. Assess for decreased pain, swollen joints, stiffness.

PATIENT/FAMILY TEACHING

- Notify physician if persistent fever, cough, abdominal pain, swelling of ankles/feet occur.

insulin HIGH ALERT

in-sull-in
Rapid-acting: INSULIN ASPART: (Novolog), **INSULIN GLULISINE:** (Apidra), **INSULIN LISPRO:** (Humalog)
Short-acting: REGULAR INSULIN: (Humulin R, Novolin R)
Intermediate-acting: NPH: (Humulin N, Novolin N)
Long-acting: INSULIN DETEMIR: (Levemir), **INSULIN GLARGINE:** (Lantus)

FIXED-COMBINATION(S)

Humalog Mix 75/25: lispro suspension 75% and lispro solution

25%. **Humulin Mix 50/50:** NPH 50% and regular 50%. **Humulin 70/30, Novolin 70/30:** NPH 70% and rapid-acting regular 30%. **Novolog Mix 70/30:** aspart suspension 70% and aspart solution 30%.

◆ CLASSIFICATION

PHARMACOTHERAPEUTIC: Exogenous insulin. **CLINICAL:** Antidiabetic (see p. 42C).

ACTION

Facilitates passage of glucose, potassium, magnesium across cellular membranes of skeletal/cardiac muscle, adipose tissue. Controls storage, metabolism of carbohydrates, protein, fats. Promotes conversion of glucose to glycogen in liver. **Therapeutic Effect:** Controls glucose levels in diabetic pts.

PHARMACOKINETICS

Rapid-Acting

	Onset (min)	Peak (hrs)	Duration (hrs)
Aspart (Novolog)	10–20	1–3	3–5
Glulisine (Apidra)	10–15	1–1.5	3–5
Lispro (Humalog)	15–30	0.5–2.5	3–6.5

Short-Acting

	Onset (min)	Peak (hrs)	Duration (hrs)
Regular (Humulin R)	30–60	1–5	6–10
Regular (Novolin R)	30–60	1–5	6–10

Intermediate-Acting

	Onset (hrs)	Peak (hrs)	Duration (hrs)
NPH (Humulin N)	1–2	6–14	16–24+
NPH (Novolin N)	1–2	6–14	16–24+

Long-Acting

	Onset (hrs)	Peak (hrs)	Duration (hrs)
Detemir (Levemir)	0.8–2	Relatively flat	12 (0.2 units/kg) 24 (0.4 units/kg)
Glargine (Lantus)	1.1	No peak	24

USES

Treatment of insulin-dependent type 1 diabetes mellitus; non–insulin-dependent type 2 diabetes mellitus (NIDDM) when diet and weight control therapy have failed to maintain satisfactory serum glucose levels or in event of pregnancy, surgery, trauma, infection, fever, severe renal, hepatic, endocrine dysfunction. Regular insulin used for emergency treatment of ketoacidosis, to promote passage of glucose across cell membrane in hyperalimentation, to facilitate intracellular shift of potassium in hyperkalemia. **OFF-LABEL:** Insulin aspart, insulin lispro, insulin regular: Gestational diabetes, mild to moderate diabetic ketoacidosis, mild to moderate hyperosmolar hyperglycemic state. Insulin NPH: Gestational diabetes.

PRECAUTIONS

Contraindications: Hypersensitivity, insulin resistance may require change of type or species source of insulin.

⌛ LIFESPAN CONSIDERATIONS

Pregnancy/Lactation: Insulin is drug of choice for diabetes in pregnancy; close medical supervision is needed. Following delivery, insulin needs may drop for 24–72 hrs, then rise to pre-pregnancy levels. Not distributed in breast milk; lactation may decrease insulin requirements. **Pregnancy Category B:** Aspart, Lispro, Regular, NPH; **Pregnancy Category C:** Detemir, Glargine, Glulisine. **Children:** No age-related precautions noted. **El-**

derly: Decreased vision, fine motor tremors may lead to inaccurate self-dosing.

INTERACTIONS

DRUG: **Alcohol** may increase effects. **Beta-adrenergic blockers** may increase risk of hyperglycemia, hypoglycemia; may mask signs, prolong periods of hypoglycemia. **Glucocorticoids, thiazide diuretics** may increase serum glucose. **HERBAL:** None significant. **FOOD:** None known. **LAB VALUES:** May decrease serum magnesium, phosphate, potassium.

AVAILABILITY

Rapid-Acting

Aspart (Novolog): 100 units/ml vial, 3 ml cartridge, 3 ml Flex-Pen. **Glulisine (Apidra):** 100 units/ml vial, 3 ml cartridge. **Lispro (Humalog):** 100 units/ml vial, 3 ml cartridge, 3 ml pen.

Short-Acting

Regular (Humulin R): 100 units/ml vial. **Regular (Novolin R):** 100 units/ml vial, 3 ml cartridge, 3 ml Innolet prefilled syringe.

Intermediate-Acting

NPH (Humulin N): 100 units/ml vial, 3 ml pen. **NPH (Novolin N):** 100 units/ml vial, 3 ml cartridge, 3 ml Innolet prefilled syringe.

Long-Acting

Detemir (Levemir): 100 units/ml vial, 3 ml Flex-Pen. **Glargine (Lantus):** 100 units/ml vial, 3 ml cartridge.

Intermediate- and Short-Acting Mixtures

Humulin 50/50, Humulin 70/30, Humalog Mix 75/25, Humalog Mix 50/50, Novolin 70/30, Novolog Mix 70/30.

ADMINISTRATION/HANDLING

IV (Regular and Insulin Glulisine [Apidra])

• Use only if solution is clear. • May give undiluted.

Rapid-Acting

Aspart (Novolog) • May give subcutaneous, IV infusion. • Can mix with NPH (draw aspart into syringe first; inject immediately after mixing). • After first use, stable at room temperature for 28 days. • Administer 5–10 min before meals.

Glulisine (Apidra) • May mix with NPH (draw glulisine into syringe first; inject immediately after mixing). • After first use, stable at room temperature for 28 days. • Administer 15 min before or within 20 min after starting a meal.

Lispro (Humalog) • For subcutaneous use only. • May mix with NPH. Stable for 28 days at room temperature; syringe is stable for 14 days if refrigerated. • After first use, stable at room temperature for 28 days. • Administer 15 min before or immediately after meals.

Short-Acting

Regular (Humulin R, Novolin R) • May give subcutaneous, IM, IV. • May mix with NPH for immediate use or for storage for future use. Stable for 1 mo at room temperature, 3 mos if refrigerated. • Can mix with Sterile Water for Injection or 0.9% NaCl. • After first use, stable at room temperature for 28 days. • Administer 30 min before meals.

Intermediate-Acting

NPH (Humulin N, Novolin N) • For subcutaneous use only. • May mix with aspart (Novolog) or lispro (Humalog). Draw aspart or lispro first and use immediately. • May mix with regular (Humulin R, Novolin R) insulin. Draw regular insulin first, use immediately or may store for future use (up to 28 days). • After first use, stable at room temperature for 28 days. • Administer 15 min before meals when mixed with aspart or lispro; 30 min before meals when mixed with regular.

Long-Acting

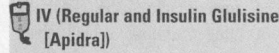

Detemir (Levemir) • For subcutaneous use only. • Do not mix with other insulins. • After first use, stable at room temperature for 42 days. • Evening dose given at dinner or at bedtime. Twice daily regimens can be given 12 hrs after morning dose.

Glargine (Lantus) • For subcutaneous use only. • Do not mix with other insulins. • After first use, stable at room temperature for 28 days. • Administer once daily at same time. Meal timing is not applicable.

Subcutaneous

• Check serum glucose concentration before administration; dosage highly individualized. • Subcutaneous injections may be given in thigh, abdomen, upper arm, buttocks, upper back if there is adequate adipose tissue. • Rotation of injection sites is essential; maintain careful record. • Prefilled syringes should be stored in vertical or oblique position to avoid plugging; plunger should be pulled back slightly and syringe rocked to remix solution before injection.

IV INCOMPATIBILITIES

Diltiazem (Cardizem), dopamine (Intropin), nafcillin (Nafcil).

IV COMPATIBILITIES

Amiodarone (Cordarone), ampicillin/sulbactam (Unasyn), cefazolin (Ancef), cimetidine (Tagamet), digoxin (Lanoxin): (physically compatible for 3 hrs in 0.9% NaCl. In D_5W, water, a slight haze develops within 1 hr), dobutamine (Dobutrex), famotidine (Pepcid), gentamicin, heparin, magnesium sulfate, metoclopramide (Reglan), midazolam (Versed), milrinone (Primacor), morphine, nitroglycerin, potassium chloride, propofol (Diprivan), vancomycin (Vancocin).

INDICATIONS/ROUTES/DOSAGE

Usual Dosage

◀ALERT▶ Adjust dosage to achieve premeal and bedtime serum glucose of 80–140 mg/dl (children younger than 5 yrs: 100–200 mg/dl).

SUBCUTANEOUS: ADULTS, ELDERLY, CHILDREN: 0.5–1 unit/kg/day. **ADOLESCENTS (DURING GROWTH SPURT):** 0.8–1.2 units/kg/day.

Diabetic Ketoacidosis

IV: ADULTS, ELDERLY: 0.1 unit/kg/hr. Titration based on serum glucose level.

SIDE EFFECTS

Occasional: Localized redness, swelling, itching (due to improper insulin injection technique), allergy to insulin cleansing solution. **Infrequent:** Somogyi effect, (rebound hyperglycemia) with chronically excessive insulin dosages. Systemic allergic reaction (rash, angioedema, anaphylaxis), lipodystrophy (depression at injection site due to breakdown of adipose tissue), lipohypertrophy (accumulation of subcutaneous tissue at injection site due to inadequate site rotation). **Rare:** Insulin resistance.

ADVERSE EFFECTS/ TOXIC REACTIONS

Severe hypoglycemia (due to hyperinsulinism) may occur with insulin overdose, decrease/delay of food intake, excessive exercise, those with brittle diabetes. Diabetic ketoacidosis may result from stress, illness, omission of insulin dose, long-term poor insulin control.

NURSING CONSIDERATIONS

BASELINE ASSESSMENT

Check serum glucose level. Discuss lifestyle to determine extent of learning, emotional needs.

INTERVENTION/EVALUATION

Assess for hypoglycemia (refer to pharmacokinetics table for peak times and duration): cool, wet skin, tremors, dizziness, headache, anxiety, tachycardia, numbness in mouth, hunger, diplopia. Check sleeping pt for restlessness, diaphoresis. Check for hyperglycemia: polyuria (excessive urine output), polyphagia (excessive food intake), polydipsia (excessive thirst), nausea/vomiting, dim vision, fatigue, deep and rapid breathing (Kussmaul respirations). Be alert to conditions altering glucose requirements: fever, increased activity/stress, surgical procedure.

PATIENT/FAMILY TEACHING

• Instruct on proper technique for drug administration, testing of glucose, signs/symptoms of hypoglycemia and hyperglycemia. • Prescribed diet is an essential part of treatment; do not skip/delay meals. • Carry candy, sugar packets, other sugar supplements for immediate response to hypoglycemia. • Wear or carry medical alert identification. • Check with physician when insulin demands are altered (e.g., fever, infection, trauma, stress, heavy physical activity). • Do not take other medication without consulting physician. • Weight control, exercise, hygiene (including foot care), not smoking are integral parts of therapy. • Protect skin, limit sun exposure. • Inform dentist, physician, surgeon of medication before any treatment is given.

Integrilin, *see eptifibatide*

interferon alfa-2b HIGH ALERT

inn-ter-**fear**-on
(Intron-A)

BLACK BOX ALERT May cause or aggravate fatal or life-threatening autoimmune disorders, ischemia, neuropsychiatric symptoms (profound depression, suicidal thoughts/behaviors), infectious disorders.

Do not confuse interferon alfa-2b with interferon alfa-2a, interferon alfa-n3, or peginterferon alfa-2b, or Intron with Peg-Intron.

FIXED-COMBINATION(S)

Rebetron: interferon alfa-2b/ribavirin (an antiviral): 3 million units/200 mg.

◆CLASSIFICATION

PHARMACOTHERAPEUTIC: Biologic response modifier. **CLINICAL:** Antineoplastic (see p. 85C).

ACTION

Inhibits viral replication in virus-infected cells, suppresses cell proliferation, augments specific cytotoxicity of lymphocytes. **Therapeutic Effect:** Prevents rapid growth of malignant cells; inhibits hepatitis virus.

PHARMACOKINETICS

Well absorbed after IM, subcutaneous administration. Undergoes proteolytic degradation during reabsorption in kidneys. **Half-life:** 2–3 hrs.

USES

Treatment of hairy cell leukemia, condylomata acuminata (genital, venereal warts), AIDS-related Kaposi's sarcoma, chronic hepatitis (non-A, non-B/C), chronic hepatitis B (including children 1 yr and older), follicular lymphoma. **OFF-LABEL:** Treatment of bladder, cervical, renal carcinoma; chronic myelocytic leukemia; laryngeal papillomatosis; multiple myeloma; mycosis fungoides; West Nile virus.

PRECAUTIONS

Contraindications: Autoimmune hepatitis. **Cautions:** Renal/hepatic impairment, seizure disorders, compromised CNS function, cardiac diseases, history of cardiac abnormalities, myelosuppression.

⌛ LIFESPAN CONSIDERATIONS

Pregnancy/Lactation: If possible, avoid use during pregnancy. Breast-feeding not recommended. **Pregnancy Category C (X in combination with ribavirin).** **Children:** Safety and efficacy not established. **Elderly:** Neurotoxicity, cardiotoxicity may occur more frequently. Age-related renal impairment may require dosage adjustment.

INTERACTIONS

DRUG: **Bone marrow depressants** may increase myelosuppression. **HERBAL:** None significant. **FOOD:** None known. **LAB VALUES:** May increase PT, aPTT, LDH, alkaline phosphatase, AST, ALT. May decrease Hgb, Hct, leukocyte, platelet counts.

AVAILABILITY (Rx)

Injection, Powder for Reconstitution: 10 million units, 18 million units, 50 million units. **Injection, Solution (Multidose Prefilled Pen):** 3 million units/0.2 ml (6 doses-18 million units), 5 million units/0.2 ml (6 doses-30 million units), 10 million units/0.2 mg (6 doses-60 million units). **Injection, Solution (Multidose Vial):** 6 million units/ml, 10 million units/ml. **Injection, Solution (Single-Dose Vial):** 10 million units/ml.

I

ADMINISTRATION/HANDLING

IV

Reconstitution • Prepare immediately before use. • Reconstitute with diluent provided by manufacturer. • Withdraw desired dose and further dilute with 100 ml 0.9% NaCl to provide final concentration of at least 10 million international units/100 ml.

Rate of administration • Administer over 20 min.

Storage • Refrigerate unopened vials. • Following reconstitution, stable for 24 hrs if refrigerated.

IM, Subcutaneous

• Do not give IM if platelets are less than 50,000/m^3; give subcutaneous. • For hairy cell leukemia, reconstitute each 3 million international units vial with 1 ml Bacteriostatic Water for Injection to provide concentration of 3 million international units/ml (1 ml to 5 million-international units vial; 2 ml to 10 million-international units vial; 5 ml to 25 million-international units vial provides concentration of 5 million international units/ml). • For condylomata acuminata, reconstitute each 10 million-international units vial with 1 ml Bacteriostatic Water for Injection to provide concentration of 10 million international units/ml. • For AIDS-related Kaposi's sarcoma, reconstitute 50 million international units vial with 1 ml Bacteriostatic Water for Injection to provide concentration of 50 million international units/ml. • Agitate vial gently, withdraw with sterile syringe.

IV INCOMPATIBILITIES

D_5W. Do not mix with other medications via Y-site administration.

IV COMPATIBILITY

0.9% NaCl, Lactated Ringer's.

INDICATIONS/ROUTES/DOSAGE

Hairy Cell Leukemia

IM, SUBCUTANEOUS: ADULTS: 2 million units/m^2 3 times a wk for 2–6 mos. If severe adverse reactions occur, modify dose or temporarily discontinue drug.

Condylomata Accuminata

INTRALESIONAL: ADULTS: 1 million units/lesion 3 times a wk for 3 wks. May administer a 2nd course at 12–16 wks. Use only 10-million-unit vial, and reconstitute with no more than 1 ml diluent. **Maximum:** 5 lesions per treatement.

AIDS-Related Kaposi's Sarcoma

IM, SUBCUTANEOUS: ADULTS: 30 million units/m^2 3 times a wk. Use only 50-million-unit vials. If severe adverse reactions occur, modify dose or temporarily discontinue drug.

Chronic Hepatitis C

IM, SUBCUTANEOUS: ADULTS: 3 million units 3 times a wk for up to 6 mos. For pts who tolerate therapy and whose ALT level normalizes within 16 wks, therapy may be extended for up to 18–24 mos. May be used in combination with ribavirin.

Chronic Hepatitis B

IM, SUBCUTANEOUS: ADULTS: 30–35 million units weekly, either as 5 million

units/day or 10 million units 3 times a wk for 16 wks.
SUBCUTANEOUS: CHILDREN 1–17 YRS: 3 million units/m² 3 times/wk for 1 wk, then 6 million units/m² 3 times/wk for 16–24 wks. **Maximum:** 10 million units 3 times/wk.

Malignant Melanoma

IV: ADULTS: Initially, 20 million units/m² 5 times a wk for 4 wks. Maintenance: 10 million units subcutaneously 3 times a wk for 48 wks.

Follicular Lymphoma

SUBCUTANEOUS: ADULTS: 5 million units 3 times a wk for up to 18 mos.

SIDE EFFECTS

Frequent: Flu-like symptoms (fever, fatigue, headache, myalgia, anorexia, chills), rash (hairy cell leukemia, Kaposi's sarcoma only). **Pts with Kaposi's sarcoma:** All previously mentioned side effects plus depression, dyspepsia, dry mouth or thirst, alopecia, rigors. Occasional: Dizziness, pruritus, dry skin, dermatitis, altered taste. Rare: Confusion, leg cramps, back pain, gingivitis, flushing, tremor, anxiety, eye pain.

ADVERSE EFFECTS/ TOXIC REACTIONS

Hypersensitivity reactions occur rarely. Severe flu-like symptoms appear dose-related.

NURSING CONSIDERATIONS

BASELINE ASSESSMENT

CBC, platelet count, blood chemistries, urinalysis, renal/hepatic function tests, Hgb, Hct should be performed before initial therapy and routinely thereafter.

INTERVENTION/EVALUATION

Offer emotional support. Monitor all levels of clinical function (numerous side effects). Encourage ample fluid intake, particularly during early therapy. Monitor for worsening depression, suicidal ideation, associated behaviors.

PATIENT/FAMILY TEACHING

• Clinical response occurs in 1–3 mos. • Flu-like symptoms tend to diminish with continued therapy. • Some symptoms may be alleviated or minimized by bedtime doses. • Do not have immunizations without physician's approval (drug lowers resistance). • Avoid contact with those who have recently received live virus vaccine. • Avoid tasks that require alertness, motor skills until response to drug is established. • Sips of tepid water may relieve dry mouth. • Notify physician if depression, thoughts of suicide, unusual behavior occur.

interferon beta-1a

inn-ter-**fear**-on
(Avonex, Avonex Prefilled Syringe, Rebif)
Do not confuse interferon beta-1a with interferon beta-1b, or Avonex with Avelox.

◆CLASSIFICATION

PHARMACOTHERAPEUTIC: Biologic response modifier. **CLINICAL:** Multiple sclerosis agent.

ACTION

Interacts with specific cell receptors found on surface of cells. **Therapeutic Effect:** Produces antiviral, immunoregulatory effects.

PHARMACOKINETICS

Peak serum levels attained 3–15 hrs after IM administration. Biologic markers increase within 12 hrs and remain elevated for 4 days. **Half-life:** 10 hrs (Avonex); 69 hrs (Rebif).

USES

Treatment of relapsing multiple sclerosis to slow progression of physical disability, decrease frequency of clinical exacerbations.

PRECAUTIONS

Contraindications: **Avonex:** Hypersensitivity to natural or recombinant interferon beta, human albumin. **Rebif:** Hypersensitivity to natural or recombinant interferon, human albumin. **Cautions:** Chronic progressive multiple sclerosis, children younger than 18 yrs, depression.

LIFESPAN CONSIDERATIONS

Pregnancy/Lactation: Has abortifacient potential. Unknown if distributed in breast milk. **Pregnancy Category C.** **Children:** Safety and efficacy not established. **Elderly:** No information available.

I

INTERACTIONS

DRUG: **Alcohol, hepatotoxic drugs** may increase risk of hepatic injury. **Myelosuppressive drugs** may increase myelosuppressant effect. **HERBAL:** None significant. **FOOD:** None known. **LAB VALUES:** May increase serum glucose, BUN, alkaline phosphatase, bilirubin, calcium, AST, ALT. May decrease Hgb, neutrophil, platelet, WBC counts.

AVAILABILITY (Rx)

Injection, Powder for Reconstitution (Avonex): 30 mcg. **Injection Solution (Prefilled Syringe):** 22 mcg/ml (Rebif), 30 mcg/0.5 ml (Avonex Prefilled Syringe), 44 mcg/0.5 ml (Rebif). **Titration Pack (Prefilled Syringe [Rebif]):** 8.8 mcg/0.2 ml, 22 mcg/0.5 ml.

ADMINISTRATION/HANDLING

IM (Avonex) Syringe

• Refrigerate syringe. • Allow to warm to room temperature before use. • May store up to 7 days at room temperature.

IM (Avonex) Vial

• Refrigerate vials (may store at room temperature up to 30 days). • Following reconstitution, may refrigerate again but use within 6 hrs if refrigerated. • Reconstitute 30-mcg *MicroPin* (6.6 million international units) vial with 1.1 ml diluent (supplied by manufacturer). • Gently swirl to dissolve medication; do not shake. • Discard if discolored or particulate forms. • Discard unused portion (contains no preservative).

Subcutaneous (Rebif)

• Refrigerate. May store at room temperature up to 30 days. Avoid heat, light. • Administer at same time of day 3 days each wk. Separate doses by at least 48 hrs.

INDICATIONS/ROUTES/DOSAGE

Relapsing Multiple Sclerosis

IM (AVONEX): ADULTS: 30 mcg once weekly.

SUBCUTANEOUS (REBIF): ADULTS: **(Target dose 44 mcg 3 times a wk)** Initially, 8.8 mcg 3 times a wk for 8 wks, then 22 mcg 3 times a wk for 8 wks, then 44 mcg 3 times a wk thereafter. **(Target dose 22 mcg 3 times a wk)** Initially, 4.4 mcg 3 times a wk for 8 wks, then 11 mcg 3 times a wk for 8 wks, then 22 mcg 3 times a wk thereafter.

Dosage in Hepatic Impairment (Rebif)

Increased hepatic function test results, leukopenia: Decrease dose 20%–50% until toxicity resolves.

SIDE EFFECTS

Frequent: Headache (67%), flu-like symptoms (61%), myalgia (34%), upper respiratory tract infection (31%), depression with suicidal thoughts (25%), generalized pain (24%), asthenia (loss of strength, energy), chills (21%), sinusitis (18%), infection (11%). **Occasional:** Abdominal pain, arthralgia (9%), chest pain, dyspnea (6%), malaise, syncope (4%). **Rare:** Injection site reaction, hypersensitivity reaction (3%).

ADVERSE EFFECTS/ TOXIC REACTIONS

Anemia occurs in 8% of pts. Hepatic failure has been reported.

NURSING CONSIDERATIONS

BASELINE ASSESSMENT

Obtain Hgb, CBC, platelet count, blood chemistries including hepatic function tests. Assess home situation for support of therapy.

INTERVENTION/EVALUATION

Assess for headache, flu-like symptoms, myalgia. Periodically monitor lab results, reevaluate injection technique. Assess for depression, suicidal ideation.

PATIENT/FAMILY TEACHING

• Do not change schedule, dosage without consulting physician. • Follow guidelines for reconstitution of product and administration, including aseptic technique. • Use puncture-resistant container for used needles, syringes; dispose of used needles, syringes properly. • Injection site reactions may occur. These do not require discontinuation of therapy, but type and extent should be carefully noted.

interferon beta-1b

inn-ter-**fear**-on
(Betaseron, Extavia)
Do not confuse interferon beta-1b with interferon beta-1a.

◆CLASSIFICATION

PHARMACOTHERAPEUTIC: Biologic response modifier. **CLINICAL:** Multiple sclerosis agent.

ACTION

Interacts with specific cell receptors found on surface of cells. **Therapeutic Effect:** Produces antiviral, immunoregulatory effects.

PHARMACOKINETICS

Slowly absorbed following subcutaneous administration. **Half-life:** 8 min–4.3 hrs.

USES

Reduces frequency of clinical exacerbations in pts with relapsing-remitting multiple sclerosis (recurrent attacks of neurologic dysfunction). Treatment of early stages of multiple sclerosis.

PRECAUTIONS

Contraindications: Hypersensitivity to albumin, interferon. **Cautions:** Chronic progressive multiple sclerosis, children younger than 18 yrs.

⌛ LIFESPAN CONSIDERATIONS

Pregnancy/Lactation: Unknown if distributed in breast milk. **Pregnancy Category C. Children:** Safety and efficacy not established. **Elderly:** No information available.

INTERACTIONS

DRUG: None significant. **HERBAL:** None significant. **FOOD:** None known. **LAB VALUES:** May increase bilirubin, AST, ALT. May decrease neutrophil, lymphocyte, WBC counts.

AVAILABILITY (Rx)

Injection, Powder for Reconstitution: 0.3 mg (9.6 million units).

ADMINISTRATION/HANDLING

Subcutaneous

• Store vials at room temperature. • After reconstitution, stable for 3 hrs if refrigerated. • Use within 3 hrs of reconstitution. • Discard if discolored or precipitate forms. • Reconstitute 0.3-mg (9.6 million international units) vial with 1.2 ml diluent (supplied by manufacturer) to provide concentration of 0.25 mg/ml (8 million units/ml). • Gently swirl to dissolve medication; do not shake. • Discard if discolored or particulate forms. • Withdraw 1 ml solution and inject subcutaneous into arms, abdomen, hips, thighs using 27-gauge needle. • Discard unused portion (contains no preservative).

INDICATIONS/ROUTES/DOSAGE

Relapsing-Remitting Multiple Sclerosis
SUBCUTANEOUS: ADULTS: Initially, 0.0625 mg (2 million units) every other day; gradually increase by 0.0625 mg every 2 weeks. Target dose: 0.25 mg (8 million units) every other day.

SIDE EFFECTS

Frequent: Injection site reaction (85%), headache (84%), flu-like symptoms (76%), fever (59%), asthenia (loss of strength, energy) (49%), myalgia (44%), sinusitis (36%), diarrhea, dizziness (35%), altered mental status (29%), constipation (24%), diaphoresis (23%), vomiting (21%). **Occasional:** Malaise (15%), drowsiness (6%), alopecia (4%).

ADVERSE EFFECTS/ TOXIC REACTIONS

Seizures occur rarely.

NURSING CONSIDERATIONS

BASELINE ASSESSMENT

Obtain Hgb, CBC, platelet count, blood chemistries (including hepatic function tests). Assess home situation for support of therapy.

INTERVENTION/EVALUATION

Periodically monitor lab results, reevaluate injection technique. Assess for nausea (high incidence). Monitor sleep pattern. Monitor daily pattern of bowel activity, stool consistency. Assist with ambulation if dizziness occurs. Monitor food intake.

PATIENT/FAMILY TEACHING

• Inform physician of flu-like symptoms (occur commonly but decrease over time). • Wear sunscreen, protective clothing if exposed to sunlight, ultraviolet light until tolerance known.

interferon gamma-1b

inn-ter-**fear**-on
(Actimmune)

◆CLASSIFICATION

PHARMACOTHERAPEUTIC: Biologic response modifier. **CLINICAL:** Immunologic agent.

ACTION

Induces activation of macrophages in blood monocytes to phagocytes (necessary in cellular immune response to intracellular, extracellular pathogens). Enhances phagocytic function, antimicrobial activity of monocytes. **Therapeutic Effect:** Decreases signs/symptoms of serious infections in chronic granulomatous disease.

PHARMACOKINETICS

Slowly absorbed after subcutaneous administration. **Half-life:** 3–6 hrs.

USES

Reduces frequency, severity of serious infections due to chronic granulomatous disease. Delays time to disease progression in pts with severe, malignant osteopetrosis.

PRECAUTIONS

Contraindications: Hypersensitivity to *Escherichia coli*-derived products. **Cautions:** Seizure disorders, compromised CNS function, preexisting cardiac disease (e.g., ischemia, CHF, arrhythmias), myelosuppression.

⌛ LIFESPAN CONSIDERATIONS

Pregnancy/Lactation: Unknown if drug crosses placenta or is distributed in breast milk. **Pregnancy Category C. Children:** Safety and efficacy not established in those younger than 1 yr. Flu-like symptoms may occur more frequently. **Elderly:** No information available.

INTERACTIONS

DRUG: Bone marrow depressants may increase myelosuppression. **HERBAL:** None significant. **FOOD:** None known. **LAB VALUES:** May increase ALT, AST, alkaline phosphatase, LDH, triglycerides, cortisol concentrations. May decrease leukocytes, neutrophils, platelets.

AVAILABILITY (Rx)

Injection Solution: 100 mcg (2 million units).

ADMINISTRATION/HANDLING

◀ALERT▶ Avoid excessive agitation of vial; do not shake.

Subcutaneous

• Refrigerate vials. Do not freeze. • Do not keep at room temperature for more than 12 hrs; discard after 12 hrs. • Vials are single dose; discard unused portion. • Solution is clear, colorless. Do not use if discolored or precipitate forms. • When given 3 times a wk, rotate injection sites.

INDICATIONS/ROUTES/DOSAGE

Chronic Granulomatous Disease; Severe, Malignant Osteopetrosis

SUBCUTANEOUS: ADULTS, ELDERLY, CHILDREN OLDER THAN 1 YR: 50 mcg/m² (1 million units/m²) in pts with body surface area (BSA) greater than 0.5 m²; 1.5 mcg/kg/dose in pts with BSA 0.5 m² or less. Give 3 times a wk.

SIDE EFFECTS

Frequent: Fever (52%), headache (33%), rash (17%), chills, fatigue, diarrhea (14%). **Occasional (13%–10%):** Vomiting, nausea. **Rare (6%–3%):** Weight loss, myalgia, anorexia.

ADVERSE EFFECTS/ TOXIC REACTIONS

May exacerbate preexisting CNS dysfunction (manifested as decreased mental status, gait disturbance, dizziness), cardiac abnormalities.

NURSING CONSIDERATIONS

BASELINE ASSESSMENT

CBC, platelet count, blood chemistries, urinalysis, renal/hepatic function tests should be performed before initial therapy and at 3-mo intervals during course of treatment.

INTERVENTION/EVALUATION

Monitor for flu-like symptoms (fever, chills, fatigue, myalgia). Assess skin for evidence of rash.

PATIENT/FAMILY TEACHING

• Flu-like symptoms (fever, chills, fatigue, muscle aches) are generally mild and tend to disappear as treatment continues. Symptoms may be minimized with bedtime administration. • Avoid tasks that require alertness, motor skills until response to drug is established. • If home use prescribed, follow guidelines for proper technique of administration; care in proper disposal of needles, syringes. • Vials should remain refrigerated.

I

interleukin-2 (aldesleukin)

HIGH ALERT

in-ter-**loo**-kin
(IL-2, Proleukin)

BLACK BOX ALERT High-dose therapy is associated with capillary leak syndrome resulting in significant hypotension and reduced organ perfusion. Use restricted to pts with normal cardiac/pulmonary function. Increased risk of disseminated infection (sepsis, bacterial endocarditis). Withhold treatment for pts developing moderate-to-severe lethargy or drowsiness (continued treatment may result in coma). Must be administered by personnel trained in administration/handling of chemotherapeutic agents.

Do not confuse aldesleukin with oprelvekin.

CLASSIFICATION

PHARMACOTHERAPEUTIC: Biologic response modifier. **CLINICAL:** Antineoplastic (see p. 79C).

ACTION

Promotes proliferation, differentiation, recruitment of T and B cells, lymphokine-activated and natural killer cells, thymocytes. **Therapeutic Effect:** Enhances cytolytic activity in lymphocytes.

PHARMACOKINETICS

Primarily distributed into plasma, lymphocytes, lungs, liver, kidney, spleen. Metabolized to amino acids in cells lining the kidneys. **Half-life:** 80–120 min.

USES

Treatment of metastatic renal cell carcinoma, metastatic melanoma. **OFF-LABEL:** Treatment of colorectal cancer, Kaposi's sarcoma, non-Hodgkin's lymphoma, multiple myeloma, HIV/AIDS.

PRECAUTIONS

Contraindications: Abnormal pulmonary function or thallium stress test results, bowel ischemia or perforation, coma or toxic psychosis lasting longer than 48 hrs, GI bleeding requiring surgery, intubation lasting more than 72 hrs, organ allografts, pericardial tamponade, renal dysfunction requiring dialysis for longer than 72 hrs, repetitive or difficult-to-control seizures; re-treatment in those who experience any of the following toxicities: angina, MI, recurrent chest pain with EKG changes, sustained ventricular tachycardia, uncontrolled or unresponsive cardiac rhythm disturbances. **Extreme Caution:** Pts with normal thallium stress tests and pulmonary function tests who have history of cardiac or pulmonary disease. **Cautions:** Pts with fixed requirements for large volumes of fluid (e.g., those with hypercalcemia), history of seizures.

LIFESPAN CONSIDERATIONS

Pregnancy/Lactation: Avoid use in those of either sex not practicing effective contraception. **Pregnancy Category C.** **Children:** Safety and efficacy not established. **Elderly:** Age-related renal impairment may require dosage adjustment; will not tolerate toxicity.

INTERACTIONS

DRUG: **Antihypertensives** may increase hypotensive effect. **Cardiotoxic, hepatotoxic, myelotoxic, nephrotoxic medications** may increase risk of toxicity. **Glucocorticoids** may decrease effects. **HERBAL:** None significant. **FOOD:** None known. **LAB VALUES:** May increase BUN, serum alkaline phosphatase, bilirubin, creatinine, AST, ALT. May decrease serum calcium, magnesium, phosphorus, potassium, sodium.

AVAILABILITY (Rx)

Injection, Powder for Reconstitution (Proleukin): 22 million units (1.3 mg) (18 million units/ml when reconstituted).

ADMINISTRATION/HANDLING

◀ALERT▶ Hold administration in pts who develop moderate to severe lethargy or drowsiness (continued administration may result in coma).

IV

Reconstitution • Reconstitute 22 million units vial with 1.2 ml Sterile Water for Injection to provide concentration of 18 million units/ml. Bacteriostatic Water for Injection or NaCl should not be used to reconstitute because of increased aggregation. • During reconstitution, direct Sterile Water for Injection at the side of vial. Swirl contents gently to avoid foaming. Do not shake.

Rate of administration • Further dilute dose in D_5W to a final concentration between 0.49 and 1.1 million international units/ml and infuse over 15 min. Do not use an in-line filter. • Solution should be warmed to room temperature before infusion. • Monitor diligently for drop in mean arterial B/P (sign of capillary leak syndrome [CLS]). Continued treatment may result in significant hypotension (less than 90 mm Hg or a 20 mm Hg drop from baseline systolic pressure), edema, pleural effusion, altered mental status.

Storage • Refrigerate vials; do not freeze. • Reconstituted solution is stable for 48 hrs refrigerated or at room temperature (refrigeration preferred).

IV INCOMPATIBILITIES

Ganciclovir (Cytovene), pentamidine (Pentam), prochlorperazine (Compazine), promethazine (Phenergan).

IV COMPATIBILITIES

Calcium gluconate, dopamine (Intropin), heparin, lorazepam (Ativan), magnesium, potassium.

INDICATIONS/ROUTES/DOSAGE

Metastatic Melanoma, Metastatic Renal Cell Carcinoma

IV: ADULTS 18 YRS AND OLDER: 600,000 units/kg q8h for 14 doses; followed by 9 days of rest, then another 14 doses for a total of 28 doses per course. Course may be repeated after rest period of at least 7 wks from date of hospital discharge.

SIDE EFFECTS

Side effects are generally self-limiting and reversible within 2–3 days after discontinuing therapy. **Frequent (89%–48%):** Fever, chills, nausea, vomiting, hypotension, diarrhea, oliguria/anuria, altered mental status, irritability, confusion, depression, sinus tachycardia, pain (abdominal, chest, back), fatigue, dyspnea, pruritus. **Occasional (47%–17%):** Edema, erythema, rash, stomatitis, anorexia, weight gain, infection (UTI, injection site, catheter tip), dizziness. **Rare (15%–4%):** Dry skin, sensory disorders (vision, speech, taste), dermatitis, headache, arthralgia, myalgia, weight loss, hematuria, conjunctivitis, proteinuria.

ADVERSE EFFECTS/ TOXIC REACTIONS

Anemia, thrombocytopenia, leukopenia occur commonly. GI bleeding, pulmonary edema occur occasionally. Capillary leak syndrome (CLS) results in hypotension (systolic pressure less than 90 mm Hg or a 20 mm Hg drop from baseline systolic pressure), extravasation of plasma proteins and fluid into extravascular space, loss of vascular tone. May result in cardiac arrhythmias, angina, MI, respiratory insufficiency. Fatal malignant hyperthermia, cardiac arrest, CVA, pulmonary emboli, bowel perforation/gangrene, severe depression leading to suicide occur in less than 1% of pts.

NURSING CONSIDERATIONS

BASELINE ASSESSMENT

Pts with bacterial infection and with indwelling central lines should be treated with antibiotic therapy before treatment begins. All pts should be neurologically stable with a negative CT scan before treatment begins. CBC, blood chemistries (including electrolytes), renal/hepatic function tests, chest X-ray should be performed before therapy begins and daily thereafter.

INTERVENTION/EVALUATION

Monitor CBC with differential, platelets, electrolytes, renal/hepatic function tests, weight, pulse oximetry. Determine serum amylase frequently during therapy. Discontinue medication at first sign of hypotension and hold for moderate to severe lethargy (physician must decide whether therapy should continue). Assess altered mental status (irritability, confusion, depression), weight gain/loss. Maintain strict I&O. Assess for extravascular fluid accumulation (rales in lungs, edema in dependent areas).

PATIENT/FAMILY TEACHING

• Nausea may decrease during therapy. • At home, increase fluid intake (protects against renal impairment). • Do not have immunizations without physician's approval (drug lowers resistance). • Avoid exposure to persons with infection. • Contact physician if fever, chills, lower back pain, difficulty with urination, unusual bleeding/bruising, black tarry stools, blood in urine, petechial rash (pinpoint red spots on skin) occur. • Report symptoms of depression or suicidal ideation immediately.

I

Invanz, *see ertapenem*

ipratropium

ih-prah-**trow**-pea-um
(Apo-Ipravent ✱, Atrovent, Atrovent HFA, Novo-Ipramide ✱, Nu-Ipratropium ✱, PMS-Ipratropium ✱)
Do not confuse Atrovent with Alupent or Serevent, or ipratropium with tiotropium.

FIXED-COMBINATION(S)

Combivent, DuoNeb: ipratropium/albuterol (a bronchodilator): *Aerosol:* 18 mcg/90 mcg per actuation. *Solution:* 0.5 mg/2.5 mg per 3 ml.

◆CLASSIFICATION

PHARMACOTHERAPEUTIC: Anticholinergic. **CLINICAL:** Bronchodilator.

ACTION

Blocks action of acetylcholine at parasympathetic sites in bronchial smooth muscle. **Therapeutic Effect:** Causes bronchodilation, inhibits nasal secretions.

PHARMACOKINETICS

Route	Onset	Peak	Duration
Inhalation	1–3 min	1.5–2 hrs	Up to 4 hrs
Nasal	5 min	1–4 hrs	4–8 hrs

Minimal systemic absorption after inhalation. Metabolized in liver (systemic absorption). Primarily eliminated in feces. **Half-life:** 1.5–4 hrs (nasal).

USES

Inhalation, Nebulization: Maintenance treatment of bronchospasm due to COPD, bronchitis, emphysema, asthma. Not to be used for immediate bronchospasm relief. **Nasal Spray:** Symptomatic relief of rhinorrhea associated with the common cold and allergic and nonallergic rhinitis.

PRECAUTIONS

Contraindications: History of hypersensitivity to atropine. **Cautions:** Narrow-angle glaucoma, prostatic hypertrophy, bladder neck obstruction.

⌛ LIFESPAN CONSIDERATIONS

Pregnancy/Lactation: Unknown if distributed in breast milk. **Pregnancy Category B. Children/Elderly:** No age-related precautions noted.

INTERACTIONS

DRUG: Anticholinergics, medications with anticholinergic properties may increase toxicity. **HERBAL:** None significant. **FOOD:** None known. **LAB VALUES:** None known.

AVAILABILITY (Rx)

Aerosol for Oral Inhalation: (Atrovent HFA): 17 mcg/actuation. **Solution, Intranasal Spray:** 0.03%; 0.06%. **Solution for Nebulization:** 0.02% (500 mcg).

ADMINISTRATION/HANDLING

Inhalation

• Shake container well. • Instruct pt to exhale completely, place mouthpiece between lips, inhale deeply through mouth while fully depressing top of canister. Hold breath as long as possible before exhaling slowly. • Allow at least 1 minute between inhalations. • Rinse mouth with water immediately after inhalation (prevents mouth/throat dryness).

Nebulization

• May be administered with or without dilution in 0.9% NaCl. • Stable for 1 hr when mixed with albuterol. • Give over 5–15 min.

Nasal

• Store at room temperature. • Initial pump priming requires 7 actuations of pump. • If used regularly as recommended, no further priming is required. If not used for more than 4 hrs, pump will require 2 actuations, or if not used for more than 7 days, the pump will require 7 actuations to reprime.

INDICATIONS/ROUTES/DOSAGE

Bronchodilator for COPD

INHALATION: ADULTS, ELDERLY, CHILDREN OLDER THAN 12 YRS: 2 inhalations 4 times a day. **Maximum:** 12 inhalations/day.
NEBULIZATION: ADULTS, ELDERLY, CHILDREN OLDER THAN 12 YRS: 500 mcg (one unit dose vial) 3–4 times a day.

Asthma Exacerbation

INHALATION: ADULTS, ELDERLY, CHILDREN OLDER THAN 12 YRS: 8 inhalations q20min as needed for up to 3 hrs. **CHILDREN 12 YRS OR LESS:** 4–8 inhalations q20min as needed for up to 3 hrs.
NEBULIZATION: ADULTS, ELDERLY, CHILDREN OLDER THAN 12 YRS: 500 mcg q20min for 3 doses, then as needed. **CHILDREN 12 YRS OR LESS:** 250–500 mg q20min for 3 doses, then as needed.

Rhinorrhea (Perennial Allergic/ Nonallergic Rhinitis)

INTRANASAL (0.03%): ADULTS, ELDERLY, CHILDREN 6 YRS AND OLDER: 2 sprays per nostril 2–3 times a day.

Rhinorrhea (Common Cold)

INTRANASAL (0.06%): ADULTS, ELDERLY, CHILDREN 12 YRS AND OLDER: 2 sprays per nostril 3–4 times a day for up to 4 days. **CHILDREN 5–11 YRS:** 2 sprays per nostril 3 times a day for up to 4 days.

Rhinorrhea (Seasonal Allergy)

INTRANASAL (0.06%): ADULTS, ELDERLY, CHILDREN 5 YRS AND OLDER: 2 sprays per nostril 4 times a day for up to 3 wks.

SIDE EFFECTS

Frequent: **Inhalation (6%–3%):** Cough, dry mouth, headache, nausea. **Nasal:** Dry nose/mouth, headache, nasal irritation. Occasional: **Inhalation (2%):** Dizziness, transient increased bronchospasm. Rare (less than 1%): **Inhalation:** Hypotension, insomnia, metallic/unpleasant taste, palpitations, urinary retention. **Nasal:** Diarrhea, constipation, dry throat, abdominal pain, nasal congestion.

ADVERSE EFFECTS/ TOXIC REACTIONS

Worsening of angle-closure glaucoma, acute eye pain, hypotension occur rarely.

NURSING CONSIDERATIONS

BASELINE ASSESSMENT

Offer emotional support (high incidence of anxiety due to difficulty in breathing, sympathomimetic response to drug).

INTERVENTION/EVALUATION

Monitor rate, depth, rhythm, type of respiration; quality, rate of pulse. Assess lung sounds for rhonchi, wheezing, rales. Monitor ABGs. Observe lips, fingernails for cyanosis (blue or dusky color in light-skinned pts; gray in dark-skinned pts). Observe for retractions (clavicular, sternal, intercostal), hand tremor. Evaluate for clinical improvement (quieter, slower respirations, relaxed facial expression, cessation of retractions). Monitor for improvement of rhinorrhea.

PATIENT/ FAMILY TEACHING

• Increase fluid intake (decreases lung secretion viscosity). • Do not take more than 2 inhalations at any one time (excessive use may produce paradoxical bronchoconstriction, decreased bronchodilating effect). • Rinsing mouth with water immediately after inhalation may prevent mouth and throat dryness. • Avoid excessive use of caffeine derivatives (chocolate, coffee, tea, cola, cocoa).

irbesartan

ir-beh-**sar**-tan
(Avapro)

BLACK BOX ALERT May cause fetal injury, mortality if used during second or third trimester of pregnancy.

Do not confuse Avapro with Anaprox.

FIXED-COMBINATION(S)

Avalide: irbesartan/hydrochlorothiazide (a diuretic): 150 mg/12.5 mg, 300 mg/12.5 mg, 300 mg/25 mg.

◆CLASSIFICATION

PHARMACOTHERAPEUTIC: Angiotensin II receptor antagonist. **CLINICAL:** Antihypertensive (see p. 10C).

ACTION

Blocks vasoconstrictor, aldosterone-secreting effects of angiotensin II, inhibiting binding of angiotensin II to AT_1 receptors. **Therapeutic Effect:** Produces vasodilation, decreases peripheral resistance, decreases B/P.

PHARMACOKINETICS

Route	Onset	Peak	Duration
PO	–	1–2 hrs	Greater than 24 hrs

Rapidly, completely absorbed after PO administration. Protein binding: 90%. Undergoes hepatic metabolism to inactive metabolite. Recovered primarily in feces and, to a lesser extent, in urine. Not removed by hemodialysis. **Half-life:** 11–15 hrs.

USES

Treatment of hypertension alone or in combination with other antihypertensives. Treatment of diabetic nephropathy. **OFF-LABEL:** Treatment of atrial fibrillation, slow rate of progression of aortic root dilation in children with Marfan's syndrome.

PRECAUTIONS

Contraindications: Bilateral renal artery stenosis, biliary cirrhosis/obstruction, primary hyperaldosteronism, severe hepatic insufficiency. **Cautions:** Mild to moderate hepatic dysfunction, sodium/water depletion, CHF, unilateral renal artery stenosis, coronary artery disease.

⧖ LIFESPAN CONSIDERATIONS

Pregnancy/Lactation: Unknown if distributed in breast milk. May cause fetal or neonatal morbidity or mortality. **Pregnancy Category C (D if used in second or third trimester). Children:** Safety and efficacy not established. **Elderly:** No age-related precautions noted.

INTERACTIONS

DRUG: Diuretics produce additive hypotensive effects. **HERBAL: Ephedra, ginseng, yohimbe** may worsen hypertension. **Garlic** may increase antihypertensive effect. **FOOD:** None known. **LAB VALUES:** May slightly increase BUN, serum creatinine. May decrease Hgb.

AVAILABILITY (Rx)

Tablets: 75 mg, 150 mg, 300 mg.

ADMINISTRATION/HANDLING

PO

- Give without regard to meals.

INDICATIONS/ROUTES/DOSAGE

Hypertension

PO: ADULTS, ELDERLY, CHILDREN 13 YRS AND OLDER: Initially, 75–150 mg/day. May increase to 300 mg/day. **CHILDREN 6–12 YRS:** Initially, 75 mg/day. May increase to 150 mg/day.

Nephropathy

PO: ADULTS, ELDERLY: 300 mg once daily.

SIDE EFFECTS

Occasional (9%–3%): Upper respiratory tract infection, fatigue, diarrhea, cough. **Rare (2%–1%):** Heartburn, dizziness, headache, nausea, rash.

ADVERSE EFFECTS/ TOXIC REACTIONS

Overdose may manifest as hypotension, tachycardia. Bradycardia occurs less often.

NURSING CONSIDERATIONS

BASELINE ASSESSMENT

Obtain B/P, apical pulse immediately before each dose, in addition to regular monitoring (be alert to fluctuations). If excessive reduction in B/P occurs, place pt in supine position, feet slightly elevated. Question possibility of pregnancy (see Pregnancy Category). Assess medication history (esp. diuretic therapy).

INTERVENTION/EVALUATION

Maintain hydration (offer fluids frequently). Assess for evidence of upper respiratory infection. Assist with ambulation if dizziness occurs. Monitor electrolytes, renal/hepatic function tests, urinalysis, B/P, pulse. Assess for hypotension.

PATIENT/ FAMILY TEACHING

• Irbesartan may cause fetal or neonatal morbidity or mortality. • Avoid tasks that require alertness, motor skills until response to drug is established (possible dizziness effect). • Report any sign of infection (sore throat, fever). • Avoid exercising during hot weather (risk of dehydration, hypotension).

irinotecan

eye-rin-**oh**-teh-can
(Camptosar)

BLACK BOX ALERT Can induce both early and late forms of severe diarrhea. Early diarrhea (during or shortly after administration) accompanied by salivation, rhinitis, lacrimation, diaphoresis, flushing. Late diarrhea (occurring more than 24 hrs after administration) can be prolonged and life-threatening. May produce severe, profound myelosuppression.

◆ CLASSIFICATION

PHARMACOTHERAPEUTIC: DNA topoisomerase inhibitor. **CLINICAL:** Antineoplastic (see p. 85C).

ACTION

Interacts with topoisomerase I, an enzyme that relieves torsional strain in DNA by inducing reversible single-strand breaks. Prevents religation of these single-stranded breaks resulting in damage to double-strand DNA, cell death. **Therapeutic Effect:** Produces cytotoxic effect on cancer cells.

PHARMACOKINETICS

Metabolized to active metabolite in liver after IV administration. Protein binding: 95% (metabolite). Excreted in urine and eliminated by biliary route. **Half-life:** 6–12 hrs; metabolite, 10–20 hrs.

USES

Treatment of metastatic carcinoma of colon, rectum in pts whose disease has recurred or progressed after 5-fluorouracil-based therapy. **OFF-LABEL:** Non–small-cell lung cancer, refractory solid tumor configuration, untreated rhabdomyosarcoma, cervical, gastric, pancreatic, breast cancer, leukemia, lymphoma, brain tumor.

PRECAUTIONS

Contraindications: None known. **Cautions:** Pt previously receiving pelvic, abdominal irradiation (increased risk of myelosuppression), elderly older than 65 yrs.

⌛ LIFESPAN CONSIDERATIONS

Pregnancy/Lactation: May cause fetal harm. Unknown if distributed in breast milk. Breast-feeding not recommended. **Pregnancy Category D. Children:** Safety and efficacy not established. **Elderly:** Risk of diarrhea significantly increased.

INTERACTIONS

DRUG: Diuretics may increase risk of dehydration (due to vomiting, diarrhea associated with irinotecan therapy). **Laxatives** may increase severity of diarrhea. **Immunosuppressants (e.g., cyclosporine, tacrolimus)** may increase risk of infection. **Live virus vaccines** may potentiate virus replication, increase vaccine side effects, decrease pt's antibody response to vaccine. **Other bone marrow depressants** may increase risk of myelosuppression. **HERBAL: St. John's wort** may decrease irinotecan effectiveness. **FOOD:** None known. **LAB**

VALUES: May increase serum alkaline phosphatase, AST. May decrease Hgb, leukocytes, platelets.

AVAILABILITY (Rx)

Injection Solution: 20 mg/ml (2 ml, 5 ml, 25 ml).

ADMINISTRATION/HANDLING

IV

Reconstitution • Dilute in D_5W (preferred) or 0.9% NaCl to concentration of 0.12–2.8 mg/ml.
Rate of administration • Administer all doses as IV infusion over 30–90 min. • Assess for extravasation (flush site with Sterile Water for Injection, apply ice if extravasation occurs).
Storage • Store vials at room temperature, protect from light. • Solution diluted with D_5W is stable for 24 hrs at room temperature or 48 hrs if refrigerated. • Solution diluted with 0.9% NaCl is stable for 24 hrs at room temperature. • Do not refrigerate solution if diluted with 0.9% NaCl.

IV INCOMPATIBILITY

Gemcitabine (Gemzar).

INDICATIONS/ROUTES/DOSAGE

Carcinoma of the Colon, Rectum
IV: ADULTS, ELDERLY: (WEEKLY REGIMEN): Initially, 125 mg/m^2 once weekly for 4 wks, followed by a rest period of 2 wks. Additional courses may be repeated q6wks. Dosage may be adjusted in 25–50 mg/m^2 increments to as high as 150 mg/m^2 or as low as 50 mg/m^2. **(THREE-WEEK REGIMEN):** 350 mg/m^2 q3wks.

SIDE EFFECTS

Expected: Nausea (64%), alopecia (49%), vomiting (45%), diarrhea (32%). **Frequent:** Constipation, fatigue (29%); fever (28%); asthenia (loss of strength, energy) (25%); skeletal pain (23%); abdominal pain, dyspnea (22%). **Occasional:** Anorexia (19%); headache, stomatitis (18%); rash (16%).

ADVERSE EFFECTS/ TOXIC REACTIONS

Myelosuppression characterized as neutropenia occurs in 97% of pts; neutrophil count less than 50/mm^3 occurs in 78% of pts. Thrombocytopenia, anemia, sepsis occur frequently.

NURSING CONSIDERATIONS

BASELINE ASSESSMENT

Offer emotional support to pt, family. Assess hydration status, electrolytes, CBC before each dose. Premedicate with antiemetics on day of treatment, starting at least 30 min before administration.

INTERVENTION/EVALUATION

Assess for early signs of diarrhea (preceded by complaints of diaphoresis, abdominal cramping). Monitor hydration status, I&O, electrolytes, CBC, Hgb, platelets, renal/hepatic function tests. Monitor infusion site for signs of inflammation. Inform pt of possibility of alopecia. Assess skin for rash.

PATIENT/ FAMILY TEACHING

• Notify physician if diarrhea, vomiting, fever, light-headedness, dizziness occur. • Do not have immunizations without physician's approval (drug lowers resistance). • Avoid contact with those who have recently received live virus vaccine. • Avoid crowds, those with infections.

iron dextran

iron **dex**-tran
(DexFerrum, Dexiron ✱, Infed, Infufer ✱)

BLACK BOX ALERT Potentially fatal anaphylactic-type reaction has been associated with parenteral administration.

Do not confuse DexFerrum with Desferal, or iron dextran with iron sucrose.

◆CLASSIFICATION

PHARMACOTHERAPEUTIC: Trace element. **CLINICAL:** Hematinic iron preparation.

ACTION

Essential component in formation of Hgb. Necessary for effective erythropoiesis, transport and utilization of oxygen. Serves as cofactor of several essential enzymes. **Therapeutic Effect:** Replenishes Hgb, depleted iron stores.

PHARMACOKINETICS

Readily absorbed after IM administration. Most absorption occurs within 72 hrs; remainder within 3–4 wks. Bound to protein to form hemosiderin, ferritin, or transferrin. No physiologic system of elimination. Small amounts lost daily in shedding of skin, hair, nails and in feces, urine, perspiration. **Half-life:** 5–20 hrs.

USES

Treatment of anemia, iron deficiency. Use only when PO administration is not feasible or when rapid replenishment of iron is warranted.

PRECAUTIONS

Contraindications: All anemias except iron deficiency anemia (pernicious, aplastic, normocytic, refractory). **Extreme Caution:** Serious hepatic impairment. **Cautions:** History of allergies, bronchial asthma, rheumatoid arthritis.

LIFESPAN CONSIDERATIONS

Pregnancy/Lactation: May cross placenta in some form (unknown). Trace distributed in breast milk. **Pregnancy Category C. Children/Elderly:** No age-related precautions noted.

INTERACTIONS

DRUG: None significant. **HERBAL:** None significant. **FOOD:** None known. **LAB VALUES:** None significant.

AVAILABILITY (Rx)

Injection Solution (DexFerrum, Infed): 50 mg/ml.

ADMINISTRATION/HANDLING

◀ALERT▶ Test dose is generally given before full dosage; monitor pt for several min after injection due to potential for anaphylactic reaction.

IV

Reconstitution • May give undiluted or dilute in 250–1,000 ml 0.9% NaCl for infusion. • Avoid dilution in dextrose (increased pain/phlebitis).

Rate of administration • Do not exceed IV administration rate of 50 mg/min (1 ml/min). Too-rapid IV rate may produce flushing, chest pain, hypotension, tachycardia, shock. • Infuse diluted solution over 1–6 hrs. • Pt must remain recumbent 30–45 min after IV administration (minimizes postural hypotension).

Storage • Store at room temperature.

IM

• Draw up medication with one needle; use new needle for injection (minimizes skin staining). • Administer deep IM in upper outer quadrant of buttock only. • Use Z-tract technique (displacement of subcutaneous tissue lateral to injection site before inserting needle) to minimize skin staining.

IV INCOMPATIBILITIES

Do not mix with other medications, TPN solutions.

INDICATIONS/ROUTES/DOSAGE

0.5-ml test dose (0.25 ml in infants). Give prior to initiating iron dextran therapy.

◀ALERT▶ Discontinue oral iron preparations before administering iron dextran. Dosage expressed in terms of milligrams of elemental iron. Dosage individualized based on degree of anemia, pt weight, presence of any bleeding. Use periodic hematologic determinations as guide to therapy.

◀ALERT▶ Not normally given in first 4 mos of life.

Iron Deficiency Anemia

IV, IM: ADULTS, ELDERLY, CHILDREN WEIGHING MORE THAN 15 KG: Dose in ml (50 mg elemental iron/ml) = 0.0442 (desired Hgb less observed Hgb) × lean body weight (in kg) + (0.26 × lean body weight). Give 2 ml or less once daily until total dose reached. **CHILDREN WEIGHING 5–15 KG:** Dose in ml (50 mg elemental iron/ml) = 0.0442 (desired Hgb less observed Hgb) × body weight (in kg) + (0.26 × body weight). Give 2 ml or less once daily until total dose reached.

Maximum Daily Dosages

ADULTS WEIGHING MORE THAN 50 KG: 100 mg. **CHILDREN WEIGHING MORE THAN 15 KG:** 100 mg. **CHILDREN WEIGHING 5–15 KG:** 50 mg. **CHILDREN WEIGHING LESS THAN 5 KG:** 25 mg.

SIDE EFFECTS

Frequent: Allergic reaction (rash, pruritus), backache, myalgia, chills, dizziness, headache, fever, nausea, vomiting, flushed skin, pain/redness at injection site, brown discoloration of skin, metallic taste.

ADVERSE EFFECTS/ TOXIC REACTIONS

Anaphylaxis occurs rarely in first few min following injection. Leukocytosis, lymphadenopathy occur rarely.

NURSING CONSIDERATIONS

BASELINE ASSESSMENT

Do not give concurrently with oral iron form (excessive iron may produce excessive iron storage [hemosiderosis]). Be alert to pts with rheumatoid arthritis (RA), iron deficiency anemia (acute exacerbation of joint pain, swelling may occur). Inguinal lymphadenopathy may occur with IM injection. Assess for adequate muscle mass before injecting medication.

INTERVENTION/EVALUATION

Monitor IM site for abscess formation, necrosis, atrophy, swelling, brownish color of skin. Question pt regarding soreness, pain, inflammation at/near IM injection site. Check IV site for phlebitis. Monitor serum ferritin.

PATIENT/FAMILY TEACHING

• Pain, brown staining may occur at injection site. • Oral iron should not be taken when receiving iron injections. • Stools often become black with iron therapy but is harmless unless accompanied by red streaking, sticky consistency of stool, abdominal pain/cramping, which should be reported to physician. • Oral hygiene, hard candy, gum may reduce metallic taste. • Notify physician immediately if fever, back pain, headache occur.

iron sucrose

iron **soo**-krose
(Venofer)
Do not confuse iron sucrose with iron dextran.

◆CLASSIFICATION

PHARMACOTHERAPEUTIC: Trace element. **CLINICAL:** Hematinic iron preparation.

ACTION

Essential component in formation of Hgb. Necessary for effective erythropoiesis, transport and utilization of oxygen. Serves as cofactor of several essential enzymes. **Therapeutic Effect:** Replenishes body iron stores in pts on chronic hemodialysis who have iron deficiency anemia and are receiving erythropoietin.

PHARMACOKINETICS

Distributed mainly in blood and to some extent in extravascular fluid. Iron sucrose is dissociated into iron and sucrose by reticuloendothelial system. Sucrose component is eliminated mainly by urinary excretion. **Half-life:** 6 hrs.

USES

Treatment of iron deficiency anemia in pts undergoing chronic hemodialysis or peritoneal dialysis who are receiving supplemental erythropoietin therapy. Treatment of iron deficiency anemia in pts with chronic kidney disease who are not undergoing dialysis (with or without erythropoietin therapy). **OFF-LABEL:** Treatment of dystrophic epidermolysis bullosa.

PRECAUTIONS

Contraindications: All anemias except iron deficiency anemia (pernicious, aplastic, normocytic, refractory anemia), evidence of iron overload. **Cautions:** History of allergies, bronchial asthma; hepatic/renal/cardiac dysfunction.

LIFESPAN CONSIDERATIONS

Pregnancy/Lactation: Unknown if drug crosses placenta or is distributed in breast milk. **Pregnancy Category B. Children:** Safety and efficacy not established. **Elderly:** Age-related renal impairment may require dosage adjustment.

INTERACTIONS

DRUG: None significant. **HERBAL:** None significant. **FOOD:** None known. **LAB VALUES:** Increases Hgb, Hct, serum ferritin, transferrin.

AVAILABILITY (Rx)

Injection Solution: 20 mg of elemental iron/ml in 5-ml, 10-ml vials.

ADMINISTRATION/HANDLING

◀ALERT▶ Administer directly into dialysis line during hemodialysis.

IV

Reconstitution • May give undiluted as slow IV injection or IV infusion. For IV infusion, dilute each vial in maximum of 100 ml 0.9% NaCl immediately before infusion. • Dilute large doses in maximum of 250 ml 0.9% NaCl.

Rate of administration • For IV injection, administer 100–200 mg (5–10 ml) over 2–5 min. • For IV infusion, administer 100 mg over at least 15 min; 300 mg over 1.5 hrs; 400 mg over 2.5 hrs; 500 mg over 3.5 hrs.

Storage • Store at room temperature. • Following dilution, stable for 48 hrs at room temperature or if refrigerated.

IV INCOMPATIBILITIES

Do not mix with other medications or add to parenteral nutrition solution for IV infusion.

INDICATIONS/ROUTES/DOSAGE

Iron Deficiency Anemia

Dosage is expressed in terms of milligrams of elemental iron.

IV: ADULTS, ELDERLY (HEMODIALYSIS-DEPENDENT PTS): 5 ml iron sucrose (100 mg elemental iron) delivered during dialysis; administer 1–3 times a wk to total dose of 1,000 mg in 10 doses. Give no more than 3 times a wk. **(PERITONEAL DIALYSIS-DEPENDENT PTS):** 300 mg over 90 min 14 days apart followed by 400 mg over 2½ hrs 14 days later. **(NON-DIALYSIS-DEPENDENT PTS):** 200 mg over 2–5 min on 5 different occasions within 14 days.

SIDE EFFECTS

Frequent (36%–23%): Hypotension, leg cramps, diarrhea.

ADVERSE EFFECTS/ TOXIC REACTIONS

Too-rapid IV administration may produce severe hypotension, headache, vomiting, nausea, dizziness, paresthesia, abdominal/muscle pain, edema, cardiovascular collapse. Hypersensitivity reaction occurs rarely.

NURSING CONSIDERATIONS

INTERVENTION/EVALUATION

Initially, monitor Hgb, Hct, serum ferritin, transferrin monthly, then q2–3mo thereafter. Reliable serum iron values can be obtained 48 hrs following administration.

isoniazid

eye-**soe**-nye-a-zid
(Isotamine, PMS Isoniazid)

BLACK BOX ALERT Severe, potentially fatal hepatitis may occur.

FIXED-COMBINATION(S)

Rifamate: isoniazid/rifampin (antitubercular): 150 mg/300 mg.
Rifater: isoniazid/pyrazinamide/rifampin (antitubercular): 50 mg/300 mg/120 mg.

CLASSIFICATION

PHARMACOTHERAPEUTIC: Isonicotinic acid derivative. **CLINICAL:** Antitubercular.

ACTION

Inhibits mycolic acid synthesis. Causes disruption of bacterial cell wall, loss of acid-fast properties in susceptible mycobacteria. Active only during bacterial cell division. **Therapeutic Effect:** Bactericidal against actively growing intracellular, extracellular susceptible mycobacteria.

PHARMACOKINETICS

Readily absorbed from GI tract. Protein binding: 10%–15%. Widely distributed (including to CSF). Metabolized in liver. Primarily excreted in urine. Removed by hemodialysis. **Half-life:** 0.5–5 hrs.

USES

Treatment of susceptible mycobacterial infection due to *M. tuberculosis*. Drug of choice in tuberculosis prophylaxis. Used in combination with one or more other antitubercular agents for treatment of active tuberculosis.

PRECAUTIONS

Contraindications: Acute hepatic disease, history of hypersensitivity reactions, hepatic injury with previous isoniazid therapy. **Cautions:** Chronic hepatic disease, alcoholism, severe renal impairment. May be cross-sensitive with nicotinic acid, other chemically related medications.

LIFESPAN CONSIDERATIONS

Pregnancy/Lactation: Prophylaxis usually postponed until after delivery. Crosses placenta. Distributed in breast milk. **Pregnancy Category C. Children:** No age-related precautions noted. **Elderly:** More susceptible to developing hepatitis.

INTERACTIONS

DRUG: **Alcohol may** increase isoniazid metabolism, risk of hepatotoxicity. May increase toxicity of **carbamazepine, phenytoin. Disulfiram** may increase CNS effects. **Hepatotoxic medications** may increase risk of hepatotoxicity. May decrease **ketoconazole** concentration. **HERBAL:** None significant. **FOOD:** **Foods containing tyramine** may cause hypertensive crisis. **LAB VALUES:** May increase serum bilirubin, AST, ALT.

AVAILABILITY (Rx)

Oral Solution: 50 mg/5 ml. **Tablets:** 100 mg, 300 mg.

ADMINISTRATION/HANDLING

PO

• Give 1 hr before or 2 hrs following meals (may give with food to decrease GI upset, but will delay absorption). • Administer at least 1 hr before antacids, esp. those containing aluminum.

INDICATIONS/ROUTES/DOSAGE

Active Tuberculosis (in Combination with One or More Antituberculars)

PO: ADULTS, ELDERLY: 5 mg/kg/day as a single daily dose. Usual dose: 300 mg/day. **CHILDREN:** 10–15 mg/kg/day as a single dose or 2 divided doses. **Maximum:** 300 mg/day.

Tuberculosis Prophylaxis

PO: ADULTS, ELDERLY: 300 mg/day as a single dose or 900 mg 2–3 times/wk. **CHILDREN:** 10 mg/kg/day as a single dose or 2 divided doses. **Maximum:** 300 mg/

day or 20–40 mg/kg 2–3 times/wk. **Maximum:** 900 mg/dose.

SIDE EFFECTS

Frequent: Nausea, vomiting, diarrhea, abdominal pain. **Rare:** Pain at injection site, hypersensitivity reaction.

ADVERSE EFFECTS/ TOXIC REACTIONS

Neurotoxicity (ataxia, paresthesia), optic neuritis, hepatotoxicity occur rarely.

NURSING CONSIDERATIONS

BASELINE ASSESSMENT

Question for history of hypersensitivity reactions, hepatic injury or disease, sensitivity to nicotinic acid or chemically related medications. Ensure collection of specimens for culture, sensitivity. Evaluate initial hepatic function results.

INTERVENTION/EVALUATION

Monitor hepatic function test results, assess for hepatitis: anorexia, nausea, vomiting, weakness, fatigue, dark urine, jaundice (hold concurrent INH therapy and inform physician promptly). Assess for paresthesia of extremities (those esp. at risk for neuropathy may be given pyridoxine prophylactically: malnourished, elderly, diabetics, pts with chronic hepatic disease [including alcoholics]). Be alert for fever, skin eruptions (hypersensitivity reaction).

PATIENT/FAMILY TEACHING

• Do not skip doses; continue taking isoniazid for full length of therapy (6–24 mos). • Take preferably 1 hr before or 2 hrs following meals (with food if GI upset). • Avoid alcohol during treatment. • Do not take any other medications, including antacids, without consulting physician. • Must take isoniazid at least 1 hr before antacid. • Avoid tuna, sauerkraut, aged cheeses, smoked fish (consult list of tyramine-containing foods) that may cause hypertensive reaction (red/itching skin, palpitations, light-headedness, hot or clammy feeling, headache). • Notify physician of any new symptom, immediately for vision difficulties, nausea/vomiting, dark urine, yellowing of skin/eyes (jaundice), fatigue, paresthesia of extremities.

isosorbide dinitrate

eye-sew-**sore**-bide
(Apo-ISDN ♣, Cedocard SR ♣, Dilatrate-SR, Isochron, Isordil)

isosorbide mononitrate

(Apo-ISMN ♣, Imdur, ISMO, Monoket)
Do not confuse Isordil with Inderal, Isuprel, or Plendil, Imdur with Imuran, Inderal, or K-Dur, or Monoket with Monopril.

FIXED-COMBINATION(S)

BiDil: isosorbide dinitrate/hydralazine (a vasodilator): 20 mg/37.5 mg.

◆ CLASSIFICATION

PHARMACOTHERAPEUTIC: Nitrate. **CLINICAL:** Antianginal (see p. 125C).

ACTION

Stimulates intracellular cyclic guanosine monophosphate. **Therapeutic Effect:** Relaxes vascular smooth muscle of arterial, venous vasculature. Decreases preload, afterload.

PHARMACOKINETICS

Route	Onset	Peak	Duration
Dinitrate			
Sublingual	2–10 min	N/A	1–2 hrs
PO (Chewable)	3 min	N/A	0.5–2 hrs
PO	45–60 min	N/A	4–6 hrs
Mononitrate			
PO (Extended-Release)	30–60 min	N/A	N/A

Dinitrate poorly absorbed and metabolized in liver to its active metabolite isosorbide mononitrate. Mononitrate well absorbed after PO administration. Excreted in urine and feces. **Half-life:** Dinitrate, 1–4 hrs; mononitrate, 4 hrs.

USES

Prophylaxis, treatment of angina pectoris, CHF. **OFF-LABEL:** Dysphagia, pain relief, relief of esophageal spasm with gastroesophageal reflux.

PRECAUTIONS

Contraindications: Closed-angle glaucoma, head trauma, hypersensitivity to nitrates, increased intracranial pressure (ICP), orthostatic hypotension, concurrent use of sildenafil, tadalafil, vardenafil. **Extended-Release Tablets:** GI hypermotility, GI malabsorption, severe anemia. **Cautions:** Acute MI, hepatic/renal disease, glaucoma (contraindicated in closed-angle glaucoma), blood volume depletion from diuretic therapy, systolic B/P less than 90 mm Hg.

LIFESPAN CONSIDERATIONS

Pregnancy/Lactation: Unknown if drug crosses placenta or is distributed in breast milk. **Pregnancy Category C. Children:** Safety and efficacy not established. **Elderly:** May be more sensitive to hypotensive effects. Age-related renal impairment may require dosage adjustment.

INTERACTIONS

DRUG: Alcohol, antihypertensives, vasodilators may increase risk of orthostatic hypotension. **Sildenafil, tadalafil, vardenafil** may potentiate hypotensive effects (concurrent use of these agents is contraindicated). **HERBAL:** None significant. **FOOD:** None known. **LAB VALUES:** May increase urine catecholamine, urine vanillylmandelic acid levels.

AVAILABILITY (Rx)

Dinitrate

Tablets: (Isordil): 5 mg, 10 mg, 20 mg, 30 mg, 40 mg.

Capsules, Sustained-Release (Dilatrate SR): 40 mg. **Tablets, Extended-Release: (Isochron):** 40 mg. **Tablets, Sublingual: (Isordil):** 2.5 mg, 5 mg.

Mononitrate

Tablets (ISMO): 20 mg. **(Monoket):** 10 mg, 20 mg.

Tablets, Extended-Release (Imdur): 30 mg, 60 mg, 120 mg.

ADMINISTRATION/HANDLING

PO

- Best if taken on an empty stomach.
- Oral tablets may be crushed.
- Do not crush/break sustained-, extended-release form.
- Do not crush chewable form before administering.

Sublingual

- Do not crush/chew sublingual tablets.
- Dissolve tablets under tongue; do not swallow.

INDICATIONS/ROUTES/DOSAGE

Angina

PO (ISOSORBIDE DINITRATE): ADULTS, ELDERLY: 5–40 mg 4 times a day.
SUBLINGUAL: ADULTS, ELDERLY: 2.5–5 mg, 5–10 min. **Maximum:** 3 doses in 15–30 min.
SUSTAINED-RELEASE: ADULTS, ELDERLY: 40 mg q8–12h.
PO (ISOSORBIDE MONONITRATE): ADULTS, ELDERLY: 5–20 mg twice a day given 7 hrs apart. **SUSTAINED-RELEASE:** Initially, 30–60 mg/day in morning as a single dose. May increase dose at 3 day intervals. **Maximum:** 240 mg/day.

CHF

PO (ISORDIL DINITRATE): ADULTS, ELDERLY: Initially, 20 mg 3–4 times/day. May increase to 120–160 mg/day in divided doses in combination with hydralazine.

SIDE EFFECTS

Frequent: Headache (may be severe) occurs mostly in early therapy, diminishes rapidly in intensity, usually disappears during continued treatment, transient flushing of face/neck, dizziness (esp. if pt is standing immobile or is in a warm environment), weakness, orthostatic hypotension, nausea, vomiting, restlessness. **Occasional:** GI upset, blurred vision, dry mouth. **Sublingual: Frequent:** Burning, tingling at oral point of dissolution.

ADVERSE REACTIONS/ TOXIC EFFECTS

Drug should be discontinued if blurred vision occurs. Severe orthostatic hypotension manifested by syncope, pulselessness, cold/clammy skin, diaphoresis. Tolerance may occur with repeated, prolonged therapy, but may not occur with extended-release form. Minor tolerance with intermittent use of sublingual tablets. High dosage tends to produce severe headache.

NURSING CONSIDERATIONS

BASELINE ASSESSMENT

Record onset, type (sharp, dull, squeezing), radiation, location, intensity, duration of anginal pain; precipitating factors (exertion, emotional stress). If headache occurs during management therapy, administer medication with meals.

INTERVENTION/EVALUATION

Assist with ambulation if light-headedness, dizziness occurs. Assess for facial/neck flushing. Monitor number of anginal episodes, orthostatic B/P.

PATIENT/FAMILY TEACHING

• Do not chew/crush sublingual, extended-release, sustained-release forms. • Take sublingual tablets while sitting down. • Rise slowly from lying to sitting position, dangle legs momentarily before standing (prevents dizziness effect). • Take oral form on empty stomach (however, if headache occurs during management therapy, take medication with meals). • Dissolve sublingual tablet under tongue; do not swallow. • Avoid alcohol (intensifies hypotensive effect). • If alcohol is ingested soon after taking nitrates, possible acute hypotensive episode (marked drop in B/P, vertigo, pallor) may occur. • Report signs/symptoms of hypotension, angina.

isotretinoin

eye-so-**tret**-ah-noyn
(Accutane, Amnesteem, Claravis, Isotrex ✦, Sotret)

BLACK BOX ALERT High risk of teratogenic effects; Pregnancy Category X. Obtain two negative pregnancy tests prior to treatment. All pts (male and female) must register and be active in the IPLEDGE™ risk management program.

Do not confuse Accutane with Accolate or Accupril, Claravis with Cleviprex, or isotretinoin with tretinoin.

◆ CLASSIFICATION

PHARMACOTHERAPEUTIC: Keratinization stabilizer. **CLINICAL:** Antiacne, antirosacea agent.

ACTION

Reduces sebaceous gland size, inhibiting gland activity. **Therapeutic Effect:** Produces antikeratinizing, anti-inflammatory effects.

USES

Treatment of severe, recalcitrant cystic acne unresponsive to conventional acne therapies. **OFF-LABEL:** Treatment of gram-negative folliculitis, severe rosacea, severe keratinization disorders. Treatment of children with metastatic neuroblastoma or leukemia not responding to conventional therapy.

PRECAUTIONS

Contraindications: Hypersensitivity to isotretinoin, parabens (component of capsules). **Cautions:** Renal/hepatic dysfunction.

I

LIFESPAN CONSIDERATIONS

Pregnancy/Lactation: Contraindicated in females who are or may become pregnant while undergoing treatment (very high risk of fetal harm, major fetal birth defects/deformities). Unknown if distributed in breast milk. Breast-feeding not recommended. **Pregnancy Category X.** **Children:** Safety and efficacy not established in those younger than 12 yrs. Careful consideration must be given to those 12–17 yrs, esp. children with known metabolic disease, structural bone disease. **Elderly:** No age-related precautions noted.

INTERACTIONS

DRUG: **Etretinate, tretinoin, vitamin A** may increase toxic effects. **Tetracycline** may increase potential for pseudotumor cerebri. HERBAL: **Dong quai, St. John's wort** may cause photosensitization. FOOD: None known. LAB VALUES: May increase serum triglycerides, cholesterol, AST, ALT, alkaline phosphatase, LDH, fasting serum glucose, uric acid, sedimentation rate. May decrease HDL.

AVAILABILITY (Rx)

Capsules: (Accutane, Amnesteem, Claravis): 10 mg, 20 mg, 40 mg; **(Sotret):** 10 mg, 20 mg, 30 mg, 40 mg.

ADMINISTRATION/HANDLING

PO

• Give with meals. • May chew or open capsule with large needle, place on applesauce or ice cream.

INDICATIONS/ROUTES/DOSAGE

Recalcitrant Cystic Acne

PO: ADULTS, CHILDREN 12–17 YRS: Initially, 0.5–1 mg/kg/day divided in 2 doses for 15–20 wks. Adults may require doses up to 2 mg/kg/day. May repeat after at least 2 mos off therapy.

Dosage in Hepatic Disease

Dose reductions recommended.

SIDE EFFECTS

Frequent: Cheilitis (inflammation of lips) (90%), skin/mucous membrane dryness (80%), skin fragility, pruritus, epistaxis, dry nose/mouth, conjunctivitis (40%), hypertriglyceridemia (25%), nausea, vomiting, abdominal pain (20%). **Occasional (16%–5%):** Musculoskeletal symptoms (16%) including bone/joint pain, arthralgia, generalized muscle aches; photosensitivity (10%–5%). **Rare:** Diminished night vision, depression.

ADVERSE EFFECTS/ TOXIC REACTIONS

Inflammatory bowel disease, pseudotumor cerebri (benign intracranial hypertension) have been associated with isotretinoin therapy.

NURSING CONSIDERATIONS

BASELINE ASSESSMENT

Assess baselines for serum glucose, lipids, triglycerides. Obtain two negative pregnancy tests prior to treatment (Pregnancy Category X).

INTERVENTION/EVALUATION

Assess acne for decreased cysts. Evaluate skin/mucous membranes for excessive dryness. Monitor serum glucose, lipids, triglycerides.

PATIENT/FAMILY TEACHING

• Transient exacerbation of acne may occur during initial period. • Must be registered and be active in the iPLEDGE risk management program (see www.ipledgeprogram.com). • May have decreased tolerance to contact lenses during and following therapy. • Do not take vitamin supplements with vitamin A due to additive effects. • Immediately notify physician of onset of abdominal pain, severe diarrhea, rectal bleeding (possible inflammatory bowel disease), headache, nausea/vomiting, visual disturbances (possible pseudotumor cerebri). • Diminished night vision may occur suddenly; take caution with night driving.

• Avoid prolonged exposure to sunlight; use sunscreens, protective clothing. • Do not donate blood during or for 1 mo following treatment. • **Women:** Explain serious risk to fetus if pregnancy occurs (give both oral and written warnings, with pt acknowledging in writing that she understands the warnings and consents to treatment). • Must have negative serum pregnancy test within 2 wks before starting therapy; therapy will begin on the second or third day of next normal menstrual period. • Effective contraception (using 2 reliable forms of contraception simultaneously) must be used for at least 1 mo before, during, and for at least 1 mo after therapy.

isradipine

is-**rah**-dih-peen
(DynaCirc, DynaCirc CR)
Do not confuse DynaCirc with Dynabac or Dynacin.

CLASSIFICATION

PHARMACOTHERAPEUTIC: Calcium channel blocker. **CLINICAL:** Antihypertensive (see p. 77C).

ACTION

Inhibits calcium movement across cardiac, vascular smooth-muscle cell membranes. Potent peripheral vasodilator (does not depress SA, AV nodes). **Therapeutic Effect:** Produces relaxation of coronary vascular smooth muscle, coronary vasodilation. Increases myocardial oxygen delivery in those with vasospastic angina.

PHARMACOKINETICS

Route	Onset	Peak	Duration
PO (immediate-release hypertension)	2–3 hrs	2–4 wks (multiple doses) 8–16 hrs (single dose)	Greater than 12 hrs

Well absorbed from GI tract. Protein binding: 95%. Metabolized in liver (undergoes first-pass effect). Primarily excreted in urine. Not removed by hemodialysis. **Half-life:** 8 hrs.

USES

Management of hypertension. May be used alone or with other antihypertensives. **OFF-LABEL:** Treatment of chronic angina pectoris, Raynaud's phenomenon, pediatric hypertension.

PRECAUTIONS

Contraindications: Cardiogenic shock, CHF, heart block, hypotension, sinus bradycardia, ventricular tachycardia. **Cautions:** Sick sinus syndrome, severe left ventricular dysfunction, hepatic disease, edema, concurrent therapy with beta-blockers.

LIFESPAN CONSIDERATIONS

Pregnancy/Lactation: Unknown if drug crosses placenta or is distributed in breast milk. **Pregnancy Category C. Children:** Safety and efficacy not established. **Elderly:** Age-related renal impairment may require dosage adjustment.

INTERACTIONS

DRUG: **Beta blockers** may have additive effect. **HERBAL:** **Ephedra, ginseng, yohimbe** may worsen hypertension. **Garlic** may increase antihypertensive effect. **FOOD:** **Grapefruit, grapefruit juice** may increase absorption. **LAB VALUES:** None significant.

AVAILABILITY (Rx)

Capsules, Immediate-Release (DynaCirc): 2.5 mg, 5 mg.

Tablets, Controlled-Release (DynaCirc CR): 5 mg, 10 mg.

ADMINISTRATION/HANDLING

PO

• May give without regard to food. • Swallow controlled-release tablet whole; do not crush, break, chew, divide.

INDICATIONS/ROUTES/DOSAGE

Hypertension

PO: ADULTS, ELDERLY: (IMMEDIATE-RELEASE): Initially 2.5 mg twice a day. May increase by 2.5 mg at 2- to 4-wk intervals. Range: 2.5–10 mg in 2 divided doses. **(CONTROLLED-RELEASE):** Initially, 5 mg once daily. May increase at 2- to 4-wk intervals in increments of 5 mg. **Maximum:** 20 mg/day.

SIDE EFFECTS

Frequent (7%–4%): Peripheral edema, palpitations (higher frequency in females). **Occasional (3%):** Facial flushing, cough. **Rare (2%–1%):** Angina, tachycardia, rash, pruritus.

ADVERSE EFFECTS/ TOXIC REACTIONS

Overdose produces nausea, drowsiness, confusion, slurred speech. CHF occurs rarely.

NURSING CONSIDERATIONS

BASELINE ASSESSMENT

Assess baseline renal/hepatic function tests. Assess B/P, apical pulse immediately before drug is administered (if pulse is 60 beats/min or less or systolic B/P is less than 90 mm Hg, withhold medication, contact physician).

INTERVENTION/EVALUATION

Assess for peripheral edema behind medial malleolus (sacral area in bedridden pts). Monitor pulse rate for bradycardia. Monitor B/P; observe for signs, symptoms of CHF. Assess skin for flushing.

PATIENT/FAMILY TEACHING

• Do not abruptly discontinue medication. Compliance with therapy regimen is essential to control hypertension. • To avoid hypotensive effect, rise slowly from lying to sitting position, wait momentarily before standing. • Contact physician if palpitations, shortness of breath, pronounced dizziness, nausea, chest pain, swelling in extremities occur. • Avoid grapefruit, grapefruit juice.

itraconazole

eye-tra-**con**-ah-zoll
(Sporanox)

BLACK BOX ALERT Serious cardiovascular events, including ventricular tachycardia, torsade de pointes, death, have occurred due to concurrent use with cisapride, pimozide, quinidine, dofetilide, or levomethadyl.

Do not confuse itraconazole with fluconazole, or Sporanox with Suprax.

◆CLASSIFICATION

CLINICAL: Antifungal.

ACTION

Inhibits synthesis of ergosterol (vital component of fungal cell formation). **Therapeutic Effect:** Damages fungal cell membrane, altering its function. Fungistatic.

PHARMACOKINETICS

Moderately absorbed from GI tract. Absorption is increased if drug is taken with food. Protein binding: 99%. Widely distributed, primarily in fatty tissue, liver, kidneys. Metabolized in liver to active metabolite. Primarily excreted in urine. Not removed by hemodialysis. **Half-life:** 16–26 hrs.

USES

Treatment of aspergillosis, blastomycosis, esophageal and oropharyngeal candidiasis, empiric treatment in febrile neutropenia, histoplasmosis, onychomycosis. **OFF-LABEL:** Suppression of histoplasmosis; treatment of disseminated sporotrichosis, fungal pneumonia/septicemia, tinea infection (ringworm) of the hand.

PRECAUTIONS

Contraindications: Hypersensitivity to fluconazole, ketoconazole, miconazole,

CHF. **Cautions:** Hepatitis, HIV-infected pts, pts with achlorhydria, hypochlorhydria (decreases absorption), hepatic impairment, left ventricular dysfunction, history of CHF.

LIFESPAN CONSIDERATIONS

Pregnancy/Lactation: Distributed in breast milk. **Pregnancy Category C. Children:** Safety and efficacy not established. **Elderly:** Age-related renal impairment may require dosage adjustment.

INTERACTIONS

DRUG: May increase concentration/toxicity of **calcium channel-blocking agents (e.g., felodipine, nifedipine), carbamazepine, cyclosporine, digoxin, ergot alkaloids, HMG-CoA reductase inhibitors (e.g., lovastatin, simvastatin), midazolam, oral antidiabetic agents (e.g., glyburide, glipizide), protease inhibitors (e.g., indinavir, ritonavir, saquinavir), sirolimus, tacrolimus, triazolam, warfarin. Carbamazepine, isoniazid, phenobarbital, phenytoin, rifampin** may decrease concentration/effect. May inhibit metabolism of **busulfan, docetaxel, vinca alkaloids. Erythromycin** may increase risk of cardiac toxicity. **Antacids, H_2 antagonists, proton pump inhibitors (e.g., omeprazole)** may decrease absorption. **HERBAL: St. John's wort** may decrease concentration. **FOOD: Grapefruit, grapefruit juice** may alter absorption. **LAB VALUES:** May increase LDH, serum alkaline phosphatase, bilirubin, AST, ALT. May decrease serum potassium.

AVAILABILITY (Rx)

Capsules: 100 mg. **Oral Solution:** 10 mg/ml.

ADMINISTRATION/HANDLING

PO

• Give capsules with food (increases absorption). • Give solution on empty stomach.

INDICATIONS/ROUTES/DOSAGE

Usual Dosage Range

PO: ADULTS, ELDERLY: 100—400 mg/day. Doses greater than 200 mg given in 2 divided doses.

Blastomycosis, Histoplasmosis

PO: ADULTS, ELDERLY: Initially, 200 mg once a day. **Maximum:** 400 mg/day in 2 divided doses.

Aspergillosis

PO: ADULTS, ELDERLY: 600 mg/day in 3 divided doses for 3–4 days, then 200–400 mg/day in 2 divided doses.

Esophageal Candidiasis

PO: ADULTS, ELDERLY: Swish 100–200 mg (10–20 ml) in mouth for several seconds, then swallow once daily for a minimum of 3 wks. Continue for 2 wks after resolution of symptoms. **Maximum:** 200 mg/day.

Oropharyngeal Candidiasis

PO: ADULTS, ELDERLY: 200 mg (10 ml) oral solution, swish and swallow once a day for 7–14 days.

Onychomycosis (Fingernail)

PO: ADULTS, ELDERLY: 200 mg twice a day for 7 days, off for 21 days, repeat 200 mg twice a day for 7 days.

Onychomycosis (Toenail)

PO: ADULTS, ELDERLY: 200 mg once daily for 12 wks.

SIDE EFFECTS

Frequent (11%–9%): Nausea, rash. **Occasional (5%–3%):** Vomiting, headache, diarrhea, hypertension, peripheral edema, fatigue, fever. **Rare (2% or less):** Abdominal pain, dizziness, anorexia, pruritus.

ADVERSE EFFECTS/ TOXIC REACTIONS

Hepatitis (anorexia, abdominal pain, unusual fatigue/weakness, jaundiced skin/ sclera, dark urine) occurs rarely.

NURSING CONSIDERATIONS

BASELINE ASSESSMENT

Determine baseline temperature, hepatic function tests. Assess allergies.

INTERVENTION/EVALUATION

Assess for signs, symptoms of hepatic dysfunction. Monitor hepatic enzyme test results in pts with preexisting hepatic dysfunction.

PATIENT/ FAMILY TEACHING

• Take capsules with food, liquids if GI distress occurs. • Therapy will continue for at least 3 mos, until lab tests, clinical presentation indicate infection is controlled. • Immediately report unusual fatigue, yellow skin, dark urine, pale stool, anorexia, nausea, vomiting. • Avoid grapefruit, grapefruit juice.

I

ixabepilone

ix-ah-**bep**-i-lone
(Ixempra)

BLACK BOX ALERT Combination therapy with capecitabine is contraindicated in pts with AST or ALT greater than 2.5 times upper limit of normal (ULN) or bilirubin greater than 1 times ULN. Increased risk of toxicity, neutropenia-related mortality.

◆CLASSIFICATION

PHARMACOTHERAPEUTIC: Epothilone microtubule inhibitor. **CLINICAL:** Antineoplastic.

ACTION

Binds directly on microtubules during active stage of G2 and M phases of cell cycle, preventing formation of microtubules, an essential part of the process of separation of chromosomes. **Therapeutic Effect:** Blocks cells in mitotic phase of cell division, leading to cell death.

PHARMACOKINETICS

Extensively metabolized in liver. Protein binding: 77%. Excreted mainly in feces, with lesser amount eliminated in urine. **Half-life:** 52 hrs.

USES

Combination therapy with capecitabine for treatment of metastatic or locally advanced breast cancer in pts after failure of anthrocycline, taxane therapy. As monotherapy, treatment of metastatic or locally advanced breast cancer in pts after failure of anthrocycline, taxane, and capecitabine therapy. **OFF-LABEL:** Treatment of endometrical cancer.

PRECAUTIONS

Contraindications: Severe hypersensitivity reaction to Cremophor, baseline neutrophil count less than 1,500/mm^3, platelet count less than 100,000 cells/mm^3. **Combination Capecitabine Therapy:** AST or ALT greater than 2.5 times normal range, bilirubin greater than 1 times normal range. **Monotherapy:** AST or ALT greater than 5 times normal range, bilirubin greater than 3 times normal range. **Cautions:** Diabetes mellitus, existing moderate to severe neuropathy.

⌛ LIFESPAN CONSIDERATIONS

Pregnancy/Lactation: May cause fetal harm. Unknown if distributed in breast milk. **Pregnancy Category D. Children:** Safety and efficacy not established. **Elderly:** Higher incidence of severe adverse reactions in those older than 65 yrs.

INTERACTIONS

DRUG: Amprenavir, atazanavir, clarithromycin, delaviridine, indinavir, itraconazole, ketaconazole, nefazodone, nelfinavir, ritonavir, saquinavir, voriconazole may increase concentration. **Carbamazepine, dexamethasone, phenobarbital, phenytoin, rifabutin, rifampin, rifapentin** may decrease concentration. **HERBAL: St. John's wort** may decrease plasma concentration. **FOOD:**

Grapefruit, grapefruit juice may increase plasma concentration. LAB VALUES: May increase ALT, AST, bilirubin. May decrease WBCs, Hgb, platelets.

AVAILABILITY (Rx)

Injection, Solution: Kit: 15 mg kit supplied with diluent for Ixempra, 8 ml; 45 mg supplied with diluent for Ixempra, 23.5 ml.

ADMINISTRATION/HANDLING

IV

Reconstitution • Withdraw diluent and slowly inject into vial. • Gently swirl and invert until powder is completely dissolved. • Further dilute with 250 ml lactated Ringer's. • Solution may be stored in vial for a maximum of 1 hr at room temperature. • Final concentration for infusion must be between 0.2 mg/ml and 0.6 mg/ml. • Mix infusion bag by manual rotation.

Rate of administration • Administer through an in-line filter of 0.2 to 1.2 microns. • Infuse over 3 hrs. Administration must be completed within 6 hrs of reconstitution.

Storage • Refrigerate kit. • Prior to reconstitution, kit should be removed from refrigerator and allowed to stand at room temperature for approximately 30 min. • When vials are initially removed from refrigerator, a white precipitate may be observed in the diluent vial. • This precipitate will dissolve to form a clear solution once diluent warms to room temperature. • Once diluted with lactated Ringer's, solution is stable at room temperature and room light for a maximum of 6 hrs.

INDICATIONS/ROUTES/DOSAGE

◀ALERT▶ An H_1 antagonist (diphenhydramine 50 mg PO or equivalent) and an H_2 antagonist (ranitidine 150–300 mg PO or equivalent) must be given prior to beginning treatment with ixabepilone. Those who experienced a previous hypersensitivity reaction to ixabepilone require pretreatment with corticosteroids (dexamethasone 20 mg IV, 30 min before infusion or PO, 1 hr before infusion) in addition to pretreatment with H_1 and H_2 antagonists.

Combination Therapy with Capecitabine

IV: ADULTS, ELDERLY: 40 mg/m² infused over 3 hrs, every 3 wks. **Maximum:** 88 mg.

Monotherapy

Mild Hepatic Impairment (AST and ALT Less Than 2.5 Times Normal Range and Bilirubin Less Than Normal Range)

IV: ADULTS, ELDERLY: 40 mg/m² infused over 3 hrs, every 3 wks.

Mild Hepatic Impairment (AST and ALT Less Than 10 Times Normal Range and Bilirubin Less Than 1.5 Times Normal Range)

IV: ADULTS, ELDERLY: 32 mg/m² infused over 3 hrs, every 3 wks.

Moderate Hepatic Impairment (AST and ALT Less Than 2.5 Times Normal Range and Bilirubin Less Than 3 Times Normal Range)

IV INFUSION: ADULTS, ELDERLY: 20–30 mg/m² infused over 3 hrs, every 3 wks.

Dose Modification

Dosage adjustment based on grade of neuropathy, hematologic conditions.

SIDE EFFECTS

Common (62%): Peripheral sensory neuropathy. Frequent (56%–46%): Fatigue, asthenia (loss of strength, energy), myalgia, arthralgia, alopecia, nausea. Occasional (29%–11%): Vomiting, stomatitis, mucositis, diarrhea, musculoskeletal pain, anorexia, constipation, abdominal pain, headache. Rare (9%–5%): Skin rash, nail disorder, edema, hand-foot syndrome (blistering/rash/peeling of skin on palms of hands, soles of feet), pyrexia, dizziness, pruritus, gastroesophageal reflux disease (GERD), hot flashes, taste disorder, insomnia.

ADVERSE EFFECTS/ TOXIC REACTIONS

Neuropathy occurs early during treatment; 75% of new onset or worsening neuropathy occurred during first 3 cycles. Pts with diabetes mellitus may be at increased risk for severe neuropathy manifested as Grade 4 neutropenia. Neutropenia, leukopenia occurs commonly; anemia, thrombocytopenia occur rarely.

NURSING CONSIDERATIONS

BASELINE ASSESSMENT

Question possibility of pregnancy. Obtain baseline CBC, serum chemistries including hepatic function tests (bilirubin, AST, ALT) before treatment begins as baseline and diligently monitor for hepatotoxicity, peripheral neuropathy (most frequent cause of drug discontinuation).

INTERVENTION/EVALUATION

Monitor for symptoms of neuropathy (burning sensation, hyperesthesia, hypoesthesia, paresthesia, discomfort, neuropathic pain). Assess hands and feet for erythema. Monitor CBC for evidence of neutropenia, thrombocytopenia; assess hepatic function tests for hepatotoxicity. Assess mouth for stomatitis, mucositis.

PATIENT/FAMILY TEACHING

• Avoid crowds, those with known infection. • Avoid contact with those who have recently received live virus vaccine. • Do not have immunizations without physician's approval (drug lowers resistance). • Promptly report fever over 100.5°F, chills, numbness, tingling, burning sensation, erythema of hands/feet.

Kadian, *see morphine*

Kaletra, *see lopinavir/ritonavir*

Kaopectate, *see bismuth*

kava kava

Also known as ava, kew, sakau, tonga, yagona.

◀ALERT▶ May be removed from market.

◆CLASSIFICATION

HERBAL: See Appendix G.

ACTION

Exact mechanism of action unknown but possesses CNS effects. **Effect:** Anxiolytic, sedative, analgesic effects.

USES

Treatment of anxiety disorders, stress, restlessness. Used for sedation, sleep enhancement.

PRECAUTIONS

Contraindications: Pregnancy, lactation (may cause loss of uterine tone). **Cautions:** Depression, history of recurrent hepatitis.

LIFESPAN CONSIDERATIONS

Pregnancy/Lactation: Contraindicated. **Children:** Safety and efficacy not established. **Elderly:** No age-related precautions noted.

INTERACTIONS

DRUG: **Alcohol, benzodiazepines** may increase risk of drowsiness. **HERBAL:** **Chamomile, ginseng, goldenseal, melatonin, St. John's wort, valerian** may increase risk of excessive drowsiness. **FOOD:** None known. **LAB VALUES:** May increase hepatic function tests.

AVAILABILITY (OTC)

Capsules: 140 mg, 150 mg, 250 mg, 300 mg, 425 mg, 500 mg. **Extract. Liquid. Tincture.**

INDICATIONS/ROUTES/DOSAGE

Usual Dosage

PO: ADULTS, ELDERLY: 100 mg 3 times a day or 1 cup of tea 3 times a day.

SIDE EFFECTS

GI upset, headache, dizziness, vision changes (blurred vision, red eyes), allergic skin reactions, dermopathy (dry, flaky skin), yellowing of skin, hair, nails, sclera of eyes, nausea, vomiting, weight loss, shortness of breath.

ADVERSE EFFECTS/ TOXIC REACTIONS

None known.

NURSING CONSIDERATIONS

BASELINE ASSESSMENT

Assess if pt is pregnant or breast-feeding (contraindicated). Determine baseline hepatic function tests. Assess for use of other CNS depressants.

INTERVENTION/EVALUATION

Monitor hepatic function tests. Assess for allergic skin reactions.

PATIENT/FAMILY TEACHING

• Avoid use if pregnant, planning to become pregnant, or breast-feeding; not for use in children 12 yrs and younger. • Avoid tasks that require alertness, motor skills until response to herbal is established. • Do not use for more than 3 mos (may be habit forming).

Keflex, *see cephalexin*

Kefzol, *see cefazolin*

Keppra, *see levetiracetam*

ketamine

HIGH ALERT

ket-ah-meen
(Ketalar)

BLACK BOX ALERT Post emergent reactions (vivid imagery, dreamlike state, hallucinations, delirium) occur in 12% of pts; less common in pts older than 65 yrs or when given IM.

Do not confuse Ketalar with Kenalog or Ketorolac.

◆CLASSIFICATION

CLINICAL: Rapid-acting general anesthetic **(Schedule III)** (see p. 5C).

ACTION

Selectively blocks afferent impulses, interacts with CNS transmitter systems. **Therapeutic Effect:** Produces anesthetic state characterized by profound analgesia, normal pharyngeal-laryngeal reflexes.

PHARMACOKINETICS

Route	Onset	Peak	Duration
IM (anesthetic)	3–8 min	N/A	12–25 min
IV (anesthetic)	1–2 min	N/A	5–15 min

Rapidly distributed. Metabolized in liver. Primarily excreted in urine. **Half-life:** 2–3 hrs.

USES

Induction, maintenance of general anesthesia (esp. when cardiovascular depression to be avoided). **OFF-LABEL:** Analgesia, sedation.

PRECAUTIONS

Contraindications: Aneurysms, angina, CHF, elevated ICP, hypertension, psychotic disorders, thyrotoxicosis. **Cautions:** Gastroesophageal reflux disease (GERD), hepatic impairment, pts with recent food intake (large meal), chronic alcoholism, acute intoxication.

⌛ LIFESPAN CONSIDERATIONS

Pregnancy/Lactation: Not recommended; safety not established. **Pregnancy Category D. Children/Elderly:** No age-related precautions noted.

K

INTERACTIONS

DRUG: **Clarithromycin, ketoconazole, NSAIDS, paroxetine, propofol, protease inhibitors, sertraline** may increase concentration/effect. **Barbiturates, narcotics** may prolong recovery from sedation. HERBAL: None significant. FOOD: None known. LAB VALUES: May increase IOP.

AVAILABILITY (Rx)

Injection Solution: 10 mg/ml, 50 mg/ml, 100 mg/ml.

ADMINISTRATION/HANDLING

IV

Reconstitution • For induction anesthesia using IV push, dilute 100 mg/ml with equal volume Sterile Water for Injection, D_5W, or 0.9% NaCl. • For maintenance IV infusion, dilute 50 mg/ml vial (10 ml) or 100 mg/ml vial (5 ml) to 250–500 ml D_5W or 0.9% NaCl to provide a concentration of 1–2 mg/ml.
Rate of administration • Administer IV push slowly over 60 sec (too-rapid IV may produce severe hypotension, respiratory depression). • Administer IV infusion at rate of 0.5 mg/kg/min.

IM
• Use 10 mg/ml vial.

IV INCOMPATIBILITY

Doxapram (Dopram).

IV COMPATIBILITIES

Bupivacaine (Marcaine), clonidine (Duraclon), fentanyl (Sublimaze), lidocaine, morphine, propofol (Diprivan).

INDICATIONS/ROUTES/DOSAGE

Induction/Maintenance of General Anesthesia

IV: ADULTS, ELDERLY, CHILDREN 16 YRS AND OLDER: 1–4.5 mg/kg. Usual induction dose: 1–2 mg/kg. **CHILDREN:** 0.5–2 mg/kg. Usual induction dose: 1–2 mg/kg.
IM: ADULTS, ELDERLY: 3–8 mg/kg. **CHILDREN:** 3–7 mg/kg.

SIDE EFFECTS

Frequent: Increased B/P, pulse. Emergence reaction occurs frequently (12%), resulting in dreamlike state, vivid imagery, hallucinations, delirium, and occasionally accompanied by confusion, excitement, irrational behavior; lasts from few hrs to 24 hrs after administration. Occasional: Pain at injection site. Rare: Rash.

ADVERSE EFFECTS/ TOXIC REACTIONS

Continuous/repeated intermittent infusion may result in extreme drowsiness, circulatory/respiratory depression. Too-rapid IV administration may produce severe hypotension, respiratory depression, irregular muscle movements.

NURSING CONSIDERATIONS

BASELINE ASSESSMENT

Resuscitative equipment, O_2 must be available. Obtain vital signs before induction.

INTERVENTION/EVALUATION

Monitor vital signs q3–5min during and after administration until recovery is achieved. Assess for emergence reaction (hypnotic or barbiturate may be needed). Keep verbal, tactile, visual stimulation at minimum during recovery.

PATIENT/FAMILY TEACHING

• Avoid tasks that require alertness, motor skills for 24 hrs after anesthesia.

ketoconazole

kee-toe-**koe**-na-zole
(Apo-Ketoconazole, Extina, Kuric, Nizoral, Nizoral AD, Nizoral Topical, Novo-Ketoconazole, Xolegel)

BLACK BOX ALERT Potentially fatal hepatotoxicity has occurred. Concurrent cisapride, terfenadine, astemizole contraindicated; serious cardiovascular events (QT prolongation, torsade de pointes, ventricular tachycardia, ventricular fibrillation, fatalities) have occurred.

Do not confuse Nizoral with Nasarel or Nitrol, or Kuric with Carac.

◆CLASSIFICATION

PHARMACOTHERAPEUTIC: Imidazole derivative. **CLINICAL:** Antifungal (see pp. 47C, 48C).

ACTION

Inhibits synthesis of ergosterol, a vital component of fungal cell formation. **Therapeutic Effect:** Damages fungal cell membrane, altering its function. Fungistatic.

PHARMACOKINETICS

Well absorbed from GI tract following PO administration. Protein binding: 93%–96%. Metabolized in liver. Primarily excreted in bile with minimal elimination in urine. Negligible systemic absorption following topical absorption. Ketoconazole is not detected in plasma after shampooing, topical administration. **Half-life:** 8 hrs.

USES

PO: Treatment of histoplasmosis, blastomycosis, candidiasis, chronic mucocutaneous candidiasis, coccidioidomycosis, paracoccidioidomycosis, chromomycosis, seborrheic dermatitis, tineas (ringworm), corporis, capitis, manus, cruris, pedis, unguium (onychomycosis), oral thrush, candiduria. **Shampoo:** Reduces scaling due to dandruff. Treatment of tinea versicolor. **Topical:** Treatment of tineas, pityriasis versicolor, cutaneous candidiasis, seborrhea dermatitis, dandruff. **Xolegel:** Treatment of seborrheic dermatitis. **OFF-LABEL:** **Systemic:** Treatment of fungal pneumonia, prostate cancer, septicemia.

PRECAUTIONS

Contraindications: Concurrent use with cisapride (ventricular arrhythmias). **Cautions:** Hepatic impairment.

⌛ LIFESPAN CONSIDERATIONS

Pregnancy/Lactation: Oral form distributed in breast milk. Unknown if topical form crosses placenta or is distributed in breast milk. **Pregnancy Category C.** **Children:** **Cream, shampoo:** Safety and efficacy not established. **Oral form:** Safety and efficacy not established in those younger than 2 yrs. **Elderly:** No age-related precautions noted.

INTERACTIONS

DRUG: May increase concentration/toxicity of **cyclosporine, digoxin, ergot alkaloids, midazolam, protease inhibitors (e.g., indinavir, ritonavir, saquinavir), sirolimus, triazolam, tacrolimus, warfarin. Isoniazid, rifampin** may decrease concentration/effect. **Erythromycin** may increase risk of cardiac toxicity. **Antacids, H_2 antagonists, proton pump inhibitors (e.g., omeprazole)** may decrease absorption. **HERBAL:** **St. John's wort** may decrease concentration. **FOOD:** None known. **LAB VALUES:** May increase serum alkaline phosphatase, bilirubin, AST, ALT. May decrease serum corticosteroid, testosterone.

AVAILABILITY (Rx)

Cream (Kuric): 2%. **Foam (Extina):** 2%. **Gel (Xolegel):** 2%. **Shampoo (Nizoral AD [OTC]):** 1%. **Tablets (Nizoral):** 200 mg.

ADMINISTRATION/HANDLING

PO

• Give with food to minimize GI irritation. • Tablets may be crushed. • Ketoconazole requires acidity; give antacids, anticholinergics, H_2 blockers **at least** 2 hrs following dosing.

Shampoo

• Apply to wet hair, massage for 1 min, rinse thoroughly, reapply for 3 min, rinse.

Topical

• Apply, rub gently into affected/surrounding area.

INDICATIONS/ROUTES/DOSAGE

Usual Dosage

PO: **ADULTS, ELDERLY:** 200–400 mg/day. **CHILDREN 2 YRS AND OLDER:** 3.3–6.6 mg/

kg/day. **Maximum:** 800 mg/day in 2 divided doses.
TOPICAL: ADULTS, ELDERLY: Apply to affected area 1–2 times a day for 2–4 wks.
SHAMPOO: ADULTS, ELDERLY: Use twice weekly for 4 wks, allowing at least 3 days between shampooing. Use intermittently to maintain control.

SIDE EFFECTS

Occasional (10%–3%): Nausea, vomiting. **Rare (less than 2%):** Abdominal pain, diarrhea, headache, dizziness, photophobia. **Topical:** Burning, irritation, pruritus.

ADVERSE EFFECTS/ TOXIC REACTIONS

Hematologic toxicity (thrombocytopenia, hemolytic anemia, leukopenia) occurs occasionally. Hepatotoxicity may occur within first wk to several mos after starting therapy. Anaphylaxis occurs rarely.

K

NURSING CONSIDERATIONS

BASELINE ASSESSMENT

Confirm that culture or histologic test was done for accurate diagnosis; therapy may begin before results known.

INTERVENTION/EVALUATION

Monitor hepatic function tests; be alert for hepatotoxicity: dark urine, pale stools, jaundice, fatigue, anorexia, nausea, or vomiting (unrelieved by giving medication with food). Monitor CBC for hematologic toxicity. Monitor daily pattern of bowel activity, stool consistency. Assess for dizziness, provide assistance as needed. Evaluate skin for rash, urticaria, pruritus. **Topical:** Check for localized burning, pruritus, irritation.

PATIENT/FAMILY TEACHING

• Prolonged therapy (wks or mos) is usually necessary. • Do not miss a dose; continue therapy as long as directed. • Avoid alcohol (potential for hepatotoxicity). • May cause dizziness; avoid tasks that require alertness, motor skills until response to drug is established. • Take antacids, antiulcer medications at least 2 hrs after ketoconazole. • Notify physician of dark urine, pale stool, yellow skin or eyes, vomiting, increased irritation in topical use, onset of other new symptoms. • **Topical:** Rub well into affected areas. • Avoid contact with eyes. • Keep skin clean, dry; wear light clothing for ventilation. • Separate personal items in direct contact with affected area. • **Shampoo:** Initially, use 2 times a wk for 4 wks with at least 3 days between shampooing; frequency then determined by response to medication.

ketoprofen

kee-toe-**proe**-fen
(Apo-Keto ✱, Novo-Keto-EC ✱, Oruvail ✱, Rhodis ✱)

BLACK BOX ALERT Increased risk of serious cardiovascular thrombotic events, including myocardial infarction, CVA. Increased risk of severe GI reactions, including ulceration, bleeding, perforation.

Do not confuse Oruvail with Clinoril or Elavil.

◆ CLASSIFICATION

PHARMACOTHERAPEUTIC: Nonsteroidal anti-inflammatory. **CLINICAL:** Antirheumatic, analgesic, antidysmenorrheal, vascular headache suppressant (see p. 128C).

ACTION

Produces analgesic, anti-inflammatory effects by inhibiting prostaglandin synthesis. **Therapeutic Effect:** Reduces inflammatory response, intensity of pain.

PHARMACOKINETICS

Immediate-release capsules are rapidly, well absorbed following PO administration; extended-release capsules are well-absorbed. Protein binding: 99%. Metabolized in liver. Excreted in urine; less than 10% excreted as unchanged (unconjugated) drug. **Half-life:** 2–4 hrs; extended-release: 3–7.5 hrs.

USES

Symptomatic treatment of acute and chronic rheumatoid arthritis (RA), osteoarthritis. Relief of mild to moderate pain, primary dysmenorrhea. **OFF-LABEL:** Treatment of acute gouty arthritis, psoriatic arthritis, ankylosing spondylitis, vascular headache.

PRECAUTIONS

Contraindications: Active peptic ulcer disease, chronic inflammation of GI tract, GI bleeding/ulceration, history of hypersensitivity to aspirin, NSAIDs. **Cautions:** Renal/hepatic impairment, history of GI tract disease, predisposition to fluid retention.

LIFESPAN CONSIDERATIONS

Pregnancy/Lactation: Crosses placenta; unknown if distributed in breast milk. Avoid during late pregnancy (ductus arteriosis). **Pregnancy Category C. (D if used in third trimester or near delivery).** **Children:** Safety and efficacy not established. **Elderly:** Age-related renal impairment may require dosage adjustment.

INTERACTIONS

DRUG: May decrease effects of **antihypertensives, diuretics. Aspirin, other salicylates** may increase risk of GI side effects, bleeding. **Bone marrow depressants** may increase risk of hematologic reactions. May increase effects of **heparin, oral anticoagulants, thrombolytics.** May increase concentration, risk of toxicity of **lithium.** May increase risk of **methotrexate** toxicity. **Probenecid** may increase concentration. **HERBAL: Cat's claw, dong quai, evening primrose, feverfew, garlic, ginkgo, ginseng, horse chestnut, red clover** may increase antiplatelet activity, risk of bleeding. **FOOD:** None known. **LAB VALUES:** May prolong bleeding time. May increase serum alkaline phosphatase, hepatic function test results. May decrease Hgb, Hct, serum sodium.

AVAILABILITY (OTC)

Capsules: 50 mg, 75 mg.

Capsules, Extended-Release: 200 mg.

ADMINISTRATION/HANDLING

PO

• May give with food, milk, full glass (8 oz) of water (minimizes potential GI distress). • Do not break, chew extended-release capsules.

INDICATIONS/ROUTES/DOSAGE

Acute or Chronic Rheumatoid Arthritis and Osteoarthritis

PO: ADULTS: Initially, 75 mg 3 times a day or 50 mg 4 times a day. **ELDERLY:** Initially, 25–50 mg 3–4 times a day. Maintenance: 150–300 mg/day in 3–4 divided doses.

PO (EXTENDED-RELEASE): ADULTS, ELDERLY: 200 mg once a day.

Mild to Moderate Pain, Dysmenorrhea

PO: ADULTS, ELDERLY: 25–50 mg q6–8h. **Maximum:** 300 mg/day.

Dosage in Renal Impairment

MILD: 150 mg/day maximum. **SEVERE (creatinine clearance less than 25 ml/min):** 100 mg/day maximum.

SIDE EFFECTS

Frequent (11%): Dyspepsia (heartburn, indigestion, epigastric pain). **Occasional (more than 3%):** Nausea, diarrhea/constipation, flatulence, abdominal cramps, headache. **Rare (less than 2%):** Anorexia, vomiting, visual disturbances, fluid retention.

ADVERSE EFFECTS/ TOXIC REACTIONS

Peptic ulcer, GI bleeding, gastritis, severe hepatic reaction (cholestasis, jaundice) occur rarely. Nephrotoxicity (dysuria, hematuria, proteinuria, nephrotic syndrome), severe hypersensitivity reaction (bronchospasm, angioedema) occur rarely.

K

NURSING CONSIDERATIONS

BASELINE ASSESSMENT

Assess onset, type, location, duration of pain/inflammation. Inspect appearance of affected joints for immobility, deformities, skin condition.

INTERVENTION/EVALUATION

Monitor for evidence of nausea, dyspepsia. Monitor for therapeutic response: Relief of pain, improved range of motion, grip strength, mobility. Monitor renal/hepatic function tests, occult blood loss, mental status.

PATIENT/FAMILY TEACHING

• Avoid aspirin, alcohol during therapy (increases risk of GI bleeding). • If GI upset occurs, take with food, milk. • Swallow capsule whole; do not crush/chew.

K

ketorolac

key-**tore**-oh-lak
(Acular, Acular LS, Acular PF, Apo-Ketorolac ✦, Novo-Ketorolac ✦, Sprix, Toradol)

BLACK BOX ALERT Increased risk of serious cardiovascular thrombotic events, including myocardial infarction, CVA. Increased risk of severe GI reactions, including ulceration, bleeding, perforation.

Do not confuse Acular with Acthar or Ocular, ketorolac with Ketalar, or Toradol with Foradil, Inderal, Tegretol, or tramadol.

◆ CLASSIFICATION

PHARMACOTHERAPEUTIC: Nonsteroidal anti-inflammatory. **CLINICAL:** Analgesic, intraocular anti-inflammatory (see p. 128C).

ACTION

Inhibits prostaglandin synthesis, reduces prostaglandin levels in aqueous humor. **Therapeutic Effect:** Reduces intensity of pain stimulus, reduces intraocular inflammation.

PHARMACOKINETICS

Readily absorbed from GI tract after IM administration. Protein binding: 99%. Largely metabolized in liver. Primarily excreted in urine. Not removed by hemodialysis. **Half-life:** 2–8 hrs (increased in renal impairment, in elderly).

USES

PO, injection: Short-term (5 days or less) relief of mild to moderate pain. **Ophthalmic:** Relief of ocular itching due to seasonal allergic conjunctivitis. Treatment postop for inflammation following cataract extraction, pain following incisional refractive surgery. **OFF-LABEL:** Prevention, treatment of ocular inflammation (ophthalmic form).

PRECAUTIONS

Contraindications: Advanced renal impairment, active peptic ulcer disease, chronic inflammation of GI tract, GI bleeding/ulceration, history of hypersensitivity to aspirin, NSAIDs. **Cautions:** Renal/hepatic impairment, history of GI tract disease, predisposition to fluid retention.

⌛ LIFESPAN CONSIDERATIONS

Pregnancy/Lactation: Unknown if distributed in breast milk. Avoid use during third trimester (may adversely affect fetal cardiovascular system: premature closure of ductus arteriosus). **Pregnancy Category C (D if used in third trimester).** **Children:** Safety and efficacy not established, but doses of 0.5 mg/kg have been used. **Elderly:** GI bleeding, ulceration more likely to cause serious adverse effects. Age-related renal impairment may increase risk of hepatic/renal toxicity; decreased dosage recommended.

INTERACTIONS

DRUG: May decrease effects of **antihypertensives, diuretics. Aspirin, NSAIDs,**

other salicylates may increase risk of GI side effects, bleeding. May increase effects of **heparin, oral anticoagulants, thrombolytics.** May increase concentration, risk of toxicity of **lithium.** May increase risk of **methotrexate** toxicity. **Probenecid** may increase concentration. HERBAL: **Cat's claw, dong quai, evening primrose, feverfew, garlic, ginkgo, ginseng, horse chestnut, red clover** may decrease antiplatelet activity, risk of bleeding. FOOD: None known. LAB VALUES: May prolong bleeding time. May increase hepatic function test results, BUN, potassium, creatinine.

AVAILABILITY (Rx)

Injection Solution (Toradol): 15 mg/ml, 30 mg/ml. Nasal Spray (Sprix): 1.7-g bottle provides 8 sprays (15.75 mg/spray). Ophthalmic Solution: 0.4% (Acular LS), 0.5% (Acular, Acular PF). Tablets (Toradol): 10 mg.

ADMINISTRATION/HANDLING

IV

• Give undiluted as IV push. • Give over at least 15 sec.

IM

• Give deep IM slowly into large muscle mass.

PO

• Give with food, milk, antacids if GI distress occurs.

Ophthalmic

• Place gloved finger on lower eyelid and pull out until pocket is formed between eye and lower lid. Place prescribed number of drops into pocket. • Instruct pt to close eye gently for 1–2 min (so medication will not be squeezed out of the sac) and to apply digital pressure to lacrimal sac at inner canthus for 1 min to minimize system absorption.

IV INCOMPATIBILITY

Promethazine (Phenergan).

IV COMPATIBILITIES

Fentanyl (Sublimaze), hydromorphone (Dilaudid), morphine, nalbuphine (Nubain).

INDICATIONS/ROUTES/DOSAGE

Short-Term Relief of Mild to Moderate Pain (Multiple Doses)

PO: ADULTS, ELDERLY: Initially, 20 mg (10 mg for elderly), then 10 mg q4–6h. **Maximum:** 40 mg/24 hrs. CHILDREN 2–16 YRS: 0.25 mg/kg q6h.

IV, IM: ADULTS YOUNGER THAN 65 YRS: 30 mg q6h. **Maximum:** 120 mg/24 hrs. ADULTS 65 YRS AND OLDER, THOSE WITH RENAL IMPAIRMENT, THOSE WEIGHING LESS THAN 50 KG: 15 mg q6h. **Maximum:** 60 mg/24 hrs. CHILDREN 2–16 YRS: 0.5 mg/kg, then 0.25–1 mg/kg q6h for up to 48 hrs. **Maximum:** 90 mg/day.

NASAL SPRAY: ADULTS, ELDERLY YOUNGER THAN 65 YRS: 31.5 mg (1 spray each nostril) q6–8hr. **Maximum daily dose:** 126 mg. ADULTS 65 YRS AND OLDER, PTS WEIGHING LESS THAN 50 KG: 15.75 mg q6–8hr. **Maximum daily dose:** 63 mg.

Short-Term Relief of Mild to Moderate Pain (Single Dose)

IV: ADULTS YOUNGER THAN 65 YRS, CHILDREN 17 YRS AND OLDER WEIGHING MORE THAN 50 KG: 30 mg. ADULTS 65 YRS AND OLDER, WITH RENAL IMPAIRMENT, WEIGHING LESS THAN 50 KG: 15 mg. CHILDREN 2–16 YRS: 0.5 mg/kg. **Maximum:** 15 mg.

IM: ADULTS YOUNGER THAN 65 YRS, CHILDREN 17 YRS AND OLDER, WEIGHING MORE THAN 50 KG: 60 mg. ADULTS 65 YRS AND OLDER, WITH RENAL IMPAIRMENT, WEIGHING LESS THAN 50 KG: 30 mg. CHILDREN 2–16 YRS: 1 mg/kg. **Maximum:** 30 mg.

Allergic Conjunctivitis

OPHTHALMIC: ADULTS, ELDERLY, CHILDREN 3 YRS AND OLDER: 1 drop 4 times a day.

Cataract Extraction

OPHTHALMIC: ADULTS, ELDERLY: 1 drop 4 times a day. Begin 24 hrs after surgery and continue for 2 wks.

K

Refractive Surgery

OPHTHALMIC: ADULTS, ELDERLY: 1 drop 4 times a day for 3 days.

SIDE EFFECTS

Frequent (17%–12%): Headache, nausea, abdominal cramps/pain, dyspepsia (heartburn, indigestion, epigastric pain). **Occasional (9%–3%):** Diarrhea. **Nasal:** Nasal discomfort, rhinalgia, increased lacrimation, throat irritation, rhinitis. **Ophthalmic:** Transient stinging, burning. **Rare (3%–1%):** Constipation, vomiting, flatulence, stomatitis. **Ophthalmic:** Ocular irritation, allergic reactions (manifested by pruritus, stinging), superficial ocular infection, keratitis.

ADVERSE EFFECTS/ TOXIC REACTIONS

Peptic ulcer, GI bleeding, gastritis, severe hepatic reaction (cholestasis, jaundice) occur rarely. Nephrotoxicity (glomerular nephritis, interstitial nephritis, nephrotic syndrome) may occur in pts with preexisting renal impairment. Acute hypersensitivity reaction (fever, chills, joint pain) occurs rarely.

NURSING CONSIDERATIONS

BASELINE ASSESSMENT

Assess onset, type, location, duration of pain. Obtain baseline renal/hepatic function tests.

INTERVENTION/EVALUATION

Monitor renal/hepatic function tests, urinary output. Monitor daily pattern of bowel activity, stool consistency. Observe for occult blood loss. Assess for therapeutic response: relief of pain, stiffness, swelling; increased joint mobility, reduced joint tenderness, improved grip strength. Be alert to signs of bleeding (may also occur with ophthalmic route due to systemic absorption).

PATIENT/ FAMILY TEACHING

• Avoid aspirin, alcohol during therapy with oral or ophthalmic ketorolac (increases tendency to bleed). • If GI upset occurs, take with food, milk. • Avoid tasks that require alertness, motor skills until response to drug is established. • **Ophthalmic:** Transient stinging, burning may occur upon instillation. • Do not administer while wearing soft contact lenses.

Klonopin, *see clonazepam*

Klor-Con, *see potassium chloride*

Kytril, *see granisetron*

labetalol

lah-**bet**-ah-lol
(Apo-Labetalol 🍁, Normodyne 🍁, Trandate)

Do not confuse labetalol with betaxolol or lamotrigine, or Trandate with tramadol or Trental.

FIXED-COMBINATION(S)

Normozide: labetalol/hydrochlorothiazide (a diuretic): 100 mg/25 mg, 200 mg/25 mg, 300 mg/25 mg.

◆CLASSIFICATION

PHARMACOTHERAPEUTIC: Alpha-, beta-adrenergic blocker. **CLINICAL:** Antihypertensive.

ACTION

Blocks alpha$_1$-, beta$_1$-, beta$_2$- (large doses) adrenergic receptor sites. Large doses increase airway resistance. **Therapeutic Effect:** Slows sinus heart rate; decreases peripheral vascular resistance, cardiac output, B/P.

PHARMACOKINETICS

Route	Onset	Peak	Duration
PO	0.5–2 hrs	2–4 hrs	8–12 hrs
IV	2–5 min	5–15 min	2–4 hrs

Completely absorbed from GI tract. Protein binding: 50%. Undergoes first-pass metabolism in liver. Primarily excreted in urine. Not removed by hemodialysis. **Half-life:** 2.5–8 hrs.

USES

Management of mild to severe hypertension. May be used alone or in combination with other antihypertensives. **OFF-LABEL:** Control of hypotension during surgery, treatment of chronic angina pectoris, pediatric hypertension.

PRECAUTIONS

Contraindications: Bronchial asthma, cardiogenic shock, overt cardiac failure, second- or third-degree heart block, severe bradycardia, uncontrolled CHF, other conditions associated with severe, prolonged hypotension. **Cautions:** Medication-controlled CHF, nonallergic bronchospastic disease (chronic bronchitis, emphysema), hepatic or cardiac impairment, pheochromocytoma, diabetes mellitus.

LIFESPAN CONSIDERATIONS

Pregnancy/Lactation: Drug crosses placenta. Small amount distributed in breast milk. **Pregnancy Category C (D if used in second or third trimester). Children:** Safety and efficacy not established. **Elderly:** Age-related peripheral vascular disease may increase susceptibility to decreased peripheral circulation.

INTERACTIONS

DRUG: Diuretics, other antihypertensives may increase hypotensive effect. **Insulin, oral hypoglycemics** may mask symptoms of hypoglycemia, prolong hypoglycemic effect of these drugs. **Sympathomimetics, xanthines** may mutually inhibit effects. **HERBAL: Ephedra, ginseng, yohimbe** may worsen hypertension. **Garlic** may increase antihypertensive effect. **Licorice** may cause water retention, increased serum sodium, decreased serum potassium. **FOOD:** None known. **LAB VALUES:** May increase serum antinuclear antibody titer (ANA), BUN, LDH, lipoprotein, alkaline phosphatase, bilirubin, creatinine, potassium, triglyceride, uric acid, AST, ALT.

AVAILABILITY (Rx)

Injection Solution (Trandate): 5 mg/ml. **Tablets (Trandate):** 100 mg, 200 mg, 300 mg.

ADMINISTRATION/HANDLING

IV

◀ALERT▶ Pt must be in supine position for IV administration and for 3 hrs after receiving medication (substantial drop in B/P upon standing should be expected).

Reconstitution • For IV infusion, dilute in D_5W to provide concentration of 1–2 mg/ml.

Rate of administration • For IV push, give over 2–3 min at 10-min intervals. • Do not administer faster than 2 mg/min. • For IV infusion, administer at rate of 2 mg/min initially. Rate is adjusted according to B/P. • Monitor B/P immediately before and q5–10min during IV administration (maximum effect occurs within 5 min).

Storage • Store at room temperature. • After dilution, IV solution is stable for 24 hrs. • Solution appears clear, colorless to light yellow. • Discard if discolored or precipitate forms.

PO

• Give without regard to food. • Tablets may be crushed.

IV INCOMPATIBILITIES

Amphotericin B complex (Abelcet, AmBisome, Amphotec), ceftriaxone (Rocephin), furosemide (Lasix), heparin, nafcillin (Nafcil), thiopental.

IV COMPATIBILITIES

Aminophylline, amiodarone (Cordarone), calcium gluconate, diltiazem (Cardizem), dobutamine (Dobutrex), dopamine (Intropin), enalapril (Vasotec), fentanyl (Sublimaze), hydromorphone (Dilaudid), lidocaine, lorazepam (Ativan), magnesium sulfate, midazolam (Versed), milrinone (Primacor), morphine, nitroglycerin, norepinephrine (Levophed), potassium chloride, potassium phosphate, propofol (Diprivan).

INDICATIONS/ROUTES/DOSAGE

Hypertension

PO: ADULTS: Initially, 100 mg twice a day adjusted in increments of 100 mg twice a day q2–3days. Maintenance: 200–400 mg twice a day. **Maximum:** 2.4 g/day. **ELDERLY:** Initially, 100 mg 1–2 times a day. May increase as needed.

Severe Hypertension, Hypertensive Crisis

IV: ADULTS: Initially, 20 mg. Additional doses of 20–80 mg may be given at 10-min intervals, up to total dose of 300 mg. **IV INFUSION: ADULTS:** Initially, 2 mg/min up to total dose of 300 mg.

SIDE EFFECTS

Frequent: Drowsiness, difficulty sleeping, excessive fatigue, weakness, diminished sexual function, transient scalp tingling. **Occasional:** Dizziness, dyspnea, peripheral edema, depression, anxiety, constipation, diarrhea, nasal congestion, nausea, vomiting, abdominal discomfort. **Rare:** Altered taste, dry eyes, increased urination, paresthesia.

ADVERSE EFFECTS/ TOXIC REACTIONS

May precipitate, aggravate CHF due to decreased myocardial stimulation. Abrupt withdrawal may precipitate myocardial ischemia, producing chest pain, diaphoresis, palpitations, headache, tremor. May mask signs, symptoms of acute hypoglycemia (tachycardia, B/P changes) in diabetic pts.

NURSING CONSIDERATIONS

BASELINE ASSESSMENT

Assess baseline renal/hepatic function tests. Assess B/P, apical pulse immediately before drug administration (if pulse is 60/min or less or systolic B/P is lower than 90 mm Hg, withhold medication, contact physician).

INTERVENTION/EVALUATION

Monitor B/P for hypotension. Assess pulse for quality, irregular rate, bradycardia. Monitor EKG for cardiac arrhythmias. Monitor daily pattern of bowel activity and stool consistency. Assist with ambulation if dizziness occurs. Assess for evidence of CHF: dyspnea (particularly on exertion or lying down), night cough, peripheral edema, distended neck veins. Monitor I&O (increase in weight, decrease in urine output may indicate CHF).

PATIENT/FAMILY TEACHING

• Do not discontinue drug except upon advice of physician (abrupt discontinuation may precipitate heart failure). • Rise slowly from sitting position. • Compliance with therapy regimen is essential to control hypertension, arrhythmias. • Avoid tasks that require alertness, motor skills until response to drug is established. • Report shortness of breath, excessive fatigue, weight gain, prolonged dizziness, headache. • Do not use nasal decongestants, OTC cold preparations (stimulants) without physician approval. • Limit alcohol.

lacosamide

lah-**coe**-sah-mide
(Vimpat)
Do not confuse lacosamide with zonisamide.

◆CLASSIFICATION

PHARMACOTHERAPEUTIC: Succinimide. **CLINICAL:** Anticonvulsant. **Schedule V.**

ACTION

Selectively enhances slow inactivation of sodium channels, stabilizing hyperexcitable neuronal membranes and inhibits

L

neuronal firing. **Therapeutic Effect:** Produces anticonvulsant effect.

PHARMACOKINETICS

Completely absorbed following PO administration. Protein binding: 15%. Maximum plasma concentration occurs 1–4 hrs after oral dosing and is reached at the end of IV infusion. Primarily excreted in urine. Steady-state levels achieved in 3 days. Removed by hemodialysis. **Half-life:** 13 hrs.

USES

Tablets used as adjunctive therapy for treatment of partial-onset seizures in pts 17 yrs and older with epilepsy. Injection form indicated as adjunctive therapy for treatment of partial-onset seizures in pts 17 years and older with epilepsy when oral administration is temporarily not feasible. **OFF-LABEL:** Treatment of fibromyalgia.

PRECAUTIONS

Contraindications: Severe hepatic impairment. **Cautions:** Renal/hepatic impairment, marked first-degree AV block, second-degree or higher AV block, sick sinus syndrome without pacemaker, myocardial ischemia, heart failure.

LIFESPAN CONSIDERATIONS

Pregnancy/Lactation: Unknown if distributed in breast milk. **Pregnancy Category C. Children:** Safety and efficacy not established in those younger than 17 yrs. **Elderly:** No age-related precautions noted.

INTERACTIONS

DRUG: None significant. **HERBAL:** None significant. **FOOD:** None known. **LAB VALUES:** May increase ALT, serum transaminase, proteinuria.

AVAILABILITY (Rx)

Injection Solution: 200 mg/20 ml.

Tablets: 50 mg, 100 mg, 150 mg, 200 mg.

ADMINISTRATION/HANDLING

PO

• Give without regard to meals. • Do not crush or break film-coated tablets.

IV

• Appears as a clear, colorless solution. • Discard unused portion or if precipitate or discoloration is present. • If mixing with diluent, may be stored for 24 hrs at room temperature. Infuse over 30–60 min.

IV COMPATIBILITIES

0.9% NaCl, D_5W, lactated Ringer's.

INDICATIONS/ROUTES/DOSAGE

Partial-Onset Seizures

PO: ADULTS, CHILDREN 17 YRS AND OLDER: Initially, 50 mg twice daily (100 mg/day). May increase by 100 mg/day at weekly intervals, given as 2 daily divided doses up to maintenance dose of 200–400 mg/day, based on pt response, tolerability.

IV: ADULTS, CHILDREN 17 YRS AND OLDER: May be given undiluted or mixed in compatible diluent and given as 30- to 60-min infusion.

Switch from IV to PO

When switching from IV to PO form, use same equivalent daily dosage and frequency of IV administration.

Switch from PO to IV

When switching from PO to IV form, initial total daily IV dosage should be equivalent to total daily dosage and frequency of PO form and should be infused IV over 30–60 min.

Severe Renal Impairment (Creatinine Clearance 30 ml/min or Less, Pts with End-Stage Renal Disease)

PO/IV: ADULTS, ELDERLY, CHILDREN 17 YRS AND OLDER: Maximum: 300 mg/day.

Mild to Moderate Hepatic Impairment

PO/IV: ADULTS, ELDERLY, CHILDREN 17 YRS AND OLDER: Maximum: 300 mg/day.

L

SIDE EFFECTS

Frequent (31%–13%): Dizziness, headache. **Occasional (11%–5%):** Nausea, double vision, vomiting, fatigue, blurred vision, ataxia (difficulty with balance, coordination, slurred speech), tremor, nystagmus (involuntary movement of eyeball). **Rare (4%–2%):** Vertigo, diarrhea, gait disturbances, memory impairment, depression, pruritus, injection site discomfort.

ADVERSE EFFECTS/ TOXIC REACTIONS

Increased risk of suicidal thoughts, behavior. Dose-dependent prolongations in PR interval noted. Leukopenia, anemia, thrombocytopenia occur rarely.

NURSING CONSIDERATIONS

BASELINE ASSESSMENT

Review history of seizure disorder (intensity, frequency, duration, level of consciousness). Initiate seizure precautions. Hepatic/renal function tests, CBC, platelet count should be performed before therapy begins and periodically during therapy.

INTERVENTION/EVALUATION

Observe frequently for recurrence of seizure activity. Assess for clinical improvement (decrease in intensity/frequency of seizures). Assist with ambulation if dizziness occurs. Assess for suicidal ideation, depression, behavioral changes. Drug should be withdrawn gradually (over a minimum of 1 wk) to minimize potential for increased seizure frequency.

PATIENT/FAMILY TEACHING

• Strict maintenance of drug therapy is essential for seizure control. • Avoid tasks that require alertness, motor skills until response to drug is established. • Avoid alcohol. • Notify physician of depression, suicidal thoughts, unusual behavioral changes.

lactulose

lak-tew-lose
(Acilac ✱, Apo-Lactulose ✱, Constulose, Enulose, Generlac, Kristalose, Laxilose ✱)
Do not confuse lactulose with lactose.

◆CLASSIFICATION

PHARMACOTHERAPEUTIC: Lactose derivative. **CLINICAL:** Hyperosmotic laxative, ammonia detoxicant (see p. 122C).

ACTION

Prevents reabsorption of ammonia, producing osmotic effect. **Therapeutic Effect:** Promotes increased peristalsis, bowel evacuation; decreases serum ammonia concentration.

PHARMACOKINETICS

Poorly absorbed from GI tract. Extensively metabolized in colon. Primarily excreted in feces.

USES

Prevention, treatment of portal-systemic encephalopathy (including hepatic precoma, coma); treatment of chronic constipation.

PRECAUTIONS

Contraindications: Abdominal pain, appendicitis, nausea, pts on galactose-free diet, vomiting. **Cautions:** Diabetes mellitus.

⌛ LIFESPAN CONSIDERATIONS

Pregnancy/Lactation: Unknown if drug crosses placenta or is distributed in breast milk. **Pregnancy Category B. Children:** Avoid use in those younger than 6 yrs (usually unable to describe symptoms). **Elderly:** No age-related precautions noted.

INTERACTIONS

DRUG: May decrease transit time of concurrently administered **oral medications,** decreasing absorption. **HERBAL:**

None significant. **FOOD:** None known. **LAB VALUES:** May decrease serum potassium.

AVAILABILITY (Rx)

Packets (Kristalose): 10 g, 20 g. **Solution, Oral (Constulose, Enulose, Generlac):** 10 g/15 ml.

ADMINISTRATION/HANDLING

PO

• Store solution at room temperature. • Solution appears pale yellow to yellow, viscous liquid. Cloudiness, darkened solution does not indicate potency loss. • Drink water, juice, milk with each dose (aids stool softening, increases palatability).

Rectal

• Lubricate anus with petroleum jelly before enema insertion. • Insert carefully (prevents damage to rectal wall) with nozzle toward navel. • Squeeze container until entire dose expelled. • Instruct pt to retain until definite lower abdominal cramping felt.

INDICATIONS/ROUTES/DOSAGE

Constipation

PO: ADULTS, ELDERLY: 15–30 ml (10–20 g)/day, up to 60 ml (40 g)/day. **CHILDREN:** 7.5 ml (5 g)/day after breakfast.

Prevention of Portal-Systemic Encephalopathy

CHILDREN: 40–90 ml/day in divided doses 3–4 times a day. **INFANTS:** 2.5–10 ml/day in 3–4 divided doses.

Treatment of Portal-Systemic Encephalopathy

PO: ADULTS, ELDERLY: Initially, 30–45 ml (20–30 g) every hr to induce rapid laxation. Then, 30–45 ml 3–4 times a day. Adjust dose q1–2days to produce 2–3 soft stools a day. Usual daily dose: 90–150 ml (60–100 g).

Rectal Administration (as Retention Enema)

200 g (300 ml) diluted with 700 ml water or NaCl via rectal balloon catheter. Retain 30–60 min q4–6hrs.

SIDE EFFECTS

Occasional: Abdominal cramping, flatulence, increased thirst, abdominal discomfort. **Rare:** Nausea, vomiting.

ADVERSE EFFECTS/ TOXIC REACTIONS

Diarrhea indicates overdose. Long-term use may result in laxative dependence, chronic constipation, loss of normal bowel function.

NURSING CONSIDERATIONS

INTERVENTION/EVALUATION

Encourage adequate fluid intake. Assess bowel sounds for peristalsis. Monitor daily pattern of bowel activity, stool consistency; record time of evacuation. Assess for abdominal disturbances. Monitor serum electrolytes in pts exposed to prolonged, frequent, excessive use of medication.

PATIENT/FAMILY TEACHING

• Evacuation occurs in 24–48 hrs of initial dose. • Institute measures to promote defecation: increase fluid intake, exercise, high-fiber diet.

Lamictal, *see lamotrigine*

Lamisil, *see terbinafine*

lamivudine

la-**miv**-ue-deen

(Epivir, Epivir-HBV, Heptovir ✦)

BLACK BOX ALERT Serious, sometimes fatal lactic acidosis, severe hepatomegaly with steatosis (fatty liver) have occurred. Pts must be monitored for chronic hepatitis B for several months following therapy.

Do not confuse lamivudine with lamotrigine, or Epivir with Combivir.

L

FIXED-COMBINATION(S)

Combivir: lamivudine/zidovudine (an antiviral): 150 mg/300 mg. **Epzicom:** lamivudine/abacavir (an antiviral): 300 mg/600 mg. **Trizivir:** lamivudine/zidovudine/abacavir (an antiviral): 150 mg/300 mg/300 mg.

◆ CLASSIFICATION

PHARMACOTHERAPEUTIC: Nucleoside reverse transcriptase inhibitors. **CLINICAL:** Antiviral (see pp. 69C, 115C).

ACTION

Inhibits HIV reverse transcriptase by viral DNA chain termination. Inhibits RNA-, DNA-dependent DNA polymerase, an enzyme necessary for HIV replication. **Therapeutic Effect:** Slows HIV replication, reduces progression of HIV infection.

L

PHARMACOKINETICS

Rapidly, completely absorbed from GI tract. Protein binding: less than 36%. Widely distributed (crosses blood-brain barrier). Primarily excreted unchanged in urine. Not removed by hemodialysis or peritoneal dialysis. **Half-life: Children:** 2 hrs. **Adults:** 5–7 hrs.

USES

Epivir: Treatment of HIV infection in combination with other antiretroviral agents. **Epivir-HBV:** Treatment of chronic hepatitis B. **OFF-LABEL:** Prophylaxis in health care workers at risk of acquiring HIV after occupational exposure to virus.

PRECAUTIONS

Contraindications: None known. **Cautions:** Peripheral neuropathy, history of peripheral neuropathy, history of pancreatitis in children, renal impairment.

⌛ LIFESPAN CONSIDERATIONS

Pregnancy/Lactation: Drug crosses placenta. Unknown if distributed in breast milk. Breast-feeding not recommended (possibility of HIV transmission). **Pregnancy Category C. Children:** Safety and efficacy not established in those younger than 3 mos. **Elderly:** Age-related renal impairment may require dosage adjustment.

INTERACTIONS

DRUG: **Co-trimoxazole** increases concentration. **Zalcitabine** may inhibit absorption of both drugs; avoid concurrent administration. **HERBAL:** **St. John's wort** may decrease concentration, effect. **FOOD:** None known. **LAB VALUES:** May increase Hgb, neutrophil count, serum amylase, AST, ALT, bilirubin.

AVAILABILITY (Rx)

Oral Solution: 5 mg/ml (Epivir-HBV), 10 mg/ml (Epivir). **Tablets:** 100 mg (Epivir-HBV), 150 mg (Epivir), 300 mg (Epivir).

ADMINISTRATION/HANDLING

PO

- Give without regard to meals.

INDICATIONS/ROUTES/DOSAGE

HIV Infection

PO: ADULTS WEIGHING 50 KG OR MORE: 150 mg twice a day or 300 mg once a day. **ADULTS WEIGHING LESS THAN 50 KG:** 4 mg/kg twice a day (up to 150 mg/dose). **CHILDREN 4 MOS–16 YRS:** 4 mg/kg twice a day (up to 150 mg/dose). **INFANTS 1–3 MOS:** 4 mg/kg twice/day. **NEONATES YOUNGER THAN 30 DAYS:** 2 mg/kg twice/day.

Chronic Hepatitis B

PO: ADULTS: 100 mg/day. **CHILDREN 2–17 YRS:** 3 mg/kg/day. **Maximum:** 100 mg/day.

Dosage in Renal Impairment

Dosage and frequency are modified based on creatinine clearance.

Creatinine Clearance	Dosage HIV	Dosage Hepatitis B
30–49 ml/min	150 mg once a day	100 mg first dose, then 50 mg once a day

Creatinine Clearance	Dosage HIV	Dosage Hepatitis B
15–29 ml/min	150 mg first dose, then 100 mg once a day	100 mg first dose, then 25 mg once a day
5–14 ml/min	150 mg first dose, then 50 mg once a day	35 mg first dose, then 15 mg once a day
Less than 5 ml/min	50 mg first dose, then 25 mg once a day	35 mg first dose, then 10 mg once a day

SIDE EFFECTS

Frequent: Headache (35%), nausea (33%), malaise, fatigue (27%), nasal disturbances (20%), diarrhea, cough (18%), musculoskeletal pain, neuropathy (12%), insomnia (11%), anorexia, dizziness, fever, chills (10%). **Occasional:** Depression (9%), myalgia (8%), abdominal cramps (6%), dyspepsia, arthralgia (5%).

ADVERSE EFFECTS/ TOXIC REACTIONS

Pancreatitis occurs in 13% of pediatric pts. Anemia, neutropenia, thrombocytopenia occur rarely. Lactic acidosis, severe hepatomegaly with steatosis have been reported.

NURSING CONSIDERATIONS

BASELINE ASSESSMENT

Establish baseline lab values, esp. renal function. Screen HIV pt for hepatitis B infection before initiating therapy.

INTERVENTION/EVALUATION

Monitor serum creatinine, amylase, lipase ALT, AST, bilirubin, BUN. Assess for headache, nausea, cough. Monitor daily pattern of bowel activity, stool consistency. Modify diet or administer laxative as needed. Assess for dizziness, sleep pattern. If pancreatitis in children occurs, movement aggravates abdominal pain; sitting up, flexing at the waist relieves the pain.

PATIENT/FAMILY TEACHING

• Continue therapy for full length of treatment. • Doses should be evenly spaced. • Lamivudine is not a cure for HIV infection, nor does it reduce risk of transmission to others. • Avoid tasks requiring alertness, motor skills until response to drug is established. • Avoid alcohol. • Closely monitor for symptoms of pancreatitis (severe, steady abdominal pain often radiating to the back, clammy skin, hypotension; nausea/vomiting may accompany abdominal pain).

lamotrigine

lam-**oh**-trih-jeen
(Apo-Lamotrigine ✤, Lamictal, Lamictal ODT, Lamictal XR, Novo-Lamotrigine ✤)

BLACK BOX ALERT Severe, potentially life-threatening skin rashes have been reported, including Stevens-Johnson syndrome. Risk increased with coadministration with valproic acid and rapid dose titration.

Do not confuse Lamictal with Lamisil or Lomotil, or lamotrigine with labetalol or lamivudine.

◆ CLASSIFICATION

CLINICAL: Anticonvulsants (see p. 35C).

ACTION

May block voltage-sensitive sodium channels, stabilizing neuronal membranes, regulating presynaptic transmitter release of excitatory amino acids. **Therapeutic Effect:** Produces anticonvulsant activity.

USES

Adjunctive therapy in adults and children with partial seizures, treatment of adults and children with generalized seizures of Lennox-Gastaut syndrome. Conversion to monotherapy in adults treated with another enzyme-inducing antiepileptic drug (EIAED). Long-term maintenance treat-

L

ment of bipolar disorder. Treatment of pts 2 yrs and older with primary generalized tonic-clonic seizures. **Extended-Release:** Adjunctive therapy for primary generalized tonic-clonic and partial-onset seizures in pts 13 yrs and older.

PRECAUTIONS

Contraindications: None known. **Cautions:** Renal, hepatic, cardiac impairment.

LIFESPAN CONSIDERATIONS

Pregnancy/Lactation: Distributed in breast milk. Breast-feeding not recommended. Increased fetal risk of oral cleft formation has been noted with use during pregnancy. **Pregnancy Category C. Children:** Safety and efficacy in those 18 yrs and younger with bipolar disorder, younger than 13 yrs with epilepsy has not been established. **Elderly:** Age-related renal impairment may require dosage adjustment.

INTERACTIONS

DRUG: **Carbamazepine, phenobarbital, primidone, valproic acid** decrease concentration. May increase concentration of **carbamazepine, valproic acid.** May decrease effect of **oral contraceptives.** **HERBAL:** **Evening primrose** may decrease seizure threshold. **FOOD:** None known. **LAB VALUES:** None significant.

AVAILABILITY (Rx)

Tablets: 25 mg, 100 mg, 150 mg, 200 mg. **Tablets (Chewable):** 2 mg, 5 mg, 25 mg. **Tablets (Orally-Disintegrating):** 25 mg, 50 mg, 100 mg, 200 mg.

Tablets (Extended-Release): 25 mg, 50 mg, 100 mg, 200 mg.

ADMINISTRATION/HANDLING

PO

• Give without regard to food. • Chewable tablets may be dispensed in water or diluted fruit juice, or swallowed whole. • Extended-release tablets must be swallowed whole; do not chew, crush or divide. • Place orally-disintegrating tablet on tongue, allow to dissolve; do not break, cut, or chew.

INDICATIONS/ROUTES/DOSAGE

Lennox-Gastaut, Primary Generalized Tonic-Clonic Seizures, Partial Seizures

PO: ADULTS, ELDERLY, CHILDREN OLDER THAN 12 YRS: Initially, 25 mg/day for 2 wks, then increase to 50 mg/day for 2 wks. After 4 wks, may increase by 50 mg/day at 1- to 2-wk intervals. Maintenance: 225–375 mg/day in 2 divided doses. **CHILDREN 2–12 YRS:** Initially, 0.3 mg/kg/day in 1–2 divided doses for 2 wks, then increase to 0.6 mg/kg/day in 1–2 divided doses for 2 wks. After 4 wks, may increase by 0.6 mg/kg/day at 1- to 2-wk intervals. Maintenance: 4.5–7.5 mg/kg/day in 2 divided doses. **Maximum:** 300 mg/day in 2 divided doses.

Adjusted Dosage with Anti-Epileptic Drugs Containing Valproic Acid

PO: ADULTS, ELDERLY, CHILDREN OLDER THAN 12 YRS: Initially, 25 mg every other day for 2 wks, then increase to 25 mg/day for 2 wks. After 4 wks, may increase by 25–50 mg/day at 1- to 2-wk intervals. Maintenance: 100–400 mg/day in 2 divided doses (100–200 mg/day when taking lamotrigine with valproic acid alone). **CHILDREN 2–12 YRS:** Initially, 0.15 mg/kg/day in 1–2 divided doses for 2 wks, then increase to 0.3 mg/kg/day in 1–2 divided doses for 2 wks. After 4 wks, may increase by 0.3 mg/kg/day at 1- to 2-wk intervals. Maintenance: 1–5 mg/kg/day in 2 divided doses. **Maximum:** 200 mg/day in 2 divided doses.

Adjusted Dosage with EIAED without Valproic Acid

PO: ADULTS, ELDERLY, CHILDREN OLDER THAN 12 YRS: Initially, 50 mg/day for 2 wks, then increase to 100 mg/day in 2 divided doses for 2 wks. After 4 wks, may increase by 100 mg/day at 1- to 2-wk intervals. Maintenance: 300–500 mg/day in 2 divided doses. **CHILDREN 2–12 YRS:** Initially, 0.6 mg/kg/day in 1–2 divided doses for 2 wks, then increase to 1.2 mg/kg/day in 1–2 divided doses for 2 wks. After 4 wks, may increase by 1.2 mg/kg/day at 1- to

2-wk intervals. Maintenance: 5–15 mg/kg/day in 2 divided doses. **Maximum:** 400 mg/day in 2 divided doses.

Usual Maintenance Range for Extended-Release Tablets
PT TAKING VALPROIC ACID: 200–250 mg once daily. **PT TAKING EIAED WITHOUT VALPROIC ADIC:** 400–600 mg once daily. **PT NOT TAKING EIAED:** 300–400 mg once daily.

Conversion to Monotherapy for Pts Receiving EIAEDs
PO: ADULTS, ELDERLY, CHILDREN 16 YRS AND OLDER: 500 mg/day in 2 divided doses. Titrate to desired dose while maintaining EIAED at fixed level, then withdraw EIAED by 20% each wk over a 4-wk period.

Conversion to Monotherapy for Pts Receiving Valproic Acid
PO: ADULTS, ELDERLY, CHILDREN 16 YRS AND OLDER: Titrate lamotrigine to 200 mg/day, maintaining valproic acid dose. Maintain lamotrigine dose and decrease valproic acid to 500 mg/day, no greater than 500 mg/day/wk, then maintain 500 mg/day for 1 wk. Increase lamotrigine to 300 mg/day and decrease valproic acid to 250 mg/day. Maintain for 1 wk, then discontinue valproic acid and increase lamotrigine by 100 mg/day each wk until maintenance dose of 500 mg/day reached.

Bipolar Disorder
PO: ADULTS, ELDERLY: Initially, 25 mg/day for 2 wks, then 50 mg/day for 2 wks, then 100 mg/day for 1 wk, then 200 mg/day begining with wk 6.

Bipolar Disorder in Pts Receiving EIAEDs
PO: ADULTS, ELDERLY: 50 mg/day for 2 wks, then 100 mg/day for 2 wks, then 200 mg/day for 1 wk, then 300 mg/day for 1 wk, then up to usual maintenance dose 400 mg/day in divided doses.

Bipolar Disorder in Pts Receiving Valproic Acid
PO: ADULTS, ELDERLY: 25 mg/day every other day for 2 wks, then 25 mg/day for 2 wks, then 50 mg/day for 1 wk, then 100 mg/day. Usual maintenance dose with valproic acid: 100 mg/day.

Discontinuation Therapy
◀ALERT▶ A dosage reduction of approximately 50% per wk over at least 2 wks is recommended.

Dosage in Renal Impairment
◀ALERT▶ Decreased dosage may be effective in pts with significant renal impairment.

SIDE EFFECTS

Frequent: Dizziness (38%), headache (29%), diplopia (double vision) (28%), ataxia (22%), nausea (19%), blurred vision (16%), drowsiness, rhinitis (14%). **Occasional (10%–5%):** Rash, pharyngitis, vomiting, cough, flu-like symptoms, diarrhea, dysmenorrhea, fever, insomnia, dyspepsia. **Rare:** Constipation, tremor, anxiety, pruritus, vaginitis, hypersensitivity reaction.

ADVERSE EFFECTS/ TOXIC REACTIONS

Abrupt withdrawal may increase seizure frequency. Serious rashes, including Stevens-Johnson syndrome, have been reported.

NURSING CONSIDERATIONS

BASELINE ASSESSMENT

Review history of seizure disorder (type, onset, intensity, frequency, duration, LOC), drug history (esp. other anticonvulsants), other medical conditions (e.g., renal impairment). Provide safety precautions; quiet, dark environment.

INTERVENTION/EVALUATION

Report to physician promptly if rash occurs (drug discontinuation may be necessary). Assist with ambulation if dizziness, ataxia occurs. Assess for clinical improvement (decreased intensity/frequency of seizures). Assess for visual abnormalities, headache. Monitor for suicidal ideation, depression, behavioral changes.

L

PATIENT/ FAMILY TEACHING

• Take medication only as prescribed; do not abruptly discontinue medication after long-term therapy. • Avoid alcohol. • Avoid tasks that require alertness, motor skills until response to drug is established. • Carry identification card/bracelet to note anticonvulsant therapy. • Strict maintenance of drug therapy is essential for seizure control. • Report to physician any rash, fever, swelling of glands, worsening depression, suicidal ideation, unusual changes in behavior, worsening of seizure control. • May cause photosensitivity reaction; avoid exposure to sunlight, artificial light.

Lanoxin, *see digoxin*

lanreotide

lan-**ree**-oh-tide
(Somatuline Depot)
Do not confuse Somatuline with somatropin or sumatriptan.

◆CLASSIFICATION

PHARMACOTHERAPEUTIC: Somatostatin analog. **CLINICAL:** Acromegaly agent.

ACTION

Inhibits synthesis of thyroid-stimulating hormone (TSH), lowers levels of growth hormone (GH) and insulin-like growth factor-1 (IGF-1). Inhibits some digestive hormones, intestinal secretions. Inhibits insulin, glucagon secretion. **Therapeutic Effect:** Normalizes IGF-1 and GH levels in acromegalic pts.

PHARMACOKINETICS

Diffuses into tissue, absorbed into bloodstream. **Half-life:** 23–30 days.

USES

Long-term treatment of acromegalic pts who have had an inadequate response to surgery/radiotherapy, or for whom surgery/radiotherapy is not an option.

PRECAUTIONS

Contraindications: None known. **Cautions:** History of cholelithiasis, hyperglycemia, hypoglycemia, bradycardia, renal impairment, hepatic impairment.

LIFESPAN CONSIDERATIONS

Pregnancy/Lactation: May cause fetal harm. Unknown if distributed in breast milk. **Pregnancy Category C. Children:** Safety and efficacy not established. **Elderly:** No age-related precautions noted.

INTERACTIONS

DRUG: May decrease **cyclosporine** concentration. May increase effects of **beta-blockers, calcium channel blockers, drugs that affect heart rate. FOOD:** None known. **HERBAL:** None significant. **LAB VALUES:** May decrease Hgb, Hct. May alter serum glucose.

AVAILABILITY (Rx)

Single-Use Syringe: 60 mg, 90 mg, 120 mg.

ADMINISTRATION/HANDLING

Deep subcutaneous • Inject into superior external quadrant of buttock. • Alternate injection sites.
Storage • Refrigerate syringes. • Remove from refrigerator 30 min prior to administration to allow contents to warm to room temperature.

INDICATIONS/ROUTES/DOSAGE

Acromegaly

DEEP SUBCUTANEOUS, DOSE RANGE: ADULTS, ELDERLY: 60–120 mg every 4 wks. **Recommended:** 90 mg every 4 wks for 3 mos.

Renal, Hepatic Impairment

DEEP SUBCUTANEOUS: ADULTS, ELDERLY: Initially, 60 mg every 4 wks for 3 mos.

SIDE EFFECTS

Frequent (37%): Diarrhea. **Occasional (19%–8%):** Abdominal pain, nausea, injection site pain, nodules, induration, pruritus; constipation. **Rare (7%–6%):** Flatulence, vomiting, arthralgia, headache, loose stools.

ADVERSE EFFECTS/ TOXIC REACTIONS

Cholelithiasis occurs in 20% of pts. Sinus bradycardia, hypertension, anemia occur in 7% of pts.

NURSING CONSIDERATIONS

BASELINE ASSESSMENT

Obtain baseline hepatic function tests before treatment begins and monthly thereafter. Serum levels of growth hormone (GH) and insulin-like growth factor-1 (IGF-1) should be assessed 3 mos after initiation of treatment.

INTERVENTION/EVALUATION

Periodic monitoring required for cholelithiasis. Monitor glucose levels and adjust antidiabetic treatment accordingly.

PATIENT/FAMILY TEACHING

- Contact physician if diarrhea, abdominal pain, constipation, vomiting, joint pain occur.

lansoprazole

lan-so-**prah**-zoll
(Apo-Lansoprazole ✤, Novo-Lansoprazole ✤, Prevacid, Prevacid Solu-Tab)

Do not confuse lansoprazole with aripiprazole or dexlansoprazole, or Prevacid with Pravachol, Prilosec, or Prinivil.

FIXED-COMBINATION(S)

Prevacid NapraPac: lansoprazole/naproxen (an NSAID): 15 mg/375 mg, 15 mg/500 mg. **Prevpac:** Combination card containing amoxicillin 500 mg (4 capsules), lansoprazole 30 mg (2 capsules), clarithromycin 500 mg (2 tablets).

◆CLASSIFICATION

CLINICAL: Proton pump inhibitor (see p. 148C).

ACTION

Selectively inhibits parietal cell membrane enzyme system (hydrogen-potassium adenosine triphosphatase), proton pump. **Therapeutic Effect:** Suppresses gastric acid secretion.

PHARMACOKINETICS

Rapid, complete absorption (food may decrease absorption) once drug has left stomach. Protein binding: 97%. Distributed primarily to gastric parietal cells and converted to two active metabolites. Extensively metabolized in liver. Eliminated in bile and urine. Not removed by hemodialysis. **Half-life:** 1.5 hrs (increased in hepatic impairment, elderly).

USES

Short-term treatment (4 wks and less) of healing, symptomatic relief of active duodenal ulcer; short-term treatment (8 wks and less) for healing, symptomatic relief of erosive esophagitis. Long-term treatment of pathologic hypersecretory conditions, including Zollinger-Ellison syndrome. Short-term treatment (8 wks and less) of active gastric ulcer, *H. pylori*–associated duodenal ulcer, maintenance treatment for healed duodenal ulcer. Treatment of gastroesophageal reflux disease (GERD), NSAID-associated gastric ulcer. **IV:** Short-term treatment of erosive esophagitis.

PRECAUTIONS

Contraindications: None known. **Cautions:** Hepatic impairment. May increase risk of hip, wrist, spine fractures.

⌛ LIFESPAN CONSIDERATIONS

Pregnancy/Lactation: Unknown if distributed in breast milk. **Pregnancy Cate-**

gory B. **Children:** Safety and efficacy not established. **Elderly:** No age-related precautions noted but doses greater than 30 mg not recommended.

INTERACTIONS

DRUG: May interfere with absorption of **ampicillin, digoxin, iron salts, ketoconazole. Sucralfate** may delay absorption. May increase effect of **warfarin.** May decrease effect of **clopidogrel.** HERBAL: None significant. FOOD: **Food** may decrease absorption. LAB VALUES: May increase LDH, serum alkaline phosphatase, bilirubin, cholesterol, creatinine, AST, ALT, triglycerides, uric acid, Hgb, Hct. May produce abnormal albumin/globulin ratio, electrolyte balance, platelet, RBC, WBC count.

AVAILABILITY (Rx)

Tablets, Orally-Disintegrating (Prevacid Solu-Tab): 15 mg, 30 mg.

Capsules (Delayed-Release [Prevacid]): 15 mg, 30 mg.

ADMINISTRATION/HANDLING

PO

• Give while fasting or before meals (food diminishes absorption). • Do not chew/crush delayed-release capsules. • If pt has difficulty swallowing capsules, open capsules, sprinkle granules on 1 tbsp of applesauce, swallow immediately.

PO (Solu-Tab)

• Place tablet on tongue; allow to dissolve, then swallow. • May give via oral syringe or nasogastric tube. • May dissolve in 4 ml (15 mg) or 10 ml (30 mg) water.

INDICATIONS/ROUTES/DOSAGE

Duodenal Ulcer

PO: ADULTS, ELDERLY: 15 mg/day, before eating, preferably in the morning, for up to 4 wks. Maintenance: 15 mg/day.

Erosive Esophagitis

PO: ADULTS, ELDERLY: 30 mg/day, before eating, for up to 8 wks. If healing does not occur within 8 wks (in 5%–10% of cases), may give for additional 8 wks. Maintenance: 15 mg/day. CHILDREN 12–17 YRS: 30 mg/day up to 8 wks. CHILDREN 1–11 YRS, WEIGHING GREATER THAN 30 KG: 30 mg/day; WEIGHING 30 KG OR LESS: 15 mg/day.

Gastric Ulcer

PO: ADULTS: 30 mg/day for up to 8 wks.

NSAID Gastric Ulcer

PO: ADULTS, ELDERLY: (Healing): 30 mg/day for up to 8 wks. (Prevention): 15 mg/day for up to 12 wks.

Gastroesophageal Reflux Disease (GERD)

PO: ADULTS: 15 mg/day for up to 8 wks.

H. Pylori Infection

PO: ADULTS, ELDERLY: (triple drug therapy) 30 mg q12h for 10–14 day.

Pathologic Hypersecretory Conditions (Including Zollinger-Ellison Syndrome)

PO: ADULTS, ELDERLY: 60 mg/day. Individualize dosage according to pt needs and for as long as clinically indicated. Administer up to 120 mg/day in divided doses.

SIDE EFFECTS

Occasional (3%–2%): Diarrhea, abdominal pain, rash, pruritus, altered appetite. Rare (1%): Nausea, headache.

ADVERSE EFFECTS/ TOXIC REACTIONS

Bilirubinemia, eosinophilia, hyperlipemia occur rarely.

NURSING CONSIDERATIONS

BASELINE ASSESSMENT

Obtain baseline lab values. Assess for epigastric/abdominal pain, evidence of bleeding, ecchymosis.

INTERVENTION/EVALUATION

Monitor ongoing laboratory results, CBC, hepatic/renal function tests. Assess for therapeutic response (relief of GI symptoms). Question if diarrhea, abdominal pain, nausea occurs.

PATIENT/ FAMILY TEACHING

• Do not chew/crush delayed-release capsules. • For pts who have difficulty swallowing capsules, open capsules, sprinkle granules on 1 tbsp of applesauce, swallow immediately.

lanthanum

lan-thah-num
(Fosrenol)
Do not confuse lanthanum with lithium.

◆CLASSIFICATION

CLINICAL: Phosphate regulator.

ACTION

Dissociates in acidic environment of upper GI tract to lanthanum ions that bind to dietary phosphate released from food during digestion, forming highly insoluble lanthanum phosphate complexes. **Therapeutic Effect:** Reduces phosphate absorption.

PHARMACOKINETICS

Very low absorption following PO administration. Protein binding: greater than 99%. Not metabolized. Phosphate complexes are eliminated in urine. **Half-life:** 53 hrs (in plasma); 2–3.6 yrs (from bone).

USES

Reduce serum phosphate levels in pts with end-stage renal disease.

PRECAUTIONS

Contraindications: None known. **Cautions:** Acute peptic ulcer disease, ulcerative colitis, Crohn's disease, bowel obstruction.

LIFESPAN CONSIDERATIONS

Pregnancy/Lactation: Unknown if drug crosses placenta or is distributed in breast milk. Breast-feeding not recommended. **Pregnancy Category C. Children:** Safety and efficacy not established; not recommended for children. **Elderly:** No age-related precautions noted.

INTERACTIONS

DRUG: Antacids interact with lanthanum carbonate; separate administration by 2 hrs. **HERBAL:** None significant. **FOOD:** None known. **LAB VALUES:** None known.

AVAILABILITY (Rx)

Tablets, Chewable: 500 mg, 750 mg, 1 g.

ADMINISTRATION/HANDLING

PO

• Tablets should be chewed thoroughly before swallowing. • Give during or immediately after meals.

INDICATIONS/ROUTES/DOSAGE

Phosphate Control

PO: ADULTS, ELDERLY: 750 mg–1,500 mg in divided doses, taken with or immediately after a meal. Dose can be titrated at 2- to 3-wk intervals in 750-mg increments, based on serum phosphate levels. Usual dosage range: 1,500–3,000 mg/day.

SIDE EFFECTS

Frequent: Nausea (11%), vomiting (9%), dialysis graft occlusion (8%), abdominal pain (5%). Nausea, vomiting decrease over time.

ADVERSE EFFECTS/ TOXIC REACTIONS

None known.

NURSING CONSIDERATIONS

BASELINE ASSESSMENT

Obtain baseline serum phosphorus level.

INTERVENTION/EVALUATION

Monitor serum phosphate (target concentration is less than 6 mg/dl).

PATIENT/FAMILY TEACHING

• Take with or immediately after a meal. • Do not take lanthanum within 2 hrs of antacids. • Nausea, vomiting usually diminish over time.

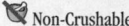

Lantus, *see insulin*

lapatinib

la-**pa**-ti-nib
(Tykerb)

BLACK BOX ALERT Hepatotoxicity, possibly severe, has occurred.

Do not confuse lapatinib with dasatinib, erlotinib, or imatinib.

◆CLASSIFICATION

PHARMACOTHERAPEUTIC: Tyrosine kinase inhibitor. **CLINICAL:** Antineoplastic.

ACTION

Inhibitory action against kinases targeting intracellular components of epidermal growth factor receptor ErbB1 and a second receptor, human epidermal receptor (HER2 [ErbB2]). **Therapeutic Effect:** Inhibits ErbB-driven tumor cell growth, produces tumor regression, inhibits metastasis.

PHARMACOKINETICS

Route	Onset	Peak	Duration
PO	30 min	4 hrs	—

Steady-state level occurs within 6–7 days. Incomplete and variable oral absorption. Undergoes extensive metabolism. Protein binding: 99%. Minimally excreted in feces and plasma. **Half-life:** 24 hrs.

USES

Combination treatment with capecitabine for advanced or metastatic breast cancer in those who have received prior therapy including an anthracycline, a taxane, and trastuzumab. Combination treatment with letrozole for treatment of postmenopausal women with hormone receptor-positive metastatic breast cancer for whom hormonal therapy is indicated. **OFF-LABEL:** Treatment of head/neck cancer.

PRECAUTIONS

Contraindications: None significant. **Cautions:** Left ventricular function abnormalities, prolonged QT interval on EKG, hepatic impairment.

LIFESPAN CONSIDERATIONS

Pregnancy/Lactation: Has potential for fetal harm. Unknown if distributed in breast milk. **Pregnancy Category D. Children:** Safety and efficacy not established. **Elderly:** No age-related precautions noted.

INTERACTIONS

DRUG: Atazanavir, clarithromycin, indinavir, itraconazole, ketoconazole, nefazodone, nelfinavir, ritonavir, saquinavir, voriconizole may increase plasma concentration. **Carbamazepine, dexamethasone, fosphenytoin, phenobarbital, phenytoin, rifabutin, rifampin, rifapentin** may decrease plasma concentration. **HERBAL: St. John's wort** may decrease plasma concentration. **FOOD: Grapefruit, grapefruit juice** may increase plasma concentration. **LAB VALUES:** May increase serum ALT, AST, bilirubin. May decrease neutrophils, Hgb, platelets.

AVAILABILITY (Rx)

Tablets: 250 mg.

ADMINISTRATION/HANDLING

PO

- Do not crush, chew, or break film-coated tablets.
- Give at least 1 hr before or 1 hr after food.

INDICATIONS/ROUTES/DOSAGE

Breast Cancer

PO: ADULTS, ELDERLY: (With capecitabine): 1,250 mg (5 tablets) once daily on days 1–21 continuously in combination with capecitabine on days 1–14 in a repeating 21-day cycle. **(With letrozole):** 1,500 mg once daily continuously with letrozole.

Dose Modification

PO: ADULTS, ELDERLY: Discontinue with decreased left ventricular ejection fraction grade 2 or more or in pts with an ejection fraction that drops to lower limit of normal. May be started at a reduced dose (1,000 mg/day) at a minimum of 2 wks when ejection fraction returns to normal and pt is asymptomatic.

SIDE EFFECTS

Common (65%–44%): Diarrhea (sometimes severe), hand-foot syndrome (blistering/rash/peeling of skin on palms of hands, soles of feet), nausea. **Frequent (28%–26%):** Rash, vomiting. **Occasional (15%–10%):** Mucosal inflammation, stomatitis, extremity pain, back pain, dry skin, insomnia.

ADVERSE EFFECTS/ TOXIC REACTIONS

Decreases in left ventricular ejection grade 3 or higher have been observed; 20% decrease relative to baseline is considered toxic.

NURSING CONSIDERATIONS

BASELINE ASSESSMENT

Question for possibility of pregnancy. Obtain baseline CBC, serum chemistries before treatment begins and monthly thereafter.

INTERVENTION/EVALUATION

Offer antiemetics to control nausea, vomiting. Monitor daily pattern of bowel activity, stool consistency. Monitor CBC, particularly Hgb, platelets, neutrophil count, hepatic function tests (AST, ALT, total bilirubin). Assess hands and feet for erythema/blistering/peeling. Monitor for shortness of breath, palpitations, fatigue (decreased cardiac ejection fraction).

PATIENT/FAMILY TEACHING

• Avoid crowds, those with known infection. • Avoid contact with those who recently received live virus vaccine. • Do not have immunizations without physician's approval (drug lowers resistance). • Promptly report fever, unusual bruising/bleeding from any site.

Lasix, *see furosemide*

leflunomide

lee-**floo**-noe-mide
(Apo-Leflunomide ✤, Arava, Novo-Leflunomide ✤)

BLACK BOX ALERT Do not use during pregnancy (Pregnancy Category X). Women of childbearing potential must be counseled regarding fetal risk, use of reliable contraceptives confirmed, possibility of pregnancy excluded.

◆ CLASSIFICATION

PHARMACOTHERAPEUTIC: Immunomodulatory agent. **CLINICAL:** Anti-inflammatory.

ACTION

Inhibits dihydro-orotate dehydrogenase, the enzyme involved in autoimmune process that leads to rheumatoid arthritis (RA). **Therapeutic Effect:** Reduces signs/symptoms of RA, retards structural damage.

PHARMACOKINETICS

Well absorbed after PO administration. Protein binding: greater than 99%. Metabolized to active metabolite in GI wall, liver. Excreted through renal, biliary systems. Not removed by hemodialysis. **Half-life:** 16 days.

USES

Treatment of active rheumatoid arthritis (RA). Improve physical function in pts with rheumatoid arthritis. **OFF-LABEL:** Treatment of cytomegalovirus (CMV) disease. Prevention of acute/chronic rejection in recipients of solid organ transplants.

PRECAUTIONS

Contraindications: Pregnancy or plans for pregnancy. **Cautions:** Hepatic/renal impairment, positive hepatitis B or C serology, those with immunodeficiency or bone marrow dysplasias, breast-feeding mothers.

LIFESPAN CONSIDERATIONS

Pregnancy/Lactation: Can cause fetal harm. Unknown if distributed in breast milk. Breast-feeding not recommended. **Pregnancy Category X. Children:** Safety and efficacy not established in those younger than 18 yrs. **Elderly:** No age-related precautions noted.

INTERACTIONS

DRUG: **Hepatotoxic medications** may increase risk of side effects, hepatotoxicity. Use of **live virus vaccine** not recommended. HERBAL: None significant. FOOD: None known. LAB VALUES: May increase serum AST, ALT, alkaline phosphatase, bilirubin.

AVAILABILITY (Rx)

Tablets: 10 mg, 20 mg.

ADMINISTRATION/HANDLING

PO

- Give without regard to food.

INDICATIONS/ROUTES/DOSAGE

Rheumatoid Arthritis (RA)

PO: ADULTS, ELDERLY: Initially, 100 mg/day for 3 days, then 10–20 mg/day.

Dosage Adjustment in Hepatic Toxicity

ALT Greater Than 2 But Less Than 3 Times Upper Limit of Normal (ULN): 10 mg/day. **ALT Levels Persist Greater Than 3 Times ULN:** Discontinue and initiate cholestyramine (8 g 3 times/day for 1–3 days) or activated charcoal (50 g q6h for 24 hrs) to accelerate elimination.

SIDE EFFECTS

Frequent (20%–10%): Diarrhea, respiratory tract infection, alopecia, rash, nausea.

ADVERSE EFFECTS/ TOXIC REACTIONS

Leflunomide may cause immunosuppression. Transient thrombocytopenia, leukopenia, hepatotoxicity occur rarely.

NURSING CONSIDERATIONS

BASELINE ASSESSMENT

Question for possibility of pregnancy (Pregnancy Category X). Obtain baseline CBC, Hgb, Hct, platelet, phosphate, hepatic function tests. Assess limitations in activities of daily living due to rheumatoid arthritis (RA).

INTERVENTION/EVALUATION

Monitor tolerance to medication. Assess symptomatic relief of RA (relief of pain; improved range of motion, grip strength, mobility). Monitor hepatic function tests.

PATIENT/FAMILY TEACHING

- May take without regard to food. • Improvement may take longer than 8 wks. • Avoid pregnancy (Pregnancy Category X).

lenalidomide

len-ah-**lid**-oh-mide
(Revlimid)

BLACK BOX ALERT Pregnancy Category X. Analogue to thalidomide. High potential for significant birth defects. Hematologic toxicity (thrombocytopenia, neutropenia) occurs in 80% of pts. Greatly increases risk for DVT, pulmonary embolism in multiple myeloma pts.

Do not confuse lenalidomide with thalidomide.

CLASSIFICATION

PHARMACOTHERAPEUTIC: Immunomodulator. CLINICAL: Immunosuppressive.

ACTION

Inhibits secretion of pro-inflammatory cytokines, increases secretion of anti-inflammatory cytokines. **Therapeutic Effect:** Prevents growth of B-cell lymphoma cell line, myeloblastic cell line.

PHARMACOKINETICS

Well absorbed following PO administration. Protein binding: 30%. Eliminated in urine. **Half-life:** 3 hrs (increased in renal impairment).

USES

Treatment of transfusion-dependent anemia due to myelodysplastic syndromes. Treatment of multiple myeloma (in combination with dexamethasone). **OFF-LABEL:** Treatment of mantle cell lymphoma, systemic amyloidosis, myelodysplastic syndrome, relapsed or refractory chronic lymphocytic leukemia (CLL).

PRECAUTIONS

Contraindications: Pregnancy **(Pregnancy Category X),** women capable of becoming pregnant. **Cautions:** Renal impairment.

LIFESPAN CONSIDERATIONS

Pregnancy/Lactation: Contraindicated in women who are or may become pregnant and who are not using two required types of birth control or who are not continually abstaining from heterosexual sexual contact. Can cause severe birth defects, fetal death. Unknown if distributed in breast milk; breast-feeding not recommended. **Pregnancy Category X. Children:** Safety and efficacy not established in those younger than 18 yrs. **Elderly:** Age-related renal impairment may require caution in dosage selection. Risk of toxic reactions greater in those with renal insufficiency.

INTERACTIONS

DRUG: None significant. **HERBAL:** None significant. **FOOD:** None known. **LAB VALUES:** May decrease WBC count, Hgb, Hct, thrombocytes, troponin I, serum creatinine, sodium, T_3, T_4. May decrease serum bilirubin, glucose, potassium, magnesium.

AVAILABILITY (Rx)

Capsules: 5 mg, 10 mg, 15 mg, 25 mg.

ADMINISTRATION/HANDLING

• Store at room temperature. • Do not crush/open capsules. • Swallow whole with water.

INDICATIONS/ROUTES/DOSAGE

Myelodysplastic Syndrome

PO: ADULTS, ELDERLY: 10 mg once daily.

Dosage Adjustments

PLATELETS:

Thrombocytopenia within 4 wks with 10 mg/day

Baseline platelets 100,000/mcl or greater: Platelets less than 50,000/mcl, hold treatment. Resume at 5 mg/day when platelets return to 50,000/mcl or greater. **Baseline platelets less than 100,000/mcl:** Platelets fall to 50% of baseline, hold treatment. Resume at 5 mg/day if baseline is 60,000/mcl or greater and platelets return to 50,000/mcl or greater. Resume at 5 mg/day if baseline is less than 60,000/mcl and platelets return to 30,000/mcl or greater.

Thrombocytopenia after 4 wks with 10 mg/day: Platelets less than 30,000/mcl OR less than 50,000/mcl with platelet transfusion, hold treatment. Resume at 5 mg/day when platelets return to 30,000/mcl or greater.

Thrombocytopenia developing with 5 mg/day: Platelets less than 30,000/mcl OR less than 50,000/mcl with platelet transfusion, hold treatment. Resume at 5 mg every other day when platelets return to 30,000/mcl or greater.

NEUTROPHILS:

Neutropenia within 4 wks with 10 mg/day

Baseline absolute neutrophil count (ANC) 1,000/mcl or greater: ANC less than 750/mcl, hold treatment. Resume at 5 mg/day when ANC 1,000/mcl or greater. **Baseline ANC less than 1,000/mcl:** ANC less than 500/mcl, hold treatment. Resume at 5 mg/day when ANC 500/mcl or greater.

Neutropenia after 4 wks with 10 mg/day: ANC less than 500/mcl for 7 days or

L

longer or associated with fever, hold treatment. Resume at 5 mg/day when ANC 500/mcl or greater.

Neutropenia developing with 5 mg/day: ANC less than 500/mcl for 7 days or longer or associated with fever, hold treatment. Resume at 5 mg every other day when ANC 500/mcl or greater.

Multiple Myeloma

PO: ADULTS, ELDERLY: 25 mg/day on days 1–21 of repeated 28-day cycle. (Dexamethasone 40 mg/day on days 1–4, 9–12, 17–20 of each 28-day cycle for first 4 cycles, then 40 mg/day on days 1–4 every 28 days.)

Dosage Adjustments

PLATELETS:

Thrombocytopenia: Platelets fall to less than 30,000/mcl, hold treatment, monitor CBC. Resume at 15 mg/day when platelets 30,000/mcl or greater. For each subsequent fall to less than 30,000/mcl, hold treatment and resume at 5 mg/day less than previous dose when platelets return to 30,000/mcl or greater. Do not dose to less than 5 mg/day.

NEUTROPHILS:

Neutropenia: Neutrophils fall to less than 1,000/mcl, hold treatment, add G-CSF, follow CBC weekly. Resume at 25 mg/day when neutrophils return to 1,000/mcl and neutropenia is the only toxicity. Resume at 15 mg/day if other toxicity is present. For each subsequent fall to less than 1,000/mcl, hold treatment and resume at 5 mg/day less than previous dose when neutrophils return to 1,000/mcl or greater. Do not dose to less than 5 mg/day.

SIDE EFFECTS

Frequent (49%–31%): Diarrhea, pruritus, rash, fatigue. **Occasional (24%–12%):** Constipation, nausea, arthralgia, fever, back pain, peripheral edema, cough, dizziness, headache, muscle cramps, epistaxis, asthenia (loss of strength, energy), dry skin, abdominal pain. **Rare (10%–5%):** Extremity pain, vomiting, generalized edema, anorexia, insomnia, night sweats, myalgia, dry mouth, ecchymosis, rigors, depression, dysgeusia, palpitations.

ADVERSE EFFECTS/ TOXIC REACTIONS

Significant increased risk of deep vein thrombosis (DVT), pulmonary embolism. Thrombocytopenia occurs in 62% of pts, neutropenia in 59% of pts, and anemia in 12% of pts. Upper respiratory infection (nasopharyngitis, pneumonia, sinusitis, bronchitis, rhinitis), UTI occur occasionally. Cellulitis, peripheral neuropathy, hypertension, hypothyroidism occur in approximately 6% of pts.

NURSING CONSIDERATIONS

BASELINE ASSESSMENT

Due to high potential for human birth defects/fetal death, female pts must avoid pregnancy 4 wks before therapy, during therapy, during dose interruptions, and 4 wks following therapy. Contraception must be used even if pt has history of infertility unless it is due to hysterectomy or menopause that has occurred for at least 24 consecutive mos. Two reliable forms of contraception must be used. Females of childbearing potential must have two negative pregnancy tests before therapy initiation.

Dosage in Renal Impairment

	Creatinine Clearance 30–49 ml/min	Creatinine Clearance Less Than 30 ml/min (Nondialysis Dependent)	Creatinine Clearance Less Than 30 ml/min (Dialysis Dependent)
Myelodysplastic syndrome	5 mg once daily	5 mg q48h	5 mg 3 times/wk (give after dialysis)
Multiple myeloma	10–15 mg once daily	15 mg q48h	15 mg 3 times/wk (give after dialysis)

INTERVENTION/EVALUATION

Perform pregnancy tests on women of childbearing potential: weekly during the first 4 wks of use, then at 4-wk intervals in those with regular menstrual cycles or q2wk in those with irregular menstrual cycles. Monitor for hematologic toxicity; obtain CBC weekly during first 8 wks of therapy and at least monthly thereafter. Observe for signs, symptoms of thromboembolism (shortness of breath, chest pain, extremity pain, swelling, stroke-like symptoms).

PATIENT/FAMILY TEACHING

• Two approved birth control methods must be used before, during, and after therapy for female pts. • A pregnancy test must be performed within 10–14 days and 24 hrs before therapy begins. • Males must always use a latex condom during any sexual contact with females of childbearing potential even if they have undergone a successful vasectomy.

lepirudin HIGH ALERT

leh-**peer**-u-din
(Refludan)

◆CLASSIFICATION

PHARMACOTHERAPEUTIC: Thrombin inhibitor. **CLINICAL:** Anticoagulant.

ACTION

Inhibits thrombogenic action of thrombin (independent of antithrombin II, not inhibited by platelet factor 4). **Therapeutic Effect:** Produces dose-dependent increases in aPTT.

PHARMACOKINETICS

Distributed primarily in extracellular fluid. Primarily eliminated by kidneys. **Half-life:** 1.3 hrs (increased in renal impairment).

USES

Anticoagulant in pts with heparin-induced thrombocytopenia or associated thromboembolic disease to prevent further thromboembolic complications. **OFF-LABEL:** Acute coronary syndromes with history of heparin-induced thrombocytopenia, acute MI, percutaneous coronary intervention with history of heparin-induced thrombocytopenia, prevention/reduction of ischemic complications associated with unstable angina.

PRECAUTIONS

Contraindications: Hypersensitivity to hirudins or to any of the components in Refludan [lepirudin (rDNA)] for injection. **Cautions:** Conditions associated with increased risk of bleeding (bacterial endocarditis, recent major bleeding, CVA, stroke, intracranial surgery, hemorrhagic diathesis, severe hypertension, severe renal/hepatic impairment, recent major surgery).

LIFESPAN CONSIDERATIONS

Pregnancy/Lactation: Unknown if drug is distributed in breast milk or crosses placenta. **Pregnancy Category B. Children:** Safety and efficacy not established. **Elderly:** Age-related renal impairment may require dosage adjustment.

INTERACTIONS

DRUG: Platelet aggregation inhibitors, thrombolytics, warfarin may increase risk of bleeding complications. **HERBAL: Cats's claw, dong quai, evening primrose, feverfew, garlic, ginkgo, ginseng, horse chestnut, red clover** may increase antiplatelet activity. **FOOD:** None known. **LAB VALUES:** Increases aPTT, thrombin time.

AVAILABILITY (Rx)

Injection, Powder for Reconstitution: 50 mg.

ADMINISTRATION/HANDLING

IV

Reconstitution • Add 1 ml Sterile Water for Injection or 0.9% NaCl to 50 mg vial. • Shake gently. • Produces a clear, colorless solution (do not use if cloudy). • For IV push, further dilute by transferring to syringe and adding sufficient Sterile Water for Injection, 0.9% NaCl, or D_5W to produce concentration of 5 mg/ml. • For IV infusion, add contents of 2 vials (100 mg) to 250 ml or 500 ml 0.9% NaCl or D_5W, providing concentration of 0.4 or 0.2 mg/ml, respectively.

Rate of administration • IV push given over 15–20 sec. • Adjust IV infusion based on aPTT or pt's body weight.

Storage • Store unreconstituted vials at room temperature. • Reconstituted solution to be used immediately. • IV infusion stable for up to 24 hrs at room temperature.

IV INCOMPATIBILITIES

Do not mix with other medications.

INDICATIONS/ROUTES/DOSAGE

Anticoagulation

ALERT Dosage adjusted according to aPTT ratio with target range of 1.5–2.5 times normal.

IV: ADULTS, ELDERLY: 0.2–0.4 mg/kg, IV slowly over 15–20 sec, followed by IV infusion of 0.1–0.15 mg/kg/hr for 2–10 days or longer.

ALERT For pts weighing more than 110 kg, maximum initial dose is 44 mg, with maximum IV rate of 16.5 mg/hr.

Dosage in Renal Impairment

Initial dose is decreased to 0.2 mg/kg, with infusion rate adjusted based on creatinine clearance.

Creatinine Clearance	Adjusted Infusion Rate	
45–60 ml/min	50% of standard	0.075 mg/kg/hr
30–44 ml/min	30% of standard	0.045 mg/kg/hr
15–29 ml/min	15% of standard	0.0225 mg/kg/hr

SIDE EFFECTS

Frequent (14%–5%): Bleeding from gums, puncture sites, wounds; hematuria; fever; GI, rectal bleeding. **Occasional (3%–1%):** Epistaxis, allergic reaction (rash, pruritus), vaginal bleeding.

ADVERSE EFFECTS/ TOXIC REACTIONS

Overdose is characterized by excessively high aPTT. Intracranial bleeding occurs rarely. Abnormal hepatic function has been reported in 6% of pts.

NURSING CONSIDERATIONS

BASELINE ASSESSMENT

Assess CBC, including platelet count. Determine initial B/P. Assess renal/hepatic function.

INTERVENTION/EVALUATION

Monitor aPTT diligently. Assess Hct, platelet count, urine/stool specimen for occult blood, AST, ALT, renal function studies. Assess for decrease in B/P, increase in pulse rate, complaint of abdominal/back pain, severe headache (may be evidence of hemorrhage). Question for increased discharge during menses. Check peripheral pulses; skin for ecchymosis, petechiae. Check for excessive bleeding from minor cuts, scratches. Assess gums for erythema, gingival bleeding. Assess urine output for hematuria.

PATIENT/FAMILY TEACHING

• Report bleeding, bruising, dizziness, light-headedness, rash, pruritus, fever, edema, breathing difficulty to physician.

Lescol, *see fluvastatin*

Lescol XL, *see fluvastatin*

letrozole

HIGH ALERT

leh-troe-zoll

(Femara)

Do not confuse Femara with Famvir, Femhrt, or Provera, or letrozole with anastrozole.

CLASSIFICATION

PHARMACOTHERAPEUTIC: Aromatase inhibitor, hormone. **CLINICAL:** Antineoplastic (see p. 85C).

ACTION

Decreases circulating estrogen by inhibiting aromatase, an enzyme that catalyzes the final step in estrogen production. **Therapeutic Effect:** Inhibits growth of breast cancers stimulated by estrogens.

PHARMACOKINETICS

Rapidly, completely absorbed. Metabolized in liver. Primarily eliminated by kidneys. Unknown if removed by hemodialysis. **Half-life:** Approximately 2 days.

USES

First-line treatment of locally advanced or metastatic breast cancer. Treatment of advanced breast cancer in postmenopausal women with disease progression following anti-estrogen therapy. Postsurgical treatment for postmenopausal women with hormone sensitive early breast cancer. Prevention of recurrent breast cancer. **OFF-LABEL:** Treatment of ovarian, endometrial cancer.

PRECAUTIONS

Contraindications: None known. **Cautions:** Renal/hepatic impairment.

LIFESPAN CONSIDERATIONS

Pregnancy/Lactation: Unknown if distributed in breast milk. **Pregnancy Category D. Children:** Safety and efficacy not established. **Elderly:** No age-related precautions noted.

INTERACTIONS

DRUG: **Tamoxifen** may reduce concentration. **HERBAL:** None significant. **FOOD:** None known. **LAB VALUES:** May increase serum calcium, cholesterol, GGT, AST, ALT, bilirubin.

AVAILABILITY (Rx)

Tablets: 2.5 mg.

ADMINISTRATION/HANDLING

PO

- Give without regard to food.

INDICATIONS/ROUTES/DOSAGE

Breast Cancer

PO: ADULTS, ELDERLY: 2.5 mg/day. Continue until tumor progression is evident.

Dosage in Severe Hepatic Impairment

PO: ADULTS, ELDERLY: 2.5 mg every other day.

SIDE EFFECTS

Frequent (21%–9%): Musculoskeletal pain (back, arm, leg), nausea, headache. **Occasional (8%–5%):** Constipation, arthralgia, fatigue, vomiting, hot flashes, diarrhea, abdominal pain, cough, rash, anorexia, hypertension, peripheral edema. **Rare (4%–1%):** Asthenia (loss of strength, energy), drowsiness, dyspepsia (heartburn, indigestion, epigastric pain), weight gain, pruritus.

ADVERSE EFFECTS/ TOXIC REACTIONS

Pleural effusion, pulmonary embolism, bone fracture, thromboembolic disorder, MI occur rarely.

NURSING CONSIDERATIONS

BASELINE ASSESSMENT

Obtain baseline CBC, chemistries, hepatic/renal function tests.

INTERVENTION/EVALUATION

Monitor for, assist with ambulation if asthenia (loss of strength, energy), dizziness occurs. Assess for headache. Offer antiemetic for nausea, vomiting. Monitor CBC, thyroid function, electrolytes, hepatic/renal function tests. Monitor for evidence of musculoskeletal pain; offer analgesics for pain relief.

PATIENT/FAMILY TEACHING

- Notify physician if nausea, asthenia (loss of strength, energy), hot flashes become unmanageable.

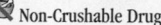

L

leucovorin calcium (folinic acid, citrovorum factor)

loo-**koe**-vor-in

Do not confuse leucovorin with Leukeran, or folinic acid with folic acid.

◆CLASSIFICATION

PHARMACOTHERAPEUTIC: Folic acid antagonist. **CLINICAL:** Antidote.

ACTION

Competes with methotrexate for same transport processes into cells (limits methotrexate action on normal cells). **Therapeutic Effect:** Reverses toxic effects of folic acid antagonists. Reverses folic acid deficiency.

L

PHARMACOKINETICS

Readily absorbed from GI tract. Widely distributed. Primarily concentrated in liver. Metabolized in liver, intestinal mucosa to active metabolite. Primarily excreted in urine. **Half-life:** 15 min; metabolite, 30–35 min.

USES

Antidote for folic acid antagonists (methotrexate, trimethoprim, pyrimethoamine). Treatment of megaloblastic anemias when folate deficient (e.g., infancy, celiac disease, pregnancy, when oral therapy not possible). Treatment of colon cancer (with fluorouracil). Methotrexate rescue, after high-dose methotrexate for osteosarcoma. **OFF-LABEL:** Treatment of Ewing's sarcoma, gestational trophoblastic neoplasms, non-Hodgkin's lymphoma; treatment adjunct for head/neck carcinoma.

PRECAUTIONS

Contraindications: Pernicious anemia, other megaloblastic anemias secondary to vitamin B_{12} deficiency. **Cautions:** History of allergies, bronchial asthma. **With 5-fluorouracil:** Those with GI toxicities (more common/severe).

⌛ LIFESPAN CONSIDERATIONS

Pregnancy/Lactation: Unknown if drug crosses placenta or is distributed in breast milk. **Pregnancy Category C. Children:** May increase risk of seizures by counteracting anticonvulsant effects of barbiturate, hydantoins. **Elderly:** Age-related renal impairment may require dosage adjustment when used for rescue from effects of high-dose methotrexate therapy.

INTERACTIONS

DRUG: May decrease effects of **anticonvulsants.** May increase **5-fluorouracil** toxicity/effect when taken in combination. **HERBAL:** None significant. **FOOD:** None known. **LAB VALUES:** None significant.

AVAILABILITY (Rx)

Injection, Powder for Reconstitution: 50 mg, 100 mg, 200 mg, 350 mg. **Injection, Solution:** 10 mg/ml. **Tablets:** 5 mg, 10 mg, 15 mg, 25 mg.

ADMINISTRATION/HANDLING

IV

◀ALERT▶ Strict adherence to timing of 5-fluorouracil following leucovorin therapy must be maintained.

Reconstitution • Reconstitute each 50-mg vial with 5 ml Sterile Water for Injection or Bacteriostatic Water for Injection containing benzyl alcohol to provide concentration of 10 mg/ml. • Due to benzyl alcohol in 1-mg ampule and in Bacteriostatic Water for Injection, reconstitute doses greater than 10 mg/m^2 with Sterile Water for Injection. • Further dilute with 100–1,000 ml D_5W or 0.9% NaCl.

Rate of administration • Do not exceed 160 mg/min if given by IV infusion (due to calcium content).

Storage • Store vials for parenteral use at room temperature. • Injection appears as clear, yellowish solution. • Use immediately if reconstituted with Sterile Water for Injection; stable for 7 days if reconstituted with Bacteriostatic Water for Injection.

PO

• Scored tablets may be crushed.

IV INCOMPATIBILITIES

Amphotericin B complex (Abelcet, AmBisome, Amphotec), droperidol (Inapsine), foscarnet (Foscavir).

IV COMPATIBILITIES

Cisplatin (Platinol AQ), cyclophosphamide (Cytoxan), doxorubicin (Adriamycin), etoposide (VePesid), filgrastim (Neupogen), 5-fluorouracil, gemcitabine (Gemzar), granisetron (Kytril), heparin, methotrexate, metoclopramide (Reglan), mitomycin (Mutamycin), piperacillin and tazobactam (Zosyn), vinblastine (Velban), vincristine (Oncovin).

INDICATIONS/ROUTES/DOSAGE

Conventional Rescue Dosage in High-Dose Methotrexate Therapy

PO, IV, IM: ADULTS, ELDERLY, CHILDREN: 10–15 mg/m^2 IM or IV one time, then PO q6h until serum methotrexate level is less than 0.05 micromole/L. If 24-hr serum creatinine level increases by 50% or greater over baseline or methotrexate level exceeds 5 micromole/L, increase to 150 mg q3h until methotrexate level is less than 1 micromole/L, then 15 mg q3h until methotrexate level is less than 0.05 micromole/L.

Folic Acid Antagonist Overdose

PO: ADULTS, ELDERLY, CHILDREN: 5–15 mg/day.

Megaloblastic Anemia Secondary to Folate Deficiency

IM: ADULTS, ELDERLY, CHILDREN: 1 mg/day.

Colon Cancer

◀ALERT▶ For rescue therapy in cancer chemotherapy, refer to specific protocols used for optimal dosage and sequence of leucovorin administration.

IV: ADULTS, ELDERLY: 200 mg/m^2 followed by 370 mg/m^2 fluorouracil daily for 5 days. Repeat course at 4-wk intervals for 2 courses, then 4- to 5-wk intervals or 20 mg/m^2 followed by 425 mg/m^2 fluorouracil daily for 5 days. Repeat course at 4-wk intervals for 2 courses, then 4- to 5-wk intervals.

SIDE EFFECTS

Frequent: When combined with chemotherapeutic agents: diarrhea, stomatitis, nausea, vomiting, lethargy, malaise, fatigue, alopecia, anorexia. **Occasional:** Urticaria, dermatitis.

ADVERSE EFFECTS/ TOXIC REACTIONS

Excessive dosage may negate chemotherapeutic effects of folic acid antagonists. Anaphylaxis occurs rarely. Diarrhea may cause rapid clinical deterioration.

NURSING CONSIDERATIONS

BASELINE ASSESSMENT

Give as soon as possible, preferably within 1 hr, for treatment of accidental overdosage of folic acid antagonists.

INTERVENTION/EVALUATION

Monitor for vomiting—may need to change from oral to parenteral therapy. Observe elderly, debilitated closely due to risk for severe toxicities. Assess CBC with differential, platelet count (also electrolytes, hepatic function tests if used in combination with chemotherapeutic agents).

PATIENT/FAMILY TEACHING

• Explain purpose of medication in treatment of cancer. • Report allergic reaction, vomiting.

leuprolide

HIGH ALERT

loo-proe-lide
(Eligard, Lupron, Lupron Depot, Lupron Depot-Ped)

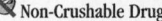

L

CLASSIFICATION

PHARMACOTHERAPEUTIC: Gonadotropin-releasing hormone (GnRH) analogue. **CLINICAL:** Antineoplastic (see pp. 85C, 105C).

ACTION

Stimulates release of luteinizing hormone (LH), follicle-stimulating hormone (FSH) from anterior pituitary gland, stimulating production of estrogen, testosterone. **Therapeutic Effect:** Produces pharmacologic castration, decreases growth of abnormal prostate tissue in males; causes endometrial tissue to become inactive, atrophic in females; decreases rate of pubertal development in children with central precocious puberty.

PHARMACOKINETICS

Rapidly, well absorbed after subcutaneous administration. Absorbed slowly after IM administration. Protein binding: 43%–49%. **Half-life:** 3–4 hrs.

USES

Palliative treatment of advanced prostate carcinoma. Initial management of endometriosis or treatment of recurrent symptoms. Preop treatment of anemia caused by uterine leiomyomata (fibroids). Treatment of central precocious puberty. **OFF-LABEL:** Treatment of breast, ovarian, endometrial cancer; infertility; prostatic hyperplasia.

PRECAUTIONS

Contraindications: Lactation, pernicious anemia, pregnancy, undiagnosed vaginal bleeding. Eligard 7.5 mg is contraindicated in pts with hypersensitivity to GnRH, GnRH agonist analogues, or any of its components. 30 mg Lupron Depot contraindicated in women. **Cautions:** Long-term use in children.

LIFESPAN CONSIDERATIONS

Pregnancy/Lactation: Depot: Contraindicated in pregnancy. May cause spontaneous abortion. **Pregnancy Category X. Children:** Long-term safety not established. **Elderly:** No age-related precautions noted.

INTERACTIONS

DRUG: None significant. **HERBAL:** None significant. **FOOD:** None known. **LAB VALUES:** May increase serum prostatic acid phosphatase (PAP). Initially increases, then decreases, serum testosterone. May increase serum ALT, AST, alkaline phosphatase, LDH, LDL, cholesterol, triglycerides. May decrease platelets, WBC.

AVAILABILITY (Rx)

Injection Depot Formulation: 3.75 mg (Lupron Depot), 7.5 mg (Eligard, Lupron Depot, Lupron Depot-Ped), 11.25 mg (Lupron Depot-Ped), 15 mg (Lupron Depot-Ped), 22.5 mg (Eligard), 30 mg (Lupron Depot), 45 mg (Eligard). **Injection Solution (Lupron):** 5 mg/ml.

ADMINISTRATION/HANDLING

◄ALERT► May be carcinogenic, mutagenic, teratogenic. Handle with extreme care during preparation/administration.

IM

Lupron Depot • Store at room temperature. • Protect from light, heat. • Do not freeze vials. • Reconstitute only with diluent provided. Follow manufacturer's instructions for mixing.
• Do not use needles less than 22 gauge; use syringes provided by the manufacturer (0.5-ml low-dose insulin syringes may be used as an alternative). • Administer immediately.
Eligard • Refrigerate. • Allow to warm to room temperature before reconstitution. • Follow manufacturer's instructions for mixing. • Following reconstitution, administer within 30 min.

Subcutaneous

Lupron • Refrigerate vials. • Injection appears clear, colorless. • Discard if discolored or precipitate forms. • Administer into deltoid muscle, anterior thigh, abdomen.

INDICATIONS/ROUTES/DOSAGE

Advanced Prostatic Carcinoma

IM (LUPRON DEPOT): ADULTS, ELDERLY: 7.5 mg every mo, 22.5 mg q3mos, or 30 mg q4mos.
SUBCUTANEOUS (ELIGARD): ADULTS, ELDERLY: 7.5 mg every mo, 22.5 mg q3mos, 30 mg q4mos, or 45 mg q6mos.
SUBCUTANEOUS (LUPRON): ADULTS, ELDERLY: 1 mg/day.

Endometriosis

IM (LUPRON DEPOT): ADULTS, ELDERLY: 3.75 mg/mo for up to 6 mos or 11.25 mg q3mo for up to 2 doses.

Uterine Leiomyomata

IM (WITH IRON [LUPRON DEPOT]): ADULTS, ELDERLY: 3.75 mg/mos for up to 3 mos or 11.25 mg as a single injection.

Precocious Puberty

IM (LUPRON DEPOT-PED): CHILDREN: 0.3 mg/kg/dose every 28 days. Minimum: 7.5 mg. If down regulation is not achieved, titrate upward in 3.75-mg increments q4wks.
SUBCUTANEOUS (LUPRON): CHILDREN: 20–45 mcg/kg/day. Titrate upward by 10 mcg/kg/day if down regulation is not achieved.

SIDE EFFECTS

Frequent: Hot flashes (ranging from mild flushing to diaphoresis). **Females:** Amenorrhea, spotting. **Occasional:** Arrhythmias; palpitations; blurred vision; dizziness; edema; headache; burning, pruritus, swelling at injection site; nausea; insomnia; weight gain. **Females:** Deepening voice, hirsutism, decreased libido, increased breast tenderness, vaginitis, altered mood. **Males:** Constipation, decreased testicle size, gynecomastia, impotence, decreased appetite, angina. **Rare:** **Males:** Thrombophlebitis.

ADVERSE EFFECTS/ TOXIC REACTIONS

Occasionally, signs/symptoms of prostatic carcinoma worsen 1–2 wks after initial dosing (subsides during continued therapy). Increased bone pain and, less frequently, dysuria, hematuria, weakness, paresthesia of lower extremities may be noted. MI, pulmonary embolism occur rarely.

NURSING CONSIDERATIONS

BASELINE ASSESSMENT

Question for possibility of pregnancy before initiating therapy (Pregnancy Category X). Obtain serum testosterone, prostatic acid phosphates (PAP) periodically during therapy. Serum testosterone, PAP should increase during first wk of therapy. Serum testosterone then should decrease to baseline level or less within 2 wks, PAP within 4 wks.

INTERVENTION/EVALUATION

Monitor for arrhythmias, palpitations. Assess for peripheral edema. Assess sleep pattern. Monitor for visual difficulties. Assist with ambulation if dizziness occurs. Offer antiemetics if nausea occurs.

PATIENT/ FAMILY TEACHING

• Hot flashes tend to decrease during continued therapy. • Temporary exacerbation of signs/symptoms of disease may occur during first few wks of therapy. • Use contraceptive measures during therapy. • Inform physician immediately if regular menstruation persists, pregnancy occurs. • Avoid tasks that require alertness, motor skills until response to drug is established (potential for dizziness).

levalbuterol

lee-val-**bue**-ter-all
(Xopenex, Xopenex HFA)
Do not confuse Xopenex with Xanax.

CLASSIFICATION

PHARMACOTHERAPEUTIC: Sympathomimetic. **CLINICAL:** Bronchodilator (see p. 74C).

L

ACTION

Stimulates beta$_2$-adrenergic receptors in lungs, resulting in relaxation of bronchial smooth muscle. **Therapeutic Effect:** Relieves bronchospasm, reduces airway resistance.

PHARMACOKINETICS

Route	Onset	Peak	Duration
Inhalation	5–10 min	1.5 hrs	5–6 hrs
Nebulization	10–17 min	1.5 hrs	5–8 hrs

Half-life: 3.3–4 hrs.

USES

Treatment, prevention of bronchospasm due to reversible obstructive airway disease (e.g., asthma, bronchitis, emphysema).

PRECAUTIONS

Contraindications: History of hypersensitivity to sympathomimetics. **Cautions:** Cardiovascular disorders (cardiac arrhythmias), seizures, hypertension, hyperthyroidism, diabetes mellitus.

LIFESPAN CONSIDERATIONS

Pregnancy/Lactation: Crosses placenta. Unknown if distributed in breast milk. **Pregnancy Category C. Children:** Safety and efficacy not established in those younger than 12 yrs. **Elderly:** Lower initial dosages recommended.

INTERACTIONS

DRUG: **Beta-adrenergic blocking agents (beta-blockers)** antagonize effects. **Digoxin** may increase risk of arrhythmias. **MAOIs, tricyclic antidepressants** may potentiate cardiovascular effects. **Diuretics** may increase hypokalemia. **HERBAL:** None significant. **FOOD:** None known. **LAB VALUES:** May increase serum potassium.

AVAILABILITY (Rx)

Inhalation Aerosol: 45 mcg/activation. **Solution for Nebulization:** 0.31 in 3-ml vials, 0.63 mg in 3-ml vials, 1.25 mg in 3-ml vials, 1.25 mg in 0.5-ml vials.

ADMINISTRATION/HANDLING

Nebulization

• No diluent necessary. • Protect from light, excessive heat. Store at room temperature. • Once foil is opened, use within 2 wks. • Use within 1 wk and protect from light after removal from pouch.• Discard if solution is not colorless. • Do not mix with other medications. • Concentrated solution (1.25 mg in 0.5 ml) should be diluted with 2.5 ml 0.9% NaCl prior to use. • Give over 5–15 min.

Inhalation

• Shake well before inhalation. • Following first inhalation, wait 2 min before inhaling second dose (allows for deeper bronchial penetration). • Rinsing mouth with water immediately after inhalation prevents mouth/throat dryness.

INDICATIONS/ROUTES/DOSAGE

Treatment/Prevention of Bronchospasm

NEBULIZATION: ADULTS, ELDERLY, CHILDREN 12 YRS AND OLDER: Initially, 0.63 mg 3 times a day 6–8 hrs apart. May increase to 1.25 mg 3 times a day with dose monitoring. **CHILDREN 6–11 YRS:** Initially 0.31 mg 3 times a day. **Maximum:** 0.63 mg 3 times a day.

INHALATION: ADULTS, ELDERLY, CHILDREN 4 YRS AND OLDER: 1–2 inhalations q4–6h.

SIDE EFFECTS

Frequent: Tremor, anxiety, headache, throat dryness or irritation. **Occasional:** Cough, bronchial irritation. **Rare:** Drowsiness, diarrhea, dry mouth, flushing, diaphoresis, anorexia.

ADVERSE EFFECTS/ TOXIC REACTIONS

Excessive sympathomimetic stimulation may produce palpitations, extrasystoles, tachycardia, chest pain, slight increase in B/P followed by substantial decrease, chills, diaphoresis, blanching of skin. Too-frequent or excessive use may decrease bronchodilating effectiveness, lead to severe, paradoxical bronchoconstriction.

NURSING CONSIDERATIONS

BASELINE ASSESSMENT

Offer emotional support (high incidence of anxiety due to difficulty in breathing, sympathomimetic response to drug). Assess lung sounds, pulse, B/P. Note color, amount of sputum.

INTERVENTION/EVALUATION

Monitor rate, depth, rhythm, type of respiration; quality/rate of pulse, EKG, serum potassium, ABG determinations. Assess lung sounds for wheezing (bronchoconstriction), rales. Observe for paradoxical bronchospasm.

PATIENT/ FAMILY TEACHING

• Increase fluid intake (decreases lung secretion viscosity). • Rinsing mouth with water immediately after inhalation may prevent mouth/throat dryness. • Avoid excessive use of caffeine derivatives (chocolate, coffee, tea, cola, cocoa). • Notify physician if palpitations, tachycardia, chest pain, tremors, dizziness, headache occurs or shortness of breath is not relieved.

Levaquin, *see levofloxacin*

levetiracetam

lev-eh-tir-**ass**-eh-tam
(Apo-Levetiracetam ✤, Keppra, Keppra XR)
Do not confuse Keppra with Kaletra or Keppra XR, or levetiracetam with levofloxacin.

◆CLASSIFICATION

CLINICAL: Anticonvulsant.

ACTION

Inhibits burst firing without affecting normal neuronal excitability. **Therapeutic Effect:** Prevents seizure activity.

PHARMACOKINETICS

Rapidly, completely absorbed following PO administration. Protein binding: less than 10%. Metabolized primarily by enzymatic hydrolysis. Primarily excreted in urine as unchanged drug. **Half-life:** 6–8 hrs.

USES

PO: Adjunctive therapy in treatment of partial-onset seizures in pts 4 yrs and older with epilepsy. Adjunctive therapy in myoclonic seizures in adults and adolescents. Adjunctive therapy in treatment of primary generalized tonic-clonic seizures in pts 6 yrs and older with idiopathic generalized seizures. **Keppra XR:** Adjunctive therapy in treatment of partial-onset seizures in pts 16 yrs of age and older. **Injection:** Treatment of partial-onset seizures in adults. **OFF-LABEL:** Bipolar disorder.

PRECAUTIONS

Contraindications: None known. **Cautions:** Renal impairment.

⌛ LIFESPAN CONSIDERATIONS

Pregnancy/Lactation: Distributed in breast milk. Breast-feeding not recommended. **Pregnancy Category C. Children:** Safety and efficacy not established in children 4 yrs or younger. **Elderly:** Age-related renal impairment may require dosage adjustment.

INTERACTIONS

DRUG: None significant. **HERBAL:** None significant. **FOOD:** None known. **LAB VALUES:** May increase Hgb, Hct, RBC, WBC counts.

AVAILABILITY (Rx)

Injection, Solution: 100 mg/ml. **Oral Solution:** 100 mg/ml. **Tablets:** 250 mg, 500 mg, 750 mg, 1,000 mg.

Tablets, Extended-Release: 500 mg, 750 mg.

ADMINISTRATION/HANDLING

IV

Rate of infusion • Infuse over 15 mins.

Reconstitution • Dilute with 100 ml 0.9% NaCl or D_5W.
Storage • Store at room temperature. • Stable for 24 hrs following dilution.

IV INCOMPATIBILITY

Data not available.

IV COMPATIBILITIES

Diazepam (Valium), lorazepam (Ativan), valproate (Depacon).

PO
• Give without regard to food. • Use oral solution for pts weighing 20 kg or less. • Use tablets or oral solution for pts weighing more than 20 kg. • Oral solution should be administered with a calibrated measuring device. • Swallow extended-release tablets whole; do not chew, break, or crush.

INDICATIONS/ROUTES/DOSAGE

Partial-Onset Seizures
IV/PO: ADULTS, ELDERLY, CHILDREN 17 YRS AND OLDER: Initially, 500 mg q12h. May increase by 1,000 mg/day q2wk. **Maximum:** 3,000 mg/day. **KEPPRA XR:** 1,000 mg once daily. May increase in increments of 1,000 mg every 2 weeks. **Maximum:** 3,000 mg daily.
PO: CHILDREN 4–16 YRS: 20 mg/kg/day in 2 divided doses. May increase at weekly intervals by 10 mg/kg/dose. **Maximum:** 60 mg/kg/day in 2 divided doses.

Myoclonic Seizures
PO: ADULTS, ELDERLY, CHILDREN 12 YRS AND OLDER: Initially, 500 mg q12h. May increase by 1,000 mg/day q2wk. **Maximum:** 3,000 mg/day.

Tonic-Clonic Seizures
PO: ADULTS, ELDERLY, CHILDREN 16 YRS AND OLDER: Initially, 500 mg twice a day. May increase by 1,000 mg/day q2wks until dose of 3,000 mg/day attained. **CHILDREN 6–15 YRS:** Initially, 10 mg/kg twice a day. May increase by 20 mg/kg/day q2wks until dose of 60 mg/kg/day attained.

Dosage in Renal Impairment
Dosage is modified based on creatinine clearance.

Creatinine Clearance	Dosage (Immediate-Release, IV)	Dosage (Extended-Release)
Greater than 80 ml/min	500–1,500 mg q12h	1,000–3,000 mg q24h
50–80 ml/min	500–1,000 mg q12h	1,000–2,000 mg q24h
30–49 ml/min	250–750 mg q12h	500–1,500 mg q24h
Less than 30 ml/min	250–500 mg q12h	500–1,000 mg q24h
End-stage renal disease using dialysis	500–1,000 mg q24h, after dialysis, a 250- to 500-mg supplemental dose is recommended	NA

SIDE EFFECTS

Frequent (15%–10%): Drowsiness, asthenia (loss of strength, energy), headache, infection. **Occasional (9%–3%):** Dizziness, pharyngitis, pain, depression, anxiety, vertigo, rhinitis, anorexia. **Rare (less than 3%):** Amnesia, emotional lability, cough, sinusitis, anorexia, diplopia.

ADVERSE EFFECTS/ TOXIC REACTIONS

Acute psychosis, seizures have been reported. Sudden discontinuance increases risk of seizure activity.

NURSING CONSIDERATIONS

BASELINE ASSESSMENT

Review history of seizure disorder (intensity, frequency, duration, LOC). Initiate seizure precautions. Assess for hypersensitivity to levetiracetam, renal function tests.

INTERVENTION/EVALUATION

Observe for recurrence of seizure activity. Assess for clinical improvement (decrease in intensity/frequency of seizures). Monitor renal function tests, suicidal ideation, depression, behavioral changes. Assist with ambulation if dizziness occurs.

PATIENT/ FAMILY TEACHING

• Drowsiness usually diminishes with continued therapy. • Avoid tasks that require alertness, motor skills until response to drug is established. • Avoid alcohol. • Do not abruptly discontinue medication (may precipitate seizures). • Strict maintenance of drug therapy is essential for seizure control. • Report mood swings, hostile behavior, suicidal ideation, unusual changes in behavior.

Levitra, *see vardenafil*

levocetirizine

lee-voe-seh-**tir**-i-zeen
(Xyzal)
Do not confuse levocetirazine with cetirazine.

◆CLASSIFICATION

PHARMACOTHERAPEUTIC: Second-generation piperazine. **CLINICAL:** Antihistamine.

ACTION

Competes with histamine for H_1-receptor sites on effector cells in GI tract, blood vessels, respiratory tract. **Therapeutic Effect:** Relieves allergic response (sneezing, rhinorrhea, postnasal discharge, nasal pruritus, ocular pruritus, tearing), allergic rhinitis (hay fever), mediated by histamine (urticaria, pruritus).

PHARMACOKINETICS

Rapidly, almost completely absorbed from GI tract. Protein binding: 92%. Excreted primarily unchanged in urine. **Half-life:** 8 hrs (increased in renal impairment).

USES

Relief of symptoms of allergic rhinitis (seasonal, perennial) and uncomplicated skin manifestations of chronic idiopathic urticaria.

PRECAUTIONS

Contraindications: Hypersensitivity to hydroxyzine, end-stage renal disease, children 6–11 yrs with renal impairment. **Cautions:** Renal impairment.

⌛ LIFESPAN CONSIDERATIONS

Pregnancy/Lactation: Distributed in breast milk. **Pregnancy Category B. Children:** Less likely to cause anticholinergic effects (e.g., dry mouth, urinary retention). Safety and efficacy not established in those younger than 6 yrs. **Elderly:** More sensitive to anticholinergic effects (e.g., dry mouth, urinary retention). Age-related renal impairment may require dosage adjustment.

INTERACTIONS

DRUG: May increase **ritonavir, theophylline** concentrations. **HERBAL:** None significant. **FOOD:** None known. **LAB VALUES:** May suppress wheal and flare reactions to antigen skin testing, unless antihistamines are discontinued 4 days before testing.

AVAILABILITY (Rx)

Oral Solution: 0.5 mg/ml. **Tablets:** 5 mg.

ADMINISTRATION/HANDLING

PO

• Give without regard to food. Tablets may be crushed.

INDICATIONS/ROUTES/DOSAGE

Allergic Rhinitis, Chronic Urticaria

PO: ADULTS, ELDERLY, CHILDREN 12 YRS AND OLDER: 5 mg once daily in the evening. **CHILDREN 6–11 YRS:** 2.5 mg once daily in the evening. **CHILDREN 6 MOS–5 YRS:** 1.25 mg once daily in the evening.

Dosage in Renal Impairment

Mild renal function impairment (creatinine clearance 50–80 ml/min): 2.5 mg once daily. **Moderate renal function**

impairment (creatinine clearance 30–49 ml/min): 2.5 mg every other day. **Severe renal function impairment (creatinine clearance 10–29 ml/min):** 2.5 mg twice weekly (once every 3–4 days).

SIDE EFFECTS

Adults: Occasional (6%–4%): Drowsiness, nasopharyngitis, fatigue. Rare (2%–1%): Dry mouth, pharyngitis. **Children 6–12 yrs:** Rare (4%–2%): Fever, cough, fatigue, epistaxis.

ADVERSE EFFECTS/ TOXIC REACTIONS

None significant.

NURSING CONSIDERATIONS

BASELINE ASSESSMENT

Assess severity of rhinitis, urticaria, other symptoms. Obtain baseline renal function tests.

INTERVENTION/EVALUATION

For upper respiratory allergies, increase fluids to maintain thin secretions and offset thirst. Monitor symptoms for therapeutic response.

PATIENT/FAMILY TEACHING

- Avoid tasks that require alertness, motor skills until response to drug is established.
- Avoid alcohol during antihistamine therapy.

L

levofloxacin

levo-**flox**-a-sin
(Iquix, Levaquin,
Novo-Levofloxacin ✦, Quixin)

BLACK BOX ALERT May increase risk of tendonitis, tendon rupture.

Do not confuse Levaquin with Levoxyl, Levsin/SL, or Lovenox, or levofloxacin with levetiracetam or levothyroxine.

CLASSIFICATION

PHARMACOTHERAPEUTIC: Fluoroquinolone. **CLINICAL:** Antibiotic (see p. 25C).

ACTION

Inhibits DNA enzyme gyrase in susceptible microorganisms, interfering with bacterial cell replication, repair. **Therapeutic Effect:** Bactericidal.

PHARMACOKINETICS

Well absorbed after PO, IV administration. Protein binding: 50%. Widely distributed. Eliminated unchanged in urine. Partially removed by hemodialysis. **Half-life:** 6–8 hrs.

USES

Treatment of susceptible infections due to *S. pneumoniae, S. aureus, E. faecalis, H. influenzae, M. catarrhalis, Serratia marcescens, K. pneumoniae, E. coli, P. mirabilis, P. aeruginosa, C. pneumoniae, Legionella pneumophila, Mycoplasma pneumoniae.* Treatment of acute bacterial exacerbation of chronic bronchitis, acute bacterial sinusitus, community-acquired pneumonia, nosocomial pneumonia, acute maxillary sinusitis, complicated UTI, acute pyelonephritis, uncomplicated mild to moderate skin/skin structure infections, prostatitis. **Ophthalmic:** Treatment of superficial infections to conjunctiva (0.5%), cornea (1.5%). **OFF-LABEL:** Anthrax, gonorrhea, pelvic inflammatory disease (PID), diverticulitis, enterocolitis, gonococcal infections, Legionnaire's disease, peritonitis.

PRECAUTIONS

Contraindications: Hypersensitivity to other fluoroquinolones, cinoxacin, nalidixic acid. **Cautions:** Suspected CNS disorders, seizure disorder, renal impairment, bradycardia, cardiomyopathy, hypokalemia, hypomagnesemia.

LIFESPAN CONSIDERATIONS

Pregnancy/Lactation: Distributed in breast milk. Avoid use in pregnancy. **Pregnancy Category C. Children:** Safety and efficacy not established in those younger than 18 yrs. **Elderly:** Age-related renal impairment may require dosage adjustment.

INTERACTIONS

DRUG: **Antacids, iron preparations, sucralfate, zinc** decrease absorption. **NSAIDs** may increase risk of CNS stimulation, seizures. May increase effects of **warfarin.** HERBAL: None significant. FOOD: None known. LAB VALUES: May alter serum glucose.

AVAILABILITY (Rx)

Infusion Premix: 250 mg/50 ml, 500 mg/100 ml, 750 mg/150 ml. **Injection, Solution:** 25 mg/ml. **Ophthalmic Solution:** (Iquix) 1.5%; (Quixin) 0.5%. **Oral Solution:** 25 mg/ml. **Tablets:** 250 mg, 500 mg, 750 mg.

ADMINISTRATION/HANDLING

IV

Reconstitution • For infusion using single-dose vial, withdraw desired amount (10 ml for 250 mg, 20 ml for 500 mg). Dilute each 10 ml (250 mg) with minimum 40 ml 0.9% NaCl, D_5W, providing a concentration of 5 mg/ml.
Rate of administration • Administer slowly, over not less than 60 min for 250 mg or 500 mg; 90 min for 750 mg.
Storage • Available in single-dose 20-ml (500-mg) vials and premixed with D_5W, ready to infuse. • Diluted vials stable for 72 hrs at room temperature, 14 days if refrigerated.

PO

• Do not administer antacids (aluminum, magnesium), sucralfate, iron or multivitamin preparations with zinc within 2 hrs of levofloxacin administration (significantly reduces levofloxacin absorption). • Give tablets without regard to food. • Give oral solution 1 hr before or 2 hrs after meals.

Ophthalmic

• Place a gloved finger on lower eyelid and pull out until a pocket is formed between eye and lower lid. • Place prescribed number of drops into pocket. • Instruct pt to close eye gently (so medication will not be squeezed out of the sac) and to apply digital pressure to lacrimal sac for 1–2 min to minimize systemic absorption.

IV INCOMPATIBILITIES

Furosemide (Lasix), heparin, insulin, nitroglycerin, propofol (Diprivan).

IV COMPATIBILITIES

Aminophylline, dobutamine (Dobutrex), dopamine (Intropin), fentanyl (Sublimaze), lidocaine, lorazepam (Ativan), morphine.

INDICATIONS/ROUTES/DOSAGE

Usual Dosage Range
IV/PO: ADULTS, ELDERLY: 250–500 mg q24h; 750 mg q24h for severe or complicated infections.

Bacterial Sinusitis
PO: ADULTS, ELDERLY: 500 mg once daily for 10 days or 750 mg once daily for 5 days.

Bronchitis
PO, IV: ADULTS, ELDERLY: 500 mg q24h for 7 days.

Community-Acquired Pneumonia
PO: ADULTS, ELDERLY: 750 mg/day for 5 days or 500 mg q24h for 7–14 days.

Pneumonia, Nosocomial
PO, IV: ADULTS, ELDERLY: 750 mg q24h for 7–14 days.

Acute Maxillary Sinusitis
PO, IV: ADULTS, ELDERLY: 500 mg q24h for 10–14 days.

Skin/Skin Structure Infections
PO, IV: ADULTS, ELDERLY: (Uncomplicated) 500 mg q24h for 7–10 days. (Complicated) 750 mg q24h for 7–14 days.

L

Prostatitis
IV, PO: ADULTS, ELDERLY: 500 mg q24h for 28 days.

Uncomplicated UTI
IV, PO: ADULTS, ELDERLY: 250 mg q24h for 3 days.

UTI, Acute Pyelonephritis
PO, IV: ADULTS, ELDERLY: 250 mg q24h for 10 days.

Bacterial Conjunctivitis
OPHTHALMIC: ADULTS, ELDERLY, CHILDREN 1 YR AND OLDER (QUIXIN): 1–2 drops q2h for 2 days (up to 8 times a day), then 1–2 drops q4h for 5 days.

Corneal Ulcer
OPHTHALMIC: ADULTS, ELDERLY, CHILDREN OLDER THAN 5 YRS (IQUIX): Days 1–3: Instill 1–2 drops q30min to 2 hrs while awake and 4–6 hrs after retiring. **Days 4 through completion:** 1–2 drops q1–4h while awake.

L

Dosage in Renal Impairment
Normal renal function dosage of 500 mg/day:

Creatinine Clearance	Dosage
50–80 ml/min	No change
20–49 ml/min	500 mg initially, then 250 mg q24h
10–19 ml/min	500 mg initially, then 250 mg q48h

For pts undergoing dialysis, 500 mg initially, then 250 mg q48h.

Normal renal function dosage of 250 mg/day:

Creatinine Clearance	Dosage
20–49 ml/min	No change
10–19 ml/min	250 mg initially, then 250 mg q48h

Normal renal function dosage of 750 mg/day:

Creatinine Clearance	Dosage
50–80 ml/min	No change
20–49 ml/min	Initially, 750 mg, then 750 mg q48h
10–19 ml/min	Initially 750 mg, then 500 mg q48h
Dialysis	500 mg q48h

SIDE EFFECTS

Occasional (3%–1%): Diarrhea, nausea, abdominal pain, dizziness, drowsiness, headache, light-headedness. **Ophthalmic:** Local burning/discomfort, margin crusting, crystals/scales, foreign body sensation, ocular itching, altered taste. **Rare (less than 1%):** Flatulence; pain, inflammation, swelling in calves, hands, shoulder; chest pain; difficulty breathing; palpitations; edema; tendon pain. **Ophthalmic:** Corneal staining, keratitis, allergic reaction, eyelid swelling, tearing, reduced visual acuity.

ADVERSE EFFECTS/ TOXIC REACTIONS

Antibiotic-associated colitis, other superinfections (abdominal cramps, severe watery diarrhea, fever) may occur. Superinfection (genital/anal pruritus, ulceration/changes in oral mucosa, moderate to severe diarrhea) may occur from altered bacterial balance. Hypersensitivity reactions, including photosensitivity (rash, pruritus, blisters, edema, sensation of burning skin) have occurred in pts receiving fluoroquinolones.

NURSING CONSIDERATIONS

BASELINE ASSESSMENT

Question for hypersensitivity to levofloxacin, other fluoroquinolones.

INTERVENTION/EVALUATION

Monitor serum glucose, renal/hepatic function tests. Monitor daily pattern of bowel activity, stool consistency. Report hypersensitivity reaction: skin rash, urticaria, pruritus, photosensitivity promptly. Be alert for superinfection: fever, vomiting, diarrhea, anal/genital pruritus, oral mucosal changes (ulceration, pain, erythema). Provide symptomatic relief for nausea. Evaluate food tolerance, altered taste.

PATIENT/ FAMILY TEACHING

• Drink 6–8 glasses of fluid a day (prevents formation of urine crystals). • Avoid tasks that require alertness, motor skills until response to drug is established (may cause dizziness, drowsiness). • Notify physician if tendon pain/ swelling, palpitations, chest pain, difficulty breathing, persistent diarrhea occurs. • Avoid exposure to direct sunlight. • Report use of warfarin.

Levothroid, *see levothyroxine*

levothyroxine

lee-voe-thye-**rox**-een
(Eltroxin ✤, Levothroid, Levoxyl, Synthroid, Unithroid)

BLACK BOX ALERT Ineffective, potentially toxic for weight reduction. High doses increase risk of serious, life-threatening toxic effects, especially when used with some anorectic drugs.

Do not confuse levothyroxine with levofloxacin or liothyronine, Levoxyl with Lanoxin, Levaquin, or Luvox, or Synthroid with Symmetrel.

FIXED-COMBINATION(S)

With liothyronine, T_3 **(Thyrolar).**

◆CLASSIFICATION

PHARMACOTHERAPEUTIC: Synthetic isomer of thyroxine. **CLINICAL:** Thyroid hormone (T_4) (see p. 159C).

ACTION

Involved in normal metabolism, growth, development, esp. of CNS in infants. Possesses catabolic, anabolic effects. **Therapeutic Effect:** Increases basal metabolic rate, enhances gluconeogenesis, stimulates protein synthesis.

PHARMACOKINETICS

Variable, incomplete absorption from GI tract. Protein binding: greater than 99%. Widely distributed. Deiodinated in peripheral tissues, minimal metabolism in liver. Eliminated by biliary excretion. **Half-life:** 6–7 days.

USES

Treatment of hypothyroidism, myxedema coma, pituitary thyroid-stimulating hormone (TSH) suppression.

PRECAUTIONS

Contraindications: Hypersensitivity to tablet components (e.g., tartrazine); allergy to aspirin; lactose intolerance; MI; thyrotoxicosis uncomplicated by hypothyroidism; treatment of obesity. **Cautions:** Elderly, angina pectoris, hypertension, other cardiovascular disease.

⌛ LIFESPAN CONSIDERATIONS

Pregnancy/Lactation: Does not cross placenta. Minimal distribution in breast milk. **Pregnancy Category A. Children:** No age-related precautions noted. Caution in neonates in interpreting thyroid function tests. **Elderly:** May be more sensitive to thyroid effects; individualized dosage recommended.

INTERACTIONS

DRUG: **Cholestyramine, colestipol** may decrease absorption. **Estrogens** may cause decrease in serum-free thyroxine. May alter effect of **oral anticoagulants. Sympathomimetics** may increase risk of coronary insufficiency, effects of levothyroxine. **H_2 antagonists, proton pump inhibitors** may decrease effect. **HERBAL:** None significant. **FOOD:** None known. **LAB VALUES:** None significant.

AVAILABILITY (Rx)

Injection, Powder for Reconstitution (Synthroid): 200 mcg, 500 mcg. **Tablets: (Le-**

vothroid, Levoxyl, Synthroid, Unithroid): 25 mcg, 50 mcg, 75 mcg, 88 mcg, 100 mcg, 112 mcg, 125 mcg, 137 mcg, 150 mcg, 175 mcg, 200 mcg, 300 mcg.

ADMINISTRATION/HANDLING

◀ALERT▶ Do not interchange brands (problems with bioequivalence between manufacturers).

IV

Reconstitution • Reconstitute 200-mcg or 500-mcg vial with 5 ml 0.9% NaCl to provide concentration of 40 or 100 mcg/ml, respectively; shake until clear.

Rate of administration • Use immediately; discard unused portions. • Give each 100 mcg or less over 1 min.

Storage • Store vials at room temperature.

PO

• Administer in the morning on an empty stomach, 30 min before food. • Administer before breakfast to prevent insomnia. • Tablets may be crushed. • Take 4 hrs apart from antacids, iron, calcium supplements.

IV INCOMPATIBILITIES

Do not use or mix with other IV solutions.

INDICATIONS/ROUTES/DOSAGE

Hypothyroidism

PO: ADULTS, ELDERLY, CHILDREN OLDER THAN 12 YRS, GROWTH AND PUBERTY COMPLETE: 1.7 mcg/kg/day as single daily dose. Usual maintenance: 100–200 mcg/day. **CHILDREN OLDER THAN 12 YRS, GROWTH AND PUBERTY INCOMPLETE:** 2–3 mcg/kg/day. **CHILDREN 6–12 YRS:** 4–5 mcg/kg/day. **CHILDREN 1–5 YRS:** 5–6 mcg/kg/day. **CHILDREN 6–12 MOS:** 6–8 mcg/kg/day. **CHILDREN 3–5 MOS:** 8–10 mcg/kg/day. **CHILDREN YOUNGER THAN 3 MOS:** 10–15 mcg/kg/day.

Myxedema Coma

IV: ADULTS, ELDERLY: Initially, 200–500 mcg, then 100–300 mcg next day if necessary.

Pituitary Thyroid-Stimulating Hormone (TSH) Suppression

PO: ADULTS, ELDERLY: Doses greater than 2 mcg/kg/day usually required to suppress TSH below 0.1 milliunits/L.

SIDE EFFECTS

Occasional: Reversible hair loss at start of therapy in children. **Rare:** Dry skin, GI intolerance, rash, urticaria, pseudotumor cerebri, severe headache in children.

ADVERSE EFFECTS/ TOXIC REACTIONS

Excessive dosage produces signs/symptoms of hyperthyroidism (weight loss, palpitations, increased appetite, tremors, anxiety, tachycardia, hypertension, headache, insomnia, menstrual irregularities). Cardiac arrhythmias occur rarely.

NURSING CONSIDERATIONS

BASELINE ASSESSMENT

Obtain baseline weight, vital signs. Signs/symptoms of diabetes mellitus, diabetes insipidus, adrenal insufficiency, hypopituitarism may become intensified. Treat with adrenocortical steroids before thyroid therapy in coexisting hypothyroidism and hypoadrenalism.

INTERVENTION/EVALUATION

Monitor pulse for rate, rhythm (report pulse of 100 or marked increase). Observe for tremors, anxiety. Assess appetite, sleep pattern. **Children: (Undertreatment):** May decrease intellectual development, linear growth. **(Overtreatment):** Adversely affects brain maturation, accelerates bone age.

PATIENT/ FAMILY TEACHING

• Do not discontinue drug therapy; replacement for hypothyroidism is lifelong. • Follow-up office visits, thyroid function tests are essential. • Take medication at the same time each day, preferably in the morning. • Monitor pulse for rate, rhythm; report irregular rhythm or pulse rate over 100 beats/min. • Do not change brands. • Notify physician promptly of chest pain, weight loss, anxiety, tremors, insomnia. • Children may have reversible hair loss, increased aggressiveness during first few mos of therapy. • Full therapeutic effect may take 1–3 wks.

Levoxyl, *see levothyroxine*

Lexapro, *see escitalopram*

Lexiva, *see fosamprenavir*

lidocaine HIGH ALERT

lye-doe-kane
(Anestacon, Betacaine ✱, Lidoderm, Xylocaine)

FIXED-COMBINATION(S)

EMLA: lidocaine/prilocaine (an anesthetic): 2.5%/2.5%. **Lidosite:** lidocaine/epinephrine (a sympathomimetic): 10%/0.1%. **Lidocaine with epinephrine:** lidocaine/epinephrine (a sympathomimetic): 2%/1:50,000, 1%/1:100,000, 1%/1:200,000, 0.5%/1:200,000. **Synéra:** lidocaine/tetracaine (an anesthetic): 70 mg/70 mg.

◆CLASSIFICATION

PHARMACOTHERAPEUTIC: Amide anesthetic. **CLINICAL:** Antiarrhythmic, anesthetic (see pp. 7C, 16C).

ACTION

Anesthetic: Inhibits conduction of nerve impulses. **Therapeutic Effect:** Causes temporary loss of feeling/sensation. **Antiarrhythmic:** Decreases depolarization, automaticity, excitability of ventricle during diastole by direct action. **Therapeutic Effect:** Inhibits ventricular arrhythmias.

PHARMACOKINETICS

Route	Onset	Peak	Duration
IV	30–90 sec	N/A	10–20 min
Local anesthetic	2.5 min	N/A	30–60 min

Completely absorbed after IM administration. Protein binding: 60%–80%. Widely distributed. Metabolized in liver. Primarily excreted in urine. Minimally removed by hemodialysis. **Half-life:** 1–2 hrs.

USES

Antiarrhythmic: Rapid control of acute ventricular arrhythmias following MI, cardiac catheterization, cardiac surgery, digitalis-induced ventricular arrhythmias. **Local Anesthetic:** Infiltration/nerve block for dental/surgical procedures, childbirth. **Topical Anesthetic:** Local skin disorders (minor burns, insect bites, prickly heat, skin manifestations of chickenpox, abrasions). Mucous membranes (local anesthesia of oral, nasal, laryngeal mucous membranes; local anesthesia of respiratory, urinary tracts; relief of discomfort of pruritus ani, hemorrhoids, pruritus vulvae). **Dermal patch:** Relief of chronic pain in post-herpetic neuralgia, allodynia (painful hypersensitivity). **OFF-LABEL:** Fentanyl-induced cough.

PRECAUTIONS

Contraindications: Adams-Stokes syndrome, hypersensitivity to amide-type local anesthetics, supraventricular arrhythmias, Wolff-Parkinson-White syndrome. Spinal anesthesia contraindicated in septicemia. **Cautions:** Hepatic disease, marked hypoxia, severe respiratory depression, hypovolemia, heart block, bradycardia, atrial fibrillation.

⌛ LIFESPAN CONSIDERATIONS

Pregnancy/Lactation: Crosses placenta. Distributed in breast milk. **Pregnancy Category B. Children:** No age-related precautions noted. **Elderly:** More sensitive to adverse effects. Dose, rate of infusion should be reduced. Age-related renal impairment may require dosage adjustment.

INTERACTIONS

DRUG: **Anticonvulsants** may increase cardiac depressant effects. **Beta-adrenergic blockers** may increase risk of toxicity. **Other antiarrhythmics** may increase cardiac effects. HERBAL: **St. John's wort** may decrease concentration. FOOD: None known. LAB VALUES: IM lidocaine may increase creatine kinase (CK) level (used to diagnose acute MI). **Therapeutic serum level:** 1.5 to 6 mcg/ml; **toxic serum level:** greater than 6 mcg/ml.

AVAILABILITY (Rx)

Cream, Topical: 4%. Infusion Premix: 0.4% (4 mg/ml in 250 ml, 500 ml); 0.8% (8 mg/ml in 250 ml, 500 ml). Injection, Solution: 0.5% (5 mg/ml), 1% (10 mg/ml), 2% (20 mg/ml). Jelly, Topical: 2%. Solution, Topical: 4%. Solution, Viscous: 2%. Transdermal, Topical (Lidoderm): 5%.

ADMINISTRATION/HANDLING

◀ALERT▶ Resuscitative equipment, drugs (including O_2) must always be readily available when administering lidocaine by any route.

IV

◀ALERT▶ Use only lidocaine without preservative, clearly marked **for IV use.**

Reconstitution • For IV infusion, prepare solution by adding 2 g to 250–500 ml D_5W or 0.9% NaCl to provide concentration of 8 mg/ml or 4 mg/ml, respectively. • Commercially available preparations of 0.4% and 0.8% may be used for IV infusion. **Maximum concentration:** 4 g/250 ml (16 mg/ml).

Rate of administration • For IV push, use 1% (10 mg/ml) or 2% (20 mg/ml). • Administer IV push at rate of 25–50 mg/min. • Administer for IV infusion at rate of 1–4 mg/min (1–4 ml); use volume control IV set.

Storage • Store premix solutions at room temperature.

IM

• Use 10% (100 mg/ml); clearly identify lidocaine that is **for IM use.** • Give in deltoid muscle (serum level is significantly higher than if injection is given in gluteus muscle or lateral thigh).

Topical

• Not for ophthalmic use. • For skin disorders, apply directly to affected area or put on gauze or bandage, which is then applied to the skin. • For mucous membrane use, apply to desired area per manufacturer's insert. • Administer lowest dosage possible that still provides anesthesia.

Dermal Patch

Patch may be cut to appropriate size.

IV INCOMPATIBILITIES

Amphotericin B complex (Abelcet, AmBisome, Amphotec), thiopental.

IV COMPATIBILITIES

Aminophylline, amiodarone (Cordarone), calcium gluconate, digoxin (Lanoxin), diltiazem (Cardizem), dobutamine (Dobutrex), dopamine (Intropin), enalapril (Vasotec), furosemide (Lasix), heparin, insulin, lipids, nitroglycerin, potassium chloride.

INDICATIONS/ROUTES/DOSAGE

Ventricular Arrhythmias

IM: ADULTS, ELDERLY: 300 mg (or 4.3 mg/kg). May repeat in 60–90 min.

IV: ADULTS, ELDERLY: Initially, 1–1.5 mg/kg. Refractory ventricular tachycardia, fibrillation: Repeat dose at 0.5–0.75 mg/kg q10–15min after initial dose for a maximum of 3 doses. Total dose not to exceed 3 mg/kg. Follow with continuous infusion (1–4 mg/min) after return of perfusion. Reappearance of arrhythmia during infusion: 0.5 mg/kg, reassess infusion. CHILDREN, INFANTS: Initially, 1 mg/kg (**maximum:** 100 mg). May repeat second dose of 0.5–1 mg/kg if start of infusion longer than 15 min. Maintenance: 20–50 mcg/kg/min as IV infusion.

Local Anesthesia

INFILTRATION, NERVE BLOCK: ADULTS: Local anesthetic dosage varies with procedure, degree of anesthesia, vascularity, duration. **Maximum dose:** 4.5 mg/kg. Do not repeat within 2 hrs.

Topical Local Anesthesia

TOPICAL: ADULTS, ELDERLY: Apply to affected areas as needed.

Treatment of Post-Herpetic Neuralgia

◀ALERT▶ Transdermal patch may contain conducting metal (e.g., aluminum). Remove patch prior to MRI.

TOPICAL (DERMAL PATCH): ADULTS, ELDERLY: Apply to intact skin over most painful area (up to 3 applications once for up to 12 hrs in a 24-hr period).

SIDE EFFECTS

CNS effects generally dose-related and of short duration. Occasional: **IM:** Pain at injection site. **Topical:** Burning, stinging, tenderness at application site. Rare: Generally with high dose: Drowsiness; dizziness; disorientation; light-headedness; tremors; apprehension; euphoria; sensation of heat, cold, numbness; blurred or double vision; tinnitus (ringing in ears); nausea.

ADVERSE EFFECTS/ TOXIC REACTIONS

Serious adverse reactions to lidocaine are uncommon, but high dosage by any route may produce cardiovascular depression, bradycardia, hypotension, arrhythmias, heart block, cardiovascular collapse, cardiac arrest. Potential for malignant hyperthermia, CNS toxicity may occur, esp. with regional anesthesia use, progressing rapidly from mild side effects to tremors, drowsiness, seizures, vomiting, respiratory depression. Methemoglobinemia (evidenced by cyanosis) has occurred following topical application of lidocaine for teething discomfort and laryngeal anesthetic spray.

NURSING CONSIDERATIONS

BASELINE ASSESSMENT

Question for hypersensitivity to lidocaine, amide anesthetics. Obtain baseline B/P, pulse, respiratory rate, EKG, serum electrolytes.

INTERVENTION/EVALUATION

Monitor EKG, vital signs closely during and following drug administration for cardiac performance. If EKG shows arrhythmias, prolongation of PR interval or QRS complex, inform physician immediately. Assess pulse for rhythm, rate, quality. Assess B/P for evidence of hypotension. Monitor for therapeutic serum level (1.5–6 mcg/ml). For lidocaine given by all routes, monitor vital signs, LOC. Drowsiness should be considered a warning sign of high serum levels of lidocaine. **Therapeutic serum level:** 1.5–6 mcg/ml; **toxic serum level:** greater than 6 mcg/ml.

PATIENT/ FAMILY TEACHING

• **Local anesthesia:** Due to loss of feeling/sensation, protective measures may be needed until anesthetic wears off (no ambulation, including special positions for some regional anesthesia). • **Oral mucous membrane anesthesia:** Do not eat, drink, chew gum for 1 hr after application (swallowing reflex may be impaired, increasing risk of aspiration; numbness of tongue, buccal mucosa may lead to bite trauma). • **IV infusions:** Report dizziness, numbness, double vision, nausea, pain/burning, respiratory difficulty. • **Topical:** Report irritation, pain, numbness, swelling, blurred vision, tinnitus, respiratory difficulty.

Lidoderm, *see lidocaine*

linezolid

lin-**ayz**-oh-lid
(Zyvox, Zyvoxam ✱)
Do not confuse Zyvox with Zosyn or Zovirax.

◆CLASSIFICATION

PHARMACOTHERAPEUTIC: Oxalodinone. **CLINICAL:** Antibiotic.

L

ACTION

Binds to site on bacterial 23S ribosomal RNA, preventing formation of a complex essential for bacterial translation. **Therapeutic Effect:** Bacteriostatic against enterococci, staphylococci; bactericidal against streptococci.

PHARMACOKINETICS

Rapidly, extensively absorbed after PO administration. Protein binding: 31%. Metabolized in liver by oxidation. Excreted in urine. **Half-life:** 4–5.4 hrs.

USES

Treatment of susceptible infections due to aerobic and facultative, gram-positive microorganisms, including *E. faecium* (vancomycin-resistant strains only), *S. aureus* (including methicillin-resistant strains), *S. agalactiae, S. pneumoniae* (including multidrug-resistant strains), *S. pyogenes.* Treatment of pneumonia, skin, soft tissue infections (including diabetic foot infections), bacteremia caused by susceptible vancomycin-resistant organisms.

PRECAUTIONS

Contraindications: None known. **Cautions:** Uncontrolled hypertension, pheochromocytoma, carcinoid syndrome, severe renal/hepatic impairment, untreated hyperthyroidism.

LIFESPAN CONSIDERATIONS

Pregnancy/Lactation: Unknown if distributed in breast milk. **Pregnancy Category C. Children:** Safety and efficacy not established. **Elderly:** No age-related precautions noted.

INTERACTIONS

DRUG: **Bone marrow depressants** may increase risk of leukopenia, thrombocytopenia. **Adrenergic medications (sympathomimetics)** may increase effect. **SSRIs** may increase risk of serotonin syndrome. **HERBAL:** None significant. **FOOD:** Excessive amounts of **tyramine-containing foods, beverages** may cause significant hypertension. **LAB VALUES:** May decrease Hgb, neutrophils, platelets, WBC. May increase serum ALT, AST, alkaline phosphatase, amylase, bilirubin, BUN, creatinine, LDH, lipase.

AVAILABILITY (Rx)

Injection Premix: 2 mg/ml in 100-ml, 300-ml bags. **Powder for Oral Suspension:** 100 mg/5 ml. **Tablets:** 600 mg.

ADMINISTRATION/HANDLING

IV

Rate of administration • Infuse over 30–120 min. • Should be administered without further dilution.

Storage • Store at room temperature. • Protect from light. • Yellow color does not affect potency.

PO

• Give without regard to meals. • Use suspension within 21 days after reconstitution. Gently invert 3–5 times before administration. • Do not shake.

IV INCOMPATIBILITIES

Amphotericin B complex (Abelcet, AmBisome, Amphotec), chlorpromazine (Thorazine), co-trimoxazole (Bactrim), diazepam (Valium), erythromycin (Erythrocin), pentamidine (Pentam IV), phenytoin (Dilantin), total parenteral nutrition (TPN).

INDICATIONS/ROUTES/DOSAGE

Vancomycin-Resistant Infections (VRI)

PO, IV: ADULTS, ELDERLY, CHILDREN OLDER THAN 11 YRS: 600 mg q12h for 14–28 days. **CHILDREN 11 YRS AND YOUNGER:** 10 mg/kg q8–12h for 14–28 days.

Nosocomial Pneumonia, Community-Acquired Pneumonia, Complicated Skin/Skin Structure Infections

PO, IV: ADULTS, ELDERLY, CHILDREN OLDER THAN 11 YRS: 600 mg q12h for 10–14 days. **CHILDREN 11 YRS AND YOUNGER:** 10 mg/kg q8h for 10–14 days.

Uncomplicated Skin/Skin Structure Infections

PO: ADULTS, ELDERLY: 400 mg q12h for 10–14 days. **CHILDREN OLDER THAN 11 YRS:** 600 mg q12h for 10–14 days. **CHILDREN 5–11 YRS:** 10 mg/kg/dose q12h for 10–14 days. **CHILDREN YOUNGER THAN 5 YRS:** 10 mg/kg q8h for 10–14 days.

MRSA

PO, IV: ADULTS, ELDERLY: 600 mg q12h.

Usual Neonate Dosage

PO, IV: NEONATES: 10 mg/kg/dose q8–12h.

SIDE EFFECTS

Occasional (5%–2%): Diarrhea, nausea, headache. **Rare (less than 2%):** Altered taste, vaginal candidiasis, fungal infection, dizziness, tongue discoloration.

ADVERSE EFFECTS/ TOXIC REACTIONS

Thrombocytopenia, myelosuppression occur rarely. Antibiotic-associated colitis, other superinfections (abdominal cramps, severe watery diarrhea, fever) may result from altered bacterial balance.

NURSING CONSIDERATIONS

INTERVENTION/EVALUATION

Monitor daily pattern of bowel activity, stool consistency. Mild GI effects may be tolerable, but increasing severity may indicate onset of antibiotic-associated colitis. Be alert for superinfection: fever, vomiting, diarrhea, anal/genital pruritus, oral mucosal changes (ulceration, pain, erythema). Monitor CBC, platelets, Hgb.

PATIENT/ FAMILY TEACHING

• Continue therapy for full length of treatment. • Doses should be evenly spaced. • May cause GI upset (may take with food, milk). • Excessive amounts of tyramine-containing foods (red wine, aged cheese) may cause severe reaction (severe headache, neck stiffness, diaphoresis, palpitations). • Avoid alcohol. • Notify physician of persistent diarrhea, nausea, vomiting.

Lipitor, *see atorvastatin*

liraglutide

lear-ah-**glue**-tide
(Victoza)

BLACK BOX ALERT Causes dose-dependent and treatment duration–dependent thyroid C-cell tumors, including medullary thyroid cancer.

◆ CLASSIFICATION

PHARMACOTHERAPEUTIC: Antihyperglycemic (glucagon-like peptide-1 [GLP-1] receptor agonist. **CLINICAL:** Antidiabetic.

ACTION

Stimulates release of insulin from pancreatic beta cells, mimics enhancement of glucose-dependent insulin secretion, suppresses elevated glucagon secretion, slows gastric emptying. **Therapeutic Effect:** Improves glycemic control by increasing postmeal insulin secretion, emptying, increasing satiety.

PHARMACOKINETICS

Maximum concentration achieved in 8–12 hrs. Protein binding: 98%. Metabolized to large proteins without a specific organ as major route of elimination. **Half-life:** 13 hrs.

USES

Adjunct to diet and exercise to improve glycemic control in adult pts with type 2 diabetes mellitus.

PRECAUTIONS

Contraindications: Personal or family history of medullary thyroid carcinoma, those with multiple endocrine neoplasia syndrome type 2 diabetic ketoacidosis.

Cautions: History of pancreatitis, renal/hepatic impairment.

LIFESPAN CONSIDERATIONS

Pregnancy/Lactation: Unknown if distributed in breast milk. **Pregnancy Category C. Children:** Safety and efficacy not established. **Elderly:** No age-related precautions noted.

INTERACTIONS

DRUG: Liraglutide has potential to alter absorption of concurrently administered **oral medications. Ethanol** increases risk of hypoglycemia. **HERBAL:** None significant. **FOOD:** None known. **LAB VALUES:** Decreases glucose serum levels (when used in combination with insulin secretagogues [e.g., sulfonylureas]).

L

AVAILABILITY (Rx)

Subcutaneous, Solution (Prefilled Pen): 0.6 mg, 1.2 mg, 1.8 mg.

ADMINISTRATION/HANDLING

Subcutaneous

• May be given in thigh, abdomen, upper arm. • Rotation of injection sites is essential; maintain careful records. • Give at any time without regard to meals.

Storage • Refrigerate prefilled pens. • Discard if freezing occurs. • Discard pen 30 days after initial use.

INDICATIONS/ROUTES/DOSAGE

Diabetes Mellitus

SUBCUTANEOUS: ADULTS, ELDERLY: Initial dose: 0.6 mg subcutaneously once per day for at least 1 wk. This dose is intended to reduce GI symptoms during initial titration; it is not effective for glycemic control. After 1 wk, increase dose to 1.2 mg. If 1.2-mg dose does not result in acceptable glycemic control, dose can be increased to 1.8 mg.

SIDE EFFECTS

Frequent (5%): Headache, nausea, diarrhea, liraglutide antibody resistance. **Occasional (13%–6%):** Diarrhea, vomiting, dizziness, jitteriness, dyspepsia. **Rare (less than 6%):** Weakness, decreased appetite.

ADVERSE EFFECTS/TOXIC REACTIONS

Serious hypoglycemia may occur when used concurrently with insulin analogue (e.g., sulfonylurea); consider lowering dose.

NURSING CONSIDERATIONS

BASELINE ASSESSMENT

Check blood glucose concentration before administration. Discuss pt's lifestyle to determine extent of learning, emotional needs. Ensure follow-up instruction if pt/family does not thoroughly understand diabetes management or glucose testing technique. Dose is gradually increased to improve GI tolerance.

INTERVENTION/EVALUATION

Monitor blood glucose level, food intake. Assess for hypoglycemia (cool wet skin, tremors, dizziness, anxiety, headache, tachycardia, numbness in mouth, hunger, diplopia) or hyperglycemia (polyuria, polyphagia, polydipsia, nausea, vomiting, dim vision, fatigue, deep rapid breathing). Be alert to conditions that alter glucose requirements (fever, increased activity/stress, surgical procedures.

PATIENT/FAMILY TEACHING

• Diabetes mellitus requires lifelong control. • Prescribed diet, exercise are principal parts of treatment; do not skip/delay meals. • Continue following dietary instructions, regular exercise program, regular testing of blood glucose level. • Serious hypoglycemia may occur when used concurrently with insulin analogue (e.g., sulfonylurea). Consider lowering dose of insulin analogue to reduce risk of hypoglycemia. • Have source of glucose available to treat symptoms of low blood sugar.

lisdexamfetamine

lis-dex-am-**fet**-ah-meen
(Vyvanse)

BLACK BOX ALERT Associated with serious cardiovascular events in pts with preexisting structural cardiac abnormalities or other serious heart problems. Potential for drug dependency exists.

Do not confuse lisdexamfetamine with dextroamphetamine, or Vyvanse with Glucovance, Vivactil, or Vytorin.

◆ CLASSIFICATION

PHARMACOTHERAPEUTIC: Amphetamine **(Schedule II). CLINICAL:** CNS stimulant.

ACTION

Enhances action of dopamine, norepinephrine by blocking reuptake from synapses, increasing levels in extraneuronal space. **Therapeutic Effect:** Improves attention span in ADHD.

PHARMACOKINETICS

Route	Onset	Peak	Duration
PO	Rapid	1 hr	24 hrs

Rapidly absorbed. Converted to dextroamphetamine. Excreted in urine. **Half-life:** Less than 1 hr.

USES

Treatment of ADHD.

PRECAUTIONS

Contraindications: Advanced arteriosclerosis, symptomatic cardiovascular disease, moderate to severe hypertension, hyperthyroidism, known hypersensitivity to sympathomimetic amines, glaucoma, agitated mental states, history of drug abuse, use of MAOIs within 14 days (hypertensive crisis may result). **Cautions:** History of preexisting psychosis, bipolar disorder, aggression, tics, Tourette's syndrome.

⌛ LIFESPAN CONSIDERATIONS

Pregnancy/Lactation: Has potential for fetal harm. Unknown if distributed in breast milk. **Pregnancy Category C. Children:** Safety and efficacy not established in those younger than 6 yrs. **Elderly:** No age-related precautions noted.

INTERACTIONS

DRUG: May increase effects of **adrenergic blockers. MAOIs** may prolong/intensify effects. May decrease sedative effect of **antihistamines.** May decrease hypotensive effects of **antihypertensives.** Effects may be decreased by **chlorpromazine, haloperidol, lithium, urinary acidifying agents (ammonium chloride, sodium acid phosphate).** May increase absorption of **phenobarbital, phenytoin. Tricyclic antidepressants** may increase cardiovascular effects. **HERBAL:** None significant. **FOOD:** None known. **LAB VALUES:** May increase plasma corticosteroid.

AVAILABILITY (Rx)

Capsules: 20 mg, 30 mg, 40 mg, 50 mg, 60 mg, 70 mg.

ADMINISTRATION/HANDLING

PO

- May be given without regard to food.
- Swallow capsule whole; do not chew.
- Capsules may be opened and dissolved in water and taken immediately.

INDICATIONS/ROUTES/DOSAGE

ADHD

PO: ADULTS, CHILDREN 6 YRS AND OLDER: Initially, 30 mg once daily in the morning. May increase dosage in increments of 10 or 20 mg/day at weekly intervals. **Maximum:** 70 mg/day.

SIDE EFFECTS

Frequent (39%): Decreased appetite. **Occasional (19%–9%):** Insomnia, upper abdominal pain, headache, irritability, vomiting, weight decrease. **Rare (6%–2%):** Nausea, dry mouth, dizziness, rash, affect change, fatigue, tic.

L

ADVERSE EFFECTS/ TOXIC REACTIONS

Abrupt withdrawal following prolonged administration of high dosage may produce extreme fatigue (may last for wks). Prolonged administration to children with ADHD may produce a suppression of weight and/or height patterns. May produce cardiac irregularities, psychotic syndrome.

NURSING CONSIDERATIONS

BASELINE ASSESSMENT

Assess attention span, impulse control, interaction with others.

INTERVENTION/EVALUATION

Monitor for CNS stimulation, increase in B/P, weight loss, pulse, sleep pattern, appetite. Observe for signs of hostility, aggression, depression.

PATIENT/FAMILY TEACHING

• Avoid tasks that require alertness, motor skills until response to drug is established. • Take early in day. • May mask extreme fatigue. • Report pronounced dizziness, decreased appetite, dry mouth, weight loss, new or worsened psychiatric problems, palpitations, dyspnea.

L

lisinopril

ly-**sin**-oh-pril
(Apo-Lisinopril ✤, Novo-Lisinopril ✤, Prinivil, Zestril)

BLACK BOX ALERT May cause fetal injury, mortality if used during second or third trimester of pregnancy.

Do not confuse lisinopril with fosinopril or Risperdal, Prinivil with Plendil, Pravachol, Prevacid, Prilosec, Proventil, or Restoril, or Zestril with Desyrel, Restoril, Vistaril, Zetia, or Zostrix. Do not confuse lisinopril's combination form Zestoretic with Prilosec.

FIXED-COMBINATION(S)

Prinzide/Zestoretic: lisinopril/hydrochlorothiazide (a diuretic): 10 mg/12.5 mg, 20 mg/12.5 mg, 20 mg/25 mg.

◆CLASSIFICATION

PHARMACOTHERAPEUTIC: ACE inhibitor. **CLINICAL:** Antihypertensive (see p. 9C).

ACTION

Suppresses renin-angiotensin-aldosterone system (prevents conversion of angiotensin I to angiotensin II, a potent vasoconstrictor; may inhibit angiotensin II at local vascular, renal sites). Decreases plasma angiotensin II, increases plasma renin activity, decreases aldosterone secretion. **Therapeutic Effect:** Reduces peripheral arterial resistance, B/P (afterload), pulmonary capillary wedge pressure (preload), pulmonary vascular resistance. In those with heart failure, decreases heart size, increases cardiac output, exercise tolerance time.

PHARMACOKINETICS

Route	Onset	Peak	Duration
PO	1 hr	6 hrs	24 hrs

Incompletely absorbed from GI tract. Protein binding: 25%. Primarily excreted unchanged in urine. Removed by hemodialysis. **Half-life:** 12 hrs (increased in renal impairment).

USES

Treatment of hypertension. Used alone or in combination with other antihypertensives. Adjunctive therapy in management of heart failure. Treatment of acute MI within 24 hrs in hemodynamically stable pts to improve survival. Treatment of left ventricular dysfunction following MI. **OFF-LABEL:** Treatment of hypertension, renal crises with scleroderma.

PRECAUTIONS

Contraindications: History of angioedema from treatment with ACE inhibitors. **Cau-**

tions: Renal impairment, those with sodium depletion or on diuretic therapy, dialysis, hypovolemia, coronary/cerebrovascular insufficiency, severe CHF.

LIFESPAN CONSIDERATIONS

Pregnancy/Lactation: Crosses placenta. Unknown if distributed in breast milk. **Pregnancy Category C (D if used in second or third trimester). Children:** Safety and efficacy not established. **Elderly:** May be more sensitive to hypotensive effects.

INTERACTIONS

DRUG: **Alcohol, diuretics, hypotensive agents** may increase effects. May increase concentration, risk of toxicity of **lithium. NSAIDs** may decrease effects. **Potassium-sparing diuretics, potassium supplements** may cause hyperkalemia. **HERBAL: Ephedra, ginseng, yohimbe** may worsen hypertension. **Garlic** may increase antihypertensive effect. **FOOD:** None known. **LAB VALUES:** May increase BUN, serum alkaline phosphatase, bilirubin, creatinine, potassium, AST, ALT. May decrease serum sodium. May cause positive ANA titer.

AVAILABILITY (Rx)

Tablets (Prinivil, Zestril): 2.5 mg, 5 mg, 10 mg, 20 mg, 30 mg, 40 mg.

ADMINISTRATION/HANDLING

PO

- Give without regard to food.
- Tablets may be crushed.

INDICATIONS/ROUTES/DOSAGE

Hypertension (Used Alone)

PO: ADULTS: Initially, 10 mg/day. May increase by 5–10 mg/day at 1- to 2-wk intervals. **Maximum:** 40 mg/day. **ELDERLY:** Initially, 2.5–5 mg/day. May increase by 2.5–5 mg/day at 1- to 2-wk intervals. **Maximum:** 40 mg/day. **CHILDREN 6 YRS OR OLDER:** Initially, 0.07 mg/kg once daily (up to 5 mg). Titrate at 1- to 2-wk intervals. **Maximum:** 40 mg/day.

Hypertension (in Combination with Other Antihypertensives)

ALERT Discontinue diuretics 48–72 hrs prior to initiating lisinopril therapy.

PO: ADULTS: Initially, 2.5–5 mg/day titrated to pt's needs. Range: 10–40 mg/day.

Adjunctive Therapy for Management of Heart Failure

PO: ADULTS, ELDERLY: Initially, 2.5–5 mg/day. May increase by no more than 10 mg/day at intervals of at least 2 wks. Maintenance: 5–40 mg/day.

Improve Survival in Pts after MI

PO: ADULTS, ELDERLY: Initially, 5 mg, then 5 mg after 24 hrs, 10 mg after 48 hrs, then 10 mg/day for 6 wks. For pts with low systolic B/P, give 2.5 mg/day for 5 days, then 2.5–5 mg/day. Pt should continue with thrombolytics, aspirin, beta-blockers.

Dosage in Renal Impairment

Titrate to pt's needs after giving the following initial dose:

Creatinine Clearance	Dosage
10–30 ml/min	5 mg
Dialysis	2.5 mg

SIDE EFFECTS

Frequent (12%–5%): Headache, dizziness, postural hypotension. **Occasional (4%–2%):** Chest discomfort, fatigue, rash, abdominal pain, nausea, diarrhea, upper respiratory infection. **Rare (1% or less):** Palpitations, tachycardia, peripheral edema, insomnia, paresthesia, confusion, constipation, dry mouth, muscle cramps.

ADVERSE EFFECTS/ TOXIC REACTIONS

Excessive hypotension ("first-dose syncope") may occur in pts with CHF, severe salt/volume depletion. Angioedema (swelling of face and lips), hyperkalemia occur rarely. Agranulocytosis, neutropenia may be noted in pts with collagen vascular disease (scleroderma, systemic lupus erythematosus). Nephrotic syndrome may be noted in pts with history of renal disease.

NURSING CONSIDERATIONS

BASELINE ASSESSMENT

Obtain B/P, apical pulse immediately before each dose, in addition to regular monitoring (be alert to fluctuations). If excessive reduction in B/P occurs, place pt in supine position, feet slightly elevated. In pts with renal impairment, autoimmune disease, taking drugs that affect leukocytes or immune response, CBC and differential count should be performed before beginning therapy and q2wks for 3 mos, then periodically thereafter.

INTERVENTION/EVALUATION

Assess for edema. Auscultate lungs for rales. Monitor I&O; weigh daily. Monitor daily pattern of bowel activity and stool consistency. Assist with ambulation if dizziness occurs. Monitor B/P, renal function tests, WBC, serum potassium.

PATIENT/ FAMILY TEACHING

• To reduce hypotensive effect, rise slowly from lying to sitting position, permit legs to dangle from bed momentarily before standing. • Limit alcohol intake. • Inform physician if vomiting, diarrhea, diaphoresis, swelling of face/lips/tongue, difficulty in breathing, persistent cough occur. • Limit salt intake.

lithium carbonate

lith-ee-um
(Apo-Lithium ✱, Duralith ✱, Lithobid)

BLACK BOX ALERT Lithium toxicity is closely related to serum lithium levels and can occur at therapeutic doses. Routine determination of serum lithium levels is essential during therapy.

lithium citrate

(Cibalith-S)

Do not confuse Lithobid with Levbid or Lithostat.

◆CLASSIFICATION

PHARMACOTHERAPEUTIC: Psychotherapeutic. **CLINICAL:** Antimanic, antidepressant, vascular headache prophylactic.

ACTION

Affects storage, release, reuptake of neurotransmitters. Antimanic effect may result from increased norepinephrine reuptake, serotonin receptor sensitivity. **Therapeutic Effect:** Produces antimanic, antidepressant effects.

PHARMACOKINETICS

Rapidly, completely absorbed from GI tract. Protein binding: None. Primarily excreted unchanged in urine. Removed by hemodialysis. **Half-life:** 18–24 hrs (increased in elderly).

USES

Prophylaxis, treatment of acute mania, manic phase of bipolar disorder (manic depressive illness). **OFF-LABEL:** Prevention of vascular headache; treatment of depression, neutropenia, aggression, posttraumatic stress disorder, conduct disorder in children.

PRECAUTIONS

Contraindications: Debilitated pts, severe cardiovascular disease, severe dehydration, severe renal disease, severe sodium depletion. **Cautions:** Cardiovascular disease, thyroid disease, elderly.

⌛ LIFESPAN CONSIDERATIONS

Pregnancy/Lactation: Freely crosses placenta. Distributed in breast milk. **Pregnancy Category D. Children:** May increase bone formation or density (alter parathyroid hormone concentrations). **Elderly:** More susceptible to develop lithium-induced goiter or clinical hypothyroidism, CNS toxicity. Increased thirst, urination noted more frequently; lower dosage recommended.

INTERACTIONS

DRUG: May increase effects of **antithyroid medications, iodinated glycerol, potassium iodide. Diuretics, NSAIDs** may increase lithium concentration, risk of toxicity. **Haloperidol** may increase extrapyramidal symptoms (EPS), risk of neurologic toxicity. **Molindone** may increase risk of neurotoxicity. May decrease absorption of **phenothiazines. Phenothiazines** may increase intracellular concentration, increase renal excretion of lithium. **Phenothiazines** may increase delirium, EPS when given concurrently with lithium. Antiemetic effect of some **phenothiazines** may mask early signs of lithium toxicity. **HERBAL:** None significant. **FOOD:** None known. **LAB VALUES:** May increase serum glucose, immunoreactive parathyroid hormone, calcium. **Therapeutic serum level:** 0.6–1.2 mEq/L; **toxic serum level:** greater than 1.5 mEq/L.

AVAILABILITY (Rx)

Capsules: 150 mg, 300 mg, 600 mg. **Oral Solution:** 300 mg/5 ml. **Syrup:** 300 mg/5 ml. **Tablets:** 300 mg.

Tablets (Controlled-Release): 450 mg.
Tablets (Slow-Release): 300 mg.

ADMINISTRATION/HANDLING

PO

• Preferable to administer with meals, milk. • Do not crush, chew, break controlled- or slow-release tablets.

INDICATIONS/ROUTES/DOSAGE

◀ALERT▶ During acute phase, a therapeutic serum lithium concentration of 1–1.4 mEq/L is required. For long-term control, desired level is 0.5–1.3 mEq/L. Monitor serum drug concentration, clinical response to determine proper dosage.

Usual Dosage

PO: ADULTS: 300 mg 3–4 times a day or 450–900 mg slow-release form twice a day. **Maximum:** 2.4 g/day. **ELDERLY:** 900–1,200 mg/day. Maintenance: 300 mg twice a day. May increase by 300 mg/day q1wk. **CHILDREN 12 YRS AND OLDER:** 600–1,800 mg/day in 3–4 divided doses (2 doses/day for slow-release). **CHILDREN 6–11 YRS:** 15–60 mg/kg/day in 3–4 divided doses not to exceed usual adult dose.

Dosage in Renal Impairment

Creatinine Clearance	Dosage
10–50 ml/min	50%–75% normal dose
Less than 10 ml/min	25%–50% normal dose

SIDE EFFECTS

◀ALERT▶ Side effects are dose related and seldom occur at lithium serum levels less than 1.5 mEq/L. **Occasional:** Fine hand tremor, polydipsia, polyuria, mild nausea. **Rare:** Weight gain, bradycardia, tachycardia, acne, rash, muscle twitching, peripheral cyanosis, pseudotumor cerebri (eye pain, headache, tinnitus, vision disturbances).

ADVERSE EFFECTS/ TOXIC REACTIONS

Lithium serum concentration of 1.5–2.0 mEq/L may produce vomiting, diarrhea, drowsiness, confusion, incoordination, coarse hand tremor, muscle twitching, T-wave depression on EKG. Lithium serum concentration of 2.0–2.5 mEq/L may result in ataxia, giddiness, tinnitus, blurred vision, clonic movements, severe hypotension. Acute toxicity may be characterized by seizures, oliguria, circulatory failure, coma, death.

NURSING CONSIDERATIONS

BASELINE ASSESSMENT

Assess mental status (e.g., mood, behavior.) Serum lithium levels should be tested q3–4days during initial phase of therapy, q1–2mos thereafter, and weekly if there is no improvement of disorder or adverse effects occur.

INTERVENTION/EVALUATION

Serum lithium testing should be performed as close as possible to 12th hr following

L

last dose. Clinical assessment of therapeutic effect, tolerance to drug effect is also necessary for correct dosing-level management. Assess behavior, appearance, emotional status, response to environment, speech pattern, thought content. Monitor serum lithium concentrations, CBC with differential, urinalysis, creatinine clearance. Monitor renal, hepatic, thyroid, cardiovascular function; serum electrolytes. Assess for increased urinary output, persistent thirst. Report polyuria, prolonged vomiting, diarrhea, fever to physician (may need to temporarily reduce or discontinue dosage). Monitor for signs of lithium toxicity. Assess for therapeutic response (interest in surroundings, improvement in self-care, increased ability to concentrate, relaxed facial expression). Monitor lithium levels q3–4days at initiation of therapy (then q1–2mos). Obtain lithium levels 8–12 hrs postdose. **Therapeutic serum level:** 0.6–1.2 mEq/L; **toxic serum level:** greater than 1.5 mEq/L.

PATIENT/ FAMILY TEACHING

• Limit alcohol, caffeine intake. • Avoid tasks requiring coordination until CNS effects of drug are known. • May cause dry mouth. • Maintain steady salt, fluid intake (avoid dehydration). • Inform physician if vomiting, diarrhea, muscle weakness, tremors, drowsiness, ataxia occur. • Serum level monitoring is necessary to determine proper dose.

Lomotil, *see diphenoxylate with atropine*

lomustine HIGH ALERT

low-**muss**-steen
(CeeNU)

BLACK BOX ALERT Must be administered by certified chemotherapy personnel. Severe myelosuppressant (notably thrombocytopenia, leukopenia). May lead to bleeding, overwhelming infection.

Do not confuse lomustine with bendamustine or carmustine.

CLASSIFICATION

PHARMACOTHERAPEUTIC: Alkylating agent (nitrosourea). **CLINICAL:** Antineoplastic (see p. 85C).

ACTION

Inhibits DNA, RNA protein synthesis by cross-linking with DNA and RNA strands, preventing cell division. Cell cycle–phase nonspecific. **Therapeutic Effect:** Interferes with DNA, RNA function.

PHARMACOKINETICS

Rapidly, completely absorbed following PO administration. Highly lipid soluble. Metabolized in liver. Excreted in urine. **Half-life:** 16–72 hrs.

USES

Treatment of primary/metastatic brain tumors, disseminated Hodgkin's lymphoma. **OFF-LABEL:** Breast, colorectal, GI, non–small-cell lung, renal carcinoma; malignant melanoma, multiple myeloma, non-Hodgkin's lymphoma.

PRECAUTIONS

Contraindications: Pregnancy. **Cautions:** Depressed platelet, leukocyte, erythrocyte counts.

LIFESPAN CONSIDERATIONS

Pregnancy/Lactation: May be harmful to fetus. Distributed in breast milk. Breast-feeding not recommended. **Pregnancy Category D. Children:** Safety and efficacy not established. **Elderly:** Age-related renal impairment may require dosage adjustment.

INTERACTIONS

DRUG: Bone marrow depressants may increase myelosuppression. **Live virus vaccines** may potentiate virus replication, increase vaccine side effects, decrease pt's antibody response to vaccine. **HERBAL:** None significant. **FOOD:** None known. LAB VALUES: May increase serum hepatic function test results.

AVAILABILITY (Rx)

Capsules: 10 mg, 40 mg, 100 mg.

ADMINISTRATION/HANDLING

PO

• Take with fluids on an empty stomach (decreases nausea, vomiting). • Do not break capsules. • No food or drink for 2 hrs after administration.

INDICATIONS/ROUTES/DOSAGE

◀ALERT▶ Lomustine dosage is individualized based on clinical response and tolerance of adverse effects. When used in combination therapy, consult specific protocols for optimum dosage, sequence of drug administration.

Usual Dosage

PO: ADULTS, ELDERLY: 100–130 mg/m^2 as single dose. Repeat dose at intervals of at least 6 wks but not until circulating blood elements have returned to acceptable levels. Adjust dose based on hematologic response to previous dose. **CHILDREN:** 75–150 mg/m^2 as a single dose every 6 wks.

Dosage in Renal Impairment

Creatinine Clearance	Dosage
10–50 ml/min	75% of normal dose
Less than 10 ml/min	25%–50% of normal dose

SIDE EFFECTS

Frequent: Nausea, vomiting (occurs 45 min–6 hrs after dose, lasts 12–24 hrs); anorexia (often follows for 2–3 days). Occasional: Neurotoxicity (confusion, slurred speech), stomatitis, darkening of skin, diarrhea, rash, pruritus, alopecia.

ADVERSE EFFECTS/ TOXIC REACTIONS

Myelosuppression may result in hematologic toxicity (principally leukopenia, mild anemia, thrombocytopenia). Leukopenia occurs about 6 wks after a dose, thrombocytopenia about 4 wks after a dose; both persist for 1–2 wks. Refractory anemia, thrombocytopenia occur commonly if lomustine therapy continues for more than 1 yr. Hepatotoxicity occurs infrequently. Large cumulative doses of lomustine may result in renal damage.

NURSING CONSIDERATIONS

BASELINE ASSESSMENT

Manufacturer recommends weekly blood counts; experts recommend first blood count obtained 2–3 wks following initial therapy, subsequent blood counts indicated by prior toxicity. Antiemetics can reduce duration, frequency of nausea, vomiting.

INTERVENTION/EVALUATION

Monitor CBC with differential; platelet count; hepatic, renal, pulmonary function tests. Monitor for stomatitis. Monitor for hematologic toxicity (fever, sore throat, signs of local infection, unusual bruising/bleeding from any site), symptoms of anemia (excessive fatigue, weakness).

PATIENT/FAMILY TEACHING

• Nausea, vomiting generally abates in less than 1 day. • Fasting before therapy can reduce frequency/duration of GI effects. • Maintain fastidious oral hygiene. • Do not have immunizations without physician's approval (drug lowers resistance). • Avoid crowds, those with known illness. • Promptly report fever, sore throat, signs of local infection, unusual bruising/bleeding from any site, swelling of legs or feet, jaundice (yellowing of eyes, skin).

L

loperamide

loe-**per**-a-mide
(Apo-Loperamide ✤, Diamode, Diarr-Eze ✤, Imodium, Imodium A-D, Loperacap ✤, Novo-Loperamide ✤)

Do not confuse Imodium with Indocin or Ionamin, or loperamide with furosemide.

FIXED-COMBINATION(S)

Imodium Advanced: loperamide/simethicone (an antiflatulant): 2 mg/125 mg.

CLASSIFICATION

CLINICAL: Antidiarrheal (see p. 45C).

ACTION

Directly affects intestinal wall muscles. **Therapeutic Effect:** Slows intestinal motility, prolongs transit time of intestinal contents by reducing fecal volume, diminishing loss of fluid, electrolytes, increasing viscosity, bulk of stool.

L

PHARMACOKINETICS

Poorly absorbed from GI tract. Protein binding: 97%. Metabolized in liver. Eliminated in feces; excreted in urine. Not removed by hemodialysis. **Half-life:** 7–14 hrs.

USES

Controls, provides symptomatic relief of acute nonspecific diarrhea, chronic diarrhea associated with inflammatory bowel disease, traveler's diarrhea. **OFF-LABEL:** Cancer treatment-induced diarrhea, chronic diarrhea caused by bowel resection.

PRECAUTIONS

Contraindications: Acute ulcerative colitis (may produce toxic megacolon), diarrhea associated with pseudomembranous enterocolitis due to broad-spectrum antibiotics or to organisms that invade intestinal mucosa (e.g., *Escherichia coli,* shigella, salmonella), pts who must avoid constipation. **Cautions:** Those with fluid or electrolyte depletion, hepatic impairment.

LIFESPAN CONSIDERATIONS

Pregnancy/Lactation: Unknown if drug crosses placenta or is distributed in breast milk. **Pregnancy Category C. Children:** Not recommended for those younger than 6 yrs (infants younger than 3 mos more susceptible to CNS effects). **Elderly:** May mask dehydration, electrolyte depletion.

INTERACTIONS

DRUG: **Opioid (narcotic) analgesics** may increase risk of constipation. **HERBAL:** None significant. **FOOD:** None known. **LAB VALUES:** None significant.

AVAILABILITY (Rx)

Caplets: 2 mg. **Capsules:** 2 mg. **Liquid:** 1 mg/5 ml, 1 mg/7.5 ml. **Tablets:** 2 mg.

ADMINISTRATION/HANDLING

Liquid

• When administering to children, use accompanying plastic dropper to measure the liquid.

INDICATIONS/ROUTES/DOSAGE

Acute Diarrhea

PO (CAPSULES): ADULTS, ELDERLY: Initially, 4 mg, then 2 mg after each unformed stool. **Maximum:** 16 mg/day. **CHILDREN 9–12 YRS, WEIGHING MORE THAN 30 KG:** Initially, 2 mg 3 times a day for 24 hrs. **CHILDREN 6–8 YRS, WEIGHING 20–30 KG:** Initially, 2 mg twice a day for 24 hrs. **CHILDREN 2–5 YRS, WEIGHING 13–20 KG:** Initially, 1 mg 3 times a day for 24 hrs. Maintenance: 1 mg/10 kg only after loose stool but not exceeding initial dose.

Chronic Diarrhea

PO: ADULTS, ELDERLY: Initially, 4 mg, then 2 mg after each unformed stool until diarrhea is controlled. Average maintenance dose: 4–8 mg/day. **Maximum:** 16 mg/day. **CHILDREN:** 0.08–0.24 mg/kg/day in 2–3 divided doses. **Maximum:** 2 mg/dose.

Traveler's Diarrhea

PO: ADULTS, ELDERLY: Initially, 4 mg, then 2 mg after each loose bowel movement (LBM). **Maximum:** 8 mg/day for 2 days.

CHILDREN 9–11 YRS: Initially, 2 mg, then 1 mg after each LBM. **Maximum:** 6 mg/day for 2 days. **CHILDREN 6–8 YRS:** Initially, 2 mg, then 1 mg after each LBM. **Maximum:** 4 mg/day for 2 days.

SIDE EFFECTS

Rare: Dry mouth, drowsiness, abdominal discomfort, allergic reaction (rash, pruritus).

ADVERSE EFFECTS/ TOXIC REACTIONS

Toxicity results in constipation, GI irritation (nausea, vomiting), CNS depression. Activated charcoal is used to treat loperamide toxicity.

NURSING CONSIDERATIONS

BASELINE ASSESSMENT

Do not administer in presence of bloody diarrhea, temperature greater than 101°F.

INTERVENTION/EVALUATION

Encourage adequate fluid intake. Assess bowel sounds for peristalsis. Monitor daily pattern of bowel activity, stool consistency. Withhold drug, notify physician promptly in event of abdominal pain, distention, fever.

PATIENT/FAMILY TEACHING

• Do not exceed prescribed dose. • May cause dry mouth. • Avoid alcohol. • Avoid tasks that require alertness, motor skills until response to drug is established. • Notify physician if diarrhea does not stop within 3 days; abdominal distention, pain occurs; fever develops.

lopinavir/ritonavir

low-**pin**-ah-veer/rit-**oh**-na-veer
(Kaletra)
Do not confuse Kaletra with Keppra.

◆ CLASSIFICATION

PHARMACOTHERAPEUTIC: Protease inhibitor combination. **CLINICAL:** Antiretroviral (see pp. 69C, 117C).

ACTION

Lopinavir inhibits activity of protease, an enzyme, late in HIV replication process; ritonavir increases plasma levels of lopinavir. **Therapeutic Effect:** Formation of immature, noninfectious viral particles.

PHARMACOKINETICS

Readily absorbed after PO administration (absorption increased when taken with food). Protein binding: 98%–99%. Metabolized in liver. Eliminated primarily in feces. Not removed by hemodialysis. **Half-life:** 5–6 hrs.

USES

In combination with other antiretroviral agents for treatment of HIV infection.

PRECAUTIONS

Contraindications: Concomitant use of ergot derivatives (causes vasospasm, peripheral ischemia of extremities), flecainide, midazolam, pimozide, propafenone (increased risk of serious cardiac arrhythmias), triazolam (increased sedation, respiratory depression); hypersensitivity to lopinavir, ritonavir. **Cautions:** Hepatic impairment, hepatitis B or C. High-dose itraconazole, ketoconazole not recommended. Metronidazole may cause disulfiram-type reaction with oral solution (contains alcohol).

⌛ LIFESPAN CONSIDERATIONS

Pregnancy/Lactation: Unknown if distributed in breast milk. Breast-feeding by HIV-infected mothers not recommended. **Pregnancy Category C. Children:** Safety and efficacy not established in those younger than 6 mos. **Elderly:** Age-related renal/hepatic/cardiac impairment requires caution.

INTERACTIONS

DRUG: May increase concentration/toxicity of **amiodarone, atorvastatin, bepridil, clarithromycin, cyclosporine, felodipine, fluticasone, itraconazole, ketoconazole, lidocaine, lovastatin, midazolam, nelfinavir, nicardipine, nifedipine, sildenafil, simvastatin, sirolimus, tacrolimus, trazodone, triazolam, warfarin.** May decrease concentration/effect of **atovaquone, oral contraceptives. Carbamazepine, phenobarbital, phenytoin, rifampin** may decrease concentration/effect. May cause acute ergot toxicity with **dihydroergotamine, ergotamine.** May cause disulfiram-like reaction with **metronidazole.** HERBAL: **St. John's wort** may decrease concentration/effect. FOOD: None known. LAB VALUES: May increase serum glucose, GGT, amylase, bilirubin, total cholesterol, triglycerides, uric acid, AST, ALT. May decrease platelets, serum sodium.

L

AVAILABILITY (Rx)

Oral Solution: 80 mg/ml lopinavir/20 mg/ml ritonavir.

Tablets: 100 mg lopinavir/25 mg ritonavir, 200 mg lopinavir/50 mg ritonavir.

ADMINISTRATION/HANDLING

PO

• Swallow tablets whole; do not chew, break, crush. • Does not require refrigeration. • Give tablets without regard to food. • Solution must be given with food.

INDICATIONS/ROUTES/DOSAGE

HIV Infection

Doses based on lopinavir component.

PO: ADULTS: 800 mg once daily or 400 mg twice daily. CHILDREN 6 MOS–18 YRS, WEIGHING GREATER THAN 40 KG: 400 mg twice daily. WEIGHING 15–40 KG: 10 mg/kg twice a day. WEIGHING LESS THAN 15 KG: 12 mg/kg twice daily. CHILDREN 14 DAYS–6 MOS: 16 mg/kg twice daily.

Dosage Adjustment for Combination Therapy

EFAVIRENZ, FOSAMPRENAVIR, NELFINAVIR, NEVIRAPINE: ADULTS, CHILDREN 6 MOS–18 YRS, WEIGHING GREATER THAN 45 KG: 500 mg (533-mg solution) twice daily. WEIGHING 15–45 KG: 11 mg/kg twice daily. WEIGHING LESS THAN 15 KG: 13 mg/kg twice daily.

MARAVIROC, SAQUINAVIR: ADULTS: 400 mg twice daily.

SIDE EFFECTS

Frequent (14%): Mild to moderate diarrhea. Occasional (6%–2%): Nausea, asthenia (loss of strength, energy), abdominal pain, headache, vomiting. Rare (less than 2%): Insomnia, rash.

ADVERSE EFFECTS/ TOXIC REACTIONS

Anemia, leukopenia, lymphadenopathy, deep vein thrombosis (DVT), Cushing's syndrome, pancreatitis, hemorrhagic colitis occur rarely.

NURSING CONSIDERATIONS

BASELINE ASSESSMENT

Obtain baseline CBC, renal/hepatic function tests, weight.

INTERVENTION/EVALUATION

Monitor daily pattern of bowel activity, stool consistency. Assess for opportunistic infections: onset of fever, oral mucosa changes, cough, other respiratory symptoms. Check weight at least 2 times a wk. Assess for nausea, vomiting. Observe for signs/symptoms of pancreatitis (nausea, vomiting, abdominal pain). Monitor electrolytes, serum glucose, cholesterol, hepatic function, CBC with differential, platelets, CD4 cell count, viral load.

PATIENT/ FAMILY TEACHING

• Explain correct administration of medication. • Eat small, frequent meals to offset nausea, vomiting. • Lopinavir/ritonavir is not a cure for HIV infection, nor does it reduce risk of transmission to others. • Pt must continue practices to prevent HIV transmission. • Illnesses, including opportunistic infections, may still occur.

Lopressor, *see metoprolol*

loratadine

low-**rat**-ah-deen
(Alavert, Claritin, Dimetapp ND, Loradamed, Tavist ND)

FIXED-COMBINATION(S)

Alavert Allergy and Sinus, Claritin-D: loratadine/pseudoephedrine (a sympathomimetic): 5 mg/120 mg, 10 mg/240 mg.

◆CLASSIFICATION

PHARMACOTHERAPEUTIC: H_1 antagonist. **CLINICAL:** Antihistamine (see p. 55C).

ACTION

Competes with histamine for H_1 receptor sites on effector cells. **Therapeutic Effect:** Prevents allergic responses mediated by histamine (e.g., rhinitis, urticaria, pruritus).

PHARMACOKINETICS

Route	Onset	Peak	Duration
PO	1–3 hrs	8–12 hrs	Longer than 24 hrs

Rapidly, almost completely absorbed from GI tract. Protein binding: 97%; metabolite, 73%–77%. Distributed mainly to liver, lungs, GI tract, bile. Metabolized in liver to active metabolite; undergoes extensive first-pass metabolism. Eliminated in urine and feces. Not removed by hemodialysis. **Half-life:** 8.4 hrs; metabolite, 28 hrs (increased in elderly, hepatic impairment).

USES

Relief of nasal, non-nasal symptoms of seasonal allergic rhinitis (hayfever). Treatment of idiopathic chronic urticaria (hives). **OFF-LABEL:** Adjunct treatment of bronchial asthma.

PRECAUTIONS

Contraindications: Hypersensitivity to loratadine or its ingredients. **Cautions:** Hepatic impairment, breast-feeding women.

LIFESPAN CONSIDERATIONS

Pregnancy/Lactation: Distributed in breast milk. **Pregnancy Category B. Children:** Safety and efficacy not established in those younger than 2 yrs. **Elderly:** More sensitive to anticholinergic effects (e.g., dry mouth, nose, throat).

INTERACTIONS

DRUG: **Clarithromycin, erythromycin, fluconazole, ketoconazole** may increase concentration. **HERBAL:** None significant. **FOOD:** **All foods** delay absorption. **LAB VALUES:** May suppress wheal, flare reactions to antigen skin testing unless drug is discontinued 4 days before testing.

AVAILABILITY (Rx)

Solution, Oral: 5 mg/5 ml. **Syrup:** 10 mg/10 ml. **Tablets (Alavert, Claritin, Loradamed, Tavist ND):** 10 mg. **Tablets, Chewable (Claritin):** 5 mg. **Tablets (Rapidly-Disintegrating [Alavert, Dimetapp ND]):** 10 mg.

ADMINISTRATION/HANDLING

PO

• Preferably give on empty stomach (food delays absorption).

Rapidly-Disintegrating Tablets

• Place under tongue. • Disintegration occurs within seconds, after which tablet contents may be swallowed with or without water.

L

INDICATIONS/ROUTES/DOSAGE

Allergic Rhinitis, Urticaria

PO: ADULTS, ELDERLY, CHILDREN 6 YRS AND OLDER: 10 mg once a day. **CHILDREN 2–5 YRS:** 5 mg once a day.

Dosage in Renal (Creatinine Clearance Less Than 30 ml/min)/Hepatic Impairment

PO: ADULTS, ELDERLY, CHILDREN 6 YRS AND OLDER: 10 mg every other day. **CHILDREN 2–5 YRS:** 5 mg every other day.

SIDE EFFECTS

Frequent (12%–8%): Headache, fatigue, drowsiness. **Occasional (3%):** Dry mouth, nose, throat. **Rare:** Photosensitivity.

ADVERSE EFFECTS/ TOXIC REACTIONS

None significant.

L

NURSING CONSIDERATIONS

BASELINE ASSESSMENT

Assess lung sounds for wheezing, skin for urticaria, other allergy symptoms.

INTERVENTION/EVALUATION

For upper respiratory allergies, increase fluids to decrease viscosity of secretions, offset thirst, replenish loss of fluids from increased diaphoresis. Monitor symptoms for therapeutic response.

PATIENT/FAMILY TEACHING

• Drink plenty of water (may cause dry mouth). • Avoid alcohol. • Avoid tasks that require alertness, motor skills until response to drug is established (may cause drowsiness). • May cause photosensitivity reactions (avoid direct exposure to sunlight).

lorazepam

low-**raz**-ah-pam
(Apo-Lorazepam ✱, Ativan, Lorazepam Intensol, Novo-Lorazem ✱)

Do not confuse Ativan with Ambien or Atarax, or lorazepam with alprazolam, diazepam, Lovaza, temazepam, or Zolpidem.

◆CLASSIFICATION

PHARMACOTHERAPEUTIC: Benzodiazepine **(Schedule IV). CLINICAL:** Antianxiety, sedative-hypnotic, antiemetic, skeletal muscle relaxant, amnesiac, anticonvulsant, antitremor (see p. 14C).

ACTION

Enhances action of inhibitory neurotransmitter gamma-aminobutyric acid (GABA) in CNS, affecting memory, motor, sensory, cognitive function. **Therapeutic Effect:** Produces anxiolytic, anticonvulsant, sedative, muscle relaxant, antiemetic effects.

PHARMACOKINETICS

Route	Onset	Peak	Duration
PO	30–60 min	N/A	6–8 hrs
IV	5–20 min	N/A	6–8 hrs
IM	20–30 min	N/A	6–8 hrs

Well absorbed after PO, IM administration. Protein binding: 85%. Widely distributed. Metabolized in liver. Primarily excreted in urine. Not removed by hemodialysis. **Half-life:** 10–20 hrs.

USES

PO: Management of anxiety disorders, short-term relief of symptoms of anxiety, anxiety associated with depressive symptoms. Treatment of nausea, vomiting. **IV:** Status epilepticus, preanesthesia for amnesia, antiemetic adjunct. **OFF-LABEL:** Treatment of alcohol withdrawal, panic disorders, skeletal muscle spasms, chemotherapy-induced nausea/vomiting, tension headache, tremors. Adjunctive treatment before endoscopic procedures (diminishes pt recall).

PRECAUTIONS

Contraindications: Narrow-angle glaucoma, preexisting CNS depression, severe hypotension, severe uncontrolled pain.

Cautions: Neonates, renal/hepatic impairment, compromised pulmonary function, concomitant CNS depressant use.

LIFESPAN CONSIDERATIONS

Pregnancy/Lactation: May cross placenta. May be distributed in breast milk. May increase risk of fetal abnormalities if administered during first trimester of pregnancy. Chronic ingestion during pregnancy may produce fetal toxicity, withdrawal symptoms, CNS depression in neonates. **Pregnancy Category D. Children:** Safety and efficacy not established in those younger than 12 yrs. **Elderly:** Use small initial doses with gradual increases to avoid ataxia, excessive sedation.

INTERACTIONS

DRUG: **Alcohol, other CNS depressants** may increase CNS depression. HERBAL: **Gotu kola, kava kava, St. John's wort, valerian** may increase CNS depression. FOOD: None significant. LAB VALUES: None significant. **Therapeutic serum level:** 50–240 ng/ml; **toxic serum level:** unknown.

AVAILABILITY (Rx)

Injection Solution: 2 mg/ml, 4 mg/ml. Oral Solution (Lorazepam Intensol): 2 mg/ml. Tablets: 0.5 mg, 1 mg, 2 mg.

ADMINISTRATION/HANDLING

IV

Reconstitution • Dilute with equal volume of Sterile Water for Injection.

Rate of administration • Give by IV push into tubing of free-flowing IV infusion (0.9% NaCl, D_5W) at a rate not to exceed 2 mg/min.

Storage • Refrigerate parenteral form. • Do not use if discolored or precipitate forms. • Avoid freezing.

IM

• Give deep IM into large muscle mass.

PO

• Give with food. • Tablets may be crushed. • Dilute oral solution in water, juice, soda, or semi-solid food.

IV INCOMPATIBILITIES

Aldesleukin (Proleukin), aztreonam (Azactam), idarubicin (Idamycin), ondansetron (Zofran), sufentanil (Sufenta).

IV COMPATIBILITIES

Bumetanide (Bumex), cefepime (Maxipime), diltiazem (Cardizem), dobutamine (Dobutrex), dopamine (Intropin), heparin, labetalol (Normodyne, Trandate), lipids, milrinone (Primacor), norepinephrine (Levophed), piperacillin and tazobactam (Zosyn), potassium, propofol (Diprivan).

INDICATIONS/ROUTES/DOSAGE

Anxiety

PO: ADULTS: 1–10 mg/day in 2–3 divided doses. Average: 2–6 mg/day. **ELDERLY:** Initially, 0.5–1 mg/day. May increase gradually. Range: 0.5–4 mg.

IV: ADULTS, ELDERLY: 0.02–0.06 mg/kg q2–6h.

IV INFUSION: ADULTS, ELDERLY: 0.01–0.1 mg/kg/h.

PO, IV: CHILDREN: 0.05 mg/kg/dose q4–8h. Range: 0.02–0.1 mg/kg. **Maximum:** 2 mg/dose.

Insomnia Due to Anxiety

PO: ADULTS: 2–4 mg at bedtime. **ELDERLY:** 0.5–1 mg at bedtime.

Antiemetic

IV: ADULTS, ELDERLY: 0.5–2 mg q4–6h as needed. **CHILDREN 2–15 YRS:** 0.05 mg/kg (up to 2 mg) prior to chemotherapy.

PO: ADULTS, ELDERLY: 0.5–2 mg q4–6h as needed.

Preop Sedation

IV: ADULTS, ELDERLY: 0.044 mg/kg 15–20 min before surgery. **Usual maximum total dose:** 2 mg.

IM: ADULTS, ELDERLY: 0.05 mg/kg 2 hrs before procedure. **Maximum total dose:** 4 mg.

Status Epilepticus

IV: ADULTS, ELDERLY: 4 mg over 2–5 min. May repeat in 10–15 min. **Usual maximum:** 8 mg in 12-hr period. **CHILDREN:** 0.05–0.1 mg/kg over 2–5 min. **Maximum:** 4 mg. May repeat in 10–15min. **NEONATES:** 0.05 mg/kg. May repeat in 10–15 min.

SIDE EFFECTS

Frequent: Drowsiness (initially in the morning), ataxia, confusion. **Occasional:** Blurred vision, slurred speech, hypotension, headache. **Rare:** Paradoxical CNS restlessness, excitement in elderly/debilitated.

ADVERSE EFFECTS/ TOXIC REACTIONS

Abrupt or too-rapid withdrawal may result in pronounced restlessness, irritability, insomnia, hand tremor, abdominal cramping, muscle cramps, diaphoresis, vomiting, seizures. Overdose results in drowsiness, confusion, diminished reflexes, coma. **Antidote:** Flumazenil (see Appendix M for dosage).

NURSING CONSIDERATIONS

BASELINE ASSESSMENT

Offer emotional support to anxious pt. Pt must remain recumbent following parenteral administration to reduce hypotensive effect. Assess motor responses (agitation, trembling, tension), autonomic responses (cold or clammy hands, diaphoresis).

INTERVENTION/EVALUATION

Monitor B/P, respiratory rate, heart rate, CBC with differential, hepatic function tests. For those on long-term therapy, hepatic/renal function tests, blood counts should be performed periodically. Assess for paradoxical reaction, particularly during early therapy. Evaluate for therapeutic response: calm facial expression, decreased restlessness, insomnia. **Therapeutic serum level:** 50–240 ng/ml; **toxic serum level:** N/A.

PATIENT/ FAMILY TEACHING

• Drowsiness usually disappears during continued therapy. • Avoid tasks that require alertness, motor skills until response to drug is established. • Smoking reduces drug effectiveness. • Do not abruptly discontinue medication after long-term therapy. • Do not use alcohol, CNS depressants. • Contraception recommended for long-term therapy. • Notify physician at once if pregnancy is suspected.

losartan

lo-**sar** tan

(Cozaar)

BLACK BOX ALERT May cause fetal injury, mortality if used during second or third trimester of pregnancy.

Do not confuse Cozaar with Colace, Coreg, Hyzaar, or Zocor, or losartan with valsartan.

FIXED-COMBINATION(S)

Hyzaar: losartan/hydrochlorothiazide (a diuretic): 50 mg/12.5 mg, 100 mg/12.5 mg, 100 mg/25 mg.

◆CLASSIFICATION

PHARMACOTHERAPEUTIC: Angiotensin II receptor antagonist. **CLINICAL:** Antihypertensive (see p. 10C).

ACTION

Potent vasodilator. Blocks vasoconstrictor, aldosterone-secreting effects of angiotensin II, inhibiting binding of angiotensin II to AT_1 receptors. **Therapeutic Effect:** Causes vasodilation, decreases peripheral resistance, decreases B/P.

PHARMACOKINETICS

Route	Onset	Peak	Duration
PO	N/A	6 hrs	24 hrs

Well absorbed after PO administration. Protein binding: 98%. Undergoes first-pass metabolism in liver to active metabolites. Excreted in urine and via the biliary system. Not removed by hemodialysis. Half-life: 2 hrs; metabolite, 6–9 hrs.

USES

Treatment of hypertension. Used alone or in combination with other antihypertensives. Treatment of diabetic nephropathy, prevention of stroke in pts with hypertension and left ventricular hypertrophy. OFF-LABEL: Slow rate of progression of aortic root dilation in children with Marfan's syndrome.

PRECAUTIONS

Contraindications: None known. Cautions: Renal/hepatic impairment, renal arterial stenosis.

⌛ LIFESPAN CONSIDERATIONS

Pregnancy/Lactation: Has caused fetal/neonatal morbidity, mortality. Potential for adverse effects on breast-fed infant. Breast-feeding not recommended. **Pregnancy Category C (D if used in second or third trimester). Children**: Safety and efficacy not established. **Elderly**: No age-related precautions noted.

INTERACTIONS

DRUG: **NSAIDs** may decrease effect. **Cyclosporine, potassium-sparing diuretics, potassium supplements** may increase serum potassium. **Diuretics, other antihypertensive medications** may produce additive hypotension. HERBAL: **Ephedra, ginseng, yohimbe** may worsen hypertension. **Garlic** may increase antihypertensive effect. FOOD: None known. LAB VALUES: May increase bilirubin, AST, ALT, Hgb, Hct.

AVAILABILITY (Rx)

Tablets: 25 mg, 50 mg, 100 mg.

ADMINISTRATION/HANDLING

PO

- May give without regard to food.

INDICATIONS/ROUTES/DOSAGE

Hypertension

PO: ADULTS, ELDERLY: Initially, 50 mg once a day. **Maximum:** May be given once or twice a day, with total daily doses ranging from 25–100 mg. **CHILDREN 6–16 YRS:** 0.7 mg/kg once daily. **Maximum:** 50 mg/day.

Nephropathy

PO: ADULTS, ELDERLY: Initially, 50 mg/day. May increase to 100 mg/day based on B/P response.

Stroke Prevention

PO: ADULTS, ELDERLY: 50 mg/day. **Maximum:** 100 mg/day.

Hepatic Impairment

PO: ADULTS, ELDERLY: Initially, 25 mg/day. May increase up to 100 mg/day.

SIDE EFFECTS

Frequent (8%): Upper respiratory tract infection. Occasional (4%–2%): Dizziness, diarrhea, cough. Rare (1% or less): Insomnia, dyspepsia, heartburn, back/leg pain, muscle cramps, myalgia, nasal congestion, sinusitis, depression.

ADVERSE EFFECTS/ TOXIC REACTIONS

Overdosage may manifest as hypotension and tachycardia. Bradycardia occurs less often. Institute supportive measures.

NURSING CONSIDERATIONS

BASELINE ASSESSMENT

Obtain B/P, apical pulse immediately before each dose, in addition to regular monitoring (be alert to fluctuations). If excessive reduction in B/P occurs, place pt in supine position, feet slightly elevated. Question for possibility of pregnancy (see Pregnancy/Lactation). Assess medication history (esp. diuretic).

INTERVENTION/EVALUATION

Maintain hydration (offer fluids frequently). Assess for evidence of upper respiratory infection, cough. Assist with ambulation if dizziness occurs. Monitor daily pattern of bowel activity and stool consistency. Monitor B/P, pulse.

PATIENT/FAMILY TEACHING

• Pts should take measures to avoid pregnancy. • Report pregnancy to physician as soon as possible. • Avoid tasks that require alertness, motor skills until response to drug is established (possible dizziness effect). • Report any sign of infection (sore throat, fever), chest pain. • Do not take OTC cold preparations, nasal decongestants. • Do not stop taking medication. • Limit salt intake.

Lotensin, *see benazepril*

Lotensin HCT, *see benazepril and hydrochlorothiazide*

Lotrel, *see amlodipine and benazepril*

lovastatin

lo-va-**sta**-tin
(Altoprev, Apo-Lovastatin ♣, Mevacor, Novo-Lovastatin ♣)
Do not confuse lovastatin with Leustatin or Lotensin, or Mevacor with Mivacron.

FIXED-COMBINATION(S)

Advicor: lovastatin/niacin: 20 mg/500 mg, 20 mg/750 mg, 20 mg/1,000 mg.

◆CLASSIFICATION

PHARMACOTHERAPEUTIC: HMG-CoA reductase inhibitor. **CLINICAL:** Antihyperlipidemic (see p. 58C).

ACTION

Inhibits HMG-CoA reductase, the enzyme that catalyzes the early step in cholesterol synthesis. **Therapeutic Effect:** Decreases LDL, VLDL, triglycerides; increases HDL.

PHARMACOKINETICS

Route	Onset	Peak	Duration
PO (LDL, cholesterol reduction)	3 days	N/A	N/A

Incompletely absorbed from GI tract (increased on empty stomach). Protein binding: 95%. Hydrolyzed in liver to active metabolite. Primarily eliminated in feces. Not removed by hemodialysis. **Half-life:** 1.1–1.7 hrs.

USES

Decreases elevated serum total and LDL cholesterol in primary hypercholesterolemia; primary prevention of coronary artery disease. Slows progression of coronary atherosclerosis in pts with coronary heart disease. Adjunct to diet in adolescent pts (10–17 yrs) with heterozygous familial hypercholesterolemia.

PRECAUTIONS

Contraindications: Active hepatic disease, pregnancy, unexplained elevated hepatic function tests. **Cautions:** History of heavy/chronic alcohol use; renal impairment; concomitant use of cyclosporine, fibrates, gemfibrozil, niacin.

⌛ LIFESPAN CONSIDERATIONS

Pregnancy/Lactation: Contraindicated in pregnancy (suppression of cholesterol biosynthesis may cause fetal toxicity) and lactation. Unknown if drug is distributed in breast milk. **Pregnancy Category X. Children:** Safety and efficacy not established. **Elderly:** No age-related precautions noted.

INTERACTIONS

DRUG: **Cyclosporine, fibrates, gemfibrozil, niacin** may increase risk of rhabdomyolysis, acute renal failure. **HERBAL:** None significant. **FOOD:** Large amounts of **grapefruit juice** may increase risk of side effects (e.g., myalgia, weakness). Red yeast rice contains approximately 2.4 mg lovastatin per 600 mg rice. **LAB VALUES:** May increase serum creatine kinase (CK), transaminase.

AVAILABILITY (Rx)

Tablets (Mevacor): 10 mg, 20 mg, 40 mg.

Tablets (Extended-Release [Altoprev]): 20 mg, 40 mg, 60 mg.

ADMINISTRATION/HANDLING

PO

• Immediate-release tablet given with meals; extended-release at bedtime. • Avoid intake of large quantities of grapefruit juice (greater than 1 quart). • Do not crush extended-release tablets.

INDICATIONS/ROUTES/DOSAGE

Atherosclerosis, Coronary Artery Disease

PO: ADULTS, ELDERLY: Initially, 20 mg/day. Maintenance: 10–80 mg once daily or in 2 divided doses. **Maximum:** 80 mg/day.

Hypercholesterolemia

PO: ADULTS, ELDERLY: Initially, 20 mg/day. Maintenance: 10–80 mg once daily or in 2 divided doses. **Maximum:** 80 mg/day.
PO (EXTENDED-RELEASE): ADULTS, ELDERLY: Initially, 20–60 mg once daily at bedtime. Maintenance: 10–60 mg once daily at bedtime.

Heterozygous Familial Hypercholesterolemia

PO: CHILDREN 10–17 YRS: Initially, 10 mg/day. May increase to 20 mg/day after 8 wks and 40 mg/day after 16 wks if needed.

SIDE EFFECTS

Generally well tolerated. Side effects usually mild and transient. **Frequent (9%–5%):** Headache, flatulence, diarrhea, abdominal pain, abdominal cramping, rash, pruritus. **Occasional (4%–3%):** Nausea, vomiting, constipation, dyspepsia. **Rare (2%–1%):** Dizziness, heartburn, myalgia, blurred vision, eye irritation.

ADVERSE EFFECTS/ TOXIC REACTIONS

Potential for cataract development. Occasionally produces myopathy manifested as muscle pain, tenderness, weakness with elevated creatine kinase (CK). Severe myopathy may lead to rhabdomyolysis.

NURSING CONSIDERATIONS

BASELINE ASSESSMENT

Obtain dietary history. Question for possibility of pregnancy before initiating therapy (Pregnancy Category X). Assess baseline lab results: serum cholesterol, triglycerides, hepatic function tests.

INTERVENTION/EVALUATION

Monitor daily pattern of bowel activity and stool consistency. Monitor for headache, dizziness, blurred vision. Assess for rash, pruritus. Monitor serum cholesterol, triglycerides for therapeutic response. Be alert for malaise, muscle cramping/weakness. Monitor hepatic function tests.

PATIENT/FAMILY TEACHING

• Follow special diet (important part of treatment). • Periodic lab tests are essential part of therapy. • Avoid grapefruit juice, alcohol. • Inform physician of severe gastric upset, vision changes, myalgia, weakness, changes in color of urine/stool, yellowing of eyes/skin, unusual bruising.

Lovenox, *see enoxaparin*

lubiprostone

loo-bi-**pros**-tone
(Amitiza)

◆CLASSIFICATION

PHARMACOTHERAPEUTIC: Chloride channel activator. **CLINICAL:** Constipation agent.

ACTION

Secretes fluid into abdominal lumen through activation of chloride channels in apical membranes of GI epithelium. **Therapeutic Effect:** Increases intestinal motility, thereby increasing passage of stool, alleviating symptoms associated with chronic idiopathic constipation.

PHARMACOKINETICS

Rapidly, extensively metabolized within stomach and jejunum. Minimal distribution beyond GI tissue. Protein binding: 94%. Excreted mainly in urine with trace amount eliminated in feces. **Half-life:** 0.9–1.4 hrs.

USES

Treatment of chronic idiopathic constipation in adults. Treatment of irritable bowel syndrome (IBS) with constipation in women 18 yrs and older.

L

PRECAUTIONS

Contraindications: History of mechanical GI obstruction. **Cautions:** Diarrhea.

LIFESPAN CONSIDERATIONS

May have potential for teratogenic effects. **Pregnancy/Lactation:** Unknown if distributed in breast milk. **Pregnancy Category C. Children:** Safety and efficacy not established. **Elderly:** No age-related precautions noted.

INTERACTIONS

DRUG: None significant. **HERBAL:** None significant. **FOOD:** None known. **LAB VALUES:** None significant.

AVAILABILITY (Rx)

Capsules: 8 mcg, 24 mcg.

ADMINISTRATION/HANDLING

PO

- Give with food.

INDICATIONS/ROUTES/DOSAGE

Chronic Idiopathic Constipation

PO: ADULTS, ELDERLY: 24 mcg twice daily with food.

IBS

PO: ADULTS, ELDERLY: 8 mcg twice daily with food.

SIDE EFFECTS

Frequent (31%): Nausea. **Occasional (13%–4%):** Headache, diarrhea, abdominal distention, abdominal pain, flatulence, vomiting, peripheral edema, dizziness. **Rare (3%–2%):** Dyspepsia (heartburn, indigestion, epigastric distress), loose stools, fatigue, dry mouth, arthralgia, back pain, cough.

ADVERSE EFFECTS/ TOXIC REACTIONS

UTI, upper respiratory tract infection occurs in 4% of pts.

NURSING CONSIDERATIONS

BASELINE ASSESSMENT

Women should have negative pregnancy test prior to beginning therapy and comply with effective contraceptive measures during therapy. Assess for diarrhea (avoid use in these pts).

INTERVENTION/EVALUATION

Assess for improvement in symptoms (relief from bloating, cramping, urgency, abdominal discomfort).

PATIENT/FAMILY TEACHING

• Inform physician of new/worsening episodes of abdominal pain, severe diarrhea. • Avoid tasks that require alertness, motor skills until response to drug is established.

Lunesta, *see eszopiclone*

Lupron, *see leuprolide*

lurasidone

lure-**ass**-ih-doan
(Latuda)

BLACK BOX ALERT Elderly pts with dementia-related psychosis are at increased risk for mortality due to cerebrovascular events, infectious diseases.

◆CLASSIFICATION

PHARMACOTHERAPEUTIC: Dopamine, serotonin receptor antagonist. **CLINICAL:** Antipsychotic.

ACTION

Antagonizes central dopamine type 2 and serotonin type 2 receptors. **Therapeutic Effect:** Diminishes symptoms of schizophrenia.

PHARMACOKINETICS

Absorbed in 1–3 hrs. Steady-state concentration occurs in 7 days. Well absorbed from GI tract (unaffected by food). Protein binding: 99%. Metabolized in liver to active and inactive metabolites. Primarily excreted in urine, with lesser amount eliminated in feces. **Half-life:** 28–36 hrs.

USES

Treatment of schizophrenia.

PRECAUTIONS

Contraindications: Strong CYP3A4 inhibitors (diltiazem, ketoconazole, ritonavir) and inducer (rifampin). **Cautions:** Cardiovascular disease (heart failure, history of MI, ischemia, conduction abnormalities), cerebrovascular disease (history of CVA in pts with dementia, seizure disorders). Those with an established diagnosis of diabetes mellitus.

⌛ LIFESPAN CONSIDERATIONS

Pregnancy/Lactation: Unknown if distributed in breast milk. Breast-feeding not recommended. **Pregnancy Category B. Children:** Safety and efficacy not established. **Elderly:** More susceptible to postural hypotension. Increased risk of cerebrovascular events, mortality, including stroke, in elderly pts with psychosis.

INTERACTIONS

DRUG: **Alcohol, CNS depressants** may increase CNS depression. **Rifampin** decreases concentration/effect. **Diltiazem, ketoconazole** may increase concentration, effect. **HERBAL:** **Gotu kola, kava kava, St. John's wort, valerian** may increase CNS depression. **FOOD:** None known. **LAB VALUES:** May increase prolactin levels.

AVAILABILITY (Rx)

Tablets: 40 mg, 80 mg.

ADMINISTRATION/HANDLING

PO

- Give with food. • Tablets may be crushed.

INDICATIONS/ROUTES/DOSAGE

Schizophrenia

PO: ADULTS, ELDERLY: 40 mg once daily with food. **Maximum:** 80 mg once daily with food. In those with moderate to severe hepatic/renal impairment, do not exceed 40 mg daily.

SIDE EFFECTS

Frequent (15%–7%): Drowsiness, sedation, insomnia (paradoxical reaction). **Occasional (6%–3%):** Nausea, vomiting, dyspepsia (heartburn, GI upset), fatigue, back pain, akathisia, dizziness, agitation, anxiety. **Rare (2%–1%):** Restlessness, salivary hypersecretion, tongue spasm, torticollis, trismus.

ADVERSE EFFECTS/ TOXIC REACTIONS

Extrapyramidal disorder (including cogwheel rigidity, drooling, bradykinesia, tremors) occurs in 5% of pts. Neuroleptic malignant syndrome (fever, muscle rigidity, irregular B/P or pulse, altered mental status) occurs rarely.

NURSING CONSIDERATIONS

BASELINE ASSESSMENT

Assess behavior, appearance, emotional status, response to environment, speech pattern, thought content. Renal/hepatic function tests should be obtained before therapy as dose adjustment is required when initiating therapy.

INTERVENTION/EVALUATION

Supervise suicidal risk pt closely during early therapy (as depression lessens, energy level improves, increasing suicide potential). Monitor for potential neuroleptic malignant syndrome (fever, muscle rigidity, irregular B/P or pulse, altered mental status, visual changes, dyspnea). Assess for therapeutic response (greater interest in surroundings, improved self-care, increased ability to concentrate, relaxed facial expression).

PATIENT/FAMILY TEACHING

• Avoid tasks that may require alertness, motor skills until response to drug is established (may cause drowsiness, dizziness). • Avoid alcohol. • Inform physician of trembling in fingers, altered gait, unusual muscle/skeletal movements, palpitations, severe dizziness, fainting, visual changes, rash, difficulty breathing. • Report suicidal ideation, unusual changes in behavior.

lymphocyte immune globulin N

lim-foe-site ih-**mewn**
glah-byew-lin N
(Atgam)

BLACK BOX ALERT Use only by physicians experienced in immunosuppressive therapy for treatment of renal transplant or aplastic anemia pts.

Do not confuse Atgam with Ativan.

◆CLASSIFICATION

PHARMACOTHERAPEUTIC: Biologic response modifier. **CLINICAL:** Immunosuppressant.

ACTION

Acts as lymphocyte selective immunosuppressant, reducing number/altering function of T lymphocytes, which are responsible for cell-mediated and humoral immunity. Stimulates release of hematopoietic growth factors. **Therapeutic Effect:** Prevents allograft rejection; treats aplastic anemia.

PHARMACOKINETICS

Unknown absorption, metabolism, elimination. **Half-life:** Approximately 5–7 days.

USES

Prevention/treatment of renal allograft rejection. Treatment of moderate to severe aplastic anemia in pts not candidates for bone marrow transplant. **OFF-LABEL:** Immunosuppressant in bone marrow, heart, liver transplants; treatment of pure red cell aplasia, multiple sclerosis, myasthenia gravis, scleroderma.

PRECAUTIONS

Contraindications: Systemic hypersensitivity reaction to previous injection of lymphocyte immune globulin N. **Cautions:** Concurrent immunosuppressive therapy.

LIFESPAN CONSIDERATIONS

Pregnancy/Lactation: Unknown if drug crosses placenta or is distributed in breast milk. **Pregnancy Category C.** **Children:** Safety and efficacy not established. **Elderly:** No age-related precautions noted.

INTERACTIONS

DRUG: **Corticosteroids, other immunosuppresants** mask reaction to lymphocyte immune globulin. **HERBAL:** None significant. **FOOD:** None known.

LAB VALUES: May alter renal function test results.

AVAILABILITY

Injection Solution: 250 mg/5 ml.

ADMINISTRATION/HANDLING

IV

Reconstitution • Total daily dose must be further diluted with 0.9% NaCl (do not use D_5W). • Gently rotate diluted solution. Do not shake. • Final concentration must not exceed 4 mg/ml.
Rate of administration • Use 0.2- to 1-micron filter. • Give total daily dose over minimum of 4 hrs.
Storage • Keep refrigerated before and after dilution. • Discard diluted solution after 24 hrs.

IV INCOMPATIBILITIES

No information is available for Y-site administration.

INDICATIONS/ROUTES/DOSAGE

Prevention of Renal Allograft Rejection
IV: ADULTS, ELDERLY, CHILDREN: 15 mg/kg/day for 14 days, then every other day for 14 days. First dose within 24 hrs before or after transplantation.

Treatment of Renal Allograft Rejection
IV: ADULTS, ELDERLY, CHILDREN: 10–15 mg/kg/day for 14 days, then every other day for 14 more days. **Maximum:** 21 doses in 28 days.

Aplastic Anemia
IV: ADULTS, ELDERLY, CHILDREN: 10–20 mg/kg once a day for 8–14 days, then every other day. **Maximum:** 21 doses.

SIDE EFFECTS

Frequent: Fever (51%), thrombocytopenia (30%), rash (22%), chills (16%), leukopenia (14%), systemic infection (13%).
Occasional (10%–5%): Serum sickness-like reaction, dyspnea, apnea, arthralgia, chest pain, back pain, flank pain, nausea, vomiting, diarrhea, phlebitis.

ADVERSE EFFECTS/TOXIC REACTIONS

Thrombocytopenia may occur but is generally transient. Severe hypersensitivity reaction, including anaphylaxis, occurs rarely.

NURSING CONSIDERATIONS

BASELINE ASSESSMENT

Use of high-flow vein (CVL, PICC, Groshong catheter) may prevent chemical phlebitis that may occur if peripheral vein is used.

INTERVENTION/EVALUATION

Monitor frequently for chills, fever, erythema, pruritus. Obtain order for prophylactic antihistamines or corticosteroids.

Lyrica, *see pregabalin*

Macrobid, *see nitrofurantoin*

magnesium

HIGH ALERT

mag-**knee**-see-um

magnesium chloride

(Mag-Delay, Slow-Mag)

magnesium citrate

(Citroma, Citro-Mag ✦)

magnesium hydroxide

(Phillips Milk of Magnesia)

magnesium oxide

(Mag-Ox 400, Uro-Mag)

M

magnesium protein complex

(Mg-PLUS)

magnesium sulfate

(Epsom salt, magnesium sulfate injection)

Do not confuse magnesium sulfate with morphine sulfate.

FIXED-COMBINATION(S)

With aluminum, an antacid **(Aludrox, Delcid, Gaviscon, Maalox)**; with aluminum and simethicone, an antiflatulent **(Di-Gel, Gelusil, Maalox Plus, Mylanta)**; with aluminum and calcium, an antacid **(Camalox)**; with mineral oil, a lubricant laxative **(Haley's MO)**; with magnesium oxide and aluminum oxide, an antacid **(Riopan)**.

M

◆CLASSIFICATION

CLINICAL: Antacid, anticonvulsant, electrolyte, laxative (see pp. 12C, 121C).

ACTION

Antacid: Acts in stomach to neutralize gastric acid. **Therapeutic Effect:** Increases pH. **Laxative:** Osmotic effect primarily in small intestine, draws water into intestinal lumen. **Therapeutic Effect:** Promotes peristalsis, bowel evacuation. **Systemic (dietary supplement replacement):** Found primarily in intracellular fluids. **Therapeutic Effect:** Essential for enzyme activity, nerve conduction, muscle contraction. Maintains and restores magnesium levels. **Anticonvulsant:** Blocks neuromuscular transmission, amount of acetylcholine released at motor end plate. **Therapeutic Effect:** Produces seizure control.

PHARMACOKINETICS

Antacid, laxative: Minimal absorption through intestine. Absorbed dose primarily excreted in urine. **Systemic:** Widely distributed. Primarily excreted in urine.

USES

Magnesium Chloride: Dietary supplement. **Magnesium Citrate:** Evacuation of bowel before surgical, diagnostic procedures. **Magnesium Hydroxide:** Short-term treatment of constipation, symptoms of hyperacidity, magnesium replacement. **Magnesium Oxide:** Magnesium replacement. **Magnesium Sulfate:** Treatment/prevention of hypomagnesemia; prevention and treatment of seizures in eclampsia; torsade de pointes (atypical ventricular tachycardia); treatment of arrhythmias due to hypomagnesemia (ventricular tachycardia/ventricular fibrillation). **OFF-LABEL: Magnesium sulfate:** Premature labor, torsade de pointes, acute asthma, MI, tocolysis.

PRECAUTIONS

Contraindications: Antacid: Appendicitis, symptoms of appendicitis, ileostomy, intestinal obstruction, severe renal impairment. **Laxative:** Appendicitis, CHF, colostomy, hypersensitivity, ileostomy, intestinal obstruction, undiagnosed rectal bleeding. **Systemic:** Heart block, myocardial damage, renal failure. **Cautions:** Safety in children younger than 6 yrs not known. **Antacids:** Undiagnosed GI/rectal bleeding, ulcerative colitis, colostomy, diverticulitis, chronic diarrhea. **Laxative:** Diabetes mellitus, pts on low-salt diet (some products contain sugar, sodium). **Systemic:** Severe renal impairment.

LIFESPAN CONSIDERATIONS

Pregnancy/Lactation: Antacid: Unknown if distributed in breast milk. **Parenteral:** Readily crosses placenta. Distributed in breast milk for 24 hrs after magnesium therapy is discontinued. Continuous IV infusion increases risk of magnesium toxicity in neonate. IV administration should not be used 2 hrs preceding delivery. **Pregnancy Category B. Children:** No age-related precautions noted. **Elderly:** Increased risk of developing magnesium deficiency (e.g., poor diet, decreased absorption, medications).

INTERACTIONS

DRUG: **Antacids** may decrease absorption of **fluoroquinolones, ketoconazole, tetracyclines.** May decrease effect of **methenamine. Antacids, laxatives** may decrease effects of **digoxin, oral anticoagulants, phenothiazines.** May decrease absorption of **ciprofloxacin. Sodium polystyrene sulfonate** may bind with magnesium, preventing neutralization of bicarbonate ions, leading to systemic alkalosis. May form nonabsorbable complex with **tetracyclines. Calcium** may neutralize effects of magnesium. **CNS depressant medications** may increase CNS depression. May alter cardiac conduction, increase degree of heart block with **digoxin.** HERBAL: None significant. FOOD: None known. LAB VALUES: **Antacid:** May increase gastrin production, pH. **Laxative:** May decrease serum potassium. **Systemic:** None significant.

AVAILABILITY

MAGNESIUM CHLORIDE
Tablets (Mag Delay, Slow-Mag): 64 mg.
MAGNESIUM CITRATE
Oral Solution (Citroma): 290 mg/5 ml.
MAGNESIUM HYDROXIDE
Oral Liquid (Phillips Milk of Magnesia): 400 mg/5 ml, 800 mg/5 ml.
Tablets (Chewable [Phillips Milk of Magnesia]): 311 mg.
MAGNESIUM OXIDE
Capsules (Uro-Mag): 140 mg. Tablets (Mag-Ox 400): 400 mg.
MAGNESIUM SULFATE
Infusion Solution: 10 mg/ml, 20 mg/ml, 40 mg/ml, 80 mg/ml. Injection Solution: 125 mg/ml, 500 mg/ml.

ADMINISTRATION/HANDLING

IV

Reconstitution • Must dilute to maximum concentration of 20%.
Rate of administration • For IV infusion, maximum rate of infusion is 2 g/hr.
Storage • Store at room temperature.

IM

• For adults, elderly, use 250 mg/ml (25%) or 500 mg/ml (50%) magnesium sulfate concentration. • For infants, children, do not exceed 200 mg/ml (20%).

PO (Antacid)

• Shake suspension well before use. • Chewable tablets should be chewed thoroughly before swallowing, followed by full glass of water.

PO (Laxative)

• Drink full glass of liquid (8 oz) with each dose (prevents dehydration). • Flavor may be improved by following with fruit juice, citrus carbonated beverage. • Refrigerate citrate of magnesia (retains potency, palatability).

IV INCOMPATIBILITIES

Amphotericin B complex (Abelcet, AmBisome, Amphotec), cefepime (Maxipime), lansoprazole (Prevacid), lipids, pantoprazole (Protonix).

IV COMPATIBILITIES

Amikacin (Amikin), cefazolin (Ancef), ciprofloxacin (Cipro), dobutamine (Dobutrex), enalapril (Vasotec), gentamicin, heparin, hydromorphone (Dilaudid), insulin, linezolid (Zyvox), metoclopramide (Reglan), milrinone (Primacor), morphine, piperacillin/tazobactam (Zosyn), potassium chloride, propofol (Diprivan), tobramycin (Nebcin), vancomycin (Vancocin).

INDICATIONS/ROUTES/DOSAGE

Hypomagnesemia
Magnesium sulfate

Mild Deficiency
IM: ADULTS, ELDERLY: 1 g q6h for 4 doses.

Severe Deficiency
IM: ADULTS, ELDERLY: Up to 250 mg/kg over 4 hrs.

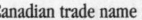

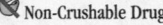

M

IV: ADULTS, ELDERLY: 1–2 g/hr for 3–6 hrs, then 0.5–1 g/hr as needed to correct deficiency.

Symptomatic Deficiency

IV: ADULTS, ELDERLY: 1–2 g over 5–60 min.

Usual Dose for Children

IM/IV: 25–50 mg/kg/dose q4–6h for 3–4 doses. **Maximum single dose:** 2 g.

Usual Dose for Neonates

IM/IV: 25–50 mg/kg/dose q8–12h for 2–3 doses.

Eclampsia

IV: ADULTS: 4–5 g infusion, then 1–2 g/hr continuous infusion. **Maximum:** 40 g/24 hrs.

Hypertension, Seizures

IV, IM (MAGNESIUM SULFATE): ADULTS, ELDERLY: 1 g q6h for 4 doses as needed. **CHILDREN:** 20–100 mg/kg/dose q4–6h as needed.

M

Arrhythmias, Torsade de Pointes

IV (MAGNESIUM SULFATE): ADULTS, ELDERLY: Initially, 1–2 g then infusion of 0.5–1 g/hr.

Constipation

PO (MAGNESIUM HYDROXIDE): ADULTS, ELDERLY, CHILDREN 12 YRS AND OLDER: 6–8 tablets or 30–60 ml/day (400 mg/5 ml). **CHILDREN 6–11 YRS:** 3–4 tablets or 15–30 ml/day (400 mg/5 ml). **CHILDREN 2–5 YRS:** 1–2 tablets or 5–15 ml/day (400 mg/5 ml).

Hyperacidity

PO (MAGNESIUM HYDROXIDE): ADULTS, ELDERLY, CHILDREN 12 YRS AND OLDER: 2–4 tablets or 5–15 ml as needed up to 4 times a day.

Magnesium Deficiency

PO (MAGNESIUM OXIDE): ADULTS, ELDERLY: 1–2 tablets 2–3 times a day.

Dietary Supplement

PO (MAGNESIUM CHLORIDE): ADULTS, ELDERLY: 2 tablets daily.

Cathartic

PO (MAGNESIUM CITRATE): ADULTS, ELDERLY, CHILDREN 12 YRS AND OLDER: 120–300 ml. **CHILDREN 6–11 YRS:** 100–150 ml. **CHILDREN YOUNGER THAN 6 YRS:** 0.5 ml/kg up to maximum of 200 ml.

SIDE EFFECTS

Frequent: **Antacid:** Chalky taste, diarrhea, laxative effect. Occasional: **Antacid:** Nausea, vomiting, stomach cramps. **Antacid, laxative:** Prolonged use or large doses in renal impairment may cause hypermagnesemia (dizziness, palpitations, altered mental status, fatigue, weakness). **Laxative:** Cramping, diarrhea, increased thirst, flatulence. **Systemic (dietary supplement, electrolyte replacement):** Reduced respiratory rate, decreased reflexes, flushing, hypotension, decreased heart rate.

ADVERSE EFFECTS/ TOXIC REACTIONS

Magnesium as antacid, laxative has no known adverse reactions. Systemic use may produce prolonged PR interval, widening of QRS interval. Magnesium toxicity may cause loss of deep tendon reflexes, heart block, respiratory paralysis, cardiac arrest. **Antidote:** 10–20 ml 10% calcium gluconate (5–10 mEq of calcium).

NURSING CONSIDERATIONS

BASELINE ASSESSMENT

Assess if pt is sensitive to magnesium. **Antacid:** Assess GI pain (duration, location, quality, time of occurrence, relief with food, causative/excacerbative factors). **Laxative:** Assess for weight loss, nausea, vomiting, history of recent abdominal surgery. **Systemic:** Assess renal function, serum magnesium.

INTERVENTION/EVALUATION

Antacid: Assess for relief of gastric distress. Monitor renal function (esp. if dosing is long term or frequent). **Laxative:** Monitor daily pattern of bowel activity, stool consistency. Maintain adequate fluid intake. **Systemic:** Monitor renal function, magnesium levels, EKG for cardiac function. Test patellar reflexes (knee jerk reflexes) before giving repeat parenteral doses (used as indication of CNS depression; suppressed reflexes may be sign of impending respiratory arrest). Patellar reflex must be present, respiratory rate should be 16/min or over before each parenteral dose. Initiate seizure precautions.

PATIENT/FAMILY TEACHING

• **Antacid:** Take at least 2 hrs apart from other medication. • Do not take longer than 2 wks unless directed by physician. • For peptic ulcer, take 1 and 3 hrs after meals and at bedtime for 4–6 wks. • Chew tablets thoroughly, followed by 8 oz of water; shake suspensions well. • Repeat dosing or large doses may have laxative effect. • **Laxative:** Drink full glass (8 oz) liquid to aid stool softening. • Use only for short term. Do not use if abdominal pain, nausea, vomiting is present. • **Systemic:** Inform physician of any signs of hypermagnesemia (dizziness, palpitations, altered mental status, fatigue, weakness).

mannitol

man-i-tall
(Osmitrol)
Do not confuse Osmitrol with esmolol.

◆CLASSIFICATION

CLINICAL: Osmotic diuretic, antiglaucoma, antihemolytic.

ACTION

Elevates osmotic pressure of glomerular filtrate, inhibiting tubular reabsorption of water and electrolytes, resulting in increased flow of water into interstitial fluid/plasma. **Therapeutic Effect:** Produces diuresis; reduces intraocular pressure (IOP), intracranial pressure (ICP), cerebral edema.

PHARMACOKINETICS

Route	Onset	Peak	Duration
IV (diuresis)	1–3 hrs	N/A	—
IV (reduced ICP)	—	N/A	1.5–6 hrs

Remains in extracellular fluid. Primarily excreted in urine unchanged. Removed by hemodialysis. **Half-life:** 1.1–1.6 hrs.

USES

Prevention, treatment of oliguric phase of acute renal failure (before evidence of permanent renal failure). Reduces increased ICP due to cerebral edema, spinal cord edema, IOP due to acute glaucoma. Promotes urinary excretion of toxic substances (aspirin, bromides, imipramine, barbiturates).

PRECAUTIONS

Contraindications: Dehydration, intracranial bleeding, severe pulmonary edema, congestion; several renal disease (anuria), increasing oliguria, azotemia. **Cautions:** None known.

⌛ LIFESPAN CONSIDERATIONS

Pregnancy/Lactation: Unknown if drug crosses placenta or is distributed in breast milk. **Pregnancy Category C. Children:** Safety and efficacy not established in those younger than 12 yrs. **Elderly:** Age-related renal impairment may require dosage adjustment.

INTERACTIONS

DRUG: May increase risk of **lithium** toxicity associated with mannitol-induced hyponatremia. **HERBAL:** None significant. **FOOD:** None known. **LAB VALUES:** May decrease serum phosphate, potassium, sodium.

M

AVAILABILITY (Rx)

Injection Solution (Osmitrol): 5%, 10%, 15%, 20%, 25%.

ADMINISTRATION/HANDLING

◀ALERT▶ Assess IV site for patency before each dose. Pain, thrombosis noted with extravasation. In-line filter (less than 5 microns) used for concentrations over 20%.

IV

Rate of administration • Administer test dose for pts with oliguria. • Give IV push over 3–5 min; over 20–30 min for cerebral edema, elevated ICP. Maximum concentration: 25%. • Do not add KCl or NaCl to mannitol 20% or greater. Do not add to whole blood for transfusion.

Storage • Store at room temperature. • If crystals are noted in solution, warm bottle in hot water, shake vigorously at intervals. Cool to body temperature before administration. Do not use if crystals remain after warming procedure.

IV INCOMPATIBILITIES

Cefepime (Maxipime), doxorubicin liposomal (Doxil), filgrastim (Neupogen) imipenem-cilastatin (Primaxin).

IV COMPATIBILITIES

Cisplatin (Platinol), furosemide (Lasix), linezolid (Zyvox), lipids, ondansetron (Zofran), propofol (Diprivan).

INDICATIONS/ROUTES/DOSAGE

Usual Dosage

TEST DOSE (to assess adequate renal function): ADULTS, ELDERLY: 12.5 g (200 mg/kg) over 3–5 min to produce urine flow of at least 30–50 ml urine/hr. **CHILDREN:** 200 mg/kg over 3–5 min to produce urine flow of at least 1 ml/kg for 1–3 hrs.

INITIAL: ADULTS, ELDERLY: 0.5–1 g/kg. **CHILDREN:** 0.25–1 g/kg.

MAINTENANCE: ADULTS, ELDERLY: 0.25–0.5 g/kg q4–6h. **CHILDREN:** 0.25–0.5 g/kg q4–6h.

SIDE EFFECTS

Frequent: Dry mouth, thirst. **Occasional:** Blurred vision, increased urinary frequency/volume, headache, arm pain, backache, nausea, vomiting, urticaria, dizziness, hypotension, hypertension, tachycardia, fever, angina-like chest pain.

ADVERSE EFFECTS/ TOXIC REACTIONS

Fluid, electrolyte imbalance may occur due to rapid administration of large doses or inadequate urine output resulting in overexpansion of extracellular fluid. Circulatory overload may produce pulmonary edema, CHF. Excessive diuresis may produce hypokalemia, hyponatremia. Fluid loss in excess of electrolyte excretion may produce hypernatremia, hyperkalemia.

NURSING CONSIDERATIONS

BASELINE ASSESSMENT

Check B/P, pulse before giving medication. Assess skin turgor, mucous membranes, mental status, muscle strength. Obtain baseline weight, chemistry studies. Assess I&O.

INTERVENTION/EVALUATION

Monitor urinary output to ascertain therapeutic response. Monitor serum electrolytes, BUN, renal/hepatic function tests. Assess vital signs, skin turgor, mucous membranes. Weigh daily. Signs of hyponatremia include confusion, drowsiness, thirst, dry mouth, cold/clammy skin. Signs of hypokalemia include changes in muscle strength, tremors, muscle cramps, altered mental status, cardiac arrhythmias. Signs of hyperkalemia include colic, diarrhea, muscle twitching followed by weakness, paralysis, arrhythmias.

PATIENT/FAMILY TEACHING

- Expect increased urinary frequency/volume.
- May cause dry mouth.

maraviroc

mar-**ah**-vir-ock
(Celsentri ♣, Selzentry)

BLACK BOX ALERT Possible drug-induced hepatotoxicity with allergic-type features reported.

◆CLASSIFICATION

PHARMACOTHERAPEUTIC: Chemokine receptor 5 (CCR5) co-receptor antagonist. **CLINICAL:** Antiretroviral.

ACTION

Binds to human chemokine receptor (CCR5), present on CD-4 and T-cell membranes, preventing interaction of HIV-1 and CCR5, necessary for HIV-1 to enter cells. **Therapeutic Effect:** Decreased invasion of HIV-1 virus into cells.

PHARMACOKINETICS

Variably absorbed following PO administration. Protein binding: 76%. Metabolized in liver. Eliminated mainly in feces, with lesser amount eliminated in urine. **Half-life:** 14–18 hrs.

USES

Treatment of HIV infection in those infected only with detectable chemokine receptor 5 (CCR5)-tropic HIV-1, with evidence of viral replication; HIV-1 strains resistant to multiple antiretroviral agents. Used in combination with other antiretroviral agents.

PRECAUTIONS

Contraindications: Severe renal impairment or ESRD (CrCl less than 30 mL/min) who are taking potent CYP3A inhibitors or inducers. **Cautions:** Hepatic/renal impairment, history of orthostatic hypotension, hepatitis B or C, concurrent medication known to lower B/P, those at increased risk for cardiovascular events.

⌛ LIFESPAN CONSIDERATIONS

Pregnancy/Lactation: Unknown if drug crosses placenta or is distributed in breast milk. Breast-feeding not recommended. **Pregnancy Category B. Children:** Safety and efficacy not established in those younger than 16 yrs. **Elderly:** Age-related hepatic/renal impairment requires close monitoring.

INTERACTIONS

DRUG: Atazanavir, atazanavir/ritonavir, ketoconazole, lopinavir, ritonavir, saquinavir/ritonavir may increase concentration. **Efavirenz, rifampin** may decrease concentration. **HERBAL: St. John's wort** may lead to loss of virologic response, potential resistance to maraviroc. **FOOD:** None known. **LAB VALUES:** May increase serum AST, ALT, total bilirubin, amylase, lipase. May decrease lymphocytes/neutrophil count, WBC count.

AVAILABILITY (Rx)

Tablets: 150 mg, 300 mg.

ADMINISTRATION/HANDLING

PO

• Give without regard to food. • Do not crush, split, chew film-coated tablets.

INDICATIONS/ROUTES/DOSAGE

HIV Infection

PO: ADULTS, ELDERLY, CHILDREN OVER 16 YRS WITH CONCURRENT ANTIRETROVIRAL AGENTS: 300 mg twice a day. **(with CYP3A inhibitors): Clarithromycin, delavirdine, itraconazole, ketoconazole, nefazodone, telethromycin:** 150 mg twice a day. **(with CYP3A inducers): Carbamazepine, efavirenz, phenobarbital, phenytoin, rifampin:** 600 mg twice a day.

SIDE EFFECTS

Common (20%): Upper respiratory tract infection. **Frequent (13%–7%):** Cough, fever, rash, musculoskeletal pain, abdominal pain, dizziness, appetite change, herpes simplex infection, sleep disturbances. **Occasional (6%–4%):** Sinusitis, joint pain, bronchitis, constipation, bladder infection, paresthesia, sensory abnormalities. **Rare (3% or less):** Sleep disturbances, pruritus, peripheral neuropathy, dermatitis, dyspepsia.

M

ADVERSE EFFECTS/ TOXIC REACTIONS

Cardiovascular events (MI, ischemia, unstable angina, coronary artery occlusion/disease), CVA, hepatic failure/cirrhosis, neoplasms occur in less than 2% of pts.

NURSING CONSIDERATIONS

BASELINE ASSESSMENT

Obtain baseline laboratory testing, esp. hepatic function tests, before beginning therapy and at periodic intervals during therapy. Offer emotional support. Obtain medication history.

INTERVENTION/EVALUATION

Closely monitor for evidence of GI discomfort. Monitor daily pattern of bowel activity, stool consistency. Assess skin for evidence of rash. Monitor serum chemistry tests for marked laboratory abnormalities, particularly hepatic profile. Assess for opportunistic infections: onset of fever, cough, or other respiratory symptoms.

PATIENT/FAMILY TEACHING

• Contact physician if fever, abdominal pain, jaundice, dark urine occur. • Avoid tasks that require alertness, motor skills until response to drug is established. • Maraviroc is not a cure for HIV infection, nor does it reduce risk of transmission to others. • May continue to experience illnesses, including opportunistic infections.

Mavik, *see trandolapril*

Maxalt, *see rizatriptan*

Maxipime, *see cefepime*

meclizine

mek-li-zeen
(Antivert, Bonamine ✦, Bonine, Dramamine Less Drowsy Formula)
Do not confuse Antivert with Alavert, Avodart, or Axert.

◆CLASSIFICATION

PHARMACOTHERAPEUTIC: Anticholinergic. **CLINICAL:** Antiemetic, antivertigo.

ACTION

Reduces labyrinthine excitability, diminishes vestibular stimulation of labyrinth, affecting chemoreceptor trigger zone. **Therapeutic Effect:** Reduces nausea, vomiting, vertigo.

PHARMACOKINETICS

Route	Onset	Peak	Duration
PO	30–60 min	N/A	8–24 hrs

Well absorbed from GI tract. Widely distributed. Metabolized in liver. Primarily excreted in urine. **Half-life:** 6 hrs.

USES

Prevention/treatment of nausea, vomiting, vertigo due to motion sickness. Treatment of vertigo associated with diseases affecting vestibular system.

PRECAUTIONS

Contraindications: None known. **Cautions:** Narrow-angle glaucoma, obstructive diseases of GI/GU tract.

⌛ LIFESPAN CONSIDERATIONS

Pregnancy/Lactation: Unknown if drug crosses placenta or is distributed in breast milk (may produce irritability in nursing infants). **Pregnancy Category B. Children/Elderly:** May be more sensitive to anticholinergic effects (e.g., dry mouth).

INTERACTIONS

DRUG: Alcohol, CNS depressants may increase CNS depressant effect. **HERBAL:**

None significant. **FOOD:** None known. **LAB VALUES:** May produce false-negative results in antigen skin testing unless meclizine is discontinued 4 days before testing.

AVAILABILITY (Rx)

Tablets (Antivert): 12.5 mg, 25 mg. **(Dramamine Less Drowsy Formula):** 25 mg. **Tablets (Chewable [Bonine]):** 25 mg.

ADMINISTRATION/HANDLING

PO

• Give without regard to meals. • Scored tablets may be crushed.

INDICATIONS/ROUTES/DOSAGE

Motion Sickness

PO: ADULTS, ELDERLY, CHILDREN 12 YRS AND OLDER: 12.5–25 mg 1 hr before travel. May repeat q12–24h. May require a dose of 50 mg.

Vertigo

PO: ADULTS, ELDERLY, CHILDREN 12 YRS AND OLDER: 25–100 mg/day in divided doses, as needed.

SIDE EFFECTS

Frequent: Drowsiness. **Occasional:** Blurred vision; dry mouth, nose, throat.

ADVERSE EFFECTS/ TOXIC REACTIONS

Hypersensitivity reaction (eczema, pruritus, rash, cardiac disturbances, photosensitivity) may occur. Overdose may vary from CNS depression (sedation, apnea, cardiovascular collapse, death) to severe paradoxical reaction (hallucinations, tremor, seizures). Children may experience paradoxical reaction (restlessness, insomnia, euphoria, anxiety, tremors). Overdose in children may result in hallucinations, seizures, death.

NURSING CONSIDERATIONS

BASELINE ASSESSMENT

Assess degree of nausea/vomiting, degree of vertigo.

INTERVENTION/EVALUATION

Monitor B/P, esp. in elderly (increased risk of hypotension). Monitor children closely for paradoxical reaction. Monitor serum electrolytes in those with severe vomiting. Assess skin turgor, mucous membranes to evaluate hydration status.

PATIENT/FAMILY TEACHING

• Tolerance to sedative effect may occur. • Avoid tasks that require alertness, motor skills until response to drug is established. • Dry mouth, drowsiness, dizziness may be an expected response of drug. • Avoid alcoholic beverages during therapy. • Sugarless gum, sips of tepid water may relieve dry mouth. • Coffee, tea may help reduce drowsiness.

*medroxy-PROGESTERone

me-**drox**-ee-proe-**jess**-te-rone (Apo-Medroxy ♣, Depo-Provera, Depo-Provera Contraceptive, Depo-SubQ-Provera 104, Novo-Medrone ♣, Provera)

BLACK BOX ALERT Prolonged use (over 2 yrs) of contraceptive injection form may result in loss of bone mineral density.

Do not confuse medroxyprogesterone with hydroxyprogesterone, methylprednisolone, or methyltestosterone, or Provera with Covera, Femara, Parlodel, or Premarin.

FIXED-COMBINATION(S)

Prempro, Premphase: medroxyprogesterone/conjugated estrogens: 1.5 mg/0.3 mg, 1.5 mg/0.45 mg, 2.5 mg/0.625 mg, 5 mg/0.625 mg.

◆CLASSIFICATION

PHARMACOTHERAPEUTIC: Hormone. **CLINICAL:** Progestin, antineoplastic.

M

ACTION

Transforms endometrium from proliferative to secretory (in estrogen-primed endometrium). Inhibits secretion of pituitary gonadotropins. Therapeutic Effect: Prevents follicular maturation, ovulation. Stimulates growth of mammary alveolar tissue; relaxes uterine smooth muscle. Corrects hormonal imbalance.

PHARMACOKINETICS

Well absorbed after PO administration. Slowly absorbed after IM administration. Protein binding: 90%, primarily albumin. Metabolized in liver. Primarily excreted in urine. Half-life: **PO:** 12–17 hrs. **IM:** 40–50 days.

USES

PO: Prevention of endometrial hyperplasia (concurrently given with estrogen to women with intact uterus), treatment of secondary amenorrhea, abnormal uterine bleeding. **IM:** Adjunctive therapy, palliative treatment of inoperable, recurrent, metastatic endometrial carcinoma, renal carcinoma; prevention of pregnancy, endometriosis-associated pain. OFF-LABEL: Hormone replacement therapy in estrogen-treated menopausal women. Treatment of endometrial carcinoma.

PRECAUTIONS

Contraindications: Carcinoma of breast; estrogen-dependent neoplasm; history of or active thrombotic disorders (cerebral apoplexy, thrombophlebitis, thromboembolic disorders), hypersensitivity to progestins; known or suspected pregnancy; missed abortion; severe hepatic dysfunction; undiagnosed abnormal genital bleeding; use as pregnancy test. **Cautions:** Those with conditions aggravated by fluid retention (asthma, seizures, migraine, cardiac/renal dysfunction), diabetes, history of mental depression.

⌛ LIFESPAN CONSIDERATIONS

Pregnancy/Lactation: Avoid use during pregnancy, esp. first 4 mos (congenital heart, limb reduction defects may occur). Distributed in breast milk. **Pregnancy Category X. Children:** Safety and efficacy not established. **Elderly:** No age-related precautions noted.

INTERACTIONS

DRUG: **Hepatic enzyme inducers (e.g., carbamazepine, phenytoin, rifampin)** may decrease effect. HERBAL: **St. John's wort** may decrease effect of progestin contraceptive. FOOD: None known. LAB VALUES: May alter serum thyroid, hepatic function tests, PT, metapyrone test, HDL, total cholesterol, triglycerides. May increase LDL.

AVAILABILITY (Rx)

Injection Suspension: 104 mg/0.65 ml prefilled syringe (Depo-SubQ-Provera 104), 150 mg/ml (Depo-Provera Contraceptive), 400 mg/ml (Depo-Provera). **Tablets (Provera):** 2.5 mg, 5 mg, 10 mg.

ADMINISTRATION/HANDLING

IM

• Shake vial immediately before administering (ensures complete suspension). • Administer deep IM into gluteal or deltoid muscle.

SUBCUTANEOUS

• Shake vigorously prior to administration. • Inject in upper thigh or abdomen (avoid bony areas and umbilicus). • Give over 5–7 sec; do not rub injection area.

PO

• Give without regard to meals.

INDICATIONS/ROUTES/DOSAGE

Endometrial Hyperplasia

PO: ADULTS: 2.5–10 mg/day for 14 days.

Secondary Amenorrhea

PO: ADULTS: 5–10 mg/day for 5–10 days, beginning at any time during menstrual cycle.

Abnormal Uterine Bleeding

PO: ADULTS: 5–10 mg/day for 5–10 days, beginning on calculated day 16 or day 21 of menstrual cycle.

Endometrial, Renal Carcinoma
IM: ADULTS, ELDERLY: Initially, 400–1,000 mg; repeat at 1-wk intervals. If improvement occurs and disease is stabilized, begin maintenance with as little as 400 mg/mo.

Pregnancy Prevention
IM (DEPO-PROVERA CONTRACEPTIVE): ADULTS: 150 mg q3mo.
SUBCUTANEOUS (DEPO-SUBQ-PROVERA 104): ADULTS: 104 mg q3mo (q12–14wk).

Endometriosis-Associated Pain
SUBCUTANEOUS (DEPO-SUBQ-PROVERA 104): ADULTS: 104 mg q3mo (q12–14 wks).

SIDE EFFECTS

Frequent: Transient menstrual abnormalities (spotting, change in menstrual flow/cervical secretions, amenorrhea) at initiation of therapy. **Occasional:** Edema, weight change, breast tenderness, anxiety, insomnia, fatigue, dizziness. **Rare:** Alopecia, depression, dermatologic changes, headache, fever, nausea.

ADVERSE EFFECTS/ TOXIC REACTIONS

Thrombophlebitis, pulmonary/cerebral embolism, retinal thrombosis occur rarely.

NURSING CONSIDERATIONS

BASELINE ASSESSMENT

Obtain usual menstrual history. Question for hypersensitivity to progestins, possibility of pregnancy before initiating therapy (Pregnancy Category X). Obtain baseline weight, serum glucose, B/P.

INTERVENTION/EVALUATION

Check weight daily; report weekly gain of 5 lb or more. Check B/P periodically. Assess skin for rash, urticaria. Report development of chest pain, sudden shortness of breath, sudden decrease in vision, migraine headache, pain (esp. with swelling, warmth, redness) in calves, numbness of arm/leg (thrombotic disorders) immediately.

PATIENT/FAMILY TEACHING

• Inform physician of sudden loss of vision, severe headache, chest pain, coughing up of blood (hemoptysis), numbness in arm/leg, severe pain/swelling in calf, unusual heavy vaginal bleeding, severe abdominal pain/tenderness. • Depo-Provera Contraceptive injection should be used as long-term birth control method (e.g., longer than 2 yrs) only if other birth control methods are inadequate.

megestrol HIGH ALERT

meh-**jess**-trol
(Apo-Megestrol ✤, Megace, Megace ES, Megace OS ✤)

◆ CLASSIFICATION

PHARMACOTHERAPEUTIC: Synthetic hormone. **CLINICAL:** Antineoplastic (see p. 86C).

ACTION

Suppresses release of luteinizing hormone (LH) from anterior pituitary gland by inhibiting pituitary function. **Therapeutic Effect:** Reduces tumor size. Increases appetite.

PHARMACOKINETICS

Well absorbed from GI tract. Metabolized in liver; excreted in urine. **Half-life:** 13–105 hrs (mean 34 hrs).

USES

Palliative management of recurrent, inoperable, metastatic endometrial or breast carcinoma. Treatment of anorexia, cachexia, unexplained significant weight loss in pts with AIDS. **OFF-LABEL:** Appetite stimulant, treatment of hormone-dependent or advanced prostate carcinoma, treatment of uterine bleeding.

M

PRECAUTIONS

Contraindications: **Suspension:** Known or suspected pregnancy. Cautions: History of thrombophlebitis.

LIFESPAN CONSIDERATIONS

Pregnancy/Lactation: If possible, avoid use during pregnancy, esp. first 4 mos. Breast-feeding not recommended. **Pregnancy Category D (tablets), X (suspension). Children:** Safety and efficacy not established. **Elderly:** No age-related precautions noted.

INTERACTIONS

DRUG: **Dofetilide** may increase risk of cardiotoxicity (QT prolongation, torsade de pointes, cardiac arrest). HERBAL: Avoid **black cohosh, dong quai** in estrogen-dependent tumors. FOOD: None known. LAB VALUES: May alter serum thyroid, hepatic function tests, PT, HDL, total cholesterol, triglycerides. May increase LDL.

M

AVAILABILITY (Rx)

Oral Suspension: 40 mg/ml (Megace), 125 mg/ml (Megace ES). Tablets (Megace): 20 mg, 40 mg.

ADMINISTRATION/HANDLING

PO

• Store tablets, oral suspension at room temperature. • Shake suspension well before use. • Administer without regard to food.

INDICATIONS/ROUTES/DOSAGE

Palliative Treatment of Advanced Breast Cancer

PO: ADULTS, ELDERLY: 160 mg/day in 4 equally divided doses.

Palliative Treatment of Advanced Endometrial Carcinoma

PO: ADULTS, ELDERLY: 40–320 mg/day in divided doses. **Maximum:** 800 mg/day in 1–4 divided doses.

Anorexia, Cachexia, Weight Loss

PO: ADULTS, ELDERLY: 800 mg (20 ml)/day.

PO (MEGACE ES): ADULTS, ELDERLY: 625 mg/day.

SIDE EFFECTS

Frequent: Weight gain secondary to increased appetite. Occasional: Nausea, breakthrough menstrual bleeding, backache, headache, breast tenderness, carpal tunnel syndrome. Rare: Feeling of coldness.

ADVERSE EFFECTS/ TOXIC REACTIONS

Thrombophlebitis, pulmonary embolism occur rarely.

NURSING CONSIDERATIONS

BASELINE ASSESSMENT

Question for possibility of pregnancy before initiating therapy (Pregnancy Category D [tablets]; X [suspension]). Provide support to pt, family, recognizing this drug is palliative, not curative.

INTERVENTION/EVALUATION

Monitor for tumor response. Monitor pt weight, caloric intake (appetite stimulant).

PATIENT/FAMILY TEACHING

• Contraception is imperative. • Report lower leg (calf) pain, difficulty breathing, vaginal bleeding. • May cause headache, nausea, vomiting, breast tenderness, backache.

melatonin

Also known as pineal hormone.

CLASSIFICATION

HERBAL: See Appendix G.

ACTION

Hormone synthesized endogenously by pineal gland. Interacts with melatonin receptors in brain. **Effect:** Regulates body's circadian rhythm, sleep patterns.

Acts as antioxidant, protecting cells from oxidative damage by free radicals.

USES

Treatment for ADHD, insomnia, jet lag. Used as an antioxidant.

PRECAUTIONS

Contraindications: Pregnancy or lactation. **Cautions:** Depression (may worsen dysphoria), seizures (may increase incidence), cardiovascular/hepatic disease.

LIFESPAN CONSIDERATIONS

Pregnancy/Lactation: Contraindicated. **Children:** Safety and efficacy not established. **Elderly:** No age-related precautions noted.

INTERACTIONS

DRUG: **Alcohol, benzodiazepines** may have additive effects. Melatonin may interfere with effects of **immunosuppressants.** May enhance effects of **isoniazid.** **HERBAL:** **Chamomile, ginseng, goldenseal, kava kava, valerian** may increase sedative effects. **FOOD:** None known. **LAB VALUES:** May increase human growth hormone levels. May decrease luteinizing hormone (LH) levels.

AVAILABILITY (OTC)

Lozenges: 3 mg. **Powder. Tablets:** 0.5 mg, 3 mg.

INDICATIONS/ROUTES/DOSAGE

Insomnia

PO: ADULTS, ELDERLY: 0.5–5 mg at bedtime.

Jet Lag

PO: ADULTS, ELDERLY: 5 mg/day beginning 3 days before flight and continuing until 3 days after flight.

SIDE EFFECTS

Headache, transient depression, fatigue, drowsiness, dizziness, abdominal cramps/irritability, decreased alertness, hypersensitivity reaction, tachycardia, nausea, vomiting, anorexia, altered sleep patterns, confusion.

ADVERSE EFFECTS/TOXIC REACTIONS

None known.

NURSING CONSIDERATIONS

BASELINE ASSESSMENT

Assess if pt is pregnant or breast-feeding (avoid use). Determine whether pt has history of seizures, depression. Assess sleep patterns if used for insomnia. Determine medication usage (esp. CNS depressants).

INTERVENTION/EVALUATION

Monitor effectiveness in improving insomnia. Assess for hypersensitivity reactions, CNS effects.

PATIENT/FAMILY TEACHING

• Do not use if pregnant, planning to become pregnant, breast-feeding. • Avoid tasks that require alertness, motor skills, until response to drug is established.

meloxicam

mel-**ocks**-ih-cam
(Apo-Meloxicam ✤, Mobic, Novo-Meloxicam ✤)

BLACK BOX ALERT Increased risk of serious cardiovascular thrombotic events, including myocardial infarction, CVA. Increased risk of severe GI reactions, including ulceration, bleeding, GI perforation.

CLASSIFICATION

PHARMACOTHERAPEUTIC: Nonsteroidal anti-inflammatory. **CLINICAL:** Anti-inflammatory, analgesic (see p. 128C).

ACTION

Produces analgesic, anti-inflammatory effects by inhibiting prostaglandin synthesis. **Therapeutic Effect:** Reduces inflammatory response, intensity of pain.

PHARMACOKINETICS

Route	Onset	Peak	Duration
PO (analgesic)	30 min	4–5 hrs	N/A

Well absorbed after PO administration. Protein binding: 99%. Metabolized in liver. Eliminated in urine, feces. Not removed by hemodialysis. **Half-life:** 15–20 hrs.

USES

Relief of signs/symptoms of osteoarthritis, rheumatoid arthritis (RA). Treatment of juvenile rheumatoid arthritis (JRA). **OFF-LABEL:** Ankylosing spondylitis.

PRECAUTIONS

Contraindications: Aspirin-induced nasal polyps associated with bronchospasm. **Cautions:** History of GI disease (e.g., ulcers), renal/hepatic impairment, CHF, dehydration, hypertension, asthma, hemostatic disease. Concurrent use of anticoagulants.

M

LIFESPAN CONSIDERATIONS

Pregnancy/Lactation: Distributed in breast milk. **Pregnancy Category C (D if used in third trimester or near delivery). Children:** Safety and efficacy not established. **Elderly:** Age-related renal impairment may require dosage adjustment. More susceptible to GI toxicity; lower dosage recommended.

INTERACTIONS

DRUG: **Aspirin** may increase risk of epigastric distress (heartburn, indigestion). May increase concentration, risk of toxicity of **lithium. HERBAL: Cat's claw, dong quai, evening primrose, feverfew, garlic, ginger, ginkgo, green tea, red clover, SAMe** may increase antiplatelet activity, risk of bleeding. **FOOD:** None known. **LAB VALUES:** May increase serum creatinine, AST, ALT.

AVAILABILITY (Rx)

Oral Suspension: 7.5 mg/5 ml. **Tablets:** 7.5 mg, 15 mg.

ADMINISTRATION/HANDLING

PO

- Give with food or milk to minimize GI irritation.

INDICATIONS/ROUTES/DOSAGE

Osteoarthritis, Rheumatoid Arthritis (RA)

PO: ADULTS, ELDERLY: Initially, 7.5 mg/day. **Maximum:** 15 mg/day.

Juvenile Rheumatoid Arthritis (JRA)

PO: CHILDREN, 2 YRS AND OLDER: 0.125 mg/kg once daily. **Maximum:** 7.5 mg.

SIDE EFFECTS

Frequent (9%–7%): Dyspepsia, headache, diarrhea, nausea. **Occasional (4%–3%):** Dizziness, insomnia, rash, pruritus, flatulence, constipation, vomiting. **Rare (less than 2%):** Drowsiness, urticaria, photosensitivity, tinnitus.

ADVERSE EFFECTS/ TOXIC REACTIONS

In those treated chronically, peptic ulcer, GI bleeding, gastritis, severe hepatic reaction (jaundice), nephrotoxicity (hematuria, dysuria, proteinuria), severe hypersensitivity reaction (bronchospasm, angioedema) occur rarely.

NURSING CONSIDERATIONS

BASELINE ASSESSMENT

Assess onset, type, location, duration of pain/inflammation. Inspect appearance of affected joints for immobility, deformities, skin condition.

INTERVENTION/EVALUATION

Monitor CBC, hepatic/renal function tests. Assess skin for petechiae. Assess for therapeutic response: relief of pain, stiffness, swelling; increased joint mobility; reduced joint tenderness; improved grip strength.

PATIENT/FAMILY TEACHING

• Take with food, milk to reduce GI upset. • Inform physician of tinnitus, persistent abdominal pain/cramping, severe nausea/vomiting, difficulty breathing, unusual bruising/bleeding, rash, peripheral edema, chest pain, palpitations.

melphalan

HIGH ALERT

mel-fah-lan
(Alkeran, Alkeran IV)

BLACK BOX ALERT Myelosuppression is common. Potentially mutagenic, leukemogenic. Hypersensitivity noted with IV administration. Must be administered by certified chemotherapy personnel.

Do not confuse Alkeran with Leukeran or Myleran, or melphalan with Mephyton or Myleran.

◆ CLASSIFICATION

PHARMACOTHERAPEUTIC: Alkylating agent. **CLINICAL:** Antineoplastic (see p. 86C).

ACTION

Inhibits protein synthesis primarily by cross-linking strands of DNA, RNA. Cell cycle–phase nonspecific. **Therapeutic Effect:** Disrupts nucleic acid function producing cell death.

PHARMACOKINETICS

Oral administration is highly variable. Incomplete intestinal absorption, variable first-pass metabolism, rapid hydrolysis may result. Protein binding: 60%–90%. Extensively metabolized in blood. Eliminated from plasma primarily by chemical hydrolysis. Partially excreted in feces; minimal elimination in urine. **Half-life: PO:** 1–1.25 hrs. **IV:** 1.5 hrs.

USES

Treatment of epithelial ovarian carcinoma, multiple myeloma. **OFF-LABEL:** Treatment of breast, endometrial, testicular carcinoma; chronic myelocytic leukemia, Hodgkin's lymphoma, malignant melanoma, neuroblastoma, rhabdomyosarcoma, induction regimen for bone marrow and stem cell transplantation.

PRECAUTIONS

Contraindications: Pregnancy, severe myelosuppression. **Cautions:** Leukocyte count less than 3,000/mm^3 or platelet count less than 100,000/mm^3, bone marrow suppression, renal impairment.

⧗ LIFESPAN CONSIDERATIONS

Pregnancy/Lactation: May cause fetal harm. Unknown if distributed in breast milk. **Pregnancy Category D. Children:** Safety and efficacy not established. **Elderly:** Age-related renal impairment may require dosage adjustment.

INTERACTIONS

DRUG: Bone marrow depressants may increase myelosuppression. **Live virus vaccines** may potentiate virus replication, increase vaccine side effects, decrease pt's antibody response to vaccine. **HERBAL:** None significant. **FOOD:** None known. **LAB VALUES:** May increase serum uric acid.

AVAILABILITY (Rx)

Injection, Powder for Reconstitution (Alkeran IV): 50 mg. **Tablets (Alkeran):** 2 mg.

ADMINISTRATION/HANDLING

IV

Reconstitution • Reconstitute 50-mg vial with diluent supplied by manufacturer to yield 5 mg/ml solution. • Further dilute with 0.9% NaCl to final concentration not exceeding 2 mg/ml (central line) or 0.45 mg/ml (peripheral line).

Rate of administration • Infuse over 15–30 min at rate not to exceed 10 mg/min (total infusion should be administered within 1 hr).

Storage • Store at room temperature; protect from light. • Once reconstituted, stable for 90 min at room temperature (do not refrigerate).

PO

• Store tablets in refrigerator; protect from light. • Give on empty stomach (1 hr before or 2 hrs after meals).

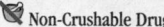

M

IV INCOMPATIBILITIES

Amphotericin B complex (Abelcet, AmBisome, Amphotec).

IV COMPATIBILITIES

Acyclovir, dexamethasone (Decadron), famotidine (Pepcid), furosemide (Lasix), lorazepam (Ativan), morphine.

INDICATIONS/ROUTES/DOSAGE

Ovarian Carcinoma

PO: ADULTS, ELDERLY: 0.2 mg/kg/day for 5 successive days. Repeat at 4- to 5-wk intervals.

Multiple Myeloma

PO: ADULTS: Initially, 6 mg once a day for 2–3 wks, followed by up to 4 wks rest, then maintenance dose of 2 mg daily; or 0.15 mg/kg/day for 7 days with 2–6 wks rest, then maintenance dose of 0.05 mg/kg/day; or 0.25 mg/kg/day for 4 days, repeat at 4- to 6-wk intervals.

IV: ADULTS: 16 mg/m^2/dose every 2 wks for 4 doses, then repeat monthly according to protocol.

Dosage in Renal Impairment

PO, IV: BUN LEVEL GREATER THAN 30 MG/DL: Decrease melphalan dosage by 50%. **SERUM CREATININE LEVEL GREATER THAN 1.5 MG/DL:** Decrease melphalan dosage by 50%.

SIDE EFFECTS

Frequent: Nausea, vomiting (may be severe with large dose). **Occasional:** Diarrhea, stomatitis, rash, pruritus, alopecia.

ADVERSE EFFECTS/ TOXIC REACTIONS

Myelosuppression manifested as hematologic toxicity (principally leukopenia, thrombocytopenia, and, to lesser extent, anemia, pancytopenia, agranulocytosis). Leukopenia may occur as early as 5 days after drug initiation. WBC, platelet counts return to normal during 5th wk after therapy, but leukopenia, thrombocytopenia may last more than 6 wks after discontinuing drug. Hyperuricemia noted by hematuria, crystalluria, flank pain.

NURSING CONSIDERATIONS

BASELINE ASSESSMENT

Obtain CBC weekly. Dosage may be decreased or discontinued if WBC falls below 3,000/mm^3 or platelet count falls below 100,000/mm^3. Antiemetics may be effective in preventing/treating nausea, vomiting.

INTERVENTION/EVALUATION

Monitor CBC with diffferential, platelet count, serum electrolytes, Hgb. Monitor for stomatitis. Monitor for hematologic toxicity (fever, sore throat, signs of local infection, unusual bruising/bleeding from any site), symptoms of anemia (excessive fatigue, weakness), signs of hyperuricemia (hematuria, flank pain). Avoid IM injections, rectal temperatures, other traumas that may induce bleeding.

PATIENT/FAMILY TEACHING

• Increase fluid intake (may protect against hyperuricemia). • Maintain fastidious oral hygiene. • Alopecia is reversible, but new hair growth may have different color, texture. • Avoid crowds, those with infections. • Inform physician if fever, shortness of breath, cough, sore throat, bleeding, bruising occurs.

memantine

meh-**man**-teen
(Ebixa, Namenda, Namenda XR)

CLASSIFICATION

PHARMACOTHERAPEUTIC: Neurotransmitter inhibitor. **CLINICAL:** Anti-Alzheimer's agent.

ACTION

Decreases effects of glutamate, the principal excitatory neurotransmitter in the brain. Persistent CNS excitation by glutamate is thought to cause symptoms of Alzheimer's disease. **Therapeutic Effect:** May inhibit clinical deterioration in moderate to severe Alzheimer's disease.

PHARMACOKINETICS

Rapidly, completely absorbed after PO administration. Protein binding: 45%. Undergoes little metabolism; most of dose is excreted unchanged in urine. **Half-life:** 60–80 hrs.

USES

Treatment of moderate to severe dementia of Alzheimer's type. **OFF-LABEL:** Treatment of mild to moderate vascular disease, mild cognitive impairment, migraine headaches.

PRECAUTIONS

Contraindications: Severe renal impairment. **Cautions:** Moderate renal impairment, seizure disorder, GU conditions that raise urine pH level.

LIFESPAN CONSIDERATIONS

Pregnancy/Lactation: Unknown if drug crosses placenta or is distributed in breast milk. **Pregnancy Category B. Children:** Not prescribed for this pt population. **Elderly:** No age-related precautions noted, but use is not recommended in those with severe renal impairment (creatinine clearance less than 9 ml/min).

INTERACTIONS

DRUG: **Carbonic anhydrase inhibitors, sodium bicarbonate** may decrease renal elimination of memantine. **Cimetidine, hydrochlorothiazide, nicotine, quinidine, ranitidine** may alter plasma levels. **HERBAL:** None significant. **FOOD:** None known. **LAB VALUES:** None significant.

AVAILABILITY (Rx)

Oral Solution: 2 mg/ml. **Tablets:** 5 mg, 10 mg.

Capsules (Extended-Release [Namenda XR]): 7 mg, 14 mg, 21 mg, 28 mg.

ADMINISTRATION/HANDLING

PO

• Give without regard to food. • Administer oral solution using syringe provided. Do not dilute or mix with other fluids. • Do not divide, chew, or crush. Swallow extended-release capsules whole. May open capsule and sprinkle on applesauce.

INDICATIONS/ROUTES/DOSAGE

Alzheimer's Disease

PO: ADULTS, ELDERLY (Immediate-Release): Initially, 5 mg once a day. May increase dosage at intervals of at least 1 wk in 5-mg increments to 10 mg/day (5 mg twice a day), then 15 mg/day (5 mg and 10 mg as separate doses), and finally 20 mg/day (10 mg twice a day). Target dose: 20 mg/day. **(Extended-Release):** Initially, 7 mg once daily. May increase at intervals of at least 7 days in increments of 7 mg. **Maximum:** 28 mg once daily. Switching from immediate-release to extended-release: Begin the day following last dose of immediate release.

10 mg twice a day: 28 mg once daily.
5 mg twice a day: 14 mg once daily.

Dosage in Renal Impairment

Creatinine Clearance	Dosage: Immediate-Release	Dosage: Extended-Release
30 ml/min or greater	No adjustments	No adjustments
5–29 ml/min	5 mg twice daily	14 mg once daily

SIDE EFFECTS

Occasional (7%–4%): Dizziness, headache, confusion, constipation, hypertension, cough. **Rare (3%–2%):** Back pain, nausea, fatigue, anxiety, peripheral edema, arthralgia, insomnia.

ADVERSE EFFECTS/ TOXIC REACTIONS

None known.

NURSING CONSIDERATIONS

BASELINE ASSESSMENT

Assess cognitive, behavioral, functional deficits of pt. Assess renal function.

INTERVENTION/EVALUATION

Monitor cognitive, behavioral, functional status of pt. Monitor urine pH (alterations of urine pH toward the alkaline condition may lead to accumulation of the drug with possible increase in side effects). Monitor BUN, creatinine clearance lab values.

PATIENT/FAMILY TEACHING

• Do not reduce or stop medication; do not increase dosage without physician direction. • Ensure adequate fluid intake. • If therapy is interrupted for several days, restart at lowest dose, titrate to current dose at minimum of 1-wk intervals. • Local chapter of Alzheimer's Disease Association can provide a guide to services.

meperidine

HIGH ALERT

me-**per**-i-deen
(Demerol)

Do not confuse Demerol with Demulen, Desyrel, Dilaudid, or Pamelor, or meperidine with meprobamate.

◆CLASSIFICATION

PHARMACOTHERAPEUTIC: Narcotic agonist. **CLINICAL:** Opiate analgesic **(Schedule II)** (see p. 142C).

ACTION

Binds to opioid receptors within CNS. **Therapeutic Effect:** Alters pain perception, emotional response to pain.

PHARMACOKINETICS

Route	Onset	Peak	Duration
PO	15 min	120 min	2–4 hrs
IV	Less than 5 min	5–7 min	2–3 hrs
IM	10–15 min	30–50 min	2–4 hrs
Subcutaneous	10–15 min	60 min	2–4 hrs

Variably absorbed from GI tract; absorption erratic and highly variable after IM administration. Protein binding: 15%–30%. Widely distributed. Metabolized in liver to active metabolite. Primarily excreted in urine. Not removed by hemodialysis. **Half-life:** 2.4–4 hrs; metabolite, 15–30 hrs (increased in hepatic impairment/disease).

USES

Relief of moderate to severe pain. **OFF-LABEL:** Reduces postop shivering. Reduces rigors from amphotericin.

PRECAUTIONS

Contraindications: Delivery of premature infant, diarrhea due to poisoning, use of MAOIs within 14 days. **Cautions:** Renal/hepatic impairment, elderly, debilitated, supraventricular tachycardia, cor pulmonale, history of seizures, acute abdominal conditions, increased intracranial pressure (ICP), respiratory abnormalities.

⌛ LIFESPAN CONSIDERATIONS

Pregnancy/Lactation: Crosses placenta. Distributed in breast milk. Respiratory depression may occur in neonate if mother received opiates during labor. Regular use of opiates during pregnancy may produce withdrawal symptoms in neonate (irritability, excessive crying, tremors, hyperactive reflexes, fever, vomiting, diarrhea, yawning, sneezing, seizures). **Pregnancy Category B (D if used for prolonged periods or at high dosages at term). Children:** Paradoxical excitement may occur. Those younger than 2 yrs more susceptible to respiratory depressant effects. **Elderly:** More susceptible to respiratory depressant effects. Age-related renal impairment may increase risk of urinary retention.

INTERACTIONS

DRUG: **Alcohol, other CNS depressants** may increase CNS, respiratory depression, hypotension. **MAOIs** may produce severe, sometimes fatal reaction; meperidine use is contraindicated. HERBAL: **Gotu kola, kava kava, St. John's wort, valerian** may increase CNS depression, sedation. FOOD: None known. LAB VALUES: May increase serum amylase, lipase. **Therapeutic serum level:** 100–550 ng/ml; **toxic serum level:** greater than 1,000 ng/ml.

AVAILABILITY (Rx)

Injection, Solution: 25 mg/ml, 50 mg/ml, 75 mg/ml, 100 mg/ml. Injection, Solution (Patient-Controlled Analgesia [PCA]): 10 mg/ml. Syrup (Demerol): 50 mg/5 ml. Tablets (Demerol): 50 mg, 100 mg.

ADMINISTRATION/HANDLING

IV

Reconstitution • May give undiluted or dilute in D_5W, dextrose-saline combination (2.5%, 5%, 10% dextrose in water—0.45%, 0.9% NaCl), Ringer's, lactated Ringer's, molar sodium lactate diluent for IV injection or infusion.

Rate of administration • IV dosage must always be administered very slowly, over 2–3 min. • Rapid IV increases risk of severe adverse reactions (chest wall rigidity, apnea, peripheral circulatory collapse, anaphylactoid effects, cardiac arrest).

Storage • Store at room temperature.

IM, Subcutaneous

◀ALERT▶ IM preferred over subcutaneous route (subcutaneous produces pain, local irritation, induration). • Administer slowly. • Those with circulatory impairment at higher risk for overdosage due to delayed absorption of repeated administration.

PO

• Give without regard to meals. • Dilute syrup in glass of water (prevents anesthetic effect on mucous membranes).

IV INCOMPATIBILITIES

Allopurinol (Aloprim), amphotericin B complex (Abelcet, AmBisome, Amphotec), cefepime (Maxipime), cefoperazone (Cefobid), doxorubicin liposomal (Doxil), furosemide (Lasix), heparin, idarubicin (Idamycin), nafcillin (Nafcil), phenytoin (Dilantin), sodium bicarbonate.

IV COMPATIBILITIES

Atropine, bumetanide (Bumex), diltiazem (Cardizem), diphenhydramine (Benadryl), dobutamine (Dobutrex), dopamine (Intropin), glycopyrrolate (Robinul), hydroxyzine (Vistaril), insulin, lidocaine, lipids, magnesium, midazolam (Versed), oxytocin (Pitocin), potassium, total parenteral nutrition (TPN).

INDICATIONS/ROUTES/DOSAGE

Analgesia

IV: ADULTS: 5–25 mg q2–4h as needed. CHILDREN: 1–1.5 mg/kg/dose q3–4h as needed.

IM, SUBCUTANEOUS: ADULTS: 50–75 mg q3–4h as needed. ELDERLY: 25 mg q4h as needed. CHILDREN: 1–1.5 mg/kg/dose q3–4h as needed.

PO: ADULTS: 50 mg q3–4h as needed. Range: 50–150 mg q2–4h as needed. ELDERLY: 50 mg q4h as needed. CHILDREN: 1–1.5 mg/kg/dose q3–4h as needed.

Patient-Controlled Analgesia (PCA)

IV: ADULTS: **Initial dose:** 10 mg. **Demand dose:** 5–25 mg. **Lockout Interval:** 5–10 min.

Dosage in Renal Impairment

Avoid use in renal impairment.

SIDE EFFECTS

Frequent: Sedation, hypotension (including orthostatic hypotension), diaphoresis, facial flushing, dizziness, nausea, vomit-

M

ing, constipation. **Occasional:** Confusion, arrhythmias, tremors, urinary retention, abdominal pain, dry mouth, headache, irritation at injection site, euphoria, dysphoria. **Rare:** Allergic reaction (rash, pruritus), insomnia.

ADVERSE EFFECTS/ TOXIC REACTIONS

Overdose results in respiratory depression, skeletal muscle flaccidity, cold/clammy skin, cyanosis, extreme drowsiness progressing to seizures, stupor, coma. **Antidote:** 0.4 mg naloxone (Narcan). Tolerance to analgesic effect, physical dependence may occur with repeated use.

NURSING CONSIDERATIONS

BASELINE ASSESSMENT

Pt should be in recumbent position before drug is administered by parenteral route. Assess onset, type, location, duration of pain. Obtain vital signs before giving medication. If respirations are 12/min or less (20/min or less in children), withhold medication, contact physician. Effect of medication is reduced if full pain recurs before next dose.

INTERVENTION/EVALUATION

Monitor vital signs 15–30 min after subcutaneous/IM dose, 5–10 min after IV dose (monitor for hypotension, change in rate/quality of pulse). Monitor pain level, sedation response. Monitor daily pattern of bowel activity, stool consistency; avoid constipation. Check for adequate voiding. Initiate deep breathing, coughing exercises, particularly in pts with pulmonary impairment. **Therapeutic serum level:** 100–550 ng/ml; **toxic serum level:** greater than 1,000 ng/ml.

PATIENT/FAMILY TEACHING

• Medication should be taken before pain fully returns, within ordered intervals. • Discomfort may occur with injection. • Change positions slowly to avoid orthostatic hypotension. • Increase fluids, bulk to prevent constipation. • Tolerance, dependence may occur with prolonged use of high doses. • Avoid alcohol, other CNS depressants. • Avoid tasks requiring mental alertness, motor skills until response to drug is established.

meropenem

mer-oh-**pen**-em
(Merrem IV)
Do not confuse meropenem with doripenem, ertapenem, or imipenem.

◆CLASSIFICATION

PHARMACOTHERAPEUTIC: Carbapenem. **CLINICAL:** Antibiotic.

ACTION

Binds to penicillin-binding proteins. Inhibits bacterial cell wall synthesis. **Therapeutic Effect:** Bactericidal.

PHARMACOKINETICS

After IV administration, widely distributed into tissues and body fluids, including CSF. Protein binding: 2%. Primarily excreted unchanged in urine. Removed by hemodialysis. **Half-life:** 1 hr.

USES

Treatment of intra-abdominal infections caused by *viridans group streptococci, E. coli, K. pneumoniae, P. aeruginosa, B. fragilis*, peptostreptococcus spp.; bacterial meningitis caused by *S. pneumoniae, H. influenzae, N. meningitidis*. **OFF-LABEL:** Lower respiratory tract infections, febrile neutropenia, gynecologic/obstetric infections, sepsis.

PRECAUTIONS

Contraindications: History of seizures, CNS abnormality, hypersensitivity to penicillins. **Cautions:** Hypersensitivity to penicillins, cephalosporins, other allergens; renal impairment; CNS disorders, particularly with history of seizures, concurrent probenecid use.

LIFESPAN CONSIDERATIONS

Pregnancy/Lactation: Unknown if distributed in breast milk. **Pregnancy Category B. Children:** Safety and efficacy not established in those younger than 3 mos. **Elderly:** Age-related renal impairment may require dosage adjustment.

INTERACTIONS

DRUG: None significant. **HERBAL:** None significant. **FOOD:** None known. **LAB VALUES:** May increase BUN, serum alkaline phosphatase, LDH, AST, ALT, bilirubin. May decrease Hgb, Hct, WBC.

AVAILABILITY (Rx)

Injection, Powder for Reconstitution: 500 mg, 1 g.

ADMINISTRATION/HANDLING

IV

Reconstitution • Reconstitute each 500 mg with 10 ml Sterile Water for Injection, 0.9% NaCl, or D_5W to provide concentration of 50 mg/ml. • Shake to dissolve until clear. • May further dilute with 0.9% NaCl or D_5W to a concentration of 1–20 mg/ml.

Rate of administration • May give by IV push or IV intermittent infusion (piggyback). • If administering as IV intermittent infusion (piggyback), give over 15–30 min (at a concentration of 1–20 mg/ml); if administered by IV push, give over 3–5 min (at a concentration not greater than 50 mg/ml).

Storage • Store vials at room temperature. • After reconstitution of vials with 0.9% NaCl, stable for 2 hrs at room temperature or 18 hrs if refrigerated (with D_5W, stable for 1 hr at room temperature, 8 hrs if refrigerated). IV infusion with 0.9% NaCl stable for 4 hrs at room temperature or 24 hrs if refrigerated (with D_5W, 1 hr at room temperature or 4 hrs if refrigerated).

IV INCOMPATIBILITIES

Acyclovir (Zovirax), amphotericin B (Fungizone), diazepam (Valium), doxycycline (Vibramycin), metronidazole (Flagyl), ondansetron (Zofran).

IV COMPATIBILITIES

Dexamethasone (Decadron), dobutamine (Dobutrex), dopamine (Intropin), furosemide (Lasix), heparin, lipids, magnesium, morphine.

INDICATIONS/ROUTES/DOSAGE

Usual Dosage

IV: ADULTS, ELDERLY: 1.5–6 g/day in divided doses q8h. **CHILDREN 3 MOS AND OLDER:** 30–120 mg/kg/day in divided doses q8h. **Maximum:** 6 g/day. **NEONATES:** 20 mg/kg/dose q8–12h.

Meningitis

IV: ADULTS, ELDERLY, CHILDREN WEIGHING 50 KG OR MORE: 2 g q8h. **CHILDREN 3 MOS AND OLDER WEIGHING LESS THAN 50 KG:** 40 mg/kg q8h. **Maximum:** 2 g/dose.

Dosage in Renal Impairment

Dosage and frequency are modified based on creatinine clearance.

Creatinine Clearance	Dosage	Interval
26–49 ml/min	Normal dose (1,000 mg)	q12h
10–25 ml/min	50% of normal dose	q12h
Less than 10 ml/min	50% of normal dose	q24h

SIDE EFFECTS

Frequent (5%–3%): Diarrhea, nausea, vomiting, headache, inflammation at injection site. **Occasional (2%):** Oral candidiasis, rash, pruritus. **Rare (less than 2%):** Constipation, glossitis.

ADVERSE EFFECTS/ TOXIC REACTIONS

Antibiotic-associated colitis, other superinfections (abdominal cramps, severe watery diarrhea, fever) may result from altered bacterial balance. Anaphylactic reactions have been reported. Seizures may occur in those with CNS disorders (e.g., brain lesions, history of seizures), bacterial meningitis, renal impairment.

NURSING CONSIDERATIONS

BASELINE ASSESSMENT

Inquire about history of seizures.

INTERVENTION/EVALUATION

Monitor daily pattern of bowel activity, stool consistency. Monitor for nausea, vomiting. Evaluate for inflammation at IV injection site. Assess skin for rash. Evaluate hydration status. Monitor I&O, renal/hepatic function tests. Check mental status; be alert to tremors, possible seizures. Assess temperature, B/P twice a day, more often if necessary. Monitor serum electrolytes, esp. potassium.

PATIENT/FAMILY TEACHING

- Inform physician of persistent diarrhea, abdominal cramps, fever.

M

Merrem IV, *see meropenem*

mesalamine (5-aminosalicylic acid, 5-ASA)

mes-**al**-a-meen
(Apriso, Asacol, Canasa, Lialda, Mesasal ❋, Pentasa, Rowasa, Salofalk ❋)

Do not confuse Asacol with Os-Cal, Lialda with Aldara, or mesalamine with megestrol, memantine, or methenamine.

◆CLASSIFICATION

PHARMACOTHERAPEUTIC: Salicylic acid derivative. **CLINICAL:** Anti-inflammatory agent.

ACTION

Locally inhibits arachidonic acid metabolite production (increased in chronic inflammatory bowel disease). **Therapeutic Effect:** Blocks prostaglandin production, diminishes inflammation in colon.

PHARMACOKINETICS

Poorly absorbed from colon. Moderately absorbed from GI tract. Metabolized in liver to active metabolite. Unabsorbed portion eliminated in feces; absorbed portion excreted in urine. Unknown if removed by hemodialysis. **Half-life:** 0.5–1.5 hrs; metabolite, 5–10 hrs.

USES

PO: Treatment, maintenance of remission of mild to moderate active ulcerative colitis. **Rectal:** Treatment of active mild to moderate distal ulcerative colitis, proctosigmoiditis or proctitis.

PRECAUTIONS

Contraindications: None known. **Cautions:** Preexisting renal disease, sulfasalazine sensitivity.

⌛ LIFESPAN CONSIDERATIONS

Pregnancy/Lactation: Unknown if drug crosses placenta or is distributed in breast milk. **Pregnancy Category B. Children:** Safety and efficacy not established. **Elderly:** Age-related renal impairment may require dosage adjustment.

INTERACTIONS

DRUG: None significant. **HERBAL:** None significant. **FOOD:** None known. **LAB VALUES:** May increase serum alkaline phosphatase, AST, ALT, bilirubin.

AVAILABILITY (Rx)

Rectal Suspension (Rowasa): 4 g/60 ml. **Suppositories (Canasa):** 1 g.

Capsules (Controlled-Release [Pentasa]): 250 mg, 500 mg. **Capsules (Extended-Release [Apriso]):** 375 mg. **Tablets (Delayed-Release [Asacol]):** 400 mg. **(Lialda):** 1.2 g.

ADMINISTRATION/HANDLING

◀ALERT▶ Store rectal suspension, suppository, oral forms at room temperature.

PO

• Have pt swallow whole; do not break outer coating of tablet. • Give without regard to food. **Apriso:** Do not administer with antacids. **Lialda:** Administer once daily with meal.

Rectal

• Shake bottle well. • Instruct pt to lie on left side with lower leg extended, upper leg flexed forward. • Knee-chest position may also be used. • Insert applicator tip into rectum, pointing toward umbilicus. • Squeeze bottle steadily until contents are emptied. • Store suppositories at room temperature. Do not refrigerate.

INDICATIONS/ROUTES/DOSAGE

Treatment of Ulcerative Colitis

PO (CAPSULE [PENTASA]): ADULTS, ELDERLY: 1 g 4 times a day. **CHILDREN:** 50 mg/kg/day divided q6–12h.
PO (TABLET [ASACOL]): ADULTS, ELDERLY: 800 mg 3 times a day. **CHILDREN:** 50 mg/kg/day divided q8–12h.
PO (TABLET [LIALDA]): ADULTS, ELDERLY: 2.4–4.8 g once daily.

Maintenance of Remission in Ulcerative Colitis

PO (CAPSULE [PENTASA]): ADULTS, ELDERLY: 1 g 4 times a day.
PO (CAPSULE, EXTENDED-RELEASE [APRISO]): ADULTS, ELDERLY: 1,500 mg once daily.
PO (TABLET [ASACOL]): ADULTS, ELDERLY: 1.6 g/day in divided doses.

Distal Ulcerative Colitis, Proctosigmoiditis, Proctitis

◀ALERT▶ Suppository should be retained for 1–3 hrs for maximum benefit.
RECTAL (RETENTION ENEMA): ADULTS, ELDERLY: 60 ml (4 g) at bedtime; retained overnight for approximately 8 hrs for 3–6 wks.
RECTAL (1 G SUPPOSITORY): ADULTS, ELDERLY: Once daily at bedtime. Continue therapy for 3–6 wks.

SIDE EFFECTS

Mesalamine is generally well tolerated, with only mild, transient effects. **Frequent (greater than 6%): PO:** Abdominal cramps/pain, diarrhea, dizziness, headache, nausea, vomiting, rhinitis, unusual fatigue. **Rectal:** Abdominal/stomach cramps, flatulence, headache, nausea. **Occasional (6%–2%): PO:** Hair loss, decreased appetite, back/joint pain, flatulence, acne. **Rectal:** Hair loss. **Rare (less than 2%): Rectal:** Anal irritation.

ADVERSE EFFECTS/ TOXIC REACTIONS

Sulfite sensitivity may occur in susceptible pts, manifested as cramping, headache, diarrhea, fever, rash, urticaria, pruritus, wheezing. Discontinue drug immediately. Hepatitis, pancreatitis, pericarditis occur rarely with oral forms.

NURSING CONSIDERATIONS

INTERVENTION/EVALUATION

Encourage adequate fluid intake. Assess bowel sounds for peristalsis. Monitor daily pattern of bowel activity, stool consistency; record time of evacuation. Assess for abdominal disturbances. Assess skin for rash, urticaria. Discontinue medication if rash, fever, cramping, diarrhea occurs.

PATIENT/FAMILY TEACHING

• Report rash, fever, abdominal pain, significant diarrhea to physician. • Avoid tasks that require alertness, motor skills until response to drug is established. • May discolor urine yellow-brown. • Suppositories stain fabrics.

mesna

mess-na
(Mesnex, Uromitexan ✱)

M

CLASSIFICATION

PHARMACOTHERAPEUTIC: Cytoprotective agent. **CLINICAL:** Antineoplastic adjunct, antidote.

ACTION

Binds with, detoxifies urotoxic metabolites of ifosfamide/cyclophosphamide. **Therapeutic Effect:** Inhibits ifosfamide/cyclophosphamide-induced hemorrhagic cystitis.

PHARMACOKINETICS

Rapidly metabolized after IV administration to mesna disulfide, which is reduced to mesna in kidneys. Protein binding. 69%–75%. Excreted in urine. **Half-life:** 24 min; metabolite: 72 min.

USES

Detoxifying agent used as protectant against hemorrhagic cystitis induced by ifosfamide. **OFF-LABEL:** Reduce incidence of cyclophosphamide-induced hemorrhagic cystitis.

M

PRECAUTIONS

Contraindications: None known. **Cautions:** None known.

LIFESPAN CONSIDERATIONS

Pregnancy/Lactation: Unknown if drug crosses placenta or is distributed in breast milk. **Pregnancy Category B. Children:** Safety and efficacy not established. **Elderly:** Information not available.

INTERACTIONS

DRUG: None significant. **HERBAL:** None significant. **FOOD:** None known. **LAB VALUES:** May produce false-positive test result for urinary ketones.

AVAILABILITY (Rx)

Injection Solution: 100 mg/ml. **Tablets:** 400 mg.

ADMINISTRATION/HANDLING

IV

Reconstitution • May dilute with D_5W or 0.9% NaCl to concentration of 1–20 mg/ml. • May add to solutions containing ifosfamide or cyclophosphamide.

Rate of administration • Administer by IV infusion over 15–30 min or by continuous infusion.

Storage • Store parenteral form at room temperature. • After dilution, in 0.9% NaCl or D_5W, stable for 48 hrs at room temperature (solutions of mesna and cyclophosphamide in D_5W stable for 48 hrs if refrigerated or 6 hrs at room temperature). Discard unused medication.

PO

• Administer orally in either tablet formulation or parenteral solution. • Dilute mesna solution before PO administration to decrease sulfur odor. Can be diluted (1:1 to 1:10) in carbonated cola drinks, fruit juices, milk.

IV INCOMPATIBILITIES

Amphotericin B complex (Abelcet, AmBisome, Amphotec), cisplatin (Platinol).

IV COMPATIBILITIES

Allopurinol (Aloprim), docetaxel (Taxotere), doxorubicin (Adriamycin), etoposide (VePesid), gemcitabine (Gemzar), granisetron (Kytril), lipids, methotrexate, ondansetron (Zofran), paclitaxel (Taxol), vinorelbine (Navelbine).

INDICATIONS/ROUTES/DOSAGE

Prevention of Hemorrhagic Cystitis in Pts Receiving Ifosfamide

IV: ADULTS, ELDERLY: 20% of ifosfamide dose at time of ifosfamide administration and 4 and 8 hrs after each dose of ifosfamide. Total dose: 60% of ifosfamide dosage. Range: 60%–160% of the daily ifosfamide dose.

IV/PO: 100% of ifosfamide dose, given as 20% at start time followed by 40% given orally 2 and 6 hrs after start of ifosfamide.

SIDE EFFECTS

Frequent (greater than 17%): Altered taste, soft stools. **Large doses:** Diarrhea, myalgia, headache, fatigue, nausea, hypotension, allergic reaction.

ADVERSE EFFECTS/ TOXIC REACTIONS

Hematuria occurs rarely.

NURSING CONSIDERATIONS

BASELINE ASSESSMENT

◀ALERT▶ Each dose must be administered with ifosfamide therapy.

INTERVENTION/EVALUATION

Assess morning urine specimen for hematuria. If such occurs, dosage reduction or discontinuation may be necessary. Monitor daily pattern of bowel activity, stool consistency; record time of evacuation. Monitor B/P for hypotension.

PATIENT/FAMILY TEACHING

- Inform physician if headache, myalgia, nausea occurs.

Metamucil, *see psyllium*

metaproterenol

met-a-proe-**ter**-e-nole
(Alupent, Apo-Orciprenaline ✤)
Do not confuse metaproterenol with metipranolol or metoprolol, or Alupent with Atrovent.

◆ CLASSIFICATION

PHARMACOTHERAPEUTIC: Sympathomimetic (an adrenergic agonist). **CLINICAL:** Bronchodilator.

ACTION

Stimulates $beta_2$-adrenergic receptors, resulting in relaxation of bronchial smooth muscle. **Therapeutic Effect:** Relieves bronchospasm, reduces airway resistance.

PHARMACOKINETICS

Systemic absorption is rapid following aerosol administration; however, serum concentrations at recommended doses are very low. Metabolized in liver. Excreted in urine primarily as glucoside metabolite. **Half-life:** Unknown.

USES

Treatment of reversible airway obstruction caused by asthma, COPD.

PRECAUTIONS

Contraindications: Narrow-angle glaucoma, preexisting arrhythmias associated with tachycardia. **Cautions:** Ischemic heart disease, hypertension, hyperthyroidism, seizure disorder, CHF, diabetes, arrhythmias.

⌛ LIFESPAN CONSIDERATIONS

Pregnancy/Lactation: Unknown if drug crosses placenta or is distributed in breast milk. **Pregnancy Category C. Children:** Safety and efficacy not established. **Elderly:** No age-related precautions noted.

INTERACTIONS

DRUG: May decrease effects of **beta-blockers. Digoxin, other sympathomimetics** may increase risk of arrhythmias. **MAOIs** may increase risk of hypertensive crisis. **Tricyclic antidepressants** may increase cardiovascular effects. **HERBAL:** None significant. **FOOD:** None known. **LAB VALUES:** May decrease serum potassium. May increase serum glucose.

AVAILABILITY (Rx)

Aerosol Oral Inhalation: 0.65 mg/inhalation. **Solution for Nebulization:** 0.4%, 0.6%. **Syrup:** 10 mg/5 ml. **Tablets:** 10 mg, 20 mg.

INDICATIONS/ROUTES/DOSAGE

Treatment of Bronchospasm

PO: ADULTS, CHILDREN 10 YRS AND OLDER: 20 mg 3–4 times a day. **ELDERLY:** 10 mg 3–4 times a day. May increase to 20 mg/dose. **CHILDREN 6–9 YRS:** 10 mg 3–4 times a day. **CHILDREN 2–5 YRS:** 1–2.6 mg/kg/day in 3–4 divided doses. **CHILDREN YOUNGER THAN 2 YRS:** 0.4 mg/kg/dose 3–4 times a day.

M

ORAL INHALATION: ADULTS, ELDERLY, CHILDREN 12 YRS AND OLDER: 2–3 inhalations q3–4h. **Maximum:** 12 inhalations/24 hrs.
NEBULIZATION: ADULTS, ELDERLY, CHILDREN 12 YRS AND OLDER: 10–15 mg (0.2–0.3 ml) of 5% q4–6h. **CHILDREN YOUNGER THAN 12 YRS, INFANTS:** 0.5–1 mg/kg (0.01–0.02 ml/kg) of 5% q4–6h. **Minimum dose:** 0.1 ml. **Maximum dose:** 0.3 ml.

SIDE EFFECTS

Frequent (greater than 10%): Rigors, tremors, anxiety, nausea, dry mouth. **Occasional (9%–1%):** Dizziness, vertigo, asthenia (loss of strength, energy), headache, GI distress, vomiting, cough, dry throat. **Rare (less than 1%):** Drowsiness, diarrhea, altered taste.

ADVERSE EFFECTS/ TOXIC REACTIONS

Excessive sympathomimetic stimulation may cause palpitations, extrasystoles, tachycardia, chest pain, slight increase in B/P followed by substantial decrease, chills, diaphoresis, blanching of skin. Too-frequent or excessive use may lead to loss of bronchodilating effectiveness and/or severe, paradoxical bronchoconstriction.

M

NURSING CONSIDERATIONS

BASELINE ASSESSMENT

Offer emotional support (high incidence of anxiety because of difficulty in breathing, sympathomimetic response to drug).

INTERVENTION/EVALUATION

Monitor rate, depth, rhythm, type of respiration; quality/rate of pulse. Assess lung sounds for rhonchi, wheezing, rales. Monitor ABGs, pulmonary function tests. Observe lips, fingernails for cyanosis (blue or dusky color in light-skinned pts; gray in dark-skinned pts). Evaluate for clinical improvement (quieter, slower respirations; relaxed facial expression; cessation of clavicular, sternal, intercostal retractions).

PATIENT/FAMILY TEACHING

• Increase fluid intake (decreases lung secretion viscosity). • Do not exceed recommended dosage. • May cause anxiety, restlessness, insomnia. • Inform physician if palpitations, tachycardia, chest pain, tremors, dizziness, headache, flushing, difficulty in breathing persists. • Avoid excessive use of caffeine derivatives (chocolate, coffee, tea, cola, cocoa).

metaxalone

meh-**tax**-ah-lone
(Skelaxin)
Do not confuse metaxalone with mesalamine or metolazone, or Skelaxin with Robaxin.

◆CLASSIFICATION

CLINICAL: Skeletal muscle relaxant.

ACTION

Skeletal muscle relaxant action may be related to its CNS depressant effects. Does not directly relax skeletal muscle, motor end plate, or nerve fiber. **Therapeutic Effect:** Relieves musculoskeletal pain.

PHARMACOKINETICS

Rapidly absorbed from GI tract. Extensively distributed in tissues. Converts to metabolites. Metabolized in liver; excreted in urine. **Half-life:** 9 hrs.

USES

Adjunct to rest and physical therapy to decrease musculoskeletal pain, muscle spasm associated with strains, sprains, other muscle injuries.

PRECAUTIONS

Contraindications: Severe renal/hepatic impairment, drug-induced anemia, hemolytic anemia. **Cautions:** Hepatic/renal impairment, elderly, debilitated.

LIFESPAN CONSIDERATIONS

Pregnancy/Lactation: Unknown if distributed in breast milk. **Pregnancy Category B. Children:** Safety and efficacy not established in those 12 yrs and younger. **Elderly:** May be more susceptible to CNS effects.

INTERACTIONS

DRUG: **CNS depressants,** including **alcohol, benzodiazepines, opioids, tricyclic antidepressants,** may increase sedative effects. HERBAL: **St. John's wort** may increase concentration. FOOD: **High-fat meal** may increase concentration. LAB VALUES: May decrease WBC, RBC, platelet count.

AVAILABILITY (Rx)

Tablets: 800 mg.

ADMINISTRATION/HANDLING

• Give without regard to food. • May crush, chew, break tablets.

INDICATIONS/ROUTES/DOSAGE

PO: ADULTS, ELDERLY, CHILDREN 12 YRS AND OLDER: 800 mg (1 tablet) 3–4 times daily.

SIDE EFFECTS

Occasional: Dizziness, drowsiness, headache, irritability, nausea, nervousness, dyspepsia (indigestion, heartburn, epigastric distress), vomiting.

ADVERSE EFFECTS/ TOXIC REACTIONS

Severe allergic reaction (rash, pruritus, urticaria, circumoral swelling). Overdosage produces progressive sedation, hypnosis, respiratory failure, but emetic action begins 15–30 min after increasingly higher doses are taken. Leukopenia, hemolytic anemia, hepatobiliary abnormalities occur rarely.

NURSING CONSIDERATIONS

BASELINE ASSESSMENT

Record onset, type, location, duration of musculoskeletal pain, inflammation. Inspect appearance of affected joints for immobility, stiffness, swelling.

INTERVENTION/EVALUATION

Assist with ambulation at all times. Evaluate for therapeutic response: relief of pain, stiffness, swelling, improved mobility, reduced joint tenderness, improved grip strength.

PATIENT/FAMILY TEACHING

• Avoid tasks that require alertness, motor skills until response to drug is established. • Avoid alcohol. • Medication intended for short-term use (3 wks). • If no improvement noted, contact physician.

metformin HIGH ALERT

met-**for**-min
(Apo-Metformin ✚, Fortamet, Glucophage, Glucophage XR, Glumetza, Glycon ✚, Novo-Metformin ✚, Riomet)

BLACK BOX ALERT Lactic acidosis occurs very rarely, but mortality rate is 50%. Risk increases with degree of renal impairment, pt's age, those with diabetes, unstable or acute CHF.

Do not confuse Glucophage with Glucotrol, or metformin with metronidazole.

FIXED-COMBINATION(S)

Actoplus Met: metformin/pioglitazone (an antidiabetic): 500 mg/15 mg, 850 mg/15 mg. **Avandamet:** metformin/rosiglitazone (an antidiabetic): 500 mg/1 mg, 500 mg/2 mg, 500 mg/4 mg, 1,000 mg/2 mg, 1,000 mg/4 mg. **Glucovance:** metformin/glyburide (an antidiabetic): 250 mg/1.25 mg, 500 mg/2.5 mg, 500 mg/5 mg. **Janumet:** metformin/sitagliptin (an antidiabetic): 500 mg/50 mg, 1,000 mg/50 mg. **Kombiglyze XR:** metformin/saxagliptin (an antidiabetic): 500 mg/5 mg, 1,000 mg/5 mg, 1,000 mg/2.5 mg. **Metaglip:** metformin/glipizide (an antidiabetic): 250 mg/2.5 mg, 500 mg/2.5 mg, 500 mg/5 mg. **PrandiMet:** metformin/repaglinide (an antidiabetic): 500 mg/1 mg, 500 mg/2 mg.

CLASSIFICATION

PHARMACOTHERAPEUTIC: Antihyperglycemic. **CLINICAL:** Antidiabetic.

ACTION

Decreases hepatic production of glucose. Decreases absorption of glucose, improves insulin sensitivity. **Therapeutic Effect:** Improves glycemic control, stabilizes/decreases body weight, improves lipid profile.

PHARMACOKINETICS

Slowly, incompletely absorbed after PO administration. Food delays, decreases extent of absorption. Protein binding: Negligible. Primarily distributed to intestinal mucosa, salivary glands. Primarily excreted unchanged in urine. Removed by hemodialysis. **Half-life:** 9–17 hrs.

USES

Management of type 2 diabetes mellitus as monotherapy or concomitantly with oral sulfonylurea or insulin. **OFF-LABEL:** Treatment of HIV lipodystrophy syndrome, metabolic complications of AIDS, polycystic ovary syndrome, prediabetes, weight reduction.

PRECAUTIONS

◀ALERT▶ Lactic acidosis is a rare but potentially severe consequence of metformin therapy. Withhold in pts with conditions that may predispose to lactic acidosis (e.g., hypoxemia, dehydration, hypoperfusion, sepsis).

Contraindications: Acute CHF, MI, cardiovascular collapse, renal disease/dysfunction, respiratory failure, septicemia. **Cautions:** Conditions delaying food absorption (e.g., diarrhea, high fever, malnutrition, gastroparesis, vomiting), causing hyperglycemia, hypoglycemia, uncontrolled hypothyroidism, hyperthyroidism, cardiovascular pts, concurrent drugs that affect renal function, hepatic impairment, elderly, malnourished/debilitated pts with renal impairment, CHF, excessive alcohol intake, chronic respiratory difficulty.

LIFESPAN CONSIDERATIONS

Pregnancy/Lactation: Insulin is drug of choice during pregnancy. Distributed in breast milk in animals. **Pregnancy Category B.** **Children:** Safety and efficacy not established. **Elderly:** Age-related renal impairment or peripheral vascular disease may require dosage adjustment or discontinuation.

INTERACTIONS

DRUG: **Cimetidine, furosemide** may increase concentration. **Cationic medications (e.g., digoxin, morphine, quinine, ranitidine, vancomycin)** may increase concentration, effect. **Contrast agents** may increase risk of metformin-induced lactic acidosis, acute renal failure (discontinue metformin 48 hrs prior to contrast exposure). **HERBAL:** **Garlic** may cause hypoglycemia. **FOOD:** None known. **LAB VALUES:** May alter cholesterol, LDL, triglycerides, HDL.

AVAILABILITY (Rx)

Oral Solution (Riomet): 100 mg/ml. **Tablets (Glucophage):** 500 mg, 850 mg, 1,000 mg.

Tablets (Extended-Release): 500 mg (Fortamet, Glucophage XR, Glumetza), 750 mg (Glucophage XR), 1,000 mg (Fortamet, Glumetza).

ADMINISTRATION/HANDLING

PO

• Swallow whole. Do not crush, break, or chew extended-release tablets. • Give with meals (to decrease GI upset). Give Fortamet with glass of water.

INDICATIONS/ROUTES/DOSAGE

◀ALERT▶ Allow 1–2 wks between dose titrations.

Diabetes Mellitus

PO (IMMEDIATE-RELEASE TABLETS, SOLUTION): ADULTS, ELDERLY: Initially, 500 mg twice a day or 850 mg once daily. Maintenance: 1,000–2,550 mg/day in 2–3 divided doses. **Maximum:** 2,550 mg/day. **CHILDREN 10–16 YRS:** Initially, 500-mg twice a day. Maintenance: Titrate in 500-mg increments weekly. **Maximum:** 2,000 mg/day.

PO (EXTENDED-RELEASE TABLETS [GLUCOPHAGE XR]): ADULTS, ELDERLY: Initially, 500 mg once daily. May increase by 500 mg at 1-wk intervals. Maintenance: 1,000–2,000 mg daily. **Maximum:** 2,000 mg/day.

PO (EXTENDED-RELEASE TABLETS [FORTAMET, GLUMETZA]): ADULTS, ELDERLY: 1,000 mg once daily. May increase by 500 mg at 1-wk intervals. Maintenance: 1–2.5 g once daily. **Maximum: (Fortamet)** 2,500 mg/day. **(Glumetza)** 2,000 mg/day.

Dosage in Renal Impairment

Contraindicated in pts with serum creatinine greater than 1.5 mg/dl (males) or greater than 1.4 mg/dl (females). Clinically not recommended in pts with creatinine clearance less than 60–70 ml/min.

SIDE EFFECTS

Occasional (greater than 3%): GI disturbances (diarrhea, nausea, vomiting, abdominal bloating, flatulence, anorexia) that are transient and resolve spontaneously during therapy. **Rare (3%–1%):** Unpleasant/metallic taste that resolves spontaneously during therapy.

ADVERSE EFFECTS/ TOXIC REACTIONS

Lactic acidosis occurs rarely (0.03 cases/1,000 pts) but is a serious and often fatal (50%) complication. Lactic acidosis is characterized by increase in blood lactate levels (greater than 5 mmol/L), decrease in blood pH, electrolyte disturbances. Symptoms include unexplained hyperventilation, myalgia, malaise, drowsiness. May advance to cardiovascular collapse (shock), acute CHF, acute MI, prerenal azotemia.

NURSING CONSIDERATIONS

BASELINE ASSESSMENT

Assess baseline glucose, renal function tests.

INTERVENTION/EVALUATION

Monitor fasting serum glucose, Hgb A_{1c}, renal function, Hgb, Hct, RBC. Monitor folic acid, renal function tests for evidence of early lactic acidosis. If pt is on concurrent oral sulfonylureas, assess for hypoglycemia (cool/wet skin, tremors, dizziness, anxiety, headache, tachycardia, numbness in mouth, hunger, diplopia). Be alert to conditions that alter glucose requirements: fever, increased activity, stress, surgical procedure.

PATIENT/FAMILY TEACHING

• Discontinue metformin, contact physician immediately if evidence of lactic acidosis appears (unexplained hyperventilation, muscle aches, extreme fatigue, unusual drowsiness). • Prescribed diet is principal part of treatment; do not skip, delay meals. • Diabetes mellitus requires lifelong control. • Avoid alcohol. • Inform physician if headache, nausea, vomiting, diarrhea persist or skin rash, unusual bruising/bleeding, change in color of urine or stool occurs.

methadone

meth-a-done
(Dolophine, Metadol ✤, Methadone Intensol, Methadose)

BLACK BOX ALERT Potential to prolong QT interval. May cause respiratory depression.

Do not confuse methadone with Mephyton, Metadate CD, Metadate ER, or methylphenidate.

M

◆CLASSIFICATION

PHARMACOTHERAPEUTIC: Narcotic agonist. **CLINICAL:** Opioid analgesic **(Schedule II)** (see p. 142C).

ACTION

Binds with opioid receptors within CNS. **Therapeutic Effect:** Alters processes affecting analgesia, emotional response to pain; reduces withdrawal symptoms from other opioid drugs.

PHARMACOKINETICS

Route	Onset	Peak	Duration
PO	0.5–1 hr	1.5–2 hrs	6–8 hrs
IM	10–20 min	1–2 hrs	4–5 hrs
IV	N/A	15–30 min	3–4 hrs

Well absorbed after IM injection. Protein binding: 85%–90%. Metabolized in liver. Primarily excreted in urine. Not removed by hemodialysis. **Half-life:** 7–59 hrs.

M

USES

Relief of severe pain, detoxification, temporary maintenance treatment of narcotic abstinence syndrome.

PRECAUTIONS

Contraindications: Delivery of premature infant, diarrhea due to poisoning, hypersensitivity to narcotics, labor. **Extreme Caution:** Renal/hepatic impairment, elderly/debilitated, supraventricular tachycardia, cor pulmonale, history of seizures, acute abdominal conditions, increased intracranial pressure (ICP), respiratory abnormalities.

⌛ LIFESPAN CONSIDERATIONS

Pregnancy/Lactation: Crosses placenta. Distributed in breast milk. Respiratory depression may occur in neonate if mother received opiates during labor. Regular use of opiates during pregnancy may produce withdrawal symptoms in neonate (irritability, excessive crying, tremors, hyperactive reflexes, fever, vomiting, diarrhea, yawning, sneezing, seizures). **Pregnancy Category B (D if used for prolonged periods or at high dosages at term). Children:** Paradoxical excitement may occur. Those younger than 2 yrs more susceptible to respiratory depressant effects. **Elderly:** More susceptible to respiratory depressant effects. Age-related renal impairment may increase risk of urinary retention.

INTERACTIONS

DRUG: Alcohol, other CNS depressants may increase CNS effects, respiratory depression, hypotension. **Clarithromycin** may increase concentration/toxicity. **Amiodarone, erythromycin** may prolong QT interval. **MAOIs** may produce severe, sometimes fatal reaction (reduce dose to ¼ of usual methadone dose). **HERBAL: Gotu kola, kava kava, St. John's wort, valerian** may increase CNS depression. **FOOD: Grapefruit, grapefruit juice** may alter concentration, effect. **LAB VALUES:** May increase serum amylase, lipase.

AVAILABILITY (Rx)

Injection Solution (Dolophine): 10 mg/ml. **Oral Concentrate (Methadone Intensol, Methadose):** 10 mg/ml. **Oral Solution:** 5 mg/5 ml, 10 mg/5 ml. **Tablets (Dispersible [Methadose]):** 40 mg. **Tablets (Dolophine, Methadose):** 5 mg, 10 mg.

ADMINISTRATION/HANDLING

IM, Subcutaneous

◀ALERT▶ IM preferred over subcutaneous route (subcutaneous produces pain, local irritation, induration). • Do not use if solution appears cloudy or contains a precipitate. • Administer slowly. • Those with circulatory impairment experience higher risk of overdosage due to delayed absorption of repeated administration.

PO

• Give without regard to meals. • Oral dose for detoxification and maintenance may be given in fruit juice or water. • Dispersible tablet should not be chewed or swallowed; add to liquid, allow to dissolve before swallowing.

INDICATIONS/ROUTES/DOSAGE

Analgesia

PO: ADULTS, ELDERLY: Initially, 2.5–10 mg q4–12h. **CHILDREN:** 0.1 mg/kg/dose q4h for 2–3 doses then q6–12h as needed. **Maximum dose:** 10 mg.

IV, IM, SUBCUTANEOUS: ADULTS, ELDERLY: Initially, 2.5–10 mg q8–12h. **CHILDREN:** 0.1 mg/kg q4–12 hrs. **Maximum:** 10 mg/dose.

Detoxification

PO: ADULTS, ELDERLY: Initially, dose should not exceed 30 mg. An additional 5–10 mg may be provided if withdrawal symptoms have not been suppressed or if symptoms reappear after 2–4 hrs. Total daily dose not to exceed 40 mg. Maintenance Range: 80–120 mg/day with titration occurring cautiously. Withdrawal should be less than 10% of the maintenance dose every 10–14 days. **Short-term:** Initially, titrate to 40 mg/day in 2 divided doses. Continue 40 mg dose for 2–3 days. Decrease dose every day or every other day.

SIDE EFFECTS

Frequent: Sedation, decreased B/P (orthostatic hypotension), diaphoresis, facial flushing, constipation, dizziness, nausea, vomiting. **Occasional:** Confusion, urinary retention, palpitations, abdominal cramps, visual changes, dry mouth, headache, decreased appetite, anxiety, insomnia. **Rare:** Allergic reaction (rash, pruritus).

ADVERSE EFFECTS/ TOXIC REACTIONS

Overdose results in respiratory depression, skeletal muscle flaccidity, cold/clammy skin, cyanosis, extreme drowsiness progressing to seizures, stupor, coma. Early sign of toxicity presents as increased sedation after being on a stable dose. Cardiac toxicity manifested as QT prolongation, torsade de pointes. Tolerance to analgesic effect, physical dependence may occur with repeated use. **Antidote:** Naloxone (see Appendix M for dosage).

NURSING CONSIDERATIONS

BASELINE ASSESSMENT

Assess type, location, intensity of pain, bowel function. **Detoxification:** Assess pt for opioid withdrawal. Pt should be in recumbent position before drug administration by parenteral route. Obtain vital signs before giving medication. If respirations are 12/min or less (20/min or less in children), withhold medication, contact physician.

INTERVENTION/EVALUATION

Monitor vital signs 15–30 min after subcutaneous/IM dose, 5–10 min following IV dose. Oral medication is 50% as potent as parenteral. Assess for adequate voiding. Assess for clinical improvement, record onset of relief of pain. Provide support to pt in detoxification program; monitor for withdrawal symptoms.

PATIENT/FAMILY TEACHING

• Methadone may produce drug dependence, has potential for being abused. • Avoid alcohol. • Do not stop taking abruptly after prolonged use. • May cause dry mouth, drowsiness. • Avoid tasks that require alertness, motor skills until response to drug is established. • Report severe drowsiness, respiratory depression.

methocarbamol

meth-oh-**car**-buh-mawl
(Robaxin)
Do not confuse Robaxin with Skelaxin.

◆CLASSIFICATION

PHARMACOTHERAPEUTIC: Carbamate derivative of guaifenesin. **CLINICAL:** Skeletal muscle relaxant.

ACTION

Skeletal muscle relaxant action may be related to its CNS depressant effects. Does

M

not directly relax skeletal muscle, motor end plate, or nerve fiber. **Therapeutic Effect:** Relieves musculoskeletal pain.

PHARMACOKINETICS

Extensively distributed in tissues. Protein binding: 46%–50%. Converts to metabolites. Metabolized by dealkylation, hydroxylation; excreted in urine. **Half-life:** 1–2 hrs.

USES

Adjunct to rest and physical therapy for relief of discomfort associated with acute, painful musculoskeletal conditions.

PRECAUTIONS

Contraindications: None significant. **Cautions:** Myasthenia gravis pts receiving anticholinesterase agents, elderly, debilitated.

LIFESPAN CONSIDERATIONS

Pregnancy/Lactation: Unknown if distributed in breast milk. **Pregnancy Category C. Children:** Safety and efficacy not established in those 16 yrs and younger. **Elderly:** May be more susceptible to CNS effects.

INTERACTIONS

DRUG: CNS depressants, including **alcohol, benzodiazepines, opioids, tricyclic antidepressants,** may increase sedative effects. May inhibit effect of **pyridostigmine. HERBAL: St. John's wort** may increase concentration. **FOOD: High-fat meal** may increase concentration. **LAB VALUES:** May decrease WBC counts.

AVAILABILITY (Rx)

Tablets, Film-Coated: 500 mg, 750 mg.

ADMINISTRATION/HANDLING

• Give without regard to food. • Do not crush or break tablets.

INDICATIONS/ROUTES/DOSAGE

Robaxin, 500 mg

PO: ADULTS, ELDERLY, CHILDREN 17 YRS AND OLDER: Initially, 500 mg (3 tablets) 4 times daily. Maintenance: 2 tablets 4 times daily.

Robaxin, 750 mg

PO: ADULTS, ELDERLY, CHILDREN 17 YRS AND OLDER: Initially, 1,500 mg (2 tablets) 4 times daily. Maintenance: 1 tablet q4h or 2 tablets 3 times daily. For first 48–72 hrs of treatment, 6 g daily is recommended; for severe conditions, 8 g daily may be given. Thereafter, dosage usually can be reduced to approximately 4 g daily.

SIDE EFFECTS

Occasional: Dizziness, drowsiness, confusion, double vision, insomnia, headache, irritability, nausea, nervousness, dyspepsia (including nausea, vomiting), vomiting, metallic taste.

ADVERSE EFFECTS/ TOXIC REACTIONS

Anaphylactic reaction (rash, pruritus, urticaria, angioneurotic edema, fever, bradycardia, hypotension, syncope) has occurred. Leukopenia, cholestatic jaundice, seizure occur rarely.

NURSING CONSIDERATIONS

BASELINE ASSESSMENT

Record onset, type, location, duration of musculoskeletal pain, inflammation. Inspect appearance of affected joints for immobility, stiffness, swelling.

INTERVENTION/EVALUATION

Assist with ambulation at all times. Evaluate for therapeutic response: relief of pain, stiffness, swelling, improved mobility, reduced joint tenderness, improved grip strength.

PATIENT/FAMILY TEACHING

• Avoid tasks that require alertness, motor skills until response to drug is established. • Avoid alcohol. • May color urine brown, black, or green. • Medication intended for short-term use (3 wks). • If no improvement noted, contact physician. • Report severe sedation.

methotrexate

HIGH ALERT

meth-oh-**trex**-ate
(Apo-Methotrexate ✦, Rheumatrex, Trexall)

BLACK BOX ALERT Pregnancy Category X. May cause fetal abnormalities, death. May produce potentially fatal chronic hepatotoxicity, dermatologic reactions, acute renal failure, pneumonitis, myelosuppression, malignant lymphoma, aplastic anemia, GI toxicity.

Do not confuse methotrexate with metolazone or mitoxantrone. MTX is an error-prone abbreviation; do not use as an abbreviation.

CLASSIFICATION

PHARMACOTHERAPEUTIC: Antimetabolite. **CLINICAL:** Antineoplastic, antiarthritic, antipsoriatic (see p. 86C).

ACTION

Competes with enzymes necessary to reduce folic acid to tetrahydrofolic acid, a component essential to DNA, RNA, protein synthesis. **Therapeutic Effect:** Inhibits DNA, RNA, protein synthesis.

PHARMACOKINETICS

Variably absorbed from GI tract. Completely absorbed after IM administration. Protein binding: 50%–60%. Widely distributed. Metabolized intracellularly in liver. Primarily excreted in urine. Removed by hemodialysis but not by peritoneal dialysis. **Half-life:** 3–10 hrs (large doses, 8–15 hrs).

USES

Treatment of breast, head/neck, non–small-cell lung, small-cell lung carcinomas, trophoblastic tumors, acute lymphocytic, meningeal leukemias, non-Hodgkin's lymphomas (lymphosarcoma, Burkitt's lymphoma), carcinoma of gastrointestinal tract, mycosis fungoides, osteosarcoma, psoriasis, rheumatoid arthritis, including juvenile rheumatoid arthritis. **OFF-LABEL:** Treatment of acute myelocytic leukemia; bladder, cervical, ovarian, prostatic, renal, testicular carcinomas; psoriatic arthritis; systemic dermatomyositis. Treatment of and maintenance of remission in Crohn's disease.

PRECAUTIONS

Contraindications: Hepatic disease, renal impairment, preexisting myelosuppression, rheumatoid arthritis with alcoholism. **Cautions:** Peptic ulcer, ulcerative colitis, myelosuppression, ascites, pleural effusion.

LIFESPAN CONSIDERATIONS

Pregnancy/Lactation: Avoid pregnancy during methotrexate therapy and minimum 3 mos after therapy in males or at least one ovulatory cycle after therapy in females. May cause fetal death, congenital anomalies. Drug is distributed in breast milk. Breast-feeding not recommended. **Pregnancy Category D (X for patients with psoriasis or rheumatoid arthritis). Children/Elderly:** Renal/hepatic impairment may require dosage adjustment.

INTERACTIONS

DRUG: **Acyclovir (parenteral)** may increase risk of neurotoxicity. **Alcohol, hepatotoxic medications** may increase risk of hepatotoxicity. **Asparaginase** may decrease effect. **Bone marrow depressants** may increase myelosuppression. **Live virus vaccines** may potentiate virus replication, increase vaccine side effects, decrease pt's antibody response to vaccine. **NSAIDs** may increase risk of toxicity. **Probenecid, salicylates** may increase concentration, risk of toxicity. **HERBAL:** **Cat's claw, echinacea** possess immunostimulant properties. **FOOD:** None known. **LAB VALUES:** May increase serum uric acid, AST.

AVAILABILITY (Rx)

Injection, Powder for Reconstitution: 1 g. **Injection Solution:** 25 mg/ml. **Tablets:** 2.5 mg (Rheumatrex), 5 mg (Trexall), 7.5 mg (Trexall), 10 mg (Trexall), 15 mg (Trexall).

M

ADMINISTRATION/HANDLING

◀ALERT▶ May be carcinogenic, mutagenic, teratogenic. Handle with extreme care during preparation/administration. Wear gloves when preparing solution. If powder or solution comes in contact with skin, wash immediately, thoroughly with soap, water. May give IM, IV, intra-arterially, intrathecally.

IV

Reconstitution • Reconstitute powder with D_5W or 0.9% NaCl to provide concentration of 50 mg/ml. • For intrathecal use, dilute with preservative-free 0.9% NaCl to provide a concentration not greater than 2 mg/ml.

Rate of administration • Give IV push at rate of 10 mg/min. • Give IV infusion at rate of 4–20 mg/hr.

Storage • Store vials at room temperature.

IV INCOMPATIBILITIES

Chlorpromazine (Thorazine), droperidol (Inapsine), gemcitabine (Gemzar), idarubicin (Idamycin), midazolam (Versed), nalbuphine (Nubain).

IV COMPATIBILITIES

Cisplatin (Platinol AQ), cyclophosphamide (Cytoxan), daunorubicin (DaunoXome), doxorubicin (Adriamycin), etoposide (VePesid), 5-fluorouracil, granisetron (Kytril), leucovorin, lipids, mitomycin (Mutamycin), ondansetron (Zofran), paclitaxel (Taxol), vinblastine (Velban), vincristine (Oncovin), vinorelbine (Navelbine).

INDICATIONS/ROUTES/DOSAGE

◀ALERT▶ Refer to individual specific protocols for optimum dosage, sequence of administration.

Trophoblastic Neoplasms

PO, IM: ADULTS, ELDERLY: 15–30 mg/day for 5 days; repeat in 7 days for 3–5 courses.

IV: 11 mg/m² on days 1–5, repeat every 3 wks.

Head/Neck Cancer

PO, IV, IM: ADULTS, ELDERLY: 25–50 mg/m² once weekly.

Breast Cancer

IV: ADULTS, ELDERLY: 30–60 mg/m² days 1 and 8 q3–4wk.

Bladder Cancer (Off Label)

IV: ADULTS, ELDERLY: 30 mg/m² days 1 and 8 q3wks.

Gastric Cancer

IV: ADULTS, ELDERLY: 1,500 mg/m² q28days.

Mycosis Fungoides

IM, PO: ADULTS, ELDERLY: 5–50 mg once weekly. If refractory, 15–37.5 mg twice a wk.

Rheumatoid Arthritis (RA)

PO: ADULTS: 7.5 mg once weekly or 2.5 mg q12h for 3 doses once weekly. **ELDERLY:** Initially, 5–7.5 mg/wk. **Maximum:** 20 mg/wk.

Juvenile Rheumatoid Arthritis (JRA)

PO, IM, SUBCUTANEOUS: CHILDREN: Initially, 10 mg/m² once weekly, then 5–15 mg/m²/wk as a single dose or in 3 divided doses given q12h.

Psoriasis

PO: ADULTS, ELDERLY: 10–25 mg once weekly or 2.5–5 mg q12h for 3 doses once weekly.

IM: ADULTS, ELDERLY: 10–25 mg once weekly.

Antineoplastic Dosage for Children

PO, IM: CHILDREN: 7.5–30 mg/m²/wk or q2wk.

IV: CHILDREN: 10–18,000 mg/m² bolus or continuous infusion over 6–42 hrs.

Dosage in Renal Impairment

Creatinine Clearance	Reduce Dose To
61–80 ml/min	75% of normal
51–60 ml/min	70% of normal
10–50 ml/min	30–50% of normal

SIDE EFFECTS

Frequent (10%–3%): Nausea, vomiting, stomatitis; burning/erythema at psoriatic site (in pts with psoriasis). **Occasional (3%–1%):** Diarrhea, rash, dermatitis, pruritus, alopecia, dizziness, anorexia, malaise, headache, drowsiness, blurred vision.

ADVERSE EFFECTS/ TOXIC REACTIONS

High potential for various, severe toxicities. GI toxicity may produce gingivitis, glossitis, pharyngitis, stomatitis, enteritis, hematemesis. Hepatotoxicity more likely to occur with frequent small doses than with large intermittent doses. Pulmonary toxicity characterized by interstitial pneumonitis. Hematologic toxicity, resulting from marked myelosuppression, may manifest as leukopenia, thrombocytopenia, anemia, hemorrhage. Dermatologic toxicity may produce rash, pruritus, urticaria, pigmentation, photosensitivity, petechiae, ecchymosis, pustules. Severe nephrotoxicity produces azotemia, hematuria, renal failure.

NURSING CONSIDERATIONS

BASELINE ASSESSMENT

Rheumatoid Arthritis: Assess pain, range of motion. **Psoriasis:** Assess skin lesions. Question for possibility of pregnancy before initiating therapy (Pregnancy Category X) in pts with psoriasis, rheumatoid arthritis (RA). Obtain all functional tests before therapy, repeat throughout therapy. Antiemetics may prevent nausea, vomiting.

INTERVENTION/EVALUATION

Monitor hepatic/renal function tests, Hgb, Hct, WBC, differential, platelet count, urinalysis, chest X-rays, serum uric acid. Monitor for hematologic toxicity (fever, sore throat, signs of local infection, unusual bruising/bleeding from any site), symptoms of anemia (excessive fatigue, weakness). Assess skin for evidence of dermatologic toxicity. Keep pt well hydrated, urine alkaline. Avoid rectal temperatures, traumas that induce bleeding. Apply 5 full min of pressure to IV sites.

PATIENT/FAMILY TEACHING

• Maintain fastidious oral hygiene. • Do not have immunizations without physician's approval (drug lowers resistance). • Avoid crowds, those with infection. • Avoid alcohol, salicylates. • Avoid sunlamp, sunlight exposure. • Use contraceptive measures during therapy and for 3 mos (males) or 1 ovulatory cycle (females) after therapy. • Promptly report fever, sore throat, signs of local infection, unusual bruising/bleeding from any site, diarrhea. • Alopecia is reversible, but new hair growth may have different color, texture. • Contact physician if nausea/vomiting continues at home.

methylergonovine

meth-ill-er-goe-**noe**-veen
(Methergine)

✚CLASSIFICATION

PHARMACOTHERAPEUTIC: Ergot alkaloid. **CLINICAL:** Uterine stimulant.

ACTION

Stimulates alpha-adrenergic, serotonin receptors, producing arterial vasoconstriction. Causes vasospasm of coronary arteries. Directly stimulates uterine muscle. **Therapeutic Effect:** Increases strength, frequency of uterine contractions, decreases uterine bleeding.

PHARMACOKINETICS

Route	Onset	Peak	Duration
PO	5–10 min	N/A	3 hrs
IV	Immediate	N/A	45 min
IM	2–5 min	N/A	3 hrs

Rapidly absorbed from GI tract after IM administration. Distributed rapidly to plasma, extracellular fluid, tissues. Metabolized in liver, undergoes first-pass

M

effect. Primarily excreted in urine. **Half-life:** 0.5–2 hrs.

USES

Prevention/treatment of postpartum, postabortion hemorrhage due to atony, involution (not for induction, augmentation of labor). **OFF-LABEL:** Treatment of incomplete abortion.

PRECAUTIONS

Contraindications: Hypertension, pregnancy, toxemia, untreated hypocalcemia. **Cautions:** Renal/hepatic impairment, coronary artery disease, occlusive peripheral vascular disease, sepsis.

LIFESPAN CONSIDERATIONS

Pregnancy/Lactation: Contraindicated during pregnancy. Small amounts distributed in breast milk. **Pregnancy Category C. Children/Elderly:** No information available.

M

INTERACTIONS

DRUG: Vasoconstrictors, vasopressors may increase effects. **HERBAL:** None significant. **FOOD:** None known. **LAB VALUES:** May decrease serum prolactin.

AVAILABILITY (Rx)

Injection Solution: 0.2 mg/ml. **Tablets:** 0.2 mg.

ADMINISTRATION/HANDLING

Reconstitution • Dilute with 0.9% NaCl to volume of 5 ml.
Rate of administration • Give over at least 1 min, carefully monitoring B/P.
Storage • Refrigerate ampules. • Initial dose may be given parenterally, followed by oral regimen. • IV use in life-threatening emergencies only.

IV INCOMPATIBILITIES

None known.

IV COMPATIBILITIES

Heparin, potassium.

INDICATIONS/ROUTES/DOSAGE

Prevention/Treatment of Postpartum, Postabortion Hemorrhage

PO: ADULTS: 0.2 mg 3–4 times a day. Continue for up to 7 days.
IV, IM: ADULTS: Initially, 0.2 mg after delivery of anterior shoulder, after delivery of placenta, or during puerperium. May repeat q2–4h as needed.

SIDE EFFECTS

Frequent: Nausea, uterine cramping, vomiting. **Occasional:** Abdominal pain, diarrhea, dizziness, diaphoresis, tinnitus, bradycardia, chest pain. **Rare:** Allergic reaction (rash, pruritus), dyspnea; severe or sudden hypertension.

ADVERSE EFFECTS/ TOXIC REACTIONS

Severe hypertensive episodes may result in CVA, serious arrhythmias, seizures. Hypertensive effects are more frequent with pt susceptibility, rapid IV administration, concurrent use of regional anesthesia, vasoconstrictors. Peripheral ischemia may lead to gangrene.

NURSING CONSIDERATIONS

BASELINE ASSESSMENT

Determine baseline serum calcium level, B/P, pulse. Assess for any evidence of bleeding before administration.

INTERVENTION/EVALUATION

Monitor uterine tone, bleeding, B/P, pulse q15min until stable (about 1–2 hrs). Assess extremities for color, warmth, movement, pain. Report chest pain promptly. Provide support with ambulation if dizziness occurs.

PATIENT/FAMILY TEACHING

• Avoid smoking because of added vasoconstriction. • Report increased cramping, bleeding, foul-smelling lochia. • Report pale, cold hands/feet (possibility of diminished circulation).

methylnaltrexone

meth-ill-nal-**trex**-own
(Relistor)
Do not confuse methylnaltrexone with naltrexone.

◆CLASSIFICATION

PHARMACOTHERAPEUTIC: Opioid receptor antagonist. **CLINICAL:** Constipation agent.

ACTION

Blocks binding of opioids to peripheral opioid receptors within GI tract. **Therapeutic Effect:** Decreases constipating effect of opioids without reducing analgesic effect.

PHARMACOKINETICS

Absorbed rapidly. Undergoes moderate tissue distribution. Protein binding: 11%–15%. Excreted primarily in urine, with lesser amount eliminated in feces. **Half-life:** 8 hrs.

USES

Treatment of opioid-induced constipation in pts with advanced illness who are receiving palliative care when response to laxative therapy is insufficient.

PRECAUTIONS

Contraindications: Known or suspected mechanical GI obstruction. **Cautions:** Severe renal impairment.

⌛ LIFESPAN CONSIDERATIONS

Pregnancy/Lactation: Unknown if distributed in breast milk. **Pregnancy Category B. Children:** Safety and efficacy not established. **Elderly:** No age-related precautions noted.

INTERACTIONS

DRUG: Benefits of **opioid-containing products (antidiarrheal preparations, cough and cold preparations, opioid analgesics)** are negated. **HERBAL:** None significant. **FOOD:** None known. **LAB VALUES:** None known.

AVAILABILITY (Rx)

Subcutaneous: 12 mg/0.6 ml single-use vial.

ADMINISTRATION/HANDLING

Subcutaneous

• Inject into upper arm, abdomen, or thigh. **Storage** • Solution appears as clear and colorless to pale yellow. • If particulate matter is noted, discard. • Once solution is drawn into syringe, may be stored at room temperature. • Administer within 24 hrs.

INDICATIONS/ROUTES/DOSAGE

Constipation

SUBCUTANEOUS: ADULTS, ELDERLY WEIGHING 38 KG TO LESS THAN 62 KG: 8 mg. **ADULTS, ELDERLY WEIGHING 62–114 KG:** 12 mg. **ADULTS, ELDERLY WHOSE WEIGHT FALLS OUTSIDE THESE RANGES:** Dose at 0.15 mg/kg. Usual schedule is once every other day, as needed, but no more frequently than once every 24 hrs.

Severe Renal Impairment (Creatinine Clearance Less Than 30 ml/min)

SUBCUTANEOUS: ADULTS, ELDERLY: Administer 50% of recommended dose.

SIDE EFFECTS

Frequent: Abdominal pain (29%), flatulence (13%), nausea (12%). **Occasional (7%–5%):** Diarrhea, dizziness.

ADVERSE EFFECTS/ TOXIC REACTIONS

None known.

NURSING CONSIDERATIONS

BASELINE ASSESSMENT

30% of pts report defecation within 30 min after drug administration.

INTERVENTION/EVALUATION

Encourage fluid intake. Assess bowel sounds for peristalsis. Monitor daily pattern of bowel activity, stool consistency. If

M

opioid medication is stopped, drug should be discontinued. Assess for abdominal disturbances.

PATIENT/FAMILY TEACHING

• Laxative effect usually occurs within 30 min but may take up to 24 hrs after medication administration. • Common side effects include transient abdominal pain, nausea, vomiting. • Contact physician if any of these symptoms persist or worsen, or if severe or persistant diarrhea occurs.

methylphenidate

meth-ill-**fen**-i-date
(Apo-Methylphenidate ♣, Concerta, Daytrana, Metadate CD, Metadate ER, Methylin, Methylin ER, PMS-Methylphenidate ♣, Riphenidate ♣, Ritalin, Ritalin LA, Ritalin SR)

BLACK BOX ALERT Chronic abuse can lead to marked tolerance, psychological dependence. Abrupt withdrawal from prolonged use may lead to severe depression, psychosis.

Do not confuse Metadate ER with Metadate CD, Methylphenidate with methadone, or Ritalin with Rifadin.

◆CLASSIFICATION

CLINICAL: (Schedule II) CNS stimulant.

ACTION

Blocks reuptake of norepinephrine, dopamine into presynaptic neurons. **Therapeutic Effect:** Decreases motor restlessness, fatigue. Increases motor activity, attention span, mental alertness. Produces mild euphoria.

PHARMACOKINETICS

Onset	Peak	Duration
Immediate-release	2 hrs	3–6 hrs
Sustained-release	4–7 hrs	8 hrs
Extended-release	N/A	12 hrs
Transdermal	2 hrs	N/A

Slowly, incompletely absorbed from GI tract. Protein binding: 15%. Metabolized in liver. Eliminated in urine, in feces by biliary system. Unknown if removed by hemodialysis. **Half-life:** 2–4 hrs.

USES

Adjunct to treatment of ADHD with moderate to severe distractibility, short attention spans, hyperactivity, emotional impulsivity in children older than 6 yrs. **Concerta:** ADHD in children 6 yrs and older, adolescents, and adults up to age 65. Management of narcolepsy in adults. **OFF-LABEL:** Treatment of disease-related fatigue, secondary mental depression (especially elderly, medically ill).

PRECAUTIONS

Contraindications: Use of MAOIs within 14 days, marked anxiety, tension, agitation, motor tics, family history or diagnosis of Tourette's syndrome, glaucoma. **Cautions:** Hypertension, seizures, acute stress reaction, emotional instability, history of drug dependence, heart failure, recent MI, hyperthyroidism, known structural cardiac abnormality, psychosis.

⌛ LIFESPAN CONSIDERATIONS

Pregnancy/Lactation: Unknown if drug crosses placenta or is distributed in breast milk. **Pregnancy Category C. Children:** May be more susceptible to developing anorexia, insomnia, stomach pain, decreased weight. Chronic use may inhibit growth. **Elderly:** No age-related precautions noted.

INTERACTIONS

DRUG: MAOIs may increase effects. **Other CNS stimulants** may have additive effect. **HERBAL: Ephedra** may cause hypertension, arrhythmias. **Yohimbe** may increase CNS stimulation. **FOOD:** None known. **LAB VALUES:** None significant.

AVAILABILITY (Rx)

Oral Solution (Methylin): 5 mg/5 ml, 10 mg/5 ml. **Tablets (Chewable [Methylin]):** 2.5 mg, 5 mg, 10 mg. **Tablets (Methylin, Ritalin):** 5 mg, 10 mg, 20 mg. **Topical Patch (Daytrana):** 10 mg/9 hrs, 15 mg/9 hrs, 20 mg/9 hrs, 30 mg/9 hrs.

Capsules (Extended-Release [Metadate CD]): 10 mg, 20 mg, 30 mg, 40 mg, 50 mg, 60 mg. **Capsules (Extended-Release [Ritalin LA]):** 10 mg, 20 mg, 30 mg, 40 mg. **Tablets (Extended-Release [Concerta]):** 18 mg, 27 mg, 36 mg, 54 mg, 72 mg. **Tablets (Extended-Release [Metadate ER, Methylin ER]):** 10 mg, 20 mg. **Tablets (Sustained-Release [Ritalin SR]):** 20 mg.

ADMINISTRATION/HANDLING

◀ALERT▶ Sustained-release, extended-release tablets may be given in place of regular tablets, once daily dose is titrated using regular tablets, and titrated dosage corresponds to sustained-release or extended-release tablet strength.

PO

• Do not give drug in afternoon or evening (may cause insomnia). • Do not crush, break extended-release capsules, extended- or sustained-release tablets. • Immediate-release tablets may be crushed. • Give dose 30–45 min before meals.
• **Concerta:** Administer once daily in morning. Must be taken with water, milk, or juice.
• **Methylin Chewable:** Give with at least 8 oz of water or other fluid.
• **Metadate CD, Ritalin LA:** • May be opened, sprinkled on applesauce. • Swallow applesauce without chewing. Do not crush or chew capsule contents.

Patch

• To be worn daily for 9 hrs. • Replace daily in morning. • Apply to dry, clean area of hip. • Avoid applying to waistline (clothing may cause patch to rub off). • Alternate application site daily. • Press firmly in place for 30 sec to ensure patch is in good contact with skin.

INDICATIONS/ROUTES/DOSAGE

ADHD

PO: ADULTS, CHILDREN 6 YRS AND OLDER: Initially, 0.3 mg/kg/dose or 2.5–5 mg before breakfast and lunch. May increase by 0.1 mg/kg/dose or by 5–10 mg/day at weekly intervals. Usual dose: 0.5–1 mg/kg/day. **Maximum:** 2 mg/kg/day or 60 mg/day.

PO (CONCERTA): CHILDREN 6 YRS AND OLDER, ADULTS UP TO 65 YRS OF AGE: Initially, 18 mg once a day; may increase by 18 mg/day at weekly intervals. **Maximum:** 72 mg/day.

PO (METADATE CD): CHILDREN 6 YRS AND OLDER: Initially, 20 mg/day. May increase by 20 mg/day at weekly intervals. **Maximum:** 60 mg/day.

PO (RITALIN LA): CHILDREN 6 YRS AND OLDER: Initially, 20 mg/day. May increase by 10 mg/day at weekly intervals. **Maximum:** 60 mg/day.

PO (METADATE ER, METHYLIN ER, RITALIN SR): CHILDREN 6 YRS AND OLDER: May replace regular tablets after daily dose is titrated and 8-hr dosage corresponds to sustained-release or extended-release tablet strength. **Maximum:** 60 mg/day.

PATCH (DAYTRANA): CHILDREN: 10–30 mg daily (applied and worn for 9 hrs). Dosage is titrated to desired effect.

Narcolepsy

PO: ADULTS, ELDERLY: 10 mg 2–3 times a day. Range: 10–60 mg/day.

SIDE EFFECTS

Frequent: Anxiety, insomnia, anorexia. **Occasional:** Dizziness, drowsiness, headache, nausea, abdominal pain, fever, rash, arthralgia, vomiting. **Rare:** Blurred vision, Tourette's syndrome (uncontrolled vocal outbursts, repetitive body movements, tics), palpitations.

ADVERSE EFFECTS/ TOXIC REACTIONS

Prolonged administration to children with ADHD may delay normal weight gain pattern. Overdose may produce tachycardia, palpitations, arrhythmias, chest pain, psychotic episode, seizures, coma. Hypersensitivity reactions, blood dyscrasias occur rarely.

NURSING CONSIDERATIONS

BASELINE ASSESSMENT

ADHD: Assess attention span, impulsivity, interaction with others, distractibility. **Narcolepsy:** Observe/assess frequency of episodes.

INTERVENTION/EVALUATION

Monitor B/P, pulse, changes in ADHD symptoms. CBC with differential, platelet count should be performed routinely during therapy. If paradoxical return of attention deficit occurs, dosage should be reduced or discontinued. Monitor growth.

PATIENT/FAMILY TEACHING

• Avoid tasks that require alertness, motor skills until response to drug is established. • Sugarless gum, sips of tepid water may relieve dry mouth. • Report any increase in seizures. • Take daily dose early in morning to avoid insomnia. • Report anxiety, palpitations, fever, vomiting, skin rash. • Report new or worsened symptoms (e.g., behavior, hostility, concentration ability). • Avoid caffeine. • Do not stop taking abruptly after prolonged use.

M

*methylPREDNISolone

(Medrol)

*methylPREDNISolone acetate

(DepoMedrol)

*methylPREDNISolone sodium succinate

(Solu-Medrol)
meth-il-pred-**niss**-oh-lone

Do not confuse methylprednisolone with medroxyprogesterone or prednisolone, Medrol with Mebaral, or DepoMedrol with SoluMedrol.

◆CLASSIFICATION

PHARMACOTHERAPEUTIC: Adrenal corticosteroid. **CLINICAL:** Anti-inflammatory (see p. 98C).

ACTION

Suppresses migration of polymorphonuclear leukocytes, reverses increased capillary permeability. **Therapeutic Effect:** Decreases inflammation.

PHARMACOKINETICS

Route	Onset	Peak	Duration
PO	Rapid	1–2 hrs	30–36 hrs
IM	Rapid	4–8 days	1–4 wks
IV	Rapid	N/A	N/A

Well absorbed from GI tract after IM administration. Widely distributed. Metabolized in liver. Excreted in urine. Removed by hemodialysis. **Half-life:** 3.5 hrs.

USES

Endocrine Disorders: Substitution therapy for deficiency states (acute or chronic adrenal insufficiency, congenital adrenal hyperplasia, adrenal insufficiency secondary to pituitary insufficiency). **Nonendocrine Disorders:** Arthritis; rheumatic carditis; allergic reaction; collagen, intestinal tract, hepatic, ocular, renal, skin diseases; bronchial asthma; cerebral edema; malignancies; spinal cord injury.

PRECAUTIONS

Contraindications: Administration of live virus vaccines, systemic fungal infection. **Cautions:** Hypothyroidism, cirrhosis, hypertension, diabetes, CHF, ulcerative colitis, thromboembolic disorders.

⌛ LIFESPAN CONSIDERATIONS

Pregnancy/Lactation: Crosses placenta. Distributed in breast milk. May cause cleft palate (chronic use in first trimester). Breast-feeding not recommended. **Pregnancy Category C. Children:** Prolonged treatment or high dosages may decrease short-term growth rate, cortisol secretion. **Elderly:** No age-related precaution noted.

INTERACTIONS

DRUG: Amphotericin may increase hypokalemia. May increase risk of **digoxin** toxicity caused by hypokalemia. May decrease effects of **diuretics, insulin, oral hypoglycemics, potassium supplements. Hepatic enzyme inducers** may decrease effects. **Live virus vaccines** may decrease pt's antibody response to vaccine, increase vaccine side effects, potentiate virus replication. **HERBAL: Cat's claw, echinacea** possess immunostimulant properties. **St. John's wort** may decrease concentration. **FOOD:** None known. **LAB VALUES:** May increase serum glucose, cholesterol, lipid, amylase, sodium. May decrease serum calcium, potassium, thyroxine, hypothalmic-pituitary-adrenal (HPA) axis.

AVAILABILITY (Rx)

Injection, Powder for Reconstitution (Solu-Medrol): 40 mg, 125 mg, 500 mg, 1 g. **Injection Suspension:** 40 mg/ml, 80 mg/ml. **Tablets (Medrol):** 2 mg, 4 mg, 8 mg, 16 mg, 32 mg. **(Medrol Dosepak):** 4 mg (21 g).

ADMINISTRATION/HANDLING

IV

Reconstitution • For infusion, add to D_5W, 0.9% NaCl.
Rate of administration • Give IV push over 3–15 min. • Give IV piggyback. Dose of 250 mg over 15–30 min; dose of 500–999 mg over at least 30 min; dose of 1g or greater over 1 hr. • Do **not** give methylprednisolone acetate IV.
Storage • Store vials at room temperature.

IM

• Methylprednisolone acetate should not be further diluted. • Methylprednisolone sodium succinate should be reconstituted with Bacteriostatic Water for Injection. • Give deep IM in gluteus maximus (avoid injection into deltoid muscle).

PO

• Give with food, milk.

IV INCOMPATIBILITIES

Ciprofloxacin (Cipro), diltiazem (Cardizem), docetaxel (Taxotere), etoposide (VePesid), filgrastim (Neupogen), gemcitabine (Gemzar), paclitaxel (Taxol), potassium chloride, propofol (Diprivan), vinorelbine (Navelbine).

IV COMPATIBILITIES

Dopamine (Intropin), heparin, lipids, midazolam (Versed), theophylline.

INDICATIONS/ROUTES/DOSAGE

Anti-Inflammatory, Immunosuppressive
IV: ADULTS, ELDERLY: 10–40 mg. May repeat as needed. **CHILDREN:** 0.5–1.7 mg/kg/day or 5–25 mg/m²/day in 2–4 divided doses.
PO: ADULTS, ELDERLY: 2–60 mg/day in 1–4 divided doses. **CHILDREN:** 0.5–1.7 mg/kg/day or 5–25 mg/m²/day in 2–4 divided doses.
IM (METHYLPREDNISOLONE ACETATE): ADULTS, ELDERLY: 10–80 mg/day. **CHILDREN:** 0.5–1.7 mg/kg/day or 5–25 mg/m²/day in 2–4 divided doses.
INTRA-ARTICULAR, INTRALESIONAL: ADULTS, ELDERLY: 20–60 mg q1–5wk.

Status Asthmaticus
IV: ADULTS, ELDERLY, CHILDREN: Initially, 2 mg/kg/dose, then 0.5–1 mg/kg/dose q6h for up to 5 days.

Spinal Cord Injury
IV BOLUS: ADULTS, ELDERLY: 30 mg/kg over 15 min, followed by 5.4 mg/kg/hr over 23 hrs, to be given within 45 min of bolus dose.

SIDE EFFECTS

Frequent: Insomnia, heartburn, anxiety, abdominal distention, diaphoresis, acne,

M

mood swings, increased appetite, facial flushing, GI distress, delayed wound healing, increased susceptibility to infection, diarrhea, constipation. **Occasional:** Headache, edema, tachycardia, change in skin color, frequent urination, depression. **Rare:** Psychosis, increased blood coagulability, hallucinations.

ADVERSE EFFECTS/ TOXIC REACTIONS

Long-term therapy: Hypocalcemia, hypokalemia, muscle wasting (esp. in arms, legs), osteoporosis, spontaneous fractures, amenorrhea, cataracts, glaucoma, peptic ulcer, CHF. **Abrupt withdrawal after long-term therapy:** Anorexia, nausea, fever, headache, severe arthralgia, rebound inflammation, fatigue, weakness, lethargy, dizziness, orthostatic hypotension.

NURSING CONSIDERATIONS

BASELINE ASSESSMENT

Question for hypersensitivity to any of the corticosteroids, components. Obtain baselines for height, weight, B/P, serum glucose, electrolytes. Check results of initial tests (tuberculosis [TB] skin test, X-rays, EKG).

INTERVENTION/EVALUATION

Monitor I&O, daily weight; assess for edema. Monitor daily pattern of bowel activity and stool consistency. Check vital signs at least twice a day. Be alert for infection (sore throat, fever, vague symptoms). Monitor serum electrolytes, including B/P, glucose. Monitor for hypocalcemia (muscle twitching, cramps, positive Trousseau's or Chvostek's signs), hypokalemia (weakness, muscle cramps, numbness, tingling [esp. lower extremities], nausea/vomiting, irritability, EKG changes). Assess emotional status, ability to sleep. Check lab results for blood coagulability, clinical evidence of thromboembolism.

PATIENT/FAMILY TEACHING

• Take oral dose with food, milk. • Do not change dose/schedule or stop taking drug; must taper off gradually under medical supervision. • Notify physician of fever, sore throat, muscle aches, sudden weight gain or loss, edema, loss of appetite, fatigue. • Maintain fastidious personal hygiene, avoid exposure to disease, trauma. • Severe stress (serious infection, surgery, trauma) may require increased dosage. • Follow-up visits, lab tests are necessary. • Children must be assessed for growth retardation. • Inform dentist, other physicians of methylprednisolone therapy now or within past 12 mos.

metoclopramide

meh-tah-**klo**-prah-myd
(Apo-Metoclop 🍁, Metozolv ODT, Reglan)

BLACK BOX ALERT Prolonged use may cause tardive dyskinesia.

Do not confuse metoclopramide with metolazone or metoprolol, or Reglan with Renagel.

◆ CLASSIFICATION

PHARMACOTHERAPEUTIC: Dopamine receptor antagonist. **CLINICAL:** GI emptying adjunct, peristaltic stimulant, antiemetic.

ACTION

Stimulates motility of upper GI tract. Decreases reflux into esophagus. Raises threshold activity in chemoreceptor trigger zone. **Therapeutic Effect:** Accelerates intestinal transit, gastric emptying. Relieves nausea, vomiting.

PHARMACOKINETICS

Route	Onset	Peak	Duration
PO	30–60 min	N/A	1–2 hrs
IV	1–3 min	N/A	1–2 hrs
IM	10–15 min	N/A	1–2 hrs

Well absorbed from GI tract. Metabolized in liver. Protein binding: 30%. Primarily excreted in urine. Not removed by hemodialysis. **Half-life:** 4–6 hrs.

USES

Facilitates placement of enteral feeding tubes; stimulates gastric emptying, intestinal transit in conjunction with radiography; treatment of gastroparesis, gastroesophageal reflux disease (GERD); prevents or treats cancer chemotherapy-induced nausea, vomiting; prevents or treats postop nausea, vomiting. **Orally-Disintegrating Tablets:** Treatment of gastroparesis, GERD. OFF-LABEL: Prevention of aspiration pneumonia; treatment of drug-related postop nausea/vomiting, gastric stasis in preterm infants, persistent hiccups, slow gastric emptying, vascular headaches.

PRECAUTIONS

Contraindications: Concurrent use of medications likely to produce extrapyramidal reactions, GI hemorrhage, GI obstruction/perforation, history of seizure disorders, pheochromocytoma. **Cautions:** Renal impairment, CHF, cirrhosis.

LIFESPAN CONSIDERATIONS

Pregnancy/Lactation: Crosses placenta. Distributed in breast milk. **Pregnancy Category B. Children:** More susceptible to having dystonic reactions. **Elderly:** More likely to have parkinsonian dyskinesias after long-term therapy.

INTERACTIONS

DRUG: **Alcohol, other CNS depressants** may increase CNS depressant effect. HERBAL: None significant. FOOD: None known. LAB VALUES: May increase serum aldosterone, prolactin.

AVAILABILITY (Rx)

Injection Solution: 5 mg/ml. **Syrup:** 5 mg/5 ml. **Tablets:** 5 mg, 10 mg.

Tablets, Orally-Disintegrating: 5 mg, 10 mg.

ADMINISTRATION/HANDLING

IV

Reconstitution • Dilute doses greater than 10 mg in 50 ml D_5W, 0.9% NaCl, or lactated Ringer's.

Rate of administration • Infuse over 15–30 min. • May give slow IV push at rate of 10 mg over 1–2 min. • Too-rapid IV injection may produce intense feeling of anxiety, restlessness, followed by drowsiness.

Storage • Store vials at room temperature. • After dilution, IV infusion (piggyback) is stable for 24 hrs.

PO

• Give 30 min before meals and at bedtime. • Tablets may be crushed. • Do not cut, divide, chew orally-disintegrating tablets. Place on tongue.

IV INCOMPATIBILITIES

Allopurinol (Aloprim), cefepime (Maxipime), doxorubicin liposomal (Doxil), furosemide (Lasix), propofol (Diprivan).

IV COMPATIBILITIES

Dexamethasone, diltiazem (Cardizem), diphenhydramine (Benadryl), fentanyl (Sublimaze), heparin, hydromorphone (Dilaudid), lipids, morphine, potassium chloride, total parenteral nutrition (TPN).

INDICATIONS/ROUTES/DOSAGE

Prevention of Chemotherapy-Induced Nausea/Vomiting

IV: ADULTS, ELDERLY, CHILDREN: 1–2 mg/kg 30 min before chemotherapy; repeat q2h for 2 doses, then q3h as needed for total of 5 doses/day.

Postop Nausea/Vomiting

IV: ADULTS, ELDERLY: 10–20 mg q4–6h as needed. **CHILDREN:** 0.1–0.2 mg/kg/dose q6–8h as needed.

Diabetic Gastroparesis

PO, IV: ADULTS: 10 mg 30 min before meals and at bedtime for 2–8 wks.

PO: ELDERLY: Initially, 5 mg 30 min before meals and at bedtime. May increase to 10 mg.

IV: ELDERLY: 5 mg over 1–2 min. May increase to 10 mg.

M

Symptomatic Gastroesophageal Reflux Disease (GERD)

PO: ADULTS: 10–15 mg up to 4 times a day, or single doses up to 20 mg as needed. **ELDERLY:** Initially, 5 mg 4 times a day. May increase to 10 mg. **CHILDREN:** 0.4–0.8 mg/kg/day in 4 divided doses.

Facilitate Small Bowel Intubation (Single Dose)

IV: ADULTS, ELDERLY: 10 mg as a single dose. **CHILDREN 6–14 YRS:** 2.5–5 mg as a single dose. **CHILDREN YOUNGER THAN 6 YRS:** 0.1 mg/kg as a single dose.

Dosage in Renal Impairment

Dosage is modified based on creatinine clearance.

Creatinine Clearance	Dosage
Less than 40 ml/min	50% of normal dose

M

SIDE EFFECTS

◀ALERT▶ Doses of 2 mg/kg or greater, or increased length of therapy, may result in a greater incidence of side effects.

Frequent (10%): Drowsiness, restlessness, fatigue, lethargy. **Occasional (3%):** Dizziness, anxiety, headache, insomnia, breast tenderness, altered menstruation, constipation, rash, dry mouth, galactorrhea, gynecomastia. **Rare (less than 3%):** Hypotension, hypertension, tachycardia.

ADVERSE EFFECTS/ TOXIC REACTIONS

Extrapyramidal reactions occur most frequently in children, young adults (18–30 yrs) receiving large doses (2 mg/kg) during chemotherapy and usually are limited to akathisia (involuntary limb movement, facial grimacing, motor restlessness). Neuroleptic malignant syndrome (diaphoresis, fever, unstable B/P, muscular rigidity).

NURSING CONSIDERATIONS

BASELINE ASSESSMENT

Antiemetic: Assess for dehydration (poor skin turgor, dry mucous membranes, longitudinal furrows in tongue). Assess for nausea, vomiting, abdominal distention, bowel sounds.

INTERVENTION/EVALUATION

Monitor for anxiety, restlessness, extrapyramidal symptoms (EPS) during IV administration. Monitor daily pattern of bowel activity and stool consistency. Assess skin for rash. Evaluate for therapeutic response from gastroparesis (nausea, vomiting, bloating). Monitor renal function, B/P, heart rate.

PATIENT/FAMILY TEACHING

• Avoid tasks that require alertness, motor skills until drug response is established. • Report involuntary eye, facial, limb movement (extrapyramidal reaction). • Avoid alcohol.

metolazone

meh-**toh**-lah-zone
(Zaroxolyn)

Do not confuse metolazone with metaxolone, methotrexate, metoclopramide, or metoprolol, or Zaroxolyn with Zarontin.

◆CLASSIFICATION

PHARMACOTHERAPEUTIC: Thiazide diuretic. **CLINICAL:** Diuretic, antihypertensive (see p. 102C).

ACTION

Diuretic: Blocks reabsorption of sodium, potassium, chloride at distal convoluted tubule, promoting delivery of sodium to potassium side, increasing sodium-potassium (Na-K) exchange. **Therapeutic Ef-**

fect: Produces renal excretion. **Antihypertensive:** Reduces plasma and extracellular fluid volume, peripheral vascular resistance. **Therapeutic Effect:** Reduces B/P.

PHARMACOKINETICS

Route	Onset	Peak	Duration
PO (diuretic)	1 hr	2 hrs	12–24 hrs

Incompletely absorbed from GI tract. Protein binding: 95%. Primarily excreted unchanged in urine. Not removed by hemodialysis. **Half-life:** 20 hrs.

USES

Treatment of mild to moderate essential hypertension, edema due to renal disease, edema due to CHF.

PRECAUTIONS

Contraindications: Anuria, hepatic coma/precoma, history of hypersensitivity to sulfonamides, thiazide diuretics, renal decompensation. **Cautions:** Severe renal disease, hepatic impairment, gout, lupus erythematosus, diabetes, elevated serum cholesterol, triglycerides.

LIFESPAN CONSIDERATIONS

Pregnancy/Lactation: Crosses placenta. Small amount distributed in breast milk. Breast-feeding not recommended. **Pregnancy Category B (D if used in pregnancy-induced hypertension). Children:** No age-related precautions noted. **Elderly:** May be more sensitive to hypotensive or electrolyte effects. Age-related renal impairment may require dosage adjustment.

INTERACTIONS

DRUG: **Cholestyramine, colestipol** may decrease absorption/effect. May increase risk of **digoxin** toxicity associated with metolazone-induced hypokalemia. May increase risk of **lithium** toxicity. **HERBAL:** **Dong quai, St. John's wort** may increase photosensitization. **Ephedra, ginseng, yohimbe** may worsen hypertension. **Garlic** may increase antihypertensive effect. **FOOD:** None known. **LAB VALUES:** May increase serum glucose, cholesterol, LDL, bilirubin, calcium, creatinine, uric acid, triglycerides. May decrease urinary calcium, serum magnesium, potassium, sodium.

AVAILABILITY (Rx)

Tablets: 2.5 mg, 5 mg, 10 mg.

ADMINISTRATION/HANDLING

PO

- May give with food, milk if GI upset occurs, preferably with breakfast (may prevent nocturia).

INDICATIONS/ROUTES/DOSAGE

Edema

PO: ADULTS: 2.5–10 mg/day. May increase to 20 mg/day in edema associated with renal disease or heart failure.

Hypertension

PO: ADULTS: 2.5–5 mg/day.

Usual Elderly Dosage

PO: Initially, 2.5 mg/day or every other day.

Usual Pediatric Dosage

PO: 0.2–0.4 mg/kg/day in 1–2 divided doses.

SIDE EFFECTS

Expected: Increased urinary frequency/volume. **Frequent (10%–9%):** Dizziness, light-headedness, headache. **Occasional (6%–4%):** Muscle cramps/spasm, drowsiness, fatigue, lethargy. **Rare (less than 2%):** Asthenia (loss of strength, energy), palpitations, depression, nausea, vomiting, abdominal bloating, constipation, diarrhea, urticaria.

ADVERSE EFFECTS/ TOXIC REACTIONS

Vigorous diuresis may lead to profound water loss and electrolyte depletion, resulting in hypokalemia, hyponatremia, dehydration. Acute hypotensive episodes may occur. Hyperglycemia may occur during prolonged therapy. Pancreatitis, paresthe-

M

sia, blood dyscrasias, pulmonary edema, allergic pneumonitis, dermatologic reactions occur rarely. Overdose can lead to lethargy, coma without changes in electrolytes, hydration.

NURSING CONSIDERATIONS

BASELINE ASSESSMENT

Check vital signs, esp. B/P for hypotension, before administration. Assess baseline serum electrolytes, particularly check for hypokalemia. Assess skin turgor, mucous membranes for hydration status. Assess for peripheral edema. Assess muscle strength, mental status. Note skin temperature, moisture. Obtain baseline weight. Monitor I&O.

INTERVENTION/EVALUATION

Continue to monitor B/P, vital signs, serum electrolytes, I&O, weight. Note extent of diuresis. Monitor for electrolyte disturbances (hypokalemia may result in weakness, tremors, muscle cramps, nausea, vomiting, altered mental status, tachycardia; hyponatremia may result in confusion, thirst, cold/clammy skin).

PATIENT/FAMILY TEACHING

• Expect increased urinary frequency/volume. • Rise slowly from lying to sitting position, permit legs to dangle momentarily before standing to reduce hypotensive effect. • Avoid tasks requiring motor skills, mental alertness until response to drug is established. • Eat foods high in potassium, such as whole grains (cereals), legumes, meat, bananas, apricots, orange juice, potatoes (white, sweet), raisins.

metoprolol

HIGH ALERT

me-**toe**-pro-lole
(Apo-Metoprolol ♣, Betaloc ♣, Lopressor, Novo-Metoprolol ♣, Nu-Metop ♣, Toprol XL)

BLACK BOX ALERT Abrupt withdrawal can produce acute tachycardia, hypertension, ischemia. Drug should be gradually tapered over 1–2 wks.

Do not confuse Lopressor with Lyrica, metoprolol with metaproterenol, metoclopramide, or metolazone, or Toprol XL with Tegretol, Tegretol XR, or Topamax.

FIXED-COMBINATION(S)

Lopressor HCT: metoprolol/hydrochlorothiazide (a diuretic): 50 mg/25 mg, 100 mg/25 mg, 100 mg/50 mg.

◆CLASSIFICATION

PHARMACOTHERAPEUTIC: Beta$_1$-adrenergic blocker. **CLINICAL:** Antianginal, antihypertensive, MI adjunct (see p. 72C).

ACTION

Selectively blocks beta$_1$-adrenergic receptors; high dosages may block beta$_2$-adrenergic receptors. Decreases oxygen requirements. Large doses increase airway resistance. **Therapeutic Effect:** Slows heart rate, decreases cardiac output, reduces B/P. Decreases myocardial ischemia severity.

PHARMACOKINETICS

Route	Onset	Peak	Duration
PO	10–15 min	1–2 hrs	N/A
PO (extended-release)	N/A	6–12 hrs	N/A
IV	Immediate	20 min	N/A

Well absorbed from GI tract. Protein binding: 12%. Widely distributed. Metabolized in liver (undergoes significant first-pass metabolism). Primarily excreted in urine. Removed by hemodialysis. **Half-life:** 3–7 hrs.

USES

Lopressor: Treatment of hemodynamically stable acute myocardial infarction (AMI), angina pectoris, hypertension.

Toprol XL: Treatment of angina pectoris, to reduce mortality or hospitalizations in pts with heart failure, hypertension. OFF-LABEL: To increase survival rate in diabetic pts with coronary artery disease (CAD). Treatment/prevention of anxiety, cardiac arrhythmias, hypertrophic cardiomyopathy, mitral valve prolapse syndrome, pheochromocytoma, tremors, thyrotoxicosis, vascular headache.

PRECAUTIONS

Contraindications: Cardiogenic shock, MI with heart rate less than 45 beats/min or systolic B/P less than 100 mm Hg, overt heart failure, second- or third-degree heart block, sinus bradycardia. Cautions: Bronchospastic disease, renal impairment, peripheral vascular disease, hyperthyroidism, diabetes mellitus, inadequate cardiac function.

LIFESPAN CONSIDERATIONS

Pregnancy/Lactation: Crosses placenta; distributed in breast milk. Avoid use during first trimester. May produce bradycardia, apnea, hypoglycemia, hypothermia during delivery, low birth-weight infants. **Pregnancy Category C (D if used in second or third trimester). Children:** Safety and efficacy not established. **Elderly:** Age-related peripheral vascular disease may increase susceptibility to decreased peripheral circulation.

INTERACTIONS

DRUG: **Diuretics, other antihypertensives** may increase hypotensive effect. May mask symptoms of hypoglycemia, prolong hypoglycemic effect of **insulin, oral hypoglycemics. NSAIDs** may decrease antihypertensive effect. **Sympathomimetics, xanthines** may mutually inhibit effects. HERBAL: **Ephedra, ginseng, yohimbe** may worsen hypertension. **Garlic** may increase antihypertensive effect. FOOD: None known. LAB VALUES: May increase serum antinuclear antibody titer (ANA), BUN, serum lipoprotein, LDH, alkaline phosphatase, bilirubin, creatinine, potassium, uric acid, AST, ALT, triglycerides.

AVAILABILITY (Rx)

Injection Solution (Lopressor): 1 mg/ml. Tablets (Lopressor): 25 mg, 50 mg, 100 mg.

Tablets (Extended-Release [Toprol XL]): 25 mg, 50 mg, 100 mg, 200 mg.

ADMINISTRATION/HANDLING

IV

Rate of administration • May give undiluted. • Administer IV injection over 1 min. • May give by IV piggyback over 30–60 min. • Monitor EKG, B/P during administration.

Storage • Store at room temperature.

PO

• Tablets may be crushed; do not crush/chew extended-release tablets. • Extended-release tablets may be divided in half. • Give at same time each day. • May be given with or immediately after meals (enhances absorption).

IV INCOMPATIBILITY

Amphotericin B complex (Abelcet, AmBisome, Amphotec).

IV COMPATIBILITIES

Alteplase (Activase), meperidine (Demerol), morphine.

INDICATIONS/ROUTES/DOSAGE

Hypertension

PO: ADULTS: Initially, 100 mg/day as single or divided dose. Increase at weekly (or longer) intervals. Maintenance: 100–450 mg/day. ELDERLY: Initially, 25 mg/day. Range: 25–300 mg/day.

PO (EXTENDED-RELEASE): ADULTS: 25–100 mg/day as single dose. May increase at least at weekly intervals until optimum B/P attained. **Maximum:** 400 mg/day. ELDERLY: Initially, 25–50 mg/day as a single dose. May increase at 1- to 2-wk intervals.

Angina Pectoris

PO: ADULTS: Initially, 100 mg/day as single or divided dose. Increase at weekly

M

(or longer) intervals. Maintenance: 100–450 mg/day.

PO (EXTENDED-RELEASE): ADULTS: Initially, 100 mg/day as single dose. May increase at least at weekly intervals until optimum clinical response achieved. **Maximum:** 400 mg/day.

CHF

PO (EXTENDED-RELEASE): ADULTS: Initially, 25 mg/day. May double dose q2wk. **Maximum:** 200 mg/day.

Early Treatment of MI

IV: ADULTS: 5 mg q5min for 3 doses, followed by 50 mg orally q6h for 48 hrs. Begin oral dose 15 min after last IV dose. In pts who do not tolerate full IV dose, give 25–50 mg orally q6h, 15 min after last IV dose.

Late Treatment, Maintenance After MI

PO: ADULTS: 100 mg twice a day for at least 3 mos.

M

SIDE EFFECTS

Metoprolol is generally well tolerated, with transient and mild side effects. **Frequent:** Diminished sexual function, drowsiness, insomnia, unusual fatigue/weakness. **Occasional:** Anxiety, diarrhea, constipation, nausea, vomiting, nasal congestion, abdominal discomfort, dizziness, difficulty breathing, cold hands/feet. **Rare:** Altered taste, dry eyes, nightmares, paresthesia, allergic reaction (rash, pruritus).

ADVERSE EFFECTS/ TOXIC REACTIONS

Overdose may produce profound bradycardia, hypotension, bronchospasm. Abrupt withdrawal may result in diaphoresis, palpitations, headache, tremulousness, exacerbation of angina, MI, ventricular arrhythmias. May precipitate CHF, MI in pts with heart disease; thyroid storm in those with thyrotoxicosis; peripheral ischemia in those with existing peripheral vascular disease. Hypoglycemia may occur in pts with previously controlled diabetes mellitus. **Antidote:** Glucagon (see Appendix M for dosage).

NURSING CONSIDERATIONS

BASELINE ASSESSMENT

Assess baseline renal/hepatic function tests. Assess B/P, apical pulse immediately before drug administration (if pulse is 60/min or less or systolic B/P is less than 90 mm Hg, withhold medication, contact physician). **Antianginal:** Record onset, type (sharp, dull, squeezing), radiation, location, intensity, duration of anginal pain, precipitating factors (exertion, emotional stress).

INTERVENTION/EVALUATION

Measure B/P near end of dosing interval (determines whether B/P is controlled throughout day). Monitor B/P for hypotension, respiration for shortness of breath. Assess pulse for quality, irregular rate, bradycardia. Assess for evidence of CHF: dyspnea (esp. on exertion, lying down), night cough, peripheral edema, distended neck veins. Monitor I&O (increased weight, decreased urinary output may indicate CHF). Therapeutic response to hypertension noted in 1–2 wks.

PATIENT/FAMILY TEACHING

• Do not abruptly discontinue medication. • Compliance with therapy regimen is essential to control hypertension, arrhythmias. • If dose is missed, take next scheduled dose (do not double dose). • To avoid hypotensive effect, rise slowly from lying to sitting position, wait momentarily before standing. • Report excessive fatigue, dizziness. • Avoid tasks that require alertness, motor skills until response to drug is established. • Do not use nasal decongestants, OTC cold preparations (stimulants) without physician approval. • Monitor B/P, pulse before taking medication. • Restrict salt, alcohol intake.

metronidazole

me-troe-**ni**-da-zole
(Apo-Metronidazole ✤, Flagyl, Flagyl ER, Flagyl 375, MetroCream, MetroGel, MetroGel-Vaginal, NidaGel ✤, Noritate, Vandazole)

Do not confuse metronidazole with meropenum, metformin, methotrexate, or miconazole.

FIXED-COMBINATION(S)

Helidac: metronidazole/bismuth/tetracycline (an anti-infective): 250 mg/262 mg/500 mg. **Pylera:** metronidazole/bismuth/tetracycline (an anti-infective): 125 mg/140 mg/125 mg.

◆ CLASSIFICATION

PHARMACOTHERAPEUTIC: Nitroimidazole derivative. **CLINICAL:** Antibacterial, antiprotozoal.

ACTION

Disrupts DNA, inhibiting nucleic acid synthesis. **Therapeutic Effect:** Produces bactericidal, antiprotozoal, amebicidal, trichomonacidal effects. Produces anti-inflammatory, immunosuppressive effects when applied topically.

PHARMACOKINETICS

Well absorbed from GI tract; minimally absorbed after topical application. Protein binding: less than 20%. Widely distributed; crosses blood-brain barrier. Metabolized in liver to active metabolite. Primarily excreted in urine; partially eliminated in feces. Removed by hemodialysis. **Half-life:** 8 hrs (increased in alcoholic hepatic disease, neonates).

USES

Treatment of anaerobic infections (skin/skin structure, CNS, lower respiratory tract, bone/joints, intra-abdominal, gynocologic, endocarditis, septicemia). Treatment of trichomoniasis, amebiasis, antibiotic-associated pseudomembranous colitis (AAPC). Topical treatment of acne rosacea. **OFF-LABEL:** Treatment of bacterial vaginosis, grade III-IV decubitus ulcers with anaerobic infection, *H. pylori*-associated gastritis and duodenal ulcer, inflammatory bowel disease.

PRECAUTIONS

Contraindications: Hypersensitivity to other nitroimidazole derivatives (also parabens with topical application). **Cautions:** Blood dyscrasias, severe hepatic dysfunction, CNS disease, predisposition to edema, concurrent corticosteroid therapy.

LIFESPAN CONSIDERATIONS

Pregnancy/Lactation: Readily crosses placenta. Distributed in breast milk. Contraindicated during first trimester in those with trichomoniasis. Topical use during pregnancy, lactation discouraged. **Pregnancy Category B. Children:** Safety and efficacy of topical administration not established in those younger than 21 yrs. **Elderly:** Age-related hepatic impairment may require dosage adjustment.

INTERACTIONS

DRUG: **Alcohol** may cause disulfiram-type reaction. **Disulfiram** may increase risk of toxicity. May increase effects of **oral anticoagulants. HERBAL:** None significant. **FOOD:** None known. **LAB VALUES:** May increase serum LDH, AST, ALT.

AVAILABILITY (Rx)

Capsules (Flagyl 375): 375 mg. **Injection (Infusion):** 500 mg/100 ml. **Tablets (Flagyl):** 250 mg, 500 mg. **Topical Cream:** 0.75% (MetroCream), 1% (Noritate). **Topical Gel (MetroGel):** 0.75%, 1%. **Vaginal Gel (MetroGel-Vaginal, Vandazole):** 0.75%.

Tablets (Extended-Release [Flagyl ER]): 750 mg.

ADMINISTRATION/HANDLING

IV

Rate of administration • Infuse IV over 30–60 min. Do not give by IV bolus.

M

Storage • Store at room temperature (ready-to-use infusion bags).

PO

• Give without regard to meals. Give with food to decrease GI irritation. • Extended-release tablet should be given on an empty stomach (1 hr before or 2 hrs after meals). • Do not crush extended-release tablets.

IV INCOMPATIBILITIES

Amphotericin B complex (Abelcet, AmBisome, Amphotec), filgrastim (Neupogen), total parenteral nutrition (TPN).

IV COMPATIBILITIES

Diltiazem (Cardizem), dopamine (Intropin), heparin, hydromorphone (Dilaudid), lipids, lorazepam (Ativan), magnesium sulfate, midazolam (Versed), morphine.

INDICATIONS/ROUTES/DOSAGE

Anaerobic Infections

PO, IV: ADULTS, ELDERLY: 500 mg q6–8h. **Maximum:** 4 g/day.

PO: CHILDREN, INFANTS: 15–35 mg/kg in divided doses q8h.

IV: CHILDREN, INFANTS: 30 mg/kg/day in divided doses q6h.

Amebiasis

PO: ADULTS, ELDERLY: 500–750 mg 3 times a day for 5–10 days. **CHILDREN:** 35–50 mg/kg/day in 3 divided doses for 10 days. **Maximum:** 750 mg/dose.

Giardiasis

PO: ADULTS, ELDERLY: 500 mg 2 times per day for 5–7 days.

Pseudomembranous Colitis

PO: ADULTS, ELDERLY: 250–500 mg 3–4 times a day. **CHILDREN:** 5 mg/kg q6h for 7–10 days. **Maximum:** 2 g/day.

Trichomoniasis

PO: ADULTS, ELDERLY: 250 mg 3 times a day or 375 mg twice a day or 500 mg twice a day or 2 g as a single dose. **CHILDREN:** 15–30 mg/kg/day in 3 divided doses for 7 days.

Bacterial Vaginosis

PO: ADULTS: (NON-PREGNANT): 500 mg twice a day for 7 days or 750 mg (extended-release) once daily for 7 days.

INTRAVAGINAL: ADULTS: 0.75% apply twice a day for 5 days.

ALERT Centers for Disease Control and Prevention (CDC) does not recommend the use of topical agents during pregnancy.

Rosacea

TOPICAL: ADULTS, ELDERLY: (1%): Apply to affected area once daily. **(0.75%):** Apply to affected area twice a day.

Dosage in Renal Impairment

Creatinine clearance less than 10 ml/min: Administer 50% of dose or q12h.

SIDE EFFECTS

Frequent: **Systemic:** Anorexia, nausea, dry mouth, metallic taste. **Vaginal:** Symptomatic cervicitis/vaginitis, abdominal cramps, uterine pain. Occasional: **Systemic:** Diarrhea, constipation, vomiting, dizziness, erythematous rash, urticaria, reddish-brown urine. **Topical:** Transient erythema, mild dryness, burning, irritation, stinging, tearing when applied too close to eyes. **Vaginal:** Vaginal, perineal, vulvar itching; vulvar swelling. Rare: Mild, transient leukopenia; thrombophlebitis with IV therapy.

ADVERSE EFFECTS/ TOXIC REACTIONS

Oral therapy may result in furry tongue, glossitis, cystitis, dysuria, pancreatitis, flattening of T waves on EKG. Peripheral neuropathy (manifested as numbness, tingling of hands/feet) usually is reversible if treatment is stopped immediately upon appearance of neurologic symptoms. Seizures occur occasionally.

M

NURSING CONSIDERATIONS

BASELINE ASSESSMENT

Question for history of hypersensitivity to metronidazole, other nitroimidazole derivatives (and parabens with topical). Obtain specimens for diagnostic tests, cultures before giving first dose (therapy may begin before results are known).

INTERVENTION/EVALUATION

Monitor daily pattern of bowel activity and stool consistency. Monitor I&O, assess for urinary problems. Be alert to neurologic symptoms (dizziness; paresthesia of extremities). Assess for rash, urticaria. Watch for onset of superinfection (ulceration/change of oral mucosa, furry tongue, vaginal discharge, genital/anal pruritus).

PATIENT/FAMILY TEACHING

• Urine may be red-brown or dark. • Avoid alcohol, alcohol-containing preparations (cough syrups, elixirs) for at least 48 hrs after last dose. • Avoid tasks that require alertness, motor skills until response to drug established. • If taking metronidazole for trichomoniasis, refrain from sexual intercourse until full treatment is completed. • For amebiasis, frequent stool specimen checks will be necessary. • **Topical:** Avoid contact with eyes. • May apply cosmetics after application. • Metronidazole acts on erythema, papules, pustules but has no effect on rhinophyma (hypertrophy of nose), telangiectasia, ocular problems (conjunctivitis, keratitis, blepharitis). • Other recommendations for rosacea include avoidance of hot/spicy foods, alcohol, extremes of hot/cold temperatures, excessive sunlight.

Mevacor, *see lovastatin*

Miacalcin, *see calcitonin*

micafungin

my-cah-**fun**-gin
(Mycamine)

CLASSIFICATION

CLINICAL: Antifungal.

ACTION

Inhibits synthesis of glucan (vital component of fungal cell formation), damaging fungal cell membrane. **Therapeutic Effect:** Decreased glucan content leads to cellular lysis.

PHARMACOKINETICS

Extensively bound to albumin. Protein binding: greater than 99%. Slowly metabolized in liver to active metabolite. Primarily excreted in feces and, to a lesser extent, in urine. Not removed by hemodialysis. **Half-life:** 11–21 hrs.

USES

Treatment of esophageal candidiasis, candidemia, candida peritonitis, abscesses, acute disseminated candidiasis, infections due to *Aspergillus*, prophylaxis of *Candida* infection in pts undergoing hematopoietic stem cell transplant. **OFF-LABEL:** Prophylaxis of HIV-related esophageal candidiasis.

PRECAUTIONS

Contraindications: None known. **Cautions:** Hepatic/renal impairment.

LIFESPAN CONSIDERATIONS

Pregnancy/Lactation: May reduce sperm count. May be embryotoxic. Unknown if distributed in breast milk. **Pregnancy Category C. Children:** Safety and efficacy not established. **Elderly:** No age-related precautions noted.

INTERACTIONS

DRUG: May increase concentration of **nifedipine, sirolimus. HERBAL:** None significant. **FOOD:** None known. **LAB VALUES:** May increase serum creatinine, alkaline phosphatase, LDH, AST, ALT.

M

AVAILABILITY (Rx)

Injection, Powder for Reconstitution: 50 mg, 100 mg.

ADMINISTRATION/HANDLING

IV

Reconstitution • Add 5 ml 0.9% NaCl (without bacteriostatic agent) to each 50-mg vial (10 ml to 100-mg vial) to yield micafungin 10 mg/ml. • Gently swirl to dissolve; do not shake. • Further dilute in 0.9% NaCl or D_5W to final concentration of 0.5–1.5 mg/ml. • Alternatively, D_5W may be used for reconstitution and dilution. • Flush existing IV line with 0.9% NaCl or D_5W before infusion.
Rate of administration • Infuse over 60 min.
Storage • Reconstituted solution is stable for 24 hrs at room temperature. • Discard if precipitate is present.

IV INCOMPATIBILITIES

Do not mix with any other medication.

INDICATIONS/ROUTES/DOSAGE

Esophageal Candidiasis
IV: ADULTS, ELDERLY: 150 mg/day for 10–30 days.

Candida Prophylaxis in Stem Cell Pts
IV: ADULTS, ELDERLY: 50 mg/day.

Candidemia, Disseminated Candidiasis, Peritonitis, Abscesses
IV: ADULTS, ELDERLY: 100 mg/day for 15 days.

SIDE EFFECTS

Occasional (3%–2%): Nausea, headache, diarrhea, vomiting, fever. **Rare (1%):** Dizziness, drowsiness, pruritus, abdominal pain, dyspepsia (heartburn, indigestion, epigastric pain).

ADVERSE EFFECTS/ TOXIC REACTIONS

Hypersensitivity reaction characterized by rash, pruritus, facial edema occurs rarely. Anaphylaxis, hemoglobinuria, hemolytic anemia have been reported.

NURSING CONSIDERATIONS

BASELINE ASSESSMENT

Determine baseline hepatic/renal function tests and periodically thereafter.

INTERVENTION/EVALUATION

Monitor serum chemistry results for evidence of hepatic/renal impairment.

Micardis, *see telmisartan*

miconazole

mih-**kon**-nah-zoll
(Baza Antifungal, Lotrimin, Micaderm, Micatin, Micozole ✦, Mitrazol, Monistat, Monistat 3, Monistat 7, Oravig)
Do not confuse miconazole with Micronase or metronidazole, Lotrimin with Lotrisone, or Micatin with Miacalcin.

◆CLASSIFICATION

PHARMACOTHERAPEUTIC: Imidazole derivative. **CLINICAL:** Antifungal (see p. 48C).

ACTION

Inhibits synthesis of ergosterol (vital component of fungal cell formation), damaging fungal cell membrane. **Therapeutic Effect:** Fungistatic; may be fungicidal, depending on concentration.

PHARMACOKINETICS

Small amounts absorbed systemically after vaginal administration. Widely distributed. Protein binding: 91%–93%. Metabolized in liver. Primarily excreted in feces. **Half-life:** 24 hrs.

USES

Buccal Tablet: Oropharyngeal candidiasis. **Vaginal:** Vulvovaginal candidiasis. **Topical:** Cutaneous candidiasis, *tinea cruris, t. corporis, t. pedis, t. versicolor.*

PRECAUTIONS

Contraindications: Avoid vaginal preparations during first trimester of pregnancy. **Cautions:** Sensitivity to other antifungals (clotrimazole, ketoconazole).

LIFESPAN CONSIDERATIONS

Pregnancy/Lactation: Unknown if drug crosses placenta or is distributed in breast milk. **Pregnancy Category C. Children:** Safety not established in those younger than 1 yr. **Elderly:** No age-related precautions noted.

INTERACTIONS

DRUG: None significant. **HERBAL:** None significant. **FOOD:** None known. **LAB VALUES:** None significant.

AVAILABILITY (Rx)

Cream (Topical): Baza, Micaderm, Micatin: 2%. **Cream (Vaginal): Monistat 7:** 2%; **Monistat 3:** 2%, 4%. **Tablet (Buccal):** 50 mg. **Topical Powder: Mitrazol:** 2%. **Vaginal Suppository: Monistat 3:** 200 mg; 1,200 mg; **Monistat 7:** 100 mg.

INDICATIONS/ROUTES/DOSAGE

Vulvovaginal Candidiasis

INTRAVAGINAL SUPPOSITORY: ADULTS, ELDERLY: 100-mg suppository at bedtime for 7 days, 200-mg suppository at bedtime for 3 days, or 1,200-mg suppository once at bedtime or during the day.
INTRAVAGINAL CREAM: ADULTS, ELDERLY: 2% cream: 1 applicatorful at bedtime for 7 days. 4% cream: 1 applicatorful at bedtime for 3 days.

Topical Fungal Infections, Cutaneous Candidiasis

TOPICAL: ADULTS, ELDERLY, CHILDREN: Apply liberally twice per day, morning and evening.

Oropharyngeal Candidiasis

BUCCAL: ADULTS, ELDERLY: 50 mg once daily to gum region for 14 consecutive days.

Diaper Rash

TOPICAL: INFANTS: As needed.

SIDE EFFECTS

Topical: Pruritus, burning, stinging, erythema, urticaria. **Vaginal (2%):** Vulvovaginal burning, pruritus, irritation; headache; skin rash.

ADVERSE EFFECTS/ TOXIC REACTIONS

None known.

NURSING CONSIDERATIONS

BASELINE ASSESSMENT

Topical: Avoid occlusive dressings. Apply only small amount to cover area completely.

INTERVENTION/EVALUATION

Topical/Vaginal: Assess for burning, pruritus, irritation.

PATIENT/FAMILY TEACHING

• **Vaginal Preparation:** Base interacts with certain latex products (e.g., condoms, contraceptive diaphram). • Ask physician about douching, sexual intercourse. • **Topical:** Rub well into affected areas. • Avoid getting in eyes. • Keep areas clean, dry; wear light clothing for ventilation. • Separate personal items in contact with affected areas.

midazolam HIGH ALERT

my-**dah**-zoe-lam
(Apo-Midazolam ✱, Versed)

BLACK BOX ALERT May cause severe respiratory depression, respiratory arrest, apnea. Avoid rapid injection, prolonged infusion (increases risk).

M

Do not confuse Versed with VePesid or Vistaril.

CLASSIFICATION

PHARMACOTHERAPEUTIC: Benzodiazepine **(Schedule IV). CLINICAL:** Sedative (see p. 5C).

ACTION

Enhances action of gamma-aminobutyric acid (GABA), one of the major inhibitory neurotransmitters in the brain. **Therapeutic Effect:** Produces anxiolytic, hypnotic, anticonvulsant, muscle relaxant, amnestic effects.

PHARMACOKINETICS

Route	Onset	Peak	Duration
PO	10–20 min	N/A	N/A
IV	1–5 min	5–7 min	20–30 min
IM	5–15 min	30–60 min	2–6 hrs

Well absorbed after IM administration. Protein binding: 97%. Metabolized in liver. Primarily excreted in urine. Not removed by hemodialysis. **Half-life:** 1–5 hrs.

USES

Sedation, anxiolytic, amnesia before procedure or induction of anesthesia, conscious sedation before diagnostic/radiographic procedure, continuous IV sedation of intubated or mechanically ventilated pts. **OFF-LABEL:** Anxiety, status epilepticus.

PRECAUTIONS

Contraindications: Acute alcohol intoxication, acute narrow-angle glaucoma, allergies to cherries, coma, shock. **Cautions:** Acute illness, severe fluid electrolyte imbalance, renal/hepatic/pulmonary impairment, CHF, treated open-angle glaucoma.

LIFESPAN CONSIDERATIONS

Pregnancy/Lactation: Crosses placenta. Unknown if drug is distributed in breast milk. **Pregnancy Category D. Children:** Neonates more likely to have respiratory depression. **Elderly:** Age-related renal impairment may require dosage adjustment.

INTERACTIONS

DRUG: Alcohol, other CNS depressants may increase CNS effects, respiratory depression, hypotensive effects. **Antihypertensives, hypotensive medications** may increase hypotensive effects. **HERBAL: Gotu kola, kava kava, St. John's wort, valerian** may increase CNS depression. **FOOD: Grapefruit, grapefruit juice** increase oral absorption, systemic availability. **LAB VALUES:** None significant.

AVAILABILITY (Rx)

Injection Solution: 1 mg/ml, 5 mg/ml. **Injection Solution (Preservative-Free):** 1 mg/ml, 5 mg/ml. **Syrup:** 2 mg/ml.

ADMINISTRATION/HANDLING

IV

Rate of administration • May give undiluted or as infusion. • Resuscitative equipment, O_2 must be readily available before IV administration. • Administer by slow IV injection over at least 2–5 min at concentration of 1–5 mg/ml. • Reduce IV rate in those older than 60 yrs, debilitated pts with chronic disease states, pulmonary impairment. • Too-rapid IV rate, excessive doses, or single large dose increases risk of respiratory depression/arrest.

Storage • Store vials at room temperature.

IM

• Give deep IM into large muscle mass. **Maximum concentration:** 1 mg/ml.

IV INCOMPATIBILITIES

Albumin, ampicillin and sulbactam (Unasyn), amphotericin B complex (Abelcet, AmBisome, Amphotec), ampicillin (Polycillin), bumetanide (Bumex), co-trimoxazole (Bactrim), dexamethasone (Decadron), fosphenytoin (Cerebyx), furosemide (Lasix), hydrocortisone (Solu-Cortef), lipids, methotrexate, nafcillin (Nafcil), sodium bicarbonate, sodium pentothal (Thiopental).

IV COMPATIBILITIES

Amiodarone (Cordarone), atropine, calcium gluconate, diltiazem (Cardizem), diphenhydramine (Benadryl), dobutamine (Dobutrex), dopamine (Intropin), etomidate (Amidate), fentanyl (Sublimaze), glycopyrrolate (Robinul), heparin, hydromorphone (Dilaudid), hydroxyzine (Vistaril), insulin, lorazepam (Ativan), milrinone (Primacor), morphine, nitroglycerin, norepinephrine (Levophed), potassium chloride, propofol (Diprivan).

INDICATIONS/ROUTES/DOSAGE

Preop Sedation

PO: CHILDREN: 0.25–0.5 mg/kg. **Maximum:** 20 mg.
IV: ADULTS, ELDERLY: 0.02–0.04 mg/kg. **CHILDREN 6–12 YRS:** 0.025–0.05 mg/kg. **CHILDREN 6 MOS–5 YRS:** 0.05–0.1 mg/kg.
IM: ADULTS, ELDERLY: 0.07–0.08 mg/kg 30–60 min before surgery. Usual dose: 5 mg. **CHILDREN:** 0.1–0.15 mg/kg 30–60 min before surgery. **Maximum:** 10 mg.

Conscious Sedation for Diagnostic, Therapeutic, Endoscopic Procedures

IV: ADULTS, ELDERLY: 0.5–2 mg over 2 min. Titrate as needed. **Maximum total dose:** 2.5–5 mg. **CHILDREN 6–12 YRS:** 0.025–0.05 mg/kg. Total dose of 0.4 mg/kg may be necessary. **Maximum total dose:** 10 mg. **CHILDREN 6 MOS–5 YRS:** 0.05–0.1 mg/kg. Total dose of 0.6 mg/kg may be necessary. **Maximum total dose:** 6 mg.

Continuous Sedation During Mechanical Ventilation

IV: ADULTS, ELDERLY: Initially, 0.02–0.08 mg/kg. May repeat at 5- to 15-min intervals or continuous infusion rate of 0.04–0.2 mg/kg/hr and titrated to desired effect. **CHILDREN:** Initially, 0.05–0.2 mg/kg followed by continuous infusion of 0.06–0.12 mg/kg/hr (1–2 mcg/kg/min) titrated to desired effect. Usual range: 0.4–6 mcg/kg/min.

SIDE EFFECTS

Frequent (10%–4%): Decreased respiratory rate, tenderness at IM or IV injection site, pain during injection, oxygen desaturation, hiccups. **Occasional (3%–2%):** Hypotension, paradoxical CNS reaction. **Rare (less than 2%):** Nausea, vomiting, headache, coughing.

ADVERSE EFFECTS/ TOXIC REACTIONS

Inadequate or excessive dosage, improper administration may result in cerebral hypoxia, agitation, involuntary movements, hyperactivity, combativeness. Too-rapid IV rate, excessive doses, or single large dose increases risk of respiratory depression/arrest. Respiratory depression/apnea may produce hypoxia, cardiac arrest.

NURSING CONSIDERATIONS

BASELINE ASSESSMENT

Resuscitative equipment, oxygen must be available. Obtain vital signs before administration.

INTERVENTION/EVALUATION

Monitor respiratory rate, oxygen saturation continuously during parenteral administration for underventilation, apnea. Monitor vital signs, level of sedation q3–5min during recovery period.

M

midodrine

my-doe-dreen
(Amatine ✦, Apo-Midodrine ✦, ProAmatine)

BLACK BOX ALERT Can cause marked rise in supine blood pressure; use in pts for whom orthostatic hypotension significantly impairs daily life.

Do not confuse Amatine or ProAmatine with amantadine or protamine, or midodrine with Midrin.

◆CLASSIFICATION

PHARMACOTHERAPEUTIC: Vasopressor. **CLINICAL:** Orthostatic hypotension adjunct.

ACTION

Forms active metabolite desglymidodrine, an alpha$_1$-agonist, activating alpha receptors of arteriolar, venous vasculature. **Therapeutic Effect:** Increases vascular tone, B/P.

PHARMACOKINETICS

Route	Onset	Peak	Duration
PO	1 hr	–	2–3 hrs

Rapid absorption from GI tract following PO administration. Protein binding: Low. Undergoes enzymatic hydrolysis (deglycination) in systemic circulation. Excreted in urine. **Half-life:** 0.5 hr.

USES

Treatment of symptomatic orthostatic hypotension. **OFF-LABEL:** Infection-related hypotension, intradialytic hypotension, psychotropic agent-induced hypotension, urinary incontinence.

PRECAUTIONS

Contraindications: Acute renal impairment, persistent hypertension, pheochromocytoma, severe cardiac disease, thyrotoxicosis, urine retention. **Cautions:** Renal/hepatic impairment, history of visual problems.

LIFESPAN CONSIDERATIONS

Pregnancy/Lactation: Unknown if drug crosses placenta or is distributed in breast milk. **Pregnancy Category C. Children:** Safety and efficacy not established. **Elderly:** Age-related renal impairment may require dosage adjustment.

INTERACTIONS

DRUG: **Digoxin** may have additive bradycardic effects. **Sodium-retaining steroids (e.g., fludrocortisone)** may increase sodium retention. **Vasoconstrictors** may have additive effects. **HERBAL:** None significant. **FOOD:** None known. **LAB VALUES:** None significant.

AVAILABILITY (Rx)

Tablets: 2.5 mg, 5 mg, 10 mg.

ADMINISTRATION/HANDLING

• Give without regard to food. • Last dose of day should be given 3–4 hrs before bedtime.

INDICATIONS/ROUTES/DOSAGE

Orthostatic Hypotension

PO: ADULTS, ELDERLY: 10 mg 3 times a day. Give during the day when pt is upright, such as upon arising, midday, and late afternoon. Do not give later than 6 PM. **Maximum:** 40 mg/day.

Dosage in Renal Impairment

For adults and elderly pts, give 2.5 mg 3 times a day; increase gradually, as tolerated.

SIDE EFFECTS

Frequent (20%–7%): Paresthesia, piloerection, pruritus, dysuria, supine hypertension. **Occasional (less than 7%–1%):** Pain, rash, chills, headache, facial flushing, confusion, dry mouth, anxiety.

ADVERSE EFFECTS/ TOXIC REACTIONS

Increased systolic arterial pressure has been noted.

NURSING CONSIDERATIONS

BASELINE ASSESSMENT

Assess sensitivity to midodrine, other medications (esp. digoxin, sodium-retaining vasoconstrictors). Assess medical history, esp. for renal impairment, severe hypertension, cardiac disease.

INTERVENTION/EVALUATION

Monitor B/P, renal, hepatic, cardiac function.

PATIENT/FAMILY TEACHING

• Do not take last dose of the day after evening meal or less than 4 hrs before bedtime. • Do not give if pt will be supine. • Use caution with OTC medications that may affect B/P (e.g., cough and cold, diet medications).

mifepristone

miff-eh-**pris**-tone
(Mifeprex)

BLACK BOX ALERT Discuss medication guide, pt agreement, and expected effects before prescribing. Serious, sometimes fatal, infections, excessive bleeding have occurred following surgical and medical abortions, including following use of misopristone.

Do not confuse Mifeprex with Mirapex, or mifepristone with misoprostol.

◆CLASSIFICATION

CLINICAL: Abortifacient.

ACTION

Has antiprogestational activity resulting from competitive interaction with progesterone. Inhibits activity of endogenous, exogenous progesterone. Has antiglucocorticoid, weak antiandrogenic activity. **Therapeutic Effect:** Terminates pregnancy.

PHARMACOKINETICS

Rapidly absorbed from GI tract. Protein binding: 98%. Metabolized in liver. Primarily eliminated in feces; minimal excretion in urine. **Half-life:** 18 hrs.

USES

Termination of intrauterine pregnancy through day 49 of pregnancy. **OFF-LABEL:** Breast/ovarian cancer, Cushing's syndrome, endometriosis, intrauterine fetal death, nonviable early pregnancy, postcoital contraception/contragestation, unresectable meningioma.

PRECAUTIONS

Contraindications: Chronic adrenal failure, concurrent long-term steroid or anticoagulant therapy, confirmed or suspected ectopic pregnancy, intrauterine device (IUD) in place, hemorrhagic disorders, concurrent anticoagulant therapy, inherited porphyria, hypersensitivity to misoprostol, other prostaglandins. **Cautions:** Treatment of women older than 35 yrs, smoking more than 10 cigarettes/day, cardiovascular disease, hypertension, hepatic/renal impairment, diabetes, severe anemia. **Pregnancy Category X.**

INTERACTIONS

DRUG: **Anticoagulants** may increase risk of bleeding. **Carbamazepine, phenobarbital, phenytoin, rifampin** may increase metabolism. **Erythromycin, itraconazole, ketoconazole** may inhibit metabolism. **HERBAL:** **St. John's wort** may increase metabolism. **FOOD:** **Grapefruit, grapefruit juice** may inhibit metabolism. **LAB VALUES:** May alter serum ALT, AST, alkaline phosphatase.

AVAILABILITY (Rx)

Tablets: 200 mg.

INDICATIONS/ROUTES/DOSAGE

Termination of Pregnancy

PO: ADULTS: Day 1: 600 mg as single dose. **Day 3:** 400 mcg misoprostol. **Day 14:** Post-treatment examination.

SIDE EFFECTS

Frequent (greater than 10%): Headache, dizziness, abdominal pain, nausea, vomiting, diarrhea, fatigue. **Occasional (10%–3%):** Uterine hemorrhage, insomnia, vaginitis, dyspepsia (heartburn, indigestion, epigastric pain), back pain, fever, viral infections, rigors. **Rare (2%–1%):** Anxiety, syncope, anemia, asthenia (loss of strength, energy), leg pain, sinusitis, leukorrhea.

ADVERSE EFFECTS/ TOXIC REACTIONS

None known.

M

NURSING CONSIDERATIONS

BASELINE ASSESSMENT

Assess for use of ketoconazole, itraconazole, erythromycin, rifampin, anticonvulsants (affects metabolism).

INTERVENTION/EVALUATION

◀ALERT▶ If mifepristone results in an incomplete abortion, surgical intervention may be necessary.

Monitor Hgb/Hct. Confirm pregnancy is completely terminated at approximately 14 days after drug administration. Assess degree of vaginal bleeding.

PATIENT/FAMILY TEACHING

• Advise pts of treatment procedure and effects, need for follow-up visit. • Vaginal bleeding, uterine cramping may occur.

milnacipran

mill-nah-**sip**-ran
(Savella)

BLACK BOX ALERT Increased risk of suicidal thinking and behavior in children, adolescents, and young adults 18–24 yrs with major depressive disorder, other psychiatric disorders.

Do not confuse Savella with cevimeline or sevelamer.

◆CLASSIFICATION

PHARMACOTHERAPEUTIC: Serotonin, norepinephrine reuptake inhibitor. **CLINICAL:** Fibromyalgia agent.

ACTION

Appears to inhibit serotonin and norepinephrine reuptake at CNS neuronal presynaptic membranes. **Therapeutic Effect:** Reduces chronic pain, fatigue, depression, sleep disorders associated with fibromyalgia syndrome; improves physical function.

PHARMACOKINETICS

Well absorbed following PO administration. Protein binding: 13%. Eliminated unchanged in urine. Steady-state levels reached in 36–48 hrs. **Half-life:** 6–8 hrs.

USES

Management of fibromyalgia.

PRECAUTIONS

Contraindications: Concomitant use of monoamine oxidase inhibitors (MAOIs), uncontrolled narrow-angle glaucoma. **Cautions:** Pts with depression, other psychiatric disorders; elevated blood pressure or heart rate; history of seizures; pts with substantial alcohol use or chronic liver disease; pts with history of dysuria (e.g., prostatic hypertrophy, prostatitis; controlled narrow-angle glaucoma).

⌛ LIFESPAN CONSIDERATIONS

Pregnancy/Lactation: Increased risk of fetal complications, including need for respiratory support, if drug is given during third trimester of pregnancy. Unknown if distributed in breast milk. **Pregnancy Category C. Children:** Safety and efficacy not established in those 17 yrs and younger. **Elderly:** Severe renal impairment requires dosage adjustment.

INTERACTIONS

DRUG: Lithium, MAOIs may impair serotonin metabolism. **Epinephrine, norepinephrine** may produce paroxysmal hypertension, arrhythmias. **Intravenous digoxin** may produce tachycardia, hypotension. May inhibit antihypertensive effect of **clonidine. NSAIDs, aspirin** may increase risk of bleeding. **HERBAL: Gotu kola, kava kava, St. John's wort, valerian** may increase CNS depression. **FOOD:** None known. **LAB VALUES:** May decrease serum sodium.

AVAILABILITY (Rx)

Tablets, Film-Coated: 12.5 mg, 25 mg, 50 mg, 100 mg.

ADMINISTRATION/HANDLING

• Give without regard to food. • Do not crush, break film-coated tablets.

INDICATIONS/ROUTES/DOSAGE

Fibromyalgia

PO: ADULTS, ELDERLY: Day 1: 12.5 mg once. **Days 2–3:** 25 mg/day (12.5 mg twice daily). **Days 4–7:** 50 mg/day (25 mg twice daily). **After Day 7:** 100 mg/day (50 mg twice daily). Dose may be increased to 200 mg/day (100 mg twice daily).

Severe Renal Impairment (Creatine Clearance 5–29 ml/min)

Reduce maintenance dose by 50% to 50 mg/day (25 mg twice daily). Based on pt response, dose may be increased to 100 mg/day (50 mg twice daily). Not recommended in end stage renal disease.

SIDE EFFECTS

Frequent (37%–10%): Nausea, headache, constipation, insomnia, hot flushing, dizziness. **Occasional (4%–2%):** Hyperhidrosis of face, underarms, hands; palpitations, vomiting, increased pulse, upper respiratory infection, migraine, dry mouth, hypertension, anxiety. **Rare (2%–1%):** Abdominal pain, increased B/P, rash, pruritus, tremor, paresthesia, blurred vision, tachycardia.

ADVERSE EFFECTS/ TOXIC REACTIONS

Abrupt discontinuation may present withdrawal symptoms (dysphoria, irritability, agitation, dizziness, paresthesia, anxiety, confusion, headache, lethargy, emotional lability, tinnitus, seizures). Serotonin syndrome symptoms may include mental status changes (agitation, hallucinations), hyperreflexia, incoordination. May increase risk of bleeding events (e.g., ecchymoses, hematomas, epistaxis).

NURSING CONSIDERATIONS

BASELINE ASSESSMENT

Obtain baseline pain intensity scale, location(s) of pain, tenderness. Obtain baseline blood pressure, heart rate. Question for history of changes in day-to-day pain intensity.

INTERVENTION/EVALUATION

Control nausea with antiemetics. Treat complaint of headache, migraine with appropriate analgesics. Monitor for increase in B/P, pulse. Question for changes in visual acuity. Assess for clinical improvement and record onset of pain control, decreased fatigue, lessening of depressive symptoms, improvement in sleep pattern. Monitor for suicidal ideation.

PATIENT/FAMILY TEACHING

• Avoid tasks that require alertness, motor skills until response to drug is established. • Do not abruptly discontinue medication. • Increase fluids, bulk to prevent constipation. • Contact physician if mental status changes occur (including thoughts of suicide, unusual behavior) or sweating, hot flushing become intolerable. • Caution about risk of bleeding associated with concomitant use of NSAIDs, aspirin.

milrinone HIGH ALERT

mill-re-none
(Primacor, Primacor I.V.)
Do not confuse Primacor with Primaxin.

◆CLASSIFICATION

PHARMACOTHERAPEUTIC: Cardiac inotropic agent. **CLINICAL:** Vasodilator.

ACTION

Inhibits phosphodiesterase, which increases cyclic adenosine monophosphate (cAMP), potentiating delivery of calcium to myocardial contractile systems. **Therapeutic Effect:** Relaxes vascular muscle, causing vasodilation. Increases cardiac output; decreases pulmonary capillary wedge pressure, vascular resistance.

M

PHARMACOKINETICS

Route	Onset	Peak	Duration
IV	5–15 min	N/A	N/A

Protein binding: 70%. Metabolized in liver. Primarily excreted in urine. **Half-life:** 1.7–2.7 hrs.

USES

Short-term management of CHF. OFF-LABEL: Inotropic therapy for pts unresponsive to other therapy, heart transplant candidates, palliation of symptoms in end-stage heart failure.

PRECAUTIONS

Contraindications: None known. **Cautions:** Severe obstructive aortic or pulmonic valvular disease, history of ventricular arrhythmias, atrial fibrillation/flutter, renal impairment.

LIFESPAN CONSIDERATIONS

Pregnancy/Lactation: Unknown if drug crosses placenta or is distributed in breast milk. **Pregnancy Category C. Children:** Safety and efficacy not established. **Elderly:** Age-related renal impairment may require dosage adjustment.

INTERACTIONS

DRUG: **Other cardiac glycosides** produce additive inotropic effects. HERBAL: None significant. FOOD: None known. LAB VALUES: None significant.

AVAILABILITY (Rx)

Injection Solution (Primacor, Primacor I.V.): 1 mg/ml, 10-ml single-dose vial, 20-ml single-dose vial, 50-ml single-dose vial. **Injection Solution (Premix [Primacor]):** 200 mcg/ml (100 ml, 200 ml).

ADMINISTRATION/HANDLING

IV

Reconstitution • For IV infusion, dilute 20-mg (20-ml) vial with 80 ml 0.9% NaCl or D_5W to provide concentration of 0.2 mg/ml.

Rate of administration • For IV injection (loading dose), administer undiluted slowly over 10 min. • Monitor for arrhythmias, hypotension during IV therapy; reduce or temporarily discontinue infusion until condition stabilizes.

Storage • Diluted solutions stable for 72 hrs at room temperature.

IV INCOMPATIBILITIES

Furosemide (Lasix), imipenem-cilastatin (Primaxin), procainamide (Pronestyl).

IV COMPATIBILITIES

Calcium gluconate, dexamethasone (Decadron), digoxin (Lanoxin), diltiazem (Cardizem), dobutamine (Dobutrex), dopamine (Intropin), heparin, hydromorphone (Dilaudid), lidocaine, magnesium, midazolam (Versed), morphine, nitroglycerin, potassium, propofol (Diprivan).

INDICATIONS/ROUTES/DOSAGE

Management of CHF

IV: ADULTS: Initially, 50 mcg/kg over 10 min. Continue with maintenance infusion rate of 0.375–0.75 mcg/kg/min based on hemodynamic and clinical response.

Dosage in Renal Impairment

Creatinine Clearance	Dosage
50 ml/min	0.43 mcg/kg/min
40 ml/min	0.38 mcg/kg/min
30 ml/min	0.33 mcg/kg/min
20 ml/min	0.28 mcg/kg/min
10 ml/min	0.23 mcg/kg/min
5 ml/min	0.2 mcg/kg/min

SIDE EFFECTS

Occasional (3%–1%): Headache, hypotension. **Rare (less than 1%):** Angina, chest pain.

ADVERSE EFFECTS/ TOXIC REACTIONS

Supraventricular/ventricular arrhythmias (12%), nonsustained ventricular tachycardia (2%), sustained ventricular tachycardia (1%) may occur.

NURSING CONSIDERATIONS

BASELINE ASSESSMENT

Obtain baseline lab studies, esp. BN peptide. Offer emotional support (difficulty breathing may produce anxiety). Assess B/P, apical pulse rate before treatment begins and during IV therapy. Assess lung sounds; observe for edema.

INTERVENTION/EVALUATION

Monitor B/P, heart rate, cardiac output, EKG, serum potassium, renal function, signs/symptoms of CHF.

minocycline

mi-noe-**sye**-kleen
(Apo-Minocycline ✱, Dynacin, Minocin, Myrac, Novo-Minocycline ✱, Solodyn)
Do not confuse Dynacin with Dyazide, DynaCirc, or Dynapen, or Minocin with Indocin, Mithracin, or niacin.

◆CLASSIFICATION

PHARMACOTHERAPEUTIC: Tetracycline. **CLINICAL:** Antibiotic.

ACTION

Inhibits bacterial protein synthesis by binding to ribosomes. **Therapeutic Effect:** Bacteriostatic.

PHARMACOKINETICS

Well absorbed from GI tract. Protein binding: 70%–75%. Partial elimination in feces; minimal excretion in urine. Not removed by hemodialysis. **Half-life:** 11–23 hrs.

USES

Treatment of susceptible infections due to *Rickettsiae, M. pneumoniae, C. trachomatis, C. psittaci, H. ducreyi, Yersinia pestis, Francisella tularensis, Vibrio cholerae, Brucella* spp., gram-negative organisms. Treatment of prostate, urinary tract, CNS infections (not meningitis), uncomplicated gonorrhea, inflammatory acne, brucellosis, skin granulomas, cholera, trachoma, nocardiasis, yaws, syphilis (when penicillins are contraindicated). **Solodyn:** Treatment of inflammatory lesions of non-nodular moderate to severe acne. **OFF-LABEL:** Treatment of atypical mycobacterial infection, rheumatoid arthritis (RA), scleroderma.

PRECAUTIONS

Contraindications: Children younger than 8 yrs, hypersensitivity to tetracyclines, last half of pregnancy. **Cautions:** Renal impairment, sun/ultraviolet exposure (severe photosensitivity reaction).

⌛ LIFESPAN CONSIDERATIONS

Pregnancy/Lactation: Readily crosses placenta; distributed in breast milk. May inhibit fetal skeletal growth. **Pregnancy Category D. Children:** May cause permanent discoloration of teeth, enamel hypoplasia. Not recommended in those younger than 8 yrs. **Elderly:** No age-related precautions noted.

INTERACTIONS

DRUG: **Antacids** may decrease absorption, effect. **Carbamazepine, phenytoin** may decrease concentration. **Cholestyramine, colestipol** may decrease absorption. **Ergot** may increase risk of ergotism. May decrease the effects of **estrogen-containing oral contraceptives.** **HERBAL:** **St. John's wort** may increase risk of photosensitivity. **FOOD:** None known. **LAB VALUES:** May increase serum alkaline phosphatase, amylase, bilirubin, AST, ALT, BUN.

AVAILABILITY (Rx)

Capsules (Dynacin, Minocin): 50 mg, 75 mg, 100 mg. **Tablets (Minocin, Myrac):** 50 mg, 75 mg, 100 mg.

Capsules (Pellet-Filled [Minocin]): 50 mg, 100 mg. **Tablets (Extended-Release [Solodyn]):** 45 mg, 90 mg, 135 mg.

ADMINISTRATION/HANDLING

PO

• Take without regard to food. • Give with adequate fluid (reduces risk of esophageal irritation and ulceration). • Swallow pellet-filled capsules, extended-release tablets whole; do not chew, crush, or split.

INDICATIONS/ROUTES/DOSAGE

Usual Dosage

PO: ADULTS, ELDERLY: Initially, 100–200 mg, then 100 mg q12h. **CHILDREN OLDER THAN 8 YRS:** Initially, 4 mg/kg, then 2 mg/kg q12h.

Acne (Solodyn)

PO: CHILDREN 12 YRS AND OLDER, WEIGHING 91–136 KG: 135 mg once daily, **WEIGHING 60–90 KG:** 90 mg once daily, **WEIGHING 45–59 KG:** 45 mg once daily.

(CAPSULE OR IMMEDIATE-RELEASE TABLET): ADULTS, ELDERLY: 50–100 mg/day.

SIDE EFFECTS

Frequent: Dizziness, light-headedness, diarrhea, nausea, vomiting, abdominal cramps, possibly severe photosensitivity, drowsiness, vertigo. **Occasional:** Altered pigmentation of skin, mucous membranes; rectal/genital pruritus, stomatitis.

ADVERSE EFFECTS/ TOXIC REACTIONS

Superinfection (esp. fungal), anaphylaxis, increased ICP may occur. Bulging fontanelles occur rarely in infants.

NURSING CONSIDERATIONS

BASELINE ASSESSMENT

Question for history of allergies, esp. tetracyclines, sulfite.

INTERVENTION/EVALUATION

Assess ability to ambulate (may cause vertigo, dizziness). Monitor daily pattern of bowel activity and stool consistency. Monitor hepatic/renal function tests with long-term therapy. Assess skin for rash. Observe for signs of increased intracranial pressure (altered LOC, widened pulse pressure). Be alert for superinfection: fever, vomiting, diarrhea, anal/genital pruritus, oral mucosal changes (ulceration, pain, erythema).

PATIENT/FAMILY TEACHING

• Continue antibiotic for full length of treatment. • Space doses evenly. • Drink full glass of water with capsules or tablets. • Avoid tasks that require alertness, motor skills until response to drug is established. • Notify physician if diarrhea, rash, other new symptom occurs. • Protect skin from sun exposure. • Advise female pts to use additional form of birth control (may decrease effectiveness of oral contraceptives).

minoxidil

min-**ox**-i-dill

(Apo-Gain ✱, Loniten, Minox ✱, Rogaine, Rogaine Extra Strength)

BLACK BOX ALERT Can cause pericarditis and pericardial effusion, occasionally progressing to tamponade; can exacerbate angina pectoris.

Do not confuse Loniten with Lipitor or Lotensin, or minoxidil with metolazone, midodrine, Minipress, Minocin, Monopril, or Noxafil.

◆CLASSIFICATION

CLINICAL: Antihypertensive, hair growth stimulant (see p. 62C).

ACTION

Acts directly on vascular smooth muscle, producing vasodilation of arterioles. **Therapeutic Effect:** Decreases peripheral vascular resistance, B/P; increases cutaneous blood flow; stimulates hair follicle epithelium, hair follicle growth.

PHARMACOKINETICS

Route	Onset	Peak	Duration
PO	0.5 hr	2–8 hrs	2–5 days

Well absorbed from GI tract; minimal absorption after topical application. Protein binding: None. Widely distributed. Metabolized in liver to active metabolite. Primarily excreted in urine. Removed by hemodialysis. **Half-life:** 3.5 hrs.

USES

Treatment of severe symptomatic hypertension, hypertension associated with organ damage. Used for pts who fail to respond to maximal therapeutic dosages of diuretic and two other antihypertensive agents. Treatment of alopecia androgenetica (**males:** baldness of vertex of scalp; **females:** diffuse hair loss or thinning of frontoparietal areas).

PRECAUTIONS

Contraindications: Pheochromocytoma. **Cautions:** Severe renal impairment, chronic CHF, coronary artery disease, recent MI (1 mo).

LIFESPAN CONSIDERATIONS

Pregnancy/Lactation: Crosses placenta; distributed in breast milk. **Pregnancy Category C. Children:** No age-related precautions noted. **Elderly:** More sensitive to hypotensive effects. Age-related renal impairment may require dosage adjustment.

INTERACTIONS

DRUG: **NSAIDs** may decrease hypotensive effects. **Nitrates, parenteral antihypertensives** may increase hypotensive effect. **HERBAL:** **Licorice** may cause increased serum sodium, water retention. **FOOD:** None known. **LAB VALUES:** May increase plasma renin activity, BUN, serum alkaline phosphatase, creatinine, sodium. May decrease Hgb, Hct, erythrocyte count.

AVAILABILITY

Tablets (Loniten): 2.5 mg, 10 mg. **Topical Solution (OTC):** 2% (20 mg/ml) (Rogaine), 5% (50 mg/ml) (Rogaine Extra Strength).

ADMINISTRATION/HANDLING

PO

• Give without regard to food. Give with food if GI upset occurs. • Tablets may be crushed.

Topical

• Shampoo, dry hair before applying medication. • Wash hands immediately after application. • Do not use hair dryer after application (reduces effectiveness).

INDICATIONS/ROUTES/DOSAGE

Hypertension

PO: ADULTS, CHILDREN 12 YRS AND OLDER: Initially, 5 mg/day. Increase in at least 3-day intervals to 10 mg, then 20 mg, then up to 40 mg/day in 1–2 doses. **ELDERLY:** Initially, 2.5 mg/day. May increase gradually. Maintenance: 10–40 mg/day. **Maximum:** 100 mg/day. **CHILDREN YOUNGER THAN 12 YRS:** Initially, 0.1–0.2 mg/kg (5 mg maximum) daily. Gradually increase at a minimum of 3-day intervals. Maintenance: 0.25–1 mg/kg/day in 1–2 doses. **Maximum:** 50 mg/day.

Hair Regrowth

TOPICAL: ADULTS: Apply to affected areas of scalp 2 times per day. Four months of therapy may be needed for hair growth.

SIDE EFFECTS

Frequent: **PO:** Edema with concurrent weight gain, hypertrichosis (elongation, thickening, increased pigmentation of fine body hair; develops in 80% of pts within 3–6 wks after beginning therapy). **Occasional:** **PO:** EKG T-wave changes (usually revert to pretreatment state with continued therapy or drug withdrawal). **Topical:** Pruritus, rash, dry/flaking skin, erythema. **Rare:** **PO:** Breast tenderness, headache, photosensitivity reaction. **Topical:** Allergic reaction, alopecia, burning sensation at scalp, soreness at hair root, headache, visual disturbances.

M

ADVERSE EFFECTS/ TOXIC REACTIONS

Tachycardia, angina pectoris may occur due to increased oxygen demands associated with increased heart rate, cardiac output. Fluid/electrolyte imbalance, CHF may occur, esp. if a diuretic is not given concurrently. Too-rapid reduction in B/P may result in syncope, CVA, MI, ocular/vestibular ischemia. Pericardial effusion, tamponade may be seen in pts with renal impairment not on dialysis.

NURSING CONSIDERATIONS

BASELINE ASSESSMENT

Assess B/P in both arms and take pulse for 1 full min immediately before giving medication. If pulse increases 20 beats/min or more over baseline or systolic or diastolic B/P decreases more than 20 mm Hg, withhold drug, contact physician.

INTERVENTION/EVALUATION

Monitor fluids/electrolytes, body weight, B/P. Assess for peripheral edema. Assess for signs of CHF (cough, rales at base of lungs, cool extremities, dyspnea on exertion). Monitor fluid, serum electrolytes. Assess for distant or muffled heart sounds by auscultation (pericardial effusion, tamponade).

PATIENT/FAMILY TEACHING

• Maximum B/P response occurs in 3–7 days. • Rise slowly from sitting/lying position. • Reversible growth of fine body hair may begin 3–6 wks following initiation of treatment. • When used topically for stimulation of hair growth, treatment must continue on a permanent basis—cessation of treatment will begin reversal of new hair growth. • Avoid exposure to sunlight, artificial light sources.

Mirapex, *see pramipexole*

mirtazapine

mir-**taz**-a-peen
(Apo-Mirtazapine 🍁, Novo-Mirtazapine 🍁, Remeron, Remeron Soltab)

BLACK BOX ALERT Increased risk of suicidal thinking and behavior in children, adolescents, young adults 18–24 yrs with major depressive disorder, other psychiatric disorders.

Do not confuse Remeron with Premarin, Rozerem, or Zemuron.

◆CLASSIFICATION

PHARMACOTHERAPEUTIC: Tetracyclic compound. **CLINICAL:** Antidepressant (see p. 40C).

ACTION

Acts as antagonist at presynaptic alpha$_2$-adrenergic receptors, increasing norepinephrine, serotonin neurotransmission. Has low anticholinergic activity. **Therapeutic Effect:** Relieves depression, produces sedative effects.

PHARMACOKINETICS

Rapidly, completely absorbed after PO administration; absorption not affected by food. Protein binding: 85%. Metabolized in liver. Primarily excreted in urine. Unknown if removed by hemodialysis. **Half-life:** 20–40 hrs (longer in males [37 hrs] than females [26 hrs]).

USES

Treatment of depression. **OFF-LABEL:** Post-traumatic stress disorder.

PRECAUTIONS

Contraindications: Use of MAOIs within 14 days. **Cautions:** Cardiovascular/GI disorders, prostatic hyperplasia, urinary retention, narrow-angle glaucoma, renal/hepatic impairment.

LIFESPAN CONSIDERATIONS

Pregnancy/Lactation: Unknown if distributed in breast milk. **Pregnancy Category C. Children:** Safety and efficacy not established. **Elderly:** Age-related renal impairment may require dosage adjustment.

INTERACTIONS

DRUG: **Alcohol, CNS depressant medications** may increase impairment of cognition, motor skills. **MAOIs** may increase risk of neuroleptic malignant syndrome, hypertensive crisis, severe seizures. HERBAL: **Gotu kola, kava kava, St. John's wort, valerian** may increase CNS depression. FOOD: None known. LAB VALUES: May increase serum cholesterol, triglycerides, ALT.

AVAILABILITY (Rx)

Tablets (Remeron): 7.5 mg, 15 mg, 30 mg, 45 mg. **Tablets (Orally-Disintegrating [Remeron Soltab]):** 15 mg, 30 mg, 45 mg.

ADMINISTRATION/HANDLING

PO

• Give without regard to food. • May crush/break scored tablets.

Orally-Disintegrating Tablets

• Do not split tablet. • Place on tongue; dissolves without water.

INDICATIONS/ROUTES/DOSAGE

Depression

PO: ADULTS: Initially, 15 mg at bedtime. May increase by 15 mg/day q1–2wk. **Maximum:** 45 mg/day. **ELDERLY:** Initially, 7.5 mg at bedtime. May increase by 7.5–15 mg/day q1–2wk. **Maximum:** 45 mg/day.

Dosage in Renal Impairment

Creatinine Clearance	
11–39 ml/min	30% decreased clearance
Less than 11 ml/min	50% decreased clearance

SIDE EFFECTS

Frequent: Drowsiness (54%), dry mouth (25%), increased appetite (17%), constipation (13%), weight gain (12%). **Occasional:** Asthenia (loss of strength, energy) (8%), dizziness (7%), flu-like symptoms (5%), abnormal dreams (4%). **Rare:** Abdominal discomfort, vasodilation, paresthesia, acne, dry skin, thirst, arthralgia.

ADVERSE EFFECTS/ TOXIC REACTIONS

Higher incidence of seizures than with tricyclic antidepressants (esp. in those with no history of seizures). Overdose may produce cardiovascular effects (severe orthostatic hypotension, dizziness, tachycardia, palpitations, arrhythmias). Abrupt discontinuation from prolonged therapy may produce headache, malaise, nausea, vomiting, vivid dreams. Agranulocytosis occurs rarely.

NURSING CONSIDERATIONS

BASELINE ASSESSMENT

Assess mental status (mood, behavior), baseline weight. For pts on long-term therapy, hepatic/renal function tests, blood counts should be performed periodically.

INTERVENTION/EVALUATION

Supervise suicidal-risk pt closely during early therapy (as depression lessens, energy level improves, increasing suicide potential). Children, adolescents are at increased risk for suicidal thoughts/behavior and worsening of depression, esp. during first few mos of therapy. Assess appearance, behavior, speech pattern, level of interest, mood. Monitor for hypotension, arrhythmias.

PATIENT/FAMILY TEACHING

• Take as single bedtime dose. • Avoid alcohol, depressant/sedating medications. • Avoid tasks requiring alertness, motor skills until response to drug established. • Report worsening depression, suicidal ideation, unusual changes in behavior.

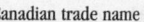

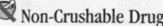

M

misoprostol

mis-oh-**pros**-toll
(Apo-Misoprostol, Cytotec, Novo-Misoprostol)

BLACK BOX ALERT Pregnancy Category X. Use during pregnancy can cause abortion, premature birth, birth defects. Not to be given to women of childbearing potential unless pt is capable of complying with effective contraception.

Do not confuse misoprostol with metoprolol or mifepristone, or Cytotec with Cytoxan.

FIXED-COMBINATION(S)

Arthrotec: misoprostol/diclofenac (an NSAID): 200 mcg/50 mg, 200 mcg/75 mg.

CLASSIFICATION

PHARMACOTHERAPEUTIC: Prostaglandin. **CLINICAL:** Antisecretory, gastric protectant.

ACTION

Replaces protective prostaglandins consumed with prostaglandin-inhibiting therapies (e.g., NSAIDs). **Therapeutic Effect:** Reduces acid secretion from gastric parietal cells, stimulates bicarbonate production from gastric/duodenal mucosa.

PHARMACOKINETICS

Route	Onset	Peak	Duration
PO	30 min	1–1.5 hrs	3–6 hrs

Rapidly absorbed from GI tract. Protein binding: 80%–90%. Rapidly converted to active metabolite. Primarily excreted in urine. Unknown if removed by hemodialysis. **Half-life:** 20–40 min.

USES

Prevention of NSAID-induced gastric ulcers and in pts at high risk for developing gastric ulcer/gastric ulcer complications. Chemical termination of pregnancy (in conjunction with mifepristone). **OFF-LABEL:** Treatment of therapeutic second-trimester abortion, cervical ripening, duodenal ulcer, treatment/prevention of NSAID-associated gastric ulcer, induction of labor.

PRECAUTIONS

Contraindications: Pregnancy (produces uterine contractions). **Cautions:** Renal impairment.

LIFESPAN CONSIDERATIONS

Pregnancy/Lactation: Unknown if distributed in breast milk. Produces uterine contractions, uterine bleeding, expulsion of products of conception (abortifacient property). **Pregnancy Category X. Children:** Safety and efficacy not established. **Elderly:** No age-related precautions noted.

INTERACTIONS

DRUG: **Antacids containing magnesium** worsen diarrhea associated with misoprostol. **HERBAL:** None significant. **FOOD:** None known. **LAB VALUES:** None significant.

AVAILABILITY (Rx)

Tablets: 100 mcg, 200 mcg.

ADMINISTRATION/HANDLING

PO

- Give with or after meals (minimizes diarrhea).

INDICATIONS/ROUTES/DOSAGE

Prevention of NSAID-Induced Gastric Ulcer

PO: ADULTS: 200 mcg 4 times a day with food (last dose at bedtime). Continue for duration of NSAID therapy. May reduce dosage to 100 mcg 4 times a day or 200 mcg 2 times a day with food. **ELDERLY:** 100–200 mcg 4 times a day with food.

Chemical Termination of Pregnancy

Refer to mifepristone monograph.

SIDE EFFECTS

Frequent (40%–20%): Abdominal pain, diarrhea. **Occasional (3%–2%):** Nausea, flatulence, dyspepsia, headache. **Rare (1%):** Vomiting, constipation.

ADVERSE EFFECTS/ TOXIC REACTIONS

Overdosage may produce sedation, tremor, seizures, dyspnea, palpitations, hypotension, bradycardia.

NURSING CONSIDERATIONS

BASELINE ASSESSMENT

Question for possibility of pregnancy before initiating therapy (Pregnancy Category X).

PATIENT/FAMILY TEACHING

- Avoid magnesium-containing antacids (minimizes potential for diarrhea).
- Women of childbearing potential must not be pregnant before or during medication therapy (may result in hospitalization, surgery, infertility, fetal death).
- Incidence of diarrhea may be lessened by taking immediately following meals.

mitomycin

HIGH ALERT

my-toe-**my**-sin
(Mutamycin)

BLACK BOX ALERT Potent vesicant. Marked myelosuppression. Infiltration produces ulceration, necrosis, cellulitis, tissue sloughing. Must be administered by certified chemotherapy personnel.

Do not confuse mitomycin with mithramycin or mitoxantrone.

CLASSIFICATION

PHARMACOTHERAPEUTIC: Antibiotic. **CLINICAL:** Antineoplastic (see p. 86C).

ACTION

Alkylating agent, cross-linking with strands of DNA. **Therapeutic Effect:** Inhibits DNA, RNA synthesis.

PHARMACOKINETICS

Widely distributed. Does not cross blood-brain barrier. Primarily metabolized in liver, excreted in urine. **Half-life:** 50 min.

USES

Treatment of disseminated adenocarcinoma of stomach, pancreas, bladder, breast or colorectal cancer. **OFF-LABEL:** Treatment of biliary, cervical, head/neck, lung carcinomas; chronic myelocytic leukemia, esophageal cancer.

PRECAUTIONS

Contraindications: Coagulation disorders, bleeding tendencies, platelet count less than 75,000/mm^3, serious infection, serum creatinine greater than 1.7 mg/dl, WBC count less than 3,000/mm^3. **Cautions:** Myelosuppression, renal/hepatic impairment.

LIFESPAN CONSIDERATIONS

Pregnancy/Lactation: If possible, avoid use during pregnancy, esp. first trimester. Breast-feeding not recommended. Safety in pregnancy not established. **Pregnancy Category D. Children:** No age-related precautions noted. **Elderly:** Age-related renal impairment may require dosage adjustment.

INTERACTIONS

DRUG: Bone marrow depressants may increase myelosuppression. **Live virus vaccines** may potentiate virus replication, increase vaccine side effects, decrease pt's antibody response to vaccine. **HERBAL:** Avoid **black cohosh, dong quai** in estrogen-dependent tumors. **FOOD:** None known. **LAB VALUES:** May increase BUN, serum creatinine.

AVAILABILITY (Rx)

Injection, Powder for Reconstitution: 5 mg, 20 mg, 40 mg.

ADMINISTRATION/HANDLING

◀ALERT▶ May be carcinogenic, mutagenic, teratogenic. Handle with extreme care during preparation/administration.

M

Give via IV push, IV infusion. Extremely irritating to vein. Injection may produce pain with induration, thrombophlebitis, paresthesia.

IV

Reconstitution • Reconstitute with Sterile Water for Injection to provide solution containing 0.5–1 mg/ml. • Do not shake vial to dissolve. • Allow vial to stand at room temperature until complete dissolution occurs. • For IV infusion, further dilute with 50–100 ml D_5W or 0.9% NaCl (concentration 20–40 mcg/ml).

Rate of administration • Extravasation may produce cellulitis, ulceration, tissue sloughing. Terminate administration immediately, inject ordered antidote. Apply ice intermittently for up to 72 hrs; keep area elevated.

Storage • Use only clear, blue-gray solutions. • Concentration of 0.5 mg/ml (reconstituted vial or syringe) is stable for 7 days at room temperature or 2 wks if refrigerated. Further diluted solution with D_5W is stable for 3 hrs, 12 hrs if diluted with 0.9% NaCl at room temperature.

IV INCOMPATIBILITIES

Aztreonam (Azactam), bleomycin (Blenoxane), cefepime (Maxipime), filgrastim (Neupogen), heparin, piperacillin/tazobactam (Zosyn), sargramostin (Leukine), vinorelbine (Navelbine).

IV COMPATIBILITIES

Cisplatin (Platinol AQ), cyclophosphamide (Cytoxan), doxorubicin (Adriamycin), 5-fluorouracil, granisetron (Kytril), leucovorin, methotrexate, ondansetron (Zofran), vinblastine (Velban), vincristine (Oncovin).

INDICATIONS/ROUTES/DOSAGE

Refer to individual protocols.

Usual Dosage

IV: ADULTS, ELDERLY, CHILDREN: Initially, 10–20 mg/m^2 as single dose. Repeat q6–8wks. Give additional courses only after platelet, WBC counts are within acceptable levels, as shown below.

Leukocytes/ mm^3	Platelets/ mm^3	% of Prior Dose to Give
4,000	More than 100,000	100%
3,000–3,999	75,000–99,000	100%
2,000–2,999	25,000–74,999	70%
1,999 or less	Less than 25,000	50%

Dosage in Renal Impairment

Creatinine clearance less than 10 ml/min: Give 75% of normal dose.

SIDE EFFECTS

Frequent (greater than 10%): Fever, anorexia, nausea, vomiting. **Occasional (10%–2%):** Stomatitis, paresthesia, purple colored bands on nails; rash, alopecia, unusual fatigue. **Rare (less than 1%):** Thrombophlebitis, cellulitis with extravasation.

ADVERSE EFFECTS/ TOXIC REACTIONS

Marked myelosuppression results in hematologic toxicity manifested as leukopenia, thrombocytopenia, and, to a lesser extent, anemia (generally occurs within 2–4 wks after initial therapy). Renal toxicity may be evidenced by increased BUN, serum creatinine levels. Pulmonary toxicity manifested as dyspnea, cough, hemoptysis, pneumonia. Long-term therapy may produce hemolytic uremic syndrome, characterized by hemolytic anemia, thrombocytopenia, renal failure, hypertension.

NURSING CONSIDERATIONS

BASELINE ASSESSMENT

Obtain CBC with differential, platelets, PT, bleeding time, before and periodically during therapy. Antiemetics before and during therapy may alleviate nausea/vomiting.

INTERVENTION/EVALUATION

Monitor hematologic status, renal function studies. Assess IV site for phlebitis, extravasation. Monitor for hematologic toxicity (fever, sore throat, signs of local infection, unusual bruising/bleeding from any site), symptoms of anemia (excessive fatigue, weakness). Assess for renal toxicity (foul odor from urine, elevated BUN, serum creatinine).

PATIENT/FAMILY TEACHING

• Maintain fastidious oral hygiene. • Immediately report any stinging, burning, pain at injection site. • Do not have immunizations without physician's approval (drug lowers resistance to infection). • Avoid contact with those who have recently received live virus vaccine. • Alopecia is reversible, but new hair growth may have different color, texture. • Contact physician if nausea/vomiting, fever, sore throat, bruising, bleeding, shortness of breath, painful urination occur.

mitoxantrone HIGH ALERT

my-toe-**zan**-trone
(Novantrone)

BLACK BOX ALERT May cause cardiotoxicity, potentially fatal CHF. Infiltration produces ulceration, necrosis, cellulitis, tissue sloughing. Secondary AML, myelodysplasia have occurred. Must be administered by certified chemotherapy personnel.

Do not confuse mitoxantrone with methotrexate, mitomycin or Mutamycin.

◆CLASSIFICATION

PHARMACOTHERAPEUTIC: Anthracenedione. **CLINICAL:** Nonvesicant, antineoplastic (see p. 86C).

ACTION

Inhibits B-cell, T-cell, macrophage proliferation, DNA, RNA synthesis. Active throughout entire cell cycle. **Therapeutic Effect:** Causes cell death.

PHARMACOKINETICS

Protein binding: greater than 95%. Widely distributed. Metabolized in liver. Primarily eliminated in feces by biliary system. Not removed by hemodialysis. **Half-life:** 2.3–13 days.

USES

Treatment of acute, nonlymphocytic leukemia (monocytic, myelogenous, promyelocytic), late-stage hormone-resistant prostate cancer, multiple sclerosis. **OFF-LABEL:** Treatment of acute lymphocytic leukemia; breast, hepatic carcinoma; non-Hodgkin's lymphoma; pediatric acute leukemias, sarcoma.

PRECAUTIONS

Contraindications: Baseline left ventricular ejection fraction less than 50%, cumulative lifetime mitoxantrone dose of 140 mg/m^2 or more, multiple sclerosis with hepatic impairment. **Cautions:** Preexisting bone marrow suppression, previous treatment with cardiotoxic medications, hepatobiliary impairment.

LIFESPAN CONSIDERATIONS

Pregnancy/Lactation: If possible, avoid use during pregnancy, esp. first trimester. May cause fetal harm. Breast-feeding not recommended. **Pregnancy Category D. Children:** Safety and efficacy not established. **Elderly:** No age-related precautions noted.

INTERACTIONS

DRUG: May decrease effect of **antigout medications. Bone marrow depressants** may increase myelosuppression. **Live virus vaccines** may potentiate virus replication, increase vaccine side effects, decrease pt's antibody response to vaccine. **HERBAL:** Avoid **black cohosh, dong quai** in estrogen-dependent tumors. **FOOD:** None known. **LAB VALUES:** May increase serum bilirubin, uric acid, AST, ALT.

M

AVAILABILITY (Rx)

Injection Solution: 2 mg/ml.

ADMINISTRATION/HANDLING

◀ALERT▶ May be carcinogenic, mutagenic, teratogenic. Handle with extreme care during preparation/administration. Give by IV injection, IV infusion. Must dilute before administration.

IV

Reconstitution • Dilute with at least 50 ml D_5W or 0.9% NaCl.

Rate of administration • Do not administer by subcutaneous, IM, intrathecal, or intra-arterial injection. • Do not give IV push over less than 3 min. • Give IV bolus over at least 3 min, IV intermittent infusion over 15–60 min, or IV continuous infusion (0.02–0.5 mg/ml) in D_5W or 0.9% NaCl.

Storage • Store vials at room temperature. • Opened vials, diluted solutions stable for 7 days at room temperature or refrigerated.

M

IV INCOMPATIBILITIES

Aztreonam (Azactam), cefepime (Maxipime), heparin, paclitaxel (Taxol), piperacillin/tazobactam (Zosyn).

IV COMPATIBILITIES

Allopurinol (Aloprim), etoposide (VePesid), gemcitabine (Gemzar), granisetron (Kytril), ondansetron (Zofran), potassium chloride.

INDICATIONS/ROUTES/DOSAGE

Refer to individual protocols.

Leukemias

IV: ADULTS, ELDERLY: 12 mg/m^2 once a day for 2–3 days. CHILDREN OLDER THAN 2 YRS: 8–12 mg/m^2 once daily for 4–5 days. CHILDREN 2 YRS AND YOUNGER: 0.4 mg/kg once a day for 3–5 days.

Solid Tumors

IV: ADULTS, ELDERLY: 12–14 mg/m^2 once q3–4wk. CHILDREN: 18–20 mg/m^2 once q3–4 wk.

Prostate Cancer

IV: ADULTS, ELDERLY: 12–14 mg/m^2 every 21 days.

Multiple Sclerosis

IV: ADULTS, ELDERLY: 12 mg/m^2/dose q3mo. **Maximum lifetime cumulative dose:** 140 mg/m^2.

SIDE EFFECTS

Frequent (greater than 10%): Nausea, vomiting, diarrhea, cough, headache, stomatitis, abdominal discomfort, fever, alopecia. Occasional (9%–4%): Ecchymosis, fungal infection, conjunctivitis, UTI. Rare (3%): Arrhythmias.

ADVERSE EFFECTS/ TOXIC REACTIONS

Myelosuppression may be severe, resulting in GI bleeding, sepsis, pneumonia. Renal failure, seizures, jaundice, CHF may occur. Cardiotoxicity has been reported.

NURSING CONSIDERATIONS

BASELINE ASSESSMENT

Evaluate left ventricular ejection fraction before initiating therapy and before administering each dose. Offer emotional support. Establish baseline for CBC with differential, temperature, pulse rate/quality, respiratory status. Obtain pregnancy test prior to each dose for females of child-bearing age.

INTERVENTION/EVALUATION

Monitor hematologic status, pulmonary function studies, hepatic/renal function tests. Monitor for stomatitis, fever, signs of local infection, unusual bruising/bleeding from any site. Extravasation produces swelling, pain, burning, blue discoloration of skin.

PATIENT/FAMILY TEACHING

• Urine will appear blue-green for 24 hrs after administration. Blue tint to sclera may appear. • Maintain adequate daily fluid intake (may protect against renal impairment). • Do not have immunizations without physician's approval (drug lowers resistance to infection). • Avoid crowds, those with infection. • Contraceptive measures recommended during therapy. • Notify physician if chills, fever, sore throat, difficulty breathing, unusual bruising/bleeding occur.

Mobic, *see meloxicam*

modafinil

mode-ah-**feen**-awl
(Alertec ✱, Apo-Modafinil ✱, Provigil)

◆CLASSIFICATION

PHARMACOTHERAPEUTIC: Alpha$_1$-agonist. **CLINICAL:** Wakefulness-promoting agent, antinarcoleptic. **(Schedule IV).**

ACTION

Binds to dopamine reuptake carrier sites, increasing alpha activity, decreasing delta, theta, beta brain wave activity. **Therapeutic Effect:** Reduces number of sleep episodes, total daytime sleep.

PHARMACOKINETICS

Well absorbed from GI tract. Protein binding: 60%. Widely distributed. Metabolized in liver. Excreted by kidneys. Unknown if removed by hemodialysis. **Half-life:** 15 hrs.

USES

Treatment of excessive daytime sleepiness associated with narcolepsy, other sleep disorders. **OFF-LABEL:** Treatment of ADHD, brain injury–related underarousal, depression, endozepine stupor, multiple sclerosis–related fatigue, parkinson-related fatigue, seasonal affective disorder.

PRECAUTIONS

Contraindications: None known. **Cautions:** History of clinically significant mitral valve prolapse, left ventricular hypertrophy, hepatic impairment, history of seizures.

LIFESPAN CONSIDERATIONS

Pregnancy/Lactation: Unknown if drug is excreted in breast milk. Use caution if given to pregnant women. **Pregnancy Category C. Children:** Safety and efficacy not established in those younger than 16 yrs. **Elderly:** Age-related renal/hepatic impairment may require decreased dosage.

INTERACTIONS

DRUG: May decrease concentrations of **cyclosporine, oral contraceptives, theophylline.** May increase concentrations of **diazepam, phenytoin, propranolol, tricyclic antidepressants, warfarin. Other CNS stimulants** may increase CNS stimulation. **HERBAL:** None significant. **FOOD:** None known. **LAB VALUES:** None known.

AVAILABILITY (Rx)

Tablets (Provigil): 100 mg, 200 mg.

ADMINISTRATION/HANDLING

PO

- Give without regard to meals.

INDICATIONS/ROUTES/DOSAGE

Narcolepsy, Other Sleep Disorders

PO: ADULTS: 200 mg/day. **ELDERLY:** Initially, 100 mg/day.

SIDE EFFECTS

Frequent: Anxiety, insomnia, nausea. **Occasional:** Anorexia, diarrhea, dizziness, dry mouth/skin, muscle stiffness, polydipsia, rhinitis, paresthesia, tremor, headache, vomiting.

ADVERSE EFFECTS/ TOXIC REACTIONS

Agitation, excitation, increased B/P, insomnia may occur. Psychiatric disturbances (anxiety, hallucinations, suicidal ideation), serious allergic reactions (an-

M

gioedema, Stevens-Johnson syndrome) may occur.

NURSING CONSIDERATIONS

BASELINE ASSESSMENT

Obtain baseline evidence of narcolepsy or other sleep disorders, including pattern, environmental situations, length of sleep episodes. Question for sudden loss of muscle tone (cataplexy) precipitated by strong emotional responses before sleep episode. Assess frequency/severity of sleep episodes before drug therapy.

INTERVENTION/EVALUATION

Monitor sleep pattern, evidence of restlessness during sleep, length of insomnia episodes at night. Assess for dizziness, anxiety; initiate fall precautions. Sugarless gum, sips of tepid water may relieve dry mouth.

PATIENT/FAMILY TEACHING

• Avoid tasks that require alertness, motor skills until response to drug is established. • Avoid alcohol. • Do not increase dose without physician approval. • Use alternative contraceptives during therapy and 1 mo after discontinuing modafinil (reduces effectiveness of oral contraceptives).

moexipril

moe-**ex**-i-pril
(Univasc)

BLACK BOX ALERT May cause fetal injury, mortality if used during second or third trimester of pregnancy.

Do not confuse moexipril with Monopril.

FIXED-COMBINATION(S)

Uniretic: moexipril/hydrochlorothiazide (a diuretic): 7.5 mg/12.5 mg, 15 mg/12.5 mg, 15 mg/25 mg.

◆CLASSIFICATION

PHARMACOTHERAPEUTIC: ACE inhibitor. **CLINICAL:** Antihypertensive (see p. 9C).

ACTION

Suppresses renin-angiotensin-aldosterone system (prevents conversion of angiotensin I to angiotensin II, a potent vasoconstrictor; may inhibit angiotensin II at local vascular, renal sites). **Therapeutic Effect:** Reduces peripheral arterial resistance, B/P.

PHARMACOKINETICS

Route	Onset	Peak	Duration
PO	1 hr	1–2 hrs	Greater than 24 hrs

Incompletely absorbed from GI tract. Food decreases drug absorption. Rapidly converted to active metabolite. Protein binding: 50%. Primarily recovered in feces, partially excreted in urine. Unknown if removed by dialysis. **Half-life:** 1 hr; metabolite, 2–9 hrs.

USES

Treatment of hypertension. Used alone or in combination with thiazide diuretics. **OFF-LABEL:** Treatment of left ventricular dysfunction after MI.

PRECAUTIONS

Contraindications: History of angioedema from previous treatment with ACE inhibitors. **Cautions:** Renal impairment, dialysis, hypovolemia, coronary or cerebrovascular insufficiency, hyperkalemia, aortic stenosis, ischemic heart disease, angina, severe CHF, cerebrovascular disease, those with sodium depletion or on diuretic therapy.

⌛ LIFESPAN CONSIDERATIONS

Pregnancy/Lactation: Crosses placenta. Unknown if distributed in breast milk. **Pregnancy Category C (D if used in second or third trimester). Children:** Safety and efficacy not established. **Elderly:** Age-related renal impairment may require dosage adjustment.

INTERACTIONS

DRUG: **Alcohol, antihypertensives, diuretics** may increase effect. May increase **lithium** concentration, risk of toxicity. **NSAIDs** may decrease effects. **Potassium-sparing diuretics, potassium supplements** may cause hyperkalemia. HERBAL: **Ephedra, ginseng, yohimbe** may worsen hypertension. **Garlic** may increase antihypertensive effect. FOOD: None known. LAB VALUES: May increase BUN, serum alkaline phosphatase, bilirubin, creatinine, potassium, AST, ALT. May cause positive serum antinuclear antibody (ANA) titer.

AVAILABILITY (Rx)

Tablets: 7.5 mg, 15 mg.

ADMINISTRATION/HANDLING

PO

• Give 1 hr before meals. • Tablets may be crushed.

INDICATIONS/ROUTES/DOSAGE

Hypertension

PO: ADULTS, ELDERLY: For pts not receiving diuretics, initial dose is 7.5 mg once a day or 3.75 mg (when combined with thiazide diuretic) 1 hr before meals. Adjust according to B/P effect. Maintenance: 7.5–30 mg a day in 1–2 divided doses 1 hr before meals.

Dosage in Renal Impairment

PO: ADULTS, ELDERLY: 3.75 mg once a day in pts with creatinine clearance of 40 ml/min or less. **Maximum:** May titrate up to 15 mg/day.

SIDE EFFECTS

Occasional: Cough, headache (6%), dizziness (4%), fatigue (3%). Rare: Flushing, rash, myalgia, nausea, vomiting.

ADVERSE EFFECTS/ TOXIC REACTIONS

Excessive hypotension ("first-dose syncope") may occur in pts with CHF, severe salt/volume depletion. Angioedema (swelling of face/lips), hyperkalemia occur rarely. Agranulocytosis, neutropenia may be noted in those with collagen vascular disease (scleroderma, systemic lupus erythematosus), renal impairment. Nephrotic syndrome may be noted in those with history of renal disease.

NURSING CONSIDERATIONS

BASELINE ASSESSMENT

Obtain B/P, apical pulse immediately before each dose, in addition to regular monitoring (be alert to fluctuations). If excessive reduction in B/P occurs, place pt in supine position, feet slightly elevated. Renal function tests should be performed before therapy begins. In pts with renal impairment, autoimmune disease, taking drugs that affect leukocytes or immune response, CBC with differential count should be performed before therapy, q2wk for 3 mos, then periodically thereafter.

INTERVENTION/EVALUATION

Monitor B/P, serum potassium, renal function, WBC count. Observe for hypotensive effect within 1–3 hrs of first dose or increase in dose. Assist with ambulation if dizziness occurs.

PATIENT/FAMILY TEACHING

• Do not abruptly stop medication. • Inform physician of sore throat, fever, difficulty breathing, chest pain, cough, signs of angioedema. • Arrhythmias may occur. • To reduce hypotensive effect, rise slowly from lying to sitting position, permit legs to dangle momentarily before standing.

mometasone

mo-**met**-a-sone
(Elocon)

mometasone furoate

(Asmanex Twisthaler, Nasonex)

M

FIXED-COMBINATION(S)

Dulera: mometasone/formoterol (beta-adrenergic agonist): 100 mcg/5 mcg, 200 mcg/5 mcg.

◆CLASSIFICATION

PHARMACOTHERAPEUTIC: Adrenocorticosteroid. **CLINICAL:** Anti-inflammatory.

ACTION

Inhibits release of inflammatory cells into nasal tissue, preventing early activation of allergic reaction. **Therapeutic Effect:** Decreases response to seasonal/perennial rhinitis.

PHARMACOKINETICS

Undetectable in plasma. Protein binding: 98%–99%. Swallowed portion undergoes extensive metabolism. Excreted primarily through bile and, to a lesser extent, urine. **Half-life:** 5 hrs.

M

USES

Nasal: Treatment of nasal symptoms of seasonal/perennial allergic rhinitis in adults, children over 2 yrs. Prophylaxis of nasal symptoms of seasonal allergic rhinitis in adults, adolescents over 12 yrs. Treatment of nasal polyps. **Inhalation:** Maintenance treatment of asthma as prophylactic therapy or supplement in pts requiring oral steroids for purpose of decreasing oral steroid requirement. **Topical:** Relief of inflammatory, pruritic manifestations of steroid-responsive dermatoses.

PRECAUTIONS

Contraindications: Hypersensitivity to any corticosteroid, persistently positive sputum cultures for *Candida albicans*, status asthmaticus (inhalation), systemic fungal infections, untreated localized infection involving nasal mucosa. **Cautions:** Adrenal insufficiency, cirrhosis, glaucoma, hypothyroidism, untreated infection, osteoporosis, tuberculosis.

⌛ LIFESPAN CONSIDERATIONS

Pregnancy/Lactation: Unknown if drug crosses placenta or is distributed in breast milk. **Pregnancy Category C. Children:** Prolonged treatment/high doses may decrease short-term growth rate, cortisol secretion. **Elderly:** No age-related precautions noted.

INTERACTIONS

DRUG: Ketoconazole may increase concentration (inhalation). **HERBAL:** None significant. **FOOD:** None known. **LAB VALUES:** None significant.

AVAILABILITY (Rx)

Cream (Elocon): 0.1%. **Lotion (Elocon):** 0.1%. **Nasal Spray (Nasonex):** 50 mcg/spray. **Ointment (Elocon):** 0.1%. **Powder for Oral Inhaler (Asmanex Twisthaler):** 110 mcg, 220 mcg.

ADMINISTRATION/HANDLING

Inhalation

• Hold twisthaler straight up with pink portion (base) on bottom, remove cap. • Exhale fully. • Firmly close lips around mouthpiece and inhale a fast, deep breath. • Hold breath for 10 sec.

Intranasal

• Instruct pt to clear nasal passages as much as possible before use. • Tilt head slightly forward. • Insert spray tip into nostril, pointing toward nasal passages, away from nasal septum. • Spray into one nostril while pt holds other nostril closed, concurrently inspires through nose to permit medication as high into nasal passages as possible.

Topical

• Apply thin layer of cream, lotion, ointment to cover affected area. Rub in gently. • Do not cover area with occlusive dressing.

INDICATIONS/ROUTES/DOSAGE

Allergic Rhinitis

NASAL SPRAY: ADULTS, ELDERLY, CHILDREN 12 YRS AND OLDER: 2 sprays in each nostril once a day. **CHILDREN 2–11 YRS:** 1 spray in each nostril once a day.

Asthma

INHALATION: ADULTS, ELDERLY, CHILDREN 12 YRS AND OLDER (Previous therapy with bronchodilators or inhaled corticosteroids): Initially, inhale 220 mcg (1 puff) once a day. **Maximum:** 440 mcg/day as single or 2 divided doses. **(Previous therapy with oral corticosteroids):** Initially, inhale 440 mcg (2 puffs) twice a day. Reduce prednisone no faster than 2.5 mg/day beginning after at least 1 wk of mometasone. **CHILDREN 4–11 YRS:** 110 mcg once daily in evening.

Skin Disease

TOPICAL: ADULTS, ELDERLY, CHILDREN 12 YRS AND OLDER: Apply cream, lotion, or ointment to affected area once a day.

Nasal Polyp

NASAL SPRAY: ADULTS, ELDERLY: 2 sprays (100 mcg) in each nostril twice a day.

SIDE EFFECTS

Occasional: Inhalation: Headache, allergic rhinitis, upper respiratory infection, muscle pain, fatigue. **Nasal:** Nasal irritation, stinging. **Topical:** Burning. **Rare: Inhalation:** Abdominal pain, dyspepsia, nausea. **Nasal:** Nasal/pharyngeal candidiasis. **Topical:** Pruritus.

ADVERSE EFFECTS/ TOXIC REACTIONS

Acute hypersensitivity reaction (urticaria, angioedema, severe bronchospasm) occurs rarely. Transfer from systemic to local steroid therapy may unmask previously suppressed bronchial asthma condition.

NURSING CONSIDERATIONS

BASELINE ASSESSMENT

Question for hypersensitivity to any corticosteroids.

INTERVENTION/EVALUATION

Teach proper use of nasal spray, oral inhaler. Instruct pt to clear nasal passages before use. Contact physician if no improvement in symptoms, sneezing, nasal irritation occur. Assess lung sounds for wheezing, rales.

PATIENT/FAMILY TEACHING

• Do not change dose schedule or stop taking drug; must taper off gradually under medical supervision. **Nasal:** Contact physician if symptoms do not improve; sneezing, nasal irritation occur. • Clear nasal passages prior to use. **Inhalation:** Inhale rapidly, deeply; rinse mouth after inhalation. • Not indicated for acute asthma attacks. **Topical:** Do not cover affected area with bandage, dressing.

Monopril, *see fosinopril*

montelukast

mon-**tee**-leu-cast
(Singulair)
Do not confuse Singulair with Sinequan.

◆ CLASSIFICATION

PHARMACOTHERAPEUTIC: Leukotriene receptor inhibitor. **CLINICAL:** Antiasthmatic (see p. 76C).

ACTION

Binds to cysteinyl leukotriene receptors, inhibiting effects of leukotrienes on bronchial smooth muscle. **Therapeutic Effect:** Decreases bronchoconstriction, vascular permeability, mucosal edema, mucus production.

PHARMACOKINETICS

Route	Onset	Peak	Duration
PO	N/A	N/A	24 hrs
PO (chewable)	N/A	N/A	24 hrs

Rapidly absorbed from GI tract. Protein binding: 99%. Extensively metabolized in liver. Excreted almost exclusively in feces. **Half-life:** 2.7–5.5 hrs (slightly longer in elderly).

USES

Prophylaxis, chronic treatment of asthma. Treatment of exercise-induced bronchoconstriction. Not for use in reversal of bronchospasm in acute asthma attacks, status asthmaticus. Treatment of seasonal allergic rhinitis (hay fever). Relief of perennial allergic rhinitis. **OFF-LABEL:** Acute asthma.

PRECAUTIONS

Contraindications: None known. **Cautions:** Systemic corticosteroid treatment reduction during montelukast therapy, hepatic impairment.

LIFESPAN CONSIDERATIONS

Pregnancy/Lactation: Unknown if distributed in breast milk. Use during pregnancy only if necessary. **Pregnancy Category B. Children/Elderly:** No age-related precautions noted in those older than 6 yrs or the elderly.

INTERACTIONS

DRUG: **Carbamazepine, phenobarbital, rifampin** may decrease levels/effect. **HERBAL:** **St. John's wort** may decrease concentration, effect. **FOOD:** None known. **LAB VALUES:** May increase serum AST, ALT, eosinophils.

AVAILABILITY (Rx)

Oral Granules: 4 mg. **Tablets:** 10 mg. **Tablets (Chewable):** 4 mg, 5 mg.

ADMINISTRATION/HANDLING

PO

• When treating asthma, administer in evening without regard to meals. • When treating allergic rhinitis, may individualize administration times. • Granules may be given directly in mouth or mixed with carrots, rice, applesauce, ice cream, baby formula, or breast milk (do not add to any other liquid or food). • Give within 15 min of opening packet.

INDICATIONS/ROUTES/DOSAGE

Bronchial Asthma

PO: ADULTS, ELDERLY, CHILDREN 15 YRS AND OLDER: One 10-mg tablet a day, taken in the evening. **CHILDREN 6–14 YRS:** One 5-mg chewable tablet a day, taken in the evening. **CHILDREN 2–5 YRS:** One 4-mg chewable tablet a day, taken in the evening. **CHILDREN 6–23 MOS:** 4 mg (oral granules) once daily in the evening.

Seasonal Allergic Rhinitis

PO: ADULTS, ELDERLY, CHILDREN 15 YRS AND OLDER: One 10-mg tablet, taken in the evening. **CHILDREN 6–14 YRS:** One 5-mg chewable tablet, taken in the evening. **CHILDREN 2–5 YRS:** One 4-mg chewable tablet, taken in the evening.

Perennial Allergic Rhinitis

PO: ADULTS, ELDERLY, CHILDREN 15 YRS AND OLDER: One 10-mg tablet, taken in the evening. **CHILDREN 6–14 YRS:** One 5-mg chewable tablet, taken in the evening. **CHILDREN 2–5 YRS:** One 4-mg chewable tablet, taken in the evening. **CHILDREN 6–23 MOS:** 4-mg oral granules, taken in the evening.

Exercise-Induced Bronchoconstriction

PO: ADULTS, ELDERLY, CHILDREN 15 YRS AND OLDER: 10 mg 2 or more hrs before exercise. No additional doses within 24 hrs.

SIDE EFFECTS

Adults, children 15 yrs and older: **Frequent (18%):** Headache. **Occasional (4%):** Influenza. **Rare (3%–2%):** Abdominal pain, cough, dyspepsia, dizziness, fatigue, dental pain. **Children 6–14 yrs:** **Rare (less than 2%):** Diarrhea, laryngitis, pharyngitis, nausea, otitis media, sinusitis, viral infection.

ADVERSE EFFECTS/ TOXIC REACTIONS

Suicidal thinking and behavior, depression has been noted.

NURSING CONSIDERATIONS

BASELINE ASSESSMENT

Chewable tablet contains phenylalanine (component of aspartame); parents of phenylketonuric pts should be informed. Assess lung sounds for wheezing, rales, rhonchi, allergy symptoms.

INTERVENTION/EVALUATION

Monitor rate, depth, rhythm, type of respirations; quality/rate of pulse. Assess lung sounds for rhonchi, wheezing, rales. Monitor for change in mood, behavior.

PATIENT/FAMILY TEACHING

• Increase fluid intake (decreases lung secretion viscosity). • Take as prescribed, even during symptom-free periods as well as during exacerbations of asthma. • Do not alter/stop other asthma medications. • Drug is not for treatment of acute asthma attacks. • Report increased use or frequency of short-acting bronchodilators, changes in behavior, suicidal ideation.

morphine HIGH ALERT

mor-feen

(Astramorph PF, Avinza, DepoDur, Duramorph PF, Infumorph, Kadian, M-Eslon ✦, MS Contin, MSIR ✦, Oramorph SR, Roxanol)

BLACK BOX ALERT Be alert for signs of abuse, misuse, diversion. ***Epidural:*** Monitor for delayed sedation. ***Sustained-release:*** Do not crush or chew. ***MS Contin:*** Use only in opioid-tolerant pts requiring over 400 mg/day. ***Kadian:*** Use only in opioid-tolerant pts. ***Avinza:*** Alcohol disrupts extended-release timing. ***Duramorph PF:*** Risk of severe and/or sustained cardiopulmonary depression.

Do not confuse Avinza with Evista or Invanz, morphine with hydromorphone, morphine sulfate with magnesium sulfate, MS Contin with Oxycontin, Roxanol with Roxicet, OxyFast, or Roxicodone. MSO_4 and MS are error-prone abbreviations.

FIXED-COMBINATION(S)

Embeda: morphine/nalaxone (an opioid antagonist): 20 mg/0.8 mg, 30 mg/1.2 mg, 50 mg/2 mg, 60 mg/2.4 mg, 80 mg/3.2 mg, 100 mg/4 mg.

◆CLASSIFICATION

PHARMACOTHERAPEUTIC: Narcotic agonist. **CLINICAL:** Opiate analgesic **(Schedule II)** (see p. 142C).

ACTION

Binds with opioid receptors within CNS. **Therapeutic Effect:** Alters pain perception, emotional response to pain.

PHARMACOKINETICS

Route	Onset	Peak	Duration
Oral solution	30 min	1 hr	3–5 hrs
Tablets	30 min	1 hr	3–5 hrs
Tablets (extended-release)	N/A	3–4 hrs	8–12 hrs
IV	Rapid	0.3 hr	3–5 hrs
IM	5–30 min	0.5–1 hr	3–5 hrs
Epidural	15–60 min	1 hr	12–20 hrs
Subcutaneous	10–30 min	1.1–5 hrs	3–5 hrs
Rectal	20–60 min	0.5–1 hr	3–7 hrs

Variably absorbed from GI tract. Readily absorbed after IM, subcutaneous administration. Protein binding: 20%–35%. Widely distributed. Metabolized in liver. Primarily excreted in urine. Removed by hemodialysis. **Half-life:** 2–4 hrs (increased in hepatic disease).

USES

Relief of moderate to severe, acute, or chronic pain; analgesia during labor. Drug of choice for pain due to MI, dyspnea from pulmonary edema not resulting from chemical respiratory irritant. **DepoDur:** Epidural (lumbar) single dose management of surgical pain. **Infumorph:** Use in devices for managing intractable chronic pain.

PRECAUTIONS

Contraindications: Acute or severe asthma, GI obstruction, paralytic ileus, severe hepatic/renal impairment, severe respiratory depression. Extreme Caution: COPD, cor pulmonale, hypoxia, hypercapnia, preexisting respiratory depression, head injury, ICP, severe hypotension. Cautions: Biliary tract disease, pancreatitis, Addison's disease, hypothyroidism, urethral stricture, prostatic hyperplasia, debilitated pts, those with CNS depression, toxic psychosis, seizure disorders, alcoholism.

LIFESPAN CONSIDERATIONS

Pregnancy/Lactation: Crosses placenta. Distributed in breast milk. May prolong labor if administered in latent phase of first stage of labor or before cervical dilation of 4–5 cm has occurred. Respiratory depression may occur in neonate if mother received opiates during labor. Regular use of opiates during pregnancy may produce withdrawal symptoms in neonate (irritability, excessive crying, tremors, hyperactive reflexes, fever, vomiting, diarrhea, yawning, sneezing, seizures). **Pregnancy Category C (D if used for prolonged periods or at high dosages at term). Children:** Paradoxical excitement may occur; those younger than 2 yrs are more susceptible to respiratory depressant effects. **Elderly:** Paradoxical excitement may occur. Age-related renal impairment may increase risk of urinary retention.

INTERACTIONS

DRUG: **Alcohol, other CNS depressants** may increase CNS effects, respiratory depression, hypotension. **MAOIs** may produce severe, sometimes fatal reaction (reduce dosage to ¼ of usual morphine dose). HERBAL: **Gotu kola, kava kava, St. John's wort, valerian** may increase CNS depression. FOOD: None known. LAB VALUES: May increase serum amylase, lipase.

AVAILABILITY (Rx)

Injection, Liposomal Suspension (DepoDur): 10 mg/ml. Injection, Solution: 2 mg/ml, 4 mg/ml, 5 mg/ml, 10 mg/ml, 15 mg/ml, 25 mg/ml, 50 mg/ml. Injection, Solution (Epidural, Intrathecal, IV Infusion) (Astramorph PF, Duramorph PF): 0.5 mg/ml, 1 mg/ml. Injection, Solution (Epidural or Intrathecal) (Infumorph): 10 mg/ml, 25 mg/ml. Injection, Solution Patient-Controlled Analgesia (PCA) Pump: 0.5 mg/ml, 1 mg/ml, 2 mg/ml, 5 mg/ml. Solution Oral (Roxanol): 20 mg/ml, 10 mg/5 ml, 20 mg/5 ml. Suppository: 5 mg, 10 mg, 20 mg, 30 mg. Tablets: 10 mg, 15 mg, 30 mg.

Capsules, Extended-Release (Avinza): 30 mg, 45 mg, 60 mg, 75 mg, 90 mg, 120 mg. Capsules, Sustained-Release (Kadian): 20 mg, 30 mg, 50 mg, 60 mg, 80 mg, 100 mg, 200 mg. Tablets, Extended-Release (MS Contin, Oramorph SR): 15 mg, 30 mg, 60 mg, 100 mg, 200 mg.

ADMINISTRATION/HANDLING

IV

Reconstitution • May give undiluted. • For IV injection, may dilute 2.5–15 mg morphine in 4–5 ml Sterile Water for Injection. • For continuous IV infusion, dilute to concentration of 0.1–1 mg/ml in D_5W and give through controlled infusion device.

Rate of administration • Always administer very slowly. Rapid IV increases risk of severe adverse reactions (apnea, chest wall rigidity, peripheral circulatory collapse, cardiac arrest, anaphylactoid effects).

Storage • Store at room temperature.

Epidural, Liposomal

• May give either diluted or undiluted. • Do not use an in-line filter. • Store solution in refrigerator; do not freeze. May store at room temperature for 7 days. • Following withdrawal from vial, use within 4 hrs. • Gently invert vial to resuspend drug; avoid aggressive agitation.

IM, Subcutaneous

• Administer slowly, rotating injection sites. • Pts with circulatory impairment experience higher risk of overdosage due to delayed absorption of repeated administration.

PO

• Mix liquid form with fruit juice to improve taste. • Do not crush, break extended-release capsule, tablets. • **Avinza, Kadian:** May mix with applesauce immediately prior to administration.

Rectal

• If suppository is too soft, chill for 30 min in refrigerator or run cold water over foil wrapper. • Moisten suppository with cold water before inserting well into rectum.

IV INCOMPATIBILITIES

Amphotericin B complex (Abelcet, AmBisome, Amphotec), cefepime (Maxipime), doxorubicin (Doxil), lipids, phenytoin (Dilantin), thiopental.

IV COMPATIBILITIES

Amiodarone (Cordarone), atropine, bumetanide (Bumex), bupivacaine (Marcaine, Sensorcaine), diltiazem (Cardizem), diphenhydramine (Benadryl), dobutamine (Dobutrex), dopamine (Intropin), glycopyrrolate (Robinul), heparin, hydroxyzine (Vistaril), lidocaine, lorazepam (Ativan), magnesium, midazolam (Versed), milrinone (Primacor), nitroglycerin, potassium, propofol (Diprivan), total parenteral nutrition (TPN).

INDICATIONS/ROUTES/DOSAGE

ALERT Dosage should be titrated to desired effect.

Analgesia

PO (IMMEDIATE-RELEASE): ADULTS, ELDERLY: 10–30 mg q3–4h as needed. **CHILDREN:** 0.15–0.3 mg/kg q3–4h as needed.

ALERT For the Avinza dosage below, be aware that this drug is to be administered once a day only.

ALERT For the Kadian dosage information below, be aware that this drug is to be administered q12h or once a day.

ALERT Be aware that pediatric dosages of extended-release preparations of Kadian and Avinza have not been established.

ALERT For the MS Contin and Oramorph SR dosage information below, be aware that the daily dosage is divided and given q8h or q12h.

PO (EXTENDED-RELEASE [AVINZA]): ADULTS, ELDERLY: Dosage requirement should be established using prompt-release formulations and is based on total daily dose. Avinza is given once a day only.

PO (EXTENDED-RELEASE [KADIAN]): ADULTS, ELDERLY: Dosage requirement should be established using prompt-release formulations and is based on total daily dose. Dose is given once a day or divided and given q12h.

PO (EXTENDED-RELEASE [MS CONTIN, ORAMORPH SR]): ADULTS, ELDERLY: Dosage requirement should be established using prompt-release formulations and is based on total daily dose. Daily dose is divided and given q8h or q12h. **CHILDREN:** 0.3–0.6 mg/kg/dose q12h.

IV: ADULTS, ELDERLY: 2.5–5 mg q3–4h as needed. Note: Repeated doses (e.g., 1–2 mg) may be given more frequently (e.g., every hr) if needed. **CHILDREN:** 0.1–0.2 mg/kg q3–4h as needed.

IV CONTINUOUS INFUSION: ADULTS, ELDERLY: 0.8–10 mg/hr. Range: Titrate up to 80 mg/hr. **CHILDREN:** 10–60 mcg/kg/hr.

IM: ADULTS, ELDERLY: 5–10 mg q3–4h as needed. **CHILDREN:** 0.1–0.2 mg/kg q3–4h as needed.

EPIDURAL: ADULTS, ELDERLY: Initially, 1–6 mg bolus, infusion rate: 0.1–2 mg/hr. **Maximum:** 10 mg/24 hrs.

INTRATHECAL: ADULTS, ELDERLY: One-tenth of the epidural dose: 0.2–0.25 mg/dose.

Patient-Controlled Analgesia (PCA)

IV: ADULTS, ELDERLY: Loading dose: 5–10 mg. **Intermittent bolus:** 0.5–3 mg. **Lockout interval:** 5–12 min. **Continuous infusion:** 1–10 mg/hr. **4-hr limit:** 20–30 mg.

M

SIDE EFFECTS

◀ALERT▶ Ambulatory pts, those not in severe pain may experience nausea, vomiting more frequently than those in supine position or who have severe pain. **Frequent:** Sedation, decreased B/P (including orthostatic hypotension), diaphoresis, facial flushing, constipation, dizziness, drowsiness, nausea, vomiting. **Occasional:** Allergic reaction (rash, pruritus), dyspnea, confusion, palpitations, tremors, urinary retention, abdominal cramps, vision changes, dry mouth, headache, decreased appetite, pain/burning at injection site. **Rare:** Paralytic ileus.

ADVERSE EFFECTS/ TOXIC REACTIONS

Overdose results in respiratory depression, skeletal muscle flaccidity, cold/clammy skin, cyanosis, extreme drowsiness progressing to seizures, stupor, coma. Tolerance to analgesic effect, physical dependence may occur with repeated use. Prolonged duration of action, cumulative effect may occur in those with hepatic/renal impairment. **Antidote:** Naloxone (see Appendix M for dosage).

NURSING CONSIDERATIONS

BASELINE ASSESSMENT

Pt should be in recumbent position before drug is given by parenteral route. Assess onset, type, location, duration of pain. Obtain vital signs before giving medication. If respirations are 12/min or less (20/min or less in children), withhold medication, contact physician. Effect of medication is reduced if full pain recurs before next dose.

INTERVENTION/EVALUATION

Monitor vital signs 5–10 min after IV administration, 15–30 min after subcutaneous, IM. Be alert for decreased respirations, B/P. Check for adequate voiding. Monitor daily pattern of bowel activity and stool consistency. Avoid constipation. Initiate deep breathing, coughing exercises, particularly in those with pulmonary impairment. Assess for clinical improvement, record onset of pain relief. Consult physician if pain relief is not adequate.

PATIENT/FAMILY TEACHING

• Discomfort may occur with injection. • Change positions slowly to avoid orthostatic hypotension. • Avoid tasks that require alertness, motor skills until response to drug is established. • Avoid alcohol, CNS depressants. • Tolerance, dependence may occur with prolonged use of high doses. • Report ineffective pain control, constipation, urinary retention.

Motrin, *see ibuprofen*

moxifloxacin

moks-i-**floks**-a-sin
(Avelox, Avelox IV, Moxeza, Vigamox)

BLACK BOX ALERT May increase risk of tendonitis, tendon rupture.

Do not confuse Avelox with Avonex.

◆CLASSIFICATION

PHARMACOTHERAPEUTIC: Fluoroquinolone. **CLINICAL:** Antibacterial (see p. 25C).

ACTION

Inhibits two enzymes, topoisomerase II and IV, in susceptible microorganisms. **Therapeutic Effect:** Interferes with bacterial DNA replication. Prevents/delays emergence of resistant organisms. Bactericidal.

PHARMACOKINETICS

Well absorbed from GI tract after PO administration. Protein binding: 50%. Widely distributed throughout body with tissue concentration often exceeding plasma concentration. Metabolized in liver. Primarily excreted in urine, with lesser amount in feces. **Half-life: PO:** 12 hrs; **IV:** 15 hrs.

USES

Treatment of susceptible infections due to *S. pneumoniae, S. pyogenes, S. aureus, H. influenzae, M. catarrhalis, K. pneumoniae, M. pneumoniae, C. pneumoniae* including acute bacterial exacerbation of chronic bronchitis, acute bacterial sinusitis, intra-abdominal infection, community-acquired pneumonia, uncomplicated skin/skin structure infections. **Ophthalmic:** Topical treatment of bacterial conjunctivitis due to susceptible strains of bacteria. **OFF-LABEL:** Legionella.

PRECAUTIONS

Contraindications: Hypersensitivity to quinolones. **Cautions:** Renal/hepatic impairment, CNS disorders, cerebral arthrosclerosis, seizures, those with prolonged QT interval, uncorrected hypokalemia, those receiving quinidine, procainamide, amiodarone, sotalol.

LIFESPAN CONSIDERATIONS

Pregnancy/Lactation: May be distributed in breast milk. May produce teratogenic effects. **Pregnancy Category C. Children:** Safety and efficacy not established. **Elderly:** No age-related precautions noted.

INTERACTIONS

DRUG: **Antacids, iron preparations, sucralfate** may decrease absorption. **HERBAL:** None significant. **FOOD:** None known. **LAB VALUES:** None significant.

AVAILABILITY (Rx)

Injection Infusion (Avelox IV): 400 mg (250 ml). **Ophthalmic Solution (Vigamox):** 0.5%. **Tablets (Avelox):** 400 mg.

ADMINISTRATION/HANDLING

IV

Reconstitution • Available in ready-to-use containers.

Rate of administration • Give by IV infusion only. • Avoid rapid or bolus IV infusion. • Infuse over 60 min.

Storage • Store at room temperature. • Do not refrigerate.

PO

• Give without regard to meals. • Oral moxifloxacin should be administered 4 hrs before or 8 hrs after antacids, multivitamins, iron preparations, sucralfate, didanosine chewable/buffered tablets, pediatric powder for oral solution.

Ophthalmic

• Place gloved finger on lower eyelid and pull out until a pocket is formed between eye and lower lid. • Place prescribed number of drops into pocket. • Instruct pt to close eye gently (so medication will not be squeezed out of the sac) and to apply digital pressure to lacrimal sac at inner canthus for 1 min to minimize systemic absorption.

IV INCOMPATIBILITIES

Do not add or infuse other drugs simultaneously through the same IV line. Flush line before and after use if same IV line is used with other medications.

INDICATIONS/ROUTES/DOSAGE

Acute Bacterial Sinusitis

PO, IV: ADULTS, ELDERLY: 400 mg q24h for 10 days.

Acute Bacterial Exacerbation of Chronic Bronchitis

PO, IV: ADULTS, ELDERLY: 400 mg q24h for 5 days.

Community-Acquired Pneumonia

PO, IV: ADULTS, ELDERLY: 400 mg q24h for 7–14 days.

Intra-Abdominal Infection

PO, IV: ADULTS, ELDERLY: 400 mg q24h for 5–14 days.

M

Skin/Skin Structure Infection
PO, IV: ADULTS, ELDERLY: 400 mg once a day for 7–21 days.

Topical Treatment of Bacterial Conjunctivitis Due to Susceptible Strains of Bacteria
OPHTHALMIC: ADULTS, ELDERLY CHILDREN 1 YR AND OLDER: (Vigamox): 1 drop 3 times a day for 7 days. **(Moxeza):** 1 drop 2 times a day for 7 days.

SIDE EFFECTS

Frequent (8%–6%): Nausea, diarrhea. **Occasional: PO, IV (3%–2%):** Dizziness, headache, abdominal pain, vomiting. **Ophthalmic (6%–1%):** Conjunctival irritation, reduced visual acuity, dry eye, keratitis, eye pain, ocular itching, swelling of tissue around cornea, eye discharge, fever, cough, pharyngitis, rash, rhinitis. **Rare (1%):** Change in sense of taste, dyspepsia (heartburn, epigastric pain, indigestion), photosensitivity.

ADVERSE EFFECTS/ TOXIC REACTIONS

Pseudomembranous colitis (severe abdominal cramps/pain, severe watery diarrhea, fever) may occur. Superinfection (anal/genital pruritus, moderate to severe diarrhea, stomatitis) may occur.

NURSING CONSIDERATIONS

BASELINE ASSESSMENT
Question for history of hypersensitivity to moxifloxacin, quinolones.

INTERVENTION/EVALUATION
Monitor daily pattern of bowel activity/stool consistency. Assist with ambulation if dizziness occurs. Assess for headache, abdominal pain, vomiting, altered taste, dyspepsia (heartburn, indigestion). Monitor WBC, signs of infection.

PATIENT/FAMILY TEACHING
• May be taken without regard to food. • Drink plenty of fluids. • Avoid exposure to direct sunlight; may cause photosensitivity reaction. • Do not take antacids 4 hrs before or 8 hrs after dosing. • Take full course of therapy. • Report abdominal cramping/pain, persistent diarrhea.

MS Contin, *see morphine*

mupirocin

mew-pie-ro-sin
(Bactroban, Bactroban Nasal)
Do not confuse Bactroban or Bactroban Nasal with bacitracin, baclofen, or Bactrim.

◆CLASSIFICATION

PHARMACOTHERAPEUTIC: Anti-infective. **CLINICAL:** Topical antibacterial.

ACTION

Inhibits bacterial protein, RNA synthesis. Less effective on DNA synthesis. **Nasal:** Eradicates nasal colonization of methicillin-resistant *Staphylococcus aureus* (MRSA). **Therapeutic Effect:** Prevents bacterial growth, replication. Bacteriostatic.

PHARMACOKINETICS

Following topical administration, penetrates outer layer of skin (minimal through intact skin). Protein binding: 95%. Metabolized in liver; excreted in urine. **Half-life:** 17–36 min.

USES

Ointment: Topical treatment of impetigo caused by *S. aureus*, *S. pyogenes;* treatment of folliculitis, furunculosis, minor wounds, burns, ulcers caused by susceptible organisms. **Cream:** Treatment of traumatic skin lesions due to *S. aureus*, *S. pyogenes,* prophylactic agent applied to IV catheter exit sites. **Intranasal ointment:** Eradication of *S. aureus* from nasal, perineal carriage sites. OFF-LABEL: Treatment of infected eczema, folliculitis, minor bacterial skin infections. Surgical prophylaxis to prevent wound infections.

PRECAUTIONS

Contraindications: None known. Cautions: Renal impairment, burn pts.

LIFESPAN CONSIDERATIONS

Pregnancy/Lactation: Unknown if distributed in breast milk. Breast-feeding not recommended. **Pregnancy Category B. Children:** Safety and efficacy not established. **Elderly:** No age-related precautions noted.

INTERACTIONS

DRUG: None significant. HERBAL: None significant. FOOD: None known. LAB VALUES: None significant.

AVAILABILITY (Rx)

Cream, Topical (Bactroban): 2%. Ointment, Intranasal (1-g single-use tube) (Bactroban Nasal): 2%. Ointment, Topical (Bactroban): 2%.

ADMINISTRATION/HANDLING

Topical

Cream, ointment • For topical use only. • May cover with gauze dressing. • Avoid contact with eyes.

Intranasal

• Apply ½ of the ointment from single-use tube into each nostril. • Avoid contact with eyes.

INDICATIONS/ROUTES/DOSAGE

Usual Topical Dosage

TOPICAL: ADULTS, ELDERLY, CHILDREN: Cream: Apply small amount 3 times a day for 10 days. **Ointment:** Apply small amount 3–5 times a day for 5–14 days.

Usual Nasal Dosage

INTRANASAL: ADULTS, ELDERLY, CHILDREN: Apply small amount 2–4 times a day for 5–14 days.

SIDE EFFECTS

Frequent: **Nasal (9%–3%):** Headache, rhinitis, upper respiratory congestion, pharyngitis, altered taste. Occasional: **Nasal (2%):** Burning, stinging, cough. **Topical (2%–1%):** Pain, burning, stinging, pruritus. Rare: **Nasal (less than 1%):** Pruritus, diarrhea, dry mouth, epistaxis, nausea, rash. **Topical (less than 1%):** Rash, nausea, dry skin, contact dermatitis.

ADVERSE EFFECTS/ TOXIC REACTIONS

Superinfection may result in bacterial, fungal infections, esp. with prolonged, repeated therapy.

NURSING CONSIDERATIONS

BASELINE ASSESSMENT

Assess skin for type, extent of lesions.

INTERVENTION/EVALUATION

Monitor healing of skin lesions. In event of skin reaction, stop applications, cleanse area gently, notify physician.

PATIENT/FAMILY TEACHING

• For external use only. • Avoid contact with eyes. • Explain precautions to avoid spread of infection; teach how to apply medication. • If skin reaction, irritation develops, notify physician. • If no improvement is noted in 3–5 days, contact physician.

Mycamine, *see micafungin*

mycophenolate

my-co-**fen**-o-late
(CellCept, Myfortic)

BLACK BOX ALERT Increased risk of congenital malformation, spontaneous abortion. Increased risk for development of lymphoma, skin malignancy.

M

◆CLASSIFICATION

PHARMACOTHERAPEUTIC: Immunologic agent. **CLINICAL:** Immunosuppressant (see p. 119C).

ACTION

Suppresses immunologically mediated inflammatory response by inhibiting inosine monophosphate dehydrogenase, an enzyme that deprives lymphocytes of nucleotides necessary for DNA, RNA synthesis, thus inhibiting proliferation of T and B lymphocytes. **Therapeutic Effect:** Prevents transplant rejection.

PHARMACOKINETICS

Rapidly, extensively absorbed after PO administration (food decreases drug plasma concentration but does not affect absorption). Protein binding: 97%. Completely hydrolyzed to active metabolite mycophenolic acid. Primarily excreted in urine. Not removed by hemodialysis. **Half-life:** 17.9 hrs.

USES

Should be used concurrently with cyclosporine and corticosteroids. **CellCept:** Prophylaxis of organ rejection in pts receiving allogeneic hepatic/renal/cardiac transplants. **Myfortic:** Renal transplants. **OFF-LABEL:** Treatment of hepatic transplant rejection, mild heart transplant rejection, moderate to severe psoriasis.

PRECAUTIONS

Contraindications: Hypersensitivity to mycophenolic acid or polysorbate 80 (IV formulation). **Cautions:** Active serious digestive disease, renal impairment, neutropenia, women of childbearing potential.

LIFESPAN CONSIDERATIONS

Pregnancy/Lactation: Unknown if drug crosses placenta or is distributed in breast milk. Breast-feeding not recommended. Increased risk of miscarriage, birth defects. **Pregnancy Category C. (Myfortic: Pregnancy Category D). Children:** Safety and efficacy not established. **Elderly:** Age-related renal impairment may require dosage adjustment.

INTERACTIONS

DRUG: May increase concentrations of **acyclovir, ganciclovir** in pts with renal impairment. **Antacids (aluminum- and magnesium-containing), cholestyramine** may decrease absorption. **Live virus vaccines** may potentiate virus replication, increase vaccine side effects, decrease pt's antibody response to vaccine. **Other immunosuppressants (e.g., cyclophosphamide, cyclosporine, tacrolimus)** may increase risk of infection, lymphomas. **Probenecid** may increase concentration. **HERBAL: Cat's claw, echinacea** may decrease effects. **FOOD: All foods** may decrease concentration. **LAB VALUES:** May increase serum cholesterol, alkaline phosphatase, creatinine, AST, ALT. May alter serum glucose, lipids, calcium, potassium, phosphate, uric acid.

AVAILABILITY (Rx)

Capsules (CellCept): 250 mg. **Injection, Powder for Reconstitution (CellCept):** 500 mg. **Oral Suspension (CellCept):** 200 mg/ml. **Tablets (CellCept):** 500 mg.

Tablets (Delayed-Release [Myfortic]): 180 mg, 360 mg.

ADMINISTRATION/HANDLING

IV

Reconstitution • Reconstitute each 500-mg vial with 14 ml D_5W. Gently agitate. • For 1-g dose, further dilute with 140 ml D_5W; for 1.5-g dose further dilute with 210 ml D_5W, providing a concentration of 6 mg/ml.

Rate of administration • Infuse over at least 2 hrs. • Begin infusion within 4 hrs of reconstitution.

Storage • Store at room temperature. • IV infusion stable for 12 hrs at room temperature.

PO

• Give on empty stomach (1 hr before or 2 hrs after food). • Do not open capsules or crush delayed-release tablets. Avoid inhalation of powder in capsules, direct contact of powder on skin/mucous membranes. If contact occurs, wash thoroughly, with soap, water. Rinse eyes profusely with plain water. • May store reconstituted suspension in refrigerator or at room temperature. • Suspension is stable for 60 days after reconstitution. • Suspension can be administered orally or via a NG tube (minimum size 8 French).

IV INCOMPATIBILITIES

Mycophenolate is compatible only with D_5W. Do not infuse concurrently with other drugs or IV solutions.

INDICATIONS/ROUTES/DOSAGE

Prevention of Renal Transplant Rejection

PO, IV (CELLCEPT): ADULTS, ELDERLY: 1 g twice a day. **CHILDREN:** 600 mg/m²/dose twice a day. **Maximum:** 1 g twice a day.

PO (MYFORTIC): ADULTS, ELDERLY: 720 mg twice a day. **CHILDREN 5–16 YRS:** 400 mg/m² twice a day. **Maximum:** 720 mg twice a day.

Prevention of Heart Transplant Rejection

PO, IV (CELLCEPT): ADULTS, ELDERLY: 1.5 g twice a day.

Prevention of Hepatic Transplant Rejection

PO (CELLCEPT): ADULTS, ELDERLY: 1.5 g twice a day.

IV (CELLCEPT): ADULTS, ELDERLY: 1 g twice a day.

SIDE EFFECTS

Frequent (37%–20%): UTI, hypertension, peripheral edema, diarrhea, constipation, fever, headache, nausea. **Occasional** (18%–10%): Dyspepsia; dyspnea; cough; hematuria; asthenia (loss of strength, energy); vomiting; edema; tremors; abdominal, chest, back pain; oral candidiasis; acne. **Rare** (9%–6%): Insomnia, respiratory tract infection, rash, dizziness.

ADVERSE EFFECTS/ TOXIC REACTIONS

Significant anemia, leukopenia, thrombocytopenia, neutropenia, leukocytosis may occur, particularly in those undergoing renal transplant rejection. Sepsis, infection occur occasionally. GI tract hemorrhage occurs rarely. There is an increased risk of developing neoplasms. Immunosuppression results in increased susceptibility to infection.

NURSING CONSIDERATIONS

BASELINE ASSESSMENT

Women of childbearing potential should have a negative serum or urine pregnancy test within 1 wk before initiation of drug therapy. Assess medical history, esp. renal function, existence of active digestive system disease, drug history, esp. other immunosuppressants.

INTERVENTION/EVALUATION

CBC should be performed weekly during first mo of therapy, twice monthly during second and third mos of treatment, then monthly throughout the first yr. If rapid fall in WBC occurs, dosage should be reduced or discontinued. Assess particularly for delayed bone marrow suppression. Report any major change in assessment of pt.

PATIENT/FAMILY TEACHING

• Effective contraception should be used before, during, and for 6 wks after discontinuing therapy, even if pt has a history of infertility, other than hysterectomy. • Two forms of contraception must be used concurrently unless abstinence is absolute. • Contact physician if unusual bleeding/bruising, sore throat, mouth sores, abdominal pain, fever occurs. • Laboratory follow-up while taking medication is important part of therapy. • Malignancies may occur.

M

nabumetone

na-**bue**-me-tone
(Apo-Nabumetone ✦, Novo-Nabumetone ✦, Relafen)

BLACK BOX ALERT Increased risk of serious cardiovascular thrombotic events, including myocardial infarction, CVA. Increased risk of severe GI reactions, including ulceration, bleeding, perforation of stomach, intestines.

CLASSIFICATION

PHARMACOTHERAPEUTIC: Nonsteroidal anti-inflammatory. **CLINICAL:** Analgesic, anti-inflammatory (see p. 129C).

ACTION

Produces analgesic anti-inflammatory effects by inhibiting prostaglandin synthesis. **Therapeutic Effect:** Reduces inflammatory response, intensity of pain.

PHARMACOKINETICS

Readily absorbed from GI tract. Protein binding: 99%. Widely distributed. Metabolized in liver to active metabolite. Primarily excreted in urine. Not removed by hemodialysis. **Half-life:** 22–30 hrs.

USES

Acute, chronic treatment of osteoarthritis, rheumatoid arthritis (RA). **OFF-LABEL:** Moderate pain.

PRECAUTIONS

Contraindications: Active peptic ulcer disease, chronic inflammation of GI tract, GI bleeding/ulceration, history of hypersensitivity to aspirin or NSAIDs, history of significant renal impairment. **Cautions:** CHF, hypertension, hepatic/renal impairment, concurrent use of anticoagulants.

LIFESPAN CONSIDERATIONS

Pregnancy/Lactation: Distributed in low concentration in breast milk. Avoid use during last trimester (may adversely affect fetal cardiovascular system: premature closing of ductus arteriosus). **Pregnancy Category C (D if used in third trimester or near delivery). Children:** Safety and efficacy not established. **Elderly:** Age-related renal impairment may increase risk of hepatic/renal toxicity; reduced dosage recommended. More likely to have serious adverse effects with GI bleeding/ulceration.

INTERACTIONS

DRUG: May decrease effects of **antihypertensives, diuretics. Aspirin, other salicylates** may increase risk of GI side effects, bleeding. **Bone marrow depressants** may increase risk of hematologic reactions. May increase concentration of **cyclosporine,** risk of cyclosporine-induced nephropathy. May increase effects of **heparin, oral anticoagulants, thrombolytics.** May increase concentration/risk of **lithium** toxicity. May increase risk of **methotrexate** toxicity. **Probenecid** may increase concentration. **HERBAL: Cat's claw, dong quai, evening primrose, feverfew, garlic, ginger, ginkgo, ginseng, horse chestnut** possess antiplatelet activity, may increase risk of bleeding. **FOOD:** None known. **LAB VALUES:** May increase urine protein levels, BUN, serum LDH, alkaline phosphatase, creatinine, potassium, AST, ALT. May decrease serum uric acid, Hgb, Hct, leukocytes, platelets.

AVAILABILITY (Rx)

Tablets (Relafen): 500 mg, 750 mg.

ADMINISTRATION/HANDLING

PO

• Give with food, milk, antacids to decrease GI irritation, increase absorption.

INDICATIONS/ROUTES/DOSAGE

Rheumatoid Arthritis (RA), Osteoarthritis

PO: ADULTS, ELDERLY: Initially, 1,000 mg as a single dose or in 2 divided doses. May increase up to 2,000 mg/day as a single dose or in 2 divided doses.

Dosage in Renal Impairment

Creatinine Clearance	Dosage
30–49 ml/min	Initially, 750 mg/day. **Maximum:** 1,500 mg/day
Less than 30 ml/min	Initially, 500 mg/day. **Maximum:** 1,000 mg/day

SIDE EFFECTS

Frequent (14%–12%): Diarrhea, abdominal cramps/pain, dyspepsia. **Occasional (9%–4%):** Nausea, constipation, flatulence, dizziness, headache. **Rare (3%–1%):** Vomiting, stomatitis, confusion.

ADVERSE EFFECTS/ TOXIC REACTIONS

Overdose may result in acute hypotension, tachycardia. Rare reactions with long-term use include peptic ulcer, GI bleeding, gastritis, nephrotoxicity (dysuria, cystitis, hematuria, proteinuria, nephrotic syndrome), severe hepatic reactions (cholestasis, jaundice), severe hypersensitivity reactions (bronchospasm, angioedema).

NURSING CONSIDERATIONS

BASELINE ASSESSMENT

Assess onset, type, location, duration of pain/inflammation. Inspect appearance of affected joints for immobility, deformities, skin condition.

INTERVENTION/EVALUATION

Monitor renal function tests in pts with renal insufficiency. Assist with ambulation if drowsiness, dizziness occurs. Monitor for evidence of dyspepsia. Monitor daily pattern of bowel activity and stool consistency. Assess for therapeutic response: relief of pain, stiffness, swelling; increase in joint mobility; reduced joint tenderness; improved grip strength.

PATIENT/FAMILY TEACHING

• May cause serious GI bleeding with or without pain. • Avoid aspirin, alcohol. • May take with food if GI upset occurs. • Avoid tasks requiring mental alertness, motor skills until response to drug is established. • Report GI symptoms.

nadolol

HIGH ALERT

nay-**doe**-lol
(Apo-Nadol ✦, Corgard, Novo-Nadolol ✦)

BLACK BOX ALERT Severe angina exacerbation, MI, ventricular arrhythmias noted in angina pts after abrupt withdrawal.

Do not confuse Corgard with Coreg.

FIXED-COMBINATION(S)

Corzide: nadolol/bendroflumethiazide (a diuretic): 40 mg/5 mg, 80 mg/5 mg.

◆CLASSIFICATION

PHARMACOTHERAPEUTIC: Beta-adrenergic blocker. **CLINICAL:** Antianginal, antihypertensive (see p. 72C).

ACTION

Blocks $beta_1$- and $beta_2$-adrenergenic receptors. Large doses increase airway resistance. **Therapeutic Effect:** Slows heart rate, decreases cardiac output, B/P. Decreases myocardial ischemia severity by decreasing oxygen requirements.

PHARMACOKINETICS

Variable absorption after PO administration. Protein binding: 28%–30%. Not metabolized. Excreted unchanged in feces. **Half-life:** 20–24 hrs.

USES

Management of mild to moderate hypertension. Used alone or in combination with diuretics, esp. thiazide type. Management of chronic stable angina pectoris. **OFF-LABEL:** Treatment of arrhythmias, hypertrophic cardiomyopathy, MI, mitral valve prolapse syndrome, neuroleptic-induced akathisia, pheochromocytoma, tremors, thyrotoxicosis, vascular headaches.

N

PRECAUTIONS

Contraindications: Bronchial asthma, cardiogenic shock, CHF secondary to tachyarrhythmias, COPD, pts receiving MAOI therapy, second- or third-degree heart block, sinus bradycardia, uncontrolled cardiac failure. **Cautions:** Inadequate cardiac function, renal/hepatic impairment, diabetes mellitus, hyperthyroidism.

⌛ LIFESPAN CONSIDERATIONS

Pregnancy/Lactation: Crosses placenta; distributed in breast milk. **Pregnancy Category C (D if used in second or third trimester). Children:** Safety and efficacy not established. **Elderly:** No age-related precautions noted.

INTERACTIONS

DRUG: **Diuretics, other antihypertensives** may increase hypotensive effect. May mask symptoms of hypoglycemia, prolong hypoglycemic effect of **insulin, oral hypoglycemics. NSAIDs** may decrease antihypertensive effect. **Sympathomimetics, xanthines** may mutually inhibit effects. **HERBAL:** **Ephedra, garlic, ginseng, yohimbe** may increase hypertension. **Licorice** may cause increased serum sodium, water retention, decreased serum potassium. **FOOD:** None known. **LAB VALUES:** May increase serum antinuclear antibody (ANA) titer, BUN, serum LDH, lipoprotein, alkaline phosphatase, bilirubin, potassium, uric acid, AST, ALT, triglycerides.

AVAILABILITY (Rx)

Tablets: 20 mg, 40 mg, 80 mg, 120 mg, 160 mg.

ADMINISTRATION/HANDLING

PO

• Give without regard to meals. • Tablets may be crushed.

INDICATIONS/ROUTES/DOSAGE

Hypertension, Angina

PO: ADULTS: Initially, 40 mg/day. May increase by 40–80 mg at 3- to 7-day intervals. **Maximum: (Hypertension)** 240–320 mg/day. **(Angina):** 160–240 mg. **ELDERLY:** Initially, 20 mg/day. May increase gradually. Range: 20–240 mg/day.

Dosage in Renal Impairment

Dosage is modified based on creatinine clearance.

Creatinine Clearance	Dosage
31–40 ml/min	q24–36 hrs or 50% of normal dose
10–30 ml/min	q24–48 hrs or 50% of normal dose
Less than 10 ml/min	q40–60 hrs or 25% of normal dose

SIDE EFFECTS

Nadolol is generally well tolerated, with transient, mild side effects. **Frequent:** Diminished sexual function, drowsiness, unusual fatigue/weakness. **Occasional:** Bradycardia, difficulty breathing, depression, cold hands/feet, diarrhea, constipation, anxiety, nasal congestion, nausea, vomiting. **Rare:** Altered taste, dry eyes, pruritus.

ADVERSE EFFECTS/ TOXIC REACTIONS

Overdose may produce profound bradycardia, hypotension. Abrupt withdrawal may result in diaphoresis, palpitations, headache, tremors, exacerbation of angina, MI, ventricular arrhythmias. May precipitate CHF, MI in pts with cardiac disease; thyroid storm in those with thyrotoxicosis; peripheral ischemia in those with existing peripheral vascular disease. Hypoglycemia may occur in pts with previously controlled diabetes.

NURSING CONSIDERATIONS

BASELINE ASSESSMENT

Assess baseline renal/hepatic function tests. Assess B/P, apical pulse immediately before drug administration (if pulse is 60/min or less or systolic B/P is less than 90 mm Hg, withhold medication, contact physician). **Antianginal:** Record onset, type (sharp, dull, squeezing), radiation, location, intensity, duration of anginal pain; precipitating factors (exertion, emotional stress).

INTERVENTION/EVALUATION

Monitor B/P for hypotension, respiratory effort for dyspnea. Assess pulse for quality, irregular rate, bradycardia. Assess hands/feet for coldness, tingling, numbness. Assess for evidence of CHF: dyspnea (particularly on exertion, lying down), night cough, peripheral edema, distended neck veins. Monitor I&O (increase in weight, decrease in urinary output may indicate CHF).

PATIENT/FAMILY TEACHING

• Do not discontinue abruptly (may precipitate angina). • Inform physician if difficulty breathing, night cough, swelling of arms/legs, slow pulse, dizziness, confusion, depression, rash, fever, sore throat, unusual bleeding/bruising occurs. • Avoid tasks that require alertness, motor skills until response to drug is established. • Limit alcohol.

nafarelin

naf-ah-**rell**-in
(Synarel)
Do not confuse nafarelin with Anafranil or enalapril, or Synarel with Symmetrel.

◆ CLASSIFICATION

PHARMACOTHERAPEUTIC: Gonadotropin inhibitor. **CLINICAL:** Hormone agonist (see p. 106C).

ACTION

Initially stimulates release of pituitary gonadotropins, luteinizing hormone (LH) and follicle-stimulating hormone (FSH). **Therapeutic Effect:** Results in temporary increase of ovarian steroidogenesis. Continued dosing abolishes stimulatory effect on pituitary gland and, after about 4 wks, leads to decreased secretion of gonadal steroids.

USES

Management of endometriosis, including dysmenorrhea, dyspareunia, pelvic pain. Treatment of central precocious puberty.

PRECAUTIONS

Contraindications: Hypersensitivity to nafarelin, other agonist analogues; undiagnosed abnormal vaginal bleeding. **Cautions:** History of osteoporosis, chronic alcohol/tobacco use, intercurrent rhinitis. **Pregnancy Category X.**

INTERACTIONS

DRUG: None significant. **HERBAL:** None significant. **FOOD:** None known. **LAB VALUES:** None significant.

AVAILABILITY (Rx)

Nasal Solution: 2 mg/ml (each spray delivers 200 mcg).

INDICATIONS/ROUTES/DOSAGE

Endometriosis

◄ALERT► Initiate treatment between days 2 and 4 of menstrual cycle. Duration of therapy is 6 mos.

INTRANASAL: ADULTS: 400 mcg/day: 200 mcg (1 spray) into 1 nostril in morning, 1 spray into other nostril in evening. For pts with persistent regular menstruation following initial treatment, increase dosage to 800 mcg/day (1 spray into each nostril in morning and evening).

Central Precocious Puberty

INTRANASAL: CHILDREN: 1,600 mcg/day: 400 mcg (2 sprays into each nostril in morning and evening; total 8 sprays). May increase dose to 1,800 mcg/day: 600 mcg (3 sprays) into alternating nostrils 3 times a day.

SIDE EFFECTS

Common (90%): Hot flashes. **Occasional (22%–10%):** Decreased libido, vaginal dryness, headache, emotional lability, acne, myalgia, decreased breast size, nasal irritation. **Rare (8%–2%):** Insomnia, edema, weight gain, seborrhea, depression.

ADVERSE EFFECTS/ TOXIC REACTIONS

None known.

NURSING CONSIDERATIONS

BASELINE ASSESSMENT

Inquire about menstrual cycle; therapy should begin between days 2 and 4 of cycle.

INTERVENTION/EVALUATION

Check for pain relief as result of therapy. Inquire about menstrual cessation, other decreased estrogen effects.

PATIENT/FAMILY TEACHING

• Pt should use nonhormonal contraceptive during therapy. • Do not take drug if pregnancy is suspected **(Pregnancy Category X)**. • Completing full length of therapy, regular visits to physician's office are important elements of therapy. • Notify physician if regular menstruation continues (menstruation should stop with therapy).

nafcillin

naf-**sill**-in
(Nallpen ❋, Unipen ❋)

◆CLASSIFICATION

PHARMACOTHERAPEUTIC: Penicillinase-resistant penicillin. **CLINICAL:** Antibiotic (see p. 28C).

ACTION

Binds to bacterial membranes. **Therapeutic Effect:** Inhibits cell wall synthesis. Bactericidal.

USES

Treatment of respiratory tract, skin/skin structure infections, osteomyelitis, endocarditis; meningitis, perioperatively, esp. in cardiovascular, orthopedic procedures. Predominant treatment of infections caused by penicillinase-producing staphylococci.

PRECAUTIONS

Contraindications: Hypersensitivity to any penicillin. **Cautions:** History of allergies, particularly cephalosporins, severe renal/hepatic impairment.

⌛ LIFESPAN CONSIDERATIONS

Pregnancy/Lactation: Readily crosses placenta; appears in cord blood, amniotic fluid. Distributed in breast milk. May lead to rash, diarrhea, candidiasis in neonate, infant. **Pregnancy Category B. Children:** Immature renal function in neonate may delay renal excretion. **Elderly:** Age-related renal impairment may require dosage adjustment.

INTERACTIONS

DRUG: **Probenecid** may increase concentration, risk of toxicity. **HERBAL:** None significant. **FOOD:** None known. **LAB VALUES:** May cause false-positive Coombs' test.

AVAILABILITY (Rx)

Injection, Powder for Reconstitution: 1 g, 2 g. **Infusion (Pre-Mix):** 1 g/50 ml, 2g/100 ml.

ADMINISTRATION/HANDLING

◀ALERT▶ Space doses evenly around the clock.

IV

Reconstitution • Reconstitute each vial with 10 ml Sterile Water for Injection or 0.9% NaCl. • For intermittent IV infusion (piggyback), further dilute with 50–100 ml 0.9% NaCl or D_5W to maximum concentration of 40 mg/ml.

Rate of administration • Infuse over 30–60 min. • Because of potential for hypersensitivity/anaphylaxis, start initial dose at few drops per min, increase slowly to ordered rate; stay with pt first 10–15 min, then check q10min. • Limit IV therapy to less than 48 hrs, if possible. Stop infusion if pt complains of pain at IV site.

Storage (IV infusion [piggyback])
• Stable for 24 hrs at room temperature, 96 hrs if refrigerated. • Discard if precipitate forms.

IM
• Reconstitute each 500 mg with 1.7 ml Sterile Water for Injection or 0.9% NaCl to provide concentration of 250 mg/ml. • Inject IM into large muscle mass.

IV INCOMPATIBILITIES

Aztreonam (Azactam), diltiazem (Cardizem), droperidol (Inapsine), fentanyl, gentamicin, insulin, labetalol (Normodyne, Trandate), methylprednisolone (Solu-Medrol), midazolam (Versed), nalbuphine (Nubain), vancomycin (Vancocin), verapamil (Isoptin).

IV COMPATIBILITIES

Acyclovir, famotidine (Pepcid), fluconazole (Diflucan), heparin, hydromorphone (Dilaudid), lidocaine, lipids, magnesium, morphine, potassium chloride, propofol (Diprivan).

INDICATIONS/ROUTES/DOSAGE

Usual Dosage
IV: ADULTS, ELDERLY: 0.5–2 g q4–6h. **CHILDREN:** 50–200 mg/kg/day in divided doses q4–6h. **Maximum:** 12 g/day. **NEONATES:** 50–140 mg/kg/day in divided doses q6–12h.
IM: ADULTS, ELDERLY: 500 mg q4–6h. **CHILDREN:** 25 mg/kg twice daily.

SIDE EFFECTS

Frequent: Mild hypersensitivity reaction (fever, rash, pruritus), GI effects (nausea, vomiting, diarrhea). **Occasional:** Hypokalemia with high IV dosages, phlebitis, thrombophlebitis (common in elderly). **Rare:** Extravasation with IV administration.

ADVERSE EFFECTS/ TOXIC REACTIONS

Potentially fatal antibiotic-associated colitis, superinfections (abdominal cramps, severe watery diarrhea, fever) may result from altered bacterial balance. Hematologic effects (esp. involving platelets, WBCs), severe hypersensitivity reactions, anaphylaxis occur rarely.

NURSING CONSIDERATIONS

BASELINE ASSESSMENT

Question for history of allergies, esp. penicillins, cephalosporins.

INTERVENTION/EVALUATION

Hold medication, promptly report rash (possible hypersensitivity), diarrhea (fever, abdominal pain, mucus/blood in stool may indicate antibiotic-associated colitis). Evaluate IV site frequently for phlebitis (heat, pain, red streaking over vein), infiltration (potential extravasation). Monitor periodic CBC, urinalysis, serum potassium, renal/hepatic function. Be alert for superinfection: fever, vomiting, diarrhea, anal/genital pruritus, oral mucosal changes (ulceration, pain, erythema). Check hematology reports (esp. WBCs), periodic serum renal/hepatic reports in prolonged therapy.

PATIENT/FAMILY TEACHING

• Continue antibiotic for full length of treatment. • Doses should be evenly spaced. • Discomfort may occur with IM injection. • Report IV discomfort immediately. • Notify physician in event of diarrhea, rash, other new symptoms.

nalbuphine HIGH ALERT

nal-byoo-feen
(Nubain)
Do not confuse Nubain with Navane.

◆CLASSIFICATION

PHARMACOTHERAPEUTIC: Narcotic agonist, antagonist. **CLINICAL:** Opioid analgesic (see p. 142C).

N

ACTION

Binds with opioid receptors within CNS. May displace opioid agonists, competitively inhibiting their action; may precipitate withdrawal symptoms. **Therapeutic Effect:** Alters pain perception, emotional response to pain.

PHARMACOKINETICS

Route	Onset	Peak	Duration
IV	2–3 min	30 min	3–4 hrs
IM	Less than 15 min	60 min	3–6 hrs
Subcutaneous	Less than 15 min	N/A	3–6 hrs

Well absorbed after IM, subcutaneous administration. Metabolized in liver. Primarily eliminated in feces by biliary secretion. **Half-life:** 3.5–5 hrs.

USES

Relief of moderate to severe pain, preop analgesia, obstetric analgesia, adjunct to anesthesia. **OFF-LABEL:** Opioid-induced pruritus.

N

PRECAUTIONS

Contraindications: Hypoventilation (respiratory rate less than 12 breaths/min). **Cautions:** Hepatic/renal impairment, respiratory depression, recent MI, recent biliary tract surgery, head trauma, increased intracranial pressure (ICP), pregnancy, those suspected of being opioid dependent.

LIFESPAN CONSIDERATIONS

Pregnancy/Lactation: Readily crosses placenta. Distributed in breast milk. Breast-feeding not recommended. May cause fetal, neonatal adverse effects during labor/delivery (e.g., fetal bradycardia). **Pregnancy Category B (D if used for prolonged periods or at high dosages at term). Children:** Paradoxical excitement may occur. Those younger than 2 yrs more susceptible to respiratory depression. **Elderly:** More susceptible to respiratory depression. Age-related renal impairment may increase risk of urinary retention.

INTERACTIONS

DRUG: **Alcohol, other CNS depressants** may increase CNS effects, respiratory depression, hypotension. **Buprenorphine** may decrease effects. **MAOIs** may produce a severe, possibly fatal reaction (reduce dose to 25% of usual nalbuphine dose). **HERBAL:** **Gotu kola, kava kava, St. John's wort, valerian** may increase CNS depression. **FOOD:** None known. **LAB VALUES:** May increase serum amylase, lipase.

AVAILABILITY (Rx)

Injection Solution: 10 mg/ml, 20 mg/ml.

ADMINISTRATION/HANDLING

IV

Reconstitution • May give undiluted.
Rate of administration • For IV push, administer each 10 mg over 3–5 min.
Storage • Store parenteral form at room temperature.

IM

• Rotate IM injection sites.

IV INCOMPATIBILITIES

Amphotericin B complex (Abelcet, AmBisome, Amphotec), cefepime (Maxipime), docetaxel (Doxil), ketorolac (Toradol), lipids, methotrexate, nafcillin (Nafcil), piperacillin and tazobactam (Zosyn), sargramostim (Leukine, Prokine), sodium bicarbonate.

IV COMPATIBILITIES

Diphenhydramine (Benadryl), droperidol (Inapsine), glycopyrrolate (Robinul), hydroxyzine (Vistaril), lidocaine, midazolam (Versed), prochlorperazine (Compazine), propofol (Diprivan).

INDICATIONS/ROUTES/DOSAGE

Analgesia

IV, IM, SUBCUTANEOUS: ADULTS, ELDERLY: 10 mg q3–6h as needed. Do not exceed maximum single dose of 20 mg or daily dose of 160 mg. For pts receiving long-term narcotic analgesics of similar duration of action, give 25% of usual dose. **CHILDREN 1 YR AND OLDER:** 0.1–0.2 mg/kg q3–6h as needed. **Maximum:** 20 mg/dose, 160 mg/day.

Supplement to Anesthesia

IV: ADULTS, ELDERLY: Induction: 0.3–3 mg/kg over 10–15 min. Maintenance: 0.25–0.5 mg/kg as needed.

SIDE EFFECTS

Frequent (35%): Sedation. **Occasional (9%–3%):** Diaphoresis, cold/clammy skin, nausea, vomiting, dizziness, vertigo, dry mouth, headache. **Rare (less than 1%):** Restlessness, emotional lability, paresthesia, flushing, paradoxical reaction.

ADVERSE EFFECTS/ TOXIC REACTIONS

Abrupt withdrawal after prolonged use may produce symptoms of narcotic withdrawal (abdominal cramping, rhinorrhea, lacrimation, anxiety, fever, piloerection [goose bumps]). Overdose results in severe respiratory depression, skeletal muscle flaccidity, cyanosis, extreme drowsiness progressing to seizures, stupor, coma. Tolerance to analgesic effect, physical dependence may occur with chronic use.

NURSING CONSIDERATIONS

BASELINE ASSESSMENT

Obtain vital signs before giving medication. If respirations are 12/min or less (20/min or less in children), withhold medication, contact physician. Assess onset, type, location, duration of pain. Effect of medication is reduced if full pain recurs before next dose. Low abuse potential.

INTERVENTION/EVALUATION

Monitor for change in respirations, B/P, rate/quality of pulse. Monitor daily pattern of bowel activity and stool consistency. Initiate deep breathing, coughing exercises, particularly in pts with pulmonary impairment. Assess for clinical improvement, record onset of relief of pain. Consult physician if pain relief is not adequate.

PATIENT/FAMILY TEACHING

• Avoid alcohol. • Avoid tasks that require alertness, motor skills until response to drug is established. • May cause dry mouth. • May be habit forming.

naloxone

nay-**lox**-own
(Narcan)

Do not confuse naloxone with Lanoxin or naltrexone, or Narcan with Marcaine or Norcuron.

FIXED-COMBINATION(S)

Embeda: naloxone/morphine (an opioid agonist): 0.8 mg/20 mg, 1.2 mg/30mg, 2 mg/50 mg, 2.4 mg/60 mg, 3.2 mg/80 mg, 4 mg/100 mg.

◆CLASSIFICATION

PHARMACOTHERAPEUTIC: Narcotic antagonist. **CLINICAL:** Antidote.

ACTION

Displaces opioids at opioid-occupied receptor sites in CNS. **Therapeutic Effect:** Reverses opioid-induced sleep/sedation, increases respiratory rate, raises B/P to normal range.

PHARMACOKINETICS

Route	Onset	Peak	Duration
IV	1–2 min	N/A	20–60 min
IM	2–5 min	N/A	20–60 min
Subcutaneous	2–5 min	N/A	20–60 min

Well absorbed after IM, subcutaneous administration. Metabolized in liver. Primarily excreted in urine. **Half-life:** 60–100 min.

USES

Complete or partial reversal of opioid depression including respiratory depression.

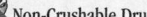

N

Diagnosis of suspected opioid tolerance or acute opioid overdose. Neonatal opiate depression. Coma of unknown origin. **OFF-LABEL:** Treatment of ethanol ingestion, *Pneumocystis jiroveci* pneumonia (PCP), opioid-induced pruritus.

PRECAUTIONS

Contraindications: Respiratory depression due to nonopioid drugs. **Cautions:** Chronic cardiac/pulmonary disease, coronary artery disease. Those suspected of being opioid dependent, postop pts (to avoid cardiovascular changes).

LIFESPAN CONSIDERATIONS

Pregnancy/Lactation: Unknown if drug crosses placenta or is distributed in breast milk. **Pregnancy Category B. Children/Elderly:** No age-related precautions noted.

INTERACTIONS

DRUG: Reverses analgesic properties, side effects, may precipitate withdrawal symptoms of **butorphanol, nalbuphine, opioid agonist analgesics, pentazocine. HERBAL:** None significant. **FOOD:** None known. **LAB VALUES:** None significant.

AVAILABILITY (Rx)

Injection Solution: 0.4 mg/ml, 1 mg/ml.

ADMINISTRATION/HANDLING

IV

Reconstitution • May dilute 1 mg/ml with 50 ml Sterile Water for Injection to provide concentration of 0.02 mg/ml. • For continuous IV infusion, dilute each 2 mg of naloxone with 500 ml of D_5W or 0.9% NaCl, producing solution containing 0.004 mg/ml (4 mcg/ml).
Rate of administration • May administer undiluted. • Give each 0.4 mg as IV push over 30 sec.
Storage • Store parenteral form at room temperature. • Use mixture within 24 hrs; discard unused solution. • Protect from light. Stable in D_5W or 0.9% NaCl at 4 mcg/ml for 24 hrs.

IM

• Give deep IM in large muscle mass.

IV INCOMPATIBILITY

Amphotericin B complex (Abelcet, AmBisome, Amphotec).

IV COMPATIBILITIES

Heparin, ondansetron (Zofran), propofol (Diprivan).

INDICATIONS/ROUTES/DOSAGE

Opioid Toxicity, Respiratory Depression

IV, IM, SUBCUTANEOUS: ADULTS, ELDERLY: 0.4–2 mg q2–3min as needed. May repeat doses q20–60min. **CHILDREN 5 YRS AND OLDER, WEIGHING 20 KG OR MORE:** 2 mg/dose; if no response, may repeat q2–3min. May need to repeat doses q20–60min. **CHILDREN YOUNGER THAN 5 YRS, WEIGHING LESS THAN 20 KG:** 0.1 mg/kg; if no response, repeat q2–3min. May need to repeat doses q20–60min.

Postanesthesia Narcotic Reversal

IV: INFANTS, CHILDREN: 0.01 mg/kg; may repeat q2–3min.

SIDE EFFECTS

None known; little or no pharmacologic effect in absence of narcotics.

ADVERSE EFFECTS/ TOXIC REACTIONS

Too-rapid reversal of narcotic-induced respiratory depression may result in nausea, vomiting, tremors, increased B/P, tachycardia. Excessive dosage in postop pts may produce significant reversal of analgesia, tremors. Hypotension or hypertension, ventricular tachycardia/fibrillation, pulmonary edema may occur in those with cardiovascular disease.

NURSING CONSIDERATIONS

BASELINE ASSESSMENT

Maintain clear airway. Obtain weight of children to calculate drug dosage.

N

INTERVENTION/EVALUATION

Monitor vital signs, esp. rate, depth, rhythm of respiration, during and frequently following administration. Carefully observe pt after satisfactory response (duration of opiate may exceed duration of naloxone, resulting in recurrence of respiratory depression). Assess for increased pain with reversal of opiate.

naltrexone

nal-**trex**-own
(Depade, ReVia, Vivitrol)

BLACK BOX ALERT Can cause hepatic injury in excessive doses.

Do not confuse naltrexone with naloxone, ReVia with Revatio or Revex, or Vivitrol with Vivactil.

◆CLASSIFICATION

PHARMACOTHERAPEUTIC: Opioid receptor antagonist. **CLINICAL:** Ethanol detoxification agent, antidote.

ACTION

Blocks effects of endogenous opioid peptides by competitively binding at opioid receptors. **Therapeutic Effect: Alcohol Deterrent:** Decreases craving, drinking days, relapse rate. **Antidote:** Blocks physical dependence of morphine, heroin, other opioids.

PHARMACOKINETICS

Route	Onset	Peak	Duration
PO	N/A	N/A	24–72 hrs
IM	N/A	2 hrs	2–4 wks

Well absorbed following PO administration. Protein binding: 21%. Metabolized in liver; undergoes first-pass metabolism. Reduction in first-pass hepatic metabolism when given by intramuscular route. Excreted primarily in urine; partial elimination in feces. **Half-life: PO:** 4 hrs; **IM:** 5–10 days.

USES

Vivitrol: Treatment of alcohol dependence in pts able to abstain from alcohol in outpatient setting prior to initiation of treatment. Prevention of relapse to opioid dependence following opioid detoxification. **ReVia:** Blocks effects of exogenously administered opioids. **OFF-LABEL:** Treatment of postconcussional syndrome unresponsive to other treatments; eating disorders, irritable bowel syndrome.

PRECAUTIONS

Contraindications: Opioid dependence, acute opioid withdrawal, failed naloxone challenge, positive urine screen for opioids, acute hepatitis, hepatic failure. **Cautions:** Active hepatic disease. History of suicide attempts, depression.

⌛ LIFESPAN CONSIDERATIONS

Pregnancy/Lactation: Unknown if drug crosses placenta or is distributed in breast milk. **Pregnancy Category C. Children:** Safety and efficacy not established in those younger than 18 yrs. **Elderly:** No age-related precautions noted.

INTERACTIONS

DRUG: Administration to pt physically dependent on **opioid drugs** will precipitate withdrawal syndrome. **HERBAL:** None significant. **FOOD:** None known. **LAB VALUES:** May increase serum transaminase, AST, ALT.

AVAILABILITY (Rx)

Injection Suspension, Extended-Release Kit (Vivitrol): 380 mg/4 ml vial. **Tablets (Depade):** 25 mg, 50 mg, 100 mg. **(ReVia):** 50 mg.

ADMINISTRATION/HANDLING

◀ALERT▶ In those with narcotic dependence, do not attempt treatment until pt has remained opioid free for 7–10 days. Test urine for opioids for verification. Pt should not be experiencing withdrawal symptoms.

N

IM

• Give in deep muscle mass of gluteal region, alternating buttocks. • Vivitrol must be suspended only in diluent supplied in kit.

Storage • Store entire diluent supplied in the kit. • All components (microspheres, diluent, preparation needle, administration needle with safety device) are required for preparation administration. Spare administration needle is provided in case of clogging.

PO

• Administer with food or antacids or after meals.

INDICATIONS/ROUTES/DOSAGE

Adjunct in Treatment of Alcohol Dependence, Prevention of Relapse to Opioid Dependence

IM: ADULTS, ELDERLY: (Vivitrol): 380 mg once every 4 wks or once/mo.

Block Effects of Opioids, Alcohol Dependence

PO: ADULTS, ELDERLY: Initially, 25 mg. Observe pt for 1 hr. If no withdrawal signs appear, give another 25 mg. Maintenance regimen is flexible, variable, and individualized. May be given as 50 mg daily, 100 mg every other day, or 150 mg every 3 days for 12 wks.

SIDE EFFECTS

Common: IM: (69%): Injection site reaction (induration, tenderness, pain, nodules, swelling, pruritus, ecchymosis). **Frequent: Alcohol Deterrent: (33%–10%):** Nausea, headache, depression. **Narcotic Addiction (10%–5%):** Insomnia, anxiety, headache, low energy, abdominal cramps, nausea, vomiting, joint/muscle pain. **Occasional: Alcohol Deterrent (4%–2%):** Dizziness, anxiety, fatigue, insomnia, vomiting, suicidal ideation. **Narcotic Addiction (5% or less):** Irritability, increased energy, dizziness, anorexia, diarrhea, constipation, rash, chills, increased thirst.

ADVERSE EFFECTS/ TOXIC REACTIONS

Signs/symptoms of opioid withdrawal include stuffy/runny nose, tearing, yawning, diaphoresis, tremor, vomiting, piloerection (goose bumps), feeling of temperature change, arthralgia, myalgia, abdominal cramps, formication (feeling of skin crawling). Accidental naltrexone overdosage produces withdrawal symptoms within 5 min of ingestion, lasts up to 48 hrs. Symptoms present as confusion, visual hallucinations, drowsiness, significant vomiting, diarrhea. Hepatotoxicity may occur with large doses.

NURSING CONSIDERATIONS

BASELINE ASSESSMENT

Treatment with naltrexone should not be instituted unless pt is opioid free for 7–10 days, alcohol free for 3–5 days before therapy begins. Obtain medication history (esp. opioids), other medical conditions (esp. hepatitis, other hepatic disease). If there is any question of opioid dependence, a naloxone challenge test (see Indications/Routes/Dosage) should be performed.

INTERVENTION/EVALUATION

Monitor closely for evidence of hepatotoxicity (abdominal pain that lasts longer than a few days, white bowel movements, dark urine, jaundice). Monitor serum AST, ALT, bilirubin.

PATIENT/FAMILY TEACHING

• If heroin, other opiates are self-administered, there will be no effect. However, any attempt to overcome naltrexone's prolonged 24- to 72-hr blockade of opioid effect by taking large amounts of opioids is dangerous and may result in coma, serious injury, fatal overdose. • Naltrexone blocks effects of opioid-containing medicine (cough/cold preparations, antidiarrheal preparations, opioid analgesics). • Contact physician if abdominal pain lasting longer than 3 days, white bowel movement, dark-colored urine, yellow eyes occur.

Namenda, *see memantine*

Naprosyn, *see naproxen*

naproxen

na-**prox**-en
(Aleve, Anaprox, Anaprox DS, Apo-Naproxen ✤, EC-Naprosyn, Naprelan, Naprosyn, Novo-Naprox ✤, Nu-Naprox ✤, Pamprin)

BLACK BOX ALERT Increased risk of serious cardiovascular thrombotic events, including myocardial infarction, CVA. Increased risk of severe GI reactions, including ulceration, bleeding, perforation of stomach, intestines.

Do not confuse Aleve with Allese, or Anaprox with Anaspaz or Avapro.

FIXED-COMBINATION(S)

Prevacid NapraPac: naproxen/lansoprazole (proton pump inhibitor): 375 mg/15 mg, 500 mg/15 mg.
Treximet: naproxen/sumatriptan (an antimigraine): 500 mg/85mg.
Vimovo: naproxen/esomeprazole (proton pump inhibitor): 375 mg/20 mg, 500 mg/20 mg.

◆CLASSIFICATION

PHARMACOTHERAPEUTIC: Nonsteroidal anti-inflammatory. **CLINICAL:** Analgesic, anti-inflammatory (see p. 129C).

ACTION

Produces analgesic, anti-inflammatory effects by inhibiting prostaglandin synthesis. **Therapeutic Effect:** Reduces inflammatory response, intensity of pain.

PHARMACOKINETICS

Route	Onset	Peak	Duration
PO (analgesic)	1 hr	2–4 hrs	7 hrs or less
PO (anti-inflammatory)	2 wks	2–4 wks	12 hrs

Completely absorbed from GI tract. Protein binding: 99%. Metabolized in liver. Primarily excreted in urine. Not removed by hemodialysis. **Half-life:** 13 hrs.

USES

Treatment of acute or long-term mild to moderate pain, primary dysmenorrhea, rheumatoid arthritis (RA), juvenile rheumatoid arthritis (JRA), osteoarthritis, ankylosing spondylitis, acute gouty arthritis, bursitis, tendinitis. **OFF-LABEL:** Treatment of vascular headaches.

PRECAUTIONS

Contraindications: Hypersensitivity to aspirin, naproxen, other NSAIDs. **Cautions:** GI/cardiac disease, renal/hepatic impairment. Concurrent use of anticoagulants.

⌛ LIFESPAN CONSIDERATIONS

Pregnancy/Lactation: Crosses placenta. Distributed in breast milk. Avoid use during third trimester (may adversely affect fetal cardiovascular system: premature closing of ductus arteriosus). **Pregnancy Category C (D if used in third trimester or near delivery). Children:** Safety and efficacy not established in those younger than 2 yrs. Children older than 2 yrs at increased risk for skin rash. **Elderly:** Age-related renal impairment may increase risk of hepatic/renal toxicity; reduced dosage recommended. More likely to have serious adverse effects with GI bleeding/ulceration.

INTERACTIONS

DRUG: May decrease effects of **antihypertensives, diuretics. Aspirin, other salicylates** may increase risk of GI side effects, bleeding. **Bone marrow depressants** may increase risk of hematologic reactions. May increase effects of **heparin, oral anticoagulants, thrombolytics.** May increase concentration, risk of toxicity of **lithium.** May increase risk of **methotrexate** toxicity. **Probenecid** may increase concentration. HERBAL: **Cat's claw, dong quai, evening primrose, feverfew, garlic, ginger, ginkgo, ginseng, horse chestnut, red clover** possess antiplatelet activity, may increase risk of bleeding. FOOD: None known. LAB VALUES: May prolong bleeding time. May increase ALT, AST, alkaline phosphatase, BUN, creatinine. May decrease Hgb, Hct, leukocytes, platelets, uric acid.

AVAILABILITY (Rx)

Gelcaps (Aleve [OTC]): 220 mg naproxen sodium (equivalent to 200 mg naproxen). **Oral Suspension (Naprosyn):** 125 mg/5 ml naproxen. **Tablets:** 220 mg naproxen sodium (equivalent to 200 mg naproxen) (Aleve [OTC]), 250 mg (Naprosyn), 275 mg naproxen sodium (equivalent to 250 mg naproxen) (Anaprox), 550 mg naproxen sodium (equivalent to 500 mg naproxen) (Anaprox DS).

Tablets (Controlled-Release): 375 mg naproxen (EC-Naprosyn), 421 mg naproxen sodium (equivalent to 375 mg naproxen) (Naprelan), 500 mg naproxen (EC-Naprosyn), 550 mg naproxen sodium (equivalent to 500 mg naproxen) (Naprelan).

ADMINISTRATION/HANDLING

PO

• Swallow controlled-release form whole. Do not break, crush, chew. • Scored tablets may be broken/crushed. • Best taken with food or milk (decreases GI irritation). • Shake suspension well.

INDICATIONS/ROUTES/DOSAGE

Rheumatoid Arthritis (RA), Osteoarthritis, Ankylosing Spondylitis

PO: ADULTS, ELDERLY: 500–1,000 mg/day in 2 divided doses.

Acute Gouty Arthritis

PO: ADULTS, ELDERLY: Initially, 750 mg naproxen (825 mg naproxen sodium), then 250 mg naproxen (275 mg naproxen sodium) q8h until attack subsides. **Naprelan:** Initially, 1,000–1,500 mg, then 1,000 mg once daily until attack subsides.

Mild to Moderate Pain, Dysmenorrhea, Bursitis, Tendinitis

PO: ADULTS, ELDERLY: Initially, 500 mg naproxen (550 mg naproxen sodium), then 250 mg naproxen (275 mg naproxen sodium) q6–8h as needed. **Maximum:** 1.25 g/day naproxen (1.375 g/day naproxen sodium). **Naprelan:** 1,000 mg once daily.

Juvenile Rheumatoid Arthritis (JRA)

PO (NAPROXEN ONLY): CHILDREN OLDER THAN 2 YRS: 10 mg/kg/day in 2 divided doses. **Maximum:** 1,000 mg/day.

OTC Uses

PO: ADULTS 65 YRS AND YOUNGER, CHILDREN 12 YRS AND OLDER: 220 mg (200 mg naproxen sodium) q8–12h. May take 440 mg (200 mg naproxen sodium) as initial dose. **ADULTS OLDER THAN 65 YRS:** 220 mg (200 mg naproxen sodium) q12h.

SIDE EFFECTS

Frequent (9%–4%): Nausea, constipation, abdominal cramps/pain, heartburn, dizziness, headache, drowsiness. **Occasional (3%–1%):** Stomatitis, diarrhea, indigestion. **Rare (less than 1%):** Vomiting, confusion.

ADVERSE EFFECTS/ TOXIC REACTIONS

Rare reactions with long-term use include peptic ulcer, GI bleeding, gastritis, severe hepatic reactions (cholestasis, jaundice), nephrotoxicity (dysuria, hematuria, proteinuria, nephrotic syndrome), and severe hypersensitivity reaction (fever, chills, bronchospasm).

NURSING CONSIDERATIONS

BASELINE ASSESSMENT

Assess onset, type, location, duration of pain/inflammation. Inspect appearance of affected joints for immobility, deformities, skin condition.

INTERVENTION/EVALUATION

Assist with ambulation if dizziness occurs. Monitor CBC, platelet count, serum renal/hepatic function tests, Hgb, daily pattern of bowel activity and stool consistency. Evaluate for therapeutic response: relief of pain, stiffness, swelling; increased joint mobility; reduced joint tenderness; improved grip strength.

PATIENT/FAMILY TEACHING

• Avoid tasks that require alertness, motor skills until response to drug is established. • Take with food, milk. • Avoid aspirin, alcohol during therapy (increases risk of GI bleeding). • Report headache, rash, visual disturbances, weight gain, black or tarry stools, bleeding, persistent headache.

naratriptan

nar-a-**trip**-tan
(Amerge)
Do not confuse Amerge with Altace or Amaryl.

◆CLASSIFICATION

PHARMACOTHERAPEUTIC: Serotonin receptor agonist. **CLINICAL:** Antimigraine (see p. 63C).

ACTION

Binds selectively to vascular receptors, producing vasoconstrictive effect on cranial blood vessels. **Therapeutic Effect:** Relieves migraine headache.

PHARMACOKINETICS

Well absorbed after PO administration. Protein binding: 28%–31%. Metabolized by liver to inactive metabolite. Eliminated primarily in urine and, to lesser extent, in feces. **Half-life:** 6 hrs (increased in hepatic/renal impairment).

USES

Treatment of acute migraine headache with or without aura in adults.

PRECAUTIONS

Contraindications: Basilar/hemiplegic migraine, cerebrovascular, peripheral vascular disease, coronary artery disease, ischemic heart disease (including angina pectoris, history of MI, silent ischemia, Prinzmetal's angina), severe hepatic impairment (Child-Pugh grade C), severe renal impairment (serum creatinine less than 15 ml/min), uncontrolled hypertension, use within 24 hrs of ergotamine-containing preparations or another serotonin receptor agonist, MAOI use within 14 days. **Cautions:** Mild to moderate renal/hepatic impairment, pt profile suggesting cardiovascular risks.

⌛ LIFESPAN CONSIDERATIONS

Pregnancy/Lactation: Unknown if drug is distributed in breast milk. **Pregnancy Category C. Children:** Safety and efficacy not established. **Elderly:** Not recommended in the elderly.

INTERACTIONS

DRUG: Ergotamine-containing medications may produce vasospastic reaction. **Fluoxetine, fluvoxamine, paroxetine, sertraline** may produce hyperreflexia, incoordination, weakness. **Oral contraceptives** decrease naratriptan clearance, volume of distribution. **HERBAL:** None significant. **FOOD:** None known. **LAB VALUES:** None significant.

AVAILABILITY (Rx)

Tablets: 1 mg, 2.5 mg.

ADMINISTRATION/HANDLING

PO

• Give without regard to food. • Do not crush, chew tablets.

N

INDICATIONS/ROUTES/DOSAGE

Acute Migraine Attack

PO: ADULTS: 1 or 2.5 mg. If headache improves but then returns, dose may be repeated after 4 hrs. **Maximum:** 5 mg/24 hrs.

Dosage in Renal/Hepatic Impairment

Hepatic Failure	Creatinine Clearance	Dosage
Mild to moderate	15–39 ml/min	Initial, 1 mg. Max: 2.5/24 hrs
Severe	Less than 15 ml/min	Do not use

SIDE EFFECTS

Occasional (5%): Nausea. **Rare** (2%): Paresthesia, dizziness, fatigue, drowsiness, feeling of pressure in throat, neck, jaw.

ADVERSE EFFECTS/ TOXIC REACTIONS

Corneal opacities, other ocular defects may occur. Cardiac events (ischemia, coronary artery vasospasm, MI), noncardiac vasospasm-related reactions (hemorrhage, cerebrovascular accident [CVA]) occur rarely, particularly in pts with hypertension, diabetes, strong family history of coronary artery disease, obese pts, smokers, males older than 40 yrs, postmenopausal women.

NURSING CONSIDERATIONS

BASELINE ASSESSMENT

Question for history of peripheral vascular disease, renal/hepatic impairment, possibility of pregnancy. Question pt regarding possible precipitating symptoms, onset, location, duration of migraine.

INTERVENTION/EVALUATION

Assess for relief of migraine headache; potential for photophobia, phonophobia (sound sensitivity), nausea, vomiting.

PATIENT/FAMILY TEACHING

• Do not crush, chew tablet; swallow whole with water. • May repeat dose after 4 hrs (maximum of 5 mg/24 hrs). • May cause dizziness, fatigue, drowsiness. • Avoid tasks that require alertness, motor skills until response to drug is established. • Inform physician of any chest pain, palpitations, tightness in throat, rash, hallucinations, anxiety, panic.

Narcan, *see naloxone*

Nasacort AQ, *see triamcinolone*

Nasonex, *see mometasone*

natalizumab

na-tah-**liz**-oo-mab
(Tysabri)

BLACK BOX ALERT Restricted distribution program (TOUCH), given only to program-qualified/enrolled pts. Increased risk of leukoencephalopathy (progressive, often fatal viral brain infection).

◆CLASSIFICATION

PHARMACOTHERAPEUTIC: Monoclonal antibody. **CLINICAL:** Multiple sclerosis agent.

ACTION

Binds to surface of leukocytes, inhibiting adhesion of leukocytes to vascular endothelial cells of GI tract, preventing migration of leukocytes across endothelium into inflamed parenchymal tissue. **Therapeutic Effect:** Inhibits inflammatory activity of activated immune cells, reduces clinical exacerbations of multiple sclerosis.

PHARMACOKINETICS

Half-life: 11 days.

USES

Treatment of relapsing forms of multiple sclerosis to reduce frequency of clinical exacerbations. Treatment of moderate to severe Crohn's disease.

PRECAUTIONS

Contraindications: None known. **Cautions:** Chronic progressive multiple sclerosis, children younger than 18 yrs. Concomitant immunosuppressants (may increase risk of infection).

LIFESPAN CONSIDERATIONS

Pregnancy/Lactation: Unknown if drug crosses placenta or is distributed in breast milk. **Pregnancy Category C. Children:** Safety and efficacy not established in those younger than 18 yrs. **Elderly:** No age-related precautions noted.

INTERACTIONS

DRUG: Antineoplastics, immunomodulating agents, immunosuppresants may increase risk of infection. **HERBAL:** None significant. **FOOD:** None known. **LAB VALUES:** Increases lymphocytes, monocytes, eosinophils, basophils, red blood cells, usually reversible within 16 wks after last dose.

AVAILABILITY (Rx)

Injection Solution: 300 mg/15 ml concentrate.

ADMINISTRATION/HANDLING

IV

Reconstitution • Withdraw 15 ml natalizumab from vial; inject concentrate into 100 ml 0.9% NaCl. • Invert solution to mix completely; do not shake. • Discard if solution is discolored or particulate forms.

Rate of administration • Infuse over 1 hr. • Following completion of infusion, flush with 0.9% NaCl.

Storage • Refrigerate vials. • Do not shake, freeze. Protect from light. • After reconstitution, solution is stable for 8 hrs if refrigerated.

IV INCOMPATIBILITIES

Do not mix with any other medications or diluent other than 0.9% NaCl.

INDICATIONS/ROUTES/DOSAGE

Relapsed Multiple Sclerosis, Crohn's Disease

IV INFUSION: ADULTS 18 YRS AND OLDER, ELDERLY: 300 mg every 4 wks.

SIDE EFFECTS

Frequent (35%–15%): Headache, fatigue, depression, arthralgia. **Occasional (10%–5%):** Abdominal discomfort, rash, urinary urgency/frequency, irregular menstruation/dysmenorrhea, dermatitis. **Rare (4%–2%):** Pruritus, chest discomfort, local bleeding, rigors, tremor, syncope.

ADVERSE EFFECTS/ TOXIC REACTIONS

UTI, lower respiratory tract infection, gastroenteritis, vaginitis, allergic reaction, tonsillitis occur occasionally.

NURSING CONSIDERATIONS

BASELINE ASSESSMENT

Obtain CBC, serum chemistries including hepatic enzyme levels. Assess home situation for support of therapy.

INTERVENTION/EVALUATION

Periodically monitor lab results and reevaluate injection technique. Assess for arthralgia, depression, urinary changes, menstrual irregularities. Assess skin for evidence of rash, pruritus, dermatitis. Monitor for signs/symptoms of UTI, respiratory infection.

nateglinide HIGH ALERT

nah-**teh**-glih-nide
(Starlix)

CLASSIFICATION

PHARMACOTHERAPEUTIC: Antihyperglycemic. **CLINICAL:** Antidiabetic.

N

ACTION

Stimulates insulin release from beta cells of pancreas by depolarizing beta cells, leading to opening of calcium channels. Resulting calcium influx induces insulin secretion. **Therapeutic Effect:** Lowers serum glucose concentration.

PHARMACOKINETICS

Route	Onset	Peak	Duration
PO	20 min	1 hr	4 hrs

Rapidly absorbed from GI tract. Protein binding: 98%, primarily to albumin. Extensive metabolism in liver. Primarily excreted in urine; minimal elimination in feces. **Half-life:** 1.5 hrs.

USES

Treatment of type 2 diabetes mellitus in pts whose disease cannot be adequately controlled with diet and exercise and in pts who have not been chronically treated with other antidiabetic agents. Used as monotherapy or in combination with other drugs.

PRECAUTIONS

Contraindications: Diabetic ketoacidosis, type 1 diabetes mellitus. **Cautions:** Hepatic/renal impairment.

LIFESPAN CONSIDERATIONS

Pregnancy/Lactation: Unknown if drug crosses placenta or is distributed in breast milk. **Pregnancy Category C. Children:** Safety and efficacy not established. **Elderly:** Increased susceptibility to hypoglycemia.

INTERACTIONS

DRUG: **Beta-blockers** may mask symptoms of hypoglycemia. **Beta-blockers, MAOIs, NSAIDs, salicylates** may increase hypoglycemic effect. **Corticosteroids, sympathomimetics, thiazide diuretics, thyroid medications** may decrease hypoglycemic effect. **HERBAL:** **Bilberry, garlic, ginger, ginseng** may increase hypoglycemic effect. **FOOD:** None known. **LAB VALUES:** None significant.

AVAILABILITY (Rx)

Tablets: 60 mg, 120 mg.

ADMINISTRATION/HANDLING

PO

- Ideally, give within 15 min of a meal, but may be given immediately before a meal to as long as 30 min before a meal.

INDICATIONS/ROUTES/DOSAGE

Diabetes Mellitus

PO: ADULTS, ELDERLY: 120 mg 3 times a day before meals. 60 mg 3 times a day may be given in pts close to HbA_{1C} goal.

SIDE EFFECTS

Frequent (10%): Upper respiratory tract infection. **Occasional (4%–3%):** Back pain, flu symptoms, dizziness, arthropathy, diarrhea. **Rare (2% or less):** Bronchitis, cough.

ADVERSE EFFECTS/ TOXIC REACTIONS

Hypoglycemia occurs in less than 2% of pts.

NURSING CONSIDERATIONS

BASELINE ASSESSMENT

Check fasting serum glucose, glycosylated Hgb (HbA_{1C}) periodically to determine minimum effective dose. Discuss lifestyle to determine extent of learning, emotional needs. Ensure follow-up instruction if pt, family do not thoroughly understand diabetes management, glucose-testing technique. At least 1 wk should elapse to assess response to drug before new dose adjustment is made.

INTERVENTION/EVALUATION

Monitor serum glucose, food intake. Assess for hypoglycemia (cool, wet skin, tremors, dizziness, anxiety, headache, tachycardia, numbness in mouth, hunger, diplopia), hyperglycemia (polyuria, polyphagia, polydipsia, nausea, vomiting, dim vision, fatigue, deep rapid breathing). Be alert to conditions that alter glucose requirements: fever, increased activity, stress, surgical procedures.

PATIENT/FAMILY TEACHING

• Diabetes mellitus requires lifelong control. • Prescribed diet, exercise are principal parts of treatment; do not skip, delay meals. • Continue to adhere to dietary instructions, regular exercise program, regular testing of serum glucose.

Natrecor, *see nesiritide*

nebivolol

neh-**biv**-oh-lol
(Bystolic)

◆CLASSIFICATION

PHARMACOTHERAPEUTIC: Beta-adrenergic blocker. **CLINICAL:** Antihypertensive.

ACTION

Predominantly blocks $beta_1$-adrenergic receptors. Large doses block both $beta_1$ and $beta_2$ receptors. **Therapeutic Effect:** Slows sinus heart rate, decreases myocardial contractility, B/P.

PHARMACOKINETICS

	Onset	Peak	Duration
PO	30 min	1.5–4 hrs	12 hrs

Completely absorbed from GI tract. Protein binding: 98%. Metabolized in liver. Primarily excreted unchanged in feces (44%), with lesser amount eliminated in urine (38%). **Half-life:** 12 hrs (increased in severe renal impairment).

USES

Management of hypertension. Used alone or in combination with other antihypertensives. **OFF-LABEL:** Heart failure.

PRECAUTIONS

Contraindications: Severe bradycardia, overt cardiac failure, cardiogenic shock, heart block greater than first degree, severe hepatic impairment. **Cautions:** Renal/hepatic impairment, peripheral vascular disease, hyperthyroidism, diabetes mellitus, inadequate cardiac function.

LIFESPAN CONSIDERATIONS

Pregnancy/Lactation: May cross placenta; appears to be distributed in breast milk. May produce small birth weight infants. **Pregnancy Category C (D in second or third trimester). Children:** Safety and efficacy not established. **Elderly:** No age-related precautions noted.

INTERACTIONS

DRUG: Diuretics, other hypotensives may increase hypotensive effect. **Sympathomimetics, xanthines** may mutually inhibit effect. May mask symptoms of hypoglycemia, prolong hypoglycemic effect of **insulin, oral hypoglycemics. NSAIDs** may decrease antihypertensive effect. **Cimetidine** may increase concentration. **HERBAL: Ephedra, ginseng, yohimbe** may worsen hypertension. **Garlic** may increase antihypertensive effect. **FOOD:** None known. **LAB VALUES:** May increase BUN, serum uric acid, AST, ALT, bilirubin, triclycerides. May decrease platelet count, serum HDL.

AVAILABILITY (Rx)

Tablets: 2.5 mg, 5 mg, 10 mg.

ADMINISTRATION/HANDLING

PO

• Give without regard to meals. • Do not crush, split, chew tablets.

INDICATIONS/ROUTES/DOSAGE

Hypertension

PO: ADULTS, ELDERLY: Initially, 5 mg once a day alone or in combination with other antihypertensives. May increase at 2-wk intervals to maximum 40 mg once a day.

Severe Renal Impairment (Creatinine Clearance Less Than 30 ml/min)

PO: ADULTS, ELDERLY: Initially, 2.5 mg once a day.

N

Moderate Hepatic Impairment
PO: ADULTS, ELDERLY: Initially, 2.5 mg once a day.

SIDE EFFECTS

Generally well tolerated, with mild and transient side effects. **Occasional (9%):** Headache. **Rare (2%–1%):** Fatigue, dizziness, diarrhea, nausea, insomnia, peripheral edema.

ADVERSE EFFECTS/ TOXIC REACTIONS

Large doses may produce bradycardia, dyspnea, rash. Acute pulmonary edema, renal failure, AV block reported. **Antidote:** Glucagon (see Appendix M for dosage).

NURSING CONSIDERATIONS

BASELINE ASSESSMENT

Assess baseline renal/hepatic function tests. Assess B/P, apical pulse immediately before drug administration (if pulse is 60/min or less, or systolic B/P is less than 90 mm Hg, withhold medication, contact physician).

INTERVENTION/EVALUATION

Measure B/P near end of dosing interval (determines whether B/P is controlled throughout day). Monitor B/P for hypotension. Assess pulse for quality, irregular rate, bradycardia. Question for evidence of headache.

PATIENT/FAMILY TEACHING

• Compliance with therapy regimen is essential to control hypertension. • Do not use nasal decongestants, OTC cold preparations (stimulants) without physician's approval. • Monitor B/P, pulse before taking medication. • Restrict salt, alcohol intake.

nelarabine

HIGH ALERT

nel-**ar**-a-bean
(Arranon, Atriance)

BLACK BOX ALERT Dose-limiting neurotoxicity (confusion, severe drowsiness, seizures, ataxia, ascending neuropathy). Must be administered by certified chemotherapy personnel.

CLASSIFICATION

PHARMACOTHERAPEUTIC: DNA demethylation agent. **CLINICAL:** Antineoplastic; antimetabolite.

ACTION

Incorporates into DNA, leading to inhibition of DNA synthesis. Exerts cytotoxic effect on rapidly dividing cells by causing demethylation of DNA. **Therapeutic Effect:** Produces cell death.

PHARMACOKINETICS

Rapidly eliminated from plasma. Extensive distribution. Protein binding: Less than 25%. Partially eliminated in urine. **Half-life:** 30 min.

USES

Treatment of T-cell acute lymphoblastic leukemia, T-cell lymphoblastic lymphoma in pts whose disease has not responded to or has relapsed following treatment with at least two chemotherapy regimens. **OFF-LABEL:** Chronic myelocytic leukemia (CML) T-cell blast phase.

PRECAUTIONS

Contraindications: None known. **Cautions:** Previous or current intrathecal chemotherapy, craniospinal radiation therapy, hepatic disease, renal impairment.

LIFESPAN CONSIDERATIONS

Pregnancy/Lactation: May cause developmental abnormalities of the fetus. Breast-feeding not recommended. **Pregnancy Category D. Children:** No age-related precautions noted. **Elderly:** Increased risk of neurologic toxicities.

INTERACTIONS

DRUG: Live virus vaccines may potentiate virus replication, increase vaccine side effects, decrease pt's antibody response to vaccine. **HERBAL:** None significant. **FOOD:** None known. **LAB VALUES:** May decrease Hgb, Hct, WBCs, RBCs, platelets, serum albumin, calcium, glucose, magnesium, potassium. May increase serum bilirubin, transaminase, creatinine, AST.

AVAILABILITY (Rx)

Injection Solution: 250 mg (5 mg/ml) in 50-ml vials (Arranon).

ADMINISTRATION/HANDLING

IV

Reconstitution • Do not dilute before administration. • Transfer appropriate dose into polyvinylchloride infusion bag or glass container before administration.
Rate of administration • Administer as 2-hr infusion for adults, 1-hr infusion for pediatric pts.
Storage • Store vials at room temperature. • Solution should appear colorless, free of precipitate.

INDICATIONS/ROUTES/DOSAGE

T-Cell Leukemia, Lymphoma
IV: ADULTS, ELDERLY: 1,500 mg/m^2 infused over 2 hrs on days 1, 3, and 5 repeated q21days. **CHILDREN:** 650 mg/m^2 infused over 1 hr daily for 5 consecutive days repeated q21days.

SIDE EFFECTS

ADULTS
Frequent (50%–41%): Fatigue, nausea. **Occasional (25%–11%):** Cough, fever, drowsiness, vomiting, dyspnea, diarrhea, constipation, dizziness, asthenia (loss of strength, energy), peripheral edema, paresthesia, headache, peripheral neuropathy, myalgia, petechiae, generalized edema. **Rare (9%–4%):** Anorexia, abdominal pain, arthralgia, hypertension, tachycardia, confusion, rigors, stomatitis, back pain, epistaxis, insomnia, dehydration, extremity pain, depression, abdominal distention, blurred vision.
CHILDREN
Frequent (17%): Headache. **Occasional (10%–6%):** Vomiting, drowsiness, asthenia (loss of strength, energy), peripheral neuropathy. **Rare (4%–2%):** Paresthesia, tremor, ataxia.

ADVERSE EFFECTS/ TOXIC REACTIONS

Overdose may result in severe neurotoxicity, myelosuppression. Hematologic toxicity manifested as thrombocytopenia, neutropenia, anemia occurs in most cases. Pleural effusion occurs in 10% of pts, pneumonia in 8% of pts, seizures in 6% of pts.

NURSING CONSIDERATIONS

BASELINE ASSESSMENT

Give emotional support to pt, family. Use strict asepsis, protect pt from infection. Hydration, urine alkalization, prophylaxis with allopurinol must be given to prevent hyperuricemia of tumor lysis syndrome. Perform blood counts as needed to monitor response and toxicity but esp. before each dosing cycle.

INTERVENTION/EVALUATION

Monitor for neurologic toxicity (severe drowsiness, confusion, seizure), hematologic toxicity (fever, sore throat, signs of local infections, unusual bruising/bleeding), symptoms of anemia (excessive fatigue, weakness). Assess response to medication; monitor and report nausea, vomiting, diarrhea. Avoid rectal temperatures, other traumas that may induce bleeding. Monitor renal/hepatic function.

PATIENT/FAMILY TEACHING

• Do not have immunizations without physician's approval (drug lowers resistance). • Avoid crowds, persons with known infections. • Report signs of infection at once (fever, flu-like symptoms). • Contact physician if nausea/vomiting continues at home. • Advise men to use barrier contraception while receiving treatment. • Measures should be taken to avoid pregnancy. • Contact physician if new or worsening symptoms of peripheral neuropathy occur.

nelfinavir

nel-**fin**-ah-veer
(Viracept)
Do not confuse nelfinavir with nevirapine, or Viracept with Viramune.

◆ CLASSIFICATION

PHARMACOTHERAPEUTIC: Protease inhibitor. **CLINICAL:** Antiviral (see pp. 69C, 117C).

ACTION

Inhibits activity of HIV-1 protease, the enzyme necessary for formation of infectious HIV. **Therapeutic Effect:** Formation of immature noninfectious viral particles rather than HIV replication.

PHARMACOKINETICS

Well absorbed after PO administration (absorption increased with food). Protein binding: 98%. Metabolized in liver. Highly bound to plasma proteins. Eliminated primarily in feces. Unknown if removed by hemodialysis. **Half-life:** 3.5–5 hrs.

USES

Treatment of HIV infection in combination with other antiretrovirals. **OFF-LABEL:** HIV, postexposure prophylaxis.

PRECAUTIONS

Contraindications: Concurrent administration with amiodarone, midazolam, rifampin, triazolam. **Cautions:** Hepatic impairment.

LIFESPAN CONSIDERATIONS

Pregnancy/Lactation: Unknown if distributed in breast milk. **Pregnancy Category B. Children:** No age-related precautions noted in those older than 2 yrs. **Elderly:** No information available.

INTERACTIONS

DRUG: **Anticonvulsants, rifabutin, rifampin** decrease concentration. Increases concentration of **fluticasone, immunosuppressants (e.g., cyclosporine, sirolimus, tacrolimus), indinavir, saquinavir, trazodone.** Decreases effects of **oral contraceptives. Ritonavir** increases concentration. **Lovastatin, simvastatin** may increase risk of adverse effects. **HERBAL:** **St. John's wort** may decrease concentration/effects. **FOOD:** **All foods** increase concentration. **LAB VALUES:** May decrease neutrophil, WBC counts.

AVAILABILITY (Rx)

Powder for Oral Suspension: 50 mg/g. **Tablets:** 250 mg, 625 mg.

ADMINISTRATION/HANDLING

PO

• Give with food (light meal, snack). • Tablets can be dissolved in water then mixed with milk or crushed and mixed with pudding. • Mix oral powder with small amount of water, milk, formula, soy formula, soy milk, dietary supplement. • Entire contents must be consumed in order to ingest full dose. • Do not mix with acidic food, orange juice, apple juice, applesauce (bitter taste), or with water in original oral powder container.

INDICATIONS/ROUTES/DOSAGE

HIV Infection

PO: ADULTS: 750 mg (three 250-mg tablets) 3 times a day or 1,250 mg twice a day in combination with other antiretrovirals. **CHILDREN 2–13 YRS:** 45–55 mg/kg twice a day or 25–35 mg/kg 3 times a day. **Maximum:** 2,500 mg/day.

SIDE EFFECTS

Frequent (20%): Diarrhea. **Occasional (7%–3%):** Nausea, rash. **Rare (2%–1%):** Flatulence, asthenia (loss of strength, energy).

ADVERSE EFFECTS/ TOXIC REACTIONS

Diabetes mellitus, hyperglycemia occur rarely.

NURSING CONSIDERATIONS

BASELINE ASSESSMENT

Check hematology, hepatic function tests for accurate baseline.

INTERVENTION/EVALUATION

Monitor daily pattern of bowel activity, stool consistency. Monitor hepatic enzyme studies for abnormalities. Be alert to development of opportunistic infections (fever, chills, cough, myalgia).

PATIENT/FAMILY TEACHING

• Take with food (optimizes absorption). • Take medication every day as prescribed. • Doses should be evenly spaced around the clock. • Do not alter dose, discontinue medication without informing physician. • Nelfinavir is not a cure for HIV infection nor does it reduce risk of transmission to others. • Illnesses, including opportunistic infections, may still occur.

neostigmine

nee-oh-**stig**-meen
(Prostigmin)
Do not confuse neostigmine or Prostigmin with physostigmine.

◆ CLASSIFICATION

PHARMACOTHERAPEUTIC: Cholinergic. **CLINICAL:** Antimyasthenic, antidote (see p. 91C).

ACTION

Prevents destruction of acetylcholine by attaching to enzyme acetylcholinesterase, enhancing impulse transmission across myoneural junction. **Therapeutic Effect:** Improves intestinal/skeletal muscle tone; stimulates salivary, sweat gland secretions.

USES

Improvement of muscle strength in control of myasthenia gravis, diagnosis of myasthenia gravis, prevention/treatment of postop bladder distention, urinary retention, antidote for reversal of effects of nondepolarizing neuromuscular blocking agents after surgery.

PRECAUTIONS

Contraindications: GI/GU obstruction, history of hypersensitivity reaction to bromides, peritonitis. **Cautions:** Epilepsy, asthma, bradycardia, hyperthyroidism, arrhythmias, peptic ulcer, recent coronary occlusion. **Pregnancy Category C.**

INTERACTIONS

DRUG: Anticholinergics reverse, prevent effects. **Cholinesterase inhibitors** may increase risk of toxicity. Antagonizes effects of **neuromuscular blockers. Procainamide, quinidine** may antagonize action. **HERBAL:** None significant. **FOOD:** None known. **LAB VALUES:** None significant.

AVAILABILITY (Rx)

Injection Solution (Prostigmin): 0.5 mg/ml, 1 mg/ml. **Tablets (Prostigmin):** 15 mg.

ADMINISTRATION/HANDLING

◀ALERT▶ Discontinue all anticholinesterase therapy at least 8 hrs prior to testing for diagnosis of myasthenia gravis. Give 0.011 mg/kg atropine sulfate IV simultaneously with neostigmine or IM 30 min before administering neostigmine to prevent adverse effects.

PO

• May administer with or without food.

IV COMPATIBILITIES

Glycopyrrolate (Robinul), heparin, ondansetron (Zofran), potassium chloride, thiopental (Pentothal).

INDICATIONS/ROUTES/DOSAGE

Myasthenia Gravis

PO: ADULTS, ELDERLY: Initially, 15–30 mg 3–4 times a day. Increase as necessary. Maintenance: 150 mg/day (range of 15–375 mg). **CHILDREN:** 2 mg/kg/day or 60 mg/m^2/day divided q3–4h.

N

IV, IM, SUBCUTANEOUS: ADULTS: 0.5–2.5 mg q1–3h up to 10 mg/24 hrs. **CHILDREN:** 0.01–0.04 mg/kg q2–4h.

Diagnosis of Myasthenia Gravis

◀ALERT▶ Discontinue all cholinesterase medications at least 8 hrs before, atropine should be given IV immediately before or IM 30 min before neostigmine.

IM: ADULTS, ELDERLY: 0.02 mg/kg as single dose. **CHILDREN:** 0.025–0.04 mg/kg as a single dose.

Prevention of Postop Bladder Distention, Urinary Retention

IM, SUBCUTANEOUS: ADULTS, ELDERLY: 0.25 mg q4–6h for 2–3 days.

Treatment of Postop Bladder Distention, Urinary Retention

IM, SUBCUTANEOUS: ADULTS, ELDERLY: 0.5–1 mg q3h for 5 doses after bladder has been emptied.

Reversal of Neuromuscular Blockade After Surgery

IV: ADULTS, ELDERLY: 0.5–2.5 mg given slowly. **CHILDREN:** 0.025–0.08 mg/kg/dose. **INFANTS:** 0.025–0.1 mg/kg/dose.

SIDE EFFECTS

Frequent: Muscarinic effects (diarrhea, diaphoresis, increased salivation, nausea, vomiting, abdominal cramps/pain). **Occasional:** Muscarinic effects (urinary urgency/frequency, increased bronchial secretions, miosis, lacrimation).

ADVERSE EFFECTS/ TOXIC REACTIONS

Overdose produces cholinergic crisis manifested as abdominal discomfort/cramps, nausea, vomiting, diarrhea, flushing, facial warmth, excessive salivation, diaphoresis, lacrimation, pallor, bradycardia, tachycardia, hypotension, bronchospasm, urinary urgency, blurred vision, miosis, fasciculation (involuntary muscular contractions visible under skin).

NURSING CONSIDERATIONS

BASELINE ASSESSMENT

Larger doses should be given at time of greatest fatigue. Avoid large doses in those with megacolon, reduced GI motility.

INTERVENTION/EVALUATION

Monitor muscle strength, vital signs. Monitor for therapeutic response to medication (increased muscle strength, decreased fatigue, improved chewing, swallowing functions).

PATIENT/FAMILY TEACHING

- Report nausea, vomiting, diarrhea, diaphoresis, increased salivary secretions, palpitations, muscle weakness, severe abdominal pain, difficulty breathing.

Neo-Synephrine, *see phenylephrine*

nesiritide

HIGH ALERT

ness-**ear**-ih-tide
(Natrecor)

◆CLASSIFICATION

PHARMACOTHERAPEUTIC: Brain natriuretic peptide. **CLINICAL:** Endogenous hormone.

ACTION

Facilitates cardiovascular homeostasis, fluid status through counterregulation of renin-angiotensin-aldosterone system, stimulating cyclic guanosine monophosphate, thereby leading to smooth muscle cell relaxation. **Therapeutic Effect:** Promotes vasodilation, natriuresis, diuresis, correcting CHF.

PHARMACOKINETICS

Route	Onset	Peak	Duration
IV	15 min	1 hr	Up to 4 hrs

Excreted primarily in heart by left ventricle. Metabolized by natriuretic neutral endopeptidase enzymes on vascular luminal surface. **Half-life:** 18–23 min.

USES

Treatment of acutely decompensated CHF in pts who have dyspnea at rest or with minimal activity.

PRECAUTIONS

Contraindications: Cardiogenic shock, systolic B/P less than 90 mm Hg. **Cautions:** Significant valvular stenosis, restrictive/obstructive cardiomyopathy, constrictive pericarditis, pericardial tamponade, suspected low cardiac filling pressures, atrial/ventricular arrhythmias/conduction defects, hypotension, hepatic/renal insufficiency.

LIFESPAN CONSIDERATIONS

Pregnancy/Lactation: Unknown if drug crosses placenta or is distributed in breast milk. **Pregnancy Category C. Children:** Safety and efficacy not established. **Elderly:** No age-related precautions noted.

INTERACTIONS

DRUG: ACE inhibitors may increase risk of hypotension. **HERBAL: Ephedra, ginger, ginseng, licorice** may increase B/P. **Black cohosh, goldenseal, hawthorne** may decrease B/P. **FOOD:** None known. **LAB VALUES:** May increase serum creatinine.

AVAILABILITY (Rx)

Injection, Powder for Reconstitution: 1.5 mg/5-ml vial.

ADMINISTRATION/HANDLING

◀ALERT▶ Do not mix with other injections, infusions. Do not give IM.

IV

Reconstitution • Reconstitute one 1.5-mg vial with 5 ml D_5W or 0.9% NaCl, 0.2% NaCl, or any combination thereof. Swirl or rock gently, add to 250-ml bag D_5W or 0.9% NaCl, 0.2% NaCl, or any combination thereof, yielding a solution of 6 mcg/ml.

Rate of administration • Give as IV bolus over approximately 60 sec initially, followed by continuous IV infusion.

Storage • Store vial at room temperature. Once reconstituted, vials are stable at 36°–77°F (2°–25°C) for up to 24 hrs. Use reconstituted solution within 24 hrs.

IV INCOMPATIBILITIES

Bumetanide (Bumex), enalapril (Vasotec), ethacrynic acid (Edecrin), furosemide (Lasix), heparin, hydralazine (Apresoline), insulin, sodium metabisulfite.

INDICATIONS/ROUTES/DOSAGE

Treatment of Acute CHF

IV BOLUS: ADULTS, ELDERLY: 2 mcg/kg followed by continuous IV infusion of 0.01 mcg/kg/min. At intervals of 3 hrs or longer, may be increased by 0.005 mcg/kg/min (preceded by bolus of 1 mcg/kg), up to maximum of 0.03 mcg/kg/min.

SIDE EFFECTS

Frequent (11%): Hypotension. **Occasional (8%–2%):** Headache, nausea, bradycardia. **Rare (1% or less):** Confusion, paresthesia, drowsiness, tremor.

ADVERSE EFFECTS/ TOXIC REACTIONS

Ventricular arrhythmias (ventricular tachycardia, atrial fibrillation, AV node conduction abnormalities), angina pectoris occur rarely.

NURSING CONSIDERATIONS

BASELINE ASSESSMENT

Obtain B/P immediately before each dose, in addition to regular monitoring (be alert to fluctuations).

INTERVENTION/EVALUATION

Monitor B/P, pulse rate for hypotension frequently during therapy. Hypotension is dose-limiting and dose-dependent. If excessive reduction in B/P occurs, place pt in supine position with legs elevated. With

N

physician, establish parameters for adjusting rate, stopping infusion. Maintain accurate I&O; measure urinary output frequently. Immediately notify physician of decreased urinary output, cardiac arrhythmias, significant decrease in B/P, heart rate.

PATIENT/FAMILY TEACHING

- Report chest pain, palpitations.

Neulasta, *see pegfilgrastim*

Neupogen, *see filgrastim*

Neurontin, *see gabapentin*

N

nevirapine

neh-**veer**-a-peen
(Viramune)

BLACK BOX ALERT Potentially severe, life-threatening dermatologic hypersensitivity, hepatic reactions may occur. Greatest risk occurs within first 6 wks of treatment.

Do not confuse nevirapine with nelfinavir, or Viramune with Viracept.

CLASSIFICATION

PHARMACOTHERAPEUTIC: Nonnucleoside reverse transcriptase inhibitor. **CLINICAL:** Antiviral (see p. 116C).

ACTION

Binds directly to HIV-1 reverse transcriptase, changing shape of enzyme, blocking RNA-, DNA-dependent polymerase activity. **Therapeutic Effect:** Interferes with HIV replication, slowing progression of HIV infection.

PHARMACOKINETICS

Readily absorbed after PO administration. Protein binding: 60%. Widely distributed. Extensively metabolized in liver. Excreted primarily in urine. **Half-life:** 45 hrs (single dose); 25–30 hrs (multiple doses).

USES

Used in combination with other antiretroviral agents for treatment of HIV-1 infected adults who have experienced clinical, immunologic deterioration. **OFF-LABEL:** Reduce risk of transmitting HIV from infected mother to newborn.

PRECAUTIONS

Contraindications: Moderate to severe hepatic impairment. **Cautions:** Elevated AST, ALT levels, history of chronic hepatitis (B or C), higher $CD4^+$ cell counts.

LIFESPAN CONSIDERATIONS

Pregnancy/Lactation: Crosses placenta. Distributed in breast milk. Breastfeeding not recommended (possibility of HIV transmission). **Pregnancy Category C. Children:** Granulocytopenia occurs more frequently. **Elderly:** No information available.

INTERACTIONS

DRUG: May alter effect of **clarithromycin.** May decrease effect of **methadone, warfarin.** Concurrent use of **prednisone** may increase incidence, severity of rash in first 6 wks of nevirapine therapy. May decrease concentrations of **ketoconazole, oral contraceptives, protease inhibitors. Rifabutin, rifampin** may decrease concentration. **HERBAL: St. John's wort** may decrease concentration, effects. **FOOD:** None known. **LAB VALUES:** May increase serum bilirubin, alkaline phosphatase, GGT, AST, ALT. May decrease Hgb, neutrophil, platelet counts.

AVAILABILITY (Rx)

Oral Suspension: 50 mg/5 ml. **Tablets:** 200 mg.

ADMINISTRATION/HANDLING

PO

• Give without regard to meals.

INDICATIONS/ROUTES/DOSAGE

HIV Infection

PO: ADULTS: 200 mg once daily for 14 days (to reduce risk of rash). Maintenance: 200 mg twice daily in combination with nucleoside analogues. **NEONATES 15 DAYS AND OLDER, INFANTS, CHILDREN:** Initially, 150 mg/m² (**Maximum dose:** 200 mg) once daily for 14 days. Increase to 150 mg/m² q12h if no rash occurs (**Maximum dose:** 200 mg).

SIDE EFFECTS

Frequent (8%–3%): Rash, fever, headache, nausea, granulocytopenia (more common in children). **Occasional (2%–1%):** Stomatitis (burning, erythema, ulceration of oral mucosa; dysphagia). **Rare (less than 1%):** Paresthesia, myalgia, abdominal pain.

ADVERSE EFFECTS/ TOXIC REACTIONS

Skin reactions, hepatitis may become severe, life-threatening.

NURSING CONSIDERATIONS

BASELINE ASSESSMENT

Establish baseline lab values, esp. hepatic function tests, before initiating therapy and at intervals during therapy. Obtain medication history (esp. use of oral contraceptives).

INTERVENTION/EVALUATION

Closely monitor for evidence of rash (usually appears on trunk, face, extremities; occurs within first 6 wks of drug initiation). Observe for rash accompanied by fever, blistering, oral lesions, conjunctivitis, swelling, muscle/joint aches, general malaise.

PATIENT/FAMILY TEACHING

• If nevirapine therapy is missed for longer than 7 days, restart by using one 200-mg tablet daily for first 14 days, followed by one 200-mg tablet twice a day. • Continue therapy for full length of treatment. • Doses should be evenly spaced. • Nevirapine is not a cure for HIV infection, nor does it reduce risk of transmission to others. • Notify physician if any rash, yellowing of skin/eyes, nausea, loss of appetite occur.

Nexium, *see esomeprazole*

niacin, nicotinic acid

nye-a-sin

(Niacor, Niaspan, Slo-Niacin)

Do not confuse niacin, Niacor, or Niaspan with minocin or Nitro-Bid.

FIXED-COMBINATION(S)

Advicor: niacin/lovastatin (HMG-CoA reductase inhibitor [statin]): 500 mg/20 mg, 750 mg/20 mg, 1,000 mg/20 mg. **Simcor:** niacin/simvastatin (HMG-CoA reductase inhibitor [statin]): 500 mg/20 mg, 500 mg/40 mg, 750 mg/20 mg, 1,000 mg/20 mg, 1,000 mg/40 mg.

◆CLASSIFICATION

CLINICAL: Antihyperlipidemic, water-soluble vitamin (see pp. 57C, 161C).

ACTION

Component of two coenzymes needed for tissue respiration, lipid metabolism, glycogenolysis. Inhibits synthesis of very-low-density lipoproteins (VLDLs). **Therapeutic Effect:** Reduces total, LDL, VLDL cholesterol levels and triglyceride levels; increases HDL cholesterol concentration.

PHARMACOKINETICS

Readily absorbed from GI tract. Widely distributed. Metabolized in liver (exten-

N

sive first pass effect). Primarily excreted in urine. **Half-life:** 45 min.

USES

Adjunct in treatment of hyperlipidemias, peripheral vascular disease; treatment of pellagra; dietary supplement.

PRECAUTIONS

Contraindications: Active peptic ulcer disease, arterial hemorrhaging, hepatic dysfunction, hypersensitivity to niacin, tartrazine (frequently seen in pts sensitive to aspirin), severe hypotension. **Cautions:** Diabetes mellitus, gallbladder disease, gout, history of jaundice/hepatic disease.

LIFESPAN CONSIDERATIONS

Pregnancy/Lactation: Not recommended for use during pregnancy/lactation. Distributed in breast milk. **Pregnancy Category A (C if used at dosages above the recommended daily allowance). Children:** No age-related precautions noted. Not recommended in those younger than 2 yrs. **Elderly:** No age-related precautions noted.

N

INTERACTIONS

DRUG: Alcohol may increase risk of side effects. May alter effect of **anticoagulants.** May increase effect of **antihypertensives. Lovastatin, pravastatin, simvastatin** may increase risk of acute renal failure, rhabdomyolysis. **Vasoactive drugs (e.g., calcium channel blockers, nitrates)** may increase hypotension. **HERBAL:** None significant. **FOOD:** None known. **LAB VALUES:** May increase serum uric acid, PT, amylase, bilirubin, fasting glucose, LDH, transaminase. May decrease platelets.

AVAILABILITY (OTC)

Tablets (Immediate-Release [Niacor]): 50 mg, 100 mg, 250 mg, 500 mg.

Capsules (Extended-Release): 250 mg, 400 mg, 500 mg. **Tablets (Controlled-Release [Slo-Niacin]):** 250 mg, 500 mg, 750 mg. **Tablets (Extended-Release [Niaspan]):** 500 mg, 750 mg, 1,000 mg.

ADMINISTRATION/HANDLING

PO

• For pts switching from immediate-release niacin to extended-release niacin, initiate extended-release form with low doses and titrate to therapeutic response. • Give with food. • Give aspirin 30 min before taking extended-release niacin to minimize flushing. • Do not crush, break, or chew long-acting forms.

INDICATIONS/ROUTES/DOSAGE

Hyperlipidemia

PO (IMMEDIATE-RELEASE): ADULTS, ELDERLY: Initially, 250 mg once a day (with evening meal). May increase dose q4–7days up to 1.5–2 g/day in 2–3 divided doses. After 2 mos may increase at 2- to 4-wk intervals to 3 g/day in 3 divided doses. **Maximum:** 6 g/day in 3 divided doses.

PO (CONTROLLED-RELEASE): ADULTS, ELDERLY: Initially, 500 mg/day at bedtime for 4 wks, then 1 g at bedtime for 4 wks. May increase by 500 mg q4wks up to maximum of 2 g/day.

Nutritional Supplement

PO: ADULTS, ELDERLY: 10–20 mg/day. **Maximum:** 100 mg/day.

Pellagra

PO (IMMEDIATE-RELEASE): ADULTS, ELDERLY: 50–100 mg 3–4 times a day. **Maximum:** 500 mg/day. **CHILDREN:** 50–100 mg 3 times a day.

SIDE EFFECTS

Frequent: Flushing (esp. face, neck) occurring within 20 min of drug administration and lasting for 30–60 min, GI upset, pruritus. **Occasional:** Dizziness, hypotension, headache, blurred vision, burning/tingling of skin, flatulence, nausea, vomiting, diarrhea. **Rare:** Hyperglycemia, glycosuria, rash, hyperpigmentation, dry skin.

ADVERSE EFFECTS/ TOXIC REACTIONS

Arrhythmias occur rarely.

NURSING CONSIDERATIONS

BASELINE ASSESSMENT

Obtain diet history, especially fat consumption. Question for history of hypersensitivity to niacin, tartrazine, aspirin. Assess serum baselines, cholesterol, triglyceride, glucose, hepatic function tests.

INTERVENTION/EVALUATION

Evaluate flushing, degree of GI discomfort. Check for headache, dizziness, blurred vision. Monitor daily pattern of bowel activity and stool consistency. Monitor hepatic function, serum cholesterol, triglycerides. Check serum glucose carefully in those on insulin, oral antihyperglycemics. Assess skin for rash, dryness. Monitor serum uric acid.

PATIENT/FAMILY TEACHING

• Transient flushing of the skin, sensation of warmth, pruritus, tingling may occur. • Notify physician if dizziness occurs (avoid sudden changes in posture). • Inform physician if nausea, vomiting, loss of appetite, yellowing of skin, dark urine, feeling of weakness occur. • If medically approved, take aspirin 30 min before taking extended-release niacin to minimize flushing. • Take at bedtime with low-fat snack. • Limit alcohol consumption.

Niaspan, *see niacin, nicotinic acid*

*niCARdipine

nye-**car**-di-peen
(Cardene, Cardene IV, Cardene SR)
Do not confuse nicardipine with nifedipine or nimodipine, Cardene with Cardizem, Cardura, or codeine, or Cardene SR with Cardizem SR or codeine.

CLASSIFICATION

PHARMACOTHERAPEUTIC: Calcium channel blocker. **CLINICAL:** Antianginal, antihypertensive (see p. 78C).

ACTION

Inhibits calcium ion movement across cell membranes, depressing contraction of cardiac, vascular smooth muscle. **Therapeutic Effect:** Increases heart rate, cardiac output. Decreases systemic vascular resistance, B/P.

PHARMACOKINETICS

Route	Onset	Peak	Duration
PO	0.5–2 hr	—	8 hrs

Rapidly, completely absorbed from GI tract. Protein binding: 95%. Undergoes first-pass metabolism in liver. Primarily excreted in urine. Not removed by hemodialysis. **Half-life:** 2–4 hrs.

USES

PO: Immediate-release: Treatment of chronic stable (effort-associated) angina, essential hypertension. **Sustained-release:** Treatment of essential hypertension. **Parenteral:** Short-term treatment of hypertension when oral therapy not feasible or desirable. **OFF-LABEL:** Treatment of Raynaud's phenomenon, subarachnoid hemorrhage, associated neurologic deficits, vasospastic angina. Prevention of migraine headaches, CHF.

PRECAUTIONS

Contraindications: Atrial fibrillation/flutter associated with accessory conduction pathways, cardiogenic shock, CHF, second- or third-degree heart block, severe hypotension, sinus bradycardia, ventricular tachycardia, within several hours of IV beta-blocker therapy. **Cautions:** Sick sinus syndrome, severe left ventricular dysfunction, renal/hepatic impairment, cardiomyopathy, edema, concomitant beta-blocker or digoxin therapy.

N

LIFESPAN CONSIDERATIONS

Pregnancy/Lactation: Unknown if distributed in breast milk. **Pregnancy Category C. Children:** Safety and efficacy not established. **Elderly:** Age-related renal impairment may require dosage adjustment.

INTERACTIONS

DRUG: **Beta-blockers** may have additive effect. **Digoxin** may increase concentration. **Hypokalemia-producing agents (e.g., furosemide, other diuretics)** may increase risk of arrhythmias. **Procainamide, quinidine** may increase risk of QT-interval prolongation. HERBAL: **Ephedra, garlic, ginseng, yohimbe** may increase hypertension. **Licorice** may cause retention of sodium, water; may increase loss of potassium. FOOD: **Grapefruit, grapefruit juice** may alter absorption. LAB VALUES: None significant.

AVAILABILITY (Rx)

Capsules (Cardene): 20 mg, 30 mg. Infusion, Ready to Use: 20 mg/200 ml, 40 mg/200 ml. Injection Solution (Cardene IV): 2.5 mg/ml (10 ml vial).

Capsules (Sustained-Release [Cardene SR]): 30 mg, 45 mg, 60 mg.

ADMINISTRATION/HANDLING

IV

Reconstitution • Dilute 25-mg vial with 240 ml D_5W, 0.45% NaCl, or 0.9% NaCl to provide concentration of 0.1 mg/ml.

Rate of administration • Give by slow IV infusion. • Change IV site q12h if administered peripherally.

Storage • Store at room temperature. • Diluted IV solution is stable for 24 hrs at room temperature.

PO

• Give without regard to food. • Do not crush/break sustained-release capsules. Swallow whole.

IV INCOMPATIBILITIES

Ampicillin (Principen), ampicillin/sulbactam (Unasyn), cefepime (Maxipime), ceftazidine (Fortaz), furosemide (Lasix), heparin, sodium bicarbonate, thiopental (Pentothal).

IV COMPATIBILITIES

Diltiazem (Cardizem), dobutamine (Dobutrex), dopamine (Intropin), epinephrine, hydromorphone (Dilaudid), labetalol (Trandate), lorazepam (Ativan), midazolam (Versed), milrinone (Primacor), morphine, nitroglycerin, norepinephrine (Levophed), potassium chloride.

INDICATIONS/ROUTES/DOSAGE

Chronic Stable Angina

PO: ADULTS, ELDERLY: Initially, 20 mg 3 times a day. Range: 20–40 mg 3 times a day (allow 3 days between dosage increases).

Essential Hypertension

PO: ADULTS, ELDERLY: Initially, 20 mg 3 times a day. Range: 20–40 mg 3 times a day (allow 3 days between dosage increases).

PO (SUSTAINED-RELEASE): ADULTS, ELDERLY: Initially, 30 mg twice a day. Range: 30–60 mg twice a day.

Short-Term Treatment of Hypertension (Parenteral Dosage as Substitute for Oral Nicardipine)

IV: ADULTS, ELDERLY: 0.5 mg/hr (for pt receiving 20 mg PO q8h), 1.2 mg/hr (for pt receiving 30 mg PO q8h), 2.2 mg/hr (for pt receiving 40 mg PO q8h).

Pts Not Already Receiving Nicardipine

IV: ADULTS, ELDERLY (GRADUAL B/P DECREASE): Initially, 5 mg/hr. May increase by 2.5 mg/hr q15min. After B/P goal is achieved, decrease rate to 3 mg/hr. **ADULTS, ELDERLY (RAPID B/P DECREASE):** Initially, 5 mg/hr. May increase by 2.5 mg/hr q5min. **Maximum:** 15 mg/hr until desired B/P attained. After B/P goal achieved, decrease rate to 3 mg/hr.

Changing From IV to Oral Antihypertensive Therapy

ADULTS, ELDERLY: Begin antihypertensives other than nicardipine when IV has been discontinued; for nicardipine, give first dose 1 hr before discontinuing IV.

Dosage in Hepatic Impairment

Adults, elderly pts: Initially give 20 mg twice a day, then titrate.

Dosage in Renal Impairment

Adults, elderly pts: Initially give 20 mg q8h (30 mg twice a day [sustained-release capsules]), then titrate.

SIDE EFFECTS

Frequent (10%–7%): Headache, facial flushing, peripheral edema, light-headedness, dizziness. **Occasional (6%–3%):** Asthenia (loss of strength, energy), palpitations, angina, tachycardia. **Rare (less than 2%):** Nausea, abdominal cramps, dyspepsia (heartburn, indigestion, epigastric pain), dry mouth, rash.

ADVERSE EFFECTS/ TOXIC REACTIONS

Overdose produces confusion, slurred speech, drowsiness, marked hypotension, bradycardia.

NURSING CONSIDERATIONS

BASELINE ASSESSMENT

Concurrent therapy of sublingual nitroglycerin may be used for relief of anginal pain. Record onset, type (sharp, dull, squeezing), radiation, location, intensity, duration of anginal pain, precipitating factors (exertion, emotional stress).

INTERVENTION/EVALUATION

Monitor B/P during and following IV infusion. Assess for peripheral edema behind medial malleolus. Assess skin for facial flushing, dermatitis, rash. Question for asthenia (loss of strength, energy), headache. Monitor serum hepatic enzyme results. Assess EKG, pulse for tachycardia.

PATIENT/FAMILY TEACHING

• May take without regard to food. Sustained-release capsule taken whole; do not crush, chew, cut. • Avoid alcohol, grapefruit juice, limit caffeine. • Inform physician if angina pains not relieved or palpitations, shortness of breath, swelling, dizziness, constipation, nausea, hypotension occur. • Avoid tasks requiring motor skills, alertness until response to drug is established.

nicotine

nik-o-teen
(Commit, Habitrol ✱, NicoDerm ✱, NicoDerm CQ, Nicorette, Nicorette Plus ✱, Nicotrol ✱, Nicotrol Inhaler, Nicotrol NS, Thrive)

Do not confuse Nicoderm with Nitroderm.

◆ CLASSIFICATION

PHARMACOTHERAPEUTIC: Cholinergic-receptor agonist. **CLINICAL:** Smoking deterrent.

ACTION

Binds to acetylcholine receptors, producing both stimulating, depressant effects on peripheral, central nervous systems. **Therapeutic Effect:** Provides source of nicotine during nicotine withdrawal, reduces withdrawal symptoms.

PHARMACOKINETICS

Absorbed slowly after transdermal administration. Protein binding: 5%. Metabolized in liver. Excreted primarily in urine. **Half-life:** 4 hrs.

USES

Alternative, less potent form of nicotine (without tar, carbon monoxide, carcinogenic substances of tobacco) used as part of smoking cessation program. **OFF-LABEL: Transdermal:** Management of ulcerative colitis.

PRECAUTIONS

Contraindications: Immediate post-MI period, life-threatening arrhythmias, severe or worsening angina. **Cautions:** Hyperthyroidism, pheochromocytoma, insulin-dependent diabetes mellitus, severe renal impairment, eczematous dermatitis, oral/pharyngeal inflammation, esophagitis, peptic ulcer (delays healing in peptic ulcer disease).

⌛ LIFESPAN CONSIDERATIONS

Pregnancy/Lactation: Distributed freely into breast milk. Use of cigarettes, nicotine gum associated with decrease in fetal breathing movements. **Pregnancy Category D. Children:** Not recommended in this pt population. **Elderly:** Age-related decrease in cardiac function may require dosage adjustment.

INTERACTIONS

DRUG: Smoking cessation, decreased dosage of nicotine may increase effects of **beta-adrenergic blockers, bronchodilators (e.g., theophylline), insulin, propoxyphene.** **HERBAL:** None significant. **FOOD:** None known. **LAB VALUES:** None significant.

AVAILABILITY (OTC)

Chewing Gum (Nicorette, Thrive): 2 mg, 4 mg. **Inhalation (Nicotrol Inhaler):** 10 mg cartridge. **Lozenges (Commit):** 2 mg, 4 mg. **Nasal Spray (Nicotrol NS):** 0.5 mg/spray. **Transdermal Patch (NicoDerm CQ):** 7 mg/24 hrs, 14 mg/24 hrs, 21 mg/24 hrs.

ADMINISTRATION/HANDLING

Gum

• Do not swallow. • Chew 1 piece when urge to smoke present. • Chew slowly and intermittently for 30 min. • Chew until distinctive nicotine taste (peppery) or slight tingling in mouth perceived, then stop; when tingling almost gone (about 1 min) repeat chewing procedure (this allows constant slow buccal absorption). • Too-rapid chewing may cause excessive release of nicotine, resulting in adverse effects similar to oversmoking (e.g., nausea, throat irritation).

Inhaler

• Insert cartridge into mouthpiece. • Puff on nicotine cartridge mouthpiece for 20 min.

Lozenge

• Do not chew or swallow. • Allow to dissolve slowly (20–30 min).

Transdermal

• Apply promptly upon removal from protective pouch (prevents evaporation, loss of nicotine). Use only intact pouch. Do not cut patch. • Apply only once daily to hairless, clean, dry skin on upper body, outer arm. • Replace daily; rotate sites; do not use same site within 7 days; do not use same patch longer than 24 hrs. • Wash hands with water alone after applying patch (soap may increase nicotine absorption). • Discard used patch by folding patch in half (sticky side together), placing in pouch of new patch, and throwing away in such a way as to prevent child or pet accessibility. • Patch may contain conducting metal; remove prior to MRI.

INDICATIONS/ROUTES/DOSAGE

Smoking Cessation Aid to Relieve Nicotine Withdrawal Symptoms

PO (CHEWING GUM): ADULTS, ELDERLY: Less than 25 cigarettes/day: Use 2 mg. 25 or more cigarettes/day: Use 4 mg. Chew 1 piece of gum when urge to smoke, up to 24/day. Use following schedule: wks 1–6: q1–2h (at least 9 pieces/day); wks 7–9: q2–4h; wks 10–12: q4–8h.

PO (LOZENGE):

◄ALERT► For those who smoke the first cigarette within 30 min of waking, administer the 4-mg lozenge; otherwise administer the 2-mg lozenge.

ADULTS, ELDERLY: One 4-mg or 2-mg lozenge q1–2h for the first 6 wks (use at least 9 lozenges/day first 6 wks); 1 lozenge q2–4h for wks 7–9; and 1 lozenge q4–8h for wks 10–12. **Maximum:** 1 lozenge at a time, 5 lozenges/6 hrs, 20 lozenges/day.

TRANSDERMAL: ◀ALERT▶ Apply 1 new patch q24h. **ADULTS, ELDERLY WHO SMOKE 10 CIGARETTES OR MORE PER DAY:** Follow the guidelines below. **Step 1:** 21 mg/day for 6 wks. **Step 2:** 14 mg/day for 2 wks. **Step 3:** 7 mg/day for 2 wks. **ADULTS, ELDERLY WHO SMOKE LESS THAN 10 CIGARETTES PER DAY:** Follow the guidelines below. **Step 1:** 14 mg/day for 6 wks. **Step 2:** 7 mg/day for 2 wks.
NASAL: ADULTS, ELDERLY: Each dose (2 sprays, 1 spray in each nostril) = 1 mg nicotine. Initially, 1–2 doses/hr. **Maximum:** 5 doses/hr (10 sprays), 40 doses/day (80 sprays). Take at least 8 doses (16 sprays) per day.
INHALER (NICOTROL): ADULTS, ELDERLY: Puff on nicotine cartridge mouthpiece for about 20 min as needed.

SIDE EFFECTS

Frequent: **All forms:** Hiccups, nausea. **Gum:** Mouth/throat soreness, nausea, hiccups. **Transdermal:** Erythema, pruritus, burning at application site. Occasional: **All forms:** Eructation, GI upset, dry mouth, insomnia, diaphoresis, irritability. **Gum:** Hiccups, hoarseness. **Inhaler:** Mouth/throat irritation, cough. Rare: **All forms:** Dizziness, myalgia, arthralgia.

ADVERSE EFFECTS/ TOXIC REACTIONS

Overdose produces palpitations, tachyarrhythmias, seizures, depression, confusion, diaphoresis, hypotension, rapid/weak pulse, dyspnea. Lethal dose for adults is 40–60 mg. Death results from respiratory paralysis.

NURSING CONSIDERATIONS

BASELINE ASSESSMENT

Screen, evaluate those with coronary heart disease (history of MI, angina pectoris), serious cardiac arrhythmias, Buerger's disease, Prinzmetal's variant angina.

INTERVENTION/EVALUATION

Monitor smoking habit, B/P, pulse, sleep pattern, skin for erythema, pruritus, burning at application site if transdermal system used.

PATIENT/FAMILY TEACHING

• Follow guidelines for proper application of transdermal system. • Chew gum slowly to avoid jaw ache, maximize benefit. • Inform physician if persistent rash, pruritus occurs with patch. • Do not smoke while wearing patches.

*NIFEdipine

nye-**fed**-i-peen
(Adalat CC, Adalat XL ✤, Apo-Nifed ✤, Nifediac CC, Nifedical XL, Novo-Nifedin ✤, Procardia, Procardia XL)
Do not confuse nifedipine with nicardipine or nimodipine, or Procardia XL with Cartia XT.

◆CLASSIFICATION

PHARMACOTHERAPEUTIC: Calcium channel blocker. **CLINICAL:** Antianginal, antihypertensive (see p. 78C).

ACTION

Inhibits calcium ion movement across cell membranes, depressing contraction of cardiac, vascular smooth muscle. **Therapeutic Effect:** Increases heart rate, cardiac output. Decreases systemic vascular resistance, B/P.

PHARMACOKINETICS

Rapidly, completely absorbed from GI tract. Protein binding: 92%–98%. Undergoes first-pass metabolism in liver. Primarily excreted in urine. Not removed by hemodialysis. **Half-life:** 2–5 hrs.

USES

Treatment of angina due to coronary artery spasm (Prinzmetal's variant angina), chronic stable angina (effort-associated angina). **Extended-release:** Treatment of essential hypertension. **OFF-LABEL:** Treatment of Raynaud's phenomenon, pulmonary hypertension, ureteral stones.

PRECAUTIONS

Contraindications: Cardiogenic shock, concomitant administration with strong CYP450 inducers. **Cautions:** Renal/hepatic impairment.

LIFESPAN CONSIDERATIONS

Pregnancy/Lactation: Insignificant amount distributed in breast milk. **Pregnancy Category C. Children:** Safety and efficacy not established. **Elderly:** Age-related renal impairment may require dosage adjustment.

INTERACTIONS

DRUG: Beta-blockers may have additive effect. May increase **digoxin** concentration, risk of toxicity. **Hypokalemia-producing agents (e.g., furosemide, other diuretics)** may increase risk of arrhythmias. **HERBAL: Ephedra, garlic, ginseng, yohimbe** may increase hypertension. **Licorice** may cause retention of sodium, water; may increase loss of potassium. **FOOD: Grapefruit, grapefruit juice** may increase concentration. **LAB VALUES:** May cause positive ANA, direct Coombs' test.

AVAILABILITY (Rx)

Capsules (Procardia): 10 mg, 20 mg.

Tablets, Extended-Release: (Adalat CC, Nifediac CC, Nifedical XL, Procardia XL): 30 mg, 60 mg, 90 mg.

ADMINISTRATION/HANDLING

PO

• Do not crush/break/chew extended-release tablets. • Give without regard to meals (Adalat CC, Nifediac CC should be taken on an empty stomach). • Grapefruit juice may alter absorption; avoid with all products.

Sublingual

• Capsules must be punctured, chewed, and/or squeezed to express liquid into mouth.

INDICATIONS/ROUTES/DOSAGE

Prinzmetal's Variant Angina, Chronic Stable (Effort-Associated) Angina

PO: ADULTS, ELDERLY: Initially, 10 mg 3 times a day. Increase at 7- to 14-day intervals. Maintenance: 10 mg 3 times a day up to 30 mg 4 times a day.

PO (EXTENDED-RELEASE): ADULTS, ELDERLY: Initially, 30–60 mg/day. May increase at 7- to 14-day intervals. **Maximum:** 120–180 mg/day.

Essential Hypertension

PO (EXTENDED-RELEASE): ADULTS, ELDERLY: Initially, 30–60 mg/day. May increase at 7- to 14-day intervals. **Maximum:** 90–120 mg/day. **CHILDREN 1–17 YRS:** Initially, 0.25–0.5 mg/kg/day. **Maximum:** 3 mg/kg/day or 120 mg/day.

SIDE EFFECTS

Frequent (30%–11%): Peripheral edema, headache, flushed skin, dizziness. **Occasional (12%–6%):** Nausea, shakiness, muscle cramps/pain, drowsiness, palpitations, nasal congestion, cough, dyspnea, wheezing. **Rare (5%–3%):** Hypotension, rash, pruritus, urticaria, constipation, abdominal discomfort, flatulence, sexual dysfunction.

ADVERSE EFFECTS/ TOXIC REACTIONS

May precipitate CHF, MI in pts with cardiac disease, peripheral ischemia. Overdose produces nausea, drowsiness, confusion, slurred speech. **Antidote:** Glucagon (see Appendix M for dosage).

NURSING CONSIDERATIONS

BASELINE ASSESSMENT

Concurrent therapy of sublingual nitroglycerin may be used for relief of anginal pain. Record onset, type (sharp, dull, squeezing), radiation, location, intensity, duration of anginal pain; precipitating factors (exertion, emotional stress). Check B/P for hypotension immediately before giving medication.

INTERVENTION/EVALUATION

Assist with ambulation if light-headedness, dizziness occurs. Assess for peripheral edema. Assess skin for flushing. Monitor serum hepatic enzymes, signs/symptoms of CHF.

PATIENT/FAMILY TEACHING

• Rise slowly from lying to sitting position, permit legs to dangle from bed momentarily before standing to reduce hypotensive effect. • Contact physician if palpitations, shortness of breath, pronounced dizziness, nausea, exacerbations of angina occur. • Avoid alcohol, concomitant grapefruit, grapefruit juice use.

nilotinib

HIGH ALERT

ni-**low**-tih-nib
(Tasigna)

BLACK BOX ALERT Prolongs QT interval; sudden deaths reported. Do not use in pts with hypokalemia, hypomagnesemia, prolonged QT syndrome.

Do not confuse nilotinib with dasatinib, erlotinib, imatinib, nilutamide, sorafenib, sunitinib.

◆CLASSIFICATION

PHARMACOTHERAPEUTIC: Protein-tyrosine kinase inhibitor. **CLINICAL:** Antineoplastic.

ACTION

Inhibits the Bcr-Abl tyrosine kinase, a translocation-created enzyme, created by the Philadelphia chromosome abnormality noted in chronic myelogenous leukemia (CML). **Therapeutic Effect:** Inhibits proliferation and tumor growth during two stages of CML: accelerated phase, chronic phase.

PHARMACOKINETICS

Well absorbed following PO administration. Protein binding: 98%. Metabolized in liver. Eliminated mainly in feces. Food increases concentration, and dose cannot be given 2 hrs before and 1 hr after food. **Half-life:** 17 hrs.

USES

Treatment of chronic phase and accelerated phase of chronic myelogenous leukemia (CML) in adult pts resistant or intolerant to prior therapy that included imatinib. Treatment of newly diagnosed Philadelphia chromosome positive chronic myeloid leukemia in chronic phase (Ph+ CML-CP). **OFF-LABEL:** Acute lymphoblastic leukemia, systemic mastocytosis hypereosinophilic syndrome.

PRECAUTIONS

Contraindications: Hypokalemia, hypomagnesemia, prolonged QT syndrome, galactose intolerance, severe lactase deficiency, glucose-galactose malabsorption. **Cautions:** Myelosuppression, QT prolongation, history of pancreatitis, hepatic impairment, electrolyte abnormalities.

⌛ LIFESPAN CONSIDERATIONS

Pregnancy/Lactation: May cause fetal harm. Breast-feeding not recommended. **Pregnancy Category D. Children:** Safety and efficacy not established in those younger than 18 yrs. **Elderly:** No age-related precautions noted.

INTERACTIONS

DRUG: Clarithromycin, erythromycin, itraconazole, ketoconazole increase concentration. **Carbamazepine, dexamethasone, phenobarbital, phenytoin, rifampicin** decrease concentration. May increase concentration of **benzodiazepines, calcium channel blockers, dihydropyridine, midazolam, simvastatin, triazolodiazepines.** May alter therapeutic effects of **cyclosporine, pimozide.** Reduces effect of **warfarin. HERBAL: St. John's wort** decreases concentration. **FOOD: Grapefruit, grapefruit juice** may alter absorption. **LAB VALUES:** May decrease WBCs, platelets, magnesium, phosphorus, albumin, sodium. May increase glucose, lipase, bilirubin, ALT, AST. May alter potassium, alkaline phosphatase, creatinine.

AVAILABILITY (Rx)

Capsules: 150 mg, 200 mg.

ADMINISTRATION/HANDLING

PO

- Give at least 2 hrs before and 1 hr after ingestion of food. • Swallow capsules whole; do not crush. • Store at room temperature.

INDICATIONS/ROUTES/DOSAGE

Chronic Myelogenous Leukemia (CML)

PO: ADULTS, ELDERLY: 400 mg twice daily every 12 hrs, without food. Dosage adjusted in hepatic impairment, hematologic toxicity, nonhematologic toxicity, QT prolongation (consult specific product labeling).

Ph+ CML-CP

PO: ADULTS, ELDERLY: 300 mg twice daily.

SIDE EFFECTS

Frequent (33%–21%): Rash, nausea, headache, pruritus, fatigue, diarrhea, constipation, vomiting. **Occasional (18%–10%):** Arthralgia, cough, pharyngitis, asthenia (loss of strength, energy), fever, myalgia, abdominal pain, peripheral edema, weight gain, bone pain, muscle spasm, back pain. **Rare (9%–1%):** Anorexia, insomnia, dizziness, paresthesia, vertigo, palpitations, flushing, hypertension, flatulence, alopecia, night sweats.

ADVERSE EFFECTS/ TOXIC REACTIONS

Prolongation of QT interval producing ventricular tachycardia (torsade de pointes) may result in seizure, sudden death. Neutropenia, thrombocytopenia, anemia are expected response to drug. Respiratory toxicity manifested as dyspnea, pneumonia.

NURSING CONSIDERATIONS

BASELINE ASSESSMENT

Obtain CBC every 2 wks for the first 2 mos and then monthly thereafter. Hypokalemia or hypomagnesemia must be corrected prior to initiating therapy. Monitor hepatic function tests (AST, ALT, bilirubin, alkaline phosphatase) before treatment begins and monthly thereafter. Obtain baseline weight.

INTERVENTION/EVALUATION

Monitor serum electrolytes periodically during therapy, particularly potassium, magnesium, sodium, lipase. Monitor for unexpected weight gain. Offer antiemetics to control nausea, vomiting. Monitor daily pattern of bowel frequency, stool consistency. Monitor CBC for evidence of neutropenia, thrombocytopenia; assess hepatic function tests for hepatotoxicity. These pts should be closely monitored for QT interval prolongation.

PATIENT/FAMILY TEACHING

- Avoid crowds, those with known infection. • Avoid contact with anyone who recently received live virus vaccine; do not receive vaccinations. • Do not ingest food at least 2 hours before and at least 1 hr after dose is taken. • Avoid grapefruit products.

nilutamide

HIGH ALERT

ni-**lute**-ah-mide
(Anandron, Nilandron)

BLACK BOX ALERT Interstitial pneumonitis reported in 2% of pts manifested as progressive exertional dyspnea, cough, chest pain, fever.

Do not confuse nilutamide with nilotinib.

CLASSIFICATION

PHARMACOTHERAPEUTIC: Hormone. **CLINICAL:** Antineoplastic (see p. 87C).

N

ACTION

Competitively inhibits androgen activity by binding to androgen receptors in target tissue. **Therapeutic Effect:** Decreases growth of abnormal prostate tissue.

PHARMACOKINETICS

Well absorbed following PO administration. Protein binding: 72%–85%. Metabolized in liver. Primarily excreted in urine. **Half-life:** 23–87 hrs.

USES

Treatment of metastatic prostatic carcinoma (stage D_2) in combination with surgical castration. For maximum benefit, begin on same day or day after surgical castration.

PRECAUTIONS

Contraindications: Severe hepatic impairment, severe respiratory insufficiency. **Cautions:** Hepatitis, marked increase in serum hepatic enzymes.

LIFESPAN CONSIDERATIONS

Pregnancy Category C. Children: Safety and efficacy not established. **Elderly:** No age-related precautions noted.

INTERACTIONS

DRUG: May increase effect of **warfarin.** May increase concentration, risk of toxicity with **fosphenytoin, phenytoin, theophylline. HERBAL: St. John's wort** may decrease concentration. **FOOD:** None known. **LAB VALUES:** May increase serum bilirubin, creatinine, AST, ALT, alkaline phosphatase, BUN, glucose. May decrease Hgb, WBC.

AVAILABILITY (Rx)

Tablets: 150 mg.

ADMINISTRATION/HANDLING

PO

- May give without regard to food.

INDICATIONS/ROUTES/DOSAGE

Prostatic Carcinoma

PO: ADULTS, ELDERLY: 300 mg once a day for 30 days, then 150 mg once a day. Begin on day of, or day after, surgical castration.

SIDE EFFECTS

Frequent (greater than 10%): Hot flashes, delay in recovering vision after bright illumination (e.g., sun, television, bright lights), decreased libido, diminished sexual function, mild nausea, gynecomastia, alcohol intolerance. **Occasional (less than 10%):** Constipation, hypertension, dizziness, dyspnea, UTI.

ADVERSE EFFECTS/ TOXIC REACTIONS

Interstitial pneumonitis occurs rarely.

NURSING CONSIDERATIONS

BASELINE ASSESSMENT

Obtain baseline chest X-ray, hepatic enzymes before beginning therapy.

INTERVENTION/EVALUATION

Monitor B/P periodically and hepatic function tests in long-term therapy.

PATIENT/FAMILY TEACHING

- Contact physician if any side effects occur at home, esp. signs of hepatic toxicity (jaundice, dark urine, fatigue, abdominal pain).
- Tinted glasses may help improve night driving.

N

nimodipine

nye-**mode**-i-peen
(Nimotop)

BLACK BOX ALERT Severe cardiovascular events, including fatalities, have resulted when capsule contents have been withdrawn by syringe and administered by IV injection rather than nasogastric tube.

Do not confuse nimodipine with nicardipine or nifedipine.

CLASSIFICATION

PHARMACOTHERAPEUTIC: Calcium channel blocker. **CLINICAL:** Cerebral vasospasm agent (see p. 78C).

ACTION

Inhibits movement of calcium ions across vascular smooth-muscle cell membranes. **Therapeutic Effect:** Produces favorable effect on severity of neurologic deficits due to cerebral vasospasm. Exerts greatest effect on cerebral arteries; may prevent cerebral spasm.

PHARMACOKINETICS

Rapidly absorbed from GI tract. Protein binding: 95%. Metabolized in liver. Excreted in urine; eliminated in feces. Not removed by hemodialysis. **Half-life:** 1–2 hrs.

USES

Improvement of neurologic deficits due to cerebral vasospasm following subarachnoid hemorrhage from ruptured congenital intracranial aneurysms in pts in satisfactory neurologic condition. **OFF-LABEL:** Treatment of chronic and classic migraine, chronic cluster headaches.

PRECAUTIONS

N

Contraindications: Atrial fibrillation/flutter, cardiogenic shock, CHF, heart block, sinus bradycardia, ventricular tachycardia, within several hours of IV beta-blocker therapy. **Cautions:** Renal/hepatic impairment.

LIFESPAN CONSIDERATIONS

Pregnancy/Lactation: Unknown if drug crosses placenta or is distributed in breast milk. **Pregnancy Category C. Children:** Safety and efficacy not established. **Elderly:** Age-related renal impairment may require dosage adjustment. May experience greater hypotensive response, constipation.

INTERACTIONS

DRUG: Beta-blockers may have additive effect, increase depression of cardiac SA/AV conduction. May increase **digoxin** concentration. **Agents inducing hypokalemia** may increase risk of arrhythmias. **Erythromycin, itraconazole, ketoconazole, protease inhibitors** may inhibit metabolism. **Rifabutin, rifampin** may increase metabolism. **HERBAL: Ephedra, garlic, ginseng, yohimbe** may increase hypertension. **Licorice** may cause retention of sodium, water; may increase loss of potassium. **FOOD: Grapefruit juice** may increase concentration, risk of toxicity. **LAB VALUES:** None significant.

AVAILABILITY (Rx)

Capsules: 30 mg.

ADMINISTRATION/HANDLING

PO

- If pt unable to swallow, place hole in both ends of capsule with 18-gauge needle to extract contents into syringe.
- Empty into NG tube; flush tube with 30 ml normal saline.

INDICATIONS/ROUTES/DOSAGE

Subarachnoid Hemorrhage

PO: ADULTS, ELDERLY: 60 mg q4h for 21 days. Begin within 96 hrs of subarachnoid hemorrhage.

Dosage in Hepatic Failure

PO: ADULTS, ELDERLY: 30 mg q4h.

SIDE EFFECTS

Occasional (6%–2%): Hypotension, peripheral edema, diarrhea, headache. **Rare (less than 2%):** Allergic reaction (rash, urticaria), tachycardia, flushing of skin.

ADVERSE EFFECTS/ TOXIC REACTIONS

Overdose produces nausea, weakness, dizziness, drowsiness, confusion, slurred speech.

NURSING CONSIDERATIONS

BASELINE ASSESSMENT

Assess LOC, neurologic response, initially and throughout therapy. Monitor baseline hepatic function tests. Assess B/P, apical pulse immediately before drug administration (if pulse is 60/min or less or systolic B/P is less than 90 mm Hg, withhold medication, contact physician).

INTERVENTION/EVALUATION

Monitor CNS response, heart rate, B/P for evidence of hypotension, signs/symptoms of CHF.

PATIENT/FAMILY TEACHING

- Do not crush, chew, split capsules.
- Inform physician if palpitations, shortness of breath, swelling, constipation, nausea, dizziness occur.

nitazoxanide

nye-tah-**zocks**-ah-nide
(Alinia)

◆CLASSIFICATION

PHARMACOTHERAPEUTIC: Antiparasitic. **CLINICAL:** Antiprotozoal.

ACTION

Interferes with body's reaction to pyruvate ferredoxin oxidoreductase, an enzyme essential for anaerobic energy metabolism. **Therapeutic Effect:** Produces antiprotozoal activity, reducing/terminating diarrheal episodes.

PHARMACOKINETICS

Rapidly hydrolyzed to active metabolite. Protein binding: 99%. Excreted in urine, bile, feces. **Half-life:** 2–4 hrs.

USES

Treatment of diarrhea caused by *Cryptosporidium parvum, Giardia lamblia* in children 12 mos and older, adults.

PRECAUTIONS

Contraindications: History of sensitivity to aspirin, salicylates. **Cautions:** GI disorders, hepatic/biliary disease, renal impairment.

LIFESPAN CONSIDERATIONS

Pregnancy/Lactation: Unknown if distributed in breast milk. **Pregnancy Category B. Children:** Safety and efficacy not established in those younger than 1 yr (suspension) and younger than 12 yrs (tablet). **Elderly:** Not for use in this age group.

INTERACTIONS

DRUG: None significant. **HERBAL:** None significant. **FOOD:** None known. **LAB VALUES:** May increase serum creatinine, ALT.

AVAILABILITY (Rx)

Powder for Oral Suspension: 100 mg/5 ml. **Tablets:** 500 mg.

ADMINISTRATION/HANDLING

PO (Oral Suspension)

- Store unreconstituted powder at room temperature. • Reconstitute oral suspension with 48 ml water to provide concentration of 100 mg/5 ml. • Shake vigorously to suspend powder. • Reconstituted solution is stable for 7 days at room temperature. • Give with food.

PO (Tablets)

- Give with food.

INDICATIONS/ROUTES/DOSAGE

Diarrhea Caused by *C. Parvum, G. Lamblia*

PO: ADULTS, ELDERLY, CHILDREN 12 YRS AND OLDER: 500 mg q12h for 3 days. **CHILDREN 4–11 YRS:** 200 mg q12h for 3 days. **CHILDREN 12–47 MOS:** 100 mg q12h for 3 days.

SIDE EFFECTS

Occasional (8%): Abdominal pain. **Rare** (2%–1%): Diarrhea, vomiting, headache.

ADVERSE EFFECTS/ TOXIC REACTIONS

None known.

NURSING CONSIDERATIONS

BASELINE ASSESSMENT

Establish baseline B/P, weight, serum glucose, electrolytes. Assess for dehydration.

INTERVENTION/EVALUATION

Evaluate serum glucose in diabetics, electrolytes (therapy generally reduces abnor-

N

malities). Weigh pt daily. Encourage adequate fluid intake. Assess bowel sounds for peristalsis. Monitor daily pattern of bowel activity, stool consistency.

PATIENT/FAMILY TEACHING

• Parents of children with diabetes should be aware that the oral suspension contains 1.48 g of sucrose per 5 ml. • Therapy should provide significant improvement of diarrhea.

Nitro-Bid, *see nitroglycerin*

nitrofurantoin

nye-tro-feur-**an**-toyn
(Apo-Nitrofurantoin, Furadantin, Macrobid, Macrodantin, Novo-Furantoin)

Do not confuse Macrobid with MicroK or Nitro-Bid, or nitrofurantoin with Neurontin or nitroglycerin.

CLASSIFICATION

PHARMACOTHERAPEUTIC: Antibacterial. **CLINICAL:** UTI prophylaxis.

ACTION

Inhibits synthesis of bacterial DNA, RNA, proteins, cell walls by altering, inactivating ribosomal proteins. **Therapeutic Effect:** Bacteriostatic (bactericidal at high concentrations).

PHARMACOKINETICS

Microcrystalline form rapidly, completely absorbed; macrocrystalline form more slowly absorbed. Food increases absorption. Protein binding: 60%. Primarily concentrated in urine, kidneys. Metabolized in most body tissues. Primarily excreted in urine. Removed by hemodialysis. **Half-life:** 20–60 min.

USES

Prevention/treatment of UTI caused by susceptible gram-negative, gram-positive organisms, including *E. coli, S. aureus, Enterococcus, Klebsiella, Enterobacter.*

PRECAUTIONS

Contraindications: Anuria, oliguria, substantial renal impairment (creatinine clearance less than 40 ml/min); infants younger than 1 mo because of risk of hemolytic anemia. **Cautions:** Renal impairment, diabetes mellitus, electrolyte imbalance, anemia, vitamin B deficiency, debilitated (greater risk of peripheral neuropathy), G6PD deficiency (greater risk of hemolytic anemia).

LIFESPAN CONSIDERATIONS

Pregnancy/Lactation: Readily crosses placenta. Distributed in breast milk. Contraindicated at term and during lactation when infant suspected of having G6PD deficiency. **Pregnancy Category B (contraindicated at term). Children:** No age-related precautions noted in those older than 1 mo. **Elderly:** More likely to develop acute pneumonitis, peripheral neuropathy. Age-related renal impairment may require dosage adjustment.

INTERACTIONS

DRUG: Hemolytics may increase risk of toxicity. **Neurotoxic medications** may increase risk of neurotoxicity. **Probenecid** may increase concentration, risk of toxicity. **HERBAL:** None significant. **FOOD:** None known. **LAB VALUES:** May increase ALT, AST, phosphorus. May decrease Hgb.

AVAILABILITY (Rx)

Capsules (Macrocrystalline, Monohydrate [Macrobid]): 100 mg. **Capsules (Macrocrystalline [Macrodantin]):** 25 mg, 50 mg, 100 mg. **Oral Suspension (Microcrystalline [Furadantin]):** 25 mg/5 ml.

ADMINISTRATION/HANDLING

PO

• Give with food, milk to enhance absorption, reduce GI upset. • May mix suspension with water, milk, fruit juice; shake well.

INDICATIONS/ROUTES/DOSAGE

UTI

PO (FURADANTIN, MACRODANTIN): ADULTS, ELDERLY: 50–100 mg q6h. **Maximum:** 400 mg/day. **CHILDREN:** 5–7 mg/kg/day in divided doses q6h. **Maximum:** 400 mg/day.
PO (MACROBID): ADULTS, ELDERLY: 100 mg twice daily. **Maximum:** 400 mg/day.

Long-Term Prevention of UTI

PO: ADULTS, ELDERLY: 50–100 mg at bedtime. **CHILDREN:** 1–2 mg/kg/day as a single dose. **Maximum:** 100 mg/day.

Dosage in Renal Impairment

Contraindicated in pts with creatinine clearance less than 60 ml/min.

SIDE EFFECTS

Frequent: Anorexia, nausea, vomiting, dark urine. **Occasional:** Abdominal pain, diarrhea, rash, pruritus, urticaria, hypertension, headache, dizziness, drowsiness. **Rare:** Photosensitivity, transient alopecia, asthmatic exacerbation in those with history of asthma.

ADVERSE EFFECTS/ TOXIC REACTIONS

Superinfection, hepatotoxicity, peripheral neuropathy (may be irreversible), Stevens-Johnson syndrome, permanent pulmonary impairment, anaphylaxis occur rarely.

NURSING CONSIDERATIONS

BASELINE ASSESSMENT

Question for history of asthma. Evaluate lab test results for renal/hepatic baseline values.

INTERVENTION/EVALUATION

Monitor I&O, renal/hepatic function tests, CBC. Monitor daily pattern of bowel activity and stool consistency. Assess skin for rash, urticaria. Be alert for numbness/tingling, esp. of lower extremities (may signal onset of peripheral neuropathy). Observe for signs of hepatotoxicity (fever, rash, arthralgia, hepatomegaly). Perform respiratory assessment: auscultate lungs, check for cough, chest pain, difficulty breathing.

PATIENT/ FAMILY TEACHING

• Urine may become dark yellow/brown. • Take with food, milk for best results, reduce GI upset. • Complete full course of therapy. • Avoid sun, ultraviolet light; use sunscreen, wear protective clothing. • Notify physician if cough, fever, chest pain, difficult breathing, numbness/tingling of fingers, toes occur. • Rare occurrence of alopecia is transient.

nitroglycerin

nye-troe-**gli**-ser-in
(Minitran, Nitro-Bid, Nitro-Dur, Nitrolingual, NitroQuick, Nitrostat, Nitro-Time, Trinipatch ✱)
Do not confuse Nitro-Bid with Macrobid or Nicobid, Nitro-Dur with Nicoderm, nitroglycerin with nitrofurantoin or nitroprusside, or Nitrostat with Nilstat or Nystatin.

◆CLASSIFICATION

PHARMACOTHERAPEUTIC: Nitrate. **CLINICAL:** Antianginal, antihypertensive, coronary vasodilator (see p. 126C).

ACTION

Decreases myocardial oxygen demand. Reduces left ventricular preload, afterload. **Therapeutic Effect:** Dilates coronary arteries, improves collateral blood flow to ischemic areas within myocardium. IV form produces peripheral vasodilation.

PHARMACOKINETICS

Route	Onset	Peak	Duration
Sublingual	1–3 min	4–8 min	30–60 min
Translingual spray	2 min	4–10 min	30–60 min
Buccal tablet	2–5 min	4–10 min	2 hrs
PO (extended-release)	20–45 min	45–120 min	4–8 hrs
Topical	15–60 min	30–120 min	2–12 hrs
Transdermal patch	40–60 min	60–180 min	18–24 hrs
IV	1–2 min	Immediate	3–5 min

Well absorbed after PO, sublingual, topical administration. Undergoes extensive first-pass metabolism. Metabolized in liver, by enzymes in bloodstream. Protein binding: 60%. Excreted in urine. Not removed by hemodialysis. **Half-life:** 1–4 min.

USES

Lingual, sublingual, buccal dose used for acute relief of angina pectoris. Extended-release, topical forms used for prophylaxis, long-term angina management. IV form used in treatment of CHF, acute MI. **OFF-LABEL:** Esophageal spastic disorders.

PRECAUTIONS

Contraindications: Allergy to adhesives (transdermal), closed-angle glaucoma, constrictive pericarditis (IV), early MI (sublingual), GI hypermotility/malabsorption (extended-release), head trauma, hypotension (IV), inadequate cerebral circulation (IV), increased ICP, nitrates, orthostatic hypotension, pericardial tamponade (IV), severe anemia, uncorrected hypovolemia (IV). **Cautions:** Acute MI, hepatic/renal disease, glaucoma (contraindicated in closed-angle glaucoma), blood volume depletion from diuretic therapy, systolic B/P less than 90 mm Hg.

LIFESPAN CONSIDERATIONS

Pregnancy/Lactation: Unknown if drug crosses placenta or is distributed in breast milk. **Pregnancy Category B. Children:** Safety and efficacy not established. **Elderly:** More susceptible to hypotensive effects. Age-related renal impairment may require dosage adjustment.

INTERACTIONS

DRUG: Alcohol, other antihypertensives, vasodilators may increase risk of orthostatic hypotension. Concurrent use of **sildenafil, tadalafil, vardenafil** produces significant hypotension. **HERBAL: Ephedra, ginger, ginseng, licorice** may increase hypertension. **Black cohosh, goldenseal, hawthorne** may cause hypotension. **FOOD:** None known. **LAB VALUES:** May increase serum methemoglobin, urine, catecholamine concentrations.

AVAILABILITY (Rx)

Infusion, Pre-Mix: 25 mg/250 ml, 50 mg/500 ml (0.1 mg/ml), 50 mg/250 ml (0.2 mg/ml), 100 mg/250 ml, 200 mg/500 ml (0.4 mg/ml). **Injection, Solution:** 5 mg/ml. **Ointment: (Nitro-Bid):** 2%. **Solution, Translingual Spray: (Nitrolingual):** 0.4 mg/spray. **Transdermal Patch: (Minitran, Nitrek, Nitro-Dur):** 0.1 mg/hr, 0.2 mg/hr, 0.3 mg/hr, 0.4 mg/hr, 0.6 mg/hr, 0.8 mg/hr.

Capsules, Extended-Release: (Nitro-Time): 2.5 mg, 6 mg, 9 mg. **Tablets, Sublingual: (NitroQuick, Nitrostat):** 0.4 mg.

ADMINISTRATION/HANDLING

◄ALERT► Cardioverter/defibrillator must not be discharged through paddle electrode overlying nitroglycerin (transdermal, ointment) system (may cause burns to pt or damage to paddle via arcing).

IV

Reconstitution • Available in ready-to-use injectable containers. • Dilute vials in D_5W or 0.9% NaCl. Maximum concentration: 400 mcg/ml. • Use glass bottles.

Rate of administration • Use micro-drop or infusion pump.

Storage • Store at room temperature. • Reconstituted solutions stable for 48 hrs at room temperature or 7 days if refrigerated.

PO

• Do not chew, crush, split extended-release capsules. • Do not shake oral aerosol canister before lingual spraying.

Sublingual

• Do not swallow. • Dissolve under tongue. • Administer while seated. • Slight burning sensation under tongue may be lessened by placing tablet in buccal pouch. • Keep sublingual tablets in original container.

Topical

• Spread thin layer on clean, dry, hairless skin of upper arm or body (not below knee or elbow), using applicator or dose-measuring papers. Do not use fingers; do not rub/massage into skin.

Transdermal

• Apply patch on clean, dry, hairless skin of upper arm or body (not below knee or elbow). • May keep patch on when bathing/showering. • Do not cut/trim to adjust dose.

IV INCOMPATIBILITIES

Alteplase (Activase), phenytoin (Dilantin).

IV COMPATIBILITIES

Amiodarone (Cordarone), diltiazem (Cardizem), dobutamine (Dobutrex), dopamine (Intropin), epinephrine, famotidine (Pepcid), fentanyl (Sublimaze), furosemide (Lasix), heparin, hydromorphone (Dilaudid), insulin, labetalol (Trandate), lidocaine, lipids, lorazepam (Ativan), midazolam (Versed), milrinone (Primacor), morphine, nicardipine (Cardene), nitroprusside (Nipride), norepinephrine (Levophed), propofol (Diprivan).

INDICATIONS/ROUTES/DOSAGE

Acute Treatment/Prophylaxis of Angina Pectoris

LINGUAL SPRAY: ADULTS, ELDERLY: 1–2 sprays onto or under tongue q3–5min until relief is noted (no more than 3 sprays in 15-min period).

SUBLINGUAL: ADULTS, ELDERLY: One tablet under tongue. If chest pain has not improved in 5 min, call 911. After the call, may take additional tablet. A third tablet may be taken 5 min after second dose (maximum of 3 tablets).

Long-Term Prophylaxis of Angina

PO (EXTENDED-RELEASE): ADULTS, ELDERLY: 2.5–9 mg 2–4 times a day. **Maximum:** 26 mg 4 times a day.

TOPICAL: ADULTS, ELDERLY: Initially, ½ inch q8h. Increase by ½ inch with each application. Range: 1–2 inches q8h up to 4–5 inches q4h.

TRANSDERMAL PATCH: ADULTS, ELDERLY: Initially, 0.2–0.4 mg/hr. Maintenance: 0.4–0.8 mg/hr. Consider patch on for 12–14 hrs, patch off for 10–12 hrs (prevents tolerance).

CHF, Acute MI

IV: ADULTS, ELDERLY: Initially, 5 mcg/min via infusion pump. Increase in 5-mcg/min increments at 3- to 5-min intervals until B/P response is noted or until dosage reaches 20 mcg/min, then increase as needed by 10 mcg/min. Dosage may be further titrated according to clinical, therapeutic response up to 200 mcg/min. **CHILDREN:** Initially, 0.25–0.5 mcg/kg/min; titrate by 0.5–1 mcg/kg/min up to 20 mcg/kg/min.

SIDE EFFECTS

Frequent: Headache (possibly severe; occurs mostly in early therapy, diminishes rapidly in intensity, usually disappears during continued treatment), transient flushing of face/neck, dizziness (esp. if pt is standing immobile or is in a warm environment), weakness, orthostatic hypotension. **Sublingual:** Burning, tingling sensation at oral point of dissolution. **Ointment:** Erythema, pruritus. **Occasional:** GI upset. **Transdermal:** Contact dermatitis.

N

ADVERSE EFFECTS/ TOXIC REACTIONS

Discontinue drug if blurred vision, dry mouth occurs. Severe orthostatic hypotension may occur, manifested by syncope, pulselessness, cold/clammy skin, diaphoresis. Tolerance may occur with repeated, prolonged therapy; minor tolerance may occur with intermittent use of sublingual tablets. High doses tend to produce severe headache.

NURSING CONSIDERATIONS

BASELINE ASSESSMENT

Record onset, type (sharp, dull, squeezing), radiation, location, intensity, duration of anginal pain; precipitating factors (exertion, emotional stress). Assess B/P, apical pulse before administration and periodically following dose. Pt must have continuous EKG monitoring for IV administration.

INTERVENTION/EVALUATION

Monitor B/P, heart rate. Assess for facial, neck flushing. Cardioverter/defibrillator must not be discharged through paddle electrode overlying nitroglycerin system (may cause burns to pt or damage to paddle via arcing).

PATIENT/FAMILY TEACHING

• Rise slowly from lying to sitting position, dangle legs momentarily before standing. • Take oral form on empty stomach (however, if headache occurs during therapy, take medication with meals). • Use spray only when lying down. • Dissolve sublingual tablet under tongue; do not swallow. • Take at first sign of angina. • May take another dose q5min if needed up to a total of 3 doses. • If not relieved within 5 min, contact physician or immediately go to emergency room. • Do not change brands. • Keep container away from heat, moisture. • Do not inhale lingual aerosol but spray onto or under tongue (avoid swallowing after spray is administered). • Expel from mouth any remaining lingual, sublingual, intrabuccal tablet after pain is completely relieved. • Place transmucosal tablets under upper lip or buccal pouch (between cheek and gum); do not chew/swallow tablet. • Avoid alcohol (intensifies hypotensive effect). If alcohol is ingested soon after taking nitroglycerin, possible acute hypotensive episode (marked drop in B/P, vertigo, diaphoresis, pallor) may occur.

nitroprusside HIGH ALERT

nye-tro-**pruss**-ide
(Nipride, Nitropress)

BLACK BOX ALERT Must dilute with D_5W. Can cause sharp decrease in B/P; may lead to irreversible ischemia, death. Unless used briefly or at low infusion rate (less than 2 mcg/kg/min), potentially lethal levels of cyanide may result. Do not use maximum dose for longer than 10 min.

Do not confuse nitroprusside with nitroglycerin or Nitrostat.

◆CLASSIFICATION

PHARMACOTHERAPEUTIC: Hypertensive emergency agent. **CLINICAL:** Antihypertensive, vasodilator, CHF/MI adjunct, antidote.

ACTION

Direct vasodilating action on arterial, venous smooth muscle. Decreases peripheral vascular resistance, preload, afterload; improves cardiac output. **Therapeutic Effect:** Dilates coronary arteries, decreases oxygen consumption, relieves persistent chest pain.

PHARMACOKINETICS

Route	Onset	Peak	Duration
IV	Less than 2 min	Dependent on infusion rate	1–10 min

Reacts with Hgb in erythrocytes, producing cyanmethemoglobin, cyanide ions. Primarily excreted in urine. **Half-life:** less than 10 min.

USES

Immediate reduction of B/P in hypertensive crisis. Produces controlled hypotension in surgical procedures to reduce bleeding. Treatment of acute CHF. **OFF-LABEL:** Control of paroxysmal hypertension before, during surgery for pheochromocytoma, peripheral vasospasm caused by ergot alkaloid overdose, treatment adjunct for MI, valvular regurgitation.

PRECAUTIONS

Contraindications: Compensatory hypertension (AV shunt, coarctation of aorta), congenital (Leber's) optic atrophy, inadequate cerebral circulation, moribund pts, tobacco amblyopia (dim vision). **Cautions:** Severe hepatic/renal impairment, hypothyroidism, hyponatremia, elderly.

LIFESPAN CONSIDERATIONS

Pregnancy/Lactation: Unknown if drug crosses placenta or is distributed in breast milk. **Pregnancy Category C. Children:** Safety and efficacy not established. **Elderly:** More sensitive to hypotensive effect. Age-related renal impairment may require dosage adjustment.

INTERACTIONS

DRUG: Dobutamine may increase cardiac output, decrease pulmonary wedge pressure. **Antihypertensives** may increase hypotensive effect. **HERBAL:** None significant. **FOOD:** None known. **LAB VALUES:** None significant.

AVAILABILITY (Rx)

Injection Solution: 25 mg/ml.

ADMINISTRATION/HANDLING

IV

Reconstitution • Dilute with 250–1,000 ml D_5W to provide concentration of 200 mcg, 50 mcg/ml, respectively. **Maximum concentration:** 200 mg/250 ml. • Wrap infusion bottle in aluminum foil immediately after mixing.

Rate of administration • Give by IV infusion only, using infusion rate chart provided by manufacturer or protocol. • Administer using IV infusion pump. • Be alert for extravasation (produces severe pain, sloughing).

Storage • Protect solution from light. • Solution should appear very faint brown. • Use only freshly prepared solution. Once prepared, do not keep or use longer than 24 hrs. • Deterioration evidenced by color change from brown to blue, green, dark red. • Discard unused portion.

IV INCOMPATIBILITY

Cisatracurium (Nimbex).

IV COMPATIBILITIES

Diltiazem (Cardizem), dobutamine (Dobutrex), dopamine (Intropin), enalapril (Vasotec), heparin, insulin, labetalol (Normodyne, Trandate), lidocaine, midazolam (Versed), milrinone (Primacor), nitroglycerin, propofol (Diprivan).

N

INDICATIONS/ROUTES/DOSAGE

Usual Parenteral Dosage

IV INFUSION: ADULTS, ELDERLY, CHILDREN: Initially, 0.3–0.5 mcg/kg/min. May increase by 0.5 mcg/kg/min to desired hemodynamic effect or appearance of headache, nausea. Usual dose: 3 mcg/kg/min. Doses greater than 4 mcg/kg/min rarely needed. **Maximum:** 10 mcg/kg/min (Children: 5 mcg/kg/min).

SIDE EFFECTS

Occasional: Flushing of skin, pruritus, pain/redness at injection site.

ADVERSE EFFECTS/ TOXIC REACTIONS

Too-rapid IV infusion rate reduces B/P too quickly. Nausea, vomiting, diaphoresis, apprehension, headache, restlessness, muscle twitching, dizziness, palpitations, retrosternal pain, abdominal pain may occur. Symptoms disappear rapidly if rate of administration is slowed or temporarily discontinued. Overdose produces metabolic acidosis, tolerance to therapeutic effect.

NURSING CONSIDERATIONS

BASELINE ASSESSMENT

Check with physician for desired B/P parameters (B/P is normally maintained approximately 30%–40% below pretreatment levels). Medication should be discontinued if therapeutic response is not achieved within 10 min after IV infusion at 10 mcg/kg/min.

INTERVENTION/EVALUATION

Monitor EKG, B/P continuously. Monitor blood acid-base balance, electrolytes, laboratory results, I&O. Assess for metabolic acidosis (weakness, disorientation, headache, nausea, hyperventilation, vomiting). Assess for therapeutic response to medication. Monitor B/P for potential rebound hypertension after infusion is discontinued.

N

nizatidine

ni-**za**-ti-deen
(Apo-Nizatidine ✦, Axid, Axid AR, Novo-Nizatidine ✦)
Do not confuse Axid with Ansaid.

◆CLASSIFICATION

PHARMACOTHERAPEUTIC: H_2 receptor antagonist. **CLINICAL:** Antiulcer, gastric acid secretion inhibitor (see p. 108C).

ACTION

Inhibits histamine action at histamine-2 (H_2) receptors of parietal cells. **Therapeutic Effect:** Inhibits basal/nocturnal gastric acid secretion.

PHARMACOKINETICS

Rapidly, well absorbed from GI tract. Protein binding: 35%. Metabolized in liver. Primarily excreted in urine. Not removed by hemodialysis. **Half-life:** 1–2 hrs (increased in renal impairment).

USES

Short-term treatment of active duodenal ulcer, active benign gastric ulcer. Prevention of duodenal ulcer recurrence. Treatment of gastroesophageal reflux disease (GERD), including erosive esophagitis. OTC for prevention of meal-induced heartburn, acid indigestion, sour stomach. **OFF-LABEL:** Gastric hypersecretory conditions, multiple endocrine adenoma, Zollinger-Ellison syndrome, weight gain reduction in pts taking Zyprexa. Part of multidrug therapy for *H. pylori* eradication used to reduce risk of duodenal ulcer recurrence.

PRECAUTIONS

Contraindications: Hypersensitivity to other H_2-antagonists. **Cautions:** Renal/hepatic impairment.

LIFESPAN CONSIDERATIONS

Pregnancy/Lactation: Unknown if drug crosses placenta or is distributed in breast milk. **Pregnancy Category B. Children:** Safety and efficacy not established in those younger than 12 yrs. **Elderly:** No age-related precautions noted.

INTERACTIONS

DRUG: Antacids may decrease absorption (do not give within 1 hr). May decrease absorption of **itraconazole, ketoconazole** (separate by 2 hrs). **HERBAL:** None significant. **FOOD:** None known. **LAB VALUES:** Interferes with skin tests using allergen extracts. May increase serum alkaline phosphatase, AST, ALT.

AVAILABILITY (Rx)

Capsules: 150 mg (Axid), 300 mg (Axid). **Oral Solution (Axid):** 15 mg/ml. **Tablets (Axid AR [OTC]):** 75 mg.

ADMINISTRATION/HANDLING

PO

• Give without regard to meals. Best given after meals or at bedtime. • Do not administer within 1 hr of magnesium- or aluminum-containing antacids (decreases absorption). • May give immediately before eating for heartburn prevention.

INDICATIONS/ROUTES/DOSAGE

Active Duodenal Ulcer

PO: ADULTS, ELDERLY: 300 mg at bedtime or 150 mg twice daily.

Prevention of Duodenal Ulcer Recurrence

PO: ADULTS, ELDERLY: 150 mg at bedtime.

Gastroesophageal Reflux Disease (GERD)

PO: ADULTS, ELDERLY: 150 mg twice a day.

Active Benign Gastric Ulcer

PO: ADULTS, ELDERLY: 150 mg twice daily or 300 mg at bedtime.

PO, ORAL SOLUTION: CHILDREN 12 YRS AND OLDER: 150 mg twice daily.

Meal-Induced Heartburn, Acid Indigestion, Sour Stomach

PO: ADULTS, ELDERLY: 75 mg 30–60 min before meals; no more than 2 tablets a day.

Dosage in Renal Impairment

Dosage adjustment is based on creatinine clearance.

Creatinine Clearance	Active Ulcer	Maintenance Therapy
20–50 ml/min	150 mg at bedtime	150 mg every other day
Less than 20 ml/min	150 mg every other day	150 mg q3days

SIDE EFFECTS

Occasional (2%): Drowsiness, fatigue. **Rare (1%):** Diaphoresis, rash.

ADVERSE EFFECTS/ TOXIC REACTIONS

Asymptomatic ventricular tachycardia, hyperuricemia not associated with gout, nephrolithiasis occur rarely.

NURSING CONSIDERATIONS

INTERVENTION/EVALUATION

Assess for abdominal pain, GI bleeding (overt blood in emesis/stool, tarry stools). Monitor blood tests for elevated AST, ALT, serum alkaline phosphatase (hepatocellular injury).

PATIENT/FAMILY TEACHING

• Avoid tasks that require alertness, motor skills until drug response is established. • Avoid alcohol, aspirin, smoking, excessive amounts of caffeine. • Inform physician if symptoms of heartburn, acid indigestion, sour stomach persist after 2 wks of continuous use of nizatidine.

Nizoral, *see ketoconazole*

Nolvadex, *see tamoxifen*

norepinephrine HIGH ALERT

nor-eh-pih-**nef**-rin
(Levophed)

BLACK BOX ALERT Extravasation may produce severe tissue necrosis, sloughing. Using fine hypodermic needle, liberally infiltrate area with 10–15 ml saline solution containing 5–10 mg phentolamine.

Do not confuse Levophed with Levaquin or levofloxacin, or norepinephrine with epinephrine.

◆CLASSIFICATION

PHARMACOTHERAPEUTIC: Sympathomimetic. **CLINICAL:** Vasopressor (see p. 158C).

ACTION

Stimulates $beta_1$-adrenergic receptors, alpha-adrenergic receptors, increasing

N

peripheral resistance. Enhances contractile myocardial force, increases cardiac output. Constricts resistance, capacitance vessels. **Therapeutic Effect:** Increases systemic B/P, coronary blood flow.

PHARMACOKINETICS

Route	Onset	Peak	Duration
IV	Rapid	1–2 min	N/A

Localized in sympathetic tissue. Metabolized in liver. Primarily excreted in urine.

USES

Corrects hypotension unresponsive to adequate fluid volume replacement (as part of shock syndrome) caused by MI, bacteremia, open heart surgery, renal failure.

PRECAUTIONS

Contraindications: Hypovolemic states (unless as an emergency measure), mesenteric/peripheral vascular thrombosis, profound hypoxia. **Cautions:** Severe cardiac disease, hypertensive or hypothyroid pts, those taking MAOIs.

LIFESPAN CONSIDERATIONS

Pregnancy/Lactation: Readily crosses placenta. May produce fetal anoxia due to uterine contraction, constriction of uterine blood vessels. **Pregnancy Category C. Children/Elderly:** No age-related precautions noted.

INTERACTIONS

DRUG: **Beta-blockers, ergot alkaloids, MAOIs, tricyclic antidepressants** may increase effect. **Atropine** may block bradycardia and enhance vasopressor response. **HERBAL:** None significant. **FOOD:** None known. **LAB VALUES:** None significant.

AVAILABILITY (Rx)

Injection Solution: 1 mg/ml.

ADMINISTRATION/HANDLING

◀ALERT▶ Blood, fluid volume depletion should be corrected before drug is administered.

IV

◀ALERT▶ Dilute only in dextrose-containing solutions (D_5W, D_5NS). Dextrose-containing fluids offer protection against significant loss of potency due to oxidation. Administration in saline solution only is not recommended.

Reconstitution • Add 4 ml (4 mg) to 250 ml D_5W (16 mcg/ml). **Maximum concentration:** 32 ml (32 mg) to 250 ml (128 mcg/ml).

Rate of administration • Closely monitor IV infusion flow rate (use infusion pump). • Monitor B/P q2min during IV infusion until desired therapeutic response is achieved, then q5min during remaining IV infusion. • Never leave pt unattended. • Maintain B/P at 80–100 mm Hg in previously normotensive pts, and 30–40 mm Hg below preexisting B/P in previously hypertensive pts. • Reduce IV infusion gradually. Avoid abrupt withdrawal. • If using peripherally inserted catheter, it is imperative to check the IV site frequently for free flow and infused vein for blanching, hardness to vein, coldness, pallor to extremity. • If extravasation occurs, area should be infiltrated with 10–15 ml sterile saline containing 5–10 mg phentolamine (does not alter pressor effects of norepinephrine).

Storage • Do not use if solution is brown or contains precipitate. • Store at room temperature.

IV INCOMPATIBILITIES

Pantoprazole (Protonix), phenobarbital, phenytoin (Dilantin), regular insulin.

IV COMPATIBILITIES

Amiodarone (Cordarone), calcium gluconate, diltiazem (Cardizem), dobutamine (Dobutrex), dopamine (Intropin), epinephrine, esmolol (Brevibloc), fentanyl (Sublimaze), furosemide (Lasix), haloperidol (Haldol), heparin, hydromorphone (Dilaudid), labetalol (Trandate), lipids, lorazepam (Ativan), magnesium, midazolam (Versed), milrinone (Primacor), morphine, nicardipine (Cardene), nitroglycerin, potassium chloride, propofol (Diprivan).

INDICATIONS/ROUTES/DOSAGE

Acute Hypotension Unresponsive to Fluid Volume Replacement

IV: ADULTS, ELDERLY: Initially, administer at 0.5–1 mcg/min. Adjust rate of flow to establish and maintain desired B/P (40 mm Hg below preexisting systolic pressure). Average maintenance dose: 8–30 mcg/min. **CHILDREN:** Initially, 0.05–0.1 mcg/kg/min; titrate to desired effect. **Maximum:** 1–2 mcg/kg/min.

SIDE EFFECTS

Norepinephrine produces less pronounced, less frequent side effects than epinephrine. **Occasional (5%–3%):** Anxiety, bradycardia, palpitations. **Rare (2%–1%):** Nausea, anginal pain, shortness of breath, fever.

ADVERSE EFFECTS/ TOXIC REACTIONS

Extravasation may produce tissue necrosis, sloughing. Overdose manifested as severe hypertension with violent headache (may be first clinical sign of overdose), arrhythmias, photophobia, retrosternal or pharyngeal pain, pallor, diaphoresis, vomiting. Prolonged therapy may result in plasma volume depletion. Hypotension may recur if plasma volume is not maintained.

NURSING CONSIDERATIONS

BASELINE ASSESSMENT

Assess EKG, B/P continuously (be alert to precipitous B/P drop). Never leave pt alone during IV infusion. Be alert to pt complaint of headache.

INTERVENTION/EVALUATION

Monitor IV flow rate diligently. Assess for extravasation characterized by blanching of skin over vein, coolness (results from local vasoconstriction); color, temperature of IV site extremity (pallor, cyanosis, mottling). Assess nailbed capillary refill. Monitor I&O; measure output hourly, report urine output less than 30 ml/hr. Once B/P parameter has been reached, IV infusion should not be restarted unless systolic B/P falls below 70–80 mm Hg.

norfloxacin

nor-**flox**-a-sin
(Apo-Norflox ✱, Norfloxacine ✱, Noroxin, Novo-Norfloxacin ✱, PMS-Norfloxacin ✱)

BLACK BOX ALERT May increase risk of tendonitis, tendon rupture.

Do not confuse norfloxacin with Norflex, or Noroxin with Neurontin.

◆CLASSIFICATION

PHARMACOTHERAPEUTIC: Quinolone. **CLINICAL:** Anti-infective (see p. 25C).

ACTION

Interferes with bacterial cell replication by inhibiting DNA-gyrase in susceptible microorganisms. **Therapeutic Effect:** Bactericidal.

USES

Treatment of susceptible infections due to *E. faecalis, E. coli, K. pneumoniae, P. mirabilis, P. aeruginosa, S. epidermidis, S. saprophyticus,* including UTIs, uncomplicated gonococcal infections, acute or chronic prostatitis.

PRECAUTIONS

Contraindications: Children younger than 18 yrs (increased risk of arthropathy), hypersensitivity to other quinolones or their components. **Cautions:** Renal impairment, predisposition to seizures.

⧖ LIFESPAN CONSIDERATIONS

Pregnancy/Lactation: Unknown if drug crosses placenta or is distributed in breast milk. **Pregnancy Category C. Children:**

Safety and efficacy not established. **Elderly:** Age-related renal impairment may require dosage adjustment.

INTERACTIONS

DRUG: **Antacids, sucralfate** may decrease absorption. May increase effects of **oral anticoagulants. Didanosine** may decrease absorption, effect. Decreases clearance of **theophylline**, may increase concentration, risk of toxicity. HERBAL: **Dong quai, St. John's wort** may increase risk of photosensitization. FOOD: None known. LAB VALUES: May increase serum alkaline phosphatase, LDH, AST, ALT, amylase.

AVAILABILITY (Rx)

Tablets: 400 mg.

ADMINISTRATION/HANDLING

PO

• Give 1 hr before or 2 hrs after meals with 8 oz of water. • Encourage additional glasses of water between meals. • Do not administer antacids with or within 2 hrs of norfloxacin dose. • Encourage cranberry juice, citrus fruits (to acidify urine).

INDICATIONS/ROUTES/DOSAGE

UTI

PO: ADULTS, ELDERLY: 400 mg twice daily for 3–21 days.

Prostatitis

PO: ADULTS: 400 mg twice daily for 4–6 wks.

Gonorrhea

PO: ADULTS, ELDERLY: 800 mg as a single dose.

Dosage in Renal Impairment

Dosage and frequency are modified based on creatinine clearance.

Creatinine Clearance	Dosage
30 ml/min or higher	400 mg twice daily
Less than 30 ml/min	400 mg once daily

SIDE EFFECTS

Frequent: Nausea, headache, dizziness. Rare: Vomiting, diarrhea, dry mouth, bitter taste, anxiety, drowsiness, insomnia, photosensitivity, tinnitus, crystalluria, rash, fever, seizures.

ADVERSE EFFECTS/ TOXIC REACTIONS

Superinfection, anaphylaxis, Stevens-Johnson syndrome, arthropathy occur rarely. Hypersensitivity reactions, including photosensitivity (rash, pruritus, blisters, edema, burning skin) may be noted.

NURSING CONSIDERATIONS

BASELINE ASSESSMENT

Question for history of hypersensitivity to norfloxacin, quinolones.

INTERVENTION/EVALUATION

Assess for nausea, headache, dizziness. Evaluate food tolerance. Assess for chest, joint pain (arthropathy).

PATIENT/FAMILY TEACHING

• Take 1 hr before or 2 hrs after meals. • Complete full course of therapy. • Take with 8 oz of water; drink several glasses of water between meals. • May cause dizziness, drowsiness. • Do not take antacids with or within 2 hrs of norfloxacin dose (reduces or destroys effectiveness).

Normodyne, *see labetalol*

Norpramin, *see desipramine*

nortriptyline

nor-**trip**-ti-leen
(Apo-Nortriptyline 🍁, Aventyl 🍁, Norventyl 🍁, Novo-Nortriptyline 🍁, Pamelor)

BLACK BOX ALERT Increased risk of suicidal thinking and behavior in children, adolescents, young adults 18–24 yrs with major depressive disorder, other psychiatric disorders.

Do not confuse Aventyl with Bentyl, or nortriptyline with amitriptyline, desipramine, or Norpramin.

CLASSIFICATION

PHARMACOTHERAPEUTIC: Tricyclic compound. **CLINICAL:** Antidepressant (see pp. 38C, 156C).

ACTION

Blocks reuptake of neurotransmitters (norepinephrine, serotonin) at neuronal presynaptic membranes, increasing their availability at postsynaptic receptor sites. **Therapeutic Effect:** Relieves depression, anxiety disorders, nocturnal enuresis.

USES

Treatment of various forms of depression, often in conjunction with psychotherapy. Treatment of nocturnal enuresis. **OFF-LABEL:** Treatment of neurogenic pain, panic disorder; prevention of migraine headache. Treatment of chronic pain, anxiety disorders, ADHD, adjunctive therapy for smoking cessation.

PRECAUTIONS

Contraindications: Acute recovery period after MI, MAOI use within 14 days. **Cautions:** Prostatic hyperplasia, history of urinary retention/obstruction, glaucoma, diabetes mellitus, history of seizures, hyperthyroidism, cardiac/hepatic/renal disease, schizophrenia, increased intraocular pressure, hiatal hernia. **Pregnancy Category C.**

INTERACTIONS

DRUG: **Alcohol, other CNS depressants** may increase CNS effects, respiratory depression, hypotensive effects. **Antithyroid agents** may increase risk of agranulocytosis. **Cimetidine** may increase concentration, risk of toxicity. May decrease effects of **clonidine. MAOIs** may increase risk of neuroleptic malignant syndrome, seizures, hyperpyrexia, hypertensive crisis. **Phenothiazines** may increase anticholinergic, sedative effects. **Sympathomimetics** may increase risk of cardiac effects. **HERBAL:** **Gotu kola, kava kava, St. John's wort, valerian** may increase CNS depression. **FOOD:** None known. **LAB VALUES:** May alter serum glucose, EKG readings. Therapeutic peak serum level: 6–10 mcg/ml; therapeutic trough serum level: 0.5–2 mcg/ml. Toxic peak serum level: greater than 12 mcg/ml; toxic trough serum level: greater than 2 mcg/ml.

AVAILABILITY (Rx)

Capsules (Pamelor): 10 mg, 25 mg, 50 mg, 75 mg. **Oral Solution (Pamelor):** 10 mg/5 ml.

ADMINISTRATION/HANDLING

◀ALERT▶ At least 14 days must elapse between use of MAOIs and nortriptyline.

PO

- Give with food, milk if GI distress occurs.

INDICATIONS/ROUTES/DOSAGE

Depression

PO: ADULTS: 25 mg 3–4 times a day up to 150 mg/day. **ELDERLY:** Initially, 10–25 mg at bedtime. May increase by 25 mg every 3–7 days. **Maximum:** 150 mg/day. **CHILDREN 12 YRS AND OLDER:** 30–50 mg/day in 3–4 divided doses. **Maximum:** 150 mg/day. **CHILDREN 6–11 YRS:** 10–20 mg/day in 3–4 divided doses.

Enuresis

PO: CHILDREN 12 YRS AND OLDER: 25–35 mg/day. **CHILDREN 8–11 YRS:** 10–20 mg/day. **CHILDREN 6–7 YRS:** 10 mg/day.

SIDE EFFECTS

Frequent: Drowsiness, fatigue, dry mouth, blurred vision, constipation, delayed mic-

N

turition, orthostatic hypotension, diaphoresis, impaired concentration, increased appetite, urinary retention. **Occasional:** GI disturbances (nausea, GI distress, metallic taste), photosensitivity. **Rare:** Paradoxical reactions (agitation, restlessness, nightmares, insomnia), extrapyramidal symptoms (particularly fine hand tremor).

ADVERSE EFFECTS/ TOXIC REACTIONS

High dosage may produce cardiovascular effects (severe orthostatic hypotension, dizziness, tachycardia, palpitations, arrhythmias), altered temperature regulation (hyperpyrexia, hypothermia). Abrupt discontinuation from prolonged therapy may produce headache, malaise, nausea, vomiting, vivid dreams.

NURSING CONSIDERATIONS

BASELINE ASSESSMENT

Assess for suicidal ideation/tendencies, behavior, thought content, appearance, baseline glucose, cholesterol levels. For pts on long-term therapy, hepatic/renal function tests, blood counts should be performed periodically.

INTERVENTION/EVALUATION

Supervise suicidal-risk pt closely during early therapy (as depression lessens, energy level improves, increasing suicide potential). Assess appearance, behavior, speech pattern, level of interest, mood. Monitor daily pattern of bowel activity and stool consistency. Avoid constipation with increased fluids, bulky foods. Monitor B/P, pulse for hypotension, arrhythmias, weight. Assess for urinary retention, including output estimate, bladder palpation if indicated. Therapeutic peak serum level: 6–10 mcg/ml; trough serum level: 0.5–2 mcg/ml. Toxic peak serum level: greater than 12 mcg/ml; toxic trough: greater than 2 mcg/ml.

PATIENT/FAMILY TEACHING

• Change positions slowly to avoid hypotensive effect. • Tolerance to postural hypotension, sedative, anticholinergic effects usually develops during early therapy. • Avoid alcohol. • Avoid tasks that require alertness, motor skills until response to drug is established. • Therapeutic effect may be noted in 2 wks or longer. • Photosensitivity to sun may occur. • Use sunscreen, protective clothing. • Dry mouth may be relieved by sugarless gum, sips of tepid water. • Report visual disturbances, worsening depression, suicidal ideation, unusual changes in behavior (esp. at initiation of therapy or with changes in dosage). • Do not abruptly discontinue medication.

Norvasc, *see amlodipine*

nystatin

nye-**stat**-in
(Bio-Statin, Mycostatin, Nilstat ✤, Nystat-Rx, Nystop, Pedi-Dri)
Do not confuse Mycostatin with Nitrostat, or nystatin with atorvastatin, fluvastatin, lovastatin, Nitrostat, pitavastatin, pravastatin, rosuvastatin, or simvastatin.

FIXED-COMBINATION(S)

Mycolog, Myco-Triacet: nystatin/triamcinolone (a steroid): 100,000 units/0.1%.

◆CLASSIFICATION

CLINICAL: Antifungal (see p. 49C).

ACTION

Binds to sterols in cell membrane, increasing fungal cell-membrane permeability, permitting loss of potassium, other cellular components. **Therapeutic Effect:** Fungistatic.

PHARMACOKINETICS

PO: Poorly absorbed from GI tract. Eliminated unchanged in feces. **Topical:** Not absorbed systemically from intact skin.

USES

Treatment of cutaneous, intestinal, oral cavity, vaginal fungal infections caused by *Candida* spp. **OFF-LABEL:** Prophylaxis, treatment of oropharyngeal candidiasis, tinea barbae, tinea capitis.

PRECAUTIONS

Contraindications: None known. **Cautions:** None known.

⌛ LIFESPAN CONSIDERATIONS

Pregnancy/Lactation: Unknown if distributed in breast milk. Vaginal applicators may be contraindicated, requiring manual insertion of tablets during pregnancy. **Pregnancy Category B (C: oral). Children:** No age-related precautions noted for suspension, topical use. Lozenges not recommended in those younger than 5 yrs. **Elderly:** No age-related precautions noted.

INTERACTIONS

DRUG: None significant. **HERBAL:** None significant. **FOOD:** None known. **LAB VALUES:** None significant.

AVAILABILITY (Rx)

Capsules (Bio-Statin): 500,000 units, 1,000,000 units. **Cream (Mycostatin Topical):** 100,000 units/g. **Ointment:** 100,000 units/g. **Oral Suspension (Mycostatin):** 100,000 units/ml. **Tablets (Mycostatin):** 500,000 units. **Topical Powder (Mycostatin Topical, Nystop, Pedi-Dri):** 100,000 units/g. **Vaginal Tablets:** 100,000 units.

ADMINISTRATION/HANDLING

PO

• Shake suspension well before administration. • Place and hold suspension in mouth or swish throughout mouth as long as possible before swallowing.

INDICATIONS/ROUTES/DOSAGE

Intestinal Infection

PO: ADULTS, ELDERLY: 500,000–1,000,000 units q8h.

Oral Candidiasis

PO: ADULTS, ELDERLY, CHILDREN: 400,000–600,000 units 4 times a day. **INFANTS:** 200,000 units 4 times a day.

Vaginal Infections

VAGINAL: ADULTS, ELDERLY: 1 tablet/day at bedtime for 14 days.

Cutaneous Candidal Infections

TOPICAL: ADULTS, ELDERLY, CHILDREN: Apply 2–4 times a day.

SIDE EFFECTS

Occasional: PO: None known. **Topical:** Skin irritation. **Vaginal:** Vaginal irritation.

ADVERSE EFFECTS/ TOXIC REACTIONS

High dosages of oral form may produce nausea, vomiting, diarrhea, GI distress.

NURSING CONSIDERATIONS

BASELINE ASSESSMENT

Confirm that cultures, histologic tests were done for accurate diagnosis. Inspect oral mucous membranes.

INTERVENTION/EVALUATION

Assess for increased irritation with topical, increased vaginal discharge with vaginal application.

PATIENT/FAMILY TEACHING

• Do not miss doses; complete full length of treatment (continue vaginal use during menses). • Notify physician if nausea, vomiting, diarrhea, stomach pain develops. • **Vaginal:** Insert high in vagina. • Check with physician regarding douching, sexual intercourse. • **Topical:** Rub well into affected areas. • Avoid contact with eyes. • Use cream (sparingly) or powder on erythematous areas. • Keep areas clean, dry; wear light clothing for ventilation. • Separate personal items in contact with affected areas.

octreotide

ok-**tree**-oh-tide
(Sandostatin, Sandostatin LAR Depot)
Do not confuse Sandostatin with Sandimmune, Sandostatin LAR, sargramostim, or simvastatin.

CLASSIFICATION

CLINICAL: Secretory inhibitory, growth hormone suppressant.

ACTION

Suppresses secretion of serotonin, gastroenteropancreatic peptides. Enhances fluid/electrolyte absorption from GI tract. **Therapeutic Effect:** Prolongs intestinal transit time.

O

PHARMACOKINETICS

Route	Onset	Peak	Duration
Subcutaneous	N/A	N/A	Up to 12 hrs

Rapidly, completely absorbed from injection site. Protein binding: 65%. Metabolized in liver. Excreted in urine. Removed by hemodialysis. **Half-life:** 1.7–1.9 hrs.

USES

Controls diarrhea in pts with metastatic carcinoid tumors, vasoactive intestinal peptic-secreting tumors (VIPomas), secretory diarrhea, acromegaly. **OFF-LABEL:** Control of bleeding esophageal varices, treatment of AIDS-associated secretory diarrhea, chemotherapy-induced diarrhea, insulinomas, small-bowel fistulas, Zollinger-Ellison syndrome.

PRECAUTIONS

Contraindications: None known. **Cautions:** Insulin-dependent diabetes, renal failure.

LIFESPAN CONSIDERATIONS

Pregnancy/Lactation: Unknown if distributed in breast milk. **Pregnancy Category B. Children:** Safety and efficacy not established. **Elderly:** No age-related precautions noted.

INTERACTIONS

DRUG: May decrease effectiveness of **cyclosporine. Glucagon, growth hormone, insulin, oral antidiabetics** may alter glucose concentrations. **HERBAL: Garlic, ginger, ginseng** may increase hypoglycemic effect. **FOOD:** None known. **LAB VALUES:** May decrease serum thyroxine (T_4). May increase ALT, AST, alkaline phosphatase, GGT.

AVAILABILITY (Rx)

Injection Solution (Sandostatin): 0.05 mg/ml, 0.1 mg/ml, 0.2 mg/ml, 0.5 mg/ml, 1 mg/ml. **Injection Suspension (Sandostatin LAR Depot):** 10-mg, 20-mg, 30-mg vials.

ADMINISTRATION/HANDLING

◀ALERT▶ Sandostatin may be given IV, IM, subcutaneous. Sandostatin LAR Depot may be given only IM.

IM

• Give immediately after mixing. • Administer deep IM in large muscle mass at 4-wk intervals. • Avoid deltoid injections.

Subcutaneous

• Do not use if discolored or particulates form. • Avoid multiple injections at same site within short periods.

IV

• Dilute in 50–100 ml 0.9% NaCl or D_5W and infuse over 15–30 min.

INDICATIONS/ROUTES/DOSAGE

Diarrhea

IV (SANDOSTATIN): ADULTS, ELDERLY: Initially, 50–100 mcg q8h. May increase by 100 mcg/dose q48h. **Maximum:** 500 mcg q8h.

SUBCUTANEOUS (SANDOSTATIN): ADULTS, ELDERLY: 50 mcg 1–2 times a day.

Carcinoid Tumor

IV, SUBCUTANEOUS (SANDOSTATIN): ADULTS, ELDERLY: Initial 2 wks, 100–600 mcg/day in 2–4 divided doses. Range: 50–1,500 mcg.
IM (SANDOSTATIN LAR DEPOT): ADULTS, ELDERLY: Must be stabilized on subcutaneous octreotide for at least 2 wks. 20 mg q4wk.

Vasoactive Intestinal Peptic-Secreting Tumor (VIPoma)

IV, SUBCUTANEOUS (SANDOSTATIN): ADULTS, ELDERLY: Initial 2 wks, 200–300 mcg/day in 2–4 divided doses. Range: 150–750 mcg.
IM (SANDOSTATIN LAR DEPOT): ADULTS, ELDERLY: Must be stabilized on subcutaneous octreotide for at least 2 wks. 20 mg q4wk.

Esophageal Varices

IV (SANDOSTATIN): ADULTS, ELDERLY: Bolus of 25–50 mcg followed by IV infusion of 25–50 mcg/hr for 48 hrs.

Acromegaly

IV, SUBCUTANEOUS (SANDOSTATIN): ADULTS, ELDERLY: 50 mcg 3 times a day. Increase as needed. Range: 300–1,500 mcg/day.
IM (SANDOSTATIN LAR DEPOT): ADULTS, ELDERLY: Must be stabilized on subcutaneous octreotide for at least 2 wks. 20 mg q4wk for 3 mos. **Maximum:** 40 mg q4wk.

SIDE EFFECTS

Frequent (10%–6%, 58%–30% in acromegaly pts): Diarrhea, nausea, abdominal discomfort, headache, injection site pain. **Occasional (5%–1%):** Vomiting, flatulence, constipation, alopecia, facial flushing, pruritus, dizziness, fatigue, arrhythmias, ecchymosis, blurred vision. **Rare (less than 1%):** Depression, diminished libido, vertigo, palpitations, dyspnea.

ADVERSE EFFECTS/ TOXIC REACTIONS

Increased risk of cholelithiasis. Prolonged high-dose therapy may produce hypothyroidism. GI bleeding, hepatitis, seizures occur rarely.

NURSING CONSIDERATIONS

BASELINE ASSESSMENT

Establish baseline B/P, weight, serum glucose, electrolytes.

INTERVENTION/EVALUATION

Monitor serum glucose, thyroid function tests; fluid, electrolyte balance; fecal fat. In acromegaly, monitor growth hormone levels. Weigh every 2–3 days, report over 5 lb gain per wk. Monitor B/P, pulse, respirations periodically during treatment. Be alert for decreased urinary output, peripheral edema (esp. ankles). Monitor daily pattern of bowel activity, stool consistency.

PATIENT/FAMILY TEACHING

- Therapy should provide significant improvement of severe, watery diarrhea.

O

ocular lubricant

ock-you-lar **lube**-rih-cant
(Hypotears, Lacrilube, Tears Naturale)

◆ CLASSIFICATION

PHARMACOTHERAPEUTIC: Topical ophthalmic. **CLINICAL:** Lubricant, toner, buffer, viscosity agent.

ACTION

Forms an occlusive film on eye surface. **Therapeutic Effect:** Lubricates/protects eye from drying.

USES

Protection/lubrication of eye in exposure keratitis, decreased corneal sensitivity, recurrent corneal erosions, keratitis sicca (particularly for nighttime use), after removal of foreign body, during and following surgery.

PRECAUTIONS

Contraindications: None known. **Cautions:** None known. **Pregnancy Category Unknown.**

INTERACTIONS

DRUG: None significant. **HERBAL:** None significant. **FOOD:** None known. **LAB VALUES:** None significant.

AVAILABILITY (OTC)

Ophthalmic Ointment. Solution.

ADMINISTRATION/HANDLING

Ophthalmic

• Do not use with contact lenses. • Place gloved finger on lower eyelid and pull out until a pocket is formed between eye and lower lid. • Place prescribed number of drops (¼-½ inch of ointment) into pocket. • Instruct pt to close eye gently (so medication will not be squeezed out of the sac).

Solution

• Instruct pt to apply digital pressure to lacrimal sac at inner canthus for 1 min to minimize systemic absorption.

Ointment

• Instruct pt to roll eyeball to increase contact area of drug to eye.

INDICATIONS/ROUTES/DOSAGE

Usual Ophthalmic Dosage

OPHTHALMIC: ADULTS, ELDERLY: Small amount in conjunctival sac as needed.

SIDE EFFECTS

Frequent: Temporary blurred vision after administration, esp. with ointment.

ADVERSE EFFECTS/ TOXIC REACTIONS

None known.

NURSING CONSIDERATIONS

PATIENT/FAMILY TEACHING

• Do not use with contact lenses. • Do not touch tip of tube or dropper to any surface (may contaminate). • Temporary blurred vision will occur, esp. with administration of ointment. • Avoid activities requiring visual acuity until blurring clears. • Notify physician if eye pain, change of vision, worsening of condition occur or if condition is unchanged after 72 hrs.

ofatumumab

oh-fah-**too**-mue-mab
(Arzerra)

◆CLASSIFICATION

PHARMACOTHERAPEUTIC: Monoclonal antibody. **CLINICAL:** Antineoplastic.

ACTION

Binds to CD20 molecule, the antigen on surface of B cell lymphocytes; inhibits early-stage B lymphocyte activation. **Therapeutic Effect:** Controls tumor growth, triggers cell death.

PHARMACOKINETICS

Eliminated through both a target-independent route and a B-cell–mediated route. Due to depletion of B cells, clearance of ofatumumab is decreased substantially after subsequent infusions compared to first infusion. **Half-life:** 12–16 days.

USES

Treatment of chronic lymphocytic leukemia (CLL) refractory to fludarabine and alemtuzumab.

PRECAUTIONS

Contraindications: None known. **Cautions:** Interstitial pneumonitis, pulmonary fibrosis, pulmonary infiltrates, COPD. Carriers of hepatitis B virus.

LIFESPAN CONSIDERATIONS

Pregnancy/Lactation: Unknown if distributed in breast milk. **Pregnancy Category C. Children:** Safety and efficacy not established. **Elderly:** No age-related precautions noted.

INTERACTIONS

DRUG: **Bone marrow depressants** may increase myelosuppression. **Live virus vaccines** may potentiate virus replication, increase vaccine side effects, decrease pt's response to vaccine. **HERBAL:** None significant. **FOOD:** None known. **LAB VALUES:** May decrease WBC count, platelets.

AVAILABILITY (Rx)

Solution for Injection: 100 mg/5 ml single-use vial.

ADMINSTRATION/HANDLING

IV

ALERT Do not give by IV push or bolus. Use in-line filter supplied with product.

Reconstitution • 300-mg dose: Withdraw and discard 15 ml from 1,000 ml 0.9% NaCl. • Withdraw 5 ml from each of 3 vials and add to bag. • Gently invert. • 2,000-mg dose: Withdraw and discard 100 ml from 1,000 ml 0.9% NaCl. • Withdraw 5 ml from each of 20 vials and add to bag. • Gently invert.

Rate of administration • Dose 1: Initiate infusion at rate of 3.6 mg/hr (12 ml/hr). • Dose 2: Initiate infusion at rate of 24 mg/hr (12 ml/hr). • Doses 3–12: Initiate infusion at rate of 50 mg/hr (25 ml/hr). • If no infusion toxicity, rate of infusion may be increased every 30 min, using following table:

Interval after start of infusion (min)	Dose 1 (ml/hr)	Dose 2 (ml/hr)	Doses 3–12 (ml/hr)
0–30	12	12	25
31–60	25	25	50
61–90	50	50	100
91–120	100	100	200
Over 120	200	200	400

Storage • Refrigerate vials. • After dilution, solution should be used within first 12 hrs; discard preparation after 24 hrs. • Discard if discoloration is present, but solution may contain visible, translucent-to-white particulates (will be removed by in-line filter).

IV COMPATIBILITY

Prepare all doses with 0.9% NaCl. Do not mix with dextrose solutions or any other medications.

INDICATIONS/ROUTES/DOSAGE

ALERT Premedicate 30 min to 2 hrs before each infusion with acetaminophen, an antihistamine, and a corticosteroid. Flush IV line with 0.9% NaCl before and after each dose.

Chronic Lymphocytic Leukemia

IV INFUSION: ADULTS, ELDERLY: Recommended dosage is 12 doses given on the following schedule: 300 mg initial dose (dose 1), followed 1 wk later by 2,000 mg weekly for 7 doses (Doses 2–8), followed 4 wks later by 2,000 mg every 4 wks for 4 doses (Doses 9–12).

SIDE EFFECTS

Frequent (20%–14%): Fever, cough, diarrhea, fatigue, rash. **Occasional (19%–5%):** Nausea, bronchitis, peripheral edema, nasopharyngitis, urticaria, insomnia, headache, sinusitis, muscle spasm, hypertension.

ADVERSE EFFECTS/ TOXIC REACTIONS

Most common serious adverse reactions were bacterial, viral, fungal infections (including pneumonia and sepsis), septic shock, neutropenia, thrombocytopenia. Infusion reactions occur more frequently with first 2 infusions. Severe infusion reactions manifested as angioedema, bronchospasm, dyspnea, fever, chills, back pain, hypotension. Progressive multifocal leukoencephalopathy may occur. Obstruction of small intestine has been noted.

O

NURSING CONSIDERATIONS

BASELINE ASSESSMENT

Screen pts at high risk of hepatitis B virus. Assess baseline CBC, platelet count prior to therapy.

INTERVENTION/EVALUATION

Monitor CBC for evidence of myelosuppression during therapy, and increase frequency of monitoring in pts who develop grade 3 or 4 cytopenia. Monitor for blood dyscrasias (fever, sore throat, signs of local infection, unusual bruising/bleeding from any site), symptoms of anemia (excessive fatigue, weakness).

PATIENT/FAMILY TEACHING

• Do not have immunizations without physician's approval (lowers body's resistance). • Avoid contact with those who have recently received live virus vaccine. • Avoid crowds, those with infection. • Promptly report fever, sore throat, signs of infection. • Report symptoms of infusion reactions (e.g., fever, chills, breathing problems, rash); bleeding, bruising, petechiae, worsening weakness or fatigue; new neurological symptoms (e.g., confusion, loss of balance, vision problems); symptoms of hepatitis (e.g., fatigue, yellow discoloration of skin/eyes); worsening abdominal pain, nausea.

O

ofloxacin

o-**flox**-a-sin
(Apo-Oflox ✦, Apo-Ofloxacin ✦, Floxin, Floxin Otic, Novo-Ofloxacin ✦, Ocuflox)

BLACK BOX ALERT May increase risk of tendonitis, tendon rupture.

Do not confuse Floxin with Flexeril, or Ocuflox with Ocufen.

◆CLASSIFICATION

PHARMACOTHERAPEUTIC: Fluoroquinolone. **CLINICAL:** Antibiotic (see p. 25C).

ACTION

Interferes with bacterial cell replication, repair by inhibiting DNA-gyrase in susceptible microorganisms. **Therapeutic Effect:** Bactericidal.

PHARMACOKINETICS

Rapidly, well absorbed from GI tract. Protein binding: 20%–25%. Widely distributed (including CSF). Metabolized in liver. Primarily excreted in urine. Removed by hemodialysis. **Half-life:** 4.7–7 hrs (increased in renal impairment, cirrhosis, elderly).

USES

Treatment of susceptible infections due to *S. pneumoniae, S. aureus, S. pyogenes, H. influenzae, P. mirabilis, N. gonorrhoeae, C. trachomatis, E. coli, K. pneumoniae, P. aeruginosa,* including infections of urinary tract, lower respiratory tract, skin/skin structure; sexually transmitted diseases; prostatitis due to *E. coli;* pelvic inflammatory disease (PID). **Ophthalmic:** Bacterial conjunctivitis, corneal ulcers. **Otic:** Otitis externa, acute or chronic otitis media. **OFF-LABEL:** Epididymitis, leprosy, traveler's diarrhea.

PRECAUTIONS

Contraindications: Children 18 yrs and younger, hypersensitivity to any quinolones. **Cautions:** Renal impairment, CNS disorders, seizures, those taking theophylline, caffeine. May mask/delay symptoms of syphilis; serologic test for syphilis should be done at diagnosis and 3 mos after treatment.

⧗ LIFESPAN CONSIDERATIONS

Pregnancy/Lactation: Distributed in breast milk; potentially serious adverse reactions in breast-feeding infants. Risk of arthropathy to fetus. **Pregnancy Category C. Children:** Safety and efficacy not established (otic not established in those younger than 1 yr). **Elderly:** No age-related precautions for otic. Age-related renal impairment may require dosage adjustment for oral administration.

INTERACTIONS

DRUG: **Antacids, sucralfate** may decrease absorption, effect. May increase effects of **caffeine. Didanosine** may decrease absorption, effect. May increase **theophylline** concentration, risk of toxicity. **HERBAL:** **Dong quai, St. John's wort** may increase photosensitization. **FOOD:** None known. **LAB VALUES:** May increase ALT, AST, alkaline phosphatase, amylase, LDH.

AVAILABILITY (Rx)

Ophthalmic Solution (Ocuflox): 0.3%. **Otic Solution (Floxin):** 0.3%. **Tablets (Floxin):** 200 mg, 300 mg, 400 mg.

ADMINISTRATION/HANDLING

PO

• Do not give with food; preferred dosing time is 1 hr before or 2 hrs following meals. • Do not administer antacids (aluminum, magnesium) or iron/zinc-containing products within 2 hrs of ofloxacin. • Encourage cranberry juice, citrus fruits (to acidify urine). • Give with 8 oz of water; encourage fluid intake.

Ophthalmic

• Place gloved finger on lower eyelid and pull out until a pocket is formed between eye and lower lid. Place prescribed number of drops into pocket. Instruct pt to close eye gently (so medication will not be squeezed out of the sac) and apply digital pressure to lacrimal sac at inner canthus for 1 min to minimize systemic absorption.

Otic

• Instruct pt to lie down with head turned so affected ear is upright. • Instill toward canal wall, not directly on eardrum. • Pull auricle down and posterior in children; up and posterior in adults.

INDICATIONS/ROUTES/DOSAGE

Usual Dosage Range

PO: ADULTS, ELDERLY: 200–400 mg q12h. **OPHTHALMIC: ADULTS, ELDERLY, CHILDREN 1 YR AND OLDER:** 1–2 drops q30min to 4 hrs. **OTIC: ADULTS, ELDERLY, CHILDREN OLDER THAN 12 YRS:** 10 drops 1–2 times/day. **CHILDREN 6 MOS–12YRS:** 5 drops once daily.

UTI

PO: ADULTS: 200 mg q12h for 3–10 days.

Pelvic Inflammatory Disease (PID)

PO: ADULTS: 400 mg q12h for 10–14 days.

Lower Respiratory Tract, Skin/Skin Structure Infection

PO: ADULTS: 400 mg q12h for 10 days.

Prostatitis, Sexually Transmitted Disease (Cervicitis, Urethritis)

PO: ADULTS: 400 mg once, then 300 mg q12h for 10 days.

Acute, Uncomplicated Gonorrhea

PO: ADULTS: 400 mg 1 time.

Usual Elderly Dosage

PO: ELDERLY: 200–400 mg q12–24h for 7 days up to 6 wks.

Bacterial Conjunctivitis

OPHTHALMIC: ADULTS, ELDERLY: 1–2 drops q2–4h for 2 days, then 4 times a day for 5 days.

Corneal Ulcer

OPHTHALMIC: ADULTS: 1–2 drops q30min while awake for 2 days, then q60min while awake for 5–7 days, then 4 times a day.

Acute Otitis Media

OTIC: CHILDREN 1–12 YRS: 5 drops into affected ear twice a day for 10 days.

Otitis Externa

OTIC: ADULTS, ELDERLY, CHILDREN 12 YRS AND OLDER: 10 drops into affected ear once daily for 7 days. **CHILDREN 6 MOS–11 YRS:** 5 drops into affected ear once daily for 7 days.

O

Dosage in Renal Impairment

After normal initial dose, dosage and frequency are based on creatinine clearance.

Creatinine Clearance	Adjusted Dose	Dosage Interval
Greater than 50 ml/min	None	q12h
20–50 ml/min	None	q24h
Less than 20 ml/min	Half	q24h

SIDE EFFECTS

Frequent (10%–7%): Nausea, headache, insomnia. **Occasional (5%–3%):** Abdominal pain, diarrhea, vomiting, dry mouth, flatulence, dizziness, fatigue, drowsiness, rash, pruritus, fever. **Rare (less than 1%):** Constipation, paresthesia.

ADVERSE EFFECTS/ TOXIC REACTIONS

Antibiotic-associated colitis, other superinfections (abdominal cramps, severe watery diarrhea, fever) may occur from altered bacterial balance. Hypersensitivity reaction (evidenced by rash, pruritus, blisters, edema, photosensitivity) occurs rarely. Arthropathy (swelling, pain, clubbing of fingers/toes, degeneration of stress-bearing portion of joint) may occur in children.

NURSING CONSIDERATIONS

BASELINE ASSESSMENT

Question for history of hypersensitivity to ofloxacin, other quinolones.

INTERVENTION/EVALUATION

Monitor signs/symptoms of infection, altered mental status. Monitor renal/hepatic function, WBC. Assess skin, discontinue medication at first sign of rash, other allergic reaction. Monitor daily pattern of bowel activity, stool consistency. Assess for insomnia. Check for dizziness, headache, visual difficulties, tremors; provide assistance with ambulation as needed. Be alert for superinfection: fever, vomiting, diarrhea, anal/genital pruritus, oral mucosal changes (ulceration, pain, erythema).

PATIENT/FAMILY TEACHING

• Do not take antacids within 2 hrs before or 2 hrs after taking ofloxacin. • Best taken 1 hr before or 2 hrs after meals. • May cause insomnia, headache, drowsiness, dizziness. • Avoid tasks requiring alertness, motor skills until response to drug is established. • Notify physician if tendon pain/swelling, persistent diarrhea occurs.

olanzapine

oh-**lan**-za-peen
(Apo-Olanzapine, Novo-Olanzapine, Zyprexa, Zyprexa Intramuscular, Zyprexa Relprevv, Zyprexa Zydis)

BLACK BOX ALERT Elderly pts with dementia-related psychosis are at increased risk for mortality due to cerebrovascular events.

Do not confuse olanzapine with olsalazine or quetiapine, or Zyprexa with Celexa, Zestril, or Zyrtec.

FIXED-COMBINATION(S)

Symbyax: olanzapine/fluoxetine (an antidepressant): 6 mg/25 mg, 6 mg/50 mg, 12 mg/25 mg, 12 mg/50 mg.

CLASSIFICATION

PHARMACOTHERAPEUTIC: Dibenzazepine derivative. **CLINICAL:** Antipsychotic (see p. 65C).

ACTION

Antagonizes alpha$_1$-adrenergic, dopamine, histamine, muscarinic, serotonin receptors. Produces anticholinergic, histaminic, CNS depressant effects. **Therapeutic Effect:** Diminishes psychotic symptoms.

PHARMACOKINETICS

Well absorbed after PO administration. Rapid absorption following IM administration. Protein binding: 93%. Extensively distributed throughout body. Undergoes extensive first-pass metabolism in liver. Excreted primarily in urine and, to lesser extent, in feces. Not removed by dialysis. **Half-life:** 21–54 hrs.

USES

PO: Management of manifestations of psychotic disorders. Treatment of acute mania associated with bipolar disorder. In combination with fluoxetine: treatment of depressive episodes associated with bipolar I disorder and treatment of treatment-resistant depression. **IM:** Controls agitation in schizophrenia, bipolar disorder. **Relprevv:** Long acting antipsychotic for IM injection for treatment of schizophrenia. **OFF-LABEL:** Treatment of anorexia, borderline personality disorder, Huntington's disease; maintenance of long-term treatment response in schizophrenic pts; nausea; vomiting; psychosis/agitation related to Alzheimer's dementia.

PRECAUTIONS

Contraindications: None known. **Cautions:** Hypersensitivity to clozapine, pts who should avoid anticholinergics (e.g., pts with benign prostatic hyperplasia), hepatic impairment, elderly, concurrent use of potentially hepatotoxic drugs, dose escalation, known cardiovascular disease (history of MI, ischemia, heart failure, conduction abnormalities), cerebrovascular disease, conditions predisposing pts to hypotension (dehydration, hypovolemia, hypertensive medications), history of seizures, conditions lowering seizure threshold (e.g., Alzheimer's dementia), those at risk for aspiration pneumonia.

⌛ LIFESPAN CONSIDERATIONS

Pregnancy/Lactation: Unknown if drug crosses placenta or is distributed in breast milk. **Pregnancy Category C. Children:** Safety and efficacy not established. **Elderly:** No age-related precautions noted.

INTERACTIONS

DRUG: Alcohol, CNS depressants may increase CNS depressant effects. **Anticholinergics** may increase anticholinergic effects. **Hepatotoxic medications** may increase hepatic function test levels. **HERBAL: Dong quai, St. John's wort** may increase photosensitization. **Gotu kola, kava kava, St. John's wort, valerian** may increase CNS depression. **FOOD:** None known. **LAB VALUES:** May increase serum GGT, cholesterol, prolactin, AST, ALT.

AVAILABILITY (Rx)

Injection, Powder for Reconstitution (Zyprexa Intramuscular): 10 mg. **Suspension for IM Injection (Relprevv):** 210 mg, 300 mg, 405 mg. **Tablets (Zyprexa):** 2.5 mg, 5 mg, 7.5 mg, 10 mg, 15 mg, 20 mg. **Tablets (Orally-Disintegrating [Zyprexa Zydis]):** 5 mg, 10 mg, 15 mg, 20 mg.

ADMINISTRATION/HANDLING

PO

• Give without regard to meals.

ORALLY DISINTEGRATING

• Remove by peeling back foil (do not push through foil). • Place in mouth immediately. • Tablet dissolves rapidly with saliva and may be swallowed with or without liquid.

IM (Zyprexa Intramuscular)

• Reconstitute 10-mg vial with 2.1 ml Sterile Water for Injection to provide concentration of 5 mg/ml. • Use within 1 hr following reconstitution. • Discard unused portion.

INDICATIONS/ROUTES/DOSAGE

Schizophrenia

PO: ADULTS: Initially, 5–10 mg once daily. May increase to 10 mg/day within 5–7 days. If further adjustments are indicated, may increase by 5 mg/day at 7-day intervals. Range: 10–30 mg/day. **ELDERLY:** Initially, 2.5 mg/day. May increase as indicated. Range: 2.5–10 mg/day. **CHILDREN:** Initially, 2.5 mg/day. Titrate as necessary up to 20 mg/day.

Depression Associated with Bipolar Disorder (with fluoxetine)

PO: ADULTS: Initially, 5 mg in evening. Range: 5–12.5 mg/day.

O

Bipolar Mania

PO: ADULTS: Initially, 10–15 mg/day. May increase by 5 mg/day at intervals of at least 24 hrs. **Maximum:** 20 mg/day. **CHILDREN:** Initially, 2.5 mg/day. Titrate as necessary up to 20 mg/day.

Dosage for Elderly, Debilitated Pts, Those Predisposed to Hypotensive Reactions

Initial dosage for these pts is 5 mg/day.

Usual Relprevv Dosage (Based on Oral Zyprexa Dose)

IM: ADULTS, ELDERLY: 210 mg q2wks or 405 mg q4wks or 300 mg q2wks for first 8 wks, then 150 mg q2wks or 300 mg q4wks or 210 mg q2wks or 405 mg q4wks thereafter.

Control of Agitation

IM: ADULTS, ELDERLY: 2.5–10 mg. May repeat 2 hrs after first dose and 4 hrs after 2nd dose. **Maximum:** 30 mg/day.

SIDE EFFECTS

Frequent: Drowsiness (26%), agitation (23%), insomnia (20%), headache (17%), nervousness (16%), hostility (15%), dizziness (11%), rhinitis (10%). **Occasional:** Anxiety, constipation (9%); nonaggressive atypical behavior (8%); dry mouth (7%); weight gain (6%); orthostatic hypotension, fever, arthralgia, restlessness, cough, pharyngitis, visual changes (dim vision) (5%). **Rare:** Tachycardia; back, chest, abdominal, or extremity pain; tremor.

ADVERSE EFFECTS/ TOXIC REACTIONS

Rare reactions include seizures, neuroleptic malignant syndrome, a potentially fatal syndrome characterized by hyperpyrexia, muscle rigidity, irregular pulse or B/P, tachycardia, diaphoresis, cardiac arrhythmias. Extrapyramidal symptoms (EPS), dysphagia may occur. Overdose (300 mg) produces drowsiness, slurred speech.

NURSING CONSIDERATIONS

BASELINE ASSESSMENT

Obtain baseline hepatic function lab values, glucose, weight, lipid profile before initiating treatment. Assess behavior, appearance, emotional status, response to environment, speech pattern, thought content.

INTERVENTION/EVALUATION

Monitor B/P, glucose, lipids, hepatic function tests. Assess for tremors, changes in gait, abnormal muscular movements, behavior. Supervise suicidal-risk pt closely during early therapy (as depression lessens, energy level improves, increasing suicide potential). Assess for therapeutic response (interest in surroundings, improvement in self-care, increased ability to concentrate, relaxed facial expression). Assist with ambulation if dizziness occurs. Assess sleep pattern. Notify physician if extrapyramidal symptoms (EPS) occur.

PATIENT/FAMILY TEACHING

• Avoid dehydration, particularly during exercise, exposure to extreme heat, concurrent use of medication causing dry mouth, other drying effects. • Sugarless gum, sips of tepid water may relieve dry mouth. • Notify physician if pregnancy occurs or if there is intention to become pregnant during olanzapine therapy. • Take medication as ordered; do not stop taking or increase dosage. • Rise slowly from sitting/lying position. • Avoid alcohol. • Avoid tasks that require alertness, motor skills until response to drug is established. • Monitor diet, exercise program to prevent weight gain.

olmesartan

ol-**mess**-er-tan
(Benicar, Olmetec)

BLACK BOX ALERT May cause fetal injury, mortality if used during second or third trimester of pregnancy.

Do not confuse Benicar with Mevacor.

FIXED-COMBINATION(S)

Azor: olmesartan/amlodipine (calcium channel blocker): 20 mg/5 mg, 40 mg/5 mg, 20 mg/10 mg, 40 mg/10 mg. **Benicar HCT:** olmesartan/hydrochlorothiazide (a diuretic): 20 mg/12.5 mg, 40 mg/12.5 mg, 40 mg/25 mg. **Tribenzor:** olmesartan/hydrochlorothiazide/amlodipine: 20 mg/12.5 mg/5 mg, 40 mg/12.5 mg/5 mg, 40 mg/25 mg/5 mg, 40 mg/12.5 mg/10 mg, 40 mg/25 mg/10 mg.

◆ CLASSIFICATION

PHARMACOTHERAPEUTIC: Angiotensin II receptor antagonist. **CLINICAL:** Antihypertensive (see p. 10C).

ACTION

Blocks vasoconstrictor, aldosterone-secreting effects of angiotensin II by inhibiting binding of angiotensin II to AT_1 receptors in vascular smooth muscle. **Therapeutic Effect:** Causes vasodilation, decreases peripheral resistance, decreases B/P.

PHARMACOKINETICS

Moderately absorbed after PO administration. Hydrolyzed in GI tract to olmesartan. Protein binding: 99%. Recovered primarily in feces and, to lesser extent, in urine. Not removed by hemodialysis. **Half-life:** 13 hrs.

USES

Treatment of hypertension alone or in combination with other antihypertensives.

PRECAUTIONS

Contraindications: Bilateral renal arterial stenosis. **Cautions:** Renal/hepatic impairment, renal arterial stenosis.

⌛ LIFESPAN CONSIDERATIONS

Pregnancy/Lactation: Unknown if distributed in breast milk. **Pregnancy Category C (D if used in second or third trimester). Children:** Safety and efficacy not established. **Elderly:** No age-related precautions noted.

INTERACTIONS

DRUG: Diuretics have additive effects on B/P, may cause hypotension. **HERBAL: Ephedra, ginseng, yohimbe** may worsen hypertension. **Garlic** may increase antihypertensive effect. **FOOD:** None known. **LAB VALUES:** May slightly decrease Hgb, Hct. May increase bilirubin, liver enzymes, BUN, serum creatinine.

AVAILABILITY (Rx)

Tablets: 5 mg, 20 mg, 40 mg.

ADMINISTRATION/HANDLING

PO

- Give without regard to meals.

INDICATIONS/ROUTES/DOSAGE

Hypertension

PO: ADULTS, ELDERLY: Initially, 20 mg/day. May increase to 40 mg/day after 2 wks. Lower initial dose may be necessary in pts receiving volume-depleting medications (e.g., diuretics). **CHILDREN 6–16 YRS, WEIGHING 20 TO LESS THAN 35 KG:** Initially, 10 mg once daily. Range: 10–20 mg once daily. **WEIGHING 35 KG OR GREATER:** Initially, 20 mg once daily. Range: 20–40 mg once daily.

SIDE EFFECTS

Occasional (3%): Dizziness. **Rare (less than 2%):** Headache, diarrhea, upper respiratory tract infection.

ADVERSE EFFECTS/ TOXIC REACTIONS

Overdosage may manifest as hypotension, tachycardia. Bradycardia occurs less often. Rare cases of rhabdomyolysis have been reported.

NURSING CONSIDERATIONS

BASELINE ASSESSMENT

Obtain B/P, apical pulse immediately before each dose in addition to regular

O

monitoring (be alert to fluctuations). If excessive reduction in B/P occurs, place pt in supine position, feet slightly elevated. Question for possibility of pregnancy (see Pregnancy Category). Assess medication history (esp. diuretics).

INTERVENTION/EVALUATION

Maintain hydration (offer fluids frequently). Assess for evidence of upper respiratory infection. Assist with ambulation if dizziness occurs. Monitor serum potassium level. Assess B/P for hypertension, hypotension.

PATIENT/FAMILY TEACHING

• Pts and/or their partner should take measures to avoid pregnancy. • Avoid tasks that require alertness, motor skills until response to drug is established (possible dizziness effect). • Report any signs of infection (sore throat, fever). • Therapy requires lifelong control, diet, exercise. • Maintain adequate hydration during hot weather (risk of dehydration, hypotension).

O

olsalazine

ohl-**sal**-ah-zeen
(Dipentum)
Do not confuse Dipentum with Dilantin, or olsalazine with olanzapine.

◆CLASSIFICATION

PHARMACOTHERAPEUTIC: Salicylic acid derivative. **CLINICAL:** Anti-inflammatory.

ACTION

Converted to mesalamine in colon by bacterial action. Blocks prostaglandin production in bowel mucosa. **Therapeutic Effect:** Reduces colonic inflammation.

PHARMACOKINETICS

Small amount absorbed. Protein binding: 99%. Metabolized by bacteria in colon. Minimal elimination in urine, feces. **Half-life:** 0.9 hr.

USES

Maintenance of remission of ulcerative colitis in pts intolerant of sulfasalazine medication. **OFF-LABEL:** Treatment of inflammatory bowel disease.

PRECAUTIONS

Contraindications: History of hypersensitivity to salicylates. **Cautions:** Preexisting renal disease.

⌛ LIFESPAN CONSIDERATIONS

Pregnancy/Lactation: Crosses placenta; distributed in breast milk. **Pregnancy Category C. Children:** Safety and efficacy not established. **Elderly:** Age-related renal impairment may require dosage adjustment.

INTERACTIONS

DRUG: **Warfarin** may increase PT. **HERBAL:** None significant. **FOOD:** None known. **LAB VALUES:** May increase AST, ALT.

AVAILABILITY (Rx)

Capsules: 250 mg.

ADMINISTRATION/HANDLING

PO

• Give with food.

INDICATIONS/ROUTES/DOSAGE

Maintenance of Controlled Ulcerative Colitis

PO: ADULTS, ELDERLY: 1 g/day in 2 divided doses, preferably q12h.

SIDE EFFECTS

Frequent (10%–5%): Headache, diarrhea, abdominal pain/cramps, nausea. **Occasional (4%–2%):** Depression, fatigue, dyspepsia, upper respiratory tract infection, decreased appetite, rash, pruritus, arthralgia. **Rare (1%):** Dizziness, vomiting, stomatitis.

ADVERSE EFFECTS/ TOXIC REACTIONS

Sulfite sensitivity may occur in susceptible pts (manifested as cramping, headache, diarrhea, fever, rash, urticaria, pruritus, wheezing). Discontinue drug immediately. Excessive diarrhea associated with extreme fatigue is rarely noted.

NURSING CONSIDERATIONS

INTERVENTION/EVALUATION

Encourage adequate fluid intake. Assess bowel sounds for peristalsis. Monitor daily pattern of bowel activity, stool consistency; record time of evacuation. Assess for abdominal disturbances. Assess skin for rash, urticaria. Medication should be discontinued if rash, fever, cramping, diarrhea occur.

PATIENT/FAMILY TEACHING

- Notify physician if diarrhea, cramping continues or worsens or if rash, fever, pruritus occur.

omalizumab

oh-mah-**liz**-oo-mab
(Xolair)

BLACK BOX ALERT Anaphylaxis (severe bronchospasm, hypotension, angioedema, syncope, urticaria) has occurred after first dose and in some cases after 1 yr of regular treatment.

Do not confuse omalizumab with ofatumumab.

◆CLASSIFICATION

PHARMACOTHERAPEUTIC: Monoclonal antibody. **CLINICAL:** Antiasthmatic.

ACTION

Selectively binds to human immunoglobulin E (IgE). Inhibits binding of IgE on surface of mast cells, basophiles. **Therapeutic Effect:** Prevents/reduces number of asthmatic attacks.

PHARMACOKINETICS

Absorbed slowly after subcutaneous administration, with peak concentration in 7–8 days. Excreted primarily via hepatic degradation. **Half-life:** 26 days.

USES

Treatment of moderate to severe persistent asthma in pts reactive to perennial allergen and inadequately controlled asthma symptoms with inhaled corticosteroids. **OFF-LABEL:** Treatment of seasonal allergic rhinitis.

PRECAUTIONS

Contraindications: None known. **Cautions:** Not for use in reversing acute bronchospasm, status asthmaticus.

LIFESPAN CONSIDERATIONS

Pregnancy/Lactation: Because IgE is present in breast milk, omalizumab is expected to be present in breast milk. Use only if clearly needed. **Pregnancy Category B. Children:** Safety and efficacy not established in those younger than 12 yrs. **Elderly:** No age-related precautions noted.

INTERACTIONS

DRUG: None significant. **HERBAL:** None significant. **FOOD:** None known. **LAB VALUES:** May increase serum IgE levels.

AVAILABILITY (Rx)

Injection, Powder for Reconstitution: 150 mg/1.2 ml after reconstitution.

ADMINISTRATION/HANDLING

Subcutaneous

Reconstitution • Use only Sterile Water for Injection to prepare for subcutaneous administration. • Medication takes 15–20 min to dissolve. • Draw 1.4 ml Sterile Water for Injection into 3-ml syringe with 1-inch, 18-gauge needle; inject contents into powdered vial. • Swirl vial for approximately 1 min (do not shake) and again swirl vial for 5–10 sec every 5 min until no gel-like particles appear in the solution. • Do not use if contents do not dissolve completely within 40 min. • In-

vert vial for 15 sec (allows solution to drain toward the stopper). • Using new 3-ml syringe with 1-inch 18-gauge needle, obtain required 1.2-ml dose, replace 18-gauge needle with 25-gauge needle for subcutaneous administration.
Rate of administration • Subcutaneous administration may take 5–10 sec to administer due to its viscosity.
Storage • Use only clear or slightly opalescent solution; solution is slightly viscous. • Refrigerate. • Reconstituted solution is stable for 8 hrs if refrigerated or within 4 hrs of reconstitution when stored at room temperature.

INDICATIONS/ROUTES/DOSAGE

◀ALERT▶ Retesting of IgE levels during treatment cannot be used as a guide for dosage determination (IgE levels remain elevated for up to 1 yr after discontinuation of treatment). Dosage is based on IgE levels obtained at initiation of treatment.

Asthma
SUBCUTANEOUS: ADULTS, ELDERLY, CHILDREN 12 YRS AND OLDER: 150–375 mg every 2 or 4 wks; dose and dosing frequency are individualized based on body weight and pretreatment IgE level (as shown below). (Consult specific product labeling.)

SIDE EFFECTS

Frequent (45%–11%): Injection site ecchymosis, redness, warmth, stinging, urticaria; viral infection; sinusitis; headache; pharyngitis. **Occasional (8%–3%):** Arthralgia, leg pain, fatigue, dizziness. **Rare (2%):** Arm pain, earache, dermatitis, pruritus.

ADVERSE EFFECTS/ TOXIC REACTIONS

Anaphylaxis, occurring within 2 hrs of first dose or subsequent doses, occurs in 0.1% of pts. Malignant neoplasms occur in 0.5% of pts.

NURSING CONSIDERATIONS

BASELINE ASSESSMENT

Obtain baseline serum total IgE levels before initiation of treatment (dosage is based on pretreatment levels). Drug is not for treatment of acute exacerbations of asthma, acute bronchospasm, status asthmaticus.

INTERVENTION/EVALUATION

Monitor rate, depth, rhythm, type of respirations, quality/rate of pulse. Assess

4-Wk Dosing Table

Pretreatment Serum IgE Levels (units/ml)	Weight 30–60 kg	Weight 61–70 kg	Weight 71–90 kg	Weight 91–150 kg
30–100	150 mg	150 mg	150 mg	300 mg
101–200	300 mg	300 mg	300 mg	See next table
201–300	300 mg	See next table	See next table	See next table

2-Week Dosing Table

Pretreatment Serum IgE Levels (units/ml)	Weight 30–60 kg	Weight 61–70 kg	Weight 71–90 kg	Weight 91–150 kg
101–200	See preceding table	See preceding table	See preceding table	225 mg
201–300	See preceding table	225 mg	225 mg	300 mg
301–400	225 mg	225 mg	300 mg	Do not dose
401–500	300 mg	300 mg	375 mg	Do not dose
501–600	300 mg	375 mg	Do not dose	Do not dose
601–700	375 mg	Do not dose	Do not dose	Do not dose

lung sounds for rhonchi, wheezing, rales. Observe lips, fingernails for cyanosis (blue/dusky color in light-skinned pts, gray in dark-skinned pts).

PATIENT/FAMILY TEACHING

• Increase fluid intake (decreases viscosity of pulmonary secretions). • Do not alter/stop other asthma medications. • Notify physician of allergic reactions (e.g., breathing difficulty, swelling of throat/tongue).

omega-3 acid ethyl esters

oh-**meg**-ah 3 **ah**-sid **eth**-ill **eh**-stirs
(Lovaza)

Do not confuse Lovaza with lorazepam.

◆CLASSIFICATION

PHARMACOTHERAPEUTIC: Omega-3 fatty acid. **CLINICAL:** Antihypertriglyceridemia.

ACTION

Inhibits esterification of fatty acids, prevents hepatic enzymes from catalyzing final step of triglyceride synthesis. **Therapeutic Effect:** Reduces serum triglyceride levels.

PHARMACOKINETICS

Well absorbed following PO administration. Incorporated into phospholipids. **Half-life:** N/A.

USES

Adjunct to diet to reduce very high (500 mg/dl or higher) serum triglyceride levels in adult pts. **OFF-LABEL:** Treatment of IgA nephropathy.

PRECAUTIONS

Contraindications: None known. **Cautions:** Known sensitivity, allergy to fish.

LIFESPAN CONSIDERATIONS

Pregnancy/Lactation: Unknown if distributed in breast milk. **Pregnancy Category C. Children:** Safety and efficacy not established in those younger than 18 yrs. **Elderly:** No age-related precautions noted.

INTERACTIONS

DRUG: May increase bleeding time with **anticoagulants. Beta-blockers, estrogens, thiazide diuretics (e.g., hydrochlorothiazide)** may increase serum triglycerides (discontinue or change drug before therapy). **HERBAL:** None significant. **FOOD:** None known. **LAB VALUES:** May increase ALT, LDL.

AVAILABILITY (Rx)

Capsules, Soft Gelatin (Oil-Filled): 1 g.

ADMINISTRATION/HANDLING

PO

• Give without regard to meals.

INDICATIONS/ROUTES/DOSAGE

ALERT Before initiating therapy, pt should be on standard cholesterol-lowering diet for minimum of 3–6 mos. Continue diet throughout therapy.

Usual Dosage

PO: ADULTS, ELDERLY: 4 g/day, given as a single dose (4 capsules) or 2 capsules twice daily.

SIDE EFFECTS

Occasional (5%–3%): Eructation, altered taste, dyspepsia. **Rare (2%–1%):** Rash, back pain.

ADVERSE EFFECTS/ TOXIC REACTIONS

None known.

NURSING CONSIDERATIONS

BASELINE ASSESSMENT

Assess baseline serum triglyceride level, hepatic function tests. Obtain diet history, esp. fat consumption.

INTERVENTION/EVALUATION

Monitor serum triglyceride levels for therapeutic response. Monitor serum ALT, LDL periodically during therapy. Discontinue therapy if no response after 2 mos of treatment.

PATIENT/FAMILY TEACHING

• Continue to adhere to lipid-lowering diet (important part of treatment). • Periodic lab tests are essential part of therapy to determine drug effectiveness.

omeprazole

oh-**mep**-rah-zole
(Apo-Omeprazole, Losec,
Prilosec, Prilosec OTC)
Do not confuse Prilosec with Plendil, prednisone, Prevacid, prilocaine, Prinivil, or Prozac.

FIXED-COMBINATION(S)

Zegerid: omeprazole/sodium bicarbonate (an antacid): 20 mg/1,100 mg, 40 mg/1,100 mg. **Zegerid Powder:** 20 mg/1,680 mg, 40 mg/1,680 mg.

CLASSIFICATION

PHARMACOTHERAPEUTIC: Benzimidazole. **CLINICAL:** Gastric acid pump inhibitor (see p. 148C).

ACTION

Converted to active metabolites that irreversibly bind to, inhibit hydrogen-potassium adenosine triphosphatase, an enzyme on the surface of gastric parietal cells. Inhibits hydrogen ion transport into gastric lumen. **Therapeutic Effect:** Increases gastric pH, reduces gastric acid production.

PHARMACOKINETICS

Route	Onset	Peak	Duration
PO	1 hr	2 hrs	72 hrs

Rapidly absorbed from GI tract. Protein binding: 95%. Primarily distributed into gastric parietal cells. Metabolized extensively in liver. Primarily excreted in urine. Unknown if removed by hemodialysis. **Half-life:** 0.5–1 hr (increased in hepatic impairment).

USES

Short-term treatment (4–8 wks) of erosive esophagitis (diagnosed by endoscopy), symptomatic gastroesophageal reflux disease (GERD) poorly responsive to other treatment. *H. pylori*–associated duodenal ulcer (with amoxicillin and clarithromycin). Long-term treatment of pathologic hypersecretory conditions; treatment of active duodenal ulcer. Maintenance healing of erosive esophagitis. **OFF-LABEL:** Prevention/treatment of NSAID-induced ulcers, treatment of active benign gastric ulcers, stress ulcer prophylaxis in critically ill pts.

PRECAUTIONS

Contraindications: None known. **Cautions:** May increase risk of fractures.

LIFESPAN CONSIDERATIONS

Pregnancy/Lactation: Unknown if drug crosses placenta or is distributed in breast milk. **Pregnancy Category C. Children:** Safety and efficacy not established. **Elderly:** No age-related precautions noted.

INTERACTIONS

DRUG: May increase concentration of **diazepam, oral anticoagulants, phenytoin.** May decrease effect of **clopidogrel. HERBAL: Ginkgo biloba** may decrease effectiveness. **St. John's wort** may decrease concentration. **FOOD:** None known. **LAB VALUES:** May increase serum alkaline phosphatase, AST, ALT.

AVAILABILITY (Rx)

Granules for oral suspension: 2.5 mg/packet, 10 mg/packet.

Capsules (Delayed-Release [Prilosec]): 10 mg, 20 mg, 40 mg. **Tablets (Delayed-Release [Prilosec OTC]):** 20 mg.

ADMINISTRATION/HANDLING

PO

• Give before meals. • Swallow whole. Do not crush or chew delayed-release forms. • May open, mix with applesauce and give immediately.

PO (Suspension)

• Following reconstitution, allow to thicken (2–3 min). • Administer within 30 min.

INDICATIONS/ROUTES/DOSAGE

Erosive Esophagitis, Poorly Responsive Gastroesophageal Reflux Disease (GERD), Active Duodenal Ulcer, Prevention/Treatment of NSAID-Induced Ulcers

PO: ADULTS, ELDERLY: 20 mg/day.

Maintenance Healing of Erosive Esophagitis

PO: ADULTS, ELDERLY: 20 mg/day for up to 12 mos.

Pathologic Hypersecretory Conditions

PO: ADULTS, ELDERLY: Initially, 60 mg/day up to 120 mg 3 times a day.

H. Pylori **Duodenal Ulcer**

PO: ADULTS, ELDERLY: 20 mg once daily or 40 mg/day as a single or in 2 divided doses in combination therapy with antibiotics. Dose varies with regimen used.

Gastric Ulcer

PO: ADULTS, ELDERLY: 40 mg/day for 4–8 wks.

OTC Use (Frequent Heartburn)

PO: ADULTS, ELDERLY: 20 mg/day for 14 days. May repeat after 4 mos if needed.

Usual Pediatric Dosage

CHILDREN 1–16 YRS, WEIGHT 20 KG OR MORE: 20 mg/day. **CHILDREN OLDER THAN 2 YRS, WEIGHT 10–19 KG:** 10 mg/day. **WEIGHT 5–9 KG:** 5 mg/day.

SIDE EFFECTS

Frequent (7%): Headache. **Occasional (3%–2%):** Diarrhea, abdominal pain, nausea. **Rare (2%):** Dizziness, asthenia (loss of strength, energy), vomiting, constipation, upper respiratory tract infection, back pain, rash, cough.

ADVERSE EFFECTS/ TOXIC REACTIONS

Pancreatitis, hepatotoxicity, interstitial nephritis occur rarely.

NURSING CONSIDERATIONS

INTERVENTION/EVALUATION

Evaluate for therapeutic response (relief of GI symptoms). Question if GI discomfort, nausea, diarrhea occurs.

PATIENT/FAMILY TEACHING

• Report headache, onset of black, tarry stools, diarrhea, abdominal pain. • Avoid alcohol. • Swallow capsules whole; do not chew/crush. • Take before eating.

Omnicef, *see cefdinir*

Oncovin, *see vincristine*

O

ondansetron

on-**dan**-sah-tron
(Apo-Ondansetron ✤, Novo-Ondansetron ✤, Zofran, Zofran ODT, Zuplenz)

Do not confuse ondansetron with dolasetron, granisetron, or palonosetron, or Zofran with Zantac or Zosyn.

◆ CLASSIFICATION

PHARMACOTHERAPEUTIC: Selective receptor antagonist. **CLINICAL:** Antinausea, antiemetic.

ACTION

Blocks serotonin, both peripherally on vagal nerve terminals and centrally in chemoreceptor trigger zone. **Therapeutic Effect:** Prevents nausea/vomiting.

PHARMACOKINETICS

Readily absorbed from GI tract. Protein binding: 70%–76%. Metabolized in liver. Primarily excreted in urine. Unknown if removed by hemodialysis. **Half-life:** 3–6 hrs (increased in hepatic impairment).

USES

Prevention/treatment of nausea/vomiting due to cancer chemotherapy (including high-dose cisplatin). Prevention of postop nausea, vomiting. Prevention of radiation-induced nausea, vomiting. Treatment of postop nausea, vomiting. **OFF-LABEL:** Postanesthetic shivering, vomiting due to viral illness. Treatment of early-onset alcoholism, hyperemesis gravidarum.

PRECAUTIONS

Contraindications: Use of apomorphine. **Cautions:** None known.

LIFESPAN CONSIDERATIONS

Pregnancy/Lactation: Unknown if drug crosses placenta or is distributed in breast milk. **Pregnancy Category B. Children:** Safety and efficacy not established. **Elderly:** No age-related precautions noted.

INTERACTIONS

DRUG: **Apomorphine** may cause profound hypotension, alter LOC. **HERBAL:** **St. John's wort** may decrease concentration. **FOOD:** None known. **LAB VALUES:** May transiently increase serum bilirubin, AST, ALT.

AVAILABILITY (Rx)

Injection (Premix): 32 mg/50 ml. **Injection Solution (Zofran):** 2 mg/ml. **Oral Soluble Film (Zuplenz):** 4 mg, 8 mg. **Oral Solution (Zofran):** 4 mg/5 ml. **Tablets (Zofran):** 4 mg, 8 mg. **Tablets (Orally-Disintegrating [Zofran ODT]):** 4 mg, 8 mg.

ADMINISTRATION/HANDLING

IV

Reconstitution • May give undiluted. • For IV infusion, dilute with 50 ml D_5W or 0.9% NaCl before administration.

Rate of administration • Give IV push over 2–5 min. • Give IV infusion over 15 min.

Storage • Store at room temperature. • Stable for 48 hrs at room temperature following dilution.

IM

• Inject undiluted into large muscle mass.

PO

• Give without regard to food.

Orally-Disintegrating Tablets

• Do not remove from blister until needed. • Peel backing off; do not push through. • Place tablet on tongue; allow to dissolve. • Swallow with saliva.

Oral Soluble Film

• Keep film in pouch until ready to use. • Remove film strip from pouch and place on top of tongue, allow to dissolve. • Swallow after film dissolves. Do not chew or swallow film whole.

IV INCOMPATIBILITIES

Acyclovir (Zovirax), allopurinol (Aloprim), aminophylline, amphotericin B (Fungizone), amphotericin B complex (Abelcet, AmBisome, Amphotec), ampicillin (Polycillin), ampicillin and sulbactam (Unasyn), cefepime (Maxipime), cefoperazone (Cefobid), 5-fluorouracil, lipids, lorazepam (Ativan), meropenem (Merrem IV), methylprednisolone (Solu-Medrol).

IV COMPATIBILITIES

Carboplatin (Paraplatin), cisplatin (Platinol), cyclophosphamide (Cytoxan), cytarabine (Cytosar), dacarbazine (DTIC-Dome), daunorubicin (Cerubidine), dexamethasone (Decadron), diphenhydramine (Benadryl), docetaxel (Taxotere), dopamine (Intropin), etoposide

(VePesid), gemcitabine (Gemzar), heparin, hydromorphone (Dilaudid), ifosfamide (Ifex), magnesium, mannitol, mesna (Mesnex), methotrexate, metoclopramide (Reglan), mitomycin (Mutamycin), mitoxantrone (Novantrone), morphine, paclitaxel (Taxol), potassium chloride, teniposide (Vumon), topotecan (Hycamtin), vinblastine (Velban), vincristine (Oncovin), vinorelbine (Navelbine).

INDICATIONS/ROUTES/DOSAGE

Chemotherapy-Induced Emesis

IV: ADULTS, ELDERLY: 0.15 mg/kg 3 times a day beginning 30 min before chemotherapy or 0.45 mg/kg once daily or 8–10 mg 1–2 times a day or 24–32 mg once daily. **CHILDREN 6 MOS AND OLDER:** 0.15 mg/kg 3 times a day beginning 30 min before chemotherapy and again 4 and 8 hrs after first dose or 0.45 mg/kg as a single dose.

PO: ADULTS, ELDERLY, CHILDREN 12 YRS AND OLDER: (highly emetogenic) 24 mg 30 min before start of chemotherapy, (moderately emetogenic) 8 mg q12h beginning 30 min before chemotherapy and continuing for 1–2 days after completion of chemotherapy. **Zuplenz:** 8 mg 30 min before chemotherapy, followed by 8 mg 8 hrs later, then continue q12h for 1–2 days after completion of chemotherapy. **CHILDREN 4–11 YRS:** 4 mg 30 min before chemotherapy, repeat 4 and 8 hrs after initial dose then q8h for 1–2 days after chemotherapy completed.

Prevention of Postop Nausea/Vomiting

IV, IM: ADULTS, ELDERLY, CHILDREN OLDER THAN 12 YRS: 4 mg as a single dose. **CHILDREN 1 MO–12 YRS, WEIGHING MORE THAN 40 KG:** 4 mg. **CHILDREN 1 MO–12 YRS, WEIGHING 40 KG AND LESS:** 0.1 mg/kg.

PO: ADULTS, ELDERLY: 16 mg 1 hr before induction of anesthesia.

Prevention of Radiation-Induced Nausea/Vomiting

PO: ADULTS, ELDERLY: (total body irradiation) 8 mg 1–2 hrs daily before each fraction of radiotherapy, (single high-dose radiotherapy to abdomen) 8 mg 1–2 hrs before irradiation, then 8 mg q8h after first dose for 1–2 days after completion of radiotherapy, (daily fractionated radiotherapy to abdomen) 8 mg 1–2 hrs before irradiation, then 8 mg 8 hrs after first dose for each day of radiotherapy. **Zuplenz:** 8 mg q8h.

SIDE EFFECTS

Frequent (13%–5%): Anxiety, dizziness, drowsiness, headache, fatigue, constipation, diarrhea, hypoxia, urinary retention. **Occasional (4%–2%):** Abdominal pain, xerostomia, fever, feeling of cold, redness/pain at injection site, paresthesia, asthenia (lack of strength, energy). **Rare (1%):** Hypersensitivity reaction (rash, pruritus), blurred vision.

ADVERSE EFFECTS/ TOXIC REACTIONS

Hypertension, acute renal failure, GI bleeding, respiratory depression, coma, extrapyramidal effects occur rarely.

NURSING CONSIDERATIONS

BASELINE ASSESSMENT

Assess degree of nausea, vomiting. Assess for dehydration if excessive vomiting occurs (poor skin turgor, dry mucous membranes, longitudinal furrows in tongue). Provide emotional support.

INTERVENTION/EVALUATION

Monitor pt in environment. Assess bowel sounds for peristalsis. Provide supportive measures. Assess mental status. Monitor daily pattern of bowel activity and stool consistency. Record time of evacuation.

PATIENT/FAMILY TEACHING

• Relief from nausea/vomiting generally occurs shortly after drug administration. • Avoid alcohol, barbiturates. • Report persistent vomiting. • Avoid tasks that require alertness, motor skills until response to drug is established (may cause drowsiness, dizziness).

O

Onxol, *see paclitaxel*

oprelvekin (interleukin-2, IL-2)

oh-**prel**-vee-kin
(Neumega)

BLACK BOX ALERT Allergic or hypersensitivity reactions, including anaphylaxis, have occurred.

Do not confuse Neumega with Neulasta or Neupogen, or oprelvekin with aldesleukin or Proleukin.

CLASSIFICATION

PHARMACOTHERAPEUTIC: Hematopoietic. **CLINICAL:** Platelet growth factor.

ACTION

Stimulates production of blood platelets, essential to blood-clotting process. **Therapeutic Effect:** Increases platelet production.

O

PHARMACOKINETICS

Renal elimination as metabolite. **Half-life:** 5–8 hrs.

USES

Prevents severe thrombocytopenia, reduces need for platelet transfusions following myelosuppressive chemotherapy in pts with nonmyeloid malignancies.

PRECAUTIONS

Contraindications: None known. **Cautions:** CHF, those susceptible to developing CHF, history of heart failure, history of atrial arrhythmia.

LIFESPAN CONSIDERATIONS

Pregnancy/Lactation: Unknown if drug crosses placenta or is distributed in breast milk. **Pregnancy Category C. Children:** Safety and efficacy not established. **Elderly:** No age-related precautions noted.

INTERACTIONS

DRUG: Diuretics may increase loss of potassium, worsen effects of hypokalemia. **HERBAL:** None significant. **FOOD:** None known. **LAB VALUES:** May decrease Hgb, Hct, usually within 3–5 days of initiation of therapy; reverses approximately 1 wk after discontinuation of therapy.

AVAILABILITY (Rx)

Injection, Powder for Reconstitution: 5 mg.

ADMINISTRATION/HANDLING

Subcutaneous

Reconstitution • Add 1 ml Sterile Water for Injection directed at side of vial; swirl contents gently (avoid excessive agitation) to provide concentration of 5 mg/ml oprelvekin. • Discard unused portion.

Storage • Store in refrigerator. Once reconstituted, use within 3 hrs. • Give single injection in abdomen, thigh, hip, upper arm.

INDICATIONS/ROUTES/DOSAGE

ALERT Give first dose 6–24 hrs after end of chemotherapy and stop at least 48 hrs before starting next cycle of chemotherapy.

Prevention of Thrombocytopenia

SUBCUTANEOUS: ADULTS: 50 mcg/kg once daily. **CHILDREN:** 25–50 mcg/kg once daily. Continue for 10–21 days or until platelet count reaches 50,000 cells/mcl after its nadir.

Dosage in Renal Impairment

ADULTS WITH CREATININE CLEARANCE LESS THAN 30 ML/MIN: 25 mcg once daily.

SIDE EFFECTS

Frequent: Nausea/vomiting (77%), fluid retention (59%), neutropenic fever (48%), diarrhea (43%), rhinitis (42%), headache (41%), dizziness (38%), fever

(36%), insomnia (33%), cough (29%), rash, pharyngitis (25%), tachycardia (20%), vasodilation (19%).

ADVERSE EFFECTS/ TOXIC REACTIONS

Transient atrial fibrillation/flutter occurs in 10% of pts (may be due to increased plasma volume; oprelvekin is not directly arrhythmogenic). Arrhythmias usually are brief in duration and spontaneously convert to normal sinus rhythm. Papilledema may occur in children.

NURSING CONSIDERATIONS

BASELINE ASSESSMENT

Obtain CBC before chemotherapy and at regular intervals thereafter.

INTERVENTION/EVALUATION

Monitor platelet counts. Closely monitor fluid and electrolyte status, esp. in pts receiving diuretic therapy. Assess for fluid retention (peripheral edema, dyspnea on exertion, generally occurs during first wk of therapy and continues for duration of treatment). Monitor platelet count periodically to assess therapeutic duration of therapy. Dosing should continue until postnadir platelet count is more than 50,000 cells/mcl. Treatment should be stopped longer than 2 days before starting next round of chemotherapy.

PATIENT/FAMILY TEACHING

• Notify physician if swelling in arms or legs, shortness of breath, irregular heartbeat, hypersensitivity reaction occur.

Orapred, *see prednisolone*

orlistat

or-lye-stat
(Alli, Xenical)

Do not confuse Xenical with Xeloda.

◆CLASSIFICATION

PHARMACOTHERAPEUTIC: Gastric/pancreatic lipase inhibitor. **CLINICAL:** Obesity management agent (see p. 137C).

ACTION

Inhibits absorption of dietary fats by inactivating gastric, pancreatic enzymes. **Therapeutic Effect:** Resulting caloric deficit may have positive effects on weight control.

PHARMACOKINETICS

Minimal absorption after administration. Protein binding: 99%. Metabolized within GI wall. Primarily eliminated in feces. Unknown if removed by hemodialysis. **Half-life:** 1–2 hrs.

USES

Management of obesity, including weight loss/maintenance, when used in conjunction with reduced-calorie diet. **OFF-LABEL:** Treatment of type 2 diabetes.

PRECAUTIONS

Contraindications: Cholestasis, chronic malabsorption syndrome. **Cautions:** None known.

⌛ LIFESPAN CONSIDERATIONS

Pregnancy/Lactation: Unknown if distributed in breast milk. Not recommended during pregnancy. Breast-feeding not recommended. **Pregnancy Category B. Children:** Safety and efficacy not established. **Elderly:** No age-related precautions noted.

INTERACTIONS

DRUG: May increase concentration of **pravastatin,** risk of rhabdomyolysis. May reduce absorption of **vitamin E.** May alter effect of **warfarin** by altering vitamin K level. **HERBAL:** None significant. **FOOD:** None known. **LAB VALUES:** Decreases serum glucose, cholesterol, LDL.

O

AVAILABILITY (Rx)

Capsules (Alli): 60 mg. **(Xenical):** 120 mg.

ADMINISTRATION/HANDLING

PO

• Multivitamin supplements containing fat soluble vitamins should be taken once daily at least 2 hrs before or after taking orlistat. • Distribute daily fat intake over 3 main meals (GI effects may increase when taken with any 1 meal very high in fat.)

INDICATIONS/ROUTES/DOSAGE

Weight Reduction

PO: ADULTS, ELDERLY, CHILDREN 12–16 YRS: (XENICAL): 120 mg 3 times a day. **(ALLI):** 60 mg 3 times a day with each main meal containing fat (do not take if meal is occasionally missed or contains no fat).

SIDE EFFECTS

Frequent (30%–20%): Headache, abdominal discomfort, flatulence, fecal urgency, fatty/oily stool. **Occasional (14%–5%):** Back pain, menstrual irregularity, nausea, fatigue, diarrhea, dizziness. **Rare (less than 4%):** Anxiety, rash, myalgia, dry skin, vomiting.

O

ADVERSE EFFECTS/ TOXIC REACTIONS

Hypersensitivity reaction occurs rarely.

NURSING CONSIDERATIONS

INTERVENTION/EVALUATION

Monitor serum cholesterol, LDL, glucose, changes in coagulation parameters.

PATIENT/FAMILY TEACHING

• Maintain nutritionally balanced, reduced-calorie diet. • Daily intake of fat, carbohydrates, protein to be distributed over 3 main meals.

oseltamivir

oh-sel-**tam**-ah-veer
(Tamiflu)
Do not confuse Tamiflu with Thera-flu.

◆CLASSIFICATION

PHARMACOTHERAPEUTIC: Neuraminidase inhibitor. **CLINICAL:** Antiviral (see p. 69C).

ACTION

Selective inhibitor of influenza virus neuraminidase, an enzyme essential for viral replication. Acts against influenza A and B viruses. **Therapeutic Effect:** Suppresses spread of infection within respiratory system, reduces duration of clinical symptoms.

PHARMACOKINETICS

Readily absorbed after PO administration. Protein binding: 3%. Extensively converted to active drug in liver. Primarily excreted in urine. **Half-life:** 6–10 hrs.

USES

Symptomatic treatment of uncomplicated acute illness caused by influenza A or B virus in adults and children 1 yr and older who are symptomatic no longer than 2 days. Prevention of influenza in adults, children 1 yr and older.

PRECAUTIONS

Contraindications: None known. **Cautions:** Renal impairment.

⌛ LIFESPAN CONSIDERATIONS

Pregnancy/Lactation: Unknown if distributed in breast milk. **Pregnancy Category C. Children:** Safety and efficacy not established in those younger than 1 yr. **Elderly:** No age-related precautions noted.

INTERACTIONS

DRUG: Probenecid increases concentration. **HERBAL:** None significant. **FOOD:** None known. **LAB VALUES:** None significant.

AVAILABILITY (Rx)

Capsules: 30 mg, 45 mg, 75 mg. **Powder for Oral Suspension:** 12 mg/ml.

ADMINISTRATION/HANDLING

PO

• Give without regard to food. • May open capsules and mix with sweetened liquid. • Oral suspension stable for 10 days following reconstitution.

INDICATIONS/ROUTES/DOSAGE

Treatment of Influenza

PO: ADULTS, ELDERLY, CHILDREN 13 YRS AND OLDER: 75 mg twice daily for 5 days. **CHILDREN 1–12 YRS, WEIGHING MORE THAN 40 KG:** 75 mg twice daily. **CHILDREN 1–12 YRS, WEIGHING 24–40 KG:** 60 mg twice daily. **CHILDREN 1–12 YRS, WEIGHING 15–23 KG:** 45 mg twice daily. **CHILDREN 1–12 YRS, WEIGHING LESS THAN 15 KG:** 30 mg twice daily.

Prevention of Influenza

PO: ADULTS, ELDERLY, CHILDREN 13 YRS AND OLDER: 75 mg once daily. **CHILDREN 1–12 YRS, WEIGHING MORE THAN 40 KG:** 75 mg once daily. **WEIGHING 24–40 KG:** 60 mg once daily. **WEIGHING 15–23 KG:** 45 mg once daily. **WEIGHING LESS THAN 25 KG:** 30 mg once daily.

Dosage in Renal Impairment

Creatinine clearance 10–30 ml/min: Treatment: 75 mg/day. Prevention: 75 mg every other day or 30 mg daily.

SIDE EFFECTS

Frequent (10%–7%): Nausea, vomiting, diarrhea. Rare (2%–1%): Abdominal pain, bronchitis, dizziness, headache, cough, insomnia, fatigue, vertigo.

ADVERSE EFFECTS/ TOXIC REACTIONS

Colitis, pneumonia, tympanic membrane disorder, fever occur rarely.

NURSING CONSIDERATIONS

INTERVENTION/EVALUATION

Monitor serum glucose, renal function in pts with diabetes, influenza symptoms.

PATIENT/FAMILY TEACHING

• Begin as soon as possible from first appearance of flu symptoms. • Avoid contact with those who are at high risk for influenza. • Not a substitute for flu shot.

Osmitrol, *see mannitol*

oxaliplatin HIGH ALERT

ox-al-ee-plah-tin
(Eloxatin)

BLACK BOX ALERT Anaphylactic-like reaction may occur within minutes of administration; may be controlled with epinephrine, corticosteroids, antihistamines.

Do not confuse oxaliplatin with Aloxi, carboplatin, or cisplatin.

◆CLASSIFICATION

PHARMACOTHERAPEUTIC: Platinum-containing complex. **CLINICAL:** Antineoplastic (see p. 87C).

ACTION

Inhibits DNA replication by cross-linking with DNA strands. Cell cycle–phase nonspecific. Therapeutic Effect: Prevents cell division.

PHARMACOKINETICS

Rapidly distributed. Protein binding: 90%. Undergoes rapid, extensive nonenzymatic biotransformation. Excreted in urine. Half-life: 391 hrs.

USES

Combination treatment of metastatic carcinoma of colon, rectum with 5-fluorouracil (5-FU)/leucovorin in pts whose disease has recurred or progressed during or within 6 mos of completion of first-line therapy with bolus 5-FU/leucovorin and irinotecan. OFF-LABEL: Treatment of germ cell cancer, ovarian cancer, pancreatic

O

cancer, renal cell cancer, solid tumors, head and neck cancer, esophageal cancer, gastric cancer, non-Hodgkin's lymphoma.

PRECAUTIONS

Contraindications: History of allergy to other platinum compounds. **Cautions:** Previous therapy with other antineoplastic agents, radiation, renal impairment, infection, pregnancy, immunosuppression, presence or history of peripheral neuropathy.

LIFESPAN CONSIDERATIONS

Pregnancy/Lactation: If possible, avoid use during pregnancy, esp. first trimester. May cause fetal harm. Breastfeeding not recommended. **Pregnancy Category D. Children:** Safety and efficacy not established. **Elderly:** Increased incidence of diarrhea, dehydration, hypokalemia, fatigue.

INTERACTIONS

DRUG: **Bone marrow depressants** may increase myelosuppression, GI effects. **Live virus vaccines** may potentiate virus replication, increase vaccine side effects, decrease pt's antibody response to vaccine. **Nephrotic medications** may decrease clearance. **HERBAL:** None significant. **FOOD:** None known. **LAB VALUES:** May increase serum creatinine, bilirubin, AST, ALT.

AVAILABILITY (Rx)

Injection, Solution: 5 mg/ml, 10 ml, 20 ml, 40 ml vials.

ADMINISTRATION/HANDLING

◄ALERT► Wear protective gloves during handling of oxaliplatin. If solution comes in contact with skin, wash skin immediately with soap, water. Do not use aluminum needles or administration sets that may come in contact with drug; may cause degradation of platinum compounds.

◄ALERT► Pt should avoid ice, drinking cold beverages, touching cold objects during infusion and for 5 days thereafter (can exacerbate acute neuropathy).

IV

Reconstitution • Dilute with 250–500 ml D_5W (never dilute with sodium chloride solution or other chloride-containing solutions) to final concentration of 0.2–0.6 mg/ml.

Rate of administration • Infuse over 2–6 hrs.

Storage • Do not freeze; protect from light. • Store vials at room temperature. • After dilution, solution is stable for 6 hrs at room temperature, 24 hrs if refrigerated.

IV INCOMPATIBILITIES

Do not infuse oxaliplatin with alkaline medications.

INDICATIONS/ROUTES/DOSAGE

Refer to individual protocols.

◄ALERT► Pretreat pt with antiemetics (should be ordered). Repeat courses should not be given more frequently than every 2 wks.

Colorectal Cancer

IV: ADULTS: Day 1: Oxaliplatin 85 mg/m^2 in 250–500 ml D_5W and leucovorin 200 mg/m^2, given simultaneously over more than 2 hrs in separate bags using a Y-line, followed by 5-FU 400 mg/m^2 IV bolus given over 2–4 min, followed by 5-FU 600 mg/m^2 in 500 ml D_5W as a 22-hr continuous IV infusion. **Day 2:** Leucovorin 200 mg/m^2 IV infusion given over more than 2 hrs, followed by 5-FU 400 mg/m^2 IV bolus given over 2–4 min, followed by 5-FU 600 mg/m^2 in 500 ml D_5W as a 22-hr continuous IV infusion. Repeat cycle every 2 wks for total of 6 mos. Prior to subsequent therapy cycles, evaluate pt for clinical toxicities and laboratory tests.

Ovarian Cancer

IV: ADULTS: Cisplatin 100 mg/m^2 and oxaliplatin 130 mg/m^2 q3wk. Prior to subsequent therapy cycles, evaluate pt for clinical toxicities and laboratory tests.

SIDE EFFECTS

Frequent (76%–20%): Peripheral/sensory neuropathy (usually occurs in hands, feet, perioral area, throat but may present as jaw spasm, abnormal tongue sensation, eye pain, chest pressure, difficulty walking, swallowing, writing), nausea (64%), fatigue, diarrhea, vomiting, constipation, abdominal pain, fever, anorexia. **Occasional (14%–10%):** Stomatitis, earache, insomnia, cough, difficulty breathing, backache, edema. **Rare (7%–3%):** Dyspepsia, dizziness, rhinitis, flushing, alopecia.

ADVERSE EFFECTS/ TOXIC REACTIONS

Peripheral/sensory neuropathy can occur without any prior event by drinking or holding a glass of cold liquid during IV infusion. Pulmonary fibrosis (characterized as nonproductive cough, dyspnea, crackles, radiologic pulmonary infiltrates) may warrant drug discontinuation. Hypersensitivity reaction (rash, urticaria, pruritus) occurs rarely.

NURSING CONSIDERATIONS

BASELINE ASSESSMENT

Pt should avoid ice or drinking, holding glass of cold liquid during IV infusion and for 5 days following completion of infusion; can precipitate/exacerbate neurotoxicity (occurs within hrs or 1–2 days of dosing, lasts up to 14 days). Assess baseline BUN, serum creatinine, WBC, platelet count.

INTERVENTION/EVALUATION

Monitor for decrease in WBC, platelets (myelosuppression is minimal). Monitor for diarrhea, GI bleeding (bright red, tarry stool), signs of neuropathy. Maintain strict I&O. Assess oral mucosa for stomatitis.

PATIENT/FAMILY TEACHING

• Promptly report fever, sore throat, signs of local infection, unusual bruising/bleeding from any site, persistent diarrhea, difficulty breathing. • Do not have immunizations without physician's approval (drug lowers resistance). • Avoid contact with those who have recently taken oral polio vaccine. • Avoid cold drinks, ice, cold objects (may produce neuropathy).

oxaprozin

ox-a-**pro**-zin
(Apo-Oxaprozin ✤, Daypro)

BLACK BOX ALERT Increased risk of serious cardiovascular thrombotic events, including myocardial infarction, CVA, new onset or worsening of preexisting hypertension. Increased risk of severe GI reactions, including ulceration, bleeding, perforation of stomach, intestines.

Do not confuse oxaprozin with oxazepam.

◆CLASSIFICATION

PHARMACOTHERAPEUTIC: Nonsteroidal anti-inflammatory. **CLINICAL:** Analgesic, anti-inflammatory (see p. 129C).

ACTION

Produces analgesic, anti-inflammatory effects by inhibiting prostaglandin synthesis. **Therapeutic Effect:** Reduces inflammatory response, intensity of pain.

PHARMACOKINETICS

Well absorbed from GI tract. Protein binding: 99%. Widely distributed. Metabolized in liver. Primarily excreted in urine; partially eliminated in feces. Not removed by hemodialysis. **Half-life:** 42–50 hrs.

USES

Acute, chronic treatment of osteoarthritis, juvenile rheumatoid arthritis (JRA), rheumatoid arthritis (RA).

PRECAUTIONS

Contraindications: Active peptic ulcer disease, chronic inflammation of GI tract, GI bleeding/ulceration, history of hypersensitivity to aspirin, NSAIDs. **Cautions:** Renal/

O

hepatic impairment, history of GI tract disease, predisposition to fluid retention.

LIFESPAN CONSIDERATIONS

Pregnancy/Lactation: Unknown if drug is distributed in breast milk. Avoid use during third trimester (may adversely affect fetal cardiovascular system: premature closure of ductus arteriosus). **Pregnancy Category C (D if used in third trimester or near delivery). Children:** Safety and efficacy not established. **Elderly:** Age-related renal impairment may increase risk of hepatic/renal toxicity; decreased dosage recommended. GI bleeding/ulceration more likely to cause serious adverse effects.

INTERACTIONS

DRUG: May decrease effects of **antihypertensives, diuretics. Aspirin, other salicylates** may increase risk of GI side effects, bleeding. **Bone marrow depressants** may increase risk of hematologic reactions. May increase effects of **heparin, oral anticoagulants, thrombolytics.** May increase concentration, risk of toxicity of **lithium.** May increase risk of **methotrexate** toxicity. **Probenecid** may increase concentration. HERBAL: **Cat's claw, dong quai, evening primrose, feverfew, garlic, ginger, ginkgo, ginseng, horse chestnut, red clover** possess antiplatelet activity, may increase risk of bleeding. FOOD: None known. LAB VALUES: May increase BUN, serum creatinine, AST, ALT, potassium, LDH, alkaline phosphatase. May decrease Hgb, Hct.

AVAILABILITY (Rx)

Tablets: 600 mg.

ADMINISTRATION/HANDLING

PO

- May give with food, milk, antacids if GI distress occurs.

INDICATIONS/ROUTES/DOSAGE

Osteoarthritis

PO: ADULTS, ELDERLY: 600–1,200 mg once a day (600 mg in pts with low body weight or mild disease).

Rheumatoid Arthritis (RA)

PO: ADULTS, ELDERLY: 1,200 mg once daily. Range: 600–1,800 mg/day. **Maximum dose:** weight greater than 50 kg: 1,800 mg; weight 50 kg or less: 1,200 mg.

Juvenile Rheumatoid Arthritis (JRA)

PO: CHILDREN WEIGHING MORE THAN 54 KG: 1,200 mg/day. **CHILDREN WEIGHING 32–54 KG:** 900 mg/day. **CHILDREN WEIGHING 22–31 KG:** 600 mg/day.

Dosage in Renal Impairment

Adults, elderly pts with renal impairment: Recommended initial dose is 600 mg/day; may be increased up to 1,200 mg/day.

SIDE EFFECTS

Occasional (9%–3%): Nausea, diarrhea, constipation, dyspepsia (heartburn, indigestion, epigastric pain), edema. Rare (less than 3%): Vomiting, abdominal cramps/pain, flatulence, anorexia, confusion, tinnitus, insomnia, drowsiness.

ADVERSE EFFECTS/ TOXIC REACTIONS

Hypertension, acute renal failure, respiratory depression, GI bleeding, coma occur rarely.

NURSING CONSIDERATIONS

BASELINE ASSESSMENT

Assess onset, type, location, duration of pain/inflammation.

INTERVENTION/EVALUATION

Observe for weight gain, edema, bleeding, ecchymoses, mental confusion. Monitor renal/hepatic function tests. Assess for therapeutic response: relief of pain, stiffness, swelling; increased joint mobility; reduced joint tenderness; improved grip strength.

PATIENT/FAMILY TEACHING

- Avoid aspirin, alcohol during therapy (increases risk of GI bleeding). • If gas-

O

tric upset occurs, take with food, milk, antacids. • If GI effects persist, inform physician. • Notify physician if blood in stool, weight gain, persistent abdominal pain occur. • Avoid tasks that require alertness, motor skills until response to drug is established.

oxcarbazepine

ox-car-**bah**-zeh-peen
(Trileptal)

Do not confuse oxcarbazepine with carbamazepine or Trileptal with TriLipix.

◆CLASSIFICATION

CLINICAL: Anticonvulsant (see p. 35C).

ACTION

Blocks sodium channels, stabilizing hyperexcited neural membranes, inhibiting repetitive neuronal firing, diminishing synaptic impulses. **Therapeutic Effect:** Prevents seizures.

PHARMACOKINETICS

Completely absorbed from GI tract. Extensively metabolized in liver to active metabolite. Protein binding: 40%. Primarily excreted in urine. **Half-life:** 2 hrs; metabolite, 6–10 hrs.

USES

Monotherapy, adjunctive therapy in adults, children 4 yrs and older for treatment of partial seizures. Adjunctive therapy in children 2 yrs and older for partial seizures. **OFF-LABEL:** Atypical panic disorder, bipolar disorder, neuralgia/neuropathy.

PRECAUTIONS

Contraindications: None significant. **Cautions:** Renal impairment, sensitivity to carbamazepine.

⌛ LIFESPAN CONSIDERATIONS

Pregnancy/Lactation: Crosses placenta. Distributed in breast milk. **Pregnancy Category C. Children:** No age-related precautions in those older than 4 yrs. **Elderly:** Age-related renal impairment may require dosage adjustment.

INTERACTIONS

DRUG: **Alcohol, CNS depressants** may have additive sedative effect. **Carbamazepine, phenobarbital, phenytoin, valproic acid, verapamil** may decrease concentration, effects. May decrease effectiveness of **felodipine, oral contraceptives, verapamil.** May increase concentration, risk of toxicity of **phenobarbital, phenytoin.** **HERBAL:** **Gotu kola, kava kava, St. John's wort, valerian** may increase CNS depression. **Evening primrose** may decrease seizure threshold. **St. John's wort** may decrease concentration. **FOOD:** None known. **LAB VALUES:** May increase hepatic function test results. May decrease serum sodium.

AVAILABILITY (Rx)

Oral Suspension: 300 mg/5 ml. **Tablets:** 150 mg, 300 mg, 600 mg.

ADMINISTRATION/HANDLING

PO

• Give without regard to food.

INDICATIONS/ROUTES/DOSAGE

Adjunctive Treatment of Seizures

PO: ADULTS, ELDERLY: Initially, 600 mg/day in 2 divided doses. May increase by up to 600 mg/day at weekly intervals. **Maximum:** 2,400 mg/day. **CHILDREN 4–16 YRS:** 8–10 mg/kg. **Maximum:** 600 mg/day. Maintenance (based on weight): 1,800 mg/day for children weighing more than 39 kg; 1,200 mg/day for children weighing 29.1–39 kg; and 900 mg/day for children weighing 20–29 kg. **CHILDREN 2–3 YRS:** 8–10 mg/kg/day. **Maximum:** 600 mg/day.

Conversion to Monotherapy

PO: ADULTS, ELDERLY: 600 mg/day in 2 divided doses (while decreasing concomitant anticonvulsant over 3–6 wks).

May increase by 600 mg/day at weekly intervals up to 2,400 mg/day. **CHILDREN 4–16 YRS:** Initially, 8–10 mg/kg/day in 2 divided doses with simultaneous initial reduction of dose of concomitant antiepileptic over 3–6 wks. May increase by maximum of 10 mg/kg/day at weekly intervals (see below for recommended daily dose by weight).

Initiation of Monotherapy

PO: ADULTS, ELDERLY: 600 mg/day in 2 divided doses. May increase by 300 mg/day every 3 days up to 1,200 mg/day. **CHILDREN 4–16 YRS:** Initially, 8–10 mg/kg/day in 2 divided doses. Increase at 3 day intervals by 5 mg/kg/day to achieve maintenance dose by weight as follows:

Weight	Dosage
70+ kg	1,500–2,100 mg/day
60–69 kg	1,200–2,100 mg/day
50–59 kg	1,200–1,800 mg/day
41–49 kg	1,200–1,500 mg/day
35–40 kg	900–1,500 mg/day
25–34 kg	900–1,200 mg/day
20–24 kg	600–900 mg/day

Dosage in Renal Impairment

Creatinine clearance less than 30 ml/min: Give 50% of normal starting dose, then titrate slowly to desired dose.

SIDE EFFECTS

Frequent (22%–13%): Dizziness, nausea, headache. **Occasional (7%–5%):** Vomiting, diarrhea, ataxia (muscular incoordination), nervousness, dyspepsia (heartburn, indigestion, epigastric pain), constipation. **Rare (4%):** Tremor, rash, back pain, epistaxis, sinusitis, diplopia.

ADVERSE EFFECTS/ TOXIC REACTIONS

Clinically significant hyponatremia may occur, manifested as leg cramping, hypotension, cold/clammy skin, increased pulse rate, headache, nausea, vomiting, diarrhea. Suicidal ideation occurs rarely.

NURSING CONSIDERATIONS

BASELINE ASSESSMENT

Review history of seizure disorder (type, onset, intensity, frequency, duration, LOC), drug history (esp. other anticonvulsants). Provide safety precautions; quiet, dark environment.

INTERVENTION/EVALUATION

Assist with ambulation if dizziness, ataxia occur. Assess for visual abnormalities, headache. Monitor serum sodium. Assess for signs of hyponatremia (nausea, malaise, headache, lethargy, confusion). Assess for clinical improvement (decrease in intensity, frequency of seizures). Monitor for suicidal ideation.

PATIENT/FAMILY TEACHING

• Do not abruptly stop taking medication (may increase seizure activity). • Inform physician if rash, nausea, headache, dizziness occurs. • May need periodic blood tests. • Avoid tasks that require alertness, motor skills until response to drug is established. • Avoid alcohol. • May decrease effectiveness of oral contraceptives.

oxybutynin

ox-i-**byoo**-ti-nin
(Apo-Oxybutynin 🍁, Ditropan, Ditropan XL, Gelnique, Novo-Oxybutynin 🍁, Oxytrol)
Do not confuse Ditropan with Detrol, diazepam, or Diprivan, or oxybutynin with OxyContin.

◆CLASSIFICATION

PHARMACOTHERAPEUTIC: Anticholinergic. **CLINICAL:** Antispasmodic.

ACTION

Exerts antispasmodic (papaverine-like), antimuscarinic (atropine-like) action on detrusor smooth muscle of bladder.

Therapeutic Effect: Increases bladder capacity, delays desire to void.

PHARMACOKINETICS

Route	Onset	Peak	Duration
PO	0.5–1 hr	3–6 hrs	6–10 hrs

Rapidly, well absorbed from GI tract. Metabolized in liver. Primarily excreted in urine. Unknown if removed by hemodialysis. **Half-life:** 1–2.3 hrs; metabolite, 7–8 hrs.

USES

Relief of symptoms (urgency, incontinence, frequency, nocturia, urge incontinence) associated with uninhibited neurogenic bladder, reflex neurogenic bladder.

PRECAUTIONS

Contraindications: GI/GU obstruction, glaucoma, myasthenia gravis, toxic megacolon, ulcerative colitis. **Cautions:** Renal/hepatic impairment, cardiovascular disease, hyperthyroidism, reflux esophagitis, hypertension, prostatic hypertrophy, neuropathy.

LIFESPAN CONSIDERATIONS

Pregnancy/Lactation: Unknown if drug crosses placenta or is distributed in breast milk. **Pregnancy Category B. Children:** No age-related precautions noted in those older than 5 yrs. **Elderly:** May be more sensitive to anticholinergic effects (e.g., dry mouth, urinary retention).

INTERACTIONS

DRUG: Medications with anticholinergic effects (e.g., antihistamines) may increase anticholinergic effects. **Clarithromycin, erythromycin, itraconazole, ketoconazole** may alter pharmacokinetic parameters. **HERBAL:** None significant. **FOOD:** None known. **LAB VALUES:** None significant.

AVAILABILITY (Rx)

Syrup (Ditropan): 5 mg/5 ml. **Tablets (Ditropan):** 5 mg. **Topical Gel (Gelnique):** 100 mg/unit dose sachet. **Transdermal (Oxytrol):** 3.9 mg.

Tablets (Extended-Release [Ditropan XL]): 5 mg, 10 mg, 15 mg.

ADMINISTRATION/HANDLING

PO

• Give without regard to meals. • Extended-release tablet must be swallowed whole; do not crush, divide, chew.

Transdermal

• Apply patch to dry, intact skin on abdomen, hip, buttock. • Use new application site for each new patch; avoid reapplication to same site within 7 days.

Topical Gel

• Apply contents of 1 sachet once daily to dry, intact skin on abdomen, upper arms/shoulders, or thighs. • Do not bathe/shower until 1 hr after gel is applied.

INDICATIONS/ROUTES/DOSAGE

Neurogenic Bladder

PO: ADULTS: 5 mg 2–3 times a day up to 5 mg 4 times a day. **ELDERLY:** 2.5–5 mg 2–3 times a day. **CHILDREN OLDER THAN 5 YRS:** 5 mg twice a day up to 5 mg 3 times a day. **CHILDREN 1–5 YRS:** 0.2 mg/kg/dose 2–4 times a day.

PO (EXTENDED-RELEASE): ADULTS, ELDERLY: 5–10 mg/day up to 30 mg/day. **CHILDREN 6 YRS AND OLDER:** Initially, 5–10 mg once a day. May increase in 5–10 mg increments. **Maximum:** 20 mg/day.

TRANSDERMAL: ADULTS: 3.9 mg applied twice a wk. Apply every 3–4 days.

TOPICAL GEL: ADULTS, ELDERLY: 100 mg once daily.

SIDE EFFECTS

Frequent: Constipation, dry mouth, drowsiness, decreased perspiration. **Occasional:** Decreased lacrimation/salivation, impotence, urinary hesitancy/retention, suppressed lactation, blurred vision, mydriasis, nausea/vomiting, insomnia.

O

ADVERSE EFFECTS/ TOXIC REACTIONS

Overdose produces CNS excitation (nervousness, restlessness, hallucinations, irritability), hypotension/hypertension, confusion, tachycardia, facial flushing, respiratory depression.

NURSING CONSIDERATIONS

BASELINE ASSESSMENT

Assess dysuria, urgency, frequency, incontinence.

INTERVENTION/EVALUATION

Monitor for symptomatic relief. Monitor I&O; palpate bladder for retention. Monitor daily pattern of bowel activity and stool consistency.

PATIENT/FAMILY TEACHING

- Avoid alcohol. • May cause dry mouth (sugarless candy/gum may reduce effect). • Avoid tasks that require alertness, motor skills until response to drug is established (may cause drowsiness).
- Avoid strenuous activity in warm environment.

O

oxycodone

HIGH ALERT

ox-ee-**koe**-done
(ETH-Oxydose, OxyContin, OxyIR, Roxicodone, Roxicodone Intensol, Supeudol ❖)

BLACK BOX ALERT **OxyContin (controlled-release):** Not intended as an "as needed" analgesic or for immediate postop pain control. Extended-release should not be crushed, broken, or chewed (otherwise leads to rapid release and absorption of potentially fatal dose). Be alert to signs of abuse, misuse, and diversion. CYP3A4 inhibitors or inducers can affect oxycodone levels.

Do not confuse oxycodone with hydrocodone, oxybutynin, or oxymorphone, OxyContin with MS Contin or oxybutynin, or Roxicodone with Roxanol.

FIXED-COMBINATION(S)

Combunox: oxycodone/ibuprofen (an NSAID): 5 mg/400 mg. **Endocet:** oxycodone/acetaminophen (a non-narcotic analgesic): 5 mg/325 mg, 7.5 mg/325 mg, 7.5 mg/500 mg, 10 mg/325 mg, 10 mg/650 mg. **Magnacet:** oxycodone/acetaminophen (a non-narcotic analgesic): 2.5 mg/400 mg, 7.5 mg/400 mg, 10 mg/400 mg. **Percocet:** oxycodone/acetaminophen: 2.5 mg/325 mg, 5 mg/325 mg, 5 mg/500 mg, 7.5 mg/325 mg, 7.5 mg/500 mg, 10 mg/325 mg, 10 mg/650 mg. **Percocet, Roxicet, Tylox:** oxycodone/acetaminophen (a non-narcotic analgesic): 5 mg/500 mg. **Percodan:** oxycodone/aspirin (a non-narcotic analgesic): 2.25 mg/325 mg, 4.5 mg/325 mg.

◆CLASSIFICATION

PHARMACOTHERAPEUTIC: Opioid analgesic **(Schedule II). CLINICAL:** Narcotic analgesic (see p. 142C).

ACTION

Binds with opioid receptors within CNS. **Therapeutic Effect:** Alters perception of and emotional response to pain.

PHARMACOKINETICS

Route	Onset	Peak	Duration
PO, Immediate-release	10–15 min	0.5–1 hr	3–6 hrs
PO, Controlled-release	10–15 min	0.5–1 hr	Up to 12 hrs

Moderately absorbed from GI tract. Protein binding: 38%–45%. Widely distributed. Metabolized in liver. Excreted in urine. Unknown if removed by hemodialysis. **Half-life:** 2–3 hrs (5 hrs controlled-release).

USES

Relief of mild to moderately severe pain.

PRECAUTIONS

Contraindications: Acute bronchial asthma, hypercarbia, paralytic ileus, respiratory depression. Extreme Caution: CNS depression, anoxia, hypercapnia, respiratory depression, seizures, acute alcoholism, shock, untreated myxedema, respiratory dysfunction. Cautions: Increased ICP, hepatic impairment, acute abdominal conditions, hypothyroidism, prostatic hypertrophy, Addison's disease, urethral stricture, COPD.

LIFESPAN CONSIDERATIONS

Pregnancy/Lactation: Readily crosses placenta. Distributed in breast milk. Respiratory depression may occur in neonate if mother received opiates during labor. Regular use of opiates during pregnancy may produce withdrawal symptoms in neonate (irritability, excessive crying, tremors, hyperactive reflexes, fever, vomiting, diarrhea, yawning, sneezing, seizures). **Pregnancy Category B (D if used for prolonged periods or at high dosages at term).** **Children:** Paradoxical excitement may occur. Those younger than 2 yrs are more susceptible to respiratory depressant effects. **Elderly:** Age-related renal impairment may increase risk of urinary retention. May be more susceptible to respiratory depressant effects.

INTERACTIONS

DRUG: **Alcohol, other CNS depressants** may increase CNS effects, respiratory depression, hypotension. **CYP3A4 inhibitors (clarithromycin, ketoconazole)** may increase concentration, toxicity. **CYP3A4 inducers (carbamazepine, rifampin)** may decrease concentration, effect. **MAOIs** may produce severe, sometimes fatal reaction (administer ¼ of usual oxycodone dose). HERBAL: **Gotu kola, kava kava, St. John's wort, valerian** may increase CNS depression. FOOD: None known. LAB VALUES: May increase serum amylase, lipase.

AVAILABILITY (Rx)

Note: New formulation of controlled-release intended to prevent medication from being cut, broken, chewed, crushed, or dissolved to reduce risk of overdose due to tampering, snorting, or injection.

Capsules (Immediate-Release [Oxyir]): 5 mg. Oral Concentrate (Oxydose, Roxicodone Intensol): 20 mg/ml. Oral Solution (Roxicodone): 5 mg/5 ml. Tablets (Roxicodone): 5 mg, 10 mg, 15 mg, 20 mg, 30 mg, 40 mg.

Tablets (Controlled-Release [Oxycontin]): 10 mg, 15 mg, 20 mg, 30 mg, 40 mg, 60 mg, 80 mg.

ADMINISTRATION/HANDLING

PO

• Give without regard to meals. • Tablets may be crushed. • **Controlled-Release:** Swallow whole; do not crush, break, chew.

INDICATIONS/ROUTES/DOSAGE

Analgesia

PO (IMMEDIATE-RELEASE): ADULTS, ELDERLY: Initially, 5–10 mg q4–6h as needed. Range: 2.5–15 mg/dose. **CHILDREN, 6–18 YRS:** 0.1–0.2 mg/kg/dose q6h as needed. **Maximum initial dose:** 5 mg for moderate pain, 10 mg for severe pain.

Opioid Naive

PO (CONTROLLED-RELEASE): ADULTS, ELDERLY: Initially, 10 mg q12h.

◀ALERT▶ To convert from other opioids or non-opioid analgesics to oxycodone controlled-release, refer to OxyContin package insert. Dosages are reduced in pts with severe hepatic disease.

SIDE EFFECTS

◀ALERT▶ Effects are dependent on dosage amount. Ambulatory pts, those not in severe pain may experience dizziness, nausea, vomiting, hypotension more frequently than those in supine position or having severe pain. Frequent: Drowsiness, dizziness, hypotension (including ortho-

O

static hypotension), anorexia. **Occasional:** Confusion, diaphoresis, facial flushing, urinary retention, constipation, dry mouth, nausea, vomiting, headache. **Rare:** Allergic reaction, depression, paradoxical CNS hyperactivity, nervousness in children, paradoxical excitement, restlessness in elderly, debilitated pts.

ADVERSE EFFECTS/ TOXIC REACTIONS

Overdose results in respiratory depression, skeletal muscle flaccidity, cold/clammy skin, cyanosis, extreme drowsiness progressing to seizures, stupor, coma. Hepatotoxicity may occur with overdose of acetaminophen component of fixed-combination product. Tolerance to analgesic effect, physical dependence may occur with repeated use. **Antidote:** Naloxone (see Appendix M for dosage).

NURSING CONSIDERATIONS

BASELINE ASSESSMENT

Assess onset, type, location, duration of pain. Effect of medication is reduced if full pain recurs before next dose. Obtain vital signs before giving medication. If respirations are 12/min or less (20/min or less in children), withhold medication, contact physician.

INTERVENTION/EVALUATION

Palpate bladder for urinary retention. Monitor daily pattern of bowel activity and stool consistency. Initiate deep breathing, coughing exercises, esp. in pts with pulmonary impairment. Monitor pain relief, respiratory rate, mental status, B/P.

PATIENT/FAMILY TEACHING

• May cause dry mouth, drowsiness. • Avoid tasks that require alertness, motor skills until response to drug is established. • Avoid alcohol. • May be habit forming. • Do not crush, chew, break controlled-release tablets. • Report severe constipation, absence of pain relief.

OxyContin, *see oxycodone*

OxyIR, *see oxycodone*

oxymorphone

HIGH ALERT

ox-ee-**more**-phone
(Opana, Opana ER, Opana Injectable)

BLACK BOX ALERT Has abuse liability. Concern about increased risk of abuse, misuse, or diversion.

Do not confuse oxymorphone with oxycodone.

◆CLASSIFICATION

PHARMACOTHERAPEUTIC: Opioid agonist **(Schedule II). CLINICAL:** Narcotic analgesic, antianxiety, preop anesthetic.

ACTION

Binds to opiate receptors sites within CNS. **Therapeutic Effect:** Reduces intensity of pain stimuli, alters pain perception, emotional response to pain. Parenterally, 1 mg oxymorphone equivalent to 10 mg morphine.

PHARMACOKINETICS

Route	Onset	Peak	Duration
Parenteral	5–10 min	N/A	3–6 hrs

Well absorbed. Protein binding: 10%. Widely distributed. Extensive hepatic metabolism. Excreted in urine. **Half-life:** 7–9 hrs; **Extended-release:** 9–11 hrs.

USES

Injection: Relief of moderate to severe pain, preop medication, anesthesia support, obstetric analgesia, relief of anxiety in those with dyspnea associated with pulmonary edema secondary to acute left ventricular dysfunction. **PO (Immedi-**

ate-Release): Relief of moderate to severe acute pain. **(Extended-Release):** Pts requiring continuous treatment for extended period of time.

PRECAUTIONS

Contraindications: Hypersensitivity to morphine, acute asthma attack, acute respiratory depression, paralytic ileus, pulmonary edema secondary to chemical respiratory irritants, moderate to severe hepatic function impairment. **Extreme Cautions:** Anoxia, hypercapnia, seizures, acute alcoholism, shock, untreated myxedema. **Cautions:** Hypothyroidism, prostatic hypertrophy, Addison's disease, urethral stricture, COPD.

LIFESPAN CONSIDERATIONS

Pregnancy/Lactation: Unknown if distributed in breast milk. May prolong labor if administered in latent phase of first stage of labor or before cervical dilation of 4–5 cm has occurred. Respiratory depression may occur in neonate if mother received opiates during labor. Regular use of opiates during pregnancy may produce withdrawal symptoms in the neonate (irritability, excessive crying, tremors, hyperactive reflexes, fever, vomiting, diarrhea, yawning, sneezing, seizures). **Pregnancy Category C.** (**Category D** if used for prolong periods or high doses at term.) **Children:** Safety and efficacy not established in those younger than 18 yrs. **Elderly:** May be more susceptible to respiratory depression, may cause paradoxical excitement. Age-related hepatic impairment, debilitation may require dosage adjustment.

INTERACTIONS

DRUG: **Alcohol, other CNS depressants** may increase CNS effects, respiratory depression, hypotension. **Anticholinergics** may increase risk of urinary retention, severe constipation (may lead to paralytic ileus). **Propofol** increases risk of bradycardia. Decreased effect when given concurrently with **phenothiazines.** **HERBAL:** **Gotu kola, kava kava, St. John's wort, valerian** may produce CNS depressant effects. **FOOD:** None known. **LAB VALUES:** May increase serum amylase, lipase.

AVAILABILITY (Rx)

Injection: 1 mg/ml. **Tablets:** 5 mg, 10 mg.

Tablets (Extended-Release): 5 mg, 7.5 mg, 10 mg, 15 mg, 20 mg, 30 mg, 40 mg.

ADMINISTRATION/HANDLING

IV

Rate of administration • Administer IV push very slowly. • Rapid IV increases risk of severe adverse reactions (chest wall rigidity, apnea, peripheral circulatory collapse, anaphylactoid effects, cardiac arrest).

IM/Subcutaneous

• Inject deep IM, preferably in upper, outer quadrant of buttock. • Use short 30-gauge needle for subcutaneous injection. • Administer slowly, rotating injection sites. • Pts with circulatory impairment experience higher risk of overdosage due to delayed absorption of repeated administration.

Storage • Store parenteral form at room temperature. Refrigerate suppository form. • Discard parenteral form if discolored or particulate forms.

PO

• Give 1 hr before or 2 hrs after meals. • Do not chew, dissolve, crush extended-release tablet.

IV COMPATIBILITIES

Glycopyrrolate, hydroxyzine, ranitidine.

INDICATIONS/ROUTES/DOSAGE

Analgesia

IV: ADULTS 18 YRS AND OLDER, ELDERLY: Initially, 0.5 mg. Dose may be cautiously increased until satisfactory response is achieved.

ALERT IM preferred over subcutaneous route (subcutaneous rate of absorption is less reliable).

O

IM/SUBCUTANEOUS: ADULTS 18 YRS AND OLDER, ELDERLY: Initially, 1–1.5 mg every 4–6 hrs as needed.

PO: ADULTS, ELDERLY: (IMMEDIATE-RELEASE): 10–20 mg q4–6hrs. **(EXTENDED-RELEASE):** Initially, 5 mg q12h. May increase by 5–10 mg q12h every 3–7 days.

Analgesia During Labor

IM/SUBCUTANEOUS: ADULTS 18 YRS AND OLDER, ELDERLY: 0.5–1 mg.

SIDE EFFECTS

Note: Effects are dependent on dosage amount, route of administration. Ambulatory pts, those not in severe pain may experience dizziness, nausea, vomiting, hypotension more frequently than those in supine position or having severe pain. **Frequent (10% or higher):** Drowsiness, hypotension, dizziness, nausea, vomiting, constipation, weakness. **Occasional (9%–2%):** Nervousness, headache, restlessness, malaise, confusion, anorexia, abdominal cramps, dry mouth, decreased urinary output, ureteral spasm, pain at injection site. **Rare (1% or less):** Depression, paradoxical CNS stimulation, hallucinations, rash, urticaria.

ADVERSE EFFECTS/ TOXIC REACTIONS

Overdose results in respiratory depression, skeletal muscle flaccidity, cold/clammy skin, cyanosis, extreme drowsiness progressing to convulsions, stupor, coma. Tolerance to analgesic effect, physical dependence may occur with repeated use. Prolonged duration of action, cumulative effect may occur in those with hepatic/renal impairment.

NURSING CONSIDERATIONS

BASELINE ASSESSMENT

Assess onset, type, location, duration of pain. Obtain vital signs before giving medication. If respirations are 12/min or lower, withhold medication, contact physician. Effect of medication is reduced if full pain recurs before next dose.

INTERVENTION/EVALUATION

Monitor vital signs 5–10 min after IV administration, 15–30 min after subcutaneous, IM. Be alert for decreased respirations, B/P. To prevent pain cycles, instruct pt to request pain medication as soon as discomfort begins. Assess for clinical improvement, record onset of pain relief. Consult physician if pain relief is not adequate.

PATIENT/FAMILY TEACHING

• Discomfort may occur with injection. • Change positions slowly to avoid postural hypotension. • Avoid tasks that require alertness, motor skills until response to drug is established. • Avoid alcohol. • Tolerance/dependence may occur with prolonged use of high doses.

oxytocin

HIGH ALERT

ox-ee-**toe**-sin
(Pitocin, Syntocinon)

BLACK BOX ALERT Not to be given for elective labor induction, but when medically indicated.

Do not confuse Pitocin with Pitressin.

CLASSIFICATION

PHARMACOTHERAPEUTIC: Uterine smooth muscle stimulant. **CLINICAL:** Oxytocic.

ACTION

Affects uterine myofibril activity, stimulates mammary smooth muscle. **Therapeutic Effect:** Contracts uterine smooth muscle. Enhances lactation.

PHARMACOKINETICS

Route	Onset	Peak	Duration
IV	Immediate	N/A	1 hr
IM	3–5 min	N/A	2–3 hrs

O

Rapidly absorbed through nasal mucous membranes. Protein binding: 30%. Distributed in extracellular fluid. Metabolized in liver, kidney. Primarily excreted in urine. **Half-life:** 1–6 min.

USES

Induction of labor at term, control of post-partum bleeding. Adjunct in management of abortion.

PRECAUTIONS

Contraindications: Adequate uterine activity that fails to progress, cephalopelvic disproportion, fetal distress without imminent delivery, grand multiparity, hyperactive or hypertonic uterus, obstetric emergencies that favor surgical intervention, prematurity, unengaged fetal head, unfavorable fetal position/presentation, when vaginal delivery is contraindicated, (e.g., active genital herpes infection, placenta previa, cord presentation). **Cautions:** Induction of labor should be for medical, not elective, reasons.

LIFESPAN CONSIDERATIONS

Pregnancy/Lactation: Used as indicated, not expected to present risk of fetal abnormalities. Small amounts in breast milk. Breast-feeding not recommended. **Pregnancy Category X. Children/Elderly:** Not used in these pt populations.

INTERACTIONS

DRUG: **Caudal block anesthetics, vasopressors** may increase pressor effects. **Other oxytocics** may cause cervical lacerations, uterine hypertonus, uterine rupture. **HERBAL:** None significant. **FOOD:** None known. **LAB VALUES:** None significant.

AVAILABILITY (Rx)

Injection (Pitocin): 10 units/ml.

ADMINISTRATION/HANDLING

IV

Reconstitution • Dilute 10–40 units (1–4 ml) in 1,000 ml of 0.9% NaCl, lactated Ringer's, or D_5W to provide concentration of 10–40 milliunits/ml solution.

Rate of administration • Give by IV infusion (use infusion device to carefully control rate of flow as ordered by physician).

Storage • Store at room temperature.

IV INCOMPATIBILITIES

No known incompatibilities via Y-site administration.

IV COMPATIBILITIES

Heparin, insulin, multivitamins, potassium chloride.

INDICATIONS/ROUTES/DOSAGE

Induction or Stimulation of Labor

IV: ADULTS: 0.5–1 milliunit/min. May gradually increase in increments of 1–2 milliunits/min. Rates of 9–10 milliunits/min are rarely required.

Abortion

IV: ADULTS: 10–20 milliunits/min. **Maximum:** 30 units/12-hr dose.

Control of Postpartum Bleeding

IV INFUSION: ADULTS: 10–40 units in 1,000 ml IV fluid at rate sufficient to control uterine atony.

IM: ADULTS: 10 units (total dose) after delivery.

SIDE EFFECTS

Occasional: Tachycardia, premature ventricular contractions, hypotension, nausea, vomiting. **Rare:** **Nasal:** Lacrimation/tearing, nasal irritation, rhinorrhea, unexpected uterine bleeding/contractions.

ADVERSE EFFECTS/ TOXIC REACTIONS

Hypertonicity may occur with tearing of uterus, increased bleeding, abruptio placentae (i.e., placental abruption), cervical/vaginal lacerations. **FETAL:** Bradycardia, CNS/brain damage, trauma due to rapid propulsion, low Apgar score at 5 min, retinal hemorrhage occur rarely. Prolonged IV infusion of oxytocin with excessive fluid volume has caused severe water intoxication with seizures, coma, death.

NURSING CONSIDERATIONS

BASELINE ASSESSMENT

Assess baselines for vital signs, B/P, fetal heart rate. Determine frequency, duration, strength of contractions.

INTERVENTION/EVALUATION

Monitor B/P, pulse, respirations, fetal heart rate, intrauterine pressure, contractions (duration, strength, frequency) q15min. Notify physician of contractions that last longer than 1 min, occur more frequently than every 2 min, or stop. Maintain careful I&O; be alert to potential water intoxication. Check for blood loss.

PATIENT/FAMILY TEACHING

- Keep pt, family informed of labor progress.

Oxytrol, *see oxybutynin*

Pacerone, *see amiodarone*

paclitaxel HIGH ALERT

pak-li-**tax**-el
(Abraxane ✦, Apo-Paclitaxel ✦, Onxol, Taxol)

BLACK BOX ALERT Myelosuppression is major dose-limiting toxicity. Must be administered by certified chemotherapy personnel. Severe hypersensitivity reactions reported.

Do not confuse paclitaxel with paroxetine or Paxil, or Taxol with Paxil or Taxotere.

◆CLASSIFICATION

PHARMACOTHERAPEUTIC: Taxoid, antimitotic agent. **CLINICAL:** Antineoplastic (see p. 87C).

ACTION

Promotes the polymerization of tubulin, disrupting normal microtubule dynamics required for cell division in late G_2, M phases of cell cycle. **Therapeutic Effect:** Inhibits cellular mitosis, replication.

PHARMACOKINETICS

Does not readily cross blood-brain barrier. Protein binding: 89%–98%. Metabolized in liver to active metabolites; eliminated by bile. Not removed by hemodialysis. **Half-life:** 3-hr infusion: 13.1–20.2 hrs; 24-hr infusion: 15.7–52.7 hrs.

USES

(Onxol, Taxol): First-line treatment of advanced ovarian cancer, treatment of metastatic ovarian cancer following failure of first-line or subsequent chemotherapy. Treatment of breast cancer, AIDS-related Kaposi's sarcoma, non–small-cell lung cancer (NSCLC). **(Abraxane):** Treatment of breast cancer after failure of combination chemotherapy or relapse within 6 mos of adjuvant chemotherapy. **OFF-LABEL:** Treatment of upper GI tract adenocarcinoma, head and neck cancer, hormone-refractory prostate cancer, metastatic breast cancer, non-Hodgkin's lymphoma, small-cell lung cancer, transitional cell cancer of urothelium.

PRECAUTIONS

Contraindications: Baseline neutropenia (neutrophil count 1,500 cells/mm^3 or less) 1,000 cells/mm^3 or less when treating AIDS-related Kaposi's sarcoma (Onxol, Taxol), hypersensitivity to drugs developed with Cremophor EL (polyoxyethylated castor oil). **Cautions:** Hepatic impairment, severe neutropenia, peripheral neuropathy.

LIFESPAN CONSIDERATIONS

Pregnancy/Lactation: May produce fetal harm. Unknown if distributed in breast milk. Avoid use in pregnancy. **Pregnancy Category D. Children:** Safety and efficacy not established. **Elderly:** No age-related precautions noted.

INTERACTIONS

Drug: **Bone marrow depressants** may increase myelosuppression. **Live virus vaccines** may potentiate virus replication, increase vaccine side effects, decrease pt's antibody response to vaccine. HERBAL: Avoid **black cohosh, dong quai** in estrogen-dependent tumors. **Gotu kola, kava kava, St. John's wort, valerian** may increase CNS depression. FOOD: None known. LAB VALUES: May elevate serum alkaline phosphatase, bilirubin, AST, ALT, triglycerides.

AVAILABILITY (Rx)

Injection, Powder for Reconstitution (Abraxane): 100-mg vial. **Injection Solution (Onxol, Taxol):** 6 mg/ml.

ADMINISTRATION/HANDLING

IV

◀ALERT▶ Wear gloves during handling; if contact with skin occurs, wash hands thoroughly with soap, water. If contact with mucous membranes occurs, flush with water.

Onxol, Taxol

Reconstitution • Dilute with 250–1,000 ml 0.9% NaCl, D_5W to final concentration of 0.3–1.2 mg/ml.

Rate of administration • Administer at rate as ordered by physician (over 1–24 hrs) through in-line filter not greater than 0.22 microns. • Monitor vital signs during infusion, esp. during first hour. • Discontinue administration if severe hypersensitivity reaction occurs.

Storage • Store unopened vials at room temperature. • Prepared solution is stable at room temperature for 48 hrs. • Store diluted solutions in bottles or plastic bags. Administer through polyethylene-lined administration sets (avoid plasticized PVC equipment or devices).

Abraxane

Reconstitution • Reconstitute each vial with 20 ml 0.9% NaCl to provide concentration of 5 mg/ml. • Slowly inject onto inside wall of vial; gently swirl over 2 min to avoid foaming. • Inject appropriate amount into empty PVC-type bag.

Rate of administration • Infuse over 30 min.

Storage • Store unopened vials at room temperature • Once reconstituted, use immediately but may refrigerate for up to 8 hrs.

IV INCOMPATIBILITIES

◀ALERT▶ IV Compatibility: Data for Abraxane not known; avoid mixing with other medication. **Onxol, Taxol:** Amphotericin B complex (Abelcet, AmBisome, Amphotec), chlorpromazine (Thorazine), doxorubicin liposomal (Doxil), hydroxyzine (Vistaril), methylprednisolone (Solu-Medrol), mitoxantrone (Novantrone).

IV COMPATIBILITIES

Onxol, Taxol: Carboplatin (Paraplatin), cisplatin (Platinol AQ), cyclophosphamide (Cytoxan), cytarabine (Cytosar), dacarbazine (DTIC-Dome), dexamethasone (Decadron), diphenhydramine (Benadryl), doxorubicin (Adriamycin), etoposide (VePesid), gemcitabine (Gemzar), granisetron (Kytril), hydromorphone (Dilaudid), lipids, magnesium sulfate, mannitol, methotrexate, morphine, ondansetron (Zofran), potassium chloride, vinblastine (Velban), vincristine (Oncovin).

INDICATIONS/ROUTES/DOSAGE

Onxol, Taxol

Ovarian Cancer

IV: ADULTS: 135–175 mg/m^2/dose over 3 hrs q3wks, 135 mg/m^2 over 24 hrs, or 50–80 mg/m^2 over 1–3 hrs weekly.

P

Breast Cancer

IV: ADULTS, ELDERLY: 175–250 mg/m^2 over 3 hrs q3wks or 50–80 mg/m^2 over 1–3 hrs weekly.

Non–Small-Cell Lung Cancer

IV: ADULTS, ELDERLY: 135 mg/m^2 over 24 hrs, followed by cisplatin 75 mg/m^2 q3wks.

Kaposi's Sarcoma

IV: ADULTS, ELDERLY: 135 mg/m^2/dose over 3 hrs q3wks or 100 mg/m^2/dose over 3 hrs q2wks.

Dosage in Hepatic Impairment

Transaminase Level	Bilirubin	Dose
24-HR INFUSION		
Less than 2 times ULN	1.5 mg/dl or less	135 mg/m^2
2 to less than 10 times ULN	1.5 mg/dl or less	100 mg/m^2
Less than 10 times ULN	1.6–7.5 mg/dl or less	50 mg/m^2
3-HR INFUSION		
Less than 10 times ULN	1.25 mg/dl or less	175 mg/m^2
Less than 10 times ULN	1.26–2 times ULN	135 mg/m^2
Less than 10 times ULN	2.01–5 times ULN	90 mg/m^2
10 times ULN or greater	Greater than 5 times ULN	Avoid use

ULN: upper limit of normal

Abraxane

Breast Cancer

IV INFUSION: ADULTS, ELDERLY: 260 mg/m^2 q3wks. For pts who experience severe neutropenia (neutrophils less than 500 cells/mm^3 for a wk or longer) or severe sensory neuropathy, reduce dosage to 220 mg/m^2 for subsequent courses. For recurrence of severe neutropenia or severe sensory neuropathy, reduce dosage to 180 mg/m^2 q3wks for subsequent courses. For grade 3 sensory neuropathy, hold until resolution to grade 1 or 2, followed by reduced dose for subsequent courses. Dosage of Abraxane for bilirubin greater than 1.5 mg/dl is not known.

SIDE EFFECTS

Expected (90%–70%): Diarrhea, alopecia, nausea, vomiting. **Frequent (48%–46%):** Myalgia, arthralgia, peripheral neuropathy. **Occasional (20%–13%):** Mucositis, hypotension during infusion, pain/redness at injection site. **Rare (3%):** Bradycardia.

ADVERSE EFFECTS/ TOXIC REACTIONS

Neutropenic nadir occurs at median of 11 days. Anemia, leukopenia occur commonly; thrombocytopenia occurs occasionally. Severe hypersensitivity reaction (dyspnea, severe hypotension, angioedema, generalized urticaria) occurs rarely.

NURSING CONSIDERATIONS

BASELINE ASSESSMENT

Offer emotional support to pt, family. Use strict asepsis, protect pt from infection. Check blood counts, particularly neutrophil, platelet count before each course of therapy or as clinically indicated.

INTERVENTION/EVALUATION

Monitor CBC, platelets, vital signs, hepatic enzymes. Monitor for hematologic toxicity (fever, sore throat, signs of local infections, unusual bleeding/bruising), symptoms of anemia (excessive fatigue, weakness). Assess response to medication; monitor, report diarrhea. Avoid IM injections, rectal temperatures, other traumas that may induce bleeding. Hold pressure to injection sites for full 5 min.

PATIENT/FAMILY TEACHING

• Alopecia is reversible, but new hair may have different color, texture. • Do not have immunizations without physician's approval (drug lowers resistance). • Avoid crowds, persons with known infections. • Report signs of infection at once (fever, flu-like symptoms). • Contact physician if nausea/vomiting continues at home. • Be alert for signs of peripheral neuropathy. • Avoid pregnancy during therapy. • Avoid tasks that may require alertness, motor skills until response to drug is established.

palifermin

pal-ee-**fer**-min
(Kepivance)

◆CLASSIFICATION

PHARMACOTHERAPEUTIC: Keratinocyte growth factor. **CLINICAL:** Antineoplastic adjunct.

ACTION

Binds to keratinocyte growth factor receptor, present on epithelial cells of buccal mucosa, tongue, resulting in proliferation, differentiation, migration of epithelial cells. Therapeutic Effect: Reduces incidence, duration of severe oral mucositis.

PHARMACOKINETICS

Clearance is higher in cancer pts compared to healthy subjects. Half-life: 4.5 hrs.

USES

Reduces incidence, duration, severity of severe stomatitis in pts with hematologic malignancies receiving myelotoxic therapy requiring hematopoietic stem cell support.

PRECAUTIONS

Contraindications: Pts allergic to *Escherichia coli*–derived proteins. **Cautions:** Pregnant and breast-feeding pts.

LIFESPAN CONSIDERATIONS

Pregnancy/Lactation: Unknown if drug crosses placenta or is excreted in breast milk. Use only if potential benefit justifies fetal risk. **Pregnancy Category C.** **Children:** Safety and efficacy not established. **Elderly:** No age-related precautions noted.

INTERACTIONS

DRUG: Binds to **heparin,** decreasing effectiveness. Administration during or within 24 hrs before or after **myelotoxic chemotherapy** results in increased severity, duration of oral mucositis. **HERBAL:** None significant. **FOOD:** None known. **LAB VALUES:** May elevate serum lipase, amylase.

AVAILABILITY (Rx)

Injection, Powder for Reconstitution: 6.25-mg vials.

ADMINISTRATION/HANDLING

IV

Reconstitution • Reconstitute only with 1.2 ml Sterile Water for Injection, using aseptic technique. • Swirl gently to dissolve. Dissolution takes less than 3 min. Do not shake/agitate solution. • Yields final concentration of 5 mg/ml.

Rate of administration • If heparin is being used to maintain an IV line, use 0.9% NaCl to rinse IV line before and after palifermin administration. • Administer by IV bolus injection.

Storage • Store intact vials in refrigerator • If reconstituted solution is not used immediately, may be refrigerated for up to 24 hrs. • Before administration, may be warmed to room temperature for up to 1 hr. • Discard if left at room temperature for more than 1 hr, if discolored or particulate forms. • Protect from light.

INDICATIONS/ROUTES/DOSAGE

Mucositis (Premyelotoxic Therapy)

IV: ADULTS, ELDERLY: 60 mcg/kg/day for 3 consecutive days, with 3rd dose 24–48 hrs before chemotherapy.

Mucositis (Postmyelotoxic Therapy)

IV: ADULTS, ELDERLY: Last 3 doses of 60 mcg/kg/day should be administered after myelotoxic therapy; first of these doses should be administered after, but on the same day of, hematopoietic stem cell infusion and at least 4 days after most recent administration of palifermin.

P

SIDE EFFECTS

Frequent: Rash (62%), fever (39%), pruritus (35%), erythema (32%), edema (28%). **Occasional:** Mouth/tongue thickness/discoloration (17%), altered taste (16%), dysesthesia manifested as hyperesthesia, hypoesthesia, paresthesia (12%), arthralgia (10%).

ADVERSE EFFECTS/ TOXIC REACTIONS

Transient hypertension occurs occasionally.

NURSING CONSIDERATIONS

BASELINE ASSESSMENT

Assess oral mucous membranes for stomatitis (erythema, white patches, ulceration, bleeding).

INTERVENTION/EVALUATION

Assess for oral inflammation, difficulty swallowing, mucosal bleeding. Offer sponge sticks to wash mouth with water. Monitor pt's pain level; medicate as necessary for improved pain control. Offer pt/family emotional support.

PATIENT/FAMILY TEACHING

• Consume bland meals; avoid eating any spicy food. • Rinse mouth often with tepid water; avoid hot, cold liquids. • Take measures to prevent pregnancy.

paliperidone

pal-ee-**per**-i-doan
(Invega, Invega Sustenna)

BLACK BOX ALERT Elderly pts with dementia-related psychosis are at increased risk for mortality due to cerebrovascular events.

◆CLASSIFICATION

PHARMACOTHERAPEUTIC: Benzisoxazole derivative. **CLINICAL:** Antipsychotic.

ACTION

May antagonize dopamine and serotonin receptors. **Therapeutic Effect:** Suppresses behavioral response in psychosis.

PHARMACOKINETICS

Absorbed from GI tract. Metabolized in liver to active metabolite. Primarily excreted in urine. **Half-life:** 23 hrs.

USES

Oral: Treatment of acute (short-term) and long-term maintenance of schizophrenia. Acute treatment of schizoaffective disorder as monotherapy or as adjunct to mood stabilizers and/or antidepressants. **Injection:** Acute and maintenance treatment of schizophrenia. **OFF-LABEL:** Psychosis/agitation related to Alzheimer's dementia.

PRECAUTIONS

Contraindications: Sensitivity to risperidone. Concomitant use with other medications that prolong QT interval (e.g., amiodarone, quinidine). **Cautions:** History of cardiac arrhythmias, renal impairment, diabetes mellitus, heart failure, seizures, pts at risk for aspiration pneumonia. May increase risk of stroke in pts with dementia-related psychosis.

⌛ LIFESPAN CONSIDERATIONS

Pregnancy/Lactation: Unknown if drug crosses placenta or is distributed in breast milk. **Pregnancy Category C. Children:** Safety and efficacy not established. **Elderly:** Potential for orthostatic hypotension. Age-related renal impairment may require dosage adjustment.

INTERACTIONS

DRUG: May decrease effects of **dopamine agonists, levodopa. Alcohol, CNS depressants** may increase CNS depression. **HERBAL:** None significant. **FOOD:** None known. **LAB VALUES:** May increase serum creatine phosphatase, uric acid, triglycerides, AST, ALT, prolactin. May decrease serum potassium, sodium, protein, glucose. May cause EKG changes (including prolonged QT interval).

AVAILABILITY (Rx)

Injection Suspension: 39 mg/0.25 ml, 78 mg/0.5 ml, 117 mg/0.75 ml, 156 mg/ml, 234 mg/1.5 ml.

Tablets, Extended-Release: 1.5 mg, 3 mg, 6 mg, 9 mg, 12 mg.

ADMINISTRATION/HANDLING

PO

• May give without regard to food. • Do not chew, divide, crush extended-release tablets.

IM

• Administer 2 initial injections in deltoid muscle. • Maintenance doses may be given in gluteal or deltoid muscle.

INDICATIONS/ROUTES/DOSAGE

Treatment of Schizophrenia

PO: ADULTS, ELDERLY: 6 mg once daily in the morning. May increase dose in increments of 3 mg/day at intervals of more than 5 days. Range: 3–12 mg/day.
IM: ADULTS, ELDERLY: 234 mg on day 1 followed by 156 mg 1 wk later. Maintenance: Initially, 117 mg monthly. Range: 39–234 mg.

Schizoaffective Disorder

PO: ADULTS, ELDERLY: 6 mg once daily in the morning. May increase in increments of 3 mg/day at intervals of more than 4 days. Range: 3–12 mg/day.

Dosage in Renal Impairment

Creatinine Clearance	Oral Dosage	IM Dosage
50–80 ml/min	6 mg/day maximum	156 mg on day 1, then 117 mg 1 wk later Maintenance: 78 mg once monthly
10–49 ml/min	3 mg/day maximum	Not recommended

SIDE EFFECTS

Occasional: Tachycardia (14%), headache (12%), drowsiness (9%), akathesia (motor restlessness), anxiety (7%), dizziness (5%), dyspepsia, nausea (4%).

ADVERSE EFFECTS/ TOXIC REACTIONS

Neuroleptic malignant syndrome (NMS), hyperpyrexia, muscle rigidity, change in mental status, irregular pulse or B/P, tachycardia, diaphoresis, cardiac arrhythmias, rhabdomyolysis, acute renal failure, tardive dyskinesia (protrusion of tongue, puffing of cheeks, chewing/puckering of mouth) may occur rarely.

NURSING CONSIDERATIONS

BASELINE ASSESSMENT

Renal function tests should be performed before therapy. Assess behavior, appearance, emotional status, response to environment, speech pattern, thought content.

INTERVENTION/EVALUATION

Monitor B/P, heart rate, weight, renal function tests, EKG. Monitor for fine tongue movement (may be first sign of tardive dyskinesia). Supervise suicidal-risk pt closely during early therapy (as depression lessons, energy level improves, increasing suicide potential). Assess for therapeutic response (greater interest in surroundings, improved self-care, increased ability to concentrate, relaxed facial expression). Monitor for potential neuroleptic malignant syndrome (fever, muscle rigidity, irregular B/P or pulse, altered mental status).

PATIENT/FAMILY TEACHING

• Avoid tasks that may require alertness, motor skills until response to drug is established. • Use caution when changing position from lying or sitting to standing. • Inform physician of trembling in fingers, altered gait, unusual muscle/skeletal movements, palpitations, severe dizziness, fainting, swelling/pain in breasts, visual changes, rash, difficulty in breathing.

P

palivizumab

pal-i-**viz**-u-mab
(Synagis)
Do not confuse Synagis with Synalgos-DC.

◆CLASSIFICATION

PHARMACOTHERAPEUTIC: Monoclonal antibody. **CLINICAL:** Antiviral.

ACTION

Exhibits neutralizing activity against respiratory syncytial virus (RSV) in infants. **Therapeutic Effect:** Inhibits RSV replication in lower respiratory tract of children.

USES

Prevention of serious lower respiratory tract disease caused by RSV in pediatric pts younger than 2 yrs at high risk for RSV disease (e.g., hemodynamically significant congenital heart disease).

PRECAUTIONS

Contraindications: Children with cyanotic congenital heart disease. **Cautions:** Thrombocytopenia, any coagulation disorder. Not to be used for treatment of established RSV disease. **Pregnancy Category C.**

INTERACTIONS

DRUG: None significant. **HERBAL:** None significant. **FOOD:** None known. **LAB VALUES:** May increase AST.

AVAILABILITY (Rx)

Injection Solution: 100 mg/ml.

ADMINISTRATION/HANDLING

IM

• Refrigerate vials. • Give undiluted in anterolateral aspect of thigh.

INDICATIONS/ROUTES/DOSAGE

Prevention of Respiratory Syncytial Virus (RSV)

IM: CHILDREN: 15 mg/kg once/mo during RSV season.

SIDE EFFECTS

Frequent (49%–22%): Upper respiratory tract infection, otitis media, rhinitis, rash. **Occasional (10%–2%):** Pain, pharyngitis. **Rare (less than 2%):** Cough, diarrhea, vomiting, injection site reaction.

ADVERSE EFFECTS/ TOXIC REACTIONS

Anaphylaxis, severe acute hypersensitivity reaction occur very rarely.

NURSING CONSIDERATIONS

BASELINE ASSESSMENT

Assess for sensitivity to palivizumab.

INTERVENTION/EVALUATION

Monitor potential side effects, esp. otitis media, rhinitis, skin rash, upper respiratory tract infection.

PATIENT/FAMILY TEACHING

• Discuss with family the purpose, potential side effects of medication.

palonosetron

pal-oh-**noe**-se-tron
(Aloxi)
Do not confuse Aloxi with Eloxatin or oxaliplatin, or palonosetron with dolesetron, granisteron, or ondansetron.

◆CLASSIFICATION

PHARMACOTHERAPEUTIC: 5-HT_3 receptor antagonist. **CLINICAL:** Antinauseant, antiemetic.

ACTION

Acts centrally in chemoreceptor trigger zone, peripherally at vagal nerve terminals. **Therapeutic Effect:** Prevents nausea/vomiting associated with chemotherapy.

PHARMACOKINETICS

Protein binding: 52%. Metabolized in liver. Eliminated in urine. **Half-life:** 40 hrs.

USES

Prevention of acute and delayed nausea/vomiting associated with initial/repeated courses of moderately or highly hematogenic cancer chemotherapy. Prevention of postop nausea/vomiting for up to 24 hrs following surgery.

PRECAUTIONS

Contraindications: None known. **Cautions:** History of cardiovascular disease.

LIFESPAN CONSIDERATIONS

Pregnancy/Lactation: Unknown if distributed in breast milk. **Pregnancy Category B. Children:** Safety and efficacy not established. **Elderly:** No age-related precautions noted.

INTERACTIONS

DRUG: Apomorphine may cause profound hypotension, altered consciousness. **HERBAL:** None significant. **FOOD:** None known. **LAB VALUES:** May transiently increase serum bilirubin, AST, ALT.

AVAILABILITY (Rx)

Capsules: 0.5 mg. **Injection Solution:** 0.05 mg/ml.

ADMINISTRATION/HANDLING

IV

Reconstitution • Give undiluted as IV push.
Rate of administration • Give IV push over 30 sec. • Flush infusion line with 0.9% NaCl before and following administration.
Storage • Store at room temperature. Solution should appear colorless, clear. Discard if cloudy precipitate forms.

IV COMPATIBILITIES

Lorazepam (Ativan), midazolam (Versed).

INDICATIONS/ROUTES/DOSAGE

Chemotherapy-Induced Nausea/Vomiting
IV: ADULTS, ELDERLY: 0.25 mg as single dose 30 min before starting chemotherapy day 1 of each cycle. May be given more frequently than once weekly.

Postop Nausea/Vomiting
IV: ADULTS, ELDERLY: 0.075 mg over 10 sec immediately before induction of anesthesia.

SIDE EFFECTS

Occasional (9%–5%): Headache, constipation. **Rare (less than 1%):** Diarrhea, dizziness, fatigue, abdominal pain, insomnia.

ADVERSE EFFECTS/TOXIC REACTIONS

Overdose may produce combination of CNS stimulation, depressant effects.

NURSING CONSIDERATIONS

BASELINE ASSESSMENT

Assess for dehydration if excessive vomiting occurs (poor skin turgor, dry mucous membranes, longitudinal furrows in tongue). Provide emotional support.

INTERVENTION/EVALUATION

Monitor pt in environment. Provide supportive measures. Assess mental status. Monitor daily pattern of bowel activity, stool consistency. Record time of evacuation.

PATIENT/FAMILY TEACHING

• Relief from nausea/vomiting generally occurs shortly after drug administration. • Avoid alcohol, barbiturates. • Report persistent vomiting.

pamidronate

pam-i-**droe**-nate
(Aredia)
Do not confuse Aredia with Adriamcyin.

CLASSIFICATION

PHARMACOTHERAPEUTIC: Bisphosphonate. **CLINICAL:** Hypocalcemic.

P

ACTION

Binds to bone, inhibits osteoclast-mediated calcium resorption. **Therapeutic Effect:** Lowers serum calcium concentration.

PHARMACOKINETICS

Route	Onset	Peak	Duration
IV	24–48 hrs	3–7 days	N/A

After IV administration, rapidly absorbed by bone. Slowly excreted unchanged in urine. Unknown if removed by hemodialysis. **Half-life:** 21–35 hrs.

USES

Treatment of moderate to severe hypercalcemia associated with malignancy (with/without bone metastases). Treatment of moderate to severe Paget's disease, osteolytic bone lesions of multiple myeloma, breast cancer. **OFF-LABEL:** Treatment of pediatric osteoporosis, osteogenesis imperfecta.

PRECAUTIONS

Contraindications: Hypersensitivity to other bisphosphonates (e.g., etidronate, tiludronate, risedronate, alendronate). **Cautions:** Cardiac failure, renal impairment.

LIFESPAN CONSIDERATIONS

Pregnancy/Lactation: No adequate, well-controlled studies in pregnant women; unknown if fetal harm can occur. Unknown if distributed in breast milk. **Pregnancy Category D. Children:** Safety and efficacy not established. **Elderly:** May become overhydrated. Careful monitoring of fluid and electrolytes indicated; recommend dilution in smaller volume.

INTERACTIONS

DRUG: **Calcium-containing medications, vitamin D** may antagonize effects in treatment of hypercalcemia. **Nephrotoxic medications** may increase potential for nephrotoxicity. **HERBAL:** None significant. **FOOD:** None known. **LAB VALUES:** None significant.

AVAILABILITY (Rx)

Injection, Powder for Reconstitution: 30 mg, 90 mg. **Injection Solution:** 3 mg/ml, 6 mg/ml, 9 mg/ml.

ADMINISTRATION/HANDLING

IV

Reconstitution • Reconstitute each vial with 10 ml Sterile Water for Injection to provide concentration of 3 mg/ml or 9 mg/ml. • Allow drug to dissolve before withdrawing. • Further dilute with 250–1,000 ml sterile 0.45% or 0.9% NaCl or D_5W (1,000 ml for hypercalcemia of malignancy, 500 ml for Paget's disease, multiple myeloma, 250 ml for breast cancer).

Rate of administration • Adequate hydration is essential in conjunction with pamidronate therapy (avoid overhydration in pts with potential for cardiac failure). • Administer as IV infusion over 2–24 hrs for treatment of hypercalcemia; over 2–4 hrs for other indications.

Storage • Store parenteral form at room temperature. • Reconstituted vial is stable for 24 hrs if refrigerated; IV solution is stable for 24 hrs after dilution.

IV INCOMPATIBILITIES

Calcium-containing IV fluids.

INDICATIONS/ROUTES/DOSAGE

Hypercalcemia

IV INFUSION: ADULTS, ELDERLY: Moderate hypercalcemia (corrected serum calcium level 12–13.5 mg/dl): 60–90 mg. Severe hypercalcemia (corrected serum calcium level greater than 13.5 mg/dl): 90 mg.

Paget's Disease

IV INFUSION: ADULTS, ELDERLY: 30 mg/day over 4 hrs for 3 days.

Osteolytic Bone Lesion

IV INFUSION: ADULTS, ELDERLY: 90 mg over 2–4 hrs once/mo.

SIDE EFFECTS

Frequent (greater than 10%): Temperature elevation (at least 1°C) 24–48 hrs after administration (27%); redness, swelling, induration, pain at catheter site in pts receiving 90 mg (18%); anorexia, nausea, fatigue. **Occasional (10%–1%):** Constipation, rhinitis.

ADVERSE EFFECTS/ TOXIC REACTIONS

Hypophosphatemia, hypokalemia, hypomagnesemia, hypocalcemia occur more frequently with higher dosages. Anemia, hypertension, tachycardia, atrial fibrillation, drowsiness occur more frequently with 90-mg doses. GI hemorrhage occurs rarely.

NURSING CONSIDERATIONS

BASELINE ASSESSMENT

Obtain corrected serum calcium level prior to therapy. Determine hydration status.

INTERVENTION/EVALUATION

Monitor serum calcium, potassium, magnesium, creatinine, Hgb, Hct, CBC. Provide adequate hydration; avoid overhydration. Monitor I&O carefully; check lungs for rales, dependent body parts for edema. Monitor B/P, temperature, pulse. Assess catheter site for redness, swelling, pain. Monitor food intake, daily pattern of bowel activity, stool consistency. Be alert for potential GI hemorrhage with 90-mg dosage.

pancrelipase

pan-kree-**lie**-pace
(Creon, Pancreaze, Zenpep)

◆ CLASSIFICATION

PHARMACOTHERAPEUTIC: Digestive enzyme. **CLINICAL:** Pancreatic enzyme replenisher.

ACTION

Replaces endogenous pancreatic enzymes. **Therapeutic Effect:** Assists in digestion of protein, starch, fats.

USES

Replacement therapy for malabsorption syndrome caused by pancreatic insufficiency due to cystic fibrosis, chronic pancreatitis, pancreactectomy, or other conditions. **OFF-LABEL:** Treatment of occluded feeding tubes.

PRECAUTIONS

Contraindications: Acute pancreatitis, exacerbation of chronic pancreatitis, hypersensitivity to pork protein. **Cautions:** Inhalation of powder may cause asthmatic attack. **Pregnancy Category C.**

INTERACTIONS

DRUG: **Antacids** may decrease effects. May decrease absorption of **iron supplements.** **HERBAL:** None significant. **FOOD:** None known. **LAB VALUES:** May increase serum uric acid.

AVAILABILITY (Rx)

Capsules, Delayed-Release: (Creon): 6,000 units lipase; 19,000 units protease; 30,000 units amylase. 12,000 units lipase; 38,000 units protease; 60,000 units amylase. 24,000 units lipase; 76,000 units protease; 120,000 units amylase. **(Pancreaze):** 4,200 units lipase; 10,000 units protease; 17,500 units amylase; 10,500 units lipase; 25,000 units protease; 43,750 units amylase; 16,800 units lipase; 40,000 units protease; 70,000 units amylase; 21,000 units lipase; 37,000 units protease; 61,000 units amylase. **(Zenpep):** 5,000 units lipase; 17,000 units protease; 27,000 units amylase. 10,000 units lipase; 34,000 units protease; 55,000 units amylase. 15,000 units lipase; 51,000 units protease; 82,000 units amylase. 20,000 units lipase; 68,000 units protease; 109,000 units amylase.

ADMINISTRATION/HANDLING

PO

• Swallow capsules whole. • If unable to swallow intact capsule, contents of Creon may be given without crushing/chewing, followed by fluid. Zenpep contents may be sprinkled on soft acidic food such as applesauce.

P

INDICATIONS/ROUTES/DOSAGE

ALERT Dosage expressed as lipase units/kg.

Pancreatic Enzyme Replacement Therapy

PO: ADULTS, ELDERLY, CHILDREN 4 YRS AND OLDER: Initially, 500 units/kg lipase/kg/meal up to 2,500 units lipase/kg/meal (or less than or equal to 10,000 lipase units/kg/day) or less than 4,000 lipase units/g of fat ingested/day. **CHILDREN OLDER THAN 12 MOS AND YOUNGER THAN 4 YRS:** Initially, 1,000 units lipase/kg/meal up to 2,500 units lipase/kg/meal (or less than or equal to 10,000 lipase units/kg/day) or less than 4,000 lipase units/g of fat ingested/day. **INFANTS UP TO 12 MOS:** 2,000–4,000 units lipase per 120 ml of formula or per breast-feeding. Do not mix Creon or Zenpep capsule contents directly into formula or breast milk prior to administration.

SIDE EFFECTS

Rare: Allergic reaction, mouth irritation, shortness of breath, wheezing.

ADVERSE EFFECTS/ TOXIC REACTIONS

Excessive dosage may produce nausea, cramping, diarrhea. Hyperuricosuria, hyperuricemia reported with extremely high dosages.

NURSING CONSIDERATIONS

INTERVENTION/EVALUATION

Question for therapeutic relief from GI symptoms. Do not change brands without consulting physician.

PATIENT/FAMILY TEACHING

• Do not chew capsules. • Instruct pts with trouble swallowing to open capsules, spread contents over applesauce, mashed fruit, rice cereal or follow with glass of water or juice to ensure swallowing.

panitumumab

pan-i-**toom**-ue-mab
(Vectibix)

BLACK BOX ALERT 90% of pts experience dermatologic toxicities (dermatitis acneiform, pruritus, erythema, rash, skin exfoliation, skin fissures, abscess). Potential for severe infusion reaction (anaphylaxis, bronchospasm, fever, chills, hypotension) (fatal reactions have occurred).

◆CLASSIFICATION

PHARMACOTHERAPEUTIC: Monoclonal antibody. **CLINICAL:** Antineoplastic.

ACTION

Binds specifically to epidermal growth factor receptor (EGFR) and competitively inhibits binding of epidermal growth factor. **Therapeutic Effect:** Prevents cell growth, proliferation, transformation, survival.

PHARMACOKINETICS

Clearance varies by body weight, gender, tumor burden. **Half-life:** 3–10 days.

USES

Treatment of EGFR-expressing metastatic colorectal carcinoma with disease progression during or following fluoropyrimidine, oxaliplatin, irinotecan-containing chemotherapy regimens.

PRECAUTIONS

Contraindications: None known. **Cautions:** Interstitial pneumonitis, pulmonary fibrosis, pulmonary infiltrates.

LIFESPAN CONSIDERATIONS

Pregnancy/Lactation: Teratogenic. Potential for fertility impairment. May decrease fetal body weight; increase risk of skeletal fetal abnormalities. Breastfeeding not recommended. **Pregnancy Category C. Children:** Safety and efficacy not established. **Elderly:** No age-related precautions noted.

INTERACTIONS

DRUG: None significant. **HERBAL:** None significant. **FOOD:** None known. **LAB VALUES:** May decrease serum magnesium, calcium.

AVAILABILITY (Rx)

Injection Solution: 20 mg/ml vial (5-ml, 10-ml, 20-ml vials).

ADMINISTRATION/HANDLING

IV

◀ALERT▶ Do not give by IV push or bolus. Use low-protein-binding 0.2- or 0.22-micron in-line filter. Flush IV line before and after chemotherapy administration with 0.9% NaCl.

Reconstitution • Dilute in 100–150 ml 0.9% NaCl to provide concentration of 10 mg/ml or less. • Do not shake solution. • Discard any unused portion.

Rate of administration • Give as IV infusion over 60 min. • Infuse doses greater than 1,000 mg over 90 min.

Storage • Refrigerate vials. • After dilution, solution may be stored for up to 6 hrs at room temperature, up to 24 hrs if refrigerated. • Discard if discolored but solution may contain visible, translucent-to-white particulates (will be removed by in-line filter).

IV INCOMPATIBILITY

Do not mix with dextrose solutions or any other medications.

INDICATIONS/ROUTES/DOSAGE

◀ALERT▶ Stop infusion immediately in pts experiencing severe infusion reactions.

Metastatic Colorectal Carcinoma

IV INFUSION: ADULTS, ELDERLY: 6 mg/kg given over 60 min once every 14 days. Doses greater than 1,000 mg should be infused over 90 min.

SIDE EFFECTS

Common (65%–57%): Erythema, acneiform dermatitis, pruritus. **Frequent (26%–20%):** Fatigue, abdominal pain, skin exfoliation, paronychia (inflammation involving folds of tissue surrounding fingernail), nausea, rash, diarrhea, constipation, skin fissures. **Occasional (19%–10%):** Vomiting, acne, cough, peripheral edema, dry skin. **Rare (7%–2%):** Stomatitis, mucosal inflammation, eyelash growth, conjunctivitis, increased lacrimation.

ADVERSE EFFECTS/TOXIC REACTIONS

Pulmonary fibrosis, severe dermatologic toxicity (complicated by infectious sequelae), sepsis occur rarely. Severe infusion reactions manifested as bronchospasm, fever, chills, hypotension occur rarely. Hypomagnesemia occurs in 39% of pts.

NURSING CONSIDERATIONS

BASELINE ASSESSMENT

Assess baseline serum magnesium, calcium prior to therapy, periodically during therapy, and for 8 wks after completion of therapy.

INTERVENTION/EVALUATION

Assess for skin, ocular, mucosal toxicity; report effects. Median time to development of skin/ocular toxicity is 14–15 days; resolution after last dosing is 84 days. Monitor serum electrolytes for hypomagnesemia, hypocalcemia. Offer antiemetic if nausea/vomiting occurs. Monitor daily pattern of bowel activity, stool consistency.

PATIENT/FAMILY TEACHING

• Do not have immunizations without physician's approval (drug lowers resistance). • Avoid contact with those who have recently received a live virus vaccine. • Avoid crowds, those with infection. • There is a potential risk for development of fetal abnormalities if pregnancy occurs; take measures to prevent pregnancy.

P

pantoprazole

pan-toe-**pra**-zole
(Apo-Pantoprazole ✱, Novo-Pantoprazole ✱, Protonix, Protonix IV)
Do not confuse pantoprazole with aripiprazole, or Protonix with Lovenox.

CLASSIFICATION

PHARMACOTHERAPEUTIC: Benzimidazole. **CLINICAL:** Proton pump inhibitor (see p. 148C).

ACTION

Irreversibly binds to, inhibits hydrogen-potassium adenosine triphosphate, an enzyme on surface of gastric parietal cells. Inhibits hydrogen ion transport into gastric lumen. **Therapeutic Effect:** Increases gastric pH, reduces gastric acid production.

PHARMACOKINETICS

Route	Onset	Peak	Duration
PO	N/A	N/A	24 hrs

Well absorbed from GI tract. Protein binding: 98% (primarily albumin). Primarily distributed into gastric parietal cells. Metabolized extensively in liver. Primarily excreted in urine. Not removed by hemodialysis. **Half-life:** 1 hr.

USES

PO: Treatment, maintenance of healing of erosive esophagitis associated with gastroesophageal reflux disease (GERD). Treatment of hypersecretory conditions including Zollinger-Ellison syndrome. **IV:** Short-term treatment of erosive esophagitis associated with GERD, treatment of hypersecretory conditions. **OFF-LABEL:** Peptic ulcer disease, active ulcer bleeding (injection), adjunct in treatment of *H. pylori,* stress ulcer prophylaxis in critically ill pts.

PRECAUTIONS

Contraindications: None known. **Cautions:** History of chronic or current hepatic disease. May increase risk of fractures.

LIFESPAN CONSIDERATIONS

Pregnancy/Lactation: Unknown if drug crosses placenta or is distributed in breast milk. **Pregnancy Category B. Children:** Safety and efficacy not established. **Elderly:** No age-related precautions noted.

INTERACTIONS

DRUG: May increase effect of **warfarin.** May decrease effects of **clopidogrel. HERBAL:** None significant. **FOOD:** None known. **LAB VALUES:** May increase serum creatinine, cholesterol, uric acid, glucose, lipoprotein, ALT.

AVAILABILITY (Rx)

Granules for Suspension: 40 mg. **Injection, Powder for Reconstitution (Protonix IV):** 40 mg.

Tablets (Delayed-Release [Protonix]): 20 mg, 40 mg.

ADMINISTRATION/HANDLING

IV

Reconstitution • Mix 40-mg vial with 10 ml 0.9% NaCl injection. • May be further diluted with 100 ml D_5W, 0.9% NaCl, or lactated Ringer's.
Rate of administration • Infuse 10 ml solution over at least 2 min. • Infuse 100 ml solution over at least 15 min.
Storage • Store undiluted vials at room temperature. • Once diluted with 10 ml 0.9% NaCl, stable for 6 hrs at room temperature; when further diluted with 100 ml, stable for 24 hrs at room temperature.

PO

• May be given without regard to food. Best given before breakfast. • Do not crush, chew, split tablets; swallow whole.

• Administer oral suspension only in apple juice or applesauce.

IV INCOMPATIBILITIES

Do not mix with other medications. Flush IV with D_5W, 0.9% NaCl, or lactated Ringer's solution before and after administration.

INDICATIONS/ROUTES/DOSAGE

Erosive Esophagitis

PO: ADULTS, ELDERLY: 40 mg/day for up to 8 wks. If not healed after 8 wks, may continue an additional 8 wks.

IV: ADULTS, ELDERLY: 40 mg/day for 7–10 days.

Maintenance of Healing of Erosive Esophagitis

PO: ADULTS, ELDERLY: 40 mg once daily.

Hypersecretory Conditions

PO: ADULTS, ELDERLY: Initially, 40 mg twicc a day. May increase to 240 mg/day.

IV: ADULTS, ELDERLY: 80 mg twice a day. May increase to 80 mg q8h.

SIDE EFFECTS

Rare (less than 2%): Diarrhea, headache, dizziness, pruritus, rash.

ADVERSE EFFECTS/ TOXIC REACTIONS

Hyperglycemia occurs rarely.

NURSING CONSIDERATIONS

BASELINE ASSESSMENT

Obtain baseline lab values, including serum creatinine, cholesterol.

INTERVENTION/EVALUATION

Evaluate for therapeutic response (relief of GI symptoms). Question if GI discomfort, nausea occur.

PATIENT/FAMILY TEACHING

• Report headache, onset of black, tarry stools, diarrhea. • Avoid alcohol. • Swallow tablets whole; do not chew, crush. • Best if given before breakfast. May give without regard to food.

Paraplatin, *see carboplatin*

paroxetine

par-**ox**-e-teen
(Apo-Paroxetine ✱, Novo-Paroxetine ✱, Paxil, Paxil CR, Pexeva)

BLACK BOX ALERT Increased risk of suicidal thinking and behavior in children, adolescents, young adults 18–24 yrs with major depressive disorder, other psychiatric disorders.

Do not confuse paroxetine with fluoxetine or pyridoxine, or Paxil with Doxil, Plavix, or Taxol.

◆ CLASSIFICATION

PHARMACOTHERAPEUTIC: Serotonin uptake inhibitor. **CLINICAL:** Antidepressant, antiobsessive-compulsive, antianxiety (see pp. 14C, 39C).

ACTION

Selectively blocks uptake of neurotransmitter serotonin at CNS neuronal presynaptic membranes, increasing its availability at postsynaptic receptor sites. **Therapeutic Effect:** Relieves depression, reduces obsessive-compulsive behavior, decreases anxiety.

PHARMACOKINETICS

Well absorbed from GI tract. Protein binding: 95%. Widely distributed. Metabolized in liver. Excreted in urine. Not removed by hemodialysis. **Half-life:** 24 hrs.

USES

Treatment of major depression exhibited as persistent, prominent dysphoria (occurring nearly every day for at least 2 wks) manifested by 4 of 8 symptoms: change in appetite, change in sleep pattern, increased fatigue, impaired concen-

P

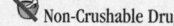

tration, feelings of guilt or worthlessness, loss of interest in usual activities, psychomotor agitation/retardation, suicidal tendencies. Treatment of panic disorder, obsessive-compulsive disorder (OCD) manifested as repetitive tasks producing marked distress, time-consuming, or significant interference with social/occupational behavior. Treatment of social anxiety disorder (SAD), generalized anxiety disorder (GAD), premenstrual dysphoric disorder, post-traumatic stress disorder (PTSD). OFF-LABEL: Eating disorders, impulse disorders, menopause symptoms, premenstrual disorders, treatment of depression and OCD in children, mild dementia-associated agitation in nonpsychotic pts.

PRECAUTIONS

Contraindications: Use of MAOIs within 14 days, use of thioridazine. Cautions: History of seizures, mania, renal/hepatic impairment, cardiac disease, pts with suicidal tendencies, impaired platelet aggregation. Those who are volume depleted or using diuretics.

LIFESPAN CONSIDERATIONS

Pregnancy/Lactation: May impair reproductive function. Not distributed in breast milk. May increase risk of congenital malformations. **Pregnancy Category D.** **Children:** Safety and efficacy not established. **Elderly:** Age-related renal impairment may require dosage adjustment.

INTERACTIONS

DRUG: May increase concentration, risk of toxicity of **tricyclic antidepressants. Aspirin, NSAIDs, warfarin** may increase risk of bleeding. **MAOIs** may cause confusion, agitation, severe seizures; increase risk of serotonin syndrome, hypertensive crises. **Thioridazine** may prolong QT interval. HERBAL: **Kava kava, St. John's wort, valerian** may increase CNS depression. **St. John's wort** may increase effects, risk of toxicity. FOOD: None known. LAB VALUES: May decrease Hgb, Hct, WBC count.

AVAILABILITY (Rx)

Oral Suspension (Paxil): 10 mg/5 ml. Tablets (Paxil, Pexeva): 10 mg, 20 mg, 30 mg, 40 mg.

Tablets (Controlled-Release [Paxil CR]): 12.5 mg, 25 mg, 37.5 mg.

ADMINISTRATION/HANDLING

PO

- Give with food, milk if GI distress occurs. • Scored tablet may be crushed.
- Do not crush controlled-release tablets.
- Best if given as single morning dose.

INDICATIONS/ROUTES/DOSAGE

Depression

PO: ADULTS: Initially, 20 mg/day. May increase by 10 mg/day at intervals of more than 1 wk. **Maximum:** 50 mg/day.

PO (CONTROLLED-RELEASE): ADULTS: Initially, 25 mg/day. May increase by 12.5 mg/day at intervals of more than 1 wk. **Maximum:** 62.5 mg/day.

Generalized Anxiety Disorder (GAD)

PO: ADULTS: Initially, 20 mg/day. May increase by 10 mg/day at intervals of more than 1 wk. Range: 20–50 mg/day.

Obsessive-Compulsive Disorder (OCD)

PO: ADULTS: Initially, 20 mg/day. May increase by 10 mg/day at intervals of more than 1 wk. Range: 20–60 mg/day.

Panic Disorder

PO: ADULTS: Initially, 10–20 mg/day. May increase by 10 mg/day at intervals of more than 1 wk. Range: 10–60 mg/day.

PO (CONTROLLED-RELEASE): ADULTS, ELDERLY: Initially, 12.5 mg once daily. May increase by 12.5 mg/day at weekly intervals. **Maximum:** 75 mg/day.

Social Anxiety Disorder (SAD)

PO: ADULTS: Initially 20 mg/day. Range: 20–60 mg/day.

PO (CONTROLLED-RELEASE): ADULTS, ELDERLY: Initially, 12.5 mg once daily. May increase by 12.5 mg/day at weekly intervals. **Maximum:** 37.5 mg/day.

Post-Traumatic Stress Disorder (PTSD)

PO: ADULTS: Initially, 20 mg/day. May increase by 10 mg/day at intervals of more than 1 wk. Range: 20–50 mg/day.

Premenstrual Dysphoric Disorder

PO (PAXIL CR): ADULTS: Initially, 12.5 mg/day. May increase by 12.5 mg at weekly intervals. **Maximum:** 25 mg/day.

Usual Elderly Dosage

PO: Initially, 10 mg/day. May increase by 10 mg/day at intervals of more than 1 wk. **Maximum:** 40 mg/day.

PO (CONTROLLED-RELEASE): Initially, 12.5 mg/day. May increase by 12.5 mg/day at intervals of more than 1 wk. **Maximum:** 50 mg/day.

SIDE EFFECTS

Frequent: Nausea (26%); drowsiness (23%); headache, dry mouth (18%); asthenia (loss of strength, energy) (15%); constipation (15%); dizziness, insomnia (13%); diarrhea (12%); diaphoresis (11%); tremor (8%). **Occasional:** Decreased appetite, respiratory disturbance (e.g., increased cough) (6%); anxiety (5%); flatulence, paresthesia, yawning (4%); decreased libido, sexual dysfunction, abdominal discomfort (3%). **Rare:** Palpitations, vomiting, blurred vision, altered taste, confusion.

ADVERSE EFFECTS/ TOXIC REACTIONS

Hyponatremia, seizures have been reported. Serotonin syndrome (agitation, confusion, diaphoresis, hallucinations, hyper-reflexia) occurs rarely.

NURSING CONSIDERATIONS

BASELINE ASSESSMENT

Assess appearance, behavior, speech pattern, level of interest, mood.

INTERVENTION/EVALUATION

For those on long-term therapy, hepatic/renal function tests, blood counts should be performed periodically. Assess mental status for depression, suicidal ideation (esp. at beginning of therapy or change in dosage), anxiety, social functioning, panic attacks. Assess appearance, behavior, speech pattern, level of interest, mood.

PATIENT/FAMILY TEACHING

• May cause dry mouth. • Avoid alcohol, St. John's wort. • Therapeutic effect may be noted within 1–4 wks. • Do not abruptly discontinue medication. • Avoid tasks that require alertness, motor skills until response to drug is established. • Inform physician of intention for pregnancy or if pregnancy occurs. • Report worsening depression, suicidal ideation, unusual changes in behavior.

Paxil, *see paroxetine*

pazopanib

paz-**oh**-pa-nib
(Votrient)

BLACK BOX ALERT Severe, fatal hepatotoxicity has been observed.

◆CLASSIFICATION

PHARMACOTHERAPEUTIC: Tyrosine kinase inhibitor. **CLINICAL:** Antineoplastic.

ACTION

Interferes with proliferation of tumor vasculature, preventing tumor growth. **Therapeutic Effect:** Inhibits angiogenesis, blocks tumor growth.

PHARMACOKINETICS

Peak concentration occurs 2–4 hrs following oral administration. Undergoes extensive hepatic metabolism. Protein binding: greater than 99%. Eliminated primarily in feces, with a lesser amount excreted in urine. **Half-life:** 31 hrs.

USES

Treatment of advanced renal cell carcinoma in adults.

P

PRECAUTIONS

Contraindications: None significant. **Cautions:** Avoid use of strong CYP3A4 inhibitors (e.g., clarithromycin, ketoconazole, ritonavir) or inducers (carbamazepine, dexamethasone, phenobarbital, phenytoin, rifabutin, rifampin) and grapefruit juice. Cautious use in those with increased risk or history of arterial thrombotic events, QT prolongation, hypertension, severe hepatic impairment, concomitant use of medications that may prolong QT interval, history of hemoptysis, cerebral or significant GI hemorrhage.

LIFESPAN CONSIDERATIONS

Pregnancy/Lactation: May cause fetal harm. Unknown if distributed in breast milk. **Pregnancy Category D. Children:** Safety and efficacy not established in those younger than 18 yrs. **Elderly:** No age-related precautions noted.

INTERACTIONS

DRUG: Concurrent use of **clarithromycin, ketoconazole, ritonavir** may increase concentration. Concomitant use of **carbamazepine, dexamethasone, phenobarbital, phenytoin, rifabutin, rifampin** may decrease concentration. **HERBAL:** **St. John's wort** decreases concentration. **FOOD:** **Food** may increase concentration. Give 1 hr before or 2 hrs after meals. **Grapefruit, grapefruit juice** may increase concentration. **LAB VALUES:** May decrease serum phosphorus, sodium, magnesium, glucose, WBC count. May increase serum ALT, AST.

AVAILABILITY (Rx)

Tablets: 200 mg, 400 mg.

ADMINISTRATION/HANDLING

PO

• Give at least 1 hr before or 2 hrs after ingestion of food. • Swallow tablets whole; do not crush, chew, or break.

INDICATIONS/ROUTES/DOSAGE

Renal Cell Carcinoma

PO: ADULTS, ELDERLY: 800 mg once daily. Initial dose reduction should be 400 mg with additional increases/decreases in 200 mg steps based on individual tolerability. Initial dose of 400 mg/day with concomitant strong CYP3A4 inhibitors.

Dosage in Hepatic Impairment

Reduce dose to 200 mg/day for moderate hepatic impairment. Not recommended in pts with severe hepatic impairment.

SIDE EFFECTS

Frequent (52%–19%): Diarrhea, hypertension, hair color changes, nausea, fatigue, anorexia, vomiting. **Occasional (14%–10%):** Asthenia, abdominal pain, headache. **Rare (less than 10%):** Alopecia, chest pain, altered taste, dyspepsia, proteinuria, rash, decreased weight.

ADVERSE EFFECTS/ TOXIC REACTIONS

Hepatotoxicity, manifested as increase in serum bilirubin, ALT, AST, has been observed and may be fatal. Hemorrhagic events (hematuria, epistaxis, hemoptysis, GI bleeding or perforation, intracranial hemorrhage) have been noted and may be fatal. Hypertension (B/P greater than 150/100 mm Hg) is common (47%), usually occurring early in the first 18 wks of treatment. Hypothyroidism has been reported occasionally. Arterial thrombotic events (MI, CVA), QT prolongation, torsade de pointes have been seen rarely.

NURSING CONSIDERATIONS

BASELINE ASSESSMENT

Assess medical history, esp. hepatic function abnormalities. Obtain baseline EKG, CBC, serum chemistries, hepatic function tests (ALT, AST, bilirubin) before beginning therapy.

INTERVENTION/EVALUATION

Monitor B/P, serum hepatic function tests periodically for elevations. Monitor CBC, serum chemistries for changes from baseline. Observe for signs of hepatotoxicity (jaundice, dark-colored urine, unusual fatigue, right upper quadrant abdominal pain). Observe EKG for QT-interval prolongation. Monitor for evidence of bleeding, hemorrhage. Monitor daily pattern of bowel activity, stool consistency.

PATIENT/FAMILY TEACHING

• Avoid crowds, those with known infection. • Avoid contact with anyone who recently received live virus vaccine; do not receive vaccinations. • No food should be taken at least 1 hr before and 2 hrs after dose is taken. Avoid grapefruit juice, grapefruit products. • Notify physician if diarrhea, abdominal pain, yellowing of skin or sclera, discolored urine, fatigue occur or diarrhea persists.

Pegasys, *see peginterferon alfa-2a*

pegfilgrastim

peg-fill-**gras**-tim
(Neulasta)
Do not confuse Neulasta with Lunesta, Neumega, or Neupogen.

◆CLASSIFICATION

PHARMACOTHERAPEUTIC: Colony-stimulating factor. **CLINICAL:** Hematopoietic, antineutropenic.

ACTION

Regulates production of neutrophils within bone marrow. A glycoprotein, primarily affects neutrophil progenitor proliferation, differentiation, selected end-cell functional activation. **Therapeutic Effect:** Increases phagocytic ability, antibody-dependent destruction; decreases incidence of infection.

PHARMACOKINETICS

Readily absorbed after subcutaneous administration. **Half-life:** 15–80 hrs.

USES

Decreases incidence of infection manifested by febrile neutropenia in cancer pts receiving moderately myelosuppressive chemotherapy. Stimulates WBC production in pts receiving myelosuppressive chemotherapy.

PRECAUTIONS

Contraindications: Hypersensitivity to *Escherichia coli*–derived protein. Do not administer within 14 days before and 24 hrs after cytotoxic chemotherapy. **Cautions:** Concurrent use with medications having mycoloid properties, sickle cell disease.

⌛ LIFESPAN CONSIDERATIONS

Pregnancy/Lactation: Unknown if drug crosses placenta or is distributed in breast milk. **Pregnancy Category C. Children:** Safety and efficacy not established in children younger than 12 yrs of age. **Elderly:** No age-related precautions noted.

INTERACTIONS

DRUG: Lithium may potentiate release of neutrophils. Do not administer within 14 days before and 24 hrs after **cytotoxic chemotherapy agents. HERBAL:** None significant. **FOOD:** None known. **LAB VALUES:** May increase serum LDH, alkaline phosphatase, uric acid.

AVAILABILITY (Rx)

Injection Solution: 6 mg/0.6 ml syringe.

ADMINISTRATION/HANDLING

Subcutaneous

Storage • Store in refrigerator. Warm to room temperature prior to administering injection. Discard if left at room temperature for more than 48 hrs. • Protect from light. • Avoid freezing; but if accidentally frozen, may allow to thaw in refrigerator before administration. Discard if freezing takes place a second time. • Discard if discolored or precipitate forms.

P

INDICATIONS/ROUTES/DOSAGE

Myelosuppression

SUBCUTANEOUS: ADULTS, ELDERLY, CHILDREN 12–17 YRS, WEIGHING MORE THAN 45 KG: Give as single 6-mg injection once per chemotherapy cycle.

◀ALERT▶ Do not administer between 14 days before and 24 hrs after cytotoxic chemotherapy. Do not use in infants, children, adolescents weighing less than 45 kg.

SIDE EFFECTS

Frequent (72%–15%): Bone pain, nausea, fatigue, alopecia, diarrhea, vomiting, constipation, anorexia, abdominal pain, arthralgia, generalized weakness, peripheral edema, dizziness, stomatitis, mucositis, neutropenic fever.

ADVERSE EFFECTS/ TOXIC REACTIONS

Allergic reactions (anaphylaxis, rash, urticaria) occur rarely. Cytopenia resulting from antibody response to growth factors occurs rarely. Splenomegaly occurs rarely. Adult respiratory distress syndrome (ARDS) may occur in septic pts.

NURSING CONSIDERATIONS

BASELINE ASSESSMENT

CBC, platelet count should be obtained before initiating therapy and routinely thereafter.

INTERVENTION/EVALUATION

Monitor for allergic-type reactions. Assess for peripheral edema, particularly behind medial malleolus (usually first area showing peripheral edema). Assess mucous membranes for evidence of stomatitis, mucositis (red mucous membranes, white patches, extreme mouth soreness). Assess muscle strength. Monitor daily pattern of bowel activity, stool consistency. Adult respiratory distress syndrome (ARDS) may occur in septic pts.

PATIENT/FAMILY TEACHING

• Inform pts of possible side effects, signs/symptoms of allergic reactions. • Counsel pt on importance of compliance with pegfilgrastim treatment, including regular monitoring of blood counts. • Notify physician of unusual fever or chills, severe bone pain, chest pain or palpitations.

peginterferon alfa-2a

peg-in-ter-**feer**-on
(Pegasys)

BLACK BOX ALERT Can cause or aggravate fatal or life-threatening autoimmune, neuropsychiatric (depression, suicidal thoughts/behaviors), ischemic, including worsening hepatic function, and infectious disorders. Combination with ribavirin can cause fetal mortality, birth defects, hemolytic anemia. May be carcinogenic.

Do not confuse peginterferon alfa-2a with interferon alfa-2b, interferon alfa-n3, or peginterferon alfa-2b.

◆CLASSIFICATION

PHARMACOTHERAPEUTIC: Immunomodulator. **CLINICAL:** Immunologic agent.

ACTION

Binds to specific membrane receptors on virus-infected cell surface, inhibiting viral replication. Suppresses cell proliferation, producing reversible decreases in leukocyte, platelet counts. **Therapeutic Effect:** Inhibits viral hepatitis.

PHARMACOKINETICS

Readily absorbed after subcutaneous administration. Excreted by kidneys. **Half-life:** 50–140 hrs.

USES

Treatment of chronic hepatitis C alone or in combination with ribavirin in pts who have compensated hepatic disease. Treatment of chronic hepatitis B.

PRECAUTIONS

Contraindications: Autoimmune hepatitis, decompensated hepatic disease, infants, neonates. **Extreme Caution:** History of neuropsychiatric disorders. **Cautions:** Renal impairment (creatinine clearance less than 50 ml/min), elderly, pulmonary disorders, compromised CNS function, cardiac diseases, autoimmune disorders, endocrine abnormalities, colitis, ophthalmologic disorders, myelosuppression.

LIFESPAN CONSIDERATIONS

Pregnancy/Lactation: May have abortifacient potential. Unknown if distributed in breast milk. **Pregnancy Category C (X when used with ribavirin). Children:** Safety and efficacy not established in those younger than 18 yrs. **Elderly:** CNS, cardiac, systemic effects may be more severe in the elderly, particularly in those with renal impairment.

INTERACTIONS

DRUG: **Didanosine** may cause hepatic failure, peripheral neuropathy, pancreatitis, lactic acidosis. May increase concentration, risk of toxicity of **methadone, theophylline.** Concurrent use of **ribavirin** may increase risk of hemolytic anemia. **HERBAL:** None significant. **FOOD:** None known. **LAB VALUES:** May increase serum ALT. May decrease absolute neutrophil, platelet, WBC counts.

AVAILABILITY (Rx)

Injection, Prefilled Syringe: 180 mcg/0.5 ml. **Injection Solution:** 180 mcg/ml.

ADMINISTRATION/HANDLING

Subcutaneous

• Refrigerate. • Vials are for single use only; discard unused portion. • Give subcutaneously in abdomen, thigh.

INDICATIONS/ROUTES/DOSAGE

Hepatitis C, Hepatitis B

SUBCUTANEOUS: ADULTS 18 YRS AND OLDER, ELDERLY: 180 mcg injected in abdomen or thigh once weekly for 48 wks.

Dosage in Renal Impairment

For pts who require hemodialysis, dosage is 135 mg injected in abdomen or thigh once weekly for 48 wks.

Dosage in Hepatic Impairment

For pts with progressive ALT increases above baseline values, dosage is 135 mcg injected in abdomen or thigh once weekly for 48 wks.

SIDE EFFECTS

Frequent (54%): Headache. **Occasional (23%–13%):** Alopecia, nausea, insomnia, anorexia, dizziness, diarrhea, abdominal pain, flu-like symptoms, psychiatric reactions (depression, irritability, anxiety), injection site reaction. **Rare (8%–5%):** Impaired concentration, diaphoresis, dry mouth, nausea, vomiting.

ADVERSE EFFECTS/ TOXIC REACTIONS

Serious, acute hypersensitivity reactions, (urticaria, angioedema, bronchoconstriction, anaphylaxis), pancreatitis, colitis, endocrine disorders (diabetes mellitus, hyperthyroidism, hypothyroidism), ophthalmologic disorders, pulmonary abnormalities occur rarely.

NURSING CONSIDERATIONS

BASELINE ASSESSMENT

CBC, platelet count, blood chemistry, urinalysis, renal/hepatic function tests, EKG should be performed before initial therapy and routinely thereafter. Pts with diabetes, hypertension should have ophthalmologic exam before treatment begins.

INTERVENTION/EVALUATION

Monitor for evidence of depression. Offer emotional support. Monitor for abdominal pain, bloody diarrhea as evidence of colitis. Monitor chest X-ray for pulmonary infiltrates. Assess for pulmonary impairment. Encourage ample fluid intake, particularly during early therapy. Assess serum hepatitis C virus RNA levels after 24 wks of treatment.

PATIENT/FAMILY TEACHING

• Clinical response occurs in 1–3 mos. • Flu-like symptoms tend to diminish with continued therapy. • Immediately report symptoms of depression, suicidal ideation. • Avoid tasks requiring alertness, motor skills until response to drug is established. • Do not drink alcohol.

peginterferon alfa-2b

peg-in-ter-**feer**-on
(PEG-Intron)

BLACK BOX ALERT Can cause or aggravate fatal or life-threatening autoimmune, neuropsychiatric (depression, suicidal thoughts/behaviors), ischemic, including worsening hepatic function, and infectious disorders. Combination with ribavirin can cause fetal mortality, birth defects, hemolytic anemia. May be carcinogenic.

Do not confuse peginterferon alfa-2b with interferon alfa-2b, interferon alfa-n3, or peginterferon alfa-2a.

CLASSIFICATION

PHARMACOTHERAPEUTIC: Immunomodulator. **CLINICAL:** Immunologic agent.

ACTION

Inhibits viral replication in virus-infected cells, suppresses cell proliferation, increases phagocytic action of macrophages, augments specific cytotoxicity of lymphocytes for target cells. **Therapeutic Effect:** Inhibits viral hepatitis.

PHARMACOKINETICS

Bioavailability is increased after multiple weekly doses. Excreted in urine. **Half-life:** 22–60 hrs.

USES

As monotherapy or in combination with ribavirin for treatment of chronic hepatitis C in pts not previously treated with interferon alfa who have compensated hepatic disease and are older than 18 yrs. **OFF-LABEL:** Treatment of advanced melanoma.

PRECAUTIONS

Contraindications: Autoimmune hepatitis, decompensated hepatic disease, history of psychiatric disorders. **Cautions:** Renal impairment (creatinine clearance less than 50 ml/min), elderly, pulmonary disorders, compromised CNS function, cardiac diseases, autoimmune disorders, endocrine disorders (diabetes, hyperthyroidism, hypothyroidism), ophthalmologic disorders, myelosuppression.

LIFESPAN CONSIDERATIONS

Pregnancy/Lactation: May have abortifacient potential. Unknown if distributed in breast milk. **Pregnancy Category C (X when used with ribavirin). Children:** Safety and efficacy not established in those younger than 18 yrs. **Elderly:** CNS, cardiac, systemic effects may be more severe in the elderly, particularly in those with renal impairment.

INTERACTIONS

DRUG: None significant. **HERBAL:** None significant. **FOOD:** None known. **LAB VALUES:** May increase serum ALT. May decrease neutrophil, platelet counts.

AVAILABILITY (Rx)

Injection, Powder for Reconstitution: 50 mcg, 80 mcg, 120 mcg, 150 mcg. **Prefilled Syringe (RediPen):** 50 mcg, 80 mcg, 120 mcg, 150 mcg.

ADMINISTRATION/HANDLING

Subcutaneous

Reconstitution • To reconstitute, add 0.7 ml Sterile Water for Injection (supplied) to vial. • Gently swirl. Use immediately; after reconstituted may be refrigerated for up to 24 hrs before use. • Prefilled Syringe (RediPen): Hold cartridge upright, press two halves together until "click" is heard. • Gently invert to mix.

Storage • Store at room temperature. • Refrigerate RediPen. Once reconstituted, both products stable for 24 hrs if refrigerated.

INDICATIONS/ROUTES/DOSAGE

Chronic Hepatitis C, Monotherapy

SUBCUTANEOUS: ADULTS 18 YRS AND OLDER, ELDERLY: Initially, 1 mcg/kg/wk. Administer appropriate dosage (see chart below) once weekly for 1 yr on same day each wk.

Vial Strength	Weight (kg)	mcg*	ml*
100 mcg/ml	37–45	40	0.4
	46–56	50	0.5
160 mcg/ml	57–72	64	0.4
	73–88	80	0.5
240 mcg/ml	89–106	96	0.4
	107–136	120	0.5
300 mcg/ml	137–160	150	0.5

*Of peginterferon alfa-2b to administer.

Chronic Hepatitis C

SUBCUTANEOUS: COMBINATION THERAPY WITH RIBAVIRIN (400 MG TWICE A DAY): ADULTS, ELDERLY: Initially, 1.5 mcg/kg/wk. **CHILDREN 3 YRS AND OLDER:** 60 mcg/m^2 once weekly.

Weight	Dosage
Less than 40 kg	50 mcg
40–50 kg	64 mcg
51–60 kg	80 mcg
61–75 kg	96 mcg
76–85 kg	120 mcg
Greater than 85 kg	150 mcg

ALERT Do not use in pts with creatinine clearance less than 50 ml/min. Dosage adjustments needed for hematologic toxicity (hemoglobin, WBCs, neutrophils, platelets).

SIDE EFFECTS

Frequent (50%–47%): Flu-like symptoms; inflammation, bruising, pruritus, irritation at injection site. **Occasional (29%–18%):** Psychiatric reactions (depression, anxiety, emotional lability, irritability), insomnia, alopecia, diarrhea. **Rare:** Rash, diaphoresis, dry skin, dizziness, flushing, vomiting, dyspepsia.

ADVERSE EFFECTS/ TOXIC REACTIONS

Serious, acute hypersensitivity reactions (urticaria, angioedema, bronchoconstriction, anaphylaxis), pulmonary disorders, endocrine disorders (diabetes mellitus, hypothyroidism, hyperthyroidism) pancreatitis occur rarely. Ulcerative colitis may occur within 12 wks of starting treatment.

NURSING CONSIDERATIONS

BASELINE ASSESSMENT

CBC, platelet count, blood chemistry, urinalysis, renal/hepatic function tests, EKG should be performed before initial therapy and routinely thereafter. Pts with diabetes, hypertension should have ophthalmologic exam before treatment begins.

INTERVENTION/EVALUATION

Monitor for abdominal pain, bloody diarrhea as evidence of colitis. Monitor chest X-ray for pulmonary infiltrates. Assess for pulmonary impairment. Encourage adequate fluid intake, particularly during early therapy. Assess serum hepatitis C virus RNA levels after 24 wks of treatment. Monitor for depression, suicidal ideation.

PATIENT/FAMILY TEACHING

• Maintain adequate hydration, avoid drinking alcohol. • May experience flu-like syndrome (nausea, body aches, headache). • Inform physician of persistent abdominal pain, bloody diarrhea, fever, signs of depression, suicidal ideation, or infection, unusual bruising/bleeding.

PEG-Intron, *see peginterferon alfa-2b*

P

pegloticase

peg-**low**-tih-case
(Krystexxa)

BLACK BOX ALERT Severe infusion reactions, anaphylaxis (bronchospasm, stridor, urticaria, hypotension, dyspnea, flushing, circumoral swelling), have occurred, especially within 2 hrs of first infusion. Pt to be premedicated with corticosteroids, antihistamines. Should be administered in healthcare setting by healthcare providers prepared to manage infusion reactions.

Do not confuse pegloticase with Activase, cholinesterase, or pegaspargase.

CLASSIFICATION

PHARMACOTHERAPEUTIC: Uric acid enzyme. **CLINICAL:** Antigout.

ACTION

Decreases uric acid production by catalyzing oxidation of uric acid to allantoin, lowering serum uric acid. **Therapeutic Effect:** Lowers serum uric acid concentration.

PHARMACOKINETICS

Catalyzes oxidation of uric acid to allantoin, an inert and water-soluble purine metabolite. Readily eliminated, primarily by renal excretion. **Half-life:** 14.5 days.

USES

Treatment of chronic gout in adult pts refractory to conventional therapy. Not recommended for treatment of asymptomatic hyperuricemia.

PRECAUTIONS

Contraindications: Glucose-6-phosphate dehydrogenase (G6PD) deficiency due to risk of hemodialysis, methemoglobinemia. **Cautions:** History of CHF, elderly, debilitated.

LIFESPAN CONSIDERATIONS

Pregnancy/Lactation: Unknown if drug crosses placenta or is distributed in breast milk. **Pregnancy Category C. Children:** Safety and efficacy not established in those younger than 18 yrs. **Elderly:** No age-related precautions noted.

INTERACTIONS

DRUG: None significant. **HERBAL:** None significant. **FOOD:** None known. **LAB VALUES:** Decreases serum uric acid (expected).

AVAILABILITY (Rx)

Injection Solution: 2-ml (8 mg/ml) single-use vials.

ADMINISTRATION/HANDLING

IV

Reconstitution • Withdraw 1 ml from single-use vial and inject into 250 ml 0.9% NaCl or 0.45% NaCl. • Invert infusion bag a number of times to ensure thorough mixing; do not shake.
Rate of administration • Infuse slowly over no less than 120 min.
Storage • Store in refrigerator. • Solution should appear clear; discard if particulate is present. • Allow diluted solution to reach room temperature prior to infusion. • Following dilution, solution remains stable for 4 hrs if refrigerated or at room temperature.

INDICATIONS/ROUTES/DOSAGE

ALERT Give by IV infusion; do not give as IV push or IV bolus. Pt to be pretreated with corticosteroids, antihistamines to reduce risk of infusion reaction, anaphylaxis.

Gout

IV INFUSION: ADULTS, ELDERLY: 8 mg every 2 wks.

SIDE EFFECTS

Occasional (12%–9%): Nausea, ecchymosis at IV site, nasopharyngitis. **Rare (6%–5%):** Constipation, vomiting.

ADVERSE EFFECTS/TOXIC REACTIONS

Exacerbation of CHF has been noted. Infusion-related reaction (urticaria, dyspnea, chest discomfort, chest pain, erythema, pruritus) occurs in 26% of pts; anaphylaxis occurs in 7% of pts. Increase in gout flares is frequently noted upon initiation of antihyperuricemic therapy due to changing serum uric acid levels.

NURSING CONSIDERATIONS

BASELINE ASSESSMENT

If gout flare occurs during treatment, prophylaxis with a nonsteroidal antiinflammatory drug (NSAID) or colchicine is recommended. Pts at higher risk for G6PD deficiency (e.g., those of African or Mediterranean ancestry) should be screened for G6PD deficiency before starting therapy. Obtain serum uric acid levels prior to each infusion. If levels reach greater than 6 mg/dl, particularly when 2 consecutive levels greater than 6 mg/dl are observed, treatment should be discontinued.

INTERVENTION/EVALUATION

Monitor closely for infusion reaction during therapy and for 2 hrs post treatment. If infusion reaction occurs during administration, infusion may be slowed, or stopped and restarted at slower rate. If severe infusion reaction occurs, discontinue infusion and institute treatment as needed. Assess for therapeutic response (reduced joint tenderness, swelling, redness, limitation of motion).

PATIENT/FAMILY TEACHING

• Educate pts on the most common signs and symptoms of infusion reaction (rash, redness of skin, difficulty breathing, flushing, chest discomfort, chest pain). • Advise pts to seek medical care immediately if they experience any symptoms of allergic reaction during or at any time after infusion.

pegvisomant

peg-**vis**-oh-mant
(Somavert)
Do not confuse Somavert with somatrem or somatropin.

◆CLASSIFICATION

PHARMACOTHERAPEUTIC: Protein. **CLINICAL:** Acromegaly agent.

ACTION

Selectively binds to growth hormone receptors on cell surfaces, blocking binding of endogenous growth hormones, interfering with growth hormone signal transduction. **Therapeutic Effect:** Decreases serum concentrations of insulin-like growth factor 1 (IGF-1) serum protein, normalizing serum IGF-1 levels.

PHARMACOKINETICS

Not distributed extensively into tissues after subcutaneous administration. Less than 1% excreted in urine. **Half-life:** 6 days.

USES

Treatment of acromegaly in pts with inadequate response to surgery, radiation, other medical therapies or those for whom these therapies are inappropriate.

PRECAUTIONS

Contraindications: Latex allergy (stopper on vial contains latex). **Cautions:** Elderly, diabetes mellitus.

LIFESPAN CONSIDERATIONS

Pregnancy/Lactation: Unknown if distributed in breast milk. **Pregnancy Category B. Children:** Safety and efficacy not established. **Elderly:** Initiation of treatment should begin at low end of dosage range.

INTERACTIONS

DRUG: May enhance effects of **insulin, oral antidiabetics** (may result in hypoglycemia). Dosage should be decreased when initiating pegvisomant therapy. **Opioids** decrease serum concentration. **HERBAL:** None significant. **FOOD:** None known. **LAB VALUES:** May increase serum alkaline phosphatase, total bilirubin, AST, ALT. Interferes with measurement of serum growth hormone concentration. Glucose tolerance test results may be elevated.

P

AVAILABILITY (Rx)

Injection, Powder for Reconstitution: 10-mg, 15-mg, 20-mg vials.

ADMINISTRATION/HANDLING

Subcutaneous

Reconstitution • Withdraw 1 ml Sterile Water for Injection, inject into vial of pegvisomant, aiming stream against glass wall. • Hold vial between palms of both hands, roll to dissolve powder (do not shake).
Rate of administration • Administer subcutaneously only 1 dose from each vial.
Storage • Refrigerate unreconstituted vials. • Administer within 6 hrs following reconstitution. • Solution should appear clear after reconstitution. Discard if cloudy or particulate forms.

INDICATIONS/ROUTES/DOSAGE

Acromegaly

SUBCUTANEOUS: ADULTS, ELDERLY: Initially, 40 mg, as a loading dose, then 10 mg daily. After 4–6 wks, adjust dosage in 5-mg increments if serum IGF-1 level is still elevated, or in 5-mg decrements if IGF-1 level has decreased below the normal range. **Maximum:** 30 mg daily.

Dosage in Hepatic Impairment

BASELINE HEPATIC FUNCTION TESTS GREATER THAN 3 TIMES UPPER LIMIT OF NORMAL (ULN): Do not initiate without comprehensive workup to determine cause.
HEPATIC FUNCTION TESTS 3 TIMES OR GREATER BUT LESS THAN 5 TIMES ULN: Continue treatment but monitor for hepatitis, hepatic injury.
HEPATIC FUNCTION TESTS 5 TIMES OR GREATER OR SERUM TRANSAMINASE GREATER THAN 3 TIMES ULN ASSOCIATED WITH ANY INCREASE IN TOTAL BILIRUBIN: Discontinue immediately, perform comprehensive hepatic workup.

SIDE EFFECTS

Frequent (23%): Infection (cold symptoms, upper respiratory tract infection, blister, ear infection). **Occasional (8%–5%):** Back pain, dizziness, injection site reaction, peripheral edema, sinusitis, nausea. **Rare (less than 4%):** Diarrhea, paresthesia.

ADVERSE EFFECTS/ TOXIC REACTIONS

May produce marked elevation of hepatic enzymes, including serum transaminase. Substantial weight gain occurs rarely.

NURSING CONSIDERATIONS

BASELINE ASSESSMENT

Obtain baseline hepatic function tests.

INTERVENTION/EVALUATION

Monitor hepatic function tests. Monitor all pts with tumors that secrete growth hormone with periodic imaging scans of sella turcica for progressive tumor growth. Monitor diabetic pts for hypoglycemia. Obtain IGF-1 serum concentrations 4–6 wks after therapy begins and periodically thereafter; dosage adjustment based on results; dosage adjustment should not be based on growth hormone assays.

PATIENT/FAMILY TEACHING

• Routine monitoring of hepatic function tests is essential during treatment. • Contact physician if jaundice (yellowing of eyes, skin) occurs.

pemetrexed

HIGH ALERT

pem-eh-**trex**-ed
(Alimta)

◆CLASSIFICATION

PHARMACOTHERAPEUTIC: Antimetabolite. **CLINICAL:** Antineoplastic.

ACTION

Disrupts folate-dependent enzymes essential for cell replication. **Therapeutic Effect:** Inhibits growth of mesothelioma cell lines.

P

PHARMACOKINETICS

Protein binding: 81%. Not metabolized. Excreted in urine. **Half-life:** 3.5 hrs.

USES

Combination chemotherapy with cisplatin for treatment of malignant pleural mesothelioma. Single agent treatment of locally advanced or metastatic non–small-cell lung cancer (NSCLC) after prior chemotherapy. Initial treatment of NSCLC in combination with cisplatin. Maintenance treatment of NSCLC in those whose disease has not progressed following 4 cycles of platinum-based first-line chemotherapy. **OFF-LABEL:** Treatment of bladder, breast, cervical, colorectal, esophageal, gastric, head and neck, ovarian, pancreatic, renal cell carcinoma.

PRECAUTIONS

Contraindications: None known. **Cautions:** Hepatic/renal impairment.

LIFESPAN CONSIDERATIONS

Pregnancy/Lactation: Unknown if drug crosses placenta or is distributed in breast milk. Breast-feeding not recommended. May cause fetal harm. Not recommended during pregnancy. **Pregnancy Category D. Children:** Safety and efficacy not established in those younger than 18 yrs. **Elderly:** Higher incidence of fatigue, leukopenia, neutropenia, thrombocytopenia in those 65 yrs and older.

INTERACTIONS

DRUG: **Bone marrow depressants** may increase risk of myelosuppression. **Live virus vaccines** may potentiate virus replication, increase vaccine side effects, decrease pt's antibody response to vaccine. **HERBAL:** None significant. **FOOD:** None known. **LAB VALUES:** May increase serum ALT, AST, creatinine.

AVAILABILITY (Rx)

Injection, Powder for Reconstitution: 100 mg, 500 mg.

ADMINISTRATION/HANDLING

IV Infusion

Reconstitution • Dilute 500-mg vial with 20 ml (4.2 ml to 100-mg vial) 0.9% NaCl to provide concentration of 25 mg/ml. • Gently swirl each vial until powder is completely dissolved. • Solution appears clear and ranges in color from colorless to yellow or green-yellow. • Further dilute reconstituted solution with 100 ml 0.9% NaCl.
Rate of administration • Infuse over 10 min.
Storage • Store at room temperature. • Diluted solution is stable for up to 24 hrs at room temperature or if refrigerated.

IV INCOMPATIBILITIES

Use only 0.9% NaCl to reconstitute; flush line prior to and following infusion. Do not add any other medications to IV line.

INDICATIONS/ROUTES/DOSAGE

Refer to individual protocols.
◀ALERT▶ Pretreatment with dexamethasone (or equivalent) will reduce risk, severity of cutaneous reaction; treatment with folic acid and vitamin B_{12} beginning 1 wk before treatment and continuing for 21 days after last pemetrexed dose will reduce risk of side effects. Do not begin new treatment cycles unless ANC 1,500/mm^3 or greater, platelets 100,000/mm^3 or greater, and CrCl 45 ml/min or greater.

Malignant Pleural Mesothelioma

IV: ADULTS, ELDERLY: 600 mg/m^2 q3wks when used as a single agent; 500 mg/m^2 q3wks when used in combination with cisplatin 75 mg/m^2.

Non–Small-Cell Lung Cancer (NSCLC)

IV: ADULTS, ELDERLY: 500 mg/m^2 q3wks.

SIDE EFFECTS

Frequent (12%–10%): Fatigue, nausea, vomiting, rash, desquamation. **Occasional (8%–4%):** Stomatitis, pharyngitis, diarrhea, anorexia, hypertension, chest pain. **Rare (less than 3%):** Constipation, depression, dysphagia.

P

ADVERSE EFFECTS/ TOXIC REACTIONS

Myelosuppression, characterized as grade 1–4 neutropenia, thrombocytopenia, anemia, has been noted.

NURSING CONSIDERATIONS

BASELINE ASSESSMENT

Question for possibility of pregnancy before initiating therapy (Pregnancy Category D). Breast-feeding not recommended once treatment has been initiated. Obtain CBC, serum chemistry tests before therapy and repeat throughout therapy.

INTERVENTION/EVALUATION

Monitor Hgb, Hct, WBC, platelet count, renal/hepatic function. Monitor for hematologic toxicity (fever, sore throat, signs of local infection, unusual bruising/bleeding from any site), symptoms of anemia (excessive fatigue, weakness). Assess skin for evidence of dermatologic toxicity. Keep pt well hydrated, urine alkaline. Monitor WBC count for nadir, recovery.

PATIENT/FAMILY TEACHING

• Maintain fastidious oral hygiene. • Do not have immunizations without physician's approval (drug lowers resistance). • Avoid crowds, those with infection. • Use contraceptive measures during therapy. • Promptly report fever, sore throat, signs of local infection, unusual bruising/bleeding from any site.

P

penicillamine

pen-ih-**sill**-ah-meen
(Cuprimine, Depen)

BLACK BOX ALERT Pt must remain under close medical supervision for signs of toxicity (fever, sore throat, chills, ecchymosis, bleeding).
Do not confuse penicillamine with penicillin.

◆CLASSIFICATION

PHARMACOTHERAPEUTIC: Heavy metal antagonist. **CLINICAL:** Chelating agent, anti-inflammatory.

ACTION

Chelates with lead, copper, mercury, iron to form soluble complexes; depresses circulating IgM rheumatoid factor levels; depresses T-cell activity; combines with cystine to form more soluble compound. **Therapeutic Effect:** Promotes excretion of heavy metals, acts as anti-inflammatory drug, prevents renal calculi (may dissolve existing stones).

USES

Promotes excretion of copper in treatment of Wilson's disease, decreases excretion of cystine, prevents renal calculi in cystinuria associated with nephrolithiasis. Treatment of active rheumatoid arthritis (RA) not controlled with conventional therapy. **OFF-LABEL:** Treatment of rheumatoid vasculitis, heavy metal toxicity, arsenic poisoning.

PRECAUTIONS

Contraindications: History of penicillamine-related aplastic anemia or agranulocytosis, rheumatoid arthritis, pts with history or evidence of renal insufficiency, pregnancy, breast-feeding. **Cautions:** Elderly, debilitated, renal/hepatic impairment, penicillin allergy.

⧖ LIFESPAN CONSIDERATIONS

Pregnancy/Lactation: Contraindicated in pregnancy. Teratogenic; may cause fetal death. **Pregnancy Category D. Children:** Efficacy not established. **Elderly:** Age-related renal/hepatic impairment may require dosage adjustment.

INTERACTIONS

DRUG: **Iron supplements** may decrease absorption. **Bone marrow depressants, gold compounds, immunosuppressants** may increase risk of adverse hematologic, renal effects. **HERBAL:** None significant. FOOD: **All foods** may decrease absorption. LAB VALUES: None known.

AVAILABILITY (Rx)

Capsules (Cuprimine): 250 mg. Tablets (Depen): 250 mg.

ADMINISTRATION/HANDLING

PO

• Administer 1 hr before or 2 hrs after meals, milk, other medication. • Contents of capsule may be mixed with fruit juice or pureed fruit. • For cystinuria, drink copious amounts of water.

INDICATIONS/ROUTES/DOSAGE

Rheumatoid Arthritis (RA)

PO: ADULTS, ELDERLY: 125–250 mg/day. **Maximum (adults):** May increase at 1- to 3-mo intervals up to 1–1.5 g/day. **Maximum (elderly):** 750 mg/day.

◄ALERT► Dose more than 500 mg/day should be in divided doses.

CHILDREN YOUNGER THAN 12 YRS: Initially, 3 mg/kg/day (**Maximum:** 250 mg) for 3 mos, then 6 mg/kg/day (**Maximum:** 500 mg) in 2 divided doses for 3 mos. **Maximum:** 10 mg/kg/day (750 mg/day) in 3–4 divided doses.

Wilson's Disease

PO: ADULTS, CHILDREN 12 YRS AND OLDER: 1 g/day in 4 divided doses. **Maximum:** 2 g/day. **ELDERLY:** 750 mg/day in 3–4 divided doses. **CHILDREN YOUNGER THAN 12 YRS:** 20 mg/kg/day in 2–4 doses. **Maximum:** 1 g/day.

◄ALERT► Titrate to maintain urinary copper excretion greater than 1 mg/day.

Cystinuria

PO: ADULTS, ELDERLY: Initially, 2 g/day in divided doses q6h. Range: 1–4 g/day. **CHILDREN:** 30 mg/kg/day in 4 divided doses. **Maximum:** 4 g/day.

◄ALERT► Titrate to maintain urinary cystine excretion at 100–200 mg/day.

SIDE EFFECTS

Frequent: Rash (pruritic, erythematous, maculopapular, morbilliform), reduced/altered sense of taste (hypogeusia), GI disturbances (anorexia, epigastric pain, nausea, vomiting, diarrhea), oral ulcers, glossitis. **Occasional:** Proteinuria, hematuria, hot flashes, drug-induced hyperthermia (drug fever). **Rare:** Alopecia, tinnitus, pemphigoid rash (water blisters).

ADVERSE EFFECTS/ TOXIC REACTIONS

Aplastic anemia, agranulocytosis, thrombocytopenia, leukopenia, myasthenia gravis, bronchiolitis, erythematous-like syndrome, evening hypoglycemia, skin friability at sites of pressure/trauma producing extravasation or white papules at venipuncture, surgical sites reported. Iron deficiency may develop, particularly in children, menstruating women.

NURSING CONSIDERATIONS

BASELINE ASSESSMENT

Baseline CBC with differential, WBC, Hgb, platelet count should be performed before beginning therapy, q2wks thereafter for first 6 mos, then monthly during therapy. Hepatic function tests (GGT, AST, ALT, LDH), CT scan for renal stones should also be ordered. A 2-hr interval is necessary between iron and penicillamine therapy. In event of upcoming surgery, dosage should be reduced to 250 mg/day until wound healing is complete.

INTERVENTION/EVALUATION

Encourage copious amounts of water in pts with cystinuria. Monitor WBC, differential, platelet count. If WBC less than 3,500, neutrophils less than 2,000/mm^3, monocytes more than 500/mm^3, or platelet counts less than 100,000, or if progressive fall in platelet count or WBC in 3 successive determinations noted, inform physician (drug withdrawal necessary). Assess for evidence of hematuria. Monitor urinalysis for hematuria, proteinuria (if proteinuria exceeds 1 g/24 hrs, inform physician).

P

PATIENT/FAMILY TEACHING

- Promptly report any missed menstrual periods/other indications of pregnancy.
- Report fever, sore throat, chills, bruising, bleeding, difficulty breathing on exertion, unexplained cough or wheezing.
- Take medication 1 hr before or 2 hrs after meals or at least 1 hr before or after any other drug, food, or milk.

penicillin G benzathine

pen-ih-**sil**-lin G **benz**-ah-theen
(Bicillin LA)
Do not confuse penicillin G benzathine with penicillin G potassium.

FIXED-COMBINATION(S)

Bicillin CR: penicillin G benzathine/penicillin procaine: 600,000 units benzathine/600,000 units procaine.

◆ CLASSIFICATION

PHARMACOTHERAPEUTIC: Penicillin. **CLINICAL:** Antibiotic (see p. 28C).

ACTION

Inhibits bacterial cell wall synthesis by binding to one or more of the penicillin-binding proteins of bacteria. **Therapeutic Effect:** Bactericidal.

USES

Treatment of mild to moderate severe infections caused by organisms susceptible to low concentrations of penicillin including streptococcal (Group A) upper respiratory infections, syphilis, yaws. Prophylaxis of infections caused by susceptible organisms (e.g., rheumatic fever prophylaxis).

PRECAUTIONS

Contraindications: Hypersensitivity to any penicillin. **Cautions:** Renal/cardiac impairment, seizure disorder, hypersensitivity to cephalosporins.

LIFESPAN CONSIDERATIONS

Pregnancy/Lactation: Readily crosses placenta; distributed in breast milk. **Pregnancy Category B. Children:** May delay renal excretion in neonates, young infants. **Elderly:** Age-related renal impairment may require dosage adjustment.

INTERACTIONS

DRUG: Probenecid increases concentration. **HERBAL:** None significant. **FOOD:** None known. **LAB VALUES:** May cause positive Coombs' test. May increase serum ALT, AST, alkaline phosphatase, LDH. May decrease WBC count.

AVAILABILITY (Rx)

Injection (Prefilled Syringe [Bicillin LA]): 600,000 units/ml.

ADMINISTRATION/HANDLING

◀ALERT▶ Do not give IV, intra-arterially, subcutaneously (may cause thrombosis, severe neurovascular damage, cardiac arrest, death).

IM

- Store in refrigerator. Do not freeze.
- Administer undiluted by deep IM injection.

INDICATIONS/ROUTES/DOSAGE

Usual Dosage Range

IM: ADULTS, ELDERLY: 1.2–2.4 million units as single dose. **CHILDREN:** 25,000–50,000 units/kg as single dose. **Maximum:** 2.4 million units.

SIDE EFFECTS

Occasional: Lethargy, fever, dizziness, rash, pain at injection site. **Rare:** Seizures, interstitial nephritis.

ADVERSE EFFECTS/ TOXIC REACTIONS

Hypersensitivity reactions, ranging from chills, fever, rash to anaphylaxis, may occur.

NURSING CONSIDERATIONS

BASELINE ASSESSMENT

Question for history of allergies, particularly penicillins, cephalosporins.

INTERVENTION/EVALUATION

Monitor CBC, urinalysis, renal function tests.

penicillin G potassium

pen-ih-**sil**-lin G
(Crystapen, Pfizerpen)
Do not confuse penicillin with penicillamine.

◆CLASSIFICATION

PHARMACOTHERAPEUTIC: Penicillin. **CLINICAL:** Antibiotic (see p. 28C).

ACTION

Inhibits bacterial cell wall synthesis by binding to one or more of the penicillin-binding proteins of bacteria. **Therapeutic Effect:** Bactericidal.

PHARMACOKINETICS

Protein binding: 60%. Widely distributed (poor CNS penetration). Metabolized in liver. Primarily excreted in urine. **Half-life:** 0.5–1 hr (increased in renal impairment).

USES

Treatment of susceptible infections due to gram-positive organisms, gram-negative organisms, actinomycosis, clostridium, diphtheria, Listeria, *N. meningitidis,* pasteurella including anthrax, endocarditis, respiratory tract infections, meningitis, neurosyphilis, skin/skin structure infections.

PRECAUTIONS

Contraindications: Hypersensitivity to any penicillin. **Cautions:** Renal/hepatic impairment, seizure disorder, hypersensitivity to cephalosporins.

⌛ LIFESPAN CONSIDERATIONS

Pregnancy/Lactation: Readily crosses placenta; distributed in breast milk. **Pregnancy Category B. Children:** May delay renal excretion in neonates, young infants. **Elderly:** Age-related renal impairment may require dosage adjustment.

INTERACTIONS

DRUG: Concurrent use of **aminoglycosides** may cause mutual inactivation (must be given at least 1 hr apart). **ACE inhibitors, potassium-sparing diuretics, potassium supplements** may increase risk of hyperkalemia. May increase **methotrexate** concentration, toxicity. **Probenecid** increases concentration. **HERBAL:** None significant. **FOOD: Food, milk** decrease absorption. **LAB VALUES:** May cause positive Coombs' test. May increase serum ALT, AST, alkaline phosphatase, LDH. May decrease WBC count.

AVAILABILITY (Rx)

Infusion (Pre-Mix): 1 million units/50 ml, 2 million units/50 ml, 3 million units/50 ml. **Injection, Powder for Reconstitution:** 5 million units.

ADMINISTRATION/HANDLING

IV

Reconstitution • Follow dilution guide per manufacturer. • After reconstitution, further dilute with 50–100 ml D_5W or 0.9% NaCl for final concentration of 100,000–500,000 units/ml (50,000 units/ml for infants, neonates).

Rate of administration • Infuse over 15–60 min (15–30 min for infants, neonates).

Storage • Reconstituted solution is stable for 7 days if refrigerated.

IV INCOMPATIBILITIES

Amikacin (Amikin), aminophylline, amphotericin B, dopamine (Intropin), gentamicin, tobramycin.

P

IV COMPATIBILITIES

Amiodarone (Cordarone), calcium gluconate, diltiazem (Cardizem), diphenhydramine (Benadryl), furosemide (Lasix), heparin, hydromorphone (Dilaudid), lidocaine, lipids, magnesium sulfate, methylprednisolone (Solu-Medrol), morphine, potassium chloride, total parenteral nutrition (TPN).

INDICATIONS/ROUTES/DOSAGE

Usual Dosage

IV, IM: ADULTS, ELDERLY: 2–30 million units/day in divided doses q4–6h. **CHILDREN:** 25,000–400,000 units/kg/day in divided doses q4–6h. **NEONATES:** 25,000–50,000 units q6–12h.

Dosage in Renal Impairment

Dosage interval is modified based on creatinine clearance.

Creatinine Clearance	Dosage
10–30 ml/min	Usual dose q8–12h
Less than 10 ml/min	Usual dose q12–18h

SIDE EFFECTS

Occasional: Lethargy, fever, dizziness, rash, electrolyte imbalance, diarrhea, thrombophlebitis. **Rare:** Seizures, interstitial nephritis.

ADVERSE EFFECTS/ TOXIC REACTIONS

Hypersensitivity reactions ranging from rash, fever, chills to anaphylaxis occur occasionally.

NURSING CONSIDERATIONS

BASELINE ASSESSMENT

Question for history of allergies, particularly penicillins, cephalosporins.

INTERVENTION/EVALUATION

Monitor CBC, urinalysis electrolytes, renal function tests.

penicillin V potassium

pen-ih-**sil**-in V
(Apo-Pen-VK ✦, Novo-Pen-VK ✦, NuPen VK ✦)

◆ CLASSIFICATION

PHARMACOTHERAPEUTIC: Penicillin. **CLINICAL:** Antibiotic (see p. 28C).

ACTION

Inhibits cell wall synthesis by binding to bacterial cell membranes. **Therapeutic Effect:** Bactericidal.

PHARMACOKINETICS

Moderately absorbed from GI tract. Protein binding: 80%. Widely distributed. Metabolized in liver. Primarily excreted in urine. **Half-life:** 1 hr (increased in renal impairment).

USES

Treatment of mild to moderate infections of respiratory tract, skin/skin structure, otitis media, necrotizing ulcerative gingivitis; prophylaxis for rheumatic fever, dental procedures.

PRECAUTIONS

Contraindications: Hypersensitivity to any penicillin. **Cautions:** Renal impairment, history of allergies (particularly cephalosporins), history of seizures.

⌛ LIFESPAN CONSIDERATIONS

Pregnancy/Lactation: Readily crosses placenta; appears in cord blood, amniotic fluid. Distributed in breast milk in low concentrations. May lead to allergic sensitization, diarrhea, candidiasis, skin rash in infant. **Pregnancy Category B.** **Children:** Use caution in neonates and young infants (may delay renal elimination). **Elderly:** Age-related renal impairment may require dosage adjustment.

INTERACTIONS

DRUG: **ACE inhibitors, potassium-sparing diuretics, potassium supplements** may increase risk of hyperkalemia. May increase **methotrexate** concentration, toxicity. **Probenecid** may increase concentration, risk of toxicity. HERBAL: None significant. FOOD: None known. LAB VALUES: May cause positive Coombs' test. May increase ALT, AST, alkaline phosphatase, LDH. May decrease WBC count.

AVAILABILITY (Rx)

Powder for Oral Solution: 125 mg/5 ml, 250 mg/5 ml. Tablets: 250 mg, 500 mg.

ADMINISTRATION/HANDLING

PO

• Give on empty stomach 1 hr before or 2 hrs after meals (increases absorption). • After reconstitution, oral solution is stable for 14 days if refrigerated. • Space doses evenly around the clock.

INDICATIONS/ROUTES/DOSAGE

Usual Dosage

PO: ADULTS, ELDERLY, CHILDREN 12 YRS AND OLDER: 125–500 mg q6–8h. **CHILDREN YOUNGER THAN 12 YRS:** 25–50 mg/kg/day in divided doses q6–8h. **Maximum:** 3 g/day.

Prophylaxis of Pneumococcal Recurrent Rheumatic Fever

PO: ADULTS, ELDERLY, CHILDREN 5 YRS AND OLDER: 250 mg twice a day. **CHILDREN YOUNGER THAN 5 YRS:** 125 mg twice a day.

Dosage in Renal Impairment

Creatinine clearance less than 10 ml/min: 250 mg q6h.

SIDE EFFECTS

Frequent: Mild hypersensitivity reaction (chills, fever, rash), nausea, vomiting, diarrhea. Rare: Bleeding, allergic reaction.

ADVERSE EFFECTS/ TOXIC REACTIONS

Severe hypersensitivity reactions, including anaphylaxis, may occur. Nephrotoxicity, antibiotic-associated colitis, other superinfections (abdominal cramps, severe watery diarrhea, fever) may result from high dosages, prolonged therapy.

NURSING CONSIDERATIONS

BASELINE ASSESSMENT

Question for history of allergies, particularly penicillins, cephalosporins.

INTERVENTION/EVALUATION

Hold medication, promptly report rash (hypersensitivity), diarrhea (with fever, abdominal pain, mucus or blood in stool may indicate antibiotic-associated colitis). Monitor I&O, urinalysis, renal function tests for nephrotoxicity. Be alert for superinfection: fever, vomiting, diarrhea, anal/genital pruritus, oral mucosal change (ulceration, pain, erythema). Review Hgb levels; check for bleeding (overt bleeding, ecchymosis, swelling of tissue).

PATIENT/FAMILY TEACHING

• Continue antibiotic for full length of treatment. • Space doses evenly. • Notify physician immediately if rash, diarrhea, bleeding, bruising, other new symptoms occur.

P

pentamidine

pen-**tam**-i-deen
(NebuPent, Pentam-300)

◆ CLASSIFICATION

PHARMACOTHERAPEUTIC: Anti-infective. **CLINICAL:** Antiprotozoal.

ACTION

Interferes with nuclear metabolism, incorporation of nucleotides, inhibiting DNA, RNA, phospholipid, protein synthesis. **Therapeutic Effect:** Produces antibacterial, antiprotozoal effects.

PHARMACOKINETICS

Well absorbed after IM administration; minimally absorbed after inhalation.

Widely distributed. Primarily excreted in urine. Minimally removed by hemodialysis. **Half-life:** 6.4–9.4 hrs (increased in renal impairment).

USES

Treatment of pneumonia caused by *Pneumocystis jiroveci* (PCP). Prevention of PCP in high-risk HIV-infected pts. **OFF-LABEL:** Treatment of African trypanosomiasis, cutaneous/visceral leishmaniasis.

PRECAUTIONS

Contraindications: Concurrent use with didanosine. **Cautions:** Diabetes mellitus, renal/hepatic impairment, hypertension/hypotension.

LIFESPAN CONSIDERATIONS

Pregnancy/Lactation: Unknown if drug crosses placenta or is distributed in breast milk. **Pregnancy Category C. Children:** No age-related precautions noted. **Elderly:** No age-related information available.

INTERACTIONS

DRUG: Delavirdine, fluconazole, fluvoxamine, gemfibrozil, isoniazid, omeprazole may increase concentration, toxicity. **Carbamazepine, phenytoin, rifampin** may decrease effect. **Didanosine** may increase risk of pancreatitis. **Foscarnet** may increase risk of hypocalcemia, hypomagnesemia, nephrotoxicity of pentamidine. **HERBAL:** None significant. **FOOD:** None known. **LAB VALUES:** May increase serum alkaline phosphatase, bilirubin, BUN, creatinine, AST, ALT. May decrease serum calcium, magnesium. May alter serum glucose.

AVAILABILITY (Rx)

Injection, Powder for Reconstitution (Pentam-300): 300 mg. **Powder for Nebulization (NebuPent):** 300 mg.

ADMINISTRATION/HANDLING

◀ALERT▶ Pt must be in supine position during IM, IV administration, with frequent B/P checks until stable (potential for life-threatening hypotensive reaction). Have resuscitative equipment immediately available.

IV

Reconstitution • For intermittent IV infusion (piggyback), reconstitute each vial with 3–5 ml D_5W or Sterile Water for Injection. • Withdraw desired dose; further dilute with 50–250 ml D_5W to concentration not to exceed 6 mg/ml.

Rate of administration • Infuse over 60–120 min. • Do not give by IV injection or rapid IV infusion (increases potential for severe hypotension).

Storage • Store vials at room temperature. • After reconstitution, IV solution is stable for 48 hrs at room temperature (24 hrs if reconstituted with D_5W). • Discard unused portion.

IM

• Reconstitute 300-mg vial with 3 ml Sterile Water for Injection to provide concentration of 100 mg/ml. • Administer deep IM.

Aerosol (Nebulizer)

• Aerosol stable for 48 hrs at room temperature. • Reconstitute 300-mg vial with 6 ml Sterile Water for Injection. Avoid NaCl (may cause precipitate). • Do not mix with other medication in nebulizer reservoir.

IV INCOMPATIBILITIES

Cefazolin (Ancef), cefotaxime (Claforan), ceftazidime (Fortaz), ceftriaxone (Rocephin), fluconazole (Diflucan), foscarnet (Foscavir), interleukin (Proleukin).

IV COMPATIBILITIES

Diltiazem (Cardizem), total parenteral nutrition (TPN), zidovudine (Retrovir).

INDICATIONS/ROUTES/DOSAGE

Treatment of *Pneumocystis Jiroveci* Pneumonia (PCP)

IV, IM: ADULTS, ELDERLY: 4 mg/kg/day once daily for 14–21 days. **CHILDREN:** 4 mg/kg/day once daily for 14–21 days.

Prevention of PCP
INHALATION: ADULTS, ELDERLY: 300 mg once q4wks.
IM, IV: CHILDREN: 4 mg/kg/dose q2–4 wks.

SIDE EFFECTS

Frequent: **Injection (greater than 10%):** Abscess, pain at injection site. **Inhalation (greater than 5%):** Fatigue, metallic taste, shortness of breath, decreased appetite, dizziness, rash, cough, nausea, vomiting, chills. Occasional: **Injection (10%–1%):** Nausea, decreased appetite, hypotension, fever, rash, altered taste, confusion. **Inhalation (5%–1%):** Diarrhea, headache, anemia, muscle pain. Rare: **Injection (less than 1%):** Neuralgia, thrombocytopenia, phlebitis, dizziness.

ADVERSE EFFECTS/ TOXIC REACTIONS

Life-threatening/fatal hypotension, arrhythmias, hypoglycemia, leukopenia, nephrotoxicity, renal failure, anaphylactic shock, Stevens-Johnson syndrome, toxic epidural necrolysis occur rarely. Hyperglycemia, insulin-dependent diabetes mellitus (often permanent) may occur even mos after therapy has stopped.

NURSING CONSIDERATIONS

BASELINE ASSESSMENT

Avoid concurrent use of nephrotoxic drugs. Establish baseline for B/P, serum glucose. Obtain specimens for diagnostic tests before giving first dose.

INTERVENTION/EVALUATION

Monitor B/P during administration until stable for both IM and IV administration (pt should remain supine). Check serum glucose levels; observe for clinical signs of hypoglycemia (diaphoresis, anxiety, tremor, tachycardia, palpitations, lightheadedness, headache, numbness of lips, double vision, incoordination), hyperglycemia (polyuria, polyphagia, polydipsia, malaise, visual changes, abdominal pain, headache, nausea/vomiting). Evaluate IM sites for pain, redness, induration; IV sites for phlebitis (heat, pain, red streaking over vein). Monitor renal, hepatic, hematology test results. Assess skin for rash. Evaluate equilibrium during ambulation. Be alert for respiratory difficulty when administering by inhalation route.

PATIENT/FAMILY TEACHING

• Remain flat in bed during administration of medication; get up slowly with assistance only when B/P stable. • Notify physician immediately of diaphoresis, shakiness, light-headedness, palpitations. • Drowsiness, increased urination, thirst, anorexia may develop in mos following therapy. • Maintain adequate fluid intake. • Inform physician if fever, cough, shortness of breath occurs. • Avoid alcohol.

Pentasa, *see mesalamine*

pentoxifylline

pen-tox-ih-**fi**-leen
(Albert ✦, Apo-Pentoxifylline SR ✦, Pentoxil, Trental)
Do not confuse pentoxifylline with tamoxifen, or Trental with Bentyl, Tegretol, or Trandate.

◆CLASSIFICATION

PHARMACOTHERAPEUTIC: Hemorrheologic agent. **CLINICAL:** Hemorrheologic.

ACTION

Alters flexibility of RBCs; inhibits production of tumor necrosis factor (TNF), neutrophil activation, platelet aggregation. **Therapeutic Effect:** Reduces blood viscosity, improves blood flow.

PHARMACOKINETICS

Well absorbed after PO administration. Undergoes first-pass metabolism in liver. Primarily excreted in urine. Unknown if removed by hemodialysis. **Half-life:** 24–48 min; metabolite, 60–90 min.

P

USES

Symptomatic treatment of intermittent claudication associated with occlusive peripheral vascular disease, diabetic angiopathies. **OFF-LABEL:** Diabetic neuropathy, gangrene, hemodialysis shunt thrombosis, septic shock, sickle cell syndrome, vascular impotence, venous leg ulcers.

PRECAUTIONS

Contraindications: History of intolerance to xanthine derivatives, such as caffeine, theophylline, theobromine; recent cerebral/retinal hemorrhage. **Cautions:** Renal/hepatic impairment, insulin-treated diabetes, chronic occlusive arterial disease, recent surgery, peptic ulcer disease.

LIFESPAN CONSIDERATIONS

Pregnancy/Lactation: Unknown if drug crosses placenta. Distributed in breast milk. **Pregnancy Category C. Children:** Safety and efficacy not established. **Elderly:** Age-related renal impairment may require dosage adjustment.

INTERACTIONS

DRUG: May increase effects of **antihypertensives. HERBAL:** None significant. **FOOD:** None known. **LAB VALUES:** None significant.

AVAILABILITY (Rx)

Tablets (Controlled-Release [Pentoxil, Trental]): 400 mg.

ADMINISTRATION/HANDLING

PO

• Do not crush/break controlled-release tablets. • Give with meals to avoid GI upset.

INDICATIONS/ROUTES/DOSAGE

Intermittent Claudication

PO: ADULTS, ELDERLY: 400 mg 3 times daily. Decrease to 400 mg twice daily if GI, CNS adverse effects occur. Continue for at least 8 wks.

SIDE EFFECTS

Occasional (5%–2%): Dizziness, nausea, altered taste, dyspepsia (heartburn, epigastric pain, indigestion). **Rare (less than 2%):** Rash, pruritus, anorexia, constipation, dry mouth, blurred vision, edema, nasal congestion, anxiety.

ADVERSE EFFECTS/ TOXIC REACTIONS

Angina, chest pain occur rarely; may be accompanied by palpitations, tachycardia, arrhythmias. Signs/symptoms of overdose (flushing, hypotension, nervousness, agitation, hand tremor, fever, drowsiness) appear 4–5 hrs after ingestion, last up to 12 hrs.

NURSING CONSIDERATIONS

INTERVENTION/EVALUATION

Assist with ambulation if dizziness occurs. Assess for hand tremor. Monitor for relief of symptoms of intermittent claudication (pain, aching, cramping in calf muscles, buttocks, thigh, feet). Symptoms generally occur while walking/exercising and not at rest or with weight bearing in absence of walking/exercising.

PATIENT/FAMILY TEACHING

• Therapeutic effect generally noted in 2–4 wks. • Avoid tasks requiring alertness, motor skills until response to drug is established. • Do not smoke (causes constriction, occlusion of peripheral blood vessels). • Limit caffeine.

Pepcid, *see famotidine*

Percocet, *see acetaminophen and oxycodone*

phenazopyridine

fen-az-o-**peer**-i-deen
(Azo-Gesic, Azo-Standard, Phenazo ✱, Pyridium, Uristat)
Do not confuse phenazopyridine with pyridoxine, or Pyridium with Dyrenium.

◆ CLASSIFICATION

PHARMACOTHERAPEUTIC: Interstitial cystitis agent. **CLINICAL:** Urinary tract analgesic.

ACTION

Exerts topical analgesic effect on urinary tract mucosa. **Therapeutic Effect:** Relieves urinary pain, burning, urgency, frequency.

PHARMACOKINETICS

Well absorbed from GI tract. Partially metabolized in liver. Primarily excreted in urine. **Half-life:** Unknown.

USES

Symptomatic relief of pain, burning, urgency, frequency resulting from lower urinary tract mucosa irritation (may be caused by infection, trauma, surgery).

PRECAUTIONS

Contraindications: Hepatic/renal insufficiency. **Cautions:** None known.

LIFESPAN CONSIDERATIONS

Pregnancy/Lactation: Unknown if drug crosses placenta or is distributed in breast milk. **Pregnancy Category B. Children:** No age-related precautions noted in those older than 6 yrs. **Elderly:** Age-related renal impairment may increase toxicity.

INTERACTIONS

DRUG: None significant. **HERBAL:** None significant. **FOOD:** None known. **LAB VALUES:** May interfere with urinalysis tests based on color reactions (e.g., urinary glucose, ketones, protein, 17-ketosteroids).

AVAILABILITY (Rx)

Tablets: **(Azo-Gesic, Azo-Standard, Uristat):** 95 mg. **(Pyridium):** 100 mg, 200 mg.

ADMINISTRATION/HANDLING

PO

- Give with meals.

INDICATIONS/ROUTES/DOSAGE

Urinary Analgesic

PO: ADULTS: (PYRIDIUM): 100–200 mg 3–4 times a day. **(AZO-STANDARD):** 95–190 mg 3 times a day. **CHILDREN 6 YRS AND OLDER:** 12 mg/kg/day in 3 divided doses for 2 days.

Dosage in Renal Impairment

Dosage interval is modified based on creatinine clearance.

Creatinine Clearance	Dosage
50–80 ml/min	Usual dose q8–16h
Less than 50 ml/min	Avoid use

SIDE EFFECTS

Occasional: Headache, GI disturbance, rash, pruritus.

ADVERSE EFFECTS/ TOXIC REACTIONS

Overdose in pts with renal impairment, severe hypersensitivity may lead to hemolytic anemia, nephrotoxicity, hepatotoxicity. Methemoglobinemia generally occurs as result of massive, acute overdose.

NURSING CONSIDERATIONS

BASELINE ASSESSMENT

Assess pt for urgency, frequency, pain on urination.

INTERVENTION/EVALUATION

Monitor for therapeutic response: relief of dysuria (pain, burning), urgency, frequency of urination.

PATIENT/FAMILY TEACHING

• Reddish orange discoloration of urine should be expected. • May stain fabric.

• Take with meals (reduces possibility of GI upset).

phenelzine

fen-ell-zeen
(Nardil)

BLACK BOX ALERT Increased risk of suicidal thinking and behavior in children, adolescents, young adults 18–24 yrs with major depressive disorder, other psychiatric disorders.

Do not confuse phenelzine with phenytoin.

◆CLASSIFICATION

PHARMACOTHERAPEUTIC: MAOI. **CLINICAL:** Antidepressant (see p. 38C).

ACTION

Inhibits activity of the enzyme monoamine oxidase at CNS storage sites, leading to increased levels of epinephrine, norepinephrine, serotonin, dopamine at neuronal receptor sites. **Therapeutic Effect:** Relieves depression.

USES

Treatment of depression refractory to other antidepressants, electroconvulsive therapy. **OFF-LABEL:** Treatment of panic disorder, selective mutism, vascular/tension headaches.

PRECAUTIONS

Contraindications: Cardiovascular/cerebrovascular disease, hepatic/renal impairment, pheochromocytoma. **Cautions:** Ingestion of tyramine-containing foods, cardiac arrhythmias, severe/frequent headaches, hypertension, suicidal tendencies.

LIFESPAN CONSIDERATIONS

Pregnancy/Lactation: Crosses placenta. Minimally distributed in breast milk. **Pregnancy Category C. Children:** Not recommended for children (increased risk of suicidal ideation). **Elderly:** Increased risk of drug toxicity may require dosage adjustment.

INTERACTIONS

DRUG: Alcohol, other CNS depressants may increase CNS depression. **Buspirone** may increase B/P. **Caffeine-containing medications** may increase risk of cardiac arrhythmias, hypertension. **Carbamazepine, cyclobenzaprine, maprotiline, other MAOIs** may precipitate hypertensive crisis. **Dopamine, tryptophan** may cause sudden, severe hypertension. **Fluoxetine, trazodone, tricyclic antidepressants** may cause serotonin syndrome. May increase effects of **insulin, oral antidiabetics. Meperidine, other opioid analgesics** may produce diaphoresis, immediate excitation, rigidity, severe hypertension/hypotension, sometimes leading to severe respiratory distress, vascular collapse, seizures, coma, death. May increase CNS stimulant effects of **methylphenidate. Sympathomimetics** may increase cardiac stimulant, vasopressor effects. **HERBAL:** None significant. **FOOD: Caffeine, chocolate, tyramine-containing foods** may cause sudden, severe hypertension. **LAB VALUES:** None significant.

AVAILABILITY (Rx)

Tablets: 15 mg.

ADMINISTRATION/HANDLING

PO

• Store tablets at room temperature. • Give with food, milk if GI distress occurs. • Tablets may be crushed.

INDICATIONS/ROUTES/DOSAGE

Depression

PO: ADULTS: 15 mg 3 times daily. May increase to 60–90 mg/day. **ELDERLY:** Initially, 7.5 mg/day. May increase by 7.5–15 mg/day q3–4days up to 60 mg/day in 3–4 divided doses.

SIDE EFFECTS

Frequent: Orthostatic hypotension, restlessness, GI upset, insomnia, dizziness, headache, lethargy, asthenia (loss of strength, energy), dry mouth, peripheral edema. **Occasional:** Flushing, diaphoresis, rash, urinary frequency, increased appetite, transient impotence. **Rare:** Visual disturbances.

ADVERSE EFFECTS/ TOXIC REACTIONS

Hypertensive crisis occurs rarely, marked by severe hypertension, occipital headache radiating frontally, neck stiffness/soreness, nausea, vomiting, diaphoresis, fever, chills, clammy skin, dilated pupils, palpitations, tachycardia or bradycardia, constricting chest pain. **Antidote for hypertensive crisis:** 5–10 mg phentolamine IV.

NURSING CONSIDERATIONS

BASELINE ASSESSMENT

Periodic hepatic function tests should be performed for pts requiring high dosage who are undergoing prolonged therapy.

INTERVENTION/EVALUATION

Assess appearance, behavior, speech pattern, level of interest, mood. Monitor for suicidal ideation, worsening depression. Monitor for occipital headache radiating frontally and/or neck stiffness/soreness (may be first signal of impending hypertensive crisis). Monitor B/P, heart rate, diet, weight.

PATIENT/FAMILY TEACHING

• Notify physician if depression worsens, suicidal ideation, or unusual changes in behavior occur. • Antidepressant relief may be noted during first wk of therapy; maximum benefit noted in 2–6 wks. • Report headache, neck stiffness/soreness immediately. • Avoid foods that require bacteria/molds for their preparation/preservation or those that contain tyramine (e.g., cheese, sour cream, beer, wine, figs, raisins, bananas, avocados, soy sauce, yeast extracts, yogurt, papaya, broad beans, meat tenderizers), excessive amounts of caffeine (coffee, tea, chocolate), OTC preparations for hay fever, colds, weight reduction.

Phenergan, *see promethazine*

phenobarbital

fee-noe-**bar**-bi-tal
(Luminal)
Do not confuse phenobarbital with pentobarbital.

FIXED-COMBINATION(S)

Bellergal-S: phenobarbital/ergotamine/belladonna (an anticholinergic): 40 mg/0.6 mg/0.2 mg. **Dilantin with PB:** phenobarbital/phenytoin (an anticonvulsant): 15 mg/100 mg, 30 mg/100 mg. **Donnatal:** phenobarbital/atropine (an anticholinergic)/hyoscyamine (an anticholinergic)/scopolamine (an anticholinergic): 16.2 mg/0.0194 mg/0.1037 mg/0.0065 mg.

◆CLASSIFICATION

PHARMACOTHERAPEUTIC: Barbiturate **(Schedule IV). CLINICAL:** Anticonvulsant, hypnotic (see p. 35C).

ACTION

Enhances activity of gamma-aminobutyric acid (GABA) by binding to GABA receptor complex. **Therapeutic Effect:** Depresses CNS activity.

PHARMACOKINETICS

Route	Onset	Peak	Duration
PO	20–60 min	N/A	6–10 hrs
IV	5 min	30 min	4–10 hrs

Well absorbed after PO, parenteral administration. Protein binding: 20%–45%. Rapidly and widely distributed. Metabolized in liver. Primarily excreted in urine. Removed by hemodialysis. **Half-life:** 53–140 hrs.

USES

Management of generalized tonic-clonic (grand mal) seizures, partial seizures,

P

control of acute seizure episodes (status epilepticus, eclampsia, febrile seizures). Used as sedative, hypnotic. **OFF-LABEL:** Prevention/treatment of febrile seizures in children, hyperbilirubinemia, management of sedative/hypnotic withdrawal.

PRECAUTIONS

Contraindications: Hypersensitivity to other barbiturates, porphyria, preexisting CNS depression, severe pain, severe respiratory disease. **Cautions:** Renal/hepatic impairment.

LIFESPAN CONSIDERATIONS

Pregnancy/Lactation: Readily crosses placenta. Distributed in breast milk. Produces respiratory depression in neonates during labor. May cause postpartum hemorrhage, hemorrhagic disease in newborn. Withdrawal symptoms may appear in neonates born to women receiving barbiturates during last trimester of pregnancy. Lowers serum bilirubin in neonates. **Pregnancy Category D. Children:** May cause paradoxical excitement. **Elderly:** May exhibit excitement, confusion, mental depression.

P

INTERACTIONS

DRUG: **Alcohol, other CNS depressants** may increase effects. May increase metabolism of **carbamazepine.** May decrease effects of **metronidazole, oral anticoagulants, quinidine. Valproic acid** increases concentration, risk of toxicity. **HERBAL:** **Evening primrose** may decrease seizure threshold. **Gotu kola, kava kava, St. John's wort, valerian** may increase CNS depression. **FOOD:** None known. **LAB VALUES:** May decrease serum bilirubin. **Therapeutic serum level:** 10–40 mcg/ml; **toxic serum level:** greater than 40 mcg/ml.

AVAILABILITY (Rx)

Elixir: 20 mg/5 ml. **Injection, Solution:** 65 mg/ml, 130 mg/ml. **Tablets:** 15 mg, 30 mg, 60 mg, 100 mg.

ADMINISTRATION/HANDLING

IV

Reconstitution • May give undiluted or may dilute with NaCl, D_5W, lactated Ringer's.

Rate of administration • Adequately hydrate pt before and immediately after drug therapy (decreases risk of adverse renal effects). • Do not inject IV faster than 1 mg/kg/min and maximum of 30 mg/min for children and 60 mg/min for adults. Too-rapid IV may produce severe hypotension, marked respiratory depression. • Inadvertent intra-arterial injection may result in arterial spasm with severe pain, tissue necrosis. Extravasation in subcutaneous tissue may produce redness, tenderness, tissue necrosis. If this occurs, treat with 0.5% procaine solution into affected area, apply moist heat.

Storage • Store vials at room temperature.

IM

• Do not inject more than 5 ml in any one IM injection site (produces tissue irritation). • Inject deep IM into large muscle mass.

PO

• Give without regard to meals. • Tablets may be crushed. • Elixir may be mixed with water, milk, fruit juice.

IV INCOMPATIBILITIES

Amphotericin B complex (Abelcet, AmBisome, Amphotec), hydrocortisone (Solu-Cortef), hydromorphone (Dilaudid), insulin, lipids.

IV COMPATIBILITIES

Calcium gluconate, enalapril (Vasotec), fentanyl (Sublimaze), fosphenytoin (Cerebyx), morphine, propofol (Diprivan).

INDICATIONS/ROUTES/DOSAGE

Status Epilepticus

IV: ADULTS, ELDERLY: 10–20 mg/kg. May repeat dose in 20-min intervals. **Maximum total dose:** 30 mg/kg. **CHILDREN,**

INFANTS: 15–20 mg/kg (**maximum:** 1,000 mg). May repeat q15–30min until seizures controlled or total dose of 40 mg/kg administered.

Seizure Control

PO, IV: ADULTS, ELDERLY, CHILDREN OLDER THAN 12 YRS: 1–3 mg/kg/day or 50–100 mg 2–3 times daily. **CHILDREN 6–12 YRS:** 4–6 mg/kg/day. **CHILDREN 1–5 YRS:** 6–8 mg/kg/day. **CHILDREN YOUNGER THAN 1 YR:** 5–6 mg/kg/day. **NEONATES:** 3–4 mg/kg/day.

Sedation

PO, IM: ADULTS, ELDERLY: 30–120 mg/day in 2–3 divided doses. **CHILDREN:** 2 mg/kg 3 times daily.

Hypnotic

PO, IV, IM, SUBCUTANEOUS: ADULTS, ELDERLY: 100–320 mg at bedtime. **CHILDREN:** 3–5 mg/kg at bedtime.

SIDE EFFECTS

Occasional (3%–1%): Drowsiness. **Rare** (less than 1%): Confusion, paradoxical CNS reactions (hyperactivity, anxiety in children; excitement, restlessness in elderly, generally noted during first 2 wks of therapy, particularly in presence of uncontrolled pain).

ADVERSE EFFECTS/ TOXIC REACTIONS

Abrupt withdrawal after prolonged therapy may produce increased dreaming, nightmares, insomnia, tremor, diaphoresis, vomiting, hallucinations, delirium, seizures, status epilepticus. Skin eruptions appear as hypersensitivity reaction. Blood dyscrasias, hepatic disease, hypocalcemia occur rarely. Overdose produces cold/clammy skin, hypothermia, severe CNS depression, cyanosis, tachycardia, Cheyne-Stokes respirations. Toxicity may result in severe renal impairment.

NURSING CONSIDERATIONS

BASELINE ASSESSMENT

Assess B/P, pulse, respirations immediately before administration. **Hypnotic:** Raise bed rails, provide environment conducive to sleep (back rub, quiet environment, low lighting). **Seizures:** Review history of seizure disorder (length, presence of auras, LOC). Observe frequently for recurrence of seizure activity. Initiate seizure precautions.

INTERVENTION/EVALUATION

Monitor CNS status, seizure activity, hepatic/renal function, respiratory rate, heart rate, B/P. Monitor for therapeutic serum level. **Therapeutic serum level:** 10–40 mcg/ml; **toxic serum level:** greater than 40 mcg/ml.

PATIENT/FAMILY TEACHING

• Avoid alcohol, limit caffeine. • May be habit forming. • Do not discontinue abruptly. • May cause dizziness/drowsiness; impair ability to perform tasks requiring mental alertness, coordination.

phentolamine

fen-**toll**-ah-meen
(OraVerse, Regitine ✦, Rogitine ✦)
Do not confuse phentolamine with phentermine.

CLASSIFICATION

PHARMACOTHERAPEUTIC: Alpha-adrenergic blocking agent. **CLINICAL:** Pheochromocytoma agent.

ACTION

Blocks presynaptic ($alpha_2$), postsynaptic ($alpha_1$) adrenergic receptors, acting on arterial tree, venous bed. **Therapeutic Effect:** Decreases total peripheral resistance, diminishes venous return to heart.

PHARMACOKINETICS

Onset	Peak	Duration
IM 15–20 min	20 min	30–45 min
IV Immediate	2 min	15–30 min

P

Metabolized in liver. Excreted in urine. Half-life: 19 min.

USES

Diagnosis of pheochromocytoma. Control/prevention of hypertensive episodes immediately before, during surgical excision. Prevention/treatment of dermal necrosis, sloughing after IV administration of alpha-adrenergic drugs (e.g., norepinephrine/dopamine). **OFF-LABEL**: Pralidoxime-induced hypertension.

PRECAUTIONS

Contraindications: Epinephrine, MI, coronary insufficiency, angina, coronary artery disease. **Cautions**: Gastritis, peptic ulcer, history of arrhythmias.

LIFESPAN CONSIDERATIONS

Pregnancy/Lactation: Unknown if drug crosses placenta or is distributed in breast milk. **Pregnancy Category C. Children**: Safety and efficacy not established. **Elderly**: No age-related precautions noted.

INTERACTIONS

DRUG: May decrease effects of **sympathomimetics (e.g., dopamine, phenylephrine)** when given with phentolamine. **HERBAL**: None significant. **FOOD**: None known. **LAB VALUES**: None significant.

AVAILABILITY (Rx)

Injection, Powder for Reconstitution: 5-mg vials. **Injection Solution (OraVerse)**: 0.4 mg/1.7 ml.

ADMINISTRATION/HANDLING

◀ALERT▶ Maintain pt in supine position (preferably in quiet, darkened room) during pheochromocytoma testing. Decrease in B/P generally noted in less than 2 min.

IV

Reconstitution • Reconstitute 5-mg vial with 1 ml Sterile Water for Injection to provide concentration of 5 mg/ml.

Rate of administration • Pheochromocytoma: Inject each 5 mg over 1 min. Monitor B/P immediately after injection, q30sec for 3 min, then q60sec for 7 min.

Storage • Store vials at room temperature. • After reconstitution, stable for 48 hrs at room temperature or 1 wk if refrigerated.

IV INCOMPATIBILITIES

None known.

IV COMPATIBILITIES

Amiodarone (Cordarone), dobutamine (Dobutrex), verapamil (Calan), papaverine.

INDICATIONS/ROUTES/DOSAGE

Diagnosis of Pheochromocytoma

IM, IV: ADULTS, ELDERLY: 2.5–5 mg. **CHILDREN**: 0.05–0.1 mg/kg/dose. **Maximum:** 5 mg.

Control/Prevention of Hypertension in Pheochromocytoma

IV: ADULTS, ELDERLY: 5 mg 1–2 hrs before surgery. May repeat q2–4h. **CHILDREN**: 0.05–0.1 mg/kg/dose 1–2 hrs before surgery. May repeat q2–4h. **Maximum single dose:** 5 mg.

Prevention/Treatment of Tissue Necrosis/Sloughing

ADULTS, ELDERLY: Infiltrate area with 1 ml of solution (reconstituted by diluting 5–10 mg in 0.9% NaCl) within 12 hrs of extravasation. Infiltrate with multiple small injections using only 27- or 30-gauge needles; change needles between each skin entry. **Maximum:** 0.1–0.2 mg/kg or 5 mg total. **CHILDREN**: 0.1–0.2 mg/kg diluted in 10 ml 0.9% NaCl infiltrated into area of extravasation within 12 hrs. If dose is effective, normal skin color should return within 1 hr.

SIDE EFFECTS

Occasional (3%–2%): Weakness, dizziness, flushing, nausea, vomiting, diarrhea, orthostatic hypotension.

ADVERSE EFFECTS/ TOXIC REACTIONS

Tachycardia, arrhythmias, acute/prolonged hypotension may occur. Do not use epinephrine (will produce further drop in B/P).

NURSING CONSIDERATIONS

BASELINE ASSESSMENT

Positive pheochromocytoma test indicated by decrease in B/P greater than 35 mm Hg systolic, greater than 25 mm Hg diastolic pressure. Negative test indicated by no change in B/P or elevation of B/P. B/P generally returns to baseline within 15–30 min following administration.

INTERVENTION/EVALUATION

Monitor B/P, heart rate. Assess for orthostatic hypotension. Monitor for extravasation (skin color streaking).

phenylephrine HIGH ALERT

fen-il-**ef**-rin
(AK-Dilate, Mydfrin, Neo-Synephrine, Sudafed PE)

BLACK BOX ALERT Intravenous use should be administered by adequately trained individuals familiar with its use.

Do not confuse Mydrin with Midrin or Sudafed PE with Sudafed.

◆CLASSIFICATION

PHARMACOTHERAPEUTIC: Sympathomimetic, alpha-receptor stimulant. **CLINICAL:** Nasal decongestant, mydriatic, vasopressor (see p. 158C).

ACTION

Acts on alpha-adrenergic receptors of vascular smooth muscle. Causes vasoconstriction of arterioles of nasal mucosa/conjunctiva, activates dilator muscle of pupil, causing contraction, producing systemic arterial vasoconstriction. **Therapeutic Effect:** Decreases mucosal blood flow, relieves congestion. Increases systolic B/P.

PHARMACOKINETICS

Route	Onset	Peak	Duration
IV	Immediate	N/A	15–20 min
IM	10–15 min	N/A	0.5–2 hrs
Subcutaneous	10–15 min	N/A	1 hr

Minimal absorption after intranasal, ophthalmic administration. Metabolized in liver, GI tract. Primarily excreted in urine. **Half-life:** 2.5 hrs.

USES

Nasal decongestant: Topical application to nasal mucosa reduces nasal secretion, promoting drainage of sinus secretions. **Ophthalmic:** Topical application to conjunctiva relieves congestion, itching, minor irritation; whitens sclera of eye. **Parenteral:** Vascular failure in shock, drug-induced hypotension. **Rectal:** Treatment of hemorrhoids.

PRECAUTIONS

Contraindications: Acute pancreatitis, heart disease, hepatitis, narrow-angle glaucoma, pheochromocytoma, severe hypertension, thrombosis, ventricular tachycardia. **Cautions:** Hyperthyroidism, bradycardia, heart block, severe arteriosclerosis.

LIFESPAN CONSIDERATIONS

Pregnancy/Lactation: Crosses placenta. Distributed in breast milk. **Pregnancy Category C. Children:** May exhibit increased absorption, toxicity with nasal preparation. No age-related precautions noted with systemic use. **Elderly:** More likely to experience adverse effects.

INTERACTIONS

DRUG: **Beta-blockers** may have mutually inhibitory effects. **Digoxin** may increase risk of arrhythmias. **Ergonovine, oxytocin** may increase vasoconstriction. **MAOIs** may increase vasopressor effects. **Mapro-**

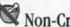

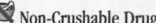

P

tiline, tricyclic antidepressants may increase cardiovascular effects. May decrease effects of **methyldopa.** HERBAL: **Ephedra, yohimbe** may increase CNS stimulation. FOOD: None known. LAB VALUES: None significant.

AVAILABILITY (OTC)

Injection, Solution: 1% (10 mg/ml). **Solution, Nasal Drops: (Neo-Synephrine):** 0.125%, 0.5%, 1%. **Solution, Nasal Spray: (Neo-Synephrine):** 0.25%, 0.5%, 1%. **Solution, Ophthalmic: (AK-Dilate, Mydfrin, Neo-Synephrine):** 0.12%, 2.5%, 10%. **Tablets: (Sudafed PE):** 10 mg.

ADMINISTRATION/HANDLING

IV

Reconstitution • For IV push, dilute 1 ml of 10 mg/ml solution with 9 ml Sterile Water for Injection to provide concentration of 1 mg/ml. • For IV infusion, dilute with 0.9% NaCl or D_5W. Usual concentration: 20–60 mcg/ml.
Rate of administration • For IV push, give over 20–30 sec. • For IV infusion, give as per physician order.
Storage • Store vials at room temperature.

P

Nasal

• Instruct pt to blow nose prior to administering medication. • With head tilted back, apply drops in 1 nostril. Wait 5 min before applying drops in other nostril. • Sprays should be administered into each nostril with head erect. • Pt should sniff briskly while squeezing container, then wait 3–5 min before blowing nose gently. • Rinse tip of spray bottle.

Ophthalmic

• Instruct pt to tilt head backward, look up. • Gently pull lower lid down to form pouch, then instill medication. • Do not touch tip of applicator to lids or any surface. • When lower lid is released, have pt keep eye open without blinking for at least 30 sec. • Apply gentle finger pressure to lacrimal sac (bridge of nose, inside corner of eye) for 1–2 min. • Remove excess solution around eye with tissue. • Wash hands immediately to remove medication on hands.

IV INCOMPATIBILITY

Thiopentothal (Pentothal).

IV COMPATIBILITIES

Amiodarone (Cordarone), dobutamine (Dobutrex), lidocaine, potassium chloride, propofol (Diprivan).

INDICATIONS/ROUTES/DOSAGE

Nasal Decongestant

INTRANASAL: ADULTS, ELDERLY, CHILDREN 12 YRS AND OLDER: 1–2 drops or 1–2 sprays of 0.25%–0.5% solution into each nostril q4h as needed. **CHILDREN 6–11 YRS:** 1–2 drops or 1–2 sprays of 0.25% solution into each nostril q4h as needed. **CHILDREN 2–5 YRS:** 1 drop of 0.125% solution (dilute 0.5% solution with 0.9% NaCl to achieve 0.125%) in each nostril. Repeat q2–4h as needed. Do not use for more than 3 days.
PO: ADULTS, ELDERLY, CHILDREN 13 YRS AND OLDER: (SUDAFED PE): 10–20 mg q12h. **CHILDREN 6–12 YRS: (SUDAFED PE):** 5–10 mg q12h.

Conjunctival Congestion, Itching, Minor Irritation

OPHTHALMIC: ADULTS, ELDERLY, CHILDREN 12 YRS AND OLDER: 1–2 drops of 0.12% solution q3–4h.

Hypotension, Shock

IV BOLUS: ADULTS, ELDERLY: 0.1–0.5 mg/dose q10–15min as needed. **CHILDREN:** 5–20 mcg/kg/dose q10–15min.
IV INFUSION: ADULTS, ELDERLY: 100–180 mcg/min. When B/P is stabilized, maintenance rate: 40–60 mcg/min. **CHILDREN:** 0.1–0.5 mcg/kg/min. Titrate to desired effect.

SIDE EFFECTS

Frequent: Nasal: Rebound nasal congestion due to overuse, esp. when used longer than 3 days. **Occasional:** Mild CNS stimulation (restlessness, nervousness, tremors, headache, insomnia, particularly in those hypersensitive to sympathomimetics, such as elderly pts). **Nasal:** Stinging, burning, drying of nasal mucosa. **Ophthalmic:** Transient burning/stinging, brow ache, blurred vision.

ADVERSE EFFECTS/ TOXIC REACTIONS

Large doses may produce tachycardia, palpitations (particularly in those with cardiac disease), light-headedness, nausea, vomiting. Overdose in those older than 60 yrs may result in hallucinations, CNS depression, seizures. Prolonged nasal use may produce chronic swelling of nasal mucosa, rhinitis.

NURSING CONSIDERATIONS

BASELINE ASSESSMENT

If phenylephine 10% ophthalmic is instilled into denuded/damaged corneal epithelium, corneal clouding may result.

INTERVENTION/EVALUATION

Monitor B/P, heart rate. For severe hypotension or shock states, monitor arterial blood gas, central venous pressure.

PATIENT/FAMILY TEACHING

• Discontinue drug if adverse reactions occur. • Do not use for nasal decongestion for longer than 5 days (rebound congestion). • Discontinue drug if insomnia, dizziness, weakness, tremor, palpitations occur. • **Nasal:** Stinging/burning of nasal mucosa may occur. • **Ophthalmic:** Blurring of vision with eye instillation generally subsides with continued therapy. • Discontinue medication if redness/swelling of eyelids, itching occurs.

phenytoin

phen-ih-toyn
(Dilantin, Phenytek)
Do not confuse Dilantin with Dilaudid or diltiazem, or phenytoin with phenelzine.

◆CLASSIFICATION

PHARMACOTHERAPEUTIC: Hydantoin. **CLINICAL:** Anticonvulsant, antiarrhythmic (see p. 35C).

ACTION

Anticonvulsant: Stabilizes neuronal membranes in motor cortex. **Therapeutic Effect:** Limits spread of seizure activity. Stabilizes threshold against hyperexcitability. Decreases post-tetanic potentiation, repetitive discharge.

PHARMACOKINETICS

Slowly, variably absorbed after PO administration. Protein binding: 90%–95%. Widely distributed. Metabolized in liver. Primarily excreted in urine. Not removed by hemodialysis. **Half-life:** 7–42 hrs.

USES

Management of generalized tonic-clonic seizures (grand mal), complex partial seizures (psychomotor), cortical focal seizures, status epilepticus. **OFF-LABEL:** Adjunctive treatment of tricyclic antidepressant toxicity; treatment of muscle hyperirritability, digoxin-induced arrhythmias, trigeminal neuralgia.

PRECAUTIONS

Contraindications: Hypersensitivity to hydantoins, seizures due to hypoglycemia. **IV:** Adam-Stokes syndrome, second- and third-degree AV block, sinoatrial block, sinus bradycardia. **EXTREME CAUTION: IV Route Only:** Respiratory depression, MI, CHF, damaged myocardium. **Cautions:** Hepatic/renal impairment, severe myocardial insufficiency, hypotension, hyperglycemia. Increased risk of suicidal behavior/thoughts.

⌛ LIFESPAN CONSIDERATIONS

Pregnancy/Lactation: Crosses placenta; distributed in small amount in breast milk. Fetal hydantoin syndrome (craniofacial abnormalities, nail/digital hypoplasia, prenatal growth deficiency) has been reported.

P

Increased frequency of seizures in pregnant women due to altered absorption of metabolism of phenytoin. May increase risk of hemorrhage in neonate, maternal bleeding during delivery. **Pregnancy Category D. Children:** More susceptible to gingival hyperplasia, coarsening of facial hair; excess body hair. **Elderly:** No age-related precautions noted but lower dosages recommended.

INTERACTIONS

DRUG: **Alcohol, other CNS depressants** may increase CNS depression. **Amiodarone, anticoagulants, cimetidine, disulfiram, fluoxetine, isoniazid, sulfonamides** may increase concentration, effects, risk of toxicity. **Antacids** may decrease absorption. **Fluconazole, ketoconazole, miconazole** may increase concentration. May decrease effects of **glucocorticoids. Lidocaine, propranolol** may increase cardiac depressant effects. **Valproic acid** may decrease metabolism, increase concentration. May increase metabolism of **xanthines.** HERBAL: **Evening primrose** may decrease seizure threshold. **Gotu kola, kava kava, St. John's wort, valerian** may increase CNS depression. FOOD: None known. LAB VALUES: May increase serum glucose, GGT, alkaline phosphatase. **Therapeutic serum level:** 10–20 mcg/ml; **toxic serum level:** greater than 20 mcg/ml.

AVAILABILITY (Rx)

Capsules, Extended-Release: (Dilantin): 30 mg, 100 mg. **(Phenytek):** 200 mg, 300 mg. **Capsules, Prompt-Release: (Dilantin):** 100 mg. **Injection, Solution: (Dilantin):** 50 mg/ml. **Suspension, Oral: (Dilantin):** 100 mg/4 ml, 125 mg/5 ml. **Tablets, Chewable: (Dilantin):** 50 mg.

ADMINISTRATION/HANDLING

IV

◀ALERT▶ Give by IV push or IV piggyback. IV push very painful (chemical irritation of vein due to alkalinity of solution). To minimize effect, flush vein with sterile saline solution through same IV needle and catheter after each IV push.

Reconstitution • May give undiluted or may dilute with 0.9% NaCl.

Rate of administration • Administer 50 mg over 2–3 min for elderly. In neonates, administer at rate not exceeding 1–3 mg/kg/min. • Severe hypotension, cardiovascular collapse occurs if rate of IV injection exceeds 50 mg/min for adults. • IV toxicity characterized by CNS depression, cardiovascular collapse.

Storage • Precipitate may form if parenteral form is refrigerated (will dissolve at room temperature). • Slight yellow discoloration of parenteral form does not affect potency, but do not use if solution is cloudy or precipitate forms.

PO

• Give with food if GI distress occurs. • Tablets may be chewed. • Shake oral suspension well before using.

IV INCOMPATIBILITIES

Diltiazem (Cardizem), dobutamine (Dobutrex), enalapril (Vasotec), heparin, hydromorphone (Dilaudid), insulin, lidocaine, morphine, nitroglycerin, norepinephrine (Levophed), potassium chloride, propofol (Diprivan).

INDICATIONS/ROUTES/DOSAGE

Status Epilepticus

IV: ADULTS, ELDERLY, CHILDREN: Loading dose: 15–20 mg/kg. Maintenance dose: 300 mg/day or 4–6 mg/kg/day in 2–3 divided doses for adults and elderly; 6–7 mg/kg/day for children 10–16 yrs; 7–8 mg/kg/day for children 7–9 yrs; 7.5–9 mg/kg/day for children 4–6 yrs; 8–10 mg/kg/day for children 6 mos–3 yrs. **NEONATES:** Loading dose: 15–20 mg/kg. Maintenance dose: 5–8 mg/kg/day.

Seizure Control

PO: ADULTS, ELDERLY, CHILDREN: Loading dose: 15–20 mg/kg in 3 divided doses 2–4 hrs apart. Maintenance dose: Same as for status epilepticus.

SIDE EFFECTS

Frequent: Drowsiness, lethargy, confusion, slurred speech, irritability, gingival hyperplasia, hypersensitivity reaction (fever, rash, lymphadenopathy), constipation, dizziness, nausea. **Occasional:** Headache, hirsutism, coarsening of facial features, insomnia, muscle twitching.

ADVERSE EFFECTS/ TOXIC REACTIONS

Abrupt withdrawal may precipitate status epilepticus. Blood dyscrasias, lymphadenopathy, osteomalacia (due to interference of vitamin D metabolism) may occur. Toxic phenytoin blood concentration (25 mcg/ml or more) may produce ataxia (muscular incoordination), nystagmus (rhythmic oscillation of eyes), diplopia. As level increases, extreme lethargy to comatose state occurs.

NURSING CONSIDERATIONS

BASELINE ASSESSMENT

Anticonvulsant: Review history of seizure disorder (intensity, frequency, duration, LOC). Initiate seizure precautions. Hepatic function tests, CBC, platelet count should be performed before beginning therapy and periodically during therapy. Repeat CBC, platelet count 2 wks following initiation of therapy and 2 wks following administration of maintenance dose.

INTERVENTION/EVALUATION

Observe frequently for recurrence of seizure activity. Assess for clinical improvement (decrease in intensity/frequency of seizures). Monitor for signs/symptoms of depression, suicidal tendencies, unusual behavior. Monitor CBC with differential, hepatic/renal function tests, B/P (with IV use). Assist with ambulation if drowsiness, lethargy occurs. Monitor for therapeutic serum level (10–20 mcg/ml). **Therapeutic serum level:** 10–20 mcg/ml; **toxic serum level:** greater than 20 mcg/ml.

PATIENT/FAMILY TEACHING

• Pain may occur with IV injection. • To prevent gingival hyperplasia (bleeding, tenderness, swelling of gums), maintain good oral hygiene, gum massage, regular dental visits. • CBC should be performed every mo for 1 yr after maintenance dose is established and q3mo thereafter. • Report sore throat, fever, glandular swelling, skin reaction (hematologic toxicity). • Drowsiness usually diminishes with continued therapy. • Avoid tasks that require alertness, motor skills until response to drug is established. • Do not abruptly withdraw medication after long-term use (may precipitate seizures). • Strict maintenance of drug therapy is essential for seizure control, arrhythmias. • Avoid alcohol. • Report any unusual changes in behavior.

PhosLo, *see calcium acetate*

phosphates

fos-fates
(Fleet Enema, Fleet Phospho-Soda, K-Phos MF, K-Phos Neutral, Neutra-Phos, Neutra-Phos-K, Uro-KP-Neutral)

◆ CLASSIFICATION

PHARMACOTHERAPEUTIC: Electrolyte. **CLINICAL:** Mineral.

ACTION

Active in bone deposition, calcium metabolism, utilization of B complex vitamins. Acts as buffers in maintaining acid-base balance. Exerts osmotic effect in small intestine. **Therapeutic Effect:** Corrects hypophosphatemia, acidifies urine, prevents calcium deposits in urinary tract, promotes peristalsis in GI tract.

P

PHARMACOKINETICS

Poorly absorbed after PO administration. PO form excreted in feces; IV form excreted in urine.

USES

Prophylactic treatment of hypophosphatemia. Short-term treatment of constipation, for evacuation of colon for exams; urinary acidifier for reduction of formation of calcium stones. OFF-LABEL: Prevention of calcium renal calculi.

PRECAUTIONS

Contraindications: Abdominal pain, fecal impaction (rectal dosage form), ascitic conditions, CHF, hyperkalemia, hypernatremia, hyperphosphatemia, hypocalcemia, hypomagnesemia, paralytic ileus, phosphate renal calculi, severe renal impairment. Cautions: Renal impairment, concomitant use of potassium-sparing drugs, adrenal insufficiency, cirrhosis.

LIFESPAN CONSIDERATIONS

Pregnancy/Lactation: Unknown if drug crosses placenta or is distributed in breast milk. **Pregnancy Category C. Children:** Increased risk of dehydration in those younger than 12 yrs. **Elderly:** No age-related precautions noted.

INTERACTIONS

DRUG: **ACE inhibitors, NSAIDs, potassium-containing medications, potassium-sparing diuretics, salt substitutes containing potassium phosphate** may increase serum potassium. **Antacids** may decrease absorption. **Calcium-containing medications** may increase risk of calcium deposition in soft tissues, decrease phosphate absorption. **Digoxin** may increase risk of heart block caused by hyperkalemia when given with potassium phosphates. **Glucocorticoids** may cause edema when given with sodium phosphate. **Phosphate-containing medications** may increase risk of hyperphosphatemia. **Sodium-containing medications** may increase risk of edema when given with sodium phosphate. HERBAL: None significant. FOOD: None known. LAB VALUES: None significant.

AVAILABILITY (Rx)

Enema (Fleet Enema): 2.25 oz, 4.5 oz. Injection Solution (Potassium Phosphate): 3 mmol phosphate and 4.4 mEq potassium per ml. Injection Solution (Sodium Phosphate): 3 mmol phosphate and 4 mEq sodium per ml. Oral Solution (Fleet Phospho-Soda): 4 mmol phosphate per ml. Powder (Neutra-Phos, Neutra-Phos-K): 250 mg (8 mmol) phosphate. Tablets: 125 mg (4 mmol) phosphate, 250 mg (8 mmol) phosphate (K-Phos MF, K-Phos Neutral, Uro-KP-Neutral).

ADMINISTRATION/HANDLING

IV

Reconstitution • Must be diluted. Soluble in all commonly used IV solutions.
Rate of administration • Infuse over minimum of 4 hrs.
Storage • Store at room temperature.

PO

• Dissolve tablets in water. • Take after meals or with food (decreases GI upset). • Maintain high fluid intake (prevents kidney stones).

Rectal

• Instruct pt to lie in left lateral Sims position. • Insert tube pointing toward navel. • Slowly squeeze and empty contents into rectum. • Pt to remain in Sims position until defecation impulse felt (usually 2–5 min).

IV INCOMPATIBILITY

Dobutamine (Dobutrex).

IV COMPATIBILITIES

Diltiazem (Cardizem), enalapril (Vasotec), famotidine (Pepcid), magnesium sulfate, metoclopramide (Reglan).

P

INDICATIONS/ROUTES/DOSAGE

Hypophosphatemia

PO (NEUTRA-PHOS, NEUTRA-PHOS-K, K-PHOS MF, K-PHOS NEUTRAL, URO-KP-NEUTRAL): ADULTS, ELDERLY: 50–150 mmol/day. **CHILDREN:** 2–3 mmol/kg/day.

IV: ADULTS, ELDERLY: 50–70 mmol/day. **CHILDREN:** 0.5–1.5 mmol/kg/day.

Laxative

PO (NEUTRA-PHOS, NEUTRA-PHOS-K, URO-KP-NEUTRAL): ADULTS, ELDERLY, CHILDREN 4 YRS AND OLDER: 1–2 capsules/packets 4 times daily. **CHILDREN YOUNGER THAN 4 YRS:** 1 capsule/packet 4 times daily.

RECTAL: ADULTS, ELDERLY, CHILDREN 12 YRS AND OLDER: 4.5-oz enema as single dose. May repeat. **CHILDREN YOUNGER THAN 12 YRS:** 2.25-oz enema as single dose. May repeat.

Urine Acidification

PO: ADULTS, ELDERLY: 8 mmol 4 times daily.

SIDE EFFECTS

Frequent: Mild laxative effect (in first few days of therapy). **Occasional:** Diarrhea, nausea, abdominal pain, vomiting. **Rare:** Headache, dizziness, confusion, heaviness of lower extremities, fatigue, muscle cramps, paresthesia, peripheral edema, arrhythmias, weight gain, thirst.

ADVERSE EFFECTS/ TOXIC REACTIONS

Hyperphosphatemia may produce extraskeletal calcification.

NURSING CONSIDERATIONS

INTERVENTION/EVALUATION

Routinely monitor serum calcium, phosphorus, potassium, sodium, AST, ALT, alkaline phosphatase, bilirubin.

PATIENT/FAMILY TEACHING

- Report diarrhea, nausea, vomiting.

pimecrolimus

pim-eh-**crow**-leh-mus
(Elidel)

BLACK BOX ALERT Rare cases of lymphoma, skin malignancy have occurred. Use only for short-term, intermittent treatment using minimum amount needed. Not recommended in children younger than 2 yrs.

Do not confuse Elidel with Elavil, or pimecrolimus with tacrolimus.

◆CLASSIFICATION

PHARMACOTHERAPEUTIC: Immunomodulator. **CLINICAL:** Anti-inflammatory.

ACTION

Inhibits release of cytokine, an enzyme that produces an inflammatory reaction. **Therapeutic Effect:** Produces anti-inflammatory activity.

USES

Treatment of mild to moderate atopic dermatitis (eczema).

PRECAUTIONS

Contraindications: None known. **Cautions:** Potential cancer risk.

LIFESPAN CONSIDERATIONS

Pregnancy/Lactation: Embryotoxic. Unknown if distributed in breast milk. **Pregnancy Category C. Children:** May be used in those 2 yrs and older. **Elderly:** No age-related precautions noted.

INTERACTIONS

DRUG: None significant. **HERBAL:** None significant. **FOOD:** None known. **LAB VALUES:** None significant.

AVAILABILITY (Rx)

Topical: 1% cream.

INDICATIONS/ROUTES/DOSAGE

Atopic Dermatitis (Eczema)

TOPICAL: ADULTS, ELDERLY, CHILDREN 2–17 YRS: Apply to affected area twice daily. Rub in gently, completely. Reevaluate if symptoms persist for more than 6 wks.

SIDE EFFECTS

Rare: Transient sensation of burning/feeling of heat at application site.

ADVERSE EFFECTS/ TOXIC REACTIONS

Lymphadenopathy, phototoxicity occur rarely.

NURSING CONSIDERATIONS

PATIENT/FAMILY TEACHING

• Wash hands after application. • May cause mild to moderate feeling of warmth, sensation of burning at application site. • Inform physician if application site reaction is severe or lasts for longer than 1 wk. • Avoid exposure to sunlight, artificial sunlight, tanning beds. • Contact physician if no improvement in atopic dermatitis is seen following 6 wks of treatment or if condition worsens.

P

pioglitazone

HIGH ALERT

pie-oh-**glit**-ah-zone
(Actos, Apo-Pioglitazone ✦, Novo-Pioglitazone ✦)

BLACK BOX ALERT May cause or exacerbate CHF.

Do not confuse Actos with Actonel.

FIXED-COMBINATION(S)

Actoplus Met: pioglitazone/metformin (an antidiabetic): 15 mg/500 mg, 15 mg/850 mg. **Duetact:** pioglitazone/glimepiride (an antidiabetic): 30 mg/2 mg, 30 mg/4 mg.

◆CLASSIFICATION

CLINICAL: Antidiabetic (see p. 44C).

ACTION

Improves target-cell response to insulin without increasing pancreatic insulin secretion. Decreases hepatic glucose output, increases insulin-dependent glucose utilization in skeletal muscle. **Therapeutic Effect:** Lowers serum glucose concentration.

PHARMACOKINETICS

Rapidly absorbed. Highly protein bound (99%), primarily to albumin. Metabolized in liver. Excreted in urine. Unknown if removed by hemodialysis. **Half-life:** 16–24 hrs.

USES

Adjunct to diet, exercise to lower serum glucose in those with type 2 non–insulin-dependent diabetes mellitus (NIDDM). Used as monotherapy or in combination with sulfonylurea, metformin, or insulin to improve glycemic control. **OFF-LABEL:** Polycystic ovary syndrome.

PRECAUTIONS

Contraindications: Active hepatic disease; diabetic ketoacidosis; increased serum transaminase, including ALT greater than 2.5 times normal serum level; type 1 diabetes mellitus; heart failure. **Cautions:** Hepatic impairment, edematous pts.

⧗ LIFESPAN CONSIDERATIONS

Pregnancy/Lactation: Unknown if drug crosses placenta or is distributed in breast milk. Not recommended in pregnant or breast-feeding women. **Pregnancy Category C. Children:** Safety and efficacy not established. **Elderly:** No age-related precautions noted.

INTERACTIONS

DRUG: Ketoconazole may significantly inhibit metabolism. May alter effects of **oral contraceptives. HERBAL: St. John's wort** may decrease concentration. **Garlic** may cause hypoglycemia. **FOOD:** None known. **LAB VALUES:** May increase serum creatine kinase (CK). May decrease Hgb (by 2%–4%), serum alkaline phosphatase, bilirubin, ALT. Less than 1% of pts experience ALT values 3 times the normal level.

AVAILABILITY (Rx)

Tablets: 15 mg, 30 mg, 45 mg.

ADMINISTRATION/HANDLING

PO

• Give without regard to meals.

INDICATIONS/ROUTES/DOSAGE

Diabetes Mellitus, Combination Therapy

PO: ADULTS, ELDERLY: With insulin: Initially, 15–30 mg once a day. Initially, continue current insulin dosage, then decrease insulin dosage by 10%–25% if hypoglycemia occurs or plasma glucose level decreases to less than 100 mg/dl. **Maximum:** 45 mg/day. **With sulfonylureas:** Initially, 15–30 mg/day. Decrease sulfonylurea dosage if hypoglycemia occurs. **With metformin:** Initially, 15–30 mg/day.

Monotherapy

Monotherapy is not to be used if pt is well controlled with diet and exercise alone. Initially, 15–30 mg/day. May increase dosage in increments until 45 mg/day is reached.

Dosage Adjustment in CHF

PO: ADULTS, ELDERLY: Initially, 15 mg once a day. May increase after several mos of treatment.

SIDE EFFECTS

Frequent (13%–9%): Headache, upper respiratory tract infection. Occasional (6%–5%): Sinusitis, myalgia, pharyngitis, aggravated diabetes mellitus.

ADVERSE EFFECTS/ TOXIC REACTIONS

Hepatotoxicity occurs rarely. May cause/worsen macular edema. Increased risk of CHF. May increase risk of fractures. Pts with ischemic heart disease are at high risk of MI.

NURSING CONSIDERATIONS

BASELINE ASSESSMENT

Obtain hepatic enzyme levels before initiating therapy and periodically thereafter. Ensure follow-up instruction if pt, family do not thoroughly understand diabetes management, glucose-testing technique.

INTERVENTION/EVALUATION

Monitor serum glucose, Hgb A_{1c}, hepatic function tests, esp. AST, ALT. Assess for hypoglycemia (cool/wet skin, tremors, dizziness, anxiety, headache, tachycardia, numbness in mouth, hunger, diplopia), hyperglycemia (polyuria, polyphagia, polydipsia, nausea, vomiting, dim vision, fatigue, deep rapid breathing). Be alert to conditions that alter serum glucose requirements: fever, increased activity, stress, surgical procedures. Monitor for signs/symptoms of CHF.

PATIENT/FAMILY TEACHING

• Be alert for signs/symptoms of hypoglycemia and take measures to manage it. • Avoid alcohol. • Inform physician of chest pain, palpitations, abdominal pain, fever, rash, hypoglycemic reactions, yellowing of skin/eyes, dark urine, light stool, nausea, vomiting. • Report any change in vision. • Report rapid weight gain, edema, difficulty breathing.

piperacillin sodium/ tazobactam sodium

pip-ur-ah-**sill**-in/tay-zoe-**back**-tam
(Tazocin ✤, Zosyn)
Do not confuse Zosyn with Zofran or Zyvox.

◆CLASSIFICATION

PHARMACOTHERAPEUTIC: Penicillin. **CLINICAL:** Antibiotic (see p. 29C).

P

ACTION

Piperacillin: Inhibits cell wall synthesis by binding to bacterial cell membranes. Therapeutic Effect: Bactericidal. **Tazobactam:** Inactivates bacterial beta-lactamase. Therapeutic Effect: Protects piperacillin from enzymatic degradation, extends its spectrum of activity, prevents bacterial overgrowth.

PHARMACOKINETICS

Protein binding: 16%–30%. Widely distributed. Primarily excreted unchanged in urine. Removed by hemodialysis. Half-life: 0.7–1.2 hrs (increased in hepatic cirrhosis, renal impairment).

USES

Treatment of appendicitis (complicated by rupture, abscess); peritonitis; uncomplicated and complicated skin/skin structure infections, including cellulitis, cutaneous abscesses, ischemic/diabetic foot infections; postpartum endometritis; pelvic inflammatory disease (PID); community-acquired pneumonia (moderate severity only); moderate to severe nosocomial pneumonia.

PRECAUTIONS

Contraindications: Hypersensitivity to any penicillin. **Cautions:** History of allergies (esp. cephalosporins, other drugs), renal impairment, preexisting seizure disorder.

LIFESPAN CONSIDERATIONS

Pregnancy/Lactation: Readily crosses placenta; appears in cord blood, amniotic fluid. Distributed in breast milk in low concentrations. May lead to allergic sensitization, diarrhea, candidiasis, skin rash in infant. **Pregnancy Category B. Children:** Dosage not established for those younger than 12 yrs. **Elderly:** Age-related renal impairment may require dosage adjustment.

INTERACTIONS

DRUG: Concurrent use of **aminoglycosides** may cause mutual inactivation (must give at least 1 hr apart). May increase concentration, toxicity of **methotrexate. Probenecid** may increase concentration, risk of toxicity. High-dose piperacillin may increase risk of bleeding with **heparin, NSAIDs, platelet inhibitors, thrombolytic agents, warfarin. HERBAL:** None significant. **FOOD:** None known. **LAB VALUES:** May increase serum sodium, alkaline phosphatase, bilirubin, LDH, AST, ALT, BUN, creatinine, PT, PTT. May decrease serum potassium. May cause positive Coombs' test.

AVAILABILITY (Rx)

ALERT Piperacillin/tazobactam is a combination product in an 8:1 ratio of piperacillin to tazobactam. **Injection Powder:** 2.25 g, 3.375 g, 4.5 g. **Premix Ready to Use:** 2.25 g, 3.375 g, 4.5 g.

ADMINISTRATION/HANDLING

IV

Reconstitution • Reconstitute each 1 g with 5 ml D_5W or 0.9% NaCl. Shake vigorously to dissolve. • Further dilute with at least 50 ml D_5W or 0.9% NaCl.

Rate of administration • Infuse over 30 min.

Storage • Reconstituted vial is stable for 24 hrs at room temperature or 48 hrs if refrigerated. • After further dilution, stable for 24 hrs at room temperature or 7 days if refrigerated.

IV INCOMPATIBILITIES

Amphotericin B (Fungizone), amphotericin B complex (Abelcet, AmBisome, Amphotec), chlorpromazine (Thorazine), dacarbazine (DTIC), daunorubicin (Cerubidine), dobutamine (Dobutrex), doxorubicin (Adriamycin), doxorubicin liposomal (Doxil), droperidol (Inapsine), famotidine (Pepcid), haloperidol (Haldol), hydroxyzine (Vistaril), idarubicin (Idamycin), minocycline (Minocin), nalbuphine (Nubain), prochlorperazine (Compazine), promethazine (Phenergan), vancomycin (Vancocin).

IV COMPATIBILITIES

Aminophylline, bumetanide (Bumex), calcium gluconate, diphenhydramine (Benadryl), dopamine (Intropin), enalapril (Vasotec), furosemide (Lasix), granisetron (Kytril), heparin, hydrocortisone (Solu-Cortef), hydromorphone (Dilaudid), lipids, lorazepam (Ativan), magnesium sulfate, methylprednisolone (Solu-Medrol), metoclopramide (Reglan), morphine, ondansetron (Zofran), potassium chloride, total parenteral nutrition (TPN).

INDICATIONS/ROUTES/DOSAGE

Severe Infections

IV: ADULTS, ELDERLY, CHILDREN 12 YRS AND OLDER: 4 g/0.5 g q8h or 3 g/0.375 g q6h. **Maximum:** 18 g/2.25 g daily.

Moderate Infections

IV: ADULTS, ELDERLY, CHILDREN 12 YRS AND OLDER: 2 g/0.25g q6–8h.

Dosage in Renal Impairment

Dosage and frequency are modified based on creatinine clearance.

Creatinine Clearance	Dosage
20–40 ml/min	2.25 g q6h (3.375 g q6h for nosocomial pneumonia)
Less than 20 ml/min	2.25 g q8h (2.25 g q6h for nosocomial pneumonia)

Dosage for Hemodialysis

IV: ADULTS, ELDERLY: 2.25 g q8–12h with additional dose of 0.75 g after each dialysis session.

SIDE EFFECTS

Frequent: Diarrhea, headache, constipation, nausea, insomnia, rash. **Occasional:** Vomiting, dyspepsia (heartburn, indigestion, epigastric pain), pruritus, fever, agitation, candidiasis, dizziness, abdominal pain, edema, anxiety, dyspnea, rhinitis.

ADVERSE EFFECTS/ TOXIC REACTIONS

Antibiotic-associated colitis, other superinfections (abdominal cramps, severe watery diarrhea, fever) may result from altered bacterial balance. Overdose, more often with renal impairment, may produce seizures, neurologic reactions. Severe hypersensitivity reactions, including anaphylaxis, occur rarely.

NURSING CONSIDERATIONS

BASELINE ASSESSMENT

Question for history of allergies, esp. to penicillins, cephalosporins.

INTERVENTION/EVALUATION

Monitor daily pattern of bowel activity, stool consistency; mild GI effects may be tolerable, but increasing severity may indicate onset of antibiotic-associated colitis. Be alert for superinfection: fever, vomiting, diarrhea, anal/genital pruritus, oral mucosal changes (ulceration, pain, erythema). Monitor I&O, urinalysis. Monitor serum electrolytes, esp. potassium, renal function tests.

P

piroxicam

peer-**ox**-i-kam
(Apo-Piroxicam ✱, Feldene, Novo-Pirocam ✱, Pexi-cam ✱)

BLACK BOX ALERT May increase risk of serious, potentially fatal cardiovascular thrombotic events, MI, stroke. Increased risk of serious GI events (bleeding, ulceration, perforation).

Do not confuse Feldene with fluoxetine.

◆CLASSIFICATION

PHARMACOTHERAPEUTIC: Nonsteroidal anti-inflammatory. **CLINICAL:** Anti-inflammatory, analgesic (see p. 129C).

ACTION

Produces analgesic, anti-inflammatory effects by inhibiting prostaglandin synthesis. **Therapeutic Effect:** Reduces inflammatory response, intensity of pain.

PHARMACOKINETICS

Route	Onset	Peak	Duration
PO	1 hr	3–5 hrs	—

Well absorbed following PO administration. Protein binding: 99%. Extensively metabolized in liver. Primarily excreted in urine; small amount eliminated in feces. **Half-life:** 50 hrs.

USES

Symptomatic treatment of acute or chronic rheumatoid arthritis (RA), osteoarthritis. **OFF-LABEL:** Treatment of acute gouty arthritis, ankylosing spondylitis, dysmenorrhea.

PRECAUTIONS

Contraindications: Active peptic ulcer disease, chronic inflammation of GI tract, GI bleeding/ulceration, history of hypersensitivity to aspirin/NSAIDs. **Cautions:** Renal/cardiac impairment, hypertension, GI disease, concomitant use of anticoagulants.

LIFESPAN CONSIDERATIONS

Pregnancy/Lactation: Crosses placenta; distributed in breast milk. Avoid use during third trimester (may adversely affect fetal cardiovascular system: premature closing of ductus arteriosus). **Pregnancy Category C (D if used in third trimester or near delivery). Children:** Safety and efficacy not established. **Elderly:** Age-related renal impairment may increase risk of hepatotoxicity, renal toxicity; reduced dosage recommended. More likely to have serious adverse effects with GI bleeding/ulceration.

INTERACTIONS

DRUG: May decrease effects of **antihypertensives, diuretics. Aspirin, other salicylates** may increase risk of GI side effects, bleeding. May increase effects of **heparin, oral anticoagulants, thrombolytics.** May increase concentration, risk of toxicity of **lithium.** May increase risk of **methotrexate** toxicity. **Probenecid** may increase concentration. **HERBAL: Cat's claw, dong quai, evening primrose, feverfew, garlic, ginger, ginkgo, ginseng, horse chestnut, red clover** possess antiplatelet activity, may increase risk of bleeding. **St. John's wort** may increase risk of phototoxicity. **FOOD:** None known. **LAB VALUES:** May increase AST, ALT, BUN, creatinine, LDH, alkaline phosphatase. May decrease serum uric acid, Hgb, Hct, platelets, leukocytes.

AVAILABILITY (Rx)

Capsules: 10 mg, 20 mg.

ADMINISTRATION/HANDLING

PO

• Do not crush/break capsules. • May give with food, milk, antacids if GI distress occurs.

INDICATIONS/ROUTES/DOSAGE

Rheumatoid Arthritis (RA), Osteoarthritis

PO: ADULTS, ELDERLY: Initially, 10–20 mg/day as a single dose or in divided doses. Some pts may require up to 30–40 mg/day. **CHILDREN:** 0.2–0.3 mg/kg/day. **Maximum:** 15 mg/day.

SIDE EFFECTS

Frequent (9%–4%): Dyspepsia (heartburn, indigestion, epigastric pain), nausea, dizziness. **Occasional (3%–1%):** Diarrhea, constipation, abdominal cramps/pain, flatulence, stomatitis. **Rare (less than 1%):** Hypertension, urticaria, dysuria, ecchymosis, blurred vision, insomnia, phototoxicity.

ADVERSE EFFECTS/ TOXIC REACTIONS

Peptic ulcer, GI bleeding, gastritis, severe hepatic reaction (cholestasis, jaundice) occur rarely. Nephrotoxicity (dysuria, hematuria, proteinuria, nephrotic syndrome), hematologic toxicity (anemia, leukopenia, eosinophilia, thrombocytopenia), severe hypersensitivity reaction (fever, chills, bronchospasm) occur rarely with long-term treatment.

NURSING CONSIDERATIONS

BASELINE ASSESSMENT

Assess onset, type, location, duration of pain/inflammation. Inspect appearance of affected joints for immobility, deformities, skin condition.

INTERVENTION/EVALUATION

Monitor daily pattern of bowel activity and stool consistency. Monitor for evidence of nausea, GI distress. Assess for therapeutic response: relief of pain, stiffness, swelling; increased joint mobility; reduced joint tenderness; improved grip strength, Monitor CBC, renal/hepatic function tests.

PATIENT/FAMILY TEACHING

• Avoid aspirin, alcohol during therapy (increases risk of GI bleeding). • If GI upset occurs, take with food, milk, antacids. • Avoid tasks that require alertness until response to drug is established.

pitavastatin

pit-ah-va-**stat**-in
(Livalo)

◆ CLASSIFICATION

PHARMACOTHERAPEUTIC: HMG-CoA reductase inhibitor. **CLINICAL:** Antihyperlipidemic.

ACTION

Interferes with cholesterol biosynthesis by inhibiting conversion of HMG-CoA reductase to a precursor to cholesterol. **Therapeutic Effect:** Lowers total cholesterol, LDL cholesterol, apolipoprotein B (Apo B), plasma triglycerides; increases HDL cholesterol.

PHARMACOKINETICS

Poorly absorbed from GI tract. Protein binding: greater than 99%. Metabolized in liver (minimal active metabolites). Primarily excreted in feces via biliary system. **Half-life:** 12 hrs.

USES

Adjunctive therapy with diet to modify lipid profiles in pts requiring intervention.

PRECAUTIONS

Contraindications: Active hepatic disease or unexplained, persistent elevations of hepatic function tests; concurrent cyclosporine use, pregnancy, breast-feeding. **Cautions:** History of hepatic disease, substantial alcohol consumption; moderate renal impairment. Withholding/discontinuing pitavastatin may be necessary when pt at risk for renal failure. Pts at risk for myopathy: advanced age, renal impairment, inadequately treated hypothyroidism.

LIFESPAN CONSIDERATIONS

Pregnancy/Lactation: Contraindicated in pregnancy (suppression of cholesterol biosynthesis may cause fetal toxicity) and lactation. Unknown if drug is distributed in breast milk (risk of serious adverse reactions in nursing infants). **Pregnancy Category X.** **Children:** Safety and efficacy not established in those younger than 18 yrs. **Elderly:** No age-related precautions noted.

INTERACTIONS:

DRUG: Increased risk of rhabdomyolysis, acute renal failure with **cyclosporine, erythromycin, gemfibrozil, niacin, other immunosuppressants. Cyclosporine, erythromycin, lopinavir/ritonavir, rifampin** significantly increase serum pitavastatin levels. **HERBAL:** None known. **FOOD:** None known. **LAB VALUES:** May increase serum creatinine kinase (CPK), AST, ALT concentrations.

AVAILABILITY (Rx)

Tablets: 1 mg, 2 mg, 4 mg.

ADMINISTRATION/HANDLING

PO

• Give without regard to meals or time of day.

INDICATIONS/ROUTES/DOSAGE

◀ALERT▶ Before initiating therapy, pt should be on standard cholesterol-lowering diet for minimum of 3–6 mos. Continue diet throughout pitavastatin therapy.

Usual Dosage

PO: ADULTS: Initially, 2 mg/day. **Maximum:** 4 mg/day. Range: 1–4 mg/day.

Dosage in Renal Impairment

CrCl 30–59: Initially, 1 mg/day. **Maximum:** 2 mg/day. CrCl less than 30: Avoid use.

SIDE EFFECTS

Generally well tolerated. Side effects usually mild and transient. **Rare (less than 4%):** Myalgia, constipation/diarrhea, back/extremity pain, arthralgia, headache, nasopharyngitis.

ADVERSE EFFECTS/ TOXIC REACTIONS

Hypersensitivity (rash, pruritus, urticaria) occurs rarely.

NURSING CONSIDERATIONS

BASELINE ASSESSMENT

Question for possibility of pregnancy before initiating therapy (Pregnancy Category X). Assess baseline lab results: cholesterol, triglycerides, hepatic function tests.

INTERVENTION/EVALUATION

Monitor cholesterol and triglyceride lab results for therapeutic response. Monitor hepatic function tests. Monitor daily pattern of bowel activity, stool consistency. Check for myalgia, arthralgia, headache. Assess for rash, pruritus. Be alert for malaise, muscle cramping/weakness.

PATIENT/FAMILY TEACHING

• Follow special diet (important part of treatment). • Periodic lab tests are essential part of therapy. • Report promptly any muscle pain/weakness. • Use nonhormonal contraception.

Pitocin, *see oxytocin*

Plavix, *see clopidogrel*

Plendil, *see felodipine*

plerixafor

pleh-**rix**-ah-for
(Mozobil)

◆CLASSIFICATION

PHARMACOTHERAPEUTIC: Chemokine receptor inhibitor. **CLINICAL:** Hematopoietic stem cell mobilizer.

ACTION

Immobilizes hematopoietic stem cells in bone marrow. Once in the marrow, acts to help anchor these cells to marrow matrix through induction of adhesion molecules. **Therapeutic Effect:** Results in leukocytosis, elevation in circulating hematopoietic progenitor cells in peripheral blood system.

PHARMACOKINETICS

Readily absorbed after subcutaneous administration. Generally confines to extravascular fluid space. Protein binding: 58%. Peak plasma concentration: 30–60 min. Eliminated in urine. Clearance reduced with renal impairment. **Half-life:** 3–5 hrs.

USES

Indicated in combination with granulocyte colony-stimulating factor (G-CSF) to mobilize stem cells to peripheral blood for collection and transplantation in pts with non-Hodgkin's lymphoma and multiple myeloma.

PRECAUTIONS

Contraindications: None significant. **Cautions:** Avoid use in leukemic pts, those with renal impairment.

LIFESPAN CONSIDERATIONS

Pregnancy/Lactation: Potential for teratogenic effects. May cause fetal harm. **Pregnancy Category D. Children:** Safety and efficacy not established. **Elderly:** Age-related renal impairment may require dosage adjustment.

INTERACTIONS

DRUG: None significant. **HERBAL:** None significant. **FOOD:** None known. **LAB VALUES:** May increase WBC count. May decrease platelet count.

AVAILABILITY (Rx)

Injection Solution: 1.2 ml of 20 mg/ml solution.

ADMINISTRATION/HANDLING

Subcutaneous

• Aspirate syringe before injection (avoid intra-arterial administration).

Storage • Store at room temperature. • Discard if particulate matter is present or if solution is discolored. • Use single dose vial; discard unused drug.

INDICATIONS/ROUTES/DOSAGE

ALERT Begin therapy after pt has received daily morning doses of G-CSF, 10 mcg/kg once daily for 4 days prior to the first evening dose of plerixafor and approximately 11 hrs prior to initiation of apheresis for up to 4 consecutive days.

Daily Dosage

SUBCUTANEOUS: ADULTS, ELDERLY: 0.24 mg/kg using following formula: 0.012 × pt's actual body weight (in kg) = volume to be administered (in ml). **Maximum:** 40 mg/day.

Moderate to Severe Renal Impairment (Creatinine Clearance Equal to or Less Than 50 ml/min):

SUBCUTANEOUS: ADULTS, ELDERLY: Decrease dose by one-third to 0.16 mg/kg, not to exceed 27 mg/day.

SIDE EFFECTS

Frequent (37%–22%): Diarrhea, nausea, injection site irritation, fatigue, headache. **Occasional (13%–7%):** Arthralgia, dizziness, vomiting, insomnia, flatulence.

ADVERSE EFFECTS/ TOXIC REACTIONS

Thrombocytopenia may occur. Dyspnea, hypoxia, vasovagal reaction, periorbital edema, urticaria has been noted; may resolve spontaneously, generally responds to antihistamines, corticosteroids.

NURSING CONSIDERATIONS

BASELINE ASSESSMENT

CBC should be obtained before initiation of therapy as baseline.

INTERVENTION/EVALUATION

Monitor WBC, platelet count during therapy. Assess for potential systemic reaction (periorbital edema, dyspnea, urticaria), orthostatic hypotension during or shortly after injection. Advise female pt with reproductive potential to use effective contraceptive method (Pregnancy Category D).

PATIENT/FAMILY TEACHING

• Manage gastrointestinal disorders; inform physician if severe diarrhea, nausea, vomiting, occur.

polyethylene glycol-electrolyte solution (PEG-ES)

poly-**eth**-ah-leen
(CoLyte, GoLYTELY, Klean-Prep ✦, MiraLax, NuLytely, Peglyte ✦, TriLyte)

Do not confuse MiraLax with Mirapex.

◆CLASSIFICATION

PHARMACOTHERAPEUTIC: Laxative. **CLINICAL:** Bowel evacuant (see p. 122C).

ACTION

Osmotic effect. **Therapeutic Effect:** Induces diarrhea, cleanses bowel without depleting electrolytes.

PHARMACOKINETICS

Route	Onset	Peak	Duration
PO (bowel cleansing)	1–2 hrs	N/A	N/A
PO (constipation)	2–4 days	N/A	N/A

USES

Bowel cleansing before GI examination, colon surgery. **MiraLax:** Treatment of occasional constipation.

PRECAUTIONS

Contraindications: Bowel perforation, gastric retention, GI obstruction, megacolon, toxic colitis, toxic ileus. **Cautions:** Ulcerative colitis.

P

⌛ LIFESPAN CONSIDERATIONS

Pregnancy/Lactation: Unknown if drug crosses placenta or is distributed in breast milk. **Pregnancy Category C. Children/Elderly:** No age-related precautions noted.

INTERACTIONS

DRUG: May decrease absorption of **oral medications** if given within 1 hr (may be flushed from GI tract). **HERBAL:** None significant. **FOOD:** None known. **LAB VALUES:** None significant.

AVAILABILITY (Rx)

Powder for Reconstitution: (CoLyte, GoLYTELY, MiraLax, NuLytely, TriLyte).

ADMINISTRATION/HANDLING

PO

• Refrigerate reconstituted solutions; use within 48 hrs. • May use tap water to prepare solution. Shake vigorously for several min to ensure complete dissolution of powder. • Fasting should occur for more than 3 hrs prior to ingestion of solution (always avoid solid food less than 2 hrs prior to administration). • Only clear liquids permitted after administration. • May give via NG tube. • Rapid drinking preferred. Chilled solution is more palatable.

INDICATIONS/ROUTES/DOSAGE

Bowel Evacuant

PO: ADULTS, ELDERLY: Before GI examination: 240 ml (8 oz) q10min until 4 liters consumed or rectal effluent clear. NG tube: 20–30 ml/min until 4 liters given. **CHILDREN:** 25–40 ml/kg/hr until rectal effluent clear.

Constipation

PO (MIRALAX): ADULTS: 17 g or 1 heaping tbsp a day.

SIDE EFFECTS

Frequent (50%): Some degree of abdominal fullness, nausea, bloating. **Occasional (10%–1%):** Abdominal cramping, vomiting, anal irritation. **Rare (less than 1%):** Urticaria, rhinorrhea, dermatitis.

ADVERSE EFFECTS/ TOXIC REACTIONS

None known.

NURSING CONSIDERATIONS

BASELINE ASSESSMENT

Do not give oral medication within 1 hr of start of therapy (may not adequately be absorbed before GI cleansing).

INTERVENTION/EVALUATION

Assess bowel sounds for peristalsis. Monitor daily pattern of bowel activity and stool consistency; record time of evacuation. Assess for abdominal disturbances.

Monitor serum electrolytes, BUN, glucose, urine osmolality.

PATIENT/FAMILY TEACHING

• May take 2–4 days to produce a bowel movement. • Report unusual cramps, bloating, diarrhea.

poractant alfa

poor-**ak**-tant
(Curosurf)

◆CLASSIFICATION

CLINICAL: Pulmonary surfactant.

ACTION

Reduces alveolar surface tension during ventilation; stabilizes alveoli against collapse that may occur at resting transpulmonary pressures. **Therapeutic Effect:** Improves lung compliance, respiratory gas exchange.

USES

Rescue treatment for respiratory distress syndrome (RDS), hyaline membrane disease in premature infants. **OFF-LABEL:** Adult RDS due to viral pneumonia or near-drowning, *Pneumocystis jiroveci* pneumonia (PCP) in HIV-infected pts, prophylaxis of RDS.

PRECAUTIONS

Contraindications: None known. **Cautions:** Pts at risk for circulatory overload. Acidosis, hypotension, anemia, hypoglycemia, hypothermia should be corrected prior to administration.

⌛ LIFESPAN CONSIDERATIONS

Pregnancy/Lactation: Neonate: No age-related precautions noted for neonates. Not used in women of child-bearing potential.

INTERACTIONS

DRUG: None significant. **HERBAL:** None significant. **FOOD:** None known. **LAB VALUES:** None significant.

AVAILABILITY (Rx)

Intratracheal Suspension: 80 mg/ml (1.5 ml, 3 ml), 1.5 ml (120 mg), 3 ml (240 mg).

ADMINISTRATION/HANDLING

Intratracheal

Administration • Attach syringe to catheter and instill through catheter inserted into infant's endotracheal tube. • Monitor for bradycardia, decreased O_2 saturation during administration. • Stop dosing procedure if these effects occur; begin appropriate measures before reinstituting therapy.

Storage • Refrigerate vials. • Warm by standing vial at room temperature for 20 min or warm in hand 8 min. • To obtain uniform suspension, turn upside down gently, swirl vial (do not shake). • After warming, may return to refrigerator one time only. • Withdraw entire contents of vial into 3- or 5-ml plastic syringe through large-gauge needle (20 gauge or larger).

P

INDICATIONS/ROUTE/DOSAGE

Respiratory Distress Syndrome (RDS)

INTRATRACHEAL: INFANTS: Initially, 2.5 ml/kg of birth weight. May give up to 2 subsequent doses of 1.25 ml/kg of birth weight at 12-hr intervals. **Maximum:** 5 ml/kg (total dose).

SIDE EFFECTS

Frequent: Transient bradycardia, oxygen (O_2) desaturation, increased carbon dioxide (CO_2) retention. **Occasional:** Endotracheal tube reflux. **Rare:** Hypotension, hypertension, apnea, pallor, vasoconstriction.

ADVERSE EFFECTS/ TOXIC REACTIONS

None known.

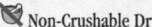

NURSING CONSIDERATIONS

BASELINE ASSESSMENT

Immediately before administration, change ventilator setting to 40–60 breaths/min, inspiratory time 0.5 sec, supplemental O_2 sufficient to maintain SaO_2 over 92%. Drug must be administered in highly supervised setting. Clinicians caring for neonate must be experienced with intubation, ventilator management. Offer emotional support to parents.

INTERVENTION/EVALUATION

Monitor infant with arterial or transcutaneous measurement of systemic O_2 and CO_2. Assess lung sounds for rales, moist breath sounds. Monitor heart rate.

posaconazole

pose-ah-**con**-ah-zole
(Noxafil, Posanol)
Do not confuse Noxafil with minoxidil.

CLASSIFICATION

PHARMACOTHERAPEUTIC: Azole derivative. **CLINICAL:** Antifungal.

ACTION

Inhibits synthesis of ergosterol, a vital component of fungal cell wall formation. **Therapeutic Effect:** Damages fungal cell wall membrane, altering its function.

PHARMACOKINETICS

Moderately absorbed following PO administration. Absorption increased if drug is taken with food. Widely distributed. Protein binding: 98%. Not significantly metabolized. Primarily excreted in feces. **Half-life:** 20–66 hrs.

USES

Prophylaxis of invasive *Aspergillosis* and *Candida* infections in pts 13 yrs and older who are at high risk for developing these infections due to severely immunocompromised conditions. Treatment of oropharyngeal candidiasis. **OFF-LABEL:** Salvage therapy of refractory invasive fungal infections.

PRECAUTIONS

Contraindications: Coadministration with pimozide, quinidine, terfenadine, astemizole, cisapride, halofantrine, ergot alkaloids (may cause QT prolongation, torsade de pointes). **Cautions:** Renal/hepatic impairment, hypersensitivity to other antifungal agents.

LIFESPAN CONSIDERATIONS

Pregnancy/Lactation: May cause fetal harm. Breast-feeding not recommended. **Pregnancy Category C. Children:** Safety and efficacy not established in those younger than 13 yrs. **Elderly:** No age-related precautions noted.

INTERACTIONS

DRUG: May increase concentrations of **atorvastatin, ergot alkaloids, felodipine, midazolam, phenytoin, pimozide, quinidine, rifabutin, sirolimus, tacrolimus, vinblastine, vincristine. Cimetidine, phenytoin** may decrease concentration. **HERBAL:** None significant. **FOOD:** Concentration higher when given with **food or nutritional supplements. LAB VALUES:** May decrease WBC, RBC, Hgb, Hct, platelets, serum calcium, potassium, magnesium. May increase serum glucose, bilirubin, ALT, AST, alkaline phosphatase.

AVAILABILITY (Rx)

Oral Suspension: 40 mg/ml.

ADMINISTRATION/HANDLING

PO

• Administer with or within 20 min of full meal, liquid nutritional supplement, or acidic carbonated beverage (e.g., ginger ale) (enhances absorption). • Store oral suspension at room temperature. • Shake suspension well before use.

INDICATIONS/ROUTES/DOSAGE

Prophylaxis of Invasive Aspergillus and Candida

PO: ADULTS, ELDERLY: 200 mg (5 ml) 3 times daily, given with full meal or liquid nutritional supplement.

Oropharyngeal Candidiasis

PO: ADULTS, ELDERLY: 100 mg twice daily for 1 day, then 100 mg once daily for 13 days.

Refractory Oropharyngeal Candidiasis

PO: ADULTS, ELDERLY: 400 mg twice daily.

SIDE EFFECTS

Common (42%–24%): Diarrhea, nausea, vomiting, headache, abdominal pain, cough. **Frequent** (20%–15%): Constipation, rigors, rash, hypertension, fatigue, insomnia, mucositis, musculoskeletal pain, edema of lower extremities, herpes simplex, anorexia. **Occasional** (14%–8%): Hypotension, epistaxis, tachycardia, pharyngitis, dizziness, pruritus, arthralgia, dyspepsia (heartburn, indigestion, epigastric pain), back pain, generalized edema, weakness.

ADVERSE EFFECTS/ TOXIC REACTIONS

Bacteremia occurs in 18% of pts; upper respiratory tract infection occurs in 7%. Allergic/hypersensitivity reactions, QT prolongation, hemolytic uremic syndrome, thrombotic thrombocytopenic purpura, pulmonary embolus have been reported.

NURSING CONSIDERATIONS

BASELINE ASSESSMENT

Obtain baselines for hepatic enzyme serum levels, CBC, serum chemistries prior to therapy.

INTERVENTION/EVALUATION

Monitor hepatic function tests periodically. Monitor daily pattern of bowel activity, stool consistency. Obtain order for antiemetic if excessive vomiting occurs. Monitor B/P for hypertension, hypotension. Assess for lower extremity edema (first sign of edema appears behind medial malleolus).

PATIENT/FAMILY TEACHING

- Take each dose with full meal or liquid nutritional supplement. • Report severe diarrhea, vomiting, chest pain, yellowing of skin/eyes. • Maintain fastidious oral hygiene.

potassium acetate

HIGH ALERT

potassium bicarbonate/citrate

(Effer-K, Klor-Con EF, K-Lyte, K-Lyte DS)

potassium chloride

(Apo-K ✤, Kaon-Cl, Kay Ciel, K-Dur, K-Lor, Klor-Con, Klor-Con M10, Klor-Con M20, Micro-K)

potassium gluconate

(Glu-K)

poe-**tah**-see-um

Do not confuse K-Dur with Cardura, K-Lor with Klor-Con, or MicroK with Macrobid or Micronase.

◆ CLASSIFICATION

PHARMACOTHERAPEUTIC: Electrolyte. **CLINICAL:** Potassium replenisher.

ACTION

Necessary for multiple cellular metabolic processes. Primary action is intracellular. **Therapeutic Effect:** Required for nerve impulse conduction, contraction of cardiac, skeletal, smooth muscle; maintains normal renal function, acid-base balance.

P

PHARMACOKINETICS

Well absorbed from GI tract. Enters cells by active transport from extracellular fluid. Primarily excreted in urine.

USES

Treatment of potassium deficiency found in severe vomiting, diarrhea, loss of GI fluid, malnutrition, prolonged diuresis, debilitated, poor GI absorption, metabolic alkalosis, prolonged parenteral alimentation. Prevention of hypokalemia in at-risk pts.

PRECAUTIONS

Contraindications: Concurrent use of potassium-sparing diuretics, digitalis toxicity, heat cramps, hyperkalemia, postop oliguria, severe burns, severe renal impairment, shock with dehydration or hemolytic reaction, untreated Addison's disease. **Cautions:** Cardiac disease, tartrazine sensitivity (mostly noted in those with aspirin hypersensitivity).

LIFESPAN CONSIDERATIONS

Pregnancy/Lactation: Unknown if drug crosses placenta or is distributed in breast milk. **Pregnancy Category C. Children:** No age-related precautions noted. **Elderly:** May be at increased risk for hyperkalemia. Age-related ability to excrete potassium is reduced.

P

INTERACTIONS

DRUG: **Angiotensin-converting enzyme (ACE) inhibitors, potassium-containing medications, potassium-sparing diuretics, salt substitutes** may increase serum potassium concentration. **HERBAL:** None significant. **FOOD:** None known. **LAB VALUES:** None significant.

AVAILABILITY (Rx)

POTASSIUM ACETATE
Injection, Solution: 2 mEq/ml.
POTASSIUM BICARBONATE AND POTASSIUM CITRATE
Tablets for Solution: 25 mEq (Klor-Con EF, Effer-K, K-Lyte), 50 mEq (K-Lyte DS).
POTASSIUM CHLORIDE
Injection, Solution: 2 mEq/ml. **Oral Solution (KAON-CL, KAY CIEL):** 20 mEq/15 ml. **Powder for Oral Solution (K-LOR, KLOR-CON):** 20 mEq/packet.

Capsules, Extended-Release (Micro-K): 8 mEq, 10 mEq. **Tablets, Extended-Release: (K-DUR):** 10 mEq, 20 mEq. **(Klor-Con M10):** 10 mEq. **(Klor-Con M20):** 20 mEq.

POTASSIUM GLUCONATE
Tablets (Glu-K): 500 mg, 610 mg.

ADMINISTRATION/HANDLING

IV

Reconstitution • For IV infusion only, must dilute before administration, mix well, infuse slowly. • Avoid adding potassium to hanging IV.
Rate of administration • Routinely, give at concentration of no more than 40 mEq/L, no faster than 10 mEq/hr for peripheral infusion, 40 mEq/hr for central infusion. • Check IV site closely during infusion for evidence of phlebitis (heat, pain, red streaking of skin over vein, hardness to vein), extravasation (swelling, pain, cool skin, little/no blood return).
Storage • Store at room temperature.

PO

• Take with or after meals, with full glass of water (decreases GI upset). • Liquids, powder, effervescent tablets: Mix, dissolve with juice, water before administering. • Do not chew, crush tablets; swallow whole.

IV INCOMPATIBILITIES

Amphotericin B complex (Abelcet, AmBisome, Amphotec), phenytoin (Dilantin).

IV COMPATIBILITIES

Aminophylline, amiodarone (Cordarone), atropine, aztreonam (Azactam), calcium gluconate, cefepime (Maxipime), ciprofloxacin (Cipro), clindamycin (Cleocin), dexamethasone (Decadron), digoxin (Lanoxin), diltiazem (Cardizem), diphenhydramine (Benadryl), dobutamine (Dobutrex), dopamine (Intropin), enalapril (Vasotec), famotidine (Pepcid), fluconazole (Diflucan), furosemide (Lasix), granisetron (Kytril), heparin, hydrocortisone (Solu-Cortef), insulin, lidocaine, lipids, lorazepam (Ativan), magnesium sulfate, methylprednisolone (Solu-Medrol), metoclopramide (Reglan), midazolam (Versed), milrinone (Primacor), morphine, norepinephrine (Levophed), ondansetron (Zofran), oxytocin (Pitocin), piperacillin and tazobactam (Zosyn), procainamide (Pronestyl), propofol (Diprivan), propranolol (Inderal).

INDICATIONS/ROUTES/DOSAGE

Prevention of Hypokalemia with Diuretic Therapy

PO: ADULTS, ELDERLY: 20–40 mEq/day in 1–2 divided doses. **CHILDREN:** 1–2 mEq/kg/day in 1–2 divided doses.

Treatment of Hypokalemia

PO: ADULTS, ELDERLY: 40–100 mEq/day in divided doses (generally limit amount per dose to 40 mEq); further doses based on laboratory values. **CHILDREN:** Initially, 1–2 mEq/kg; further doses based on laboratory values.

IV: ADULTS, ELDERLY: 5–10 mEq/hr. **Maximum:** 400 mEq/day. **CHILDREN:** 0.5–1 mEq/kg per dose. **Maximum dose:** 40 mEq per dose.

SIDE EFFECTS

Occasional: Nausea, vomiting, diarrhea, flatulence, abdominal discomfort with distention, phlebitis with IV administration (particularly when potassium concentration of greater than 40 mEq/L is infused). **Rare:** Rash.

ADVERSE EFFECTS/ TOXIC REACTIONS

Hyperkalemia (more common in elderly, those with renal impairment) manifested as paresthesia, feeling of heaviness in lower extremities, cold skin, grayish pallor, hypotension, confusion, irritability, flaccid paralysis, cardiac arrhythmias.

NURSING CONSIDERATIONS

BASELINE ASSESSMENT

Assess for hypokalemia (weakness, fatigue, polyuria, polydipsia). PO should be given with food or after meals with full glass of water, fruit juice (minimizes GI irritation).

INTERVENTION/EVALUATION

Monitor serum potassium (particularly in renal impairment). If GI disturbance is noted, dilute preparation further or give with meals. Be alert to decreased urinary output (may be indication of renal insufficiency). Monitor daily pattern of bowel activity and stool consistency. Assess I&O diligently during diuresis, IV site for extravasation, phlebitis. Be alert to evidence of hyperkalemia (skin pallor/coldness, complaints of paresthesia, feeling of heaviness of lower extremities).

PATIENT/FAMILY TEACHING

- Foods rich in potassium include beef, veal, ham, chicken, turkey, fish, milk, bananas, dates, prunes, raisins, avocados, watermelon, cantaloupe, apricots, molasses, beans, yams, broccoli, Brussels sprouts, lentils, potatoes, spinach.
- Report paresthesia, feeling of heaviness of lower extremities, tarry or bloody stools, weakness, unusual fatigue.

pralatrexate

pra-la-**trex**-ate
(Folotyn)
Do not confuse pralatrexate with methotrexate or pemetrexed, or Folotyn with Focalin.

◆CLASSIFICATION

PHARMACOTHERAPEUTIC: Antimetabolite. **CLINICAL:** Antineoplastic.

ACTION

Folate analogue metabolic inhibitor that competes with enzymes necessary for tu-

P

mor cell reproduction. **Therapeutic Effect:** Inhibits tumor growth.

PHARMACOKINETICS

Protein binding: 67%. Partially excreted in urine. **Half-life:** 12–18 hrs.

USES

Treatment of relapsed or refractory peripheral T-cell lymphoma (PTCL).

PRECAUTIONS

Contraindications: None known. **Cautions:** Moderate to severe renal impairment.

LIFESPAN CONSIDERATIONS

Pregnancy/Lactation: May cause fetal harm. Unknown if drug is distributed in breast milk. **Pregnancy Category D. Children:** Safety and efficacy not established. **Elderly:** No age-related precautions noted.

INTERACTIONS

DRUG: **NSAIDs, probenecid, trimethoprim/sulfamethoxazole** may delay clearance, increase concentration. **HERBAL:** **Cat's claw, echinacea** possess immunostimulant properties. **FOOD:** None known. **LAB VALUES:** May decrease RBC, WBC, Hgb, Hct, serum potassium, platelet count. May increase ALT, AST.

AVAILABILITY (Rx)

Injection Solution: 20 mg/ml, 40 mg/2 ml single-use vials.

ADMINISTRATION/HANDLING

◀ALERT▶ May be carcinogenic, mutagenic, teratogenic. Handle with extreme care during preparation/administration. Wear gloves when preparing solution. If powder or solution comes in contact with skin, wash immediately, thoroughly with soap, water.

◀ALERT▶ Pt should begin taking oral folic acid (1 mg) daily starting 10 days prior to first IV pralatrexate dose and continue for 30 days after last dose. Pt should also receive vitamin B_{12} (1 mg) IM injection no more than 10 wks prior to first IV pralatrexate dose and every 8–10 wks thereafter.

IV

Reconstitution • Withdraw calculated dose into syringe for immediate use. • Intended for single use only. • Do not dilute.

Rate of administration • Administer as IV push over 3–5 min into IV infusion of 0.9% NaCl.

Storage • Refrigerate vials until use, protect from light. Stable at room temperature for 72 hrs. • Discard vial if solution is discolored (solution should appear clear to yellow) or particulate matter is present.

IV INCOMPATIBILITY

Do not mix with any other medication.

INDICATIONS/ROUTES/DOSAGE

Refractory/Relapsed Peripheral T-Cell Lymphoma

IV: ADULTS, ELDERLY: 30 mg/m² administered once weekly for 6 wks in 7-wk cycles. Dose may be decreased to 20 mg/m² to manage adverse reactions.

SIDE EFFECTS

Common (70%–36%): Mucositis, nausea, fatigue. **Frequent (34%–10%):** Constipation/diarrhea, pyrexia, edema, cough, epistaxis, vomiting, dyspnea, anorexia, rash, throat/abdominal/back pain, night sweats, asthenia, tachycardia, upper respiratory infection.

ADVERSE EFFECTS/ TOXIC REACTIONS

Hematologic toxicity, resulting from blood dyscrasias, may manifest as thrombocytopenia (41%), anemia (34%), neutropenia (24%), leukopenia (11%). High potential for development of mucositis (70%). Mucositis is less severe when folic acid, vitamin B_{12} therapy is ongoing. Sepsis, pyrexia, febrile neutropenia, dehydration have been known to occur. Overdosage requires general supportive care. Prompt administration of leucovorin should be

P

considered in case of overdose, based on mechanism of action of pralatrexate.

NURSING CONSIDERATIONS

BASELINE ASSESSMENT

Question for possibility of pregnancy before initiating therapy (Pregnancy Category D). Assess baseline vital signs, temperature. Evaluate baseline CBC with differential, hepatic/renal function, serum potassium level. Antiemetics before and during therapy may alleviate nausea/vomiting. Initiate folic acid, vitamin B_{12} administration prior to and throughout therapy.

INTERVENTION/EVALUATION

Prior to any dose: mucositis should be grade 1 or less. Platelet count 100,000 or greater for 1st dose (50,000 or greater for all subsequent doses). Absolute neutrophil count (ANC) 1,000 or greater. Assess for signs of mucositis (oropharyngeal ulcers, oral/throat pain, local infection). Monitor for signs of hematologic toxicity, sepsis (fever, signs of local infection, altered CBC results). Monitor hepatic/renal function. Monitor for hypokalemia (muscle cramps, weakness, EKG changes).

PATIENT/FAMILY TEACHING

• Explain importance of folic acid, vitamin B_{12} therapy to reduce adverse effects. • Maintain fastidious oral hygiene. • Do not have immunizations without physician's approval (drug lowers body's resistance). • Avoid crowds, those with infection. • Promptly report fever, sore throat, signs of local infection, unusual bruising/bleeding from any site. • Use nonhormonal contraception. • Contact physician if nausea/vomiting continues at home.

pramipexole

pram-eh-**pex**-ol
(Apo-Pramipexole ✤, Mirapex, Mirapex ER, Novo-Pramipexole ✤)

Do not confuse Mirapex with Mifeprex or MiraLax.

◆ CLASSIFICATION

PHARMACOTHERAPEUTIC: Dopamine receptor agonist. **CLINICAL:** Antiparkinson agent.

ACTION

Stimulates dopamine receptors in striatum. **Therapeutic Effect:** Relieves signs/symptoms of Parkinson's disease.

PHARMACOKINETICS

Rapidly, extensively absorbed after PO administration. Protein binding: 15%. Widely distributed. Steady-state concentrations achieved within 2 days. Primarily eliminated in urine. Not removed by hemodialysis. **Half-life:** 8 hrs (12 hrs in pts older than 65 yrs).

USES

Treatment of signs/symptoms of idiopathic Parkinson's disease, restless legs syndrome. **Mirapex ER:** Treatment of Parkinson's disease. **OFF-LABEL:** Depression (due to bipolar disorder), fibromyalgia.

PRECAUTIONS

Contraindications: History of hypersensitivity to pramipexole. **Cautions:** History of orthostatic hypotension, syncope, hallucinations, renal impairment, concomitant use of CNS depressants.

LIFESPAN CONSIDERATIONS

Pregnancy/Lactation: Unknown if drug is distributed in breast milk. **Pregnancy Category C. Children:** Safety and efficacy not established. **Elderly:** Increased risk of hallucinations.

INTERACTIONS

DRUG: May increase plasma concentrations of **carbidopa, levodopa. HERBAL: Gotu kola, kava kava, St. John's wort, SAMe, valerian** may increase CNS depression. **FOOD: All foods** delay peak drug plasma levels by 1 hr (extent of absorption not affected). **LAB VALUES:** None significant.

AVAILABILITY (Rx)

Tablets: 0.125 mg, 0.25 mg, 0.5 mg, 0.75 mg, 1 mg, 1.5 mg.

Tablets (Extended-Release [Mirapex ER]): 0.375 mg, 0.75 mg, 1.5 mg, 3 mg, 4.5 mg.

ADMINISTRATION/HANDLING

PO (Mirapex)
- Give without regard to food.

PO (Mirapex ER)
- Give once daily, without regard to food.
- Swallow whole; do not crush, chew, or divide tablets.

INDICATIONS/ROUTES/DOSAGE

Parkinson's Disease (Mirapex)

PO: ADULTS, ELDERLY: Initially, 0.375 mg/day in 3 divided doses. Increase dosage by 0.125 mg/dose no more frequently than every 5–7 days. Maintenance: 1.5–4.5 mg/day in 3 equally divided doses.

Parkinson's Disease (Mirapex ER)

Initially, 0.375 mg once daily. May increase to 0.75 mg, then by 0.75 mg increments no more frequently than 5–7 days. Note: May switch overnight from immediate-release to extended-release at same daily dose.

Dosage in Renal Impairment

Dosage and frequency are modified based on creatinine clearance.

Creatinine Clearance	Dosage Initial	Dosage Maximum
Greater than 60 ml/min	0.125 mg 3 times a day	1.5 mg 3 times a day
35–60 ml/min	0.125 mg twice daily	1.5 mg twice daily
15–34 ml/min	0.125 mg once daily	1.5 mg once daily

Restless Legs Syndrome

PO: ADULTS, ELDERLY: Initially, 0.125 mg once daily 2–3 hrs before bedtime. May increase to 0.25 mg after 4–7 days, then to 0.5 mg after 4–7 days (interval is 14 days in pts with renal impairment).

SIDE EFFECTS

Frequent: **Early Parkinson's disease (28%–10%):** Nausea, asthenia (loss of strength, energy), dizziness, drowsiness, insomnia, constipation. **Advanced Parkinson's disease (53%–17%):** Orthostatic hypotension, extrapyramidal reactions, insomnia, dizziness, hallucinations. **Occasional:** **Early Parkinson's disease (5%–2%):** Edema, malaise, confusion, amnesia, akathisia, anorexia, dysphagia, peripheral edema, vision changes, impotence. **Advanced Parkinson's disease (10%–7%):** Asthenia (loss of strength, energy), drowsiness, confusion, constipation, abnormal gait, dry mouth. **Rare:** **Advanced Parkinson's disease (6%–2%):** General edema, malaise, angina, amnesia, tremor, urinary frequency/incontinence, dyspnea, rhinitis, vision changes. **Restless legs syndrome:** **Frequent (16%):** Headache, nausea. **Occasional (13%–9%):** Insomnia, fatigue. **Rare (6%–3%):** Drowsiness, constipation, diarrhea, dry mouth.

ADVERSE EFFECTS/ TOXIC REACTIONS

Vascular disease, atrial fibrillation, arrhythmias, pulmonary embolism, impulsive/compulsive behavior (pathological gambling, hypersexuality, binge eating) have been reported.

NURSING CONSIDERATIONS

BASELINE ASSESSMENT

Parkinson's Disease: Assess for tremor, muscle weakness and rigidity, ataxia. **Restless Legs Syndrome:** Assess frequency of symptoms, sleep pattern.

INTERVENTION/EVALUATION

Instruct pt to rise from lying to sitting or sitting to standing position slowly to prevent risk of postural hypotension. Assess for clinical improvement. Assist with ambulation if dizziness occurs. Assess for constipation; encourage fiber, fluids, exercise.

PATIENT/FAMILY TEACHING

• Inform pt that hallucinations may occur, esp. in the elderly. • Postural hypotension may occur more frequently during initial therapy (rise slowly from sitting or lying position). • Avoid tasks that require alertness, motor skills until response to drug is established. • If nausea occurs, take medication with food. • Avoid abrupt withdrawal. • Avoid alcohol. • Report new/increased need for gambling, sexual urges, compulsive eating or buying.

pramlintide HIGH ALERT

pram-lin-tide
(Symlin)

BLACK BOX ALERT Increased risk of severe hypoglycemia; usually occurs within 3 hrs of injection.

◆CLASSIFICATION

PHARMACOTHERAPEUTIC: Antihyperglycemic. **CLINICAL:** Antidiabetic.

ACTION

Co-secreted with insulin by pancreatic beta cells, reduces postprandial glucose increases by slowing gastric emptying time, reducing postprandial glucagon secretion, reducing caloric intake through centrally mediated appetite suppression. **Therapeutic Effect:** Improves glycemic control by reducing postprandial glucose concentrations in pts with type 1, type 2 diabetes mellitus.

PHARMACOKINETICS

	Onset	Peak	Duration
Subcutaneous	NA	20 min	3 hrs

Metabolized primarily by kidneys. Protein binding: 60%. Excreted in urine. **Half-life:** 48 min.

USES

Adjunctive treatment with mealtime insulin in type 1, type 2 diabetes mellitus pts who have failed to achieve desired glucose control despite optimal insulin therapy, with/without concurrent sulfonylurea and/or metformin in type 2 diabetes mellitus.

PRECAUTIONS

Contraindications: Diagnosed gastroparesis, presence of hypoglycemia or recurrent severe hypoglycemic episodes in the past 6 mos, poor compliance with insulin monitoring or current insulin therapy, those with hemoglobin A_{1c} greater than 9%, pts with conditions or taking concurrent medications likely to impair gastric motility (e.g., anticholinergics), pts requiring medication to stimulate gastric emptying. **Cautions:** Coadministration with insulin may induce severe hypoglycemia (usually within 3 hrs following administration); concurrent use of other glucose-lowering agents may increase risk of hypoglycemia.

⌛ LIFESPAN CONSIDERATIONS

Pregnancy/Lactation: Unknown if distributed in breast milk. **Pregnancy Category C. Children:** Safety and efficacy not established. **Elderly:** No age-related precautions noted.

INTERACTIONS

DRUG: **ACE inhibitors, fibrates, fluoxetine, MAOIs, salicylates, sulfonamide antibiotics** may increase effect. **Anticholinergics** may cause additive impairment of gastric motility. **Beta-blockers, clonidine** may mask early symptoms of hypoglycemia. **HERBAL:** **Garlic** may increase hypoglycemia. **FOOD:** **Ethanol** increases risk of hypoglycemia. **LAB VALUES:** None significant.

P

AVAILABILITY (Rx)

Injection, Solution: 0.6 mg/ml in 5-ml vials (Symlin). **Symlin Pen 120:** Delivers fixed doses of 60 mcg and 120 mcg.

ADMINISTRATION/HANDLING

Subcutaneous

• Administer immediately before each major meal (350 or more kcal or containing 30 g or more carbohydrate). • Give in abdomen or thigh; do not give in arm (variable absorption). • Injection site should be distinct from insulin injection site. • Rotation of injection sites is essential. • Use U-100 insulin syringe for accuracy. • Always give pramlintide and insulin as separate injections.

Storage • Store unopened vials in refrigerator. • Discard if freezing occurs. • Vials that have been opened (punctured) may be stored in refrigerator or kept at room temperature for up to 30 days.

INDICATIONS/ROUTES/DOSAGE

◀ALERT▶ Initially, current insulin dosage in all pts with type 1, type 2 diabetes mellitus should be reduced by 50%. This includes preprandial, rapid-acting, short-acting, fixed-mixed insulins.

Type 1 Diabetes Mellitus

SUBCUTANEOUS: ADULTS, ELDERLY: Initially, 15 mcg immediately before major meal. Titrate in 15-mcg increments every 3 days (if no significant nausea occurs) to target dose of 30–60 mcg.

Type 2 Diabetes Mellitus

SUBCUTANEOUS: ADULTS, ELDERLY: Initially, 60 mcg immediately before major meal. After 3–7 days, increase to 120 mcg if no significant nausea occurs (if nausea occurs at 120 mcg dose, reduce to 60 mcg).

SIDE EFFECTS

TYPE 1 DIABETES MELLITUS

Frequent (48%): Nausea. **Occasional (17%–11%):** Anorexia, vomiting. **Rare (7%–5%):** Fatigue, arthralgia, allergic reaction, dizziness.

TYPE 2 DIABETES MELLITUS

Frequent (28%): Nausea. **Occasional (13%–8%):** Headache, anorexia, vomiting, abdominal pain. **Rare (7%–5%):** Fatigue, dizziness, cough, pharyngitis.

ADVERSE EFFECTS/ TOXIC REACTIONS

Overdose produces severe nausea, vomiting, diarrhea, vasodilation, dizziness. No hypoglycemia was reported. Increased risk of severe hypoglycemia when given concurrently with nontitrated insulin.

NURSING CONSIDERATIONS

BASELINE ASSESSMENT

Check serum glucose concentration before administration, both before and after meals and at bedtime. Discuss lifestyle to determine extent of learning, emotional needs. Ensure follow-up instruction if pt, family does not thoroughly understand diabetes management, glucose testing technique.

INTERVENTION/EVALUATION

Risk for hypoglycemia occurs within first 3 hrs following drug administration if given concurrently with insulin. Assess for hypoglycemia (diaphoresis, tremors, dizziness, anxiety, headache, tachycardia, numbness in mouth, hunger, diplopia, difficulty concentrating). Be alert to conditions that alter glucose requirements (fever, increased activity, stress, surgical procedures).

PATIENT/FAMILY TEACHING

• Diabetes mellitus requires lifelong control. • Prescribed diet, exercise are principal parts of treatment; do not skip/delay meals. • Continue to adhere to dietary instructions, regular exercise program, regular testing of serum glucose. • When taking combination drug therapy, have source of glucose available to treat symptoms of low blood sugar.

Prandin, *see repaglinide*

prasugrel

pra-soo-grel
(Effient)

BLACK BOX ALERT Serious, sometimes fatal, hemorrhage may occur.

Do not confuse prasugrel with praziquantel, or Effient with Effexor.

◆ CLASSIFICATION

PHARMACOTHERAPEUTIC: Thienopyridine derivative inhibitor. **CLINICAL:** Antiplatelet agent.

ACTION

Inhibits binding of the enzyme adenosine phosphate (ADP) to its platelet receptor and subsequent ADP-mediated activation of a glycoprotein complex. **Therapeutic Effect:** Inhibits platelet aggregation.

PHARMACOKINETICS

Rapidly absorbed, with peak concentration occurring 30 min following administration. Undergoes extensive hepatic metabolism. Protein binding: 98%. Eliminated primarily in urine, with a lesser amount excreted in feces. **Half-life:** 7 hrs.

USES

Reduction of thrombotic cardiovascular events (MI, CVA, stent thrombosis) in pts with acute coronary syndrome (unstable angina, non–ST-segment elevation MI, ST-segment MI) who are to be managed with percutaneous coronary intervention (PCI).

PRECAUTIONS

Contraindications: Active bleeding, prior transient ischemic attack (TIA), CVA. **Cautions:** Pts who undergo coronary artery bypass graft (CABG) after receiving prasugrel, those at risk for bleeding (age 75 yrs or older, body weight less than 60 kg, recent trauma/surgery, recent GI bleeding or active peptic ulcer disease, severe hepatic impairment).

⧗ LIFESPAN CONSIDERATIONS

Pregnancy/Lactation: Unknown if drug crosses placenta or is distributed in breast milk. **Pregnancy Category B. Children:** Safety and efficacy not established. **Elderly:** May have increased risk for intracranial hemorrhage; caution advised in pts 75 yrs and older.

INTERACTIONS

DRUG: Aspirin, NSAIDs, warfarin may increase risk of bleeding. **HERBAL: Cat's claw, dong quai, evening primrose, feverfew, garlic, ginger, ginseng, green tea, horse chestnut, red clover** may have additive platelet effects. **Ginkgo biloba** may increase risk of bleeding. **FOOD:** None known. **LAB VALUES:** May decrease Hgb, Hct, WBC, platelet count. May increase bleeding time, serum cholesterol, AST, ALT.

AVAILABILITY (Rx)

Tablets: 5 mg, 10 mg.

ADMINSTRATION/HANDLING

PO

• Give without regard to food. • Do not crush tablet.

INDICATIONS/ROUTES/DOSAGE

Acute Coronary Syndrome

◀ALERT▶ Consider 5 mg once daily for pts weighing less than 60 kg.

PO: ADULTS, ELDERLY: Initially, 60-mg loading dose, then 10 mg once daily (in combination with aspirin).

SIDE EFFECTS

Occasional (8%–4%): Hypertension, headache, back pain, dyspnea, nausea, dizziness. **Rare (less than 4%):** Cough, hypotension, fatigue, non-cardiac chest pain, bradycardia, rash, pyrexia, peripheral edema, extremity pain, minor bleeding, diarrhea.

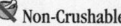

P

ADVERSE EFFECTS/ TOXIC REACTIONS

Major bleeding (intracranial hemorrhage, epistaxis, GI bleeding, hemoptysis, subcutaneous hematoma, postprocedural hemorrhage, retroperitoneal hemorrhage, retinal hemorrhage) has been reported. Severe thrombocytopenia, anemia, abnormal hepatic function, anaphylactic reaction, angioedema, atrial fibrillation occur rarely. Overdosage may require platelet transfusion to restore clotting ability.

NURSING CONSIDERATIONS

BASELINE ASSESSMENT

Obtain baseline vital signs, CBC, platelet count, EKG, hepatic function tests.

INTERVENTION/EVALUATION

Monitor vital signs for changes in B/P, pulse. Assess for signs of unusual bleeding or hemorrhage, pain. Monitor CBC, platelet count, hepatic function tests, EKG for changes from baseline.

PATIENT/FAMILY TEACHING

• It may take longer to stop minor bleeding during drug therapy. Report unusual bleeding/bruising, blood noted in stool or urine, chest/back pain, extremity pain. • Monitor for dyspnea. • Report fever, weakness, extreme skin paleness, purple skin patches, yellowing of skin or eyes, changes in mental status. • Do not discontinue drug therapy without physician approval. • Inform physicians, dentists before undergoing any invasive procedure or surgery.

P

Pravachol, *see pravastatin*

pravastatin

pra-vah-sta-tin
(Apo-Pravastatin ✤, Novo-Pravastatin ✤, Pravachol)

Do not confuse pravastatin with nystatin or pitavastatin, or Pravachol with Prevacid, Prinivil, or propranolol.

FIXED-COMBINATION(S)

Pravigard: pravastatin/aspirin (anticoagulant): 20 mg/81 mg, 40 mg/81 mg, 80 mg/81 mg, 20 mg/325 mg, 40 mg/325 mg, 80 mg/325 mg.

◆CLASSIFICATION

PHARMACOTHERAPEUTIC: Hydroxymethylglutaryl CoA (HMG-CoA) reductase inhibitor. **CLINICAL:** Antihyperlipidemic (see p. 58C).

ACTION

Interferes with cholesterol biosynthesis by preventing conversion of HMG-CoA reductase to mevalonate, a precursor to cholesterol. **Therapeutic Effect:** Lowers LDL, VLDL cholesterol, plasma triglycerides; increases HDL.

PHARMACOKINETICS

Rapidly absorbed from GI tract. Protein binding: 50%. Metabolized in liver (minimal active metabolites). Primarily excreted in feces via biliary system. Not removed by hemodialysis. **Half-life:** 2–3 hrs.

USES

Treatment of hyperlipidemias to reduce total cholesterol, LDL cholesterol, apolipoprotein B, triglycerides; increase HDL cholesterol. Primary preventive therapy to reduce risk of recurrent MI, myocardial revascularization procedures, stroke, transient ischemic attack (TIA) in pts with previous MI and normal cholesterol levels. Secondary prevention of coronary events in pts with established coronary artery disease (CAD) to slow progression of coronary atherosclerosis. Treatment of heterozygous familial hypercholesterolemia in pediatric pts 8–18 yrs.

PRECAUTIONS

Contraindications: Active hepatic disease or unexplained, persistent elevations of hepatic function test results. **Cautions:** History of hepatic disease, substantial alcohol consumption. Withholding/discontinuing pravastatin may be necessary when pt is at risk for renal failure secondary to rhabdomyolysis. Severe metabolic, endocrine, electrolyte disorders.

LIFESPAN CONSIDERATIONS

Pregnancy/Lactation: Contraindicated in pregnancy (suppression of cholesterol biosynthesis may cause fetal toxicity) and lactation. Unknown if drug is distributed in breast milk, but there is risk of serious adverse reactions in breast-feeding infants. **Pregnancy Category X. Children:** Safety and efficacy not established. **Elderly:** No age-related precautions noted.

INTERACTIONS

DRUG: **Cyclosporine, erythromycin, gemfibrozil, immunosuppressants, niacin** increase risk of acute renal failure, rhabdomyolysis. **HERBAL:** **St. John's wort** may decrease concentration. **FOOD:** **Red yeast rice** contains 2.4 mg **lovastatin** per 600 mg rice. **LAB VALUES:** May increase serum creatine kinase (CK), transaminase.

AVAILABILITY (Rx)

Tablets: 10 mg, 20 mg, 40 mg, 80 mg.

ADMINISTRATION/HANDLING

PO

• Give without regard to meals. • Administer in evening.

INDICATIONS/ROUTES/DOSAGE

ALERT Prior to initiating therapy, pt should be on standard cholesterol-lowering diet for 3–6 mos. Low-cholesterol diet should be continued throughout pravastatin therapy.

Usual Dosage

PO: ADULTS, ELDERLY: Initially, 40 mg/day. Titrate to desired response. Range: 10–80 mg/day. **CHILDREN 14–18 YRS:** 40 mg/day. **CHILDREN 8–13 YRS:** 20 mg/day.

Dosage in Hepatic/Renal Impairment

For adults, give 10 mg/day initially. Titrate to desired response.

SIDE EFFECTS

Pravastatin is generally well tolerated. Side effects are usually mild and transient. **Occasional (7%–4%):** Nausea, vomiting, diarrhea, constipation, abdominal pain, headache, rhinitis, rash, pruritus. **Rare (3%–2%):** Heartburn, myalgia, dizziness, cough, fatigue, flu-like symptoms, depression, photosensitivity.

ADVERSE EFFECTS/ TOXIC REACTIONS

Potential for malignancy, cataracts. Hypersensitivity, myopathy occur rarely. Rhabdomyolysis has been reported.

NURSING CONSIDERATIONS

BASELINE ASSESSMENT

Obtain dietary history, esp. fat consumption. Question for possibility of pregnancy before initiating therapy (Pregnancy Category X). Assess baseline serum lab results (cholesterol, triglycerides, hepatic function tests).

INTERVENTION/EVALUATION

Monitor serum cholesterol, triglyceride lab results for therapeutic response. Monitor hepatic function tests, CPK. Monitor daily pattern of bowel activity and stool consistency. Check for headache, dizziness (provide assistance as needed). Assess for rash, pruritus. Be alert for malaise, muscle cramping/weakness; if accompanied by fever, may require discontinuation of medication.

PATIENT/FAMILY TEACHING

• Follow special diet (important part of treatment). • Periodic lab tests are essential part of therapy. • Report promptly any muscle pain/weakness, esp. if accompanied by fever, malaise. • Avoid

P

tasks that require alertness, motor skills until response to drug is established (potential for dizziness). • Use nonhormonal contraception. • Avoid direct exposure to sunlight.

prazosin

pra-zoe-sin
(Apo-Prazo, Minipress, Novo-Prazin)
Do not confuse prazosin with prednisone.

◆ CLASSIFICATION

PHARMACOTHERAPEUTIC: Alpha-adrenergic blocker. **CLINICAL:** Antihypertensive, antidote, vasodilator (see p. 60C).

ACTION

Selectively blocks $alpha_1$-adrenergic receptors, decreasing peripheral vascular resistance. **Therapeutic Effect:** Produces vasodilation of veins, arterioles; decreases total peripheral resistance; relaxes smooth muscle in bladder neck, prostate.

PHARMACOKINETICS

Route	Onset	Peak	Duration
PO (B/P reduction)	2 hrs	2–4 hrs	10–24 hrs

Well absorbed following PO administration. Protein binding: 92%–97%. Metabolized in liver. Primarily excreted in feces. **Half-life:** 2–4 hrs.

USES

Treatment of mild to moderate hypertension. Used alone or in combination with other antihypertensives. **OFF-LABEL:** Treatment of benign prostate hyperplasia, CHF, ergot alkaloid toxicity, pheochromocytoma, Raynaud's phenomenon, post-traumatic stress disorder.

PRECAUTIONS

Contraindications: Hypersensitivity to quinazolines. **Cautions:** Chronic renal failure, hepatic impairment.

⌛ LIFESPAN CONSIDERATIONS

Pregnancy/Lactation: Unknown if drug crosses placenta; is distributed in breast milk. **Pregnancy Category C. Children:** Safety and efficacy not established. **Elderly:** May be more sensitive to hypotensive effects.

INTERACTIONS

DRUG: **NSAIDs** may decrease effects. **Antihypertensives, diuretics, hypotension-producing medications** may increase effects. **HERBAL:** **Ephedra, ginseng, yohimbe** may worsen hypertension. Avoid **saw palmetto. Garlic** may increase antihypertensive effect. **Licorice** causes sodium and water retention, potassium loss. **FOOD:** None known. **LAB VALUES:** None significant.

AVAILABILITY (Rx)

Capsules: 1 mg, 2 mg, 5 mg.

ADMINISTRATION/HANDLING

PO

• Give without regard to food. • Administer first dose at bedtime (minimizes risk of fainting due to "first-dose syncope").

INDICATIONS/ROUTES/DOSAGE

Hypertension

PO: ADULTS, ELDERLY: Initially, 1 mg 2–3 times a day. Maintenance: 3–15 mg/day in divided doses. **Maximum:** 20 mg/day. **CHILDREN:** Initially, 0.05–0.1 mg/kg/day in 3 divided doses. **Maximum:** 0.5 mg/kg/day or 20 mg.

SIDE EFFECTS

Frequent (10%–7%): Dizziness, drowsiness, headache, asthenia (loss of strength, energy). **Occasional (5%–4%):** Palpitations, nausea, dry mouth, nervousness. **Rare (less than 1%):** Angina, urinary urgency.

ADVERSE EFFECTS/ TOXIC REACTIONS

First-dose syncope (hypotension with sudden loss of consciousness) may occur 30–90 min following initial dose of more than 2 mg, too-rapid increase in dosage, addition of another antihypertensive agent to therapy. May be preceded by tachycardia (pulse rate of 120–160 beats/min).

NURSING CONSIDERATIONS

BASELINE ASSESSMENT

Give first dose at bedtime. If initial dose is given during daytime, pt must remain recumbent for 3–4 hrs. Assess B/P, pulse immediately before each dose and q15–30min until stabilized (be alert to B/P fluctuations).

INTERVENTION/EVALUATION

Monitor B/P, pulse diligently (first-dose syncope may be preceded by tachycardia). Monitor daily pattern of bowel activity and stool consistency. Assist with ambulation if dizziness occurs.

PATIENT/FAMILY TEACHING

• Avoid tasks that require alertness, motor skills until response to drug is established. • Use caution when rising from sitting or lying position. • Report continued dizziness, palpitations.

*prednisoLONE

pred-**niss**-oh-lone
(Millipred, Novo-Prednisolone ✦, Orapred, Orapred ODT, Pediapred, Pred Forte, Pred Mild, Prelone)
Do not confuse Pediapred with Pediazole, prednisolone with prednisone or primidone, or Prelone with Prozac.

FIXED-COMBINATION(S)

Blephamide: prednisolone/sulfacetamide (an anti-infective): 0.2%/10%. **Vasocidin:** prednisolone/sulfacetamide: 0.25%/10%.

◆CLASSIFICATION

PHARMACOTHERAPEUTIC: Adrenal corticosteroid. **CLINICAL:** Glucocorticoid (see pp. 98C, 140C).

ACTION

Inhibits accumulation of inflammatory cells at inflammation sites, phagocytosis, lysosomal enzyme release/synthesis, release of mediators of inflammation. **Therapeutic Effect:** Prevents/suppresses cell-mediated immune reactions. Decreases/prevents tissue response to inflammatory process.

PHARMACOKINETICS

Protein binding: 65%–91%. Metabolized in liver. Excreted in urine. **Half-life:** 3.6 hrs.

USES

Substitution Therapy in Deficiency States: Acute or chronic adrenal insufficiency, congenital adrenal hyperplasia, adrenal insufficiency secondary to pituitary insufficiency. **Nonendocrine Disorders:** Allergic, collagen, intestinal tract, hepatic, ocular, renal, skin diseases; bronchial asthma; arthritis; rheumatic carditis; cerebral edema; malignancies. **Ophthalmic:** Treatment of conjunctivitis, corneal injury (from chemical/thermal burns, foreign body).

PRECAUTIONS

Contraindications: Acute superficial herpes simplex keratitis, systemic fungal infections, varicella. **Cautions:** Hyperthyroidism, cirrhosis, ocular herpes simplex, peptic ulcer disease, osteoporosis, myasthenia gravis, hypertension, CHF, ulcerative colitis, thromboembolic disorders.

⌛ LIFESPAN CONSIDERATIONS

Pregnancy/Lactation: Crosses placenta. Distributed in breast milk. Fetal cleft palate often occurs with chronic,

P

first-trimester use. Breast-feeding not recommended. **Pregnancy Category C (D if used in first trimester). Children:** Prolonged treatment or high dosages may decrease short-term growth rate, cortisol secretion. **Elderly:** May be more susceptible to developing hypertension or osteoporosis.

INTERACTIONS

DRUG: **Amphotericin** may worsen hypokalemia. May increase risk of **digoxin** toxicity (due to hypokalemia). May decrease effects of **diuretics, insulin, oral hypoglycemics, potassium supplements. Hepatic enzyme inducers** may decrease effects. **Live virus vaccines** increase vaccine side effects, potentiate virus replication, decrease pt's antibody response to vaccine. HERBAL: **St. John's wort** may decrease concentration. **Cat's claw, echinacea** have immunostimulant properties. FOOD: None known. LAB VALUES: May increase serum glucose, lipids, sodium, uric acid. May decrease serum calcium, WBC, hypothalamic, pituitary adrenal (HPA) axis function, potassium.

AVAILABILITY (Rx)

Solution, Ophthalmic: 1%. **Solution, Oral (Orapred):** 15 mg/5 ml. **(Pediapred):** 5 mg/5 ml. **(Millipred):** 10 mg/5 ml. **Suspension, Ophthalmic: (Pred Forte)** 1%; **(Pred Mild)** 0.12%. **Syrup (Prelone):** 5 mg/5 ml, 15 mg/5 ml. **Tablets:** 5 mg.

Tablets, Orally-Disintegrating: 10 mg, 15 mg, 30 mg.

ADMINISTRATION/HANDLING

PO

• Give with food or fluids.

Orally-Disintegrating Tablets

• Do not cut, split, break or use partial tablets. • Remove from blister just prior to giving, place on tongue. • May swallow whole or allow to dissolve in mouth with/without water.

Ophthalmic

• For ophthalmic solution, shake well before using. • Instill drops into conjunctival sac, as prescribed. • Avoid touching applicator tip to conjunctiva to avoid contamination.

INDICATIONS/ROUTES/DOSAGE

Usual Dosage

PO: ADULTS, ELDERLY: 5–60 mg/day in divided doses. CHILDREN: 0.1–2 mg/kg/day in 1–4 divided doses.

Treatment of Conjunctivitis, Corneal Injury

OPHTHALMIC: ADULTS, ELDERLY: 1–2 drops every hr during day and q2h during night. After response, decrease dosage to 1 drop q4h, then 1 drop 3–4 times a day.

SIDE EFFECTS

Frequent: Insomnia, heartburn, nervousness, abdominal distention, diaphoresis, acne, mood swings, increased appetite, facial flushing, delayed wound healing, increased susceptibility to infection, diarrhea, constipation. **Occasional:** Headache, edema, change in skin color, frequent urination. **Rare:** Tachycardia, allergic reaction (rash, urticaria), psychological changes, hallucinations, depression. **Ophthalmic:** Stinging/burning, posterior subcapsular cataracts.

ADVERSE EFFECTS/ TOXIC REACTIONS

LONG-TERM THERAPY: Hypocalcemia, hypokalemia, muscle wasting (esp. arms, legs) osteoporosis, spontaneous fractures, amenorrhea, cataracts, glaucoma, peptic ulcer, CHF. **ABRUPT WITHDRAWAL FOLLOWING LONG-TERM THERAPY:** Anorexia, nausea, fever, headache, severe/sudden joint pain, rebound inflammation, fatigue, weakness, lethargy, dizziness, orthostatic hypotension. Sudden discontinuance may be fatal.

NURSING CONSIDERATIONS

BASELINE ASSESSMENT

Obtain baselines for height, weight, B/P, serum glucose, electrolytes. Check results of initial tests (tuberculosis [TB] skin test, X-rays, EKG). Never give live virus vaccine (e.g., smallpox).

INTERVENTION/EVALUATION

Monitor B/P, weight, serum electrolytes, glucose, results of bone mineral density test, height, weight in children. Be alert to infection (sore throat, fever, vague symptoms); assess oral cavity daily for signs of candida infection (white patches, painful tongue/mucous membranes).

PATIENT/FAMILY TEACHING

• Notify physician if fever, sore throat, muscle aches, sudden weight gain, swelling, loss of appetite, fatigue occurs. • Avoid alcohol, limit caffeine. • Do not abruptly discontinue without physician's approval. • Avoid exposure to chickenpox, measles.

*predniSONE

pred-ni-sone
(Apo-Prednisone ♣, Novo-Prednisone ♣, Prednisone Intensol, Sterapred, Sterapred DS, Winpred ♣)
Do not confuse prednisone with prazosin, prednisolone, Prilosec, primidone, or promethazine.

◆ CLASSIFICATION

PHARMACOTHERAPEUTIC: Adrenal corticosteroid. **CLINICAL:** Glucocorticoid (see p. 98C).

ACTION

Inhibits accumulation of inflammatory cells at inflammation sites, phagocytosis, lysosomal enzyme release/synthesis, release of mediators of inflammation. **Therapeutic Effect:** Prevents/suppresses cell-mediated immune reactions. Decreases/prevents tissue response to inflammatory process.

PHARMACOKINETICS

Well absorbed from GI tract. Protein binding: 70%–90%. Widely distributed. Metabolized in liver, converted to prednisolone. Primarily excreted in urine. Not removed by hemodialysis. **Half-life:** 2.5–3.5 hrs.

USES

Substitution Therapy in Deficiency States: Acute or chronic adrenal insufficiency, congenital adrenal hyperplasia, adrenal insufficiency secondary to pituitary insufficiency. **Nonendocrine Disorders:** Arthritis; rheumatic carditis; allergic, collagen, intestinal tract, liver, ocular, renal, skin diseases; bronchial asthma; cerebral edema; malignancies. **OFF-LABEL:** Prevention of postherpetic neuralgia, relief of acute pain.

PRECAUTIONS

Contraindications: Acute superficial herpes simplex keratitis, systemic fungal infections, varicella. **Cautions:** Hyperthyroidism, cirrhosis, ocular herpes simplex, peptic ulcer disease, osteoporosis, myasthenia gravis, hypertension, CHF, ulcerative colitis, thromboembolic disorders.

⌛ LIFESPAN CONSIDERATIONS

Pregnancy/Lactation: Crosses placenta. Distributed in breast milk. Fetal cleft palate often occurs with chronic, first trimester use. Breast-feeding not recommended. **Pregnancy Category C (D if used in first trimester). Children:** Prolonged treatment or high dosages may decrease short-term growth rate, cortisol secretion. **Elderly:** May be more susceptible to developing hypertension or osteoporosis.

INTERACTIONS

DRUG: **Antacids** may decrease absorption, effect. **Amphotericin** may increase hypokalemia. May increase risk of **digoxin** toxicity (due to hypokalemia). May decrease effects of **diuretics, insulin, oral hypoglycemics, potassium supplements. Hepatic enzyme inducers** may decrease effects. **Live virus vaccines** may increase vaccine side effects, potentiate virus replication, de-

P

crease pt's antibody response to vaccine. **HERBAL:** **St. John's wort** may decrease concentration. **Cat's claw, echinacea** have immunostimulant properties. **FOOD:** None known. **LAB VALUES:** May increase serum glucose, lipids, sodium, uric acid. May decrease serum calcium, potassium, WBC, hypothalamic pituitary adrenal (HPA) axis function.

AVAILABILITY (Rx)

Solution, Oral: 1 mg/ml. **Solution, Oral Concentrate (Prednisone Intensol):** 5 mg/ml. **Tablets:** 1 mg, 2.5 mg, 5 mg, 10 mg, 20 mg, 50 mg.

ADMINISTRATION/HANDLING

PO

• Give with food or fluids. • Give single doses before 9 AM, multiple doses at evenly spaced intervals.

INDICATIONS/ROUTES/DOSAGE

Usual Dosage

PO: ADULTS, ELDERLY: 5–60 mg/day in divided doses. **CHILDREN:** 0.05–2 mg/kg/day in 1–4 divided doses.

SIDE EFFECTS

Frequent: Insomnia, heartburn, nervousness, abdominal distention, diaphoresis, acne, mood swings, increased appetite, facial flushing, delayed wound healing, increased susceptibility to infection, diarrhea, constipation. **Occasional:** Headache, edema, change in skin color, frequent urination. **Rare:** Tachycardia, allergic reaction (rash, urticaria), psychological changes, hallucinations, depression.

ADVERSE EFFECTS/ TOXIC REACTIONS

LONG-TERM THERAPY: Muscle wasting (esp. in arms, legs), osteoporosis, spontaneous fractures, amenorrhea, cataracts, glaucoma, peptic ulcer, CHF. **ABRUPT WITHDRAWAL FOLLOWING LONG-TERM THERAPY:** Anorexia, nausea, fever, headache, rebound inflammation, fatigue, weakness, lethargy, dizziness, orthostatic hypotension. Sudden discontinuance may be fatal.

NURSING CONSIDERATIONS

BASELINE ASSESSMENT

Obtain baselines for height, weight, B/P, serum glucose, electrolytes. Check results of initial tests (tuberculosis [TB] skin test, X-rays, EKG). Never give live virus vaccine (e.g., smallpox).

INTERVENTION/EVALUATION

Monitor B/P, serum electrolytes, glucose, results of bone mineral density test, height, weight in children. Be alert to infection (sore throat, fever, vague symptoms); assess oral cavity daily for signs of candida infection (white patches, painful tongue/mucous membranes).

PATIENT/FAMILY TEACHING

• Notify physician if fever, sore throat, muscle aches, sudden weight gain, swelling, loss of appetite, or fatigue occurs. • Avoid alcohol, minimize use of caffeine. • Do not abruptly discontinue without physician's approval. • Avoid exposure to chickenpox, measles.

pregabalin

pre-**gab**-ah-lin
(Lyrica)
Do not confuse Lyrica with Lopressor.

◆CLASSIFICATION

CLINICAL: Anticonvulsant, antineuralgic, analgesic **(Schedule V).**

ACTION

Binds to calcium channel sites in CNS tissue, inhibiting excitatory neurotransmitter release. Exerts antinociceptive, anticonvulsant activity. **Therapeutic Effect:** Decreases symptoms of painful peripheral neuropathy; decreases frequency of partial seizures.

PHARMACOKINETICS

Well absorbed following PO administration. Eliminated in urine unchanged. **Half-life:** 6 hrs.

USES

Adjunctive therapy in treatment of partial-onset seizures. Management of neuropathic pain associated with diabetic peripheral neuropathy. Management of postherpetic neuralgia. Management of fibromyalgia.

PRECAUTIONS

Contraindications: None known. Cautions: CHF, renal impairment.

⌛ LIFESPAN CONSIDERATIONS

Pregnancy/Lactation: Increased risk of fetal skeletal abnormalities. Unknown if distributed in breast milk. **Pregnancy Category C. Children:** Safety and efficacy not established. **Elderly:** Age-related renal impairment may require dosage adjustment.

INTERACTIONS

DRUG: **Alcohol, barbiturates, narcotic analgesics, other sedative agents** may increase sedative effect. Additive effects on weight gain, edema with **pioglitazone, rosiglitazone.** HERBAL: **Gotu kola, kava kava, St. John's wort, valerian** may increase CNS depression. FOOD: None known. LAB VALUES: May increase CPK. May cause mild PR interval prolongation. May decrease platelet count.

AVAILABILITY (Rx)

Capsules (Lyrica): 25 mg, 50 mg, 75 mg, 100 mg, 150 mg, 200 mg, 225 mg, 300 mg.

ADMINISTRATION/HANDLING

• Give without regard to food. • Do not open/crush capsule.

INDICATIONS/ROUTES/DOSAGE

Partial-Onset Seizures

PO: ADULTS, ELDERLY: Initially, 75 mg twice a day or 50 mg 3 times a day. **Maximum:** 600 mg/day.

Neuropathic Pain

PO: ADULTS, ELDERLY: Initially, 50 mg 3 times a day. **Maximum:** 300 mg/day, based on efficacy and tolerability.

Postherpetic Neuralgia

PO: ADULTS, ELDERLY: Initially, 75 mg twice a day or 50 mg 3 times a day. May increase to 300 mg/day within 1 wk. May further increase to 600 mg/day after 2–4 wks. **Maximum:** 600 mg/day.

Fibromyalgia

PO: ADULTS, ELDERLY: Initially, 75 mg twice a day. May increase to 150 mg twice a day within one wk. **Maximum:** 225 mg twice a day.

Dosage in Renal Impairment

◄ALERT► Dosage based on renal function and daily dosage.

Creatinine Clearance	Daily Dosage
30–60 ml/min	75–300 mg in 2–3 divided doses
15–29 ml/min	25–150 mg in 1 or 2 doses
Less than 15 ml/min	25–75 mg once daily

Dosage for Hemodialysis

◄ALERT► Take supplemental dose immediately following dialysis.

Daily Dosage	Supplemental Dosage
25 mg	Single dose of 25 mg or 50 mg
25–50 mg	Single dose of 50 mg or 75 mg
75 mg	Single dose of 100 mg or 150 mg

SIDE EFFECTS

Frequent (32%–12%): Dizziness, drowsiness, ataxia, peripheral edema. Occasional (12%–5%): Weight gain, blurred vision, diplopia, difficulty with concentration, attention, cognition; tremor, dry mouth, headache, constipation, asthenia (loss of strength, energy). Rare (4%–2%): Abnormal gait, confusion, incoordination, twitching, flatulence, vomiting, edema, myopathy.

ADVERSE EFFECTS/ TOXIC REACTIONS

Abrupt withdrawal increases risk of seizure frequency in pts with seizure disorders; withdraw gradually over a minimum of 1 wk.

NURSING CONSIDERATIONS

BASELINE ASSESSMENT

Seizure: Review history of seizure disorder (type, onset, intensity, frequency, duration, LOC). **Pain:** Assess onset, type, location, and duration of pain.

INTERVENTION/EVALUATION

Provide safety measures as needed. Assess for seizure activity. Assess for clinical improvement; record onset of relief of pain. Assess for evidence of peripheral edema behind medial malleolus (usually first area of edema). Question for changes in visual acuity.

PATIENT/FAMILY TEACHING

• Do not abruptly stop taking drug because seizure frequency may be increased. • Do not drive, operate machinery, perform activities requiring mental acuity due to potential dizziness, drowsiness, ataxia. • Avoid alcohol. • Carry identification card, bracelet to note anticonvulsant therapy.

Premarin, *see conjugated estrogens*

Prempro, *see conjugated estrogens and medroxyprogesterone*

Prevacid, *see lansoprazole*

Prilosec, *see omeprazole*

Primacor, *see milrinone*

Primaxin, *see imipenem/cilastatin*

primidone

pri-mi-done
(Apo-Primidone ✤, Mysoline)
Do not confuse primidone with prednisone.

◆ CLASSIFICATION

PHARMACOTHERAPEUTIC: Barbiturate. **CLINICAL:** Anticonvulsant (see p. 36C).

ACTION

Decreases motor activity from electrical/chemical stimulation, stabilizes seizure threshold against hyperexcitability. **Therapeutic Effect:** Reduces seizure activity.

PHARMACOKINETICS

Rapidly, usually completely absorbed following PO administration. Protein binding: 99%. Extensively metabolized in liver to phenobarbital and phenylethylmalonamide (PEMA). Minimal excretion in urine. **Half-life:** 10–12 hrs.

USES

Management of partial seizures with complex symptomatology (psychomotor seizures), generalized tonic-clonic (grand mal) seizures, focal seizures. **OFF-LABEL:** Treatment of essential tremor.

PRECAUTIONS

Contraindications: History of bronchopneumonia, hypersensitivity to phenobarbital, porphyria. **Cautions:** Renal/hepatic impairment.

LIFESPAN CONSIDERATIONS

Pregnancy/Lactation: Crosses placenta; distributed in breast milk. **Pregnancy Category D. Children, Elderly:** May produce paradoxical excitement, restlessness.

INTERACTIONS

DRUG: Alcohol, other CNS depressants may increase effects. May increase metabolism of **carbamazepine.** May decrease effects of **glucosteroids, metronidazole, oral anticoagulants, quinidine, tricyclic antidepressants. MAOIs** may prolong effects. **Valproic acid** increases concentration, risk of toxicity. **HERBAL: Evening primrose** may decrease seizure threshold. **Gotu kola, kava kava, St. John's wort, valerian** may increase CNS depression. **FOOD:** None known. **LAB VALUES:** May decrease serum bilirubin. **Therapeutic serum level:** 4–12 mcg/ml; **toxic serum level:** greater than 12 mcg/ml.

AVAILABILITY (Rx)

Tablets: 50 mg, 250 mg.

INDICATIONS/ROUTES/DOSAGE

Seizure Control

PO: ADULTS, ELDERLY, CHILDREN 8 YRS AND OLDER: Initially, 125–250 mg/day at bedtime. May increase by 125–250 mg/day every 3–7 days. Usual dose: 750–1,500 mg/day. **Maximum:** 2 g/day. **CHILDREN YOUNGER THAN 8 YRS:** Initially, 50–125 mg/day at bedtime. May increase by 50–125 mg/day every 3–7 days. Usual dose: 10–25 mg/kg/day in divided doses. **NEONATES:** 12–20 mg/kg/day in divided doses 2–4 times a day.

Dosage Interval in Renal Impairment

Creatine Clearance	Interval
50–80 ml/min	q8h
10–49 ml/min	q8–12h
<10 ml/min	q12–24h

SIDE EFFECTS

Frequent: Ataxia, dizziness. **Occasional:** Anorexia, drowsiness, altered mental status, nausea, vomiting, paradoxical excitement. **Rare:** Rash.

ADVERSE EFFECTS/ TOXIC REACTIONS

Abrupt withdrawal after prolonged therapy may produce effects ranging from markedly increased dreaming, nightmares, insomnia, tremor, diaphoresis, vomiting to hallucinations, delirium, seizures, status epilepticus. Skin eruptions may appear as hypersensitivity reaction. Blood dyscrasias, hepatic disease, hypocalcemia occur rarely. Overdose produces cold/clammy skin, hypothermia, severe CNS depression, followed by high fever, coma.

NURSING CONSIDERATIONS

BASELINE ASSESSMENT

Review history of seizure disorder (intensity, frequency, duration, LOC). Observe frequently for recurrence of seizure activity. Initiate seizure precautions.

INTERVENTION/EVALUATION

Monitor for changes in behavior, depression, suicidal ideation. Monitor serum primidone concentrations; CBC; neurologic status (frequency, duration, severity of seizures). Monitor for **therapeutic serum level:** 4–12 mcg/ml; **toxic serum level:** more than 12 mcg/ml.

PATIENT/FAMILY TEACHING

• Do not abruptly discontinue medication after long-term use (may precipitate seizures). • Strict maintenance of drug therapy is essential for seizure control. • Drowsiness usually disappears during continued therapy. • If dizziness occurs, change positions slowly from recumbent to sitting position before standing. • Avoid tasks that require alertness, motor skills until response to drug is established. • Avoid alcohol. • Notify physician if depression, thoughts of suicide occur.

P

Prinivil, *see lisinopril*

probenecid

pro-**ben**-e-sid
(Benuryl)
Do not confuse probenecid with procainamide or Procanbid.

CLASSIFICATION

PHARMACOTHERAPEUTIC: Uricosuric. **CLINICAL:** Antigout.

ACTION

Competitively inhibits reabsorption of uric acid at proximal convoluted tubule. Inhibits renal tubular secretion of weak organic acids (e.g., penicillins). **Therapeutic Effect:** Promotes uric acid excretion, reduces serum uric acid level, increases plasma levels of penicillins, cephalosporins.

PHARMACOKINETICS

Rapidly, completely absorbed following PO administration. Extensively metabolized in liver. Excreted in urine. Excretion is dependent upon urinary pH, is increased in alkaline urine. **Half-life:** 6–12 hrs.

USES

Treatment of hyperuricemia associated with gout, gouty arthritis. Adjunctive therapy with penicillins, cephalosporins to elevate/prolong antibiotic plasma levels.

PRECAUTIONS

Contraindications: Blood dyscrasias, children younger than 2 yrs, concurrent high-dose aspirin therapy, severe renal impairment, uric acid calculi. **Cautions:** Peptic ulcer, hematuria, renal colic.

LIFESPAN CONSIDERATIONS

Pregnancy/Lactation: Unknown if drug crosses placenta or is distributed in breast milk. **Pregnancy Category C. Children:** Safety and efficacy not established in those younger than 2 yrs. **Elderly:** No age-related precautions noted.

INTERACTIONS

DRUG: Increases effect, toxicity of **methotrexate.** Increases concentration of **cephalosporins, ketorolac, NSAIDs.** **HERBAL:** None significant. **FOOD:** None known. **LAB VALUES:** May inhibit renal excretion of serum PSP (phenolsulfonphthalein), 17-ketosteroids, BSP (sulfobromophthalein).

AVAILABILITY (Rx)

Tablets: 500 mg.

ADMINISTRATION/HANDLING

PO

- Give with or immediately after meals, milk.
- Instruct pt to drink at least 6–8 glasses (8 oz) of water/day (prevents kidney stone development).

INDICATIONS/ROUTES/DOSAGE

Gout

PO: ADULTS, ELDERLY: Initially, 250 mg twice daily for 1 wk, then 500 mg twice daily. May increase by 500 mg q4wks. **Maximum:** 2–3 g/day. Maintenance: Dosage that maintains normal uric acid level.

Adjunct to Penicillin, Cephalosporin Therapy

PO: ADULTS, ELDERLY, CHILDREN OLDER THAN 14 YRS: 2 g/day in 4 divided doses. **CHILDREN 2–14 YRS:** Initially, 25 mg/kg. Maintenance: 40 mg/kg/day in 4 divided doses. **Maximum:** 500 mg dose.

Dosage in Renal Impairment

Creatinine clearance less than 30 ml/min: Avoid use.

SIDE EFFECTS

Frequent (10%–6%): Headache, anorexia, nausea, vomiting. **Occasional (5%–1%):** Lower back or side pain, rash, urticaria, pruritus, dizziness, flushed face, urinary urgency, gingivitis.

ADVERSE EFFECTS/ TOXIC REACTIONS

Severe hypersensitivity reactions, including anaphylaxis, occur rarely (usually within few hrs after administration following previous use); discontinue drug immediately, contact physician. Pruritic maculopapular rash should be considered a toxic reaction. May be accompanied by malaise, fever, chills, arthralgia, nausea, vomiting, leukopenia, aplastic anemia.

NURSING CONSIDERATIONS

BASELINE ASSESSMENT

Do not initiate therapy until acute gouty attack has subsided. Question for hypersensitivity to probenecid or if taking penicillin, cephalosporin antibiotics.

INTERVENTION/EVALUATION

If exacerbation of gout recurs after therapy, use other agents for gout. Discontinue medication immediately if rash, other evidence of allergic reaction appears. Encourage high fluid intake (3,000 ml/day). Monitor I&O (output should be at least 2,000 ml/day). Assess CBC, serum uric acid levels. Assess urine for cloudiness, unusual color, odor. Assess for therapeutic response (reduced joint tenderness, swelling, redness, limitation of motion).

PATIENT/FAMILY TEACHING

• Drink plenty of fluids to decrease risk of uric acid kidney stones. • Avoid alcohol, large doses of aspirin, other salicylates. • Consume low-purine food (reduce/omit meat, fowl, fish; use eggs, cheese, vegetables). Foods high in purine: kidney, liver, sweetbreads, sardines, anchovies, meat extracts. • May take over 1 wk for full therapeutic effect. • Drink 6–8 glasses (8 oz) of fluid daily while on medication.

procainamide HIGH ALERT

pro-**cane**-ah-mide
(Apo-Procainamide ✤, Procanbid, Procan-SR, Pronestyl-SR ✤)

BLACK BOX ALERT Prolonged use results in positive ANA tests in 50% of pts, may lead to lupus erythematosus-like syndrome. Agranulocytosis, neutropenia, hypoplastic anemia, thrombocytopenia reported; 20%–25% mortality with agranulocytosis.

Do not confuse Procanbid with probenecid, or Pronestyl with Ponstel.

◆ CLASSIFICATION

CLINICAL: Antiarrhythmic (see p. 16C).

ACTION

Increases electrical stimulation threshold of ventricles, His-Purkinje system. Decreases myocardial excitability, conduction velocity; depresses myocardial contractility. Exerts direct cardiac effects. **Therapeutic Effect:** Suppresses arrhythmias.

PHARMACOKINETICS

Rapidly, completely absorbed from GI tract. Protein binding: 15%–20%. Widely distributed. Metabolized in liver to active metabolite. Primarily excreted in urine. Removed by hemodialysis. **Half-life:** 2.5–4.5 hrs; metabolite, 6–8 hrs.

USES

Prophylactic therapy to maintain normal sinus rhythm after conversion of atrial fibrillation/flutter. Treatment of premature ventricular contractions, paroxysmal atrial tachycardia, atrial fibrillation, ventricular tachycardia. **OFF-LABEL:** Conversion, management of atrial fibrillation.

PRECAUTIONS

Contraindications: Complete heart block, myasthenia gravis, preexisting QT prolongation, second-degree heart block,

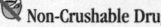

P

systemic lupus erythematosus, torsade de pointes. **Cautions:** Marked AV conduction disturbances, bundle-branch block, severe digoxin toxicity, CHF, supraventricular tachyarrhythmias, renal/hepatic impairment.

LIFESPAN CONSIDERATIONS

Pregnancy/Lactation: Crosses placenta. Unknown if distributed in breast milk. **Pregnancy Category C. Children:** No age-related precautions noted. **Elderly:** More susceptible to hypotensive effect. Age-related renal impairment may require dosage adjustment.

INTERACTIONS

DRUG: May increase effects of **antihypertensives (IV procainamide), neuromuscular blockers. Other antiarrhythmics, pimozide** may increase cardiac effects. **HERBAL: Ephedra** may worsen arrhythmias. **FOOD:** None known. **LAB VALUES:** May cause EKG changes, positive ANA titers, Coombs' test. May increase AST, ALT, serum alkaline phosphatase, bilirubin, LDH. **Therapeutic serum level:** 4–8 mcg/ml; **toxic serum level:** greater than 10 mcg/ml.

P

AVAILABILITY (Rx)

Injection Solution: 100 mg/ml, 500 mg/ml.

ADMINISTRATION/HANDLING

IV, IM

◀ALERT▶ May give by IM injection, IV push, IV infusion.

Reconstitution • For IV push, dilute with 5–10 ml D_5W. Maximum concentration: 20 mg/ml. • For initial loading infusion, add 1 g to 50 ml D_5W to provide concentration of 20 mg/ml. • For IV infusion, add 1 g to 250–500 ml D_5W to provide concentration of 2–4 mg/ml. Maximum concentration: 4 g/250 ml.

Rate of administration • For IV push, with pt in supine position, administer at rate not exceeding 25–50 mg/min. • For initial loading infusion, infuse 1 ml/min for up to 25–30 min. • For IV infusion, infuse at 1–3 ml/min. • Check B/P q5–10 min during infusion. If fall in B/P exceeds 15 mm Hg, discontinue drug, contact physician. Notify physician of any significant interval changes. • B/P, EKG should be monitored continuously during IV administration and rate of infusion adjusted to eliminate arrhythmias.

Storage • Solution appears clear, colorless to light yellow. • Discard if solution darkens or is discolored or if precipitate forms. • When diluted with 0.9% NaCl or D_5W, solution is stable for 24 hrs at room temperature, for 7 days if refrigerated.

IV INCOMPATIBILITY

Milrinone (Primacor).

IV COMPATIBILITIES

Amiodarone (Cordarone), dobutamine (Dobutrex), heparin, lidocaine, potassium chloride.

INDICATIONS/ROUTES/DOSAGE

Management of Arrhythmias

IV: ADULTS, ELDERLY: Loading dose: 50–100 mg. May repeat q5–10min or 15–18 mg/kg given as slow infusion over 25–30 min (**Maximum:** 1–1.5 g). Maintenance infusion: 3–4 mg/min. Range: 1–6 mg/min. **CHILDREN:** Loading dose: 3–6 mg/kg over 5 min (**Maximum:** 100 mg). May repeat q5–10min to maximum total dose of 15 mg/kg. Maintenance dose: 20–80 mcg/kg/min. **Maximum:** 2 g/day.

SIDE EFFECTS

Frequent: Transient, but at times, marked hypotension. **Rare:** Confusion, mental depression, psychosis.

ADVERSE EFFECTS/ TOXIC REACTIONS

Paradoxical, extremely rapid ventricular rate may occur during treatment of atrial fibrillation/flutter. Systemic lupus erythematosus-like syndrome (fever, myalgia, pleuritic chest pain) may occur with prolonged therapy. Cardiotoxic effects occur most commonly with IV administration and appear as conduction changes (50% widening of QRS complex, frequent ventricular premature contractions, ventricular tachycardia, complete AV block). Prolonged PR and QT intervals, flattened T waves occur less frequently.

NURSING CONSIDERATIONS

BASELINE ASSESSMENT

Check B/P, pulse for 1 full min (unless pt is on continuous monitor) before giving medication.

INTERVENTION/EVALUATION

Check B/P q5–10 min during infusion. If fall in B/P exceeds 15 mm/Hg, discontinue drug, contact physician. Monitor EKG for cardiac changes, particularly widening of QRS, prolongation of PR and QT intervals. Assess pulse for strength/weakness, irregular rate. Monitor I&O, serum electrolyte levels (potassium, chloride, sodium). Assess for complaints of GI upset, headache, arthralgia. Monitor daily pattern of bowel activity, stool consistency. Assess for dizziness. Assess skin for evidence of hypersensitivity reaction (esp. in pts on high-dose therapy). Monitor for therapeutic serum level. **Therapeutic serum level:** 4–8 mcg/ml; **toxic serum level:** greater than 10 mcg/ml.

procarbazine HIGH ALERT

pro-**car**-bah-zeen
(Matulane, Natulan ✦)

BLACK BOX ALERT Must be administered by personnel trained in administration/handling of chemotherapeutic agents.

Do not confuse procarbazine with dacarbazine.

◆CLASSIFICATION

PHARMACOTHERAPEUTIC: Methylhydrazine derivative. **CLINICAL:** Antineoplastic (see p. 87C).

ACTION

Inhibits DNA, RNA, protein synthesis. May directly damage DNA. Cell cycle–phase specific for S phase of cell division. **Therapeutic Effect:** Causes cell death.

PHARMACOKINETICS

Rapidly, completely absorbed from GI tract. Crosses blood-brain barrier. Metabolized primarily in liver, kidneys. Excreted in urine, feces. **Half-life:** 1 hr.

USES

Treatment of Hodgkin's disease. **OFF-LABEL:** Treatment of lung carcinoma, malignant melanoma, multiple myeloma, non-Hodgkin's lymphoma, polycythemia vera, primary brain tumors.

PRECAUTIONS

Contraindications: Myelosuppression. **Cautions:** Renal/hepatic impairment.

⌛ LIFESPAN CONSIDERATIONS

Pregnancy/Lactation: Unknown if distributed in breast milk. May cause fetal harm. **Pregnancy Category D. Children:** Safety and efficacy not established. **Elderly:** Age-related renal impairment may require dosage adjustment.

INTERACTIONS

DRUG: **Alcohol** may cause disulfiram-like reaction. May increase anticholinergic effects of **anticholinergics, antihistamines. Bone marrow depressants** may increase myelosuppression. **Buspirone, caffeine-containing medications** may increase B/P. **Carbamazepine, cyclobenzaprine, MAOIs, maprotiline** may cause hyperpyretic crisis, seizures, death. **CNS depressants** may increase CNS depression. May increase effects of **insulin, oral antidiabetics. Meperidine** may produce coma, seizures, immediate excitation, rigidity, severe hypertension/hypotension, severe respiratory distress, diaphoresis, vascular collapse. **Sympathomimetics** may increase cardiac stimulant, vasopressor effects. **Tricyclic antidepres-**

P

sants may increase anticholinergic effects; may cause seizures, hyperpyretic crisis. **Live virus vaccines** may potentiate virus replication, increase vaccine side effects, decrease pt's antibody response to vaccine. HERBAL: None significant. FOOD: **Caffeine** may increase B/P. **Foods containing tyramine** may cause clinically severe (possibly life-threatening) hypertension. LAB VALUES: None significant.

AVAILABILITY (Rx)

Capsules: 50 mg.

ADMINISTRATION/HANDLING

PO

- Administer with food or immediately after meals.

INDICATIONS/ROUTES/DOSAGE

◀ALERT▶ Base dosage on ideal body weight.

Advanced Hodgkin's Disease

PO: ADULTS, ELDERLY: Initially, 2–4 mg/kg/day as single dose or in divided doses for 1 wk, then 4–6 mg/kg/day. Maintenance: 1–2 mg/kg/day. **CHILDREN:** 50–100 mg/m²/day for 10–14 days of a 28-day cycle. Continue until maximum response occurs, leukocyte count falls below 4,000/mm³, or platelet count falls below 100,000/mm³. Maintenance: 1–2 mg/kg/day.

SIDE EFFECTS

Frequent: Severe nausea, vomiting, respiratory disorders (cough, effusion), myalgia, arthralgia, drowsiness, nervousness, insomnia, nightmares, diaphoresis, hallucinations, seizures. Occasional: Hoarseness, tachycardia, nystagmus, retinal hemorrhage, photophobia, photosensitivity, urinary frequency, nocturia, hypotension, diarrhea, stomatitis, paresthesia, unsteadiness, confusion, decreased reflexes, foot drop. Rare: Hypersensitivity reaction (dermatitis, pruritus, rash, urticaria), hyperpigmentation, alopecia.

ADVERSE EFFECTS/ TOXIC REACTIONS

Major toxic effects are myelosuppression manifested as hematologic toxicity (principally leukopenia, thrombocytopenia, anemia), hepatotoxicity manifested as jaundice, ascites. UTIs secondary to leukopenia may occur.

NURSING CONSIDERATIONS

BASELINE ASSESSMENT

Obtain bone marrow tests, Hgb, Hct, leukocyte, differential, reticulocyte, platelet, urinalysis, serum transaminase, alkaline phosphatase, BUN results before therapy and periodically thereafter. Therapy should be interrupted if WBC falls below 4,000/mm³ or platelet count falls below 100,000/mm³.

INTERVENTION/EVALUATION

Monitor hematologic status, renal/hepatic function studies. Assess for stomatitis. Monitor for hematologic toxicity (fever, sore throat, signs of local infection, unusual bruising/bleeding from any site), symptoms of anemia (excessive fatigue, weakness).

PATIENT/FAMILY TEACHING

- Inform physician of fever, sore throat, bleeding, bruising. • Avoid alcohol (may cause disulfiram reaction: nausea, vomiting, headache, sedation, visual disturbances).

prochlorperazine

pro-klor-**per**-a-zeen
(Apo-Prochlorperazine 🍁, Compazine, Compro, Stemetil 🍁)

BLACK BOX ALERT Increased risk for death in elderly with dementia-related psychosis.

Do not confuse Compazine with Copaxone or Coumadin, or prochlorperazine with chlorpromazine.

◆CLASSIFICATION

PHARMACOTHERAPEUTIC: Phenothiazine. **CLINICAL:** Antiemetic.

ACTION

Acts centrally to inhibit/block dopamine receptors in chemoreceptor trigger zone, peripherally to block vagus nerve in GI tract. Therapeutic Effect: Relieves nausea/vomiting, improves psychosis.

PHARMACOKINETICS

Route	Onset*	Peak	Duration
PO	30–40 min	N/A	3–4 hrs
IM	10–20 min	N/A	4–6 hrs
Rectal	60 min	N/A	12 hrs

*As an antiemetic.

Variably absorbed after PO administration. Widely distributed. Metabolized in liver, GI mucosa. Primarily excreted in urine. Unknown if removed by hemodialysis. Half-life: **PO:** 3–5 hrs, **IV:** 7 hrs.

USES

Management of nausea/vomiting. Treatment of acute or chronic psychosis. OFF-LABEL: Behavior syndromes in dementia, headache. Psychosis/agitation related to Alzheimer's dementia.

PRECAUTIONS

Contraindications: Narrow-angle glaucoma, CNS depression, coma, myelosuppression, severe cardiac/hepatic impairment, severe hypotension/hypertension. Cautions: Seizures, Parkinson's disease, children younger than 2 yrs.

⌛ LIFESPAN CONSIDERATIONS

Pregnancy/Lactation: Crosses placenta. Distributed in breast milk. **Pregnancy Category C. Children:** Safety and efficacy not established in those weighing less than 9 kg or younger than 2 yrs. **Elderly:** More susceptible to orthostatic hypotension, anticholinergic effects (e.g., dry mouth), sedation, extrapyramidal symptoms (EPS); lower dosage recommended.

INTERACTIONS

DRUG: **Alcohol, other CNS depressants** may increase CNS, respiratory depression, hypotensive effects. **Antihypertensives** may increase hypotension. **Antithyroid agents** may increase risk of agranulocytosis. **Extrapyramidal symptom (EPS)–producing medications** may increase EPS. May decrease effects of **levodopa. Lithium** may decrease absorption, produce adverse neurologic effects. **MAOIs, tricyclic antidepressants** may increase anticholinergic, sedative effects. HERBAL: **Dong quai, St. John's wort** may increase photosensitization. **Gotu kola, kava kava, St. John's wort, valerian** may increase CNS depression. FOOD: None known. LAB VALUES: None significant.

AVAILABILITY (Rx)

Injection Solution (Compazine): 5 mg/ml. Suppositories (Compazine, Compro): 25 mg. Tablets (Compazine): 5 mg, 10 mg.

ADMINISTRATION/HANDLING

IV

Rate of administration • May give by IV push slowly. Maximum rate: 5 mg/min. **Storage** • Store at room temperature. • Protect from light. • Clear or slightly yellow solutions may be used.

PO

• Should be administered with food or water.

Rectal

• Moisten suppository with cold water before inserting well into rectum.

IV INCOMPATIBILITIES

Atropine, furosemide (Lasix), hydrocortisone, hydromorphone (Dilaudid), midazolam (Versed).

IV COMPATIBILITIES

Calcium gluconate, diphenhydramine (Benadryl), fentanyl, glycopyrrolate (Robi-

P

nul), heparin, morphine, metoclopramide (Reglan), nalbuphine (Nubain), potassium chloride, promethazine (Phenergan), propofol (Diprivan).

INDICATIONS/ROUTES/DOSAGE

Nausea/Vomiting

PO: ADULTS, ELDERLY: 5–10 mg 3–4 times a day. **CHILDREN:** 0.4 mg/kg/day in 3–4 divided doses.
IV: ADULTS, ELDERLY: 2.5–10 mg. May repeat q3–4h.
IM: ADULTS, ELDERLY: 5–10 mg q3–4h. **CHILDREN:** 0.1–0.15 mg/kg/dose q8–12h. **Maximum:** 40 mg/day.
RECTAL: ADULTS, ELDERLY: 25 mg twice a day.

Psychosis

PO: ADULTS, ELDERLY: 5–10 mg 3–4 times a day. **Maximum:** 150 mg/day. **CHILDREN 2–12 YRS:** 2.5 mg 2–3 times a day. **Maximum Daily Dose:** 25 mg for children 6–12 yrs; 20 mg for children 2–5 yrs.
IM: ADULTS, ELDERLY: 10–20 mg q4h. **CHILDREN:** 0.13 mg/kg/dose.

SIDE EFFECTS

Frequent: Drowsiness, hypotension, dizziness, fainting (commonly occurring after first dose, occasionally after subsequent doses, rarely with oral form). **Occasional:** Dry mouth, blurred vision, lethargy, constipation, diarrhea, myalgia, nasal congestion, peripheral edema, urinary retention.

ADVERSE EFFECTS/ TOXIC REACTIONS

Extrapyramidal symptoms (EPS) appear dose related and are divided into three categories: akathisia (inability to sit still, tapping of feet), parkinsonian symptoms (mask-like face, tremors, shuffling gait, hypersalivation), acute dystonias (torticollis [neck muscle spasm], opisthotonos [rigidity of back muscles], oculogyric crisis [rolling back of eyes]). Dystonic reaction may produce diaphoresis, pallor. Tardive dyskinesia (tongue protrusion, puffing of cheeks, puckering of mouth) occurs rarely and may be irreversible. Abrupt withdrawal after long-term therapy may precipitate nausea, vomiting, gastritis, dizziness, tremors. Blood dyscrasias, particularly agranulocytosis, mild leukopenia, may occur. May lower seizure threshold.

NURSING CONSIDERATIONS

BASELINE ASSESSMENT

Avoid skin contact with solution (contact dermatitis). **Antiemetic:** Assess for dehydration (poor skin turgor, dry mucous membranes, longitudinal furrows in tongue). **Antipsychotic:** Assess behavior, appearance, emotional status, response to environment, speech pattern, thought content.

INTERVENTION/EVALUATION

Monitor B/P for hypotension. Assess for EPS. Monitor WBC, differential count for blood dyscrasias. Monitor for fine tongue movement (may be early sign of tardive dyskinesia). Supervise suicidal-risk pt closely during early therapy (as depression lessens, energy level improves, increasing suicide potential). Assess for therapeutic response (interest in surroundings, improvement in self-care, increased ability to concentrate, relaxed facial expression).

PATIENT/FAMILY TEACHING

• Limit caffeine. • Avoid alcohol. • Avoid tasks requiring alertness, motor skills until response to drug is established (may cause drowsiness, impairment).

Procrit, *see epoetin alfa*

see epoetin alfa

progesterone

pro-**jes**-ter-one
(Crinone, Endometrin Vaginal Insert, Prochieve, Prometrium)

BLACK BOX ALERT Not to be used to prevent coronary heart disease. Risk of dementia may be increased in postmenopausal women.

◆CLASSIFICATION

PHARMACOTHERAPEUTIC: Progestin. **CLINICAL:** Hormone.

ACTION

Promotes mammary gland development, relaxes uterine smooth muscle. **Therapeutic Effect:** Decreases abnormal uterine bleeding; transforms endometrium from proliferative to secretory in estrogen-primed endometrium.

PHARMACOKINETICS

Protein binding: 96%–99%. Metabolized in liver. Excreted in bile, urine. **Half-life (vaginal gel):** 5–20 min.

USES

PO: Prevent endometrial hyperplasia, secondary amenorrhea. **IM:** Amenorrhea, abnormal uterine bleeding. **Vaginal Gel (8%):** Treatment of infertility. **Vaginal Insert:** Support of embryo implantation and early pregnancy. **OFF-LABEL:** Treatment of corpus luteum dysfunction.

PRECAUTIONS

Contraindications: Allergy to peanut oil (oral), breast cancer, history of active cerebral apoplexy, thromboembolic disorders, thrombophlebitis, missed abortion, severe hepatic dysfunction, undiagnosed vaginal bleeding, use as a pregnancy test. **Cautions:** Diabetes, conditions aggravated by fluid retention (e.g., asthma, epilepsy, migraine, cardiac/renal dysfunction), history of mental depression.

LIFESPAN CONSIDERATIONS

Pregnancy/Lactation: Distributed in breast milk. Avoid use during pregnancy. **Pregnancy Category B (Prometrium).** None established for vaginal gel, vaginal insert, or injection. **Children:** Safety and efficacy not established. **Elderly:** No age-related precautions noted.

INTERACTIONS

DRUG: **Carbamazepine, phenobarbital, phenytoin, rifampin** may decrease effects of progesterone. **HERBAL:** **Red clover** may decrease effect. **FOOD:** None known. **LAB VALUES:** May alter HDL, cholesterol, triglycerides, LDL. May increase hepatic function tests.

AVAILABILITY (Rx)

Capsules (Prometrium): 100 mg, 200 mg. **Injection Oil:** 50 mg/ml. **Vaginal Gel (Crinone):** 8% (90 mg/dose). **(Prochieve):** 4% (45 mg/dose). **Vaginal Insert (Endometrin Vaginal Insert):** 100 mg.

ADMINISTRATION/HANDLING

IM

• Store at room temperature. • Administer only deep IM in large muscle mass.

PO

• If given in morning, administer 2 hrs after breakfast.

Vaginal Gel

• Remove applicator from sealed wrapper. Do not remove twist-off tab at this time. • Hold applicator by thick end. Shake down several times like a thermometer to ensure contents are at thin end. • Hold applicator by flat section of thick end and twist off tab at other end. Do not squeeze thick end while twisting tab (could force some gel to be released before insertion). • Insert applicator into vagina either in sitting position or lying on back with knees bent. • Insert thin end well into vagina. • Squeeze thick end of applicator to deposit gel. • Remove applicator, discard.

INDICATIONS/ROUTES/DOSAGE

Amenorrhea

PO: ADULTS: 400 mg daily in evening for 10 days.

IM: ADULTS: 5–10 mg for 6–8 days. Withdrawal bleeding expected in 48–72 hrs if ovarian activity produced proliferative endometrium.

VAGINAL: ADULTS: Apply 45 mg (4% gel) every other day for 6 or fewer doses.

Abnormal Uterine Bleeding
IM: ADULTS: 5–10 mg/day for 6 days. When estrogen given concomitantly, begin progesterone after 2 wks of estrogen therapy; discontinue when menstrual flow begins.

Prevention of Endometrial Hyperplasia
PO: ADULTS: 200 mg in evening for 12 days per 28-day cycle in combination with daily conjugated estrogen.

Infertility
VAGINAL: ADULTS: 90 mg (8% gel) once a day (twice a day in women with partial or complete ovarian failure). May continue up to 10–12 wks.

Support of Embryo/Early Pregnancy
VAGINAL INSERT: 100 mg 2–3 times a day for up to 10 wks.

SIDE EFFECTS

Frequent: Breakthrough bleeding/spotting at beginning of therapy, amenorrhea, change in menstrual flow, breast tenderness. **Gel:** Drowsiness. Occasional: Edema, weight gain/loss, rash, pruritus, photosensitivity, skin pigmentation. Rare: Pain/swelling at injection site, acne, depression, alopecia, hirsutism.

ADVERSE EFFECTS/ TOXIC REACTIONS

Thrombophlebitis, cerebrovascular disorders, retinal thrombosis, pulmonary embolism occur rarely.

NURSING CONSIDERATIONS

BASELINE ASSESSMENT

Question for possibility of pregnancy, hypersensitivity to progestins before initiating therapy. Obtain baseline weight, serum glucose level, B/P.

INTERVENTION/EVALUATION

Check weight daily; report weekly gain over 5 lbs. Assess skin for rash, urticaria. Immediately report development of chest pain, sudden shortness of breath, sudden decrease in vision, migraine headache, pain (esp. with swelling, warmth, redness) in calves, numbness of arm/leg (thrombotic disorders). Check B/P periodically. Note progesterone therapy on pathology specimens.

PATIENT/FAMILY TEACHING

• Use sunscreen, protective clothing to protect from sunlight, ultraviolet light until tolerance determined. • Notify physician of abnormal vaginal bleeding, other symptoms. • Stop taking medication, contact physician at once if pregnancy suspected. • If using vaginal gel, avoid tasks that require alertness, motor skills until response to drug is established.

Prograf, *see tacrolimus*

Proleukin, *see aldesleukin*

promethazine

proe-**meth**-a-zeen
(Phenadoz, Phenergan, Promethegan)

BLACK BOX ALERT Fatalities due to respiratory depression reported in children 2 yrs and younger. Severe tissue injury, including gangrene, may occur with intravenous injection (preferred route is deep intramuscular). Be alert for signs and symptoms of tissue injury including burning or pain at injection site, phlebitis, swelling, blistering. Risk reduced by diluting promethazine with 10–20 ml 0.9% NaCl or diluting in a mini-bag (piggyback); administer slowly over 10–15 min; use large veins or central venous site (no hand or wrist veins).

Do not confuse promethazine with chlorpromazine or prednisone.

FIXED-COMBINATION(S)

Phenergan with codeine: promethazine/codeine (a cough suppressant):

6.25 mg/10 mg/5 ml. **Phenergan VC:** promethazine/phenylephrine (a vasoconstrictor): 6.25 mg/5 mg/5 ml. **Phenergan VC with codeine:** promethazine/phenylephrine/codeine: 6.25 mg/5 mg/10 mg/5 ml.

◆CLASSIFICATION

PHARMACOTHERAPEUTIC: Phenothiazine. **CLINICAL:** Antihistamine, antiemetic, sedative-hypnotic (see p. 55C).

ACTION

Antihistamine: Inhibits histamine at histamine receptor sites. **Antiemetic:** Diminishes vestibular stimulation, depresses labyrinthine function, acts on chemoreceptor trigger zone. **Sedative-hypnotic:** Produces CNS depression by decreasing stimulation to brain stem reticular formation. Therapeutic Effect: Prevents allergic responses mediated by histamine (urticaria, pruritus). Prevents, relieves nausea/vomiting. Produces mild sedative effect.

PHARMACOKINETICS

Route	Onset	Peak	Duration
PO	20 min	N/A	2–8 hrs
IV	3–5 min	N/A	2–8 hrs
IM	20 min	N/A	2–8 hrs
Rectal	20 min	N/A	2–8 hrs

Well absorbed from GI tract after IM administration. Protein binding: 83%. Widely distributed. Metabolized in liver. Primarily excreted in urine. Not removed by hemodialysis. Half-life: 9–16 hrs.

USES

Treatment of allergic conditions, motion sickness, nausea, vomiting. May be used as mild sedative.

PRECAUTIONS

Contraindications: Narrow-angle glaucoma, children 2 yrs and younger (may cause fatal respiratory depression), GI/GU obstruction, hypersensitivity to phenothiazines, severe CNS depression, coma. **Cautions:** Cardiovascular/hepatic impairment, asthma, peptic ulcer, history of seizures, sleep apnea, pts suspected of Reye's syndrome.

⌛ LIFESPAN CONSIDERATIONS

Pregnancy/Lactation: Readily crosses placenta. Unknown if drug is distributed in breast milk. May inhibit platelet aggregation in neonates if taken within 2 wks of birth. May produce jaundice, extrapyramidal symptoms (EPS) in neonates if taken during pregnancy. **Pregnancy Category C. Children:** May experience increased excitement. Not recommended for those younger than 2 yrs. **Elderly:** More sensitive to dizziness, sedation, confusion, hypotension, hyperexcitability, anticholinergic effects (e.g., dry mouth).

INTERACTIONS

DRUG: Alcohol, CNS depressants may increase CNS depressant effects. **Anticholinergics** may increase anticholinergic effects. **MAOIs** may prolong, intensify anticholinergic, CNS depressant effects. **HERBAL: Gotu kola, kava kava, St. John's wort, valerian** may increase CNS depression. **FOOD:** None known. **LAB VALUES:** May suppress wheal/flare reactions to antigen skin testing unless discontinued 4 days before testing.

AVAILABILITY (Rx)

Injection Solution (Phenergan): 25 mg/ml, 50 mg/ml. **Suppositories (Phenadoz, Phenergan, Promethegan):** 12.5 mg, 25 mg, 50 mg. **Syrup (Phenergan):** 6.25 mg/5 ml. **Tablets (Phenergan):** 12.5 mg, 25 mg, 50 mg.

ADMINISTRATION/HANDLING

◀ALERT▶ IM is preferred route; avoid IV if possible. Significant tissue necrosis may occur if given subcutaneously. Inadvertent intra-arterial injection may produce severe arteriospasm, resulting in severe circulation impairment.

IV

Reconstitution • Dilute with 10–20 ml 0.9% NaCl or prepare minibag.

Rate of administration • Administer slowly over 10–15 min. • Use large vein or central venous site (no hand or wrist veins). • Too-rapid rate of infusion may result in transient fall in B/P, producing orthostatic hypotension, reflex tachycardia, serious tissue injury.

Storage • Store at room temperature.

IM

• Inject deep IM.

PO

• Give with food or fluids to reduce GI distress. • Scored tablets may be crushed.

Rectal

• Refrigerate suppository. • Moisten suppository with cold water before inserting well into rectum.

IV INCOMPATIBILITIES

Allopurinol (Aloprim), amphotericin B complex (Abelcet, AmBisome, Amphotec), heparin, ketorolac (Toradol), nalbuphine (Nubain), piperacillin and tazobactam (Zosyn).

IV COMPATIBILITIES

Atropine, diphenhydramine (Benadryl), glycopyrrolate (Robinul), hydromorphone (Dilaudid), hydroxyzine (Vistaril), meperidine (Demerol), midazolam (Versed), morphine, prochlorperazine (Compazine).

INDICATIONS/ROUTES/DOSAGE

ALERT Contraindicated in children 2 yrs and younger.

Allergic Symptoms

PO: ADULTS, ELDERLY: 6.25–12.5 mg 3 times a day plus 25 mg at bedtime. **CHILDREN:** 0.1 mg/kg/dose (**Maximum:** 12.5 mg) 3 times a day plus 0.5 mg/kg/dose (**Maximum:** 25 mg) at bedtime.

IV, IM: ADULTS, ELDERLY: 6.25–25 mg. May repeat in 2 hrs.

Motion Sickness

PO: ADULTS, ELDERLY: 25 mg 30–60 min before departure; may repeat in 8–12 hrs, then every morning on rising and before evening meal. **CHILDREN:** 0.5 mg/kg 30–60 min before departure; may repeat in 8–12 hrs, then every morning on rising and before evening meal. **Maximum:** 25 mg twice a day.

Prevention of Nausea/Vomiting

PO, IV, IM, RECTAL: ADULTS, ELDERLY: 6.25–25 mg q4–6h as needed. **CHILDREN:** 0.25–1 mg/kg q4–6h as needed.

Preop/Postop Sedation, Adjunct to Analgesics

IV, IM: ADULTS, ELDERLY: 25–50 mg. **CHILDREN:** 12.5–25 mg. **Maximum:** 25 mg/dose.

Sedative

PO, IV, IM, RECTAL: ADULTS, ELDERLY: 25–50 mg/dose. May repeat q4–6h as needed. **CHILDREN:** 0.5–1 mg/kg/dose q6h as needed. **Maximum:** 50 mg/dose.

SIDE EFFECTS

Expected: Drowsiness, disorientation; hypotension, confusion, syncope in elderly. **Frequent:** Dry mouth, nose, throat; urinary retention; thickening of bronchial secretions. **Occasional:** Epigastric distress, flushing, visual disturbances, hearing disturbances, wheezing, paresthesia, diaphoresis, chills. **Rare:** Dizziness, urticaria, photosensitivity, nightmares.

ADVERSE EFFECTS/ TOXIC REACTIONS

Paradoxical reaction (particularly in children) manifested as excitation, anxiety, tremor, hyperactive reflexes, seizures. Long-term therapy may produce extrapyramidal symptoms (EPS) noted as dystonia (abnormal movements), pronounced motor restlessness (most frequently in children), parkinsonism (esp. noted in elderly). Blood dyscrasias, particularly agranulocytosis, occur rarely.

NURSING CONSIDERATIONS

BASELINE ASSESSMENT

Assess allergy symptoms. Assess B/P, pulse for bradycardia, tachycardia if pt is given parenteral form. If used as antiemetic, assess for dehydration (poor skin turgor, dry mucous membranes, longitudinal furrows in tongue).

INTERVENTION/EVALUATION

Monitor serum electrolytes in pts with severe vomiting. Assist with ambulation if drowsiness, light-headedness occurs. Monitor for relief of nausea, vomiting, allergic symptoms.

PATIENT/FAMILY TEACHING

• Drowsiness, dry mouth may be expected response to drug. • Avoid tasks that require alertness, motor skills until response to drug is established. • Sugarless gum, sips of tepid water may relieve dry mouth. • Coffee, tea may help reduce drowsiness. • Report visual disturbances, involuntary movements, restlessness. • Avoid alcohol, other CNS depressants. • Avoid prolonged exposure to sunlight.

Prometrium, *see progesterone*

propafenone

proe-**pa**-fen-one
(Rythmol, Rythmol SR)

BLACK BOX ALERT Mortality or nonfatal cardiac arrest rate (7.7%) in asymptomatic non–life-threatening ventricular arrhythmia pts with recent MI (more than 6 days but less than 2 years prior) reported.

◆ CLASSIFICATION

CLINICAL: Antiarrhythmic (see p. 17C).

ACTION

Decreases fast sodium current in Purkinje/myocardial cells. Decreases excitability, automaticity; prolongs conduction velocity, refractory period. **Therapeutic Effect:** Suppresses arrhythmias.

PHARMACOKINETICS

Nearly completely absorbed following PO administration. Protein binding: 85%–97%. Metabolized in liver; undergoes first-pass metabolism. Primarily excreted in feces. **Half-life:** 2–10 hrs.

USES

Treatment of documented, life-threatening ventricular arrhythmias (e.g., sustained ventricular tachycardias). **Rythmol SR:** Maintenance of normal sinus rhythm in pts with symptomatic atrial fibrillation. **OFF-LABEL:** Treatment of supraventricular arrhythmias.

PRECAUTIONS

Contraindications: Bradycardia; bronchospastic disorders; cardiogenic shock; electrolyte imbalance; sinoatrial, AV, intraventricular impulse generation or conduction disorders (e.g., sick sinus syndrome, AV block) without pacemaker; uncontrolled CHF. **Cautions:** Renal/hepatic impairment, recent MI, CHF, conduction disturbances.

⧖ LIFESPAN CONSIDERATIONS

Pregnancy/Lactation: Unknown if drug crosses placenta or is distributed in breast milk. **Pregnancy Category C. Children:** Safety and efficacy not established. **Elderly:** No age-related precautions noted.

INTERACTIONS

DRUG: **Amiodarone** may affect conduction, repolarization. May increase **digoxin** concentration. May increase **warfarin** effects. **HERBAL:** **St. John's wort** may decrease concentration, effect. **Ephedra** may worsen arrhythmias. **FOOD:** None known. **LAB VALUES:** May cause EKG changes (e.g., QRS widening,

P

PR interval prolongation), positive ANA titers.

AVAILABILITY (Rx)

Tablets (Rythmol): 150 mg, 225 mg, 300 mg.

Capsules (Extended-Release [Rythmol SR]): 225 mg, 325 mg, 425 mg.

ADMINISTRATION/HANDLING

PO

- May take without regard to meals.
- Swallow capsules whole; do not open, crush, chew.

INDICATIONS/ROUTES/DOSAGE

Documented, Life-Threatening Ventricular Arrhythmias (Sustained Ventricular Tachycardia)

PO: ADULTS, ELDERLY: Initially, 150 mg q8h. May increase at 3- to 4-day intervals to 225 mg q8h, then to 300 mg q8h. **Maximum:** 900 mg/day.

PO (EXTENDED-RELEASE): ADULTS, ELDERLY: Initially, 225 mg q12h. May increase at 5-day intervals. **Maximum:** 425 mg q12h.

SIDE EFFECTS

Frequent (13%–7%): Dizziness, nausea, vomiting, altered taste, constipation. Occasional (6%–3%): Headache, dyspnea, blurred vision, dyspepsia (heartburn, indigestion, epigastric pain). Rare (less than 2%): Rash, weakness, dry mouth, diarrhea, edema, hot flashes.

ADVERSE EFFECTS/ TOXIC REACTIONS

May produce/worsen existing arrhythmias. Overdose may produce hypotension, drowsiness, bradycardia, atrioventricular conduction disturbances.

NURSING CONSIDERATIONS

BASELINE ASSESSMENT

Correct electrolyte imbalance before administering medication.

INTERVENTION/EVALUATION

Assess pulse for quality, irregular rate. Monitor EKG for cardiac performance or changes, particularly widening of QRS, prolongation of PR interval. Question for visual disturbances, headache, GI upset. Monitor fluid, serum electrolyte levels. Monitor daily pattern of bowel activity, stool consistency. Assess for dizziness, unsteadiness. Monitor hepatic enzymes results. Monitor for therapeutic serum level (0.06–1 mcg/ml).

PATIENT/FAMILY TEACHING

- Compliance with therapy regimen is essential to control arrhythmias. • Altered taste sensation may occur. • Report headache, blurred vision. • Avoid tasks that require alertness, motor skills until response to drug is established.

propofol

HIGH ALERT

pro-poe-fall
(Diprivan)

Do not confuse Diprivan with Diflucan or Ditropan, or propofol with fospropofol.

CLASSIFICATION

PHARMACOTHERAPEUTIC: Rapid-acting general anesthetic. **CLINICAL:** Sedative-hypnotic (see p. 5C).

ACTION

Inhibits sympathetic vasoconstrictor nerve activity; decreases vascular resistance. **Therapeutic Effect:** Produces hypnosis rapidly.

PHARMACOKINETICS

Route	Onset	Peak	Duration
IV	40 sec	N/A	3–10 min

Rapidly, extensively distributed. Protein binding: 97%–99%. Metabolized in liver.

Primarily excreted in urine. Unknown if removed by hemodialysis. **Half-life:** 3–12 hrs.

USES

Induction/maintenance of anesthesia. Continuous sedation in intubated and respiratory controlled adult pts in ICU. **OFF-LABEL:** Postop antiemetic, refractory delirium tremens, conscious sedation.

PRECAUTIONS

Contraindications: Impaired cerebral circulation, increased ICP. **Cautions:** Debilitated; impaired respiratory, circulatory, renal, hepatic, lipid metabolism disorders; history of epilepsy, seizure disorder.

LIFESPAN CONSIDERATIONS

Pregnancy/Lactation: Unknown if drug crosses placenta. Distributed in breast milk. Not recommended for obstetrics, breast-feeding mothers. **Pregnancy Category B. Children:** Safety and efficacy not established. FDA approved for use in those 2 mos and older. **Elderly:** No age-related precautions noted; lower dosages recommended.

INTERACTIONS

DRUG: **Alcohol, CNS depressants** may increase CNS, respiratory depression, hypotensive effects. **HERBAL:** None significant. **FOOD:** None known. **LAB VALUES:** None significant.

AVAILABILITY (Rx)

Injection Emulsion: 10 mg/ml.

ADMINISTRATION/HANDLING

IV

◄ALERT► Do not give through same IV line with blood or plasma.

Reconstitution • May give undiluted, or dilute only with D_5W. • Do not dilute to concentration less than 2 mg/ml (4 ml D_5W to 1 ml propofol yields 2 mg/ml).

Rate of administration • Too-rapid IV may produce marked severe hypotension, respiratory depression, irregular muscular movements. • Observe for signs of intra-arterial injection (pain, discolored skin patches, white or blue color to peripheral IV site area, delayed onset of drug action).

Storage • Store at room temperature. • Discard unused portions. • Do not use if emulsion separates. • Shake well before using.

IV INCOMPATIBILITIES

Amikacin (Amikin), amphotericin B complex (Abelcet, AmBisome, Amphotec), bretylium (Bretylol), calcium chloride, ciprofloxacin (Cipro), diazepam (Valium), digoxin (Lanoxin), doxorubicin (Adriamycin), gentamicin (Garamycin), methylprednisolone (Solu-Medrol), minocycline (Minocin), phenytoin (Dilantin), tobramycin (Nebcin), verapamil (Isoptin).

IV COMPATIBILITIES

Acyclovir (Zovirax), bumetanide (Bumex), calcium gluconate, ceftazidime (Fortaz), dobutamine (Dobutrex), dopamine (Intropin), enalapril (Vasotec), fentanyl, heparin, insulin, labetalol (Normodyne, Trandate), lidocaine, lorazepam (Ativan), magnesium, milrinone (Primacor), nitroglycerin, norepinephrine (Levophed), potassium chloride, vancomycin (Vancocin).

INDICATIONS/ROUTES/DOSAGE

Anesthesia

IV: ADULTS, ELDERLY: Induction, 20–40 mg every 10 sec until induction onset, then infusion of 50–200 mcg/kg/min with 20–50 mg bolus as needed. **CHILDREN 3–16 YRS:** Induction, 2.5–3.5 mg/kg over 20–30 sec, then infusion of 125–300 mcg/kg/min.

Sedation in ICU

IV: ADULTS, ELDERLY: Initially, 5 mcg/kg/min (0.3 mg/kg/hr) for 5 min, then titrate to 5–80 mcg/kg/min (0.3–4.8 mg/kg/hr) in 5–10 mcg/kg/min (0.3–0.6 mg/kg/hr) increments allowing minimum of 5 min between dose adjustments. Usual maintenance: 5–50 mcg/kg/min (0.3–3 mg/kg/hr).

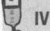

P

SIDE EFFECTS

Frequent: Involuntary muscle movements, apnea (common during induction; lasts longer than 60 sec), hypotension, nausea, vomiting, IV site burning/stinging. **Occasional:** Twitching, bucking, jerking, thrashing, headache, dizziness, bradycardia, hypertension, fever, abdominal cramps, paresthesia, coldness, cough, hiccups, facial flushing, greenish-colored urine. **Rare:** Rash, dry mouth, agitation, confusion, myalgia, thrombophlebitis.

ADVERSE EFFECTS/ TOXIC REACTIONS

Continuous infusion or repeated intermittent infusions of propofol may result in extreme drowsiness, respiratory depression, circulatory depression. Too-rapid IV administration may produce severe hypotension, respiratory depression, involuntary muscle movements. Pt may experience acute allergic reaction, characterized by abdominal pain, anxiety, restlessness, dyspnea, erythema, hypotension, pruritus, rhinitis, urticaria.

NURSING CONSIDERATIONS

BASELINE ASSESSMENT

Resuscitative equipment, suction, O_2 must be available. Obtain vital signs before administration.

INTERVENTION/EVALUATION

Monitor respiratory rate, B/P, heart rate, O_2 saturation, ABGs, depth of sedation, serum lipid, triglycerides if used longer than 24 hrs. May change urine color to green.

propranolol HIGH ALERT

proe-**pran**-oh-lole
(Apo-Propranolol ✦, Inderal, Inderal LA, InnoPran XL, Nu-Propranolol ✦)

BLACK BOX ALERT Severe angina exacerbation, MI, ventricular arrhythmias may occur in angina pts after abrupt discontinuation; must taper gradually over 1–2 wks.

Do not confuse Inderal with Adderall, Imdur, Isordil, or Toradol, or propranolol with Pravachol.

FIXED-COMBINATION(S)

Inderide: propranolol/hydrochlorothiazide (a diuretic): 40 mg/25 mg, 80 mg/25 mg. **Inderide LA:** propranolol/hydrochlorothiazide (a diuretic): 80 mg/50 mg, 120 mg/50 mg, 160 mg/50 mg.

◆ CLASSIFICATION

PHARMACOTHERAPEUTIC: Beta-adrenergic blocker. **CLINICAL:** Antihypertensive, antianginal, antiarrhythmic, antimigraine (see pp. 17C, 72C).

ACTION

Blocks $beta_1$-, $beta_2$-adrenergic receptors. Decreases oxygen requirements. Slows AV conduction, increases refractory period in AV node. Large doses increase airway resistance. **Therapeutic Effect:** Slows heart rate; decreases cardiac output, B/P, myocardial ischemia severity. Exhibits antiarrhythmic activity.

PHARMACOKINETICS

Route	Onset	Peak	Duration
PO	1–2 hrs	N/A	6 hrs

Well absorbed from GI tract. Protein binding: 93%. Widely distributed. Metabolized in liver. Primarily excreted in urine. Not removed by hemodialysis. **Half-life:** 4–6 hrs.

USES

Treatment of angina pectoris, arrhythmias, essential tremors, hypertension, hypertrophic subaortic stenosis, migraine headache, pheochromocytoma, post-MI. **OFF-LABEL:** Treatment adjunct for anxiety, mitral valve prolapse syndrome, thyrotoxicosis. Tremor due to

Parkinson's disease, alcohol withdrawal, gastric bleeding.

PRECAUTIONS

Contraindications: Asthma, bradycardia, cardiogenic shock, COPD, heart block, Raynaud's syndrome, uncompensated CHF. **Cautions:** Diabetes, renal/hepatic impairment, concurrent use of calcium blockers when using IV form.

LIFESPAN CONSIDERATIONS

Pregnancy/Lactation: Crosses placenta. Distributed in breast milk. Avoid use during first trimester. May produce low birth-weight infants, bradycardia, apnea, hypoglycemia, hypothermia during delivery. **Pregnancy Category C (D if used in second or third trimester). Children:** No age-related precautions noted. **Elderly:** Age-related peripheral vascular disease may increase susceptibility to decreased peripheral circulation.

INTERACTIONS

DRUG: Diuretics, other antihypertensives may increase hypotensive effect. May mask symptoms of hypoglycemia, prolong hypoglycemic effect of **insulin, oral hypoglycemics. IV phenytoin** may increase cardiac depressant effect. **NSAIDs** may decrease antihypertensive effect. **HERBAL: Ephedra, ginseng, yohimbe** may worsen hypertension. **Licorice** may increase water retention. **Garlic** has antihypertensive effects. **FOOD:** None known. **LAB VALUES:** May increase serum antinuclear antibody (ANA) titer, BUN, serum LDH, lipoprotein, alkaline phosphatase, potassium, uric acid, AST, ALT, triglycerides.

AVAILABILITY (Rx)

Injection Solution (Inderal): 1 mg/ml. **Oral Solution (Inderal):** 20 mg/5 ml, 40 mg/5 ml. **Tablets (Inderal):** 10 mg, 20 mg, 40 mg, 60 mg, 80 mg.

Capsules (Extended-Release [Innopran XL]): 80 mg, 120 mg. **Capsules (Sustained-Release [Inderal LA]):** 60 mg, 80 mg, 120 mg, 160 mg.

ADMINISTRATION/HANDLING

IV

Reconstitution • Give undiluted for IV push. • For IV infusion, may dilute each 1 mg in 10 ml D_5W.

Rate of administration • Do not exceed 1 mg/min injection rate. • For IV infusion, give over 30 min.

Storage • Store at room temperature. • Once diluted, stable for 24 hrs at room temperature.

PO

• May crush scored tablets. • Do not crush extended- or sustained-release capsules. • Give immediate-release tablets on empty stomach. • Give extended-release, sustained-release without regard to food.

IV INCOMPATIBILITY

Amphotericin B complex (Abelcet, AmBisome, Amphotec).

IV COMPATIBILITIES

Alteplase (Activase), heparin, milrinone (Primacor), potassium chloride, propofol (Diprivan).

INDICATIONS/ROUTES/DOSAGE

Hypertension

PO: ADULTS, ELDERLY: Initially, 40 mg twice daily. May increase dose q3–7days. **Maximum:** Up to 320 mg/day in divided doses. 640 mg/day. **CHILDREN:** Initially, 0.5–1 mg/kg/day in divided doses q6–12h. May increase at 3- to 5-day intervals. Usual dose: 1–5 mg/kg/day. **Maximum:** 16 mg/kg/day.

PO (LONG-ACTING): Initially, 80 mg once daily. May increase up to 120–160 mg once daily.

Angina

PO: ADULTS, ELDERLY: 80–320 mg/day in 2–4 divided doses.

PO (LONG-ACTING): Initially, 80 mg/day. **Maximum:** 320 mg/day.

P

Arrhythmia

IV: ADULTS, ELDERLY: 1–3 mg. Repeat q5min up to total of 5 mg. **CHILDREN:** 0.01–0.1 mg/kg. **Maximum:** Infants, 1 mg; children, 3 mg.

PO: ADULTS, ELDERLY: Initially, 10–30 mg q6–8h. May gradually increase dose. Range: 40–320 mg/day. **CHILDREN:** Initially, 0.5–1 mg/kg/day in divided doses q6–8h. May increase q3days. Usual dosage: 2–4 mg/kg/day. **Maximum:** 16 mg/kg/day or 60 mg/day.

Hypertrophic Subaortic Stenosis

PO: ADULTS, ELDERLY: 20–40 mg 3–4 times/day or 80–160 mg once daily as extended-release capsule.

Adjunct to Alpha-Blocking Agents to Treat Pheochromocytoma

PO: ADULTS, ELDERLY: 30–60 mg/day in divided doses.

Migraine Headache

PO: ADULTS, ELDERLY: 80 mg/day in divided doses or 80 mg once daily as extended-release capsule. Increase up to 160–240 mg/day in divided doses. **CHILDREN WEIGHING 35 KG OR LESS:** 10–20 mg 3 times a day. **CHILDREN WEIGHING OVER 35 KG:** 20–40 mg 3 times a day.

P

Reduction of Cardiovascular Mortality, Reinfarction in Pts with Previous MI

PO: ADULTS, ELDERLY: Initially, 40 mg 3 times/day. Range: 180–240 mg/day in 3–4 divided doses.

Essential Tremor

PO: ADULTS, ELDERLY: Initially, 40 mg twice daily increased up to 120–320 mg/day in 3 divided doses.

SIDE EFFECTS

Frequent: Diminished sexual function, drowsiness, difficulty sleeping, unusual fatigue/weakness. **Occasional:** Bradycardia, depression, sensation of coldness in extremities, diarrhea, constipation, anxiety, nasal congestion, nausea, vomiting. **Rare:** Altered taste, dry eyes, pruritus, paresthesia.

ADVERSE EFFECTS/ TOXIC REACTIONS

Overdose may produce profound bradycardia, hypotension. Abrupt withdrawal may result in diaphoresis, palpitations, headache, tremulousness. May precipitate CHF, MI in pts with cardiac disease; thyroid storm in those with thyrotoxicosis; peripheral ischemia in those with existing peripheral vascular disease. Hypoglycemia may occur in pts with previously controlled diabetes. **Antidote:** Glucagon (see Appendix M for dosage).

NURSING CONSIDERATIONS

BASELINE ASSESSMENT

Assess baseline renal/hepatic function tests. Assess B/P, apical pulse immediately before administering drug (if pulse is 60/min or less or systolic B/P is less than 90 mm Hg, withhold medication, contact physician). **Anginal:** Record onset, quality, radiation, location, intensity, duration of anginal pain, precipitating factors (exertion, emotional stress).

INTERVENTION/EVALUATION

Assess pulse for quality, irregular rate, bradycardia. Monitor EKG for cardiac arrhythmias. Assess fingers for color, numbness (Raynaud's). Assess for evidence of CHF (dyspnea [particularly on exertion or lying down], night cough, peripheral edema, distended neck veins). Monitor I&O (increase in weight, decrease in urinary output may indicate CHF). Assess for rash, fatigue, behavioral changes. Therapeutic response ranges from a few days to several wks. Measure B/P near end of dosing interval (determines if B/P is controlled throughout day).

PATIENT/FAMILY TEACHING

• Do not abruptly discontinue medication. • Compliance with therapy regimen is essential to control hypertension, arrhythmia, anginal pain. • To avoid hypotensive effect, rise slowly from lying to sitting position, wait momentarily before standing. • Avoid tasks that require alertness, motor skills until response to drug is established. • Report excessively slow pulse rate (less than 50 beats/min), peripheral numbness, dizziness. • Do not use nasal decongestants, OTC cold preparations (stimulants) without physician approval. • Restrict salt, alcohol intake.

propylthiouracil

proe-pill-thye-oh-**yoor**-a-sill
(Propylthiouracil, Propyl-Thyracil ✦)

BLACK BOX ALERT May cause severe hepatic injury, acute hepatic failure, death.

Do not confuse propylthiouracil with purinethol.

◆CLASSIFICATION

PHARMACOTHERAPEUTIC: Thiourea derivative. **CLINICAL:** Antithyroid.

ACTION

Blocks oxidation of iodine in thyroid gland, blocks synthesis of thyroxine, triiodothyronine. **Therapeutic Effect:** Inhibits synthesis of thyroid hormone.

PHARMACOKINETICS

Readily absorbed from GI tract. Protein binding: 80%. Metabolized in liver. Excreted in urine. **Half-life:** 1.5–5 hrs.

USES

Palliative treatment of hyperthyroidism; adjunct to ameliorate hyperthyroidism in preparation for surgical treatment, radioactive iodine therapy.

PRECAUTIONS

Contraindications: Breast-feeding mothers. **Cautions:** Pts older than 40 yrs or in combination with other agranulocytosis-inducing drugs. **Pregnancy Category D.**

INTERACTIONS

DRUG: **Amiodarone, iodinated glycerol, iodine, potassium iodide** may decrease response. May increase concentration of **digoxin** (as pt becomes euthyroid). May decrease thyroid uptake of ^{131}**I.** May decrease effect of **oral anticoagulants.** **HERBAL:** None significant. **FOOD:** None known. **LAB VALUES:** May increase LDH, serum alkaline phosphatase, bilirubin, AST, ALT, prothrombin time.

AVAILABILITY (Rx)

Tablets: 50 mg.

ADMINISTRATION/HANDLING

PO

- Give with food.

INDICATIONS/ROUTES/DOSAGE

Hyperthyroidism

PO: ADULTS, ELDERLY: Initially: 300–400 mg/day (**ELDERLY:** 150–300 mg/day) in divided doses q8h. Maintenance: 100–150 mg/day in divided doses q8–12h. **CHILDREN:** Initially: 5–7 mg/kg/day in divided doses q8h. Maintenance: 33%–66% of initial dose in divided doses q8–12h. **NEONATES:** 5–10 mg/kg/day in divided doses q8h.

SIDE EFFECTS

Frequent: Urticaria, rash, pruritus, nausea, skin pigmentation, hair loss, headache, paresthesia. **Occasional:** Drowsiness, lymphadenopathy, vertigo. **Rare:** Drug fever, lupus-like syndrome.

ADVERSE EFFECTS/ TOXIC REACTIONS

Agranulocytosis (may occur as long as 4 mos after therapy), pancytopenia, fatal hepatitis have occurred.

NURSING CONSIDERATIONS

BASELINE ASSESSMENT

Obtain baseline weight, pulse.

P

INTERVENTION/EVALUATION

Monitor pulse, weight daily. Check for skin eruptions, pruritus, swollen lymph glands. Be alert to hepatitis (nausea, vomiting, drowsiness, jaundice). Monitor for signs, symptoms of hepatic injury. Monitor hematology results for bone marrow suppression; check for signs of infection, bleeding.

PATIENT/FAMILY TEACHING

• Space doses evenly around the clock. • Take resting pulse daily. • Report pulse rate less than 60 beats/min. • Seafood, iodine products may be restricted. • Report fever, sore throat, yellowing of skin/eyes, unusual bleeding/bruising immediately. • Inform physician of sudden or continuous weight gain, cold intolerance, depression.

Proscar, *see finasteride*

protamine

proe-ta-meen
(Protamine, Protamine sulfate)

BLACK BOX ALERT May cause severe hypotension, cardiovascular collapse, noncardiogenic pulmonary edema, pulmonary hypertension.

Do not confuse protamine with ProAmatine or Protonix.

CLASSIFICATION

PHARMACOTHERAPEUTIC: Protein. **CLINICAL:** Heparin antagonist.

ACTION

Combines with heparin to form stable salt. **Therapeutic Effect:** Reduces anticoagulant activity of heparin.

PHARMACOKINETICS

Metabolized by fibrinolysin. **Half-life:** 7.4 min. Heparin neutralized in 5 min.

USES

Treatment of severe heparin overdose (causing hemorrhage). Neutralizes effects of heparin administered during extracorporeal circulation. **OFF-LABEL:** Treatment of low molecular weight heparin toxicity.

PRECAUTIONS

Contraindications: None known. **Cautions:** History of allergy to fish, seafood; vasectomized/infertile men; those on isophane (NPH) insulin, previous protamine therapy (propensity to hypersensitivity reaction).

LIFESPAN CONSIDERATIONS

Pregnancy/Lactation: Unknown if drug crosses placenta or is distributed in breast milk. **Pregnancy Category C. Children:** Safety and efficacy not established. **Elderly:** No age-related precautions noted.

INTERACTIONS

DRUG: None significant. **HERBAL:** None significant. **FOOD:** None known. **LAB VALUES:** None significant.

AVAILABILITY (Rx)

Injection Solution: 10 mg/ml.

ADMINISTRATION/HANDLING

IV

Rate of administration • May give undiluted over 10 min. Do not exceed 5 mg/min (50 mg in any 10-min period).
Storage • Store vials at room temperature.

INDICATIONS/ROUTES/DOSAGE

Heparin Overdose (Antidote, Treatment)
IV: ADULTS, ELDERLY: 1–1.5 mg protamine neutralizes 100 units heparin. Heparin disappears rapidly from circulation, reducing dosage demand for protamine as time elapses.

SIDE EFFECTS

Frequent: Decreased B/P, dyspnea. **Occasional:** Hypersensitivity reaction (urticaria, angioedema); nausea/vomiting, which generally occur in those sensitive to fish/seafood, vasectomized men, infertile men, those on isophane (NPH) insulin, those previously on protamine therapy. **Rare:** Back pain.

ADVERSE EFFECTS/ TOXIC REACTIONS

Too-rapid IV administration may produce acute hypotension, bradycardia, pulmonary hypertension, dyspnea, transient flushing, feeling of warmth. Heparin rebound may occur several hrs after heparin has been neutralized by protamine (usually evident 8–9 hrs after protamine administration). Heparin rebound occurs most often after arterial/cardiac surgery.

NURSING CONSIDERATIONS

BASELINE ASSESSMENT

Check PT, aPTT, Hct; assess for bleeding.

INTERVENTION/EVALUATION

Monitor coagulation tests, aPTT or ACT, B/P, cardiac function.

Protonix, *see pantoprazole*

Proventil HFA, *see albuterol*

Provigil, *see modafinil*

Prozac, *see fluoxetine*

pseudoephedrine

soo-doe-e-**fed**-rin
(Balminil Decongestant ✤, Genaphed, PMS-Pseudoephedrine ✤, Robidrine ✤, Sudafed, Sudafed 12 Hour, Sudafed 24 Hour, Sudafed Children's)

FIXED-COMBINATION(S)

Advil Cold, Motrin Cold: pseudoephedrine/ibuprofen (NSAID): 30 mg/200 mg, 15 mg/100 mg per 5 ml. **Allegra-D:** pseudoephedrine/fexofenadine (an antihistamine): 120 mg/60 mg. **Allegra-D 24 Hour:** pseudoephedrine/fexofenadine: 240 mg/180 mg. **Claritin-D:** pseudoephedrine/loratadine (an antihistamine): 120 mg/5 mg, 240 mg/10 mg. **Clarinex-D 24-Hour:** pseudoephedrine/desloratadine (an antihistamine): 240 mg/5 mg. **Clarinex-D 12-Hour:** pseudoephedrine/desloratadine: 120 mg/2.5 mg. **Zyrtec-D:** pseudoephedrine/cetirizine (an antihistamine): 120 mg/5 mg.

◆CLASSIFICATION

PHARMACOTHERAPEUTIC: Sympathomimetic. **CLINICAL:** Nasal decongestant.

ACTION

Directly stimulates alpha-adrenergic, beta-adrenergic receptors. **Therapeutic Effect:** Produces vasoconstriction of respiratory tract mucosa; shrinks nasal mucous membranes; reduces edema, nasal congestion.

PHARMACOKINETICS

Route	Onset	Peak	Duration
PO (tablets, syrup)	15–30 min	30–60 min	4–6 hrs
PO (extended-release)	N/A	N/A	8–12 hrs

Well absorbed from GI tract. Partially metabolized in liver. Primarily excreted in urine. Not removed by hemodialysis. **Half-life:** 9–16 hrs.

USES

Temporary relief of nasal congestion due to common cold, upper respiratory allergies, sinusitis. Enhances nasal, sinus drainage.

PRECAUTIONS

Contraindications: Breast-feeding women, coronary artery disease, severe hypertension, use of MAOIs within 14 days. **Extended-release:** Children younger than 12 yrs. **Cautions:** Elderly, hyperthyroidism, diabetes, ischemic heart disease, prostatic hypertrophy.

LIFESPAN CONSIDERATIONS

Pregnancy/Lactation: Crosses placenta. Distributed in breast milk. **Pregnancy Category C. Children:** Safety and efficacy not established in those younger than 2 yrs. **Elderly:** Age-related prostatic hypertrophy may require dosage adjustment.

INTERACTIONS

DRUG: May decrease effects of **antihypertensives, beta-blockers, diuretics. MAOIs** may increase cardiac stimulant, vasopressor effects. **HERBAL: Ephedra, yohimbe** may cause hypertension. **FOOD:** None known. **LAB VALUES:** None significant.

AVAILABILITY (OTC)

Liquid (Sudafed Children's): 15 mg/5 ml, 30 mg/5 ml. **Tablets (Genaphed, Sudafed):** 30 mg, 60 mg.

Caplets, Extended-Release: (Sudafed 12 Hour): 120 mg. **Tablets, Extended-Release: (Sudafed 24 Hour):** 240 mg.

◀ALERT▶ Pseudoephedrine is key ingredient in synthesizing methamphetamine. Many pharmacies have moved pseudoephedrine behind the counter due to concerns about its purchase and theft for purposes of methamphetamine manufacture.

ADMINISTRATION/HANDLING

PO

- Do not crush, chew extended-release forms; swallow whole.

INDICATIONS/ROUTES/DOSAGE

Decongestant

PO: ADULTS, ELDERLY, CHILDREN 12 YRS AND OLDER: 30–60 mg q4–6h. **Maximum:** 240 mg/day. **CHILDREN 6–11 YRS:** 30 mg q4–6h. **Maximum:** 120 mg/day. **CHILDREN 2–5 YRS:** 15 mg q4–6h. **Maximum:** 60 mg/day. **CHILDREN YOUNGER THAN 2 YRS:** 4 mg/kg/day in divided doses q6h.

PO (EXTENDED-RELEASE): ADULTS, CHILDREN 12 YRS AND OLDER: 120 mg q12h or 240 mg once daily.

SIDE EFFECTS

Occasional (10%–5%): Nervousness, restlessness, insomnia, tremor, headache. **Rare (4%–1%):** Diaphoresis, weakness.

ADVERSE EFFECTS/ TOXIC REACTIONS

Large doses may produce tachycardia, palpitations (particularly in pts with cardiac disease), light-headedness, nausea, vomiting. Overdose in those older than 60 yrs may result in hallucinations, CNS depression, seizures.

NURSING CONSIDERATIONS

PATIENT/FAMILY TEACHING

- Discontinue drug if adverse reactions occur.
- Report insomnia, dizziness, tremors, tachycardia, palpitations.

psyllium

sill-ee-yum
(Fiberall, Hydrocil, Konsyl, Metamucil)
Do not confuse Fiberall with Feverall.

CLASSIFICATION

PHARMACOTHERAPEUTIC: Bulk-forming laxative (see p. 121C).

ACTION

Dissolves and swells in water providing increased bulk, moisture content in stool. **Therapeutic Effect:** Promotes peristalsis, bowel motility.

PHARMACOKINETICS

Route	Onset	Peak	Duration
PO	12–24 hrs	2–3 days	N/A

Acts in small, large intestines.

USES

Treatment of chronic constipation, constipation associated with rectal disorders, management of irritable bowel syndrome (IBS).

PRECAUTIONS

Contraindications: Fecal impaction, GI obstruction, undiagnosed abdominal pain. **Cautions:** Esophageal strictures, ulcers, stenosis, intestinal adhesions.

⌛ LIFESPAN CONSIDERATIONS

Pregnancy/Lactation: Safe for use in pregnancy. **Pregnancy Category B. Children:** Safety and efficacy not established in those younger than 6 yrs. **Elderly:** No age-related precautions noted.

INTERACTIONS

DRUG: May decrease effect of **digoxin, oral anticoagulants, salicylates** by decreasing absorption. May interfere with effects of **potassium-sparing diuretics, potassium supplements. HERBAL:** None significant. **FOOD:** None known. **LAB VALUES:** May increase serum glucose. May decrease serum potassium.

AVAILABILITY (OTC)

Capsules (Konsyl, Metamucil): 0.52 g. **Powder (Fiberall, Hydrocil, Konsyl, Metamucil). Wafer (Metamucil):** 3.4 g/dose.

ADMINISTRATION/HANDLING

PO

• Administer at least 2 hrs before or after other medication. • All doses should be followed with 8 oz liquid. • Drink 6–8 glasses of water/day (aids stool softening). • Do not swallow in dry form; mix with at least 1 full glass (8 oz) of liquid.

INDICATIONS/ROUTES/DOSAGE

Constipation, Irritable Bowel Syndrome (IBS)

Refer to specific dosing guidelines on product labeling.

PO: ADULTS, ELDERLY: (2.5–30g/day in divided doses) 2–5 capsules/dose up to 3 times daily. 1 rounded tsp or 1 tbsp of powder up to 3 times daily. 2 wafers up to 3 times daily. **CHILDREN 6–11 YRS:** (1.25–15g/day in divided doses) Approximately ½ adult dose up to 3 times daily.

SIDE EFFECTS

Rare: Some degree of abdominal discomfort, nausea, mild abdominal cramps, griping, faintness.

ADVERSE EFFECTS/ TOXIC REACTIONS

Esophageal/bowel obstruction may occur if administered with insufficient liquid (less than 250 ml).

NURSING CONSIDERATIONS

INTERVENTION/EVALUATION

Encourage adequate fluid intake. Assess bowel sounds for peristalsis. Monitor daily pattern of bowel activity and stool consistency. Monitor serum electrolytes in pts exposed to prolonged, frequent, excessive use of medication.

PATIENT/FAMILY TEACHING

• Take each dose with full glass (250 ml) of water. • Inadequate fluid intake may cause GI obstruction. • Institute measures to promote defecation (increase fluid intake, exercise, high-fiber diet).

Pulmicort, *see budesonide*

pyrazinamide

pye-ra-**zin**-a-mide
(Pyrazinamide, Tebrazid ✤)

P

FIXED-COMBINATION(S)

Rifater: pyrazinamide/isoniazid/rifampin (an antitubercular): 300 mg/50 mg/120 mg.

◆CLASSIFICATION

CLINICAL: Antitubercular.

ACTION

May disrupt mycobacterium tuberculosis membrane transport. **Therapeutic Effect:** Bacteriostatic or bactericidal, depending on drug concentration at infection site, susceptibility of infecting bacteria.

PHARMACOKINETICS

Well absorbed from GI tract. Protein binding: 5%–10%. Widely distributed. Metabolized in liver. Excreted in urine. **Half-life:** 9–10 hrs.

USES

Treatment of clinical tuberculosis in conjunction with at least one other antitubercular agent.

PRECAUTIONS

Contraindications: Severe hepatic dysfunction. **Cautions:** Diabetes mellitus, renal impairment, history of gout, children (safety not established). Possible cross-sensitivity with isoniazid, ethionamide, niacin.

P

⌛ LIFESPAN CONSIDERATIONS

Pregnancy/Lactation: Unknown if drug crosses placenta or is distributed in breast milk. **Pregnancy Category C.** **Children:** Safety and efficacy not established. **Elderly:** No age-related precautions noted.

INTERACTIONS

DRUG: May decrease effects of **allopurinol, colchicine, probenecid, sulfinpyrazone.** **HERBAL:** None significant. **FOOD:** None known. **LAB VALUES:** May increase AST, ALT, serum uric acid.

AVAILABILITY (Rx)

Tablets: 500 mg.

INDICATIONS/ROUTES/DOSAGE

Tuberculosis (in Combination with Other Antituberculars)

PO: ADULTS: 15–30 mg/kg/day in 1–4 doses. **Maximum:** 2 g/day. **CHILDREN:** 15–30 mg/kg/day in 1 or 2 doses. **Maximum:** 2 g/day.

Dosage in Renal/Hepatic Impairment

Creatinine clearance less than 50 ml/min: 12–20 mg/kg/day or avoid use. Reduce dose in hepatic impairment.

SIDE EFFECTS

Frequent: Arthralgia, myalgia (usually mild, self-limiting). **Rare:** Hypersensitivity reaction (rash, pruritus, urticaria), photosensitivity, gouty arthritis.

ADVERSE EFFECTS/TOXIC REACTIONS

Hepatotoxicity, gouty arthritis, thrombocytopenia, anemia occur rarely.

NURSING CONSIDERATIONS

BASELINE ASSESSMENT

Question for hypersensitivity to pyrazinamide, isoniazid, ethionamide, niacin. Ensure collection of specimens for culture, sensitivity. Evaluate results of initial CBC, hepatic function tests, serum uric acid levels.

INTERVENTION/EVALUATION

Monitor hepatic function test results; be alert for hepatic reactions: jaundice, malaise, fever, liver tenderness, anorexia, nausea, vomiting (stop drug, notify physician promptly). Check serum uric acid levels; assess for hot, painful, swollen joints, esp. big toe, ankle, knee (gout). Evaluate serum blood glucose levels, diabetic status carefully (pyrazinamide makes management difficult). Assess for rash, skin eruptions. Monitor CBC for thrombocytopenia, anemia.

PATIENT/FAMILY TEACHING

• Do not skip doses; complete full length of therapy (may be mos or yrs). • Office visits, lab tests are essential part of treatment. • Take with food to reduce GI upset. • Avoid excessive exposure to sun, ultraviolet light until photosensitivity is determined. • Notify physician of any new symptom, immediately for jaundice (yellow sclera of eyes/skin); unusual fatigue; fever; loss of appetite; hot, painful, swollen joints.

pyridostigmine

peer-id-oh-**stig**-meen
(Mestinon, Mestinon SR ✦,
Mestinon Timespan, Regonol)
Do not confuse pyridostigmine with physostigmine, or Regonol with Reglan or Renagel.

◆ CLASSIFICATION

PHARMACOTHERAPEUTIC: Anticholinesterase. **CLINICAL:** Cholinergic muscle stimulant (see p. 91C).

ACTION

Prevents destruction of acetylcholine by inhibiting the enzyme acetylcholinesterase, enhancing impulse transmission across myoneural junction. **Therapeutic Effect:** Produces miosis; increases intestinal, skeletal muscle tone; stimulates salivary, sweat gland secretions.

PHARMACOKINETICS

Poorly absorbed from GI tract. Metabolized in liver. Excreted primarily unchanged in urine. **Half-life:** 1–2 hrs.

USES

Improvement of muscle strength in control of myasthenia gravis, reversal of effects of nondepolarizing neuromuscular blocking agents after surgery.

PRECAUTIONS

Contraindications: Mechanical GI/urinary tract obstruction, hypersensitivity to anticholinesterase agents. **Cautions:** Bronchial asthma, bradycardia, epilepsy, recent coronary occlusion, vagotonia, hyperthyroidism, cardiac arrhythmias, peptic ulcer.

LIFESPAN CONSIDERATIONS

Pregnancy/Lactation: Unknown if drug crosses placenta or is distributed in breast milk. **Pregnancy Category B. Children:** Safety and efficacy not established. **Elderly:** No age-related precautions noted.

INTERACTIONS

DRUG: Anticholinergics prevent, reverse effects. **Cholinesterase inhibitors** may increase risk of toxicity. Antagonizes effects of **neuromuscular blockers. Procainamide, quinidine** may antagonize action. **HERBAL:** None significant. **FOOD:** None known. **LAB VALUES:** None significant.

AVAILABILITY (Rx)

Injection Solution (Regonol): 5 mg/ml. **Syrup (Mestinon):** 60 mg/5 ml. **Tablets (Mestinon):** 60 mg.

Tablets (Extended-Release [Mestinon Timespan]): 180 mg.

ADMINISTRATION/HANDLING

IV, IM

• Give large parenteral doses concurrently with 0.6–1.2 mg atropine sulfate IV to minimize side effects.

PO

• Give with food, milk. • Tablets may be crushed; do not chew, crush extended-release tablets (may be broken). • Give larger dose at times of increased fatigue (e.g., for those with difficulty in chewing, 30–45 min before meals).

IV INCOMPATIBILITIES

Do not mix with any other medications.

INDICATIONS/ROUTES/DOSAGE

Myasthenia Gravis

PO: ADULTS, ELDERLY: Initially, 60 mg 3 times a day. Dosage increased at 48-hr

P

intervals. Maintenance: 60 mg–1.5 g a day. **CHILDREN:** 7 mg/kg/24 hr divided into 5–6 doses. **NEONATES:** 5 mg q4–6h. **PO (EXTENDED-RELEASE): ADULTS, ELDERLY:** 180–540 mg 1–2 times a day with at least a 6-hr interval between doses. **IV, IM: ADULTS, ELDERLY:** 2 mg or 1/30th of oral dose q2–3h. **CHILDREN, NEONATES:** 0.05–0.15 mg/kg/dose. **Maximum single dose:** 10 mg.

Reversal of Nondepolarizing Neuromuscular Blockade

IV: ADULTS, ELDERLY: 10–20 mg with, or shortly after, 0.6–1.2 mg atropine sulfate or 0.3–0.6 mg glycopyrrolate. **CHILDREN:** 0.1–0.25 mg/kg/dose preceded by atropine or glycopyrrolate.

SIDE EFFECTS

Frequent: Miosis, increased GI/skeletal muscle tone, bradycardia, constriction of bronchi/ureters, diaphoresis, increased salivation. **Occasional:** Headache, rash, temporary decrease in diastolic B/P with mild reflex tachycardia, short periods of atrial fibrillation (in hyperthyroid pts), marked drop in B/P (in hypertensive pts).

ADVERSE EFFECTS/ TOXIC REACTIONS

Overdose may produce cholinergic crisis, manifested as increasingly severe muscle weakness (appears first in muscles involving chewing, swallowing, followed by muscle weakness of shoulder girdle, upper extremities), respiratory muscle paralysis, followed by pelvis girdle/leg muscle paralysis. Requires withdrawal of all cholinergic drugs and immediate use of 1–4 mg atropine sulfate IV for adults, 0.01 mg/kg for infants and children younger than 12 yrs.

NURSING CONSIDERATIONS

BASELINE ASSESSMENT

Larger doses should be given at time of greatest fatigue. Assess muscle strength before testing for diagnosis of myasthenia gravis and following drug administration. Avoid large doses in pts with megacolon, reduced GI motility.

INTERVENTION/EVALUATION

Have tissues readily available at pt's bedside. Monitor respirations closely during myasthenia gravis testing or if dosage is increased. Assess diligently for cholinergic reaction, bradycardia in myasthenic pt in crisis. Coordinate dosage time with periods of fatigue and increased/decreased muscle strength. Monitor for therapeutic response to medication (increased muscle strength, decreased fatigue, improved chewing/swallowing functions).

PATIENT/FAMILY TEACHING

- Report nausea, vomiting, diarrhea, diaphoresis, profuse salivary secretions, palpitations, muscle weakness, severe abdominal pain, difficulty breathing.

pyridoxine (vitamin B_6)

peer-i-**dox**-een
(Aminoxin)

Do not confuse pyridoxine with paroxetine, pralidoxime, or Pyridium.

◆CLASSIFICATION

PHARMACOTHERAPEUTIC: Coenzyme. **CLINICAL:** Vitamin (B_6) (see p. 161C).

ACTION

Coenzyme for various metabolic functions, including metabolism of proteins, carbohydrates, fats. Aids in breakdown of glycogen and in synthesis of gamma-aminobutyric acid (GABA) in CNS. **Therapeutic Effect:** Prevents pyridoxine deficiency. Increases excretion of certain drugs (e.g., isoniazid) that are pyridoxine antagonists.

PHARMACOKINETICS

Readily absorbed primarily in jejunum. Stored in liver, muscle, brain. Metabolized in liver. Primarily excreted in urine.

Removed by hemodialysis. **Half-life:** 15–20 days.

USES

Prevention/treatment of vitamin B_6 deficiency, pyridoxine-dependent seizures in infants, drug-induced neuritis (e.g., isoniazid).

PRECAUTIONS

Contraindications: None known. **Cautions:** None known.

LIFESPAN CONSIDERATIONS

Pregnancy/Lactation: Crosses placenta. Distributed in breast milk. High dosages in utero may produce seizures in neonates. **Pregnancy Category A. Children/Elderly:** No age-related precautions noted.

INTERACTIONS

DRUG: Decreases effects of **levodopa. HERBAL:** None significant. **FOOD:** None known. **LAB VALUES:** None significant.

AVAILABILITY (OTC)

Capsules: 50 mg, 250 mg. **Injection Solution (Vitamin B_6):** 100 mg/ml. **Tablets:** 25 mg, 50 mg, 100 mg, 250 mg, 500 mg.

ADMINISTRATION/HANDLING

ALERT Give PO unless nausea, vomiting, malabsorption occurs. Avoid IV use in cardiac pts.

IV

- Give undiluted or may be added to IV solutions and given as infusion.

IV INCOMPATIBILITIES

Do not mix with any other medications.

INDICATIONS/ROUTES/DOSAGE

Pyridoxine Deficiency

PO: ADULTS, ELDERLY: 10–20 mg/day for 3 wks. **CHILDREN:** Initially, 5–25 mg/day for 3 wks, then 1.5–2.5 mg/day.

Drug-Induced Neuritis

PO (TREATMENT): ADULTS, ELDERLY: 100–200 mg/day in divided doses. **CHILDREN:** 10–50 mg/day.

PO (PROPHYLAXIS): ADULTS, ELDERLY: 25–100 mg/day. **CHILDREN:** 1–2 mg/kg/day.

SIDE EFFECTS

Occasional: Stinging at IM injection site. **Rare:** Headache, nausea, drowsiness, sensory neuropathy (paresthesia, unstable gait, clumsiness of hands) with high doses.

ADVERSE EFFECTS/ TOXIC REACTIONS

Long-term megadoses (2–6 g for longer than 2 mos) may produce sensory neuropathy (reduced deep tendon reflexes, profound impairment of sense of position in distal limbs, gradual sensory ataxia). Toxic symptoms subside when drug is discontinued. Seizures have occurred after IV megadoses.

NURSING CONSIDERATIONS

INTERVENTION/EVALUATION

Observe for improvement of deficiency symptoms, glossitis. Evaluate for nutritional adequacy.

PATIENT/FAMILY TEACHING

- Discomfort may occur with IM injection.
- Consume foods rich in pyridoxine (legumes, soybeans, eggs, sunflower seeds, hazelnuts, organ meats, tuna, shrimp, carrots, avocados, bananas, wheat germ, bran).

quetiapine

kwe-**tye**-a-peen
(Apo-Quetiapine ✤, Novo-Quetiapine ✤, Seroquel, Seroquel XR)

BLACK BOX ALERT Increased risk of suicidal thinking and behavior in children, adolescents, young adults 18–24 yrs with major depressive disorder, other psychiatric disorders. Elderly with dementia-related psychosis are at increased risk for death.

Do not confuse quetiapine with olanzapine, or Seroquel with Sinequan.

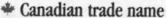

Q

CLASSIFICATION

PHARMACOTHERAPEUTIC: Dibenzapine derivative. **CLINICAL:** Antipsychotic (see p. 65C).

ACTION

Antagonizes dopamine, serotonin, histamine, $alpha_1$-adrenergic receptors. **Therapeutic Effect:** Diminishes psychotic disorders. Produces moderate sedation, few extrapyramidal effects. No anticholinergic effects.

PHARMACOKINETICS

Rapidly, well absorbed after PO administration. Protein binding: 83%. Widely distributed in tissues; CNS concentration exceeds plasma concentration. Undergoes extensive first-pass metabolism in liver. Primarily excreted in urine. **Half-life:** 6 hrs.

USES

Treatment of schizophrenia. Treatment of acute manic episodes with bipolar disorder (alone or in combination with lithium or valproate). Treatment of depressive episodes associated with bipolar disorder. Adjunctive treatment in major depressive disorder (MDD). **OFF-LABEL:** Autism, psychosis (children), psychosis/agitation related to Alzheimer's dementia.

Q

PRECAUTIONS

Contraindications: None known. **Cautions:** Alzheimer's dementia, history of breast cancer, cardiovascular disease (e.g., CHF, history of MI), cerebrovascular disease, hepatic impairment, dehydration, hypovolemia, history of drug abuse/dependence, seizures, hypothyroidism.

LIFESPAN CONSIDERATIONS

Pregnancy/Lactation: Unknown if drug is distributed in breast milk. Not recommended for breast-feeding mothers. **Pregnancy Category C. Children:** Safety and efficacy not established. **Elderly:** No age-related precautions noted, but lower initial and target dosages may be necessary.

INTERACTIONS

DRUG: Alcohol, other CNS depressants may increase CNS depression. May increase hypotensive effects of **antihypertensives. Hepatic enzyme inducers (e.g., phenytoin)** may increase clearance. **Clarithromycin, diltiazem, erythromycin, fluconazole, itraconazole, verapamil** may increase effects. **HERBAL: St. John's wort** may decrease concentration. **Gotu kola, kava kava, St. John's wort, valerian** may increase CNS depression. **FOOD:** None known. **LAB VALUES:** May decrease total free thyroxine (T_4) serum levels. May increase serum cholesterol, triglycerides, AST, ALT, WBC, GGT. May produce false-positive pregnancy test result.

AVAILABILITY (Rx)

Tablets: 25 mg, 50 mg, 100 mg, 150 mg, 200 mg, 300 mg, 400 mg.

Tablets, Extended-Release: 50 mg, 150 mg, 200 mg, 300 mg, 400 mg.

ADMINISTRATION/HANDLING

PO

• Give immediate-release tablets without regard to food. • Do not crush, split, chew extended-release tablets. • Extended-release tablets should be given without regard to food or with a light meal in evening.

INDICATIONS/ROUTES/DOSAGE

Note: When restarting pts who have been off quetiapine for less than 1 wk, titration is not required and maintenance dose can be reinstituted. • When restarting pts who have been off quetiapine for longer than 1 wk, follow initial titration schedule.

Psychotic Disorders

PO: ADULTS, ELDERLY: Initially, 25 mg twice a day, then 25–50 mg 2–3 times a day on the second and third days, up to 300–400 mg/day in divided doses 2–3 times a day by the fourth day. Further adjustments of 25–50 mg twice a day may be made at intervals of 2 days or longer. Maintenance: 300–800 mg/day (adults); 50–200 mg/day (elderly). **Seroquel XR:** Initially, 300 mg/day in evening. May increase at intervals as short as 1 day up to 300 mg/day. Range: 400–800 mg/day.

Mania in Bipolar Disorder

PO: ADULTS, ELDERLY: Initially, 50 mg twice a day for 1 day. May increase in increments of 100 mg/day to 200 mg twice a day on day 4. May increase in increments of 200 mg/day to 800 mg/day on day 6. Range: 400–800 mg/day. **Seroquel XR:** Initially, 300 mg on day 1 in the evening; 600 mg on day 2 and adjust between 400–800 mg/day thereafter.

Depression in Bipolar Disorder

PO: ADULTS, ELDERLY: Initially, 50 mg/day on day 1, increase to 100 mg/day on day 2, then increase by 100 mg/day up to target dose of 300 mg/day. **Seroquel XR:** Initially, 50 mg on day 1 in the evening, 100 mg on day 2, 200 mg on day 3, 300 mg on day 4 and thereafter.

Adjunctive Therapy in MDD

PO: ADULTS, ELDERLY: (SEROQUEL XR): Initially, 50 mg on days 1 and 2; then 150 mg on days 3 and 4; then 150–300 mg/day thereafter.

SIDE EFFECTS

Frequent (19%–10%): Headache, drowsiness, dizziness. **Occasional (9%–3%):** Constipation, orthostatic hypotension, tachycardia, dry mouth, dyspepsia (heartburn, indigestion, epigastric pain), rash, asthenia (loss of strength, energy), abdominal pain, rhinitis. **Rare (2%):** Back pain, fever, weight gain.

ADVERSE EFFECTS/ TOXIC REACTIONS

Overdose may produce heart block, hypotension, hypokalemia, tachycardia.

NURSING CONSIDERATIONS

BASELINE ASSESSMENT

Assess behavior, appearance, emotional status, response to environment, speech pattern, thought content. Obtain baseline CBC, hepatic enzyme levels before initiating treatment and periodically thereafter.

INTERVENTION/EVALUATION

Monitor mental status, onset of extrapyramidal symptoms. Assist with ambulation if dizziness occurs. Supervise suicidal-risk pt closely during early therapy (as psychosis, depression lessens, energy level improves, increasing suicide potential). Monitor B/P for hypotension, lipid profile, blood glucose, CBC, or worsening depression, unusual behavior. Assess pulse for tachycardia (esp. with rapid increase in dosage). Assess bowel activity for evidence of constipation. Assess for therapeutic response (improved thought content, increased ability to concentrate, improvement in self-care). Eye exam to detect cataract formation should be obtained q6mo during treatment.

PATIENT/ FAMILY TEACHING

• Avoid exposure to extreme heat. • Drink fluids often, esp. during physical activity. • Take medication as ordered; do not stop taking or increase dosage. • Drowsiness generally subsides during continued therapy. • Avoid tasks that require alertness, motor skills until response to drug is established. • Avoid alcohol. • Change positions slowly to reduce hypotensive effect. • Report suicidal ideation, unusual changes in behavior.

quinapril

kwin-na-pril
(Accupril)

BLACK BOX ALERT May cause fetal injury, mortality if used during second or third trimester of pregnancy.

Do not confuse Accupril with Accolate, Accutane, Aciphex, or Monopril.

FIXED-COMBINATION(S)

Accuretic: quinapril/hydrochlorothiazide (a diuretic): 10 mg/12.5 mg, 20 mg/12.5 mg, 20 mg/25 mg.

◆CLASSIFICATION

PHARMACOTHERAPEUTIC: Angiotensin-converting enzyme (ACE) inhibitor. **CLINICAL:** Antihypertensive (see p. 9C).

ACTION

Suppresses renin-angiotensin-aldosterone system, preventing conversion of angiotensin I to angiotensin II, a potent vasoconstrictor; may inhibit angiotensin II at local vascular renal sites. **Therapeutic Effect:** Reduces peripheral arterial resistance, B/P, pulmonary capillary wedge pressure; improves cardiac output.

PHARMACOKINETICS

Route	Onset	Peak	Duration
PO	1 hr	N/A	24 hrs

Readily absorbed from GI tract. Protein binding: 97%. Rapidly hydrolyzed to active metabolite. Primarily excreted in urine. Minimal removal by hemodialysis. **Half-life:** 1–2 hrs; metabolite, 3 hrs (increased in renal impairment).

USES

Treatment of hypertension. Used alone or in combination with other antihypertensives. Adjunctive therapy in management of heart failure. **OFF-LABEL:** Treatment of pediatric hypertension, renal crisis in scleroderma, treatment of left ventricular dysfunction following MI.

PRECAUTIONS

Contraindications: Bilateral renal artery stenosis, history of angioedema from previous treatment with ACE inhibitors. **Cautions:** Renal impairment, CHF, collagen vascular disease, hypovolemia, renal stenosis, hyperkalemia.

⌛ LIFESPAN CONSIDERATIONS

Pregnancy/Lactation: Crosses placenta. Unknown if distributed in breast milk. May cause fetal, neonatal mortality or morbidity. **Pregnancy Category C (D if used in second or third trimester). Children:** Safety and efficacy not established. **Elderly:** May be more sensitive to hypotensive effects.

INTERACTIONS

DRUG: **Alcohol, antihypertensives, diuretics** may increase effects. May increase concentration, risk of toxicity of **lithium. NSAIDs** may decrease effects. **Potassium-sparing diuretics, potassium supplements** may cause hyperkalemia. **HERBAL:** **Garlic** may increase antihypertensive effect. **Ginseng, yohimbe** may worsen hypertension. **FOOD:** None known. **LAB VALUES:** May increase BUN, serum alkaline phosphatase, bilirubin, creatinine, potassium, AST, ALT. May decrease serum sodium. May cause positive antinuclear antibody (ANA) titer.

AVAILABILITY (Rx)

Tablets: 5 mg, 10 mg, 20 mg, 40 mg.

ADMINISTRATION/HANDLING

PO

• Give without regard to food. • Tablets may be crushed.

INDICATIONS/ROUTES/DOSAGE

Hypertension (Monotherapy)

PO: ADULTS: Initially, 10–20 mg/day. May adjust dosage at intervals of at least 2 wks or longer. Maintenance: 10–40 mg/day as single dose or 2 divided doses. **Maximum:** 40 mg/day. **ELDERLY:** Initially, 2.5–5 mg/day. May increase by 2.5–5 mg q1–2wk.

Hypertension (Combination Therapy)

PO: ADULTS: Initially, 5 mg/day titrated to pt's needs. **ELDERLY:** Initially, 2.5–5 mg/day. May increase by 2.5–5 mg q1–2wk.

Adjunct to Manage Heart Failure

PO: ADULTS, ELDERLY: Initially, 5 mg once or twice a day. Titrate at weekly intervals. Range: 20–40 mg/day.

Dosage in Renal Impairment

Dosage is titrated to pt's needs after the following initial doses:

Hypertension

Creatinine Clearance	Initial Dose
More than 60 ml/min	10 mg
30–60 ml/min	5 mg
10–29 ml/min	2.5 mg

CHF

Creatinine Clearance	Initial Dose
Greater than 30 ml/min	5 mg
10–30 ml/min	2.5 mg

SIDE EFFECTS

Frequent (7%–5%): Headache, dizziness. **Occasional (4%–2%):** Fatigue, vomiting, nausea, hypotension, chest pain, cough, syncope. **Rare (less than 2%):** Diarrhea, cough, dyspnea, rash, palpitations, impotence, insomnia, drowsiness, malaise.

ADVERSE EFFECTS/ TOXIC REACTIONS

Excessive hypotension ("first-dose syncope") may occur in pts with CHF, those who are severely salt/volume depleted. Angioedema, hyperkalemia occur rarely. Agranulocytosis, neutropenia may be noted in those with collagen vascular disease (scleroderma, systemic lupus erythematosus), renal impairment. Nephrotic syndrome may be noted in those with history of renal disease.

NURSING CONSIDERATIONS

BASELINE ASSESSMENT

Obtain B/P immediately before each dose in addition to regular monitoring (be alert to fluctuations). If excessive reduction in B/P occurs, place pt in supine position with legs slightly elevated. Renal function tests should be performed before beginning therapy. In pts with prior renal disease, urine test for protein by dipstick method should be made with first urine of day before beginning therapy and periodically thereafter. In those with renal impairment, autoimmune disease, or taking drugs that affect leukocytes or immune response, CBC, differential count should be performed before beginning therapy and q2wk for 3 mos, then periodically thereafter.

INTERVENTION/EVALUATION

Monitor B/P, renal function, serum potassium, WBC. Assist with ambulation if dizziness occurs. Question for evidence of headache. Noncola carbonated beverage, unsalted crackers, dry toast may relieve nausea.

PATIENT/ FAMILY TEACHING

• Rise slowly from lying to sitting position, permit legs to dangle from bed momentarily before standing to reduce hypotensive effect. • Full therapeutic effect may take 1–2 wks. • Report any sign of infection (sore throat, fever). • Skipping doses or voluntarily discontinuing drug may produce severe rebound hypertension. • Avoid tasks that require alertness, motor skills until response to drug is established. • Avoid alcohol.

quinidine

kwin-ih-deen
(Apo-Quinidine ✤, BioQuin Durules ✤, Novo-Quinidine ✤, Quinidex Extentabs)

BLACK BOX ALERT Increased rate of mortality when used for non–life-threatening arrhythmias, structural heart disease.

Do not confuse quinidine with clonidine or quinine.

◆CLASSIFICATION

CLINICAL: Antiarrhythmic (see p. 16C).

ACTION

Decreases sodium influx during depolarization, potassium efflux during repolarization. Reduces calcium transport across myocardial cell membrane. Decreases myocardial excitability, conduction velocity, contractility. **Therapeutic Effect:** Suppresses arrhythmias.

Q

PHARMACOKINETICS

Almost completely absorbed after PO administration. Protein binding: 80%–90%. Metabolized in liver. Excreted in urine. Removed by hemodialysis. **Half-life:** 6–8 hrs.

USES

Prophylactic therapy to maintain normal sinus rhythm following conversion of atrial fibrillation/flutter. Prevention of premature atrial, AV, ventricular contractions, paroxysmal atrial tachycardia, paroxysmal AV junctional rhythm, atrial fibrillation, atrial flutter, paroxysmal ventricular tachycardia not associated with complete heart block. **OFF-LABEL:** Treatment of malaria.

PRECAUTIONS

Contraindications: Complete AV block, development of thrombocytopenic purpura during prior therapy with quinidine or quinine, intraventricular conduction defects (widening of QRS complex). **Cautions:** Myocardial depression, sick sinus syndrome, incomplete AV block, digoxin toxicity, renal/hepatic impairment, myasthenia gravis.

LIFESPAN CONSIDERATIONS

Pregnancy/Lactation: Crosses placenta; distributed in breast milk. **Pregnancy Category C. Children:** Safety and efficacy not established. **Elderly:** No age-related precautions noted.

INTERACTIONS

DRUG: Effects may be additive with medications (**e.g., amiodarone, erythromycin, phenothiazines, tricyclic antidepressants**) that prolong QT interval. May increase **digoxin** concentration, risk of toxicity. **HERBAL: Ephedra** may worsen arrhythmias. **St. John's wort** may decrease concentration. **FOOD:** None known. **LAB VALUES:** None known. **Therapeutic serum level:** 2–5 mcg/ml; **toxic serum level:** greater than 5 mcg/ml.

AVAILABILITY (Rx)

Injection Solution: 80 mg/ml. **Tablets:** 200 mg, 300 mg.

Tablets (Extended-Release): 324 mg.

ADMINISTRATION/HANDLING

IV

ALERT B/P, EKG should be monitored continuously during IV administration and rate of infusion adjusted to minimize arrhythmias, hypotension.

Reconstitution • For IV infusion, dilute 800 mg with 40 ml D_5W to provide concentration of 16 mg/ml.

Rate of administration • Administer with pt in supine position. • For IV infusion, give at rate of 1 ml (16 mg)/min (too-rapid rate may markedly decrease arterial pressure). • Monitor EKG for cardiac changes, particularly prolongation of PR, QT intervals, widening of QRS complex. Notify physician of any significant interval changes.

Storage • Use only clear, colorless solution. • Solution is stable for 24 hrs at room temperature when diluted with D_5W.

PO

• Do not crush/chew extended-release tablets. • GI upset can be reduced if given with food.

IV INCOMPATIBILITIES

Furosemide (Lasix), heparin.

IV COMPATIBILITY

Milrinone (Primacor).

INDICATIONS/ROUTES/DOSAGE

Arrhythmias

PO: ADULTS, ELDERLY: 100–600 mg q4–6h. (**Extended-Release**): 324–972 mg q8–12h. **CHILDREN:** 15–60 mg/kg/day in divided doses q4–6h.

IV: ADULTS, ELDERLY: 200–400 mg. May require 500–750 mg. **CHILDREN:** 2–10 mg/kg/dose in divided doses q3–6h as needed.

SIDE EFFECTS

Frequent: Abdominal pain/cramps, nausea, diarrhea, vomiting (can be immediate, intense). **Occasional:** Mild cinchonism (tinnitus, blurred vision, hearing loss), severe cinchonism (headache, vertigo, diaphoresis, light-headedness, photophobia, confusion, delirium). **Rare:** Hypotension (particularly with IV administration), hypersensitivity reaction (fever, anaphylaxis, photosensitivity reaction).

ADVERSE EFFECTS/ TOXIC REACTIONS

Cardiotoxic effects occur most commonly with IV administration, particularly at high concentrations, observed as conduction changes (50% widening of QRS complex, prolonged QT interval, flattened T waves, disappearance of P wave), ventricular tachycardia/flutter, frequent premature ventricular contractions (PVCs), complete AV block. Quinidine-induced syncope may occur with usual dosage. Severe hypotension may result from high dosages. Pts with atrial flutter/fibrillation may experience a paradoxical, extremely rapid ventricular rate (may be prevented by prior digitalization). Hepatotoxicity with jaundice due to drug hypersensitivity may occur.

NURSING CONSIDERATIONS

BASELINE ASSESSMENT

Check B/P, pulse (for 1 full min unless pt is on continuous monitor) before giving medication. For those on long-term therapy, CBC, hepatic/renal function tests should be performed periodically.

INTERVENTION/EVALUATION

Monitor EKG for cardiac changes, particularly prolongation of PR, QT intervals, widening of QRS complex. Monitor I&O, CBC, serum potassium, hepatic/renal function tests. Monitor daily pattern of bowel activity, stool consistency. Monitor B/P for hypotension (esp. in pts on high-dose therapy). If cardiotoxic effect occurs (see Adverse Effects/Toxic Reactions), notify physician immediately. **Therapeutic serum level:** 2–5 mcg/ml; **toxic serum level:** greater than 5 mcg/ml.

PATIENT/FAMILY TEACHING

• Inform physician of fever, tinnitus, visual disturbances. • May cause photosensitivity reaction; avoid direct sunlight, artificial light.

quinupristin-dalfopristin

kwin-yoo-pris-tin **dal**-foh-pris-tin
(Synercid)

◆CLASSIFICATION

PHARMACOTHERAPEUTIC: Streptogramin. **CLINICAL:** Antimicrobial.

ACTION

Two chemically distinct compounds that, when given together, bind to different sites on bacterial ribosomes, inhibiting protein synthesis. **Therapeutic Effect:** Bactericidal.

PHARMACOKINETICS

After IV administration, both are extensively metabolized in liver, with dalfopristin to active metabolite. Protein binding: quinupristin, 23%–32%; dalfopristin, 50%–56%. Primarily eliminated in feces. **Half-life:** quinupristin, 0.85 hr; dalfopristin, 0.7 hr.

USES

Treatment of serious or life-threatening infections caused by vancomycin-resistant *Enterococcus faecium* (VRE), complicated skin/skin structure infections caused by *S. aureus, S. pyogenes*.

PRECAUTIONS

Contraindications: Hypersensitivity to pristinamycin, virginiamycin. **Cautions:** Hepatic/renal dysfunction.

⌛ LIFESPAN CONSIDERATIONS

Pregnancy/Lactation: Unknown if drug crosses placenta or is distributed in breast milk. **Pregnancy Category B. Chil-**

Q

dren: Safety and efficacy not established. **Elderly:** No age-related precautions noted.

INTERACTIONS

DRUG: May increase concentration, risk of toxicity of **cyclosporine, diazepam, diltiazem, midazolam, nifedipine, tacrolimus, verapamil.** **HERBAL:** None significant. **FOOD:** None known. **LAB VALUES:** May increase serum bilirubin, creatinine, LDH, AST, ALT, BUN, alkaline phosphatase, glucose. May decrease Hgb, Hct; alter platelets.

AVAILABILITY (Rx)

Injection, Powder for Reconstitution: 500-mg vial (150 mg quinupristin/350 mg dalfopristin).

ADMINISTRATION/HANDLING

IV

Reconstitution • Reconstitute vial by slowly adding 5 ml D_5W or Sterile Water for Injection to make 100 mg/ml solution. • Gently swirl vial contents to minimize foaming. • Further dilute with D_5W to final concentration of 2 mg/ml (5 mg/ml using central line).

Rate of administration • Infuse over 60 min. • After infusion, flush line with D_5W to minimize vein irritation. Do not flush with 0.9% NaCl (incompatible).

Storage • Refrigerate unopened vials. • Reconstituted vials are stable for 1 hr at room temperature. Diluted infusion bag is stable for 5 hrs at room temperature or 54 hrs if refrigerated.

IV INCOMPATIBILITIES

Heparin, sodium chloride.

IV COMPATIBILITIES

Aztreonam (Azactam), ciprofloxacin (Cipro), fluconazole (Diflucan), haloperidol (Haldol), metoclopramide (Reglan), morphine, potassium chloride.

INDICATIONS/ROUTES/DOSAGE

Infections Due to Vancomycin-Resistant *Enterococcus Faecium* (VRE)

IV: ADULTS, ELDERLY: 7.5 mg/kg/dose q8h.

Skin/Skin Structure Infections

IV: ADULTS, ELDERLY: 7.5 mg/kg/dose q12h.

SIDE EFFECTS

Frequent: Mild erythema, pruritus, pain/burning at infusion site (with doses greater than 7 mg/kg). **Occasional:** Headache, diarrhea. **Rare:** Vomiting, arthralgia, myalgia.

ADVERSE EFFECTS/ TOXIC REACTIONS

Antibiotic-associated colitis, other superinfections (abdominal cramps, severe watery diarrhea, fever) may result from altered bacterial balance. Hepatic function abnormalities, severe venous pain, inflammation may occur.

NURSING CONSIDERATIONS

BASELINE ASSESSMENT

Assess temperature, B/P, respiratory rate, pulse. Obtain baseline hepatic function tests, BUN, CBC, urinalysis.

INTERVENTION/EVALUATION

Monitor CBC, hepatic function tests. Observe infusion site for redness, vein irritation. Hold medication, promptly inform physician of diarrhea (with fever, abdominal pain, mucus/blood in stool may indicate antibiotic-associated colitis). Evaluate IV site for erythema, pruritus, pain, burning. Be alert for superinfection: fever, vomiting, diarrhea, anal/genital pruritus, oral mucosal changes (ulceration, pain, erythema).

rabeprazole

rah-**bep**-rah-zole
(Aciphex, Novo-Rabeprazole ✦, Pariet ✦)

Do not confuse Aciphex with Accupril or Aricept, or rabeprazole with aripiprazole, lansoprazole, omeprazole, or raloxifene.

◆CLASSIFICATION

PHARMACOTHERAPEUTIC: Proton pump inhibitor. **CLINICAL:** Gastric acid inhibitor (see p. 148C).

ACTION

Converts to active metabolites that irreversibly bind to, inhibit hydrogen-potassium adenosine triphosphate, an enzyme on surface of gastric parietal cells. Actively secretes hydrogen ions for potassium ions, resulting in accumulation of hydrogen ions in gastric lumen. **Therapeutic Effect:** Increases gastric pH, reducing gastric acid production.

PHARMACOKINETICS

Rapidly absorbed from GI tract after passing through stomach relatively intact as delayed-release tablet. Protein binding: 96%. Metabolized extensively in liver. Primarily excreted in urine. Unknown if removed by hemodialysis. **Half-life:** 1–2 hrs (increased with hepatic impairment).

USES

Short-term treatment (4–8 wks) in healing, maintenance of erosive or ulcerative gastroesophageal reflux disease (GERD). Treatment of daytime/nighttime heartburn, other symptoms of GERD. Short-term treatment (4 wks or less) in healing, symptomatic relief of duodenal ulcers. Long-term treatment of pathologic hypersecretory conditions, including Zollinger-Ellison syndrome. Treatment of NSAID-induced ulcers. Treatment of *H. pylori* (in combination with other medication). **OFF-LABEL:** Maintenance treatment of duodenal ulcers.

PRECAUTIONS

Contraindications: None known. **Cautions:** Hepatic impairment. May increase risk of fractures.

⌛ LIFESPAN CONSIDERATIONS

Pregnancy/Lactation: Unknown if drug crosses placenta or is distributed in breast milk. **Pregnancy Category B. Children:** Safety and efficacy not established. **Elderly:** No age-related precautions noted.

INTERACTIONS

DRUG: May increase concentration, toxicity of **cyclosporine, digoxin, warfarin.** May decrease concentration of **ketoconazole.** May decrease effects of **clopidogrel. HERBAL:** None significant. **FOOD:** None known. **LAB VALUES:** May increase serum AST, ALT, thyroid stimulating hormone (TSH).

AVAILABILITY (Rx)

Tablets (Delayed-Release): 20 mg.

ADMINISTRATION/HANDLING

PO

• May give without regard to meals; best taken before breakfast. • Do not crush, chew, split tablet; swallow whole.

INDICATIONS/ROUTES/DOSAGE

Gastroesophageal Reflux Disease (GERD)
PO: ADULTS, ELDERLY: 20 mg/day for 4–8 wks. Maintenance: 20 mg/day.

Short-Term Treatment of GERD in Children 12 Yrs and Older
PO: 20 mg/day for up to 8 wks.

Duodenal Ulcer
PO: ADULTS, ELDERLY: 20 mg/day after morning meal for 4 wks.

NSAID-Induced Ulcer
PO: ADULTS, ELDERLY: 20 mg/day.

Pathologic Hypersecretory Conditions
PO: ADULTS, ELDERLY: Initially, 60 mg once a day. May increase to 60 mg twice a day.

R

***H. Pylori* Infection**

PO: ADULTS, ELDERLY: 20 mg twice a day for 7 days (given with amoxicillin 1,000 mg and clarithromycin 500 mg).

SIDE EFFECTS

Rare (less than 2%): Headache, nausea, dizziness, rash, diarrhea, malaise.

ADVERSE EFFECTS/ TOXIC REACTIONS

Hyperglycemia, hypokalemia, hyponatremia, hyperlipemia occur rarely.

NURSING CONSIDERATIONS

BASELINE ASSESSMENT

Obtain baseline lab values, esp. serum chemistries.

INTERVENTION/EVALUATION

Monitor ongoing laboratory results. Evaluate for therapeutic response (relief of GI symptoms). Question if GI discomfort, nausea, diarrhea, headache occurs. Assess skin for evidence of rash. Observe for evidence of dizziness; utilize appropriate safety precautions.

PATIENT/FAMILY TEACHING

• Swallow tablets whole; do not chew, split, crush tablets. • Report headache.

R

raloxifene

ra-**lox**-i-feen
(Evista)

BLACK BOX ALERT Increases risk of deep vein thrombosis, pulmonary embolism. Women with coronary heart disease or those at risk for coronary events are at increased risk for death due to stroke.

Do not confuse Evista with Avinza, or raloxifene with propoxyphene.

◆CLASSIFICATION

PHARMACOTHERAPEUTIC: Selective estrogen receptor modulator. **CLINICAL:** Osteoporosis preventive.

ACTION

Selective estrogen receptor modulator that binds to estrogen receptors, increasing bone mineral density. **Therapeutic Effect:** Reduces bone resorption, decreases bone turnover, prevents bone loss.

PHARMACOKINETICS

Rapidly absorbed after PO administration. Highly bound to plasma proteins (greater than 95%) and albumin. Undergoes extensive first-pass metabolism in liver. Excreted mainly in feces and, to a lesser extent, in urine. Unknown if removed by hemodialysis. **Half-life:** 27.7–32.5 hrs.

USES

Prevention/treatment of osteoporosis in postmenopausal women. Reduces risk of invasive breast cancer in postmenopausal women with osteoporosis and postmenopausal women at high risk for invasive breast cancer. **OFF-LABEL:** Prevention of fractures, treatment of breast cancer in postmenopausal women.

PRECAUTIONS

Contraindications: Active or history of venous thromboembolic events, such as deep vein thrombosis (DVT), pulmonary embolism, retinal vein thrombosis; women who are or may become pregnant. **Cautions:** Cardiovascular disease, history of cervical/uterine cancer, renal/hepatic impairment.

LIFESPAN CONSIDERATIONS

Pregnancy/Lactation: Unknown if distributed in breast milk. Not recommended for breast-feeding mothers. **Pregnancy Category X. Children:** Not used in this population. **Elderly:** No age-related precautions noted.

INTERACTIONS

DRUG: Cholestyramine reduces peak levels, extent of absorption. Do not use concurrently with **hormone replacement therapy, systemic estrogen.**

May decrease effect of **warfarin** (decreases PT). **HERBAL:** None significant. **FOOD:** None known. **LAB VALUES:** Lowers serum total cholesterol, LDL. Slightly decreases platelet count, serum inorganic phosphate, albumin, calcium, protein.

AVAILABILITY (Rx)

Tablets: 60 mg.

ADMINISTRATION/HANDLING

PO

- Give without regard to meals.

INDICATIONS/ROUTES/DOSAGE

Prophylaxis/Treatment of Osteoporosis, Breast Cancer Risk Reduction

PO: ADULTS, ELDERLY: 60 mg a day.

SIDE EFFECTS

Frequent (25%–10%): Hot flashes, flu-like symptoms, arthralgia, sinusitis. **Occasional (9%–5%):** Weight gain, nausea, myalgia, pharyngitis, cough, dyspepsia, leg cramps, rash, depression. **Rare (4%–3%):** Vaginitis, UTI, peripheral edema, flatulence, vomiting, fever, migraine, diaphoresis.

ADVERSE EFFECTS/ TOXIC REACTIONS

Pneumonia, gastroenteritis, chest pain, vaginal bleeding, breast pain occur rarely.

NURSING CONSIDERATIONS

BASELINE ASSESSMENT

Question for possibility of pregnancy (Pregnancy Category X). Drug should be discontinued 72 hrs before and during prolonged immobilization (postop recovery, prolonged bed rest). Therapy may be resumed only after pt is fully ambulatory. Determine serum total, LDL cholesterol before therapy and routinely thereafter.

INTERVENTION/EVALUATION

Monitor serum total, LDL cholesterol, total calcium, inorganic phosphate, total protein, albumin, bone mineral density, platelet count.

PATIENT/FAMILY TEACHING

- Avoid prolonged restriction of movement during travel (increased risk of venous thromboembolic events). • Take supplemental calcium, vitamin D if daily dietary intake is inadequate. • Engage in regular weight-bearing exercise. • Modify, discontinue habits of cigarette smoking, alcohol consumption.

raltegravir

ral-**teg**-rah-veer
(Isentress)

◆CLASSIFICATION

PHARMACOTHERAPEUTIC: Integrase inhibitor. **CLINICAL:** Antiviral.

ACTION

Inhibits activity of HIV-1 integrase, an enzyme required for viral replication. **Therapeutic Effect:** Prevents integration and replication of viral HIV-1.

PHARMACOKINETICS

Variably absorbed following PO administration. Protein binding: 83%. Metabolized in liver. Eliminated mainly in feces (51%) with a lesser amount eliminated in urine (32%). **Half-life:** 9 hrs.

USES

Treatment of HIV-1 infection in both treatment-experienced and treatment-naïve adult pts. Used in combination with other antiretroviral agents.

PRECAUTIONS

Contraindications: None known. **Cautions:** Elderly, those at increased risk for myopathy, rhabdomyolysis.

LIFESPAN CONSIDERATIONS

Pregnancy/Lactation: May cross placenta. Breast-feeding not recommended. **Pregnancy Category C. Children:** Safety and efficacy not established in those younger than 16 yrs. **Elderly:** Age-related hepatic, renal, cardiac impairment requires close monitoring.

INTERACTIONS

DRUG: **Atazanavir, atazanavir/ritonavir** may increase raltegravir concentration. **Rifampin, tipranavir/ritonavir** may decrease raltegravir concentration. HERBAL: **St. John's wort** may decrease concentration, effects. FOOD: None known. LAB VALUES: May increase serum glucose, bilirubin, aminotransferase, alkaline phosphatase, amylase, lipase, creatine kinase. May decrease lymphocytes/neutrophil count (ANC), WBC count, Hgb, platelets.

AVAILABILITY (Rx)

Tablets, Film-Coated: 400 mg.

ADMINISTRATION/HANDLING

PO

• Give without regard to food. • Do not crush, split, chew film-coated tablets.

INDICATIONS/ROUTES/DOSAGE

HIV Infection

PO: ADULTS, ELDERLY, CHILDREN OVER 16 YRS: 400 mg twice a day. Dosage increased to 800 mg twice a day when given with rifampin.

SIDE EFFECTS

Frequent (17%–10%): Diarrhea, nausea, headache. Occasional (5%): Fever. Rare (2%–1%): Vomiting, abdominal pain, fatigue, dizziness.

ADVERSE EFFECTS/ TOXIC REACTIONS

Hypersensitivity, anemia, neutropenia, MI, gastritis, hepatitis, herpes simplex, toxic nephropathy, renal failure, chronic renal failure, renal tubular necrosis occur rarely.

NURSING CONSIDERATIONS

BASELINE ASSESSMENT

Obtain baseline laboratory testing before beginning therapy and at periodic intervals during therapy. Offer emotional support. Obtain medication history.

INTERVENTION/EVALUATION

Closely monitor for evidence of GI discomfort. Monitor daily pattern of bowel activity, stool consistency. Monitor serum chemistry tests for marked laboratory abnormalities. Assess for opportunistic infections: onset of fever, cough, other respiratory symptoms.

PATIENT/FAMILY TEACHING

• Contact physician if fever, abdominal pain, yellowing of skin/eyes, dark urine occurs. • Avoid tasks that require alertness, motor skills until response to drug is established. • Raltegravir is not a cure for HIV infection, nor does it reduce risk of transmission to others. • Pt may continue to experience illnesses, including opportunistic infections.

ramelteon

ra-**mel**-tee-on
(Rozerem)
Do not confuse ramelteon with Remeron, or Rozerem with Razadyne or Remeron.

◆CLASSIFICATION

PHARMACOTHERAPEUTIC: Melatonin receptor agonist. CLINICAL: Hypnotic.

ACTION

Selectively targets melatonin receptors thought to be involved in maintenance of circadian rhythm underlying normal sleep-wake cycle. **Therapeutic Effect:** Prevents insomnia characterized by difficulty with sleep onset.

PHARMACOKINETICS

Rapidly absorbed following PO administration. Protein binding: 82%. Substantial tissue distribution. Metabolized in liver.

R

Excreted mainly in urine, with small amount eliminated in feces. **Half-life:** 2–5 hrs.

USES

Long-term treatment of insomnia in pts who experience difficulty with sleep onset.

PRECAUTIONS

Contraindications: Severe hepatic impairment, concurrent fluvoxamine therapy. **Cautions:** Clinical depression, alcohol consumption, moderate hepatic impairment.

LIFESPAN CONSIDERATIONS

Pregnancy/Lactation: Unknown if distributed in breast milk. Breast-feeding not recommended. **Pregnancy Category C. Children:** Safety and efficacy not established. **Elderly:** Age-related hepatic impairment may require dosage adjustment.

INTERACTIONS

DRUG: Concurrent use with **alcohol** produces additive effect. **Fluconazole, ketoconazole** may increase serum concentration, effect. **Fluvoxamine** may cause marked increase in serum level, toxicity. **Rifampin** may decrease serum level, effect. **HERBAL: Gotu kola, kava kava, St. John's wort, valerian** may increase CNS depression. **FOOD:** Onset of action may be reduced if taken with or immediately after a **high-fat meal. LAB VALUES:** May decrease serum cortisol.

AVAILABILITY (Rx)

Tablets, Film-Coated: 8 mg (Rozerem).

ADMINISTRATION/HANDLING

PO

• Administer within 30 min before bedtime. • Do not give with, or immediately following, a high-fat meal. • Do not crush/break tablet.

INDICATIONS/ROUTES/DOSAGE

Insomnia

PO: ADULTS, ELDERLY: 8 mg 30 min before bedtime.

SIDE EFFECTS

Frequent (7%–5%): Headache, dizziness, drowsiness (expected effect). **Occasional (4%–3%):** Fatigue, nausea, exacerbated insomnia. **Rare (2%):** Diarrhea, myalgia, depression, altered taste, arthralgia.

ADVERSE EFFECTS/ TOXIC REACTIONS

May affect reproductive hormones in adults (decreased testosterone levels, increased prolactin levels), resulting in unexplained amenorrhea, galactorrhea, decreased libido, impaired fertility.

NURSING CONSIDERATIONS

BASELINE ASSESSMENT

Assess B/P, pulse, respirations. Raise bed rails, provide call light. Provide environment conducive to sleep (quiet environment, low/no lighting, TV off).

INTERVENTION/EVALUATION

Assess sleep pattern of pt. Evaluate for therapeutic response: rapid induction of sleep onset, decrease in number of nocturnal awakenings.

PATIENT/FAMILY TEACHING

• Take within 30 min before going to bed; confine activities to those necessary to prepare for bed. • Avoid tasks that require alertness, motor skills until response to drug is established. • Avoid alcohol. • Do not take medication with or immediately after a high-fat meal.

ramipril

ram-i-pril
(Altace, Apo-Ramipril ✦, Novo-Ramipril ✦)

R

BLACK BOX ALERT May cause fetal injury, mortality if used during second or third trimester of pregnancy.

Do not confuse Altace with alteplase, Amaryl, Amerge, or Artane, or ramipril with enalapril or Monopril.

CLASSIFICATION

PHARMACOTHERAPEUTIC: Renin-angiotensin system antagonist. **CLINICAL:** Antihypertensive (see p. 9C).

ACTION

Suppresses renin-angiotensin-aldosterone system. Decreases plasma angiotensin II, increases plasma renin activity, decreases aldosterone secretion. **Therapeutic Effect:** Reduces peripheral arterial resistance, decreasing B/P.

PHARMACOKINETICS

Route	Onset	Peak	Duration
PO	1–2 hrs	3–6 hrs	24 hrs

Well absorbed from GI tract. Protein binding: 73%. Metabolized in liver to active metabolite. Primarily excreted in urine. Not removed by hemodialysis. **Half-life:** 5.1 hrs.

USES

Treatment of hypertension. Used alone or in combination with other antihypertensives. Treatment of left ventricular dysfunction following MI. Prevention of heart attack, stroke. **OFF-LABEL:** Treatment of pediatric hypertension, renal crisis in scleroderma, CHF. Delay progression of nephropathy, reduce risks of cardiovascular events in hypertensive pts with type 1 or type 2 diabetes.

PRECAUTIONS

Contraindications: Bilateral renal artery stenosis. **Cautions:** Renal impairment, collagen vascular disease, hypovolemia, renal stenosis, hyperkalemia.

LIFESPAN CONSIDERATIONS

Pregnancy/Lactation: Crosses placenta. Distributed in breast milk. May cause fetal or neonatal mortality or morbidity. **Pregnancy Category C (D if used in second or third trimester). Children:** Safety and efficacy not established. **Elderly:** May be more sensitive to hypotensive effects.

INTERACTIONS

DRUG: **Alcohol, antihypertensives, diuretics** may increase effects. May increase **lithium** concentration, risk of toxicity. **NSAIDs** may decrease effects. **Potassium-sparing diuretics, potassium supplements** may cause hyperkalemia. **HERBAL:** **Garlic** may increase antihypertensive effect. **Ginseng, yohimbe** may worsen hypertension. **FOOD:** None known. **LAB VALUES:** May increase BUN, serum alkaline phosphatase, bilirubin, creatinine, potassium, AST, ALT. May decrease serum sodium. May cause positive antinuclear antibody (ANA) titer.

AVAILABILITY (Rx)

Capsules: 1.25 mg, 2.5 mg, 5 mg, 10 mg.

ADMINISTRATION/HANDLING

PO

• Give without regard to food. • May mix with water, apple juice/sauce.

INDICATIONS/ROUTES/DOSAGE

Hypertension (Monotherapy)

PO: ADULTS, ELDERLY: Initially, 2.5 mg/day. Maintenance: 2.5–20 mg/day as single dose or in 2 divided doses.

Hypertension (in Combination with Other Antihypertensives)

PO: ADULTS, ELDERLY: Initially, 1.25 mg/day titrated to pt's needs.

Left Ventricular Dysfunction Following MI

PO: ADULTS, ELDERLY: Initially, 1.25–2.5 mg twice a day. **Maximum:** 5 mg twice a day.

Risk Reduction for MI/Stroke

PO: ADULTS, ELDERLY: Initially, 2.5 mg/day for 7 days, then 5 mg/day for 21 days, then 10 mg/day as a single dose or in divided doses.

Dosage in Renal Impairment

Creatinine clearance equal to or less than 40 ml/min: 25% of normal dose.

Renal Failure

HYPERTENSION: Initially, 1.25 mg/day titrated upward.

CHF: Initially, 1.25 mg/day, titrated up to 2.5 mg twice a day.

SIDE EFFECTS

Frequent (12%–5%): Cough, headache. **Occasional (4%–2%):** Dizziness, fatigue, nausea, asthenia (loss of strength, energy). **Rare (less than 2%):** Palpitations, insomnia, nervousness, malaise, abdominal pain, myalgia.

ADVERSE EFFECTS/ TOXIC REACTIONS

Excessive hypotension ("first-dose syncope") may occur in pts with CHF, severely salt or volume depleted. Angioedema, hyperkalemia occur rarely. Agranulocytosis, neutropenia may be noted in those with collagen vascular disease (scleroderma, systemic lupus erythematosus), renal impairment. Nephrotic syndrome may be noted in those with history of renal disease.

NURSING CONSIDERATIONS

BASELINE ASSESSMENT

Obtain B/P immediately before each dose, in addition to regular monitoring (be alert to fluctuations). If excessive reduction in B/P occurs, place pt in supine position with legs elevated. Renal function tests should be performed before beginning therapy. In pts with prior renal disease, urine test for protein (by dipstick method) should be made with first urine of day before beginning therapy and periodically thereafter. In those with renal impairment, autoimmune disease, or taking drugs that affect leukocytes or immune response, CBC, differential count should be performed before beginning therapy and q2wk for 3 mos periodically thereafter.

INTERVENTION/EVALUATION

Monitor B/P, renal function, serum potassium, WBC. Assess for cough (frequent effect). Assist with ambulation if dizziness occurs. Assess lung sounds for rales, wheezing in pts with CHF. Monitor urinalysis for proteinuria. Monitor serum potassium in those on concurrent diuretic therapy.

PATIENT/FAMILY TEACHING

• Do not discontinue medication without physician's approval. • Rise slowly from sitting/lying position to reduce hypotensive effect. • Report palpitations, cough, chest pain. • Dizziness, light-headedness may occur in first few days. • Avoid tasks that require alertness, motor skills until response to drug is established. • Avoid alcohol.

ranitidine

ra-**ni**-ti-dine

(Apo-Ranitidine ✦, Novo-Ranitidine ✦, Zantac, Zantac-75, Zantac-150, Zantac EFFERdose)

Do not confuse ranitidine with amantadine or rimantadine, or Zantac with Xanax, Ziac, Zofran, or Zyrtec.

◆CLASSIFICATION

PHARMACOTHERAPEUTIC: Histamine H_2 receptor antagonist. **CLINICAL:** Antiulcer (see p. 108C).

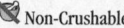

R

ACTION

Inhibits histamine action at histamine 2 receptors of gastric parietal cells. **Therapeutic Effect:** Inhibits gastric acid secretion (fasting, nocturnal, when stimulated by food, caffeine, insulin). Reduces volume, hydrogen ion concentration of gastric juice.

PHARMACOKINETICS

Rapidly absorbed from GI tract. Protein binding: 15%. Widely distributed. Metabolized in liver. Primarily excreted in urine. Not removed by hemodialysis. **Half-life: PO:** 2.5 hrs; **IV:** 2–2.5 hrs (increased with renal impairment).

USES

Short-term treatment of active duodenal ulcer. Prevention of duodenal ulcer recurrence. Treatment of active benign gastric ulcer, pathologic GI hypersecretory conditions, acute gastroesophageal reflux disease (GERD), including erosive esophagitis. Maintenance of healed erosive esophagitis. Part of regimen for *H. pylori* eradication to reduce risk of duodenal ulcer recurrence. **OTC:** Relieve heartburn, acid indigestion, sour stomach. **OFF-LABEL:** Prevention of aspiration pneumonia, treatment of recurrent postop ulcer, upper GI bleeding, prevention of acid aspiration pneumonitis during surgery, prevention of stress-induced ulcers.

PRECAUTIONS

Contraindications: History of acute porphyria. **Cautions:** Renal/hepatic impairment, elderly.

LIFESPAN CONSIDERATIONS

Pregnancy/Lactation: Unknown if drug crosses placenta or is distributed in breast milk. **Pregnancy Category B. Children:** No age-related precautions noted. **Elderly:** Confusion more likely with hepatic/renal impairment.

INTERACTIONS

DRUG: Magnesium or aluminum antacids may decrease absorption. May decrease absorption of **itraconazole, ketoconazole. HERBAL:** None significant. **FOOD:** None known. **LAB VALUES:** Interferes with skin tests using allergen extracts. May increase hepatic serum enzymes, gamma-glutamyl transpeptidase, creatinine.

AVAILABILITY (Rx)

Capsules (Zantac): 150 mg, 300 mg. **Injection Solution (Zantac):** 25 mg/ml. **Syrup (Zantac):** 15 mg/ml. **Tablets (Effervescent):** 25 mg (Zantac EFFERdose). **Tablets (Hydrochloride):** 75 mg (OTC), 150 mg, 300 mg.

ADMINISTRATION/HANDLING

IV

Reconstitution • For IV push, dilute each 50 mg with 20 ml 0.9% NaCl, D_5W. • For intermittent IV infusion (piggyback), dilute each 50 mg with 0.9% NaCl, D_5W to a maximum concentration of 0.5 mg/ml. • For IV infusion, dilute with 0.9% NaCl, D_5W to a maximum concentration of 2.5 mg/ml.

Rate of administration • Administer IV push over minimum of 5 min (prevents arrhythmias, hypotension). • Infuse IV piggyback over 15–20 min. • Infuse IV infusion over 24 hrs.

Storage • IV solutions appear clear, colorless to yellow (slight darkening does not affect potency). • IV infusion (piggyback) is stable for 48 hrs at room temperature (discard if discolored or precipitate forms).

IM

• May be given undiluted. • Give deep IM into large muscle mass.

PO

• Give without regard to meals (best given after meals or at bedtime). • Do not administer within 1 hr of magnesium- or aluminum-containing antacids (decreases absorption).

IV INCOMPATIBILITY

Amphotericin B complex (Abelcet, AmBisome, Amphotec).

IV COMPATIBILITIES

Diltiazem (Cardizem), dobutamine (Dobutrex), dopamine (Intropin), heparin, hydromorphone (Dilaudid), insulin, lidocaine, lipids, lorazepam (Ativan), morphine, norepinephrine (Levophed), potassium chloride, propofol (Diprivan).

INDICATIONS/ROUTES/DOSAGE

Duodenal Ulcer, Gastric Ulcer, GERD

PO: ADULTS, ELDERLY: 150 mg twice a day or 300 mg at bedtime. Maintenance: 150 mg at bedtime. **CHILDREN:** 2–4 mg/kg/day in divided doses twice a day. **Maximum:** 300 mg/day.

Duodenal Ulcer Associated with *H. Pylori* Infection

PO: ADULTS, ELDERLY: 150 mg twice a day for 4 wks in combination with amoxicillin and clarithromycin.

Erosive Esophagitis

PO: ADULTS, ELDERLY: 150 mg 4 times a day. Maintenance: 150 mg twice a day or 300 mg at bedtime. **CHILDREN:** 5–10 mg/kg/day in 2 divided doses. **Maximum:** 600 mg/day.

Hypersecretory Conditions

PO: ADULTS, ELDERLY: 150 mg twice a day. May increase up to 6 g/day.

OTC Use

PO: ADULTS, ELDERLY: 75 mg 30–60 min before eating food, drinking beverages that cause heartburn. **Maximum:** 150 mg per 24-hr period and/or longer than 14 days.

Usual Parenteral Dosage

IV, IM: ADULTS, ELDERLY: 50 mg/dose q6–8h. **Maximum:** 400 mg/day. **CONTINUOUS IV INFUSION:** 6.25 mg/hr. **CHILDREN:** 2–4 mg/kg/day in divided doses q6–8h. **Maximum:** 200 mg/day.

Usual Neonatal Dosage

PO: NEONATES: 2 mg/kg/day in divided doses q12h.

IV: NEONATES: Initially, 1.5 mg/kg/dose, then 1.5–2 mg/kg/day in divided doses q12h.

Dosage in Renal Impairment

Creatinine clearance less than 50 ml/min: Give 150 mg PO q24h or 50 mg IV or IM q18–24h.

SIDE EFFECTS

Occasional (2%): Diarrhea. **Rare** (1%): Constipation, headache (may be severe).

ADVERSE EFFECTS/ TOXIC REACTIONS

Reversible hepatitis, blood dyscrasias occur rarely.

NURSING CONSIDERATIONS

BASELINE ASSESSMENT

Obtain history of epigastric/abdominal pain. Obtain baseline hepatic/renal function tests.

INTERVENTION/EVALUATION

Monitor serum AST, ALT levels, creatinine, BUN. Assess mental status in elderly. Question present abdominal pain, GI distress.

PATIENT/FAMILY TEACHING

• Smoking decreases effectiveness of medication. • Do not take medicine within 1 hr of magnesium- or aluminum-containing antacids. • Transient burning/pruritus may occur with IV administration. • Report headache. • Avoid alcohol, aspirin.

ranolazine

rah-**noe**-la-zeen
(Ranexa)
Do not confuse Ranexa with Celexa.

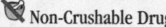

◆ CLASSIFICATION

PHARMACOTHERAPEUTIC: Sodium current inhibitor. **CLINICAL:** Antianginal, anti-ischemic.

ACTION

Thought to elicit changes in cardiac metabolism. Does not reduce heart rate, B/P. **Therapeutic Effect:** Exerts antianginal, anti-ischemic effects on cardiac tissue.

PHARMACOKINETICS

Route	Onset	Peak	Duration
PO	N/A	2–5 hrs	N/A

Absorption highly variable. Rapidly, extensively metabolized in intestine, liver. Protein binding: 62%. Eliminated mainly in urine, with lesser amount excreted in feces. **Half-life:** 7 hrs.

USES

Treatment of chronic angina, used alone or in combination with beta-blockers, calcium channel blockers, or nitrates.

PRECAUTIONS

Contraindications: Preexisting QT prolongation, hepatic impairment, concurrent use with medications known to cause QT interval prolongation, concurrent use of potent CYP3A inhibitors (ketoconazole, itraconazole, fluconazole, clarithromycin, erythromycin). **Cautions:** Renal impairment.

R

⌛ LIFESPAN CONSIDERATIONS

Pregnancy/Lactation: Unknown if drug crosses placenta or is distributed in breast milk. **Pregnancy Category C. Children:** Safety and efficacy not established. **Elderly:** No age-related precautions noted.

INTERACTIONS

DRUG: **Diltiazem, paroxetine, verapamil** may increase serum concentration. May increase concentration of **digoxin, simvastatin. Antiarrhythmic agents, dofetilide, quinidine, sotalol, thioridazine, ziprasidone** may increase risk of QT prolongation. **HERBAL:** None significant. **FOOD:** **Grapefruit, grapefruit juice** may increase plasma concentration, risk of QT prolongation. **LAB VALUES:** May slightly elevate BUN, serum creatinine.

AVAILABILITY (Rx)

Tablets (Extended-Release): 500 mg, 1,000 mg.

ADMINISTRATION/HANDLING

PO

• May give without regard to food. • Limit use of grapefruit, grapefruit juice. • Do not crush, chew, break extended-release tablets.

INDICATIONS/ROUTES/DOSAGE

Chronic Angina

PO: ADULTS, ELDERLY: Initially, 500 mg twice daily. May increase to 1,000 mg twice daily, based on clinical response. Dose should not exceed 500 mg twice daily when used concurrently with moderate CYP3A inhibitors (e.g., diltiazem, verapamil).

SIDE EFFECTS

Occasional (6%–4%): Dizziness, headache, constipation, nausea. **Rare (2%–1%):** Peripheral edema, abdominal pain, dry mouth, vomiting, tinnitus, vertigo, palpitations.

ADVERSE EFFECTS/ TOXIC REACTIONS

Overdose manifested as confusion, diplopia, dizziness, paresthesia, syncope.

NURSING CONSIDERATIONS

BASELINE ASSESSMENT

Record onset, type (sharp, dull, squeezing), radiation, location, intensity, duration of anginal pain, precipitating factors (exertion, emotional stress). Obtain baseline EKG.

INTERVENTION/EVALUATION

Assist with ambulation if dizziness occurs. Give with food if nausea occurs. Monitor daily pattern of bowel activity, stool consistency. Assess for relief of anginal pain. Monitor EKG, pulse for irregularities.

PATIENT/FAMILY TEACHING

• Limit use of grapefruit, grapefruit juice. • Do not chew/crush extended-release tablets. • Avoid tasks requiring alertness, motor skills until response to drug is established.

Rapamune, *see sirolimus*

rasagiline

rah-**sa**-jih-leen
(Azilect)
Do not confuse Azilect with Aricept.

◆CLASSIFICATION

PHARMACOTHERAPEUTIC: MAOI. **CLINICAL:** Antiparkinson agent.

ACTION

Inhibits monoamine oxidase, an enzyme that plays a major role in catabolism of dopamine. Inhibition of dopamine depletion reduces symptomatic motor deficits of Parkinson's disease. Appears to possess neuroprotective effects, delaying onset of symptoms, progression of neuronal deterioration. **Therapeutic Effect:** Reduces symptoms of Parkinson's disease, appears to delay disease progression.

PHARMACOKINETICS

Route	Onset	Peak	Duration
PO	1 hr	N/A	1 wk

Rapidly absorbed following PO administration. Protein binding: 88%–94%. Metabolized in liver. Mainly eliminated in urine, with lesser amount excreted in feces. **Half-life:** 1.3–3 hrs.

USES

Treatment of signs/symptoms of Parkinson's disease as initial monotherapy or as adjunct therapy to levodopa.

PRECAUTIONS

Contraindications: Pheochromocytoma, concurrent use with meperidine, methadone, propoxyphene, tramadol, dextromethorphan, St. John's wort, mirtazapine, cyclobenzaprine, sympathomimetic amines (including amphetamines, nasal/oral decongestants, cold products, weight-reducing preparations), other MAOIs, cocaine, local or general anesthetic agents. **Cautions:** Hepatic impairment, ingestion of tyramine-rich foods, beverages, dietary supplements or amines contained in cough/cold medications.

⌛ LIFESPAN CONSIDERATIONS

Pregnancy/Lactation: Unknown if distributed in breast milk. **Pregnancy Category C. Children:** Safety and efficacy not established. **Elderly:** No age-related precautions noted.

INTERACTIONS

DRUG: Amphetamines, other MAOIs (phenelzine, tranylcypromine), sympathomimetics (dopamine, metaraminol, phenylephrine, pseudoephedrine) may cause hypertensive crisis. **Anorexiants (dexfenfluramine, fenfluramine, sibutramine), CNS stimulants (methylphenidate), cyclobenzaprine, dextromethorphan, meperidine, methadone, mirtazapine, propoxyphene, serotonin or norepinephrine reuptake inhibitors, sibutramine, tramodol, trazodone, tricyclic antidepressants, venlafaxine** may cause serotonin syndrome. May increase risk of **atomoxetine, bupropion** toxicity. **Buspirone** may cause increase in B/P. **Ciprofloxacin, entacapone, tolcapone** may increase concentration (reduced dosage recommended). **Amino-**

R

glutethimide, carbamazepine, phenobarbital, rifampin may decrease concentration. **Levodopa** may cause hypertensive/hypotensive reaction. **Lithium** may result in malignant hyperpyrexia. **Reserpine** may result in hypertensive reaction. **Tramadol** may increase risk of seizures. HERBAL: **Kava kava, SAMe, St. John's wort, valerian** may increase risk of serotonin syndrome, excessive sedation. FOOD: **Caffeine, foods/beverages containing tyramine** may result in hypertensive reaction, hypertensive crisis. LAB VALUES: May increase serum alkaline phosphatase, bilirubin, ALT, AST. May cause leukopenia.

AVAILABILITY (Rx)

Tablets: 0.5 mg, 1 mg.

ADMINISTRATION/HANDLING

PO

• Give without regard to food. • Avoid food, beverages containing tyramine (cheese, sour cream, yogurt, pickled herring, liver, canned figs, raisins, bananas, avocados, soy sauce, broad beans, yeast extracts, meats prepared with tenderizers, red wine, beer).

INDICATIONS/ROUTES/DOSAGE

◀ALERT▶ When used in combination with levodopa, dosage reduction of levodopa should be considered.

R

Parkinson's Disease

PO: ADULTS, ELDERLY, MONOTHERAPY: 1 mg once daily.

PO: ADULTS, ELDERLY, ADJUNCTIVE THERAPY: Initially, 0.5 mg once daily. If therapeutic response is not achieved, dose may be increased to 1 mg once daily.

Mild Hepatic Impairment, Concurrent Use of Ciprofloxacin, Other CYP1A2 Inhibitors

PO: ADULTS, ELDERLY: 0.5 mg once daily.

SIDE EFFECTS

Frequent (14%–12%): Headache, nausea. Occasional (9%–5%): Orthostatic hypotension, weight loss, dyspepsia (heartburn, indigestion, epigastric pain), dry mouth, arthralgia, depression, hallucinations, constipation. Rare (4%–2%): Fever, vertigo, ecchymosis, rhinitis, neck pain, arthritis, paresthesia.

ADVERSE EFFECTS/ TOXIC REACTIONS

Increase in dyskinesia (impaired voluntary movement), dystonia (impaired muscular tone) occur in 18% of pts, angina occurs in 9%. Gastroenteritis, conjunctivitis occur rarely (3%).

NURSING CONSIDERATIONS

BASELINE ASSESSMENT

Obtain baseline hepatic enzyme levels.

INTERVENTION/EVALUATION

Give with food if nausea occurs. Monitor B/P. Instruct pt to rise from lying to sitting or sitting to standing position slowly to prevent orthostatic hypotension. Assess for clinical reversal of symptoms (improvement of tremor of head/hands at rest, mask-like facial expression, shuffling gait, muscular rigidity). If hallucinations or dyskinesia occur, symptoms may be eliminated if levodopa dosage is reduced. Hallucinations generally are accompanied by confusion and, to a lesser extent, insomnia.

PATIENT/FAMILY TEACHING

Orthostatic hypotension may occur more frequently during initial therapy. Avoid tasks that require alertness, motor skills until response to drug is established. Hallucinations may occur (more so in the elderly than in younger pts with Parkinson's disease), typically within first 2 wks of therapy. Avoid foods that contain tyramine (cheese, sour cream, beer, wine, pickled herring, liver, figs, raisins, bananas, avocados, soy sauce, yeast extracts, yogurt, papaya, broad beans, meat tenderizers), excessive amounts of caffeine (coffee, tea, chocolate), OTC preparations for hay fever, colds, weight reduction (may produce significant rise in B/P).

Rebetol, *see ribavirin*

Reglan, *see metoclopramide*

Relpax, *see eletriptan*

Remeron, *see mirtazapine*

Remicade, *see infliximab*

RenaGel, *see sevelamer*

ReoPro, *see abciximab*

repaglinide HIGH ALERT

re-**pag**-li-nide
(GlucoNorm ✱, Prandin)
Do not confuse Prandin with Avandia.

FIXED-COMBINATION(S)

Prandimet: repaglinide/metformin (an antidiabetic): 1 mg/500 mg, 2 mg/500 mg.

◆ CLASSIFICATION

PHARMACOTHERAPEUTIC: Antidiabetic. **CLINICAL:** Antihyperglycemic (see p. 44C).

ACTION

Stimulates release of insulin from beta cells of pancreas by depolarizing beta cells, leading to opening of calcium channels. Resulting calcium influx induces insulin secretion. **Therapeutic Effect:** Lowers serum glucose concentration.

PHARMACOKINETICS

Rapidly, completely absorbed from GI tract. Protein binding: 98%. Metabolized in liver to inactive metabolites. Excreted primarily in feces, with lesser amount in urine. Unknown if removed by hemodialysis. **Half-life:** 1 hr.

USES

Adjunct to diet, exercise to lower serum glucose in pts with type 2 diabetes mellitus. Used as monotherapy or in combination with metformin, pioglitazone, rosiglitazone. Used primarily to reduce postprandial glucose levels in pts taking another medication.

PRECAUTIONS

Contraindications: Diabetic ketoacidosis, type 1 diabetes mellitus. **Cautions:** Hepatic/renal impairment.

LIFESPAN CONSIDERATIONS

Pregnancy/Lactation: Unknown if drug is distributed in breast milk. **Pregnancy Category C. Children:** Safety and efficacy not established. **Elderly:** No age-related precautions noted, but hypoglycemia may be more difficult to recognize.

INTERACTIONS

DRUG: **Beta-adrenergic blocking agents (beta-blockers), gemfibrozil, MAOIs, NSAIDs, probenecid, salicylates, sulfonamides** may increase effects. **HERBAL:** **St. John's wort** may decrease concentration. **Garlic, ginger, ginseng** may cause hypoglycemia. **FOOD:** **Food** decreases concentration. **LAB VALUES:** Hepatic enzymes may be elevated.

AVAILABILITY (Rx)

Tablets: 0.5 mg, 1 mg, 2 mg.

R

ADMINISTRATION/HANDLING

PO

• Ideally, give within 15 min of a meal but may be given immediately before a meal to as long as 30 min before a meal.

INDICATIONS/ROUTES/DOSAGE

Diabetes Mellitus

PO: ADULTS, ELDERLY: 0.5–4 mg 2–4 times daily. **Maximum:** 16 mg/day.

SIDE EFFECTS

Frequent (10%–6%): Upper respiratory tract infection, headache, rhinitis, bronchitis, back pain. Occasional (5%–3%): Diarrhea, dyspepsia (heartburn, indigestion, epigastric pain), sinusitis, nausea, arthralgia, UTI. Rare (2%): Constipation, vomiting, paresthesia, allergy.

ADVERSE EFFECTS/ TOXIC REACTIONS

Hypoglycemia occurs in 16% of pts. Chest pain occurs rarely.

NURSING CONSIDERATIONS

BASELINE ASSESSMENT

Check fasting serum glucose, glycosylated Hgb (Hb_{A1C}) levels periodically to determine minimum effective dose. Ensure follow-up instruction if pt, family do not thoroughly understand diabetes management, glucose-testing technique. At least 1 wk should elapse to assess response to drug before new dosage adjustment is made.

INTERVENTION/EVALUATION

Monitor fasting serum glucose, glycosylated Hgb (Hb_{A1C}) levels, food intake. Assess for hypoglycemia (cool/wet skin, tremors, dizziness, anxiety, headache, tachycardia, numbness in mouth, hunger, diplopia), hyperglycemia (polyuria, polyphagia, polydipsia, nausea, vomiting, dim vision, fatigue, deep or rapid breathing). Be alert to conditions that alter glucose requirements (fever, increased activity/stress, surgical procedures).

PATIENT/FAMILY TEACHING

• Diabetes mellitus requires lifelong control. • Prescribed diet, exercise is principal part of treatment; do not skip, delay meals. • Continue to adhere to dietary instructions, regular exercise program, regular testing of urine or serum glucose. • When taking combination drug therapy with a sulfonylurea or insulin, have source of glucose available to treat symptoms of low blood sugar.

Requip, *see ropinirole*

Restasis, *see cyclosporine*

Restoril, *see temazepam*

reteplase

HIGH ALERT

reh-te-place

(Retavase)

Do not confuse reteplase or Retavase with Restasis.

◆ CLASSIFICATION

PHARMACOTHERAPEUTIC: Tissue plasminogen activator. **CLINICAL:** Thrombolytic (see p. 33C).

ACTION

Activates fibrinolytic system by directly cleaving plasminogen to generate plasmin, an enzyme that degrades fibrin clot within a thrombus. **Therapeutic Effect:** Exerts thrombolytic action.

PHARMACOKINETICS

Rapidly cleared from plasma. Onset: 30–90 min. Eliminated primarily by liver, kidney. **Half-life:** 13–16 min.

USES

Management of acute myocardial infarction (AMI), improvement of ventricular function following AMI, reduction of incidence of CHF, reduction of mortality associated with AMI. OFF-LABEL: Occluded indwelling venous catheters.

PRECAUTIONS

Contraindications: Active internal bleeding, AV malformation/aneurysm, bleeding diathesis, history of CVA, intracranial neoplasm, recent intracranial/intraspinal surgery or trauma, severe uncontrolled hypertension. **Cautions:** Recent major surgery (coronary artery bypass graft, OB delivery, organ biopsy), cerebrovascular disease, recent GI/GU bleeding, hypertension, mitral stenosis with atrial fibrillation, acute pericarditis, bacterial endocarditis, hepatic/renal impairment, diabetic retinopathy, ophthalmic hemorrhage, septic thrombophlebitis, occluded AV cannula at infected site, advanced age, pts receiving oral anticoagulants.

LIFESPAN CONSIDERATIONS

Pregnancy/Lactation: Unknown if drug is distributed in breast milk. **Pregnancy Category C. Children:** Safety and efficacy not established. **Elderly:** More susceptible to bleeding; caution advised.

INTERACTIONS

DRUG: **Heparin, platelet aggregation antagonists (e.g., abciximab, aspirin, dipyridamole), warfarin** increase risk of bleeding. HERBAL: **Cat's claw, dong quai, evening primrose, feverfew, garlic, ginger, ginkgo, ginseng, red clover** possess antiplatelet action, may increase bleeding. FOOD: None known. LAB VALUES: May decrease serum fibrinogen, plasminogen.

AVAILABILITY (Rx)

Injection, Powder for Reconstitution: 10.4 units (18.1 mg) (packaged with Sterile Water for Injection).

ADMINISTRATION/HANDLING

IV

Reconstitution • Reconstitute only with Sterile Water for Injection immediately before use. Use diluent, syringe, needle, dispensing pin provided with each kit. • Reconstituted solution contains 1 unit/ml. • Do not shake. • Slight foaming may occur; let stand for a few minutes to allow bubbles to dissipate.

Rate of administration • Give through dedicated IV line. • Give each IV bolus administered over 2-min period. • Give second bolus 30 min after first bolus injection. • Do not add other medications to bolus injection solution. • Do not give second bolus if serious bleeding occurs after first IV bolus is given.

Storage • Use within 4 hrs of reconstitution. • Discard any unused portion.

IV INCOMPATIBILITIES

Do not mix with other medications.

INDICATIONS/ROUTES/DOSAGE

Acute MI, CHF

IV BOLUS: ADULTS, ELDERLY: 10 units over 2 min; repeat in 30 min.

SIDE EFFECTS

Frequent: Bleeding at superficial sites, such as venous injection sites, catheter insertion sites, venous cutdowns, arterial punctures, sites of recent surgical procedures, gingival bleeding.

ADVERSE EFFECTS/ TOXIC REACTIONS

Bleeding at internal sites (intracranial, retroperitoneal, GI, GU, respiratory) occurs occasionally. Lysis of coronary thrombi may produce atrial or ventricular arrhythmias, stroke.

NURSING CONSIDERATIONS

BASELINE ASSESSMENT

Obtain baseline B/P, apical pulse. Evaluate 12-lead EKG, CPK, CPK-MB, serum

R

electrolytes. Assess Hct, platelet count, thrombin time (TT), aPTT, PT, serum plasminogen, fibrinogen levels before therapy is instituted. Type, hold blood.

INTERVENTION/EVALUATION

Carefully monitor all needle puncture sites, catheter insertion sites for bleeding. Observe continuous cardiac monitoring for arrhythmias; monitoring B/P, pulse, respiration is essential until pt is stable. Check peripheral pulses, lung sounds. Monitor for chest pain relief; notify physician of continuation/recurrence of chest pain (note location, type, intensity). Avoid any trauma that may increase risk of bleeding (injections, shaving).

Revlimid, *see lenalidomide*

Reyataz, *see atazanavir*

Rhinocort Aqua, *see budesonide*

R

Rh_o (D) immune globulin

row D ih-**mewn glah**-bue-lin (Hyper-RHO S/D Full Dose, Hyper-RHO S/D Mini Dose, MICRhoGAM, RhoGAM, Rhophylac, WinRho SDF)

◆**CLASSIFICATION**

CLINICAL: Immune globulin.

ACTION

Suppresses active antibody response, formation of anti-Rh_o(D) in Rh_o(D)-negative women exposed to Rh_o-positive blood from pregnancy with Rh_o(D)-positive fetus or transfusion with Rh_o(D)-positive blood. Injection of Rh_o(D) immune globulin into Rh-positive pt with idiopathic thrombocytopenic purpura (ITP) coats pt's own D-positive RBCs with antibody; as RBCs are cleared by spleen, they saturate capacity of spleen to clear antibody-coated cells. **Therapeutic Effect:** Prevents antibody response, hemolytic disease of newborn in women who previously conceived Rh_o(D)-positive fetus. Prevents Rh_o(D) sensitization in pts who have received Rh_o(D)-positive blood. Decreases bleeding in pts with ITP.

PHARMACOKINETICS

	Onset	Peak	Duration
ITP (increase platelets)	1–2 days	7–14 days	30 days

Half-life: 21–30 days.

USES

Treatment of Rh_o(D)-positive children, adults (without splenectomy) with chronic idiopathic thrombocytopenic purpura (ITP), children with acute ITP, children, adults with ITP secondary to HIV infection; prevention of isoimmunization in Rh-negative individuals exposed to Rh-positive blood during delivery of an Rh-positive infant, within 72 hrs of an abortion, following amniocentesis or abdominal trauma, following transfusion accident; prevention of hemolytic disease of newborn if there is a subsequent pregnancy with Rh-positive infant.

PRECAUTIONS

Contraindications: Hypersensitivity to any component, IgA deficiency, mothers whose Rh group or immune status is uncertain, prior sensitization to Rh_o(D), Rh_o(D)-positive mother or pregnant woman, transfusion of Rh_o(D)-positive blood in previous 3 mos. **Cautions:** Thrombocytopenia, bleeding disorders. Hgb less than 8 g/dl.

LIFESPAN CONSIDERATIONS

Pregnancy/Lactation: Does not appear to harm fetus. **Pregnancy Category C.** **Children/Elderly:** No age-related precautions noted.

INTERACTIONS

DRUG: May interfere with pt's immune response to **live virus vaccines.** **HERBAL:** None significant. **FOOD:** None known. **LAB VALUES:** None significant.

AVAILABILITY (Rx)

Injection Solution: (Hyper-RHO): 50 mcg, 300 mcg. **(MICRhoGAM):** 50 mcg. **(RhoGAM):** 300 mcg. **(Rhophylac):** 300 mcg/2 ml. **(WinRhO SDF):** 120 mcg/0.5 ml, 300 mcg/1.3 ml, 500 mcg/2.2 ml, 1,000 mcg/4.4 ml, 3,000 mcg/13 ml.

ADMINISTRATION/HANDLING

IM

- Administer into deltoid muscle of upper arm, anterolateral aspect of upper thigh.

INDICATIONS/ROUTES/DOSAGE

Idiopathic Thrombocytopenic Purpura (ITP)

IV (WinRho SDF): ADULTS, ELDERLY, CHILDREN: Initially, 50 mcg/kg as single dose (reduce to 25–40 mcg/kg if Hgb is less than 10 g/dl). Maintenance: 25–60 mcg/kg based on platelet count and Hgb level. **(Rhophylac):** 50 mcg/kg.

Suppression of Active Antibody Response in Pregnancy

IM (Hyper-RHO Full Dose, RhoGAM): ADULTS: 300 mcg preferably within 72 hrs of delivery.

IV, IM (WinRho SDF): ADULTS: 300 mcg at 28 wks' gestation. After delivery: 120 mcg preferably within 72 hrs.

Suppression of Active Antibody Response in Threatened Abortion

IM (Hyper-RHO Full Dose, RhoGAM): ADULTS: 300 mcg as soon as possible.

Suppression of Active Antibody Response in Abortion, Miscarriage, Termination of Ectopic Pregnancy

IM (Hyper-RHO, RhoGAM): ADULTS: 300 mcg if more than 13 wks' gestation, 50 mcg if less than 13 wks' gestation.

IV, IM (WinRho SDF): ADULTS: 120 mcg after 34 wks gestation.

Transfusion Incompatibility

ALERT Must give within 72 hrs after exposure to incompatible blood transfusion, massive fetal hemorrhage. Dose is calculated based on exposure to Rh_o(D)-positive whole blood or red blood cells.

IV: ADULTS: 3,000 units (600 mcg) q8h until total dose given.

IM: ADULTS: 6,000 units (1,200 mcg) q12h until total dose given.

SIDE EFFECTS

Hypotension, pallor, vasodilation (IV formulation), fever, headache, chills, dizziness, drowsiness, lethargy, rash, pruritus, abdominal pain, diarrhea, discomfort/swelling at injection site, back pain, myalgia, arthralgia, asthenia (loss of strength, energy).

ADVERSE EFFECTS/ TOXIC REACTIONS

Acute renal failure occurs rarely.

NURSING CONSIDERATIONS

BASELINE ASSESSMENT

Determine existence of bleeding disorders. Assess pt's Hgb level; give drug cautiously to pts with Hgb level less than 8 g/dl.

INTERVENTION/EVALUATION

Monitor CBC (esp. Hgb, platelet count), BUN, serum creatinine, reticulocyte count, urinalysis results. Assess for signs/symptoms of hemolysis.

PATIENT/FAMILY TEACHING

- This drug is given only by injection, which may be painful. • Notify physician if chills, dizziness, fever, headache, rash occur.

R

ribavirin

rye-ba-**vye**-rin
(Copegus, Rebetol, RibaPak, Ribasphere, Virazole)

BLACK BOX ALERT Pregnancy Category X. Significant teratogenic/embryocidal effects. Hemolytic anemia is significant toxicity, usually occurring within 1–2 wks. May worsen cardiac disease and lead to fatal or nonfatal MI.

Do not confuse ribavirin with riboflavin, rifampin, or Robaxin.

FIXED-COMBINATION(S)

With interferon alfa 2b (**Rebetron**). Individually packaged.

◆CLASSIFICATION

PHARMACOTHERAPEUTIC: Synthetic nucleoside. **CLINICAL:** Antiviral (see p. 69C).

ACTION

Inhibits replication of viral RNA, DNA, influenza virus RNA polymerase activity, interferes with expression of messenger RNA. **Therapeutic Effect:** Inhibits viral protein synthesis.

USES

Inhalation: Treatment of respiratory syncytial virus (RSV) infections (esp. in pts with underlying compromising conditions such as chronic lung disorders, congenital heart disease, recent transplant recipients). **Capsule/Tablet/Oral Solution:** Treatment of chronic hepatitis C in pts with compensated hepatic disease. **OFF-LABEL:** Treatment of influenza A or B, West Nile virus.

PRECAUTIONS

Contraindications: Autoimmune hepatitis, creatinine clearance less than 50 ml/min, hemoglobinopathies, hepatic decompensation, hypersensitivity to ribavirin products, pregnancy, significant or unstable cardiac disease, women of childbearing age who do not use contraception reliably. **Cautions: Inhalation:** Pts requiring assisted ventilation, COPD, asthma. **PO:** Cardiac, pulmonary disease, elderly, history of psychiatric disorders. **Pregnancy Category X.**

INTERACTIONS

DRUG: **Didanosine** may increase risk of pancreatitis, peripheral neuropathy. May decrease effects of **didanosine. Nucleoside analogues (e.g., adefovir, didanosine, lamivudine, stavudine, zalcitabine, zidovudine)** may increase risk of lactic acidosis. **HERBAL:** None significant. **FOOD:** None known. **LAB VALUES:** None significant.

AVAILABILITY (Rx)

Capsules (Rebetol, Ribasphere): 200 mg. **Powder for Aerosol (Virazole):** 6 g. **Powder for Solution, Inhalation (Virazole):** 6 g. **Solution, Oral: (Rebetol)** 40 mg/ml. **Tablet (Copegus):** 200 mg. **(RibaPak, Ribasphere):** 400 mg, 600 mg.

ADMINISTRATION/HANDLING

PO

• Capsules may be taken without regard to food. • Do not open, crush, chew or break capsules. • Use oral solution in children 5 yrs or younger, those 25 kg or less, or those unable to swallow. • Give capsules with food when combined with peginterferon alfa 2b. • Tablets should be given with food.

Inhalation

◄ALERT► May be given via nasal or oral inhalation.

• Solution appears clear, colorless; is stable for 24 hrs at room temperature. • Discard solution for nebulization after 24 hrs. • Discard if discolored or cloudy. • Add 50–100 ml Sterile Water for Injection or Inhalation to 6-g vial. • Transfer to a flask, serving as reservoir for aerosol generator. • Further dilute to final volume of 300 ml, giving solution concentration of 20 mg/ml. • Use only aerosol generator available from manufacturer of drug. • Do not give concomitantly with other drug solutions for nebulization. • Discard reservoir solution when fluid levels are low and at least q24h. • Controversy exists over safety in ventilator-dependent pts; only experienced personnel should administer drug.

INDICATIONS/ROUTES/DOSAGE

Chronic Hepatitis C

PO (CAPSULE COMBINATION WITH INTERFERON ALFA-2B): ADULTS, ELDERLY: 1,000–1,200 mg/day in 2 divided doses. **CHILDREN WEIGHING 61 KG OR MORE:** Use adult dosage. **CHILDREN WEIGHING 50–60 KG:** 400 mg twice a day. **CHILDREN WEIGHING 37–49 KG:** 200 mg in morning, 400 mg in evening. **CHILDREN WEIGHING 24–36 KG:** 200 mg twice a day.
PO (CAPSULES IN COMBINATION WITH PEGINTERFERON ALFA-2B): ADULTS, ELDERLY: 800 mg/day (with food) in 2 divided doses.
PO (TABLETS IN COMBINATION WITH PEGINTERFERON ALFA-2B): ADULTS, ELDERLY: 800–1,200 mg/day in 2 divided doses.

Severe Lower Respiratory Tract Infection Caused by Respiratory Syncytial Virus (RSV)

INHALATION: CHILDREN, INFANTS: Use with Viratek small-particle aerosol generator at concentration of 20 mg/ml (6 g reconstituted with 300 ml Sterile Water for Injection) over 12–18 hrs/day for 3–7 days.

SIDE EFFECTS

Frequent (greater than 10%): Dizziness, headache, fatigue, fever, insomnia, irritability, depression, emotional lability, impaired concentration, alopecia, rash, pruritus, nausea, anorexia, dyspepsia, vomiting, decreased hemoglobin, hemolysis, arthralgia, musculoskeletal pain, dyspnea, sinusitis, flu-like symptoms. **Occasional (10%–1%):** Nervousness, altered taste, weakness.

ADVERSE EFFECTS/ TOXIC REACTIONS

Cardiac arrest, apnea, ventilator dependence, bacterial pneumonia, pneumonia, pneumothorax occur rarely. If treatment exceeds 7 days, anemia may occur.

NURSING CONSIDERATIONS

BASELINE ASSESSMENT

Obtain sputum specimens before giving first dose or at least during first 24 hrs of therapy. Assess respiratory status for baseline. **PO:** CBC with differential, pretreatment and monthly pregnancy test for women of childbearing age.

INTERVENTION/EVALUATION

Monitor HgB, Hct, platelets, hepatic function tests, I&O, fluid balance carefully. Check hematology reports for anemia due to reticulocytosis when therapy exceeds 7 days. For ventilator-assisted pts, watch for "rainout" in tubing and empty frequently; be alert to impaired ventilation/gas exchange due to drug precipitate. Assess skin for rash. Monitor B/P, respirations; assess lung sounds.

PATIENT/FAMILY TEACHING

- Report immediately any difficulty breathing, itching/swelling/redness of eyes, severe abdominal pain, bloody diarrhea, unusual bleeding/bruising.
- Female pts should take measures to avoid pregnancy.
- Male pts should take contraceptive measures.

rifabutin

rif-a-**bue**-tin
(Mycobutin)
Do not confuse rifabutin with rifampin.

CLASSIFICATION

PHARMACOTHERAPEUTIC: Antitubercular. **CLINICAL:** Antibacterial (antimycobacterial).

ACTION

Inhibits DNA-dependent RNA polymerase, an enzyme in susceptible strains of *Escherichia coli, Bacillus subtilis*. Broad-spectrum of activity, including my-

R

cobacteria such as *Mycobacterium avium* complex (MAC). **Therapeutic Effect:** Prevents MAC disease.

PHARMACOKINETICS

Readily absorbed from GI tract (high-fat meals delay absorption). Protein binding: 85%. Widely distributed. Crosses blood-brain barrier. Extensive intracellular tissue uptake. Metabolized in liver to active metabolite. Excreted in urine; eliminated in feces. Unknown if removed by hemodialysis. **Half-life:** 16–69 hrs.

USES

Prevention of disseminated *Mycobacterium avium* complex (MAC) disease in those with advanced HIV infection. **OFF-LABEL:** Part of multidrug regimen for treatment of MAC. Prophylaxis for latent tuberculosis infection, part of multidrug regimen for treatment of active tuberculosis infection.

PRECAUTIONS

Contraindications: Active tuberculosis; hypersensitivity to other rifamycins (e.g., rifampin). **Cautions:** Safety in children not established. Renal/hepatic impairment.

⌛ LIFESPAN CONSIDERATIONS

Pregnancy/Lactation: Unknown if drug crosses placenta or is distributed in breast milk. **Pregnancy Category B. Children/Elderly:** No age-related precautions noted.

INTERACTIONS

DRUG: May decrease effectiveness of **oral contraceptives.** May decrease concentration, effect of **non-nucleoside reverse transcriptase inhibitors (e.g., delavirdine, efavirenz, nevirapine), protease inhibitors (e.g., amprenavir, indinavir, ritonavir, saquinavir). Protease inhibitors** may increase concentration, toxicity. May decrease concentration of **zidovudine** (does not affect inhibition of HIV). **HERBAL:** None significant. **FOOD:** None known. **LAB VALUES:** May increase serum alkaline phosphatase, AST, ALT.

AVAILABILITY (Rx)

Capsules: 150 mg.

ADMINISTRATION/HANDLING

PO

• Give without regard to food. Give with food if GI irritation occurs. • May mix with applesauce if pt is unable to swallow capsules whole.

INDICATIONS/ROUTES/DOSAGE

Prophylaxis of MAC Disease

PO: ADULTS, ELDERLY: 300 mg as single dose or in 2 divided doses if GI upset occurs. 150 mg/day when given concurrently with nelfinavir or indinavir; 450–600 mg/day when given concurrently with efavirenz. **CHILDREN:** 5 mg/kg daily. **Maximum dose:** 300 mg.

Dosage in Renal Impairment

Dosage is modified based on creatinine clearance. If creatinine clearance is less than 30 ml/min, reduce dosage by 50%.

SIDE EFFECTS

Frequent (30%): Red-orange or red-brown discoloration of urine, feces, saliva, skin, sputum, sweat, tears. **Occasional (11%–3%):** Rash, nausea, abdominal pain, diarrhea, dyspepsia, belching, headache, altered taste, uveitis, corneal deposits. **Rare (less than 2%):** Anorexia, flatulence, fever, myalgia, vomiting, insomnia.

ADVERSE EFFECTS/ TOXIC REACTIONS

Hepatitis, anemia, thrombocytopenia, neutropenia occur rarely.

NURSING CONSIDERATIONS

BASELINE ASSESSMENT

Obtain chest X-ray; sputum, blood cultures. Biopsy of suspicious node(s) must be done to rule out active tuberculosis. Obtain baseline CBC, serum hepatic function tests.

INTERVENTION/EVALUATION

Monitor serum hepatic function tests, CBC, platelet count, Hgb, Hct. Avoid IM injections, rectal temperatures, other trauma that may induce bleeding. Check temperature; notify physician of flu-like syndrome, rash, GI intolerance.

PATIENT/FAMILY TEACHING

• Urine, feces, saliva, sputum, perspiration, tears, skin may be discolored brown-orange. • Soft contact lenses may be permanently discolored. • Rifabutin may decrease efficacy of oral contraceptives; nonhormonal methods should be considered. • Avoid crowds, those with infection. • Report flu-like symptoms, nausea, vomiting, dark urine, unusual bruising/bleeding from any site, any visual disturbances.

rifampin

riff-**am**-pin
(Rifadin, Rifadin IV, Rofact ✱)

Do not confuse rifampin with ribavirin, rifabutin, Rifamate, rifapentine, rifaximin, or Ritalin, or Rifadin with Rifater or Ritalin.

FIXED-COMBINATION(S)

Rifamate: rifampin/isoniazid (an antitubercular): 300 mg/150 mg. **Rifater:** rifampin/isoniazid/pyrazinamide (an antitubercular): 120 mg/50 mg/300 mg.

◆CLASSIFICATION

PHARMACOTHERAPEUTIC: Antitubercular. **CLINICAL:** Antibiotic, miscellaneous.

ACTION

Interferes with bacterial RNA synthesis by binding to DNA-dependent RNA polymerase, preventing attachment to DNA, thereby blocking RNA transcription. **Therapeutic Effect:** Bactericidal in susceptible microorganisms.

PHARMACOKINETICS

Well absorbed from GI tract (food delays absorption). Protein binding: 80%. Widely distributed. Metabolized in liver to active metabolite. Primarily eliminated by biliary system. Not removed by hemodialysis. **Half-life:** 3–5 hrs (increased in hepatic impairment).

USES

In conjunction with at least one other antitubercular agent for initial treatment, retreatment of clinical tuberculosis. Eliminates *Neisseria* meningococci from nasopharynx of asymptomatic carriers in situations with high risk for meningococcal meningitis (prophylaxis, not cure). **OFF-LABEL:** Prophylaxis of *Haemophilus influenzae* type b infection, treatment of atypical mycobacterial infection, serious infections caused by *Staphylococcus* spp.

PRECAUTIONS

Contraindications: Concomitant therapy with amprenavir, hypersensitivity to other rifamycins. **Cautions:** Hepatic dysfunction, active or treated alcoholism.

LIFESPAN CONSIDERATIONS

Pregnancy/Lactation: Crosses placenta. Distributed in breast milk. **Pregnancy Category C. Children/Elderly:** No age-related precautions noted.

INTERACTIONS

DRUG: **Alcohol, hepatotoxic medications, ritonavir, saquinavir** may increase risk of hepatotoxicity. May increase clearance of **aminophylline, theophylline.** May decrease effects of **digoxin, disopyramide, fluconazole, methadone, mexiletine, oral anticoagulants, oral antidiabetics, phenytoin, quinidine, tocainide, verapamil.** May decrease **oral contraceptive** effectiveness. **HERBAL:** **St. John's wort** may decrease concentration. **FOOD:** **Food** decreases extent of absorption.

LAB VALUES: May increase serum alkaline phosphatase, bilirubin, uric acid, AST, ALT.

AVAILABILITY (Rx)

Capsules (Rifadin): 150 mg, 300 mg. **Injection, Powder for Reconstitution (Rifadin IV):** 600 mg.

ADMINISTRATION/HANDLING

IV

Reconstitution • Reconstitute 600-mg vial with 10 ml Sterile Water for Injection to provide concentration of 60 mg/ml. • Withdraw desired dose and further dilute with 0.9% NaCl or D_5W to concentration not to exceed 6 mg/ml.

Rate of administration • For IV infusion only. Avoid IM, subcutaneous administration. • Avoid extravasation (local irritation, inflammation). • Infuse over 3 hrs.

Storage • Reconstituted vial is stable for 24 hrs. • Once reconstituted vial is further diluted, it is stable for 4 hrs in D_5W or 24 hrs in 0.9% NaCl.

PO

• Preferably give 1 hr before or 2 hrs following meals with 8 oz of water (may give with food to decrease GI upset; will delay absorption). • For those unable to swallow capsules, contents may be mixed with applesauce, jelly. • Administer at least 1 hr before antacids, esp. those containing aluminum.

R

IV INCOMPATIBILITY

Diltiazem (Cardizem).

IV COMPATIBILITY

D_5W if infused within 4 hrs (risk of precipitation beyond this time period).

INDICATIONS/ROUTES/DOSAGE

Usual Dosage Range

ADULTS, ELDERLY: 600 mg once or twice daily. **CHILDREN, INFANTS:** 10–20 mg/kg/day. **Maximum:** 600 mg/day.

Tuberculosis

PO, IV: ADULTS, ELDERLY: 10 mg/kg/day. **Maximum:** 600 mg/day. **CHILDREN:** 10–20 mg/kg/day in divided doses q12–24h. **Maximum:** 600 mg/day.

Prevention of Meningococcal Infections

PO, IV: ADULTS, ELDERLY: 600 mg q12h for 2 days. **CHILDREN 1 MO AND OLDER:** 20 mg/kg/day in divided doses q12–24h. **Maximum:** 600 mg/dose. **INFANTS YOUNGER THAN 1 MO:** 10 mg/kg/day in divided doses q12h for 2 days.

Staphylococcal Infections

PO, IV: ADULTS, ELDERLY: 600 mg once daily for 5–10 days. **CHILDREN:** 15 mg/kg/day in divided doses q12h for 5–10 days.

Staphylococcus Aureus Infections (in Combination with Other Anti-Infectives)

PO: ADULTS, ELDERLY: 300–600 mg twice daily. **NEONATES:** 5–20 mg/kg/day in divided doses q12h.

H. Influenzae Prophylaxis

PO: ADULTS, ELDERLY: 600 mg/day for 4 days. **CHILDREN 1 MO AND OLDER:** 20 mg/kg/day q24h for 4 days. **Maximum:** 600 mg. **CHILDREN YOUNGER THAN 1 MO:** 10 mg/kg/day q24h for 4 days.

SIDE EFFECTS

Expected: Red-orange or red-brown discoloration of urine, feces, saliva, skin, sputum, sweat, tears. **Occasional (5%–3%):** Hypersensitivity reaction (flushing, pruritus, rash). **Rare (2%–1%):** Diarrhea, dyspepsia, nausea, oral candida (sore mouth, tongue).

ADVERSE EFFECTS/ TOXIC REACTIONS

Hepatotoxicity (risk is increased when rifampin is taken with isoniazid), hepatitis, blood dyscrasias, Stevens-Johnson syndrome, antibiotic-associated colitis occur rarely.

NURSING CONSIDERATIONS

BASELINE ASSESSMENT

Question for hypersensitivity to rifampin, rifamycins. Ensure collection of diagnostic specimens. Evaluate initial serum hepatic/renal function, CBC results.

INTERVENTION/EVALUATION

Assess IV site at least hourly during infusion; restart at another site at the first sign of irritation or inflammation. Monitor hepatic function tests, assess for hepatitis: jaundice, anorexia, nausea, vomiting, fatigue, weakness (hold rifampin, inform physician at once). Report hypersensitivity reactions promptly: any type of skin eruption, pruritus, flu-like syndrome with high dosage. Monitor daily pattern of bowel activity, stool consistency (potential for antibiotic-associated colitis). Monitor CBC results for blood dyscrasias, be alert for infection (fever, sore throat), unusual bruising/bleeding, unusual fatigue/weakness.

PATIENT/FAMILY TEACHING

• Preferably take on empty stomach with 8 oz of water 1 hr before or 2 hrs after meal (with food if GI upset). • Avoid alcohol during treatment. • Do not take **any** other medications without consulting physician, including antacids; must take rifampin at least 1 hr before antacid. • Urine, feces, sputum, sweat, tears may become red-orange; soft contact lenses may be permanently stained. • Notify physician of **any** new symptom, immediately for yellow eyes/skin, fatigue, weakness, nausea/vomiting, sore throat, fever, flu, unusual bruising/bleeding. • If taking oral contraceptives, check with physician (reliability may be affected).

rifaximin

rif-**ax**-i-min
(Xifaxan)

Do not confuse rifaximin with rifampin.

◆CLASSIFICATION

PHARMACOTHERAPEUTIC: Antiinfective. **CLINICAL:** Site-specific antibiotic.

ACTION

Inhibits bacterial RNA synthesis by binding to a subunit of bacterial DNA-dependent RNA polymerase. **Therapeutic Effect:** Bactericidal.

PHARMACOKINETICS

Less than 0.4% absorbed after PO administration. Primarily eliminated in feces; minimal excretion in urine. **Half-life:** 5.85 hrs.

USES

Treatment of traveler's diarrhea caused by noninvasive strains of *E. coli*. Reduction of risk for recurrence of overt hepatic encephalopathy. **OFF-LABEL:** Treatment of hepatic encephalopathy. Treatment of *C. difficile*–associated diarrhea.

PRECAUTIONS

Contraindications: Hypersensitivity to other rifamycin antibiotics. **Cautions:** Pseudomembranous colitis.

⌛ LIFESPAN CONSIDERATIONS

Pregnancy/Lactation: Unknown if drug is distributed in breast milk. **Pregnancy Category C. Children:** Safety and efficacy not established in those younger than 12 yrs. **Elderly:** No age-related precautions noted.

INTERACTIONS

DRUG: None significant. **HERBAL:** None significant. **FOOD:** None known. **LAB VALUES:** None significant.

AVAILABILITY (Rx)

Tablets: 200 mg, 550 mg.

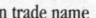

R

ADMINISTRATION/HANDLING

PO

• Give without regard to food. • Store at room temperature. • Do not break/crush film-coated tablets.

INDICATIONS/ROUTES/DOSAGE

Traveler's Diarrhea

PO: ADULTS, ELDERLY, CHILDREN 12 YRS AND OLDER: 200 mg 3 times daily for 3 days.

Hepatic Encephalopathy

PO: ADULTS, ELDERLY: 550 mg 2 times a day.

SIDE EFFECTS

Occasional (11%–5%): Flatulence, headache, abdominal discomfort, rectal tenesmus, defecation urgency, nausea. **Rare (4%–2%):** Constipation, fever, vomiting.

ADVERSE EFFECTS/ TOXIC REACTIONS

Hypersensitivity reaction, superinfection occur rarely.

NURSING CONSIDERATIONS

BASELINE ASSESSMENT

Check baseline hydration status: skin turgor, mucous membranes for dryness, urinary status.

INTERVENTION/EVALUATION

Encourage adequate fluid intake. Assess bowel sounds for peristalsis. Monitor daily pattern of bowel activity, stool consistency. Assess for GI disturbances, blood in stool.

PATIENT/FAMILY TEACHING

• Notify physician if diarrhea worsens or if blood occurs in stool, fever develops within 48 hrs.

rimantadine

ri-**man**-ti-deen
(Flumadine)

Do not confuse rimantadine with ranitidine or amantadine, or Flumadine with fludarabine, flunisolide, or flutamide.

◆ CLASSIFICATION

PHARMACOTHERAPEUTIC: Antiviral. **CLINICAL:** Antiviral.

ACTION

Exerts inhibitory effect early in viral replication cycle. May inhibit uncoating of virus. **Therapeutic Effect:** Prevents replication of influenza A virus.

PHARMACOKINETICS

Well absorbed following PO administration. Protein binding: 40%. Metabolized in liver. Excreted in urine. **Half-life:** 19–36 hrs.

USES

Adults: Prophylaxis, treatment of illness due to influenza A virus. **Children:** Prophylaxis against influenza A virus.

PRECAUTIONS

Contraindications: Hypersensitivity to amantadine. **Cautions:** Hepatic disease, seizures, history of recurrent eczematoid dermatitis, uncontrolled psychosis, renal impairment, concomitant use of CNS stimulant medications.

⌛ LIFESPAN CONSIDERATIONS

Pregnancy/Lactation: Unknown if drug crosses placenta or is distributed in breast milk. **Pregnancy Category C. Children:** Safety and efficacy not established in infants. **Elderly:** May be more susceptible to CNS side effects.

INTERACTIONS

DRUG: Acetaminophen, aspirin may decrease concentration. **HERBAL:** None significant. **FOOD:** None known. **LAB VALUES:** None significant.

AVAILABILITY (Rx)

Syrup: 50 mg/5 ml. **Tablets:** 100 mg.

ADMINISTRATION/HANDLING

PO

• Give without regard to food.

INDICATIONS/ROUTES/DOSAGE

Treatment of Influenza A Virus

PO: ADULTS: 100 mg twice a day for 7 days. **ELDERLY, DEBILITATED PTS, PTS WITH SEVERE HEPATIC/RENAL IMPAIRMENT:** 100 mg once a day for 7 days.

Prevention of Influenza A Virus

PO: ADULTS, CHILDREN 10 YRS AND OLDER: 100 mg twice a day for at least 10 days after known exposure (usually for 6–8 wks). **CHILDREN YOUNGER THAN 10 YRS:** 5 mg/kg once a day. **Maximum:** 150 mg. **ELDERLY, DEBILITATED PTS, PTS WITH SEVERE HEPATIC/RENAL IMPAIRMENT:** 100 mg once a day.

SIDE EFFECTS

Occasional (3%–2%): Insomnia, nausea, nervousness, impaired concentration, dizziness. **Rare (less than 2%):** Vomiting, anorexia, dry mouth, abdominal pain, asthenia (loss of strength, energy), fatigue.

ADVERSE EFFECTS/ TOXIC REACTIONS

None known.

NURSING CONSIDERATIONS

INTERVENTION/EVALUATION

Assess for anxiety, nervousness; evaluate sleep pattern for insomnia. Provide assistance if dizziness occurs.

PATIENT/FAMILY TEACHING

• Avoid contact with those who are at high risk for influenza A (rimantadine-resistant virus may be shed during therapy). • Avoid tasks that require alertness, motor skills until response to drug is established. • Do not take aspirin, acetaminophen, compounds containing these drugs. May cause dry mouth.

risedronate

rize-droe-nate

(Actonel)

Do not confuse Actonel with Actos, or risedronate with alendronate.

FIXED-COMBINATION(S)

Actonel with Calcium: risedronate/calcium: 35 mg/6 × 500 mg.

◆CLASSIFICATION

PHARMACOTHERAPEUTIC: Bisphosphonate. **CLINICAL:** Calcium regulator.

ACTION

Binds to bone hydroxyapatite, inhibits osteoclasts. **Therapeutic Effect:** Reduces bone turnover (number of sites at which bone is remodeled), bone resorption.

PHARMACOKINETICS

Rapidly absorbed following PO administration. Bioavailability decreased when administered with food. Protein binding: 24%. Not metabolized. Excreted unchanged in urine, feces. Not removed by hemodialysis. **Half-life:** 1.5 hrs (initial); 480 hrs (terminal).

USES

Treatment of Paget's disease of bone (osteitis deformans). Treatment/prophylaxis for postmenopausal, glucocorticoid-induced osteoporosis. Used to increase bone mass in men with osteoporosis.

PRECAUTIONS

Contraindications: Hypersensitivity to other bisphosphonates, including etidronate, tiludronate, alendronate; hypocalcemia; inability to stand or sit upright for at least 30 min; renal impairment when serum creatinine clearance is greater than 5 mg/dl; abnormalities that delay esophageal emptying. **Cautions:** GI diseases (duodenitis, dysphagia, esophagi-

R

tis, gastritis, ulcers [drug may exacerbate these conditions]), severe renal impairment. **Pregnancy Category C.**

INTERACTIONS

DRUG: **Antacids containing aluminum, calcium, magnesium; vitamin D** may decrease absorption. **HERBAL:** None significant. **FOOD:** None known. **LAB VALUES:** None significant.

AVAILABILITY (Rx)

Tablets: 5 mg, 30 mg, 35 mg, 75 mg, 150 mg.

ADMINISTRATION/HANDLING

PO

• Administer 30–60 min before any food, drink, other oral medications to avoid interference with absorption. • Give on empty stomach with full glass of plain water (not mineral water). • Pt must avoid lying down for 30 min after swallowing tablet (assists with delivery to stomach, reduces risk of esophageal irritation). • Swallow whole; do not crush, chew tablet.

INDICATIONS/ROUTES/DOSAGE

Paget's Disease

PO: ADULTS, ELDERLY: 30 mg/day for 2 mos. Retreatment may occur after 2-mo post-treatment observation period.

Prophylaxis, Treatment of Postmenopausal Osteoporosis

PO: ADULTS, ELDERLY: 5 mg/day or 35 mg once weekly or 75 mg daily for 2 consecutive days once per mo or 150 mg once per mo.

Treatment of Male Osteoporosis

PO: ADULTS, ELDERLY: 35 mg once weekly.

Glucocorticoid-Induced Osteoporosis

PO: ADULTS, ELDERLY: 5 mg/day.

Dosage in Renal Impairment

Not recommended with creatinine clearance less than 30 ml/min.

SIDE EFFECTS

Frequent (30%): Arthralgia. **Occasional (12%–8%):** Rash, diarrhea, constipation, nausea, abdominal pain, dyspepsia, flu-like symptoms, peripheral edema. **Rare (5%–3%):** Bone pain, sinusitis, asthenia (loss of strength, energy), dry eye, tinnitus.

ADVERSE EFFECTS/ TOXIC REACTIONS

Overdose produces hypocalcemia, hypophosphatemia, significant GI disturbances, osteonecrosis of jaw.

NURSING CONSIDERATIONS

BASELINE ASSESSMENT

Assess symptoms of Paget's disease (bone pain, bone deformities). Hypocalcemia, vitamin D deficiency must be corrected before therapy. Obtain lab baselines, esp. serum electrolytes, renal function.

INTERVENTION/EVALUATION

Check serum electrolytes (esp. calcium, phosphorus, alkaline phosphatase levels). Monitor I&O, BUN, creatinine in pts with renal impairment.

PATIENT/FAMILY TEACHING

• Expected benefits occur only when medication is taken with full glass (6–8 oz) of plain water, first thing in the morning and at least 30 min before first food, beverage, medication of the day. Any other beverage (mineral water, orange juice, coffee) significantly reduces absorption of medication. • Do not lie down for at least 30 min after taking medication (potentiates delivery to stomach, reduces risk of esophageal irritation). • Consider weight-bearing exercises, modify behavioral factors (cigarette smoking, alcohol consumption). • Report jaw pain, incapacitating bone, joint, or muscle pain.

Risperdal, *see risperidone*

risperidone

ris-**per**-i-done
(Apo-Risperidone ♣, Novo-Risperidone ♣, Risperdal, Risperdal Consta, Risperdal M-Tabs)

BLACK BOX ALERT Increased risk of mortality in elderly pts with dementia-related psychosis, mainly due to pneumonia, heart failure.

Do not confuse Risperdal with lisinopril or Restoril, or risperidone with ropinirole.

◆CLASSIFICATION

PHARMACOTHERAPEUTIC: Benzisoxazole derivative. **CLINICAL:** Antipsychotic (see p. 66C).

ACTION

May antagonize dopamine, serotonin receptors. **Therapeutic Effect:** Suppresses psychotic behavior.

PHARMACOKINETICS

Well absorbed from GI tract; unaffected by food. Protein binding: 90%. Extensively metabolized in liver to active metabolite. Primarily excreted in urine. **Half-life:** 3–20 hrs; metabolite, 21–30 hrs (increased in elderly). **Injection:** 3–6 days.

USES

Management of manifestations of psychotic disorders (e.g., schizophrenia), irritability associated with autistic disease in children. Treatment of acute mania associated with bipolar disorder. Short-term treatment of bipolar disorder in pediatric and adolescent pts. **OFF-LABEL:** Behavioral symptoms associated with dementia, Tourette's syndrome. Psychosis/agitation associated with Alzheimer's dementia.

PRECAUTIONS

Contraindications: None known. **Cautions:** Renal/hepatic impairment, seizure disorders, cardiac disease, recent MI, breast cancer, suicidal pts, those at risk for aspiration pneumonia. May increase risk of stroke in pts with dementia. May increase risk of hyperglycemia.

⌛ LIFESPAN CONSIDERATIONS

Pregnancy/Lactation: Unknown if drug crosses placenta or is distributed in breast milk. Breast-feeding not recommended. **Pregnancy Category C. Children:** Safety and efficacy not established. **Elderly:** More susceptible to postural hypotension. Age-related renal/hepatic impairment may require dosage adjustment.

INTERACTIONS

DRUG: Alcohol, other CNS depressants may increase CNS depression. **Carbamazepine** may decrease concentration. **Clozapine** may increase concentration. May decrease effects of **dopamine agonists, levodopa. Paroxetine** may increase concentration, risk of extrapyramidal symptoms (EPS). **Antihypertensives, hypotension-producing medications** may increase hypotensive effect. **Medications that prolong QT interval** may increase occurrence of ventricular tachycardia, torsade de pointes. **HERBAL: Gotu kola, kava kava, St. John's wort, valerian** may increase CNS depression. **FOOD:** None known. **LAB VALUES:** May increase serum prolactin. May cause EKG changes.

AVAILABILITY (Rx)

Injection, Powder for Reconstitution (Risperdal Consta): 12.5 mg, 25 mg, 37.5 mg, 50 mg. **Oral Solution (Risperdal):** 1 mg/ml. **Tablets (Risperdal):** 0.25 mg, 0.5 mg, 1 mg, 2 mg, 3 mg, 4 mg.

Tablets (Orally-Disintegrating [Risperdal M-Tabs]): 0.5 mg, 1 mg, 2 mg, 3 mg, 4 mg.

ADMINISTRATION/HANDLING

◀ALERT▶ Do not administer via IV route.

IM

Reconstitution • Use only diluent and needle supplied in dose pack. • Prepare

R

suspension according to manufacturer's directions. • May be given up to 6 hrs after reconstitution, but immediate administration is recommended. • If 2 min pass between reconstitution and injection, shake upright vial vigorously back and forth to resuspend solution.

Rate of administration • Inject IM into upper outer quadrant of gluteus maximus or into deltoid muscle in upper arm.

Storage • Store at room temperature.

PO

• Give without regard to food. • May mix oral solution with water, coffee, orange juice, low-fat milk. Do not mix with cola, tea.

Orally-Disintegrating Tablet

• Remove from blister pak immediately before administration. • Using dry hands, place immediately on tongue. • Tablet dissolves in seconds. • May swallow with or without liquid. • Do not split or chew.

INDICATIONS/ROUTES/DOSAGE

Psychotic Disorders

PO: ADULTS: Initially, 0.5–1 mg twice a day. May increase gradually to target dose of 6 mg/day. Range: 4–8 mg/day. Maintenance: Target dose of 4 mg once a day (range: 2–8 mg/day). **ELDERLY:** Initially, 0.5 mg twice a day. May increase slowly at increments of no more than 0.5 mg twice a day. Range: 2–6 mg/day. **CHILDREN 13–17 YRS:** Initially, 0.5 mg/day (as single daily dose). May increase by 0.5–1 mg/day at intervals of greater than 24 hrs to recommended dose of 3 mg/day.

IM: ADULTS, ELDERLY: 25 mg q2wk. **Maximum:** 50 mg q2wk. Dosage adjustments should not be made more frequently than every 4 wks.

Mania

PO: ADULTS, ELDERLY: Initially, 2–3 mg as a single daily dose. May increase by 1 mg/day at 24-hr intervals. Range: 1–6 mg/day. **IM: ADULTS, ELDERLY:** 25 mg q2wk. **Maximum:** 50 mg q2wk. Dosage adjustments should not be made more frequently than every 4 wks.

Irritability with Autistic Disease

PO: CHILDREN 5 YRS AND OLDER: Initially, 0.25 mg/day (0.5 mg in children weighing 20 kg or greater). May increase to 0.5 mg/day (1 mg/day in children weighing 20 kg or greater) after minimum of 4 days. Dose should be maintained for at least 14 days, after which dose may be increased by 0.25 mg/day (0.5 mg/day in children weighing 20 kg or more). **Maximum:** 1 mg (2.5 mg in children weighing 20 kg or more).

Bipolar Disorder

PO: CHILDREN 10–17 YRS: Initially, 0.5 mg/day. May increase by 0.5 mg/day at intervals of greater than 24 hrs to recommended dose of 2.5 mg/day.

Dosage in Renal Impairment

Initial dosage for adults, elderly pts is 0.25–0.5 mg twice a day. Dosage is titrated slowly to desired effect.

SIDE EFFECTS

Frequent (26%–13%): Agitation, anxiety, insomnia, headache, constipation. **Occasional (10%–4%):** Dyspepsia, rhinitis, drowsiness, dizziness, nausea, vomiting, rash, abdominal pain, dry skin, tachycardia. **Rare (3%–2%):** Visual disturbances, fever, back pain, pharyngitis, cough, arthralgia, angina, aggressive behavior, orthostatic hypotension, breast swelling.

ADVERSE EFFECTS/ TOXIC REACTIONS

Rare reactions include tardive dyskinesia (characterized by tongue protrusion, puffing of the cheeks, chewing or puckering of mouth), neuroleptic malignant syndrome (marked by hyperpyrexia, muscle rigidity, altered mental status, irregular pulse or B/P, tachycardia, diaphoresis, cardiac arrhythmias, rhabdomyolysis, acute renal failure). Hyperglycemia, in some cases extreme and associated with ketoacidosis, hyperosmolar coma, death, has been reported.

NURSING CONSIDERATIONS

BASELINE ASSESSMENT

Serum renal/hepatic function tests should be performed before therapy. Assess behavior, appearance, emotional status, response to environment, speech pattern, thought content, baseline weight. Obtain fasting serum glucose value.

INTERVENTION/EVALUATION

Monitor B/P, heart rate, weight, hepatic function tests, EKG. Monitor for fine tongue movement (may be first sign of tardive dyskinesia, which may be irreversible). Monitor for suicidal ideation. Assess for therapeutic response (greater interest in surroundings, improved self-care, increased ability to concentrate, relaxed facial expression). Monitor for potential neuroleptic malignant syndrome: fever, muscle rigidity, irregular B/P or pulse, altered mental status. Monitor fasting serum glucose periodically during therapy.

PATIENT/FAMILY TEACHING

• Avoid tasks that may require alertness, motor skills until response to drug is established (may cause dizziness/drowsiness). • Avoid alcohol. • Use caution when changing position from lying or sitting to standing. • Inform physician of trembling in fingers, altered gait, unusual muscular/skeletal movements, palpitations, severe dizziness/fainting, swelling/pain in breasts, visual changes, rash, difficulty breathing.

Ritalin, *see methylphenidate*

ritonavir

rit-**oh**-na-veer
(Norvir, Norvir SEC ✦)

BLACK BOX ALERT Concurrent use with other medications (nonsedating antihistamines, sedative hypnotics, antiarrhythmics, ergot alkaloids) may result in potentially serious, life-threatening events.

Do not confuse ritonavir with Retrovir, or Norvir with Norvasc.

◆CLASSIFICATION

PHARMACOTHERAPEUTIC: Protease inhibitor. **CLINICAL:** Antiviral (see pp. 69C, 117C).

ACTION

Inhibits HIV-1 and HIV-2 proteases, rendering these enzymes incapable of processing polypeptide precursors leading to production of noninfectious, immature HIV particles. **Therapeutic Effect:** Slows HIV replication, reducing progression of HIV infection.

PHARMACOKINETICS

Well absorbed after PO administration (absorption increased with food). Protein binding: 98%–99%. Extensively metabolized in liver to active metabolite. Primarily eliminated in feces. Unknown if removed by hemodialysis. **Half-life:** 2.7–5 hrs.

USES

Treatment of HIV infection in combination with other antiretroviral agents.

PRECAUTIONS

Contraindications: Due to potential serious and/or life-threatening drug interactions (e.g., arrhythmias, hematologic abnormalities, seizures), the following medications should not be given concomitantly with ritonavir: alfuzosin, amiodarone, bepridil, dihydroergotamine, lovastatin, midazolam, propafenone, quinidine, saquinavir, simvastatin, St. John's wort, trizolam, voriconazole; concurrent use of alprazolam, clorazepate, diazepam, estazolam, flurazepam, midazolam, triazolam, zolpidem may produce extreme sedation and respiratory depression. **Cautions:** Hepatic impairment.

R

LIFESPAN CONSIDERATIONS

Pregnancy/Lactation: Breast-feeding not recommended (possibility of HIV transmission). **Pregnancy Category B. Children:** No age-related precautions noted in those older than 2 yrs. **Elderly:** None known.

INTERACTIONS

DRUG: May increase concentration, toxicity of **clarithromycin, desipramine, fluticasone, indinavir, ketoconazole, meperidine, saquinavir, sildenafil.** May decrease concentration, effects of **didanosine, methadone, oral contraceptives, theophylline. Rifampin** may decrease concentration, effect. **HERBAL: St. John's wort** may decrease concentration, effect. **FOOD:** None known. **LAB VALUES:** May increase serum creatine kinase (CK), GGT, triglycerides, uric acid, AST, ALT, glucose. May decrease Hgb, Hct, WBC, neutrophils.

AVAILABILITY (Rx)

Capsules: 100 mg. **Oral Solution:** 80 mg/ml.

Tablets: 100 mg.

ADMINISTRATION/HANDLING

PO

• Store capsules, solution in refrigerator. Store tablets at room temperature. • Protect from light. • Refrigeration of oral solution is recommended but not necessary if used within 30 days and stored below 77°F. • Give without regard to meals (preferably give with food). • Swallow tablets whole; do not chew, break, crush. • May improve taste of oral solution by mixing with chocolate milk, Ensure, Advera, Boost within 1 hr of dosing.

INDICATIONS/ROUTES/DOSAGE

Treatment of HIV Infection

PO: ADULTS, CHILDREN 12 YRS AND OLDER: 600 mg twice daily. If nausea occurs at this dosage, give 300 mg twice daily for 1 day, then increase by 100 mg twice daily every 2–3 days to recommended dose of 600 mg twice daily. **CHILDREN 1 MO–11 YRS:** Initially, 250 mg/m^2/dose twice daily. Increase by 50 mg/m^2/dose up to 350–400 mg/m^2/dose. **Maximum:** 600 mg/dose twice daily.

Dosage Adjustments in Combination Therapy

Indinavir: Indinavir 800 mg twice daily and ritonavir 100–200 mg twice daily or indinavir 400 mg twice daily and ritonavir 400 mg twice daily. **Nelfinavir or saquinavir:** Ritonavir 400 mg twice daily. **Rifabutin:** Decrease rifabutin dosage to 150 mg every other day.

SIDE EFFECTS

Frequent: GI disturbances (abdominal pain, anorexia, diarrhea, nausea, vomiting), circumoral and peripheral paresthesias, altered taste, headache, dizziness, fatigue, asthenia (loss of strength, energy). **Occasional:** Allergic reaction, flu-like symptoms, hypotension. **Rare:** Diabetes mellitus, hyperglycemia.

ADVERSE EFFECTS/ TOXIC REACTIONS

Hepatitis, pancreatitis occur rarely.

NURSING CONSIDERATIONS

BASELINE ASSESSMENT

Pts beginning combination therapy with ritonavir and nucleosides may promote GI tolerance by beginning ritonavir alone and subsequently adding nucleosides before completing 2 wks of ritonavir monotherapy. Obtain baseline laboratory testing, esp. serum hepatic function tests, triglycerides before beginning ritonavir therapy and at periodic intervals during therapy. Offer emotional support to pt/family.

INTERVENTION/EVALUATION

Closely monitor for evidence of GI disturbances, neurologic abnormalities (particularly paresthesias). Monitor serum hepatic function tests, serum glucose, CD4 cell count, plasma levels of HIV RNA.

R

PATIENT/FAMILY TEACHING

• Continue therapy for full length of treatment. • Doses should be evenly spaced. • Ritonavir is not a cure for HIV infection, nor does it reduce risk of transmission to others. • Pts may continue to acquire illnesses associated with advanced HIV infection. • If possible, take ritonavir with food. • Taste of solution may be improved when mixed with chocolate milk, Ensure, Advera, Boost. • Inform physician of increased thirst, frequent urination, nausea, vomiting, abdominal pain.

Rituxan, *see rituximab*

rituximab HIGH ALERT

ri-**tux**-i-mab
(Rituxan)

BLACK BOX ALERT Profound, occasionally fatal infusion-related reactions reported during first 30–120 min of first infusion. Tumor lysis syndrome leading to acute renal failure may occur 12–24 hrs following first dose. Severe, sometimes fatal mucocutaneous reactions reported.

Do not confuse rituximab with bevacizumab or infliximab, or Rituxan with Remicade.

◆CLASSIFICATION

PHARMACOTHERAPEUTIC: Monoclonal antibody. **CLINICAL:** Antineoplastic (see p. 87C).

ACTION

Binds to CD20, the antigen found on surface of B lymphocytes, B-cell non-Hodgkin's lymphoma (NHL). **Therapeutic Effect:** Produces cytotoxicity, reduces tumor size.

PHARMACOKINETICS

Rapidly depletes B cells. **Half-life:** 59.8 hrs after first infusion, 174 hrs after fourth infusion.

USES

Treatment of relapsed or refractory low-grade or follicular B-cell non-Hodgkin's lymphoma (NHL). First-line treatment for diffuse large B-cell, CD20-positive, NHL. First-line treatment of previously untreated pts with follicular NHL in combination with cyclophosphamide, vincristine, and prednisolone (CVP therapy). Treatment of low-grade NHL in pts with stable disease or who achieve partial or complete response following CVP therapy, chronic lymphocytic leukemia (CLL), maintenance treatment for advanced follicular lymphoma in those responding to initial treatment of rituximab plus chemotherapy, moderate to severe rheumatoid arthritis (RA). **OFF-LABEL:** Treatment of autoimmune hemolytic anemia, chronic immune thrombocytopenic purpura (ITP), systemic autoimmune disease (other than rheumatoid arthritis), Burkitt's lymphoma, CNS lymphoma, Hodgkin's lymphoma.

PRECAUTIONS

Contraindications: Hypersensitivity to murine proteins. **Cautions:** Those with history of cardiac disease.

⌛ LIFESPAN CONSIDERATIONS

Pregnancy/Lactation: Has potential to cause fetal B-cell depletion. Unknown if distributed in breast milk. Those with childbearing potential should use contraceptive methods during treatment and up to 12 mos following therapy. **Pregnancy Category C. Children:** Safety and efficacy not established. **Elderly:** No age-related precautions noted.

INTERACTIONS

DRUG: **Cisplatin** may enhance renal toxicity. **HERBAL:** **Garlic, ginger, ginseng** may increase hypoglycemic effect. **FOOD:** None known. **LAB VALUES:** May increase creatinine, LDH. May decrease Hgb, Hct, neutrophils, platelets, B-cell counts, immunoglobulin concentrations.

AVAILABILITY (Rx)

Injection Solution: 10 mg/ml.

R

ADMINISTRATION/HANDLING

IV

◀ALERT▶ Do not give by IV push or bolus.

Reconstitution • Dilute with 0.9% NaCl or D_5W to provide final concentration of 1–4 mg/ml into infusion bag.

Rate of administration • Infuse at rate of 50 mg/hr. If no hypersensitivity or infusion related reaction, may increase infusion rate in 50 mg/hr increments q30min to maximum 400 mg/hr. • Subsequent infusion can be given at 100 mg/hr and increased by 100 mg/hr increments q30min to maximum 400 mg/hr.

Storage • Refrigerate vials. • Diluted solution is stable for 24 hrs if refrigerated or at room temperature.

IV INCOMPATIBILITIES

Do not mix with any other medications.

INDICATIONS/ROUTES/DOSAGE

Non-Hodgkin's Lymphoma (NHL)

IV: ADULTS: 375 mg/m^2 once weekly for 4–8 wks. May administer a second 4-wk course.

Rheumatoid Arthritis

IV: ADULTS: 1,000 mg every 2 wks times 2 doses with methotrexate.

R

CLL

IV: ADULTS: 375 mg/m^2 in first cycle and 500 mg/m^2 in cycles 2–6, administered every 28 days. (Dose as component of ibritumomab is 250 mg/m^2.)

SIDE EFFECTS

Frequent: Fever (49%), chills (32%), nausea (18%), asthenia (loss of strength, energy) (16%), headache (14%), angioedema (13%), hypotension (10%), rash/pruritus (10%). **Occasional (less than 10%):** Myalgia, dizziness, weakness, abdominal pain, throat irritation, vomiting, neutropenia, rhinitis, bronchospasm, urticaria.

ADVERSE EFFECTS/TOXIC REACTIONS

Hypersensitivity reaction produces hypotension, bronchospasm, angioedema. Arrhythmias may occur, particularly in those with history of preexisting cardiac conditions.

NURSING CONSIDERATIONS

BASELINE ASSESSMENT

Pretreatment with acetaminophen and diphenhydramine before each infusion may prevent infusion-related effects. CBC, platelet count should be obtained at regular intervals during therapy.

INTERVENTION/EVALUATION

Monitor for an infusion-related symptoms complex consisting mainly of fever, chills, rigors that generally occurs within 30 min–2 hrs of beginning first infusion. Slowing infusion resolves symptoms. Monitor renal/hepatic function, CBC, platelet count.

PATIENT/FAMILY TEACHING

- Notify physician if fever, sore throat, abdominal pain, yellowing of eyes/skin, unusual bruising/bleeding occur.

rivastigmine

riv-a-**stig**-meen
(Exelon)

◆CLASSIFICATION

PHARMACOTHERAPEUTIC: Cholinesterase inhibitor. **CLINICAL:** Anti-Alzheimer's dementia agent.

ACTION

Inhibits the enzyme acetylcholinesterase, increasing acetylcholine concentration at cholinergic synapses, enhancing cholinergic function. **Therapeutic Effect:** Slows progression of symptoms of Alzheimer's disease.

PHARMACOKINETICS

Rapidly, completely absorbed. Protein binding: 40%. Widely distributed throughout body. Rapidly, extensively metabolized. Primarily excreted in urine. **Half-life:** 1.5 hrs.

USES

Treatment of mild to moderate dementia of the Alzheimer's type. Treatment of dementia associated with Parkinson's disease. OFF-LABEL: Severe dementia associated with Alzheimer's disease, Lewy body dementia.

PRECAUTIONS

Contraindications: Hypersensitivity to other carbamate derivatives. **Cautions:** Peptic ulcer disease, concurrent use of NSAIDs, sick sinus syndrome, bradycardia, urinary obstruction, seizure disorders, asthma, COPD.

⌛ LIFESPAN CONSIDERATIONS

Pregnancy/Lactation: Unknown if distributed in breast milk. **Pregnancy Category B. Children:** Not indicated for use in this pt population. **Elderly:** No age-related precautions noted.

INTERACTIONS

DRUG: May interfere with **anticholinergics** effects. May have additive effect with **bethanecol. NSAIDs** may increase GI effects, irritation. HERBAL: **Ginkgo biloba** may increase cholinergic effects. FOOD: None known. LAB VALUES: None significant.

AVAILABILITY (Rx)

Capsules: 1.5 mg, 3 mg, 4.5 mg, 6 mg. **Oral Solution:** 2 mg/ml. **Transdermal Patch:** 4.6 mg/24 hrs, 9.5 mg/24 hrs.

ADMINISTRATION/HANDLING

PO

• Give with food in divided doses morning and evening. • Swallow capsule whole.

Oral Solution

• Using oral syringe provided by manufacturer; withdraw prescribed amount from container. • May be swallowed directly from syringe or mixed in small glass of water, cold fruit juice, soda (use within 4 hrs of mixing).

Transdermal Patch

• May apply the day following the last oral dose. • Apply to upper or lower back, upper arm, or chest. • Avoid reapplication to same spot of skin for 14 days. • Do not apply to red, irritated, or broken skin. • Avoid eye contact. • After removal, fold patch to press adhesive together and discard.

INDICATIONS/ROUTES/DOSAGE

Alzheimer's Disease

PO: ADULTS, ELDERLY: Initially, 1.5 mg twice daily. May increase at intervals of at least 2 wks to 3 mg twice daily, then 4.5 mg twice daily, and finally 6 mg twice daily. **Maximum:** 6 mg twice daily.

Parkinson's Disease

PO: ADULTS, ELDERLY: Initially, 1.5 mg twice daily. May increase at intervals of at least 4 wks to 3 mg twice daily, then 4.5 mg twice daily, and finally 6 mg twice daily. **Maximum:** 6 mg twice daily.

TRANSDERMAL: ADULTS, ELDERLY: Initially, 4.6 mg/24h. May increase after 4 wks to 9.5 mg/24h. Pts currently on oral rivastigmine, use 4.6 mg/24h for those taking less than 6 mg/day and 9.5 mg/24h for those taking 6–12 mg/day.

SIDE EFFECTS

Frequent (47%–17%): Nausea, vomiting, dizziness, diarrhea, headache, anorexia. **Occasional** (13%–6%): Abdominal pain, insomnia, dyspepsia (heartburn, indigestion, epigastric pain), confusion, UTI, depression. **Rare** (5%–3%): Anxiety, drowsiness, constipation, malaise, hallucinations, tremor, flatulence, rhinitis, hypertension, flu-like symptoms, weight loss, syncope.

ADVERSE EFFECTS/ TOXIC REACTIONS

Overdose can produce cholinergic crisis, characterized by severe nausea/vomiting, increased salivation, diaphoresis, bradycardia, hypotension, respiratory depression, seizures.

NURSING CONSIDERATIONS

BASELINE ASSESSMENT

Obtain baseline vital signs. Assess history for peptic ulcer, urinary obstruction, asthma, COPD. Assess cognitive, behavioral, functional deficits.

INTERVENTION/EVALUATION

Monitor for cholinergic reaction: GI discomfort/cramping, feeling of facial warmth, excessive salivation, diaphoresis, lacrimation, pallor, urinary urgency, dizziness. Monitor for nausea, diarrhea, headache, insomnia.

PATIENT/ FAMILY TEACHING

• Take with meals (at breakfast, dinner). • Swallow capsule whole. Do not chew, break, crush capsules. • Report nausea, vomiting, diarrhea, diaphoresis, increased salivary secretions, severe abdominal pain, dizziness.

R

rizatriptan

rye-zah-**trip**-tan
(Maxalt, Maxalt-MLT, Maxalt RPD ✦)

◆CLASSIFICATION

PHARMACOTHERAPEUTIC: Serotonin receptor agonist. **CLINICAL:** Antimigraine (see p. 63C).

ACTION

Binds selectively to vascular receptors, producing vasoconstrictive effect on cranial blood vessels. **Therapeutic Effect:** Relieves migraine headache.

PHARMACOKINETICS

Well absorbed after PO administration. Protein binding: 14%. Crosses blood-brain barrier. Metabolized by liver to inactive metabolite. Eliminated primarily in urine and, to a lesser extent, in feces. **Half-life:** 2–3 hrs.

USES

Treatment of acute migraine headache with or without aura.

PRECAUTIONS

Contraindications: Basilar or hemiplegic migraine, coronary artery disease, ischemic heart disease (including angina pectoris, history of MI, silent ischemia, and Prinzmetal's angina), uncontrolled hypertension, use within 24 hrs of ergotamine-containing preparations or another serotonin receptor agonist, MAOI use within 14 days. **Cautions:** Mild to moderate renal/hepatic impairment, pt profile suggesting cardiovascular risks.

⌛ LIFESPAN CONSIDERATIONS

Pregnancy/Lactation: Unknown if drug is distributed in breast milk. **Pregnancy Category C. Children:** Safety and efficacy not established. **Elderly:** No age-related precautions noted.

INTERACTIONS

DRUG: Ergotamine-containing medications may produce vasospastic reaction. **Fluoxetine, fluvoxamine, paroxetine, sertraline** may produce hyperreflexia, incoordination, weakness. **MAOIs, propranolol** may dramatically increase concentration. **HERBAL:** None significant. **FOOD: All foods** delay peak drug concentration by 1 hr. **LAB VALUES:** None significant.

AVAILABILITY (Rx)

Tablets (Maxalt): 5 mg, 10 mg. **Tablets (Orally-Disintegrating [Maxalt-MLT]):** 5 mg, 10 mg.

ADMINISTRATION/HANDLING

PO

• Orally-disintegrating tablet is packaged in individual aluminum pouch. • Open packet with dry hands. • Place tablet onto tongue, allow to dissolve, swallow with saliva. Administration with water is not necessary.

INDICATIONS/ROUTES/DOSAGE

Acute Migraine Headache

PO: ADULTS OLDER THAN 18 YRS, ELDERLY: 5–10 mg. If headache improves but then returns, dose may be repeated after 2 hrs. **Maximum:** 30 mg/24 hrs. (Use 5 mg/dose in pts taking propranolol with maximum of 15 mg/24 hrs.)

SIDE EFFECTS

Frequent (9%–7%): Dizziness, drowsiness, paresthesia, fatigue. **Occasional (6%–3%):** Nausea, chest pressure, dry mouth. **Rare (2%):** Headache; neck, throat, jaw pressure; photosensitivity.

ADVERSE EFFECTS/ TOXIC REACTIONS

Cardiac reactions (ischemia, coronary artery vasospasm, MI), noncardiac vasospasm-related reactions (hemorrhage, CVA) occur rarely, particularly in pts with hypertension, diabetes, strong family history of coronary artery disease; obesity, smokers; males older than 40 yrs; postmenopausal women.

NURSING CONSIDERATIONS

BASELINE ASSESSMENT

Question for history of peripheral vascular disease, renal/hepatic impairment. Question pt regarding onset, location, duration of migraine, possible precipitating symptoms.

INTERVENTION/EVALUATION

Monitor for evidence of dizziness. Assess for photophobia, phonophobia (sound sensitivity, nausea, vomiting) relief of migraine headache.

PATIENT/FAMILY TEACHING

• Take single dose as soon as symptoms of an actual migraine headache appear. • Medication is intended to relieve migraine, not to prevent or reduce number of attacks. • Avoid tasks that require alertness, motor skills until response to drug is established. • Contact physician immediately if palpitations, pain/tightness in chest/throat, pain/weakness of extremities occurs. • Do not remove orally-disintegrating tablet from blister pack until just before dosing. • Use protective measures (sunscreen, protective clothing) against exposure to UV light, sunlight.

Rocephin, *see ceftriaxone*

romidepsin

roe-mi-**dep**-sin
(Istodax)

Do not confuse romidepsin with romiplostim.

◆CLASSIFICATION

PHARMACOTHERAPEUTIC: Histone deacetylase inhibitor. **CLINICAL:** Antineoplastic.

ACTION

Inhibits activity of specific enzymes that catalyze removal of acetyl groups of proteins, causing accumulation of acetylated histones. **Therapeutic Effect:** Induces cell cycle arrest, cell death.

PHARMACOKINETICS

Extensively metabolized. Protein binding: 92%–94%. **Half-life:** 3 hrs.

USES

Treatment of cutaneous T-cell lymphoma in pts who have received at least 1 prior systemic therapy.

PRECAUTONS

Contraindications: None known. **Cautions:** Moderate or severe hepatic impairment, end-stage renal impairment, those with QT interval prolongation, concomitant administration of medications prolonging QT interval.

LIFESPAN CONSIDERATIONS:

Pregnancy/Lactation: May cause fetal harm. Unknown if distributed in breast milk. **Pregnancy Category D. Children:** Safety and efficacy not established. **Elderly:** No age-related precautions noted.

INTERACTIONS

DRUG: Coumarin-derivative anticoagulants prolong PT, INR. Strong CYP3A4 inhibitors **(atazanavir, clarithromycin, indinavir, itraconazole, ketoconazole, nefazodone, nelfinavir, ritonavir, saquinavir, voriconazole)** may increase concentration. Potent CYP3A4 inducers **(carbamazepine, dexamethasone, phenobarbital, phenytoin, rifabutin, rifampin, rifapentine)** may decrease concentration. **HERBAL: St. John's wort** may increase concentration. **FOOD:** None known. **LAB VALUES:** May decrease Hgb, Hct, WBC count, platelets, serum magnesium, calcium, potassium, sodium, albumin, phosphates. May increase serum glucose, AST, ALT, uric acid. May alter serum magnesium.

R

AVAILABILITY (Rx)

Injection, Powder for Reconstitution, 2-Vial Kit: 10 mg.

ADMINISTRATION/HANDLING

Reconstitution • Reconstitute powder with 2 ml of supplied diluent (80% propylene glycol, 20% dehydrated alcohol). • Swirl contents gently to dissolve powder. • Reconstituted solution provides 5 mg/ml. Further dilute in 500 ml 0.9% NaCl.

Rate of administration • Infuse over 4 hrs.

Storage • Reconstituted solution is stable for at least 24 hrs at room temperature. • Solution appears clear, colorless. Discard if precipitate is present or is discolored.

INDICATIONS/ROUTES/DOSAGE

Cutaneous T-Cell Lymphoma

IV: ADULTS, ELDERLY: 14 mg/m^2 administered over 4 hrs on days 1, 8, and 15 of a 28-day cycle. Repeat cycles every 28 days if pt continues to benefit from and tolerates therapy. Dose medication with both hematologic and non-hematologic toxicities.

SIDE EFFECTS

Frequent (57%–23%): Nausea, fatigue, vomiting, anorexia. **Occasional (20%–7%):** Diarrhea, fever, distorted sense of taste, constipation, hypotension, pruritus. **Rare (4%–2%):** Dermatitis, T-wave and ST-wave changes.

ADVERSE EFFECTS/ TOXIC REACTIONS

Infection is very common (47%), including sepsis, arrhythmias, acute respiratory distress syndrome, acute renal failure. Anemia occurs in 19% of pts, thrombocytopenia in 17%, neutropenia in 11%.

NURSING CONSIDERATIONS

BASELINE ASSESSMENT

Provide emotional support to pt, family. Baseline PT, INR, CBC, chemistry tests, esp. potassium, sodium, calcium, magnesium, glucose, hepatic enzymes, renal function tests, EKG, should be obtained prior to therapy at baseline and routinely thereafter. Inform women of childbearing potential of risk to fetus if pregnancy occurs.

INTERVENTION/EVALUATION

Calculate daily absolute neutrophil count (ANC) using the formula: % neutrophils + % bands × WBC = ANC. Closely monitor hematologic, chemistry parameters, EKG; assess Hgb, administer blood transfusions per protocol. Diligently monitor for fever and obtain blood cultures 2 times from separate injection sites. Provide antiemetics to control nausea/vomiting.

PATIENT/FAMILY TEACHING

• Diarrhea may cause dehydration, electrolyte depletion. • Do not have immunizations without physician's approval (lowers body's resistance). • Avoid contact with those who recently received live virus vaccine. • Avoid crowds, those with infection. • May reduce effectiveness of estrogen-containing contraceptives. • Report excessive nausea or vomiting, abnormal heartbeat, chest pain, shortness of breath. Seek immediate medical attention if unusual bleeding occurs.

romiplostim

roe-mi-**ploe**-stim
(Nplate)
Do not confuse romiplostim with romidepsin.

CLASSIFICATION

PHARMACOTHERAPEUTIC: Recombinant fusion protein (hematologic agent). **CLINICAL:** Thrombopoietin receptor agonist.

ACTION

Binds and activates thrombopoietin (TPO) receptors on hematopoietic cells. **Therapeutic Effect:** Increases platelet production.

PHARMACOKINETICS

Concentration is dependent on dose and baseline platelet count. Peak concentration occurs in 7–50 hrs (median, 14 hrs). **Half-life:** 1–34 days (median, 3.5 days).

USES

Treatment of thrombocytopenia in pts with chronic immune (idiopathic) thrombocytopenic purpura (ITP) who have had an insufficient response to corticosteroids, immunoglobulins, or splenectomy.

PRECAUTIONS

Contraindications: None known. **Cautions:** Myelodysplastic syndrome, hematologic malignancy, pregnancy, hepatic impairment, renal impairment.

LIFESPAN CONSIDERATIONS:

Pregnancy/Lactation: Studies suggest drug crosses placenta, is distributed in breast milk. **Pregnancy Category C. Children:** Safety and efficacy not established in those younger than 18 yrs. **Elderly:** Age-related renal, hepatic, cardiac abnormalities may require dosage adjustment.

INTERACTIONS

DRUG: None significant. **HERBAL:** None significant. **FOOD:** None known. **LAB VALUES:** Increases platelet count.

AVAILABILITY (Rx)

Injection, Powder for Reconstitution: 250-mcg, 500-mcg single-use vial.

ADMINISTRATION/HANDLING

ALERT Use syringe with 0.01-ml graduations for reconstitution.

Subcutaneous

Reconstitution • Reconstitute 0.72 ml Sterile Water for Injection to 250-mcg single-use vial for final concentration of 500 mcg/ml. • Reconstitute 1.2 ml Sterile Water for Injection to 500-mcg single-use vial for final concentration of 500 mcg/ml. • Gently swirl and invert vial to reconstitute; do not shake. • Dissolution takes less than 2 min. • Inject at abdomen, thigh, upper arm. • Do not inject at sites that are bruised, red, tender, or hard.

Storage • Refrigerate unreconstituted vial. • Reconstituted solution can be kept at room temperature or refrigerated for up to 24 hrs. Protect reconstituted solution from light. • Do not use if discolored or particulate is present. • Discard unused portion.

R

INDICATIONS/ROUTES/DOSAGE

Thrombocytopenia

SUBCUTANEOUS: ADULTS, ELDERLY: Initially, 1 mcg/kg once weekly based on actual body weight. Adjust weekly doses by increments of 1 mcg/kg to achieve platelet count 50,000/mm^3 or greater and reduce risk of bleeding. **Maximum:** 10 mcg/kg weekly.

Dosage Adjustments

Platelet Count	Dose
Less than 50,000/mm^3	Increase by 1 mcg/kg
Less than 200,000/mm^3 for 2 consecutive wks	Reduce by 1 mcg/kg
Less than 400,000/mm^3	Hold dose

SIDE EFFECTS

Frequent (35%–26%): Headache, arthralgia. **Occasional (17%–6%):** Dizziness, insomnia, myalgia, extremity pain, abdominal pain, shoulder pain, paresthesia, dyspepsia.

ADVERSE EFFECTS/ TOXIC REACTIONS

Reticulin fiber deposits within the bone marrow, progressing to bone marrow fibrosis may occur. Worsening thrombocytopenia may be noted. Discontinuation of therapy may result in thrombocytopenia of greater severity than was present prior to drug therapy, increasing risk of bleeding. Thromboembolic effects may occur. Increases risk of hematologic malignancies.

NURSING CONSIDERATIONS

BASELINE ASSESSMENT

Establish baseline CBC, including platelet count, differential count prior to initiation, weekly during therapy and for 2 wks following discontinuation of therapy. Assess extent of RBC, WBC abnormalities.

INTERVENTION/EVALUATION

Monitor CBC, including platelet count, differential count weekly during dose adjustment phase and then monthly following establishment of a stable romiplostim dose.

PATIENT/FAMILY TEACHING

• Contact physician if bruising, bleeding occur. • Essential to receive drug therapy at scheduled times or risk of bleeding may occur.

ropinirole

ro-**pin**-i-role
(Requip, Requip XL)
Do not confuse Requip with Reglan, or ropinirole with risperidone.

◆CLASSIFICATION

PHARMACOTHERAPEUTIC: Dopamine agonist. **CLINICAL:** Antiparkinson agent.

ACTION

Stimulates dopamine receptors in striatum. **Therapeutic Effect:** Relieves signs/symptoms of Parkinson's disease.

PHARMACOKINETICS

Rapidly absorbed after PO administration. Protein binding: 40%. Extensively distributed throughout body. Extensively metabolized. Steady-state concentrations achieved within 2 days. Eliminated in urine. Unknown if removed by hemodialysis. **Half-life:** 6 hrs.

USES

Treatment of signs/symptoms of idiopathic Parkinson's disease. Treatment of restless legs syndrome.

PRECAUTIONS

Contraindications: None known. **Cautions:** History of orthostatic hypotension, syncope, hallucinations, esp. in elderly. Concurrent use of CNS depressants.

LIFESPAN CONSIDERATIONS

Pregnancy/Lactation: Distributed in breast milk. Drug activity possible in

R

breast-feeding infant. **Pregnancy Category C. Children:** Safety and efficacy not established. **Elderly:** No age-related precautions noted, but hallucinations appear to occur more frequently.

INTERACTIONS

DRUG: **Ciprofloxacin** increases concentration. **Alcohol, CNS depressants** may increase CNS depressant effects. Increases concentration of **levodopa.** HERBAL: **Gotu kola, kava kava, St. John's wort, valerian** may increase CNS depression. FOOD: **All foods** delay peak plasma levels by 1 hr but do not affect drug absorption. LAB VALUES: May increase serum alkaline phosphatase.

AVAILABILITY (Rx)

Tablets: 0.25 mg, 0.5 mg, 1 mg, 2 mg, 3 mg, 4 mg, 5 mg.

Tablets, Extended-Release: 2 mg, 4 mg, 8 mg, 12 mg.

ADMINISTRATION/HANDLING

PO

• May give without regard to meals. • Do not chew, crush, divide extended-release tablets.

INDICATIONS/ROUTES/DOSAGE

Parkinson's Disease

PO: ADULTS, ELDERLY (IMMEDIATE-RELEASE): Initially, 0.25 mg 3 times a day based on individual pt response. Dosage should be titrated with weekly increments as noted:

Week 1: 0.25 mg 3 times a day; total daily dose: 0.75 mg.

Week 2: 0.5 mg 3 times a day; total daily dose: 1.5 mg.

Week 3: 0.75 mg 3 times a day; total daily dose: 2.25 mg.

Week 4: 1 mg 3 times a day; total daily dose: 3 mg.

After week 4, may increase dose by 1.5 mg/day on weekly basis up to dose of 9 mg/day. May then further increase by 3 mg/day on weekly basis up to total dose of 24 mg/day.

(EXTENDED-RELEASE): Initially, 2 mg once daily for 1–2 wks. May increase by 2 mg/day at 1 wk or longer interval. **Maximum:** 24 mg/day.

Discontinuation Taper

Gradually taper over 7 days as follows: Decrease frequency from 3 times a day to twice a day for 4 days, then decrease from twice a day to once daily for remaining 3 days.

Restless Legs Syndrome

PO: ADULTS, ELDERLY: 0.25 mg for days 1 and 2; 0.5 mg for days 3–7; 1 mg for wk 2; 1.5 mg for wk 3; 2 mg for wk 4; 2.5 mg for wk 5; 3 mg for wk 6; 4 mg for wk 7. Give all doses 1–3 hrs before bedtime.

SIDE EFFECTS

Frequent (60%–40%): Nausea, dizziness, extreme drowsiness. **Occasional (12%–5%):** Syncope, vomiting, fatigue, viral infection, dyspepsia, diaphoresis, asthenia (loss of strength, energy), orthostatic hypotension, abdominal discomfort, pharyngitis, abnormal vision, dry mouth, hypertension, hallucinations, confusion. **Rare (less than 4%):** Anorexia, peripheral edema, memory loss, rhinitis, sinusitis, palpitations, impotence.

ADVERSE EFFECTS/ TOXIC REACTIONS

Dyskinesia, impulsive/compulsive behavior (pathological gambling, hypersexuality, binge eating) occur rarely.

R

NURSING CONSIDERATIONS

BASELINE ASSESSMENT

Parkinson's Disease: Assess signs/symptoms (e.g., tremor, gait). **Restless Legs Syndrome:** Assess frequency of symptoms, sleep pattern.

INTERVENTION/EVALUATION

Assess for clinical improvement, clinical reversal of symptoms (improvement of tremors of head/hands at rest, mask-like facial expression, shuffling gait, muscular rigidity). Assist with ambulation if dizziness occurs. Monitor B/P, daytime alertness.

PATIENT/FAMILY TEACHING

• Drowsiness, dizziness may be an initial response to drug. • Postural hypotension may occur more frequently during initial therapy. Rise from lying to sitting or sitting to standing position slowly to prevent risk of postural hypotension. • Avoid tasks that require alertness, motor skills until response to drug is established. • If nausea occurs, take medication with food. • Hallucinations may occur, more so in the elderly than in younger pts with Parkinson's disease. • Report occurrence of falling asleep during activities of daily living; new or worsening symptoms, changes in B/P, fainting, unusual urges. • Avoid alcohol.

rosiglitazone

HIGH ALERT

roe-zi-**glit**-a-zone
(Avandia)

BLACK BOX ALERT May cause or exacerbate congestive heart failure.

Do not confuse Avandia with Avalide or Avinza, or Avandaryl with Benadryl.

FIXED-COMBINATION(S)

Avandamet: rosiglitazone/metformin: 1 mg/500 mg, 2 mg/500 mg, 4 mg/500 mg, 2 mg/1 g, 4 mg/1 g. **Avandaryl:** rosiglitazone/glimepiride (an antidiabetic): 4 mg/1 mg, 4 mg/2 mg, 4 mg/4 mg.

◆CLASSIFICATION

PHARMACOTHERAPEUTIC: Thiazolidinedione. **CLINICAL:** Antidiabetic (see p. 44C).

ACTION

Improves target-cell response to insulin without increasing pancreatic insulin secretion. Decreases hepatic glucose output, increases insulin-dependent glucose utilization in skeletal muscle. **Therapeutic Effect:** Lowers serum glucose concentration.

PHARMACOKINETICS

Rapidly absorbed. Protein binding: 99%. Metabolized in liver. Excreted primarily in urine, with lesser amount in feces. Not removed by hemodialysis. **Half-life:** 3–4 hrs.

USES

Adjunct to diet/exercise to lower serum glucose in those with type 2 non–insulin-dependent diabetes mellitus (NIDDM). Used as monotherapy or in combination with metformin, sulfonylurea to improve glycemic control. **OFF-LABEL:** Polycystic ovary syndrome.

PRECAUTIONS

Contraindications: Active hepatic disease, diabetic ketoacidosis, increased serum transaminase levels, including ALT greater than 2.5 times the normal serum level; type 1 diabetes mellitus; heart failure. **Cautions:** Hepatic impairment, edematous pts.

LIFESPAN CONSIDERATIONS

Pregnancy/Lactation: Unknown if drug crosses placenta or is distributed in breast milk. Not recommended in pregnant or breast-feeding women. **Pregnancy Category C. Children:** Safety and efficacy not established. **Elderly:** No age-related precautions noted.

INTERACTIONS

DRUG: **Rifampin** may decrease concentration, effect. **Gemfibrozil** may increase concentration, toxicity. **HERBAL:** **Garlic** may cause hypoglycemia. **FOOD:** None known. **LAB VALUES:** May increase serum ALT, AST, cholesterol, HDL, LDL. May decrease Hgb, Hct.

AVAILABILITY (Rx)

Tablets: 2 mg, 4 mg, 8 mg.

ADMINISTRATION/HANDLING

PO

• Give without regard to meals.

R

INDICATIONS/ROUTES/DOSAGE

Diabetes Mellitus, Combination Therapy

PO (WITH SULFONYLUREAS, METFORMIN): ADULTS, ELDERLY: Initially, 4 mg as single daily dose or in divided doses twice a day. May increase to 8 mg/day after 12 wks of therapy if fasting glucose level is not adequately controlled.

Diabetes Mellitus, Monotherapy

ADULTS, ELDERLY: Initially, 4 mg as single daily dose or in divided doses twice a day. May increase to 8 mg/day after 12 wks of therapy.

SIDE EFFECTS

Frequent (9%): Upper respiratory tract infection. **Occasional (4%–2%):** Headache, edema, back pain, fatigue, sinusitis, diarrhea.

ADVERSE EFFECTS/ TOXIC REACTIONS

Hepatotoxicity occurs rarely. Increased risk of CHF. May cause or worsen macular edema. May increase risk of fractures. Pts with ischemic heart disease are at high risk of MI.

NURSING CONSIDERATIONS

BASELINE ASSESSMENT

Obtain hepatic enzyme levels before initiation of therapy and periodically thereafter. Ensure follow-up instruction if pt, family do not thoroughly understand diabetes management, glucose-testing technique.

INTERVENTION/EVALUATION

Monitor serum glucose, Hgb, serum hepatic function tests, esp. AST, ALT. Assess for hypoglycemia (cool/wet skin, tremors, dizziness, anxiety, headache, tachycardia, numbness in mouth, hunger, diplopia), hyperglycemia (polyuria, polyphagia, polydipsia, nausea, vomiting, dim vision, fatigue, deep/rapid breathing). Be alert to conditions that alter glucose requirements (fever, increased activity/stress, surgical procedures).

PATIENT/ FAMILY TEACHING

• Diabetes mellitus requires lifelong control. • Prescribed diet, exercise are principal parts of treatment; do not skip/delay meals. • Wear medical alert identification. • Continue to adhere to dietary instructions, regular exercise program, regular testing of urine or blood glucose. • When taking combination drug therapy with a sulfonylurea or insulin, have source of glucose available to treat symptoms of low blood sugar. • Notify physician of rapid increase in weight, edema, shortness of breath, chest pain, abdominal pain, yellowing of skin/eyes.

rosuvastatin

ross-uh-vah-**stah**-tin
(Crestor)

Do not confuse rosuvastatin with atorvastatin, nystatin, or pitavastatin.

◆CLASSIFICATION

PHARMACOTHERAPEUTIC: HMG-CoA reductase inhibitor. **CLINICAL:** Antihyperlipidemic.

ACTION

Interferes with cholesterol biosynthesis by inhibiting conversion of the enzyme HMG-CoA to mevalonate, a precursor to cholesterol. **Therapeutic Effect:** Decreases LDL, VLDL, plasma triglyceride levels; increases HDL concentration.

PHARMACOKINETICS

Protein binding: 88%. Minimal hepatic metabolism. Primarily eliminated in feces. **Half-life:** 19 hrs (increased in severe renal dysfunction).

USES

Adjunct to diet therapy to decrease elevated total, LDL cholesterol concentrations in pts with primary hypercholesterolemia (types IIa, IIb), lowers serum triglyceride

R

levels, increases HDL. Adjunct to diet to slow progression of atherosclerosis in pts with elevated cholesterol. Treatment of primary dysbetalipoproteinemia, homozygous familial hypercholesterolemia (FH). Treatment of pts age 10–17 yrs with heterozygous familial hypercholesterolemia (HeFH) to reduce elevated total cholesterol, LDL cholesterol, and apolipoprotein B. Primary prevention of cardiovascular disease.

PRECAUTIONS

Contraindications: Active hepatic disease, breast-feeding, pregnancy, unexplained, persistent elevations of serum transaminase levels. **Cautions:** Anticoagulant therapy, history of hepatic disease, substantial alcohol consumption, major surgery, severe acute infection, trauma, hypotension, severe metabolic or endocrine disorders, severe electrolyte imbalances, uncontrolled seizures.

LIFESPAN CONSIDERATIONS

Pregnancy/Lactation: Contraindicated in pregnancy (suppression of cholesterol biosynthesis may cause fetal toxicity), lactation. Risk of serious adverse reactions in breast-feeding infants. **Pregnancy Category X. Children:** Safety and efficacy not established. **Elderly:** No age-related precautions noted.

R

INTERACTIONS

DRUG: **Aluminum- and magnesium-containing antacids** may decrease concentration, effect. Increased risk of myopathy with **cyclosporine, gemfibrozil, fibrate, niacin.** Increases concentrations of **estradiol, ethinyl, norgestrel. Warfarin** enhances anticoagulant effect. **HERBAL:** None significant. **FOOD:** **Red yeast rice** contains 2.4 mg **lovastatin** per 600 mg rice. **LAB VALUES:** May increase alkaline phosphatase, bilirubin, creatinine phosphokinase, glucose, transaminases. May produce hematuria, proteinuria.

AVAILABILITY (Rx)

Tablets: 5 mg, 10 mg, 20 mg, 40 mg.

ADMINISTRATION/HANDLING

PO

- Give without regard to meals. May give at any time of day.

INDICATIONS/ROUTES/DOSAGE

Hyperlipidemia, Dyslipidemia, Atherosclerosis, Dysbetalipoproteinemia, Primary Prevention of Cardiovascular Disease

PO: ADULTS, ELDERLY: Usual starting dosage is 10 mg/day, with adjustments based on lipid levels; monitor q2–4wk until desired level is achieved. Lower starting dose of 5 mg is recommended in Asians. **Maximum:** 40 mg/day. Range: 5–40 mg/day.

FH

PO: ADULTS, ELDERLY: Initially, 20 mg/day. **Maximum:** 40 mg/day.

HeFH

PO: CHILDREN 10–17 YRS: Initially, 20 mg once daily. Range: 5–20 mg once daily.

Renal Impairment (Creatinine Clearance Less Than 30 ml/min)

PO: ADULTS, ELDERLY: 5 mg/day; do not exceed 10 mg/day.

Concurrent Cyclosporine Use

PO: ADULTS, ELDERLY: 5 mg/day.

Concurrent Gemfibrozil Therapy

PO: ADULTS, ELDERLY: 10 mg/day.

SIDE EFFECTS

Generally well tolerated. Side effects are usually mild, transient. **Occasional (9%–3%):** Pharyngitis, headache, diarrhea, dyspepsia (heartburn, epigastric distress, indigestion), nausea, depression. **Rare (less than 3%):** Myalgia, asthenia (loss of strength, energy), back pain.

ADVERSE EFFECTS/ TOXIC REACTIONS

Potential for lens opacities. Hypersensitivity reaction, hepatitis, rhabdomyolysis occur rarely.

NURSING CONSIDERATIONS

BASELINE ASSESSMENT

Obtain dietary history, esp. fat consumption. Question for possibility of pregnancy before initiating therapy (Pregnancy Category X). Assess baseline lab results: serum cholesterol, triglycerides, hepatic function tests.

INTERVENTION/EVALUATION

Monitor serum cholesterol, triglycerides for therapeutic response. Lipid levels should be monitored within 2–4 wks of initiation of therapy or change in dosage. Monitor hepatic function tests. Hepatic function tests should be performed at 12 wks following initiation of therapy, at any elevation of dose, and periodically (e.g., semiannually) thereafter. Monitor CPK if myopathy is suspected. Monitor daily pattern of bowel activity and stool consistency. Assess for headache, sore throat. Be alert for myalgia, weakness.

PATIENT/FAMILY TEACHING

• Use appropriate contraceptive measures (Pregnancy Category X). • Periodic lab tests are essential part of therapy. • Maintain appropriate diet (important part of treatment). • Report unexplained muscle pain, tenderness, weakness, esp. if associated with fever, malaise.

Roxanol, *see morphine*

Roxicet, *see acetaminophen and oxycodone*

Rozerem, *see ramelteon*

rufinamide

roo-**fin**-a-mide
(Banzel)

◆ CLASSIFICATION

PHARMACOTHERAPEUTIC: Anticonvulsant. **CLINICAL:** Anticonvulsant.

ACTION

Modulates activity of sodium channels. Prolongs inactive state of the sodium channel in cortical neurons, limits sustained repetitive firing of sodium-dependent action potential, inhibiting excitatory neurotransmitter release. **Therapeutic Effect:** Exerts anticonvulsant activity.

PHARMACOKINETICS

Well absorbed following PO administration. Protein binding: 34%. Extensively metabolized. Eliminated in urine. **Half-life:** 6–10 hrs.

USES

Adjunctive therapy in treatment of seizures associated with Lennox-Gastaut syndrome in adults and children 4 yrs and older.

PRECAUTIONS

Contraindications: Familial short QT syndrome, severe hepatic impairment. **Cautions:** Other drugs that shorten QT interval, clinical depression, renal impairment, mild to moderate hepatic impairment.

⌛ LIFESPAN CONSIDERATIONS

Pregnancy/Lactation: May produce fetal skeletal abnormalities. May be distributed in breast milk. **Pregnancy Category C. Children:** Safety and efficacy not established in those younger than 4 yrs. **Elderly:** Age-related renal, hepatic, or cardiac impairment may require initiation of therapy at low end of dosing range.

INTERACTIONS

DRUG: May increase concentration of **phenobarbital, phenytoin.** May decrease concentration of **carbamazepine, lamotrigine. Valproate** may increase concentration. May decrease effect of **estradiol, norethidrone. Alcohol, CNS depressants** may increase CNS depressant effect. HERBAL: **Evening primrose** may decrease seizure threshhold. FOOD: None known. LAB VALUES: May decrease WBC count.

AVAILABILITY (Rx)

Tablets, Film-Coated: 200 mg, 400 mg.

ADMINISTRATION/HANDLING

PO

• Give with food. • Film-coated tablets may be scored or crushed for dosing flexibility.

INDICATIONS/ROUTES/DOSAGE

Lennox-Gastaut Seizures

PO: ADULTS, ELDERLY: Initially, 400–800 mg/day, given in 2 equally divided doses. Dose should be increased by 400–800 mg/day increased every 2 days. **Maximum:** 3,200 mg/day, administered in 2 equally divided doses. CHILDREN 4 YRS AND OLDER: Treatment should be initiated at a daily dose of approximately 10 mg/kg/day, given in 2 equally divided doses. Increase by approximately 10 mg/kg increments every other day to a target dose of 45 mg/kg/day or 3,200 mg/day, whichever is less, administered in 2 equally divided doses. Renal impairment pts with creatinine clearance less than 30 ml/min do not require any dosage change.

R

SIDE EFFECTS

Children: Frequent (27%–11%): Headache, dizziness, fatigue, nausea, drowsiness, diplopia. Occasional (6%–4%): Tremor, nystagmus, blurred vision, vomiting. Rare (3%): Ataxia, upper abdominal pain, anxiety, constipation, dyspepsia, back pain, gait disturbance, vertigo.
Adults: Frequent (17%–7%): Lethargy, vomiting, headache, fatigue, dizziness, nausea. Occasional (5%–4%): Influenza, nasopharyngitis, anorexia, rash, ataxia, diplopia. Rare (3%): Bronchitis, sinusitis, psychomotor hyperactivity, upper abdominal pain, aggression, ear infection, inattention, pruritus.

ADVERSE EFFECTS/ TOXIC REACTIONS

Suicidal thoughts or behavior occur rarely, noted as early as 1 wk after initiation of therapy and persisting for at least 24 wks. Shortening of the QT interval (up to 20 msec), hypersensitivity reaction (rash, fever, urticaria) has been noted. Abrupt withdrawal may precipitate seizure, status epilepticus.

NURSING CONSIDERATIONS

BASELINE ASSESSMENT

Review history of seizure disorder (intensity, frequency, duration, level of consciousness). Initiate seizure precautions.

INTERVENTION/EVALUATION

Provide safety measures as needed. Observe frequently for recurrence of seizure activity. Assess for clinical improvement (decrease in intensity, frequency of seizures). Assist with ambulation if drowsiness, lethargy occur. Question for evidence of headache.

PATIENT/FAMILY TEACHING

• Do not abruptly withdraw medication (may precipitate seizures). • Avoid tasks that require alertness, motor skills until response to drug is established. • Strict maintenance of drug therapy is essential for seizure control. • Avoid alcohol. • Female pts of childbearing age should be informed that concurrent use of rufinamide with hormonal contraceptives may render contraceptive less effective; nonhormonal forms of contraception are recommended. • Be alert for any unusual changes in mood/behavior (may increase risk of suicidal thoughts/behavior).

salmeterol

sal-**met**-er-all
(Serevent ✦, Serevent Diskus)

BLACK BOX ALERT Long-acting $beta_2$-adrenergic agonists may increase risk of asthma-related deaths.

Do not confuse salmeterol with Solu-Medrol, or Serevent with Atrovent, Combivent, Serentil, or Sinemet.

FIXED-COMBINATION(S)

Advair Diskus: salmeterol/fluticasone (a corticosteroid): 50 mcg/100 mcg, 50 mcg/250 mcg, 50 mcg/500 mcg. **Advair HFA:** salmeterol/fluticasone (a corticosteroid): 21 mcg/45 mcg, 21 mcg/115 mcg, 21 mcg/230 mcg.

◆ CLASSIFICATION

PHARMACOTHERAPEUTIC: Sympathomimetic (adrenergic agonist). **CLINICAL:** Bronchodilator (see pp. 74C, 75C, 76C).

ACTION

Stimulates $beta_2$-adrenergic receptors in lungs, resulting in relaxation of bronchial smooth muscle. **Therapeutic Effect:** Relieves bronchospasm, reducing airway resistance.

PHARMACOKINETICS

Route	Onset	Peak	Duration
Inhalation (asthma)	30–45 min	2–4 hrs	12 hrs
Inhalation (COPD)	2 hrs	3.25–4.75 hrs	12 hrs

Low systemic absorption; acts primarily in lungs. Protein binding: 95%. Metabolized in liver by hydroxylation. Primarily eliminated in feces. **Half-life:** 5.5 hrs.

USES

Maintenance therapy for asthma; prevention of exercise-induced bronchospasm, bronchospasm in pts with reversible obstructive airway disease. Long-term maintenance treatment of bronchospasm associated with COPD, including emphysema, chronic bronchitis.

PRECAUTIONS

Contraindications: History of hypersensitivity to sympathomimetics. **Cautions:** Not for acute symptoms; may cause paradoxical bronchospasm, severe asthma. Pts with cardiovascular disorders (coronary insufficiency, arrhythmias, hypertension), seizure disorders, thyrotoxicosis.

⌛ LIFESPAN CONSIDERATIONS

Pregnancy/Lactation: Unknown if distributed in breast milk. **Pregnancy Category C. Children:** No age-related precautions in those older than 4 yrs. **Elderly:** Lower dosages may be needed (may be more susceptible to tachycardia, tremors).

INTERACTIONS

DRUG: May decrease effects of **beta-adrenergic blocking agents (beta-blockers). MAOIs, tricyclic antidepressants** may increase concentration, effect, toxicity (wait 14 days after stopping MAOIs, tricyclic antidepressants before starting salmeterol). **HERBAL:** None significant. **FOOD:** None known. **LAB VALUES:** May decrease serum potassium. May increase serum glucose.

AVAILABILITY (Rx)

Powder for Oral Inhalation: 50 mcg/inhalation.

ADMINISTRATION/HANDLING

Inhalation

• Shake container well, instruct pt to exhale completely through mouth; place mouthpiece between lips, holding inhaler upright. • Inhale deeply through mouth while fully depressing top of canister. Pt should hold breath as long as possible before exhaling slowly. • Allow at least 2 min before second dose (allows for deeper bronchial penetration). • Rinse mouth with water immediately after inhalation (prevents mouth/throat dryness).

S

INDICATIONS/ROUTES/DOSAGE

Maintenance and Prevention Therapy for Asthma

INHALATION (DISKUS): ADULTS, ELDERLY, CHILDREN 4 YRS AND OLDER: 1 inhalation (50 mcg) q12h.

Prevention of Exercise-Induced Bronchospasm

INHALATION (DISKUS): ADULTS, ELDERLY, CHILDREN 4 YRS AND OLDER: 1 inhalation at least 30 min before exercise. Additional doses should not be given for 12 hrs. Do not administer if already giving salmeterol twice daily.

Maintenance Therapy for COPD

INHALATION (DISKUS): ADULTS, ELDERLY: 1 inhalation q12h.

SIDE EFFECTS

Frequent (28%): Headache. **Occasional (7%–3%):** Cough, tremor, dizziness, vertigo, throat dryness/irritation, pharyngitis. **Rare (less than 3%):** Palpitations, tachycardia, nausea, heartburn, GI distress, diarrhea.

ADVERSE EFFECTS/ TOXIC REACTIONS

May prolong QT interval (can precipitate ventricular arrhythmias). Hypokalemia, hyperglycemia may occur.

NURSING CONSIDERATIONS

BASELINE ASSESSMENT

Obtain baseline EKG and monitor for changes.

INTERVENTION/EVALUATION

Monitor rate, depth, rhythm, type of respiration; quality/rate of pulse, B/P. Assess lungs for wheezing, rales, rhonchi. Periodically evaluate serum potassium levels.

PATIENT/FAMILY TEACHING

• Not for relief of acute episodes. • Keep canister at room temperature (cold decreases effects). • Do not stop medication or exceed recommended dosage. • Notify physician promptly of chest pain, dizziness. • Wait at least 1 full min before second inhalation. • Administer dose 30–60 min before exercise when used to prevent exercise-induced bronchospasm. • Avoid excessive use of caffeine derivatives (coffee, tea, colas, chocolate).

saquinavir

sa-**kwin**-a-veer
(Invirase)

BLACK BOX ALERT Invirase is not interchangeable; must use Invirase in combination with ritonavir (provides saquinavir plasma levels at least equal to those achieved with Fortovase).

Do not confuse saquinavir with Sinequan.

◆ CLASSIFICATION

PHARMACOTHERAPEUTIC: Protease inhibitor. **CLINICAL:** Antiretroviral (see pp. 69C, 117C).

ACTION

Inhibits HIV protease, rendering the enzyme incapable of processing polyprotein precursors needed to generate functional proteins in HIV-infected cells. **Therapeutic Effect:** Interferes with HIV replication, slowing progression of HIV infection.

PHARMACOKINETICS

Poorly absorbed after PO administration (absorption increased with high-calorie, high-fat meals). Protein binding: 99%. Metabolized in liver to inactive metabolite. Primarily eliminated in feces. Unknown if removed by hemodialysis. **Half-life:** 13 hrs.

USES

Treatment of HIV infection in combination with other antiretroviral agents.

PRECAUTIONS

Contraindications: Concurrent use with amiodarone, bepridil, ergot derivatives, midazolam, propafenone, quinidine, rifampin, ritonavir, triazolam. **Cautions:** Diabetes mellitus, hepatic impairment.

LIFESPAN CONSIDERATIONS

Pregnancy/Lactation: Breast-feeding not recommended (possibility of HIV transmission). **Pregnancy Category B. Children:** Safety and efficacy not established. **Elderly:** Age-related renal/hepatic/cardiac impairment may require dosage adjustment.

INTERACTIONS

DRUG: May increase concentration, toxicity of **calcium channel-blocking agents, rifabutin, sildenafil, tadalafil, vardenafil.** May decrease concentration, effects of **efavirenz, methadone, oral contraceptives. Carbamazepine, dexamethasone, efavirenz, phenobarbital, phenytoin, rifabutin** may decrease concentration, effect. **Delavirdine, nevirapine, ritonavir** may increase concentration, toxicity. **HERBAL: Garlic, St. John's wort** may decrease concentration, effect. **FOOD: Grapefruit, grapefruit juice** may increase concentration. **LAB VALUES:** May increase serum ALT, AST, amylase, creatine kinase, GGT, LDH, bilirubin, calcium, potassium, sodium, cholesterol, triglycerides. May decrease neutrophils, platelets, WBC count.

AVAILABILITY (Rx)

Capsules (Invirase): 200 mg. **Tablets (Invirase):** 500 mg.

ADMINISTRATION/HANDLING

PO

• Give within 2 hrs after a full meal (if taken without food in stomach, may result in no antiviral activity).

INDICATIONS/ROUTES/DOSAGE

HIV Infection in Combination with Other Antiretrovirals

PO: ADULTS, ELDERLY: 1,000 mg (5 × 200 mg or 2 × 500 mg) twice a day in combination with ritonavir 100 mg twice a day.

SIDE EFFECTS

Occasional: Diarrhea, abdominal discomfort/pain, nausea, photosensitivity, stomatitis. **Rare:** Confusion, ataxia, asthenia (loss of strength, energy), headache, rash.

ADVERSE EFFECTS/TOXIC REACTIONS

None known.

NURSING CONSIDERATIONS

BASELINE ASSESSMENT

Obtain baseline laboratory testing, esp. hepatic function tests, before beginning saquinavir therapy and at periodic intervals during therapy. Offer emotional support. Obtain medication history.

INTERVENTION/EVALUATION

Monitor serum hepatic function tests, triglycerides, glucose, CD4 cell count, HIV RNA levels. Closely monitor for evidence of GI discomfort. Monitor daily pattern of bowel activity, stool consistency. Inspect mouth for signs of mucosal ulceration. Monitor serum chemistry tests for marked laboratory abnormalities. If serious or severe toxicities occur, interrupt therapy, contact physician.

PATIENT/FAMILY TEACHING

• Report persistent abdominal pain, nausea, vomiting. • Avoid exposure to sunlight, artificial light sources. • Continue therapy for full length of treatment. • Doses should be evenly spaced. • Saquinavir is not a cure for HIV infection, nor does it reduce risk of transmission to others. • Pts may continue to acquire illnesses associated with advanced HIV infection. • Take within 2 hrs after a full meal. • Avoid administration with grapefruit products.

sargramostim (granulocyte macrophage colony-stimulating factor, GM-CSF)

sar-gra-**moe**-stim
(Leukine)
Do not confuse Leukine with leucovoran or Leukeran.

CLASSIFICATION

PHARMACOTHERAPEUTIC: Colony-stimulating factor. **CLINICAL:** Hematopoietic, antineutropenic.

ACTION

Stimulates proliferation/differentiation of hematopoietic cells to activate mature granulocytes and macrophages. **Therapeutic Effect:** Assists bone marrow in making new WBCs, increases their chemotactic, antifungal, antiparasitic activity. Increases cytoneoplastic cells, activates neutrophils to inhibit tumor cell growth.

PHARMACOKINETICS

Route	Onset	Peak	Duration
IV (increase WBCs)	7–14 days	N/A	1 wk

Detected in serum within 5 min after subcutaneous administration. **Half-life: IV:** 1 hr; **Subcutaneous:** 3 hrs.

USES

Accelerates myeloid recovery in pts undergoing autologous or allogeneic bone marrow transplant or in pts who have undergone hematopoietic stem cell transplant following myeloablative chemotherapy. Prolongs survival in pts following bone marrow transplant in whom engraftment has been delayed or has failed. Enhances peripheral progenitor cell yield in autologous hematopoietic stem cell transplant. Shortens time to neutrophil recovery following induction chemotherapy of acute myelogenous leukemia (AML). **OFF-LABEL:** Treatment of AIDS-related neutropenia; chronic, severe neutropenia; drug-induced neutropenia; myelodysplastic syndrome.

PRECAUTIONS

Contraindications: 12 hrs before or after radiation therapy; 24 hrs before or after chemotherapy; excessive leukemic myeloid blasts in bone marrow or peripheral blood (greater than 10%); known hypersensitivity to yeast-derived products. **Cautions:** Preexisting cardiac disease, hypoxia, preexisting fluid retention, pulmonary infiltrates, CHF, renal/hepatic impairment.

LIFESPAN CONSIDERATIONS

Pregnancy/Lactation: Unknown if drug crosses placenta or is distributed in breast milk. **Pregnancy Category C. Children:** Safety and efficacy not established. **Elderly:** No age-related precautions noted.

INTERACTIONS

DRUG: None significant. **HERBAL:** None significant. **FOOD:** None known. **LAB VALUES:** May increase serum bilirubin, creatinine, hepatic enzyme. May decrease serum albumin.

AVAILABILITY (Rx)

Injection, Powder for Reconstitution: 250 mcg. **Injection Solution:** 500 mcg/ml.

ADMINISTRATION/HANDLING

IV

Reconstitution • To 250-mcg vial, add 1 ml Sterile Water for Injection (preservative free). • Direct Sterile Water for Injection to side of vial, gently swirl contents to avoid foaming; do not shake or vigorously agitate. • After reconstitution, further dilute with 0.9% NaCl. If final concentration less than 10 mcg/ml, add 1 mg albumin/ml 0.9% NaCl to provide a final albumin concentration of 0.1%.

◀ALERT▶ Albumin is added before addition of sargramostim (prevents drug adsorption to components of drug delivery system).

Rate of administration • Give each single dose over 30 min, 2 hr, 6 hr, or continuous infusion.

Storage • Refrigerate powder, reconstituted solution, diluted solution for injection. • Do not shake. • Reconstituted solutions are clear, colorless. • Use within 6 hrs; discard unused portions. • Use 1 dose per vial; do not reenter vial.

IV INCOMPATIBILITIES

Amphotericin B complex (Abelcet, AmBisome, Amphotec), chlorpromazine (Thorazine).

IV COMPATIBILITIES

Cimetidine (Tagamet), dexamethasone (Decadron), diphenhydramine (Benadryl), famotidine (Pepcid), heparin, meperidine (Demerol), metoclopramide (Reglan), promethazine (Phenergan), total parenteral nutrition (TPN).

INDICATIONS/ROUTES/DOSAGE

Neutrophil Recovery Following Chemotherapy in AML

IV INFUSION: ADULTS, ELDERLY: 250 mcg/m²/day (as 4-hr infusion) starting approximately 4 days following completion of induction chemotherapy.

Myeloid Recovery Following Bone Marrow Transplant (BMT)

IV INFUSION: ADULTS, ELDERLY: Usual parenteral dosage: 250 mcg/m²/day (as 2-hr infusion). Begin 2–4 hrs after autologous bone marrow infusion and not less than 24 hrs after last dose of chemotherapy or not less than 12 hrs after last radiation treatment. Continue until ANC is over 1,500 cells/mm³ for 3 consecutive days. Discontinue if blast cells appear or underlying disease progresses.

Bone Marrow Transplant Failure, Engraftment Delay

IV INFUSION: ADULTS, ELDERLY: 250 mcg/m²/day for 14 days. Infuse over 2 hrs. May repeat after 7 days off therapy if engraftment has not occurred with 500 mcg/m²/day for 14 days.

Stem Cell Transplant, Mobilization of Peripheral Blood Proginitor Cells

IV, SUBCUTANEOUS: ADULTS: 250 mcg/m²/day (IV as 24-hr infusion). Continue until ANC is over 1,500 cells/mm³ for 3 consecutive days.

SIDE EFFECTS

Frequent: GI disturbances (nausea, diarrhea, vomiting, stomatitis, anorexia, abdominal pain), arthralgia or myalgia, headache, malaise, rash, pruritus. **Occasional:** Peripheral edema, weight gain, dyspnea, asthenia (loss of strength, energy), fever, leukocytosis, capillary leak syndrome (fluid retention, irritation at local injection site, peripheral edema). **Rare:** Rapid/irregular heartbeat, thrombophlebitis.

ADVERSE EFFECTS/ TOXIC REACTIONS

Pleural/pericardial effusion occurs rarely after infusion.

NURSING CONSIDERATIONS

BASELINE ASSESSMENT

Obtain baseline pulmonary function testing, weight, vital signs. Obtain baseline chemistry studies (CBC with differential, platelet count, serum renal/hepatic function tests).

INTERVENTION/EVALUATION

Monitor CBC with differential, platelets, serum renal/hepatic function, pulmonary function, vital signs, weight. Monitor for supraventricular arrhythmias during administration (particularly in pts with history of cardiac arrhythmias). Assess closely for dyspnea during and immediately following infusion (particularly in pts with history of lung disease). If dys-

S

pnea occurs during infusion, cut infusion rate by half. If dyspnea continues, stop infusion immediately. If neutrophil count exceeds 20,000 cells/mm^3 or platelet count exceeds 500,000/mm^3, stop infusion or reduce dose by half, based on clinical condition of pt. Blood counts return to normal or baseline 3–7 days after discontinuation of therapy.

saw palmetto

Also known as American dwarf palm tree, cabbage palm, sabal, zuzhong.

CLASSIFICATION

HERBAL: See Appendix G.

ACTION

Appears to inhibit 5-alpha-reductase, prevent conversion of testosterone to dihydrotestosterone (DHT). **Effect:** Reduces prostate growth. Contains antiandrogenic, antiproliferative, anti-inflammatory properties.

USES

Symptoms of benign prostate hyperplasia (BPH). Used as a mild diuretic, sedative, anti-inflammatory agent, antiseptic.

PRECAUTIONS

Contraindications: Pregnancy, lactation due to antiandrogenic and estrogenic activity. **Cautions:** None known.

LIFESPAN CONSIDERATIONS

Pregnancy/Lactation: Contraindicated. **Children:** Safety and efficacy not established. **Elderly:** No age-related precautions noted.

INTERACTIONS

DRUG: May interfere with effects of **hormone therapy, oral contraceptives.** **HERBAL:** None significant. **FOOD:** None known. **LAB VALUES:** None significant.

AVAILABILITY (OTC)

Berries. Capsules: 80 mg, 160 mg, 500 mg. **Fluid Extract. Tea.**

INDICATIONS/ROUTES/DOSAGE

Benign Prostate Hyperplasia (BPH)

PO: ADULTS, ELDERLY: 160 mg twice daily or 320 mg once daily using liquid extract or 1–2 g of whole berries.

Diuretic, Sedative, Anti-Inflammatory, Antiseptic

PO: ADULTS, ELDERLY: 0.6–1.5 ml liquid extract or 0.5–1 g dried berries 3 times daily.

SIDE EFFECTS

Mild anorexia, dizziness, nausea, vomiting, constipation, diarrhea, headache, impotence, hypersensitivity reactions, back pain.

ADVERSE EFFECTS/TOXIC REACTIONS

None known.

NURSING CONSIDERATIONS

BASELINE ASSESSMENT

Question for use of oral contraceptives, hormone replacement therapy (herbal may interfere). Assess pt's urinary patterns. Obtain prostate-specific antigen (PSA) level before using.

INTERVENTION/EVALUATION

Assess for hypersensitivity reactions. Monitor symptoms of benign prostate hyperplasia (frequent/painful urination, hesitancy, urgency). Observe for decreased nocturia, improved urinary flow, decreased residual urine volume.

PATIENT/FAMILY TEACHING

- Should be taken with food.
- Contraindicated in pregnancy, breast-feeding.

saxagliptin

sax-a-**glip**-tin
(Onglyza)

Do not confuse saxagliptin with sitagliptin or sumatriptan.

FIXED-COMBINATION(S)

Kombiglyze XR: saxagliptin/metformin (an antidiabetic): 2.5 mg/1,000 mg, 5 mg/500 mg, 5 mg/1,000 mg.

◆CLASSIFICATION

PHARMACOTHERAPEUTIC: DDP-4 inhibitor (gliptins). **CLINICAL:** Antidiabetic.

ACTION

Slows the inactivation of incretin hormones by inhibiting DDP-4 enzyme. Incretin hormones increase insulin synthesis/release from pancreas and decrease glucagon secretion. **Therapeutic Effect:** Regulates glucose homeostasis.

PHARMACOKINETICS

Route	Onset	Peak	Duration
Oral	—	—	24 hrs

Rapidly absorbed following PO administration. Extensively metabolized (metabolite is active). Eliminated by both renal and hepatic pathways. **Half-life:** 2.5 hrs; metabolite, 3.1 hrs.

USES

Adjunctive treatment to diet and exercise to improve glycemic control in pts with type 2 diabetes mellitus.

PRECAUTIONS

Contraindications: Type 1 diabetes mellitus, diabetic ketoacidosis. **Cautions:** Concurrent use of other glucose-lowering agents may increase risk of hypoglycemia, mild renal impairment.

LIFESPAN CONSIDERATIONS

Pregnancy/Lactation: Unknown if distributed in breast milk. **Pregnancy Category B. Children:** Safety and efficacy not established. **Elderly:** Age-related renal impairment may require dosage adjustment.

INTERACTIONS

DRUG: CYP3A4 inhibitors (e.g., clarithromycin, itraconazole, ketoconazole) may increase concentration. **CYP3A4 inducers (e.g., rifampin)** may decrease concentration. **HERBAL:** None significant. **FOOD: Grapefruit juice** may increase concentration. **LAB VALUES:** May slightly decrease WBCs, particularly lymphocyte count. May increase serum creatinine.

AVAILABILITY (Rx)

Tablets, Film-Coated: 2.5 mg, 5 mg.

ADMINISTRATION/HANDLING

PO

• May give without regard to food. • Do not crush, break, chew film-coated tablets.

INDICATIONS/ROUTES/DOSAGE

Type 2 Diabetes Mellitus

PO: ADULTS OVER 18 YRS, ELDERLY: 2.5 or 5 mg once daily. **Moderate to Severe Renal Impairment (CrCl Less Than 50 ml/min):** 2.5 mg once daily. **Concurrent Strong CYP3A4 Inhibitors (e.g., Ketoconazole):** 2.5 mg once daily. **Hemodialysis:** Give dose after dialysis.

SIDE EFFECTS

Occasional (7%): Headache. **Rare (3%–1%):** Peripheral edema, sinusitis, abdominal pain, gastroenteritis, vomiting, rash.

ADVERSE EFFECTS/ TOXIC REACTIONS

Lymphopenia, rash occur rarely. Upper respiratory tract infection, urinary tract infection occur in approximately 7% of pts.

NURSING CONSIDERATIONS

BASELINE ASSESSMENT

Check blood glucose concentration before administration. Discuss lifestyle to determine extent of learning, emotional needs. Assure follow-up instruction if pt or family does not thoroughly under-

S

stand diabetes management or glucose-testing technique.

INTERVENTION/EVALUATION

Assess for hypoglycemia (diaphoresis, tremors, dizziness, anxiety, headache, tachycardia, perioral numbness, hunger, diplopia, difficulty concentrating), hyperglycemia (polyuria, polyphagia, polydipsia, nausea, vomiting, dim vision, fatigue, deep, rapid breathing). Be alert to conditions that alter glucose requirements (fever, increased activity or stress, surgical procedures).

PATIENT/FAMILY TEACHING

• Diabetes mellitus requires lifelong control. Prescribed diet and exercise are principal parts of treatment; do not skip or delay meals. • Continue to adhere to dietary instructions, regular exercise program, regular testing of blood glucose. • When taking combination drug therapy or when glucose demands are altered (fever, infection, trauma, stress, heavy physical activity), have a source of glucose available to treat symptoms of hypoglycemia.

scopolamine

skoe-**pol**-a-meen
(Trans-Derm Scop, Transderm-V🍁)

FIXED-COMBINATION(S)

Donnatal: scopolamine/atropine (anticholinergic)/hyoscyamine (anticholinergic)/phenobarbital (sedative): 0.0065 mg/0.0194 mg/0.1037 mg/16.2 mg.

◆ CLASSIFICATION

PHARMACOTHERAPEUTIC: Anticholinergic. **CLINICAL:** Antinausea, antiemetic.

ACTION

Competitively inhibits action of acetylcholine at muscarinic receptors. Reduces excitability of labyrinthine receptors, depressing conduction in vestibular cerebellar pathway. **Therapeutic Effect:** Prevents motion-induced nausea/vomiting.

USES

Prevention of motion sickness, postop nausea/vomiting.

PRECAUTIONS

Contraindications: Angle-closure glaucoma, GI/GU obstruction, myasthenia gravis, paralytic ileus, tachycardia, thyrotoxicosis. **Cautions:** Hepatic/renal impairment, cardiac disease, seizures, psychoses.

⌛ LIFESPAN CONSIDERATIONS

Pregnancy/Lactation: Crosses placenta; unknown if distributed in breast milk. **Pregnancy Category C. Children:** Safety and efficacy not established. **Elderly:** Dizziness, hallucinations, confusion may require dosage adjustment.

INTERACTIONS

DRUG: **Anticholinergics, antihistamines, tricyclic antidepressants** may increase anticholinergic effects. **CNS depressants** may increase CNS depression. **HERBAL:** None significant. **FOOD:** None known. **LAB VALUES:** May interfere with gastric secretion test.

AVAILABILITY (Rx)

Transdermal System (Trans-Derm Scop): 1.5 mg.

ADMINISTRATION/HANDLING

Transdermal

• Apply patch to hairless area behind one ear. • If dislodged or on for more than 72 hrs, replace with fresh patch.

INDICATIONS/ROUTES/DOSAGE

Prevention of Motion Sickness

TRANSDERMAL: ADULTS: One system at least 4 hrs prior to exposure and q72h as needed.

Postop Nausea/Vomiting

TRANSDERMAL: ADULTS, ELDERLY: 1 system no sooner than 1 hr before surgery and removed 24 hrs after surgery.

SIDE EFFECTS

Frequent (greater than 15%): Dry mouth, drowsiness, blurred vision. Rare (5%–1%): Dizziness, restlessness, hallucinations, confusion, difficulty urinating, rash.

ADVERSE EFFECTS/ TOXIC REACTIONS

None known.

NURSING CONSIDERATIONS

BASELINE ASSESSMENT

Obtain baseline hepatic function tests. Assess for use of other CNS depressants, drugs with anticholinergic action, history of narrow-angle glaucoma.

INTERVENTION/EVALUATION

Monitor serum hepatic/renal function tests. Observe for improvement of symptoms.

PATIENT/FAMILY TEACHING

• Avoid tasks requiring alertness, motor skills until response to drug is established (may cause drowsiness, disorientation, confusion). • Use only 1 patch at a time; do not cut. • Wash hands after administration.

selegiline

se-**le**-ji-leen
(Apo-Selegiline ✱, Eldepryl, Emsam, Novo-Selegiline ✱, Zelapar)

BLACK BOX ALERT **Transdermal:** Increased risk of suicidal thinking and behavior in children, adolescents, young adults 18–24 yrs with major depressive disorder, other psychiatric disorders.

Do not confuse selegiline with Salagen, sertraline, or Stelazine, Eldepryl with Elavil or enalapril, or Zelapar with Zemplar.

◆CLASSIFICATION

PHARMACOTHERAPEUTIC: Monoamine oxidase inhibitor (MAOI). CLINICAL: Antiparkinson agent.

ACTION

Irreversibly inhibits activity of monoamine oxidase type B (enzyme that breaks down dopamine), thereby increasing dopaminergic action. Therapeutic Effect: Relieves signs/symptoms of Parkinson's disease (tremor, akinesia, posture/equilibrium disorders, rigidity).

PHARMACOKINETICS

Route	Onset	Peak	Duration
PO	1 hr	—	24–72 hrs

Rapidly absorbed from GI tract. Crosses blood-brain barrier. Protein binding: 90%. Metabolized in liver to active metabolites. Primarily excreted in urine. Half-life: **PO:** 10 hrs. **Transdermal:** 18–25 hrs.

USES

Adjunct to levodopa/carbidopa in treatment of Parkinson's disease. **Transdermal:** Treatment of major depressive disorder (MDD). OFF-LABEL: Treatment of ADHD, Alzheimer's disease, depression, early Parkinson's disease, extrapyramidal symptoms (EPS), negative symptoms of schizophrenia.

PRECAUTIONS

Contraindications: Concurrent use with meperidine, tricyclic antidepressants. Cautions: History of peptic ulcer disease, dementia, psychosis, tardive dyskinesia, profound tremor, cardiac dysrhythmias.

⌛ LIFESPAN CONSIDERATIONS

Pregnancy/Lactation: Unknown if drug crosses placenta or is distributed in breast milk. **Pregnancy Category C. Children:** Safety and efficacy not established. **Elderly:** No age-related precautions noted.

INTERACTIONS

DRUG: **Fluoxetine, fluvoxamine, paroxetine, sertraline, venlafaxine** may cause mania, serotonin syndrome (altered mental status, restlessness, diaphoresis, diarrhea, fever). **Meperidine** may

S

cause potentially fatal reaction (e.g., excitation, diaphoresis, rigidity, hypertension/hypotension, coma, death). **Tricyclic antidepressants** may cause asystole, diaphoresis, hypertension, syncope, altered mental status, hyperpyrexia, seizures, tremors (wait 14 days between stopping selegiline and starting tricyclic antidepressants). HERBAL: **Kava kava, SAMe, St. John's wort, valerian** may increase risk of serotonin syndrome, excessive sedation. FOOD: **Tyramine-rich foods** may produce hypertensive reactions. LAB VALUES: None significant.

AVAILABILITY (Rx)

Capsules (Eldepryl): 5 mg. Tablets (Eldepryl): 5 mg. Tablets (Orally-Disintegrating [Zelapar]): 1.25 mg. Transdermal (Emsam): 6 mg/24 hrs, 9 mg/24 hrs, 12 mg/24 hrs.

ADMINISTRATION/HANDLING

PO

• Give without regard to meals. • Avoid tyramine-containing foods, large quantities of caffeine-containing beverages.

PO (Orally-Disintegrating Tablets)

• Give in morning before breakfast and without liquid. • Peel off backing with dry hands (do not push tablets through foil). • Immediately place on top of tongue, allow to disintegrate. • Avoid food, liquids for 5 min before and after taking selegiline.

Transdermal

• Apply to dry, intact skin on upper torso or thigh, outer surface of upper arm.

INDICATIONS/ROUTES/DOSAGE

Adjunctive Treatment of Parkinson's Disease

PO: ADULTS (ELDEPRYL): 10 mg/day in divided doses, such as 5 mg at breakfast and lunch, given concomitantly with each dose of carbidopa and levodopa. ELDERLY: Initially, 5 mg in the morning. May increase up to 10 mg/day. ADULTS, ELDERLY (ZELAPAR): Initially, 1.25 mg daily for at least 6 wks. May increase to 2.5 mg/day.

Major Depressive Disorder

TRANSDERMAL: ADULTS: Initially, 6 mg/24 hrs. May increase in 3 mg/24 hrs increments at minimum of 2 wks. **Maximum:** 12 mg/24 hrs. ELDERLY: 6 mg/24 hrs.

SIDE EFFECTS

Frequent (10%–4%): Nausea, dizziness, light-headedness, syncope, abdominal discomfort. Occasional (3%–2%): Confusion, hallucinations, dry mouth, vivid dreams, dyskinesia. Rare (1%): Headache, myalgia, anxiety, diarrhea, insomnia.

ADVERSE EFFECTS/ TOXIC REACTIONS

Symptoms of overdose may vary from CNS depression (sedation, apnea, cardiovascular collapse, death) to severe paradoxical reactions (hallucinations, tremor, seizures). Impaired motor coordination, (loss of balance, blepharospasm [uncontrolled blinking], facial grimaces, feeling of heaviness in lower extremities), depression, nightmares, delusions, overstimulation, sleep disturbance, anger, hallucinations, confusion may occur.

NURSING CONSIDERATIONS

INTERVENTION/EVALUATION

Be alert to neurologic effects (headache, lethargy, mental confusion, agitation). Monitor for evidence of dyskinesia (difficulty with movement). Assess for clinical reversal of symptoms (improvement of tremors of head/hands at rest, mask-like facial expression, shuffling gait, muscular rigidity). Monitor for unusual behavior, worsening depression, suicidal ideation, especially at initiation of therapy or with changes in dosage.

PATIENT/FAMILY TEACHING

• Tolerance to feeling of light-headedness develops during therapy. • To reduce hypotensive effect, rise slowly from lying to sitting position, permit legs to dangle momentarily before standing. • Avoid tasks that require alertness, motor skills until response to drug is established. • Dry mouth, drowsiness, dizziness may be an expected response of drug. • Avoid alcohol during therapy. • Coffee, tea may help reduce drowsiness. • Notify physician of worsening depression, unusual behavior, thoughts of suicide.

senna

sen-na
(Ex-Lax, Senexon, Senna-Gen, Senokot)

FIXED-COMBINATION(S)

Gentlax-S, Senokot-S: senna/docusate (a laxative): 8.6 mg/50 mg.

◆CLASSIFICATION

PHARMACOTHERAPEUTIC: GI stimulant. **CLINICAL:** Laxative (see p. 122C).

ACTION

Direct effect on intestinal smooth musculature (stimulates intramural nerve plexi). **Therapeutic Effect:** Increases peristalsis, promotes laxative effect.

PHARMACOKINETICS

Route	Onset	Peak	Duration
PO	6–12 hrs	N/A	N/A
Rectal	0.5–2 hrs	N/A	N/A

Minimal absorption after PO administration. Hydrolyzed to active form by enzymes of colonic flora. Absorbed drug metabolized in the liver. Eliminated in feces via biliary system.

USES

Short-term use for constipation, to evacuate colon before bowel/rectal examinations.

PRECAUTIONS

Contraindications: Abdominal pain, appendicitis, intestinal obstruction, nausea, vomiting. **Cautions:** Prolonged use (longer than 1 wk).

⌛ LIFESPAN CONSIDERATIONS

Pregnancy/Lactation: Unknown if distributed in breast milk. **Pregnancy Category C. Children:** Safety and efficacy not established in those younger than 6 yrs. **Elderly:** No age-related precautions noted; monitor for signs of dehydration, electrolyte loss.

INTERACTIONS

DRUG: May decrease transit time of concurrently administered **oral medications,** decreasing absorption. **HERBAL:** None significant. **FOOD:** None known. **LAB VALUES:** May increase serum glucose. May decrease serum potassium.

AVAILABILITY (OTC)

Granules (Senokot): 15 mg/tsp. **Syrup (Senokot):** 8.8 mg/5 ml. **Tablets (Ex-Lax, Senexon, Senna-Gen, Senokot):** 8.6 mg, 15 mg.

ADMINISTRATION/HANDLING

PO

• Give on an empty stomach (decreases time to effect). • Offer at least 6–8 glasses of water/day (aids stool softening). • Avoid giving within 1 hr of other oral medication (decreases drug absorption). • Syrup can be mixed with juice, milk, ice cream.

INDICATIONS/ROUTES/DOSAGE

Constipation

PO (TABLETS): ADULTS, ELDERLY, CHILDREN 12 YRS AND OLDER: 2 tablets at bedtime. **Maximum:** 4 tablets twice daily. **CHILDREN 6–11 YRS:** 1 tablet at bedtime. **Maximum:** 2 tablets twice daily. **CHILDREN 2–5 YRS:** ½ tablet at bedtime. **Maximum:** 1 tablet twice daily.

PO (SYRUP): ADULTS, ELDERLY, CHILDREN 12 YRS AND OLDER: 10–15 ml at bedtime. **Maximum:** 15 ml twice daily. **CHILDREN 6–11 YRS:** 5–7.5 ml at bedtime. **Maximum:** 7.5 ml twice daily. **CHILDREN 2–5 YRS:** 2.5–3.75 ml at bedtime. **Maximum:** 3.75 ml twice daily.

Bowel Evacuation

PO: ADULTS, ELDERLY, CHILDREN OLDER THAN 1 YR: 75 ml between 2 PM and 4 PM on day prior to procedure.

SIDE EFFECTS

Frequent: Pink-red, red-violet, red-brown, or yellow-brown discoloration of urine. **Occasional:** Some degree of abdominal discomfort, nausea, mild cramping, faintness.

ADVERSE EFFECTS/ TOXIC REACTIONS

Long-term use may result in laxative dependence, chronic constipation, loss of normal bowel function. Prolonged use/ overdose may result in electrolyte, metabolic disturbances (e.g., hypokalemia, hypocalcemia, metabolic acidosis or alkalosis), vomiting, muscle weakness, persistent diarrhea, malabsorption, weight loss.

NURSING CONSIDERATIONS

INTERVENTION/EVALUATION

Encourage adequate fluid intake. Assess bowel sounds for peristalsis. Monitor daily pattern of bowel activity, stool consistency. Assess for GI disturbances. Monitor serum electrolytes in pts exposed to prolonged, frequent, excessive use of medication.

PATIENT/FAMILY TEACHING

• Urine may turn pink-red, red-violet, red-brown, yellow-brown (only temporary and not harmful). • Institute measures to promote defecation (increase fluid intake, exercise, high-fiber diet). • Laxative effect generally occurs in 6–12 hrs but may take 24 hrs. • Do not take other oral medication within 1 hr of taking senna (decreased effectiveness).

sertraline

sir-trah-leen
(Apo-Sertraline, Novo-Sertraline, PMS-Sertraline, Zoloft)

BLACK BOX ALERT Increased risk of suicidal thinking and behavior in children, adolescents, young adults 18–24 yrs with major depressive disorder, other psychiatric disorders.

Do not confuse sertraline with selegiline, Serentil, or Serevent, or Zoloft with Zocor.

CLASSIFICATION

PHARMACOTHERAPEUTIC: Serotonin reuptake inhibitor. **CLINICAL:** Antidepressant, anxiolytic, obsessive-compulsive disorder adjunct (see p. 39C).

ACTION

Blocks reuptake of the neurotransmitter serotonin at CNS neuronal presynaptic membranes, increasing availability at postsynaptic receptor sites. **Therapeutic Effect:** Relieves depression, reduces obsessive-compulsive behavior, decreases anxiety.

PHARMACOKINETICS

Incompletely, slowly absorbed from GI tract; food increases absorption. Protein binding: 98%. Widely distributed. Undergoes extensive first-pass metabolism in liver to active compound. Excreted in urine, feces. Not removed by hemodialysis. **Half-life:** 26 hrs.

USES

Treatment of major depressive disorders, panic disorder, obsessive-compulsive disorder (OCD), post-traumatic stress disorder (PTSD), premenstrual dysphoric disorder (PMDD), social anxiety disorder. **OFF-LABEL:** Eating disorders, generalized anxiety disorder (GAD), impulse control disorders, hot flashes (men), mild dementia-associated agitation in non-psychotic pts.

PRECAUTIONS

Contraindications: MAOI use within 14 days. **Cautions:** Seizure disorders, cardiac disease, recent MI, hepatic impairment, suicidal pts.

LIFESPAN CONSIDERATIONS

Pregnancy/Lactation: Unknown if drug crosses placenta or is distributed in breast milk. **Pregnancy Category C. Children:** Children and adolescents are at increased risk for suicidal ideation and behavior or worsening of depression, esp. during the first few mos of therapy. **Elderly:** No age-related precautions noted, but lower initial dosages recommended.

INTERACTIONS

DRUG: May increase concentration, risk of toxicity of **highly protein-bound medications (e.g., digoxin, warfarin). MAOIs** may cause neuroleptic malignant syndrome, hypertensive crisis, hyperpyrexia, seizures, serotonin syndrome (diaphoresis, diarrhea, fever, mental changes, restlessness, shivering). May increase concentration, toxicity of tricyclic antidepressants. HERBAL: **Gotu kola, kava kava, St. John's wort, valerian** may increase CNS depression. FOOD: None known. LAB VALUES: May increase total serum cholesterol, triglycerides, AST, ALT. May decrease serum uric acid.

AVAILABILITY (Rx)

Oral Concentrate: 20 mg/ml. Tablets: 25 mg, 50 mg, 100 mg.

ADMINISTRATION/HANDLING

PO

• Give with food, milk if GI distress occurs. • Oral concentrate must be diluted before administration. Mix with 4 oz water, ginger ale, lemon/lime soda, or orange juice *only.* Give immediately after mixing.

INDICATIONS/ROUTES/DOSAGE

Depression

PO: ADULTS: Initially, 50 mg/day. May increase by 50 mg/day at 7-day intervals up to 200 mg/day. **ELDERLY:** Initially, 25 mg/day. May increase by 25–50 mg/day at 7-day intervals up to 200 mg/day.

Obsessive-Compulsive Disorder (OCD)

PO: ADULTS, CHILDREN 13–17 YRS: Initially, 50 mg/day with morning or evening meal. May increase by 50 mg/day at 7-day intervals. **ELDERLY, CHILDREN 6–12 YRS:** Initially, 25 mg/day. May increase by 25–50 mg/day at 7-day intervals. **Maximum:** 200 mg/day.

Panic Disorder, Post-Traumatic Stress Disorder (PTSD), Social Anxiety Disorder (SAD)

PO: ADULTS, ELDERLY: Initially, 25 mg/day. May increase by 50 mg/day at 7-day intervals. Range: 50–200 mg/day. **Maximum:** 200 mg/day.

Premenstrual Dysphoric Disorder (PMDD)

PO: ADULTS: Initially, 50 mg/day. May increase up to 150 mg/day in 50-mg increments.

SIDE EFFECTS

Frequent (26%–12%): Headache, nausea, diarrhea, insomnia, drowsiness, dizziness, fatigue, rash, dry mouth. Occasional (6%–4%): Anxiety, nervousness, agitation, tremor, dyspepsia (heartburn, indigestion, epigastric pain), diaphoresis, vomiting, constipation, sexual dysfunction, visual disturbances, altered taste. Rare (less than 3%): Flatulence, urinary frequency, paresthesia, hot flashes, chills.

ADVERSE EFFECTS/ TOXIC REACTIONS

Serotonin syndrome (seizures, arrhythmias, high fever), neuroleptic malignant syndrome (muscle rigidity, cognitive changes), suicidal ideation have occurred.

NURSING CONSIDERATIONS

BASELINE ASSESSMENT

Assess appearance, behavior, speech patterns, level of interest, mood. For those on long-term therapy, serum hepatic/renal function tests, blood counts should be performed periodically.

INTERVENTION/EVALUATION

Assess mental status for depression, suicidal ideation (esp. at beginning of therapy or change in dosage), anxiety, social

S

function, panic attack. Monitor daily pattern of bowel activity and stool consistency. Assist with ambulation if dizziness occurs.

PATIENT/FAMILY TEACHING

• Dry mouth may be relieved by sugarless gum, sips of tepid water. • Report headache, fatigue, tremor, sexual dysfunction. • Avoid tasks that require alertness, motor skills until response to drug is established (may cause dizziness, drowsiness). • Take with food if nausea occurs. • Inform physician if pregnancy occurs. • Avoid alcohol. • Do not take OTC medications without consulting physician. • Report worsening of depression, suicidal ideation.

sevelamer

seh-**vel**-a-mer
(Renagel, Renvela)
Do not confuse Renagel with Reglan or Regonol, or sevelamer with Savella.

◆ CLASSIFICATION

PHARMACOTHERAPEUTIC: Polymeric phosphate binder. **CLINICAL:** Antihyperphosphatemia.

ACTION

Binds with dietary phosphorus in GI tract, allowing phosphorus to be eliminated through normal digestive process, decreasing serum phosphorus level. **Therapeutic Effect:** Decreases incidence of hypercalcemic episodes in pts receiving calcium acetate treatment.

PHARMACOKINETICS

Not absorbed systemically. Unknown if removed by hemodialysis.

USES

Reduction of serum phosphorus in pts with chronic renal disease on hemodialysis.

PRECAUTIONS

Contraindications: Bowel obstruction, hypophosphatemia. **Cautions:** Dysphagia, severe GI tract motility disorders, major GI tract surgery, swallowing disorders.

LIFESPAN CONSIDERATIONS

Pregnancy/Lactation: Not distributed in breast milk. **Pregnancy Category C.** **Children:** Safety and efficacy not established. **Elderly:** No age-related precautions noted.

INTERACTIONS

DRUG: May decrease absorption of **oral medications** (take at least 1 hr before or 3 hrs after a dose of sevelamer). **HERBAL:** None significant. **FOOD:** None known. **LAB VALUES:** None significant.

AVAILABILITY (Rx)

Tablets (Renagel): 400 mg, 800 mg. **(Renvela):** 800 mg.

ADMINISTRATION/HANDLING

PO

• Give with meals. • Space other medication by at least 1 hr before or 3 hrs after sevelamer. • Swallow tablets whole; do not crush, chew, break.

INDICATIONS/ROUTES/DOSAGE

Note: 667 mg calcium acetate equivalent to 800 mg sevelamer.

Hyperphosphatemia

PO: ADULTS, ELDERLY: (RENAGEL): 800–1,600 mg with each meal, depending on severity of hyperphosphatemia (5.5–7.4 mg/dl: 800 mg 3 times daily; 7.5–8.9 mg/dl: 1,200–1,600 mg 3 times daily; 9 mg/dl or greater: 1,600 mg 3 times daily). **(RENVELA):** 800–1,600 mg 3 times daily with meals. Adjust by 1 tablet per meal q2wks to obtain serum phosphorus at 3.5–5.5 mg/dl. Maintenance dose adjustment based on serum phosphorous concentration. Goal (range): 3.5–5.5 mg/dl.

SIDE EFFECTS

Frequent (20%–11%): Infection, pain, hypotension, diarrhea, dyspepsia, nausea, vomiting. **Occasional (10%–1%):** Headache, constipation, hypertension, increased cough.

ADVERSE EFFECTS/ TOXIC REACTIONS

Thrombosis occurs rarely.

NURSING CONSIDERATIONS

BASELINE ASSESSMENT

Obtain baseline serum phosphorus; assess for bowel obstruction.

INTERVENTION/EVALUATION

Monitor serum phosphorus, bicarbonate, chloride, calcium.

PATIENT/FAMILY TEACHING

- Take with meals, swallow whole.
- Report persistent headache, nausea, vomiting, diarrhea, hypotension.

sildenafil

sill-**den**-a-fill
(Revatio, Viagra)
Do not confuse Revatio with ReVia, sildenafil with tadalafil or vardenafil, or Viagra with Allegra or Vaniqa.

CLASSIFICATION

PHARMACOTHERAPEUTIC: Phosphodiesterase-5 enzyme (PDE5) inhibitor. **CLINICAL:** Erectile dysfunction adjunct.

ACTION

Inhibits type 5 cyclic guanosine monophosphate (a specific phosphodiesterase), a predominant isoenzyme of pulmonary vascular smooth muscle, corpus cavernosum of penis. **Therapeutic Effect:** Relaxes smooth muscle, increases blood flow, facilitating erection.

USES

Viagra: Treatment of male erectile dysfunction. **Revatio:** Treatment of pulmonary arterial hypertension. **OFF-LABEL:** Treatment of diabetic gastroparesis, sexual dysfunction associated with use of selective serotonin reuptake inhibitors, Raynaud's phenomenon, pulmonary arterial hypertension in children.

PHARMACOKINETICS

Route	Onset	Peak	Duration
PO	1 hr	—	2–4 hrs

Rapidly absorbed. Protein binding: 96%. Metabolized in liver. Primarily eliminated in feces. **Half-life:** 4 hrs.

PRECAUTIONS

Contraindications: Concurrent use of sodium nitroprusside, nitrates in any form. **Cautions:** Renal, cardiac, hepatic impairment; anatomic deformation of penis; pts who may be predisposed to priapism (sickle cell anemia, multiple myeloma, leukemia). **Pregnancy Category B.**

INTERACTIONS

DRUG: **Alpha-adrenergic blocking agents** increase symptomatic hypotension. **Ritonavir** may increase concentration, toxicity. **Cimetidine, erythromycin, itraconazole, ketoconazole** may increase concentration. Potentiates hypotensive effects of **nitrates.** **HERBAL:** **St. John's wort** may decrease concentration. **FOOD:** **High-fat meals** delay maximum effectiveness by 1 hr. **LAB VALUES:** None significant.

AVAILABILITY (Rx)

Tablets: (Revatio): 20 mg. **(Viagra):** 25 mg, 50 mg, 100 mg.

ADMINISTRATION/HANDLING

PO

- May take approximately 1 hr before sexual activity but may be taken any time from 30 min–4 hrs before sexual activity.
- Revatio may be given without regard to meals.
- Give tablets at least 4–6 hrs apart.

INDICATIONS/ROUTES/DOSAGE

Erectile Dysfunction

PO: ADULTS: 50 mg (30 min–4 hrs before sexual activity). Range: 25–100 mg. Maximum dosing frequency is once a day. **ELDERLY OLDER THAN 65 YRS, CREATININE CLEARANCE LESS THAN 30 ML/MIN:** Consider starting dose of 25 mg.

Pulmonary Arterial Hypertension

PO: ADULTS, ELDERLY: 20 mg 3 times daily taken 4–6 hrs apart.

SIDE EFFECTS

Frequent: Headache (16%), flushing (10%). **Occasional (7%–3%):** Dyspepsia (heartburn, indigestion, epigastric pain), nasal congestion, UTI, abnormal vision, diarrhea. **Rare (2%):** Dizziness, rash.

ADVERSE EFFECTS/ TOXIC REACTIONS

Prolonged erections (lasting over 4 hrs), priapism (painful erections lasting over 6 hrs) occur rarely. Sudden hearing decrease or loss; sudden loss of vision in one or both eyes noted.

NURSING CONSIDERATIONS

BASELINE ASSESSMENT

Viagra: Determine if pt has other medical conditions, including angina, cardiac disease, benign prostatic hyperplasia (BPH). Assess pt's baseline serum renal/hepatic function. **Revatio:** Obtain baseline ABGs; assess pulmonary function, cardiovascular status.

INTERVENTION/EVALUATION

Monitor pulse, B/P, oxygen saturation, PaO_2.

PATIENT/FAMILY TEACHING

• Sildenafil has no effect in absence of sexual stimulation. • Seek treatment immediately if erection lasts longer than 4 hrs. • Avoid nitrate drugs while taking sildenafil. • Inform pt that Revatio is not to be taken with Viagra or other PDE5 inhibitors. • Seek medical attention in event of sudden loss of vision or sudden decrease or loss of hearing (may be accompanied by tinnitus or dizziness).

silodosin

sill-oh-**doe**-sin
(Rapaflo)

◆CLASSIFICATION

PHARMACOTHERAPEUTIC: Alpha$_1$-adrenergic blocker. **CLINICAL:** Benign prostatic hyperplasia agent.

ACTION

Blocks alpha-adrenergic receptors. Produces vasodilation, decreases peripheral resistance, targets receptors around bladder neck, prostate. **Therapeutic Effect:** Relaxes smooth muscle, improves urinary flow.

PHARMACOKINETICS

Well absorbed following PO administration. Widely distributed. Protein binding 97%. Metabolized in liver. Primarily excreted in feces with a lesser amount eliminated in urine. **Half-life:** 9–13 hrs.

USES

Treatment of signs and symptoms of benign prostatic hyperplasia.

PRECAUTIONS

Contraindications: Severe renal impairment (creatinine clearance less than 30 ml/min), severe hepatic impairment (Child-Pugh score equal to or less than 10), concurrent administration with ketoconazole, clarithromycin, itraconazole, ritonavir. **Cautions:** Moderate renal/hepatic impairment.

⌛ LIFESPAN CONSIDERATIONS:

Pregnancy/Lactation: Not indicated for use in women. **Pregnancy Category B. Children:** Not indicated in this pt popula-

S

tion. **Elderly:** No age-related precautions noted.

INTERACTIONS

DRUG: **Other alpha-adrenergic blocking agents (alfuzosin, doxazosin, prazosin, tamsulosin, terazosin)** may have additive effect. **Diltiazem, erythromycin, verapamil** may increase concentration. **Clarithromycin, itraconazole, ketoconazole, ritonavir** significantly increase concentration (concurrent use contraindicated). HERBAL: None significant. FOOD: None known. LAB VALUES: None significant.

AVAILABILITY (Rx)

Capsules: 4 mg, 8 mg.

ADMINISTRATION/HANDLING

PO
- Give with a meal.

INDICATIONS/ROUTES/DOSAGE

Benign Prostatic Hyperplasia

PO: ADULTS, MILD RENAL IMPAIRMENT: 8 mg once daily, with a meal.

Moderate Renal Impairment (Creatinine Clearance 30–50 ml/min)

PO: ADULTS: 4 mg once daily, with a meal.

SIDE EFFECTS

Frequent: (28%): Retrograde ejaculation. Occasional (3%–2%): Dizziness, diarrhea, orthostatic hypotension, headache nasopharyngitis, nasal congestion. Rare: (1% and less): Insomnia, sinusitis, abdominal pain, asthenia (lack of strength, energy).

ADVERSE EFFECTS/ TOXIC REACTIONS

First-dose syncope (orthostatic hypotension with sudden loss of consciousness) may occur shortly after giving initial dose. May be preceded by tachycardia (120–160 beats/min). Recovery occurs spontaneously.

NURSING CONSIDERATIONS

BASELINE ASSESSMENT

Obtain baseline renal/hepatic function tests. Give first dose at bedtime. If initial dose is given during daytime, assess B/P, pulse immediately before dose, and q15–30 min after (be alert to B/P fluctuations, postural hypotensions).

INTERVENTION/EVALUATION

Assist with ambulation if dizziness occurs. Monitor renal/hepatic function. Monitor daily pattern of bowel activity, stool consistency.

PATIENT/FAMILY TEACHING

• Use caution when getting up from sitting or lying position. • Avoid tasks that require alertness, motor skills until response to drug is established. • Do not chew, crush, or open capsule.

silver sulfadiazine

sul-fah-**dye**-ah-zeen
(Flamazine ✤, Silvadene, SSD, SSD AF, Thermazene)

◆CLASSIFICATION

PHARMACOTHERAPEUTIC: Anti-infective. **CLINICAL:** Burn preparation.

ACTION

Acts on cell wall/cell membrane in concentrations selectively toxic to bacteria. **Therapeutic Effect:** Produces bactericidal effect.

USES

Prevention, treatment of infection in second- and third-degree burns; protection against conversion from partial- to full-thickness wounds (infection causing extended tissue destruction). OFF-LABEL: Treatment of minor bacterial skin infection, dermal ulcer.

PRECAUTIONS

Contraindications: None known. **Cautions:** Renal/hepatic impairment, G6PD deficiency, premature neonates, infants younger than 2 mos. **Pregnancy Category B.**

INTERACTIONS

DRUG: Concurrent use may inactivate **collagenase, papain, sutilains.** **HERBAL:** None significant. **FOOD:** None known. **LAB VALUES:** None significant.

AVAILABILITY (Rx)

Topical Cream (Silvadene, SSD, SSD AF, Thermazene): 1% (10 mg/g).

ADMINISTRATION/HANDLING

Topical

• Apply to cleansed, debrided burns using sterile glove. • Keep burn areas covered with silver sulfadiazine cream at all times; reapply to areas where removed by pt activity. • Dressings may be ordered on individual basis.

INDICATIONS/ROUTES/DOSAGE

Usual Topical Dosage

TOPICAL: ADULTS, ELDERLY, CHILDREN: Apply 1–2 times daily.

SIDE EFFECTS

Side effects characteristic of all sulfonamides may occur when systemically absorbed (extensive burn areas [over 20% of body surface]): anorexia, nausea, vomiting, headache, diarrhea, dizziness, photosensitivity, arthralgia. **Frequent:** Burning, stinging sensation at treatment site. **Occasional:** Brown-gray skin discoloration, rash, itching. **Rare:** Increased sensitivity of skin to sunlight.

ADVERSE EFFECTS/ TOXIC REACTIONS

Hemolytic anemia, hypoglycemia, diuresis, peripheral neuropathy, Stevens-Johnson syndrome, agranulocytosis, disseminated lupus erythematosus, anaphylaxis, hepatitis, toxic nephrosis possible with significant systemic absorption. Fungal superinfections may occur. Interstitial nephritis occurs rarely.

NURSING CONSIDERATIONS

BASELINE ASSESSMENT

Determine initial CBC, serum renal/hepatic function test results.

INTERVENTION/EVALUATION

Monitor serum electrolytes, urinalysis, renal function, CBC if burns are extensive, therapy prolonged.

PATIENT/FAMILY TEACHING

• For external use only; may discolor skin.

simethicone

si-**meth**-i-kone
(Gas-X, Genasyme, Infant Mylicon, Mylanta Gas, Ovol 🍁, Phazyme)
Do not confuse simethicone with cimetidine.

FIXED-COMBINATION(S)

Mylanta, Extra Strength Maalox, Aludrox: simethicone/magnesium and aluminum hydroxide (antacids): 20 mg/200 mg/200 mg, 40 mg/400 mg/400 mg.

◆ CLASSIFICATION

PHARMACOTHERAPEUTIC: Antiflatulent. **CLINICAL:** Antiflatulent.

ACTION

Changes surface tension of gas bubbles, allowing easier elimination of gas. **Therapeutic Effect:** Disperses, prevents formation of gas pockets in GI tract.

PHARMACOKINETICS

Does not appear to be absorbed from GI tract. Excreted unchanged in feces.

USES

Treatment of flatulence, gastric bloating, postop gas pain, when gas retention may be problem (i.e., peptic ulcer, spastic colon, air swallowing). OFF-LABEL: Adjunct to bowel radiography, gastroscopy.

PRECAUTIONS

Contraindications: None known. **Cautions:** None known.

LIFESPAN CONSIDERATIONS

Pregnancy/Lactation: Unknown if drug crosses placenta or is distributed in breast milk. **Pregnancy Category C. Children/Elderly:** No age-related precautions noted.

INTERACTIONS

DRUG: None significant. **HERBAL:** None significant. **FOOD:** None known. **LAB VALUES:** None significant.

AVAILABILITY (OTC)

Oral Drops (Infant Mylicon): 40 mg/0.6 ml. **Softgel:** 125 mg (Gas-X, Mylanta Gas), 180 mg (Phazyme). **Tablets (Chewable):** 80 mg (Gas-X, Genasyme, Mylanta Gas), 125 mg (Gas-X, Mylanta Gas).

ADMINISTRATION/HANDLING

PO

• Give after meals and at bedtime as needed. • Chewable tablets are to be chewed thoroughly before swallowing. • Shake suspension well before using.

INDICATIONS/ROUTES/DOSAGE

Antiflatulent

PO: ADULTS, ELDERLY, CHILDREN 12 YRS AND OLDER: 40–125 mg after meals and at bedtime. **Maximum:** 500 mg/day. **CHILDREN 2–11 YRS:** 40 mg 4 times a day.

CHILDREN YOUNGER THAN 2 YRS: 20 mg 4 times a day.

SIDE EFFECTS

None known.

ADVERSE EFFECTS/ TOXIC REACTIONS

None known.

NURSING CONSIDERATIONS

INTERVENTION/EVALUATION

Evaluate for therapeutic response (relief of flatulence, abdominal bloating).

PATIENT/FAMILY TEACHING

• Avoid carbonated beverages. • To reduce air swallowing, take after meals and at bedtime for best results.

simvastatin

sim-vah-**stat**-tin
(Apo-Simvastatin ✤, Novo-Simvastatin ✤, Zocor)
Do not confuse Zocor with Cozaar or Zoloft.

FIXED-COMBINATION(S)

Simcor: simvastatin/niacin (an antilipemic agent): 20 mg/500 mg, 40 mg/500 mg, 20 mg/750 mg, 20 mg/1,000 mg, 40 mg/1,000 mg. **Vytorin:** simvastatin/ezetimibe (a cholesterol absorption inhibitor): 10 mg/10 mg, 20 mg/10 mg, 40 mg/10 mg, 80 mg/10 mg.

CLASSIFICATION

PHARMACOTHERAPEUTIC: Hydroxymethylglutaryl-CoA (HMG-CoA) reductase inhibitor. **CLINICAL:** Antihyperlipidemic (see p. 58C).

ACTION

Interferes with cholesterol biosynthesis by inhibiting conversion of the enzyme HMG-CoA to mevalonate. **Therapeutic Effect:** Decreases LDL, cholesterol, VLDL, triglyceride levels; slight increase in HDL concentration.

PHARMACOKINETICS

Well absorbed from GI tract. Protein binding: 95%. Undergoes extensive first-pass metabolism. Hydrolyzed to active metabolite. Primarily eliminated in feces. Unknown if removed by hemodialysis.

S

Route	Onset	Peak	Duration
PO (to reduce cholesterol)	3 days	14 days	N/A

USES

Secondary prevention of cardiovascular events in pts with hypercholesterolemia and coronary heart disease (CHD) or at high risk for CHD. Hyperlipidemias to reduce elevations in total serum cholesterol. Treatment of homozygous familial hypercholesterolemia. Treatment of heterozygous familial hypercholesterolemia in adolescents (10–17 yrs, females more than 1 yr post-menarche).

PRECAUTIONS

Contraindications: Active hepatic disease or unexplained, persistent elevations of hepatic function test results, pregnancy, breast feeding. **Cautions:** History of hepatic disease, substantial alcohol consumption. Severe metabolic, endocrine, electrolyte disorders. Withholding or discontinuing simvastatin may be necessary when pt is at risk for renal failure secondary to rhabdomyolysis.

LIFESPAN CONSIDERATIONS

Pregnancy/Lactation: Contraindicated in pregnancy (suppression of cholesterol biosynthesis may cause fetal toxicity), lactation. Risk of serious adverse reactions in breast-feeding infants. **Pregnancy Category X. Children:** Safety and efficacy not established in children less than 10 yrs of age or in premenarcheal girls. **Elderly:** No age-related precautions noted.

INTERACTIONS

DRUG: **Cyclosporine, erythromycin, gemfibrozil, immunosuppressants, niacin** increase risk of acute renal failure, rhabdomyolysis. May increase concentration, toxicity of **digoxin. HIV protease inhibitors** may increase risk of rhabdomyolysis, acute renal failure. **Verapamil** may increase risk of myopathy. **HERBAL:** **St. John's wort** may decrease concentration. **FOOD:** **Grapefruit, grapefruit juice** may increase concentration, toxicity. **Red yeast rice** contains 2.4 mg **lovastatin** per 600 mg rice. **LAB VALUES:** May increase serum creatine kinase (CK), transaminase.

AVAILABILITY (Rx)

Tablets: 5 mg, 10 mg, 20 mg, 40 mg, 80 mg.

ADMINISTRATION/HANDLING

PO

• Give without regard to meals. • Administer in evening for maximum efficacy.

INDICATIONS/ROUTES/DOSAGE

Prevention of Cardiovascular Events, Hyperlipidemias

PO: ADULTS, ELDERLY: 20–40 mg once a day. Range: 5–80 mg/day.

Homozygous Familial Hypercholesterolemia

PO: ADULTS, ELDERLY: 40 mg once a day in evening or 80 mg/day in divided doses.

Heterozygous Familial Hypercholesterolemia

PO: CHILDREN 10–17 YRS: 10 mg once a day in evening. Range: 10–40 mg/day.

SIDE EFFECTS

Generally well tolerated. Side effects are usually mild and transient. **Occasional (3%–2%):** Headache, abdominal pain/cramps, constipation, upper respiratory tract infection. **Rare (less than 2%):** Diarrhea, flatulence, asthenia (loss of strength, energy), nausea/vomiting, depression.

ADVERSE EFFECTS/ TOXIC REACTIONS

Potential for lens opacities. Hypersensitivity reaction, hepatitis occur rarely. Myopathy (muscle pain, tenderness, weakness with elevated serum creatine kinase [CK], sometimes taking the form of rhabdomyolysis) has occurred.

NURSING CONSIDERATIONS

BASELINE ASSESSMENT

Obtain dietary history, esp. fat consumption. Question for possibility of pregnancy before initiating therapy (Pregnancy Category X). Question for history of hypersensitivity to simvastatin. Assess baseline lab results: serum cholesterol, triglycerides, hepatic function tests.

INTERVENTION/EVALUATION

Monitor serum cholesterol, triglyceride lab results for therapeutic response. Monitor hepatic function tests. Monitor daily pattern of bowel activity and stool consistency. Assess for headache, myopathy.

PATIENT/FAMILY TEACHING

• Use appropriate contraceptive measures (Pregnancy Category X). • Periodic lab tests are essential part of therapy. • Maintain appropriate diet. • Report unexplained muscle pain, tenderness, weakness.

sipuleucel-T

sa-**pull**-ew-cell-tee
(Provenge)
Do not confuse Provenge with Provigil or Provera.

CLASSIFICATION

PHARMACOTHERAPEUTIC: Autologous cellular immunotherapy. **CLINICAL:** Antineoplastic.

ACTION

Activates T-cell immunity by combining antigen-presenting cells (APC) with prostatic acid phosphate (PAP) antigen and granulocyte-macrophage colony-stimulating factor (GMC-SF). **Therapeutic Effect:** Induces T-cell immunity against PAP antigen.

USES

Treatment of asymptomatic or minimally symptomatic metastatic castrate-resistant (hormone-refractory) prostate cancer.

PRECAUTIONS

Contraindications: None known. **Cautions:** Concomitant use of chemotherapy, immunosuppressive agents.

LIFESPAN CONSIDERATIONS

Pregnancy/Lactation: Not used in this pt population. **Children:** Safety and efficacy not established. **Elderly:** No age-related precautions noted.

INTERACTIONS

DRUG: None significant (no studies of drug interactions performed). **HERBAL:** None significant. **FOOD:** None known. **LAB VALUES:** None significant.

AVAILABILITY (Rx)

Infusion, Premixed: 50 million autologous $CD54^+$ cells activated with PAP-GM-CSF in 250 ml lactated Ringer's.

ADMINISTRATION/HANDLING

ALERT Do not use cell filter.

IV

Rate of administration • Infuse over 60 min.

Storage • Solution should be cloudy, cream-to-pink in color. • Gently swirl infusion bag to resuspend contents. • Discard solution if clumps remain after mixing. • Do not keep solution at room temperature for more than 3 hrs.

INDICATIONS/ROUTES/DOSAGE

ALERT Leukapheresis required 3 days before each infusion. Must strictly adhere to dosing schedule. If dose is missed, pt must undergo additional leukapheresis to continue treatment. Premedicate with antipyretics and/or antihistamines to reduce acute infusion reactions.

Metastatic Castrate-Resistant (Hormone-Refractory) Prostate Cancer
IV: ADULTS: 3 doses at 2-wk intervals

SIDE EFFECTS

Frequent (15% or greater): Chills, fatigue, pyrexia, nausea, backache, joint pain,

S

muscle spasm, constipation, rash, diaphoresis, weakness, paresthesia.

ADVERSE EFFECTS/ TOXIC REACTIONS

Infusion reactions (ischemic or hemorrhagic CVA, dyspnea, anemia, eosinophilia, rhabdomyolysis, myasthenia gravis, myositis, citrate toxicity, tumor flare, bronchospasm, hypoxia, hypertension) occur in 3.5% of pts.

NURSING CONSIDERATIONS

BASELINE ASSESSMENT

Screen for concomitant chemotherapy, immunosuppressive agents. Evaluate for preexisting cardiac/pulmonary conditions, prior blood infusion reactions, prior vaccine reactions, history of myasthenia gravis or stroke. Central venous access may be considered if peripheral access is inadequate.

INTERVENTION/EVALUATION

Monitor for reactions at least 30 min after completion of infusion. Assess for any change in cardiopulmonary, neurological status. Evaluate for inflammation, infiltration at injection site. Stop infusion and notify physician if adverse reactions occur.

PATIENT/FAMILY TEACHING

• Educate on central venous catheter care if applicable. • Report signs/symptoms of heart abnormalities, shortness of breath, angina pectoris, dizziness, nausea, vomiting, fever equal to or greater than 100°F. • Report any immunosuppressive therapies prior to treatment. • Council pts on leukapheresis procedures and side effects.

sirolimus

sir-oh-**li**-mus
(Rapamune)

BLACK BOX ALERT Increased susceptibility to infection and potential for development of lymphoma. Not recommended for liver or lung transplant pts.

Do not confuse sirolimus with everolimus, tacrolimus, or temsirolimus, or Rapamune with Rapaflo.

◆CLASSIFICATION

PHARMACOTHERAPEUTIC: Immunosuppressant. **CLINICAL:** Immunosuppressant.

ACTION

Inhibits T-lymphocyte proliferation induced by stimulation of cell surface receptors, mitogens, alloantigens, lymphokines. Prevents activation of enzyme target of rapamycin (TOR), a key regulatory kinase in cell cycle progression. **Therapeutic Effect:** Inhibits proliferation of T and B cells (essential components of immune response), prevents organ transplant rejection.

PHARMACOKINETICS

Rapidly absorbed from GI tract. Protein binding: 92%. Extensively metabolized in liver. Primarily eliminated in feces; minimal excretion in urine. **Half-life:** 57–63 hrs.

USES

Prophylaxis of organ rejection in pts after renal transplant in combination with cyclosporine and corticosteroids, including treatment of high immunologic risk in renal transplant recipient. **OFF-LABEL:** Immunosuppression in peripheral stem cell/bone marrow transplantation. Prophylaxis of organ rejection in heart transplant recipients.

PRECAUTIONS

Contraindications: Hypersensitivity to sirolimus, active malignancy. **Cautions:** Chickenpox, herpes zoster, hepatic impairment, infection.

LIFESPAN CONSIDERATIONS

Pregnancy/Lactation: Unknown if drug crosses placenta or is distributed in breast milk. **Pregnancy Category C. Children:** Safety and efficacy not established in those

S

younger than 13 yrs. **Elderly:** No age-related precautions noted.

INTERACTIONS

DRUG: **Carbamazepine, phenobarbital, phenytoin, rifabutin, rifampin, rifapentine** may decrease concentration, effect. **Clarithromycin, diltiazem, erythromycin, itraconazole, ketoconazole, verapamil, voriconazole** may increase concentration, toxicity. May increase risk of infection, lymphomas with **cyclosporine.** May increase mortality, graft loss, hepatic artery thrombosis with **tacrolimus** in liver transplant pts. HERBAL: **St. John's wort** may decrease concentration. **Cat's claw, echinacea** possess immunostimulant properties. FOOD: **Grapefruit, grapefruit juice** may decrease metabolism. LAB VALUES: May increase serum ALT, AST, alkaline phosphatase, LDH, BUN, creatine phosphate, cholestrol, triglycerides, creatinine. May alter WBC, serum glucose, calcium. May decrease Hgb, Hct.

AVAILABILITY (Rx)

Oral Solution: 1 mg/ml.

Tablets: 1 mg, 2 mg.

ADMINISTRATION/HANDLING

• Doses should be taken 4 hrs after cyclosporine. • Take consistently with or without food. • Do not crush, chew, break tablets. • Oral solution: mix with only water or orange juice, stir vigorously, drink immediately.

INDICATIONS/ROUTES/DOSAGE

Prevention of Organ Transplant Rejection (Low to Moderate Risk)

PO: ADULTS, CHILDREN 13 YRS AND OLDER WEIGHING MORE THAN 40 KG: Loading dose: 6 mg. Maintenance: 2 mg/day. **ADULTS, CHILDREN 13 YRS AND OLDER WEIGHING LESS THAN 40 KG:** Loading dose: 3 mg/m^2. Maintenance: 1 mg/m^2/day.

Prevention of Organ Transplant Rejection (High Risk)

PO: ADULTS: Loading dose: Up to 15 mg on day 1. Maintenance: 5 mg/day.

Dosage in Hepatic Impairment

Loading Dose: No change. Maintenance dose: Mild to moderate impairment: reduce dose by 33%; severe impairment: reduce dose by 50%.

SIDE EFFECTS

Occasional: Hypercholesterolemia, hyperlipidemia, hypertension, rash. **High doses (5 mg/day):** Anemia, arthralgia, diarrhea, hypokalemia, thrombocytopenia. **Rare:** Peripheral edema, hypertension.

ADVERSE EFFECTS/ TOXIC REACTIONS

Hepatotoxicity occurs rarely. Skin carcinoma (including basal cell, squamous cell, melanoma) has been observed.

NURSING CONSIDERATIONS

BASELINE ASSESSMENT

Obtain baseline serum hepatic profile. Assess for pregnancy, lactation. Question for medication usage (esp. cyclosporine, diltiazem, ketoconazole, rifampin). Determine if pt has chickenpox, herpes zoster, malignancy, infection.

INTERVENTION/EVALUATION

Monitor serum renal/hepatic function periodically. Monitor cholesterol, triglycerides, platelets, Hgb.

PATIENT/FAMILY TEACHING

• Avoid those with colds, other infections. • Avoid grapefruit juice, grapefruit. • Avoid exposure to sunlight, artificial light sources. • Strict monitoring is essential in identifying, preventing symptoms of organ rejection.

sitagliptin

HIGH ALERT

sit-ah-**glip**-tin
(Januvia)

Do not confuse Januvia with Enjuvia, Jantoven, or Janumet, or sitagliptin with saxagliptin or sumatriptan.

FIXED-COMBINATION(S)

Janumet: sitagliptin/metformin (an antidiabetic): 50 mg/500 mg, 50 mg/1,000 mg.

◆CLASSIFICATION

PHARMACOTHERAPEUTIC: DPP-4 inhibitors (gliptins). **CLINICAL:** Antidiabetic.

ACTION

Slows inactivation of incretin hormones (involved in regulation of glucose homeostasis). **Therapeutic Effect:** Increases synthesis, postmeal release of insulin from pancreatic cells; lowers postmeal glucagon secretion leading to reduced glucose output from liver.

PHARMACOKINETICS

Route	Onset	Peak	Duration
PO	N/A	1–4 hrs	24 hrs

Rapidly absorbed following PO administration. Protein binding: 38%. Eliminated mainly in urine, with lesser amount excreted in feces. **Half-life:** 12 hrs.

USES

Adjunctive treatment to diet, exercise to improve glycemic control in pts with type 2 diabetes mellitus as monotherapy or in combination with metformin or glimepiride when a single agent alone, with diet and exercise, does not provide glycemic control.

PRECAUTIONS

Contraindications: Type I diabetes, diabetic ketoacidosis. **Cautions:** Concurrent use of other glucose-lowering agents may increase risk of hypoglycemia.

⌛ LIFESPAN CONSIDERATIONS

Pregnancy/Lactation: Unknown if distributed in breast milk. **Pregnancy Category B. Children:** Safety and efficacy not established. **Elderly:** No age-related precautions noted.

INTERACTIONS

DRUG: None significant. **HERBAL:** None significant. **FOOD:** None known. **LAB VALUES:** May slightly increase WBCs, particularly neutrophil count. May increase serum creatinine.

AVAILABILITY (Rx)

Tablets (Film-Coated): 25 mg, 50 mg, 100 mg.

ADMINISTRATION/HANDLING

PO

• May give without regard to food. • Do not crush, break, chew film-coated tablets.

INDICATIONS/ROUTES/DOSAGE

Type 2 Diabetes

PO: ADULTS OVER 18 YRS, ELDERLY: 100 mg once daily.

Moderate Renal Impairment

Creatinine clearance equal to or greater than 30 ml/min to less than 50 ml/min: 50 mg once daily.

Severe Renal Impairment

Creatinine clearance less than 30 ml/min: 25 mg once daily.

SIDE EFFECTS

Occasional (5% and greater): Headache, nasopharyngitis. **Rare (3%–1%):** Diarrhea, abdominal pain, nausea.

ADVERSE EFFECTS/ TOXIC REACTIONS

Hypersensitivity reactions including angioedema, Stevens-Johnson syndrome reported. Acute pancreatitis occurs rarely.

NURSING CONSIDERATIONS

BASELINE ASSESSMENT

Check serum glucose concentration before administration. Assess renal function. Discuss lifestyle to determine extent of learning, emotional needs. Assure follow-up instruction if pt, family does not thoroughly understand diabetes management, glucose-testing technique.

INTERVENTION/EVALUATION

Monitor serum glucose, $HbgA_{1C}$, BUN, creatinine. Assess for hypoglycemia (diaphoresis, tremor, dizziness, anxiety, headache, tachycardia, perioral numbness, hunger, diplopia, difficulty concentrating), hyperglycemia (polyuria, polyphagia, polydipsia, nausea, vomiting, dim vision, fatigue, deep, rapid breathing). Be alert to conditions that alter glucose requirements (fever, increased activity, stress, surgical procedures).

PATIENT/FAMILY TEACHING

• Diabetes mellitus requires lifelong control. • Prescribed diet, exercise are principal part of treatment; do not skip, delay meals. • Continue to adhere to dietary instructions, regular exercise program, regular testing of serum glucose. • When taking combination drug therapy or when glucose demands are altered (fever, infection, trauma, stress, heavy physical activity), have source of glucose available to treat symptoms of hypoglycemia. • Report nausea, vomiting, anorexia, severe abdominal pain, pancreatitis.

sodium bicarbonate

so-dee-um bye-**car**-bon-ate
(Neut)

CLASSIFICATION

PHARMACOTHERAPEUTIC: Alkalinizing agent. **CLINICAL:** Antacid.

ACTION

Dissociates to provide bicarbonate ion. **Therapeutic Effect:** Neutralizes hydrogen ion concentration, raises blood, urinary pH.

PHARMACOKINETICS

Route	Onset	Peak	Duration
PO	15 min	N/A	1–3 hrs
IV	Immediate	N/A	8–10 min

Well absorbed following PO administration, sodium bicarbonate dissociates to sodium and bicarbonate ions. With increased hydrogen ion concentrations, bicarbonate ions combine with hydrogen ions to form carbonic acid, which then dissociates to CO_2, which is excreted by the lungs. Plasma concentration regulated by kidney (ability to form, excrete bicarbonate).

USES

Management of metabolic acidosis, antacid, alkalinization of urine, stabilizes acid-base balance, cardiac arrest, life-threatening hyperkalemia. **OFF-LABEL:** Prevention of contrast-induced nephropathy.

PRECAUTIONS

Contraindications: Excessive chloride loss due to diarrhea, diuretics, GI suctioning, vomiting; hypocalcemia; metabolic, respiratory alkalosis. **Cautions:** CHF, edematous states, renal insufficiency, pts on corticosteroid therapy.

LIFESPAN CONSIDERATIONS

Pregnancy/Lactation: May produce hypernatremia, increase tendon reflexes in neonate or fetus whose mother is administered chronically high doses. May be distributed in breast milk. **Pregnancy Category C. Children:** No age-related precautions noted. Do not use as antacid in those younger than 6 yrs. **Elderly:** Age-related renal impairment may require dosage adjustment.

INTERACTIONS

DRUG: May increase concentration, toxicity of **pseudoephedrine, quinidine, quinine.** May decrease effect of **lithium, salicylates.** **HERBAL:** None significant. **FOOD:** **Milk, other dairy products** may result in milk-alkali syndrome.

S

LAB VALUES: May increase serum, urinary pH.

AVAILABILITY

Injection Solution (Rx): 0.5 mEq/ml (4.2%), 0.9 mEq/ml (7.5%), 1 mEq/ml (8.4%). **Tablets (OTC):** 325 mg, 650 mg.

ADMINISTRATION/HANDLING

IV

◀ALERT▶ For direct IV administration in neonates or infants, use 0.5 mEq/ml concentration.

Reconstitution • May give undiluted.

Rate of administration • For IV push, give up to 1 mEq/kg over 1–3 min for cardiac arrest. • For IV infusion, do not exceed rate of infusion of 50 mEq/hr. • For children younger than 2 yrs, premature infants, neonates, administer by slow infusion, up to 10 mEq/min.

Storage • Store at room temperature.

PO

• Do not give other PO medication within 1–2 hrs of antacid administration. • Give 1–3 hrs after meals.

IV INCOMPATIBILITIES

Amiodarone (Cordarone), ascorbic acid, calcium chloride, diltiazem (Cardizem), dobutamine (Dobutrex), dopamine (Intropin), hydromorphone (Dilaudid), magnesium sulfate, midazolam (Versed), norepinephrine (Levophed), total parenteral nutrition (TPN).

IV COMPATIBILITIES

Aminophylline, furosemide (Lasix), heparin, insulin, lidocaine, lipids, mannitol, milrinone (Primacor), morphine, phenylephrine (Neo-Synephrine), potassium chloride, propofol (Diprivan), vancomycin (Vancocin).

INDICATIONS/ROUTES/DOSAGE

◀ALERT▶ May give by IV push, IV infusion, or orally. Dose individualized based on severity of acidosis, laboratory values, pt age, weight, clinical conditions. Do not fully correct bicarbonate deficit during the first 24 hrs (may cause metabolic alkalosis).

Cardiac Arrest

◀ALERT▶ Routine use not recommended.

IV: ADULTS, ELDERLY: Initially, 1 mEq/kg (as 7.5%–8.4% solution). May repeat with 0.5 mEq/kg q10min during continued cardiopulmonary arrest. Use in postresuscitation phase is based on arterial blood pH, partial pressure of carbon dioxide in arterial blood ($PaCO_2$), base deficit calculation. **CHILDREN, INFANTS:** Initially, 0.5–1 mEq/kg. Repeat q10min or as indicated by ABGs.

Metabolic Acidosis (Mild to Moderate)

IV: ADULTS, ELDERLY, CHILDREN: 2–5 mEq/kg over 4–8 hrs. May repeat based on laboratory values.

Prevention of Contrast-Induced Nephropathy

IV INFUSION: ADULTS, ELDERLY: 154 mEq/L sodium bicarbonate in D_5W solution: 3 ml/kg/hr 1 hr immediately before contrast injection, then 1 ml/kg/hr during contrast exposure and for 6 hrs after procedure.

Metabolic Acidosis (Associated with Chronic Renal Failure)

PO: ADULTS, ELDERLY: Initially, 20–36 mEq/day in divided doses. Titrate to bicarbonate level of 18–20 mEq/L. **CHILDREN:** 1–3 mEq/kg/day.

Renal Tubular Acidosis (Distal)

PO: ADULTS, ELDERLY: 0.5–2 mEq/kg/day in 4–6 divided doses. **CHILDREN:** 2–3 mEq/kg/day in divided doses.

Renal Tubular Acidosis (Proximal)

PO: ADULTS, ELDERLY, CHILDREN: 5–10 mEq/kg/day in divided doses.

Urine Alkalinization

PO: ADULTS, ELDERLY: Initially, 4 g, then 1–2 g q4h. **Maximum:** 16 g/day (8g/day in adults older than 60 yrs). **CHILDREN:** 84–840 mg/kg/day in divided doses q4–6hr.

Antacid

PO: ADULTS, ELDERLY: 300 mg–2 g 1–4 times a day.

Hyperkalemia

IV: ADULTS, ELDERLY: 1 mEq/kg over 5 min.

SIDE EFFECTS

Frequent: Abdominal distention, flatulence, belching.

ADVERSE EFFECTS/ TOXIC REACTIONS

Excessive, chronic use may produce metabolic alkalosis (irritability, twitching, paresthesias, cyanosis, slow or shallow respirations, headache, thirst, nausea). Fluid overload results in headache, weakness, blurred vision, behavioral changes, incoordination, muscle twitching, elevated B/P, bradycardia, tachypnea, wheezing, coughing, distended neck veins. Extravasation may occur at the IV site, resulting in tissue necrosis, ulceration.

NURSING CONSIDERATIONS

BASELINE ASSESSMENT

Assess for signs and symptoms of acidosis, alkalosis. Do not give PO medication within 1 hr of antacids.

INTERVENTION/EVALUATION

Monitor serum, urinary pH, CO_2 level, serum electrolytes, plasma bicarbonate levels. Watch for signs of metabolic alkalosis, fluid overload. Assess for clinical improvement of metabolic acidosis (relief from hyperventilation, weakness, disorientation). Monitor daily pattern of bowel activity, stool consistency. Monitor serum phosphate, calcium, uric acid levels. Assess for relief of gastric distress.

sodium chloride HIGH ALERT

so-dee-um **klor**-ide
(Muro 128, Nasal Moist, Ocean, SalineX)

◆CLASSIFICATION

CLINICAL: Electrolyte, ophthalmic adjunct, bronchodilator.

ACTION

Sodium is a major cation of extracellular fluid. **Therapeutic Effect:** Controls water distribution, fluid and electrolyte balance, osmotic pressure of body fluids; maintains acid-base balance.

PHARMACOKINETICS

Well absorbed from GI tract. Widely distributed. Primarily excreted in urine and, to a lesser degree, in sweat, tears, saliva.

USES

Parenteral: Source of hydration; prevention/treatment of sodium, chloride deficiencies (hypertonic for severe deficiencies). Prevention of muscle cramps, heat prostration occurring with excessive perspiration. **Nasal:** Restores moisture, relieves dry, inflamed nasal membranes. **Ophthalmic:** Therapy in reduction of corneal edema, diagnostic aid in ophthalmoscopic exam.

PRECAUTIONS

Contraindications: Fluid retention, hypernatremia. **Cautions:** CHF, renal impairment, cirrhosis, hypertension. Do not use sodium chloride preserved with benzyl alcohol in neonates.

LIFESPAN CONSIDERATIONS

Pregnancy Category C. Children/Elderly: No age-related precautions noted.

INTERACTIONS

DRUG: May decrease effect of **lithium.** **HERBAL:** None significant. **FOOD:** None known. **LAB VALUES:** None significant.

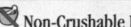

S

AVAILABILITY

Injection (Concentrate) (Rx): 23.4% (4 mEq/ml). **Injection Solution (Rx):** 0.45%, 0.9%, 3%. **Irrigation (Rx):** 0.45%, 0.9%. **Nasal Gel (Nasal Moist) (OTC):** 0.65%. **Nasal Solution (OTC):** 0.4% (SalineX), 0.65% (Nasal Moist, Ocean). **Ophthalmic Ointment (OTC [Muro 128]):** 5%. **Ophthalmic Solution (OTC [Muro 128]):** 2%, 5%.

Tablets (OTC): 1 g.

ADMINISTRATION/HANDLING

IV

• Hypertonic solutions (3% or 5%) are administered via large vein; avoid infiltration; do not exceed 100 ml/hr. • Vials containing 2.5–4 mEq/ml (concentrated NaCl) must be diluted with D_5W or $D_{10}W$ before administration.

PO

• Do not crush/break enteric-coated or extended-release tablets. • Administer with full glass of water.

Nasal

• Instruct pt to begin inhaling slowly just before releasing medication into nose. • Instruct pt to inhale slowly, then release air gently through mouth. • Continue technique for 20–30 sec.

Ophthalmic

• Place gloved finger on lower eyelid and pull out until pocket is formed between eye and lower lid. • Place prescribed number of drops (or ¼–½ inch of ointment) into pocket. • Instruct pt to close eye gently for 1–2 min so that medication will not be squeezed out of sac. • When lower lid is released, have pt keep eye open without blinking for at least 30 sec for solution; for ointment have pt close eye, roll eyeball around to distribute medication. • When using drops, apply gentle finger pressure to lacrimal sac at inner canthus for 1 min to minimize systemic absorption.

INDICATIONS/ROUTES/DOSAGE

◄ALERT► Dosage based on age, weight, clinical condition; fluid, electrolyte, acid-base balance status.

Usual Parenteral Dosage

IV: ADULTS, ELDERLY, CHILDREN: Determined by laboratory determinations (mEq). Dosage varies widely based on clinical conditions.

Usual Oral Dosage

PO: ADULTS, ELDERLY: 1–2 g 3 times a day.

Usual Nasal Dosage

INTRANASAL: ADULTS, ELDERLY, CHILDREN: 2–3 sprays as needed.

Usual Ophthalmic Dosage

OPHTHALMIC SOLUTION: ADULTS, ELDERLY: Apply 1–2 drops q3–4h.
OPHTHALMIC OINTMENT: ADULTS, ELDERLY: Apply once a day or as directed.

SIDE EFFECTS

Frequent: Facial flushing. **Occasional:** Fever; irritation, phlebitis, extravasation at injection site. **Ophthalmic:** Temporary burning, irritation.

ADVERSE EFFECTS/ TOXIC REACTIONS

Too-rapid administration may produce peripheral edema, CHF, pulmonary edema. Excessive dosage may produce hypokalemia, hypervolemia, hypernatremia.

NURSING CONSIDERATIONS

BASELINE ASSESSMENT

Obtain baseline serum electrolyte studies. Assess fluid balance (I&O, daily weight, lung sounds, edema).

INTERVENTION/EVALUATION

Monitor fluid balance (I&O, daily weight, lung sounds, edema), IV site for extravasation. Monitor serum electrolytes, acid-base balance, B/P. Hypernatremia associated with edema, weight gain, elevated B/P; hyponatremia associated with muscle cramps, nausea, vomiting, dry mucous membranes.

PATIENT/FAMILY TEACHING

• Temporary burning, irritation may occur upon instillation of eye medication. • Discontinue eye medication and contact physician if severe pain, headache, rapid change in vision (peripheral, direct), sudden appearance of floating spots, acute redness of eyes, pain on exposure to light, double vision occurs.

sodium ferric gluconate complex

so-**dee**-um **fair**-ick **glue**-koe-nate **com**-plex
(Ferrlecit)

CLASSIFICATION

PHARMACOTHERAPEUTIC: Trace element. **CLINICAL:** Hematinic.

ACTION

Repletes total iron content in body. Replaces iron found in Hgb, myoglobin, specific enzymes; allows oxygen transport via Hgb. **Therapeutic Effect:** Prevents, corrects iron deficiency.

PHARMACOKINETICS

Half-life: 1 hr.

USES

Treatment of iron deficiency anemia in pts undergoing chronic hemodialysis who are receiving supplemental erythropoietin therapy.

PRECAUTIONS

Contraindications: All anemias not associated with iron deficiency, hypersensitivity to iron products. **Cautions:** Pts with iron overload, significant allergies, asthma, hepatic impairment, rheumatoid arthritis (RA).

LIFESPAN CONSIDERATIONS

Pregnancy/Lactation: Unknown if distributed in breast milk. **Pregnancy Category B. Children:** Safety and efficacy not established. **Elderly:** No age-related precautions noted; lower initial dosages recommended.

INTERACTIONS

DRUG: May decrease absorption of **oral iron. HERBAL:** None significant. **FOOD:** None known. **LAB VALUES:** None significant.

AVAILABILITY (Rx)

Injection Solution: 12.5 mg/ml elemental iron.

ADMINISTRATION/HANDLING

IV

Reconstitution • Must be diluted. • Test dose: dilute 25 mg (2 ml) with 50 ml 0.9% NaCl. • Recommended dose: dilute 125 mg (10 ml) with 100 ml 0.9% NaCl.
Rate of administration • Infuse both test dose, recommended dose over 1 hr.
Storage • Store at room temperature. • Use immediately after dilution.

IV INCOMPATIBILITIES

Do not mix with any other medications.

INDICATIONS/ROUTES/DOSAGE

Iron Deficiency Anemia

IV INFUSION: ADULTS, ELDERLY: 125 mg in 100 ml 0.9% NaCl infused over 1 hr. Minimum cumulative dose 1 g elemental iron given over 8 sessions at sequential dialysis treatments. May be given during dialysis session. **CHILDREN 6 YRS AND OLDER:** 1.5 mg/kg diluted in 25 ml 0.9% NaCl administered over 60 min at sequential dialysis sessions. **Maximum:** 125 mg/dose.

SIDE EFFECTS

Frequent (greater than 3%): Flushing, hypotension, hypersensitivity reaction. Oc-

casional (3%–1%): Injection site reaction, headache, abdominal pain, chills, flu-like syndrome, dizziness, leg cramps, dyspnea, nausea, vomiting, diarrhea, myalgia, pruritus, edema.

ADVERSE EFFECTS/ TOXIC REACTIONS

Potentially fatal hypersensitivity reaction occurs rarely, characterized by cardiovascular collapse, cardiac arrest, dyspnea, bronchospasm, angioedema, urticaria. Rapid administration may cause hypotension associated with flushing, light-headedness, fatigue, weakness, severe pain in chest, back, groin.

NURSING CONSIDERATIONS

BASELINE ASSESSMENT

Do not give concurrently with oral iron form (excessive iron may produce excessive iron storage [hemosiderosis]). Be alert to pts with rheumatoid arthritis (RA), iron deficiency anemia (acute exacerbation of joint pain, swelling may occur).

INTERVENTION/EVALUATION

Monitor vital signs, lab tests, esp. CBC, serum iron concentrations (may not be accurate until 3 wks after administration).

PATIENT/FAMILY TEACHING

• Stools frequently become black with iron therapy (condition is harmless). Report to physician any red streaking, sticky consistency of stool, abdominal pain/cramping.

S

sodium polystyrene sulfonate

so-dee-um pol-ee-**stye**-reen (Kayexelate, Kionex, PMS-Sodium Polystyrene Sulfonate, SPS)
Do not confuse Kayexelate with Kaopectate.

◆CLASSIFICATION

PHARMACOTHERAPEUTIC: Cation exchange resin. **CLINICAL:** Antihyperkalemic.

ACTION

Releases sodium ions in exchange primarily for potassium ions. **Therapeutic Effect:** Moves potassium from blood into intestine to be expelled from the body.

PHARMACOKINETICS

Onset: 2–24 hrs. Eliminated only in feces.

USES

Treatment of hyperkalemia.

PRECAUTIONS

Contraindications: Hypokalemia, hypernatremia, intestinal obstruction/perforation. **Cautions:** Severe CHF, hypertension, edema.

LIFESPAN CONSIDERATIONS

Pregnancy/Lactation: Unknown if drug crosses placenta or is distributed in breast milk. **Pregnancy Category C. Children:** No age-related precautions noted. **Elderly:** Increased risk for fecal impaction.

INTERACTIONS

DRUG: Cation-donating antacids, laxatives (e.g., magnesium hydroxide) may decrease effect; may cause systemic alkalosis in pts with renal impairment. **HERBAL:** None significant. **FOOD:** None known. **LAB VALUES:** May decrease serum calcium, magnesium, potassium. May increase serum sodium.

AVAILABILITY (Rx)

Powder for Suspension (Kayexalate, Kionex): 15 g/4 level tsp (480 g). **Rectal Enema:** 15 g/60 ml. **Suspension (SPS):** 15 g/60 ml.

ADMINISTRATION/HANDLING

PO

• Give with 20–100 ml sorbitol (facilitates passage of resin through intestinal tract, prevents constipation, aids in potassium removal, increases palatability). • Do not mix with foods, liquids containing potassium.

Rectal
• After initial cleansing enema, insert large rubber tube into rectum well into sigmoid colon, tape in place. • Introduce suspension (with 100 ml sorbitol) via gravity. • Flush with 50–100 ml fluid and clamp. • Pt must retain for several hrs if possible. • Irrigate colon with non–sodium-containing solution to remove resin.

INDICATIONS/ROUTES/DOSAGE

Hyperkalemia
PO: ADULTS, ELDERLY: 60 ml (15 g) 1–4 times daily. **CHILDREN:** 1 g/kg/dose q6h. **RECTAL: ADULTS, ELDERLY:** 30–50 g as needed q6h. **CHILDREN:** 1 g/kg/dose q2–6h.

SIDE EFFECTS

Frequent: High dosage: Anorexia, nausea, vomiting, constipation. **High dosage in elderly:** Fecal impaction (severe stomach pain with nausea/vomiting). **Occasional:** Diarrhea, sodium retention (decreased urination, peripheral edema, increased weight).

ADVERSE EFFECTS/ TOXIC REACTIONS

Potassium deficiency may occur. Early signs of hypokalemia include confusion, delayed thought processes, extreme weakness, irritability, EKG changes (often associated with prolonged QT interval; widening, flattening, or inversion of T wave; prominent U waves). Hypocalcemia, manifested by abdominal/muscle cramps, occurs occasionally. Arrhythmias, severe muscle weakness may be noted.

NURSING CONSIDERATIONS

BASELINE ASSESSMENT

Does not rapidly correct severe hyperkalemia (may take hrs to days). Consider other measures in medical emergency (IV calcium, IV sodium bicarbonate/glucose/insulin, dialysis).

INTERVENTION/EVALUATION

Monitor serum potassium levels frequently. Assess pt's clinical condition, EKG (valuable in determining when treatment should be discontinued). Also monitor serum magnesium, calcium levels. Monitor daily pattern of bowel activity, stool consistency (fecal impaction may occur in pts on high dosages, particularly in elderly).

solifenacin

sol-ih-**fen**-ah-sin
(VESIcare)

◆CLASSIFICATION

PHARMACOTHERAPEUTIC: Anticholinergic agent. **CLINICAL:** Urinary antispasmodic.

ACTION

Acts as direct antagonist at muscarinic acetylcholine receptors in cholinergically innervated organs. Reduces tonus (elastic tension) of smooth muscle in bladder, slows parasympathetic contractions. **Therapeutic Effect:** Decreases urinary bladder contractions, increases residual urine volume, decreases detrusor muscle pressure.

PHARMACOKINETICS

Well absorbed following PO administration. Protein binding: 98%. Metabolized in liver. Excreted in feces, urine. **Half-life:** 40–68 hrs.

USES

Treatment of overactive bladder with symptoms of urinary incontinence, urgency, frequency.

PRECAUTIONS

Contraindications: Breast-feeding, GI obstruction, uncontrolled angle-closure

S

glaucoma, urinary retention. **Cautions:** Bladder outflow obstruction, GI obstructive disorders, decreased GI motility, controlled narrow-angle glaucoma, renal/hepatic impairment, congenital or acquired QT prolongation, pregnancy.

LIFESPAN CONSIDERATIONS

Pregnancy/Lactation: Unknown if drug crosses placenta or is distributed is breast milk. **Pregnancy Category C.** **Children:** Safety and efficacy not established. **Elderly:** No age-related precautions noted.

INTERACTIONS

DRUG: **Carbamazepine, nafcillin, nevirapine, phenobarbital, phenytoin** may decrease concentration, effects. **Azole antifungals, ciprofloxacin, clarithromycin, diclofenac, doxycycline, erythromycin, imatinib, isoniazid, nefazodone, nicardipine, propofol, protease inhibitors, quinidine, verapamil** may increase concentration, effects. **Ketoconazole** may increase concentration. **HERBAL:** **St. John's wort** may decrease concentration, effects. **FOOD:** **Grapefruit, grapefruit juice** may increase effects. **LAB VALUES:** None significant.

AVAILABILITY (Rx)

Tablets: 5 mg, 10 mg.

ADMINISTRATION/HANDLING

PO

• Give without regard to food. Swallow tablets whole, with liquids.

INDICATIONS/ROUTES/DOSAGE

Overactive Bladder

PO: ADULTS, ELDERLY: 5 mg/day; if tolerated, may increase to 10 mg/day.

Dosage in Renal/Hepatic Impairment

Severe renal impairment (creatinine clearance less than 30 ml/min) or moderate hepatic impairment: Maximum dosage is 5 mg/day.

SIDE EFFECTS

Frequent (11%–6%): Dry mouth, constipation, blurred vision. **Occasional (5%–3%):** UTI, dyspepsia (heartburn, indigestion, epigastric pain), nausea. **Rare (2%–1%):** Dizziness, dry eyes, fatigue, depression, edema, hypertension, epigastric pain, vomiting, urinary retention.

ADVERSE EFFECTS/ TOXIC REACTIONS

Angioneurotic edema, GI obstruction occur rarely. Overdose can result in severe anticholinergic effects.

NURSING CONSIDERATIONS

BASELINE ASSESSMENT

Assess symptoms of overactive bladder before beginning the drug.

INTERVENTION/EVALUATION

Monitor I&O, anticholinergic effects, creatinine clearance. Assess for decrease in symptoms.

PATIENT/FAMILY TEACHING

• Avoid tasks requiring alertness, motor skills until response to drug is known. • Anticholinergic side effects include constipation, urinary retention, blurred vision, heat prostration in hot environment. • Use caution during exercise, exposure to heat.

somatropin

soe-mah-**troe**-pin
(Genotropin, Genotropin Miniquick, Humatrope, Norditropin, Nutropin, Nutropin AQ, Omnitrope, Saizen, Serostim, Zorbitive)
Do not confuse somatropin with sumatriptan.

CLASSIFICATION

PHARMACOTHERAPEUTIC: Polypeptide hormone. **CLINICAL:** Growth hormone.

ACTION

Stimulates cartilaginous growth areas of long bones; increases number, size of skeletal muscle cells; influences size of organs; increases RBC mass by stimulating erythropoietin. Influences metabolism of carbohydrates (decreases insulin sensitivity), fats (mobilizes fatty acids), minerals (retains phosphorus, sodium, potassium by promotion of cell growth), proteins (increases protein synthesis). **Therapeutic Effect:** Stimulates growth.

PHARMACOKINETICS

Well absorbed after subcutaneous, IM administration. Localized primarily in kidneys, liver. **Half-life: IV:** 20–30 min; **Subcutaneous, IM:** 3–5 hrs.

USES

Long-term treatment of growth failure in children caused by pituitary growth hormone (GH) deficiency. Treatment of growth failure in adults caused by GH deficiency, treatment of growth failure in children caused by chronic renal insufficiency, long-term treatment of short stature associated with Turner's syndrome, treatment of AIDS-related cachexia/weight loss, treatment of short bowel syndrome. OFF-LABEL: Treatment of CHF, pediatric HIV pts with wasting/cachexia; HIV adipose redistribution syndrome.

PRECAUTIONS

Contraindications: Active neoplasia (newly diagnosed or recurrent), critical illness, hypersensitivity to growth hormone. Cautions: Diabetes mellitus, untreated hypothyroidism, malignancy.

LIFESPAN CONSIDERATIONS

Pregnancy/Lactation: Unknown if drug is distributed in breast milk. **Pregnancy Category B (Genotropin, Genotropin Miniquick, Omnitrope, Saizen, Serostim, Zorbitive); C (Humatrope, Norditropin, Nutropin, Nutropin AQ). Children/Elderly:** No age-related precautions noted.

INTERACTIONS

DRUG: **Corticosteroids** may inhibit growth response. HERBAL: None significant. FOOD: None known. LAB VALUES: May increase serum alkaline phosphatase, inorganic phosphorus, parathyroid hormone. May decrease glucose tolerance. May slightly decrease thyroid function.

AVAILABILITY (Rx)

Injection, Powder for Reconstitution (Genotropin): 5.8 mg, 13.8 mg. **(Genotropin Miniquick):** 0.2 mg, 0.4 mg, 0.6 mg, 0.8 mg, 1 mg, 1.2 mg, 1.4 mg, 1.6 mg, 1.8 mg, 2 mg. **(Humatrope):** 5 mg, 6 mg, 12 mg, 24 mg. **(Nutropin):** 5 mg, 10 mg. **(Omnitrope):** 5.8 mg. **(Saizen):** 5 mg, 8.8 mg. **(Serostim):** 4 mg, 5 mg, 6 mg. **(Zorbitive):** 8.8 mg. **Injection Solution: (Norditropin):** 5 mg/1.5 ml, 15 mg/1.5 ml. **(Nutropin AQ):** 5 mg/ml. **(Omnitrope):** 5 mg/1.5 ml, 10 mg/1.5 ml. **(Norditropin FlexPro Pen):** 5 mg/1.5 ml.

ADMINISTRATION/HANDLING

◀ALERT▶ **Neonate:** Benzyl alcohol as a preservative has been associated with fatal toxicity (gasping syndrome) in premature infants. Reconstitute with Sterile Water for Injection only. Use only 1 dose per vial. Discard unused portion.

Reconstitution

Gentropin, Genotropin Miniquick: reconstitute with diluent provided.
Humatrope: reconstitute with 1.5–5 ml diluent provided, swirl gently, do not shake.
Humatrope Cartridge: dilute with solution provided with cartridge only.
Nutropin: reconstitute each 5 mg with 1.5–5 ml diluent, swirl gently, do not shake.
Omnitrope: reconstitute with diluents provided, swirl gently, do not shake.
Saigen: 5 mg: reconstitute with 1–3 ml diluent provided, swirl gently, do not shake. 8.8 mg: reconstitute with 2–3 ml diluent provided, swirl gently, do not shake.
Serostim: reconstitute with Sterile Water for Injection.

S

Zorbitive: reconstitute with 1–2 ml bacteriostatic water for injection.

Storage

Long term storage: refrigerate all products except Zorbitive. Once reconstituted Humatrope, Nutropin, Saigen, Zorbitive stable for 14 days, Genotrope for 21 days, Humatrope Cartridge for 28 days. **Genotropine Miniquick:** refrigerate, use within 24 hrs.

INDICATIONS/ROUTES/DOSAGE

Growth Hormone Deficiency

SUBCUTANEOUS (GENOTROPIN, OMNITROPE): ADULTS: 0.04 mg/kg weekly divided into 6–7 equal doses/wk. May increase at 4- to 8-wk intervals to maximum of 0.08 mg/kg/wk. **CHILDREN:** 0.16–0.24 mg/kg weekly divided into daily doses.

SUBCUTANEOUS (HUMATROPE): ADULTS: 0.006 mg/kg once daily. May increase to maximum of 0.0125 mg/kg/day. **CHILDREN:** 0.18–0.3 mg/kg weekly divided into alternate-day doses or 6 doses/wk.

SUBCUTANEOUS (NORDITROPIN): ADULTS: 0.004 mg/kg/day. May increase after 6 wks up to 0.016 mg/kg/day. **CHILDREN:** 0.024–0.036 mg/kg/dose 6–7 times a wk.

SUBCUTANEOUS (NUTROPIN): ADULTS: 0.006 mg/kg once daily. May increase to maximum of 0.025 mg/kg/day (younger than 35 yrs) or 0.0125/kg/day (35 yrs and older). **CHILDREN:** 0.3–0.7 mg/kg weekly divided into daily doses.

SUBCUTANEOUS (NUTROPIN AQ): ADULTS: 0.006 mg/kg once daily. May increase to maximum of 0.0125 mg/kg/day.

SUBCUTANEOUS (SAIZEN): ADULTS: 0.005 mg/kg/day. May increase up to 0.01 mg/kg/day after 4 wks. **CHILDREN:** 0.06 mg/kg 3 times a wk.

Chronic Renal Insufficiency

SUBCUTANEOUS (NUTROPIN, NUTROPIN AQ): CHILDREN: 0.35 mg/kg weekly divided into daily doses.

Turner's Syndrome

SUBCUTANEOUS (HUMATROPE, NUTROPIN, NUTROPIN AQ): CHILDREN: 0.375 mg/kg weekly divided into equal doses 3–7 times a wk. **(GENOTROPIN):** 0.33 mg/kg weekly divided into 6–7 doses.

AIDS-Related Wasting

SUBCUTANEOUS (SEROSTIN): ADULTS WEIGHING MORE THAN 55 KG: 6 mg once daily at bedtime. **ADULTS WEIGHING 45–55 KG:** 5 mg once daily at bedtime. **ADULTS WEIGHING 35–44 KG:** 4 mg once daily at bedtime. **ADULTS WEIGHING LESS THAN 35 KG:** 0.1 mg/kg once daily at bedtime.

Short Bowel Syndrome

SUBCUTANEOUS (ZORBITIVE): ADULTS: 0.1 mg/kg/day. **Maximum:** 8 mg/day.

SIDE EFFECTS

Frequent: Otitis media, other ear disorders (with Turner's syndrome). **Occasional:** Carpal tunnel syndrome, gynecomastia, myalgia, peripheral edema, fatigue, asthenia (loss of strength, energy). **Rare:** Rash, pruritus, visual changes, headache, nausea, vomiting, injection site pain/swelling, abdominal pain, hip/knee pain.

ADVERSE EFFECTS/ TOXIC REACTIONS

Pancreatitis occurs rarely.

NURSING CONSIDERATIONS

BASELINE ASSESSMENT

Obtain baseline lab chemistries, thyroid function, serum glucose level.

INTERVENTION/EVALUATION

Monitor bone growth, growth rate in relation to pt's age. Monitor serum calcium, glucose, phosphorus levels; renal, parathyroid, thyroid function. Observe for decreased muscle wasting in AIDS pts.

PATIENT/FAMILY TEACHING

• Follow correct procedure to reconstitute drug for administration, safe handling/disposal of needles. • Regular follow-up with physician is important part of therapy. • Report development of severe headache, visual changes, pain in hip/knee, limping.

sorafenib

sor-ah-**fen**-ib
(Nexavar)
Do not confuse Nexavar with Nexium, or sorafenib with imatinib or sunitinib.

◆CLASSIFICATION

PHARMACOTHERAPEUTIC: Multikinase inhibitor. **CLINICAL:** Antineoplastic.

ACTION

Decreases tumor cell proliferation by interacting with multiple intracellular, cell surface kinases. **Therapeutic Effect:** Inhibits tumor growth.

PHARMACOKINETICS

Metabolized in liver. Protein binding: 99.5%. Eliminated mainly in feces, with lesser amount excreted in urine. **Half-life:** 25–48 hrs.

USES

Treatment of advanced renal cell carcinoma, unresectable hepatocellular carcinoma. **OFF-LABEL:** Treatment of non–small-cell lung, ovarian, pancreatic cancer, melanoma, advanced thyroid cancer, resistant gastrointestinal stromal tumor.

PRECAUTIONS

Contraindications: None known. **Cautions:** Hepatic/renal impairment, dialysis pts.

⌛ LIFESPAN CONSIDERATIONS

Pregnancy/Lactation: May cause fetal harm. Adequate contraception should be used during therapy and for at least 2 wks after therapy completion. Unknown if distributed in breast milk. Breast-feeding not recommended. **Pregnancy Category D. Children:** Safety and efficacy not established. **Elderly:** No age-related precautions noted.

INTERACTIONS

DRUG: **Carbamazine, dexamethasone, phenobarbital, phenytoin, rifampin** may decrease concentration. May increase concentration, effects of **doxorubicin. Warfarin** may increase risk of bleeding. **HERBAL:** **St. John's wort** may decrease concentration. **FOOD:** **High-fat meals** decrease effectiveness. **LAB VALUES:** May increase serum lipase, amylase, bilirubin, alkaline phosphatase, transaminases. May decrease serum phosphorus, lymphocytes, WBCs, Hgb, Hct.

AVAILABILITY (Rx)

Tablets: 200 mg (Nexavar).

ADMINISTRATION/HANDLING

PO

• Give 1 hr before or 2 hrs after eating (high-fat meal reduces effectiveness). • Swallow tablet whole.

INDICATIONS/ROUTES/DOSAGE

Renal Cell Carcinoma, Hepatocellular Carcinoma

PO: ADULTS, ELDERLY: 400 mg (2 tablets) twice daily without food.

SIDE EFFECTS

Frequent (43%–16%): Diarrhea, rash, fatigue, exfoliative dermatitis, alopecia, nausea, pruritus, hypertension, anorexia, vomiting. **Occasional (15%–10%):** Constipation, minor bleeding, dyspnea, sensory neuropathy, cough, abdominal pain, dry skin, weight loss, joint pain, headache. **Rare (9%–1%):** Acne, flushing, stomatitis, mucositis, dyspepsia (heartburn, indigestion, epigastric pain), arthralgia, myalgia, hoarseness.

ADVERSE EFFECTS/ TOXIC REACTIONS

Anemia, neutropenia, thrombocytopenia, leukopenia occur in less than 10% of pts.

S

Pancreatitis, gastritis, erectile dysfunction occur occasionally. Hemorrhage, cardiac ischemia/infarction, hypertensive crisis occur rarely.

NURSING CONSIDERATIONS

BASELINE ASSESSMENT

Monitor B/P weekly during first 6 wks of therapy and routinely thereafter. CBC, serum chemistries including electrolytes, renal/hepatic function tests, chest X-ray should be performed before therapy begins and routinely thereafter.

INTERVENTION/EVALUATION

Determine serum amylase, lipase, phosphorus concentrations frequently during therapy. Monitor CBC for evidence of myelosuppression. Monitor for blood dyscrasias (fever, sore throat, signs of local infection, unusual bruising/bleeding from any site), symptoms of anemia (excessive fatigue, weakness). Monitor for signs of neuropathy (gait disturbances, fine motor control, difficulties, numbness).

PATIENT/FAMILY TEACHING

• Report any episode of chest pain. • Do not have immunizations without physician's approval (drug lowers resistance). Avoid contact with those who have recently taken live virus vaccine. • Promptly report fever, sore throat, signs of local infection, unusual bruising/bleeding from any site.

S

sotalol

HIGH ALERT

soe-ta-lol
(Apo-Sotalol ✦, Betapace, Betapace AF, Novo-Sotalol ✦, PMS-Sotalol ✦, Sorine)

BLACK BOX ALERT Initiation, titration to occur in a hospital setting with continuous EKG to monitor potential onset of life-threatening arrhythmias. Betapace should not be substituted for Betapace AF.

Do not confuse sotalol with Stadol, or Betapace with Betapace AF.

◆ CLASSIFICATION

PHARMACOTHERAPEUTIC: Beta-adrenergic blocking agent. **CLINICAL:** Antiarrhythmic (see pp. 18C, 72C).

ACTION

Prolongs cardiac action potential, effective refractory period, QT interval. Decreases heart rate, AV node conduction; increases AV node refractoriness. **Therapeutic Effect:** Produces antiarrhythmic activity.

PHARMACOKINETICS

Route	Onset	Peak	Duration
PO	1–2 hrs	2.5–4 hrs	8–16 hrs

Well absorbed from GI tract. Protein binding: None. Widely distributed. Primarily excreted unchanged in urine. Removed by hemodialysis. **Half-life:** 12 hrs (increased in elderly, renal impairment).

USES

Betapace, Sorine: Treatment of documented, life-threatening ventricular arrhythmias. **Betapace AF:** Maintain normal sinus rhythm in pts with symptomatic atrial fibrillation/flutter. **OFF-LABEL:** Maintenance of normal heart rhythm in chronic or recurring atrial fibrillation/flutter; treatment of anxiety, chronic angina pectoris, hypertension, hypertrophic cardiomyopathy, MI, mitral valve prolapse syndrome, pheochromocytoma, thyrotoxicosis, tremors.

PRECAUTIONS

Contraindications: Bronchial asthma, cardiogenic shock, prolonged QT syndrome (unless functioning pacemaker is present), second- or third-degree heart block, sinus bradycardia, uncontrolled cardiac failure. **Cautions:** Pts with history of ventricular tachycardia, ventricular fibrillation, cardiomegaly, CHF, diabetes mellitus; excessive prolongation of QT interval; hypokalemia; hypomagnesemia. Severe, prolonged diarrhea. Pts with sick sinus syndrome, pts at risk for developing thyrotoxicosis. Avoid abrupt withdrawal.

LIFESPAN CONSIDERATIONS

Pregnancy/Lactation: Crosses placenta. Distributed in breast milk. **Pregnancy Category B (D if used in second or third trimester). Children:** Safety and efficacy not established. **Elderly:** Age-related peripheral vascular disease may increase susceptibility to decreased peripheral circulation. Age-related renal impairment may require dosage adjustment.

INTERACTIONS

DRUG: **Calcium channel blockers** may increase effect on AV conduction, B/P. May mask symptoms of hypoglycemia, prolong hypoglycemic effects of **insulin, oral hypoglycemics.** May inhibit effects of **sympathomimetics, theophylline.** HERBAL: **Ephedra** may worsen arrhythmias. FOOD: None known. LAB VALUES: May increase serum glucose, alkaline phosphatase, LDH, lipoprotein, AST, ALT, triglycerides, BUN, potassium, uric acid.

AVAILABILITY (Rx)

Tablets: 80 mg (Betapace, Betapace AF, Sorine), 120 mg (Betapace, Betapace AF, Sorine), 160 mg (Betapace, Betapace AF, Sorine), 240 mg (Betapace, Sorine).

ADMINISTRATION/HANDLING

PO

• Give without regard to food. • Give at same time each day.

INDICATIONS/ROUTES/DOSAGE

Documented, Life-Threatening Arrhythmias

PO (BETAPACE, SORINE): ADULTS, ELDERLY: Initially, 80 mg twice daily. May increase gradually at 2- to 3-day intervals. Range: 240–320 mg/day.

Atrial Fibrillation, Atrial Flutter

PO (BETAPACE AF): ADULTS, ELDERLY: 80 mg twice daily. May increase up to 160 mg twice daily.

Dosage in Renal Impairment

Dosage interval is modified based on creatinine clearance.

BETAPACE, SORINE

Creatinine Clearance	Dosage
31–60 ml/min	24 hrs
10–30 ml/min	36–48 hrs
Less than 10 ml/min	Individualized

BETAPACE AF

Creatinine Clearance	Dosage
Greater than 60 ml/min	12 hrs
40–60 ml/min	24 hrs
Less than 40 ml/min	Contraindicated

SIDE EFFECTS

Frequent: Diminished sexual function, drowsiness, insomnia, asthenia (loss of strength, energy). Occasional: Depression, cold hands/feet, diarrhea, constipation, anxiety, nasal congestion, nausea, vomiting. Rare: Altered taste, dry eyes, pruritus, paresthesia of fingers, toes, scalp.

ADVERSE EFFECTS/ TOXIC REACTIONS

Bradycardia, CHF, hypotension, bronchospasm, hypoglycemia, prolonged QT interval, torsade de pointes, ventricular tachycardia, premature ventricular complexes may occur.

NURSING CONSIDERATIONS

BASELINE ASSESSMENT

Pt must be on continuous cardiac monitoring upon initiation of therapy. Do not administer without consulting physician if pulse is 60 beats/min or less. Assess creatinine clearance before dosing.

INTERVENTION/EVALUATION

Diligently monitor for arrhythmias. Assess B/P for hypotension, pulse for bradycardia. Assess for CHF: dyspnea, peripheral edema, jugular vein distention, increased weight, rales in lungs, decreased urinary output.

PATIENT/FAMILY TEACHING

• Do not discontinue, change dose without physician approval. • Avoid tasks requiring alertness, motor skills until response to drug is established (may cause drowsiness). • Periodic lab tests, EKGs are necessary part of therapy. • Notify physician of rapid heartbeat, chest pain, swelling of ankles/legs, difficulty breathing.

spironolactone

speer-on-oh-**lak**-tone
(Aldactone, Novo-Spiroton)

BLACK BOX ALERT Has been shown to produce tumors in chronic toxicity studies.

Do not confuse Aldactone with Aldactazide.

FIXED-COMBINATION(S)

Aldactazide: spironolactone/hydrochlorothiazide (a thiazide diuretic): 25 mg/25 mg, 50 mg/50 mg.

◆CLASSIFICATION

PHARMACOTHERAPEUTIC: Aldosterone antagonist. **CLINICAL:** Potassium-sparing diuretic, antihypertensive, antihypokalemic (see p. 102C).

ACTION

Interferes with sodium reabsorption by competitively inhibiting action of aldosterone in distal tubule, promoting sodium and water excretion, increasing potassium retention. **Therapeutic Effect:** Produces diuresis, lowers B/P.

PHARMACOKINETICS

Well absorbed from GI tract (absorption increased with food). Protein binding: 91%–98%. Metabolized in liver to active metabolite. Primarily excreted in urine. Unknown if removed by hemodialysis. **Half-life:** 78–84 min.

USES

Management of edema associated with CHF, cirrhosis, nephrotic syndrome. Treatment of hypertension, male hirsutism, hypokalemia, CHF. Diagnosis/treatment of primary hyperaldosteronism. **OFF-LABEL:** Treatment of edema, hypertension in children, female acne, female hirsutism, polycystic ovary disease.

PRECAUTIONS

Contraindications: Acute renal insufficiency, anuria, BUN and serum creatinine levels more than twice normal values, hyperkalemia. **Cautions:** Dehydration, hyponatremia, renal/hepatic impairment, concurrent use of supplemental potassium.

LIFESPAN CONSIDERATIONS

Pregnancy/Lactation: Active metabolite excreted in breast milk. Breast-feeding not recommended. **Pregnancy Category C (D if used in pregnancy-induced hypertension). Children:** No age-related precautions noted. **Elderly:** May be more susceptible to developing hyperkalemia. Age-related renal impairment may require dosage adjustment.

INTERACTIONS

DRUG: **ACE inhibitors (e.g., captopril), cyclosporine, potassium-containing medications, potassium supplements** may increase risk of hyperkalemia. May decrease effects of **anticoagulants, heparin.** May increase half-life of **digoxin.** May decrease clearance, increase risk of toxicity of **lithium. NSAIDs** may decrease antihypertensive effect. **HERBAL:** Avoid **natural licorice** (possesses mineralocorticoid activity). **FOOD:** **Food** increases absorption. **LAB VALUES:** May increase urinary calcium excretion, BUN, serum glucose, creatinine, magnesium, potassium, uric acid. May decrease serum sodium.

AVAILABILITY (Rx)

Tablets: 25 mg, 50 mg, 100 mg.

ADMINISTRATION/HANDLING

PO

• Oral suspension containing crushed tablets in cherry syrup is stable for up to 30

S

days if refrigerated. • Drug absorption enhanced if taken with food. • Scored tablets may be crushed.

INDICATIONS/ROUTES/DOSAGE

Edema

PO: ADULTS, ELDERLY: 25–200 mg/day as single dose or in 2 divided doses. **CHILDREN:** 1–3.3 mg/kg/day in divided doses. **Maximum:** 100 mg. **NEONATES:** 1–3 mg/kg/day in 1–2 divided doses.

Hypertension

PO: ADULTS, ELDERLY: 25–50 mg/day in 1–2 doses/day. **CHILDREN:** 1–3.3 mg/kg/day in divided doses. **Maximum:** 100 mg.

Hypokalemia

PO: ADULTS, ELDERLY: 25–200 mg/day as single dose or in 2 divided doses.

Hirsutism

PO: ADULTS, ELDERLY: 50–200 mg/day as single dose or in 2 divided doses.

Primary Aldosteronism

PO: ADULTS, ELDERLY: 100–400 mg/day as single dose or in 2 divided doses. **CHILDREN:** 125–375 mg/m^2/day as single dose or in 2 divided doses.

CHF

PO: ADULTS, ELDERLY: 12.5–25 mg/day adjusted based on pt response, evidence of hyperkalemia. **Maximum:** 50 mg.

Dosage in Renal Impairment

Dosage interval is modified based on creatinine clearance.

Creatinine Clearance	Dosage
10–50 ml/min	Usual dose q12–24h
Less than 10 ml/min	Avoid use

SIDE EFFECTS

Frequent: Hyperkalemia (in pts with renal insufficiency, those taking potassium supplements), dehydration, hyponatremia, lethargy. **Occasional:** Nausea, vomiting, anorexia, abdominal cramps, diarrhea, headache, ataxia, drowsiness, confusion, fever. **Male:** Gynecomastia, impotence, decreased libido. **Female:** Menstrual irregularities (amenorrhea, postmenopausal bleeding), breast tenderness. **Rare:** Rash, urticaria, hirsutism.

ADVERSE EFFECTS/ TOXIC REACTIONS

Severe hyperkalemia may produce arrhythmias, bradycardia, EKG changes (tented T waves, widening QRS complex, ST segment depression). May proceed to cardiac standstill, ventricular fibrillation. Cirrhosis pts at risk for hepatic decompensation if dehydration, hyponatremia occurs. Pts with primary aldosteronism may experience rapid weight loss, severe fatigue during high-dose therapy.

NURSING CONSIDERATIONS

BASELINE ASSESSMENT

Weigh pt; initiate strict I&O. Evaluate hydration status by assessing mucous membranes, skin turgor. Obtain baseline serum electrolytes, renal/hepatic function, urinalysis. Assess for edema; note location, extent. Check baseline vital signs, note pulse rate/regularity.

INTERVENTION/EVALUATION

Monitor serum electrolyte values, esp. for increased potassium, BUN, creatinine. Monitor B/P. Monitor for hyponatremia: mental confusion, thirst, cold/clammy skin, drowsiness, dry mouth. Monitor for hyperkalemia: colic, diarrhea, muscle twitching followed by weakness/paralysis, arrhythmias. Obtain daily weight. Note changes in edema, skin turgor.

PATIENT/FAMILY TEACHING

• Expect increase in volume, frequency of urination. • Therapeutic effect takes several days to begin and can last for several days when drug is discontinued. This may not apply if pt is on a potassium-losing drug concomitantly (diet, use of supplements should be established by physician). • Notify physician of irregular or slow pulse, electrolyte imbalance (see previous Intervention/Evaluation). • Avoid foods high in potassium, such as whole grains (cereals), legumes, meat, bananas, apricots, orange juice, potatoes (white, sweet), raisins. • Avoid alcohol. • Avoid tasks that require alertness, motor skills until response to drug is established (may cause drowsiness).

St. John's wort

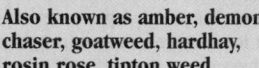

Also known as amber, demon chaser, goatweed, hardhay, rosin rose, tipton weed.

CLASSIFICATION

HERBAL: See Appendix G.

ACTION

Inhibits COMT (catechol-*O*-methyl transferase), MAO (monoamine oxidase); modulates effects of serotonin by inhibiting serotonin reuptake and 5-HT_3, 5-HT_4 antagonism. **Effect:** Relieves depression.

USES

Treatment of depression, including secondary effects of depression (fatigue, loss of appetite, anxiety, nervousness, insomnia).

PRECAUTIONS

Contraindications: Pregnancy, breast-feeding (may cause increased muscle tone of uterus; infants may experience colic, drowsiness, lethargy). **Cautions:** Bipolar disorder, schizophrenia.

LIFESPAN CONSIDERATIONS

Pregnancy/Lactation: Contraindicated. **Pregnancy Category C. Children:** Safety and efficacy not established. Avoid use. **Elderly:** No age-related precautions noted.

INTERACTIONS

DRUG: **Angiotensin-converting enzyme (ACE) inhibitors** may cause hypertension. May decrease concentration, effect of **indinavir. Antidepressants** may increase therapeutic effect. May decrease effectiveness of **cyclosporine,** resulting in organ rejection. **Digoxin** may cause CHF exacerbation. **HERBAL:** **Chamomile, ginseng, goldenseal, kava kava, valerian** may increase therapeutic, adverse effects. **FOOD:** **Tyramine-containing food may** cause hypertensive crisis with high doses of St. John's wort. **LAB VALUES:** May decrease PT/INR in pts treated with warfarin.

AVAILABILITY (Rx)

Capsules: 150 mg, 300 mg. **Extract. Liquid Tincture.**

INDICATIONS/ROUTES/DOSAGE

Depression

PO: ADULTS, ELDERLY: 300 mg 3 times a day is most common.

SIDE EFFECTS

Abdominal cramps, insomnia, vivid dreams, restlessness, anxiety, agitation, irritability, fatigue, dry mouth, headache, dizziness, photosensitivity, confusion.

ADVERSE EFFECTS/ TOXIC REACTIONS

None known.

NURSING CONSIDERATIONS

BASELINE ASSESSMENT

Assess if pt is pregnant or breast-feeding, has history of psychiatric disease. Determine medication usage (many potential interactions). Assess mental status: mood, memory, anxiety level.

INTERVENTION/EVALUATION

Monitor changes in depressive state, behavior, signs of side effects.

PATIENT/FAMILY TEACHING

• Do not abruptly discontinue drug (may increase adverse effects). • Check with physician before taking other medications (many interactions). • Avoid foods high in tyramine (aged cheese, pickled products, beer, wine). • Therapeutic effect may take 4–6 wks. • Avoid sunlight; use sunscreen/protective clothing (increased photosensitivity).

stavudine (d4T)

stav-ue-deen
(Zerit)

BLACK BOX ALERT Lactic acidosis, severe hepatomegaly with steatosis (fatty liver), pancreatitis have occurred. Fatalities reported.

Do not confuse Zerit with Zestril, Ziac, or Zyrtec.

CLASSIFICATION

PHARMACOTHERAPEUTIC: Nucleoside reverse transcriptase inhibitor. **CLINICAL:** Antiviral (see pp. 67C, 115C).

ACTION

Inhibits HIV reverse transcriptase by terminating viral DNA chain. Inhibits RNA-, DNA-dependent DNA polymerase, an enzyme necessary for HIV replication. **Therapeutic Effect:** Impedes HIV replication, slowing progression of HIV infection.

PHARMACOKINETICS

Rapidly, completely absorbed after PO administration. Undergoes intracellular phosphorylation to an active metabolite. Excreted in urine. **Half-life:** 1–1.6 hrs (increased in renal impairment).

USES

Treatment of HIV infection in combination with other agents.

PRECAUTIONS

Contraindications: None known. **Cautions:** History of peripheral neuropathy, renal/hepatic impairment.

LIFESPAN CONSIDERATIONS

Pregnancy/Lactation: Breast-feeding not recommended (possibility of HIV transmission). **Pregnancy Category C.** **Children:** No age-related precautions noted. **Elderly:** Information not available.

INTERACTIONS

DRUG: **Didanosine, ethambutol, isoniazid, lithium, metronidazole, nitrofurantoin, phenytoin, zalcitabine** may increase risk of peripheral neuropathy development. **Didanosine, hydroxyurea** may increase risk of hepatotoxicity. **Zidovudine** may have antagonistic antiviral effect. **HERBAL:** None significant. **FOOD:** None known. **LAB VALUES:** May increase serum ALT, AST, alkaline phosphatase, GGT, amylase, bilirubin.

AVAILABILITY (Rx)

Capsules: 15 mg, 20 mg, 30 mg, 40 mg. **Powder for Oral Solution:** 1 mg/ml.

ADMINISTRATION/HANDLING

PO

• Give without regard to meals.

INDICATIONS/ROUTES/DOSAGE

HIV Infection

PO: ADULTS, ELDERLY, CHILDREN WEIGHING 60 KG AND MORE: 40 mg q12h. **ADULTS, ELDERLY, CHILDREN WEIGHING 30–59 KG:** 30 mg q12h. **NEONATES 14 DAYS AND OLDER, INFANTS, CHILDREN WEIGHING LESS THAN 30 KG:** 1 mg/kg/dose q12h. **Maximum:** 30 mg q12h. **NEONATES 0–13 DAYS:** 0.5 mg/kg/dose q12h.

Dosage in Renal Impairment

Dosage and frequency are modified based on creatinine clearance and pt weight.

Creatinine Clearance	Weight 60 kg or More	Weight Less Than 60 kg
Greater than 50 ml/min	40 mg q12h	30 mg q12h
26–50 ml/min	20 mg q12h	15 mg q12h
10–25 ml/min	20 mg q24h	15 mg q24h

SIDE EFFECTS

Frequent: Headache (55%), diarrhea (50%), chills, fever (38%), nausea, vomiting, myalgia (35%), rash (33%), asthenia (loss of strength, energy) (28%), insomnia, abdominal pain (26%), anxiety (22%), back pain (20%), diaphoresis (19%), arthralgia (18%), malaise (17%), depression (14%). **Occasional:** Anorexia, weight loss, nervousness, dizziness, conjunctivitis, dyspepsia, dyspnea. **Rare:** Constipation, vasodilation, confusion, migraine, urticaria, abnormal vision.

ADVERSE EFFECTS/ TOXIC REACTIONS

Peripheral neuropathy (numbness, tingling, pain in hands/feet) occurs in 15%–21% of pts. Ulcerative stomatitis (erythema, ulcers of oral mucosa, glossitis, gingivitis), pneumonia, benign skin neoplasms occur occasionally. Pancreatitis, hepatomegaly, lactic acidosis have been reported.

NURSING CONSIDERATIONS

BASELINE ASSESSMENT

Obtain baseline laboratory testing, esp. serum hepatic function tests, before beginning stavudine therapy and at periodic intervals during therapy. Offer emotional support to pt, family. Question for history of peripheral neuropathy.

INTERVENTION/EVALUATION

Monitor for peripheral neuropathy (characterized by paresthesia in extremities). Symptoms resolve promptly if therapy is discontinued (symptoms may worsen temporarily after drug is withdrawn). If symptoms resolve completely, reduced dosage may be resumed. Assess for headache, nausea, vomiting, myalgia. Monitor skin for evidence of rash, signs of fever. Monitor daily pattern of bowel activity, stool consistency. Assess for myalgia, arthralgia, dizziness. Monitor sleep patterns. Assess eating pattern; monitor for weight loss. Check eyes for signs of conjunctivitis. Monitor CBC, Hgb, serum hepatic/renal function, CD4 cell count, HIV RNA levels.

PATIENT/FAMILY TEACHING

• Continue therapy for full length of treatment. • Doses should be evenly spaced. • Do not take any medications, including OTC drugs, without consulting physician. • Stavudine is not a cure for HIV infection, nor does it reduce risk of transmission to others. • Pt may continue to experience illnesses, including opportunistic infections. • Report tingling, burning, pain, numbness, abdominal discomfort, nausea, vomiting, fatigue, dyspnea, weakness.

sucralfate

soo-**kral**-fate
(Apo-Sucralate ✱, Carafate, Novo-Sucralate ✱)
Do not confuse Carafate with Cafergot, or sucrafate with salsalate.

◆CLASSIFICATION

PHARMACOTHERAPEUTIC: Gastrointestinal agent. **CLINICAL:** Antiulcer.

ACTION

Forms ulcer-adherent complex with proteinaceous exudate (e.g., albumin) at ulcer site. Forms viscous, adhesive barrier on surface of intact mucosa of stomach, duodenum. **Therapeutic Effect:** Protects damaged mucosa from further destruction by absorbing gastric acid, pepsin, bile salts.

PHARMACOKINETICS

Minimally absorbed from GI tract. Eliminated in feces, with small amount excreted in urine. Not removed by hemodialysis.

USES

Short-term treatment (up to 8 wks) of duodenal ulcer. Maintenance therapy of duodenal ulcer after healing of acute ulcers. **OFF-LABEL:** Prevention, treatment of stress-related mucosal damage, esp. in acutely or critically ill pts; treatment of gastric ulcer, rheumatoid arthritis (RA); relief of GI symptoms associated with NSAIDs; treatment of gastroesophageal reflux disease (GERD).

PRECAUTIONS

Contraindications: None known. **Cautions:** None known.

⌛ LIFESPAN CONSIDERATIONS

Pregnancy/Lactation: Unknown if drug crosses placenta or is distributed in breast milk. **Pregnancy Category B. Children:** Safety and efficacy not established. **Elderly:** No age-related precautions noted.

INTERACTIONS

DRUG: **Antacids** may interfere with binding. May decrease absorption of **digoxin, ketoconazole, levothyroxine, phenytoin, quinidine, quinolones (e.g., ciprofloxacin), ranitidine, tetracycline, theophylline. HERBAL:** None significant. **FOOD:** None known. **LAB VALUES:** None significant.

AVAILABILITY (Rx)

Oral Suspension: 1 g/10 ml. **Tablets:** 1 g.

ADMINISTRATION/HANDLING

PO

• Administer 1 hr before meals and at bedtime. • Tablets may be crushed and dissolved in water. • Avoid antacids for 30 min before or after giving sucralfate. • Shake suspension well before using.

INDICATIONS/ROUTES/DOSAGE

Active Duodenal Ulcers

PO: ADULTS, ELDERLY: 1 g 4 times a day (before meals and at bedtime) for up to 8 wks.

Maintenance Therapy of Duodenal Ulcers

PO: ADULTS, ELDERLY: 1 g twice a day.

SIDE EFFECTS

Frequent (2%): Constipation. **Occasional (less than 2%):** Dry mouth, backache, diarrhea, dizziness, drowsiness, nausea, indigestion, rash, urticaria, pruritus, abdominal discomfort.

ADVERSE EFFECTS/ TOXIC REACTIONS

Bezoars (compacted, undigestible material that does not pass into intestine) have been reported.

NURSING CONSIDERATIONS

INTERVENTION/EVALUATION

Monitor daily pattern of bowel activity, stool consistency.

PATIENT/FAMILY TEACHING

• Take medication on an empty stomach. • Antacids may be given as an adjunct but should not be taken for 30 min before or after sucralfate (formation of sucralfate gel is activated by stomach acid). • Dry mouth may be relieved by sour hard candy, sips of tepid water.

sulfasalazine

sul-fa-**sal**-a-zeen
(Alti-Sulfasalazine ♣, Azulfidine, Azulfidine EN-tabs, Salazopyrin ♣, Salazopyrin EN-Tabs ♣)

Do not confuse Azulfidine with Augmentin or azathioprine, or sulfasalazine with sulfadiazine or sulfisoxazole.

◆ CLASSIFICATION

PHARMACOTHERAPEUTIC: Sulfonamide. **CLINICAL:** Anti-inflammatory.

ACTION

Inhibits prostaglandin synthesis, acting locally in colon. **Therapeutic Effect:** Decreases inflammatory response, interferes with GI secretion. Effect may be result of antibacterial action with change in intestinal flora.

PHARMACOKINETICS

Poorly absorbed from GI tract. Cleaved, absorbed in colon by intestinal bacteria, forming sulfapyridine and mesalamine (5-ASA). Widely distributed. Metabolized via colonic intestinal flora. Primarily excreted in urine. Half-life: 5.7–10 hrs.

USES

Treatment of ulcerative colitis, rheumatoid arthritis (RA), juvenile rheumatoid arthritis. OFF-LABEL: Treatment of ankylosing spondylitis, collagenous colitis, Crohn's disease, inflammatory bowel disease, juvenile chronic arthritis, psoriasis, psoriatic arthritis.

PRECAUTIONS

Contraindications: Children younger than 2 yrs; hypersensitivity to carbonic anhydrase inhibitors, local anesthetics, salicylates, sulfonamides, sulfonylureas, sunscreens containing PABA, thiazide or loop diuretics; intestinal, urinary tract obstruction; porphyria; pregnancy at term; severe hepatic/renal dysfunction. Cautions: Severe allergies, bronchial asthma, impaired hepatic/renal function, G6PD deficiency.

LIFESPAN CONSIDERATIONS

Pregnancy/Lactation: May produce infertility, oligospermia in men while taking medication. Readily crosses placenta; if given near term, may produce jaundice, hemolytic anemia, kernicterus in newborn. Distributed in breast milk. Pt should not breast-feed premature infant or those with hyperbilirubinemia or G6PD deficiency. **Pregnancy Category B (D if given near term). Children:** No age-related precautions noted in those older than 2 yrs. **Elderly:** No age-related precautions noted.

INTERACTIONS

DRUG: May increase effects of **anticonvulsants, methotrexate, oral anticoagulants, oral antidiabetics. Hemolytics** may increase toxicity. **Hepatotoxic medications** may increase risk of hepatotoxicity. HERBAL: **Dong quai, St. John's wort** may increase photosensitization. FOOD: None known. LAB VALUES: None significant.

AVAILABILITY (Rx)

Tablets (Azulfidine): 500 mg.

Tablets (Delayed-Release [Azulfidine EN-Tabs]): 500 mg.

ADMINISTRATION/HANDLING

PO

• Space doses evenly (intervals not to exceed 8 hrs). • Administer after meals if possible (prolongs intestinal passage). • Swallow enteric-coated tablets whole; do not chew. • Give with 8 oz of water; encourage several glasses of water between meals.

INDICATIONS/ROUTES/DOSAGE

Ulcerative Colitis

PO: ADULTS, ELDERLY: 1 g 3–4 times a day in divided doses q4–6h. Maintenance: 2 g/day in divided doses q6–12h. **Maximum:** 6 g/day. **CHILDREN 2 YRS AND OLDER:** Initially, 40–60 mg/kg/day in 3–6 divided doses. Maintenance: 20–30 mg/kg/day in 4 divided doses.

Rheumatoid Arthritis (RA)

PO: (DELAYED-RELEASE TABLETS): ADULTS, ELDERLY: Initially, 0.5–1 g/day for 1 wk. Increase by 0.5 g/wk, up to 2 g/day. **Maximum:** 3 g/day.

Juvenile Rheumatoid Arthritis (JRA)

PO: (DELAYED-RELEASE TABLETS): CHILDREN: Initially, 10 mg/kg/day. May increase by 10 mg/kg/day at weekly intervals. Range: 30–50 mg/kg/day. **Maximum:** 2 g/day.

Dosage in Renal Impairment

Creatinine Clearance	Dosing
10–30 ml/min	Twice daily
Less than 10 ml/min	Once daily

Dosage in Hepatic Impairment

Avoid use.

SIDE EFFECTS

Frequent (33%): Anorexia, nausea, vomiting, headache, oligospermia (generally reversed by withdrawal of drug). **Occasional (3%):** Hypersensitivity reaction (rash, urticaria, pruritus, fever, anemia). **Rare (less than 1%):** Tinnitus, hypoglycemia, diuresis, photosensitivity.

ADVERSE EFFECTS/ TOXIC REACTIONS

Anaphylaxis, Stevens-Johnson syndrome, hematologic toxicity (leukopenia, agranulocytosis), hepatotoxicity, nephrotoxicity occur rarely.

NURSING CONSIDERATIONS

BASELINE ASSESSMENT

Question for hypersensitivity to medications. Check initial urinalysis, CBC, serum hepatic/renal function tests.

INTERVENTION/EVALUATION

Monitor I&O, urinalysis, renal function tests; ensure adequate hydration (minimum output 1,500 ml/24 hrs) to prevent nephrotoxicity. Assess skin for rash (discontinue drug, notify physician at first sign). Monitor daily pattern of bowel activity, stool consistency. (Dosage increase may be needed if diarrhea continues, recurs.) Monitor CBC closely; assess for and report immediately any hematologic effects (bleeding, ecchymoses, fever, pharyngitis, pallor, weakness, purpura). Monitor hepatic function tests; observe for jaundice.

PATIENT/FAMILY TEACHING

• May cause orange-yellow discoloration of urine, skin. • Space doses evenly around the clock. • Take after food with 8 oz of water; drink several glasses of water between meals. • Continue for full length of treatment; may be necessary to take drug even after symptoms relieved. • Follow-up, lab tests are essential. • Inform dentist, surgeon of sulfasalazine therapy. • Avoid exposure to sun, ultraviolet light until photosensitivity determined (may last for mos after last dose).

sulindac

sul-**in**-dak
(Apo-Sulin ✤, Clinoril, Novo-Sundac ✤)

BLACK BOX ALERT Increased risk of serious cardiovascular thrombotic events, including myocardial infarction, CVA. Increased risk of severe GI reactions, including ulceration, bleeding, perforation of stomach, intestines.

Do not confuse Clinoril with Cleocin or Clozaril.

◆ CLASSIFICATION

PHARMACOTHERAPEUTIC: Nonsteroidal anti-inflammatory. **CLINICAL:** Anti-inflammatory, antigout (see p. 129C).

ACTION

Produces analgesic, anti-inflammatory effects by inhibiting prostaglandin synthesis. **Therapeutic Effect:** Reduces inflammatory response, intensity of pain.

PHARMACOKINETICS

Route	Onset	Peak	Duration
PO (antirheumatic)	7 days	2–3 wks	N/A
Analgesic	1 hr	—	12–24 hrs

Well absorbed from GI tract. Protein binding: 93%–98%. Metabolized in liver to active metabolite. Primarily excreted in urine. Not removed by hemodialysis. **Half-life:** 7.8 hrs; metabolite, 16.4 hrs.

USES

Treatment of pain of rheumatoid arthritis (RA), osteoarthritis, ankylosing spondylitis, acute painful shoulder, bursitis, tendinitis, acute gouty arthritis.

PRECAUTIONS

Contraindications: Active peptic ulcer disease, chronic inflammation of GI tract, GI bleeding/ulceration, history of hypersensitivity to aspirin, NSAIDs. **Cautions:** Renal/

S

hepatic impairment, history of GI tract disease, predisposition to fluid retention, concurrent anticoagulant use.

LIFESPAN CONSIDERATIONS

Pregnancy/Lactation: Unknown if drug is distributed in breast milk. Avoid use during third trimester (may adversely affect fetal cardiovascular system: premature closure of ductus arteriosus). **Pregnancy Category C (D if used in third trimester near delivery). Children:** Safety and efficacy not established. **Elderly:** GI bleeding/ulceration more likely to cause serious adverse effects. Age-related renal impairment may increase risk of hepatic/renal toxicity; lower dosage recommended.

INTERACTIONS

DRUG: **Antacids** may decrease concentration. May decrease effects of **antihypertensives, diuretics. Aspirin, other salicylates** may increase risk of GI side effects, bleeding. **Bone marrow depressants** may increase risk of hematologic reactions. May increase effects of **heparin, oral anticoagulants, thrombolytics.** May increase concentration, risk of toxicity of **lithium.** May increase risk of **methotrexate** toxicity. **Probenecid** may increase concentration. HERBAL: **Cat's claw, dong quai, evening primrose, feverfew, garlic, ginkgo, ginseng** possess antiplatelet activity, may increase bleeding. FOOD: None known. LAB VALUES: May increase serum alkaline phosphatase, AST, ALT, bleeding time.

AVAILABILITY (Rx)

Tablets: 150 mg, 200 mg.

ADMINISTRATION/HANDLING

PO

• Give with food, milk, antacids if GI distress occurs.

INDICATIONS/ROUTES/DOSAGE

Rheumatoid Arthritis (RA), Osteoarthritis, Ankylosing Spondylitis

PO: ADULTS, ELDERLY: Initially, 150 mg twice a day. May increase up to 400 mg/day.

Acute Shoulder Pain, Gouty Arthritis, Bursitis, Tendinitis

PO: ADULTS, ELDERLY: 200 mg twice a day for 7–14 days.

SIDE EFFECTS

Frequent (9%–4%): Diarrhea, constipation, indigestion, nausea, maculopapular rash, dermatitis, dizziness, headache. Occasional (3%–1%): Anorexia, abdominal cramps, flatulence.

ADVERSE EFFECTS/ TOXIC REACTIONS

Rare reactions with long-term use include peptic ulcer disease, GI bleeding, gastritis, nephrotoxicity (glomerular nephritis, interstitial nephritis, nephrotic syndrome), severe hepatic reactions (cholestasis, jaundice), severe hypersensitivity reactions (fever, chills, joint pain).

NURSING CONSIDERATIONS

BASELINE ASSESSMENT

Obtain baseline renal/hepatic function tests. Assess onset, type, location, duration of pain, fever, inflammation. Inspect affected joints for immobility, deformities, skin condition.

INTERVENTION/EVALUATION

Assist with ambulation if dizziness occurs. Monitor daily pattern of bowel activity, stool consistency. Assess for evidence of rash. Evaluate for therapeutic response (relief of pain, stiffness, swelling; increased joint mobility; reduced joint tenderness; improved grip strength). Monitor serum hepatic/renal function, CBC, platelets.

PATIENT/FAMILY TEACHING

• Therapeutic antiarthritic effect noted 1–3 wks after therapy begins. • Avoid aspirin, alcohol during therapy (increases risk of GI bleeding). • Take with food, milk if GI upset occurs. • Avoid tasks that require alertness, motor skills until response to drug is established (may cause dizziness).

sumatriptan

soo-ma-**trip**-tan
(Alsuma, Apo-Sumatriptan ✱, Imitrex, Novo-Sumatriptan ✱, Sumavel DosePro)
Do not confuse sumatriptan with saxagliptin, sitagliptin, somatropin, or zolmitriptan.

FIXED-COMBINATION(S)

Treximet: Sumatriptan/naproxen (an NSAID): 85 mg/500 mg.

◆CLASSIFICATION

PHARMACOTHERAPEUTIC: Serotonin receptor agonist. **CLINICAL:** Antimigraine (see p. 63C).

ACTION

Binds selectively to vascular receptors, producing vasoconstrictive effect on cranial blood vessels. **Therapeutic Effect:** Relieves migraine headache.

PHARMACOKINETICS

Route	Onset	Peak	Duration
Nasal	15 min	N/A	24–48 hrs
PO	30 min	2 hrs	24–48 hrs
Subcutaneous	10 min	1 hr	24–48 hrs

Rapidly absorbed after subcutaneous administration. Absorption after PO administration is incomplete; significant amounts undergo hepatic metabolism, resulting in low bioavailability (about 14%). Protein binding: 10%–21%. Widely distributed. Undergoes first-pass metabolism in liver. Excreted in urine. **Half-life:** 2 hrs.

USES

PO, Subcutaneous: Acute treatment of migraine headache with or without aura. **Subcutaneous:** Treatment of cluster headaches.

PRECAUTIONS

Contraindications: CVA, ischemic heart disease (including angina pectoris, history of MI, silent ischemia, Prinzmetal's angina), severe hepatic impairment, transient ischemic attack, uncontrolled hypertension, MAOI use within 14 days, use within 24 hrs of ergotamine preparations. **Cautions:** Hepatic/renal impairment, epilepsy, hypersensitivity to sulfonamides.

⌛ LIFESPAN CONSIDERATIONS

Pregnancy/Lactation: Unknown if distributed in breast milk. **Pregnancy Category C. Children:** Safety and efficacy not established. **Elderly:** No age-related precautions noted.

INTERACTIONS

DRUG: Ergotamine-containing medications may produce vasospastic reaction. **MAOIs** may increase concentration, half-life. **SSRIs** and **SNRI antidepressants** may increase risk of serotonin syndrome. **HERBAL:** None significant. **FOOD:** None known. **LAB VALUES:** None significant.

AVAILABILITY (Rx)

Injection, Pre-Filled Auto-Injector (Alsuma): 6 mg/0.5 ml. **Injection Solution (Imitrex):** 4 mg/0.5 ml, 6 mg/0.5 ml. **Sumavel DosePro:** 6 mg/0.5 ml. **Nasal Spray (Imitrex Nasal):** 5 mg/0.1 ml, 20 mg/0.1 ml. **Tablets (Imitrex):** 25 mg, 50 mg, 100 mg.

ADMINISTRATION/HANDLING

Subcutaneous
• Follow manufacturer's instructions for autoinjection device use.

PO
• Swallow tablets whole. • Take with full glass of water.

Nasal
• Unit contains only one spray—do not test before use. • Instruct pt to gently blow nose to clear nasal passages. • With head upright, close one nostril with index finger, breathe out gently through mouth. • Have pt insert nozzle into open nostril about ½ inch, close mouth and, while taking a breath through nose, release spray dosage by firmly pressing

S

plunger. • Instruct pt to remove nozzle from nose and gently breathe in through nose and out through mouth for 10–20 sec; do not breathe in deeply.

INDICATIONS/ROUTES/DOSAGE

Acute Migraine Headache

PO: ADULTS, ELDERLY: 25–100 mg. Dose may be repeated after at least 2 hrs. **Maximum:** 100 mg/single dose; 200 mg/24 hrs.

SUBCUTANEOUS: ADULTS, ELDERLY: Up to 6 mg. **Maximum:** Up to two 6-mg injections/24 hrs (separated by at least 1 hr).

INTRANASAL: ADULTS, ELDERLY: 5–20 mg; may repeat in 2 hrs. **Maximum:** 40 mg/24 hrs.

SIDE EFFECTS

Frequent: PO (10%–5%): Tingling, nasal discomfort. **Subcutaneous (greater than 10%):** Injection site reactions, tingling, warm/hot sensation, dizziness, vertigo. **Nasal (greater than 10%):** Altered taste, nausea, vomiting. **Occasional: PO (5%–1%):** Flushing, asthenia (loss of strength, energy), visual disturbances. **Subcutaneous (10%–2%):** Burning sensation, numbness, chest discomfort, drowsiness, asthenia (loss of strength, energy). **Nasal (5%–1%):** Nasopharyngeal discomfort, dizziness. **Rare: PO (less than 1%):** Agitation, eye irritation, dysuria. **Subcutaneous (less than 2%):** Anxiety, fatigue, diaphoresis, muscle cramps, myalgia. **Nasal (less than 1%):** Burning sensation.

ADVERSE EFFECTS/ TOXIC REACTIONS

Excessive dosage may produce tremor, redness of extremities, reduced respirations, cyanosis, seizures, paralysis. Serious arrhythmias occur rarely, esp. in pts with hypertension, obesity, smokers, diabetes, strong family history of coronary artery disease. Serotonin syndrome may occur (agitation, confusion, hallucinations, hyper-reflexia, myoclonus, shiver, tachycardia).

NURSING CONSIDERATIONS

BASELINE ASSESSMENT

Question for history of peripheral vascular disease, renal/hepatic impairment, possibility of pregnancy. Question regarding onset, location, duration of migraine, possible precipitating symptoms.

INTERVENTION/EVALUATION

Evaluate for relief of migraine headache and resulting photophobia, phonophobia (sound sensitivity), nausea, vomiting.

PATIENT/FAMILY TEACHING

• Follow proper technique for loading of autoinjector, injection technique, discarding of syringe. • Do not use more than 2 injections during any 24-hr period and allow at least 1 hr between injections. • Contact physician immediately if wheezing, palpitations, skin rash, facial swelling, pain/tightness in chest/throat occur.

sunitinib

HIGH ALERT

soo-**nit**-ih-nib
(Sutent)

BLACK BOX ALERT Hepatotoxicity may be severe and/or result in fatal liver failure.

Do not confuse sunitinib with imatinib or sorafenib.

◆CLASSIFICATION

PHARMACOTHERAPEUTIC: Tyrosine kinase inhibitor, vascular endothelial growth factor. **CLINICAL:** Antineoplastic.

ACTION

Inhibitory action against multiple kinases, growth factor receptors, stem cell factor receptors, colony-stimulating factor receptors, glial cell-line neurotrophic factor receptors. **Therapeutic Effect:** Prevents tumor cell growth, produces tumor regression, inhibits metastasis.

PHARMACOKINETICS

Metabolized in liver. Protein binding: 95%. Excreted mainly in feces, with lesser amount eliminated in urine. **Half-life:** 40–60 hrs.

USES

Treatment of GI stromal tumor after disease progression while on or demonstrating intolerance to imatinib. Treatment of advanced renal cell carcinoma. **OFF-LABEL:** Treatment of acute myeloid leukemia (AML), advanced thyroid cancer.

PRECAUTIONS

Contraindications: None significant. **Cautions:** Cardiac abnormalities, bleeding tendencies, hypertension.

LIFESPAN CONSIDERATIONS

Pregnancy/Lactation: Has potential for embryotoxic, teratogenic effects. Breast-feeding not recommended. **Pregnancy Category D. Children:** Safety and efficacy not established. **Elderly:** No age-related precautions noted.

INTERACTIONS

DRUG: **Atazanavir, clarithromycin, indinavir, itraconazole, ketoconazole, nefazodone, nelfinavir, ritonavir, saquinavir, voriconizole** may increase concentration, toxicity. **Carbamazepine, dexamethasone, phenobarbital, phenytoin, rifabutin, rifampin, rifapentin** may decrease concentration, effect. **HERBAL:** **St. John's wort** may decrease concentration. **FOOD:** **Grapefruit, grapefruit juice** may increase concentration. **LAB VALUES:** May increase serum alkaline phosphatase, bilirubin, amylase, lipase, creatinine, AST, ALT. May alter serum potassium, sodium, uric acid. May produce thrombocytopenia, neutropenia. May decrease serum phosphates, thyroid function.

AVAILABILITY (Rx)

Capsules: 12.5 mg, 25 mg, 50 mg.

ADMINISTRATION/HANDLING

PO

- Give without regard to food.

INDICATIONS/ROUTES/DOSAGE

GI Stromal Tumor, Renal Cell Carcinoma

PO: ADULTS, ELDERLY: 50 mg once daily for 4 wks, followed by 2 wks off.

Dose Modification

PO: ADULTS, ELDERLY: Dosage increase or reduction in 12.5-mg increments is recommended based on safety and tolerability.

SIDE EFFECTS

Stromal tumor: Common (42%–30%): Fatigue, diarrhea, anorexia, abdominal pain, nausea, hyperpigmentation. **Frequent (29%–18%):** Mucositis/stomatitis, vomiting, asthenia (loss of strength, energy), altered taste, constipation, fever. **Occasional (15%–8%):** Hypertension, rash, myalgia, headache, arthralgia, back pain, dyspnea, cough. **Renal carcinoma: Common (74%–43%):** Fatigue, diarrhea, nausea, mucositis/stomatitis, dyspepsia (heartburn, indigestion, epigastric pain), altered taste. **Frequent (38%–20%):** Rash, vomiting, constipation, hyperpigmentation, anorexia, arthralgia, dyspnea, hypertension, headache, abdominal pain. **Occasional (18%–11%):** Limb pain, peripheral/periorbital edema, dry skin, hair color change, myalgia, cough, back pain, dizziness, fever, tongue pain, flatulence, alopecia, dehydration.

ADVERSE EFFECTS/ TOXIC REACTIONS

Hand-foot syndrome occurs occasionally (14%), manifested as blistering/rash/ peeling of skin on palms of hands, soles of feet. Bleeding, decrease in left ventricular ejection fraction, deep vein thrombosis (DVT), pancreatitis, neutropenia, seizures occur rarely.

S

NURSING CONSIDERATIONS

BASELINE ASSESSMENT

Question possibility of pregnancy. Obtain baseline CBC, platelets, serum chemistries including electrolytes, renal/hepatic function tests (alkaline phosphatase, bilirubin, ALT, AST) before beginning therapy and prior to each treatment. Obtain baseline EKG, thyroid function tests.

INTERVENTION/EVALUATION

Assess eye area, lower extremities for early evidence of fluid retention. Offer antiemetics to control nausea, vomiting. Monitor daily pattern of bowel activity, stool consistency. Monitor CBC for evidence of neutropenia, thrombocytopenia; assess hepatic function tests for hepatotoxicity.

PATIENT/FAMILY TEACHING

• Avoid crowds, those with known infection. • Avoid contact with anyone who recently received live virus vaccine. • Do not have immunizations without physician's approval (drug lowers resistance). • Promptly report fever, unusual bruising/bleeding from any site.

tacrolimus

tak-roe-**li**-mus
(Prograf, Protopic)

BLACK BOX ALERT Increased susceptibility to infection and potential for development of lymphoma. Topical form associated with rare cases of malignancy. Should be used only for short-term and intermittent treatment.

Do not confuse Protopic with Protonix, Prograf with Prozac, or tacrolimus with everolimus, pimcrolimus, sirolimus, or temsirolimus.

◆CLASSIFICATION

PHARMACOTHERAPEUTIC: Immunologic agent. **CLINICAL:** Immunosuppressant (see p. 119C).

ACTION

Inhibits T-lymphocyte activation by binding to intracellular proteins, forming a complex, inhibiting phosphatase activity. **Therapeutic Effect:** Suppresses immunologically mediated inflammatory response; prevents organ transplant rejection.

PHARMACOKINETICS

Variably absorbed after PO administration (food reduces absorption). Protein binding: 99%. Extensively metabolized in liver. Primarily eliminated in feces. Not removed by hemodialysis. **Half-life:** 21–61 hrs.

USES

PO/injection: Prophylaxis of organ rejection in pts receiving allogeneic liver, kidney, heart transplant. Should be used concurrently with adrenal corticosteroids. In heart and kidney transplants pts, should be used in conjunction with azathioprine or mycophenolate. **Topical:** Atopic dermatitis. **OFF-LABEL:** Prevention of organ rejection in pts receiving allogeneic bone marrow, heart, pancreas, pancreatic island cell, small bowel transplant; treatment of autoimmune disease; severe recalcitrant psoriasis.

PRECAUTIONS

Contraindications: Concurrent use with cyclosporine (increases risk of nephrotoxicity), hypersensitivity to HCO-60 polyoxyl 60 hydrogenated castor oil (used in solution for injection). **Cautions:** Immunosuppressed pts, renal/hepatic impairment.

⌛ LIFESPAN CONSIDERATIONS

Pregnancy/Lactation: Crosses placenta. Hyperkalemia, renal dysfunction noted in neonates. Distributed in breast milk. Breast-feeding not recommended. **Pregnancy Category C. Children:** May require higher dosages (decreased bioavailability, increased clearance). May make post-transplant lymphoproliferative disorder more common, esp. in those younger than 3 yrs. **Elderly:** Age-related renal impairment may require dosage adjustment.

INTERACTIONS

DRUG: **Aluminium-containing antacids** may decrease absorption of tacrolimus. **Erythromycin, fluconazole, itraconazole, ketoconazole, lansoprazole** may increase concentration, risk of toxicity. **Rifampin** may decrease concentration, effect. **Potassium-sparing diuretics** may increase risk of hyperkalemia. **Cyclosporine** increases risk of nephrotoxicity. **Live virus vaccines** may potentiate virus replication, increase vaccine side effects, decrease pt's antibody response to vaccine. HERBAL: **St. John's wort** may decrease concentration, effect. FOOD: **Food** decreases rate/extent of absorption. **Grapefruit, grapefruit juice** may increase concentration, toxicity. LAB VALUES: May increase serum glucose, BUN, creatinine, potassium, triglycerides, cholesterol, bilirubin, amylase, AST, ALT. May decrease serum magnesium, Hgb, Hct, platelets. May alter leukocytes.

AVAILABILITY (Rx)

Capsules (Prograf): 0.5 mg, 1 mg, 5 mg. **Injection Solution (Prograf):** 5 mg/ml. **Ointment (Protopic):** 0.03%, 0.1%.

ADMINISTRATION/HANDLING

IV

Reconstitution • Dilute with appropriate amount (250–1,000 ml, depending on desired dose) 0.9% NaCl or D_5W to provide concentration between 0.004 and 0.02 mg/ml.

Rate of administration • Give as continuous IV infusion. • Continuously monitor pt for anaphylaxis for at least 30 min after start of infusion. • Stop infusion immediately at first sign of hypersensitivity reaction.

Storage • Store diluted infusion solution in glass or polyethylene containers and discard after 24 hrs. • Do not store in PVC container (decreased stability, potential for extraction).

PO

• Administer on empty stomach. • Do not give with grapefruit, grapefruit juice or within 2 hrs of antacids.

Topical

• For external use only. • Do not cover with occlusive dressing. • Rub gently, completely onto clean, dry skin.

IV INCOMPATIBILITIES

No known drug incompatibilities.

IV COMPATIBILITIES

Calcium gluconate, dexamethasone (Decadron), diphenhydramine (Benadryl), dobutamine (Dobutrex), dopamine (Intropin), furosemide (Lasix), heparin, hydromorphone (Dilaudid), insulin, leucovorin, lipids, lorazepam (Ativan), morphine, nitroglycerin, potassium chloride.

INDICATIONS/ROUTES/DOSAGE

Prevention of Liver Transplant Rejection

PO: ADULTS, ELDERLY: 0.1–0.15 mg/kg/day in 2 divided doses 12 hrs apart. Begin oral therapy no sooner than 6 hrs post-transplant. **CHILDREN:** 0.15–0.2 mg/kg/day in 2 divided doses 12 hrs apart. Begin oral therapy no sooner than 6 hrs post-transplant.

IV: ADULTS, ELDERLY, CHILDREN: 0.03–0.05 mg/kg/day as continuous infusion.

Prevention of Kidney Transplant Rejection

PO: ADULTS, ELDERLY: 0.2 mg/kg/day in 2 divided doses 12 hrs apart. May be given within 24 hrs of transplant.

IV: ADULTS, ELDERLY: 0.03–0.05 mg/kg/day as continuous infusion.

Prevention of Heart Transplant Rejection

PO: ADULTS, ELDERLY: Initially, 0.075 mg/kg/day in 2 divided doses 12 hrs apart. Begin oral therapy no sooner than 6 hrs post-transplant.

IV: ADULTS, ELDERLY: 0.01 mg/kg/day as continuous infusion.

T

Atopic Dermatitis

TOPICAL: ADULTS, ELDERLY, CHILDREN 2 YRS AND OLDER: Apply 0.03% or 0.1% ointment to affected area twice daily. Continue treatment for 1 wk after symptoms have resolved. If no improvement within 6 wks, re-examine to confirm diagnosis.

SIDE EFFECTS

Frequent (greater than 30%): Headache, tremor, insomnia, paresthesia, diarrhea, nausea, constipation, vomiting, abdominal pain, hypertension. **Occasional (29%–10%):** Rash, pruritus, anorexia, asthenia (loss of strength, energy), peripheral edema, photosensitivity.

ADVERSE EFFECTS/ TOXIC REACTIONS

Nephrotoxicity (characterized by increased serum creatinine, decreased urinary output), neurotoxicity (tremor, headache, altered mental status), pleural effusion occur commonly. Thrombocytopenia, leukocytosis, anemia, atelectasis, sepsis, infection occur occasionally.

NURSING CONSIDERATIONS

BASELINE ASSESSMENT

Assess medical, drug history, esp. renal function, use of other immunosuppressants. Have aqueous solution of epinephrine 1:1,000 available at bedside as well as O_2 before beginning IV infusion. Assess pt continuously for first 30 min following start of infusion and at frequent intervals thereafter.

INTERVENTION/EVALUATION

Closely monitor pts with renal impairment. Monitor lab values, esp. serum creatinine, potassium levels, CBC with differential, serum hepatic function tests. Monitor I&O closely. CBC should be performed weekly during first mo of therapy, twice monthly during second and third mos of treatment, then monthly throughout the first yr. Report any major change in pt assessment.

PATIENT/FAMILY TEACHING

• Take dose at same time each day. • Avoid crowds, those with infection. • Inform physician if decreased urination, chest pain, headache, dizziness, respiratory infection, rash, unusual bleeding/bruising occur. • Avoid exposure to sun, artificial light (may cause photosensitivity reaction).

tadalafil

tah-**dal**-ah-fill
(Adcirca, Cialis)
Do not confuse Adcirca with Advair or Advicor, or tadalafil with sildenafil or vardenafil.

◆CLASSIFICATION

PHARMACOTHERAPEUTIC: Phosphodiesterase inhibitor. **CLINICAL:** Erectile dysfunction adjunct.

ACTION

Inhibits phosphodiesterase type 5, the enzyme responsible for degrading cyclic guanosine monophosphate in corpus cavernosum of penis, pulmonary vascular smooth muscle, resulting in smooth muscle relaxation, increased blood flow. **Therapeutic Effect:** Facilitates erection, improves exercise ability.

PHARMACOKINETICS

Route	Onset	Peak	Duration
PO	60 min	—	36 hrs

Rapidly absorbed after PO administration. Protein binding: 94% Metabolized in liver. Primarily eliminated in feces. Drug has no effect on penile blood flow without sexual stimulation. **Half-life:** 17.5 hrs.

USES

Treatment of erectile dysfunction. Treatment of pulmonary arterial hypertension (PAH). **OFF-LABEL:** Raynaud's phenomenon.

PRECAUTIONS

Contraindications: Concurrent use of alpha-adrenergic blockers (other than minimum dose tamsulosin), concurrent use of sodium nitroprusside or nitrates in any form, severe hepatic impairment. **Cautions:** Renal/hepatic impairment, anatomical deformation of penis, pts who may be predisposed to priapism (sickle cell anemia, multiple myeloma, leukemia).

LIFESPAN CONSIDERATIONS

Pregnancy/Lactation: Pregnancy Category B. Children: Not indicated in this pt population. **Elderly:** No age-related precautions noted.

INTERACTIONS

DRUG: Alcohol increases risk of orthostatic hypotension. Potentiates hypotensive effects of **alpha-adrenergic blockers, nitrates. Erythromycin, itraconazole, ketoconazole, ritonavir, saquinavir** may increase concentration. **HERBAL:** None significant. **FOOD: Grapefruit, grapefruit juice** may increase concentration, toxicity. **LAB VALUES:** May alter hepatic function tests, increase GGTP.

AVAILABILITY (Rx)

Tablets (Cialis): 2.5 mg, 5 mg, 10 mg, 20 mg. **(Adcirca):** 20 mg.

ADMINISTRATION/HANDLING

PO

• May give without regard to food. • Take at least 30 min before anticipated sexual activity. • Administer Adcirca dose all at same time.

INDICATIONS/ROUTES/DOSAGE

Erectile Dysfunction

PO: ADULTS, ELDERLY: 2.5–5 mg once daily or 10 mg 30 min before sexual activity, as needed. Dose may be increased to 20 mg or decreased to 5 mg, based on pt tolerance. **Maximum dosing frequency:** Once daily.

PAH

PO: ADULTS, ELDERLY: 40 mg once daily.

Dosage in Renal Impairment

Creatinine clearance 31–50 ml/min: As needed dosing: Starting dose is 5 mg before sexual activity once daily. **Maximum dose:** 10 mg no more frequently than once q48h. No dose adjustment for once daily dosing. **Creatinine clearance less than 31 ml/min:** Starting dose is 5 mg before sexual activity. Not to be given more often than q72h. Daily dosing not recommended.

Dosage in Mild to Moderate Hepatic Impairment

Pts with Child-Pugh class A or B hepatic impairment should take no more than 10 mg once daily. Not recommended in severe hepatic impairment.

SIDE EFFECTS

Occasional: Headache, dyspepsia (heartburn, indigestion, epigastric pain), back pain, myalgia, nasal congestion, flushing, sudden hearing loss, visual field loss, postural hypotension.

ADVERSE EFFECTS/ TOXIC REACTIONS

Prolonged erections (lasting over 4 hrs), priapism (painful erections lasting over 6 hrs) occur rarely. Angina, chest pain, MI have been reported.

NURSING CONSIDERATIONS

BASELINE ASSESSMENT

Assess cardiovascular status before initiating treatment for erectile dysfunction. Assess renal/hepatic function tests.

INTERVENTION/EVALUATION

Monitor B/P.

PATIENT/FAMILY TEACHING

• Has no effect in absence of sexual stimulation. • Seek treatment immediately if erection persists for over 4 hrs. • Report sudden decrease or loss of hearing or vision. • Avoid alcohol (may increase risk of postural hypotension).

T

tamoxifen

HIGH ALERT

tam-**ox**-ih-fen
(Apo-Tamox 🍁, Nolvadex-D 🍁, Novo-Tamoxifen 🍁, Tamofen 🍁)

BLACK BOX ALERT Serious, possibly life-threatening stroke, pulmonary emboli, uterine malignancy (endometrial adenocarcinoma, uterine sarcoma) have occurred.

Do not confuse tamoxifen with pentoxifylline, tamsulosin, or temazepam.

CLASSIFICATION

PHARMACOTHERAPEUTIC: Nonsteroidal antiestrogen. **CLINICAL:** Antineoplastic (see p. 88C).

ACTION

Competes with estradiol for estrogen-receptor binding sites in breast, uterus, vaginal cells. **Therapeutic Effect:** Inhibits DNA synthesis, estrogen response.

PHARMACOKINETICS

Well absorbed from GI tract. Metabolized in liver. Primarily eliminated in feces by biliary system. **Half-life:** 7 days.

USES

Adjunct treatment in advanced breast cancer, reduce risk of breast cancer in pts at high risk, reduce risk of invasive breast cancer in women with ductal carcinoma *in situ* (DCIS), metastatic breast cancer in women and men. **OFF-LABEL:** Induction of ovulation, treatment of melanoma, desmoid tumors. Treatment of gynecomastia, pancreatic carcinoma, precocious puberty in females.

PRECAUTIONS

Contraindications: Concomitant coumarin-type therapy when used in treatment of breast cancer in high-risk women, history of deep vein thrombosis (DVT) or pulmonary embolism in high-risk women. **Cautions:** Leukopenia, thrombocytopenia, pregnancy.

LIFESPAN CONSIDERATIONS

Pregnancy/Lactation: If possible, avoid use during pregnancy, esp. first trimester. May cause fetal harm. Unknown if distributed in breast milk. Breast-feeding not recommended. **Pregnancy Category D.** **Children:** Safe and effective in girls 2–10 yrs with McCune Albright syndrome, precocious puberty. **Elderly:** No age-related precautions noted.

INTERACTIONS

DRUG: **Anticoagulants** may increase risk of bleeding. **Cytotoxic agents** may increase risk of thromboembolic events. **HERBAL:** Avoid **black cohosh, dong quai** in estrogen-dependent tumors. **St. John's wort** may decrease concentration, effect. **FOOD:** None known. **LAB VALUES:** May increase serum cholesterol, calcium, triglycerides, hepatic enzymes.

AVAILABILITY (Rx)

Tablets: 10 mg, 20 mg.

ADMINISTRATION/HANDLING

PO

- Give without regard to food.

INDICATIONS/ROUTES/DOSAGE

Adjunctive Treatment of Breast Cancer

PO: ADULTS, ELDERLY: 20–40 mg/day. Give doses greater than 20 mg/day in divided doses.

Prevention of Breast Cancer in High-Risk Women, Ductal Carcinoma *in Situ*

PO: ADULTS, ELDERLY: 20 mg/day for 5 yrs.

SIDE EFFECTS

Frequent: **Women (greater than 10%):** Hot flashes, nausea, vomiting. **Occasional:** **Women (9%–1%):** Changes in menstruation, genital itching, vaginal discharge, endometrial hyperplasia, polyps. **Men:** Impotence, decreased libido. **Men and women:** Headache, nausea, vomiting, rash, bone pain, confusion, weakness, drowsiness.

T

ADVERSE EFFECTS/ TOXIC REACTIONS

Retinopathy, corneal opacity, decreased visual acuity noted in pts receiving extremely high dosages (240–320 mg/day) for longer than 17 mos.

NURSING CONSIDERATIONS

BASELINE ASSESSMENT

Obtain estrogen receptor assay prior to therapy. Obtain baseline breast and gynecologic exams, mammogram results. CBC, platelet count, serum calcium levels should be checked before and periodically during therapy.

INTERVENTION/EVALUATION

Be alert to increased bone pain, ensure adequate pain relief. Monitor I&O, weight. Observe for edema, esp. of dependent areas, signs and symptoms of DVT. Assess for hypercalcemia (increased urinary volume, excessive thirst, nausea, vomiting, constipation, hypotonicity of muscles, deep bone/flank pain, renal stones).

PATIENT/FAMILY TEACHING

• Report vaginal bleeding/discharge/itching, leg cramps, weight gain, shortness of breath, weakness. • May initially experience increase in bone, tumor pain (appears to indicate good tumor response). • Contact physician if nausea, vomiting continue at home. • Nonhormonal contraceptives are recommended during treatment.

tamsulosin

tam-**sool**-o-sin
(Flomax, Novo-Tamsulosin ✤)
Do not confuse Flomax with Flonase, Flovent, Foltx, Fosamax, or Volmax, or tamsulosin with tacrolimus, tamoxifen, or terazosin.

FIXED-COMBINATION(S)

Tamsulosin/dutasteride: (an androgen hormone inhibitor): 0.4 mg/0.5 mg.

◆CLASSIFICATION

PHARMACOTHERAPEUTIC: Alpha$_1$-adrenergic blocker. **CLINICAL:** Benign prostatic hyperplasia agent.

ACTION

Targets receptors around bladder neck, prostate capsule. **Therapeutic Effect:** Relaxes smooth muscle, improves urinary flow, symptoms of prostatic hyperplasia.

PHARMACOKINETICS

Well absorbed, widely distributed. Protein binding: 94%–99%. Metabolized in liver. Primarily excreted in urine. Unknown if removed by hemodialysis. **Half-life:** 9–13 hrs.

USES

Treatment of symptoms of benign prostatic hyperplasia (BPH), alone or in combination with dutasteride (Avodart). **OFF-LABEL:** Treatment of bladder outlet obstruction or dysfunction.

PRECAUTIONS

Contraindications: None significant. **Cautions:** Concurrent use of phosphodiesterase (PDE$_5$) inhibitors (sildenafil, tadalafil, vardenafil), renal impairment.

LIFESPAN CONSIDERATIONS

Pregnancy/Lactation: Not indicated for use in women. **Pregnancy Category B. Children:** Not indicated in this pt population. **Elderly:** No age-related precautions noted.

INTERACTIONS

DRUG: **Other alpha-adrenergic blocking agents (e.g., doxazosin, prazosin, terazosin)** may increase alpha-blockade effects of both drugs. **Sildenafil, tadafil, vardenafil** may cause severe hypotension. May alter ef-

T

fects of **warfarin.** HERBAL: Avoid **saw palmetto** (limited experience with this combination). FOOD: None known. LAB VALUES: None significant.

AVAILABILITY (Rx)

Capsules: 0.4 mg.

ADMINISTRATION/HANDLING

PO

• Give at same time each day, 30 min after the same meal. • Do not crush/open or chew capsule.

INDICATIONS/ROUTES/DOSAGE

Benign Prostatic Hyperplasia (BPH)

PO: ADULTS: 0.4 mg once a day, approximately 30 min after same meal each day. May increase dosage to 0.8 mg if inadequate response in 2–4 wks.

SIDE EFFECTS

Frequent (9%–7%): Dizziness, drowsiness. **Occasional (5%–3%):** Headache, anxiety, insomnia, orthostatic hypotension. **Rare (less than 2%):** Nasal congestion, pharyngitis, rhinitis, nausea, vertigo, impotence.

ADVERSE EFFECTS/ TOXIC REACTIONS

First-dose syncope (hypotension with sudden loss of consciousness) may occur within 30–90 min after initial dose. May be preceded by tachycardia (pulse rate of 120–160 beats/min).

NURSING CONSIDERATIONS

BASELINE ASSESSMENT

Assess history of prostatic hyperplasia (difficulty initiating urine stream, dribbling, sense of urgency, leaking). Question for sensitivity to tamsulosin, use of other alpha-adrenergic blocking agents, warfarin.

INTERVENTION/EVALUATION

Assist with ambulation if dizziness occurs. Monitor renal function, I&O, weight changes, peripheral edema, B/P. Monitor for first-dose syncope.

PATIENT/FAMILY TEACHING

• Take at same time each day, 30 min after the same meal. • Use caution when getting up from sitting or lying position. • Avoid tasks that require alertness, motor skills until response to drug is established. • Do not chew, crush, open capsule.

tapentadol

tah-**pen**-tah-doll
(Nucynta)

Do not confuse tapentadol with tramadol.

◆CLASSIFICATION

CLINICAL: Analgesic.

ACTION

Binds to and activates mu-opioid receptors in the central nervous system, increases norepinephrine by inhibiting its reabsorption into nerve cells. **Therapeutic Effect:** Produces analgesia.

PHARMACOKINETICS

Metabolized in liver. Primarily excreted in the urine. Widely distributed. Protein binding: 20%. **Half-life:** 4 hrs.

USES

Relief of moderate to severe acute pain in adults 18 yrs and older.

PRECAUTIONS

Contraindications: Significant respiratory depression, acute or severe bronchial asthma or hypercapnia, paralytic ileus, concurrent use or ingestion within 14 days of monoamine oxidase inhibitor (MAOI) use. **Cautions:** Conditions accompanied by hypoxia, hypercapnia or decreased respiratory reserve (asthma, COPD, severe obesity, sleep apnea syndrome, myxedema, CNS depression), those with head injury, intracranial lesions, pancreatic or biliary disease, renal or hepatic impairment, history of seizures, conditions that increase risk of seizures.

LIFESPAN CONSIDERATIONS

Pregnancy/lactation: Unknown if drug crosses placenta or is distributed in breast milk. **Pregnancy Category C. Children:** Not recommended for use in this pt population. **Elderly:** Age-related renal impairment may increase risk of side effects.

INTERACTIONS

DRUG: **Alcohol, CNS depressants** may increase CNS depression, respiratory depression. Serotonin syndrome may occur with use of **MAOIs, SSRIs** (e.g., **fluoxetine**), **tricyclic antidepressants** (e.g., **amitriptyline**), **triptans** (e.g., **sumatriptan**). HERBAL: **Kava kava, St. John's wort, valerian** may increase CNS depression. FOOD: None known. LAB VALUES: None known.

AVAILABILITY (RX)

Tablets: 50 mg, 75 mg, 100 mg.

ADMINISTRATION/HANDLING

PO

• Give without regard to food. • Tablets may be crushed.

INDICATIONS/ROUTES/DOSAGE

Note: Not recommended in severe renal or hepatic impairment.

Pain Control

PO: ADULTS, ELDERLY: 50–100 mg every 4–6 hrs as needed. **Maximum:** 600 mg/day.

Dosage in Hepatic Impairment

Moderate impairment: 50 mg q8h (**Maximum:** 3 doses/24 hrs).

SIDE EFFECTS

Frequent (greater than 10%): Nausea, dizziness, vomiting, sleepiness, headache.

ADVERSE EFFECTS/ TOXIC REACTIONS

Respiratory depression, serotonin syndrome.

NURSING CONSIDERATIONS

BASELINE ASSESSMENT

Assess onset, type, location, and duration of pain. Obtain vital signs before giving medication. If respirations are 12/min or lower, withhold medication, contact physician.

INTERVENTION/EVALUATION

Be alert for decreased respirations or B/P. Initiate deep breathing and coughing exercises, particularly in those with impaired pulmonary function. Assess for clinical improvement and record onset of pain relief.

PATIENT/FAMILY TEACHING

• Avoid tasks that require alertness, motor skills until response to drug is established. • Avoid alcohol, CNS depressants. • Report nausea, vomiting, shortness of breath, difficulty breathing.

telavancin

tell-ah-**van**-sin
(Vibativ)

BLACK BOX ALERT May cause fetal harm (low birth weight, limb malformations). Women of childbearing potential should have pregnancy test before treatment; avoid use during pregnancy unless benefit to pt outweighs fetal risk.

Do not confuse Vibativ with Vibramycin, Vibra-Tabs, or vigabatrin.

CLASSIFICATION

PHARMACOTHERAPEUTIC: Lipoglycopeptide antibacterial. **CLINICAL:** Antibiotic.

ACTION

Inhibits bacterial cell wall synthesis by blocking polymerization and crosslinking of peptidoglycan. Also disrupts membrane potential and changes cell wall

T

permeability. **Therapeutic Effect:** Bactericidal. Antibiotic.

PHARMACOKINETICS

Not metabolized in liver. Protein binding: 93%. Primarily excreted unchanged in urine. Not removed by hemodialysis. **Half-life:** 8–9 hrs.

USES

Treatment of complicated skin, soft tissue infections caused by gram-positive microorganisms, including methicillin susceptible or resistant *S. aureus,* vancomycin susceptible *Enterococcus.* **OFF-LABEL:** Treatment of hospital-acquired pneumonia (nosocomial infection), including methicillin-sensitive or methicillin-resistant *S. aureus,* vancomycin-susceptible *Enterococcus faecalis* and *S. pyogenes.*

PRECAUTIONS

Contraindications: None. **Cautions:** Renal dysfunction, concurrent therapy with other nephrotoxic medications. Avoid use in pts with history of congenital QT syndrome, known prolongation of QT interval, uncompensated heart failure, severe left ventricular hypertrophy, or receiving treatment with other drugs known to prolong QT interval.

LIFESPAN CONSIDERATIONS

Pregnancy/Lactation: May cause fetal harm at regular dosage. Unknown if distributed in breast milk. **Pregnancy Category C. Children:** Safety and efficacy not established. **Elderly:** Age-related renal impairment may increase risk of nephrotoxicity; dosage adjustment recommended.

INTERACTIONS

DRUG: Telavancin may increase levels/effects of **dronedarone, nilotinib, pimozide, quinine, tetrabenazene, thioridazine, ziprasidone. Ciprofloxacin** may increase levels/effect. **HERBAL:** None significant. **FOOD:** None known. **LAB VALUES:** May alter serum potassium. May increase AST, ALT, serum bilirubin, BUN, creatinine, PT, aPTT, INR. May decrease Hgb, Hct, WBC count.

AVAILABILITY (Rx)

Injection, Powder for Reconstitution: 250-mg, 750-mg single-dose vial.

ADMINISTRATION/HANDLING

IV

◀ALERT▶ Give by intermittent IV infusion (piggyback). Do not give by IV push (may result in exaggerated hypotension).

Reconstitution • **250-mg vial:** Reconstitute with 15 ml Sterile Water for Injection, D_5W, or 0.9% NaCl to provide concentration of 15 mg/ml (total volume approximately 17 ml). • **750-mg vial:** Reconstitute with 45 ml Sterile Water for Injection, D_5W, or 0.9% NaCl to provide concentration of 15 mg/ml (total volume approximately 50 ml). • Prior to administration, further dilute with D_5W or 0.9% NaCl to final concentration of 0.6–8 mg/ml.

Rate of administration • Infuse over at least 60 min.

Storage • Discard if particulate is present. • Following reconstitution, drug is stable for 4 hrs at room temperature or 72 hrs if refrigerated in vial or infusion bag.

IV COMPATIBILITY

Do not mix with any other medication.

INDICATIONS/ROUTES/DOSAGE

Usual Parenteral Dosage

IV INFUSION: ADULTS, ELDERLY: 10 mg/kg once every 24 hrs for 7–14 days. Duration based on severity and infection site and clinical progress of pt.

Dosage in Renal Impairment

Creatinine Clearance	Dosage
50 ml/min or greater	10 mg/kg every 24 hrs
30–49 ml/min	7.5 mg/kg every 24 hrs
10–29 ml/min	10 mg/kg every 48 hrs

SIDE EFFECTS

Frequent (33%–27%): Taste disturbance (metallic or soapy), nausea. **Occasional** (14%–6%): Vomiting, foamy urine, diarrhea, dizziness, pruritus. **Rare** (4%–2%): Rigors, rash, infusion site pain, anorexia, infusion site erythema.

ADVERSE EFFECTS/ TOXIC REACTIONS

Nephrotoxicity (change in amount/frequency of urination, increased thirst), diarrhea due to *C. difficile* may occur. "Red-neck syndrome" characterized by erythema on face, neck, upper torso, tachycardia, hypotension, myalgia, angioedema may occur from too-rapid rate of infusion.

NURSING CONSIDERATIONS

BASELINE ASSESSMENT

Pregnancy test should be obtained prior to treatment. Obtain baseline serum creatinine, creatinine clearance prior to initiating telavancin therapy, every 48–72 hrs, and after treatment is completed. Obtain culture and sensitivity test before giving first dose (therapy may begin before results are known).

INTERVENTION/EVALUATION

Monitor renal function tests, I&O. Assess skin for rash. Avoid administering infusion at too-rapid rate ("red-neck syndrome"). Monitor daily pattern of bowel activity, stool consistency.

PATIENT/FAMILY TEACHING

• Use effective contraception during treatment. • Notify physician if rash, signs/symptoms of nephrotoxicity, diarrhea occur. • Lab tests are important part of total therapy.

telmisartan

tel-meh-**sar**-tan
(Micardis)

BLACK BOX ALERT May cause fetal injury, mortality if used during second or third trimester of pregnancy.

FIXED-COMBINATION(S)

Micardis HCT: telmisartan/hydrochlorothiazide (a diuretic): 40 mg/12.5 mg, 80 mg/12.5 mg. **Twinsta:** telmisartan/amlodipine (a calcium channel blocker): 40 mg/5 mg, 40 mg/10 mg, 80 mg/5 mg, 80 mg/10 mg.

◆CLASSIFICATION

PHARMACOTHERAPEUTIC: Angiotensin II receptor antagonist. **CLINICAL:** Antihypertensive (see p. 10C).

ACTION

Blocks vasoconstrictor and aldosterone-secreting effects of angiotensin II, inhibiting binding of angiotensin II to AT_1 receptors. **Therapeutic Effect:** Causes vasodilation, decreases peripheral resistance, decreases B/P.

PHARMACOKINETICS

Route	Onset	Peak	Duration
PO (reduce B/P)	1–2 hrs	—	24 hrs

Rapidly, completely absorbed after PO administration. Protein binding: greater than 99%. Undergoes metabolism in liver to inactive metabolite. Excreted in feces. Unknown if removed by hemodialysis. **Half-life:** 24 hrs.

USES

Treatment of hypertension alone or in combination with other antihypertensives. Reduces risk of stroke, MI, death in pts 55 yrs of age or older with cardiovascular abnormalities (e.g., coronary artery disease, high-risk diabetes mellitus). **OFF-LABEL:** Treatment of CHF.

PRECAUTIONS

Contraindications: None known. **Cautions:** Volume-depleted pts, hepatic/renal impairment, renal artery stenosis (unilateral, bilateral).

T

LIFESPAN CONSIDERATIONS

Pregnancy/Lactation: May cause fetal harm. Unknown if drug is distributed in breast milk. **Pregnancy Category C (D if used in second or third trimester). Children:** Safety and efficacy not established. **Elderly:** No age-related precautions noted.

INTERACTIONS

DRUG: Increases **digoxin** concentration, risk of toxicity. Slightly decreases **warfarin** concentration. HERBAL: **Ephedra, ginseng, yohimbe** may worsen hypertension. **Garlic** may increase antihypertensive effect. FOOD: None known. LAB VALUES: May increase serum creatinine, BUN, uric acid, cholesterol. May decrease Hgb, Hct.

AVAILABILITY (Rx)

Tablets: 20 mg, 40 mg, 80 mg.

ADMINISTRATION/HANDLING

PO

- Give without regard to meals.

INDICATIONS/ROUTES/DOSAGE

Hypertension

PO: ADULTS, ELDERLY: 40 mg once daily. Range: 20–80 mg/day.

Risk Reduction

PO: ADULTS, ELDERLY: 80 mg once daily.

SIDE EFFECTS

Occasional (7%–3%): Upper respiratory tract infection, sinusitis, back/leg pain, diarrhea. Rare (1%): Dizziness, headache, fatigue, nausea, heartburn, myalgia, cough, peripheral edema.

ADVERSE EFFECTS/ TOXIC REACTIONS

Overdosage may manifest as hypotension, tachycardia; bradycardia occurs less often.

NURSING CONSIDERATIONS

BASELINE ASSESSMENT

Obtain B/P, apical pulse immediately before each dose, in addition to regular monitoring (be alert to fluctuations). If excessive reduction in B/P occurs, place pt in supine position, feet slightly elevated. Assess medication history (esp. diuretics). Question for history of hepatic/renal impairment, renal artery stenosis. Obtain BUN, serum creatinine, Hgb, Hct, vital signs (particularly B/P, pulse rate).

INTERVENTION/EVALUATION

Monitor B/P, pulse, serum electrolytes, renal function. Monitor for hypotension when initiating therapy.

PATIENT/FAMILY TEACHING

- Avoid tasks that require alertness, motor skills until response to drug is established (possible dizziness effect). • Maintain proper fluid intake. • Pts should take measures to avoid pregnancy. • Inform physician as soon as possible if pregnancy occurs. • Report any sign of infection (sore throat, fever). • Avoid excessive exertion during hot weather (risk of dehydration, hypotension).

temazepam

tem-**az**-eh-pam
(Apo-Temazepam ✦, Novo-Temazepam ✦, PMS-Temazepam ✦, Restoril)

Do not confuse Restoril with Risperdal, Vistaril, or Zestril, or temazepam with flurazepam, lorazepam, or tamoxifen.

CLASSIFICATION

PHARMACOTHERAPEUTIC: Benzodiazepine **(Schedule IV). CLINICAL:** Sedative-hypnotic (see p. 149C).

ACTION

Enhances action of inhibitory neurotransmitter gamma-aminobutyric acid (GABA), resulting in CNS depression. **Therapeutic Effect:** Induces sleep.

PHARMACOKINETICS

Well absorbed from GI tract. Protein binding: 96%. Widely distributed. Crosses blood-brain barrier. Metabolized in liver. Primarily excreted in urine. Not removed by hemodialysis. Half-life: 9.5–12.4 hrs.

USES

Short-term treatment of insomnia (5 wks or less). Reduces sleep-induction time, number of nocturnal awakenings; increases length of sleep. OFF-LABEL: Treatment of anxiety, depression, panic attacks.

PRECAUTIONS

Contraindications: Angle-closure glaucoma; CNS depression; pregnancy, breast-feeding; severe, uncontrolled pain; sleep apnea. Cautions: Mental impairment, pts with drug dependence potential.

LIFESPAN CONSIDERATIONS

Pregnancy/Lactation: Crosses placenta. May be distributed in breast milk. Chronic ingestion during pregnancy may produce withdrawal symptoms, CNS depression in neonates. **Pregnancy Category X. Children:** Not recommended in those younger than 18 yrs. **Elderly:** Use small initial doses with gradual dosage increases to avoid ataxia, excessive sedation.

INTERACTIONS

DRUG: **Alcohol, other CNS depressants** may increase CNS depression. HERBAL: **St. John's wort** may decrease concentration. **Gotu kola, kava kava, St. John's wort, valerian** may increase CNS depression. FOOD: None known. LAB VALUES: None significant.

AVAILABILITY (Rx)

Capsules: 7.5 mg, 15 mg, 30 mg.

ADMINISTRATION/HANDLING

PO

• Give without regard to meals. • Capsules may be emptied and mixed with food.

INDICATIONS/ROUTES/DOSAGE

Insomnia

PO: ADULTS, CHILDREN 18 YRS AND OLDER: 15–30 mg at bedtime. ELDERLY, DEBILITATED: 7.5–15 mg at bedtime.

SIDE EFFECTS

Frequent: Drowsiness, sedation, rebound insomnia (may occur for 1–2 nights after drug is discontinued), dizziness, confusion, euphoria. Occasional: Asthenia (loss of strength, energy), anorexia, diarrhea. Rare: Paradoxical CNS excitement, restlessness (particularly in elderly, debilitated pts).

ADVERSE EFFECTS/ TOXIC REACTIONS

Abrupt or too-rapid withdrawal may result in pronounced restlessness, irritability, insomnia, hand tremor, abdominal/muscle cramps, vomiting, diaphoresis, seizures. Overdose results in drowsiness, confusion, diminished reflexes, respiratory depression, coma. **Antidote:** Flumazenil (see Appendix M for dosage).

NURSING CONSIDERATIONS

BASELINE ASSESSMENT

Question for possibility of pregnancy before initiating therapy (Pregnancy Category X). Assess B/P, pulse, respirations immediately before administration. Raise bed rails. Provide environment conducive to sleep (back rub, quiet environment, low lighting). Assess mental status, sleep patterns.

INTERVENTION/EVALUATION

Assess elderly or debilitated pts for paradoxical reaction, particularly during early therapy. Monitor respiratory, cardiovascular, mental status. Evaluate for therapeutic response: decrease in number of nocturnal awakenings, increase in length of sleep.

PATIENT/FAMILY TEACHING

• Avoid alcohol, other CNS depressants. • May cause daytime drowsiness. • Avoid tasks that require alertness, motor skills until response to drug is established.

• Take approximately 30 min before bedtime. • Inform physician if pregnant or planning to become pregnant.

temozolomide

HIGH ALERT

teh-moe-**zoll**-oh-mide
(Temodal, Temodar)
Do not confuse Temodar with Tambocor.

CLASSIFICATION

PHARMACOTHERAPEUTIC: Imidazotetrazine derivative. **CLINICAL:** Antineoplastic (see p. 88C).

ACTION

Acts as prodrug and is converted to highly active cytotoxic metabolite. Cytotoxic effect is associated with methylation of DNA. **Therapeutic Effect:** Inhibits DNA replication, causing cell death.

PHARMACOKINETICS

Rapidly, completely absorbed after PO administration. Protein binding: 15%. Peak plasma concentration occurs in 1 hr. Penetrates blood-brain barrier. Eliminated primarily in urine and, to much lesser extent, in feces. **Half-life:** 1.6–1.8 hrs.

USES

Treatment of adults with refractory anaplastic astrocytoma; newly diagnosed glioblastoma multiforme (concomitantly with radiotherapy, then as maintenance therapy). **OFF-LABEL:** Malignant glioma, metastatic melanoma.

PRECAUTIONS

Contraindications: Hypersensitivity to dacarbazine, pregnancy. **Cautions:** Severe renal/hepatic impairment, bacterial/viral infection, elderly.

LIFESPAN CONSIDERATIONS

Pregnancy/Lactation: May cause fetal harm. May produce malformation of external organs, soft tissue, skeleton. If possible, avoid use during pregnancy. Unknown if drug is distributed in breast milk. **Pregnancy Category D. Children:** Safety and efficacy not established. **Elderly:** Those older than 70 yrs may experience higher risk of developing grade 4 neutropenia, grade 4 thrombocytopenia.

INTERACTIONS

DRUG: Medications causing blood dyscrasias (altering blood cell counts) may increase leukopenic, thrombocytopenic effects. **Bone marrow depressants** may increase myelosuppression. **Live virus vaccines** may potentiate virus replication, increase vaccine side effects, decrease pt's antibody response to vaccine. **HERBAL:** None significant. **FOOD: All foods** decrease rate, extent of drug absorption. **LAB VALUES:** May decrease Hgb, neutrophil, platelet, WBC counts.

AVAILABILITY (Rx)

Capsules: 5 mg, 20 mg, 100 mg, 140 mg, 180 mg, 250 mg. **Injection, Powder for Reconstitution:** 100 mg.

ADMINISTRATION/HANDLING

IV

• Reconstitute each 100-mg vial with 41 ml Sterile Water for Injection to provide concentration of 2.5 mg/ml. • Swirl gently; do not shake. • Do NOT further dilute. • Infuse over 90 min. • Stable for 14 hrs (includes infusion time).

PO

• Food reduces rate, extent of absorption; increases risk of nausea, vomiting. • For best results, administer at bedtime. • Swallow capsule whole with glass of water. Do not open, chew capsules. • If unable to swallow, may open capsule and dissolve in apple juice, applesauce (avoid exposure to cytotoxic agent).

INDICATIONS/ROUTES/DOSAGE

Anaplastic Astrocytoma

IV INFUSION, PO: ADULTS, ELDERLY: Initially, 150 mg/m^2/day for 5 consecutive days of 28-day treatment cycle. Subsequent doses based on platelet count, absolute neurophil count (ANC) during previous cycle. ANC greater than 1,500 per microliter and platelets more than 100,000 per microliter. Maintenance: 200 mg/m^2/day for 5 days q4wk. Continue until disease progression is observed. Minimum: 100 mg/m^2/day for 5 days q4wk.

Glioblastoma Multiforme

IV INFUSION, PO: ADULTS, ELDERLY: 75 mg/m^2 daily for 42 days. Maintenance: (Cycle 1): 150 mg/m^2 once daily for 5 days followed by 23 days without treatment. (Cycles 2–6): 200 mg/m^2 once daily for 5 days followed by 23 days without treatment.

SIDE EFFECTS

Frequent (53%–33%): Nausea, vomiting, headache, fatigue, constipation, seizure. **Occasional (16%–10%):** Diarrhea, asthenia (loss of strength, energy), fever, dizziness, peripheral edema, incoordination, insomnia. **Rare (9%–5%):** Paresthesia, drowsiness, anorexia, urinary incontinence, anxiety, pharyngitis, cough.

ADVERSE EFFECTS/ TOXIC REACTIONS

Myelosuppression is characterized by neutropenia and thrombocytopenia, with elderly and women showing higher incidence of developing severe myelosuppression. Usually occurs within first few cycles; is not cumulative. Nadir occurs in approximately 26–28 days, with recovery within 14 days of nadir.

NURSING CONSIDERATIONS

BASELINE ASSESSMENT

Before dosing, absolute neutrophil count (ANC) must be greater than 1,500 and platelet count greater than 100,000. Potential for nausea, vomiting readily controlled with antiemetic therapy.

INTERVENTION/EVALUATION

Obtain CBC on day 22 (21 days after first dose) or within 48 hrs of that day and weekly until ANC is greater than 1,500 and platelet count is greater than 100,000. Monitor for hematologic toxicity (fever, sore throat, signs of local infection, unusual bruising/bleeding from any site), symptoms of anemia (excessive fatigue, weakness).

PATIENT/FAMILY TEACHING

• To reduce nausea/vomiting, take on an empty stomach. • Promptly report fever, sore throat, signs of local infection, unusual bruising/bleeding from any site. • Avoid crowds, those with infection. • Do not have immunizations without physician's approval. • Avoid pregnancy.

temsirolimus HIGH ALERT

tem-sir-o-**le**-mus
(Torisel)
Do not confuse temsirolimus with everolimus, sirolimus, or tacrolimus.

CLASSIFICATION

PHARMACOTHERAPEUTIC: Kinase inhibitor. **CLINICAL:** Antineoplastic (see p. 88C).

ACTION

Prevents activation of mTOR (mammalian target of rapamycin), preventing tumor cell division. **Therapeutic Effect:** Inhibits tumor cell growth, produces tumor regression.

PHARMACOKINETICS

Undergoes extensive hepatic metabolism. Eliminated primarily in feces. **Half-life:** 17 hrs.

USES

Treatment of advanced renal cell carcinoma.

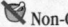

T

PRECAUTIONS

Contraindications: None significant. **Cautions:** Hypersensitivity to sirolimus, any antihistamine, those who cannot receive an antihistamine for other medical reasons, diabetes mellitus, immunosuppression.

LIFESPAN CONSIDERATIONS

Pregnancy/Lactation: May cause fetal harm. Unknown if distributed in breast milk. **Pregnancy Category D. Children:** Safety and efficacy not established. **Elderly:** No age-related precautions noted.

INTERACTIONS

DRUG: Atazanavir, clarithromycin, indinavir, itraconazole, ketoconazole, nefazodone, nelfinavir, ritonavir, saquinavir, voriconazole may increase concentration. **Carbamazepine, dexamethasone, phenobarbital, phenytoin, rifabutin, rifampin, rifapentin** may decrease concentration. **FOOD: Grapefruit, grapefruit juice** may increase plasma concentration. **HERBAL: St. John's wort** may decrease plasma concentration. **LAB VALUES:** May increase AST, serum bilirubin, alkaline phosphatase, creatinine, glucose, cholesterol, triglycerides. May decrease WBCs, neutrophils, Hgb, platelets, serum phosphorus, potassium.

AVAILABILITY (Rx)

Injection Solution Kit: 25 mg/ml supplied with 1.8-ml diluent vial.

ADMINISTRATION/HANDLING

IV

Reconstitution • Inject 1.8 ml of diluent into vial. • The vial contains an overfill of 0.2 ml (30 mg/1.2 ml). • Due to the overfill, the drug concentration of resulting solution will be 10 mg/ml. • A total volume of 3 ml will be obtained, including the overfill. • Mix well by inverting the vial. Allow sufficient time for air bubbles to subside. • Mixture must be injected rapidly into 250 ml 0.9% NaCl. • Invert bag to mix; avoid excessive shaking (may cause foaming).

Rate of administration • Administer through an in-line filter not greater than 5 microns; infuse over 30–60 min. • Final diluted infusion solution should be completed within 6 hrs from the time drug solution and diluent mixture is added to the 250 ml 0.9% NaCl.

Storage • Refrigerate kit • Reconstituted solution appears clear to slightly turbid, colorless to yellow, and free from visual particulates. • The 10 mg/ml drug solution/diluent mixture is stable for up to 24 hrs at room temperature. • Discard after 8 hrs.

IV INCOMPATIBILITIES

Both acids and bases degrade solution; combinations of temsirolimus with agents capable of modifying solution pH should be avoided.

INDICATIONS/ROUTES/DOSAGE

ALERT Pre-treat with diphenhydramine, IV, 25–50 mg 30 min before infusion.

Renal Cancer

IV: ADULTS/ELDERLY: 25 mg infused over 30–60 minutes once weekly. Treatment should continue until disease progresses or unacceptable toxicity occurs.

SIDE EFFECTS

Common (51%–32%): Asthenia (loss of strength, energy), rash, mucositis, nausea, edema (includes facial edema and peripheral edema), anorexia. **Frequent (28%–20%):** Generalized pain, dyspnea, diarrhea, cough, fever, abdominal pain, constipation, back pain, impaired taste. **Occasional (19%–8%):** Weight loss, vomiting, pruritus, chest pain, headache, nail disorder, insomnia, nosebleed, dry skin, acne, chills, myalgia.

ADVERSE EFFECTS/ TOXIC REACTIONS

UTI occurs in 15% of pts, hypersensitivity reaction in 9%, pneumonia in 8%, upper respiratory tract infection, hypertension, conjunctivitis in 7%.

NURSING CONSIDERATIONS

BASELINE ASSESSMENT

Question possibility of pregnancy. Obtain baseline CBC, serum chemistries including hepatic function tests (bilirubin, AST, alkaline phosphatase), renal function tests before treatment begins and routinely thereafter.

INTERVENTION/EVALUATION

Offer antiemetics to control nausea, vomiting. Monitor daily pattern of bowel frequency, stool consistency. Assess skin for evidence of rash, edema. Monitor CBC, particularly Hgb, platelets, neutrophil count, hepatic function tests (AST, ALT, total bilirubin), renal function tests. Monitor for shortness of breath, fatigue, hypertension. Assess mouth for stomatitis, mucositis.

PATIENT/FAMILY TEACHING

• Avoid crowds, those with known infection. • Avoid contact with anyone who recently received live virus vaccine. • Do not have immunizations without physician's approval (drug lowers body resistance). • Promptly report fever, unusual bruising/bleeding from any site.

tenecteplase HIGH ALERT

te-**neck**-teh-place
(TNKase)
Do not confuse TNKase with tPA.

◆CLASSIFICATION

PHARMACOTHERAPEUTIC: Tissue plasminogen activator. **CLINICAL:** Thrombolytic (see p. 33C).

ACTION

Produced by recombinant DNA that binds to fibrin and converts plasminogen to plasmin. Initiates fibrinolysis by degrading fibrin clots, fibrinogen, other plasma proteins. **Therapeutic Effect:** Exerts thrombolytic action.

PHARMACOKINETICS

Extensively distributed to tissues. Completely eliminated by hepatic metabolism. **Half-life:** 90–130 min.

USES

Treatment, reduction of mortality associated with acute myocardial infarction (AMI).

PRECAUTIONS

Contraindications: Active internal bleeding, aneurysm, AV malformation, bleeding diathesis, history of CVA, intracranial or intraspinal surgery or trauma within past 2 mos, intracranial neoplasm, severe uncontrolled hypertension. **Cautions:** Pts who previously received tenecteplase, severe hepatic impairment.

LIFESPAN CONSIDERATIONS

Pregnancy/Lactation: Unknown if distributed in breast milk. **Pregnancy Category C. Children:** Safety and efficacy not established. **Elderly:** May have increased risk of intracranial hemorrhage, stroke, major bleeding; caution advised.

INTERACTIONS

DRUG: **Anticoagulants (e.g., heparin, warfarin), aspirin, dipyridamole, glycoprotein IIb/IIIa inhibitors** increase risk of bleeding. **HERBAL:** **Ginkgo biloba** may increase risk of bleeding. **FOOD:** None known. **LAB VALUES:** Decreases plasminogen, fibrinogen levels during infusion, decreasing clotting time (confirms presence of lysis). Decreases Hgb, Hct.

AVAILABILITY (Rx)

Injection, Powder for Reconstitution: 50 mg.

ADMINISTRATION/HANDLING

IV

Reconstitution • Add 10 ml Sterile Water for Injection without preservative

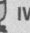

T

to vial to provide concentration of 5 mg/ml. • Gently swirl until dissolved. Do not shake. • If foaming occurs, leave vial undisturbed for several min.

Rate of administration • Administer as IV push over 5 sec.

Storage • Store at room temperature. • If possible, use immediately, but may refrigerate up to 8 hrs after reconstitution. • Appears as colorless to pale yellow solution. • Do not use if discolored or contains particulates. • Discard after 8 hrs.

IV INCOMPATIBILITIES

Do not mix with dextrose-containing solutions or any other medications.

INDICATIONS/ROUTES/DOSAGE

◀ALERT▶ Give as single IV bolus over 5 sec. Precipitate may occur when given in IV line containing dextrose. Flush line with saline before and after administration.

Acute MI

IV: ADULTS: Dosage is based on pt's weight. Treatment should be initiated as soon as possible after onset of symptoms.

Weight (kg)	(mg)	(ml)
90 or more	50	10
80–less than 90	45	9
70–less than 80	40	8
60–less than 70	35	7
Less than 60	30	6

SIDE EFFECTS

Frequent: Bleeding (minor, 21.8%; major, 4.7%).

ADVERSE EFFECTS/ TOXIC REACTIONS

Bleeding at internal sites, including intracranial, retroperitoneal, GI, GU, respiratory sites, may occur. Lysis of coronary thrombi may produce atrial or ventricular arrhythmias, stroke.

NURSING CONSIDERATIONS

BASELINE ASSESSMENT

Obtain baseline B/P, apical pulse. Record weight. Evaluate 12-lead EKG, cardiac enzymes, serum electrolytes. Assess Hgb, Hct, platelet count, thrombin time, aPTT, PT, fibrinogen level before therapy is instituted. Type and hold blood.

INTERVENTION/EVALUATION

Monitor continuous EKG for arrhythmias, B/P, pulse, respirations q15min until stable, then hourly. Check peripheral pulses, heart and lung sounds. Monitor for chest pain relief; notify physician of continuation/recurrence (note location, type, intensity). Assess for overt or occult blood in any body substance. Monitor aPTT per protocol. Maintain B/P. Avoid any trauma that might increase risk of bleeding (e.g., injections, shaving). Assess neurologic status with vital signs.

tenofovir

ten-**oh**-foh-veer
(Viread)

BLACK BOX ALERT Lactic acidosis, severe hepatomegaly with steatosis (fatty liver), including fatalities, have occurred.

FIXED-COMBINATION(S)

Atripla: tenofovir/efavirenz/emtricitabine (antiretroviral agents): 300 mg/600 mg/200 mg. **Truvada:** tenofovir/emtricitabine (an antiretroviral agent): 300 mg/200 mg.

CLASSIFICATION

PHARMACOTHERAPEUTIC: Nucleotide analogue. **CLINICAL:** Antiviral (see pp. 69C, 116C).

ACTION

Inhibits HIV reverse transcriptase by being incorporated into viral DNA, resulting in DNA chain termination. **Therapeutic Effect:** Slows HIV replication, reduces HIV RNA levels (viral load).

PHARMACOKINETICS

Bioavailability in fasted pts is approximately 25%. High-fat meals increase bio-

T

availability. Protein binding: 0.7%–7.2%. Excreted in urine. Removed by hemodialysis. **Half-life:** 17 hrs.

USES

Treatment of HIV-1 infection in combination with other antiretroviral agents. Treatment of chronic hepatitis B in adults.

PRECAUTIONS

Contraindications: None known. **Cautions:** Hepatic/renal impairment.

LIFESPAN CONSIDERATIONS

Pregnancy/Lactation: Unknown if drug crosses placenta or is distributed in breast milk. **Pregnancy Category B. Children:** Safety and efficacy not established. **Elderly:** No age-related precautions noted.

INTERACTIONS

DRUG: May increase **didanosine** concentration. May decrease concentrations of **atazanavir, indinavir, lamivudine, lopinavir, ritonavir. HERBAL:** None significant. **FOOD: High-fat food** increases bioavailability. **LAB VALUES:** May increase ALT, AST, creatinine, glucose (urine), phosphate (urine), protein (urine). May decrease neutrophils.

AVAILABILITY (Rx)

Tablets: 300 mg.

ADMINISTRATION/HANDLING

PO

• May be given without regard to meals.

INDICATIONS/ROUTES/DOSAGE

HIV Infection, Hepatitis B

PO: ADULTS, ELDERLY, CHILDREN 18 YRS AND OLDER: 300 mg once daily.

Dosage in Renal Impairment

Creatinine Clearance	Dosage
30–49 ml/min	300 mg q48h
10–29 ml/min	300 mg twice a wk
Less than 10 ml/min	Not recommended

SIDE EFFECTS

Occasional: GI disturbances (diarrhea, flatulence, nausea, vomiting).

ADVERSE EFFECTS/ TOXIC REACTIONS

Lactic acidosis, hepatomegaly with steatosis (excess fat in liver) occur rarely, may be severe.

NURSING CONSIDERATIONS

BASELINE ASSESSMENT

Obtain baseline laboratory testing, esp. serum hepatic/renal function tests, triglycerides before beginning tenofovir therapy and at periodic intervals during therapy. Offer emotional support to pt and family.

INTERVENTION/EVALUATION

Closely monitor for evidence of GI discomfort. Monitor daily pattern of bowel activity, stool consistency. Monitor CBC, Hgb, reticulocyte count, serum hepatic/ renal function, CD4 cell count, HIV, RNA plasma levels.

PATIENT/FAMILY TEACHING

• Continue therapy for full length of treatment. • Tenofovir is not a cure for HIV infection, nor does it reduce risk of transmission to others. • Take with a high-fat meal (increases absorption). • Inform physician if persistent abdominal pain, nausea, vomiting occurs.

T

terazosin

ter-**a**-zoe-sin
(Apo-Terazosin ✤, Hytrin,
Novo-Terazosin ✤)

CLASSIFICATION

PHARMACOTHERAPEUTIC: Alpha-adrenergic blocker. **CLINICAL:** Antihypertensive, benign prostatic hyperplasia agent (see p. 60C).

ACTION

Blocks alpha-adrenergic receptors. Produces vasodilation, decreases peripheral resistance, targets receptors around bladder neck, prostate. **Therapeutic Effect:** In hypertension, decreases B/P. In benign prostatic hyperplasia (BPH), relaxes smooth muscle, improves urine flow.

PHARMACOKINETICS

Route	Onset	Peak	Duration
PO	15 min	2–3 hrs	12–24 hrs

Rapidly, completely absorbed from GI tract. Protein binding: 90%–94%. Metabolized in liver to active metabolite. Primarily eliminated in feces via biliary system; excreted in urine. Not removed by hemodialysis. **Half-life:** 9.2–12 hrs.

USES

Treatment of mild to moderate hypertension. Used alone or in combination with other antihypertensives. Treatment of benign prostatic hyperplasia (BPH). **OFF-LABEL:** Pediatric hypertension.

PRECAUTIONS

Contraindications: None known. **Cautions:** Confirmed or suspected coronary artery disease.

LIFESPAN CONSIDERATIONS

Pregnancy/Lactation: Unknown if drug crosses placenta or is distributed in breast milk. **Pregnancy Category C. Children:** Safety and efficacy not established. **Elderly:** No age-related precautions noted but may be more sensitive to hypotensive effects.

T

INTERACTIONS

DRUG: **NSAIDs, sympathomimetics** may decrease effects. **Hypotensive medications (e.g., antihypertensives, diuretics)** may increase effects. **HERBAL:** **Ephedra, ginseng, yohimbe** may worsen hypertension. **Garlic** may increase antihypertensive effect. **FOOD:** None known. **LAB VALUES:** May decrease Hgb, Hct, serum albumin, total serum protein, WBC count.

AVAILABILITY (Rx)

Capsules: 1 mg, 2 mg, 5 mg, 10 mg.

ADMINISTRATION/HANDLING

PO

• Give without regard to food. • Administer first dose at bedtime (minimizes risk of fainting due to "first-dose syncope").

INDICATIONS/ROUTES/DOSAGE

◀ALERT▶ If medication has been discontinued for several days, retitrate initially using 1-mg dose at bedtime.

Mild to Moderate Hypertension

PO: ADULTS, ELDERLY: Initially, 1 mg at bedtime. Slowly increase dosage to desired levels. Range: 1–5 mg/day as single or 2 divided doses. **Maximum:** 20 mg.

Benign Prostatic Hyperplasia (BPH)

PO: ADULTS, ELDERLY: Initially, 1 mg at bedtime. May increase up to 10 mg/day if no response in 4–6 wks. **Maximum:** 20 mg/day.

SIDE EFFECTS

Frequent (9%–5%): Dizziness, headache, fatigue. **Rare (less than 2%):** Peripheral edema, orthostatic hypotension, myalgia, arthralgia, blurred vision, nausea, vomiting, nasal congestion, drowsiness.

ADVERSE EFFECTS/ TOXIC REACTIONS

First-dose syncope (hypotension with sudden loss of consciousness) generally occurs 30–90 min after initial dose of 2 mg or more, too-rapid increase in dosage, or addition of another antihypertensive agent to therapy. First-dose syncope may be preceded by tachycardia (pulse rate of 120–160 beats/min).

NURSING CONSIDERATIONS

BASELINE ASSESSMENT

Assess history of prostatic hyperplasia (difficulty initiating urine stream, dribbling, sense of urgency, leaking). Give first dose at bedtime. If initial dose is given during daytime, pt must remain recumbent for 3–4 hrs. Assess B/P, pulse immediately before each dose, and q15–30min until stabilized (be alert to B/P fluctuations).

INTERVENTION/EVALUATION

Monitor pulse diligently (first-dose syncope may be preceded by tachycardia). Assist with ambulation if dizziness occurs. Assess for peripheral edema. Monitor B/P, GU function.

PATIENT/FAMILY TEACHING

• Noncola carbonated beverage, unsalted crackers, dry toast may relieve nausea. • Nasal congestion may occur. • Full therapeutic effect may not occur for 3–4 wks. • Avoid tasks requiring alertness, motor skills until response to drug is established. • Use caution rising from sitting position. • Report dizziness, palpitations. • Avoid alcohol.

terbinafine

ter-**been**-a-feen
(Apo-Terbinafine ✤, Lamisil, Lamisil AT, Lamisil Oral Granule, Novo-Terbinafine ✤)
Do not confuse Lamisil with Lamictal or Lomotil, or terbinafine with terbutaline.

◆ CLASSIFICATION

CLINICAL: Antifungal (see p. 49C).

ACTION

Inhibits the enzyme squalene epoxidase, thereby interfering with fungal biosynthesis. **Therapeutic Effect:** Results in death of fungal cells.

PHARMACOKINETICS

Well absorbed following PO administration. Protein binding: 99%. Metabolized in liver. Primarily excreted in urine; minimal elimination in feces. **Half-life:** PO, 36 hrs; topical, 22–26 hrs.

USES

Systemic: Treatment of onychomycosis (fungal disease of nails due to dermatophytes). Treatment of tinea capitis. **Topical:** Treatment of *tinea cruris* (jock itch), *t. pedis* (athlete's foot), *t. corporis* (ringworm), tinea versicolor.

PRECAUTIONS

Contraindications: Preexisting hepatic/renal impairment (creatinine clearance 50 ml/min or less). **Cautions:** None known.

⌛ LIFESPAN CONSIDERATIONS

Pregnancy/Lactation: Distributed in breast milk. **Pregnancy Category B. Children:** Safety and efficacy not established. **Elderly:** Age-related renal impairment may require dosage adjustment.

INTERACTIONS

DRUG: **Alcohol, other hepatotoxic medications** may increase risk of hepatotoxicity. **Hepatic enzyme inducers (e.g., rifampin)** may increase clearance. **Hepatic enzyme inhibitors (e.g., cimetidine)** may decrease clearance. **HERBAL:** None significant. **FOOD:** None known. **LAB VALUES:** May increase AST, ALT.

AVAILABILITY (Rx)

Cream (Lamisil AT): 1%. **Oral Granules (Lamisil Oral Granule):** 125 mg/packet. **Tablets (Lamisil):** 250 mg. **Topical Solution (Lamisil, Lamisil AT):** 1%.

ADMINISTRATION/HANDLING

• Tablets may be given without regard to food. • Granules should be sprinkled on a spoonful of nonacidic food (e.g., mashed potatoes); swallow without chewing.

INDICATIONS/ROUTES/DOSAGE

Tinea Pedis

TOPICAL: ADULTS, ELDERLY, CHILDREN 12 YRS AND OLDER: Apply twice daily until signs/symptoms significantly improve, not to exceed 4 wks.

T

Tinea Cruris, Tinea Corporis

TOPICAL: ADULTS, ELDERLY, CHILDREN 12 YRS AND OLDER: Apply 1–2 times daily until signs/symptoms significantly improve, not to exceed 4 wks.

Onychomycosis

PO: ADULTS, ELDERLY, CHILDREN 12 YRS AND OLDER: 250 mg/day for 6 wks (fingernails) or 12 wks (toenails).

Tinea Versicolor

TOPICAL SOLUTION: ADULTS, ELDERLY: Apply to the affected area twice daily for 7 days.

Systemic Mycosis

PO: ADULTS, ELDERLY: 250–500 mg/day for up to 16 mos.

Tinea Capitis

PO: CHILDREN 4 YRS AND OLDER: (Use granules). **WEIGHING GREATER THAN 35 KG:** 250 mg once daily. **WEIGHING 25–35 KG:** 187.5 mg once daily. **WEIGHING LESS THAN 25 KG:** 125 mg once daily.

SIDE EFFECTS

Frequent (13%): PO: Headache. **Occasional (6%–3%): PO:** Abdominal pain, flatulence, urticaria, visual disturbance. **Rare: PO:** Diarrhea, rash, dyspepsia (heartburn, indigestion, epigastric pain), pruritus, altered taste, nausea. **Topical:** Irritation, burning, pruritus, dryness.

ADVERSE EFFECTS/ TOXIC REACTIONS

Hepatobiliary dysfunction (including cholestatic hepatitis), serious skin reactions, severe neutropenia occur rarely. Ocular lens, retinal changes have been noted.

NURSING CONSIDERATIONS

BASELINE ASSESSMENT

Serum hepatic function tests should be obtained in pts receiving treatment for longer than 6 wks.

INTERVENTION/EVALUATION

Check for therapeutic response. Discontinue medication, notify physician if local reaction occurs (irritation, redness, swelling, pruritus, oozing, blistering, burning). Monitor serum hepatic function in pts receiving treatment for longer than 6 wks.

PATIENT/FAMILY TEACHING

• Keep areas clean, dry; wear light clothing to promote ventilation. • Avoid topical cream contact with eyes, nose, mouth, other mucous membranes. • Rub well into affected, surrounding area. • Do not cover with occlusive dressing. • Report rash, dark urine, abdominal pain, anorexia, yellowing of skin.

terbutaline

ter-**bue**-ta-leen
(Brethine, Bricanyl 🍁)

Do not confuse terbutaline with terbinafine.

CLASSIFICATION

PHARMACOTHERAPEUTIC: Sympathomimetic (adrenergic agonist). **CLINICAL:** Bronchodilator, premature labor inhibitor.

ACTION

Stimulates $beta_2$-adrenergic receptors, resulting in relaxation of uterine, bronchial smooth muscle. **Therapeutic Effect:** Inhibits uterine contractions. Relieves bronchospasm, reduces airway resistance.

PHARMACOKINETICS

Partially absorbed in GI tract following PO administration. Protein binding: 14%–25%. Metabolized in liver. Excreted in feces, urine. **Half-life:** 11–16 hrs.

USES

Symptomatic relief of reversible bronchospasm due to bronchial asthma, bronchitis, emphysema. Delays premature labor in pregnancies between 20 and 34 wks.

PRECAUTIONS

Contraindications: History of hypersensitivity to sympathomimetics. **Cautions:** Cardiac impairment, diabetes mellitus, hypertension, hyperthyroidism, history of seizures.

LIFESPAN CONSIDERATIONS

Pregnancy/Lactation: Crosses placenta; distributed in breast milk. **Pregnancy Category B. Children:** Safety and efficacy not established in those younger than 6 yrs. **Elderly:** Increased risk of tremors, tachycardia due to sympathomimetic sensitivity.

INTERACTIONS

DRUG: May decrease effects of **beta-blockers. Digoxin, sympathomimetics** may increase risk of arrhythmias. **MAOIs** may increase risk of hypertensive crisis. **Tricyclic antidepressants** may increase cardiovascular effects. May increase effects of **thyroid hormones. HERBAL: Ephedra, yohimbe** may cause CNS stimulation. **FOOD:** None known. **LAB VALUES:** May decrease serum potassium. May increase serum glucose.

AVAILABILITY (Rx)

Injection Solution: 1 mg/ml. **Tablets:** 2.5 mg, 5 mg.

ADMINISTRATION/HANDLING

IV

• May administer undiluted, direct IV over 5–10 min or continuous infusion diluted in D_5W or 0.9% NaCl.

Subcutaneous

• Do not use if solution appears discolored. • Inject subcutaneously into lateral deltoid region.

PO

• Give without regard to food (give with food if GI upset occurs). • Tablets may be crushed.

INDICATIONS/ROUTES/DOSAGE

Bronchospasm

PO: ADULTS, ELDERLY, CHILDREN 15 YRS AND OLDER: Initially, 2.5 mg 3–4 times a day. Maintenance: 2.5–5 mg 3 times a day q6h while awake. **Maximum:** 15 mg/day. **CHILDREN 12–14 YRS:** 2.5 mg 3 times a day. **Maximum:** 7.5 mg/day. **CHILDREN YOUNGER THAN 12 YRS:** Initially, 0.05 mg/kg/dose q8h. May increase up to 0.15 mg/kg/dose. **Maximum:** 5 mg/24 hr.
SUBCUTANEOUS: ADULTS, CHILDREN 12 YRS AND OLDER: Initially, 0.25 mg. Repeat in 15–30 min if substantial improvement does not occur. **Maximum:** 0.5 mg/4 hrs. **CHILDREN YOUNGER THAN 12 YRS:** 0.005–0.01 mg/kg/dose to a maximum of 0.4 mg/dose q15–20min for 3 doses. May repeat q2–6h as needed.

Preterm Labor

PO: ADULTS: MAINTENANCE: 2.5–10 mg q4–6h.
IV: ADULTS: ACUTE: 2.5–10 mcg/min. May increase gradually q15–20min up to 17.5–30 mcg/min.

Dosage in Renal Impairment

Creatinine Clearance	Dosage
10–50 ml/min	50% of normal
Less than 10 ml/min	Avoid use

SIDE EFFECTS

Frequent (38%–23%): Tremor, anxiety. **Occasional (11%–10%):** Drowsiness, headache, nausea, heartburn, dizziness. **Rare (3%–1%):** Flushing, asthenia (loss of strength, energy), oropharyngeal dryness, irritation (with inhalation therapy).

ADVERSE EFFECTS/ TOXIC REACTIONS

Too-frequent or excessive use may lead to decreased drug effectiveness and/or severe, paradoxical bronchoconstriction. Excessive sympathomimetic stimulation may cause palpitations, extrasystoles, tachycardia, chest pain, slight increase in B/P followed by a substantial decrease, chills, diaphoresis, skin blanching.

NURSING CONSIDERATIONS

BASELINE ASSESSMENT

Bronchospasm: Offer emotional support (high incidence of anxiety due to difficulty in breathing, sympathomimetic response to drug). **Preterm labor:** Assess baseline maternal pulse, B/P, frequency and duration of contractions, fetal heart rate.

INTERVENTION/EVALUATION

Bronchospasm: Monitor rate, depth, rhythm, type of respiration; quality, rate of pulse. Assess lung sounds for rhonchi, wheezing, rales. Monitor ABGs. Observe lips, fingernails for cyanosis (blue or dusky color in light-skinned pts; gray in dark-skinned pts). Observe for clavicular retractions, hand tremor. Evaluate for clinical improvement (quieter, slower respirations, relaxed facial expression, cessation of clavicular retractions). **Preterm labor:** Monitor for frequency, duration, strength of contractions. Diligently monitor fetal heart rate.

PATIENT/FAMILY TEACHING

- Inform physician if palpitations, chest pain, muscle tremor, dizziness, headache, flushing, breathing difficulties continue.
- May cause nervousness, anxiety, shakiness.
- Avoid excessive use of caffeine derivatives (chocolate, coffee, tea, cola, cocoa).

terconazole

ter-**con**-ah-zole
(Terazol ✦, Terazol 3, Terazol 7, Zazole)
Do not confuse terconazole with tioconazole.

◆CLASSIFICATION

CLINICAL: Antifungal (vaginal).

ACTION

Disrupts fungal cell membrane permeability. **Therapeutic Effect:** Produces antifungal activity.

PHARMACOKINETICS

Minimal systemic absorption.

USES

Treatment of vulvovaginal candidiasis (moniliasis).

PRECAUTIONS

Contraindications: Allergy to azole antifungals. **Cautions:** None significant.

⌛ LIFESPAN CONSIDERATIONS

Pregnancy/Lactation: Unknown if distributed in breast milk. **Pregnancy Category C. Children:** Safety and efficacy not established. **Elderly:** No age-related precautions noted.

INTERACTIONS

DRUG: None significant. **HERBAL:** None significant. **FOOD:** None known. **LAB VALUES:** None significant.

AVAILABILITY (Rx)

Vaginal Cream: 0.4% **(Terazol 7, Zazole),** 0.8% **(Terazol 3). Vaginal Suppository (Terazol 3):** 80 mg.

INDICATIONS/ROUTES/DOSAGE

Vulvovaginal Candidiasis

TABLET (INTRAVAGINAL): ADULTS, ELDERLY: 1 suppository vaginally at bedtime for 3 days.

CREAM: ADULTS, ELDERLY: (0.4%): 1 applicatorful at bedtime for 7 days; **(0.8%):** 1 applicatorful at bedtime for 3 days.

SIDE EFFECTS

Frequent (greater than 10%): Headache, vulvovaginal burning. **Occasional (10%–1%):** Dysmenorrhea, pain in female genitalia, abdominal pain, fever, pruritus. **Rare (less than 1%):** Chills.

ADVERSE EFFECTS/ TOXIC REACTIONS

None known.

NURSING CONSIDERATIONS

BASELINE ASSESSMENT

Assess for allergy to azoles, pt's ability to self-administer.

INTERVENTION/EVALUATION

Watch for local irritation. Assist, provide education to pt regarding administration.

PATIENT/FAMILY TEACHING

• Notify physician of recurrence of symptoms following treatment. • Comply with full course of therapy. • Staining of clothes may occur with azole medications; use protective liners.

teriparatide

tear-ee-**pear**-ah-tide
(Forteo)

BLACK BOX ALERT Increased risk of osteosarcoma; risk dependent on dose and duration.

◆CLASSIFICATION

PHARMACOTHERAPEUTIC: Synthetic hormone. **CLINICAL:** Osteoporosis agent.

ACTION

Acts on bone to mobilize calcium; acts on kidney to reduce calcium clearance, increase phosphate excretion. **Therapeutic Effect:** Increases rate of release of calcium from bone into blood; stimulates new bone formation.

PHARMACOKINETICS

Extensively absorbed following subcutaneous injection. Metabolized in liver. Excreted in urine. **Half-life:** 1 hr.

USES

Treatment of postmenopausal women with osteoporosis who are at increased risk for fractures, increase bone mass in men with primary or hypogonadal osteoporosis who are at high risk for fractures. High-risk pts include those with a history of osteoporotic fractures, who have failed previous osteoporosis therapy, or were intolerant of previous osteoporosis therapy. Treatment of glucocorticoid-induced osteoporosis.

PRECAUTIONS

Contraindications: Conditions that increase risk of osteosarcoma (e.g., Paget's disease, unexplained elevations of alkaline phosphatase level, open epiphyses, prior skeletal radiation therapy, implant therapy), hypercalcemia, hypercalcemic disorders (e.g., hyperparathyroidism). **Cautions:** Bone metastases, history of skeletal malignancies, metabolic bone diseases other than osteoporosis, concurrent therapy with digoxin.

⌛ LIFESPAN CONSIDERATIONS

Pregnancy/Lactation: Unknown if drug crosses placenta or is distributed in breast milk. **Pregnancy Category C. Children:** Safety and efficacy not established. **Elderly:** No age-related precautions noted.

INTERACTIONS

DRUG: None significant. **HERBAL:** None significant. **FOOD:** None known. **LAB VALUES:** May increase serum calcium (transient).

AVAILABILITY (Rx)

Injection Solution: 750 mcg in 3-ml prefilled pen delivers 20 mcg/dose.

ADMINISTRATION/HANDLING

Subcutaneous

• Refrigerate, but minimize time out of refrigerator. Do not freeze; discard if frozen. • Administer into thigh, abdominal wall.

INDICATIONS/ROUTES/DOSAGE

Osteoporosis

SUBCUTANEOUS: ADULTS, ELDERLY: 20 mcg once daily into thigh, abdominal wall.

SIDE EFFECTS

Occasional: Leg cramps, nausea, dizziness, headache, orthostatic hypotension, tachycardia.

T

ADVERSE EFFECTS/ TOXIC REACTIONS

Angina pectoris has been reported.

NURSING CONSIDERATIONS

BASELINE ASSESSMENT

Check urinary, serum calcium levels, serum parathyroid hormone levels.

INTERVENTION/EVALUATION

Monitor bone mineral density, urinary/serum calcium levels, serum parathyroid hormone levels. Observe for symptoms of hypercalcemia. Monitor B/P for hypotension, pulse for tachycardia.

PATIENT/FAMILY TEACHING

- Immediately sit or lie down if symptoms of orthostatic hypotension occur.
- Inform physician if persistent symptoms of hypercalcemia (nausea, vomiting, constipation, lethargy, asthenia [loss of strength, energy]) occur.

testosterone

tess-**toss**-ter-one
(Andriol ✤, Androderm, AndroGel, Andropository ✤, Axiron, Delatestryl, Depotest ✤, Depo-Testosterone, Everone ✤, FIRST-Testosterone, FIRST-Testosterone MC, Striant, Testim, Testopel, Virilon IM ✤)

BLACK BOX ALERT Virilization in children and women can occur following secondary exposure to testosterone gel.

Do not confuse testosterone with testolactone.

◆CLASSIFICATION

PHARMACOTHERAPEUTIC: Androgen.
CLINICAL: Sex hormone.

ACTION

Promotes growth, development of male sex organs, maintains secondary sex characteristics in androgen-deficient males. **Therapeutic Effect:** Relieves androgen deficiency.

PHARMACOKINETICS

Well absorbed after IM administration. Protein binding: 98%. Undergoes first-pass metabolism in liver. Primarily excreted in urine. Unknown if removed by hemodialysis. **Half-life:** 10–100 min.

USES

Injection: Treatment of delayed male puberty, male hypogonadism, inoperable female breast cancer. **Pellet:** Treatment of delayed male puberty, male hypogonadism. **Buccal, transdermal:** Male hypogonadism.

PRECAUTIONS

Contraindications: Breast-feeding, cardiac impairment, hypercalcemia, pregnancy, prostate or breast cancer in males, severe hepatic/renal disease. **Cautions:** Renal/hepatic dysfunction, diabetes.

LIFESPAN CONSIDERATIONS

Pregnancy/Lactation: Contraindicated during lactation. **Pregnancy Category X.** **Children:** Safety and efficacy not established; use with caution. **Elderly:** May increase risk of hyperplasia, stimulate growth of occult prostate carcinoma.

INTERACTIONS

DRUG: May decrease serum glucose, requiring **insulin** adjustments. May increase effects of **oral anticoagulants.** **HERBAL:** None significant. **FOOD:** None known. **LAB VALUES:** May increase Hgb, Hct, LDL, serum alkaline phosphatase, bilirubin, calcium, potassium, sodium, AST. May decrease HDL.

AVAILABILITY (Rx)

Gel, Topical: (Androgel, Testim): 1%. **Injection: (Cypionate [Depo-Testosterone]):** 100 mg/ml, 200 mg/ml. **(Enanthate [Delatestryl]):** 200 mg/ml. **Mucoadhesive, for Buccal Application: (Striant):** 30 mg. **Pellet, for Subcutaneous Implantation: (Testo-**

pel): 75 mg. **Solution (Metered Dose Pump [Axiron]):** 30 mg/activation. **Transdermal System: (Androderm):** 2.5 mg/day, 5 mg/day.

ADMINISTRATION/HANDLING

IM

• Give deep in gluteal muscle. • Do not give IV. • Warming or shaking redissolves crystals that may form in long-acting preparations. • Wet needle of syringe may cause solution to become cloudy; this does not affect potency.

Buccal

Striant • Apply to gum area (above incisor tooth). • Hold firmly in place for 30 sec to ensure adhesion; do not chew or swallow. • Not affected by food, toothbrushing, gum, chewing, alcoholic beverages. • Remove before placing new system.

Transdermal

Androderm • Apply to clean, dry area on skin on back, abdomen, upper arms, thighs. • Do not apply to bony prominences (e.g., shoulder) or oily, damaged, irritated skin. Do not apply to scrotum. • Rotate application site with 7-day interval to same site.

Transdermal Gel

(Androgel, Testim) • Apply (morning preferred) to clean, dry, intact skin of shoulder, upper arms (Androgel may also be applied to abdomen). • Upon opening packet(s), squeeze entire contents into palm of hand, immediately apply to application site. • Allow to dry. • Do not apply to genitals.

INDICATIONS/ROUTES/DOSAGE

Male Hypogonadism

IM: ADULTS: 50–400 mg q2–4wk. **ADOLESCENTS:** Initiation of pubertal growth: 40–50 mg/m²/dose monthly until growth rate falls to prepubertal levels. Terminal growth phase: 100 mg/m²/dose until growth ceases.

MAINTENANCE VIRILIZING DOSE: 100 mg/m²/dose twice a mo.

SUBCUTANEOUS (Pellets): ADULTS, ADOLESCENTS: 150–450 mg q3–6mo.

TOPICAL SOLUTION (AXIRON): ADULTS, ELDERLY: 60 mg (1 pump activation of 30 mg to each axilla).

TRANSDERMAL PATCH (Androderm): ADULTS, ELDERLY: Start therapy with 5 mg/day patch applied at night. Apply patch to abdomen, back, thighs, upper arms.

TRANSDERMAL GEL (Androgel): ADULTS, ELDERLY: Initial dose of 5 g delivers 50 mg testosterone and is applied once daily to abdomen, shoulders, upper arms. May increase to 7.5 g, then to 10 g, if necessary.

TRANSDERMAL GEL (Testim): ADULTS, ELDERLY: Initial dose of 5 g delivers 50 mg testosterone and is applied once daily to the shoulders, upper arms. May increase to 10 g.

BUCCAL (Striant): ADULTS, ELDERLY: 30 mg q12h.

Delayed Male Puberty

IM: ADOLESCENTS: 40–50 mg/m²/dose every mo for 6 mos.

SUBCUTANEOUS (Pellets): ADULTS, ADOLESCENTS: 150–450 mg q3–6mo.

Breast Carcinoma

IM (Testosterone Cypionate, Testosterone Ethanate): ADULTS: 200–400 mg q2–4wk.

SIDE EFFECTS

Frequent: Gynecomastia, acne. **Females:** Hirsutism, amenorrhea, other menstrual irregularities; deepening of voice; clitoral enlargement (may not be reversible when drug is discontinued). **Occasional:** Edema, nausea, insomnia, oligospermia, priapism, male-pattern baldness, bladder irritability, hypercalcemia (in immobilized pts, those with breast cancer), hypercholesterolemia, inflammation/pain at IM injection site. **Transdermal:** Pruritus, erythema, skin irritation. **Rare:** Polycythemia (with high dosage), hypersensitivity.

ADVERSE EFFECTS/ TOXIC REACTIONS

Peliosis hepatitis (presence of blood-filled cysts in parenchyma of liver), hepatic neoplasms, hepatocellular carcinoma have been associated with prolonged high-dose therapy. Anaphylactic reactions occur rarely.

NURSING CONSIDERATIONS

BASELINE ASSESSMENT

Establish baseline weight, B/P, Hgb, Hct. Check serum hepatic function, electrolytes, cholesterol. Wrist X-rays may be ordered to determine bone maturation in children.

INTERVENTION/EVALUATION

Weigh daily, report weekly gain of more than 5 lb; evaluate for edema. Monitor I&O. Check B/P at least twice daily. Assess serum electrolytes, cholesterol, Hgb, Hct (periodically for high dosage), hepatic function test results, radiologic exam of wrist, hand (when using in prepubertal children). With breast cancer or immobility, check for hypercalcemia (lethargy, muscle weakness, confusion, irritability). Ensure adequate intake of protein, calories. Assess for virilization. Monitor sleep patterns. Check injection site for redness, swelling, pain.

PATIENT/FAMILY TEACHING

• Regular visits to physician and monitoring tests are necessary. • Do not take any other medication without consulting physician. • Maintain diet high in protein, calories. • Food may be better tolerated in small, frequent feedings. • Weigh daily, report 5 lb/wk gain. • Notify physician if nausea, vomiting, acne, pedal edema occur. • **Females:** Promptly report menstrual irregularities, hoarseness, deepening of voice. • **Males:** Report frequent erections, difficulty urinating, gynecomastia.

tetrabenazine

teh-tra-**benz**-ah-zeen
(Nitoman ✱, Xenazine)

BLACK BOX ALERT Increased risk of depression, suicidal thoughts, and behavior.

◆CLASSIFICATION

PHARMACOTHERAPEUTIC: Monoamine depletory, dopamine receptor blocker. **CLINICAL:** Huntington's disease agent.

ACTION

Depletes presynaptic dopamine, norepinephrine, serotonin storage and blocks postsynaptic dopamine receptors at nerve terminals. **Therapeutic Effect:** Relieves signs and symptoms of chorea effect of Huntington's disease, improves motor function.

PHARMACOKINETICS

Rapidly distributed to the brain. Extensive hepatic metabolism. Protein binding: 82%–85%. Primarily excreted in urine (75%), with lesser amount eliminated in feces (16%). **Half-life:** 6 hrs.

USES

Treatment of chorea associated with Huntington's disease. **OFF-LABEL:** Dyskinesia, Tourette's syndrome, dystonia.

PRECAUTIONS

Contraindications: Actively suicidal pts, pts with untreated or inadequately treated depression, impaired hepatic function, those taking MAO inhibitors or pts taking Reserpine within the past 20 days. Pts with congenital long QT syndrome and those with a history of arrhythmias. **Cautions:** Those taking concurrent neuroleptic drugs, concurrent Parkinsonism, akathisia, dysphagia, tardive dyskinesia, depression.

⧖ LIFESPAN CONSIDERATIONS

Pregnancy/Lactation: Unknown if distributed in breast milk. **Pregnancy**

T

Category C. Children: Safety and efficacy not established. **Elderly:** Parkinsonian-like adverse reactions may be dose-limiting.

INTERACTIONS

DRUG: **Amiodarone, chlorpromazine, haloperidol, levofloxacin, moxifloxacin, olanzapine, paliperidone, risperidone, sotalol, ziprasidone** may increase QT prolongation. **Fluoxetine, paroxetine, quinidine** may greatly increase concentration. Concurrent use of **chlorpromazine, haloperidol, MAO inhibitors, olanzapine, risperidone** may increase risk of neuroleptic malignant syndrome, extrapyramidal effects. **Reserpine** may increase effect. **Alcohol** may increase risk of CNS depressant effects. HERBAL: None significant. FOOD: None known. LAB VALUES: May increase AST, ALT prolactin concentration.

AVAILABILITY (Rx)

Tablets: 12.5 mg, 25 mg.

ADMINISTRATION/HANDLING

PO

• Give without regard to food. • May crush or split tablets.

INDICATIONS/ROUTES/DOSAGE

Chorea Associated with Huntington's Disease

PO: ADULTS, ELDERLY: Initially, 12.5 mg daily in the morning. After 1 wk, increase dose to 12.5 mg twice daily. Titrate dose by 12.5 mg at weekly intervals, as needed. Doses greater than 37 mg/day should be divided into 3 doses. **Maximum single dose:** 25 mg. **Maximum:** 25 mg three times daily.

SIDE EFFECTS

Frequent (31%–22%): Sedation, fatigue, insomnia. **Occasional** (19%–9%): Depression, akathisia (inability to sit still), anxiety, nausea, upper respiratory tract infection, irritability, bradykinesia, balance difficulty. **Rare** (6%–2%): Vomiting, dizziness, headache, arthralgia.

ADVERSE EFFECTS/ TOXIC REACTIONS

There is an increased risk for the emergence or worsening of depression, suicidal thoughts, unusual changes in behavior.

NURSING CONSIDERATIONS

BASELINE ASSESSMENT

Obtain baseline hepatic function tests (hepatic impairment is contraindication for drug therapy). Question current medication use, particularly MAOIs, reserpine.

INTERVENTION/EVALUATION

Supervise pt closely during early therapy for onset of depression, suicidal thoughts. Assist with ambulation if dizziness, difficulty with balance occurs. Assess for clinical improvement, reversal of symptoms of akathisia (inability to sit still, nervous pacing), bradykinesia (slow, deliberate movements), or rapid jerking motion that interrupts normal coordinated movement.

PATIENT/FAMILY TEACHING

• Pts, caregivers, families should be informed of potential for depression, suicidal thoughts and should be instructed to report behaviors of concern promptly to the treating physician. • Avoid tasks that require alertness, motor skills until response to drug is established.

tetracycline

tet-ra-**sye**-kleen
(Apo-Tetra ✱, Nu-Tetra ✱)

FIXED-COMBINATION(S)

Pylera: tetracycline/bismuth/metronidazole (an anti-infective): 125 mg/ 140 mg/125 mg.

◆ CLASSIFICATION

PHARMACOTHERAPEUTIC: Tetracycline. **CLINICAL:** Antibiotic.

T

ACTION

Inhibits bacterial protein synthesis by binding to ribosomes. **Therapeutic Effect:** Bacteriostatic.

PHARMACOKINETICS

Readily absorbed from GI tract. Protein binding: 30%–60%. Widely distributed. Excreted in urine; eliminated in feces through biliary system. Not removed by hemodialysis. **Half-life:** 6–11 hrs (increased in renal impairment).

USES

Treatment of susceptible infections due to *Rickettsiae, M. pneumoniae, C. trachomatis, C. psittaci, H. ducreyi, Yersinia pestis, Francisella tularensis, Vibrio cholerae, Brucella* spp.; treatment of susceptible infections due to gram-negative organisms including inflammatory acne vulgaris, Lyme disease, mycoplasma disease, *Legionella,* Rocky Mountain spotted fever, chlamydial infection in pts with gonorrhea. Part of multidrug regimen of *H. pylori* eradication to reduce risk of duodenal ulcer recurrence.

PRECAUTIONS

Contraindications: Children 8 yrs or younger, hypersensitivity to sulfites. **Cautions:** Sun, ultraviolet light exposure (severe photosensitivity reaction).

LIFESPAN CONSIDERATIONS

Pregnancy/Lactation: Readily crosses placenta. Distributed in breast milk. Avoid use in women during last half of pregnancy. **Pregnancy Category D. Children:** Not recommended in those 8 yrs or younger; may cause permanent staining of teeth, enamel hypoplasia, decreased linear skeletal growth rate. **Elderly:** No age-related precautions noted.

INTERACTIONS

DRUG: Cholestyramine may decrease absorption. May decrease effects of **oral contraceptives. Antacids, calcium or iron supplements, laxatives containing magnesium** may form nonabsorbable, undigestable complexes. **HERBAL: Dong quai, St. John's wort** may increase risk of photosensitivity. **FOOD: Dairy products** inhibit absorption. **LAB VALUES:** May increase BUN, serum alkaline phosphatase, amylase, bilirubin, AST, ALT.

AVAILABILITY (Rx)

Capsules: 250 mg, 500 mg.

ADMINISTRATION/HANDLING

PO

• Give with full glass of water 1 hr before or 2 hrs after meals. • Avoid antacids, dairy products within 3 hrs of tetracycline.

INDICATIONS/ROUTES/DOSAGE

ALERT Space doses evenly around the clock.

Usual Dosage

PO: ADULTS, ELDERLY: 250–500 mg q6–12h. **CHILDREN 8 YRS AND OLDER:** 25–50 mg/kg/day in 4 divided doses. **Maximum:** 3 g/day.

***H. Pylori* Infection**

PO: ADULTS, ELDERLY: 500 mg 2–4 times a day (in combination).

Dosage in Renal Impairment

Dosage interval is modified based on creatinine clearance.

Creatinine Clearance	Dosage
50–80 ml/min	Usual dose q8–12h
10–49 ml/min	Usual dose q12–24h
Less than 10 ml/min	Usual dose q24h

SIDE EFFECTS

Frequent: Dizziness, light-headedness, diarrhea, nausea, vomiting, abdominal cramps, photosensitivity (may be severe). **Occasional:** Pigmentation of skin, mucous membranes, anal/genital pruritus, stomatitis.

ADVERSE EFFECTS/ TOXIC REACTIONS

Superinfection (esp. fungal), anaphylaxis, increased ICP may occur. Bulging fontanelles occur rarely in infants.

NURSING CONSIDERATIONS

BASELINE ASSESSMENT

Question for history of allergies, esp. tetracyclines, sulfite.

INTERVENTION/EVALUATION

Assess skin for rash. Monitor daily pattern of bowel activity, stool consistency. Monitor food intake, tolerance. Be alert for superinfection (diarrhea, stomatitis, anal/genital pruritus). Monitor B/P, level of consciousness (potential for ICP).

PATIENT/FAMILY TEACHING

• Continue antibiotic for full length of treatment. • Space doses evenly. • Take oral doses on empty stomach (1 hr before or 2 hrs after food, beverages). • Avoid antacids, dairy products within 3 hrs of tetracycline. • Drink full glass of water with capsules; avoid bedtime doses. • Notify physician if diarrhea, rash, other new symptom occurs. • Protect skin from sun, ultraviolet light exposure. • Consult physician before taking any other medication. • Avoid tasks that require alertness, motor skills until response to drug is established (may cause dizziness, light-headedness).

thalidomide

thal-**id**-o-mide
(Thalomid)

BLACK BOX ALERT Significant risk of severe birth defects, fetal death, even with one dose. Increased risk of deep vein thrombosis, pulmonary embolism in multiple myeloma pts. Two methods of contraception must be used 4 wks before, during, and after therapy.

Do not confuse thalidomide with flutamide or lenalidomide.

◆CLASSIFICATION

PHARMACOTHERAPEUTIC: Immunomodulator. **CLINICAL:** Immunosuppressive agent.

ACTION

Has sedative, anti-inflammatory, immunosuppressive activity. Action may be due to selective inhibition of production of tumor necrosis factor-alpha. **Therapeutic Effect:** Reduces muscle wasting in HIV pts; reduces local and systemic effects of leprosy.

PHARMACOKINETICS

Protein binding: 55%–66%. Metabolized by nonenzymatic hydrolysis in plasma. Excreted in urine. **Half-life:** 5–7 hrs.

USES

Treatment of leprosy, multiple myeloma. **OFF-LABEL:** Prevention/treatment of discoid lupus erythematosus, erythema multiforme graft vs. host reactions following bone marrow transplantation, rheumatoid arthritis (RA). Treatment of Behcet's syndrome, Crohn's disease, GI bleeding, pruritus, recurrent aphthous stomatitis in HIV pts, wasting syndrome associated with HIV infection, cancer.

PRECAUTIONS

Contraindications: Neutropenia, peripheral neuropathy, pregnancy. **Cautions:** History of seizures.

⌛ LIFESPAN CONSIDERATIONS

Pregnancy/Lactation: Contraindicated in women who are or may become pregnant and who are not using two required types of birth control or who are not continually abstaining from heterosexual sexual contact. Can cause severe birth defects, fetal death. Unknown if distributed in breast milk. **Pregnancy Category X. Children:** Safety and efficacy not established in those younger than 12 yrs. **Elderly:** No age-related precautions noted.

T

INTERACTIONS

DRUG: **Alcohol, other CNS depressants** may increase sedative effects. **Medications associated with peripheral neuropathy (e.g., isoniazid, lithium, metronidazole, phenytoin)** may increase peripheral neuropathy. May decrease effect of **oral contraceptives. Carbamazepine, phenytoin** may decrease concentration. **HERBAL:** **Cat's claw, echinacea** possess immunostimulant properties. **FOOD:** None known. **LAB VALUES:** None significant.

AVAILABILITY (Rx)

Capsules: 50 mg, 100 mg, 200 mg.

ADMINISTRATION/HANDLING

◀ALERT▶ Thalidomide may be prescribed only by licensed prescribers who are registered in the S.T.E.P.S. program and understand the risk of teratogenicity if thalidomide is used during pregnancy.

• Administer thalidomide with water at least 1 hr after evening meal and, if possible, at bedtime due to risk of drowsiness.

INDICATIONS/ROUTES/DOSAGE

AIDS-Related Muscle Wasting, Aphthous Stomatitis

PO: ADULTS: 200 mg twice daily for 5 days, then 200 mg once daily for up to 8 wks.

Leprosy

PO: ADULTS, ELDERLY: Initially, 100–300 mg/day as single bedtime dose, at least 1 hr after evening meal. Continue until active reaction subsides, then reduce dose q2–4wks in 50-mg increments.

Multiple Myeloma

PO: ADULTS, ELDERLY: 200 mg once daily, preferably at bedtime, with dexamethasone 40 mg on days 1–4, 9–12, 17–20 of each 28-day cycle.

SIDE EFFECTS

Frequent: Drowsiness, dizziness, mood changes, constipation, dry mouth, peripheral neuropathy. **Occasional:** Increased appetite, weight gain, headache, loss of libido, edema of face/limbs, nausea, alopecia, dry skin, rash, hypothyroidism.

ADVERSE EFFECTS/ TOXIC REACTIONS

Neutropenia, peripheral neuropathy, thromboembolism occur rarely.

NURSING CONSIDERATIONS

BASELINE ASSESSMENT

Assess for hypersensitivity to thalidomide. Assess for pregnancy 24 hrs before beginning thalidomide therapy (contraindicated). Determine use of other medications (many interactions).

INTERVENTION/EVALUATION

Monitor WBC, nerve conduction studies, HIV viral load. Observe for signs/symptoms of peripheral neuropathy. Perform pregnancy tests on women of childbearing potential weekly during the first 4 wks of use, then at 4-wk intervals in women with regular menstrual cycles or q2wks in women with irregular menstrual cycles.

PATIENT/FAMILY TEACHING

• Avoid tasks requiring alertness, motor skills until response to drug is established. • Avoid use of alcoholic beverages, other drugs causing drowsiness. • Pregnancy test within 24 hrs before starting thalidomide, then q2–4wks in women of childbearing age. • Discontinue and call physician if symptoms of peripheral neuropathy occur. • Male pts receiving thalidomide should always use a latex condom during any sexual contact with women of childbearing potential.

theophylline

(Elixophyllin, Theo-24, Theochron, Uniphyl)

◆CLASSIFICATION

PHARMACOTHERAPEUTIC: Xanthine derivative. **CLINICAL:** Bronchodilator.

ACTION

Directly relaxes smooth muscle of bronchial airways and pulmonary blood vessels. **Therapeutic Effect:** Relieves bronchospasm, increases vital capacity.

USES

Symptomatic relief, prevention of bronchial asthma, reversible bronchospasm due to chronic bronchitis, emphysema, or chronic obstructive pumonary disease (COPD). **OFF-LABEL:** Treatment of apnea in neonates.

PRECAUTIONS

Contraindications: History of hypersensitivity to caffeine or xanthine. **Cautions:** Cardiac, renal, hepatic impairment; hypertension; hyperthyroidism; diabetes mellitus; peptic ulcer; glaucoma; severe hypoxemia; underlying seizure disorder. **Pregnancy Category C.**

INTERACTIONS

DRUG: **Phenytoin, primidone, rifampin** may increase metabolism. **Beta-blockers** may decrease effects. **Cimetidine, ciprofloxacin, clarithromycin, erythromycin, norfloxacin** may increase concentration, toxicity. **Smoking** may decrease concentration. **HERBAL:** None significant. **FOOD:** **Charcoal-broiled foods, high-protein/low-carbohydrate diet** may decrease serum level. **LAB VALUES:** None significant.

AVAILABILITY (Rx)

Capsules (Extended-Release [Theo-24]): 100 mg, 200 mg, 300 mg, 400 mg. **Elixir (Elixophyllin):** 80 mg/15 ml. **Infusion (Theophylline):** 0.8 mg/ml, 1.6 mg/ml, 2 mg/ml, 3.2 mg/ml, 4 mg/ml.

Tablets (Controlled-Release) (Uniphyl): 400 mg, 600 mg. **Tablets, Extended-Release:** 100 mg, 200 mg, 300 mg, 450 mg.

ADMINISTRATION/HANDLING

IV

Rate of administration • Do not exceed flow rate of 1 ml/min (25 mg/min) for either piggyback or infusion. • Administer loading dose over 20–30 min. • Use infusion pump or microdrip to regulate IV administration.

Storage • Store at room temperature. • Discard if solution contains precipitate.

PO

• Give with food to prevent GI distress. • Do not crush/break controlled-release, extended-release forms.

IV INCOMPATIBILITIES

Amiodarone (Cordarone), ciprofloxacin (Cipro), dobutamine (Dobutrex), ondansetron (Zofran).

IV COMPATIBILITIES

Aztreonam (Azactam), ceftazidime (Fortaz), diphenhydramine (Benadryl), fluconazole (Diflucan), heparin, lipids, morphine, potassium chloride, total parenteral nutrition (TPN).

INDICATIONS/ROUTES/DOSAGE

Doses are based on ideal body weight.

Acute Symptoms (Loading Dose)

IV, PO: ADULTS, CHILDREN: 5 mg/kg orally (4.6 mg/kg IV). If theophylline is given within 24 hrs, loading dose not recommended without obtaining serum theophylline concentration.

Acute Symptoms (Maintenance Dose)

IV: ADULTS OLDER THAN 60 YRS: 0.3 mg/kg/hr. **Maximum:** 400 mg/day. **ADULTS 16–60 YRS:** 0.4 mg/kg/hr. **Maximum:** 900 mg/day. **CHILDREN 12–16 YRS (NONSMOKERS):** 0.5 mg/kg/hr. **Maximum:** 900 mg/day. **CHILDREN 12–16 YRS (SMOKERS):** 0.7 mg/kg/hr. **CHILDREN 9–11 YRS:** 0.7 mg/kg/hr. **CHILDREN 1–8 YRS:** 0.8 mg/kg/hr. **CHILDREN YOUNGER THAN 1 YR:** 1–1.5 mg/kg/q12h.

T

Chronic Treatment

PO: ADULTS 16–60 YRS: 300 mg/day in divided doses for 3 days, then 400 mg/day in divided doses for 3 days, then 600 mg/day in divided doses thereafter. **ELDERLY OLDER THAN 60 YRS: Maximum:** 400 mg/day. **CHILDREN 1–15 YRS:** 12–14 mg/kg/day in divided doses for 3 days (**Maximum:** 300 mg/day), then 16 mg/kg/day in divided doses for 3 days (**Maximum:** 400 mg/day), then 20 mg/kg/day in divided doses (**Maximum:** 600 mg/day). **CHILDREN 6 MOS–YOUNGER THAN 1 YR:** 12–18 mg/kg/day in divided doses. **CHILDREN 6 WKS–YOUNGER THAN 6 MOS:** 10 mg/kg/day in divided doses. **CHILDREN YOUNGER THAN 6 WKS:** 4 mg/kg/day in divided doses.

SIDE EFFECTS

Frequent: Altered smell (during IV administration), restlessness, tachycardia, tremor. **Occasional:** Heartburn, vomiting, headache, mild diuresis, insomnia, nausea.

ADVERSE EFFECTS/ TOXIC REACTIONS

Too-rapid IV administration may produce marked hypotension with accompanying syncope, light-headedness, palpitations, tachycardia, hyperventilation, nausea, vomiting, angina-like pain, seizures, ventricular fibrillation, cardiac standstill.

NURSING CONSIDERATIONS

BASELINE ASSESSMENT

Offer emotional support (high incidence of anxiety due to difficulty in breathing and sympathomimetic response to drug). Peak serum concentration should be drawn 1 hr following IV dose, 1–2 hrs after immediate-release dose, 3–8 hrs after extended-release dose. Draw trough level just before next dose.

INTERVENTION/EVALUATION

Monitor rate, depth, rhythm, type of respiration; quality/rate of pulse. Assess lung sounds for rhonchi, wheezing, rales. Monitor ABGs. Observe lips, fingernails for cyanosis (blue or dusky color in light-skinned pts; gray in dark-skinned pts). Observe for clavicular retractions, hand tremor. Evaluate for clinical improvement (quieter, slower respirations, relaxed facial expression, cessation of clavicular retractions). Monitor serum theophylline levels (**therapeutic serum level range:** 10–20 mcg/ml).

PATIENT/FAMILY TEACHING

• Increase fluid intake (decreases lung secretion viscosity). • Avoid excessive caffeine derivatives (chocolate, coffee, tea, cola, cocoa). • Smoking, charcoal-broiled food, high-protein/low-carbohydrate diet may decrease serum theophylline level. • Notify physician if nausea, vomiting, persistent headache, palpitations occur.

thiamine (vitamin B_1)

thy-a-min
(Betaxin ✦, Vitamin B_1)
Do not confuse thiamine with Tenormin or Thorazine.

◆CLASSIFICATION

PHARMACOTHERAPEUTIC: Water-soluble vitamin. **CLINICAL:** Vitamin B complex (see p. 161C).

ACTION

Combines with adenosine triphosphate in liver, kidneys, leukocytes to form thiamine diphosphate, a coenzyme necessary for carbohydrate metabolism. **Therapeutic Effect:** Prevents, reverses thiamine deficiency.

PHARMACOKINETICS

Rapidly and completely absorbed from GI tract, primarily in duodenum, after IM administration. Widely distributed. Primarily excreted in urine.

USES

Prevention/treatment of thiamine deficiency (e.g., beriberi, Wernicke's encephalopathy syndrome, peripheral neuritis associated with pellegra, alcoholic

T

pts with altered sensorium), metabolic disorders.

PRECAUTIONS

Contraindications: None known. **Cautions:** Wernicke's encephalopathy.

LIFESPAN CONSIDERATIONS

Pregnancy/Lactation: Crosses placenta. Unknown if drug is distributed in breast milk. **Pregnancy Category A (C if used in doses above recommended daily allowance). Children/Elderly:** No age-related precautions noted.

INTERACTIONS

DRUG: None significant. **HERBAL:** None significant. **FOOD:** None known. **LAB VALUES:** None significant.

AVAILABILITY

Injection Solution (Vitamin B_1): 100 mg/ml. **Tablets (OTC):** 50 mg, 100 mg, 250 mg, 500 mg.

ADMINISTRATION/HANDLING

◄ALERT► IV, IM administration used only in acutely ill or those unresponsive to PO route (GI malabsorption syndrome). IM route preferred to IV use. Give by IV push, or add to most IV solutions and give as infusion.

IV INCOMPATIBILITY

Sodium bicarbonate.

IV COMPATIBILITIES

Famotidine (Pepcid), multivitamins.

INDICATIONS/ROUTES/DOSAGE

Dietary Supplement

PO: ADULTS, ELDERLY: 1–2 mg/day. **CHILDREN:** 0.5–1 mg/day. **INFANTS:** 0.3–0.5 mg/day.

Thiamine Deficiency (Beriberi)

PO: ADULTS, ELDERLY: 5–30 mg/dose IM or IV 3 times/day, then 5–30 mg/day, as a single dose or in 3 divided doses, for 1 mo. **CHILDREN:** 10–50 mg/day in 3 divided doses for 2 wks, then 5–10 mg/day for 1 mo.

Alcohol Withdrawal Syndrome

IV, IM: ADULTS, ELDERLY: 100 mg/day for several days, then **PO:** 50–100 mg/day.

Wernicke's Encephalopathy

IV: ADULTS, ELDERLY: Initially, 100 mg then **IV/IM:** 50–100 mg/day until consuming a regular, balanced diet.

SIDE EFFECTS

Frequent: Pain, induration, tenderness at IM injection site.

ADVERSE EFFECTS/ TOXIC REACTIONS

IV administration may result in rare, severe hypersensitivity reaction marked by feeling of warmth, pruritus, urticaria, weakness, diaphoresis, nausea, restlessness, tightness in throat, angioedema, cyanosis, pulmonary edema, GI tract bleeding, cardiovascular collapse.

NURSING CONSIDERATIONS

INTERVENTION/EVALUATION

Monitor EKG readings, lab values for erythrocyte activity. Assess for clinical improvement (improved sense of well-being, weight gain). Observe for reversal of deficiency symptoms (**neurologic:** peripheral neuropathy, hyporeflexia, nystagmus, ophthalmoplegia, ataxia, muscle weakness; **cardiac:** venous hypertension, bounding arterial pulse, tachycardia, edema; **mental:** confused state).

PATIENT/FAMILY TEACHING

• Discomfort may occur with IM injection. • Foods rich in thiamine include pork, organ meats, whole grain and enriched cereals, legumes, nuts, seeds, yeast, wheat germ, rice bran. • Urine may appear bright yellow.

thioridazine

thy-o-**rid**-a-zeen
(Mellaril)

BLACK BOX ALERT Dose-related prolongation of QT interval may cause arrhythmias, sudden death.

Do not confuse thioridazine with thiothixene or Thorazine, or Mellaril with Elavil or Mebaral.

CLASSIFICATION

PHARMACOTHERAPEUTIC: Phenothiazine. **CLINICAL:** Antipsychotic, sedative, antidyskinetic (see p. 66C).

ACTION

Blocks dopamine at postsynaptic receptor sites. Possesses strong anticholinergic, sedative effects. **Therapeutic Effect:** Suppresses behavioral response in psychosis; reduces locomotor activity, aggressiveness.

PHARMACOKINETICS

Absorption may be erratic. Protein binding: Very high. Metabolized in liver. Excreted in urine. **Half-life:** 21–24 hrs.

USES

Treatment of refractory schizophrenic pts. **OFF-LABEL:** Treatment of behavioral problems in children, dementia, depressive neurosis, psychosis/agitation related to Alzheimer's dementia.

PRECAUTIONS

Contraindications: Angle-closure glaucoma, blood dyscrasias, cardiac arrhythmias, cardiac/hepatic impairment, concurrent use of drugs that prolong QT interval, severe CNS depression. **Cautions:** Seizures, decreased GI motility, urinary retention, benign prostatic hypertrophy, visual problems.

LIFESPAN CONSIDERATIONS

Pregnancy/Lactation: Drug crosses placenta; is distributed in breast milk. **Pregnancy Category C. Children:** Increased risk for development of extrapyramidal symptoms (EPS), neuromuscular symptoms, esp. dystonias. **Elderly:** Prone to anticholinergic effects (dry mouth, EPS, orthostatic hypotension, sedation).

INTERACTIONS

DRUG: **Alcohol, other CNS depressants** may increase respiratory depression, hypotensive effects. **Antithyroid agents** may increase risk of agranulocytosis. **Extrapyramidal symptoms (EPS)-producing medications** may increase risk of EPS. **Hypotensive medications (e.g., antihypertensives, diuretics)** may worsen hypotension. May decrease effects of **levodopa. Lithium** may decrease absorption, produce adverse neurologic effects. **Tricyclic antidepressants** may increase anticholinergic, sedative effects. **Medications causing QT interval prolongation (e.g., erythromycin, procainamide, quinidine)** may lengthen QT interval. **HERBAL:** **Gotu kola, kava kava, St. John's wort, valerian** may increase CNS depression. **Dong quai, St. John's wort** may increase photosensitization. **FOOD:** None known. **LAB VALUES:** May cause EKG changes. **Therapeutic serum level:** 0.2–2.6 mcg/ml; **toxic serum level:** not established.

AVAILABILITY (Rx)

Tablets (Mellaril): 10 mg, 15 mg, 25 mg, 50 mg, 100 mg, 150 mg, 200 mg.

ADMINISTRATION/HANDLING

PO

- May give without regard to food.

INDICATIONS/ROUTES/DOSAGE

Psychosis

PO: ADULTS, ELDERLY, CHILDREN 12 YRS AND OLDER: Initially, 25–100 mg 3 times daily; dosage increased gradually. **Maximum:** 800 mg/day. **CHILDREN 2–11 YRS:** Initially, 0.5–3 mg/kg/day in 2–3 divided doses. **Maximum:** 3 mg/kg/day.

SIDE EFFECTS

Generally well tolerated with only mild, transient side effects. **Occasional:** Drowsiness during early therapy, dry mouth, blurred vision, lethargy, constipation, diarrhea, nasal congestion, peripheral edema, urinary retention. **Rare:** Ocular changes, altered skin pigmentation (in those taking high doses for prolonged periods), photosensitivity, darkening of urine.

ADVERSE EFFECTS/ TOXIC REACTIONS

Prolonged QT interval may produce torsade de pointes, a form of ventricular tachycardia, sudden death.

NURSING CONSIDERATIONS

BASELINE ASSESSMENT

Assess behavior, appearance, emotional status, response to environment, speech pattern, thought content.

INTERVENTION/EVALUATION

Assess for EPS. Monitor EKG, CBC, B/P, serum potassium, hepatic function, eye exams. Monitor for fine tongue movement (may be early sign of tardive dyskinesia). Supervise suicidal-risk pt closely during early therapy (as depression lessens, energy level improves, increasing suicide potential). Assess for therapeutic response (interest in surroundings, improvement in self-care, increased ability to concentrate, relaxed facial expression). **Therapeutic serum level:** 0.2–2.6 mcg/ml; **toxic serum level:** not established.

PATIENT/FAMILY TEACHING

• Full therapeutic effect may take up to 6 wks. • Urine may darken. • Do not abruptly withdraw from long-term drug therapy. • Report visual disturbances. • Sugarless gum, sips of tepid water may relieve dry mouth. • Drowsiness generally subsides during continued therapy. • Avoid tasks that require alertness, motor skills until response to drug is established. • Avoid alcohol. • Avoid exposure to sunlight, artificial light.

thiotepa HIGH ALERT

thy-oh-**teh**-pah
(Thioplex)

◆CLASSIFICATION

PHARMACOTHERAPEUTIC: Alkylating agent. **CLINICAL:** Antineoplastic (see p. 88C).

ACTION

Inhibits DNA, RNA protein synthesis by cross-linking with DNA, RNA strands, preventing cell growth. Cell cycle–phase nonspecific. **Therapeutic Effect:** Produces cell death.

PHARMACOKINETICS

Incompletely absorbed from GI tract. Metabolized in liver. Excreted in urine. **Half-life:** 2.3–2.4 hrs.

USES

Treatment of superficial papillary carcinoma of urinary bladder, adenocarcinoma of breast and ovary, Hodgkin's disease, lymphosarcoma. Intracavitary injection to control pleural, pericardial, peritoneal effusions due to metastatic tumors. **OFF-LABEL:** Treatment of lung carcinoma, neoplastic meningitis.

PRECAUTIONS

Contraindications: Pregnancy, severe myelosuppression (leukocyte count less than $3{,}000/mm^3$ or platelet count less than $150{,}000/mm^3$). **Cautions:** Hepatic/renal impairment, bone marrow dysfunction.

LIFESPAN CONSIDERATIONS

Pregnancy/Lactation: May cause fetal harm. Unknown if drug is distributed in breast milk. **Pregnancy Category D. Children:** Safety and efficacy not established. **Elderly:** No age-related precautions noted.

INTERACTIONS

DRUG: May decrease effects of **antigout medications. Bone marrow depressants** may increase myelosuppression. **Live virus vaccines** may potentiate virus replication, increase vaccine side effects, decrease pt's antibody response to vaccine. **HERBAL:** Avoid **black cohosh, dong quai** in estrogen-dependent tu-

T

mors. **St. John's wort** may increase photosensitization. **Echinacea** may decrease effects. FOOD: None known. LAB VALUES: May increase serum uric acid.

AVAILABILITY (Rx)

Injection, Powder for Reconstitution: 15 mg, 30 mg.

ADMINISTRATION/HANDLING

◀ALERT▶ May be carcinogenic, mutagenic, teratogenic. Handle with extreme caution during preparation/administration.

IV

◀ALERT▶ Give by IV, intrapleural, intraperitoneal, intrapericardial, or intratumor injection; intravesical instillation.

Reconstitution • Reconstitute 15-mg vial with 1.5 ml Sterile Water for Injection to provide concentration of 10 mg/ml. Shake solution gently; let stand to clear. • May further dilute with 0.9% NaCl at concentration 1 mg/ml or greater. • For intravesicular lavage, dilute in 30–60 ml Sterile Water for Injection or 0.9% NaCl.

Rate of administration • Withdraw reconstituted drug through 0.22-micron filter before administration. • For IV push, give over 1–2 min at concentration of 10 mg/ml. • Give IV infusion over 10–60 min. • For intravesical lavage, instill directly into bladder and retain for at least 2 hrs.

Storage • Refrigerate unopened vials. • Reconstituted solution appears clear to slightly opaque; is stable for 28 days if refrigerated. Discard if solution appears grossly opaque or precipitate forms.

IV INCOMPATIBILITIES

Cisplatin (Platinol-AQ), filgrastim (Neupogen).

IV COMPATIBILITIES

Allopurinol (Aloprim), bumetanide (Bumex), calcium gluconate, carboplatin (Paraplatin), cyclophosphamide (Cytoxan), dexamethasone (Decadron), diphenhydramine (Benadryl), doxorubicin (Adriamycin), etoposide (VePesid), fluorouracil, gemcitabine (Gemzar), granisetron (Kytril), heparin, hydromorphone (Dilaudid), leucovorin, lorazepam (Ativan), magnesium sulfate, morphine, ondansetron (Zofran), paclitaxel (Taxol), potassium chloride, vincristine (Oncovin), vinorelbine (Navelbine).

INDICATIONS/ROUTES/DOSAGE

◀ALERT▶ Dosage individualized based on clinical response, tolerance to adverse effects. When used in combination therapy, consult specific protocols for optimum dosage, sequence of drug administration.

Initial Therapy

IV: ADULTS, ELDERLY: Initially, 0.3–0.4 mg/kg every 1–4 wks. Maintenance dose adjusted weekly based on blood counts. **CHILDREN:** 25–65 mg/m^2 as single dose every 3–4 wks.

Control of Effusions

INTRACAVITARY INJECTION: ADULTS, ELDERLY: 0.6–0.8 mg/kg (or 30–60 mg) every 1–4 wks.

SIDE EFFECTS

Occasional: Pain at injection site, headache, dizziness, urticaria, rash, nausea, vomiting, anorexia, stomatitis. **Rare:** Alopecia, cystitis, hematuria (following intravesical administration).

ADVERSE EFFECTS/ TOXIC REACTIONS

Hematologic toxicity (leukopenia, anemia, thrombocytopenia, pancytopenia) may occur due to bone marrow depression. Although WBC count falls to its lowest point 10–14 days after initial therapy, bone marrow effect may not be evident for 30 days. Stomatitis, ulceration of intestinal mucosa may occur.

NURSING CONSIDERATIONS

BASELINE ASSESSMENT

Obtain hematologic tests at least weekly during therapy and for 3 wks after therapy discontinued.

INTERVENTION/EVALUATION

Interrupt therapy if WBC falls below 3,000/mm³, platelet count below 150,000/mm³, WBC or platelet count declines rapidly. Monitor serum uric acid levels, hematology tests. Assess for stomatitis. Monitor for hematologic toxicity: infection (fever, sore throat, signs of local infection), unusual bruising/bleeding from any site, symptoms of anemia (excessive fatigue, weakness). Assess skin for rash, urticaria.

PATIENT/FAMILY TEACHING

• Maintain fastidious oral hygiene. • Do not have immunizations without physician's approval (drug lowers resistance). • Avoid crowds, those with infection. • Promptly report fever, sore throat, signs of local infection, unusual bruising/bleeding from any site.

thiothixene

thy-oh-**thix**-een
(Navane)

BLACK BOX ALERT Elderly pts with dementia related psychosis are at increased risk for death.

Do not confuse thiothixene with fluoxetine or thioridazine, or Navane with Norvasc or Nubain.

◆CLASSIFICATION

CLINICAL: Antipsychotic (see p. 66C).

ACTION

Blocks postsynaptic dopamine receptor sites in brain. Has alpha-adrenergic blocking effects, depresses release of hypothalamic, hypophyseal hormones. **Therapeutic Effect:** Suppresses psychotic behavior.

PHARMACOKINETICS

Well absorbed from GI tract after IM administration. Widely distributed. Metabolized in liver. Primarily excreted in urine. Unknown if removed by hemodialysis. **Half-life:** 34 hrs.

USES

Symptomatic management of schizophrenia. **OFF-LABEL:** Psychosis (children), psychosis/agitation related to Alzheimer's dementia. Rapid tranquilization.

PRECAUTIONS

Contraindications: Blood dyscrasias, circulatory collapse, CNS depression, coma, history of seizures. **Cautions:** Severe cardiovascular disorders, alcohol withdrawal, pt exposure to extreme heat, glaucoma, prostatic hypertrophy.

⌛ LIFESPAN CONSIDERATIONS

Pregnancy/Lactation: Drug crosses placenta; is distributed in breast milk. **Pregnancy Category C. Children:** May develop neuromuscular or extrapyramidal symptoms (EPS), esp. dystonias. **Elderly:** More prone to orthostatic hypotension, anticholinergic effects (e.g., dry mouth), sedation, EPS.

INTERACTIONS

DRUG: **Alcohol, other CNS depressants** may increase CNS, respiratory depression, hypotensive effects. **Extrapyramidal symptoms (EPS)–producing medications** may increase risk of EPS. May inhibit effects of **levodopa. Quinidine** may increase cardiac effects. **HERBAL:** **Kava kava, St. John's wort, valerian** may increase CNS depression. **FOOD:** None known. **LAB VALUES:** May decrease serum uric acid.

AVAILABILITY (Rx)

Capsules: 1 mg, 2 mg, 5 mg, 10 mg, 20 mg.

ADMINISTRATION/HANDLING

PO

• Give without regard to meals.

INDICATIONS/ROUTES/DOSAGE

Mild to Moderate Psychosis

PO: ADULTS, ELDERLY, CHILDREN 12 YRS AND OLDER: 2 mg 3 times daily up to 20–30 mg/day.

Severe Psychosis

PO: ADULTS, ELDERLY, CHILDREN 12 YRS AND OLDER: Initially, 5 mg twice daily. May increase gradually up to 60 mg/day.

Rapid Tranquilization of Agitated Pt

PO: ADULTS, ELDERLY: 5–10 mg q30–60 min. **Average total dose:** 15–30 mg.

SIDE EFFECTS

Frequent: Transient drowsiness, dry mouth, constipation, blurred vision, nasal congestion. **Occasional:** Diarrhea, peripheral edema, urinary retention, nausea. **Rare:** Ocular changes, altered skin pigmentation (in those taking high doses for prolonged periods), photosensitivity, hypotension, dizziness, syncope.

ADVERSE EFFECTS/ TOXIC REACTIONS

Most common extrapyramidal reaction is akathisia, characterized by motor restlessness, anxiety. Akinesia, marked by rigidity, tremor, increased salivation, mask-like facial expression, reduced voluntary movements, occurs less frequently. Dystonias, including torticollis (neck muscle spasm), opisthotonos (rigidity of back muscles), oculogyric crisis (rolling back of eyes), occur rarely. Tardive dyskinesia, characterized by tongue protrusion, puffing of cheeks, chewing/puckering of mouth, occurs rarely but may be irreversible. Elderly female pts have greater risk of developing this reaction. Grand mal seizures may occur in epileptic pts. Neuroleptic malignant syndrome occurs rarely.

NURSING CONSIDERATIONS

BASELINE ASSESSMENT

Assess behavior, appearance, emotional status, response to environment, speech pattern, thought content.

INTERVENTION/EVALUATION

Supervise suicidal-risk pt closely during early therapy (as depression lessens, energy level improves, increasing suicide potential). Monitor B/P for hypotension. Assess for peripheral edema. Monitor daily pattern of bowel activity, stool consistency. Prevent constipation. Observe for extrapyramidal symptoms (EPS), tardive dyskinesia; monitor for potentially fatal, rare neuroleptic malignant syndrome. Assess for therapeutic response (interest in surroundings, improvement in self-care, increased ability to concentrate, relaxed facial expression).

PATIENT/FAMILY TEACHING

• Full therapeutic effect may take up to 6 wks. • Report visual disturbances. • Sugarless gum, sips of tepid water may relieve dry mouth. • Drowsiness generally subsides during continued therapy. • Avoid tasks that require alertness, motor skills until response to drug is established. • Avoid alcohol, other CNS depressants. • Avoid exposure to direct sunlight, artificial light.

tiagabine

tye-**ag**-ah-bean
(Gabitril)
Do not confuse tiagabine with tizanidine.

◆CLASSIFICATION

CLINICAL: Anticonvulsant (see p. 36C).

ACTION

Blocks reuptake in presynaptic neurons of gamma-aminobutyric acid (GABA), the major inhibitory neurotransmitter in the CNS, in the presynaptic neurons, increasing GABA levels at postsynaptic neurons. **Therapeutic Effect:** Inhibits seizures.

USES

Adjunctive therapy for treatment of partial seizures. **OFF-LABEL:** Bipolar disorder.

PHARMACOKINETICS

Rapidly absorbed from GI tract. Protein binding: 96%. Metabolized in liver. Primarily eliminated in feces. **Half-life:** 2–5 hrs.

PRECAUTIONS

Contraindications: None known. **Cautions:** Hepatic impairment. Concurrent use of alcohol, other CNS depressants may cause seizures.

LIFESPAN CONSIDERATIONS

Pregnancy/Lactation: May produce teratogenic effects. Distributed in breast milk. **Pregnancy Category C. Children:** Safety and efficacy not established in those younger than 12 yrs. **Elderly:** Age-related hepatic impairment may require dosage adjustment.

INTERACTIONS

DRUG: **Carbamazepine, phenobarbital, phenytoin** may increase clearance. May alter effects of **valproic acid.** **HERBAL:** **Ginkgo biloba** may increase seizure threshold. **St. John's wort** may decrease concentration. **Gotu kola, kava kava, St. John's wort, valerian** may increase CNS depression. **FOOD:** None known. **LAB VALUES:** None significant.

AVAILABILITY (Rx)

Tablets: 2 mg, 4 mg, 12 mg, 16 mg.

ADMINISTRATION/HANDLING

- Give with food.

INDICATIONS/ROUTES/DOSAGE

Partial Seizures

PO: ADULTS, ELDERLY: Initially, 4 mg once daily. May increase by 4–8 mg/day at weekly intervals. **Maximum:** 56 mg/day. **CHILDREN 12–18 YRS:** Initially, 4 mg once daily. May increase by 4 mg at wk 2 and by 4–8 mg at weekly intervals thereafter. **Maximum:** 32 mg/day.

SIDE EFFECTS

Frequent (34%–20%): Dizziness, asthenia (loss of strength, energy), drowsiness, nervousness, confusion, headache, infection, tremor. **Occasional:** Nausea, diarrhea, abdominal pain, impaired concentration.

ADVERSE EFFECTS/ TOXIC REACTIONS

Overdose characterized by agitation, confusion, hostility, weakness. Full recovery occurs within 24 hrs.

NURSING CONSIDERATIONS

BASELINE ASSESSMENT

Review history of seizure disorder (intensity, frequency, duration, LOC). Observe frequently for recurrence of seizure activity. Initiate seizure precautions.

INTERVENTION/EVALUATION

For those on long-term therapy, serum hepatic/renal function tests, CBC should be performed periodically. Assist with ambulation if dizziness occurs. Assess for clinical improvement (decrease in intensity, frequency of seizures). Monitor for depression, unusual behavior, suicidal ideation or thoughts.

PATIENT/FAMILY TEACHING

- If dizziness occurs, change positions slowly from recumbent to sitting position before standing. • Avoid tasks that require alertness, motor skills until response to drug is established. • Avoid alcohol. • Notify physician of worsening seizure activity, thoughts of suicide, increased depression.

ticlopidine HIGH ALERT

tye-**klo**-pye-deen
(Apo-Ticlopidine ✤, Novo-Ticlopidine ✤, Ticlid)

BLACK BOX ALERT Risk of neutropenia, agranulocytosis, thrombotic thrombocytopenia purpura, aplastic anemia.

CLASSIFICATION

PHARMACOTHERAPEUTIC: Aggregation inhibitor. **CLINICAL:** Antiplatelet (see p. 33C).

ACTION

Inhibits release of adenosine diphosphate from activated platelets, preventing fibrinogen from binding to glycoprotein IIb/IIIa receptors on surface of activated platelets. **Therapeutic Effect:** Inhibits platelet aggregation, thrombus formation.

PHARMACOKINETICS

Route	Onset	Peak	Duration
PO (platelet inhibition)	2 days	8–11 days	1–2 wks

Rapidly absorbed following PO administration. Protein binding: 98%. Extensively metabolized in liver. Primarily excreted in urine; partially eliminated in feces. **Half-life:** 7.9–12.6 hrs.

USES

To reduce risk of stroke in those who have experienced stroke-like symptoms (transient ischemic attacks) or with history of thrombotic stroke. **OFF-LABEL:** Prevention of postop deep vein thrombosis (DVT), protection of aortocoronary bypass grafts, reduction of graft loss after renal transplant, treatment of intermittent claudication, sickle cell disease, subarachnoid hemorrhage, diabetic microangiopathy, ischemic heart disease.

PRECAUTIONS

Contraindications: Active pathologic bleeding (e.g., bleeding peptic ulcer, intracranial bleeding), hematopoietic disorders (neutropenia, thrombocytopenia), presence of hemostatic disorder, severe hepatic impairment. **Cautions:** Those at increased risk for bleeding, severe hepatic/renal disease.

LIFESPAN CONSIDERATIONS

Pregnancy/Lactation: Unknown if drug crosses placenta or is distributed in breast milk. **Pregnancy Category B. Children:** Safety and efficacy not established. **Elderly:** No age-related precautions noted.

INTERACTIONS

DRUG: Aspirin, heparin, NSAIDs, oral anticoagulants, thrombolytics may increase risk of bleeding. May increase concentration, risk of toxicity of **phenytoin, theophylline. HERBAL: Cat's claw, dong quai, evening primrose, feverfew, garlic, ginger, ginkgo biloba, ginseng, horse chestnut, red clover** possess antiplatelet activity, may increase risk of bleeding. **FOOD: All foods** increase bioavailability. **LAB VALUES:** May increase serum cholesterol, alkaline phosphatase, bilirubin, triglycerides, AST, ALT. May prolong bleeding time. May decrease neutrophil, platelet counts.

AVAILABILITY (Rx)

Tablets: 250 mg.

ADMINISTRATION/HANDLING

PO

• Give with food or just after meals (bioavailability increased, GI discomfort decreased).

INDICATIONS/ROUTES/DOSAGE

Prevention of Stroke

PO: ADULTS, ELDERLY: 250 mg twice a day.

SIDE EFFECTS

Frequent (13%–5%): Diarrhea, nausea, dyspepsia (heartburn, indigestion, epigastric pain, bloating). **Rare (2%–1%):** Vomiting, flatulence, pruritus, dizziness.

ADVERSE EFFECTS/ TOXIC REACTIONS

Neutropenia occurs in approximately 2% of pts. Thrombotic thrombocytopenia purpura, agranulocytosis, hepatitis, cholestatic jaundice, tinnitus occur rarely.

NURSING CONSIDERATIONS

BASELINE ASSESSMENT

Drug should be discontinued 10–14 days before surgery if antiplatelet effect is not desired.

INTERVENTION/EVALUATION

Monitor daily pattern of bowel activity, stool consistency. Assist with ambulation if dizziness occurs. Observe, monitor neurologic status for changes. Assess skin for flushing, rash. Observe for signs of bleeding. Monitor CBC, serum hepatic/renal function tests.

PATIENT/FAMILY TEACHING

• Take with food to decrease GI symptoms. • Periodic blood tests are essential. • Inform physician if fever, sore throat, chills, unusual bleeding occurs.

tigecycline

tye-ge-**sye**-kleen
(Tygacil)

◆CLASSIFICATION

PHARMACOTHERAPEUTIC: Glycylcycline. **CLINICAL:** Antibiotic.

ACTION

Blocks protein synthesis by binding to ribosomal receptor sites of bacterial cell wall. **Therapeutic Effect:** Bacteriostatic effect.

PHARMACOKINETICS

Extensive tissue distribution, minimally metabolized. Eliminated mainly by biliary/fecal route, with lesser amount excreted in urine. Protein binding: 71%–89%. **Half-life:** Single dose: 27 hrs, following multiple doses: 42 hrs.

USES

Treatment of susceptible infections due to *E. coli, E. faecalis, S. aureus, S. agalactiae, S. anginosus* group (includes *S. anginosus, S. intermedius, S. constellatus*), *S. pyogenes, B. fragilis, Citrobacter freundii, E. cloacae, K. oxytoca, K. pneumoniae, B. thetaiotaomicron, B. uniformis, B. vulgatus, C. perfringens, Peptostreptococcus micros* including complicated skin/skin structure infections, complicated intra-abdominal infections, community-acquired bacterial pneumonia.

PRECAUTIONS

Contraindications: Children younger than 18 yrs. **Cautions:** Hypersensitivity to tetracyclines, last half of pregnancy, hepatic impairment.

⌛ LIFESPAN CONSIDERATIONS

Pregnancy/Lactation: May cause fetal harm. May be distributed in breast milk. Permanent discoloration of the teeth (brown-gray) may occur if used during tooth development. **Pregnancy Category D. Children:** Safety and efficacy not established in those younger than 18 yrs. **Elderly:** No age-related precautions noted.

INTERACTIONS

DRUG: Effects of **oral contraceptives** may be decreased. **Warfarin** may increase risk of hypoprothrombinemia. **HERBAL:** None significant. **FOOD:** None known. **LAB VALUES:** May increase BUN, serum alkaline phosphatase, amylase, bilirubin, glucose, LDH, ALT, AST. May decrease Hgb, WBCs, thrombocytes, serum potassium, protein.

AVAILABILITY (Rx)

Injection, Powder for Reconstitution (**Tygacil**): 50-mg vial.

ADMINISTRATION/HANDLING

IV

Reconstitution • Add 5.3 ml 0.9% NaCl or D_5W to each 50-mg vial. Swirl gently to dissolve. Resulting solution is 10 mg/ml. • Immediately withdraw 5 ml reconstituted solution and add to 100 ml 0.9% NaCl or D_5W bag for infusion (final concentration should not exceed 1 mg/ml). • Reconstituted solution appears yellow to red-orange.

T

Rate of administration • Administer over 30–60 min every 12 hrs. • May be given through a dedicated line or by Y-site piggyback. If same line is used for sequential infusion of several different drugs, line should be flushed before and after infusion of tigecycline with either 0.9% NaCl or D_5W.
Storage • Reconstituted solution is stable for up to 6 hrs at room temperature or up to 24 hrs if refrigerated. • Discard if solution is discolored (green, black) or precipitate forms.

IV INCOMPATIBILITIES

Amphotericin B, chlorpromazine, methylprednisolone, voriconazole.

IV COMPATIBILITIES

Dobutamine, dopamine, lactated Ringer's, lidocaine, potassium chloride, ranitidine, theophylline.

INDICATIONS/ROUTES/DOSAGE

Systemic Infections

IV: ADULTS OVER 18 YRS, ELDERLY: Initially, 100 mg, followed by 50 mg every 12 hrs for 5–14 days.

Dosage in Severe Hepatic Impairment

IV: ADULTS OVER 18 YRS, ELDERLY: Initially, 100 mg, followed by 25 mg every 12 hrs.

SIDE EFFECTS

Frequent (29%–13%): Nausea, vomiting, diarrhea. **Occasional (7%–4%):** Headache, hypertension, dizziness, increased cough, delayed healing. **Rare (3%–2%):** Peripheral edema, pruritus, constipation, dyspepsia (heartburn, indigestion, epigastric pain), asthenia (loss of strength, energy), hypotension, phlebitis, insomnia, rash, diaphoresis.

ADVERSE EFFECTS/ TOXIC REACTIONS

Dyspnea, abscess, pseudomembranous colitis (abdominal cramps, severe watery diarrhea, fever) ranging from mild to life-threatening may result from altered bacterial balance.

NURSING CONSIDERATIONS

BASELINE ASSESSMENT

Question for history of allergies, esp. tetracyclines, before therapy.

INTERVENTION/EVALUATION

Monitor daily pattern of bowel activity, stool consistency. Be alert for superinfection: fever, anal/genital pruritus, oral mucosal changes (ulceration, pain, erythema). Nausea, vomiting may be controlled by antiemetics.

PATIENT/FAMILY TEACHING

• Notify physician if diarrhea, rash, mouth soreness, other new symptoms occur.

tiludronate

tye-**loo**-dro-nate
(Skelid)

CLASSIFICATION

PHARMACOTHERAPEUTIC: Bone resorption inhibitor. **CLINICAL:** Calcium regulator.

ACTION

Inhibits functioning osteoclasts through disruption of cytoskeletal ring structure, inhibition of osteoclastic proton pump. **Therapeutic Effect:** Inhibits bone resorption.

PHARMACOKINETICS

Route	Onset	Peak	Duration
PO (platelet inhibition)	2 days	8–11 days	1–2 wks

Well absorbed following PO administration. Protein binding: 90%. Minimally metabolized in liver. Excreted in urine. **Half-life:** 150 hrs.

USES

Treatment of Paget's disease of bone (osteitis deformans).

PRECAUTIONS

Contraindications: GI disease (e.g., dysphagia, gastric ulcer), renal impairment, inability to stand or sit upright for at least 30 min. **Cautions:** Hyperparathyroidism, hypocalcemia, vitamin D deficiency.

LIFESPAN CONSIDERATIONS

Pregnancy/Lactation: Unknown if drug crosses placenta or is distributed in breast milk. **Pregnancy Category C. Children:** Safety and efficacy not established. **Elderly:** No age-related precautions noted.

INTERACTIONS

DRUG: Antacids containing aluminum or magnesium, calcium, salicylates may interfere with absorption. **HERBAL:** None significant. **FOOD:** None known. **LAB VALUES:** None significant.

AVAILABILITY (Rx)

Tablets: 200 mg.

ADMINISTRATION/HANDLING

PO

- Must take with 6–8 oz plain water.
- Do not give within 2 hrs of food intake.
- Avoid giving aspirin, calcium supplements, mineral supplements, antacids within 2 hrs of tiludronate administration.

INDICATIONS/ROUTES/DOSAGE

Paget's Disease

PO: ADULTS, ELDERLY: 400 mg once a day for 3 mos. Not recommended in pts with creatinine clearance less than 30 ml/min.

SIDE EFFECTS

Frequent (9%–6%): Nausea, diarrhea, generalized body pain, back pain, headache. **Occasional (less than 6%):** Rash, dyspepsia (heartburn, indigestion, epigastric pain), vomiting, rhinitis, sinusitis, dizziness.

ADVERSE EFFECTS/ TOXIC REACTIONS

Dysphagia, esophagitis, esophageal ulcer, gastric ulcer occur rarely.

NURSING CONSIDERATIONS

BASELINE ASSESSMENT

Assess if pt is using other medications (esp. aluminum, magnesium, calcium, salicylates). Determine baseline renal function. Assess for GI disease.

INTERVENTION/EVALUATION

Monitor serum osteocalcin, alkaline phosphatase, adjusted calcium, urinary hydroxyproline to assess effectiveness of medication.

PATIENT/FAMILY TEACHING

• Take with 6–8 oz water. • Avoid other medication for 2 hrs before or after taking tiludronate. • Check with physician if calcium, vitamin D supplements are necessary.

timolol

HIGH ALERT

tim-oh-lole
(Apo-Timol ✦, Apo-Timop ✦, Betimol, Gen-Timolol ✦, Istalol, Novo-Timol ✦, PMS-Timolol ✦, Timoptic, Timoptic OccuDose, Timoptic XE).

BLACK BOX ALERT Abrupt withdrawal can produce acute tachycardia, hypertension, ischemia; must be gradually tapered over 1–2 wks.

Do not confuse timolol with atenolol or Tylenol, or Timoptic with Betoptic or Viroptic.

FIXED-COMBINATION(S)

Combigan: timolol/brimonidine (an alpha$_2$ agonist): 0.5%/0.2%. **Cosopt:** timolol/dorzolamide (a carbonic anhydrase inhibitor): 0.5%/2%. **Timolide:** timolol/hydrochlorothiazide (a diuretic): 10 mg/25 mg.

CLASSIFICATION

PHARMACOTHERAPEUTIC: Beta-adrenergic blocker. **CLINICAL:** Antihypertensive, antimigraine, antiglaucoma (see pp. 52C, 72C).

T

ACTION

Blocks $beta_1$-, $beta_2$-adrenergic receptors. Therapeutic Effect: Reduces intraocular pressure (IOP) by reducing aqueous humor production, lowers B/P, slows heart rate, decreases myocardial contractility.

PHARMACOKINETICS

Route	Onset	Peak	Duration
PO	15–45 min	0.5–2.5 hrs	4 hrs
Ophthalmic	30 min	1–2 hrs	12–24 hrs

Well absorbed from GI tract. Protein binding: 60%. Minimal absorption after ophthalmic administration. Metabolized in liver. Primarily excreted in urine. Not removed by hemodialysis. **Half-life:** 2–2.7 hrs. Systemic absorption may occur with ophthalmic administration.

USES

Management of mild to moderate hypertension. Used alone or in combination with diuretics, esp. thiazide type. Reduces cardiovascular mortality in those with definite or suspected acute MI. Prophylaxis of migraine headache. **Ophthalmic:** Reduces IOP in management of open-angle glaucoma, aphakic glaucoma, ocular hypertension, secondary glaucoma. OFF-LABEL: **Systemic:** Treatment of anxiety, cardiac arrhythmias, chronic angina pectoris, hypertrophic cardiomyopathy, migraine, pheochromocytoma, thyrotoxicosis, tremors. **Ophthalmic:** Decreases IOP in acute or chronic angle-closure glaucoma, treatment of angle-closure glaucoma during and after iridectomy, malignant glaucoma, secondary glaucoma.

T

PRECAUTIONS

Contraindications: Bronchial asthma, cardiogenic shock, CHF (unless secondary to tachyarrhythmias), COPD, pts receiving MAOI therapy, second- or third-degree heart block, sinus bradycardia, uncontrolled cardiac failure. **Cautions:** Inadequate cardiac function, renal/hepatic impairment, hyperthyroidism. Precautions also apply to ophthalmic administration (due to systemic absorption of ophthalmic solution).

LIFESPAN CONSIDERATIONS

Pregnancy/Lactation: Distributed in breast milk; not for use in breast-feeding women because of potential for serious adverse effect on breast-feeding infant. Avoid use during first trimester. May produce bradycardia, apnea, hypoglycemia, hypothermia in infant during delivery; low birth-weight infants. **Pregnancy Category C (D if used in second or third trimester).** **Children:** Safety and efficacy not established. **Elderly:** Age-related peripheral vascular disease increases susceptibility to decreased peripheral circulation.

INTERACTIONS

DRUG: **Diuretics, other antihypertensives** may increase hypotensive effect. May mask symptoms of hypoglycemia, prolong hypoglycemic effects of **insulin, oral hypoglycemics. NSAIDs** may decrease antihypertensive effect. **Sympathomimetics, xanthines** may mutually inhibit effects. HERBAL: None significant. FOOD: None known. LAB VALUES: May increase antinuclear antibody titer (ANA), BUN, serum LDH, alkaline phosphatase, bilirubin, creatinine, potassium, uric acid, AST, ALT, triglycerides, lipoproteins.

AVAILABILITY (Rx)

Ophthalmic Gel (Timoptic-XE): 0.25%, 0.5%. Ophthalmic Solution (Betimol, Istalol, Timoptic, Timoptic Occudose): 0.25%, 0.5%. Tablets: 5 mg, 10 mg, 20 mg.

ADMINISTRATION/HANDLING

PO

• Give without regard to meals. • Tablets may be crushed.

Ophthalmic

ALERT When using gel, invert container, shake once prior to each use. • Place gloved finger on lower eyelid and pull out until pocket is formed between eye and lower lid. • Place prescribed number of drops or amount of prescribed gel into pocket. • Instruct pt to close eye gently so that medication will not be squeezed out of sac. • Apply gentle finger pressure to the lacrimal sac at inner canthus for 1 min following instillation (lessens risk of systemic absorption).

INDICATIONS/ROUTES/DOSAGE

Mild to Moderate Hypertension

PO: ADULTS, ELDERLY: Initially, 10 mg twice daily, alone or in combination with other therapy. Gradually increase at intervals of not less than 1 wk. Maintenance: 20–60 mg/day in 2 divided doses.

Reduction of Cardiovascular Mortality in Acute MI

PO: ADULTS, ELDERLY: 10 mg twice daily, within 1–4 wks after infarction.

Migraine Prevention

PO: ADULTS, ELDERLY: Initially, 10 mg twice daily. Range: 10–30 mg/day.

Reduction of Intraocular Pressure (IOP)

OPHTHALMIC: ADULTS, ELDERLY, CHILDREN: 1 drop of 0.25% solution in affected eye(s) twice daily. May be increased to 1 drop of 0.5% solution in affected eye(s) twice daily. When IOP is controlled, dosage may be reduced to 1 drop once daily. If pt is switched to timolol from another antiglaucoma agent, administer concurrently for 1 day. Discontinue other agent on following day.

OPHTHALMIC (Timoptic XE): ADULTS, ELDERLY: 1 drop/day (0.25% or 0.5%).

OPHTHALMIC (Istalol): ADULTS, ELDERLY: Apply 1 drop (0.5%) once daily in the morning.

SIDE EFFECTS

Frequent: Diminished sexual function, drowsiness, difficulty sleeping, asthenia (loss of strength, energy), fatigue. Ophthalmic: Eye irritation, visual disturbances. **Occasional:** Depression, cold hands/feet, diarrhea, constipation, anxiety, nasal congestion, nausea, vomiting. **Rare:** Altered taste, dry eyes, pruritus, numbness of fingers, toes, scalp.

ADVERSE EFFECTS/ TOXIC REACTIONS

Overdose may produce profound bradycardia, hypotension, bronchospasm. Abrupt withdrawal may result in diaphoresis, palpitations, headache, tremors. May precipitate CHF, MI in those with cardiac disease; thyroid storm in those with thyrotoxicosis; peripheral ischemia in those with existing peripheral vascular disease. Hypoglycemia may occur in pts with previously controlled diabetes. Ophthalmic overdose may produce bradycardia, hypotension, bronchospasm, acute cardiac failure.

NURSING CONSIDERATIONS

BASELINE ASSESSMENT

Assess B/P, apical pulse immediately before drug is administered (if pulse is 60 min or less or systolic B/P is less than 90 mm Hg, withhold medication, contact physician).

INTERVENTION/EVALUATION

Assess pulse for quality, rate, rhythm. Monitor pulse for irregular rate, bradycardia. Monitor EKG for cardiac arrhythmias, particularly PVCs. Monitor daily pattern of bowel activity, stool consistency. Monitor heart rate, B/P, serum hepatic/renal function, IOP (ophthalmic preparation).

PATIENT/FAMILY TEACHING

• Do not abruptly discontinue medication. • Compliance with therapy regimen is essential to control glaucoma, hypertension, angina, arrhythmias. • Avoid tasks that require alertness, motor skills until response to drug is established. • Report shortness of breath, unusual fatigue, prolonged dizziness, headache. • Do not use nasal decongestants, OTC cold preparations (stimulants) without physician approval. • Restrict salt, alcohol intake. • **Ophthalmic:** Instill drops correctly following guidelines. • Transient stinging, discomfort may occur upon instillation.

tinzaparin

HIGH ALERT

tin-**zap**-a-rin
(Innohep)

BLACK BOX ALERT Pts with recent epidural or spinal anesthesia are at risk for spinal or epidural hematoma, subsequent paralysis.

◆CLASSIFICATION

PHARMACOTHERAPEUTIC: Low-molecular-weight heparin. **CLINICAL:** Anticoagulant (see p. 31C).

ACTION

Inhibits factor Xa. Causes less inactivation of thrombin, inhibition of platelets, bleeding than with standard heparin. Does not significantly influence bleeding time, PT, aPTT. **Therapeutic Effect:** Produces anticoagulation.

PHARMACOKINETICS

Well absorbed after subcutaneous administration. Partially metabolized. Primarily eliminated in urine. **Half-life:** 3–4 hrs.

USES

Treatment of acute symptomatic deep vein thrombosis (DVT) with or without pulmonary embolism, when given in conjunction with warfarin.

PRECAUTIONS

Contraindications: Active major bleeding, concurrent heparin therapy, hypersensitivity to heparin, sulfites, benzyl alcohol, pork products, thrombocytopenia associated with positive in vitro test for antiplatelet antibody. **Cautions:** Conditions with increased risk of hemorrhage, history of heparin-induced thrombocytopenia, renal impairment, elderly, uncontrolled arterial hypertension, history of recent GI ulceration, hemorrhage.

⧗ LIFESPAN CONSIDERATIONS

Pregnancy/Lactation: Use with caution, particularly during last trimester, immediate postpartum period (increased risk of maternal hemorrhage). Unknown if distributed in breast milk. **Pregnancy Category B. Children:** Safety and efficacy not established. **Elderly:** May be more susceptible to bleeding.

INTERACTIONS

DRUG: **Anticoagulants, NSAIDs, platelet aggregation inhibitors** may increase risk of bleeding. **HERBAL:** None significant. **FOOD:** None known. **LAB VALUES:** May increase AST, ALT.

AVAILABILITY (Rx)

Injection Solution: 20,000 anti-Xa international units/ml.

ADMINISTRATION/HANDLING

◀ALERT▶ Do not mix with other injections or infusions. Do not give IM.

Subcutaneous

• Parenteral form appears clear and colorless to pale yellow. • Store at room temperature. • Instruct pt to lie down before administering by deep subcutaneous injection.

INDICATIONS/ROUTES/DOSAGE

Deep Vein Thrombosis (DVT)

SUBCUTANEOUS: ADULTS, ELDERLY: 175 anti-Xa international units/kg once a day. Continue for at least 6 days and until pt is sufficiently anticoagulated with warfarin (international normalized ratio [INR] of 2 or more for 2 consecutive days). Use with caution in pts with creatinine clearance 50 ml/min or less.

SIDE EFFECTS

Frequent (16%): Injection site reaction (e.g., inflammation, oozing, nodules,

T

skin necrosis). Rare (less than 2%): Nausea, asthenia (loss of strength, energy), constipation, epistaxis.

ADVERSE EFFECTS/ TOXIC REACTIONS

Overdose may lead to bleeding complications ranging from local ecchymoses to major hemorrhage. **Antidote:** Dose of protamine sulfate (1% solution) should be equal to dose of tinzaparin injected. One mg protamine sulfate neutralizes 100 units of tinzaparin. Second dose of 0.5 mg protamine sulfate per 100 units tinzaparin may be given if aPTT tested 2–4 hrs after initial infusion remains prolonged.

NURSING CONSIDERATIONS

BASELINE ASSESSMENT

Assess CBC, including platelet count. Determine baseline B/P.

INTERVENTION/EVALUATION

Periodically monitor CBC, platelet count. Assess for any sign of bleeding: bleeding at surgical site, hematuria, blood in stool, bleeding from gums, petechiae, bruising, bleeding from injection sites. Administer only subcutaneously.

PATIENT/FAMILY TEACHING

• May have tendency to bleed easily, use precautions (e.g., use electric razor, soft toothbrush). • Inform physician if chest pain, unusual bleeding/bruising, pain, numbness, tingling, swelling in joints, injection site reaction (oozing, nodules, inflammation) occur.

tiotropium

tee-oh-**trow**-pea-um
(Spiriva)
Do not confuse Spiriva with Inspra or Serevent, or tiotropium with ipratropium.

CLASSIFICATION

PHARMACOTHERAPEUTIC: Anticholinergic. **CLINICAL:** Bronchodilator.

ACTION

Binds to recombinant human muscarinic receptors at smooth muscle, resulting in long-acting bronchial smooth-muscle relaxation. **Therapeutic Effect:** Relieves bronchospasm.

PHARMACOKINETICS

Route	Onset	Peak	Duration
Inhalation	N/A	N/A	24–36 hrs

Binds extensively to tissue. Protein binding: 72%. Metabolized by oxidation. Excreted in urine. **Half-life:** 5–6 days.

USES

Long-term maintenance treatment of bronchospasm associated with COPD, including chronic bronchitis, emphysema, and for reducing COPD exacerbations.

PRECAUTIONS

Contraindications: History of hypersensitivity to atropine or its derivatives. **Cautions:** Narrow-angle glaucoma, prostatic hypertrophy, bladder neck obstruction.

LIFESPAN CONSIDERATIONS

Pregnancy/Lactation: Unknown if distributed in breast milk. **Pregnancy Category C. Children:** Safety and efficacy not established. **Elderly:** Higher frequency of dry mouth, constipation, UTI noted with increasing age.

INTERACTIONS

DRUG: Concurrent administration with **ipratropium** is not recommended. **HERBAL:** None significant. **FOOD:** None known. **LAB VALUES:** None significant.

AVAILABILITY (Rx)

Powder for Inhalation: 18 mcg/capsule (in blister packs).

T

ADMINISTRATION/HANDLING

Inhalation
• Open dustcap of *HandiHaler* by pulling it upward, then open mouthpiece. • Place capsule in center chamber and firmly close mouthpiece until a click is heard, leaving the dustcap open. • Hold *HandiHaler* device with mouthpiece upward, press piercing button completely in once, and release. • Instruct pt to breathe out completely before breathing in slowly and deeply but at rate sufficient to hear the capsule vibrate. • Have pt hold breath as long as it is comfortable until exhaling slowly. • Instruct pt to repeat once again to ensure full dose is received.

Storage • Store at room temperature. Do not expose capsules to extreme temperature, moisture. • Do not store capsules in *HandiHaler* device. • Use immediately once foil is peeled back or removed.

INDICATIONS/ROUTES/DOSAGE

COPD (Maintenance Treatment, Reduction of COPD Exacerbations)
INHALATION: ADULTS, ELDERLY: 18 mcg (1 capsule)/day via *HandiHaler* inhalation device.

SIDE EFFECTS

Frequent (16%–6%): Dry mouth, sinusitis, pharyngitis, dyspepsia, UTI, rhinitis. **Occasional (5%–4%):** Abdominal pain, peripheral edema, constipation, epistaxis, vomiting, myalgia, rash, oral candidiasis.

ADVERSE EFFECTS/ TOXIC REACTIONS

Angina pectoris, depression, flu-like symptoms, glaucoma, increased intraocular pressure occur rarely.

NURSING CONSIDERATIONS

BASELINE ASSESSMENT

Offer emotional support (high incidence of anxiety due to difficulty in breathing, sympathomimetic response to drug).

INTERVENTION/EVALUATION

Monitor rate, depth, rhythm, type of respiration; quality, rate of pulse. Assess lung sounds for rhonchi, wheezing, rales. Monitor ABGs. Observe lips, fingernails for cyanosis (blue or dusky color in light-skinned pts; gray in dark-skinned pts). Observe for clavicular retractions, hand tremor. Evaluate for clinical improvement (quieter, slower respirations, relaxed facial expression, cessation of clavicular retractions).

PATIENT/FAMILY TEACHING

• Increase fluid intake (decreases lung secretion viscosity). • Do not use more than 1 capsule for inhalation at any one time. • Rinsing mouth with water immediately after inhalation may prevent mouth/throat dryness, moniliasis. • Avoid excessive use of caffeine derivatives (chocolate, coffee, tea, cola, cocoa). • Report eye pain/discomfort, blurred vision, visual halos.

tipranavir

ti-**pran**-ah-veer
(Aptivus)

BLACK BOX ALERT May cause hepatitis (including fatalities), hepatic dysfunction. Intracranial hemorrhage has occurred.

◆CLASSIFICATION

PHARMACOTHERAPEUTIC: Antiretroviral. **CLINICAL:** Protease inhibitor.

ACTION

Prevents virus-specific processing of polyproteins, HIV-1 infected cells. **Therapeutic Effect:** Prevents formation of mature viral cells.

PHARMACOKINETICS

Incompletely absorbed following PO administration. Protein binding: 98%–99%. Metabolized in liver. Eliminated mainly in feces, with lesser amount eliminated in urine. **Half-life:** 6 hrs.

USES

Treatment of HIV infection in combination with ritonavir and other antiretroviral agents.

PRECAUTIONS

Contraindications: Moderate to severe hepatic insufficiency, concurrent use of tipranavir/ritonavir with alfuzosin, amiodarone, bepridil, dihydroergotamine, ergonovine, ergotamine, flecainide, lovastatin, methylergonovine, midazolam, propafenone, quinidine, simvastatin, St. John's wort, triazolam, voriconazole. **Cautions:** Diabetes mellitus, hemophilia, known sulfonamide allergy, mild hepatic impairment, pts at increased risk for bleeding from trauma, surgery, concurrent antiplatelet/anticoagulant therapy.

⌛ LIFESPAN CONSIDERATIONS

Pregnancy/Lactation: Unknown if drug crosses placenta or is distributed in breast milk. **Pregnancy Category C. Children:** Safety and efficacy not established. **Elderly:** Age-related hepatic impairment may require dosage adjustment.

INTERACTIONS

DRUG: May interfere with metabolism of **amiodarone, bepridil, ergotamine, lidocaine, midazolam, oral contraceptives, quinidine, triazolam, tricyclic antidepressants.** May increase concentration of **antiarrhythmics, antihistamines, GI motility medications. Benzodiazepines** may increase sedation, risk of respiratory depression. **Carbamazepine, phenobarbital, phenytoin, rifampin** may decrease concentration. May increase concentration of **clozapine, HMG-CoA reductase inhibitors, warfarin. Ergot derivatives** may cause ergot toxicity. **HMG-CoA reductase inhibitors** may increase risk of myopathy including rhabdomyolysis. **HERBAL: St. John's wort** may lead to loss of virologic response, potential resistance to tipranavir. **FOOD: High-fat meals** may increase bioavailability. **LAB VALUES:** May increase serum cholesterol, triglycerides, amylase, ALT, AST. May decrease WBC count.

AVAILABILITY (Rx)

Capsules: 250 mg. **Oral Solution:** 100 mg/ml.

ADMINISTRATION/HANDLING

PO

• Best given with food (should be given with a high-fat meal). • Store unopened bottles of capsules in refrigerator. • Do not freeze/refrigerate oral solution. • Once bottle is opened, capsules may be stored at room temperature for 60 days. Use oral solution within 60 days after opening.

INDICATIONS/ROUTES/DOSAGE

HIV Infection

PO: ADULTS, ELDERLY: 500 mg (2 capsules) administered with 200 mg of ritonavir twice a day. **CHILDREN 2–18 YRS:** 14 mg/kg with 6 mg/kg ritonavir twice daily. **Maximum:** 500 mg with 200 mg ritonavir twice daily.

SIDE EFFECTS

Frequent (11%): Diarrhea. **Occasional (7%–2%):** Nausea, fever, fatigue, headache, depression, vomiting, abdominal pain, weakness, rash. **Rare (less than 2%):** Abdominal distention, anorexia, flatulence, dizziness, insomnia, myalgia.

ADVERSE EFFECTS/ TOXIC REACTIONS

Bronchitis occurs in 3% of pts. Anemia, neutropenia, thrombocytopenia, diabetes mellitus, hepatic failure, hepatitis, peripheral neuropathy, pancreatitis occur rarely.

NURSING CONSIDERATIONS

BASELINE ASSESSMENT

Obtain baseline laboratory testing, esp. hepatic function tests, before beginning therapy and at periodic intervals during therapy. Offer emotional support. Obtain medication history.

T

INTERVENTION/EVALUATION

Closely monitor for evidence of GI discomfort. Monitor daily pattern of bowel activity, stool consistency. Assess skin for evidence of rash. Monitor serum chemistry tests for marked laboratory abnormalities, particularly hepatic profile, CD4 cell count, HIV, RNA plasma levels. Assess for opportunistic infections (onset of fever, oral mucosa changes, cough, other respiratory symptoms).

PATIENT/FAMILY TEACHING

• Eat small, frequent meals to offset nausea, vomiting. • Continue therapy for full length of treatment. • Doses should be evenly spaced. • Tipranavir is not a cure for HIV infection, nor does it reduce risk of transmission to others. • Pt may continue to experience illnesses, including opportunistic infections. • Diarrhea can be controlled with OTC medication.

tizanidine

tye-**zan**-i-deen
(Apo-Tizanidine, Zanaflex, Zanaflex Capsules)
Do not confuse tizanidine with tiagabine.

◆CLASSIFICATION

PHARMACOTHERAPEUTIC: Skeletal muscle relaxant. **CLINICAL:** Antispastic.

ACTION

Increases presynaptic inhibition of spinal motor neurons mediated by alpha$_2$-adrenergic agonists, reducing facilitation to postsynaptic motor neurons. **Therapeutic Effect:** Reduces muscle spasticity.

PHARMACOKINETICS

Metabolized in liver. Primarily excreted in urine. **Half-life:** 2 hrs.

USES

Acute and intermittent management of muscle spasticity (spasms, stiffness, rigidity). **OFF-LABEL:** Low back pain, spasticity associated with multiple sclerosis or spinal cord injury, tension headaches, trigeminal neuralgia.

PRECAUTIONS

Contraindications: None significant. **Cautions:** Renal/hepatic disease, hypotension, cardiac disease. **Pregnancy Category C.**

INTERACTIONS

DRUG: **Alcohol, other CNS depressants** may increase CNS depressant effects. **Antihypertensives** may increase hypotensive potential. **Oral contraceptives** may reduce clearance. May increase concentration, risk of toxicity of **phenytoin. HERBAL: Gotu kola, kava kava, St. John's wort, valerian** may increase CNS depression. **Black cohosh, hawthorn, periwinkle** may increase hypotensive effect. **FOOD:** None known. **LAB VALUES:** May increase serum alkaline phosphatase, AST, ALT.

AVAILABILITY (Rx)

Capsules: 2 mg, 4 mg, 6 mg. **Tablets:** 2 mg, 4 mg.

ADMINISTRATION/HANDLING

PO

• Capsules may be opened and sprinkled on food. • May give without regard to food. • Administration should be consistent and not switched between giving with or without food.

INDICATIONS/ROUTES/DOSAGE

Muscle Spasticity

PO: ADULTS, ELDERLY: Initially, 2–4 mg, gradually increased in 2- to 4-mg increments q6–8h. **Maximum:** 3 doses/day or 36 mg/24 hrs.

Dosage in Renal Impairment

May require dose reduction/less frequent dosing.

Dosage in Hepatic Impairment

Avoid use if possible. If used, monitor for adverse affects (e.g., hypotension).

SIDE EFFECTS

Frequent (49%–41%): Dry mouth, drowsiness, asthenia (loss of strength, energy). **Occasional (16%–4%):** Dizziness, UTI, constipation. **Rare (3%):** Nervousness, amblyopia, pharyngitis, rhinitis, vomiting, urinary frequency.

ADVERSE EFFECTS/ TOXIC REACTIONS

Hypotension may be associated with bradycardia, orthostatic hypotension, and, rarely, syncope. Risk of hypotension increases as dosage increases; hypotension is noted within 1 hr after administration.

NURSING CONSIDERATIONS

BASELINE ASSESSMENT

Record onset, type, location, duration of muscular spasm. Check for immobility, stiffness, swelling. Obtain baseline serum hepatic function tests, alkaline phosphatase, total bilirubin.

INTERVENTION/EVALUATION

Assist with ambulation at all times. For those on long-term therapy, serum hepatic/renal function tests should be performed periodically. Evaluate for therapeutic response (decreased intensity of skeletal muscle pain/tenderness, improved mobility, decrease in spasticity). To reduce risk of orthostatic hypotension, instruct pt to move slowly from lying to sitting and from sitting to supine position.

PATIENT/FAMILY TEACHING

• Avoid tasks that require alertness, motor skills until response to drug is established. • Avoid sudden changes in posture. • May cause hypotension, sedation, impaired coordination. • Avoid alcohol.

tobramycin

tow-bra-**my**-sin
(AK-Tob, PMS-Tobramycin ✦, TOBI, Tobrex)

BLACK BOX ALERT May cause neurotoxicity, nephrotoxicity, ototoxicity. Ototoxicity usually is irreversible. Increased risk of neuromuscular blockade, including respiratory paralysis, particularly when given after anesthesia or muscle relaxants.

Do not confuse Tobrex with TobraDex.

FIXED-COMBINATION(S)

TobraDex: tobramycin/dexamethasone (a steroid): 0.3%/0.1% per ml or per g. **Zylet:** tobramycin/loteprednol: 0.3%/0.5%.

◆ CLASSIFICATION

PHARMACOTHERAPEUTIC: Aminoglycoside. **CLINICAL:** Antibiotic (see p. 21C).

ACTION

Irreversibly binds to protein on bacterial ribosomes. **Therapeutic Effect:** Interferes with protein synthesis of susceptible microorganisms.

PHARMACOKINETICS

Rapid, complete absorption after IM administration. Protein binding: less than 30%. Widely distributed (does not cross blood-brain barrier; low concentrations in CSF). Excreted unchanged in urine. Removed by hemodialysis. **Half-life:** 2–4 hrs (increased in renal impairment, neonates; decreased in cystic fibrosis, febrile or burn pts).

USES

Treatment of susceptible infections due to *P. aeruginosa,* other gram-negative organisms including skin/skin structure, bone, joint, respiratory tract infections; postop, burn, intra-abdominal infections; complicated UTI; septicemia; meningitis. **Ophthalmic:** Superficial eye infections: blepharitis, conjunctivitis, keratitis, cor-

T

neal ulcers. **Inhalation:** Bronchopulmonary infections in pts with cystic fibrosis.

PRECAUTIONS

Contraindications: Hypersensitivity to other aminoglycosides (cross-sensitivity) and their components. **Cautions:** Renal impairment, preexisting auditory or vestibular impairment, concomitant use of neuromuscular blocking agents.

LIFESPAN CONSIDERATIONS

Pregnancy/Lactation: Drug readily crosses placenta; is distributed in breast milk. May cause fetal nephrotoxicity. Ophthalmic form should not be used in breast-feeding mothers and only when specifically indicated in pregnancy. **Pregnancy Category D (B for ophthalmic form). Children:** Immature renal function in neonates, premature infants may increase risk of toxicity. **Elderly:** Age-related renal impairment may increase risk of toxicity; dosage adjustment recommended.

INTERACTIONS

DRUG: **Nephrotoxic medications, ototoxic medications** may increase risk of nephrotoxicity, ototoxicity. **Neuromuscular blockers** may increase neuromuscular blockade. **HERBAL:** None significant. **FOOD:** None known. **LAB VALUES:** May increase BUN, serum bilirubin, creatinine, alkaline phosphatase, LDH, AST, ALT. May decrease serum calcium, magnesium, potassium, sodium. Therapeutic peak serum level: 5–20 mcg/ml; therapeutic trough serum level: 0.5–2 mcg/ml. Toxic peak serum level: greater than 20 mcg/ml; toxic trough serum level: greater than 2 mcg/ml.

AVAILABILITY (Rx)

Infusion, Premix: 60 mg/50 ml, 80 mg/100 ml. **Injection, Powder for Reconstitution:** 1.2 g. **Injection, Solution:** 10 mg/ml, 40 mg/ml. **Ointment, Ophthalmic (Tobrex):** 0.3%. **Solution, Nebulization (TOBI):** 60 mg/ml. **Solution, Ophthalmic (AK-Tob, Tobrex):** 0.3%.

ADMINISTRATION/HANDLING

◄ALERT► Coordinate peak and trough lab draws with administration times.

IV

Reconstitution • Dilute with 50–200 ml D_5W or 0.9% NaCl. Amount of diluent for infants, children depends on individual need.

Rate of administration • Infuse over 30–60 min.

Storage • Store vials at room temperature. • Solutions may be discolored by light or air (does not affect potency). • Reconstituted solution stable for 24 yrs at room temperature or 96 hrs if refrigerated.

IM

• To minimize discomfort, give deep IM slowly. • Less painful if injected into gluteus maximus rather than lateral aspect of thigh.

Inhalation

• Refrigerate. • May store at room temperature up to 28 days after removing from refrigerator. • Do not use if cloudy or contains particulates.

Ophthalmic

• Place gloved finger on lower eyelid, pull out until pocket is formed between eye and lower lid. • Place correct number of drops (¼–½ inch ointment) into pocket. • **Solution:** Apply digital pressure to lacrimal sac for 1–2 min (minimizes drainage into nose/throat, reducing risk of systemic effects). • **Ointment:** Instruct pt to close eye for 1–2 min, rolling eyeball (increases contact area of drug to eye). • Remove excess solution/ointment around eye with tissue.

IV INCOMPATIBILITIES

Amphotericin B complex (Abelcet, AmBisome, Amphotec), cephalosporins, heparin, hetastarch (Hespan), indomethacin (Indocin), penicillins, propofol (Diprivan), sargramostim (Leukine, Prokine).

IV COMPATIBILITIES

Amiodarone (Cordarone), calcium gluconate, diltiazem (Cardizem), furosemide (Lasix), hydromorphone (Dilaudid), insulin, lipids, magnesium sulfate, midazolam (Versed), morphine, theophylline, total parenteral nutrition (TPN).

INDICATIONS/ROUTES/DOSAGE

ALERT Space parenteral doses evenly around the clock. Dosage based on ideal body weight. Peak, trough levels determined periodically to maintain desired serum concentrations (minimizes risk of toxicity). Recommended peak level: 4–10 mcg/ml; trough level: 1–2 mcg/ml.

Usual Parenteral Dosage

IV: ADULTS, ELDERLY: 3–7.5 mg/kg/day in 3 divided doses. Once daily dosing: 4–7 mg/kg every 24 hrs. **CHILDREN 5 YRS AND OLDER:** 2–2.5 mg/kg/dose q8h. **CHILDREN YOUNGER THAN 5 YRS:** 2.5 mg/kg/dose q8h. **NEONATES OLDER THAN 7 DAYS:** 2.5 mg/kg/dose q8–12h; **NEONATES 7 DAYS OR YOUNGER:** 2.5 mg/kg/dose q12h; **PRETERM NEONATES:** 2.5 mg/kg/dose q18h or 3.5 mg/kg/dose q24h.

Usual Ophthalmic Dosage

OPHTHALMIC OINTMENT: ADULTS, ELDERLY, CHILDREN 2 MOS AND OLDER: Apply ½ inch to conjunctiva q8–12h (q3–4h for severe infections).

OPHTHALMIC SOLUTION: ADULTS, ELDERLY, CHILDREN 2 MOS AND OLDER: 1–2 drops in affected eye q4h (2 drops/hr for severe infections).

Usual Inhalation Dosage

INHALATION SOLUTION: ADULTS: 60–80 mg 3 times daily. **CHILDREN:** 40–80 mg 2–3 times a day.

HIGH DOSE: ADULTS, CHILDREN 6 YRS AND OLDER: 300 mg q12h 28 days on, 28 days off.

Dosage in Renal Impairment

Dosage and frequency modified based on degree of renal impairment, serum drug concentration. After loading dose of 1–2 mg/kg, maintenance dose and frequency are based on serum creatinine levels, creatinine clearance.

Creatinine Clearance	Dosing Interval
41–60 ml/min	q12h
21–40 ml/min	q24h
10–20 ml/min	q48h
Less than 10 ml/min	q72h

SIDE EFFECTS

Occasional: IM: Pain, induration. **IV:** Phlebitis, thrombophlebitis. **Topical:** Hypersensitivity reaction (fever, pruritus, rash, urticaria). **Ophthalmic:** Tearing, itching, redness, eyelid swelling. **Rare:** Hypotension, nausea, vomiting.

ADVERSE EFFECTS/ TOXIC REACTIONS

Nephrotoxicity (evidenced by increased BUN, serum creatinine, decreased creatinine clearance) may be reversible if drug is stopped at first sign of symptoms. Irreversible ototoxicity (dizziness, ringing/roaring in ears, hearing loss), neurotoxicity (headache, dizziness, lethargy, tremor, visual disturbances) occur occasionally. Risk increases with higher dosages or prolonged therapy or if solution is applied directly to mucosa. Superinfections, particularly fungal infections, may result from bacterial imbalance with any administration route. Anaphylaxis may occur.

NURSING CONSIDERATIONS

BASELINE ASSESSMENT

Dehydration must be treated before beginning parenteral therapy. Question for history of allergies, esp. aminoglycosides, sulfite (and parabens for topical, ophthalmic routes). Establish baseline for hearing acuity. Obtain baseline lab tests, esp. renal function.

INTERVENTION/EVALUATION

Monitor I&O (maintain hydration), urinalysis (casts, RBCs, WBCs, decrease in specific gravity), renal function. Monitor

T

results of peak/trough blood tests. **Therapeutic serum level:** peak: 5–20 mcg/ml; trough: 0.5–2 mcg/ml. **Toxic serum level:** peak: greater than 20 mcg/ml; trough: greater than 2 mcg/ml. Be alert to ototoxic, neurotoxic symptoms. Evaluate IV site for phlebitis (heat, pain, red streaking over vein). Assess for rash. Be alert for superinfection, particularly anal/genital pruritus, changes of oral mucosa, diarrhea. When treating pts with neuromuscular disorders, assess respiratory response carefully. **Ophthalmic:** Assess for redness, swelling, itching, tearing.

PATIENT/FAMILY TEACHING

• Notify physician in event of any hearing, visual, balance, urinary problems, even after therapy is completed. • **Ophthalmic:** Blurred vision, tearing may occur briefly after application. • Contact physician if tearing, redness, irritation continue.

tocilizumab

toe-si-**liz**-oo-mab
(Actemra)

BLACK BOX ALERT Tuberculosis, serious, invasive fungal infections, other opportunistic infections have occurred. Test for tuberculosis prior to and during treatment, regardless of initial result.

◆CLASSIFICATION

PHARMACOTHERAPEUTIC: Interleukin (IL)-6 receptor inhibitor. **CLINICAL:** Rheumatoid arthritis agent.

ACTION

Binds to IL-6 receptors, inhibiting signals of proinflammatory cytokines. **Therapeutic Effect:** Reduces inflammation, alters immune response.

PHARMACOKINETICS

Distributed in steady state of plasma and tissues compartments. Undergoes biphasic elimination from circulation. **Half-life:** 11–13 days.

USES

Treatment of moderate to severe rheumatoid arthritis. Used for inadequate response to prior tumor necrosis factor (TNF) antagonist therapy. May be used as monotherapy, in combination with methotrexate or other disease-modifying antirheumatic drugs (DMARDs).

PRECAUTIONS

Contraindications: None significant. **Cautions:** Concurrent live vaccinations, low platelet count equal to or less than 100,000/mm^3, ANC less than 2,000/mm^3, AST/ALT greater than 1.5 times upper normal limit (UNL) prior to treatment. History of opportunistic infections (bacterial, mycobacterial, invasive fungal, viral, protozoal), esp. tuberculosis, histoplasmosis, aspergillosis, candidiasis, coccidioidomycosis, listeriosis, pneumocystosis; preexisting or recent-onset CNS demyelinating disorders, including multiple sclerosis; those with chronic or recurrent infection or who have been exposed to tuberculosis; hematologic cytopenia, hepatic impairment, HIV, gastric ulcers, perforation.

⧖ LIFESPAN CONSIDERATIONS

Pregnancy/Lactation: Unknown if distributed in breast milk. **Pregnancy Category C. Children:** Safety and efficacy not established. **Elderly:** Cautious use due to increased risk of serious infections, malignancy.

INTERACTIONS

DRUG: May increase levels/effects of **leflunomide, natalizumab.** May decrease levels/effects of **sipuleucel-T. Live vaccines** not recommended. **Abciximab, denosumab, pimecrolimus, tacrolimus, trastuzumab** may increase levels/effects. **HERBAL: Echinacea** may alter levels/effects. **FOOD:** None known. **LAB VALUES:** May increase ALT,

AST (up to 48% of pts), lipids. May decrease platelets, neutrophils.

AVAILABILITY (Rx)

Injection Solution: 20 mg/ml (80 mg/4 ml, 200 mg/10 ml, 400 mg/20 ml).

ADMINISTRATION/HANDLING

◀ALERT▶ Do not infuse IV push or bolus.

IV

Reconstitution • Dilute in 100 ml 0.9% NaCl. • Prior to mixing, withdraw and discard volume of NaCl equal to volume of patient-dosed solution. • Invert bag to avoid foaming. • Inject solution and dilute for mixture that equals 100 ml in NaCl bag.
Rate of administration • Infuse over 1 hr.
Storage • Refrigerate vials; do not freeze. • Solution must be at room temperature before administration, but not for longer than 24 hrs. • Protect from light until time of use. • Solution appears colorless. Discard solution if appears cloudy, discolored, or contains particulate.

INDICATIONS/ROUTES/DOSAGE

Note: Do not infuse concomitantly in same IV line with other drugs.

Moderate to Severely Active Rheumatoid Arthritis

IV INFUSION: ADULTS, ELDERLY: 4 mg/kg every 4 wks initially. May increase to 8 mg/kg every 4 wks. **Maximum:** 800 mg per dose.

Dosage Modification

Hepatic enzyme levels greater than UNL.

Lab Value	Recommendation
1–3 × UNL	Dose modify concomitant DMARDs or reduce dose to 4 mg/kg until ALT/AST normalized
Greater than 3–5 × UNL	Interrupt treatment until ALT/AST less than 3 × UNL, then follow guidelines for 1–3 × UNL
Greater than 5 × UNL	Discontinue treatment

SIDE EFFECTS

Occasional (8%–6%): Upper respiratory tract infection, nasopharyngitis, headache, hypertension. **Rare (5%–3%):** Infusion reaction, dizziness, bronchitis, rash, oral ulceration.

ADVERSE EFFECTS/ TOXIC REACTIONS

Up to 48% of pts experience elevated ALT, AST. Neutropenia, thrombocytopenia occur in 4% of pts. Serious infections noted, including sepsis, pneumonia, tuberculosis, invasive fungal infections, hepatitis B. Anaphylactic reaction, rash, pruritus, urticaria, bronchospasm, swelling, dyspnea occur in less than 0.2% of pts; hypersensitivity reactions (hypertension, headaches, flushing) occur more frequently. Increased risk of lymphoma, melanoma. New onset or exacerbation of CNS demyelinating disorders, including multiple sclerosis. Risk of gastric perforation with concomitant use of NSAIDs, corticosteroids.

NURSING CONSIDERATIONS

BASELINE ASSESSMENT

Evaluate pt for active tuberculosis and test for latent infection prior to initiating treatment and periodically during therapy. Induration of 5 mm or greater with tuberculin skin testing should be considered a positive test result when assessing whether treatment for latent tuberculosis is necessary. Antifungal therapy should be considered for those who reside or travel to regions where mycoses are endemic. Do not initiate therapy during an active infection. Viral reactivation can occur in cases of herpes zoster, HIV. Assess baseline lab results (hepatic en-

T

zymes, cholesterol, triglycerides, platelets, neutrophils) every 4–8 weeks during treatment. Pts should report history of diverticulitis, weakened immune system, HIV, hepatic disease, GI bleeding, coughing up blood, diarrhea, weight loss, cancer, prior cancer treatment, use of NSAIDS, glucocorticosteroids.

INTERVENTION/EVALUATION

Monitor hepatitis B carriers during and several months following therapy. If reactivation occurs, reconsider interrupting treatment. Monitor pts for signs/symptoms of tuberculosis regardless of baseline PPD. Discontinue treatment if pt develops acute infection, opportunistic infection, or sepsis and initiate appropriate antimicrobial therapy. Monitor warfarin, theophylline, cyclosporine levels for therapeutic ranges. Modify, interrupt, or discontinue treatment if AST/ALT is 1–5 times UNL.

PATIENT/FAMILY TEACHING

• Inform pt that therapy may lower immune system response. • Detail any concomitant immunosuppressive therapy, methotrexate. • Report any history of HIV, fungal infections, hepatitis B, multiple sclerosis, hemoptysis, tuberculosis, or close relatives with active tuberculosis. • Report any travel plans to possible endemic areas. • Report signs/symptoms of stomach pain to evaluate risk of gastric perforation or history of taking NSAIDS, corticosteroids, methotrexate. • Pt will need blood levels drawn every 4–8 weeks during treatment along with routine tuberculosis screening. • Seek immediate medical attention if adverse reaction occurs. • Do not receive live vaccines during therapy. • Notify physician if pregnant or planning on becoming pregnant. • During treatment, report any signs of liver problems, such as stomach pains, yellowing of skin/eyes, dark-amber urine, clay-colored or bloody stools, fatigue, reduced appetite, coffee ground emesis. • Pt must adhere to strict dosing schedule. • Decreased platelet count may lead to risk of bleeding.

tolterodine

tol-**tare**-oh-deen
(Detrol, Detrol LA, Unidel 🍁)
Do not confuse Detrol with Ditropan, or tolterodine with fesoterodine.

◆CLASSIFICATION

PHARMACOTHERAPEUTIC: Muscarinic receptor antagonist. **CLINICAL:** Antispasmodic.

ACTION

Exhibits potent antimuscarinic activity by interceding via cholinergic muscarinic receptors, thereby inhibiting urinary bladder contraction. **Therapeutic Effect:** Decreases urinary frequency, urgency.

PHARMACOKINETICS

Immediate-release form rapidly, well absorbed after PO administration. Protein binding: 96%. Extensively metabolized in liver to active metabolite. Primarily excreted in urine. Unknown if removed by hemodialysis. **Half-life:** Immediate-release: 2–10 hrs. Extended-release: 7–18 hrs.

USES

Treatment of overactive bladder in pts with symptoms of urinary frequency, urgency, incontinence.

PRECAUTIONS

Contraindications: Gastric retention, uncontrolled angle-closure glaucoma, urinary retention. **Cautions:** Renal impairment, clinically significant bladder outflow obstruction (risk of urinary retention), GI obstructive disorders (e.g., pyloric stenosis [risk of gastric retention]), treated narrow-angle glaucoma.

⌛ LIFESPAN CONSIDERATIONS

Pregnancy/Lactation: Unknown if drug is distributed in breast milk. Breastfeeding not recommended. **Pregnancy**

Category C. Children: Safety and efficacy not established. **Elderly:** No age-related precautions noted.

INTERACTIONS

DRUG: **Clarithromycin, erythromycin, itraconazole, ketoconazole, miconazole** may increase concentration. **Fluoxetine** may inhibit metabolism. **HERBAL:** None significant. **FOOD:** None known. **LAB VALUES:** None significant.

AVAILABILITY (Rx)

Tablets (Detrol): 1 mg, 2 mg.

Capsules (Extended-Release [Detrol LA]): 2 mg, 4 mg.

ADMINISTRATION/HANDLING

PO

• May give without regard to food. • Do not crush, chew, open extended-release capsules; swallow whole.

INDICATIONS/ROUTES/DOSAGE

Overactive Bladder

PO: ADULTS, ELDERLY (IMMEDIATE-RELEASE): 1–2 mg twice a day. **(EXTENDED-RELEASE):** 2–4 mg once a day.

Dosage in Severe Renal/Hepatic Impairment

PO: ADULTS, ELDERLY (IMMEDIATE-RELEASE): 1 mg twice a day. **(EXTENDED-RELEASE):** 2 mg once a day.

SIDE EFFECTS

Frequent (40%): Dry mouth. **Occasional (11%–4%):** Headache, dizziness, fatigue, constipation, dyspepsia (heartburn, indigestion, epigastric pain), upper respiratory tract infection, UTI, dry eyes, abnormal vision (accommodation problems), nausea, diarrhea. **Rare (3%):** Drowsiness, chest/back pain, arthralgia, rash, weight gain, dry skin.

ADVERSE EFFECTS/ TOXIC REACTIONS

Overdose can result in severe anticholinergic effects, including abdominal cramps, facial warmth, excessive salivation/lacrimation, diaphoresis, pallor, urinary urgency, blurred vision, prolonged QT interval.

NURSING CONSIDERATIONS

BASELINE ASSESSMENT

Assess degree of overactive bladder (urinary urgency, frequency, incontinence).

INTERVENTION/EVALUATION

Assist with ambulation if dizziness occurs. Question for visual changes. Monitor incontinence, postvoid residuals.

PATIENT/FAMILY TEACHING

• May cause blurred vision, dry eyes/ mouth, constipation. • Inform physician of any confusion, altered mental status. • Avoid tasks that require alertness, motor skills until response to drug is established.

tolvaptan

toll-**vap**-tan
(Samsca)

BLACK BOX ALERT Osmotic demyelination (dysphagia, lethargy, slurred speech or inability to speak, seizures, coma, death) may occur with too-rapid correction of hyponatremia; slow rate of correction is essential. Should be initiated and re-initiated only in a hospital where serum sodium is monitored closely.

◆CLASSIFICATION

PHARMACOTHERAPEUTIC: Vasopressin antagonist. **CLINICAL:** Hyponatremia adjunct.

ACTION

Promotes excretion of free water (without loss of serum electrolytes), resulting in net fluid loss, increased urine output, decreased urine osmolarity and increase

T

in serum sodium concentration. **Therapeutic Effect:** Restores normal serum sodium levels.

PHARMACOKINETICS

Route	Onset	Peak	Duration
PO	N/A	2–4 hrs	N/A

Readily absorbed following oral administration. Metabolized in liver. Protein binding: 99%. Eliminated entirely by non-renal routes. **Half-life:** 5 hrs.

USES

Treatment of symptomatic hypervolemic or euvolemic hyponatremia resistant to correction with fluid restriction, including those with heart failure, cirrhosis, and syndrome of inappropriate antidiuretic hormone (SIADH).

PRECAUTIONS

Contraindications: Hypovolemic hyponatremia; concurrent use with strong CYP3A4 inhibitors (clarithromycin, indinavir, itraconazole, ketoconazole, nefazodone, nelfinavir, ritonavir, saquinavir), those with urgent need to raise sodium level, pt with inability to sense or respond to thirst. **Cautions:** Hepatic/renal impairment, GI bleeding in pts with cirrhosis, dehydration, hypovolemia, concurrent use with hypertonic saline.

LIFESPAN CONSIDERATIONS

Pregnancy/Lactation: Systemic exposure to fetus likely. Potential for decreased neonatal viability, delayed growth/development. Unknown if distributed in breast milk. **Pregnancy Category C. Children:** Safety and efficacy not established. **Elderly:** No age-related precautions noted.

INTERACTIONS

DRUG: CYP3A inhibitors: Aprepitant, clarithromycin, diltiazem, erythromycin, fluconazole, indinavir, itraconazole, ketoconazole, nefazodone, nelfinavir, ritonavir, saquinavir, verapamil may increase levels, effects. **CYP3A inducers: Barbiturates, carbamazepine, phenytoin, rifabutin, rifampin, rifapentine** may reduce concentration. **Cyclosporine** may increase concentration. **HERBAL: St. John's wort** may reduce concentration. **FOOD: Grapefruit, grapefruit juice** may increase absorption, concentration. **LAB VALUES:** May increase serum potassium, magnesium. May alter serum glucose.

AVAILABILITY (Rx)

Tablets: 15 mg, 30 mg.

ADMINISTRATION/HANDLING

- Give without regard to meals.

INDICATIONS/ROUTES/DOSAGE

Usual Dosage

PO: ADULTS, ELDERLY: 15 mg once daily. Increase dose to 30 mg once daily, after at least 24 hrs (**Maximum:** 60 mg once daily), to achieve desired level of serum sodium.

SIDE EFFECTS

Frequent (16%–13%): Thirst, dry mouth. **Occasional (11%–4%):** Increase in urine output/urgency, loss of strength (asthenia), nausea, constipation, hyperglycemia, anorexia.

ADVERSE EFFECTS/ TOXIC REACTIONS

Dysphagia, lethargy, slurred speech or inability to speak, affective changes, spastic quadriparesis, seizures, coma, death may occur with too-rapid correction of hyponatremia.

NURSING CONSIDERATIONS

BASELINE ASSESSMENT

Initiate only in hospital setting with serum sodium monitoring. Obtain baseline serum sodium, hepatic enzyme levels, BUN, creatinine, CBC. Assess for increased pulse rate, poor skin turgor, nausea, diarrhea (signs of hyponatremia).

INTERVENTION/EVALUATION

During initiation and titration, frequently monitor for changes in serum electrolytes and volume. Avoid fluid restriction during first 24 hrs of therapy. Monitor for improvement in signs/symptoms of hyponatremia, hypernatremia (flushing, edema, restlessness, dry mucous membranes, fever).

PATIENT/FAMILY TEACHING

• Continue ingesting fluids in response to thirst. • Notify physician if urinary changes, loss of strength, unusual fatigue occur. • Report immediately symptoms of osmotic demyelination (e.g., trouble speaking/swallowing, confusion, mood changes, trouble controlling body movements, seizures).

topiramate

toe-**peer**-a-mate
(Apo-Topiramate ✤, Novo-Topiramate ✤, Topamax)
Do not confuse topiramate or Topamax with Tegretol, Tegretol XR, or Toprol XL.

◆CLASSIFICATION

CLINICAL: Anticonvulsant (see p. 36C).

ACTION

Blocks repetitive, sustained firing of neurons by enhancing ability of gamma-aminobutyric acid (GABA) to induce influx of chloride ions into neurons; may block sodium channels. **Therapeutic Effect:** Decreases seizure activity.

PHARMACOKINETICS

Rapidly absorbed after PO administration. Protein binding: 15%–41%. Partially metabolized in liver. Primarily excreted unchanged in urine. Removed by hemodialysis. **Half-life:** 21 hrs.

USES

Adjunctive therapy for treatment of partial-onset seizures, tonic-clonic seizures, seizures associated with Lennox-Gastaut syndrome. Prevention of migraine. Initial monotherapy in pts 10 yrs and older with partial or primary generalized tonic-clonic seizures. **OFF-LABEL:** Treatment of alcohol dependence, neuropathic pain, cluster headaches, infantile spasms.

PRECAUTIONS

Contraindications: Bipolar disorder. **Cautions:** Sensitivity to topiramate, hepatic/renal impairment, predisposition to renal calculi.

⌛ LIFESPAN CONSIDERATIONS

Pregnancy/Lactation: Unknown if distributed in breast milk. **Pregnancy Category C. Children:** No age-related precautions noted in those older than 2 yrs. **Elderly:** Age-related renal impairment may require dosage adjustment.

INTERACTIONS

DRUG: Alcohol, other CNS depressants may increase CNS depression. **Carbamazepine, phenytoin, valproic acid** may decrease concentration. **Carbonic anhydrase inhibitors** may increase risk of renal calculi formation. May decrease effectiveness of **oral contraceptives. HERBAL: Evening primrose** may decrease seizure threshold. **FOOD:** None known. **LAB VALUES:** May reduce serum bicarbonate, increase AST, ALT.

AVAILABILITY (Rx)

Capsules (Sprinkle): 15 mg, 25 mg.
Tablets: 25 mg, 50 mg, 100 mg, 200 mg.

ADMINISTRATION/HANDLING

PO

• Do not break tablets (bitter taste).
• Give without regard to meals. • Capsules may be swallowed whole or contents sprinkled on teaspoonful of soft food and swallowed immediately; do not chew.

T

INDICATIONS/ROUTES/DOSAGE

Adjunctive Treatment of Partial-Onset Seizures, Lennox-Gastaut Syndrome, Tonic-Clonic Seizures

PO: ADULTS, ELDERLY, CHILDREN 17 YRS AND OLDER: Initially, 25–50 mg for 1 wk. May increase by 25–50 mg/day at weekly intervals. Usual maintenance dose: 100–200 mg twice daily. **Maximum:** 1,600 mg/day. **CHILDREN 2–16 YRS:** Initially, 1–3 mg/kg/day to maximum of 25 mg at night for 1 wk. May increase by 1–3 mg/kg/day at weekly intervals given in 2 divided doses. Maintenance: 5–9 mg/kg/day in 2 divided doses.

Monotherapy with Partial-Onset, Tonic-Clonic Seizures

PO: ADULTS, ELDERLY, CHILDREN 10 YRS AND OLDER: Initially, 25 mg twice a day. Increase at weekly intervals up to 400 mg/day according to the following schedule: Wk 1, 25 mg twice a day. Wk 2, 50 mg twice a day. Wk 3, 75 mg twice a day. Wk 4, 100 mg twice a day. Wk 5, 150 mg twice a day. Wk 6, 200 mg twice a day.

Migraine Prevention

PO: ADULTS, ELDERLY: Initially, 25 mg/day. May increase by 25 mg/day at 7-day intervals up to a total daily dose of 100 mg/day in 2 divided doses.

Dosage in Renal Impairment

Reduce drug dosage by 50% and titrate more slowly in pts who have creatinine clearance less than 70 ml/min.

SIDE EFFECTS

Frequent (30%–10%): Drowsiness, dizziness, ataxia, nervousness, nystagmus, diplopia, paresthesia, nausea, tremor. **Occasional (9%–3%):** Confusion, breast pain, dysmenorrhea, dyspepsia (heartburn, indigestion, epigastric pain), depression, asthenia (loss of strength, energy), pharyngitis, weight loss, anorexia, rash, musculoskeletal pain, abdominal pain, difficulty with coordination, sinusitis, agitation, flu-like symptoms. **Rare (3%–2%):** Mood disturbances (e.g., irritability, depression), dry mouth, aggressive behavior, impaired heat regulation.

ADVERSE EFFECTS/ TOXIC REACTIONS

Psychomotor slowing, impaired concentration, language problems (esp. word-finding difficulties), memory disturbances occur occasionally. Metabolic acidosis, suicidal ideation occur rarely.

NURSING CONSIDERATIONS

BASELINE ASSESSMENT

Seizures: Review history of seizure disorder (intensity, frequency, duration, level of consciousness). Initiate seizure precautions. Provide quiet, dark environment. Question for sensitivity to topiramate, pregnancy, use of other anticonvulsant medication (esp. carbamazepine, valproic acid, phenytoin). **Migraine:** Assess pain location, duration, intensity. Assess renal function.

INTERVENTION/EVALUATION

Observe frequently for recurrence of seizure activity. Assess for clinical improvement (decrease in intensity/frequency of seizures). Monitor renal function tests (BUN, creatinine), hepatic function tests (AST, ALT). Assist with ambulation if dizziness occurs.

PATIENT/FAMILY TEACHING

• Avoid tasks that require alertness, motor skills until response to drug is established (may cause dizziness, drowsiness, impaired concentration). • Drowsiness usually diminishes with continued therapy. • Avoid use of alcohol, other CNS depressants. • Do not abruptly discontinue drug (may precipitate seizures). • Strict maintenance of drug therapy is essential for seizure control. • Do not break tablets (bitter taste). • Maintain adequate fluid intake (decreases risk of renal stone formation). • Inform physician if blurred vision, eye pain occurs. • Report suicidal ideation, depression, unusual behavior. • Use caution with activities that may increase core temperature (exposure to extreme heat, dehydration). • Instruct pt to use alternative/additional means of contraception (topiramate decreases effectiveness of oral contraceptives).

topotecan

HIGH ALERT

toe-**poh**-teh-can
(Hycamtin)

BLACK BOX ALERT Must be administered by personnel trained in administration/handling of chemotherapeutic agents. Potent immunosuppressant; severe neutropenia (absolute neutrophil count [ANC] less than 500 cells/mm^3) occurs in 60% of pts.

Do not confuse Hycamtin with Hycomine or Mycamine.

CLASSIFICATION

PHARMACOTHERAPEUTIC: DNA topoisomerase inhibitor. **CLINICAL:** Antineoplastic (see p. 89C).

ACTION

Interacts with topoisomerase I, an enzyme that relieves torsional strain in DNA by inducing reversible single-strand breaks. Prevents religation of DNA strand, resulting in damage to double-strand DNA, cell death. **Therapeutic Effect:** Produces cytotoxic effect.

PHARMACOKINETICS

Hydrolyzed to active form after IV administration. Protein binding: 35%. Excreted in urine. **Half-life:** 2–3 hrs (increased in renal impairment).

USES

Treatment of metastatic carcinoma of ovary after failure of initial or recurrent chemotherapy. Treatment of sensitive, relapsed small-cell lung cancer. Treatment of late-stage cervical cancer. **OFF-LABEL:** Treatment of solid tumors including osteosarcoma, neuroblastoma, pediatric leukemia, rhabdomyosarcoma, myelodysplastic disorders.

PRECAUTIONS

Contraindications: Baseline neutrophil count less than 1,500 cells/mm^3, breast-feeding, pregnancy, severe myelosuppression. **Cautions:** Mild myelosuppression, hepatic/renal impairment.

LIFESPAN CONSIDERATIONS

Pregnancy/Lactation: May cause fetal harm. Avoid pregnancy; breast-feeding not recommended. **Pregnancy Category D. Children:** Safety and efficacy not established. **Elderly:** Age-related renal impairment may require dosage adjustment.

INTERACTIONS

DRUG: Immunosuppressants (e.g., azathioprine, cyclosporine, glucocorticoids, tacrolimus) may increase risk of infection. **Live virus vaccines** may potentiate virus replication, increase vaccine side effects, decrease pt's antibody response to vaccine. **Other bone marrow depressants** may increase risk of myelosuppression. **HERBAL:** None significant. **FOOD:** None known. **LAB VALUES:** May increase serum bilirubin, AST, ALT, alkaline phosphatase. May decrease RBC, leukocyte, neutrophil, platelet counts, Hgb, Hct.

AVAILABILITY (Rx)

Injection, Powder for Reconstitution: 4 mg (single-dose vial).

Capsule: 0.25 mg, 1 mg.

ADMINISTRATION/HANDLING

ALERT Because topotecan may be carcinogenic, mutagenic, teratogenic, handle drug with extreme care during preparation/administration.

PO

• May take with or without food. • Swallow whole; do not crush, chew, divide capsule. • Do not take replacement dose if vomiting occurs.

IV

Reconstitution • Reconstitute each 4-mg vial with 4 ml Sterile Water for Injection. • Further dilute with 50–100 ml 0.9% NaCl or D_5W.

Rate of administration • Administer as IV infusion over 30 min or by continuous infusion. • Extravasation associated with only mild local reactions (erythema, ecchymosis).

Storage • Store vials at room temperature in original cartons. • Reconstituted vials diluted for infusion stable at room temperature, ambient lighting for 24 hrs, or 7 days if refrigerated.

IV INCOMPATIBILITIES

Dexamethasone (Decadron), 5-fluorouracil, mitomycin (Mutamycin).

IV COMPATIBILITIES

Carboplatin (Paraplatin), cisplatin (Platinol AQ), cyclophosphamide (Cytoxan), doxorubicin (Adriamycin), etoposide (VePesid), gemcitabine (Gemzar), granisetron (Kytril), ondansetron (Zofran), paclitaxel (Taxol), vincristine (Oncovin).

INDICATIONS/ROUTES/DOSAGE

◀ALERT▶ Do not give topotecan if baseline neutrophil count is less than 1,500 cells/mm^3 and platelet count is less than 100,000/mm^3.

Ovarian Carcinoma, Small-Cell Lung Cancer

IV: ADULTS, ELDERLY: 1.5 mg/m^2/day over 30 min for 5 consecutive days, beginning on day 1 of 21-day course. Minimum of four courses recommended. If severe neutropenia (neutrophil count less than 1,500/mm^2) occurs during treatment, reduce dose for subsequent courses by 0.25 mg/m^2 or administer filgrastim (G-CSF) no sooner than 24 hrs after last dose of topotecan.

IV INFUSION (OVARIAN CANCER): ADULTS, ELDERLY: 0.2–0.7 mg/m^2/day for 7–21 days.

PO (SMALL-CELL LUNG CANCER): ADULTS, ELDERLY: 2.3 mg/m^3/day for 5 days; repeat q21days (dose rounded to nearest 0.25 mg).

Cervical Cancer

IV: ADULTS, ELDERLY: 0.75 mg/m^2/day for 3 days (followed by cisplatin 50 mg/m^2 on day 1 only). Repeat q21days (baseline neutrophil count greater than 1,500/mm^3 and platelet count greater than 100,000 mm^3).

Dosage in Renal Impairment

No dosage adjustment is necessary in pts with mild renal impairment (creatinine clearance 40–60 ml/min). For moderate renal impairment (creatinine clearance 20–39 ml/min), give 0.75 mg/m^2.

SIDE EFFECTS

Frequent: Nausea (77%), vomiting (58%), diarrhea, total alopecia (42%), headache (21%), dyspnea (21%). **Occasional:** Paresthesia (9%), constipation, abdominal pain (3%). **Rare:** Anorexia, malaise, arthralgia, asthenia (loss of strength, energy), myalgia.

ADVERSE EFFECTS/ TOXIC REACTIONS

Severe neutropenia (absolute neutrophil count [ANC] less than 500 cells/mm^3) occurs in 60% of pts (develops at median of 11 days after day 1 of initial therapy). Thrombocytopenia (platelet count less than 25,000/mm^3) occurs in 26% of pts. Severe anemia (RBC count less than 8 g/dl) occurs in 40% of pts (develops at median of 15 days after day 1 of initial therapy).

NURSING CONSIDERATIONS

BASELINE ASSESSMENT

Offer emotional support to pt and family. Assess CBC with differential, Hgb, platelet count before each dose. Myelosuppression may precipitate life-threatening hemorrhage, infection, anemia. If platelet count drops, minimize trauma to pt (e.g., IM injections, pt positioning). Premedicate with antiemetics on day of

T

treatment, starting at least 30 min before administration.

INTERVENTION/EVALUATION

Assess for bleeding, signs of infection, anemia. Monitor hydration status, I&O, serum electrolytes (diarrhea, vomiting are common side effects). Monitor CBC with differential, Hgb, platelets for evidence of myelosuppression. Monitor renal/hepatic function tests. Assess response to medication; provide interventions (e.g., small, frequent meals; antiemetics for nausea/vomiting). Question for complaints of headache. Assess breathing pattern for evidence of dyspnea.

PATIENT/FAMILY TEACHING

• Alopecia is reversible but new hair may have different color, texture. • Diarrhea may cause dehydration, electrolyte depletion. • Antiemetic and antidiarrheal medications may reduce side effects. • Notify physician if diarrhea, vomiting, persistent fever, bruising/bleeding, yellowing of eyes/skin occur. • Do not have immunizations without physician's approval (drug lowers resistance). • Avoid contact with those who have recently received live virus vaccine.

toremifene HIGH ALERT

tore-**em**-ih-feen
(Fareston)

◆CLASSIFICATION

PHARMACOTHERAPEUTIC: Nonsteroidal antiestrogen. **CLINICAL:** Antineoplastic (see p. 89C).

ACTION

Binds to estrogen receptors on tumors, producing complex that decreases DNA synthesis, inhibits estrogen effects. **Therapeutic Effect:** Blocks growth-stimulating effects of estrogen in breast cancer.

PHARMACOKINETICS

Well absorbed after PO administration. Protein binding: greater than 99%. Metabolized in liver. Eliminated in feces. **Half-life:** Approximately 5 days.

USES

Treatment of metastatic breast cancer in postmenopausal women with estrogen receptor–positive or estrogen receptor unknown. **OFF-LABEL:** Treatment of desmoid tumors, endometrial carcinoma.

PRECAUTIONS

Contraindications: History of thromboembolic disease. **Cautions:** Preexisting endometrial hyperplasia, leukopenia, thrombocytopenia.

LIFESPAN CONSIDERATIONS

Pregnancy/Lactation: Unknown if distributed in breast milk. **Pregnancy Category D. Children:** Safety and efficacy not established. Not prescribed in this pt population. **Elderly:** No age-related precautions noted.

INTERACTIONS

DRUG: **Carbamazepine, phenobarbital, phenytoin** may decrease concentration. **Warfarin** may increase PT, risk of bleeding. **HERBAL:** None significant. **FOOD:** None known. **LAB VALUES:** May increase serum alkaline phosphatase, bilirubin, calcium, AST.

AVAILABILITY (Rx)

Tablets: 60 mg.

ADMINISTRATION/HANDLING

PO

• Give without regard to food.

INDICATIONS/ROUTES/DOSAGE

Breast Cancer

PO: ADULTS: 60 mg/day as a single dose until disease progression is observed.

SIDE EFFECTS

Frequent: Hot flashes (35%), diaphoresis (20%), nausea (14%), vaginal discharge

(13%), dizziness, dry eyes (9%). **Occasional (5%–2%):** Edema, vomiting, vaginal bleeding. **Rare:** Fatigue, depression, lethargy, anorexia.

ADVERSE EFFECTS/ TOXIC REACTIONS

Ocular toxicity (cataracts, glaucoma, decreased visual acuity), hypercalcemia may occur.

NURSING CONSIDERATIONS

BASELINE ASSESSMENT

Estrogen receptor assay should be done before beginning therapy. CBC, platelet count, serum calcium levels should be checked before and periodically during therapy.

INTERVENTION/EVALUATION

Assess for hypercalcemia (increased urinary volume, excessive thirst, nausea, vomiting, constipation, hypotonicity of muscles, deep bone/flank pain, renal stones). Monitor CBC, leukocyte, platelet counts, serum calcium, hepatic function tests.

PATIENT/FAMILY TEACHING

• May have initial flare of symptoms (bone pain, hot flashes) that will subside. • Report vaginal bleeding/discharge/itching, leg cramps, weight gain, shortness of breath, weakness. • Contact physician if nausea/vomiting continue. • Nonhormone contraceptives are recommended during treatment.

T

torsemide

tore-se-myde
(Demadex)
Do not confuse torsemide with furosemide.

◆CLASSIFICATION

PHARMACOTHERAPEUTIC: Loop diuretic. **CLINICAL:** Antihypertensive, antiedema (see p. 102C).

ACTION

Enhances excretion of sodium, chloride, potassium, water at ascending limb of loop of Henle. Reduces plasma, extracellular fluid volume. **Therapeutic Effect:** Produces diuresis; lowers B/P.

PHARMACOKINETICS

Route	Onset	Peak	Duration
PO, IV (diuresis)	30–60 min	1–4 hrs	6 hrs

Rapidly, well absorbed from GI tract. Protein binding: 97%–99%. Metabolized in liver. Primarily excreted in urine. Not removed by hemodialysis. **Half-life:** 2–4 hrs.

USES

Treatment of hypertension either alone or in combination with other antihypertensives. Edema associated with CHF, renal disease, hepatic cirrhosis, chronic renal failure. Use IV form when rapid onset is desired.

PRECAUTIONS

Contraindications: Anuria, hepatic coma, severe electrolyte depletion. **Extreme Caution:** Hypersensitivity to sulfonamides. **Cautions:** Elderly, cardiac pts, pts with history of ventricular arrhythmias, pts with hepatic cirrhosis, ascites, renal impairment, systemic lupus erythematosus.

⌛ LIFESPAN CONSIDERATIONS

Pregnancy/Lactation: Unknown if drug is distributed in breast milk. **Pregnancy Category B. Children:** Safety and efficacy not established. **Elderly:** No age-related precautions noted.

INTERACTIONS

DRUG: Amphotericin B, nephrotoxic medications, ototoxic medications may increase risk of nephrotoxicity, ototoxicity. May decrease effects of **anticoagulants, heparin, thrombolytics.** May increase risk of **digoxin** toxicity associated with torsemide-induced hypokalemia. May increase risk of **lithium** toxicity. **Other hypokalemia-causing medications** may increase risk of hypokalemia. HERBAL: **Ephedra, ginseng, yohimbe** may worsen hypertension. **Garlic** may increase antihypertensive effect. FOOD: None known. LAB VALUES: May increase BUN, serum creatinine, uric acid. May decrease serum calcium, chloride, magnesium, potassium, sodium.

AVAILABILITY (Rx)

Injection Solution: 10 mg/ml. **Tablets:** 5 mg, 10 mg, 20 mg, 100 mg.

ADMINISTRATION/HANDLING

IV

Rate of administration

◀ALERT▶ Flush IV line with 0.9% NaCl before and following administration. • May give undiluted as IV push over minimum of 2 min. • For continuous IV infusion, dilute with 0.9% or 0.45% NaCl or D_5W and infuse over 24 hrs. • Too-rapid IV rate, high dosages may cause ototoxicity; administer IV rate **slowly.**

Storage • Store at room temperature. IV infusion stable for 24 hrs at room temperature.

PO

• Give without regard to food. Give with food to avoid GI upset, preferably with breakfast (prevents nocturia).

IV COMPATIBILITY

Milrinone (Primacor).

INDICATIONS/ROUTES/DOSAGE

Hypertension

PO: ADULTS, ELDERLY: Initially, 2.5–5 mg/day. May increase to 10 mg/day if no response in 4–6 wks. If no response, additional antihypertensive added.

Edema Associated with CHF

PO, IV: ADULTS, ELDERLY: Initially, 10–20 mg/day. May increase by approximately doubling dose until desired therapeutic effect is attained. **Maximum dose:** PO: 200 mg; IV: 100–200 mg.

Chronic Renal Failure

PO, IV: ADULTS, ELDERLY: Initially, 20 mg/day. May increase by approximately doubling dose until desired therapeutic effect is attained. **Maximum dose:** PO: 200 mg; IV: 100–200 mg.

Hepatic Cirrhosis

PO, IV: ADULTS, ELDERLY: Initially, 5 mg/day given with aldosterone antagonist or potassium-sparing diuretic. May increase by approximately doubling dose until desired therapeutic effect is attained. **Maximum single dose:** 40 mg.

SIDE EFFECTS

Frequent (10%–4%): Headache, dizziness, rhinitis. **Occasional (3%–1%):** Asthenia (loss of strength, energy), insomnia, nervousness, diarrhea, constipation, nausea, dyspepsia (heartburn, indigestion, epigastric pain), edema, EKG changes, pharyngitis, cough, arthralgia, myalgia. **Rare (less than 1%):** Syncope, hypotension, arrhythmias.

ADVERSE EFFECTS/TOXIC REACTIONS

Ototoxicity may occur with too-rapid IV administration or with high doses; must be given slowly. Overdose produces acute, profound water loss; volume/electrolyte depletion; dehydration; decreased blood volume; circulatory collapse.

NURSING CONSIDERATIONS

BASELINE ASSESSMENT

Check serum electrolyte levels, esp. potassium. Obtain baseline weight; check for edema. Assess for rales in lungs, signs of CHF.

INTERVENTION/EVALUATION

Monitor B/P, serum electrolytes (esp. potassium), I&O, weight. Notify physician of any hearing abnormality. Note extent of

T

diuresis. Assess lungs for rales. Check for signs of edema, particularly of dependent areas. Although less potassium is lost with torsemide than with furosemide, assess for signs of hypokalemia (change of muscle strength, tremor, muscle cramps, altered mental status, cardiac arrhythmias).

PATIENT/FAMILY TEACHING

• Take medication in morning to prevent nocturia. • Expect increased urinary volume, frequency. • Report palpitations, muscle weakness, cramps, nausea, dizziness. • Do not take other medications (including OTC drugs) without consulting physician. • Eat foods high in potassium such as whole grains (cereals), legumes, meat, bananas, apricots, orange juice, potatoes (white, sweet), raisins.

tositumomab and iodine ^{131}I-tositumomab

HIGH ALERT

toe-sit-**two**-mo-mab
(Bexxar)

BLACK BOX ALERT Hypersensitivity, including anaphylaxis, can occur. Severe thrombocytopenia and neutropenia occur in majority of pts. Should be administered only by physicians/health professionals qualified in safe handling of radionuclides.

◆CLASSIFICATION

PHARMACOTHERAPEUTIC: Monoclonal antibody. **CLINICAL:** Antineoplastic.

ACTION

Composed of an antibody conjoined with a radiolabeled antitumor antibody. The antibody portion binds specifically to the CD20 antigen, found on pre-B, B lymphocytes and on more than 90% of B-cell non-Hodgkin's lymphomas, resulting in formation of a complex. **Therapeutic Effect:** Induces cytotoxicity associated with ionizing radiation from radioisotope. Depletes circulating $CD20^{+}$ cells.

PHARMACOKINETICS

Elimination of iodine 131 (^{131}I) occurs by decay, excretion in urine. **Half-life:** 36–48 hrs. Pts with high tumor burden, splenomegaly, bone marrow involvement have faster clearance, shorter half-life, larger volume of distribution.

USES

Treatment of pts with CD20 antigen-expressing non-Hodgkin's lymphoma, whose disease has relapsed following chemotherapy.

PRECAUTIONS

Contraindications: Hypersensitivity to murine proteins, pregnancy. **Cautions:** Renal impairment, active systemic infection, immunosuppression.

⧗ LIFESPAN CONSIDERATIONS

Pregnancy/Lactation: ^{131}I-tositumomab component is contraindicated during pregnancy (severe, possibly irreversible hypothyroidism in neonates). Radioiodine is excreted in breast milk; do not breast-feed. **Pregnancy Category X. Children:** Safety and efficacy not established. **Elderly:** Response rate, duration of severe hematologic toxicity are lower in those older than 65 yrs.

INTERACTIONS

DRUG: **Anticoagulants, medications that interfere with platelet function** increase risk of bleeding, hemorrhage. **Bone marrow depressants** may increase myelosuppression. **HERBAL:** None significant. **FOOD:** None known. **LAB VALUES:** May decrease Hgb, Hct, platelet count, WBC count, thyroid stimulating hormone (TSH), neutrophils.

AVAILABILITY (Rx)

Kit (Dosimetric): tositumomab 225 mg/16.1 ml (2 vials), tositumomab 35 mg/2.5 ml (1 vial), and iodine ^{131}I-tositumomab 0.1 mg/ml (1 vial). **Kit (Thera-**

peutic): tositumomab 225 mg/16.1 ml (2 vials), tositumomab 35 mg/2.5 ml (1 vial), and iodine ^{131}I-tositumomab 1.1 mg/ml (1 or 2 vials).

ADMINISTRATION/HANDLING

◀ALERT▶ Regimen consists of 4 components given in 2 separate steps: the dosimetric step, followed 7–14 days later by a therapeutic step. When infusing, use IV tubing with in-line 0.22-micron filter (use same tubing throughout entire dosimetric or therapeutic step; changing filter results in drug loss). Reduce infusion rate by 50% for mild to moderate infusion toxicity; interrupt infusion for severe infusion toxicity (may resume when resolution of toxicity occurs). Resume at 50% reduction rate of infusion.

IV

Reconstitution

◀ALERT▶ Reconstitution amounts and rates of administration are the same for both dosimetric and therapeutic steps.

TOSITUMOMAB • Reconstitute 450 mg tositumomab in 50 ml 0.9% NaCl.

IODINE ^{131}I-TOSITUMOMAB • Reconstitute iodine ^{131}I-tositumomab in 30 ml 0.9% NaCl.

Rate of administration

TOSITUMOMAB • Infuse over 60 min.

IODINE ^{131}I-TOSITUMOMAB • Infuse over 20 min.

Storage

TOSITUMOMAB • Refrigerate vials before dilution. Protect from strong light. • Following dilution, solution is stable for 24 hrs if refrigerated, up to 8 hrs at room temperature. • Discard any unused portion left in the vial. • Do not shake.

IODINE ^{131}I-TOSITUMOMAB • Store frozen until vial is removed for thawing before administration. Thawed doses are stable for 8 hrs if refrigerated. • Discard any unused portion.

INDICATIONS/ROUTES/DOSAGE

◀ALERT▶ Initiate thyroid protective agents (potassium iodide) 24 hrs prior to administration of iodine ^{131}I-tositumomab dosimetric step and continue until 2 wks following administration of iodine ^{131}I-tositumomab therapeutic step. Pretreat against infusion reactions with acetaminophen and diphenhydramine 1 hr prior to beginning therapy.

Non-Hodgkin's Lymphoma

◀ALERT▶ **PRETREATMENT:** Diphenhydramine 50 mg and acetaminophen 650–1,000 mg given 1 hr prior to administering, followed by acetaminophen 650–1,000 mg q4h for 2 doses, then q4h prn. Full recovery from hematologic toxicities is not a requirement for giving second dose.

IV: ADULTS, ELDERLY: Dosage contains 4 components in 2 steps. **Day 0:** Tositumomab 450 mg/50 NaCl over 60 min, then iodine ^{131}I-tositumomab 35 mg in 30 ml NaCl over 20 min. **Day 7:** Tositumomab 450 mg/50 NaCl over 60 min, then iodine ^{131}I-tositumomab to deliver 65–75 cGy total body irradiation and tositumomab 35 mg over 20 min.

SIDE EFFECTS

Frequent (46%–18%): Asthenia (loss of strength, energy), fever, nausea, cough, chills. **Occasional (17%–10%):** Rash, headache, abdominal pain, vomiting, anorexia, myalgia, diarrhea, pharyngitis, arthralgia, rhinitis, pruritus. **Rare (9%–5%):** Peripheral edema, diaphoresis, constipation, dyspepsia (heartburn, indigestion, epigastric pain), back pain, hypotension, vasodilation, dizziness, drowsiness.

ADVERSE EFFECTS/ TOXIC REACTIONS

Infusion toxicity, characterized by fever, rigors, diaphoresis, hypotension, dyspnea, nausea, may occur during or within 48 hrs of infusion. Severe, prolonged myelosuppression, characterized by neutropenia, anemia, thrombocytopenia, occurs in 71% of pts. Sepsis occurs in 45% of pts, hemorrhage in 12%, myelodysplastic syndrome in 8%.

T

NURSING CONSIDERATIONS

BASELINE ASSESSMENT

Pretreatment with acetaminophen and diphenhydramine before administering infusion may prevent infusion-related effects. Obtain baseline CBC before therapy and at least weekly following administration for minimum of 10 wks. Use strict aseptic technique to protect pt from infection. Follow radiation safety protocols. Time to nadir is 4–7 wks, duration of cytopenias is approximately 30 days.

INTERVENTION/EVALUATION

Diligently monitor lab values for possibly severe, prolonged thrombocytopenia, neutropenia, anemia. Monitor for hematologic toxicity (fever, chills, unusual bruising/bleeding from any site), symptoms of anemia (excessive fatigue, weakness). Assess for signs of hypothyroidism.

PATIENT/FAMILY TEACHING

• Avoid pregnancy (Pregnancy Category X). • Do not have immunizations without physician's approval (drug lowers resistance). • Avoid contact with those who have recently received live virus vaccine. • Promptly report fever, sore throat, signs of local infection, unusual bruising/bleeding from any site.

tramadol

tray-mah-doal
(Ralivia ER ✦, Ryzolt, Tridural ✦, Ultram, Ultram ER)
Do not confuse tramadol with tapentadol, Toradol, Trandate, trazodone, or Voltaren, or Ultram with Ultracet.

FIXED-COMBINATION(S)

Ultracet: tramadol/acetaminophen (a non-narcotic analgesic): 37.5 mg/325 mg.

◆CLASSIFICATION

CLINICAL: Analgesic.

ACTION

Binds to μ-opioid receptors, inhibits reuptake of norepinephrine, serotonin. Reduces intensity of pain stimuli incoming from sensory nerve endings. **Therapeutic Effect:** Reduces pain.

PHARMACOKINETICS

Route	Onset	Peak	Duration
PO	Less than 1 hr	2–3 hrs	9 hrs

Rapidly, almost completely absorbed after PO administration. Protein binding: 20%. Extensively metabolized in liver to active metabolite (reduced in pts with advanced cirrhosis). Primarily excreted in urine. Minimally removed by hemodialysis. **Half-life:** 6–7 hrs.

USES

Management of moderate to moderately severe pain. **OFF-LABEL:** Premature ejaculation.

PRECAUTIONS

Contraindications: Acute alcohol intoxication, concurrent use of centrally acting analgesics, hypnotics, opioids, psychotropic drugs, hypersensitivity to opioids. **Extreme Caution:** CNS depression, anoxia, advanced hepatic cirrhosis, epilepsy, respiratory depression, acute alcoholism, shock. **Cautions:** Sensitivity to opioids, increased ICP, hepatic/renal impairment, acute abdominal conditions, opioid-dependent pts.

LIFESPAN CONSIDERATIONS

Pregnancy/Lactation: Crosses placenta. Distributed in breast milk. **Pregnancy Category C. Children:** Safety and efficacy not established. **Elderly:** Age-related renal impairment may require dosage adjustment.

INTERACTIONS

DRUG: Alcohol, other CNS depressants may increase CNS, respiratory depression, hypotension. **Carbamazepine** decreases concentration. **MAOIs** may increase concentration, increase risk of seizures. **Neuroleptics, opioids, selective serotonin reuptake inhibitors (SSRIs), tricyclic antidepressants** may increase risk of seizures, risk of serotonin syndrome. HERBAL: **Gotu kola, kava kava, St. John's wort, valerian** may increase CNS depression. FOOD: None known. LAB VALUES: May increase serum creatinine, AST, ALT. May decrease Hgb. May cause proteinuria.

AVAILABILITY (Rx)

Tablets (Immediate-Release): 50 mg.

Tablets (Extended-Release): 100 mg, 200 mg, 300 mg.

ADMINISTRATION/HANDLING

PO

• Give without regard to meals but consistently with or without meals. • Do not chew, crush, split; swallow extended-release tablets whole.

INDICATIONS/ROUTES/DOSAGE

Moderate to Moderately Severe Pain

PO (IMMEDIATE-RELEASE): ADULTS, ELDERLY: 50–100 mg q4–6h. **Maximum:** 400 mg/day for pts 75 yrs and younger; 300 mg/day for pts older than 75 yrs.

PO (EXTENDED-RELEASE): ADULTS, ELDERLY: 100–300 mg once a day.

Dosage in Renal Impairment

IMMEDIATE-RELEASE: For pts with creatinine clearance less than 30 ml/min, increase dosing interval to q12h. **Maximum:** 200 mg/day. Do not use extended-release.

Dosage in Hepatic Impairment

IMMEDIATE-RELEASE: Dosage is decreased to 50 mg q12h. Do not use extended-release with severe hepatic impairment.

SIDE EFFECTS

Frequent (25%–15%): Dizziness, vertigo, nausea, constipation, headache, drowsiness. Occasional (10%–5%): Vomiting, pruritus, CNS stimulation (e.g., nervousness, anxiety, agitation, tremor, euphoria, mood swings, hallucinations), asthenia (loss of strength, energy), diaphoresis, dyspepsia (heartburn, indigestion, epigastric pain), dry mouth, diarrhea. Rare (less than 5%): Malaise, vasodilation, anorexia, flatulence, rash, blurred vision, urinary retention/frequency, menopausal symptoms.

ADVERSE EFFECTS/ TOXIC REACTIONS

Seizures reported in those receiving tramadol within recommended dosage range. May have prolonged duration of action, cumulative effect in pts with hepatic/renal impairment, serotonin syndrome (agitation, hallucinations, tachycardia, hyperreflexia).

NURSING CONSIDERATIONS

BASELINE ASSESSMENT

Assess onset, type, location, duration of pain. Assess drug history, esp. carbamazepine, analgesics, CNS depressants, MAOIs. Review past medical history, esp. epilepsy, seizures. Assess renal/hepatic function lab values.

INTERVENTION/EVALUATION

Monitor pulse, B/P, renal/hepatic function. Assist with ambulation if dizziness, vertigo occurs. Dry crackers, cola may relieve nausea. Palpate bladder for urinary retention. Monitor daily pattern of bowel activity and stool consistency. Sips of tepid water may relieve dry mouth. Assess for clinical improvement, record onset of relief of pain.

PATIENT/FAMILY TEACHING

• May cause dependence. • Avoid alcohol, OTC medications (analgesics, sedatives). • May cause drowsiness, dizziness, blurred vision. • Avoid tasks requiring alertness, motor skills until response to drug is established. • Inform physician if severe constipation, difficulty breathing, excessive seda-

T

tion, seizures, muscle weakness, tremors, chest pain, palpitations occur.

trandolapril

tran-**doe**-la-pril
(Mavik)

BLACK BOX ALERT May cause fetal injury, mortality if used during second or third trimester of pregnancy.

Do not confuse trandolapril with tramadol.

FIXED-COMBINATION(S)

Tarka: trandolapril/verapamil (a calcium channel blocker): 1 mg/240 mg, 2 mg/180 mg, 2 mg/240 mg, 4 mg/240 mg.

CLASSIFICATION

PHARMACOTHERAPEUTIC: Angiotensin-converting enzyme (ACE) inhibitor. **CLINICAL:** Antihypertensive, CHF agent (see p. 9C).

ACTION

Suppresses renin-angiotensin-aldosterone system (prevents conversion of angiotensin I to angiotensin II, a potent vasoconstrictor; may inhibit angiotensin II at local vascular, renal sites). Decreases plasma angiotensin II, increases plasma renin activity, decreases aldosterone secretion. Therapeutic Effect: Reduces peripheral arterial resistance, pulmonary capillary wedge pressure; improves cardiac output, exercise tolerance.

PHARMACOKINETICS

Rapidly absorbed from GI tract. Protein binding: 80%. Metabolized in liver, GI mucosa to active metabolite. Primarily excreted in urine. Removed by hemodialysis. **Half-life:** 24 hrs.

USES

Treatment of left ventricular dysfunction following MI. Treatment of hypertension, alone or in combination with other antihypertensives. OFF-LABEL: Treatment of CHF. Delay progression of nephropathy, reduce risks of cardiovascular events in hypertensive pts with type 1 or type 2 diabetes.

PRECAUTIONS

Contraindications: History of angioedema from previous treatment with ACE inhibitors, pregnancy. **Cautions:** Renal impairment, CHF, hypovolemia, valvular stenosis, hyperkalemia.

LIFESPAN CONSIDERATIONS

Pregnancy/Lactation: Drug crosses placenta; is distributed in breast milk. May cause fetal, neonatal mortality or morbidity. **Pregnancy Category C (D if used in second or third trimester). Children:** Safety and efficacy not established. **Elderly:** No age-related precautions noted.

INTERACTIONS

DRUG: **Alcohol, antihypertensives, diuretics** may increase effects. **NSAIDs** may decrease effects. **Potassium-sparing diuretics, potassium supplements** may cause hyperkalemia. HERBAL: **Ephedra, ginseng, yohimbe** may worsen hypertension. **Garlic** may increase antihypertensive effect. FOOD: None known. LAB VALUES: May increase BUN, serum alkaline phosphatase, bilirubin, creatinine, potassium, glucose, AST, ALT. May decrease serum sodium. May cause positive antinuclear antibody (ANA) titer.

AVAILABILITY (Rx)

Tablets: 1 mg, 2 mg, 4 mg.

ADMINISTRATION/HANDLING

PO

• Give without regard to meals. • Tablets may be crushed.

INDICATIONS/ROUTES/DOSAGE

Hypertension (without Diuretic)

PO: ADULTS, ELDERLY: Initially, 1 mg once daily in nonblack pts, 2 mg once daily in black pts. Adjust dosage at least at 7-day intervals. Maintenance: 2–4 mg/day. **Maximum:** 8 mg/day.

Congestive Heart Failure, Left Ventricular Dysfunction Post-MI

PO: ADULTS, ELDERLY: Initially, 1 mg/day, titrated to target dose of 4 mg/day.

Dosage in Renal/Hepatic Failure

Creatinine clearance 30 ml/min or less, cirrhosis: Recommended starting dose: 0.5 mg/day.

SIDE EFFECTS

Frequent (35%–23%): Dizziness, cough. **Occasional (11%–3%):** Hypotension, dyspepsia (heartburn, indigestion, epigastric pain), syncope, asthenia (loss of strength, energy), tinnitus. **Rare (less than 1%):** Palpitations, insomnia, drowsiness, nausea, vomiting, constipation, flushed skin.

ADVERSE EFFECTS/ TOXIC REACTIONS

Excessive hypotension ("first-dose syncope") may occur in pts with CHF or severely salt/volume depleted. Angioedema, hyperkalemia occur rarely. Agranulocytosis, neutropenia may be noted in those with collagen vascular disease, including scleroderma, systemic lupus erythematosus, renal impairment. Nephrotic syndrome may be noted in those with history of renal disease.

NURSING CONSIDERATIONS

BASELINE ASSESSMENT

Obtain B/P immediately before each dose, in addition to regular monitoring (be alert to fluctuations). Serum renal function tests should be performed before therapy begins. In pts with renal impairment, autoimmune disease, or taking drugs that affect leukocytes or immune response, CBC, differential count should be performed before therapy begins and q2wks for 3 mos, then periodically thereafter.

INTERVENTION/EVALUATION

If excessive reduction in B/P occurs, place pt in supine position with legs elevated. Assist with ambulation if dizziness occurs. Assess for urinary frequency. Auscultate lung sounds for rales, wheezing in those with CHF. Monitor urinalysis for proteinuria. Monitor serum potassium levels in those on concurrent diuretic therapy. Monitor daily pattern of bowel activity, stool consistency.

PATIENT/FAMILY TEACHING

• Do not discontinue medication. • Inform physician if sore throat, fever, swelling, palpitations, cough, chest pain, difficulty swallowing, facial swelling, vomiting, diarrhea occur. • To reduce hypotensive effect, rise slowly from lying to sitting position and permit legs to dangle from bed momentarily before standing. • Avoid tasks that require alertness, motor skills until response to drug is established (potential for dizziness, drowsiness). • Avoid potassium supplements, salt substitutes.

tranexamic acid

tran-ex-**am**-ick acid
(Lysteda)

◆CLASSIFICATION

PHARMACOTHERAPEUTIC: Systemic hemostatic. **CLINICAL:** Antifibrinolytic agent.

ACTION

Diminishes dissolution of hemostatic fibrin by plasmin, preserving and stabilizing fibrin's matrix structure. **Therapeutic Effect:** Prevents formation of fibrin clots (antifibrinolytic).

PHARMACOKINETICS

Only small amount metabolized. No effect on platelet count, coagulation time. Protein binding: 3%. Excreted in urine. **Half-life:** 18 hrs.

USES

Treatment of cyclic excessive menstrual bleeding.

T

PRECAUTIONS

Contraindications: Evidence of active thromboembolic disease (DVT, pulmonary embolism, cerebral thrombosis), history of thrombosis, thromboembolism, including retinal vein or artery occlusion, thrombogenic valvular disease, cardiac rhythm disease, hypercoagulopathy. **Extreme Caution:** Concurrent hormonal contraceptives, women with acute promyelocytic leukemia taking retinoic acid for remission induction, history of allergies, women with subarachnoid hemorrhage.

LIFESPAN CONSIDERATIONS

Pregnancy/Lactation: Crosses placenta; distributed in breast milk. Not indicated for use in pregnant women. **Pregnancy Category B. Children:** Safety and efficacy not established in those younger than 18 yrs. **Elderly:** Not for use in postmenopausal women.

INTERACTIONS

DRUG: Anti-inhibitor coagulants, factor IX complex medications, hormonal contraceptives may increase risk of thrombosis. **HERBAL:** None significant. **FOOD:** None known. **LAB VALUES:** May prolong thrombin time.

AVAILABILITY (Rx)

Tablets: 650 mg.

ADMINISTRATION/HANDLING

PO

• Give without regard to meals. • Swallow whole; do not chew, break tablets.

INDICATIONS/ROUTES/DOSAGE

Acute Bleeding

PO: ADULTS: 2 tablets 3 times daily for maximum of 5 days during monthly menstruation.

Dosage in Renal Impairment

Serum Creatinine	Dosage
1.4–2.8 mg/dl	2 tablets twice daily
2.7–5.7 mg/dl	2 tablets once daily
Greater than 5.7 mg/dl	1 tablet once daily

SIDE EFFECTS

Frequent (50%–21%): Headache, nasal congestion, back pain. **Occasional (20%–10%):** Abdominal pain, myalgia, arthralgia. **Rare (7%–5%):** Muscle cramps and spasms, migraine headache, fatigue.

ADVERSE EFFECTS/ TOXIC REACTIONS

Venous and arterial thrombosis or thromboembolism, cases of retinal artery and retinal vein occlusions have been reported. Hypersensitivity reaction occurs rarely.

NURSING CONSIDERATIONS

BASELINE ASSESSMENT

Obtain gynecologic, obstetric history. Assess current methods of birth control.

INTERVENTION/EVALUATION

Assess for decrease in B/P, increase in pulse rate, abdominal or back pain, severe headache (may be evidence of hemorrhage). Question for change in amount of discharge during menses. Question and treat headache as appropriate.

PATIENT/FAMILY TEACHING

• Take medication only during monthly period (not meant to treat menstrual symptoms). • Stop medication and report immediately any eye symptoms or change in vision. • Report if heavy menstrual bleeding symptoms persist or worsen.

tranylcypromine

tran-ill-**sip**-roe-meen
(Parnate)

BLACK BOX ALERT Increased risk of suicidal thinking and behavior in children, adolescents, young adults 18–24 yrs with major depressive disorder, other psychiatric disorders.

CLASSIFICATION

PHARMACOTHERAPEUTIC: MAOI. **CLINICAL:** Antidepressant (see p. 38C).

ACTION

Inhibits activity of the enzyme monoamine oxidase at CNS storage sites, leading to increasing levels of neurotransmitters epinephrine, norepinephrine, serotonin, dopamine at neuronal receptor sites. **Therapeutic Effect:** Relieves depression.

USES

Treatment of depression in pts refractory to, intolerant of other therapy. **OFF-LABEL:** Post-traumatic stress disorder.

PRECAUTIONS

Contraindications: CHF, children younger than 16 yrs, pheochromocytoma, severe hepatic/renal impairment, uncontrolled hypertension, cerebrovascular defects, history of headache, history of liver disease or abnormal liver function tests. **Cautions:** Within several hrs of ingestion of contraindicated substance (e.g., tyramine-containing food). Cardiac arrhythmias, severe/frequent headaches, hypertension, suicidal tendencies.

LIFESPAN CONSIDERATIONS

Pregnancy/Lactation: Crosses placenta. Minimally distributed in breast milk. **Pregnancy Category C. Children:** Not recommended for this pt population (increased risk of suicidal ideation). **Elderly:** Increased risk of drug toxicity may require dosage adjustment.

INTERACTIONS

DRUG: Alcohol, other CNS depressants may increase CNS depressant effects. **Buspirone** may increase B/P. **Caffeine-containing medications** may increase risk of cardiac arrhythmias, hypertension. **Carbamazepine, cyclobenzaprine, MAOIs, maprotiline** may precipitate hypertensive crisis. **Dopamine, tryptophan** may cause sudden, severe hypertension. **Fluoxetine, trazodone, tricyclic antidepressants** may cause serotonin syndrome, neuroleptic malignant syndrome. May increase effects of **insulin, oral antidiabetics. Meperidine, other opioid analgesics** may produce diaphoresis, immediate excitation, rigidity, severe hypertension/hypotension, sometimes leading to severe respiratory distress, vascular collapse, seizures, coma, death. **HERBAL: Ephedra, yohimbe** may increase hypertension. Large quantities of **ginkgo, SAMe, St. John's wort, tryptophan, valerian** may increase risk of severe side effects. **FOOD: Foods containing pressor amines (aged cheese, caffeine, red wine), tyramine** may cause sudden, severe hypertension. **LAB VALUES:** None known.

AVAILABILITY (Rx)

Tablets: 10 mg.

ADMINISTRATION/HANDLING

◀ALERT▶ At least 14 days must elapse between tranylcypromine and selective serotonin reuptake inhibitors (SSRIs). Avoid foods containing tryptophan and caffeine; tyramine-containing foods/beverages (e.g., aged cheese, air-dried or cured meats, fava, soy sauce, soybean condiments, tap/draft beer).

INDICATIONS/ROUTES/DOSAGE

Depression

PO: ADULTS, ELDERLY: Initially, 10 mg twice daily. May increase by 10 mg/day at 1- to 3-wk intervals up to 60 mg/day in divided doses. Usual effective dose: 30 mg/day.

SIDE EFFECTS

Frequent: Orthostatic hypotension, restlessness, GI upset, insomnia, dizziness, lethargy, weakness, dry mouth, peripheral edema. **Occasional:** Flushing, diaphoresis, rash, urinary frequency, increased appetite, transient impotence. **Rare:** Visual disturbances.

ADVERSE EFFECTS/ TOXIC REACTIONS

Hypertensive crisis occurs rarely, marked by severe hypertension, occipital headache radiating frontally, neck stiffness/soreness, nausea, vomiting, diaphoresis, fever/chills, clammy skin, dilated pupils, palpitations, tachycardia, bradycardia, constricting

T

chest pain. Intracranial bleeding may be associated with severe hypertension.

NURSING CONSIDERATIONS

BASELINE ASSESSMENT

Perform baseline serum hepatic/renal function tests. Assess sensitivity to tranylcypromine. Assess for other medical conditions, esp. alcoholism, CHF, pheochromocytoma, arrhythmias, cardiovascular disease, hypertension, suicidal tendencies. Question for other medications, including CNS depressants, meperidine, other antidepressants. Do not use in combination with or within 14 days of taking selective serotonin reuptake inhibitors (SSRIs).

INTERVENTION/EVALUATION

Assess appearance, behavior, speech pattern, level of interest, mood. Supervise suicidal-risk pt closely during early therapy (as depression lessens, energy level improves, increasing suicide potential). Monitor for occipital headache radiating frontally, neck stiffness/soreness (may be first signal of impending hypertensive crisis). Monitor B/P diligently for hypertension. Assess skin, temperature for fever. Discontinue medication immediately if palpitations, frequent headaches occur. Monitor weight.

PATIENT/FAMILY TEACHING

• Take second daily dose no later than 4 PM to avoid insomnia. • Antidepressant relief may be noted during first wk of therapy; maximum benefit noted within 3 wks. • Notify physician of worsening depression, unusual behavior, suicidal thoughts or ideation. • Report headache, neck stiffness/soreness immediately. • To avoid orthostatic hypotension, change from lying to sitting position slowly and dangle legs momentarily before standing. • Avoid foods that require bacteria/molds for their preparation/preservation, those that contain tyramine (e.g., cheese, sour cream, beer, wine, pickled herring, liver, figs, raisins, bananas, avocados, soy sauce, yeast extracts, yogurt, papaya, broad beans, meat tenderizers), excessive amounts of caffeine (coffee, tea, chocolate), OTC cold/allergy preparations, weight reduction medications.

T

trastuzumab

HIGH ALERT

traz-**too**-zoo-mab
(Herceptin)

BLACK BOX ALERT Anaphylactic reaction, infusion reaction, acute respiratory distress syndrome have been associated with fatalities. Reduction in left ventricular ejection fraction, severe heart failure may result in thrombus formation, stroke, cardiac death.

◆CLASSIFICATION

PHARMACOTHERAPEUTIC: Monoclonal antibody. **CLINICAL:** Antineoplastic (see p. 89C).

ACTION

Binds to HER-2 protein, overexpressed in 25%–30% of primary breast cancers, inhibiting proliferation of tumor cells. **Therapeutic Effect:** Inhibits growth of tumor cells, mediates antibody-dependent cellular cytotoxicity.

PHARMACOKINETICS

Half-life: 5.8 days (range: 1–32 days).

USES

Treatment of metastatic breast cancer in pts whose tumors overexpress HER-2 protein and who have received one or more chemotherapy regimens. May be used with paclitaxel without previous treatment for metastatic disease. Postsurgical treatment of HER-2–positive, node-positive breast cancer in combination with doxorubicin, cyclophosphamide, paclitaxel. Adjuvant monotherapy for treatment of early stage HER-2–positive breast cancer. Treatment for HER-2 positive metastatic stomach cancer. **OFF-LABEL:** Treatment of ovarian, gastric, colorectal, endometrial, lung, bladder, prostate, salivary gland tumors.

PRECAUTIONS

Contraindications: Preexisting cardiac disease. **Cautions:** Previous cardiotoxic drug, radiation therapy to chest wall, those with known hypersensitivity to trastuzumab.

LIFESPAN CONSIDERATIONS

Pregnancy/Lactation: Unknown if distributed in breast milk. **Pregnancy Category D. Children:** Safety and efficacy not established. **Elderly:** Age-related cardiac dysfunction may require dosage adjustment.

INTERACTIONS

DRUG: Cyclophosphamide, doxorubicin, epirubicin may increase risk of cardiac dysfunction. **HERBAL:** None significant. **FOOD:** None known. **LAB VALUES:** None significant.

AVAILABILITY (Rx)

Injection, Powder for Reconstitution: 440 mg.

ADMINISTRATION/HANDLING

IV

Reconstitution • Reconstitute with 20 ml Bacteriostatic Water for Injection to yield concentration of 21 mg/ml. • Add calculated dose to 250 ml 0.9% NaCl (do not use D_5W). • Gently mix contents in bag.

Rate of administration • Do not give IV push or bolus. • Give loading dose (4 mg/kg) over 90 min. Give maintenance infusion (2 mg/kg) over 30 min.

Storage • Refrigerate. • Reconstituted solution appears colorless to pale yellow. • Reconstituted solution in vial is stable for 28 days if refrigerated after reconstitution with Bacteriostatic Water for Injection (if using Sterile Water for Injection without preservative, use immediately; discard unused portions). • Solution diluted in 250 ml 0.9% NaCl stable for 24 hrs if refrigerated.

IV INCOMPATIBILITIES

Do not mix with D_5W or any other medications.

INDICATIONS/ROUTES/DOSAGE

Breast Cancer

IV: ADULTS, ELDERLY: Initially, 4 mg/kg as 30- to 90-min infusion, then 2 mg/kg weekly as 30-min infusion for a total of 12 wks with concurrent pacitaxel or docetaxel or 18 wks with docetaxel/carboplatin followed 1 wk later (when concurrent chemotherapy completed) by 6 mg/kg infusion over 30–60 min q3wks for total therapy duration of 52 wks.

Stomach Cancer

IV: ADULTS, ELDERLY: Initially, 8 mg/kg over 90 min, then 6 mg/kg over 30–90 min q3wks.

Dosage Adjustment in Cardiotoxicity

Left ventricular ejection fraction (LVEF) 16% or greater decrease from baseline WNL (within normal limits) or LVEF below normal limits and 10% or greater decrease from baseline: Hold treatment for 4 wks. Repeat LVEF q4wks. Resume therapy if LVEF returns to normal limits in 4–8 wks and remains at 15% or less decrease from baseline.

SIDE EFFECTS

Frequent (greater than 20%): Pain, asthenia (loss of strength, energy), fever, chills, headache, abdominal pain, back pain, infection, nausea, diarrhea, vomiting, cough, dyspnea. **Occasional (15%–5%):** Tachycardia, CHF, flu-like symptoms, anorexia, edema, bone pain, arthralgia, insomnia, dizziness, paresthesia, depression, rhinitis, pharyngitis, sinusitis. **Rare (less than 5%):** Allergic reaction, anemia, leukopenia, neuropathy, herpes simplex.

ADVERSE EFFECTS/ TOXIC REACTIONS

Cardiomyopathy, ventricular dysfunction, CHF occur rarely. Pancytopenia may occur.

NURSING CONSIDERATIONS

BASELINE ASSESSMENT

Evaluate left ventricular function. Obtain baseline echocardiogram, EKG, multigated acquisition (MUGA) scan. Obtain CBC, platelet count at baseline and at regular intervals during therapy.

INTERVENTION/EVALUATION

Frequently monitor for deteriorating cardiac function. Assess for asthenia (loss of strength, energy). Assist with ambulation if asthenia occurs. Monitor for fever, chills, abdominal pain, back pain. Offer antiemetics if nausea, vomiting occur. Monitor daily pattern of bowel activity, stool consistency.

PATIENT/FAMILY TEACHING

• Do not have immunizations without physician's approval (lowers resistance). • Avoid contact with those who have recently taken oral polio vaccine. • Avoid crowds, those with infection.

trazodone

tray-zoe-done
(Apo-Trazodone 🍁, Desyrel, Novo-Trazodone 🍁, Oleptro, PMS-Trazodone 🍁)

BLACK BOX ALERT Increased risk of suicidal thinking and behavior in children, adolescents, young adults 18–24 yrs with major depressive disorder, other psychiatric disorders.

Do not confuse Desyrel with Demerol or Zestril, or trazodone with tramadol.

◆CLASSIFICATION

PHARMACOTHERAPEUTIC: Serotonin reuptake inhibitor. **CLINICAL:** Antidepressant (see pp. 14C, 40C).

ACTION

Blocks reuptake of serotonin at neuronal presynaptic membranes, increasing its availability at postsynaptic receptor sites. **Therapeutic Effect:** Relieves depression.

PHARMACOKINETICS

Well absorbed from GI tract. Protein binding: 85%–95%. Metabolized in liver. Primarily excreted in urine. Unknown if removed by hemodialysis. **Half-life:** 5–9 hrs.

USES

Treatment of depression exhibited as persistent, prominent dysphoria (occurring nearly daily for at least 2 wks) manifested by 4 of 8 symptoms: appetite change, sleep pattern change, increased fatigue, impaired concentration, feelings of guilt or worthlessness, loss of interest in usual activities, psychomotor agitation or retardation, suicidal tendencies. **OFF-LABEL:** Treatment of neurogenic pain, hypnotic.

PRECAUTIONS

Contraindications: None known. **Cautions:** Cardiac disease, arrhythmias.

⌛ LIFESPAN CONSIDERATIONS

Pregnancy/Lactation: Drug crosses placenta; minimally distributed in breast milk. **Pregnancy Category C. Children:** Safety and efficacy not established in those younger than 6 yrs. **Elderly:** More likely to experience sedative, hypotensive effects; lower dosage recommended.

INTERACTIONS

DRUG: Alcohol, CNS depression-producing medications may increase CNS depression. May increase effects of **antihypertensives.** May increase concentration of **digoxin, phenytoin. HERBAL: Gotu kola, kava kava, St. John's wort, valerian** may increase CNS depression. **FOOD:** None known. **LAB VALUES:** May decrease WBC, neutrophil counts.

AVAILABILITY (Rx)

Tablets: 50 mg, 100 mg, 150 mg, 300 mg.

Tablets: (Extended-Release [Oleptro]): 150 mg, 300 mg.

ADMINISTRATION/HANDLING

PO

• Give shortly after snack, meal (reduces risk of dizziness, light-headedness). • Tablets may be crushed. • Do not crush or chew extended-release tablets. Swallow whole or break in half along score line. • Best taken at bedtime.

INDICATIONS/ROUTES/DOSAGE

ALERT Therapeutic effect may take up to 6 wks to occur.

Depression

PO: ADULTS: Initially, 150 mg/day in 3 equally divided doses. Increase by 50 mg/day at 3- to 7-day intervals until therapeutic response is achieved. **Maximum:** 600 mg/day. **ELDERLY:** Initially, 25–50 mg at bedtime. May increase by 25–50 mg every 3–7 days. Range: 75–150 mg/day. **Tablets (extended-release):** Initially, 150 mg once daily. May increase by 75 mg q3days. **Maximum:** 375 mg/day. **ADOLESCENTS 13–18 YRS:** Initially, 25–50 mg/day. May increase to 100–150 mg/day in divided doses. **CHILDREN 6–12 YRS:** Initially, 1.5–2 mg/kg/day in divided doses. May increase gradually to 6 mg/kg/day in 3 divided doses.

SIDE EFFECTS

Frequent (9%–3%): Drowsiness, dry mouth, light-headedness, dizziness, headache, blurred vision, nausea, vomiting. **Occasional** (3%–1%): Nervousness, fatigue, constipation, myalgia/arthralgia, mild hypotension. **Rare:** Photosensitivity reaction.

ADVERSE EFFECTS/ TOXIC REACTIONS

Priapism, altered libido, retrograde ejaculation, impotence occur rarely. Appears to be less cardiotoxic than other antidepressants, although arrhythmias may occur in pts with preexisting cardiac disease.

NURSING CONSIDERATIONS

BASELINE ASSESSMENT

Assess mental status, mood, behavior. For those on long-term therapy, serum hepatic/renal function tests, blood counts should be performed periodically. Elderly are more likely to experience sedative, hypotensive effects.

INTERVENTION/EVALUATION

Monitor suicidal ideation (esp. at beginning of therapy or dosage change). Assess appearance, behavior, speech pattern, level of interest, mood. Monitor WBC, neutrophil count, hepatic enzymes. Assist with ambulation if dizziness, light-headedness occurs.

PATIENT/FAMILY TEACHING

• Immediately discontinue medication, consult physician if priapism occurs. • May take after meal, snack. • May take at bedtime if drowsiness occurs. • Change positions slowly to avoid hypotensive effect. • Tolerance to sedative, anticholinergic effects usually develops during early therapy. • Avoid tasks that require alertness, motor skills until response to drug is established. • Photosensitivity to sun may occur. • Dry mouth may be relieved by sugarless gum, sips of tepid water. • Report visual disturbances, worsening depression, suicidal ideation, unusual changes in behavior. • Do not abruptly discontinue medication. • Avoid alcohol.

treprostinil

tre-**pros**-tin-il
(Remodulin, Tyvaso)

CLASSIFICATION

PHARMACOTHERAPEUTIC: Aggregation inhibitor, vasodilator. **CLINICAL:** Antiplatelet.

ACTION

Directly dilates pulmonary, systemic arterial vascular beds, also inhibits platelet aggregation. **Therapeutic Effect:** Reduces symptoms of pulmonary arterial hypertension associated with exercise.

PHARMACOKINETICS

Rapidly, completely absorbed after subcutaneous infusion; protein binding: 91%. Metabolized by liver. Excreted mainly in urine, with lesser amount eliminated in feces. **Half-life:** 2–4 hrs.

USES

Injection: Treatment of pulmonary arterial hypertension (PAH) in pts with NYHA Class II–IV symptoms to decrease exercise associated symptoms; diminish clinical deterioration when transitioning from epoprostenol (Flolan). **Inhalation:** Treatment of PAH in pts with NYHA Class III symptoms to increase walk distance.

PRECAUTIONS

Contraindications: None known. **Cautions:** Hepatic/renal impairment in those older than 65 yrs. Pts with significant underlying lung disease (e.g., COPD); low systemic arterial pressure, concomitant use of anticoagulants, inducers of CYP2C8 (e.g., rifampin), inhibitors of CYP2C8 (e.g., celecoxib).

LIFESPAN CONSIDERATIONS

Pregnancy/Lactation: Unknown if distributed in breast milk. **Pregnancy Category B. Children:** Safety and efficacy not established. **Elderly:** Consider dose selection carefully because of increased incidence of diminished organ function, concurrent disease, other drug therapy.

INTERACTIONS

DRUG: **Anticoagulants, aspirin, heparin, thrombolytics** may increase risk of bleeding. **CYP2C8 inhibitors** may increase concentration/effects. **CYP2C8 inducers** may decrease concentration/effects. **HERBAL:** None significant. **FOOD:** None known. **LAB VALUES:** None significant.

AVAILABILITY (Rx)

Injection Solution (Remodulin): 1 mg/ml, 2.5 mg/ml, 5 mg/ml, 10 mg/ml. **Solution for Oral Inhalation (Tyvaso):** 0.6 mg/ml (2.9-ml ampoule) delivers 6 mcg per inhalation.

ADMINISTRATION/HANDLING

Inhalation

• Use only with supplied inhalation system. Refer to product information. Give undiluted. • Wait 1 min before inhaling next dose (allows for deeper bronchial penetration). • Administer 4 times daily 4 hrs apart, during waking hrs.

IV

Reconstitution • Dilute with either Sterile Water for Injection or 0.9% NaCl to final volume of 50 ml or 100 ml.

Rate of administration • Give as continuous IV infusion via indwelling central venous catheter.

Storage • Store unopened vials at room temperature. • Diluted solutions stable for 48 hrs at room temperature.

Subcutaneous

Reconstitution • Intended to be administered without further dilution using an appropriately designed infusion pump. • To avoid potential interruptions in drug delivery, pt must have immediate access to backup infusion pump, subcutaneous infusion sets.

Rate of administration • Give as continuous subcutaneous infusion via subcutaneous catheter, using infusion pump designed for subcutaneous drug delivery.

Storage • Store unopened vials at room temperature.

INDICATIONS/ROUTES/DOSAGE

Pulmonary Arterial Hypertension (PAH)

Continuous subcutaneous infusion, IV infusion: ADULTS, ELDERLY: Initially, 1.25 ng/kg/min. Reduce infusion rate to 0.625 ng/kg/min if initial dose cannot be tolerated. Increase infusion rate in increments of no more than 1.25 ng/kg/min per wk for first 4 wks, then no more than 2.5 ng/kg/min per wk for duration of infusion.

T

Inhalation: **ADULTS, ELDERLY:** 3 breaths (18 mcg) per treatment session. Reduce to 1 or 2 breaths if 3 breaths are not tolerated. Increase by 3 breaths at 1- to 2-wk intervals. Titrate to target dose of 9 breaths (54 mcg) per treatment session.

Hepatic Impairment (Mild to Moderate)
ADULTS, ELDERLY (IV/SUBCUTANEOUS): Decrease initial dose to 0.625 ng/kg/min based on ideal body weight; increase cautiously.

SIDE EFFECTS

IV: Frequent: Infusion site pain, erythema, induration, rash. **Occasional:** Headache, diarrhea, jaw pain, vasodilation, nausea. **Rare:** Dizziness, hypotension, pruritus, edema. **Inhalation: Common** (54%–25%): Cough, headache, throat irritation. **Occasional** (19%–6%): Nausea, flushing, syncope.

ADVERSE EFFECTS/ TOXIC REACTIONS

Abrupt withdrawal, sudden large reductions in dosage may result in worsening of pulmonary arterial hypertension symptoms. Inhalation may produce symptomatic hypotension.

NURSING CONSIDERATIONS

INTERVENTION/EVALUATION

Monitor for dyspnea, fatigue, decreased activity, symptoms of excessive dose (e.g., headache, nausea, vomiting). Monitor for changes in B/P.

PATIENT/FAMILY TEACHING

• Delivery occurs via self-inserted subcutaneous catheter using ambulatory subcutaneous pump; carefully follow instructions for drug administration. • Follow guidelines for care of subcutaneous catheter, troubleshooting infusion pump problems. • Avoid skin or eye contact with Tyvaso (rinse immediately with water).

tretinoin HIGH ALERT

tret-ih-noyn
(Atralin, Avita, Rejuva-A ✱, Refissa, Renova, Retin-A, Retin-A Micro, Tretin X, Vesanoid)

BLACK BOX ALERT High risk for teratogenicity; major fetal abnormalities, spontaneous abortions. Pts with acute promyelocytic leukemia (APL) are at severe risk for reactions (fever, dyspnea, acute respiratory distress syndrome [pulmonary infiltrates, pleural effusions, pericardial effusions]), edema, hepatic, renal, and/or multiorgan failure; 40% develop leukocytosis.

Do not confuse tretinoin with isotretinoin, phenytoin, Tenormin, or triamcinolone.

FIXED-COMBINATION(S)

With octyl methoxycinnamate and oxybenzone, moisturizers, and SPF-12, a sunscreen **(Retin-A Regimen Kit).**

◆CLASSIFICATION

PHARMACOTHERAPEUTIC: Retinoid. **CLINICAL:** Antiacne, transdermal, antineoplastic (see p. 88C).

ACTION

Antiacne: Decreases cohesiveness of follicular epithelial cells. Increases turnover of follicular epithelial cells. **Therapeutic Effect:** Causes expulsion of blackheads. Bacterial skin counts are not altered. **Transdermal:** Exerts effects on growth/differentiation of epithelial cells. **Therapeutic Effect:** Alleviates fine wrinkles, hyperpigmentation. **Antineoplastic:** Induces maturation, decreases proliferation of acute promyelocytic leukemia (APL) cells. **Therapeutic Effect:** Repopulation of bone marrow, blood by normal hematopoietic cells.

PHARMACOKINETICS

Topical: Minimally absorbed. **PO:** Well absorbed following PO administration. Protein binding: greater than 95%. Me-

T

tabolized in liver. Primarily excreted in urine. Half-life: 0.5–2 hrs.

USES

Topical: Treatment of acne vulgaris, esp. grades I–III in which blackheads, papules, pustules predominate. **PO:** Induction of remission in pts with acute promyelocytic leukemia. OFF-LABEL: Treatment of disorders of keratinization, including photo-aged skin, liver spots.

PRECAUTIONS

Contraindications: Sensitivity to parabens (used as preservative in gelatin capsule). Extreme Caution: **Topical:** Eczema, sun exposure. Cautions: **Topical:** Those with considerable sun exposure in their occupation, hypersensitivity to sun. **PO:** Elevated serum cholesterol/triglycerides.

LIFESPAN CONSIDERATIONS

Pregnancy/Lactation: **Topical:** Use during pregnancy only if clearly necessary. Unknown if distributed in breast milk; exercise caution in breast-feeding mother. **Topical:** Pregnancy Category C. **PO:** Teratogenic, embryotoxic effect. **Pregnancy Category D. Children/Elderly:** Safety and efficacy not established.

INTERACTIONS

DRUG: **TOPICAL: Retinoids (e.g., acitretin, oral tretinoin)** may increase drying, irritative effects. **PO: Tetracyclines** may increase risk of pseudotumor cerebri, intracranial hypertension. **Aminocaproic acid** may increase risk of thrombotic complications. **Phenobarbital, rifampin** may alter kinetics of tretinoin. **Ketoconazole** may increase concentration, risk of toxicity. HERBAL: **St. John's wort** may decrease concentration, effect. **Dong quai, St. John's wort** may increase photosensitization. **Vitamin A** supplementation may increase vitamin A toxicity. FOOD: None known. LAB VALUES: **PO:** Leukocytosis occurs commonly (40%). May elevate serum hepatic function tests, cholesterol, triglycerides.

AVAILABILITY (Rx)

Cream: 0.02% (Renova), 0.025% (Avita, Retin-A, Tretin X), 0.05% (Refissa, Retin-A, Tretin X), 0.1% (Retin-A). Gel: 0.01% (Retin-A, Tretin X), 0.025% (Avita, Retin-A, Tretin X), 0.04% (Retin-A, Micro), 0.1% (Retin-A Micro).

Capsules: (Vesanoid): 10 mg.

ADMINISTRATION/HANDLING

PO

• Do not crush/break capsule. • Administer with a meal.

Topical

• Thoroughly cleanse area before applying tretinoin. • Lightly cover only affected area. Liquid may be applied with fingertip, gauze, cotton, do not rub onto unaffected skin. • Keep medication away from eyes, mouth, angles of nose, mucous membranes. • Wash hands immediately after application.

INDICATIONS/ROUTES/DOSAGE

Acne

TOPICAL: ADULTS, CHILDREN 12 YRS AND OLDER: Apply once daily at bedtime or on alternate days.

Acute Promyelocytic Leukemia (APL)

PO: ADULTS: REMISSION INDUCTION: 45 mg/m^2/day given as 2–3 evenly divided doses until complete remission is documented. Discontinue therapy 30 days after complete remission or after 90 days of treatment, whichever comes first.

Remission Maintenance in APL

PO: ADULTS, ELDERLY, CHILDREN: 45–200 mg/m^2/day in 2–3 divided doses for up to 12 mos.

SIDE EFFECTS

Topical: Temporary change in pigmentation, photosensitivity. Local inflammatory reactions (peeling, dry skin, stinging, erythema, pruritus) are to be expected and are reversible with discontinuation of tretinoin. Frequent: **PO (87%–54%):** Headache, fever, dry skin/oral mucosa, bone pain, nausea, vomiting, rash. Occasional: **PO (26%–6%):** Mucositis, earache or feeling of fullness in ears, flushing, pruritus, diaphoresis, visual disturbances, hypotension/hypertension, dizziness, anxiety, insomnia, alopecia, skin changes. Rare (less than 6%): Altered visual acuity, temporary hearing loss.

ADVERSE EFFECTS/ TOXIC REACTIONS

PO: Retinoic acid syndrome (fever, dyspnea, weight gain, abnormal chest auscultatory findings [pulmonary infiltrates, pleural/pericardial effusions], episodic hypotension) occurs commonly (25%), as does leukocytosis (40%). Syndrome generally occurs during first month of therapy (sometimes after first dose). High-dose steroids (dexamethasone 10 mg IV) at first suspicion of syndrome reduce morbidity, mortality. Pseudotumor cerebri may be noted, esp. in children (headache, nausea, vomiting, visual disturbances). **Topical:** Possible tumorigenic potential when combined with ultraviolet radiation.

NURSING CONSIDERATIONS

BASELINE ASSESSMENT

PO: Inform women of childbearing potential of risk to fetus if pregnancy occurs. Instruct on need for use of 2 reliable forms of contraceptives concurrently during therapy and for 1 mo after discontinuation of therapy, even in infertile women. Pregnancy test should be obtained within 1 wk before institution of therapy. Obtain initial serum hepatic function tests, cholesterol, triglyceride levels.

INTERVENTION/EVALUATION

PO: Monitor serum hepatic function tests, hematologic, coagulation profiles, cholesterol, triglycerides. Monitor for signs/symptoms of pseudotumor cerebri in children.

PATIENT/FAMILY TEACHING

• **Topical:** Avoid exposure to sunlight, tanning beds; use sunscreens, protective clothing. • Protect affected areas from wind, cold. • If skin is already sunburned, do not use drug until fully healed. • Keep tretinoin away from eyes, mouth, angles of nose, mucous membranes. • Do not use medicated, drying, abrasive soaps; wash face no more than 2–3 times a day with gentle soap. • Avoid use of preparations containing alcohol, menthol, spice, lime (e.g., shaving lotions, astringents, perfume). • Mild redness, peeling are expected; decrease frequency or discontinue medication if excessive reaction occurs. • Nonmedicated cosmetics may be used; however, cosmetics must be removed before tretinoin application. • Improvement noted during first 24 wks of therapy. • **Anti-acne:** Therapeutic results noted in 2–3 wks; optimal results in 6 wks. **Oral:** • Avoid tasks requiring motor skills, alertness until response to drug is established. • Avoid alcohol. • Avoid exposure to sunlight, tanning beds. • Notify physician of persistent vomiting, diarrhea, unusual bleeding/bruising, acute abdominal pain, vision changes, or if pregnancy is suspected.

triamcinolone

trye-am-**sin**-oh-lone

triamcinolone acetonide

(AllerNaze, Azmacort, Kenalog, Kenalog in Orabase, Kenalog-10, Kenalog-40, Nasacort AQ, Triderm, Tri-Nasal)

triamcinolone hexacetonide

(Aristospan)

Do not confuse Nasacort with Nasalcrom.

T

FIXED-COMBINATION(S)

Myco-II, Mycolog II, Myco-Triacet: triamcinolone/nystatin (an antifungal): 0.1%/100,000 units/g.

◆CLASSIFICATION

PHARMACOTHERAPEUTIC: Adrenocortical steroid. **CLINICAL:** Anti-inflammatory (see pp. 3C, 76C, 98C, 100C).

ACTION

Inhibits accumulation of inflammatory cells at inflammation sites, phagocytosis, lysosomal enzyme release, synthesis/release of mediators of inflammation. **Therapeutic Effect:** Prevents/suppresses cell-mediated immune reactions. Decreases/prevents tissue response to inflammatory process.

USES

Oral inhalation: Long-term control of bronchial asthma. **Nasal inhalation:** Seasonal, perennial rhinitis. **Intra-articular:** Acute gouty arthritis, bursitis, tenosynovitis, epicondylitis, rheumatoid arthritis, synovitis of osteoarthritis. **Intralesional:** Alopecia areata, discoid lupus erythematosus, keloids, lichen plaques, psoriatic plaques. **Topical:** Relief of inflammation, pruritus associated with corticoid-responsive dermatoses.

PRECAUTIONS

Contraindications: Administration of live virus vaccines, esp. smallpox vaccine; hypersensitivity to corticosteroids, tartrazine; IM injection, oral inhalation in children younger than 6 yrs; peptic ulcer disease (except life-threatening situations); systemic fungal infection. **Topical:** Marked circulation impairment. **Cautions:** History of tuberculosis (may reactivate disease), hypothyroidism, cirrhosis, non-specific ulcerative colitis, CHF, hypertension, psychosis, renal insufficiency. Prolonged therapy should be discontinued slowly. **Pregnancy Category C (D if used in first trimester).**

INTERACTIONS

DRUG: **Amphotericin** may worsen hypokalemia. May increase risk of **digoxin** toxicity (due to hypokalemia). May decrease effects of **diuretics, insulin, oral hypoglycemics, potassium supplements. Hepatic enzyme inducers** may decrease effects. **Live virus vaccines** may potentiate virus replication, increase virus side effects, decrease pt's antibody response to vaccine. **HERBAL:** **Cat's claw, echinacea** possess immunostimulant properties. **FOOD:** None known. **LAB VALUES:** May increase serum glucose, lipid, amylase, sodium. May decrease serum calcium, potassium, thyroxine.

AVAILABILITY (Rx)

Aerosol, Oral Inhalation (Azmacort): 75 mcg/actuation. **Cream:** 0.025%, 0.1%, 0.5%. **Injection, Suspension (Kenalog-10):** 10 mg/ml. **(Kenalog-40):** 40 mg/ml. **Ointment:** 0.025%, 0.1%, 0.5%. **Paste, Oral, Topical:** 0.1%. **Solution, Spray Nasal Inhalation: (Tri-Nasal):** 50 mcg/inhalation. **Suspension, Spray Nasal Inhalation: (Nasacort AQ):** 55 mcg/inhalation. **(AllerNaze):** 50 mcg/inhalation.

ADMINISTRATION/HANDLING

Inhalation

• Shake container well. Instruct pt to exhale as completely as possible, place mouthpiece fully into mouth, holding inhaler upright, inhale deeply and slowly while pressing top of canister. Hold breath as long as possible before exhaling, then exhale slowly. • Allow at least 1 min between inhalations when multiple inhalations are ordered (allows for deeper bronchial penetration). • Rinse mouth with water immediately after inhalation (prevents mouth/throat dryness).

Topical

• Gently cleanse area before application. • Use occlusive dressings only as ordered. • Apply sparingly, rub into area thoroughly.

INDICATIONS/ROUTES/DOSAGE

Triamcinolone Hexacetonide

INTRALESIONAL: Up to 0.5 mg/square inch. Range: 2–48 mg.
INTRA-ARTICULAR: Average dose: 2–20 mg q3–4 wks.

Triamcinolone Acetonide

INTRA-ARTICULAR: ADULTS, ELDERLY: Initially: 2–20 mg/day. Doses can be adjusted between 20–80 mg as needed.

Control of Bronchial Asthma

INHALATION: ADULTS, ELDERLY, CHILDREN OLDER THAN 12 YRS: 150 mcg (2 inhalations) 3–4 times a day or 300 mcg (4 inhalations) twice daily. **Maximum:** 1,200 mcg/day. **CHILDREN 6–12 YRS:** 75–150 mcg (1–2 inhalations) 3–4 times a day or 150–300 mcg (2–4 inhalations) 2 times daily. **Maximum:** 900 mcg/day.

Rhinitis

INTRANASAL: ADULTS, ELDERLY, CHILDREN 12 YRS AND OLDER: 2 sprays in each nostril once daily. **Maximum:** 4 sprays in each nostril once daily or 2 sprays in each nostril twice daily. **CHILDREN 6–11 YRS:** Initially, 1 spray in each nostril once daily. **Maximum:** 2 sprays in each nostril once daily. **CHILDREN 2–5 YRS:** 1 spray in each nostril once daily.

Usual Topical Dosage

TOPICAL: ADULTS, ELDERLY: 2–4 times a day. May give 1–2 times a day or as intermittent therapy.

SIDE EFFECTS

Frequent: Insomnia, dry mouth, heartburn, nervousness, abdominal distention, diaphoresis, acne, mood swings, increased appetite, facial flushing, delayed wound healing, increased susceptibility to infection, diarrhea, constipation. **Occasional:** Headache, edema, change in skin color, frequent urination. **Rare:** Tachycardia, allergic reaction (rash, urticaria), altered mental status, hallucinations, depression. **Topical:** Allergic contact dermatitis.

ADVERSE EFFECTS/ TOXIC REACTIONS

Long-term therapy: Muscle wasting (arms, legs), osteoporosis, spontaneous fractures, amenorrhea, cataracts, glaucoma, peptic ulcer, CHF. **Abrupt withdrawal following long-term therapy:** Anorexia, nausea, fever, headache, arthralgia, rebound inflammation, fatigue, weakness, lethargy, dizziness, orthostatic hypotension. Anaphylaxis occurs rarely with parenteral administration. Sudden discontinuation may be fatal. Blindness has occurred rarely after intralesional injection around face, head.

NURSING CONSIDERATIONS

BASELINE ASSESSMENT

Question for hypersensitivity to any corticosteroids. Obtain baselines for height, weight, B/P, serum glucose, electrolytes.

INTERVENTION/EVALUATION

Oral Inhalation, Intranasal: Check mucous membranes for signs of fungal infection. Monitor growth in children. Monitor B/P.

PATIENT/FAMILY TEACHING

• Notify physician if condition being treated persists or worsens. • Avoid exposure to chickenpox or measles. • Avoid alcohol. • **Inhalation:** Do not take for acute asthma attack. • Rinse mouth to decrease risk of mouth soreness. • Inform physician if mouth lesions, sore mouth occurs (stomatitis). • **Nasal:** Report unusual cough/spasm, persistent nasal bleeding, burning, infection.

triamterene

try-**am**-ter-een
(Dyrenium)

BLACK BOX ALERT Hyperkalemia risk, potentially fatal if uncorrected; increased incidence in renal impairment, diabetes (even without evidence of diabetic nephropathy), elderly, severely ill pts.

T

Do not confuse Dyrenium with Pyridium, or triamterene with trimipramine.

FIXED-COMBINATION(S)

Dyazide, Maxzide: triamterene/hydrochlorothiazide (a diuretic): 37.5 mg/25 mg, 50 mg/25 mg, 75 mg/50 mg.

CLASSIFICATION

PHARMACOTHERAPEUTIC: Potassium-sparing diuretic. **CLINICAL:** Antiedema (see p. 102C).

ACTION

Inhibits sodium, potassium, ATPase. Interferes with sodium/potassium exchange in distal tubule, cortical collecting tubule, collecting duct. Increases sodium, decreases potassium excretion. Increases magnesium, decreases calcium loss. **Therapeutic Effect:** Produces diuresis, lowers B/P.

PHARMACOKINETICS

Route	Onset	Peak	Duration
PO	2–4 hrs	N/A	7–9 hrs

Incompletely absorbed from GI tract. Widely distributed. Metabolized in liver. Primarily eliminated in feces via biliary route. **Half-life:** 1.5–2.5 hrs (increased in renal impairment).

USES

Treatment of edema, hypertension. **OFF-LABEL:** Treatment adjunct for hypertension, prevention/treatment of hypokalemia.

PRECAUTIONS

Contraindications: Anuria, drug-induced or preexisting hyperkalemia, progressive or severe renal disease, severe hepatic disease. **Cautions:** Hepatic/renal impairment, history of renal calculi, diabetes mellitus.

LIFESPAN CONSIDERATIONS

Pregnancy/Lactation: Drug crosses placenta; distributed in breast milk. Breast-feeding not recommended. **Pregnancy Category B (D if used in pregnancy-induced hypertension). Children:** Safety and efficacy not established. **Elderly:** May be at increased risk for developing hyperkalemia.

INTERACTIONS

DRUG: **ACE inhibitors (e.g., captopril), cyclosporine, potassium-containing medications, potassium supplements** may increase risk of hyperkalemia. May decrease effects of **anticoagulants, heparin.** May decrease clearance, increase risk of toxicity of **lithium. NSAIDs** may decrease antihypertensive effect. **HERBAL:** None significant. **FOOD:** None known. **LAB VALUES:** May increase urinary calcium excretion, BUN, serum glucose, calcium, magnesium, creatinine, potassium, uric acid. May decrease sodium.

AVAILABILITY (Rx)

Capsules: 50 mg, 100 mg.

ADMINISTRATION/HANDLING

PO

• Give with food if GI disturbance occurs.

INDICATIONS/ROUTES/DOSAGE

Edema, Hypertension

PO: ADULTS, ELDERLY: 25–100 mg/day as single dose or in 2 divided doses. **Maximum:** 300 mg/day. **CHILDREN:** 1–2 mg/kg/day as single dose or in 2 divided doses. **Maximum:** 3–4 mg/kg/day or 300 mg/day.

SIDE EFFECTS

Occasional: Fatigue, nausea, diarrhea, abdominal pain, leg cramps, headache. **Rare:** Anorexia, asthenia (loss of strength, energy), rash, dizziness.

ADVERSE EFFECTS/ TOXIC REACTIONS

May result in hyponatremia (drowsiness, dry mouth, increased thirst, lack of energy), severe hyperkalemia (irritability, anxiety, heaviness of legs, paresthesia, hypotension, bradycardia, EKG changes [tented T waves, widening QRS complex, ST segment depression]), particularly in those with renal impairment, diabetes, elderly, severely ill. Agranulocytosis, nephrolithiasis, thrombocytopenia occur rarely.

NURSING CONSIDERATIONS

BASELINE ASSESSMENT

Assess baseline serum electrolytes, particularly check for hypokalemia. Assess serum renal/hepatic function tests. Assess for edema (note location, extent), skin turgor, mucous membranes for hydration status. Assess muscle strength, mental status. Note skin temperature, moisture. Obtain baseline weight. Initiate strict I&O. Note pulse rate, regularity.

INTERVENTION/EVALUATION

Monitor B/P, vital signs, serum electrolytes (particularly potassium), I&O, weight. Watch for changes from initial assessment (hyperkalemia may result in muscle strength changes, tremor, muscle cramps), altered mental status (orientation, alertness, confusion), cardiac arrhythmias. Weigh daily. Note extent of diuresis. Assess lung sounds for rhonchi, wheezing.

PATIENT/FAMILY TEACHING

• Take medication in morning. • Expect increased urinary volume, frequency. • Therapeutic effect takes several days to begin and can last for several days when drug is discontinued. • Avoid prolonged exposure to sunlight. • Report severe, persistent weakness, headache, dry mouth, nausea, vomiting, fever, sore throat, unusual bleeding/bruising. • Avoid excessive intake of food high in potassium, salt substitutes.

trifluoperazine

trye-floo-oh-**per**-a-zeen
(Apo-Trifluoperazine ✤, Novo-Trifluzine ✤, PMS-Trifluoperazine ✤, Stelazine)

BLACK BOX ALERT Elderly pts with dementia-related psychosis are at increased risk for death.

Do not confuse trifluoperazine with triflupromazine or trihexyphenidyl, or Stelazine with selegiline.

◆ CLASSIFICATION

PHARMACOTHERAPEUTIC: Phenothiazine derivative. **CLINICAL:** Antipsychotic, antianxiety (see p. 66C).

ACTION

Blocks dopamine at postsynaptic receptor sites. Possesses strong extrapyramidal, antiemetic effects, weak anticholinergic, sedative effects. **Therapeutic Effect:** Suppresses behavioral response in psychosis; reduces locomotor activity, aggressiveness.

PHARMACOKINETICS

Readily absorbed following PO administration. Protein binding: 90%–99%. Metabolized in liver. Excreted in urine. **Half-life:** 24 hrs.

USES

Treatment of schizophrenia, non-psychotic anxiety. **OFF-LABEL:** Psychotic disorders, behavioral symptoms, psychosis/agitation related to Alzheimer's dementia.

PRECAUTIONS

Contraindications: Angle-closure glaucoma, circulatory collapse, myelosuppression, severe cardiac/hepatic disease, severe hypertension/hypotension. **Cautions:** Seizure disorders, Parkinson's disease.

LIFESPAN CONSIDERATIONS

Pregnancy/Lactation: Drug crosses placenta; is distributed in breast milk. **Pregnancy Category C. Children:** Safety and efficacy not established in those younger than 2 yrs. **Elderly:** Higher risk of sedative, anticholinergic, extrapyramidal, hypotensive effects.

INTERACTIONS

DRUG: **Alcohol, other CNS depressants** may increase CNS, respiratory depression, hypotensive effects. **Antacids** may inhibit absorption if given within 2 hrs of drug. **Antithyroid agents** may increase risk of agranulocytosis. **Extrapyramidal symptom (EPS)–producing medications** may increase extrapyramidal symptoms. **Hypotensive agents** may increase hypotension. May decrease effects of **levodopa. Lithium** may decrease absorption, produce adverse neurologic effects. **MAOIs, tricyclic antidepressants** may increase anticholinergic, sedative effects. HERBAL: **Gotu kola, kava kava, St. John's wort, valerian** may increase CNS depression. **Dong quai, St. John's wort** may increase photosensitization. FOOD: None known. LAB VALUES: May cause EKG changes.

AVAILABILITY (Rx)

Tablets: 1 mg, 2 mg, 5 mg, 10 mg.

ADMINISTRATION/HANDLING

PO

• May give with food to decrease GI effects. • Do not take within 2 hrs of any antacids.

INDICATIONS/ROUTES/DOSAGE

Schizophrenia

PO: ADULTS, ELDERLY, CHILDREN 12 YRS AND OLDER: Initially, 2–5 mg 1–2 times a day. Range: 15–20 mg/day. **Maximum:** 40 mg/day. **CHILDREN 6–11 YRS:** Initially, 1 mg 1–2 times a day. Maintenance: Up to 15 mg/day.

Non-Psychotic Anxiety

PO: ADULTS, ELDERLY: 1–2 mg 2 times/day. **Maximum:** 6 mg/day. Therapy should not exceed 12 wks.

SIDE EFFECTS

Frequent: Hypotension, dizziness, syncope (occur frequently after first injection, occasionally after subsequent injections, rarely with oral form). Occasional: Drowsiness during early therapy, dry mouth, blurred vision, lethargy, constipation, diarrhea, nasal congestion, peripheral edema, urinary retention. Rare: Ocular changes, altered skin pigmentation (in those taking high doses for prolonged periods), photosensitivity.

ADVERSE EFFECTS/ TOXIC REACTIONS

Extrapyramidal symptoms appear to be dose-related (particularly high doses) and are divided into 3 categories: akathisia (inability to sit still, tapping of feet); parkinsonian symptoms (mask-like face, tremors, shuffling gait, hypersalivation); acute dystonias: torticollis (neck muscle spasm), opisthotonos (rigidity of back muscles), oculogyric crisis (rolling back of eyes). Dystonic reaction may produce diaphoresis, pallor. Tardive dyskinesia (tongue protrusion, puffing of cheeks, chewing/puckering of the mouth) occurs rarely (may be irreversible). Abrupt withdrawal after long-term therapy may precipitate nausea, vomiting, gastritis, dizziness, tremors. Blood dyscrasias, particularly agranulocytosis, mild leukopenia may occur. May lower seizure threshold.

NURSING CONSIDERATIONS

BASELINE ASSESSMENT

Assess behavior, appearance, emotional status, response to environment, speech pattern, thought content.

INTERVENTION/EVALUATION

Monitor B/P for hypotension. Assess for EPS. Monitor WBC for blood dyscrasias.

Monitor for fine tongue movement (may be early sign of tardive dyskinesia); tremor, gait changes; abnormal movement in trunk, neck, extremities. Supervise suicidal-risk pt closely during early therapy (as depression lessens, energy level improves, increasing suicide potential). Monitor target behaviors. Assess for therapeutic response (interest in surroundings, improvement in self-care, increased ability to concentrate, relaxed facial expression).

PATIENT/FAMILY TEACHING

• Do not take antacids within 2 hrs of trifluoperazine. • Avoid alcohol. • Avoid excessive exposure to sunlight, artificial light. • Avoid tasks that require alertness, motor skills until response to drug is established (may cause drowsiness). • Rise slowly from lying or sitting position (prevents hypotension).

trihexyphenidyl

trye-hex-eh-**fen**-ih-dill
(Apo-Trihex ✱, Artane)
Do not confuse Artane with Altace or Anturane, or trihexiphenidyl with trifluoperazine.

◆CLASSIFICATION

PHARMACOTHERAPEUTIC: Anticholinergic. **CLINICAL:** Antiparkinson agent.

ACTION

Blocks central cholinergic receptors (aids in balancing cholinergic and dopaminergic activity). **Therapeutic Effect:** Decreases salivation, relaxes smooth muscle.

USES

Adjunctive treatment for all forms of Parkinson's disease, including postencephalitic, arteriosclerotic, idiopathic types. Controls symptoms of drug-induced extrapyramidal symptoms (EPS).

PRECAUTIONS

Contraindications: Angle-closure glaucoma, GI obstruction, paralytic ileus, intestinal atony, severe ulcerative colitis, prostatic hypertrophy, myasthenia gravis, megacolon. **Cautions:** Hyperthyroidism, renal/hepatic impairment, hypertension, hiatal hernia, tachycardia, arrhythmias, GI ulcer, esophageal reflux, excessive activity during hot weather, exercise. **Pregnancy Category C.**

INTERACTIONS

DRUG: **Alcohol, CNS depressants** may increase sedative effect. **Amantadine, anticholinergics, MAOIs** may increase anticholinergic effects. **Antacids, antidiarrheals** may decrease absorption, effects. **HERBAL:** None significant. **FOOD:** None known. **LAB VALUES:** None significant.

AVAILABILITY (Rx)

Elixir: 2 mg/5 ml. **Tablets:** 2 mg, 5 mg.

ADMINISTRATION/HANDLING

PO

• Administer with food, water to decrease GI irritation.

INDICATIONS/ROUTES/DOSAGE

Parkinsonism

PO: ADULTS, ELDERLY: Initially, 1 mg on first day. May increase by 2 mg/day at 3- to 5-day intervals up to 6–10 mg/day (12–15 mg/day in pts with postencephalitic parkinsonism).

Drug-Induced Extrapyramidal Symptoms

PO: ADULTS, ELDERLY: Initially, 1 mg/day. Range: 5–15 mg/day in 3–4 divided doses.

SIDE EFFECTS

◀ALERT▶ Those older than 60 yrs tend to develop mental confusion, disorientation, agitation, psychotic-like symptoms. **Frequent:** Drowsiness, dry mouth. **Occasional:** Blurred vision, urinary retention, constipation, dizziness, head-

T

ache, muscle cramps. **Rare:** Skin rash, seizures, depression.

ADVERSE EFFECTS/ TOXIC REACTIONS

Hypersensitivity reaction (eczema, pruritus, rash, cardiac arrhythmias, photosensitivity) may occur. Overdosage may vary from CNS depression (sedation, apnea, cardiovascular collapse, death) to severe paradoxical reaction (hallucinations, tremor, seizures).

NURSING CONSIDERATIONS

INTERVENTION/EVALUATION

Be alert to neurologic effects (headache, lethargy, mental confusion, agitation). Monitor elderly closely for paradoxical reaction. Assess for clinical reversal of symptoms (improvement of tremor of head/ hands at rest, mask-like facial expression, shuffling gait, muscular rigidity).

PATIENT/FAMILY TEACHING

• Take after meals or with food. • Do not stop medication abruptly. • Inform physician if GI effects, palpitations, eye pain, rash, fever, heat intolerance occur. • Avoid alcohol, other CNS depressants. • May cause dry mouth, drowsiness. • Avoid tasks that require alertness, motor skills until response to drug is established. • Difficulty urinating, constipation may occur (inform physician if they persist).

trimethoprim

trye-**meth**-oh-prim
(Apo-Tremethoprim ✦, Primsol, Proloprim)
Do not confuse Proloprim with Prolixin.

FIXED-COMBINATION(S)

Bactrim, Septra: trimethoprim/sulfamethoxazole (a sulfonamide): 16 mg/80 mg/ml (injection), 40 mg/200 mg/5 ml (suspension), 80 mg/400 mg, 160 mg/800 mg (tablets).

◆CLASSIFICATION

PHARMACOTHERAPEUTIC: Folate antagonist. **CLINICAL:** Antibacterial.

ACTION

Blocks bacterial biosynthesis of nucleic acids, proteins by interfering with metabolism of folinic acid. **Therapeutic Effect:** Bacteriostatic.

PHARMACOKINETICS

Rapidly, completely absorbed from GI tract. Protein binding: 42%–46%. Widely distributed, including to CSF. Metabolized in liver. Primarily excreted in urine. Moderately removed by hemodialysis. **Half-life:** 8–10 hrs (increased in renal impairment, newborns; decreased in children).

USES

Treatment of uncomplicated UTI caused by susceptible strains of *E. coli, P. mirabilis, K. pneumoniae.* Treatment of otitis media due to *H. influenzae, S. pneumoniae*. **OFF-LABEL:** Acute exacerbation of bronchitis in adults, treatment of toxoplasmosis. Treatment of pneumonia caused by *Pneumocystis jiroveci*.

PRECAUTIONS

Contraindications: Infants younger than 2 mos, megaloblastic anemia due to folic acid deficiency. **Cautions:** Renal/hepatic impairment, pts with folic acid deficiency.

LIFESPAN CONSIDERATIONS

Pregnancy/Lactation: Drug readily crosses placenta; is distributed in breast milk. **Pregnancy Category C. Children:** Safety and efficacy not established. **Elderly:** No age-related precautions noted. May increase incidence of thrombocytopenia.

INTERACTIONS

DRUG: **Folate antagonists (including methotrexate)** may increase risk of megaloblastic anemia. **HERBAL:** None significant. **FOOD:** None known. **LAB VALUES:** May increase BUN, serum bilirubin, creatinine, AST, ALT.

AVAILABILITY (Rx)

Oral Solution (Primsol): 50 mg/5 ml. **Tablets (Proloprim):** 100 mg.

ADMINISTRATION/HANDLING

PO

• Space doses evenly to maintain constant therapeutic level. • Give without regard to meals (if GI upset occurs, give with food).

INDICATIONS/ROUTES/DOSAGE

Uncomplicated UTI

PO: ADULTS, ELDERLY, CHILDREN 12 YRS AND OLDER: 100 mg q12h or 200 mg once daily for 10 days. **CHILDREN YOUNGER THAN 12 YRS:** 4–6 mg/kg/day in 2 divided doses for 10 days.

Otitis Media

PO: CHILDREN, 6 MOS AND OLDER: 10 mg/kg/day in divided doses q12h for 10 days.

***Pneumocystis Jiroveci* Pneumonia (PCP)**

ADULTS, ELDERLY, CHILDREN 12 YRS AND OLDER: 15–20 mg/kg/day in 4 divided doses for 21 days.

Dosage in Renal Impairment

Dosage and frequency are modified based on creatinine clearance.

Creatinine Clearance	Dosage
Greater than 30 ml/min	No change
15–30 ml/min	50% of normal dose
Less than 15 ml/min	Avoid use

SIDE EFFECTS

Occasional: Nausea, vomiting, diarrhea, decreased appetite, abdominal cramps, headache. **Rare:** Hypersensitivity reaction (pruritus, rash), methemoglobinemia (bluish fingernails, lips, skin; fever; pale skin; sore throat; asthenia [loss of strength, energy]), photosensitivity.

ADVERSE EFFECTS/ TOXIC REACTIONS

Stevens-Johnson syndrome, erythema multiforme, exfoliative dermatitis, anaphylaxis occur rarely. Hematologic toxicity (thrombocytopenia, neutropenia, leukopenia, megaloblastic anemia) more likely to occur in elderly, debilitated, alcoholics, those with renal impairment or receiving prolonged high dosage.

NURSING CONSIDERATIONS

BASELINE ASSESSMENT

Assess hematology baseline reports, serum renal function tests.

INTERVENTION/EVALUATION

Assess skin for rash. Evaluate food tolerance. Monitor serum hematology reports, renal/hepatic function test results. Check for developing signs of hematologic toxicity (pallor, fever, sore throat, malaise, bleeding/bruising).

PATIENT/FAMILY TEACHING

• Space doses evenly. • Complete full length of therapy (10–14 days). • May take on empty stomach or with food if stomach upset occurs. • Avoid sun, ultraviolet light; use sunscreen, wear protective clothing. • Immediately report pallor, fatigue, sore throat, bruising/bleeding, discoloration of skin, fever, rash to physician.

T

triptorelin

trip-toe-**rel**-in
(Trelstar Depot, Trelstar LA)

◆ CLASSIFICATION

PHARMACOTHERAPEUTIC: Gonadotropin-releasing hormone analogue. **CLINICAL:** Antineoplastic.

ACTION

Through a negative feedback mechanism, inhibits gonadotropin hormone secretion. Circulating levels of luteinizing hormone (LH), follicle-stimulating hormone (FSH), testosterone, estradiol rise initially, then subside with continued therapy. Therapeutic Effect: Suppresses growth of abnormal prostate tissue.

USES

Treatment of advanced prostate cancer (alternate to orchiectomy or estrogen administration). OFF-LABEL: Treatment of endometriosis, growth hormone deficiency, hyperandrogenism, ovarian, pancreatic carcinomas, precocious puberty, uterine leiomyomata.

PRECAUTIONS

Contraindications: Hypersensitivity to luteinizing hormone-releasing hormone (LHRH), LHRH agonists, pregnancy. Cautions: None known.

LIFESPAN CONSIDERATIONS

Pregnancy/Lactation: Unknown if distributed in breast milk. **Pregnancy Category X. Children:** Safety and efficacy not established. **Elderly:** No age-related precautions noted.

INTERACTIONS

DRUG: **Hyperprolactinemic drugs (e.g., metoclopramide)** reduce number of pituitary gonadotropin-releasing hormone (GnRH) receptors. HERBAL: None significant. FOOD: None known. LAB VALUES: May alter serum pituitary-gonadal function test results. May cause transient increase in serum testosterone, usually during first wk of treatment.

AVAILABILITY (Rx)

Injection, Powder for Reconstitution (Trelstar Depot): 3.75 mg. Injection, Powder for Reconstitution (Trelstar LA): 11.25 mg, 22.5 mg.

ADMINISTRATION/HANDLING

IM

• Reconstitute with 2 ml Sterile Water for Injection. • Administer into large muscle mass, esp. gluteus muscle, alternating injection sites.

INDICATIONS/ROUTES/DOSAGE

Prostate Cancer

IM (TRELSTAR DEPOT): ADULTS, ELDERLY: 3.75 mg once q28days.
IM (TRELSTAR LA): ADULTS, ELDERLY: 11.25 mg q84days, 22.5 mg q24wks.

SIDE EFFECTS

Frequent (greater than 5%): Hot flashes, skeletal pain, headache, impotence. Occasional (5%–2%): Insomnia, vomiting, leg pain, fatigue. Rare (less than 2%): Dizziness, emotional lability, diarrhea, urinary retention, UTI, anemia, pruritus.

ADVERSE EFFECTS/ TOXIC REACTIONS

Bladder outlet obstruction, skeletal pain, hematuria, spinal cord compression with weakness, paralysis of lower extremities may occur.

NURSING CONSIDERATIONS

INTERVENTION/EVALUATION

Obtain serum testosterone, prostate-specific antigen (PSA), prostatic acid phosphatase (PAP) levels periodically during therapy. Serum testosterone, PAP levels should increase during first wk of therapy. Testosterone level then should decrease to baseline level or less within 2 wks, PAP level within 4 wks. Monitor pt closely for worsening signs and symptoms of prostatic cancer, esp. during first wk of therapy (due to transient increase in testosterone).

PATIENT/FAMILY TEACHING

• Do not miss monthly injections. • May experience increased skeletal pain, blood in urine, urinary retention initially (subsides within 1 wk). • Hot flashes may occur. • Inform physician if tachycardia, persistent nausea/vomiting, numbness of

T

arms/legs, pain/swelling of breasts, difficulty breathing, infection at injection site occurs.

trospium

trow-spee-um
(Sanctura, Sanctura XR, Trosec ✦)

◆ CLASSIFICATION

PHARMACOTHERAPEUTIC: Anticholinergic. **CLINICAL:** Antispasmotic.

ACTION

Antagonizes effect of acetylcholine on muscarinic receptors, producing parasympatholytic action. **Therapeutic Effect:** Reduces smooth muscle tone in bladder.

PHARMACOKINETICS

Minimally absorbed after PO administration. Protein binding: 50%–85%. Distributed in plasma. Excreted mainly in feces and, to lesser extent, in urine. **Half-life:** 20 hrs.

USES

Treatment of overactive bladder with symptoms of urge urinary incontinence, urgency, urinary frequency.

PRECAUTIONS

Contraindications: Decreased GI motility, gastric retention, uncontrolled angle-closure glaucoma, urinary retention. **Cautions:** Renal/hepatic impairment, obstructive GI disorders, ulcerative colitis, intestinal atony, myasthenia gravis, narrow-angle glaucoma, significant bladder obstruction.

LIFESPAN CONSIDERATIONS

Pregnancy/Lactation: Unknown if drug crosses placenta or is distributed in breast milk. **Pregnancy Category C. Children:** Safety and efficacy not established. **Elderly:** Higher incidence of dry mouth, constipation, dyspepsia, UTI, urinary retention in those 75 yrs and older.

INTERACTIONS

DRUG: Other anticholinergic agents increase severity, frequency of side effects, may alter absorption of other drugs due to anticholinergic effects on GI motility. **Digoxin, metformin, morphine, pancuronium, procainamide, tenofovir, vancomycin** may increase concentration. **HERBAL:** None significant. **FOOD: High-fat meals** may reduce absorption. **LAB VALUES:** None significant.

AVAILABILITY (Rx)

Tablets (Sanctura): 20 mg. **Capsules, Extended-Release (Sanctura XR):** 60 mg.

ADMINISTRATION/HANDLING

PO

• Store at room temperature. • Give at least 1 hr before meals or on an empty stomach. • Do not crush, chew tablet, extended-release capsule; swallow whole. • Administer tablets at bedtime, capsules in morning with full glass of water, 1 hr before eating.

INDICATIONS/ROUTES/DOSAGE

Overactive Bladder

PO: ADULTS: 20 mg twice daily. **ELDERLY 75 YRS AND OLDER:** 20 mg once daily at bedtime. **Extended-release:** 60 mg once daily.

Dosage in Renal Impairment

For pts with creatinine clearance less than 30 ml/min, dosage reduced to 20 mg once daily at bedtime. Extended-release not recommended.

SIDE EFFECTS

Frequent (20%): Dry mouth. **Occasional (10%–4%):** Constipation, headache. **Rare (less than 2%):** Fatigue, upper abdominal pain, dyspepsia (heartburn, indigestion, epigastric pain), flatulence, dry eyes, urinary retention.

T

ADVERSE EFFECTS/ TOXIC REACTIONS

Overdose may result in severe anticholinergic effects, characterized by nervousness, restlessness, nausea, vomiting, confusion, diaphoresis, facial flushing, hypertension, hypotension, respiratory depression, irritability, lacrimation. Supraventricular tachycardia and hallucinations occur rarely.

NURSING CONSIDERATIONS

BASELINE ASSESSMENT

Assess for presence of dysuria, urinary urgency, frequency, incontinence.

INTERVENTION/EVALUATION

Monitor for symptomatic relief. Monitor I&O; palpate bladder for retention. Monitor daily pattern of bowel activity, stool consistency. Dry mouth may be relieved by sips of tepid water.

PATIENT/FAMILY TEACHING

• Report nausea, vomiting, diaphoresis, increased salivary secretions, palpitations, severe abdominal pain.

ustekinumab

ue-stay-**kin**-ue-mab
(Stelara)

Do not confuse ustekinumab with infliximab or rituximab, or Stelara with Aldara.

◆CLASSIFICATION

PHARMACOTHERAPEUTIC: Monoclonal antibody. **CLINICAL:** Antipsoriasis agent.

ACTION

Strongly binds with cellular components involved in responses to inflammation and immune system, thereby decreasing likelihood of aggravating psoriatic eruptions. **Therapeutic Effect:** Significantly slows growth, migration of circulating total lymphocytes (predominant in psoriatic lesions).

PHARMACOKINETICS

Following subcutaneous injections, clearance is affected by body weight, is not affected by gender or race. Degraded into small peptides and amino acids via catabolic pathways. Serum concentration reaches steady state at 28 wks. **Half-life:** 10–126 days.

USES

Treatment of adults 18 yrs or older with moderate to severe plaque psoriasis who are candidates for systemic therapy or phototherapy.

PRECAUTIONS

Contraindications: None known. **Cautions:** History of chronic infection, recurrent infection, active tuberculosis.

⌛ LIFESPAN CONSIDERATIONS

Pregnancy/Lactation: Unknown if distributed in breast milk. **Pregnancy Category B.** **Children:** Not indicated for use in this pt population. **Elderly:** Age-related increased incidence of infection requires cautious use.

INTERACTIONS:

DRUG: **Immunosuppressive agents** increase risk of infection. **Live virus vaccine** decreases immune response. **Abciximab, trastuzumab** may increase concentration/effect. **HERBAL:** **Echinacea** may decrease concentration/effect. **FOOD:** None known. **LAB VALUES:** May increase lymphocyte count.

AVAILABILITY (Rx)

Injection Solution: 45 mg/0.5 ml, 90 mg/1 ml single-use vials.

ADMINISTRATION/HANDLING

Subcutaneous

• Do not inject into areas where skin is tender, bruised, erythematous, indurated. • Administer into thigh, abdomen, buttocks, upper arm. • Refrigerate unopened vial. • Solution appears colorless to light yellow. Discard if solution contains more than a few small translucent or white particles or is cloudy.

INDICATIONS/ROUTES/DOSAGE

Psoriasis

SUBCUTANEOUS: ADULTS, ELDERLY WEIGHING 100 KG OR LESS: Initially, 45 mg, then 45 mg 4 wks later, followed by 45 mg every 12 wks. **WEIGHING MORE THAN 100 KG:** Initially, 90 mg, then 90 mg 4 wks later, followed by 90 mg every 12 wks.

SIDE EFFECTS

Occasional (8%–4%): Nasopharyngitis, upper respiratory tract infection, headache. **Rare (3%–1%):** Fatigue, diarrhea, back pain, dizziness, pruritus, injection site erythema, myalgia, depression.

ADVERSE EFFECTS/ TOXIC REACTIONS

Worsening of psoriasis, thrombocytopenia, malignancies, serious infections (cellulitis, diverticulitis, gastroenteritis, pneumonia, osteomyelitis, urinary tract infections, postoperative wound infection) have been noted. Reversible posterior leukoencephalopathy syndrome (headache, seizures, confusion, visual disturbances) occurs rarely.

NURSING CONSIDERATIONS

BASELINE ASSESSMENT

Pts should not receive live vaccines during treatment, 1 yr prior to initiating treatment, or 1 yr following discontinuation of treatment. Inform pt of duration of treatment and required monitoring procedures. Assess skin prior to therapy; document extent and location of psoriasis lesions. Test pt for tuberculosis infection prior to initiating treatment.

INTERVENTION/EVALUATION

Closely monitor for signs/symptoms of active tuberculosis during and after treatment. Assess skin throughout therapy for evidence of improvement of psoriasis lesions. Monitor for worsening of lesions.

PATIENT/FAMILY TEACHING

• If appropriate, pt may self-inject after proper training in preparation and injection technique. • Inform physician if onset of signs of infection occurs. • If new diagnosis of malignancy occurs, inform physician of current treatment with ustekinumab.

valacyclovir

val-a-**sye**-kloe-ver
(Apo-Valacyclovir ✱, Valtrex)
Do not confuse valacyclovir with acyclovir, valganciclovir, or Valtrex with Valcyte.

◆CLASSIFICATION

PHARMACOTHERAPEUTIC: Antiviral. **CLINICAL:** Antiherpetic agent (see p. 70C).

ACTION

Converted to acyclovir triphosphate, becoming part of viral DNA chain. **Therapeutic Effect:** Interferes with DNA synthesis, replication of herpes simplex, varicella-zoster virus.

PHARMACOKINETICS

Rapidly absorbed after PO administration. Protein binding: 13%–18%. Rapidly converted by hydrolysis to active compound acyclovir. Widely distributed to tissues, body fluids (including CSF). Primarily eliminated in urine. Removed by hemodialysis. **Half-life:** (acyclovir) 2.5–3.3 hrs (increased in renal impairment).

USES

Treatment of herpes zoster (shingles) in immunocompetent adults. Episodic treatment of recurrent genital herpes in immunocompetent adults. Prevention of recurrent genital herpes. Treatment of initial genital herpes. Treatment of cold

V

sores. OFF-LABEL: Reduce risk of heterosexual transmission of genital herpes.

PRECAUTIONS

Contraindications: Hypersensitivity to or intolerance of acyclovir, valacyclovir, or their components. **Cautions:** Bone marrow or renal transplantation, advanced HIV infections, renal/hepatic impairment, dehydration, fluid or electrolyte imbalance, concurrent use of nephrotoxic agents, neurologic abnormalities.

LIFESPAN CONSIDERATIONS

Pregnancy/Lactation: May cross placenta. May be distributed in breast milk. **Pregnancy Category B. Children:** Safety and efficacy not established. **Elderly:** Age-related renal impairment may require dosage adjustment.

INTERACTIONS

DRUG: **Cimetidine, probenecid** may increase acyclovir concentration. HERBAL: None significant. FOOD: None known. LAB VALUES: None significant.

AVAILABILITY (Rx)

Caplets: 500 mg, 1,000 mg.

ADMINISTRATION/HANDLING

PO

- Give without regard to meals.
- If GI upset occurs, give with meals.

INDICATIONS/ROUTES/DOSAGE

Herpes Zoster (Shingles)

PO: ADULTS, ELDERLY: 1 g 3 times a day for 7 days.

Herpes Simplex (Cold Sores)

PO: ADULTS, ELDERLY: 2 g twice a day for 1 day (separate by 12 hrs).

Initial Episode of Genital Herpes

PO: ADULTS, ELDERLY: 1 g twice a day for 10 days.

Recurrent Episodes of Genital Herpes

PO: ADULTS, ELDERLY: 500 mg twice a day for 3 days.

Prevention of Genital Herpes

PO: ADULTS, ELDERLY: 500–1,000 mg/day.

Dosage in Renal Impairment

Dosage and frequency are modified based on creatinine clearance.

Cold Sores/Herpes Zoster

Creatinine Clearance	Herpes Zoster	Cold Sores
30–49 ml/min	1 g q12h	1 g q12h × 2 doses
10–29 ml/min	1 g q24h	500 mg q12h × 2 doses
Less than 10 ml/min	500 mg q24h	500 mg as single dose

Genital Herpes

Creatinine Clearance	Initial Episode	Recurrent Episode	Suppressive Therapy
10–29 ml/min	1 g q24h	500 mg q24h	500 mg q24–48h
Less than 10 ml/min	500 mg q24h	500 mg q24h	500 mg q24–48h

SIDE EFFECTS

Frequent: Herpes zoster (17%–10%): Nausea, headache. **Genital herpes (17%):** Headache. **Occasional: Herpes zoster (7%–3%):** Vomiting, diarrhea, constipation (50 yrs and older), asthenia (loss of strength, energy), dizziness (50 yrs and older). **Genital herpes (8%–3%):** Nausea, diarrhea, dizziness. **Rare: Herpes zoster (3%–1%):** Abdominal pain, anorexia. **Genital herpes (3%–1%):** Asthenia (loss of strength, energy), abdominal pain.

ADVERSE EFFECTS/ TOXIC REACTIONS

Neutropenia, thrombocytopenia, renal failure occur rarely.

NURSING CONSIDERATIONS

BASELINE ASSESSMENT

Question for history of allergies, particularly to valacyclovir, acyclovir. Tissue cultures for herpes zoster, herpes simplex should be done before giving first dose (therapy may proceed before results are known). Assess medical history, esp. advanced HIV infection, bone marrow or renal transplantation, hepatic/renal impairment.

INTERVENTION/EVALUATION

Evaluate cutaneous lesions. Monitor serum renal/hepatic function tests, CBC, urinalysis. Provide analgesics, comfort measures for herpes zoster (esp. exhausting to elderly). Encourage fluids. Keep pt's fingernails short, hands clean.

PATIENT/FAMILY TEACHING

• Drink adequate fluids. • Do not touch lesions with fingers to avoid spreading infection to new site. • **Genital Herpes:** Continue therapy for full length of treatment. • Space doses evenly. • Avoid sexual intercourse during duration of lesions to prevent infecting partner. • Valacyclovir does not cure herpes. • Notify physician if lesions recur or do not improve. • Pap smears should be done at least annually due to increased risk of cervical cancer in women with genital herpes. • Initiate treatment at first sign of recurrent episode of genital herpes or herpes zoster (early treatment within first 24–48 hrs is imperative for therapeutic results).

valerian

Also known as all-heal, amantilla, garden heliotrope, valeriana.

CLASSIFICATION

HERBAL: See Appendix G.

ACTION

Appears to inhibit enzyme system responsible for catabolism of gamma-aminobutyric acid (GABA), increasing GABA concentration, decreasing CNS activity. **Effect:** Produces sedative effects. Has anxiolytic, antidepressant, anticonvulsant effects.

USES

Used as sedative for insomnia, sleeping disorders associated with anxiety, restlessness. Used for depression, ADHD.

PRECAUTIONS

Contraindications: Insufficient data on pregnancy or lactation (avoid use); hepatic disease. **Cautions:** None known.

LIFESPAN CONSIDERATIONS

Pregnancy/Lactation: Contraindicated; unknown if drug crosses placenta or is distributed in breast milk. **Pregnancy Category C. Children:** Safety and efficacy not established in those younger than 16 yrs. **Elderly:** Increased risk of motor/cognitive function impairment.

INTERACTIONS

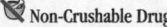

DRUG: **Alcohol, barbiturates, benzodiazepines** may cause additive effect, increase adverse effects. HERBAL: **Chamomile, ginseng, kava kava, melatonin, St. John's wort** may enhance therapeutic effect, adverse effects. FOOD: None known. LAB VALUES: None significant.

AVAILABILITY (OTC)

Capsules. Extract. Tablets. Tea. Tincture.

INDICATIONS/ROUTES/DOSAGE

Sedation

PO: ADULTS, ELDERLY: (Extract): 400–900 mg ½–1 hr before bedtime or 1 cup tea taken several times a day.

SIDE EFFECTS

Headache, hangover, cardiac arrhythmias.

V

ADVERSE EFFECTS/ TOXIC REACTIONS

Ataxia (difficulty walking), hypothermia, increased muscle relaxation, excitability, insomnia.

NURSING CONSIDERATIONS

BASELINE ASSESSMENT

Determine whether pt is using other CNS depressants, esp. benzodiazepines. Assess baseline serum hepatic function.

INTERVENTION/EVALUATION

Monitor effectiveness in decreasing insomnia. Assess for hypersensitivity reaction; monitor serum hepatic function tests.

PATIENT/FAMILY TEACHING

• Up to 4 wks may be needed for significant relief. • Avoid tasks that require alertness, motor skills until response to drug is established. • Inform physician if pregnant or breast-feeding. • Taper doses slowly; do not discontinue abruptly.

valganciclovir

val-gan-**sye**-kloh-veer
(Valcyte)

BLACK BOX ALERT May adversely affect spermatogenesis, fertility. Risk for granulocytopenia, anemia, thrombocytopenia.

Do not confuse Valcyte with Valium or Valtrex, or valganciclovir with valacyclovir.

◆CLASSIFICATION

PHARMACOTHERAPEUTIC: Synthetic nucleoside. **CLINICAL:** Antiviral (see p. 70C).

ACTION

Competes with viral DNA esterases, is incorporated directly into growing viral DNA chains. **Therapeutic Effect:** Interferes with DNA synthesis, viral replication.

PHARMACOKINETICS

Well absorbed, rapidly converted to ganciclovir by intestinal mucosal cells and hepatocytes. Widely distributed including CSF, ocular tissue. Slowly metabolized intracellularly. Primarily excreted in urine. Removed by hemodialysis. **Half-life:** Ganciclovir: 4 hrs (increased in renal impairment).

USES

Adults: Treatment of cytomegalovirus (CMV) retinitis in AIDS. Prevention of CMV disease in high-risk, renal, cardiac, renal-pancreas transplant pts. **Children:** Prevention of CMV disease in high-risk renal and cardiac transplant pts.

PRECAUTIONS

Contraindications: Hypersensitivity to acyclovir, ganciclovir. **Cautions:** Extreme caution in children because of long-term carcinogenicity, reproductive toxicity. Renal impairment, preexisting cytopenias, history of cytopenic reactions to other drugs; elderly (at greater risk for renal impairment).

⌛ LIFESPAN CONSIDERATIONS

Pregnancy/Lactation: Effective contraception should be used during therapy; valganciclovir should not be used during pregnancy. Avoid breast-feeding during therapy; may be resumed no sooner than 72 hrs after last dose of valganciclovir. **Pregnancy Category C. Children:** Safety and efficacy not established in those younger than 12 yrs. **Elderly:** Age-related renal impairment may require dosage adjustment.

INTERACTIONS

DRUG: **Bone marrow depressants** may increase myelosuppression. May increase risk of toxicity of **didanosine, mycophenolate. Probenecid** decreases renal clearance. **Zidovudine (AZT)** may increase risk of hematologic toxicity. **HERBAL:** None significant. **FOOD:** **All foods** maximize drug bioavailability. **LAB VALUES:** May decrease Hgb, creatinine clearance, serum creatinine, platelet count, absolute neutrophil count.

AVAILABILITIES (Rx)

Powder for Oral Solution: 50 mg/ml (100 ml).

Tablets: 450 mg.

ADMINISTRATION/HANDLING

PO

• Do not break, crush tablets; swallow whole (potential carcinogen). • Avoid contact with skin. • Wash skin with soap, water if contact occurs. • Give with food. • Store oral suspension in refrigerator. Discard after 49 days.

INDICATIONS/ROUTES/DOSAGE

Cytomegalovirus (CMV) Retinitis

PO: ADULTS: Initially, 900 mg (two 450-mg tablets) twice daily for 21 days. Maintenance: 900 mg once daily.

Prevention of CMV After Transplant

PO: ADULTS, ELDERLY: 900 mg once daily beginning within 10 days of transplant and continuing until 200 days post-transplant. **CHILDREN 4 MOS–16 YRS:** Once daily based on body surface area (BSA) and creatinine clearance (CrCl) using formula: (Dose = 7 × BSA × CrCl).

Dosage in Renal Impairment

Dosage and frequency are modified based on creatinine clearance.

Creatinine Clearance	Induction Dosage	Maintenance Dosage
60 ml/min or higher	900 mg twice daily	900 mg once daily
40–59 ml/min	450 mg twice daily	450 mg once daily
25–39 ml/min	450 mg once daily	450 mg every 2 days
10–24 ml/min	450 mg every 2 days	450 mg twice a wk

SIDE EFFECTS

Frequent (16%–9%): Diarrhea, neutropenia, headache. **Occasional (8%–3%):** Nausea. **Rare (less than 3%):** Insomnia, paresthesia, vomiting, abdominal pain, fever.

ADVERSE EFFECTS/ TOXIC REACTIONS

Hematologic toxicity, including severe neutropenia (most common), anemia, thrombocytopenia may occur. Retinal detachment occurs rarely. Overdose may result in renal toxicity. May decrease sperm production, fertility.

NURSING CONSIDERATIONS

BASELINE ASSESSMENT

Evaluate hematologic, serum chemistry baselines, serum creatinine.

INTERVENTION/EVALUATION

Monitor I&O, ensure adequate hydration (minimum 1,500 ml/24 hrs). Diligently evaluate CBC for decreased WBCs, Hgb, Hct, decreased platelets. Question pt regarding vision, therapeutic improvement, complications.

PATIENT/FAMILY TEACHING

• Valganciclovir provides suppression, not cure, of CMV retinitis. • Frequent blood tests are necessary during therapy because of toxic nature of drug. • Ophthalmologic exam q4–6wk during treatment is advised. • Report any new symptom promptly. • May temporarily or permanently inhibit sperm production in men, suppress fertility in women. • Barrier contraception should be used during and for 90 days after therapy because of mutagenic potential. • Avoid handling broken/crushed tablets, oral solution. • Notify physician of fever, chills, unusual bleeding/bruising.

valproic acid

val-**pro**-ick

(Apo-Divalproex ✱, Depacon, Depakene, Depakote, Depakote ER, Depakote Sprinkle, Novo-Divalproex ✱, Stavzor)

BLACK BOX ALERT Embryo, fetal neural tube defects (spina bifida) have occurred. Life-threatening pancreatitis, complete hepatic failure have occurred.

Do not confuse Depakene with Depakote.

CLASSIFICATION

CLINICAL: Anticonvulsant, antimanic, antimigraine (see p. 36C).

ACTION

Directly increases concentration of inhibitory neurotransmitter gamma-aminobutyric acid (GABA). **Therapeutic Effect:** Produces anticonvulsant effect.

PHARMACOKINETICS

Well absorbed from GI tract. Protein binding: 80%–90%. Metabolized in liver. Primarily excreted in urine. Not removed by hemodialysis. **Half-life:** 9–16 hrs (may be increased in hepatic impairment, elderly, children younger than 18 mos).

USES

Treatment of simple and complex absence (petit mal) seizures (monotherapy preferred due to unpredictable interactions, increased risk of hepatotoxicity). Adjunctive therapy of multiple seizures. Treatment of manic episodes with bipolar disorders, complex partial seizures. Prophylaxis of migraine headaches. OFF-LABEL: Treatment of behavior disorders in Alzheimer's disease; chorea, myoclonic, simple partial, tonic-clonic seizures; organic brain syndrome; schizophrenia; status epilepticus; tardive dyskinesia.

PRECAUTIONS

Contraindications: Active hepatic disease, urea cycle disorders. **Cautions:** History of hepatic disease, bleeding abnormalities.

LIFESPAN CONSIDERATIONS

Pregnancy/Lactation: Drug crosses placenta; is distributed in breast milk. **Pregnancy Category D. Children:** Increased risk of hepatotoxicity in those younger than 2 yrs. **Elderly:** No age-related precautions, but lower dosages recommended.

INTERACTIONS

DRUG: **Alcohol, other CNS depressants** may increase CNS depressant effects. May increase concentration of **amitriptyline, primidone. Anticoagulants, heparin, platelet aggregation inhibitors, thrombolytics** may increase risk of bleeding. **Carbamazepine** may decrease concentration. **Hepatotoxic medications** may increase risk of hepatotoxicity. May increase risk of dermatologic reaction with **lamotrigine.** May increase risk of **phenytoin** toxicity, decrease effects. HERBAL: **Evening primrose** may decrease seizure threshold. FOOD: None known. LAB VALUES: May increase serum LDH, bilirubin, AST, ALT. **Therapeutic serum level:** 50–100 mcg/ml; **toxic serum level:** greater than 100 mcg/ml.

AVAILABILITY (Rx)

Capsules (Depakene): 250 mg. **Capsules, Sprinkle (Depakote Sprinkle):** 125 mg. **Injection, Solution (Depacon):** 100 mg/ml. **Syrup (Depakene):** 250 mg/5 ml.

Capsules, Delayed-Release (Stavzor): 125 mg, 250 mg, 500 mg. **Tablets, Delayed-Release (Depakote):** 125 mg, 250 mg, 500 mg. **Tablets, Extended-Release (Depakote ER):** 250 mg, 500 mg.

ADMINISTRATION/HANDLING

IV

Reconstitution • Dilute each single dose with at least 50 ml D_5W, 0.9% NaCl, or lactated Ringer's.

Rate of administration • Infuse over 60 min at rate of 20 mg/min or less. • Alternatively, single doses of up to 45 mg/kg given over 5–10 min (1.5–6 mg/kg/min).

Storage • Store vials at room temperature. • Diluted solutions stable for 24 hrs. • Discard unused portion.

PO

• May give without regard to food. Do not mix oral solution with carbonated beverages (may cause mouth/throat irritation). • May sprinkle capsule (Depakote Sprinkle) contents on applesauce and give immediately (do not chew sprinkle beads). • Give delayed-release/extended-release tablets whole. Do not crush, chew, open delayed-release capsule (Stavzor). • Regular-release and delayed-release formulations usually given in 2–4 divided doses/day. Extended-release formulation (Depakote ER) usually given once daily.

IV INCOMPATIBILITIES

Do not mix with any other medications.

INDICATIONS/ROUTES/DOSAGE

Seizures

PO: ADULTS, ELDERLY, CHILDREN 10 YRS AND OLDER: Initially, 10–15 mg/kg/day in 1–3 divided doses. May increase by 5–10 mg/kg/day at weekly intervals up to 30–60 mg/kg/day. Usual adult dosage: 1,000–2,500 mg/day. **(STAVZOR):** Initially, 10–15 mg/kg/day, may increase by 5–10 mg/kg/day at 1-wk intervals to achieve desired response. **Maximum:** 60 mg/kg/day.
IV: ADULTS, ELDERLY, CHILDREN: Same as oral dose but given q6h.

Manic Episodes

PO (DEPAKOTE): ADULTS, ELDERLY: Initially, 750–1,500 mg/day in divided doses. **Maximum:** 60 mg/kg/day.
PO (EXTENDED-RELEASE [DEPAKOTE ER]): Initially, 25 mg/kg/day once daily. **Maximum:** 60 mg/kg/day. **(DELAYED-RELEASE [STAVZOR]):** Initially, 750 mg/day in divided dose. Titrate to lowest therapeutic dose. **Maximum:** 60 mg/kg/day.

Prevention of Migraine Headaches

PO (EXTENDED-RELEASE [DEPAKOTE ER]): ADULTS, ELDERLY: Initially, 500 mg/day for 7 days. May increase up to 1,000 mg/day.
PO (DELAYED-RELEASE [DEPAKOTE]): ADULTS, ELDERLY: Initially, 250 mg twice a day. May increase up to 1,000 mg/day. **(STAVZOR):** 250 mg twice a day.

SIDE EFFECTS

Frequent: **Epilepsy:** Abdominal pain, irregular menses, diarrhea, transient alopecia, indigestion, nausea, vomiting, tremors, fluctuations in body weight. **Mania (22%–19%):** Nausea, drowsiness. Occasional: **Epilepsy:** Constipation, dizziness, drowsiness, headache, skin rash, unusual excitement, restlessness. **Mania (12%–6%):** Asthenia (loss of strength, energy), abdominal pain, dyspepsia (heartburn, indigestion, epigastric distress), rash. Rare: **Epilepsy:** Mood changes, diplopia, nystagmus, spots before eyes, unusual bleeding/bruising.

ADVERSE EFFECTS/ TOXIC REACTIONS

Hepatotoxicity may occur, particularly in first 6 mos of therapy. May be preceded by loss of seizure control, malaise, weakness, lethargy, anorexia, vomiting rather than abnormal serum hepatic function test results. Blood dyscrasias may occur.

NURSING CONSIDERATIONS

BASELINE ASSESSMENT

Anticonvulsant: Review history of seizure disorder (intensity, frequency, duration, level of consciousness). Initiate safety measures, quiet dark environment. CBC, platelet count should be performed before and 2 wks after therapy begins, then 2 wks following maintenance dose. **Antimanic:** Assess behavior, appearance, emotional status, response to environment, speech pattern, thought content. **Antimigraine:** Question pt regarding onset, location, duration of migraine, possible precipitating symptoms.

INTERVENTION/EVALUATION

Monitor serum hepatic function tests, bilirubin, ammonia, CBC, platelets. **Anticonvulsant:** Observe frequently for recurrence of seizure activity. Monitor serum hepatic function tests, CBC, platelet count. Assess skin for ecchymoses, petechiae. Monitor for clinical improvement (decrease in intensity/frequency of seizures). **Antimanic:** Question for suicidal

V

ideation. Assess for therapeutic response (interest in surroundings, increased ability to concentrate, relaxed facial expression). **Antimigraine:** Evaluate for relief of migraine headache and resulting photophobia, phonophobia, nausea, vomiting. **Therapeutic serum level:** 50–100 mcg/ml; **toxic serum level:** greater than 100 mcg/ml.

PATIENT/ FAMILY TEACHING

• Do not abruptly discontinue medication after long-term use (may precipitate seizures). • Strict maintenance of drug therapy is essential for seizure control. • Drowsiness usually disappears during continued therapy. • Avoid tasks that require alertness, motor skills until response to drug is established. • Avoid alcohol. • Carry identification card, bracelet that notes anticonvulsant therapy. • Inform physician if nausea, vomiting, lethargy, altered mental status, weakness, loss of appetite, abdominal pain, yellowing of skin, unusual bruising/bleeding occurs. • Report if seizure control worsens, suicidal ideation (depression, unusual changes in behavior, suicidal thoughts) occurs.

valsartan

val-**sar**-tan
(Diovan)

BLACK BOX ALERT May cause fetal injury, mortality if used during second or third trimester of pregnancy.

Do not confuse Diovan with Darvon or Zyban, or valsartan with losartan or Valstar.

FIXED-COMBINATION(S)

Diovan HCT: valsartan/hydrochlorothiazide (a diuretic): 80 mg/12.5 mg, 160 mg/12.5 mg, 160 mg/25 mg, 320 mg/12.5 mg, 320 mg/25 mg. **Exforge:** valsartan/amlodipine (a calcium channel blocker): 160 mg/5 mg, 160 mg/10 mg, 320 mg/5 mg, 320 mg/10 mg. **Exforge HCT:** valsartan/amlodipine (a calcium channel blocker)/hydrochlorothiazide (a diuretic): 160 mg/5 mg/12.5 mg, 160 mg/5 mg/25 mg, 160 mg/10 mg/12.5 mg, 160 mg/10 mg/25 mg, 320 mg/10 mg/25 mg. **Valturna:** valsartan/aliskiren (a direct renin inhibitor): 160 mg/150 mg, 320 mg/300 mg.

◆CLASSIFICATION

PHARMACOTHERAPEUTIC: Angiotensin II receptor antagonist. **CLINICAL:** Antihypertensive (see p. 10C).

ACTION

Potent vasodilator. Blocks vasoconstrictor, aldosterone-secreting effects of angiotensin II, inhibiting binding of angiotensin II to AT_1 receptors. **Therapeutic Effect:** Produces vasodilation, decreases peripheral resistance, decreases B/P.

PHARMACOKINETICS

Poorly absorbed after PO administration. Food decreases peak plasma concentration. Protein binding: 95%. Metabolized in liver. Recovered primarily in feces and, to lesser extent, in urine. Unknown if removed by hemodialysis. **Half-life:** 6 hrs.

USES

Treatment of hypertension alone or in combination with other antihypertensives. Treatment of heart failure. Reduce mortality in high-risk pts (left ventricular failure/dysfunction) following MI. **OFF-LABEL:** Diabetic nephropathy.

PRECAUTIONS

Contraindications: Bilateral renal artery stenosis, biliary cirrhosis/obstruction, hypoaldosteronism, severe hepatic impairment. **Cautions:** Concurrent use of potassium-sparing diuretics or potassium supplements, mild to moderate hepatic impairment, CHF, unilateral renal artery stenosis, coronary artery disease.

V

LIFESPAN CONSIDERATIONS

Pregnancy/Lactation: May cause fetal harm. Unknown if distributed in breast milk. **Pregnancy Category C (D if used in second or third trimester). Children:** Safety and efficacy not established. **Elderly:** No age-related precautions noted.

INTERACTIONS

DRUG: **ACE inhibitors, beta-blockers** may worsen CHF. **Potassium-sparing drugs, potassium supplements** may increase serum potassium. **Diuretics** produce additive hypotensive effects. HERBAL: None significant. FOOD: None significant. LAB VALUES: May increase AST, ALT, serum bilirubin, BUN, creatinine, potassium. May decrease Hgb, Hct, WBC.

AVAILABILITY (Rx)

Tablets: 40 mg, 80 mg, 160 mg, 320 mg.

ADMINISTRATION/HANDLING

PO

- Give without regard to meals.

INDICATIONS/ROUTES/DOSAGE

Hypertension

PO: ADULTS, ELDERLY: Initially, 80–160 mg/day in pts who are not volume depleted. **Maximum:** 320 mg/day. **CHILDREN 6–16 YRS:** Initially, 1.3 mg/kg once a day (**Maximum:** 40 mg). May increase up to 2.7 mg/kg once a day (**Maximum:** 160 mg/day).

CHF

PO: ADULTS, ELDERLY: Initially, 40 mg twice a day. May increase up to 160 mg twice a day. **Maximum:** 320 mg/day.

Post-MI

PO: ADULTS, ELDERLY: May initiate 12 hrs or longer following MI. Initially, 20 mg twice a day. May increase within 7 days to 40 mg twice a day. May further increase up to target dose of 160 mg twice a day.

SIDE EFFECTS

Rare (2%–1%): Insomnia, fatigue, heartburn, abdominal pain, dizziness, headache, diarrhea, nausea, vomiting, arthralgia, edema.

ADVERSE EFFECTS/ TOXIC REACTIONS

Overdosage may manifest as hypotension, tachycardia. Bradycardia occurs less often. Viral infection, upper respiratory tract infection (cough, pharyngitis, sinusitis, rhinitis) occur rarely.

NURSING CONSIDERATIONS

BASELINE ASSESSMENT

Obtain B/P, apical pulse immediately before each dose, in addition to regular monitoring (be alert to fluctuations). If excessive reduction in B/P occurs, place pt in supine position, feet slightly elevated. Question for possibility of pregnancy. Assess medication history (esp. diuretic). Question for history of hepatic/ renal impairment, renal artery stenosis, history of severe CHF. Obtain BUN, AST, ALT, serum creatinine, alkaline phosphatase, bilirubin, Hgb, Hct.

INTERVENTION/EVALUATION

Maintain hydration (offer fluids frequently). Assess for evidence of upper respiratory infection. Monitor serum electrolytes, renal/ hepatic function tests, urinalysis, B/P, pulse. Observe for symptoms of hypotension.

PATIENT/ FAMILY TEACHING

- Pts should take measures to avoid pregnancy
- Inform physician as soon as possible if pregnancy occurs.
- Report any sign of infection (sore throat, fever).
- Do not stop taking medication.
- Report swelling of extremities, chest pain, palpitations.

V

vancomycin

van-koe-**mye**-sin
(Vancocin)

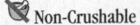

Do not confuse IV vancomycin with Invanz, or vancomycin with clindamycin, gentamicin, tobramycin, or Vibramycin.

CLASSIFICATION

CLINICAL: Tricyclic glycopeptide antibiotic.

ACTION

Binds to bacterial cell walls, altering cell membrane permeability, inhibiting RNA synthesis. **Therapeutic Effect:** Bactericidal.

PHARMACOKINETICS

PO: Poorly absorbed from GI tract. Primarily eliminated in feces. **Parenteral:** Widely distributed (except CSF). Protein binding: 10%–50%. Primarily excreted unchanged in urine. Not removed by hemodialysis. **Half-life:** 4–11 hrs (increased in renal impairment).

USES

Systemic: Treatment of infections caused by staphylococcal, streptococcal spp. bacteria. **PO:** Treatment of antibiotic colitis, pseudomembranous colitis, antibiotic-associated diarrhea, staphylococcal enterocolitis. **OFF-LABEL:** Treatment of brain abscess, perioperative infections, staphylococcal/streptococcal meningitis.

PRECAUTIONS

Contraindications: None known. **Cautions:** Renal dysfunction, preexisting hearing impairment, concurrent therapy with other ototoxic, nephrotoxic medications.

LIFESPAN CONSIDERATIONS

Pregnancy/Lactation: Drug crosses placenta. Unknown if distributed in breast milk. **Pregnancy Category C (injection), B (PO). Children:** Close monitoring of serum levels recommended in premature neonates, young infants. **Elderly:** Age-related renal impairment may increase risk of ototoxicity, nephrotoxicity; dosage adjustment recommended.

INTERACTIONS

DRUG: Aminoglycosides, amphotericin B, aspirin, bumetanide, carmustine, cisplatin, cyclosporine, ethacrynic acid, furosemide, streptozocin may increase risk of ototoxicity, nephrotoxicity of parenteral vancomycin. **Cholestyramine, colestipol** may decrease effects of oral vancomycin. **HERBAL:** None significant. **FOOD:** None known. **LAB VALUES:** May increase BUN. **Therapeutic peak serum level:** (Not routinely obtained) 20–40 mcg/ml; **therapeutic trough serum level:** 10–20 mcg/ml. **Toxic peak serum level:** greater than 40 mcg/ml; **toxic trough serum level:** greater than 20 mcg/ml.

AVAILABILITY (Rx)

Capsules (Vancocin): 125 mg, 250 mg. **Infusion (Premix [Vancocin HCl]):** 500 mg/100 ml, 1 g/200 ml. **Injection, Powder for Reconstitution (Vancocin HCl):** 500 mg, 1 g.

ADMINISTRATION/HANDLING

IV

◀ALERT▶ Give by intermittent IV infusion (piggyback) or continuous IV infusion. Do not give IV push (may result in exaggerated hypotension).

Reconstitution • For intermittent IV infusion (piggyback), reconstitute each 500-mg vial with 10 ml Sterile Water for Injection (20 ml for 1-g vial) to provide concentration of 50 mg/ml. • Further dilute with D_5W or 0.9% NaCl to final concentration not to exceed 5 mg/ml.

Rate of administration • Administer over 60 min or longer (30 min for each 500 mg recommended). • Monitor B/P closely during IV infusion.

Storage • Reconstituted vials are stable for 14 days at room temperature or if refrigerated. • Diluted solutions are stable for 14 days if refrigerated or 7 days at room temperature. • Discard if precipitate forms.

PO

• May give with food. • Powder for injection may be reconstituted and diluted for oral administration.

IV INCOMPATIBILITIES

Albumin, amphotericin B complex (Abelcet, AmBisome, Amphotec), aztreonam (Azactam), cefazolin (Ancef), cefepime (Maxipime), cefotaxime (Claforan), cefotetan (Cefotan), cefoxitin (Mefoxin), ceftazidime (Fortaz), ceftriaxone (Rocephin), cefuroxime (Zinacef), foscarnet (Foscavir), heparin, idarubicin (Idamycin), nafcillin (Nafcil), piperacillin and tazobactam (Zosyn), ticarcillin and clavulanate (Timentin).

IV COMPATIBILITIES

Amiodarone (Cordarone), calcium gluconate, diltiazem (Cardizem), hydromorphone (Dilaudid), insulin, lipids, lorazepam (Ativan), magnesium sulfate, midazolam (Versed), morphine, potassium chloride, propofol (Diprivan), total parenteral nutrition (TPN).

INDICATIONS/ROUTES/DOSAGE

Usual Parenteral Dosage

IV: ADULTS, ELDERLY: 10–20 mg/kg/dose q8–12h. Dosage requires adjustment in renal impairment. **CHILDREN OLDER THAN 1 MO:** 40 mg/kg/day in divided doses q6–8h. **NEONATES:** 15 mg/kg q24h up to 20 mg/kg/dose q8h.

Staphylococcal Enterocolitis, Antibiotic-Associated Pseudomembranous Colitis Caused by *Clostridium Difficile*

PO: ADULTS, ELDERLY: 125–250 mg 4 times a day for 7–10 days. **CHILDREN:** 40 mg/kg/day in 3–4 divided doses for 7–10 days. **NEONATES:** 10 mg/kg/day in divided doses.

Dosage in Renal Impairment

After loading dose, subsequent dosages and frequency are modified based on creatinine clearance, severity of infection, and serum concentration of drug.

SIDE EFFECTS

Frequent: PO: Bitter/unpleasant taste, nausea, vomiting, mouth irritation (with oral solution). **Rare: Parenteral:** Phlebitis, thrombophlebitis, pain at peripheral IV site, dizziness, vertigo, tinnitus, chills, fever, rash, necrosis with extravasation. **PO:** Rash.

ADVERSE EFFECTS/ TOXIC REACTIONS

Nephrotoxicity (change in amount/frequency of urination, nausea, vomiting, increased thirst, anorexia), ototoxicity (temporary or permanent hearing loss) may occur. "Red neck syndrome" (RNS) is common adverse reaction characterized by pruritus, urticaria, erythema, angioedema, tachycardia, hypotension, myalgia, maculopapular rash (usually appears on face, neck, upper torso). Cardiovascular toxicity (cardiac depression, arrest) occurs rarely. Onset of RNS usually occurs within 30 min of start of infusion, resolves within hrs following infusion. May result from too-rapid rate of infusion.

NURSING CONSIDERATIONS

BASELINE ASSESSMENT

Avoid other ototoxic, nephrotoxic medications if possible. Obtain culture, sensitivity test before giving first dose (therapy may begin before results are known).

INTERVENTION/EVALUATION

Monitor serum renal function tests, I&O. Assess skin for rash. Check hearing acuity, balance. Monitor B/P carefully during infusion. Evaluate IV site for phlebitis (heat, pain, red streaking over vein). **Therapeutic serum level: peak:** 20–40 mcg/ml; **trough:** 10–20 mcg/ml. **Toxic serum level: peak:** greater than 40 mcg/ml; **trough:** greater than 20 mcg/ml.

PATIENT/ FAMILY TEACHING

• Continue therapy for full length of treatment. • Doses should be evenly spaced. • Notify physician in event of tinnitus, rash, signs/symptoms of nephrotoxicity. • Lab tests are important part of total therapy.

vardenafil

var-**den**-ah-fill
(Levitra, Staxyn)
Do not confuse Levitra with Kaletra or Lexiva, or vardenafil with sildenafil or tadalafil.

◆CLASSIFICATION

PHARMACOTHERAPEUTIC: Phosphodiesterase inhibitor. **CLINICAL:** Erectile dysfunction adjunct.

ACTION

Inhibits phosphodiesterase type 5, the enzyme responsible for degrading cyclic guanosine monophosphate in corpus cavernosum of penis, resulting in smooth muscle relaxation, increased blood flow. **Therapeutic Effect:** Facilitates erection.

PHARMACOKINETICS

Rapidly absorbed after PO administration. Extensive tissue distribution. Protein binding: 95%. Metabolized in liver. Excreted primarily in feces, with lesser amount eliminated in urine. Drug has no effect on penile blood flow without sexual stimulation. **Half-life:** 4–5 hrs.

USES

Treatment of erectile dysfunction.

PRECAUTIONS

Contraindications: Concurrent use of alpha-adrenergic blockers, sodium nitroprusside, nitrates in any form. **Cautions:** Renal/hepatic impairment, anatomical deformation of penis, pts who may be predisposed to priapism (sickle cell anemia, multiple myeloma, leukemia).

⌛ LIFESPAN CONSIDERATIONS

Pregnancy/Lactation: Not indicated for use in women, newborns. **Pregnancy Category B. Children:** Not indicated for use in children. **Elderly:** No age-related precautions noted, but initial dose should be 5 mg.

INTERACTIONS

DRUG: Alpha-adrenergic blockers (e.g., alfuzosin, doxazosin, prazosin, tamsulosin, terazosin), nitrates may significantly lower B/P. **Erythromycin, indinavir, itraconazole, ketoconazole, ritonavir** may increase concentration. **HERBAL:** None significant. **FOOD: High-fat meals** delay maximum effectiveness. **Grapefruit juice** may increase concentration, risk of toxicity. **LAB VALUES:** May increase creatinine kinase, GGTP. May alter hepatic function tests.

AVAILABILITY (Rx)

Tablets (Levitra): 2.5 mg, 5 mg, 10 mg, 20 mg.

Tablets, Orally-Disintegrating (Staxyn): 10 mg.

ADMINISTRATION/HANDLING

PO

• May take approximately 1 hr before sexual activity. • May give without regard to food.

Orally-Disintegrating

• Take 1 hr before sexual activity. • Take without regard to meals. • Place on tongue, do not crush, split. • Do not take with liquid.

INDICATIONS/ROUTES/DOSAGE

Erectile Dysfunction

PO: ADULTS: 10 mg approximately 1 hr before sexual activity. Dose may be increased to 20 mg or decreased to 5 mg, based on pt tolerance. **Maximum dosing frequency:** Once daily. **ELDERLY OLDER THAN 65 YRS:** 5 mg. **Orally-disintegrating tablet:** 10 mg once daily at least 24 hrs apart.

Dosage in Moderate Hepatic Impairment

PO: For pts with Child-Pugh class B hepatic impairment, dosage is 5 mg 60 min before sexual activity.

Dosage with Concurrent Ritonavir

PO: ADULTS: 2.5 mg in 72-hr period.

Dosage with Concurrent Atanzavir, Clarithromycin, Ketoconazole, Itraconazole (at 400 mg/day), Indinavir, Saquinavir

PO: ADULTS: 2.5 mg in 24-hr period.

Dosage with Concurrent Ketoconazole, Itraconazole (at 200 mg/day), Erythromycin

PO: ADULTS: 5 mg in 24-hr period.

SIDE EFFECTS

Occasional: Headache, flushing, rhinitis, indigestion, sudden hearing loss. **Rare (less than 2%):** Dizziness, changes in color vision, blurred vision, postural hypotension.

ADVERSE EFFECTS/ TOXIC REACTIONS

Prolonged erections (lasting over 4 hrs), priapism (painful erections lasting over 6 hrs) occur rarely.

NURSING CONSIDERATIONS

BASELINE ASSESSMENT

Assess cardiovascular status, medication history (esp. alpha-adrenergic blockers, nitrates) before initiating treatment for erectile dysfunction.

INTERVENTION/EVALUATION

Monitor B/P.

PATIENT/FAMILY TEACHING

• Has no effect in absence of sexual stimulation. • Seek treatment immediately if erection persists for over 4 hrs. • Avoid grapefruit juice. • Report sudden decrease or loss of hearing or vision.

varenicline

vah-**ren**-neh-clean
(Champix ♣, Chantix)

BLACK BOX ALERT Risk of psychiatric symptoms and suicidal behavior. Agitation, hostility, depressed mood have been reported.

◆CLASSIFICATION

PHARMACOTHERAPEUTIC: Selective partial agonist nicotine acetylcholine receptors. **CLINICAL:** Smoking deterrent.

ACTION

Binds to acetylcholine receptors, producing agonist activity, preventing nicotine binding to specific receptors. Blocks ability of nicotine to stimulate central dopamine system, believed to be mechanism underlying reinforcement/reward experienced with smoking.

PHARMACOKINETICS

Completely absorbed following PO administration. Absorption unaffected by food, time of day dosing. Maximum plasma concentration: 3–4 hrs; steady-state condition: within 4 days. Protein binding: 20%. Minimal metabolism. Removed by hemodialysis. Primarily excreted unchanged in urine. **Half-life:** 24 hrs.

USES

Aid to smoking cessation treatment.

PRECAUTIONS

Contraindications: None known. **Cautions:** Renal impairment.

LIFESPAN CONSIDERATIONS

Pregnancy/Lactation: Unknown if distributed in breast milk. **Pregnancy Category C. Children:** Not recommended. **Elderly:** Age-related renal impairment may require dosage adjustment.

INTERACTIONS

DRUG: None significant. **HERBAL:** None significant. **FOOD:** None known. **LAB VALUES:** None significant.

AVAILABILITY

Tablets (Film-Coated): 0.5 mg, 1 mg.

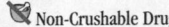

ADMINISTRATION/HANDLING

• Give with food and with full glass of water. • Do not crush, chew, break film-coated tablets.

INDICATIONS/ROUTES/DOSAGE

◀ALERT▶ Therapy should start 1 wk before stopping smoking.

Smoking Deterrent

PO: ADULTS, ELDERLY: Days 1–3: 0.5 mg once daily. Days 4–7: 0.5 mg twice daily. Day 8–end of treatment: 1 mg twice daily. Therapy should last for 12 wks. Those who have successfully stopped smoking at the end of 12 wks should continue with an additional 12 wks of treatment to increase likelihood of long-term abstinence.

Severe renal impairment (creatinine clearance less than 30 ml/min): 0.5 mg once daily. **Maximum:** 0.5 mg twice daily.

End-stage renal disease, undergoing hemodialysis: Maximum: 0.5 mg once daily.

SIDE EFFECTS

Frequent: Nausea (30%), insomnia (18%), headache (15%), abnormal dreams (13%). **Occasional (8%–5%):** Constipation, abdominal discomfort, fatigue, dry mouth, flatulence, altered taste, dyspepsia (heartburn, indigestion, epigastric pain), vomiting, anxiety, depression, irritability. **Rare (3%–1%):** Drowsiness, rash, increased appetite, lethargy, nightmares, gastroesophageal reflux disease, rhinorrhea, agitation, mood swings.

ADVERSE EFFECTS/ TOXIC REACTIONS

Hypertension, angina pectoris, arrhythmia, bradycardia, coronary artery disease, gingivitis, anemia, lymphadenopathy occur rarely. Abrupt withdrawal may cause irritability, sleep disturbances in 3% of pts. May cause bizarre behavior, suicidal ideation.

NURSING CONSIDERATIONS

BASELINE ASSESSMENT

Screen, evaluate those with coronary heart disease (history of MI, angina pectoris), serious cardiac arrhythmias.

INTERVENTION/EVALUATION

Discontinue use if increase in cardiovascular symptoms occurs. Monitor behavioral changes, psychiatric symptoms.

PATIENT/FAMILY TEACHING

• Initiate treatment 1 wk before quit smoking date. • Take with food and with full glass of water. • With twice-daily dosing, take 1 tablet in morning, 1 in evening. • Contact physician if nausea, insomnia persist. • Report change in behavior.

vasopressin

vay-soe-**press**-in
(Pitressin, Pressyn 🍁, Pressyn AR 🍁)
Do not confuse Pitressin with Pitocin.

◆CLASSIFICATION

PHARMACOTHERAPEUTIC: Posterior pituitary hormone. **CLINICAL:** Vasopressor, antidiuretic.

ACTION

Increases reabsorption of water by renal tubules. Directly stimulates smooth muscle in GI tract. **Therapeutic Effect:** Causes peristalsis, vasoconstriction.

PHARMACOKINETICS

Route	Onset	Peak	Duration
IV	N/A	N/A	0.5–1 hr
IM, subcutaneous	1–2 hrs	N/A	2–8 hrs

Distributed throughout extracellular fluid. Metabolized in liver, kidney. Primarily excreted in urine. **Half-life:** 10–20 min.

USES

Treatment of adult shock-refractory ventricular fibrillation (class IIb). Prevention/control of polydipsia, polyuria, dehydration in pts with neurogenic diabetes insipidus. Stimulates peristalsis in prevention/treatment of postop abdominal distention, intestinal paresis. Treatment of vasodilatory shock with hypotension unresponsive to fluids, catecholamines. **OFF-LABEL:** Adjunct in treatment of acute, massive hemorrhage, GI hemorrhage, esophageal varices.

PRECAUTIONS

Contraindications: None known. **Cautions:** Seizures, migraine, asthma, vascular disease, renal/cardiac disease, goiter (with cardiac complications), arteriosclerosis, nephritis.

LIFESPAN CONSIDERATIONS

Pregnancy/Lactation: Caution in giving to breast-feeding women. **Pregnancy Category C. Children/Elderly:** Caution due to risk of water intoxication/hyponatremia.

INTERACTIONS

DRUG: **Alcohol, demeclocycline, lithium, norepinephrine** may decrease antidiuretic effect. **Carbamazepine, chlorpropamide, clofibrate** may increase antidiuretic effect. **HERBAL:** None significant. **FOOD:** None known. **LAB VALUES:** None significant.

AVAILABILITY (Rx)

Injection Solution: 20 units/ml (0.5 ml, 1 ml).

ADMINISTRATION/HANDLING

IV

Reconstitution • Dilute with D_5W or 0.9% NaCl to concentration of 0.1–1 unit/ml (usual concentration: 100 units/500 ml D_5W).

Rate of administration • Give as IV infusion.

Storage • Store at room temperature.

IM, Subcutaneous

• Give with 1–2 glasses of water to reduce side effects.

IV INCOMPATIBILITIES

Amphotericin B complex (Abelcet, AmBisome, Amphotec), diazepam (Valium), etomidate (Amidate), furosemide (Lasix), thiopentothal.

IV COMPATIBILITIES

Dobutamine (Dobutrex), dopamine (Intropin), heparin, lorazepam (Ativan), midazolam (Versed), milrinone (Primacor), verapamil (Calan, Isoptin).

INDICATIONS/ROUTES/DOSAGE

Cardiac Arrest

IV: ADULTS, ELDERLY: 40 units as one-time bolus.

Diabetes Insipidus

ALERT May be administered intranasally by nasal spray or on cotton pledgets; dosage is individualized.

IV INFUSION: ADULTS, CHILDREN: 0.5 milliunits/kg/hr. May double dose q30min. **Maximum:** 10 milliunits/kg/hr.

IM, SUBCUTANEOUS: ADULTS, ELDERLY: 5–10 units 2–3 times a day. Range: 5–60 units/day. **CHILDREN:** 2.5–10 units, 2–4 times a day.

Abdominal Distention, Intestinal Paresis

IM: ADULTS, ELDERLY: Initially, 5 units. Subsequent doses, 10 units q3–4h.

GI Hemorrhage

IV INFUSION: ADULTS, ELDERLY: Initially, 0.2–0.4 unit/min progressively increased to 0.9 unit/min. **CHILDREN:** 0.002–0.005 unit/kg/min. Titrate as needed. **Maximum:** 0.01 unit/kg/min.

Vasodilatory Shock

IV INFUSION: ADULTS, ELDERLY: Initially, 0.01–0.04 units/min. Titrate to desired effect.

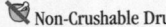

V

SIDE EFFECTS

Frequent: Pain at injection site (with vasopressin tannate). **Occasional:** Abdominal cramps, nausea, vomiting, diarrhea, dizziness, diaphoresis, pale skin, circumoral pallor, tremors, headache, eructation, flatulence. **Rare:** Chest pain, confusion, allergic reaction (rash, urticaria, pruritus, wheezing, difficulty breathing, facial/peripheral edema), sterile abscess (with vasopressin tannate).

ADVERSE EFFECTS/ TOXIC REACTIONS

Anaphylaxis, MI, water intoxication have occurred. Elderly, very young are at higher risk for water intoxication.

NURSING CONSIDERATIONS

BASELINE ASSESSMENT

Establish baselines for weight, B/P, pulse, serum electrolytes, Hgb, Hct, urine specific gravity.

INTERVENTION/EVALUATION

Monitor I&O closely, restrict intake as necessary to prevent water intoxication. Weigh daily if indicated. Check B/P, pulse twice daily. Monitor serum electrolytes, Hgb, Hct, urine specific gravity. Evaluate injection site for erythema, pain, abscess. Report side effects to physician for dose reduction. Be alert for early signs of water intoxication (drowsiness, listlessness, headache). Observe for evidence of GI bleeding. Withhold medication, report immediately any chest pain, allergic symptoms.

PATIENT/FAMILY TEACHING

• Promptly report headache, chest pain, shortness of breath, other symptoms. • Stress importance of I&O. • Avoid alcohol.

V

venlafaxine

ven-la-**fax**-een
(Effexor, Effexor XR, Novo-Venlafaxine ✤)

BLACK BOX ALERT Increased risk of suicidal thinking and behavior in children, adolescents, young adults 18–24 yrs with major depressive disorder, other psychiatric disorders.

◆CLASSIFICATION

PHARMACOTHERAPEUTIC: Phenethylamine derivative. **CLINICAL:** Antidepressant (see pp. 14C, 40C).

ACTION

Potentiates CNS neurotransmitter activity by inhibiting reuptake of serotonin, norepinephrine, and, to lesser degree, dopamine. **Therapeutic Effect:** Relieves depression.

PHARMACOKINETICS

Well absorbed from GI tract. Protein binding: 25%–30%. Metabolized in liver to active metabolite. Primarily excreted in urine. Not removed by hemodialysis. **Half-life:** 3–7 hrs; metabolite, 9–13 hrs (increased in hepatic/renal impairment).

USES

Treatment of depression exhibited as persistent, prominent dysphoria (occurring nearly every day for at least 2 wks) manifested by 4 of 8 symptoms: change in appetite, change in sleep pattern, increased fatigue, impaired concentration, feelings of guilt or worthlessness, loss of interest in usual activities, psychomotor agitation or retardation, suicidal tendencies. Psychotherapy augments therapeutic result. Treatment of generalized anxiety disorder (GAD), social anxiety disorder (SAD). Treatment of panic disorder, with or without agoraphobia. **OFF-LABEL:** Prevention of relapses of depression; treatment of ADHD, autism, chronic fatigue syndrome, obsessive-compulsive disorder.

PRECAUTIONS

Contraindications: Use of MAOIs within 14 days. **Cautions:** Seizure disorder, renal/hepatic impairment, suicidal pts, recent MI, mania, volume-depleted pts, narrow-angle glaucoma, CHF, hyperthyroidism, abnormal platelet function.

LIFESPAN CONSIDERATIONS

Pregnancy/Lactation: Unknown if distributed in breast milk. **Pregnancy Category C. Children:** Children, adolescents are at increased risk for suicidal ideation and behavior, worsening depression, esp. during first few mos of therapy. **Elderly:** No age-related precautions noted.

INTERACTIONS

DRUG: **MAOIs** may cause neuroleptic malignant syndrome, autonomic instability (including rapid fluctuations of vital signs), extreme agitation, hyperthermia, altered mental status, myoclonus, rigidity, coma. **Meperidine, selegiline, SSRIs, trazodone, tricyclic antidepressants** may increase risk of serotonin syndrome. May increase risk of bleeding with **warfarin.** HERBAL: **Gotu kola, kava kava, St. John's wort, valerian** may increase CNS depression. FOOD: None known. LAB VALUES: May increase cholesterol CPK, LDH, prolactin, GGT.

AVAILABILITY (Rx)

Tablets (Effexor): 25 mg, 37.5 mg, 50 mg, 75 mg, 100 mg.

Capsules (Extended-Release [Effexor XR]): 37.5 mg, 75 mg, 150 mg. Tablets (Extended-Release): 37.5 mg, 75 mg, 150 mg, 225 mg.

ADMINISTRATION/HANDLING

PO

• Give with food. • Scored tablet may be crushed. • Do not crush/chew extended-release capsules. • May open, sprinkle on applesauce. Give immediately without chewing and follow with full glass of water.

INDICATIONS/ROUTES/DOSAGE

Depression

PO: ADULTS, ELDERLY: Initially, 75 mg/day in 2–3 divided doses with food. May increase by 75 mg/day at intervals of 4 days or longer. **Maximum:** 375 mg/day in 3 divided doses.

PO (EXTENDED-RELEASE): ADULTS, ELDERLY: 37.5–75 mg/day as single dose with food. May increase by 75 mg/day at intervals of 4 days or longer. **Maximum:** 225 mg/day.

Generalized Anxiety Disorder (GAD), Social Anxiety Disorder (SAD)

PO (EXTENDED-RELEASE): ADULTS, ELDERLY: Initially, 37.5–75 mg/day. May increase by 75 mg/day at 4-day intervals up to 225 mg/day.

Panic Disorder

PO (EXTENDED-RELEASE): Initially, 37.5 mg/day. May increase to 75 mg after 7 days followed by increases of 75 mg/day at 7-day intervals up to 225 mg/day.

Dosage in Renal/Hepatic Impairment

Expect to decrease venlafaxine dosage by 50% in pts with moderate hepatic impairment, 25% in pts with mild to moderate renal impairment, 50% in pts on dialysis (withhold dose until completion of dialysis). When discontinuing therapy, taper dosage slowly over 2 wks.

SIDE EFFECTS

Frequent (greater than 20%): Nausea, drowsiness, headache, dry mouth. Occasional (20%–10%): Dizziness, insomnia, constipation, diaphoresis, nervousness, asthenia (loss of strength, energy), ejaculatory disturbance, anorexia. Rare (less than 10%): Anxiety, blurred vision, diarrhea, vomiting, tremor, abnormal dreams, impotence.

ADVERSE EFFECTS/ TOXIC REACTIONS

Sustained increase in diastolic B/P of 10–15 mm Hg occurs occasionally. Serotonin syndrome (agitation, confusion, hallucinations, hyper-reflexia), neuroleptic malignant syndrome (muscular rigidity, fever, cognitive changes), suicidal ideation have occurred.

NURSING CONSIDERATIONS

BASELINE ASSESSMENT

Obtain initial weight, B/P. Assess appearance, behavior, speech pattern, level of interest, mood.

INTERVENTION/EVALUATION

Monitor signs/symptoms of depression, B/P, weight. Assess sleep pattern for evidence of insomnia. Check during waking hours for drowsiness, dizziness, anxiety; provide assistance as necessary. Monitor for suicidal ideation (esp. at initiation of therapy or changes in dosage). Assess appearance, behavior, speech pattern, level of interest, mood for therapeutic response.

PATIENT/ FAMILY TEACHING

• Take with food to minimize GI distress. • Do not increase, decrease, suddenly stop medication. • Avoid tasks that require alertness, motor skills until response to drug is established. • Inform physician if breast-feeding, pregnant, or planning to become pregnant. • Avoid alcohol. • Report worsening depression, suicidal ideation, unusual changes in behavior.

verapamil

ver-**ap**-a-mill
(Apo-Verap, Calan, Calan SR, Chronovera, Covera-HS, Isoptin SR, Novo-Veramil SR, Verelan, Verelan PM)

Do not confuse Covera-HS with Provera, or Verelan with Voltaren.

FIXED-COMBINATION(S)

Tarka: verapamil/trandolapril (an ACE inhibitor): 240 mg/1 mg, 180 mg/2 mg, 240 mg/2 mg, 240 mg/4 mg.

◆CLASSIFICATION

PHARMACOTHERAPEUTIC: Calcium channel blocker. **CLINICAL:** Antihypertensive, antianginal, antiarrhythmic, hypertropic cardiomyopathy therapy adjunct (see pp. 18C, 78C).

ACTION

Inhibits calcium ion entry across cardiac, vascular smooth-muscle cell membranes, dilating coronary arteries, peripheral arteries, arterioles. **Therapeutic Effect:** Decreases heart rate, myocardial contractility, slows SA, AV conduction. Decreases total peripheral vascular resistance by vasodilation.

PHARMACOKINETICS

Route	Onset	Peak	Duration
PO	30 min	1–2 hrs	6–8 hrs
IV	1–2 min	1–5 min	10–20 min

Well absorbed from GI tract. Protein binding: 90% (60% in neonates). Undergoes first-pass metabolism in liver to active metabolite. Primarily excreted in urine. Not removed by hemodialysis. **Half-life: (single dose):** 2–8 hrs, **(multiple doses):** 4.5–12 hrs.

USES

Parenteral: Management of supraventricular tachyarrhythmias (SVT), temporary control of rapid ventricular rate in atrial flutter/fibrillation. **PO:** Management of spastic (Prinzmetal's variant) angina, unstable (crescendo, preinfarction) angina, chronic stable angina (effort-associated angina), hypertension, prophylaxis of recurrent paroxysmal supraventricular tachycardia (PSVT) (with digoxin), control of ventricular resting pulse rate in those with atrial flutter/fibrillation. **OFF-LABEL:** Treatment of bipolar disorder, hypertrophic cardiomyopathy, vascular headaches.

PRECAUTIONS

Contraindications: Atrial fibrillation/flutter in presence of accessory bypass tract (e.g., Wolff-Parkinson-White, Lown-Ganong-Levine syndromes), cardiogenic shock, second- or third-degree heart block, hypotension, sick sinus syndrome, sinus bradycardia, ventricular tachycardia. **Cautions:** CHF, renal/hepatic impairment, concomitant use of beta-blockers, digoxin.

LIFESPAN CONSIDERATIONS

Pregnancy/Lactation: Drug crosses placenta; is distributed in breast milk. Breast-feeding not recommended. **Pregnancy Category C. Children:** No age-related precautions noted. **Elderly:** Age-related renal impairment may require dosage adjustment.

INTERACTIONS

DRUG: Beta-adrenergic blockers may have additive effect. **Carbamazepine, cyclosporine, quinidine, theophylline** may increase concentration, risk of toxicity. May increase **digoxin** concentration. **Disopyramide** may increase negative inotropic effect. **Procainamide, quinidine** may increase risk of QT-interval prolongation. **Rifampin** may decrease concentration, effect. **HERBAL: St. John's wort** may decrease concentration, effect. **Ephedra, ginseng, yohimbe** may worsen hypertension. **Garlic** may increase antihypertensive effect. **FOOD: Grapefruit, grapefruit juice** may increase concentration. **LAB VALUES:** EKG may show increased PR interval. **Therapeutic serum level:** 0.08–0.3 mcg/ml. **Toxic serum level:** N/A.

AVAILABILITY (Rx)

Caplets (Sustained-Release [Calan SR]): 120 mg, 180 mg, 240 mg. **Injection Solution:** 2.5 mg/ml. **Tablets (Calan):** 40 mg, 80 mg, 120 mg.

Capsules (Extended-Release [Verelan PM]): 100 mg, 200 mg, 300 mg. **Capsules (Sustained-Release [Verelan]):** 120 mg, 180 mg, 240 mg, 360 mg. **Tablets (Extended-Release [Covera-HS]):** 180 mg, 240 mg. **Tablets (Sustained-Release [Isoptin SR]):** 120 mg, 180 mg, 240 mg.

ADMINISTRATION/HANDLING

IV

Reconstitution • May give undiluted.
Rate of administration • Administer IV push over 2 min for adults, children; give over 3 min for elderly. • Continuous EKG monitoring during IV injection is required for children, recommended for adults. • Monitor EKG for rapid ventricular rate, extreme bradycardia, heart block, asystole, prolongation of PR interval. Notify physician of any significant changes. • Monitor B/P q5–10min. • Pt should remain recumbent for at least 1 hr after IV administration.
Storage • Store vials at room temperature.

PO

• Do not give with grapefruit, grapefruit juice. • Non–sustained-release tablets may be given without regard to food. • Swallow extended-release, sustained-release preparations whole; do not chew, crush. • Sustained-release capsules may be opened and sprinkled on applesauce, then swallowed immediately (do not chew).

IV INCOMPATIBILITIES

Amphotericin B complex (Abelcet, AmBisome, Amphotec), nafcillin (Nafcil), propofol (Diprivan), sodium bicarbonate.

IV COMPATIBILITIES

Amiodarone (Cordarone), calcium chloride, calcium gluconate, dexamethasone (Decadron), digoxin (Lanoxin), dobutamine (Dobutrex), dopamine (Intropin), furosemide (Lasix), heparin, hydromorphone (Dilaudid), lidocaine, magnesium sulfate, metoclopramide (Reglan), milrinone (Primacor), morphine, multivitamins, nitroglycerin, norepinephrine (Levophed), potassium chloride, potassium phosphate, procainamide (Pronestyl), propranolol (Inderal).

INDICATIONS/ROUTES/DOSAGE

Supraventricular Tachyarrhythmias (SVT)
IV: ADULTS, ELDERLY: Initially, 2.5–5 mg over 2 min. May give 5–10 mg 30 min

after initial dose. **Maximum initial dose:** 20 mg. **CHILDREN 1–15 YRS:** 0.1–0.3 mg/kg over 2 min. **Maximum initial dose:** 5 mg. May repeat in 15 min. **Maximum second dose:** 10 mg. **CHILDREN YOUNGER THAN 1 YR:** 0.1–0.2 mg/kg over 2 min. May repeat 30 min after initial dose.

Angina, Unstable Angina, Chronic Stable Angina

PO: ADULTS: Initially, 80–120 mg 3 times a day. For elderly pts, those with hepatic dysfunction, 40 mg 3 times a day. Titrate to optimal dose. Maintenance: 240–480 mg/day in 3–4 divided doses.

Hypertension

PO (IMMEDIATE-RELEASE): ADULTS, ELDERLY: 80 mg 3 times a day. Range: 80–320 mg/day in 2 divided doses.
PO (SUSTAINED-RELEASE): ADULTS, ELDERLY: 120–240 mg/day. Range: 120–360 mg/day as single dose or in 2 divided doses.
PO (EXTENDED-RELEASE [COVERA-HS]): ADULTS, ELDERLY: 120–360 mg once a day at bedtime.
PO (EXTENDED-RELEASE [VERELAN PM]): ADULTS, ELDERLY: 200–400 mg once a day at bedtime.

Dosage for Renal Impairment

Creatinine clearance less than 10 ml/min: Give 50%–75% normal dose.

SIDE EFFECTS

Frequent (7%): Constipation. **Occasional (4%–2%):** Dizziness, light-headedness, headache, asthenia (loss of strength, energy), nausea, peripheral edema, hypotension. **Rare (less than 1%):** Bradycardia, dermatitis, rash.

ADVERSE EFFECTS/ TOXIC REACTIONS

Rapid ventricular rate in atrial flutter/fibrillation, marked hypotension, extreme bradycardia, CHF, asystole, second- or third-degree AV block occur rarely. **Antidote:** Glucagon (see Appendix M for dosage).

NURSING CONSIDERATIONS

BASELINE ASSESSMENT

Record onset, type (sharp, dull, squeezing), radiation, location, intensity, duration of anginal pain, precipitating factors (exertion, emotional stress). Check B/P for hypotension, pulse for bradycardia immediately before giving medication.

INTERVENTION/EVALUATION

Assess pulse for quality, irregular rate. Monitor B/P. Monitor EKG for cardiac changes, particularly prolongation of PR interval. Notify physician of any significant EKG interval changes. Assist with ambulation if dizziness occurs. Assess for peripheral edema behind medial malleolus (sacral area in bedridden pts). For those taking oral form, monitor daily pattern of bowel activity and stool consistency. **Therapeutic serum level:** 0.08–0.3 mcg/ml; **toxic serum level:** N/A.

PATIENT/FAMILY TEACHING

• Do not abruptly discontinue medication. • Compliance with therapy regimen is essential to control anginal pain. • To avoid hypotensive effect, rise slowly from lying to sitting position, wait momentarily before standing. • Avoid tasks that require alertness, motor skills until response to drug is established. • Limit caffeine. • Avoid or limit alcohol. • Inform physician if angina pain not reduced, irregular heartbeats, shortness of breath, swelling, dizziness, constipation, nausea, hypotension occur. • Avoid concomitant grapefruit, grapefruit juice.

vigabatrin

vye-**gab**-uh-trin
(Sabril)

BLACK BOX ALERT Progressive, permanent vision loss ranging in severity from mild to severe may occur in 30% or more of pts in all age groups. Onset of vision loss is unpredictable and may occur at any time during therapy. Risk increases with total dose and duration of use.

Do not confuse vigabatrin with Viagra, Vibativ, or Vigamox.

◆CLASSIFICATION

CLINICAL: Anticonvulsant.

ACTION

May increase accumulation of gamma-aminobutyric acid (GABA) by inhibiting GABA transaminase, the enzyme responsible for metabolism of GABA. **Therapeutic Effect:** Reduces seizure activity.

PHARMACOKINETICS

Well absorbed from GI tract (not affected by food). Does not bind to plasma proteins. Widely distributed. Primarily excreted unchanged in urine. **Half-life:** 5.7 hours in infants, 7.5 hours in adults.

USES

Treatment of infantile spasms (West syndrome) in children 1 mo to 2 yrs. Adjunct in treatment of refractory complex partial seizures (CPS) in adults not responding to multiple alternative treatments. **OFF-LABEL:** Treatment of substance dependence (cocaine, methamphetamine), spasticity, tardive dyskinesias.

PRECAUTIONS

Contraindications: None known. **Cautions:** Discontinue anticonvulsant therapy gradually (reduces loss of seizure control). Preexisting ophthalmologic conditions, history of depression, suicidal tendencies, impaired renal function.

LIFESPAN CONSIDERATIONS

Pregnancy/Lactation: Distributed in breast milk. **Pregnancy Category C. Children:** Progressive, permanent vision loss may occur in those 1 mo to 2 yrs with infantile spasms after therapy begins. **Elderly:** Progressive, permanent vision loss may occur in adult pts with refractory CPS after therapy begins. Age-related renal impairment may require dosage adjustment.

INTERACTIONS

DRUG: May decrease effect of **phenytoin, warfarin. Sevelamer** may decrease anticonvulsant effects. **HERBAL: Evening primrose** may decrease seizure threshold. **Gotu kola, kava kava, St. John's wort, valerian** may increase CNS depression. **FOOD:** None known. **LAB VALUES:** May decrease ALT, AST.

AVAILABILITY (Rx)

Powder for Oral Solution: 500-mg packet. **Tablets:** 500 mg.

ADMINISTRATION/HANDLING

PO

• Give without regard to meals. • If treatment is discontinued, gradually decrease dose at rate of 25–50 mg/kg every 3–4 days (reduces risk of loss of seizure control). • Dissolve entire contents of packet in 10 ml cold or room temperature water to provide final concentration of 50 mg/ml. • Prepare dose immediately before use.

INDICATIONS/ROUTES/DOSAGE

◀ALERT▶ Only available through a special restricted distribution program called SHARE (1-888-45-SHARE).

Infantile Spasms (West Syndrome)

PO: INFANTS, CHILDREN 1 MO TO 2 YRS: Initially, 50 mg/kg/day in 2 divided doses. May increase dose by 25–50 mg/kg/day every 3 days. **Maximum:** 150 mg/kg/day.

Adjunctive Therapy for Refractory Complex Partial Seizures

PO: ADULTS, ELDERLY: Initially, 500 mg twice a day. May increase dose by 500 mg/day each wk, based on response. **Maximum:** 1,500 mg twice daily.

Dosage in Renal Impairment

Dosage is modified based on creatinine clearance.

V

Creatinine Clearance	Dosage
10–30 ml/min	Decrease dose by 75%
31–50 ml/min	Decrease dose by 50%
51–80 ml/min	Decrease dose by 25%

SIDE EFFECTS

Frequent (18%–10%): Headache, drowsiness, fatigue, dizziness, seizures, nasopharyngitis, weight gain, upper respiratory infection, otitis media. **Occasional (9%–6%):** Visual field defect, depression, tremor, nystagmus, nausea, diarrhea, memory impairment, insomnia, irritability, abnormal gait, blurred vision, diplopia, vomiting, pyrexia, rash. **Rare (less than 2%):** Emotional lability, speech disorder, abdominal pain, constipation, dyspepsia, asthenia, edema.

ADVERSE EFFECTS/ TOXIC REACTIONS

Progressive, permanent vision loss has occurred in up to 30% of pts. Abrupt withdrawal of medication may increase seizure frequency (status epilepticus). MRI abnormalities, neurotoxicity (seizure, hypomyelination, vacuolization) have been observed in animal studies. Antiepileptic drugs increase risk of suicidal thoughts, behavior. Clinically significant cases of anemia, peripheral neuropathy have been reported. Overdose may result in altered mental status, drowsiness, psychosis, hypotension, apnea, coma. Treatment is aimed at supportive measures.

NURSING CONSIDERATIONS

BASELINE ASSESSMENT

Review history of seizure disorder (type, onset, intensity, frequency, duration, level of consciousness), previous alternative treatment therapies. Arrange for baseline ophthalmologic exam. Obtain baseline CBC.

INTERVENTION/EVALUATION

Provide safety measures as needed. Assess for seizure activity. Obtain ophthalmologic exams every 3 mos during therapy and 3–6 mos after drug is discontinued. Monitor routine CBC.

PATIENT/FAMILY TEACHING

• Advise pt/family of risk of progressive, permanent vision loss at any time during or after taking drug. • Stress importance of routine eye examinations. Notify physician of any change in vision • Avoid tasks that require alertness, motor skills until response to drug is established. • Do not abruptly discontinue medication (may increase seizure frequency). • Advise doctor if pregnant or planning to become pregnant during therapy. • Carry medical alert identification to note seizure disorder, antiepileptic therapy. • Report worsening depression, suicidal ideation or unusual behavior change.

*vinBLAStine

HIGH ALERT

vin-**blass**-teen
(Velban)

BLACK BOX ALERT Must be administered by personnel trained in administration/handling of chemotherapeutic agents. Fatal if given intrathecally (ascending paralysis, death). Vesicant; avoid extravasation.

Do not confuse vinblastine with vincristine or vinorelbine.

◆CLASSIFICATION

PHARMACOTHERAPEUTIC: Vinca alkaloid. **CLINICAL:** Antineoplastic (see p. 89C).

ACTION

Binds to microtubular protein of mitotic spindle, causing metaphase arrest. **Therapeutic Effect:** Inhibits cell division.

PHARMACOKINETICS

Does not cross blood-brain barrier. Protein binding: 99%. Metabolized in liver to active metabolite. Primarily eliminated in feces by biliary system. **Half-life:** 24.8 hrs.

USES

Treatment of disseminated Hodgkin's disease, non-Hodgkin's lymphoma, advanced stage of mycosis fungoides, advanced testicular carcinoma, Kaposi's sarcoma, Letterer-Siwe disease, breast carcinoma, choriocarcinoma. OFF-LABEL: Treatment of bladder, head/neck, kidney, lung carcinoma; chronic myelocytic leukemia; germ cell ovarian tumors; neuroblastoma, non–small-cell lung cancer, prostate, renal cancer, soft tissue sarcoma.

PRECAUTIONS

Contraindications: Bacterial infection, severe leukopenia, significant granulocytopenia (unless a result of disease being treated). Cautions: Hepatic impairment, neurotoxicity, recent exposure to radiation therapy, chemotherapy.

LIFESPAN CONSIDERATIONS

Pregnancy/Lactation: If possible, avoid use during pregnancy, esp. during first trimester. Breast-feeding not recommended. **Pregnancy Category D. Children/Elderly:** No age-related precautions noted.

INTERACTIONS

DRUG: May decrease effects of **antigout medications. Bone marrow depressants** may increase myelosuppression. **Live virus vaccines** may potentiate virus replication, increase vaccine side effects, decrease pt's antibody response to vaccine. HERBAL: **St. John's wort** may decrease concentration. Avoid **black cohosh, dong quai** in estrogen-dependent tumors. FOOD: None known. LAB VALUES: May increase serum uric acid.

AVAILABILITY (Rx)

Injection, Powder for Reconstitution: 10 mg. Injection Solution: 1 mg/ml.

ADMINISTRATION/HANDLING

◀ALERT▶ May be carcinogenic, mutagenic, teratogenic. Handle with extreme care during preparation and administration. Give by IV injection. Leakage from IV site into surrounding tissue may produce extreme irritation. Avoid eye contact with solution (severe eye irritation, possible corneal ulceration may result). If eye contact occurs, immediately irrigate eye with water.

IV

Reconstitution • Reconstitute 10-mg vial with 10 ml 0.9% NaCl preserved with phenol or benzyl alcohol to provide concentration of 1 mg/ml.

Rate of administration • Inject into tubing of running IV infusion or directly into vein over 1 min. • Do not inject into extremity with impaired, potentially impaired circulation caused by compression or invading neoplasm, phlebitis, varicosity. • Rinse syringe, needle with venous blood before withdrawing needle (minimizes possibility of extravasation). • Extravasation may result in cellulitis, phlebitis. Large amount of extravasation may result in tissue sloughing. If extravasation occurs, give local injection of hyaluronidase, apply warm compresses.

Storage • Refrigerate unopened vials. • Solution appears clear, colorless. • Following reconstitution, solution is stable for 30 days if refrigerated. • Discard if solution is discolored or precipitate forms.

IV INCOMPATIBILITIES

Cefepime (Maxipime), furosemide (Lasix).

IV COMPATIBILITIES

Allopurinol (Aloprim), cisplatin (Platinol AQ), cyclophosphamide (Cytoxan), doxorubicin (Adriamycin), etoposide (VePesid), 5-fluorouracil, gemcitabine (Gemzar), granisetron (Kytril), heparin, leucovorin, methotrexate, ondansetron (Zofran), paclitaxel (Taxol), vinorelbine (Navelbine).

INDICATIONS/ROUTES/DOSAGE

◀ALERT▶ Dosage individualized based on clinical response, tolerance to adverse effects. When used in combination therapy, consult specific protocols for optimum dosage, sequence of drug administration.

V

Usual Dosage

IV: ADULTS, ELDERLY: 5.5–7.4 mg/m^2 q7days. **Maximum:** 18.5 mg/m^2. **CHILDREN:** 2.5–6 mg/m^2 q7–14 days. **Maximum:** 12.5 mg/m^2/wk.

Dosage in Hepatic Impairment

Direct serum bilirubin concentration greater than 3 mg/dl: Reduce dose by 50%.

SIDE EFFECTS

Frequent: Nausea, vomiting, alopecia. **Occasional:** Constipation, diarrhea, rectal bleeding, headache, paresthesia (occur 4–6 hrs after administration, persist for 2–10 hrs), malaise, asthenia (loss of strength, energy), dizziness, pain at tumor site, jaw/face pain, depression, dry mouth. **Rare:** Dermatitis, stomatitis, phototoxicity, hyperuricemia.

ADVERSE EFFECTS/ TOXIC REACTIONS

Hematologic toxicity manifested most commonly as leukopenia, less frequently as anemia. WBC reaches its nadir 4–10 days after initial therapy, recovers within 7–14 days (high dosage may require 21-day recovery period). Thrombocytopenia is usually mild and transient, with recovery occurring in few days. Hepatic insufficiency may increase risk of toxicity. Acute shortness of breath, bronchospasm may occur, particularly when administered concurrently with mitomycin.

NURSING CONSIDERATIONS

BASELINE ASSESSMENT

Nausea, vomiting easily controlled by antiemetics. Discontinue therapy if WBC, thrombocyte counts fall abruptly (unless drug is clearly destroying tumor cells in bone marrow). Obtain CBC weekly or before each dosing.

INTERVENTION/EVALUATION

If WBC falls below 2,000/mm^3, assess diligently for signs of infection. Assess for stomatitis; maintain fastidious oral hygiene. Monitor for hematologic toxicity: infection (fever, sore throat, signs of local infection), unusual bruising/bleeding from any site, symptoms of anemia (excessive fatigue, weakness). Monitor daily pattern of bowel activity, stool consistency. Avoid constipation.

PATIENT/FAMILY TEACHING

• Immediately report any pain/burning at injection site during administration. • Pain at tumor site may occur during or shortly after injection. • Do not have immunizations without physician approval (drug lowers resistance). • Avoid crowds, those with infection. • Promptly report fever, sore throat, signs of local infection, unusual bruising/bleeding from any site. • Alopecia is reversible, but new hair growth may have different color, texture. • Contact physician if nausea/vomiting continues. • Avoid constipation by increasing fluids, bulk in diet, exercise as tolerated.

*vinCRIStine

HIGH ALERT

vin-**cris**-teen
(Vincasar PFS)

BLACK BOX ALERT Must be administered by personnel trained in administration/handling of chemotherapeutic agents. Fatal if given intrathecally (ascending paralysis, death). Vesicant; avoid extravasation.

Do not confuse vincristine with vinblastine.

◆CLASSIFICATION

PHARMACOTHERAPEUTIC: Vinca alkaloid. **CLINICAL:** Antineoplastic (see p. 89C).

ACTION

Binds to microtubular protein of mitotic spindle, causing metaphase arrest. **Therapeutic Effect:** Inhibits cell division.

V

PHARMACOKINETICS

Does not cross blood-brain barrier. Protein binding: 75%. Metabolized in liver. Primarily eliminated in feces by biliary system. **Half-life:** 24 hrs.

USES

Treatment of acute leukemia, disseminated Hodgkin's disease, advanced non-Hodgkin's lymphomas, neuroblastoma, rhabdomyosarcoma, Wilms tumor. **OFF-LABEL:** Treatment of breast, cervical, colorectal, lung, ovarian carcinomas; chronic lymphocytic and chronic myelocytic leukemias; germ cell ovarian tumors; idiopathic thrombocytopenic purpura; malignant melanoma; multiple myeloma; mycosis fungoides.

PRECAUTIONS

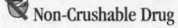

Contraindications: Demyelinating form of Charcot-Marie-Tooth syndrome, pts receiving radiation therapy through ports including liver. **Caution:** Hepatic impairment, neurotoxicity, preexisting neuromuscular disease.

LIFESPAN CONSIDERATIONS

Pregnancy/Lactation: If possible, avoid use during pregnancy, esp. first trimester. May cause fetal harm. Breast-feeding not recommended. **Pregnancy Category D. Children:** No age-related precautions noted. **Elderly:** More susceptible to neurotoxic effects.

INTERACTIONS

DRUG: Asparaginase, neurotoxic medications may increase risk of neurotoxicity. May decrease effects of **antigout medications. Doxorubicin** may increase risk of myelosuppression. **Live virus vaccines** may potentiate virus replication, increase vaccine side effects, decrease pt's antibody response to vaccine. **HERBAL: St. John's wort** may decrease concentration. **FOOD:** None known. **LAB VALUES:** May increase serum uric acid.

AVAILABILITY (Rx)

Injection Solution: 1 mg/ml.

ADMINISTRATION/HANDLING

IV

◀ALERT▶ May be carcinogenic, mutagenic, teratogenic. Handle with extreme care during preparation and administration. Give by IV injection. Use extreme caution in calculating, administering vincristine. Overdose may result in serious or fatal outcome.

Reconstitution • May give undiluted.

Rate of administration • Inject dose into tubing of running IV infusion or directly into vein over 1 min. • Do not inject into extremity with impaired, potentially impaired circulation caused by compression or invading neoplasm, phlebitis, varicosity. • Extravasation produces stinging, burning, edema at injection site. Terminate injection immediately, locally inject hyaluronidase, apply heat (disperses drug, minimizes discomfort, cellulitis).

Storage • Refrigerate unopened vials. • Solution appears clear, colorless. • Discard if solution is discolored or precipitate forms.

IV INCOMPATIBILITIES

Cefepime (Maxipime), furosemide (Lasix), idarubicin (Idamycin).

IV COMPATIBILITIES

Allopurinol (Aloprim), cisplatin (Platinol AQ), cyclophosphamide (Cytoxan), cytarabine (Ara-C, Cytosar), doxorubicin (Adriamycin), etoposide (VePesid), 5-fluorouracil, gemcitabine (Gemzar), granisetron (Kytril), leucovorin, methotrexate, ondansetron (Zofran), paclitaxel (Taxol), vinorelbine (Navelbine).

INDICATIONS/ROUTES/DOSAGE

Usual Dosage

IV: ADULTS, ELDERLY: 0.4–1.4 mg/m^2 once a wk. **CHILDREN:** 1–2 mg/m^2 once a wk. **CHILDREN WEIGHING LESS THAN 10 KG OR WITH BODY SURFACE AREA LESS THAN 1 M^2:** 0.05 mg/kg. **Maximum:** 2 mg.

V

Hepatic Impairment

Bilirubin/AST	Dosage
Bilirubin 1.5–3 mg/dl or AST 60–180 units	50% of normal
Bilirubin greater than 3 to 5 mg/dl	25% of normal
Bilirubin greater than 5 mg/dl or AST greater than 180 units	Omit dose

SIDE EFFECTS

Expected: Peripheral neuropathy (occurs in nearly every pt; first clinical sign is depression of Achilles tendon reflex). **Frequent:** Peripheral paresthesia, alopecia, constipation/obstipation (upper colon impaction with empty rectum), abdominal cramps, headache, jaw pain, hoarseness, diplopia, ptosis/drooping of eyelid, urinary tract disturbances. **Occasional:** Nausea, vomiting, diarrhea, abdominal distention, stomatitis, fever. **Rare:** Mild leukopenia, mild anemia, thrombocytopenia.

ADVERSE EFFECTS/ TOXIC REACTIONS

Acute shortness of breath, bronchospasm may occur, esp. when administered concurrently with mitomycin. Prolonged or high-dose therapy may produce foot/wrist drop, difficulty walking, slapping gait, ataxia, muscle wasting. Acute uric acid nephropathy may occur.

NURSING CONSIDERATIONS

BASELINE ASSESSMENT

Obtain baseline lab tests: CBC, WBC, Hgb, Hct, hepatic function studies. Offer pt/family emotional support.

V

INTERVENTION/EVALUATION

Monitor serum uric acid levels, renal/hepatic function studies, hematologic status. Assess Achilles tendon reflex. Monitor daily pattern of bowel activity, stool consistency. Monitor for ptosis, diplopia, blurred vision. Question pt regarding urinary changes.

PATIENT/FAMILY TEACHING

• Immediately report any pain/burning at injection site during administration. • Alopecia is reversible, but new hair growth may have different color/texture. • Contact physician if nausea/vomiting continues. • Report signs of peripheral neuropathy (burning/numbness of bottom of feet, palms of hands). • Report fever, sore throat, unusual bleeding/bruising, shortness of breath.

vinorelbine

HIGH ALERT

vin-oh-**rell**-bean
(Navelbine)

BLACK BOX ALERT Must be administered by personnel trained in administration/handling of chemotherapeutic agents. Fatal if given intrathecally (ascending paralysis, death). Extravasation produces thrombophlebitis, local tissue necrosis. May produce severe granulocytopenia.

Do not confuse vinorelbine with vinblastine.

◆CLASSIFICATION

CLINICAL: Antineoplastic (see p. 89C).

ACTION

Interferes with mitotic microtubule assembly. **Therapeutic Effect:** Prevents cellular division.

PHARMACOKINETICS

Widely distributed after IV administration. Protein binding: 80%–90%. Metabolized in liver. Primarily eliminated in feces by biliary system. **Half-life:** 28–43 hrs.

USES

Single agent or in combination with cisplatin for treatment of unresectable, advanced, non–small-cell lung cancer (NSCLC). **OFF-LABEL:** Treatment of breast cancer, cervical carcinoma, cisplatin-resistant ovarian carcinoma, Hodgkin's disease, non-Hodgkin's lymphoma.

PRECAUTIONS

Contraindications: Granulocyte count before treatment of less than 1,000 cells/mm^3. **Extreme Caution:** Immunocompromised pts. **Cautions:** Existing or recent chickenpox, herpes zoster, infection, leukopenia, pulmonary impairment, severe hepatic injury/impairment.

LIFESPAN CONSIDERATIONS

Pregnancy/Lactation: If possible, avoid use during pregnancy, esp. during first trimester. May cause fetal harm. Unknown if distributed in breast milk. Breast-feeding not recommended. **Pregnancy Category D. Children:** Safety and efficacy not established. **Elderly:** No age-related precautions noted.

INTERACTIONS

DRUG: **Bone marrow depressants** may increase risk of myelosuppression. **Cisplatin** significantly increases risk of granulocytopenia. **Live virus vaccines** may potentiate virus replication, increase vaccine side effects, decrease pt's antibody response to vaccine. **Mitomycin** may produce an acute pulmonary reaction. **Paclitaxel** may increase neuropathy. **HERBAL:** **St. John's wort** may decrease concentration. **FOOD:** None known. **LAB VALUES:** May increase serum bilirubin, AST, ALT, alkaline phosphatase.

AVAILABILITY (Rx)

Injection Solution: 10 mg/ml (1-ml, 5-ml vials).

ADMINISTRATION/HANDLING

IV

◀ALERT▶ IV needle, catheter must be correctly positioned before administration. Leakage into surrounding tissue produces extreme irritation, local tissue necrosis, thrombophlebitis. Handle drug with extreme care during administration; wear protective clothing per protocol. If solution comes in contact with skin/mucosa, immediately wash thoroughly with soap, water.

Reconstitution • Must be diluted and administered via syringe or IV bag.
SYRINGE DILUTION • Dilute calculated vinorelbine dose with D_5W or 0.9% NaCl to concentration of 1.5–3 mg/ml.
IV BAG DILUTION • Dilute calculated vinorelbine dose with D_5W, 0.45% or 0.9% NaCl, 5% dextrose and 0.45% NaCl, Ringer's or lactated Ringer's to concentration of 0.5–2 mg/ml.

Rate of administration • Administer diluted vinorelbine over 6–10 min into side port of free-flowing IV closest to IV bag followed by flushing with 75–125 ml of one of the solutions. • If extravasation occurs, stop injection immediately; give remaining portion of dose into another vein.

Storage • Refrigerate unopened vials. • Protect from light. • Unopened vials are stable at room temperature for 72 hrs. • Do not administer if particulate has formed. • Diluted vinorelbine may be used for up to 24 hrs under normal room light when stored in polypropylene syringes or polyvinyl chloride bags at room temperature.

IV INCOMPATIBILITIES

Acyclovir (Zovirax), allopurinol (Aloprim), amphotericin B (Fungizone), amphotericin B complex (Abelcet, AmBisome, Amphotec), ampicillin (Omnipen), cefazolin (Ancef), cefoperazone (Cefobid), cefotetan (Cefotan), ceftriaxone (Rocephin), cefuroxime (Zinacef), 5-fluorouracil (5-FU), furosemide (Lasix), ganciclovir (Cytovene), methylprednisolone (Solu-Medrol), sodium bicarbonate.

IV COMPATIBILITIES

Calcium gluconate, carboplatin (Paraplatin), cisplatin (Platinol AQ), cyclophosphamide (Cytoxan), cytarabine (ARA-C, Cytosar), dacarbazine (DTIC), daunorubicin (Cerubidine), dexamethasone (Decadron), diphenhydramine (Benadryl), doxorubicin (Adriamycin), etoposide (VePesid), gemcitabine (Gemzar), granisetron (Kytril), hydromorphone (Dilaudid), idarubicin (Idamycin),

V

methotrexate, morphine, ondansetron (Zofran), teniposide (Vumon), vinblastine (Velban), vincristine (Oncovin).

INDICATIONS/ROUTES/DOSAGE

◀ALERT▶ Dosage adjustments should be based on granulocyte count obtained on the day of treatment, as follows:

Granulocyte Count (cells/mm^3) on day of treatment	Dosage
1,500 or higher	100% of starting dose
1,000–1,499	50% of starting dose
Less than 1,000	Do not administer

Non–Small-Cell Lung Cancer

IV INJECTION: ADULTS, ELDERLY: 30 mg/m^2 administered weekly over 6–10 min.

Combination Therapy with Cisplatin

IV INJECTION: ADULTS, ELDERLY: 25–30 mg/m^2 every wk.

Dosage in Hepatic Impairment

Bilirubin	Dosage
2 mg/dl or less	100% of dose
2.1–3 mg/dl	50% of dose
Greater than 3 mg/dl	25% of dose

SIDE EFFECTS

Frequent: Asthenia (loss of strength, energy) (35%), nausea (34%), constipation (29%), erythema, pain, vein discoloration at injection site (28%), fatigue (27%), peripheral neuropathy manifested as paresthesia, hyperesthesia (25%), diarrhea (17%), alopecia (12%). **Occasional:** Phlebitis (10%), dyspnea (7%), loss of deep tendon reflexes (5%). **Rare:** Chest pain, jaw pain, myalgia, arthralgia, rash.

ADVERSE EFFECTS/ TOXIC REACTIONS

Bone marrow depression is manifested mainly as granulocytopenia (may be severe). Other hematologic toxicities (neutropenia, thrombocytopenia, leukopenia, anemia) increase risk of infection, bleeding. Acute shortness of breath, severe bronchospasm occur infrequently, particularly in pts with preexisting pulmonary dysfunction.

NURSING CONSIDERATIONS

BASELINE ASSESSMENT

Review medication history. Assess hematology (CBC, platelet count, Hgb, differential) values before giving each dose. Granulocyte count should be at least 1,000 cells/mm^3 before vinorelbine administration. Granulocyte nadirs occur 7–10 days following dosing. Do not give hematologic growth factors within 24 hrs before administration of chemotherapy or earlier than 24 hrs following cytotoxic chemotherapy. Advise women of childbearing potential to avoid pregnancy during drug therapy.

INTERVENTION/EVALUATION

Diligently monitor injection site for swelling, redness, pain. Frequently monitor for myelosuppression during and following therapy (infection [fever, sore throat, signs of local infection], unusual bleeding/bruising, anemia [excessive fatigue, weakness]). Monitor pts developing severe granulocytopenia for evidence of infection, fever. Crackers, dry toast, sips of cola may help relieve nausea. Monitor daily pattern of bowel activity, stool consistency. Question for tingling, burning, numbness of hands/feet (peripheral neuropathy). Pt complaint of "walking on glass" is sign of hyperesthesia.

PATIENT/FAMILY TEACHING

• Notify physician immediately if redness, swelling, pain occur at injection site. • Avoid crowds, those with infection. • Do not have immunizations without physician's approval. • Promptly report fever, signs of infection, unusual bruising/bleeding from any site, difficulty breathing. • Avoid pregnancy. • Alopecia is reversible, but new hair growth may have different color, texture.

vitamin A

vight-ah-myn A
(Aquasol A, Palmitate A)
Do not confuse Aquasol A with Anusol.

◆CLASSIFICATION

PHARMACOTHERAPEUTIC: Fat-soluble vitamin. **CLINICAL:** Nutritional supplement (see p. 161C).

ACTION

May act as cofactor in biochemical reactions. **Therapeutic Effect:** Essential for normal function of retina, visual adaptation to darkness, bone growth, testicular and ovarian function, embryonic development; preserves integrity of epithelial cells.

PHARMACOKINETICS

Rapidly absorbed from GI tract if bile salts, pancreatic lipase, protein, dietary fat are present. Transported in blood to liver, where it is metabolized; stored in parenchymal hepatic cells, then transported in plasma as retinol, as needed. Excreted primarily in bile and, to lesser extent, in urine.

USES

Treatment of vitamin A deficiency (biliary tract, pancreatic disease, sprue, colitis, hepatic cirrhosis, celiac disease, regional enteritis, extreme dietary inadequacy, partial gastrectomy, cystic fibrosis).

PRECAUTIONS

Contraindications: Hypervitaminosis A, oral use in malabsorption syndrome. **Cautions:** Renal impairment.

LIFESPAN CONSIDERATIONS

Pregnancy/Lactation: Crosses placenta. Distributed in breast milk. **Pregnancy Category A (X if used in doses above recommended daily allowance).** **Children/Elderly:** Caution with higher dosages.

INTERACTIONS

DRUG: **Cholestyramine, colestipol, mineral oil** may decrease absorption. **Isotretinoin** may increase risk of toxicity. **HERBAL:** None significant. **FOOD:** None known. **LAB VALUES:** None significant.

AVAILABILITY (Rx)

Injection Solution (Aquasol A): 50,000 units/ml. **Tablets (Palmitate A):** 5,000 units, 15,000 units.

Capsules: 10,000 units, 25,000 units.

ADMINISTRATION/HANDLING

◀ALERT▶ IM administration used only in acutely ill or pts unresponsive to oral route (GI malabsorption syndrome).

IM

• For IM injection in adults, if dosage is 1 ml (50,000 international units), may give in deltoid muscle; if dosage is over 1 ml, give in large muscle mass. Anterolateral thigh is site of choice for infants, children younger than 7 mos.

PO

• Do not crush, break capsules. • Give without regard to food.

INDICATIONS/ROUTES/DOSAGE

Severe Vitamin A Deficiency (with Xerophthalmia)

PO: ADULTS, ELDERLY, CHILDREN 8 YRS AND OLDER: 500,000 units/day for 3 days, then 50,000 units/day for 14 days, then 10,000–20,000 units/day for 2 mos. **CHILDREN 1–7 YRS:** 5,000–10,000 units/kg/day for 5 days or until recovery occurs.
IM: ADULTS, ELDERLY, CHILDREN 8 YRS AND OLDER: 100,000 units/day for 3 days, then 50,000 units/day for 14 days. **CHILDREN 1–7 YRS:** 17,500–35,000 units/day for 10 days. **INFANTS YOUNGER THAN 1 YR:** 7,500–15,000 units/day.

Vitamin A Deficiency (without Corneal Changes)

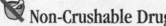

PO: ADULTS, ELDERLY, CHILDREN 8 YRS AND OLDER: 100,000 units/day for 3 days, then

50,000 units/day for 14 days. **CHILDREN 1–7 YRS:** 200,000 units every 4–6 mos. **INFANTS YOUNGER THAN 1 YR:** 100,000 units every 4–6 mos.

Malabsorption Syndrome

PO: ADULTS, ELDERLY, CHILDREN 8 YRS AND OLDER: 10,000–50,000 units/day.

Dietary Supplement

PO: ADULTS, ELDERLY: 4,000–5,000 units/day. **CHILDREN 7–10 YRS:** 3,300–3,500 units/day. **CHILDREN 4–6 YRS:** 2,500 units/day. **CHILDREN 6 MOS–3 YRS:** 1,500–2,000 units/day. **NEONATES YOUNGER THAN 5 MOS:** 1,500 units/day.

SIDE EFFECTS

None known.

ADVERSE EFFECTS/ TOXIC REACTIONS

Chronic overdose produces malaise, nausea, vomiting, drying/cracking of skin/lips, inflammation of tongue/gums, irritability, alopecia, night sweats. Bulging fontanelles have occurred in infants.

NURSING CONSIDERATIONS

INTERVENTION/EVALUATION

Closely supervise for overdosage symptoms during prolonged daily administration over 25,000 international units. Monitor for therapeutic serum vitamin A levels (80–300 international units/ml).

PATIENT/FAMILY TEACHING

• Foods rich in vitamin A include cod, halibut, tuna, shark (naturally occurring vitamin A found only in animal sources). • Avoid taking mineral oil, cholestyramine (Questran) while taking vitamin A.

vitamin D (vitamin D analogues)

calcitriol

cal-**sit**-tree-oll
(Calcijex, Rocaltrol, Vectical)

doxercalciferol

docks-err-cal-**siff**-err-oll
(Hectorol)

ergocalciferol

err-go-cal-**siff**-err-oll
(Drisdol)

paricalcitol

pear-ee-cal-**sit**-toll
(Zemplar)

◆CLASSIFICATION

PHARMACOTHERAPEUTIC: Fat-soluble vitamin. **CLINICAL:** Vitamin D analogue.

ACTION

Calcitriol: Stimulates calcium transport in intestines, resorption in bones, and tubular reabsorption in kidney; suppress parathyroid hormone (PTH) secretion/synthesis. **Doxercalciferol:** Regulates blood calcium levels, stimulates bone growth, suppresses PTH secretion/synthesis. **Ergocalciferol:** Promotes active absorption of calcium and phosphorus, increasing serum levels to allow bone mineralization; mobilizes calcium and phosphate from bone, increases reabsorption of calcium and phosphate by renal tubules. **Paricalcitol:** Suppresses PTH secretion/synthesis. **Therapeutic Effect:** Essential for absorption, utilization of calcium, phosphate, control of PTH levels.

V

PHARMACOKINETICS

Calcitriol: Rapidly absorbed. Protein binding: 99.9%. Metabolized to active metabolite (ergocalciferol). Primarily excreted in feces/urine. **Half-life:** 5–8 hrs. **Doxercalciferol:** Metabolized in liver. **Half-life:** 32–37 hrs. **Ergocalciferol:** Metabolized in liver. **Paricalcitol:** Readily absorbed. Protein binding: 99.8%. Metabolized in liver. Primarily excreted in feces. **Half-life:** 5–7 hrs.

USES

Calcitriol: Manage hypocalcemia in pts on chronic renal dialysis, secondary hypoparathyroidism in chronic kidney disease (CKD), manage hypocalcemia in hypoparathyroidism. **(Topical):** Treatment of mild to moderate plaque psoriasis. **Doxercalciferol:** Treatment of secondary hyperparathyroidism in CKD on dialysis and predialysis. **Ergocalciferol:** Treatment of refractory rickets, hypophosphatemia, hypoparathyroidism, dietary supplement. **Paricalcitol: (Intravenous):** Treatment/prevention of secondary hyperparathyroidism associated with stage 5 CKD. **(PO):** Treatment/prevention of secondary hyperparathyroidism associated with stage 3 and 4 CKD. **OFF-LABEL: Calcitriol:** Vitamin D-dependent rickets. **Ergocalciferol:** Prevention/treatment of vitamin D deficiency in pts with CKD.

PRECAUTIONS

Contraindications: Vitamin D toxicity, hypercalcemia, malabsorption syndrome. **Cautions:** Immobilization (increases risk of hypercalcemia), dehydration (increases serum creatinine, risk of hypercalcemia, dialysis pts (increases risk of hypermagnesemia/hyperphosphatemia), preexisting renal failure (ectopic calcification may occur), impaired hepatic function, renal osteodystrophy with hyperphosphatemia.

LIFESPAN CONSIDERATIONS

Pregnancy/Lactation: Unknown if drug crosses placenta. Infant risk cannot be ruled out. **Pregnancy category: (Calcitriol): A (C if used in doses above recommended daily allowance). (Doxercalciferol): B. (Ergocalciferol): A (C if used in doses above recommended daily allowance). (Paricalcitol): C. Children/Elderly:** No age-related precautions noted.

INTERACTIONS

DRUG: Magnesium-containing antacids may increase risk of hypermagnesemia, **calcium-containing products, concurrent vitamin D (or derivatives)** may increase risk of hypercalcemia, may increase **digoxin** toxicity due to hypercalcemia (may cause arrhythmias). **HERBAL:** None significant. **FOOD:** None known. **LAB VALUES:** May increase serum cholesterol, calcium, magnesium, phosphate, ALT, AST, BUN, creatinine.

AVAILABILITY (Rx)

Calcitriol

Capsules, Softgel (Rocaltrol): 0.25 mcg, 0.5 mcg. **Injection Solution (Calcijex):** 1 mcg/ml. **Oral Solution (Rocaltrol):** 1 mcg/ml.

Doxercalciferol

Capsules, Softgel (Hectorol): 0.5 mcg, 2.5 mcg. **Injection Solution (Hectorol):** 2 mcg/ml.

Ergocalciferol

Capsules (Drisdol): 50,000 units (1.25 mg). **Liquid, Oral (Drisdol):** 8,000 units/ml (200 mcg/ml). **Tablets:** 400 units.

Paricalcitol

Capsules, Gelatin (Zemplar): 1 mcg, 2 mcg, 4 mcg. **Injection Solution (Zemplar):** 2 mcg/ml.

ADMINISTRATION/HANDLING

Calcitriol

PO

- May take without regard to food.

IV

- May give as IV bolus via catheter at end of dialysis.

V

Doxercalciferol
PO
• May take without regard to food.

IV
• May give as IV bolus via catheter at end of dialysis.

Ergocalciferol
PO
• May take without regard to food.

Paricalcitol
PO
• May take without regard to food. • For 3 times/wk dosing, give no more frequently than every other day.

IV
• Give bolus anytime during dialysis. • Do not give more frequently than every other day.

INDICATIONS/ROUTES/DOSAGE

Calcitriol
Hypocalcemia on Chronic Renal Dialysis
PO: ADULTS, ELDERLY: (ROCALTROL): Initially, 0.25 mcg/day or every other day. May increase by 0.25 mcg/day at 4- to 8-wk intervals. Range: 0.5–1 mcg/day.
IV: ADULTS, ELDERLY: (CALCIJEX): 1–2 mcg 3 times/wk. Adjust dose at 2- to 4-wk intervals. Range: 0.5–4 mcg 3 times/wk.

Hypocalcemia in Hypoparathyroidism
PO: ADULTS, CHILDREN 6 YRS AND OLDER: (ROCALTROL): Initially, 0.25 mcg/day. May increase at 2- to 4-wk intervals. Range: 0.5–2 mcg/day. **CHILDREN 1–5 YRS:** 0.25–0.75 mcg once daily. **CHILDREN YOUNGER THAN 1 YR:** 0.04–0.08 mcg/kg once daily.

Secondary Hyperparathyroidism Associated with Moderate to Severe CKD Not on Dialysis
PO: ADULTS, ELDERLY, CHILDREN 3 YRS AND OLDER: (ROCALTROL): Initially, 0.25 mcg/day. May increase to 0.5 mcg/day. **CHILDREN YOUNGER THAN 3 YRS:** Initially, 0.01–0.015 mcg/kg/day.

Doxercalciferol
Secondary Hyperparathyroidism (Dialysis)
PO: ADULTS, ELDERLY: Initial dose (intact parathyroid hormone [iPTH] greater than 400 pg/ml): 10 mcg 3 times/wk at dialysis. Dose titrated to lower iPTH to 150–300 pg/ml, with dosage adjustments made at 8-wk intervals. **Maximum:** 20 mcg 3 times/wk.
IV: ADULTS, ELDERLY: Initial dose (iPTH greater than 400 pg/ml): 4 mcg 3 times/wk after dialysis, given as bolus dose. Dose titrated to lower iPTH to 150–300 pg/ml, with dosage adjustments made at 8-wk intervals. **Maximum:** 18 mcg/wk.

Secondary Hyperparathyroidism (Predialysis)
PO: ADULTS, ELDERLY: Initially, 1 mcg/day. Titrate dose to lower iPTH to 35–70 pg/ml for stage 3 CKD and 70–110 pg/ml for stage 4 CKD. **Maximum:** 3.5 mcg/day.

Ergocalciferol
Dietary Supplement
PO: ADULTS, ELDERLY, CHILDREN: 10 mcg (400 units)/day. **NEONATES:** 10–20 mcg (400–800 units)/day.

Hypoparathyroidism
PO: ADULTS, ELDERLY: 625 mcg–5 mg (25,000–200,000 units)/day (with calcium supplements). **CHILDREN:** 1.25–5 mg (50,000–200,000 units)/day (with calcium supplements).

Nutritional Rickets, Osteomalacia
PO: ADULTS, ELDERLY, CHILDREN: 25–125 mcg (1,000–5,000 units)/day for 8–12 wks. **ADULTS, ELDERLY (WITH MALABSORPTION SYNDROME):** 250–7,500 mcg (10,000–300,000 units)/day. **CHILDREN (WITH MALABSORPTION SYNDROME):** 250–625 mcg (10,000–25,000 units)/day.

Vitamin D-Dependent Rickets
PO: ADULTS, ELDERLY: 250 mcg–1.5 mg (10,000–60,000 units)/day. **CHILDREN:** 75–125 mcg (3,000–5,000 units)/day.

Maximum: 1,500 mcg (60,000 units)/day.

Vitamin D-Resistant Rickets
PO: ADULTS, ELDERLY, CHILDREN: 300 mcg–12.5 mg (12,000–500,000 units)/day.

Hypophosphatemia
PO: ADULTS, ELDERLY: 250–1,500 mcg (10,000–60,000 units)/day with phosphate supplements. **CHILDREN:** 1,000–2,000 mcg (40,000–80,000 units)/day with phosphate supplements.

Plaque Psoriasis
TOPICAL: ADULTS, ELDERLY: Apply to affected area twice daily.

Paricalcitol
Secondary Hyperparathyroidism in Stage 5 CKD
IV: ADULTS, ELDERLY, CHILDREN 5 YRS AND OLDER: Initially, 0.04–0.1 mcg/kg given as bolus dose no more frequently than every other day at any time during dialysis. May increase by 2–4 mcg every 2–4 wks. Dose is based on serum iPTH levels.

Secondary Hyperparathyroidism in Stages 3 and 4 CKD
Note: Initial dose based on baseline serum iPTH levels. Dose adjusted q2wks based on iPTH levels relative to baseline.
PO: ADULTS, ELDERLY: (iPTH 500 PG/ML OR LESS): 1 mcg/day or 2 mcg 3 times/wk. **(iPTH GREATER THAN 500 PG/ML):** 2 mcg/day or 4 mcg 3 times/wk.

SIDE EFFECTS

Frequencies not defined. **Calcitriol:** Cardiac arrhythmias, headache, pruritus, hypercalcemia, polydipsia, abdominal pain, metallic taste, nausea, vomiting, myalgia, soft tissue calcification. **Doxercalciferol:** Edema, pruritus, nausea, vomiting, headache, dizziness, dyspnea, malaise, hypercalcemia. **Ergocalciferol:** Hypercalcemia, hypervitaminosis D, decreased renal function, soft tissue calcification, bone demineralization, nausea, constipation, weight loss. **Paricalcitol:** Edema, nausea, vomiting, hypercalcemia.

ADVERSE EFFECTS/ TOXIC REACTIONS

Early signs of overdose manifested as weakness, headache, drowsiness, nausea, vomiting, dry mouth, constipation, muscle/bone pain, metallic taste. Later signs of overdose evidenced by polyuria, polydipsia, anorexia, weight loss, nocturia, photophobia, rhinorrhea, pruritus, disorientation, hallucinations, hyperthermia, hypertension, cardiac dysrhythmias.

NURSING CONSIDERATIONS

BASELINE ASSESSMENT

Obtain baseline serum calcium, phosphorus, alkaline phosphatase, creatinine, serum or plasma iPTH.

INTERVENTION/EVALUATION

Monitor serum, urinary calcium levels, serum phosphate, magnesium, creatine, alkaline phosphatase, BUN determinations (therapeutic calcium level: 9–10 mg/dl), PTH measurements. Estimate daily dietary calcium intake. Encourage adequate fluid intake. Monitor for signs/symptoms of vitamin D intoxication.

PATIENT/FAMILY TEACHING

• Adequate calcium intake should be maintained. • Dietary phosphorus may need to be restricted (foods high in phosphorus include beans, dairy products, nuts, peas, whole-grain products). • Oral formulations may cause hypersensitivity reactions. Avoid excessive doses. • Report signs/symptoms of hypercalcemia (headache, weakness, drowsiness, nausea, vomiting, dry mouth, constipation, metallic taste, muscle or bone pain). • Maintain adequate hydration. • Avoid changes in diet or supplemental calcium intake (unless directed by health care professional). • Avoid magnesium-containing antacids in pts with renal failure.

vitamin E

vight-ah-myn E
(Aquasol E, E-Gems, Key-E, Key-E Kaps)
Do not confuse Aquasol E with Anusol.

◆CLASSIFICATION

PHARMACOTHERAPEUTIC: Fat-soluble vitamin. **CLINICAL:** Nutritional supplement (see p. 162C).

ACTION

Prevents oxidation of vitamins A and C, protects fatty acids from attack by free radicals, protects RBCs from hemolysis by oxidizing agents. **Therapeutic Effect:** Prevents/treats vitamin E deficiency.

PHARMACOKINETICS

Variably absorbed from GI tract (requires bile salts, dietary fat, normal pancreatic function). Primarily concentrated in adipose tissue. Metabolized in liver. Primarily eliminated by biliary system.

USES

Dietary supplement. **OFF-LABEL:** Prevention/treatment of Alzheimer's disease, tardive dyskinesia; reduces risk of bronchopulmonary dysplasia, retrolental fibroplasia in infants exposed to high concentrations of oxygen. Treatment of hemolytic anemia secondary to vitamin E deficiency.

PRECAUTIONS

Contraindications: None known. **Cautions:** None known.

LIFESPAN CONSIDERATIONS

Pregnancy/Lactation: Unknown if drug crosses placenta or is distributed in breast milk. **Pregnancy Category A (C if used in doses above recommended daily allowance). Children/Elderly:** No age-related precautions noted in normal dosages.

INTERACTIONS

DRUG: May alter effects of **vitamin K** on clotting factors, increase effects of **warfarin.** May decrease response of **iron** in children with iron-deficiency anemia. **HERBAL:** None significant. **FOOD:** None known. **LAB VALUES:** None significant.

AVAILABILITY (OTC)

Capsules: 100 units (E-Gems), 200 units (Key-E Kaps), 400 units (Key-E Kaps), 600 units (E-Gems), 800 units (E-Gems), 1,000 units (E-Gems), 1,200 units (E-Gems). **Tablets (Key-E):** 100 units, 200 units, 400 units, 500 units.

ADMINISTRATION/HANDLING

PO

- Do not crush, break tablets/capsules.
- Give without regard to food.

INDICATIONS/ROUTES/DOSAGE

Vitamin E Deficiency

PO: ADULTS, ELDERLY: 60–75 units/day. **CHILDREN:** 1 unit/kg/day. Patients with cystic fibrosis, beta-thalassemia, sickle cell anemia may require higher maintenance doses.

Prevention of Vitamin E Deficiency

PO: ADULTS, ELDERLY: 30 units/day.

SIDE EFFECTS

Rare: Contact dermatitis, sterile abscess.

ADVERSE EFFECTS/ TOXIC REACTIONS

Chronic overdose may produce fatigue, weakness, nausea, headache, blurred vision, flatulence, diarrhea.

NURSING CONSIDERATIONS

PATIENT/FAMILY TEACHING

• Swallow tablets/capsules whole; do not crush, chew. • Toxicity consists of blurred vision, diarrhea, dizziness, nausea, headache, flu-like symptoms. • Consume foods rich in vitamin E, including vegetable oils, vegetable shortening, margarine, leafy vegetables, milk, eggs, meat.

vitamin K

vight-ah-myn K

phytonadione (vitamin K_1)

(AquaMEPHYTON, Konakion ✤, Mephyton, Vitamin K1)

Do not confuse Mephyton with melphalan or methadone.

◆CLASSIFICATION

PHARMACOTHERAPEUTIC: Fat-soluble vitamin. **CLINICAL:** Nutritional supplement, antidote (drug-induced hypoprothrombinemia), antihemorrhagic.

ACTION

Promotes hepatic formation of coagulation factors II, VII, IX, X. **Therapeutic Effect:** Essential for normal clotting of blood.

PHARMACOKINETICS

Readily absorbed from GI tract (duodenum) after IM, subcutaneous administration. Metabolized in liver. Excreted in urine; eliminated by biliary system. Onset of action (increased coagulation factors): **PO:** 6–10 hrs; **IV:** 1–2 hrs. Peak effect (INR values return to normal): **PO:** 24–48 hrs; **IV:** 12–14 hrs.

USES

Prevention, treatment of hemorrhagic states in neonates; antidote for hemorrhage induced by oral anticoagulants, hypoprothrombinemic states due to vitamin K deficiency. Will not counteract anticoagulation effect of heparin.

PRECAUTIONS

Contraindications: None known. **Cautions:** None known.

⌛ LIFESPAN CONSIDERATIONS

Pregnancy/Lactation: Crosses placenta. Distributed in breast milk. **Pregnancy Category C. Children/Elderly:** No age-related precautions noted.

INTERACTIONS

DRUG: **Broad-spectrum antibiotics, high-dose salicylates** may increase vitamin K requirements. **Cholestyramine, colestipol, mineral oil, sucralfate** may decrease absorption. May decrease effects of **oral anticoagulants.** **HERBAL:** None significant. **FOOD:** None known. **LAB VALUES:** None significant.

AVAILABILITY (Rx)

Injection Solution (AquaMEPHYTON, Vitamin K_1): 1 mg/0.5 ml, 10 mg/ml. **Tablets (Mephyton):** 5 mg.

ADMINISTRATION/HANDLING

IV

◀ALERT▶ Restrict to emergency use only.

Reconstitution • May dilute with preservative-free NaCl or D_5W immediately before use. Do not use other diluents. • Discard unused portions.

Rate of administration • Administer slow IV at rate of 1 mg/min. • Monitor continuously for hypersensitivity, anaphylactic reaction during and immediately following IV administration.

Storage • Store at room temperature.

IM, Subcutaneous

• Inject into anterolateral aspect of thigh, deltoid region.

PO

• Scored tablets may be crushed. • May give without regard to food.

IV INCOMPATIBILITY

None known.

IV COMPATIBILITIES

Heparin, potassium chloride.

INDICATIONS/ROUTES/DOSAGE

◀ALERT▶ PO/subcutaneous route preferred; IV/IM use restricted to emergent situations.

V

Oral Anticoagulant Overdose
PO, IV, SUBCUTANEOUS: ADULTS, ELDERLY: 2.5–10 mg/dose. May repeat in 12–48 hrs if given orally, in 6–8 hrs if given by IV or subcutaneous route. **CHILDREN:** 0.5–5 mg depending on need for further anticoagulation, severity of bleeding.

Vitamin K Deficiency
PO: ADULTS, ELDERLY: 2.5–25 mg/24 hrs. **CHILDREN:** 2.5–5 mg/24 hrs.
IV, IM, SUBCUTANEOUS: ADULTS, ELDERLY: 10 mg/dose. **CHILDREN:** 1–2 mg/dose.

Hemorrhagic Disease of Newborn
IM, SUBCUTANEOUS: NEONATE: Treatment: 1 mg/dose/day. May increase to 2 mg. **Prophylaxis:** 0.5–1 mg within 1 hr of birth.

SIDE EFFECTS

◄ALERT► PO/subcutaneous administration less likely to produce side effects than IV/IM routes.
Occasional: Pain, soreness, swelling at IM injection site, pruritic erythema (with repeated injections), facial flushing, altered taste.

ADVERSE EFFECTS/ TOXIC REACTIONS

Newborns (esp. premature infants) may develop hyperbilirubinemia. Severe reaction (cramp-like pain, chest pain, dyspnea, facial flushing, dizziness, rapid/weak pulse, rash, diaphoresis, hypotension progressing to shock, cardiac arrest) occurs rarely, immediately after IV administration.

NURSING CONSIDERATIONS

INTERVENTION/EVALUATION

Monitor PT, international normalized ratio (INR) routinely in those taking anticoagulants. Assess skin for ecchymoses, petechiae. Assess gums for gingival bleeding, erythema. Assess urine for hematuria. Assess Hct, platelet count, urine/stool culture for occult blood. Assess for decrease in B/P, increase in pulse rate, complaint of abdominal/back pain, severe headache (may be evidence of hemorrhage). Question for increase in amount of discharge during menses. Assess peripheral pulses. Check for excessive bleeding from minor cuts, scratches.

PATIENT/FAMILY TEACHING

• Discomfort may occur with parenteral administration. • **Adults:** Use electric razor, soft toothbrush to prevent bleeding. • Report any sign of red or dark urine, black or red stool, coffee-ground vomitus, red-speckled mucus from cough. • Do not use any OTC medication without physician approval (may interfere with platelet aggregation). • Consume foods rich in vitamin K_1, including leafy green vegetables, meat, cow's milk, vegetable oil, egg yolks, tomatoes.

voriconazole

vohr-ee-**con**-ah-zole
(Vfend)

◆CLASSIFICATION

PHARMACOTHERAPEUTIC: Triazole derivative. **CLINICAL:** Antifungal.

ACTION

Inhibits synthesis of ergosterol (vital component of fungal cell wall formation). **Therapeutic Effect:** Damages fungal cell wall membrane.

PHARMACOKINETICS

Rapidly, completely absorbed after PO administration. Widely distributed. Protein binding: 58%. Metabolized in liver. Primarily excreted as metabolite in urine. **Half-life:** Variable, dose dependent.

USES

Treatment of invasive aspergillosis, esophageal candidiasis. Treatment of serious fungal infections caused by *Scedosporium apiospermum, Fusarium* spp.

Treatment of candidemia in non-neutropenic pts. OFF-LABEL: Fungal infection prophylaxis, empiric therapy for persistent neutropenic fever.

PRECAUTIONS

Contraindications: Concurrent administration of carbamazepine; ergot alkaloids; pimozide, quinidine (may cause prolonged QT interval, torsade de pointes); rifabutin; rifampin; ritonavir; sirolimus. Cautions: Renal/hepatic impairment, hypersensitivity to other antifungal agents.

LIFESPAN CONSIDERATIONS

Pregnancy/Lactation: May cause fetal harm. **Pregnancy Category D. Children:** Safety and efficacy not established in those younger than 12 yrs. **Elderly:** No age-related precautions noted.

INTERACTIONS

DRUG: May increase concentration, risk of toxicity of **alprazolam, calcium channel blockers, cyclosporine, efavirenz, ergot alkaloids, HMG-CoA reductase inhibitors (e.g., lovastatin), methadone, midazolam, protease inhibitors (e.g., amprenavir, saquinavir), rifabutin, sirolimus, tacrolimus, triazolam, warfarin. Carbamazepine, rifabutin, rifampin, ritonavir** may decrease concentration, effect. HERBAL: **St. John's wort** may decrease concentration. FOOD: **Grapefruit juice** may increase concentration. LAB VALUES: May increase serum alkaline phosphatase, ALT, AST, bilirubin, creatinine. May decrease potassium.

AVAILABILITY (Rx)

Injection, Powder for Reconstitution: 200 mg. Powder for Oral Suspension: 200 mg/5 ml. Tablets: 50 mg, 200 mg.

ADMINISTRATION/HANDLING

IV

Reconstitution • Reconstitute 200-mg vial with 19 ml Sterile Water for Injection to provide concentration of 10 mg/ml. Further dilute with 0.9% NaCl or D_5W to provide concentration of 0.5–5 mg/ml.

Rate of administration • Infuse over 1–2 hrs at a rate not to exceed 3 mg/kg/hr.

Storage • Store powder for injection at room temperature. • Use reconstituted solution immediately. • Do not use after 24 hrs when refrigerated.

PO

• Give 1 hr before or 1 hr after a meal.
• Do not mix oral suspension with any other medication or flavoring agent.

IV INCOMPATIBILITY

Total parenteral nutrition (TPN).

INDICATIONS/ROUTES/DOSAGE

Invasive Aspergillosis, Other Serious Fungal Infection

IV: ADULTS, ELDERLY, CHILDREN 12 YRS AND OLDER: Initially, 6 mg/kg q12h × 2 doses, then 4 mg/kg q12h.

Candidemia, Other Deep Tissue Candida Infections

IV: ADULTS, ELDERLY, CHILDREN 12 YRS AND OLDER: Initially, 6 mg/kg q12h × 2 doses, then 3–4 mg/kg q12h.

Esophageal Candidiasis

PO: ADULTS, ELDERLY WEIGHING 40 KG OR MORE: 200 mg q12h for minimum of 14 days, then at least 7 days following resolution of symptoms. **Maximum:** 600 mg/day. **ADULTS, ELDERLY WEIGHING LESS THAN 40 KG:** 100 mg q12h for minimum of 14 days, then at least 7 days following resolution of symptoms. **Maximum:** 300 mg/day.

Dosage in Pts Receiving Phenytoin

IV: Increase maintenance dose to 5 mg/kg q12h.
PO: Increase 200 mg q12h to 400 mg q12h (pts weighing 40 kg or more) or 100 mg q12h to 200 mg q12h (pts weighing less than 40 kg).

Dosage in Pts Receiving Cyclosporine

Reduce cyclosporine dose by 50%.

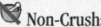

V

Dosage in Pts Receiving Efavirenz
Increase dose to 400 mg q12h and reduce efavirenz to 300 mg/day.

Dosage in Hepatic Impairment
MILD TO MODERATE: Reduce maintenance dose by 50%.
SEVERE: Use only if benefits outweigh risks. Monitor closely for toxicity.

SIDE EFFECTS

Frequent (20%–6%): Abnormal vision, fever, nausea, rash, vomiting. **Occasional (5%–2%):** Headache, chills, hallucinations, photophobia, tachycardia, hypertension.

ADVERSE EFFECTS/ TOXIC REACTIONS

Hepatotoxicity (jaundice, hepatitis, hepatic failure), acute renal failure have occurred in severely ill pts.

NURSING CONSIDERATIONS

BASELINE ASSESSMENT

Obtain baseline serum hepatic/renal function tests.

INTERVENTION/EVALUATION

Monitor serum hepatic/renal function tests. Monitor visual function (visual acuity, visual field, color perception) for drug therapy lasting longer than 28 days.

PATIENT/FAMILY TEACHING

• Take at least 1 hr before or 1 hr after a meal. • Avoid grapefruit juice. • Avoid driving at night. • Notify physician of visual changes (blurred vision, photophobia, yellowing of skin/eyes). • Avoid performing hazardous tasks if changes in vision occur. • Avoid direct sunlight. • Women of childbearing potential should use effective contraception.

vorinostat

vor-**in**-oh-stat
(Zolinza)

◆CLASSIFICATION

PHARMACOTHERAPEUTIC: Histone deacetylase inhibitor. **CLINICAL:** Antineoplastic.

ACTION

Inhibits activity of specific enzymes that catalyze removal of acetyl groups of proteins, causing accumulation of acetylated histones. **Therapeutic Effect:** Induces cell arrest.

PHARMACOKINETICS

Protein binding: 71%. Metabolized to inactive metabolites. Excreted in urine. **Half-life:** 2 hrs.

USES

Treatment of cutaneous manifestations in pts with cutaneous T-cell lymphoma (CTCL) with progressive, persistent, or recurrent disease, on or following two systemic therapies.

PRECAUTIONS

Contraindications: None significant. **Cautions:** History of deep vein thrombosis (DVT), diabetes mellitus, hepatic impairment, preexisting renal impairment, those with QT prolongation.

LIFESPAN CONSIDERATIONS

Pregnancy/Lactation: May cause fetal harm. Unknown if distributed in breast milk. **Pregnancy Category D. Children:** Safety and efficacy not established. **Elderly:** No age-related precautions noted.

INTERACTIONS

DRUG: May increase effect of **warfarin. Valproic acid** increases risk of GI bleeding, thrombocytopenia. **Concomitant QT-prolonging agents** may increase risk of arrhythmia. **HERBAL:** None significant. **FOOD:** None known. **LAB VALUES:** May decrease serum calcium, potassium, sodium, phosphate, platelet count. May increase serum glucose, creatinine, urine protein.

AVAILABILITY (Rx)

Capsules: 100 mg.

ADMINISTRATION/HANDLING

PO

• Do not open, crush capsules. • Give with food.

INDICATIONS/ROUTES/DOSAGE

Cutaneous T-Cell Lymphoma (CTCL)

PO: ADULTS, ELDERLY: 400 mg once daily with food. Dose may be reduced to 300 mg once daily with food. May be further reduced to 300 mg once daily with food for 5 consecutive days each wk.

SIDE EFFECTS

Frequent: Fatigue, diarrhea (52%), nausea (40%), altered taste (28%), anorexia (24%). **Occasional** (21%–11%): Weight decrease, muscle spasms, alopecia, dry mouth, chills, vomiting, constipation, dizziness, peripheral edema, headache, pruritus, cough, fever.

ADVERSE EFFECTS/ TOXIC REACTIONS

Thrombocytopenia occurs in 25% of pts, anemia in 15%. Pulmonary embolism occurs in 4% of pts. Deep vein thrombosis (DVT) occurs rarely.

NURSING CONSIDERATIONS

BASELINE ASSESSMENT

Baseline PT, international normalized ratio (INR), CBC, chemistry tests, esp. serum potassium, calcium, magnesium, glucose, creatinine should be obtained prior to therapy and every 2 wks during first 2 mos of therapy and monthly thereafter. Inform women of childbearing potential of risk to fetus if pregnancy occurs.

INTERVENTION/EVALUATION

Monitor platelet count, PT, INR, serum electrolytes during first 2 mos of therapy. Monitor signs/symptoms of DVT. Encourage fluid intake, approximately 2 L/day input, electrolytes, CBC. Assess for evidence of dehydration. Provide antiemetics to control nausea/vomiting. Monitor daily pattern of bowel activity, stool consistency.

PATIENT/FAMILY TEACHING

• Drink at least 2 L/day of fluids to prevent dehydration. • Report excessive vomiting, diarrhea. • Contact physician if shortness of breath, pain in any extremity occur.

warfarin

HIGH ALERT

war-far-in

(Apo-Warfarin ✤, Coumadin, Gen-Warfarin ✤, Jantoven, Novo-Warfarin ✤)

BLACK BOX ALERT May cause major or fatal bleeding. Risk factors include history of GI bleeding, hypertension, cerebrovascular disease, heart disease, malignancy, trauma, anemia, renal insufficiency, age 65 yrs and older, high anticoagulation factor (INR greater than 4).

Do not confuse Coumadin with Avandia, Cardura, or Kemadrin, or Jantoven with Janumet or Januvia.

◆CLASSIFICATION

PHARMACOTHERAPEUTIC: Coumarin derivative. **CLINICAL:** Anticoagulant (see p. 32C).

ACTION

Interferes with hepatic synthesis of vitamin K–dependent clotting factors, resulting in depletion of coagulation factors II, VII, IX, X. **Therapeutic Effect:** Prevents further extension of formed existing clot; prevents new clot formation, secondary thromboembolic complications.

PHARMACOKINETICS

Route	Onset	Peak	Duration
PO	1.5–3 days	5–7 days	2–5 days

Well absorbed from GI tract. Protein binding: 99%. Metabolized in liver. Primarily excreted in urine. Not removed by hemodialysis. **Half-life:** 20–60 hrs.

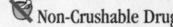

USES

Anticoagulant, prophylaxis, treatment of venous thrombosis, pulmonary embolism. Treatment of thromboembolism associated with chronic atrial fibrillation. Adjunct in treatment of coronary occlusion. Prophylaxis, treatment of thromboembolic complications associated with cardiac valve replacement. Reduces risk of death, recurrent MI, stroke, embolization after MI. OFF-LABEL: Prevention of MI, recurrent cerebral embolism; treatment adjunct in transient ischemic attacks.

PRECAUTIONS

Contraindications: Neurosurgical procedures, open wounds, pregnancy, severe hypertension, severe hepatic/renal damage, spinal puncture, uncontrolled bleeding, ulcers. **Cautions:** Active tuberculosis, diabetes, heparin-induced thrombocytopenia, those at risk for hemorrhage, necrosis, gangrene.

LIFESPAN CONSIDERATIONS

Pregnancy/Lactation: Contraindicated in pregnancy (fetal, neonatal hemorrhage, intrauterine death). Crosses placenta; distributed in breast milk. **Pregnancy Category X. Children:** More susceptible to effects. **Elderly:** Increased risk of hemorrhage; lower dosage recommended.

INTERACTIONS

DRUG: **Amiodarone, anabolic steroids, antithyroid medications, azole antifungals, cimetidine, clofibrate, diflunisal, disulfiram, fluvoxamine, lepirudin, levothyroxine, metronidazole, NSAIDs, omeprazole, paroxetine, platelet aggregation inhibitors, salicylates, sertraline, thrombolytic agents, thyroid hormones, ticlopidine, zafirlukast** may increase effects. **Griseofulvin, hepatic enzyme inducers, vitamin K** may decrease effects. **Alcohol** may enhance anticoagulant effect. HERBAL: **Cat's claw, dong quai, evening primrose, feverfew, garlic, ginger, ginkgo biloba, ginseng, horse chestnut, red clover** possess antiplatelet activity, may increase risk of bleeding. FOOD: None known. LAB VALUES: None significant.

AVAILABILITY (Rx)

Tablets (Coumadin, Jantoven): 1 mg, 2 mg, 2.5 mg, 3 mg, 4 mg, 5 mg, 6 mg, 7.5 mg, 10 mg.

ADMINISTRATION/HANDLING

PO

• Scored tablets may be crushed. • Give without regard to food. Give with food if GI upset occurs. • Give at same time each day.

INDICATIONS/ROUTES/DOSAGE

ALERT Initial dosing must be individualized.

Anticoagulant

PO: ADULTS, ELDERLY: Initially, 5–10 mg/day for 2–5 days, then adjust based on international normalized ratio (INR). Maintenance: 2–10 mg/day. **CHILDREN:** Initially, 0.05–0.2 mg/kg/day. **Maximum:** 10 mg. Maintenance: 0.05–0.34 mg/kg/day, then adjust based on INR.

SIDE EFFECTS

Occasional: GI distress (nausea, anorexia, abdominal cramps, diarrhea). **Rare:** Hypersensitivity reaction (dermatitis, urticaria), esp. in those sensitive to aspirin.

ADVERSE EFFECTS/ TOXIC REACTIONS

Bleeding complications ranging from local ecchymoses to major hemorrhage may occur. **Antidote:** Vitamin K. Amount based on INR, significance of bleeding. Range: 2.5–10 mg given orally or slow IV infusion (see Appendix M for dosage). Hepatotoxicity, blood dyscrasias, necrosis, vasculitis, local thrombosis occur rarely.

NURSING CONSIDERATIONS

BASELINE ASSESSMENT

Cross-check dose with coworker. Determine INR before administration and daily following therapy initiation. When stabilized, follow with INR determination q4–6wk. Genotyping prior to initiating therapy if available.

INTERVENTION/EVALUATION

Monitor INR reports diligently. Assess Hct, platelet count, urine/stool culture for occult blood, AST, ALT. Be alert to complaints of abdominal/back pain, severe headache (may be signs of hemorrhage). Decrease in B/P, increase in pulse rate may be signs of hemorrhage. Question for increase in amount of menstrual discharge. Assess area of thromboembolus for color, temperature. Assess peripheral pulses; skin for ecchymoses, petechiae. Check for excessive bleeding from minor cuts, scratches. Assess gums for erythema, gingival bleeding. Assess urinary output for hematuria.

PATIENT/ FAMILY TEACHING

• Take medication at same time each day. • Do not take, discontinue any other medication except on advice of physician. • Avoid alcohol, salicylates, drastic dietary changes. • Do not change from one brand to another. • Consult with physician before surgery, dental work. • Urine may become red-orange. • Notify physician if bleeding, bruising, red or brown urine, black stools occur. • Use electric razor, soft toothbrush to prevent bleeding. • Report coffee-ground vomitus, blood-tinged mucus from cough. • Do not use any OTC medication without physician approval (may interfere with platelet aggregation).

yohimbe

Also known as aphrodien, corynine, johimbi.

CLASSIFICATION

HERBAL: See Appendix G.

ACTION

Produces genital blood vessel dilation, improves nerve impulse transmission to genital area. Increases penile blood flow, central sympathetic excitation impulses to genital tissues. **Effect:** Improves sexual function, affects impotence.

USES

Used as aphrodisiac by some cultures. Used to improve libido, enhance sexual function in male. Used to manage symptoms associated with diabetic neuropathy, postural hypotension.

PRECAUTIONS

Contraindications: Pregnancy, lactation (may have uterine relaxant effect, cause fetal toxicity), angina, heart disease, benign prostatic hyperplasia (BPH), depression, renal/hepatic disease. **Cautions:** Anxiety, diabetes mellitus, hypertension, post-traumatic stress disorder (PSTD), schizophrenia.

LIFESPAN CONSIDERATIONS

Pregnancy/Lactation: Contraindicated; avoid use. **Children:** Safety and efficacy not established; avoid use. **Elderly:** Age-related renal/hepatic impairment may require discontinuation.

INTERACTIONS

DRUG: May interfere with **antidiabetic agents, antihypertensives.** May antagonize effects of **clonidine. MAOIs, sympathomimetics, tricyclic antidepressants** may have additive effects. **HERBAL:** **Ginkgo biloba, St. John's wort** may have additive therapeutic, adverse effects. **FOOD:** **Foods containing caffeine, tyramine** may increase risk of hypertensive crises. **LAB VALUES:** None significant.

AVAILABILITY (OTC)

Liquid: 5 mg/5 ml. **Tablets:** 5 mg.

INDICATIONS/ROUTES/DOSAGE

Impotence

PO: ADULTS, ELDERLY: 15–30 mg/day in divided doses.

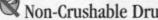

SIDE EFFECTS

Excitement, tremor, insomnia, anxiety, hypertension, tachycardia, dizziness, headache, irritability, salivation, dilated pupils, nausea, vomiting, hypersensitivity reaction.

ADVERSE EFFECTS/ TOXIC REACTIONS

Paralysis, severe hypotension, irregular heartbeat, cardiac failure may occur. Overdose can be fatal.

NURSING CONSIDERATIONS

BASELINE ASSESSMENT

Assess if pt is pregnant or breast-feeding (contraindicated). Determine other medical conditions, including angina, heart disease, benign prostatic hyperplasia (BPH). Assess baseline serum renal/hepatic function, medications (see Interactions).

INTERVENTION/EVALUATION

Monitor serum renal/hepatic function, B/P. Assess for hypersensitivity reaction.

PATIENT/FAMILY TEACHING

• Do not use other OTC or prescribed medications before checking with physician. • Inform physician if pregnant or breast-feeding.

zafirlukast

za-**feer**-loo-kast
(Accolate)
Do not confuse Accolate with Accupril, Accutane, or Aclovate.

◆CLASSIFICATION

PHARMACOTHERAPEUTIC: Leukotriene receptor antagonist. **CLINICAL:** Antiasthma (see p. 76C).

ACTION

Binds to leukotriene receptors, inhibiting bronchoconstriction due to sulfur dioxide, cold air, specific antigens (grass, cat dander, ragweed). **Therapeutic Effect:** Reduces airway edema, smooth muscle constriction; alters cellular activity associated with inflammatory process.

PHARMACOKINETICS

Rapidly absorbed after PO administration (food reduces absorption). Protein binding: 99%. Extensively metabolized in liver. Primarily excreted in feces. Unknown if removed by hemodialysis. **Half-life:** 10 hrs.

USES

Prophylaxis, chronic treatment of bronchial asthma in adults and children 5 yrs and older. **OFF-LABEL:** Exercise-induced bronchospasm.

PRECAUTIONS

Contraindications: None known. **Cautions:** Hepatic impairment.

LIFESPAN CONSIDERATIONS

Pregnancy/Lactation: Drug is distributed in breast milk. Do not administer to breast-feeding women. **Pregnancy Category B. Children:** Safety and efficacy not established in those younger than 5 yrs. **Elderly:** No age-related precautions noted.

INTERACTIONS

DRUG: Aspirin increases concentration. **Erythromycin, theophylline** decrease concentration. **Warfarin** increases prothrombin time (PT). **HERBAL:** None significant. **FOOD: Food** decreases bioavailability by 40%. **LAB VALUES:** None significant.

AVAILABILITY (Rx)

Tablets: 10 mg, 20 mg.

ADMINISTRATION/HANDLING

PO

• Give 1 hr before or 2 hrs after meals.

INDICATIONS/ROUTES/DOSAGE

Bronchial Asthma

PO: ADULTS, ELDERLY, CHILDREN 12 YRS AND OLDER: 20 mg twice daily. **CHILDREN 5–11 YRS:** 10 mg twice daily.

SIDE EFFECTS

Frequent (13%): Headache. **Occasional (3%):** Nausea, diarrhea. **Rare (less than 3%):** Generalized pain, asthenia (loss of strength, energy), myalgia, fever, dyspepsia (heartburn, indigestion, epigastric pain), vomiting, dizziness.

ADVERSE EFFECTS/ TOXIC REACTIONS

Concurrent administration of inhaled corticosteroids increases risk of upper respiratory tract infection.

NURSING CONSIDERATIONS

BASELINE ASSESSMENT

Obtain medication history. Assess serum hepatic function lab values.

INTERVENTION/EVALUATION

Monitor rate, depth, rhythm, type of respiration; quality, rate of pulse. Assess lung sounds for rhonchi, wheezing, rales. Observe for cyanosis (lips, fingernails appear blue or dusky color in light-skinned pts; gray in dark-skinned pts). Monitor serum hepatic function tests.

PATIENT/FAMILY TEACHING

• Increase fluid intake (decreases lung secretion viscosity). • Take as prescribed, even during symptom-free periods. • Do not use for acute asthma episodes. • Do not alter, stop other asthma medications. • Do not breastfeed. • Report nausea, jaundice, abdominal pain, flu-like symptoms, worsening of asthma.

zaleplon

zal-e-plon
(Sonata)
Do not confuse zaleplon with zolpidem.

◆CLASSIFICATION

PHARMACOTHERAPEUTIC: Nonbenzodiazepine. **CLINICAL:** Hypnotic **(Schedule IV)** (see p. 150C).

ACTION

Enhances action of inhibitory neurotransmitter gamma-aminobutyric acid (GABA). **Therapeutic Effect:** Induces sleep.

PHARMACOKINETICS

Route	Onset	Peak	Duration
PO	Rapid	1 hr	6–8 hrs

Rapidly, almost completely absorbed following PO administration. Protein binding: 45%–75%. Metabolized in liver. Primarily excreted in urine. Partially eliminated in feces. **Half-life:** 1 hr.

USES

Short-term treatment of insomnia (7–10 days). Decreases sleep onset time (no effect on number of nocturnal awakenings, total sleep time).

PRECAUTIONS

Contraindications: Severe hepatic impairment. **Cautions:** Mild to moderate hepatic impairment in pts experiencing signs/symptoms of depression, those hypersensitive to aspirin (allergic-type reaction).

LIFESPAN CONSIDERATIONS

Pregnancy/Lactation: Unknown if drug crosses placenta; distributed in breast milk. **Pregnancy Category C. Children:** Safety and efficacy not established. **Elderly:** May be more sensitive to zaleplon effects.

INTERACTIONS

DRUG: Alcohol, other CNS depressants may increase CNS depression. **Cimetidine** may increase effect. **Carbamazepine, phenobarbital, phenytoin, rifampin** may decrease concentration. **HERBAL: Gotu kola, kava kava, St. John's wort, valerian** may increase CNS depression. **FOOD: High-fat, heavy meals** may delay onset of sleep by approximately 2 hrs. **LAB VALUES:** None significant.

AVAILABILITY (Rx)

Capsules: 5 mg, 10 mg.

ADMINISTRATION/HANDLING

PO

• Give immediately before bedtime. • Giving drug with or immediately after high-fat meal results in slower absorption. • Capsules may be emptied and mixed with food.

INDICATIONS/ROUTES/DOSAGE

Insomnia

PO: ADULTS: 10 mg at bedtime. Range: 5–20 mg. **ELDERLY:** 5 mg at bedtime. **Maximum:** 10 mg.

Dosage in Hepatic Impairment

Mild to moderate: 5 mg. Severe: Not recommended.

SIDE EFFECTS

Expected: Drowsiness, sedation, mild rebound insomnia (on first night after drug is discontinued). **Frequent (28%–7%):** Nausea, headache, myalgia, dizziness. **Occasional (5%–3%):** Abdominal pain, asthenia (loss of strength, energy), dyspepsia (heartburn, indigestion, epigastric pain), eye pain, paresthesia. **Rare (2%):** Tremor, amnesia, hyperacusis (acute sense of hearing), fever, dysmenorrhea.

ADVERSE EFFECTS/ TOXIC REACTIONS

May produce altered concentration/behavior changes, impaired memory. Taking medication while ambulating may result in hallucinations, impaired coordination, dizziness, light-headedness. Overdose results in drowsiness, confusion, diminished reflexes, coma.

NURSING CONSIDERATIONS

BASELINE ASSESSMENT

Provide for safety; raise bed rails. Provide environment conducive to sleep (back rub, quiet environment, low lighting).

INTERVENTION/EVALUATION

Assess sleep pattern.

PATIENT/FAMILY TEACHING

• Take right before bedtime or when in bed and not falling asleep. • Avoid tasks requiring alertness, motor skills until response to drug is established. • Do not exceed prescribed dosage. • Do not take with or immediately after a high-fat or heavy meal. • Rebound insomnia may occur when drug is discontinued after short-term therapy. • Avoid alcohol, other CNS depressants.

zanamivir

zah-**nam**-ih-veer
(Relenza)

◆CLASSIFICATION

PHARMACOTHERAPEUTIC: Antiviral. **CLINICAL:** Anti-influenza (see p. 70C).

ACTION

Appears to inhibit influenza virus enzyme neuraminidase, essential for viral replication. **Therapeutic Effect:** Prevents viral release from infected cells.

PHARMACOKINETICS

Systemically absorbed, approximately 4%–17%. Protein binding: Less than 10%. Not metabolized. Partially excreted unchanged in urine. **Half-life:** 2.5–5.1 hrs.

USES

Treatment of uncomplicated acute illness due to influenza virus A and B in adults, children 7 yrs and older who have been symptomatic for less than 2 days. Prevention of influenza A and B in adults and children 5 yrs and older. **OFF-LABEL:** Influenza prophylaxis and treatment of novel influenza A (H1N1) virus.

PRECAUTIONS

Contraindications: None known. **Cautions:** COPD, asthma.

LIFESPAN CONSIDERATIONS

Pregnancy/Lactation: Unknown if drug crosses placenta or is distributed in breast milk. **Pregnancy Category C. Children:** Safety and efficacy not established in those younger than 7 yrs. **Elderly:** No age-related precautions noted.

INTERACTIONS

DRUG: None significant. **HERBAL:** None significant. **FOOD:** None known. **LAB VALUES:** None significant.

AVAILABILITY (Rx)

Powder for Inhalation: 5 mg/blister.

ADMINISTRATION/HANDLING

Inhalation

• Instruct pt to use Diskhaler device provided, exhale completely; then, holding mouthpiece 1 inch away from lips, inhale and hold breath as long as possible before exhaling. • Rinse mouth with water immediately after inhalation (prevents mouth/throat dryness). • Store at room temperature.

INDICATIONS/ROUTES/DOSAGE

Treatment of Influenza Virus

INHALATION: ADULTS, ELDERLY, CHILDREN 7 YRS AND OLDER: 2 inhalations (one 5-mg blister per inhalation for total dose of 10 mg) twice daily (approximately 12 hrs apart) for 5 days.

Prevention of Influenza Virus

INHALATION: ADULTS, ELDERLY, CHILDREN 5 YRS AND OLDER: 2 inhalations (10 mg) once daily for duration of exposure period.

SIDE EFFECTS

Occasional (3%–2%): Diarrhea, sinusitis, nausea, bronchitis, cough, dizziness, headache. **Rare (less than 1.5%):** Malaise, fatigue, fever, abdominal pain, myalgia, arthralgia, urticaria.

ADVERSE EFFECTS/ TOXIC REACTIONS

May produce neutropenia. Bronchospasm may occur in those with history of COPD, bronchial asthma.

NURSING CONSIDERATIONS

BASELINE ASSESSMENT

Pts requiring an inhaled bronchodilator at same time as zanamivir should use the bronchodilator before zanamivir administration.

INTERVENTION/EVALUATION

Provide assistance if dizziness occurs. Monitor daily pattern of bowel activity, stool consistency.

PATIENT/FAMILY TEACHING

• Follow manufacturer guidelines for use of delivery device. • Avoid contact with those who are at high risk for influenza. • Continue treatment for full 5-day course. • Doses should be evenly spaced. • In pts with respiratory disease, an inhaled bronchodilator should be readily available.

zidovudine

zye-**doe**-vyoo-deen
(Apo-Zidovudine ✦, AZT, Retrovir)

BLACK BOX ALERT Neutropenia, severe anemia may occur. Lactic acidosis, severe hepatomegaly with steatosis (fatty liver), including fatalities, have occurred. Symptomatic myopathy, myositis associated with prolonged use.

Do not confuse Retrovir with acyclovir or ritonavir.

FIXED-COMBINATION(S)

Combivir: zidovudine/lamivudine (an antiviral): 300 mg/150 mg. **Trizivir:** zidovudine/lamivudine/abacavir (an antiviral): 300 mg/150 mg/300 mg.

◆CLASSIFICATION

PHARMACOTHERAPEUTIC: Nucleoside reverse transcriptase inhibitors. **CLINICAL:** Antivirals (see pp. 70C, 115C).

ACTION

Interferes with viral RNA-dependent DNA polymerase, an enzyme necessary for viral HIV replication. **Therapeutic Effect:** Slows HIV replication, reducing progression of HIV infection.

PHARMACOKINETICS

Rapidly, completely absorbed from GI tract. Protein binding: 25%–38%. Undergoes first-pass metabolism in liver. Crosses blood-brain barrier and is widely distributed, including to CSF. Primarily excreted in urine. Minimal removal by hemodialysis. **Half-life:** 0.5–3 hrs (increased in renal impairment).

USES

Treatment of HIV infection in combination with other antiretroviral agents. Prevention of maternal/fetal HIV transmission. **OFF-LABEL:** Prophylaxis in health care workers at risk for acquiring HIV after occupational exposure.

PRECAUTIONS

Contraindications: Life-threatening allergic reactions to zidovudine or its components. **Cautions:** Bone marrow compromise, renal/hepatic dysfunction, decreased hepatic blood flow.

LIFESPAN CONSIDERATIONS

Pregnancy/Lactation: Unknown if drug crosses placenta or is distributed in breast milk. Unknown if fetal harm or effects on fertility can occur. **Pregnancy Category C.** **Children:** No age-related precautions noted. **Elderly:** Information not available.

INTERACTIONS

DRUG: **Bone marrow depressants, ganciclovir** may increase myelosuppression. **Clarithromycin** may decrease concentration. May be antagonistic with **doxorubicin.** Hematologic toxicities may occur with **interferon alfa. Probenecid** may increase concentration, risk of toxicity. **HERBAL:** None significant. **FOOD:** None known. **LAB VALUES:** May increase mean corpuscular volume (MCV).

AVAILABILITY (Rx)

Capsules (Retrovir): 100 mg. **Injection Solution (Retrovir):** 10 mg/ml. **Syrup (Retrovir):** 50 mg/5 ml. **Tablets (Retrovir):** 300 mg.

ADMINISTRATION/HANDLING

IV

Reconstitution • Must dilute before administration. • Remove calculated dose from vial and add to D_5W to provide concentration no greater than 4 mg/ml.

Rate of administration • Infuse over 1 hr. May infuse over 30 min in neonates.

Storage • After dilution, IV solution is stable for 24 hrs at room temperature; 48 hrs if refrigerated. • Use within 8 hrs if stored at room temperature or 24 hrs if refrigerated. • Do not use if solution is discolored or precipitate forms.

PO

• Keep capsules in cool, dry place. Protect from light. • Food, milk do not affect GI absorption. • Space doses evenly around the clock. • Pt should be in upright position when giving medication to prevent esophageal ulceration.

IV INCOMPATIBILITY

None known.

IV COMPATIBILITIES

Dexamethasone (Decadron), dobutamine (Dobutrex), dopamine (Intropin), heparin, lipids, lorazepam (Ativan), morphine, potassium chloride.

INDICATIONS/ROUTES/DOSAGE

HIV Infection

PO: ADULTS, ELDERLY, CHILDREN OLDER THAN 12 YRS: 200 mg q8h or 300 mg q12h. **CHILDREN 12 YRS AND YOUNGER:**

160 mg/m²/dose q8h or 240 mg/m² q12h. **NEONATES:** 2 mg/kg/dose q6h.
IV: ADULTS, ELDERLY, CHILDREN OLDER THAN 12 YRS: 1 mg/kg/dose q4h around the clock. **CHILDREN 12 YRS AND YOUNGER:** 120 mg/m²/dose q6h. **NEONATES:** 1.5 mg/kg/dose q6h.

Prevention of Maternal/Fetal HIV Transmission

PO: ADULTS: 100 mg 5 times/day, 200 mg 3 times/day, or 300 mg 2 times/day. Begin at 14–34 wks' gestation and continue until start of labor.
IV (DURING LABOR AND DELIVERY): 2 mg/kg loading dose, then IV infusion of 1 mg/kg/hr until umbilical cord clamped. **NEONATAL:** Begin 6–12 hrs after birth and continue for first 6 wks of life. Use IV route only until oral therapy can be administered.
PO: FULL-TERM INFANTS: 2 mg/kg/dose q6h (IV: 1.5 mg/kg/dose q6h). **INFANTS 30–34 WKS' GESTATION:** 2 mg/kg/dose q12h; increase to q8h at 2 wks of age (IV: 1.5 mg/kg/dose q12h; increase to q8h at 2 wks of age). **INFANTS LESS THAN 30 WKS' GESTATION:** 2 mg/kg/dose q12h; increase to q8h at 4 wks of age (IV: 1.5 mg/kg/dose q12h; increase to 8qh at 4 wks of age).

Dosage in Renal Impairment

Creatinine clearance less than 15 ml/min, including hemodialysis or peritoneal dialysis: 100 mg PO or 1 mg/kg IV q6–8h.

SIDE EFFECTS

Expected (46%–42%): Nausea, headache. **Frequent (20%–16%):** Abdominal pain, asthenia (loss of strength, energy), rash, fever, acne. **Occasional (12%–8%):** Diarrhea, anorexia, malaise, myalgia, drowsiness. **Rare (6%–5%):** Dizziness, paresthesia, vomiting, insomnia, dyspnea, altered taste.

ADVERSE EFFECTS/ TOXIC REACTIONS

Anemia (occurring most commonly after 4–6 wks of therapy), granulocytopenia are particularly significant in pts with pre-therapy low baselines. Neurotoxicity (ataxia, fatigue, lethargy, nystagmus, seizures) may occur.

NURSING CONSIDERATIONS

BASELINE ASSESSMENT

Avoid drugs that are nephrotoxic, cytotoxic, myelosuppressive; may increase risk of toxicity. Obtain specimens for viral diagnostic tests before starting therapy (therapy may begin before results are obtained). Check hematology reports for accurate baseline.

INTERVENTION/EVALUATION

Monitor CBC, Hgb, MCV, reticulocyte count, CD4 cell count, HIV RNA plasma levels. Check for bleeding. Assess for headache, dizziness. Monitor daily pattern of bowel activity, stool consistency. Evaluate skin for acne, rash. Be alert to development of opportunistic infections (fever, chills, cough, myalgia). Monitor I&O, serum renal/hepatic function tests. Check for insomnia.

PATIENT/FAMILY TEACHING

• Doses should be evenly spaced around the clock. • Zidovudine is not a cure for HIV infection, nor does it reduce risk of transmission to others. Acts to reduce symptoms and slows or arrests progress of disease. • Do not take any medications without physician's approval. • Bleeding from gums, nose, rectum may occur and should be reported to physician immediately. • Blood counts are essential because of bleeding potential. • Dental work should be done before therapy or after blood counts return to normal (often wks after therapy has stopped). • Inform physician if muscle weakness, difficulty breathing, headache, inability to sleep, unusual bleeding, rash, signs of infection occur.

zileuton

zye-**lew**-ton
(Zyflo CR)

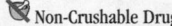

CLASSIFICATION

PHARMACOTHERAPEUTIC: Leukotriene inhibitor. **CLINICAL:** Antiasthma.

ACTION

Inhibits the enzyme responsible for producing inflammatory response. Prevents formation of leukotrienes (leukotrienes induce bronchoconstriction response, enhance vascular permeability, stimulate mucus secretion). **Therapeutic Effect:** Prevents airway edema, smooth muscle contraction, inflammatory process, relieving signs/symptoms of bronchial asthma.

PHARMACOKINETICS

Rapidly, completely absorbed following oral administration. Protein binding: 93%. Metabolized in liver. Eliminated in feces. Not removed by dialysis. **Half-life:** 2.5 hrs.

USES

Prophylaxis and chronic treatment of asthma. Not for use in reversal of bronchospasm in acute asthma attacks, status asthmaticus, exercise-induced bronchospasm.

PRECAUTIONS

Contraindications: Active hepatic disease, hepatic impairment. **Cautions:** History of alcoholism, history of hepatic disease.

LIFESPAN CONSIDERATIONS

Pregnancy/Lactation: Unknown if distributed in breast milk. **Pregnancy Category C.** **Children:** Safety and efficacy not established in those younger than 12 yrs. **Elderly:** No age-related precautions noted.

INTERACTIONS

DRUG: May increase concentration/toxicity of **calcium channel blockers (e.g., nifedipine), cyclosporine, theophylline.** Increases PT in those receiving **warfarin.** May increase effects of **beta-blockers (e.g., propranolol).** **HERBAL:** None significant. **FOOD:** None known. **LAB VALUES:** May increase ALT.

AVAILABILITY (Rx)

Tablets, Extended-Release: 600 mg.

ADMINISTRATION/HANDLING

• Give without regard to food. • Do not crush, chew extended-release tablets.

INDICATIONS/ROUTES/DOSAGE

Bronchial Asthma

PO: ADULTS, ELDERLY, CHILDREN 12 YRS AND OLDER: 1,200 mg twice daily within 1 hr after morning and evening meal. Total daily dosage: 2,400 mg.

SIDE EFFECTS

Frequent (25%): Headache. **Occasional (8–3%):** Dyspepsia, nausea, abdominal pain, asthenia (loss of strength, energy), myalgia. **Rare (1%):** Conjunctivitis, constipation, dizziness, flatulence, insomnia.

ADVERSE EFFECTS/ TOXIC REACTIONS

Hepatic dysfunction occurs rarely and may be manifested as right upper quadrant pain, nausea, fatigue, lethargy, pruritus, jaundice, or flulike symptoms.

NURSING CONSIDERATIONS

BASELINE ASSESSMENT

Obtain baseline hepatic function tests before therapy begins, monthly for the first 3 mos, and q2–3mos for the remainder of the first yr and periodically thereafter during long-term therapy.

INTERVENTION/EVALUATION

Monitor rate, depth, rhythm, type of respirations; quality, rate of pulse. Assess lung sounds for rhonchi, wheezing, rales. Observe lips, fingernails for blue or dusky color in light-skinned pts, gray in dark-skinned pts. Monitor hepatic function test results.

PATIENT/FAMILY TEACHING

• Increase fluid intake (decreases lung secretion, viscosity). • Take as prescribed, even during symptom-free periods and during worsening asthma. • Do not alter/stop other asthma medications. • Drug is not for treatment of acute asthma attacks. • Report right upper quadrant pain, nausea, fatigue, yellowing of skin/eyes, flulike symptoms.

ziprasidone

zye-**pray**-za-done
(Geodon, Zeldox ✱)

BLACK BOX ALERT Increased risk of mortality in elderly pts with dementia-related psychosis, mainly due to pneumonia, heart failure.

CLASSIFICATION

PHARMACOTHERAPEUTIC: Piperazine derivative. **CLINICAL:** Antipsychotic (see p. 66C).

ACTION

Antagonizes alpha-adrenergic, dopamine, histamine, serotonin receptors; inhibits reuptake of serotonin, norepinephrine. **Therapeutic Effect:** Diminishes symptoms of schizophrenia, depression.

PHARMACOKINETICS

Well absorbed after PO administration. Food increases bioavailability. Protein binding: 99%. Extensively metabolized in liver. Eliminated in feces. Not removed by hemodialysis. **Half-life: PO:** 7 hrs; **IM:** 2–5 hrs.

USES

Treatment of schizophrenia, acute bipolar mania, acute agitation in pts with schizophrenia. **OFF-LABEL:** Tourette's syndrome, psychosis/agitation related to Alzheimer's dementia.

PRECAUTIONS

Contraindications: Conditions associated with risk of prolonged QT interval, congenital long QT syndrome. **Cautions:** Pts with bradycardia, hypokalemia, hypomagnesemia may be at greater risk for torsade de pointes (atypical ventricular tachycardia).

LIFESPAN CONSIDERATIONS

Pregnancy/Lactation: Unknown if drug crosses placenta or is distributed in breast milk. **Pregnancy Category C. Children:** Safety and efficacy not established. **Elderly:** No age-related precautions noted.

INTERACTIONS

DRUG: Alcohol, other CNS depressants may increase CNS depression. **Carbamazepine** may decrease concentration. **Ketoconazole** may increase concentration. **Medications causing prolongation of QT interval (e.g., amiodarone, dofetilide, sotalol)** may increase effects on cardiac conduction leading to malignant arrhythmias (e.g., torsade de pointes). **HERBAL: Gotu kola, kava kava, St. John's wort, valerian** may increase CNS depression. **FOOD: All foods** enhance bioavailability. **LAB VALUES:** May prolong QT interval. May increase serum glucose, prolactin levels.

AVAILABILITY (Rx)

Capsules: 20 mg, 40 mg, 60 mg, 80 mg. **Injection, Powder for Reconstitution:** 20 mg.

ADMINISTRATION/HANDLING

IM

• Store vials at room temperature; protect from light. • Reconstitute each vial with 1.2 ml Sterile Water for Injection to provide concentration of 20 mg/ml. • Reconstituted solution stable for 24 hrs at room temperature or 7 days if refrigerated.

PO

• Give with food (increases bioavailability).

INDICATIONS/ROUTES/DOSAGE

Schizophrenia

PO: ADULTS, ELDERLY: Initially, 20 mg twice daily with food. Titrate at intervals of no less than 2 days. Range: 20–100 mg twice daily.

Acute Agitation (Schizophrenia)

IM: ADULTS, ELDERLY: 10 mg q2h or 20 mg q4h. **Maximum:** 40 mg/day.

Mania in Bipolar Disorder

PO: ADULTS, ELDERLY: Initially, 40 mg twice daily. May increase to 60–80 mg twice daily on second day of treatment. Range: 40–80 mg twice daily.

SIDE EFFECTS

Frequent (30%–16%): Headache, drowsiness, dizziness. **Occasional:** Rash, orthostatic hypotension, weight gain, restlessness, constipation, dyspepsia (heartburn, indigestion, epigastric pain). **Rare:** Hyperglycemia, priapism.

ADVERSE EFFECTS/ TOXIC REACTIONS

Prolongation of QT interval (as seen on EKG) may produce torsade de pointes, a form of ventricular tachycardia. Pts with bradycardia, hypokalemia, hypomagnesemia are at increased risk.

NURSING CONSIDERATIONS

BASELINE ASSESSMENT

Assess pt's behavior, appearance, emotional status, response to environment, speech pattern, thought content. EKG should be obtained to assess for QT prolongation before instituting medication. Blood chemistry for serum magnesium, potassium should be obtained before beginning therapy and routinely thereafter.

INTERVENTION/EVALUATION

Assess for therapeutic response (greater interest in surroundings, improved self-care, increased ability to concentrate, relaxed facial expression). Monitor weight.

PATIENT/FAMILY TEACHING

• Avoid tasks that require alertness, motor skills until response to drug is established. • Avoid alcohol.

zoledronic acid

zoe-le-dron-ik
(Aclasta, Reclast, Zometa)
Do not confuse Zometa with Zofran or Zoladex.

◆CLASSIFICATION

PHARMACOTHERAPEUTIC: Bisphosphonate. **CLINICAL:** Calcium regulator, bone resorption inhibitor.

ACTION

Inhibits resorption of mineralized bone, cartilage; inhibits increased osteoclastic activity, skeletal calcium release induced by stimulatory factors released by tumors. **Therapeutic Effect:** Increases urinary calcium, phosphorus excretion; decreases serum calcium, phosphorus levels.

USES

Zometa: Treatment of hypercalcemia of malignancy, bone metastases of solid tumors. Treatment of multiple myeloma. **Reclast:** Treatment and prevention of postmenopausal osteoporosis, glucocorticoid-induced osteoporosis, treatment of Paget's disease. Treatment of osteoporosis in men to increase bone mass. **OFF-LABEL:** Prophylaxis of bone metastases from breast, prostate cancer, treatment of bone diseases.

PRECAUTIONS

Contraindications: Hypersensitivity to other bisphosphonates, including alendronate, etidronate, pamidronate, risedronate, tiludronate. **Cautions:** History of aspirin-sensitive asthma, renal impairment, hypoparathyroidism, risk of hypocalcemia.

LIFESPAN CONSIDERATIONS

Pregnancy/Lactation: Unknown if drug crosses placenta or is distributed in breast milk. **Pregnancy Category D. Children:** Safety and efficacy not established.

Elderly: Age-related renal impairment may require dosage adjustment.

INTERACTIONS

DRUG: None significant. **HERBAL:** None significant. **FOOD:** None known. **LAB VALUES:** May decrease serum magnesium, calcium, phosphate.

AVAILABILITY (Rx)

Injection Solution (Zometa): 4 mg/5 ml. **(Reclast):** 5 mg diluted in 100 ml.

ADMINISTRATION/HANDLING

◀ALERT▶ Pt should be adequately rehydrated before administration of zoledronic acid.

IV

Reconstitution • Further dilute Zometa with 100 ml 0.9% NaCl or D_5W.

Rate of administration • Adequate hydration is essential in conjunction with zoledronic acid. • Administer as IV infusion over not less than 15 min (increases risk of deterioration in renal function).

Storage • Store intact vials at room temperature. • Infusion of solution must be completed within 24 hrs.

IV INCOMPATIBILITIES

Do not mix with other medications.

INDICATIONS/ROUTES/DOSAGE

Hypercalcemia

IV INFUSION: ADULTS, ELDERLY: 4 mg IV infusion given over no less than 15 min. Retreatment may be considered, but at least 7 days should elapse to allow for full response to initial dose.

Multiple Myeloma, Bone Metastases of Solid Tumors

IV: ADULTS, ELDERLY: 4 mg q3–4wk.

Paget's Disease

IV: ADULTS, ELDERLY: 5 mg as a single dose. Data about retreatment not available.

Osteoporosis Treatment

IV: ADULTS, ELDERLY: 5 mg once yearly.

Prevention of Glucocorticoid-Induced Osteoporosis

IV: ADULTS, ELDERLY: 5 mg once yearly.

Prevention of Postmenopausal Osteoporosis

IV: ADULTS, ELDERLY: 5 mg once q2yrs.

Dosage in Renal Impairment

Reclast: **Creatinine clearance less than 35 ml/min:** Not recommended.

Zometa:

Creatinine Clearance	Dosage
50–60 ml/min	3.5 mg
40–49 ml/min	3.3 mg
30–39 ml/min	3 mg
Less than 30 ml/min	Not recommended

SIDE EFFECTS

Frequent (44%–26%): Fever, nausea, vomiting, constipation. **Occasional (15%–10%):** Hypotension, anxiety, insomnia, flulike symptoms (fever, chills, bone pain, myalgia, arthralgia). **Rare:** Conjunctivitis.

ADVERSE EFFECTS/ TOXIC REACTIONS

Renal toxicity may occur if IV infusion is administered in less than 15 min.

NURSING CONSIDERATIONS

BASELINE ASSESSMENT

Prior to initiation, obtain dental exam for pts at risk for osteonecrosis. Establish baseline serum electrolytes, creatinine.

INTERVENTION/EVALUATION

Monitor serum renal function, CBC, Hgb, Hct. Assess vertebral bone mass (document stabilization, improvement). Monitor serum calcium, phosphate, magnesium, creatinine levels. Assess for fever. Monitor food intake, daily pattern of bowel activity, stool consistency. Check I&O, BUN, serum creatinine in pts with renal impairment.

zolmitriptan

zole-mih-**trip**-tan
(Zomig, Zomig Rapimelt ♣, Zomig-ZMT)
Do not confuse zolmitriptan with sumatriptan.

CLASSIFICATION

PHARMACOTHERAPEUTIC: Serotonin receptor agonist. **CLINICAL:** Antimigraine (see p. 63C).

ACTION

Binds selectively to vascular receptors, producing vasoconstrictive effect on cranial blood vessels. **Therapeutic Effect:** Relieves migraine headache.

PHARMACOKINETICS

Well absorbed after PO administration. Protein binding: 25%. Undergoes first-pass metabolism in liver to active metabolite. Eliminated primarily in urine (60%) and, to lesser extent, in feces (30%). **Half-life:** 2.8–3.7 hrs.

USES

Treatment of acute migraine attack with or without aura.

PRECAUTIONS

Contraindications: Arrhythmias associated with conduction disorders (e.g., Wolff-Parkinson-White syndrome), basilar or hemiplegic migraine, coronary artery disease, ischemic heart disease (including angina pectoris, history of MI, silent ischemia, Prinzmetal's angina), uncontrolled hypertension, use within 24 hrs of ergotamine-containing preparations or another serotonin receptor agonist, MAOI used within 14 days. **Cautions:** Mild to moderate renal/hepatic impairment, pt profile suggesting cardiovascular risks, controlled hypertension, history of CVA.

LIFESPAN CONSIDERATIONS

Pregnancy/Lactation: Unknown if drug is distributed in breast milk. **Pregnancy Category C. Children:** Safety and efficacy not established in those younger than 12 yrs. **Elderly:** No age-related precautions noted.

INTERACTIONS

DRUG: Ergotamine-containing medications may produce vasospastic reaction. **Fluoxetine, fluvoxamine, paroxetine, sertraline** may produce hyperreflexia, incoordination, weakness. **MAOIs** may dramatically increase concentration. **Oral contraceptives** decrease clearance, volume of distribution. **HERBAL:** None significant. **FOOD:** None known. **LAB VALUES:** None significant.

AVAILABILITY (Rx)

Nasal Spray (Zomig): 5 mg/0.1 ml. **Tablets (Zomig):** 2.5 mg, 5 mg.

Tablets (Orally-Disintegrating [Zomig-ZMT]): 2.5 mg, 5 mg.

ADMINISTRATION/HANDLING

PO

• Give without regard to food. Tablets may be crushed.

Orally-Disintegrating Tablet

• Must take whole; do not break, cut, chew. • Place on tongue, allow to dissolve. • Not necessary to administer with liquid.

Nasal

• Instruct pt to clear nasal passages as much as possible before use. • With head upright, pt should close one nostril with index finger, breathe out gently through mouth. • Instruct pt to insert nozzle into open nostril about ½ inch, close mouth, and while taking a breath through nose, release spray dosage by firmly pressing plunger. • Have pt remove nozzle from nose, gently breathe in through nose and out through mouth for 15–20 sec. Tell pt to avoid breathing in deeply.

INDICATIONS/ROUTES/DOSAGE

Acute Migraine Attack

PO: ADULTS, ELDERLY, CHILDREN OLDER THAN 18 YRS: Initially, 2.5 mg or less (may break tablet). If headache returns, may repeat dose after 2 hrs. **Maximum:** 10 mg/24 hrs.
ORALLY-DISINTEGRATING TABLET: ADULTS, ELDERLY: 2.5 mg at onset of migraine headache. If headache returns, may repeat dose after 2 hrs. **Maximum:** 10 mg/24 hrs.
INTRANASAL: ADULTS, ELDERLY: 5 mg (one spray). If headache returns, may repeat dose after 2 hrs. **Maximum:** 10 mg/24 hrs.

SIDE EFFECTS

Frequent (8%–6%): PO: Dizziness; paresthesia, neck/throat/jaw pressure; drowsiness. **Nasal:** Altered taste, paresthesia. **Occasional (5%–3%): PO:** Warm/hot sensation, asthenia (loss of strength, energy), chest pressure. **Nasal:** Nausea, drowsiness, nasal discomfort, dizziness, asthenia (loss of strength, energy), dry mouth. **Rare (2%–1%):** Diaphoresis, myalgia.

ADVERSE EFFECTS/ TOXIC REACTIONS

Cardiac events (ischemia, coronary artery vasospasm, MI), noncardiac vasospasm-related reactions (hemorrhage, stroke) occur rarely, particularly in pts with hypertension, diabetes, strong family history of coronary artery disease; obesity, smokers; males older than 40 yrs; postmenopausal women.

NURSING CONSIDERATIONS

BASELINE ASSESSMENT

Question for history of peripheral vascular disease, coronary artery disease, renal/hepatic impairment, MAOI use. Question pt regarding onset, location, duration of migraine, possible precipitating symptoms.

INTERVENTION/EVALUATION

Monitor for evidence of dizziness. Monitor B/P, esp. in pts with hepatic impairment. Assess for relief of migraine headache, migraine potential for photophobia, phonophobia (sound sensitivity, light sensitivity, nausea, vomiting).

PATIENT/FAMILY TEACHING

• Take single dose as soon as symptoms of actual migraine attack appear. • Medication is intended to relieve migraine, not to prevent or reduce number of attacks. • Lie down in quiet dark room for additional benefit after taking medication. • Avoid tasks that require alertness, motor skills until response to drug is established. • Report chest pain, palpitations, tightness in throat, edema of face, lips, eyes, rash, easy bruising, blood in urine/stool, pain/numbness in arms/legs.

zolpidem

zole pi dem
(Ambien, Ambien CR, Edluar)
Do not confuse Ambien with Abilify or ativan, or zolpidem with lorazepam or zaleplon.

◆CLASSIFICATION

PHARMACOTHERAPEUTIC: Nonbenzodiazepine. **CLINICAL:** Sedative-hypnotic **(Schedule IV)** (see p. 150C).

ACTION

Enhances action of inhibitory neurotransmitter gamma-aminobutyric acid (GABA). **Therapeutic Effect:** Induces sleep with fewer nightly awakenings, improves sleep quality.

PHARMACOKINETICS

Route	Onset	Peak	Duration
PO	30 min	N/A	6–8 hrs

Rapidly absorbed from GI tract. Protein binding: 92%. Metabolized in liver; excreted in urine. Not removed by hemodialysis. **Half-life:** 1.4–4.5 hrs (increased in hepatic impairment).

USES

Short-term treatment of insomnia. Reduces sleep-induction time, number of nocturnal awakenings; increases length of sleep; improves sleep quality.

PRECAUTIONS

Contraindications: None known. **Cautions:** Hepatic impairment, pts with depression, history of drug dependence.

LIFESPAN CONSIDERATIONS

Pregnancy/Lactation: Unknown if drug crosses placenta or is distributed in breast milk. **Pregnancy Category C.** **Children:** Safety and efficacy not established. **Elderly:** More likely to experience falls or confusion; decreased initial doses recommended. Age-related hepatic impairment may require dosage adjustment.

INTERACTIONS

DRUG: **Alcohol, other CNS depressants** may increase CNS depression. **HERBAL:** **Gotu kola, kava kava, St. John's wort, valerian** may increase CNS depression. **FOOD:** None known. **LAB VALUES:** None significant.

AVAILABILITY (Rx)

Tablets (Ambien): 5 mg, 10 mg. **Tablets (Sublingual [Edluar]):** 5 mg, 10 mg.

Tablets (Extended-Release [Ambien CR]): 6.25 mg, 12.5 mg.

ADMINISTRATION/HANDLING

PO

• For faster sleep onset, do not give with or immediately after a meal. • Do not split, crush, chew Ambien CR tablets. Swallow whole. • Edluar sublingual tablets to be placed under tongue and allowed to disintegrate. Do not swallow or administer with water.

INDICATIONS/ROUTES/DOSAGE

Insomnia

PO, SUBLINGUAL: ADULTS: 10 mg immediately before bedtime. **ELDERLY, DEBILITATED:** 5 mg immediately before bedtime.

PO (EXTENDED-RELEASE): ADULTS: 12.5 mg immediately before bedtime. **ELDERLY, DEBILITATED:** 6.25 mg immediately before bedtime.

SIDE EFFECTS

Occasional (7%): Headache. **Rare (less than 2%):** Dizziness, nausea, diarrhea, muscle pain.

ADVERSE EFFECTS/ TOXIC REACTIONS

Overdose may produce severe ataxia (clumsiness, unsteadiness), bradycardia, diplopia, severe drowsiness, nausea, vomiting, difficulty breathing, unconsciousness. Abrupt withdrawal following long-term use may produce weakness, facial flushing, diaphoresis, vomiting, tremor. Drug tolerance/dependence may occur with prolonged use of high dosages.

NURSING CONSIDERATIONS

BASELINE ASSESSMENT

Assess B/P, pulse, respirations, mental status, sleep patterns. Raise bed rails, provide call light. Provide environment conducive to sleep (back rub, quiet environment, low lighting).

INTERVENTION/EVALUATION

Monitor sleep pattern of pt. Evaluate for therapeutic response to insomnia: decrease in number of nocturnal awakenings, increase in length of sleep. Monitor daytime alertness, respiratory rate, behavior profile.

PATIENT/FAMILY TEACHING

• Do not abruptly discontinue medication after long-term use. • Avoid alcohol, tasks that require alertness, motor skills until response to drug is established. • Tolerance, dependence may occur with prolonged use of high dosages.

zonisamide

zoh-**nis**-a-mide
(Zonegran)
Do not confuse Zonegran with Sinequan or zonisamide with lacosamide.

◆CLASSIFICATION

PHARMACOTHERAPEUTIC: Succinimide. **CLINICAL:** Anticonvulsant (see p. 36C).

ACTION

May stabilize neuronal membranes, suppress neuronal hypersynchronization by blocking sodium, calcium channels. **Therapeutic Effect:** Reduces seizure activity.

PHARMACOKINETICS

Well absorbed after PO administration. Metabolized in liver. Extensively bound to RBCs. Protein binding: 40%. Primarily excreted in urine. **Half-life:** 63 hrs (plasma), 105 hrs (RBCs).

USES

Adjunctive therapy in treatment of partial seizures in adults, children older than 16 yrs with epilepsy. **OFF-LABEL:** Treatment of bulimia, bipolar disorder, obesity.

PRECAUTIONS

Contraindications: Allergy to sulfonamides. **Cautions:** Renal/hepatic impairment.

LIFESPAN CONSIDERATIONS

Pregnancy/Lactation: Unknown if distributed in breast milk. **Pregnancy Category C. Children:** Safety and efficacy not established in those younger than 16 yrs. **Elderly:** No age-related precautions noted, but lower dosages recommended.

INTERACTIONS

DRUG: Alcohol, other CNS depressants may increase sedative effect. **Carbamazepine, phenobarbital, phenytoin, valproic acid** may increase metabolism, decrease effect. **HERBAL:** None significant. **FOOD:** None known. **LAB VALUES:** May increase BUN, serum creatinine.

AVAILABILITY (Rx)

Capsules: 25 mg, 50 mg, 100 mg.

ADMINISTRATION/HANDLING

PO

• May give with or without food. • Do not crush, break capsules. Swallow capsules whole. • Do not give to pts allergic to sulfonamides.

INDICATIONS/ROUTES/DOSAGE

Partial Seizures

PO: ADULTS, ELDERLY, CHILDREN OLDER THAN 16 YRS: Initially, 100 mg/day. May increase to 200 mg/day after 2 wks. Further increases to 300 mg/day and 400 mg/day can be made with minimum of 2 wks between adjustments. Range: 100–600 mg/day.

SIDE EFFECTS

Frequent (17%–9%): Drowsiness, dizziness, anorexia, headache, agitation, irritability, nausea. **Occasional (8%–5%):** Fatigue, ataxia, confusion, depression, impaired memory/concentration, insomnia, abdominal pain, diplopia, diarrhea, speech difficulty. **Rare (4%–3%):** Paresthesia, nystagmus, anxiety, rash, dyspepsia (heartburn, indigestion, epigastric pain), weight loss.

ADVERSE EFFECTS/ TOXIC REACTIONS

Overdose characterized by bradycardia, hypotension, respiratory depression, coma. Leukopenia, anemia, thrombocytopenia occur rarely.

NURSING CONSIDERATIONS

BASELINE ASSESSMENT

Review history of seizure disorder (intensity, frequency, duration, LOC). Initiate seizure precautions. Serum hepatic function tests, CBC, platelet count should be performed before therapy begins and periodically during therapy.

INTERVENTION/EVALUATION

Observe frequently for recurrence of seizure activity. Assess for clinical improvement (decrease in intensity, frequency of seizures). Assist with ambulation if dizziness occurs.

PATIENT/FAMILY TEACHING

• Strict maintenance of drug therapy is essential for seizure control. • Avoid tasks that require alertness, motor skills until response to drug is established. • Avoid alcohol. • Report if rash, back/abdominal pain, blood in urine, fever, sore throat, ulcers in mouth, easy bruising occur. • Notify physician of worsening depression, unusual behavior, suicidal thoughts.

Appendixes

Appendix A
Calculation of Doses

Appendix B
Controlled Drugs (United States)

Appendix C
Drip Rates for Critical Care Medications

Appendix D
Drugs of Abuse

Appendix E
Equianalgesic Dosing

Appendix F
FDA Pregnancy Categories

Appendix G
Herbal Therapies and Interactions

Appendix H
Lifespan, Cultural Aspects, and Pharmacogenomics of Drug Therapy

Appendix I
Non-Crushable Drugs

Appendix J
Normal Laboratory Values

Appendix K
Orphan Drugs

Appendix L
Cytochrome P450 (CYP) Enzymes

Appendix M
Poison Antidote Chart

Appendix N
Preventing Medication Errors and Improving Medication Safety

Appendix O
Recommended Childhood and Adult Immunizations

Appendix P
Signs and Symptoms of Electrolyte Imbalance

Appendix Q
Parenteral Fluid Administration

Appendix R
Spanish Phrases Often Used in Clinical Settings

Appendix S
Techniques of Medication Administration

Appendix T
Chronic Wound Care

Appendix U
QT-Interval Prolongation and Medication Safety

Appendix A

CALCULATION OF DOSES

Frequently, dosages ordered do not correspond exactly to what is available and must be calculated.

RATIO/PROPORTION:
A pt is to receive 65 mg of a medication. It is available as 80 mg/2 ml. What volume (ml) needs to be administered to the patient?

STEP 1: Set up ratio.

$$\frac{80 \text{ mg}}{2 \text{ ml}} = \frac{65 \text{ mg}}{\text{x (ml)}}$$

STEP 2: Cross multiply and divide each side by the number with x to determine volume to be administered.

$$80 \text{ mg} \times (\text{x}) \text{ ml} = 65 \text{ mg} \times 2 \text{ ml}$$
$$80 \text{ x} = 130$$
$$\text{x} = \frac{130}{80} = 1.625 \text{ ml}$$

CALCULATIONS IN MICROGRAMS PER KILOGRAM PER MINUTE (mcg/kg/min):
A 63-year-old pt (weight 165 lb) is to receive medication A at a rate of 8 mcg/kg/min. Given a solution containing medication A in a concentration of 500 mg/250 ml, at what rate (ml/hr) would you infuse this medication?

STEP 1: Convert to same units. In this problem, the dose is expressed in mcg/kg; therefore, convert weight to kg (2.2 lb = 1 kg) and drug concentration to mcg/ml (1 mg = 1,000 mcg)

$$165 \text{ lb divided by } 2.2 = 75 \text{ kg}$$
$$\frac{500 \text{ mg}}{250 \text{ ml}} = \frac{2 \text{ mg}}{\text{ml}} = \frac{2{,}000 \text{ mcg}}{\text{ml}}$$

STEP 2: Number of mcg/hr.

$$(75 \text{ kg}) \times 8 \text{ mcg/kg/min} = 600 \text{ mcg/min or } 36{,}000 \text{ mcg/hr}$$

STEP 3: Number of ml/hr.

$$36{,}000 \text{ mcg/hr divided by } 2{,}000 \text{ mcg/ml} = 18 \text{ ml/hr}$$

Appendix B

CONTROLLED DRUGS (UNITED STATES)

Schedule I: Medications having no legal medical use. These substances may be used for research purposes with proper registration (e.g., heroin, LSD).

Schedule II: Medications having a legitimate medical use but are characterized by a very high abuse potential and/or potential for severe physical and psychic dependency. Emergency telephone orders for limited quantities of these drugs are authorized, but the prescriber must provide a written, signed prescription order (e.g., morphine, amphetamines).

Schedule III: Medications having significant abuse potential (less than Schedule II). Telephone orders are permitted (e.g., opiates in combination with other substances such as acetaminophen).

Schedule IV: Medications having a low abuse potential. Telephone orders are permitted (e.g., benzodiazepines, propoxyphene).

Schedule V: Medications having the lowest abuse potential of the controlled substances. Some Schedule V products may be available without a prescription (e.g., certain cough preparations containing limited amounts of an opiate).

Appendix C

DRIP RATES FOR CRITICAL CARE MEDICATIONS

Dobutamine

Dopamine

Heparin

Nitroglycerin

Norepinephrine

Propofol

Sodium Nitroprusside

DOBUTAMINE (Dobutrex)
Mix 250 mg in 250 ml D_5W (1,000 mcg/ml)

	Body Weight														
lb	88	99	110	121	132	143	154	165	176	187	198	209	220	231	242
kg	40	45	50	55	60	65	70	75	80	85	90	95	100	105	110
Dose ordered in mcg/kg/min	***Amount to infuse in mcgtts/min or ml/hr***														
2.5	6	7	8	8	9	10	11	11	12	13	14	14	15	16	17
5	12	14	15	17	18	20	21	23	24	26	27	29	30	32	33
7.5	18	20	23	25	27	29	32	34	36	38	41	43	45	47	50
10	24	27	30	33	36	39	42	45	48	51	54	57	60	63	66
12.5	30	34	38	41	45	49	53	56	60	64	68	71	75	79	83
15	36	41	45	50	54	59	63	68	72	77	81	86	90	95	99
20	48	54	60	66	72	78	84	90	96	102	108	114	120	126	132
25	60	68	75	83	90	98	105	113	120	128	135	143	150	158	165
30	72	81	90	99	108	117	126	135	144	153	162	171	180	189	198
35	84	95	105	116	126	137	147	158	168	179	189	200	210	221	231
40	96	108	120	132	144	156	168	180	192	204	216	228	240	252	264

- Administer 2.5–10 mcg/kg/min initially.
- Increase in increments of 5–10 mcg up to 40 mcg/kg/min as needed.
- Do not mix with sodium bicarbonate.

DOPAMINE (Intropin)
Mix 400 mg in 250 ml D_5W (1,600 mcg/ml)

Body Weight

Dose ordered in mcg/kg/min														
lb	88	99	110	121	132	143	154	165	176	187	198	209	220	231
kg	40	45	50	55	60	65	70	75	80	85	90	95	100	105
	Amount to infuse in mcgtts/min or ml/hr													
2.5	4	4	5	5	6	6	7	7	8	8	8	9	9	10
5	8	8	9	10	11	12	13	14	15	16	17	18	19	20
7.5	11	13	14	15	17	18	20	21	23	24	25	27	28	30
10	15	17	19	21	23	24	26	28	30	32	34	36	38	39
12.5	19	21	23	26	28	30	33	35	38	40	42	45	47	49
15	23	25	28	31	34	37	39	42	45	48	51	53	56	59
20	30	34	38	41	45	49	53	56	60	64	68	71	75	79
25	38	42	47	52	56	61	66	70	75	80	84	89	94	98
30	45	51	56	62	67	73	79	84	90	96	101	107	113	118
35	53	59	66	72	79	85	92	98	105	112	118	125	131	138
40	60	68	75	83	90	98	105	113	120	128	135	143	150	158
45	68	76	84	93	101	110	118	127	135	143	152	160	169	177
50	75	84	94	103	113	122	131	141	150	159	169	178	188	197

- Administer 2.5–5 mcg/kg/min initially.
- Increase in increments of 5–10 mcg to 50 mcg/kg/min as needed.
- Do not mix with sodium bicarbonate.

HEPARIN DRIP RATE CHART

ACT (sec)	aPTT (sec)	Bolus Dose (ml)	Stop Infusion (min)	Rate Change (ml/hr)	Repeat PTT (hr)	Repeat aPTT (hr)
1–200	1–49	5,000	0	+3 ml/hr (increase by 150 units/hr)	4	4
201–239	50–59	0	0	+2 ml/hr (increase by 100 units/hr)	4	4
240–300	60–85	0	0	0 (no change)	8	8
301–400	86–95	0	0	−1 ml/hr (decrease by 50 units/hr)	8	8
401–500	96–120	0	30	−2 ml/hr (decrease by 100 units/hr)	4	4
501+	121+	0	60	−3 ml/hr (decrease by 150 units/hr)	4	4

NITROGLYCERIN (Tridil)

Dose Ordered in mcg/min	50 mg/ 250 cc 100 mg/ 500 cc NTG/D_5W	100 mg/ 250 cc 200 mg/ 500 cc NTG/D_5W	Dose Ordered in mcg/min	50 mg/ 250 cc 100 mg/ 500 cc NTG/D_5W	100 mg/ 250 cc 200 mg/ 500 cc NTG/D_5W
10	3	—	210	63	32
20	6	3	220	66	33
30	9	5	230	69	35
40	12	6	240	72	36
50	15	8	250	75	38
60	18	9	260	78	39
70	21	10	270	81	41
80	24	12	280	84	42
90	27	14	290	87	44
100	30	15	300	90	45
110	33	17	310	93	47
120	36	18	320	96	48
130	39	19	330	99	50
140	42	21	340	102	51
150	45	23	350	105	53
160	48	24	360	108	54
170	51	26	370	111	56
180	54	27	380	114	57
190	57	29	390	117	59
200	60	30	400	120	60
	Amt to infuse in mcgtts/min or ml/hr			***Amt to infuse in mcgtts/min or ml/hr***	

- Administer 10–20 mcg/min initially.
- Increase in increments of 6–10 mcg/min every 5–10 min until desired response.

NOREPINEPHRINE (Levophed)
Mix: 4 mg in 250 ml D_5W
Norepinephrine 4 mg in 250 ml D_5W (rate is ml/hr)

	mcg/kg/min											
kg	0.01	0.02	0.03	0.04	0.05	0.06	0.07	0.08	0.09	0.10	0.20	0.30
50	1.9	3.8	5.7	7.6	9.5	11.4	13.3	15.2	17.1	19.0	38.0	57.0
55	2.1	4.2	6.3	8.4	10.5	12.6	14.7	16.8	18.9	21.0	42.0	63.0
60	2.3	4.6	6.9	9.2	11.5	13.8	16.1	18.4	20.7	23.0	46.0	69.0
65	2.4	4.8	7.2	9.6	12.0	14.4	16.8	19.2	21.6	24.0	48.0	72.0
70	2.6	5.2	7.8	10.4	13.0	15.6	18.2	20.8	23.4	26.0	52.0	78.0
75	2.8	5.6	8.4	11.2	14.0	16.8	19.6	22.4	25.2	28.0	56.0	84.0
80	3.0	6.0	9.0	12.0	15.0	18.0	21.0	24.0	27.0	30.0	60.0	90.0
85	3.2	6.4	9.6	12.8	16.0	19.2	22.4	25.6	28.8	32.0	64.0	96.0
90	3.4	6.8	10.2	13.6	17.0	20.4	23.8	27.2	30.6	34.0	68.0	102
95	3.6	7.2	10.8	14.4	18.0	21.6	25.2	28.8	32.4	36.0	72.0	108
100	3.8	7.6	11.4	15.2	19.0	22.8	26.6	30.4	34.2	38.0	76.0	114

Use: Hypotension, shock
Dose: 2–40 mcg/min or 0.05–0.25 mcg/kg/min; doses greater than 75 mcg/min or 1 mcg/kg/min have been used
Mechanism: Primary α_1 vasoconstriction effect (minor β_1 inotropic)
Elimination: Hepatic **Half-life:** Minutes
Adverse events: Tachyarrhythmias, hypertension at high doses

PROPOFOL (Diprivan)
Mix: Undiluted (10 mg/ml) 100-ml vial
Propofol 10 mg/ml (premixed) (rate is ml/hr)

	mcg/kg/min											
kg	10	15	20	25	30	35	40	45	50	55	60	65
50	3	5	6	8	9	11	12	14	15	17	18	20
55	3	5	7	8	10	12	13	15	17	18	20	21
60	4	5	7	9	11	13	14	16	18	20	22	23
65	4	6	8	10	12	14	16	18	20	21	23	25
70	4	6	8	11	13	15	17	19	21	23	25	27
75	5	7	9	11	14	16	18	20	23	25	27	29
80	5	7	10	12	14	17	19	22	24	26	29	31
85	5	8	10	13	15	18	20	23	26	28	31	33
90	5	8	11	14	16	19	22	24	27	30	32	35
95	6	9	11	14	17	20	23	26	29	31	34	37
100	6	9	12	15	18	21	24	27	30	33	36	39

Use: Nonamnestic sedation
Dose: Load 1–2 mg/kg IV push; **do not load if pt is hypotensive or volume depleted**
Maintenance: Initial dose of 5–20 mcg/kg/min, may titrate to effect (20–65 mcg/kg/min)
Mechanism: Di-isopropyl phenolic compound with intravenous general anesthetic properties unrelated to opiates, barbiturates, benzodiazepines
Elimination: Hepatic **Half-life:** 30 min
Adverse events: Hypotension, nausea, vomiting, seizures, hypertriglyceridemia, hyperlipidemia

SODIUM NITROPRUSSIDE (Nipride)
Mix: 50 mg in 250 ml D_5W (200 mcg/ml)

	Body Weight														
lb	88	99	110	121	132	143	154	165	176	187	198	209	220	231	242
kg	40	45	50	55	60	65	70	75	80	85	90	95	100	105	110
Dose ordered in mcg/kg/min	***Amount to infuse in mcgtts/min or ml/hr***														
0.5	6	7	8	8	9	10	11	11	12	13	14	14	15	16	17
1	12	14	15	17	18	20	21	23	24	26	27	29	30	32	33
1.5	13	20	23	25	27	29	32	34	36	38	41	43	45	47	50
2	24	27	30	33	36	39	42	45	48	51	54	57	60	63	66
3	36	41	45	50	54	59	63	68	72	77	81	86	90	95	99
4	48	54	60	66	72	78	84	90	96	102	108	114	120	126	132
5	60	68	75	83	90	98	105	113	120	128	135	143	150	158	165
6	72	81	90	99	108	117	126	135	144	153	162	171	180	189	198
7	84	95	105	116	126	137	147	158	168	179	189	200	210	221	231
8	96	108	120	132	144	156	168	180	192	204	216	228	240	252	264
9	108	122	135	149	162	176	189	203	216	230	243	257	270	284	297
10	120	135	150	165	180	195	210	225	240	255	270	285	300	315	330

- Administer 0.5–10 mcg/kg/min initially.
- Increase in increments of 1 mcg/kg/min until desired response.
- Do not leave solution exposed to light.

Appendix D

DRUGS OF ABUSE

Name (Brand)	Class	Signs and Symptoms	Treatment
Acid (see LSD)			
Adam (see MDMA)			
Amphetamine (Adderall, Dexedrine)	Stimulant	Tachycardia, hypertension, diaphoresis, agitation, headache, seizures, dehydration, hypokalemia, lactic acidosis. Severe overdose: hyperthermia, dysrhythmia, shock, rhabdomyolysis, hepatic necrosis, acute renal failure.	Control agitation, reverse hyperthermia, support hemodynamic function. **Antidote:** No specific antidote.
Angel dust (see phencyclidine)			
Apache (see fentanyl)			
Barbiturates (Nembutal, Seconal)	Depressant	Hypotension, hypothermia, apnea, nystagmus, ataxia, hyporeflexia, drowsiness, stupor, coma.	Airway management, decontamination, supportive care. **Antidote:** No specific antidote.
Barbs (see barbiturates)			
Benzodiazepines (Halcion, Librium, Valium, Xanax)	Depressant	Respiratory depression, hypothermia, hypotension, nystagmus, miosis, diplopia, bradycardia, nausea, vomiting, impaired speech and coordination, amnesia, ataxia, drowsiness, confusion, depressed deep tendon reflexes.	**Antidote:** Flumazenil (Romazicon).
Black tar (see heroin)			
Boomers (see LSD)			
Buttons (see mescaline)			
Cactus (see mescaline)			
Candy (see benzodiazepines)			
China girl (see fentanyl)			

Name (Brand)	Class	Signs and Symptoms	Treatment
China white (see heroin)			
Cocaine	Stimulant	Hypertension, tachycardia, mild hyperthermia, mydriasis, pallor, diaphoresis, psychosis, paranoid delusions, mania, agitation, seizures.	Control agitation, seizures, hyperthermia; support hemodynamic function. **Antidote:** No specific antidote.
Codeine	Opioid	Miosis, respiratory depression, decreased mental status, hypotension, cardiac dysrhythmia, hypoxia, bronchoconstriction, constipation, decreased intestinal motility, ileus, lethargy, coma.	Airway management, hemodynamic support. **Antidote:** Naloxone, nalmefene.
Coke (see cocaine)			
Crank (see amphetamine)			
Crank (see heroin)			
Crystal (see amphetamine)			
Crystal meth (see methamphetamine)			
Cubes (see LSD)			
Downers (see benzodiazepines)			
Ecstasy (see MDMA)			
Fentanyl (Sublimaze)	Opioid	Miosis, respiratory depression, decreased mental status, hypotension, cardiac dysrhythmia, hypoxia, bronchoconstriction, constipation, decreased intestinal motility, ileus, lethargy, coma.	Airway management, hemodynamic support. **Antidote:** Naloxone, nalmefene.
Flunitrazepam (Rohypnol)	Depressant	Drowsiness, slurred speech, impaired judgment and motor skills, hypothermia, hypotension, bradycardia, diplopia, blurred vision, nystagmus, respiratory depression, nausea, constipation, depression, lethargy, headache, ataxia, coma, amnesia, incoordination, tremors, vertigo.	Supportive care, airway control. **Antidote:** Flumazenil (Romazicon).
Forget me pill (see flunitrazepam)			

(continued)

Name (Brand)	Class	Signs and Symptoms	Treatment
GHB (gamma-hydroxybutyrate)	CNS depressant	Dose-related CNS depression, amnesia, hypotonia, drowsiness, dizziness, euphoria. Other effects: bradycardia, hypotension, hypersalivation, vomiting, hypothermia. Higher dosages: Cheyne-Stokes respiration, seizures, coma, death. Users may become highly agitated.	Supportive care. Severe intoxication may require airway support, including intubation. **Antidote:** No specific antidote.
Gib (see GHB)			
Goodfellas (see fentanyl)			
Grass (see marijuana)			
Hashish (see marijuana)			
Heroin	Opioid	Miosis, coma, apnea, pulmonary edema, bradycardia, hypotension, pinpoint pupils, CNS depression, seizures.	Airway management. **Antidote:** Naloxone, nalmefene.
Horse (see heroin)			
Ice (see amphetamine)			
Keets (see ketamine)			
Ketamine (Ketalar)	Anesthetic	Feeling of dissociation from one's self (sense of floating over one's body), visual hallucinations, lack of coordination, hypertension, tachycardia, palpitations, respiratory depression, apnea, confusion, negativism, hostility, delirium, reduced awareness.	Supportive care, esp. respiratory and cardiac function. **Antidote:** No specific antidote.
Kit-kat (see ketamine)			
Liquid ecstasy (see GHB)			
Liquid X (see GHB)			
LSD	Hallucinogen	Diaphoresis, mydriasis, dizziness, muscle twitching, flushing, hyperreflexia, hypertension, psychosis, behavioral changes, emotional lability, euphoria or dysphoria, paranoia, vomiting, diarrhea, anorexia, restlessness, incoordination, tremors, ataxia.	Airway management, control activity associated with hallucinations, psychosis, panic reaction. **Antidote:** No specific antidote.

Name (Brand)	Class	Signs and Symptoms	Treatment
Ludes (see methaqualone)			
Magic mushroom (see psilocybin)			
Marijuana	Cannabinoid	Increased appetite, reduced motility, constipation, urinary retention, seizures, euphoria, drowsiness, heightened awareness, relaxation, altered time perception, short-term memory loss, poor concentration, mood alterations, disorientation, decreased strength, ataxia, slurred speech, respiratory depression, coma.	Airway management, supportive care. **Antidote:** No specific antidote.
MDMA (Methylenedioxymethamphetamine)	Stimulant	Euphoria, intimacy, closeness to others, loss of appetite, tachycardia, jaw tension, bruxism, diaphoresis.	Airway management, supportive care. **Antidote:** No specific antidote.
Mescaline	Hallucinogen	Diaphoresis, mydriasis, dizziness, twitching, flushing, hyperreflexia, hypertension, psychosis, behavioral changes, emotional instability, euphoria or dysphoria, paranoia, vomiting, diarrhea, anorexia, restlessness, incoordination, tremors, ataxia.	Airway management, control activity associated with hallucinations, psychosis, panic reaction. **Antidote:** No specific antidote.
Meth (see methamphetamine)			
Methamphetamine (Desoxyn)	Stimulant	Hypertension, hyperthermia, hyperpyrexia, agitation, hyperactivity, fasciculation, seizures, coma, tachycardia, dysrhythmias, pale skin, diaphoresis, restlessness, talkativeness, insomnia, headache, coma, delusions, paranoia, aggressive behavior, visual, tactile, or auditory hallucinations.	Airway control, hyperthermia, seizures, dysrhythmias. **Antidote:** No specific antidote.

(continued)

Name (Brand)	Class	Signs and Symptoms	Treatment
Methaqualone (Quaalude)	Depressant	Slurred speech, impaired judgment and motor skills, hypothermia, hypotension, bradycardia, diplopia, blurred vision, nystagmus, mydriasis, respiratory depression, depression, lethargy, headache, ataxia, coma, amnesia, incoordination, hypertonicity, myoclonus, tremors, vertigo.	Airway management, supportive care. **Antidote:** No specific antidote.
Methylphenidate (Ritalin)	Stimulant	Agitation, hypertension, tachycardia, hyperthermia, mydriasis, dry mouth, nausea, vomiting, anorexia, abdominal pain, agitation, hyperactivity, insomnia, euphoria, dizziness, paranoid ideation, social withdrawal, delirium, hallucinations, psychosis, tremors, seizures.	Control agitation, hyperthermia, seizures; support hemodynamic function. **Antidote:** No specific antidote.
Miss Emma (see morphine)			
Mister blue (see morphine)			
Morphine (MS-Contin, Roxanol)	Opioid	Miosis, respiratory depression, decreased mental status, hypotension, cardiac dysrhythmia, hypoxia, bronchoconstriction, constipation, decreased intestinal motility, ileus, lethargy, coma.	Airway management, hemodynamic support. **Antidote:** Naloxone, nalmefene.
Oxy (see oxycodone)			
Oxycodone (OxyContin)	Opioid	Miosis, respiratory depression, decreased mental status, hypotension, cardiac dysrhythmia, hypoxia, bronchoconstriction, constipation, decreased intestinal motility, ileus, lethargy, coma.	Airway management, hemodynamic support. **Antidote:** Naloxone, nalmefene.
OxyContin (see oxycodone)			
Peace pill (see phencyclidine)			

Name (Brand)	Class	Signs and Symptoms	Treatment
Phencyclidine (PCP)	Hallucinogen	Nystagmus, hypertension, tachycardia, agitation, hallucinations, violent behavior, impaired judgment, delusions, psychosis.	Support B/P, manage airway, control agitation. **Antidote:** No specific antidote.
Phennies (see barbiturates)			
Pot (see marijuana)			
Psilocybin	Hallucinogen	Diaphoresis, mydriasis, dizziness, twitching, flushing, hyperreflexia, hypertension, psychosis, behavioral changes, emotional lability, euphoria or dysphoria, paranoia, vomiting, diarrhea, anorexia, restlessness, incoordination, tremors, ataxia.	Manage airway, control activity associated with hallucinations, psychosis, panic reaction. **Antidote:** No specific antidote.
Purple passion (see psilocybin)			
Quay (see methaqualone)			
Reefer (see marijuana)			
Rock (see cocaine)			
Rocket fuel (see phencyclidine)			
Roofies (see flunitrazepam)			
Rope (see flunitrazepam)			
Rophies (see flunitrazepam)			
Salty water (see GHB)			
Schoolboy (see codeine)			
Scoop (see GHB)			
Snow (see cocaine)			
Special K (see ketamine)			
Speed (see amphetamine)			
STP (see MDMA)			
Super acid (see ketamine)			
Super K (see ketamine)			
Tranks (see benzodiazepines)			

(continued)

Name (Brand)	Class	Signs and Symptoms	Treatment
Uppers (see amphetamine)			
White girl (see cocaine)			
Yellow jackets (see barbiturates)			
Yellow sunshine (see LSD)			

"CLUB DRUG" WEB SITES

www.drugfree.org	Partnership for a Drug-Free America
www.clubdrugs.org	Consumer-oriented site sponsored by the National Institute on Drug Abuse
www.health.org	Substance Abuse and Mental Health Services Administration
www.projectghb.org	Independent site devoted to risks and dangers of GHB use
www.nida.nih.gov	National Institute on Drug Abuse
www.dea.gov	Drug Enforcement Administration
www.whitehousedrugpolicy.org	Office of National Drug Control Policy

Appendix E

EQUIANALGESIC DOSING

Guidelines for equianalgesic dosing of commonly used analgesics are presented in the following table. The dosages are approximate to 10 mg of morphine intramuscularly. These guidelines are for the management of acute pain in the opioid-naive pt. Dosages may vary for the opioid-tolerant pt and for the management of chronic pain. Dosing adjustments for renal or hepatic insufficiency may also be necessary. Clinical response is the criterion that must be applied for each pt with titration to desired response.

Name	Equianalgesic Oral Dose	Equianalgesic Parenteral Dose (IV, IM, Subcutaneous)
Butorphanol (Stadol)	Not available	2 mg
Codeine	200 mg	100–130 mg
Fentanyl	Not available	0.1 mg (100 micrograms)
Hydrocodone	30–45 mg	Not available
Hydromorphone (Dilaudid)	7.5–8 mg	1.5–2 mg
Meperidine (Demerol)	300 mg	75–100 mg
Methadone (Dolophine)	10–20 mg	10 mg
Morphine	30 mg	10 mg
Nalbuphine (Nubain)	Not available	10 mg
Oxycodone (OxyContin)	20–30 mg	Not available
Oxymorphone	10 mg	1 mg

Appendix F

FDA PREGNANCY CATEGORIES

◀ALERT▶ Medications should be used during pregnancy only if clearly needed.

A: Adequate and well-controlled studies have failed to show a risk to the fetus in the first trimester of pregnancy (also, no evidence of risk has been seen in later trimesters). Possibility of fetal harm appears remote.

B: Animal reproduction studies have failed to show a risk to the fetus, and there are no adequate/well-controlled studies in pregnant women.

C: Animal reproduction studies have shown an adverse effect on the fetus, and there are no adequate/well-controlled studies in humans. However, the benefits may warrant use of the drug in pregnant women despite potential risks.

D: There is positive evidence of human fetal risk based on data from investigational or marketing experience or from studies in humans, but the potential benefits may warrant use of the drug despite potential risks (e.g., use in life-threatening situations in which other medications cannot be used or are ineffective).

X: Animal or human studies have shown fetal abnormalities and/or there is evidence of human fetal risk based on adverse reaction data from investigational or marketing experience where the risks of using the medication clearly outweigh potential benefits.

Appendix G

HERBAL THERAPIES AND INTERACTIONS

The use of herbal therapies is increasing in the United States. Because of the rise in the use of herbal therapy in the United States, the following is presented to provide some basic information on some of the more popular herbs. Please note this is not an all-inclusive list, which is beyond the scope of this handbook.

Name	Uses	Interactions	Precautions
Acai	Anti-inflammatory, reduces cholesterol, treats osteoarthritis, antibacterial, antioxidant.	None known.	None reported.
Aloe	***Topical:*** Promotes burn/wound healing, treatment of cold sores. ***Oral:*** Osteoarthritis, inflammatory bowel disease (e.g., ulcerative colitis).	***Topical:*** None known. ***Oral:*** Additive effect with antidiabetic agents, may increase adverse effects of digoxin, diuretics (due to hypokalemia).	***Topical:*** None known. ***Oral:*** Abdominal pain, diarrhea, reduced serum potassium.
Artichoke	Irritable bowel syndrome (IBS), dyspepsia, hangover due to alcohol, nausea, reduce cholesterol levels.	None known.	Well tolerated, may cause flatulence, allergic reactions.
Astaxanthin	***Oral:*** Macular degeneration, Alzheimer's disease, Parkinson's disease, stroke, cancer, hypercholesterolemia. ***Topical:*** Sunburn.	None known.	May cause visual disturbances.
Astragalus	Common cold, upper respiratory tract infections, strengthen and regulate immune system, fibromyalgia, anemia, chronic fatigue syndrome.	May reduce immunosuppression caused by cyclophosphamide. May decrease effects of immunosuppressive agents (e.g., azathioprine, cyclosporine, mycophenolate, sirolimus, tacrolimus).	May exacerbate autoimmune diseases (e.g., multiple sclerosis, rheumatoid arthritis). Avoid use in pregnancy (insufficient reliable information available).

(continued)

Name	Uses	Interactions	Precautions
Avocado	Reduces serum cholesterol, stimulates menstrual flow, treatment of osteoarthritis.	May reduce effects of warfarin.	Pts allergic to latex should avoid eating avocado due to possibility of cross sensitivity.
Bifidobacteria	Prevent acute diarrhea in children, necrotizing enterocolitis in neonates, traveler's diarrhea, improve immune function, replenish normal flora depleted by diarrhea, antibiotics.	Antibiotics may decrease effectiveness.	May cause pathogenic colonization in pts who are immunocompromised. Avoid use in pregnancy (insufficient reliable information available).
Bilberry	***Topical:*** Mild inflammation of mouth/throat. ***Oral:*** Improves visual acuity (e.g., night vision). Treatment of degenerative retinal conditions, atherosclerosis, hemorrhoids.	May require adjustment of antidiabetic drugs (reduces glucose effect).	May decrease serum glucose, triglycerides.
Bitter orange	Appetite stimulant, treatment of dyspepsia, weight loss, nasal congestion.	Can inhibit cytochrome P450 metabolism of drugs, causing increased drug levels, risk of adverse effects (e.g., felodipine [Plendil], indinavir [Crixivan], midazolam [Versed]).	Contains synephrine and octopamine, which may cause hypertension, cardiovascular toxicity. Avoid use in pregnancy when used for medicinal purposes. Safe when used orally in amounts found in foods.
Black cohosh*	Manages menopause symptoms, premenstrual syndrome (PMS), dysmenorrheal, dyspepsia, mild sedative.	May decrease effects of cisplatin in breast cancer. May increase risk of hepatic damage with hepatotoxic drugs (e.g., acetaminophen, amiodarone).	May cause nausea, dizziness, visual changes, migraine.
Blackberry	Diarrhea, edema, gout, inflammation. Interferes with processes contributing to skin wrinkling.	None known.	Well tolerated, no adverse reactions noted.

* See full herb entry in the A to Z section.

Name	Uses	Interactions	Precautions
Boldo	Mild GI spasms, dyspepsia, anti-inflammatory agent, laxative, gallstones.	May have additive effects when used with anticoagulant or antiplatelet medications.	***Oral:*** Seizures. ***Topical:*** Skin irritation.
Butterbur	Abdominal pain, back pain, gallbladder pain, bladder spasms, tension headache, migraine headache, asthma.	Cytochrome P450 inducers (e.g., carbamazepine, phenytoin, rifampin) may increase risk of hepatotoxicity.	May cause headache, itchy eyes, diarrhea, asthma, abdominal discomfort, fatigue, drowsiness.
Calendula	Abdominal cramps, constipation, reduces fever, inflammation of oral/pharyngeal mucosa.	May increase sedation with CNS depressants.	Well tolerated, may cause allergic reactions.
Capsicum	***Topical:*** Postherpetic, trigeminal, diabetic neuralgias; HIV-associated peripheral neuropathy. ***Oral:*** Dyspepsia, diarrhea, cramps, toothache, hyperlipidemia, prevents arteriosclerosis, heart disease.	May increase effects/adverse effects of antiplatelet medication.	Burning, urticaria, irritation to eyes, mucous membranes.
Cat's claw	Diverticulitis, peptic ulcer, colitis, hemorrhoids, Alzheimer's disease.	May increase effect of antihypertensives. May interfere with immunosuppressant therapy (e.g., cyclosporine, tacrolimus, sirolimus) due to immunostimulating activity.	Headache, dizziness, vomiting.
Catnip	***Topical:*** Arthritis, hemorrhoids. ***Oral:*** Insomnia, migraine, cold, flu, hives, indigestion, cramping, flatulence.	May be additive with other CNS depressants.	Headache, malaise, vomiting (large doses).
Cha de bugre	Weight loss, obesity, diuretic, cardiovascular disease.	None known.	None reported.

* See full herb entry in the A to Z section.

(continued)

Name	Uses	Interactions	Precautions
Chamomile*	Antispasmodic, sedative, anti-inflammatory, astringent, antibacterial.	May increase bleeding with anticoagulants. May increase sedative effect with benzodiazepines.	Anaphylactic reaction if allergic; avoid use if allergic to chrysanthemums, ragweed, and/or asters; delays absorption of medications.
Chastberry	***Oral:*** Control of menstrual irregularities, painful menstruation.	May interfere with oral contraceptives, hormone replacement therapy, dopamine antagonists (e.g., antipsychotics), pramipexole, ropinirole, metoclopramide.	GI disturbances, rash, pruritus, headache, increased menstrual flow.
Co-enzyme Q-10	***Oral:*** CHF, angina, diabetes, hypertension; reduces symptoms of chronic fatigue; stimulates immune system in those with AIDS.	May decrease effect of warfarin. May have additive effects with antihypertensives.	Reduced appetite, gastritis, nausea, diarrhea.
Conjugated linoleic acid	Obesity, bodybuilding, atherosclerosis.	May increase vitamin A storage in liver and breast tissues.	May cause GI upset, diarrhea, nausea, loose stools, dyspepsia, fatigue. Avoid use in pregnancy when used for medicinal purposes. Safe when used orally in amounts found in foods.
Cranberry	***Oral:*** Prevention, treatment of UTI, neurogenic bladder, urinary deodorizer.	May increase effect of warfarin.	Large doses may cause diarrhea.
Devil's claw	Osteoarthritis, rheumatoid arthritis, gout, myalgia, lumbago, tendonitis, GI upset, dyspepsia, migraine headache.	May increase effect of antihypertensives, warfarin. May decrease effect of antacids, H_2 blockers (e.g., cimetidine), proton pump inhibitors (e.g., lansoprazole, omeprazole).	Diarrhea, nausea, vomiting, abdominal pain. May cause skin reactions.

* See full herb entry in the A to Z section.

Name	Uses	Interactions	Precautions
DHEA*	Slows aging, boosts energy, controls weight.	May interfere with antiestrogen effects of aromatase inhibitors (e.g., anastrozole). May interfere with estrogen receptor antagonist activity of tamoxifen in estrogen receptor-positive cancer cells (e.g., breast, ovarian cancer).	Side effects: May increase risk of breast/prostate cancer. Women may develop acne, hair growth on face/body.
Dong quai*	Dysmenorrhea, PMS, menopause symptoms.	May increase effects of warfarin, antiplatelet medications.	Diarrhea, photosensitivity, skin cancer. Avoid use in pregnancy/lactation. Essential oil may contain the carcinogen safrole.
Echinacea*	Treats/prevents common cold, other upper respiratory tract infections.	May interfere with immunosuppressive therapy.	Not to be used with weakened immune system (e.g., HIV/AIDS, tuberculosis, multiple sclerosis). Habitual or continued use may suppress the immune system (should only be taken for 2–3 mos or alternating schedule of q2–3wk).
Elderberry	Treatment of influenza, laxative, diuretic, allergic rhinitis, sinusitis, neuralgia.	May interfere with immunosuppressant therapy (e.g., azathioprine [Imuran], cyclosporine [Neoral], mycophenolate [CellCept]).	Avoid using during pregnancy and lactation. Well tolerated. May cause nausea, vomiting, severe diarrhea.
Emu oil	***Oral:*** Hypercholesterolemia, weight loss, cough syrup. ***Topical:*** Relief from sore muscles, arthralgia, pain, inflammation, carpal tunnel syndrome.	None known.	None reported.
Evening primrose oil	***Oral:*** PMS, symptoms of menopause (e.g., hot flashes), psoriasis, rheumatoid arthritis.	Antipsychotics may increase risk of seizures. May increase risk of bleeding with anticoagulants/antiplatelets.	Indigestion, nausea, headache. Large doses may cause diarrhea, abdominal pain.

* See full herb entry in the A to Z section.

(continued)

Name	Uses	Interactions	Precautions
Fenugreek	Lowered blood glucose, gastritis, constipation, atherosclerosis, elevated serum cholesterol and triglyceride levels.	May have additive effects with antidiabetic, anticoagulant, antiplatelet medications.	Nasal congestion, wheezing. Large doses may cause hypoglycemia.
Feverfew*	Relieves migraine. Treatment of fever, headache, menstrual irregularities.	May increase bleeding time with aspirin, dipyridamole, warfarin.	Headache, oral ulcers. Avoid use in pregnancy (stimulates menstruation), nursing mothers, children younger than 2 yrs.
Fish oils	***Oral:*** Hypertension, hyperlipidemia, coronary artery disease, rheumatoid arthritis, psoriasis.	May increase risk of bleeding with antiplatelets, anticoagulants. Additive effect with antihypertensives. Contraceptive medications may decrease triglyceride lowering effect.	Belching, heartburn, epistaxis. Large doses may cause nausea, diarrhea.
Flaxseed/ Flaxseed oil	Chronic constipation, diverticulitis, IBS, menopausal symptoms, bladder inflammation, protection against cancer.	May increase risk of bleeding with anticoagulants, antiplatelet drugs (e.g., aspirin, Plavix, Lovenox, heparin, warfarin).	May increase risk for diarrhea; allergic reactions.
Garlic*	Reduces serum cholesterol, LDL, triglycerides, increases serum HDL, lowers B/P, inhibits platelet aggregation.	May increase effects of warfarin, aspirin, clopidogrel, enoxaparin. May decrease effects of oral contraceptives, cyclosporine, protease inhibitors.	Side effects: Altered taste, offensive odor. Large doses may cause heartburn, flatulence, other GI distress.
Ginger*	Motion sickness, morning sickness, dyspepsia, rheumatoid arthritis, osteoarthritis, loss of appetite, migraine headache.	May increase risk of bleeding with warfarin, aspirin, clopidogrel, heparin, low molecular weight heparins. May increase effect of antidiabetic agents, calcium channel blockers.	Avoid use during pregnancy when bleeding is a concern. Large overdose could potentially depress the CNS, cause cardiac arrhythmias.

* See full herb entry in the A to Z section.

Name	Uses	Interactions	Precautions
Ginkgo*	Improves memory, concentration; pt may think more clearly. Overcomes sexual dysfunction occurring with SSRI antidepressants.	May increase risk of bleeding with aspirin, warfarin, clopidogrel, heparin. May decrease effect of anticonvulsants, alter effect of insulin.	Avoid use in those taking anticoagulants or those hypersensitive to poison ivy, cashews, mangos. Side effects: GI disturbances, headache, dizziness, vertigo.
Ginseng*	Boosts energy, sexual stamina; decreases stress, effects of aging.	May increase effect of antidiabetic medications. May decrease effect of antipsychotics, warfarin.	Avoid in pts receiving anticoagulants, medications that increase B/P. Side effects: Breast tenderness, anxiety, headache, increased B/P, abnormal vaginal bleeding.
Glucosamine and chondroitin*	Osteoarthritis.	No known interactions but monitor anticoagulant effects.	None known.
Goldenrod	Diuretic, anti-inflammatory, antispasmodic. Prevents urinary tract inflammation, urinary calculi, kidney stones.	May interfere with diuretics.	Allergic reactions.
Goldenseal	***Topical:*** Eczema, itching, acne. ***Oral:*** UTI, hemorrhoids, gastritis, colitis, mucosal inflammation.	May decrease effect of antacids, H_2 blockers, proton pump inhibitors, antihypertensives.	Constipation, hallucinations. Large doses may cause nausea, vomiting, diarrhea, CNS stimulation, respiratory failure.
Gotu kola	Improves memory, intelligence, venous insufficiency (including varicose veins), wound or burn healing.	May increase effects/adverse effects of CNS depressants.	GI upset, nausea, pruritus, photosensitivity.
Grapefruit	Hyperlipidemia, atherosclerosis, psoriasis, weight loss, obesity.	May increase concentration/adverse effects of benzodiazepines, calcium channel blockers, carbamazepine, carvedilol, cyclosporine, statins.	None known.

* See full herb entry in the A to Z section.

(continued)

Name	Uses	Interactions	Precautions
Green tea	Improves cognition function, treats nausea, vomiting, headache, weight loss.	May increase risk of bleeding with anticoagulants, antiplatelets. May alter effect of antidiabetic medications. May increase effects/ adverse effects of cimetidine, clozapine, theophylline.	GI upset, constipation.
Guarana (also known as cola, caffeine)	Weight loss, enhance athletic performance, decrease mental/ physical fatigue, hypotension, chronic fatigue syndrome, stimulant, aphrodisiac.	May increase risk of bleeding with anticoagulants/ antiplatelets (e.g., aspirin, clopidogrel), cimetidine, estrogen, fluvoxamine, quinolones, verapamil. May increase risk of side effects of caffeine. May increase effects/toxicity of clozapine. May increase risk of CNS effects with amphetamines, ephedrine, nicotine. Abrupt withdrawal may increase lithium concentration, large amounts with MAOIs may cause hypertensive crisis.	May aggravate anxiety disorders, bleeding disorders. May induce arrhythmias in sensitive individuals. May alter glucose, use caution in diabetes. Side effects related to caffeine (e.g., insomnia, restlessness, nausea, vomiting, tachycardia).
Guggul	Lowers serum cholesterol, treatment of acne, skin disease, weight loss.	May increase risk of bleeding with anticoagulants/ antiplatelets. May decrease effect of dilitiazem, propranolol, tamoxifen.	May cause headache, nausea, vomiting, loose stools, bloating.
Gymnema	Treatment of diabetes, cough.	May enhance effects of insulin, oral antidiabetics.	None reported.
Hawthorn	Cardiovascular conditions (e.g., atherosclerosis), GI conditions (diarrhea, indigestion, abdominal pain), sleep disorders.	May increase effect of beta-blockers, calcium channel blockers, digoxin, nitrates. May increase vasodilation/ hypotension with sildenafil, tadalafil, vardenafil.	Nausea, GI complaints, headache, dizziness, insomnia, agitation.

* See full herb entry in the A to Z section.

Name	Uses	Interactions	Precautions
Hoodia	Appetite suppressant for obesity, weight loss.	None known.	None reported.
Horse chestnut	Treat varicose veins, hemorrhoids, phlebitis.	May enhance effects of insulin, oral antidiabetics, antiplatelet medications.	Muscle cramps, pruritus, GI irritation.
Kava kava*	Anxiety disorders, ADHD, insomnia, restlessness.	Increases CNS depression with alcohol, sedatives.	GI upset, headache, dizziness, drowsiness, enlarged pupils, disturbances of accommodation, dry mouth, allergic skin reactions.
Kombucha	Memory loss, strengthen immune system, arthritis, premenstrual syndrome.	May cause disulfiram reaction due to alcohol in fermented tea.	Those with stabilized alcoholism, compromised immunity. May cause stomach problems, yeast infection, nausea, vomiting, head/neck pain.
L-Carnitine	Treatment of primary L-carnitine deficiency, post-myocardial infarction protection, dementia, angina, CHF, intermittent claudication.	None known.	Abdominal discomfort, diarrhea, nausea, vomiting, heartburn.
Licorice	Inflammation of upper respiratory tract, mucous membranes, ulcers, expectorant.	May decrease effect of antihypertensives. May increase potassium loss with thiazides.	Large doses may cause pseudoaldosteronism (hypertension, headache, lethargy, edema).
Mangosteen	Diarrhea, UTI, gonorrhea, stimulates immune system.	None known.	None reported.
Meadowsweet	Fevers, colds, inflammation, pain relief, peptic ulcer disease, rheumatic disorders including gout.	May be additive with aspirin. May potentiate effects of narcotics.	May cause nausea, bronchospastic activity.
Melatonin*	Aids sleep, prevents jet lag.	May decrease effect of oral antidiabetic agents, immunosuppressants. May have additive effect with CNS depressants.	Headache, confusion, fatigue. Does not lengthen total sleep time.

* See full herb entry in the A to Z section.

(continued)

Name	Uses	Interactions	Precautions
Milk thistle	Hepatoprotective, antioxidant, hepatic disorders, including poisoning (e.g., mushroom), cirrhosis, hepatitis.	None known.	Mild allergic reactions, laxative effect.
Morinda	Antiviral, antifungal, reduces B/P, antibacterial, diabetes mellitus.	May increase potassium levels with ACE inhibitors (e.g., lisinopril), angiotensin receptor blockers (e.g., losartan), potassium-sparing diuretics. May decrease effectiveness of warfarin.	None reported, but may be associated with hepatotoxicity.
MSM (methyl sulfonyl methane)	***Oral/topical:*** Chronic pain, arthritis, inflammation, osteoporosis, muscle cramps/ pain, wrinkles, protection against windburn or sunburn.	None known.	May cause nausea, diarrhea, headache, pruritus, increase in allergic symptoms.
Omega-6 fatty acid	Coronary artery disease, decreases total serum LDL cholesterol, increases serum HDL.	None known.	Increases serum triglycerides.
Peppermint	Colds, cough, fever, sinusitis, IBS, upper gastrointestinal cramps, dyspepsia.	May increase concentration of cyclosporine, propranolol, verapamil, theophylline, proton pump inhibitors (e.g., omeprazole, pantoprazole), NSAIDs (e.g., ibuprofen).	Can cause nausea, vomiting, heartburn, allergic reactions (e.g., headache, flushing).
Phellodendron	Weight loss, obesity, antifungal, anti-inflammatory, treatment of osteoarthritis, diabetes mellitus, pneumonia, diarrhea, stomach problems.	May increase serum levels of cyclosporine, lovastatin, clarithromycin, indinavir, sildenafil.	Decrease in B/P, malaise reported.

* See full herb entry in the A to Z section.

Name	Uses	Interactions	Precautions
Policosanol	Hyperlipidemia, intermittent claudication, reducing myocardial ischemia.	Can inhibit platelet aggregation. May increase risk of bruising and bleeding with aspirin, Plavix, NSAIDs, heparin, warfarin.	Usually well tolerated. Avoid using during pregnancy and lactation. May cause erythema, migraines, insomnia, irritability, upset stomach, weight loss, skin rash.
Pomegranate	Hypertension, CHF, atherosclerosis, tapeworm manifestations.	May have additive effects with ACE inhibitors, antihypertensives.	Avoid using during pregnancy and breast-feeding. May cause allergic reactions, GI disturbances.
Prickly pear cactus	Hypercholesterolemia, obesity, alcohol-induced hangover.	None known.	Usually well tolerated. May cause mild diarrhea, nausea, increased stool volume/frequency, abdominal fullness, headache.
Red clover	***Oral:*** Menopausal symptoms, hot flashes, prevention of cancer, indigestion, asthma. ***Topical:*** Skin sores, burns, chronic skin disease (e.g., eczema, psoriasis).	May increase anticoagulant effects of warfarin. May interfere with hormone replacement therapy, oral contraceptives, tamoxifen.	Rash, myalgia, headache, nausea, vaginal spotting.
Red yeast	Maintain or reduce cholesterol levels, indigestion, diarrhea, improve circulation, contains statin-like drugs including lovastatin.	May increase risk of myopathy with cyclosporine, gemfibrozil, high-dose niacin. Cytochrome P450 3A4 inhibitors (e.g., clarithromycin, ketoconazole), HMG-CoA reductase inhibitors (e.g., atorvastatin, simvastatin) may increase risk of potential adverse effects. Alcohol, hepatotoxic drugs may increase risk of liver damage. Grapefruit may increase levels of lovastatin.	May cause abdominal discomfort, heartburn, flatulence, dizziness. May elevate liver enzymes, cause myopathy. Caution in those with hepatic impairment. Avoid use in pregnancy (insufficient reliable information available).

* See full herb entry in the A to Z section.

(continued)

Name	Uses	Interactions	Precautions
SAMe	Depression, heart disease, osteoarthritis, Alzheimer's disease, Parkinson's disease; slows aging process.	May increase adverse effects with antidepressants.	Nausea, vomiting, diarrhea, flatulence; headache.
Saw palmetto*	Eases symptoms of enlarged prostate (frequency, dysuria, nocturia).	May increase risk of bleeding with anticoagulants/antiplatelets. May interfere with oral contraceptives, estrogen.	Side effects: Abdominal discomfort, headache, erectile dysfunction. Does not reduce size of enlarged prostate. Obtain baseline PSA levels before initiating. Large doses can cause diarrhea.
Schisandra	Increases energy, physical performance, endurance, stimulates immune system, treats common cold, hay fever.	May increase serum levels of lovastatin, clarithromycin, cyclosporine, indinavir, diltiazem.	Abdominal upset, decreased appetite, skin rash, heartburn, acid indigestion.
Shark cartilage	Cancer, arthritis, psoriasis, wound healing.	None known.	Nausea, vomiting, constipation, dyspepsia, altered taste.
Soy	Menopausal symptoms; prevents osteoporosis and cardiovascular disease in postmenopausal women; hypertension, hyperlipidemia.	May decrease effects of estrogen replacement therapy.	Constipation, bloating, nausea, allergic reaction.
Soybean oil	Lowers total and LDL cholesterol	None known	May cause allergic reactions.
St. John's wort*	Relieves mild to moderate depression.	May decrease effect of alprazolam, oral contraceptives, cyclosporine, calcium channel blockers, antifungals, digoxin, phenytoin, protease inhibitors, atorvastatin, lovastatin, simvastatin, tacrolimus, warfarin. May increase side effects with triptans, antidepressants, MAOIs, paroxetine, sertraline.	Dizziness, dry mouth, increased sensitivity to sunlight. Report symptoms of "serotonin syndrome."

* See full herb entry in the A to Z section.

Name	Uses	Interactions	Precautions
Turmeric	Antioxidant, anti-inflammatory, stimulates immune system, treats diarrhea, dyspepsia, abdominal bloating.	May increase risk of bleeding with antiplatelets (e.g., aspirin, clopidogrel) and anticoagulants (e.g., enoxaparin, heparin, warfarin).	Nausea, diarrhea, stomach discomfort.
Tyrosine	PMS, depression, attention deficit disorder (ADD), ADHD, improve alertness.	May decrease effects of L-dopa. May have additive effects with thyroid hormone.	May cause nausea, headache, fatigue, heartburn, arthralgia.
Valerian*	Aids sleep, relieves restlessness and anxiety.	May increase sedative effects with alcohol, CNS depressants.	Palpitations, upset stomach, headache, excitability, uneasiness. May cause increased morning drowsiness.
Whey protein	Alternative to milk in those with lactose intolerance, treatment of hyperlipidemia, obesity and weight loss.	May decrease absorption of alendronate (Fosamax), levodopa, quinolone antibiotics (e.g., levofloxacin).	Well tolerated. High doses may cause increased stool frequency, nausea, thirst, bloating, cramps, decreased appetite, fatigue, headache.
Wild yam	Alternative for estrogen replacement therapy, postmenopausal vaginal dryness, PMS, osteoporosis, increases energy/libido, breast enlargement.	None known.	Large amounts may cause vomiting (tincture).
Willow bark	Headache, pain, myalgia, rheumatoid arthritis, gout, osteoarthritis.	May increase risk of bleeding with anticoagulant or antiplatelet medications (e.g., aspirin, warfarin, enoxaparin, clopidogrel).	May cause itching, rash, GI effects (e.g., nausea, dyspepsia).
Yohimbe*	Male aphrodisiac. Treatment of impotence, erectile dysfunction, orthostatic hypotension.	May decrease effect of antihypertensives. May have additive effects with MAOIs, CNS stimulants.	Large doses linked to weakness, paralysis.

* See full herb entry in the A to Z section.

Appendix H

LIFESPAN, CULTURAL ASPECTS, AND PHARMACOGENOMICS OF DRUG THERAPY

LIFESPAN

Drug therapy is unique to pts of different ages. Age-specific competencies involve understanding the development and health needs of the various age groups. Pregnant pts, children, and the elderly represent different age groups with important considerations during drug therapy.

CHILDREN

In pediatric drug therapy, drug administration is guided by the age of the child, weight, level of growth and development, and height. The dosage ordered is to be given either by kilogram of body weight or by square meter of body surface area, which is based on the height and weight of the child. Many dosages based on these calculations must be individualized based on pediatric response.

If the oral route of administration is used, often syrup or chewable tablets are given. Additionally, sometimes medication is added to liquid or mixed with foods. Remember to never force a child to take oral medications because choking or emotional trauma may ensue.

If an intramuscular injection is ordered, the vastus lateralis muscle in the mid-lateral thigh is used, because the gluteus maximus is not developed until walking occurs and the deltoid muscle is too small. For intravenous medications, administer very slowly in children. If given too quickly, high serum drug levels will occur with the potential for toxicity.

PREGNANCY

Women of childbearing years should be asked about the possibility of pregnancy before any drug therapy is initiated. Advise a woman who is either planning a pregnancy or believes she may be pregnant to inform her physician immediately. During pregnancy, medications given to the mother pass to the fetus via the placenta. Teratogenic (fetal abnormalities) effects may occur. Breast-feeding while the mother is taking certain medications may not be recommended due to the potential for adverse effects on the newborn.

The choice of drug ordered for pregnant women is based on the stage of pregnancy, because the fetal organs develop during the first trimester. Cautious use of drugs in women of reproductive age who are sexually active and who are not using contraceptives is essential to prevent the potential for teratogenic or embryotoxic effects. Refer to the different pregnancy categories (found in Appendix F) to determine the relative safety of a medication during pregnancy.

ELDERLY

The elderly are more likely to experience an adverse drug reaction owing to physiologic changes (e.g., visual, hearing, mobility changes, chronic diseases) and cognitive changes (short-term memory loss or alteration in the thought process) that may lead to multiple medication dosing. In chronic disease states such as hypertension, glaucoma, asthma, or arthritis, the daily ingestion of multiple medications increases the potential for adverse reactions and toxic effects.

Decreased renal or hepatic function may lower the metabolism of medications in the liver and reduce excretion of medications, thus prolonging the half-life of the drug and the potential for toxicity. Dosages in the elderly should initially be smaller than for the general adult population and then slowly titrated based on pt response and therapeutic effect of the medication.

CULTURE

The term *ethnopharmacology* was first used to describe the study of medicinal plants used by indigenous cultures. More recently, it is being used as a reference to the action and effects of drugs in people from diverse racial, ethnic, and cultural backgrounds. Although there are insufficient data from investigations involving people from diverse backgrounds that would provide reliable information on ethnic-specific responses to all medications, there is growing evidence that modifications in dosages are needed for some members of racial and ethnic groups. There are wide variations in the perception of side effects by pts from diverse cultural backgrounds. These differences may be related to metabolic differences that result in higher or lower levels of the drug, individual differences in the amount of body fat, or cultural differences in the way individuals perceive the meaning of side effects and toxicity. Nurses and other health care providers need to be aware that variations can occur with side effects, adverse reactions, and toxicity so that pts from diverse cultural backgrounds can be monitored.

Some cultural differences in response to medications include the following:

African Americans: Generally, African Americans are less responsive to beta-blockers (e.g., propranolol [Inderal]) and angiotensin-converting enzyme (ACE) inhibitors (e.g., enalapril [Vasotec]).

Asian Americans: On average, Asian Americans have a lower percentage of body fat, so dosage adjustments must be made for fat-soluble vitamins and other drugs (e.g., vitamin K used to reverse the anticoagulant effect of warfarin).

Hispanic Americans: Hispanic Americans may require lower dosages and may experience a higher incidence of side effects with tricyclic antidepressants (e.g., amitriptyline).

Native Americans: Alaskan Eskimos may suffer prolonged muscle paralysis with the use of succinylcholine when administered during surgery.

There has been a desire to exert more responsibility over one's health and, as a result, a resurgence of self-care practices. These practices are often influenced by folk remedies and the use of medicinal plants. In the United States, there are several major ethnic population subgroups (white, black, Hispanic, Asian, and Native Americans). Each of these ethnic groups has a wide range of practices that influence beliefs and interventions related to health and illness. At any given time, in any group, treatment may consist of the use of traditional herbal therapy, a combination of ritual and prayer with medicinal plants, customary dietary and environmental practices, or the use of Western medical practices.

African Americans

Many African Americans carry the traditional health beliefs of their African heritage. Health denotes harmony with nature of the body, mind, and spirit, whereas illness is seen as disharmony that results from natural causes or divine punishment. Common practices to the art of healing include treatments with herbals and rituals known empirically to restore health. Specific forms of healing include using home remedies, obtaining medical advice from a physician, and seeking spiritual healing.

Examples of healing practices include the use of hot baths and warm compresses for rheumatism, the use of herbal teas for respiratory illnesses, and the use of kitchen condiments in folk remedies. Lemon, vinegar, honey, saltpeter, alum, salt, baking soda, and Epsom salt are common kitchen ingredients used. Goldenrod, peppermint, sassafras, parsley, yarrow, and rabbit tobacco are a few of the herbals used.

Hispanic Americans

The use of folk healers, medicinal herbs, magic, and religious rituals and ceremonies are included in the rich and varied customs of Hispanic Americans. This ethnic group believes that God is responsible for allowing health or illness to occur. Wellness may be viewed as good luck, a reward for good behavior, or a blessing from God. Praying, using herbals and spices, wearing religious objects such as medals, and maintaining a balance in diet and physical activity are methods considered appropriate in preventing evil or poor health.

Hispanic ethnopharmacology is more complementary to Western medical practices. After the illness is identified, appropriate treatment may consist of home remedies (e.g., use of vegetables and herbs), use of over-the-counter patent medicines, and use of physician-prescribed medications.

Asian Americans

For Asian Americans, harmony with nature is essential for physical and spiritual well-being. Universal balance depends on harmony among the elemental forces: fire, water, wood, earth, and metal. Regulating these universal elements are two forces that maintain physical and spiritual harmony in the body: the *yin* and the *yang*. Practices shared by most Asian cultures include meditation, special nutritional programs, herbology, and martial arts.

Therapeutic options available to traditional Chinese physicians include prescribing herbs, meditation, exercise, nutritional changes, and acupuncture.

Native Americans

The theme of total harmony with nature is fundamental to traditional Native American beliefs about health. It is dependent on maintaining a state of equilibrium among the physical body, the mind, and the environment. Health practices reflect this holistic approach. The method of healing is determined traditionally by the medicine man, who diagnoses the ailment and recommends the appropriate intervention.

Treatment may include heat, herbs, sweat baths, massage, exercise, diet changes, and other interventions performed in a curing ceremony.

European Americans

Europeans often use home treatments as the front-line interventions. Traditional remedies practiced are based on the magical or empirically validated experience of ancestors. These cures are often practiced in combination with religious rituals or spiritual ceremonies.

Household products, herbal teas, and patent medicines are familiar preparations used in home treatments (e.g., salt water gargle for sore throat).

PHARMACOGENOMICS

Traditionally, medications are prescribed using a "one size fits all". In general, the genetic makeup is similar in all humans, regardless of race or sex. However, people inherit variations in their genes, which can affect the way a person responds to a medication. A genetic variation may make a medication stay in the body longer, causing serious side effects, or a variation may make the medication less potent.

For example, two people taking the same cancer medication may have very different responses. One may have severe, life-threatening side effects while the second may have few, if any, side effects. The drug may shrink a tumor in one person but not in another.

Pharmacogenomics examines how a person's genetic makeup affects response to medications. Although widespread application still lies in the future, pharmacogenomics has the potential to personalize medical therapies. Physicians eventually will be able to prescribe medications based on an individual's genotype, thereby maximizing effectiveness and minimizing side effects. A few tests are available today.

Cytochrome P450 genotyping test. Cytochrome (CYP) 450 enzymes CYP2D6 and CYP2C19 are involved in the metabolism of many cardiovascular, antidepressant, and antipsychotic agents. More than 1% of the human population has a genetic variation that affects CYP2D6 and CYP2C19. These patients may eliminate drugs metabolized by the CYP2D6 and CYP2C19 enzyme systems "normally" (extensive metabolizers), too quickly (ultra-rapid metabolizers), too slowly (intermediate metabolizers), or not at all (poor metabolizers). Clinical effect would be a greater likelihood of adverse reactions in people who are poor metabolizers and a greater likelihood of treatment failure in people who are rapid metabolizers. Poor metabolizers include 5%–10% Caucasians, whereas rapid metabolizers include 10% Spaniards and 39% Ethiopians.

Thiopurine methyltransferase test. An enzyme called thiopurine methyltransferase (TPMT) breaks down a type of chemotherapy medication called thiopurine (e.g., mercaptopurine, thioguanine, azathioprine), which is used in the treatment of some leukemias and autoimmune disorders. Some people have genetic variations that prevent them from producing this enzyme, resulting in the buildup of thiopurine levels in the body and leading to severe toxic reactions, including profound myelosuppression, with normal doses. Data on the frequency of occurrence in specific populations groups are not available.

UGT1A1 TA repeat genotype test. This test, commonly known as the UFT1A1 test, detects a variation in a gene that affects the UGT1A1 enzyme. This enzyme determines how the body breaks down irinotecan (Camptosar), a chemotherapy medications used in the treatment of colorectal cancer. A deficiency of this enzyme allows the medication to build up to toxic levels, possibly causing bone marrow suppression, gastrointestinal toxicities, infection, and death. Deficiency of this enzyme occurs in 16% of Chinese and 40% of European and East Indian individuals.

Dihydropyrimidine dehydrogenase test. The medication 5-fluorouracil (5-FU) and its related compounds (e.g., capecitabine) are commonly used chemotherapy medications. Some people have a genetic variation that results in a decrease in the dihydropyrimidine dehydrogenase enzyme, which is responsible for breaking down 5-FU. As a result of the deficiency, some people may develop severe or even fatal reactions to 5-FU. This deficiency occurs in 0.9% of Caucasians.

By utilizing the information provided by pharmacogenomic testing, drug therapy is changing to a more individualized approach. Anticipated benefits of pharmacogenomics include creation of better vaccines, safer medications targeted to specific diseases, and more appropriate dosing of medications at the onset of therapy. Ultimately, we may see a decrease of healthcare costs due to more efficient clinical trials, reduced adverse drug reactions, and less time needed to find effective therapy for patients.

Appendix I

NON-CRUSHABLE DRUGS

NON-CRUSHABLE MEDICATIONS

Introduction

There are instances when crushing tablets or capsules prior to administration may be indicated. For example, pts having a nasogastric tube, pts needing an oral liquid formulation that is not commercially available, or pts having difficulty swallowing tablets or capsules may require medications to be crushed.

Certain dosage forms generally should not be crushed. These include the following:

- **Extended-release tablets/capsules** are formulated to allow medication to be slowly released into the body. Capsules may contain beads that are slowly dissolved over time.
- Medication irritating to the stomach may be **enteric-coated,** delaying release of the medication until it reaches the small intestine. An example of this formulation is enteric-coated aspirin.
- **Sublingual or orally-disintegrating tablets** are designed to dissolve.

The following pages list examples of medication forms that should not be crushed. This list is not all-inclusive. Please refer to individual monographs for further information about non-crushable formulations.

Name (Brand/Generic)	Dosage Form	Comments
Aciphex (rabeprazole)	Tablet: 20 mg	Extended release, enteric coated
Actonel (risedronate)	Tablet: 5 mg, 30 mg, 35 mg, 75 mg, 150 mg	Irritant
Adalat CC (nifedipine)	Tablet: 30 mg, 60 mg, 90 mg	Extended release
Adderall XR (amphetamine)	Capsule: 5 mg, 10 mg, 15 mg, 20 mg, 25 mg, 30 mg	Extended release
Afeditab CR (nifedipine)	Tablet: 30 mg, 60 mg	Extended release
Afinitor (everolimus)	Tablet: 5 mg, 10 mg	Mucous membrane irritant
Aggrenox (combination)	Capsule	Extended release
Allegra-D (combination)	Tablet	Extended release
Alophen (bisacodyl)	Tablet: 5 mg	Enteric coated
Altoprev (lovastatin)	Tablet: 20 mg, 40 mg, 60 mg	Extended release
Ambien CR (zolpidem)	Tablet: 6.25 mg, 12.5 mg	Extended release
Amitiza (lubiprostone)	Capsule: 250 mg	Extended release, soft gel
Amrix (cyclobenzaprine)	Capsule: 15 mg, 30 mg	Extended release
Aplenzin (bupropion)	Tablet: 174 mg, 348 mg, 522 mg	Extended release

Name (Brand/Generic)	Dosage Form	Comments
Apriso (mesalamine)	Capsule: 375 mg	Extended release
Aptivus (tipranavir)	Capsule: 250 mg	Oil emulsion, taste
Arthrotec (combination)	Tablet	Enteric coated
Asacol (mesalamine)	Tablet: 400 mg	Extended release
Augmentin XR (combination)	Tablet: 1,000 mg	Extended release
Avinza (morphine)	Capsule: 30 mg, 60 mg, 90 mg, 120 mg	Extended release
Azulfidine EN (sulfasalazine)	Tablet: 500 mg	Extended release, enteric coated
Biaxin XL (clarithromycin)	Tablet: 500 mg	Extended release
Boniva (ibandronate)	Tablet: 150 mg	Irritant
Budeprion SR (bupropion)	Tablet: 100 mg, 150 mg	Extended release
Calan SR (verapamil)	Tablet: 120 mg, 180 mg, 240 mg	Extended release
Carbatrol (carbamazine)	Capsule: 100 mg, 200 mg, 300 mg	Extended release
Cardizem CD (diltiazem)	Capsule: 120 mg, 180 mg, 240 mg, 300 mg, 360 mg	Extended release
Cardizem LA (diltiazem)	Tablet: 120 mg, 180 mg, 240 mg, 300 mg, 360 mg, 420 mg	Extended release
Cardura XL (doxazosin)	Tablet: 4 mg, 8 mg	Extended release
Cartia XT (Diltiazem)	Capsule: 120 mg, 180 mg, 240 mg, 300 mg	Extended release
Cefaclor ER	Tablet: 500 mg	Extended release
Cipro XR (ciprofloxacin)	Tablet: 500 mg, 1,000 mg	Extended release
Claritin-D (combination)	Tablet	Extended release
Concerta (methylphenidate)	Tablet: 18 mg, 24 mg, 36 mg, 54 mg	Extended release
Covera-HS (verapamil)	Tablet: 180 mg, 240 mg	Extended release
Cymbalta (duloxetine)	Capsule: 20 mg, 30 mg, 60 mg	Extended release
Depakote (valproic acid)	Tablet: 125 mg, 250 mg, 500 mg	Extended release
Depakote ER (valproic acid)	Tablet: 250 mg, 500 mg	Extended release
Detrol LA (tolterodine)	Capsule: 2 mg, 4 mg	Extended release
Dexilant (dexlansoprazole)	Capsule: 30 mg, 60 mg	Extended release
Dilacor XR (diltiazem)	Capsule: 120 mg, 180 mg, 240 mg	Extended release

(continued)

Name (Brand/Generic)	Dosage Form	Comments
Dilatrate SR (isosorbide)	Capsule: 40 mg	Extended release
Dilt XR (diltiazem)	Capsule: 120 mg, 180 mg, 240 mg	Extended release
Ditropan XL (oxybutin)	Tablet: 5 mg, 10 mg, 15 mg	Extended release
Dulcolax (bisacodyl)	Tablet: 5 mg	Enteric coated
DynaCirc CR (isradipine)	Tablet: 5 mg, 10 mg	Extended release
EC-Naprosyn (naproxen)	Tablet, 375 mg, 500 mg	Enteric coated
Ecotrin (aspirin)	Tablet: 325 mg	Enteric coated
Effexor XR (venlafaxine)	Capsule: 37.5 mg, 75 mg, 150 mg	Extended release
Embeda (morphine combination)	Capsule	Extended release (do not give via NG tube)
Enablex (darifenacin)	Tablet: 7.5 mg, 15 mg	Extended release
Entocort EC (budesonide)	Capsule: 3 mg	Enteric coated
Equetro (carbamazepine)	Capsule: 100 mg, 200 mg, 300 mg	Extended release
Ery-Tab (erythromycin)	Tablet: 250 mg, 333 mg, 500 mg	Enteric coated
Feldene (piroxicam)	Capsule: 10 mg, 20 mg	Mucous membrane irritant
Fentora (fentanyl)	Tablet (buccal): 100 mcg, 200 mcg, 300 mcg, 400 mcg, 600 mcg, 800 mcg	Buccal tablet, swallow whole
Feosol (ferrous sulfate)	Tablet: 160 mg	Enteric coated
Fergon (ferrous gluconate)	Tablet: 300 mg	Enteric coated
Flagyl ER (metronidazole)	Tablet: 750 mg	Extended release
Flomax (tamsulosin)	Capsule: 0.4 mg	Extended release
Focalin XR (dexmethylphenidate)	Capsule: 5 mg, 10 mg, 15 mg, 20 mg	Extended release
Fosamax (alendronate)	Tablet: 5 mg, 10 mg, 35 mg, 40 mg, 70 mg	Irritant
Glucophage XR (metformin)	Tablet: 500 mg	Extended release
Glucotrol XL (Glipizide)	Tablet: 2.5 mg, 5 mg, 10 mg	Extended release
Glumetza (metformin)	Tablet: 500 mg, 1,000 mg	Extended release
Halfprin 81 (aspirin)	Tablet: 81 mg	Enteric coated
Imdur (isosorbide)	Tablet: 30 mg, 60 mg	Extended release
Inderal LA (propranolol)	Capsule: 60 mg, 80 mg, 120 mg, 160 mg	Extended release
Innopran XL (propranolol)	Capsule: 80 mg, 120 mg	Extended release

Name (Brand/Generic)	Dosage Form	Comments
Intuniv (guanfacine)	Tablet: 1 mg, 2 mg, 3 mg, 4 mg	Extended release
Invega (paliperidone)	Tablet: 1.5 mg, 3 mg, 6 mg, 9 mg	Extended release
Isoptin SR (verapamil)	Tablet: 120 mg, 180 mg, 240 mg	Extended release
K-Dur (potassium chloride)	Tablet: 20 mEq	Extended release
Kadian (morphine)	Capsule: 10 mg, 20 mg, 30 mg, 50 mg, 60 mg, 80 mg, 100 mg, 120 mg	Extended release
Kaletra (combination)	Tablet	Film coated
Keppra XL (levetiracetam)	Tablet: 500 mg	Extended release
Klor-Con (potassium chloride)	Tablet: 8 mEq	Extended release
Lamictal XR (lomotrigine)	Tablet: 25 mg, 50 mg, 100 mg, 200 mg	Extended release
Lescol XL (fluvastatin)	Tablet: 80 mg	Extended release
Letairis (ambrisentan)	Tablet: 5 mg, 10 mg	Extended release
Levbid (hyoscyamine)	Tablet: 0.375 mg	Extended release
Liaida (mesalamine)	Tablet: 1.2 g	Extended release
Lithobid (lithium)	Tablet: 450 mg	Extended release
Luvox CR (fluvoxamine)	Capsule: 100 mg, 150 mg	Extended release
Metadate CD (methylphenidate)	Capsule: 10 mg, 20 mg, 30 mg, 40 mg, 50 mg, 60 mg	Extended release
Metadate ER (methylphenidate)	Tablet: 10 mg, 20 mg	Extended release
Methylin ER (methylphenidate)	Tablet: 10 mg, 20 mg	Extended release
Micro K (potassium chloride)	Capsule: 8 mEq, 10 mEq	Extended release
Moxatag (amoxicillin)	Tablet: 775 mg	Extended release
MS Contin (morphine)	Tablet: 15 mg, 30 mg, 60 mg, 100 mg, 200 mg	Extended release
Mucinex (guaifenesin)	Tablet: 600 mg	Extended release
Myfortic (mycophenolate)	Tablet: 180 mg, 360 mg	Extended release
Namenda XR (memantine)	Capsule: 28 mg	Extended release (may open and mix with soft food)
Naprelan (naproxen)	Tablet: 375 mg, 500 mg	Extended release
Nexium (esomeprazole)	Capsule: 20 mg, 40 mg	Extended release

(continued)

Name (Brand/Generic)	Dosage Form	Comments
Niaspan (nicotinic acid)	Tablet: 500 mg, 750 mg, 1,000 mg	Extended release
Nifediac CC (nifedipine)	Tablet: 30 mg, 60 mg, 90 mg	Extended release
Nifedical XL (nifedipine)	Tablet: 30 mg, 60 mg	Extended release
Oramorph SR (morphine)	Tablet: 15 mg, 30 mg, 60 mg, 100 mg	Extended release
OxyContin (oxycodone)	Tablet: 10 mg, 15 mg, 20 mg, 30 mg, 40 mg, 60 mg, 80 mg, 160 mg	Extended release
Paxil CR (paroxetine)	Tablet: 12.5 mg, 25 mg, 37.5 mg	Extended release
Pentasa (mesalamine)	Capsule: 250 mg, 500 mg	Extended release
Plendil (felodipine)	Tablet: 2.5 mg, 5 mg	Extended release
Prevacid (lansoprazole)	Capsule: 15 mg, 30 mg	Extended release
Prevacid SoluTab (lansoprazole)	Tablet: 15 mg, 30 mg	Orally-disintegrating
Prilosec (omeprazole)	Capsule: 10 mg, 20 mg, 40 mg	Extended release
Prilosec OTC (omeprazole)	Tablet: 20 mg	Extended release
Procardia XL (nifedipine)	Tablet: 30 mg, 60 mg, 90 mg	Extended release
Proquin XR (ciprofloxacin)	Tablet: 500 mg	Extended release
Protonix (pantoprazole)	Tablet: 20 mg, 40 mg	Extended release
Prozac Weekly (fluoxetine)	Tablet: 90 mg	Enteric coated
Ranexa (ranolazine)	Tablet: 500 mg, 1,000 mg	Extended release
Razadyne ER (galantamine)	Capsule: 8 mg, 16 mg, 24 mg	Extended release
Requip XL (ropinirole)	Tablet: 2 mg, 4 mg, 8 mg	Extended release
Ritalin LA (methylphenidate)	Capsule: 10 mg, 20 mg, 30 mg, 40 mg	Extended release
Seroquel XR (quetiapine)	Tablet: 50 mg, 200 mg, 300 mg, 400 mg	Extended release
Sinemet CR (levodopa/carbidopa)	Tablet: 25 mg/100 mg, 50 mg/200 mg	Extended release (scored; may break)
Slo-Niacin (nicotinic acid)	Tablet: 250 mg, 500 mg, 750 mg	Extended release
Sprycel (dasatinib)	Tablet: 20 mg, 50 mg, 70 mg, 100 mg	Film coated
Strattera (atomoxetine)	Capsule: 10 mg, 18 mg, 25 mg, 40 mg, 60 mg, 80 mg, 100 mg	Contents can cause ocular irritation

Name (Brand/Generic)	Dosage Form	Comments
Tegretol XR (carbamazepine)	Tablet: 100 mg, 200 mg, 400 mg	Extended release
Temodar (temozolomide)	Capsule: 5 mg, 20 mg, 100 mg, 140 mg, 180 mg, 250 mg	Extended release
Tiazac (diltiazem)	Capsule: 120 mg, 180 mg, 240 mg, 300 mg, 360 mg, 420 mg	Extended release
Toprol XL (metoprolol)	Tablet: 25 mg, 50 mg, 100 mg, 200 mg	Extended release
Toviaz (fesoterodine)	Tablet: 4 mg, 8 mg	Extended release
Tylenol Arthritis (acetaminophen)	Tablet: 650 mg	Extended release
Ultram ER (tramadol)	Tablet: 100 mg, 200 mg, 300 mg	Extended release
Uroxatral (alfuzosin)	Tablet: 10 mg	Extended release
Verelan (verapamil)	Capsule: 120 mg, 180 mg, 240 mg, 360 mg	Extended release
Verelan PM (verapamil)	Capsule: 100 mg, 200 mg, 300 mg	Extended release
VesiCare (solifenacin)	Tablet: 5 mg, 10 mg	Enteric coated
Videx EC (didanosine)	Capsule: 125 mg, 200 mg, 250 mg, 400 mg	Extended release
Voltaren XR (diclofenac)	Tablet: 100 mg	Extended release
VoSpire ER (albuterol)	Tablet: 4 mg, 8 mg	Extended release
Wellbutrin SR	Tablet: 150 mg, 300 mg	Extended release
Wellbutrin XL	Tablet: 150 mg, 300 mg	Extended release
Xanax XR (alprazolam)	Tablet: 0.5 mg, 1 mg, 2 mg, 3 mg	Extended release
Zenpep (pancrelipase)	Capsules	Extended release (may open and mix with soft food)
Zolinza (vorinostat)	Capsule: 100 mg	Irritant (avoid contact with skin, mucous membranes; avoid contact with crushed/broken tablets)
Zortress (everolimus)	Tablet: 0.25 mg, 0.5 mg, 0.75 mg	Crushed powder may cause irritant effects to mucous membranes
Zyban (bupropion)	Tablet: 150 mg	Extended release
Zyflo CR (zileuton)	Tablet: 600 mg	Extended release

Appendix J

NORMAL LABORATORY VALUES

HEMATOLOGY/COAGULATION

Test	Normal Range
Activated partial thromboplastin time (aPTT)	25–35 sec
Erythrocyte count (RBC count)	M: 4.5–5.5 million cells/mm^3 F: 4.0–4.9 million cells/mm^3
Hematocrit (HCT, Hct)	M: 41%–50% F: 36%–44%
Hemoglobin (Hb, Hgb)	M: 13.5–16.5 g/dl F: 12.0–15.0 g/dl
Leukocyte count (WBC count)	4.5–10.0 thousand cells/mm^3
Leukocyte differential count	
Basophils	0%–0.75%
Eosinophils	1%–3%
Lymphocytes	25%–33%
Monocytes	3%–7%
Neutrophils-bands	3%–5%
Neutrophils-segmented	54%–62%
Mean corpuscular hemoglobin (MCH)	26–34 pg/cell
Mean corpuscular hemoglobin concentration (MCHC)	31%–37% Hb/cell
Mean corpuscular volume (MCV)	80–100 fL
Partial thromboplastin time (PTT)	60–85 sec
Platelet count (thrombocyte count)	100–450 thousand/mm^3
Prothrombin time (PT)	11–13.5 sec
RBC count (see Erythrocyte count)	

CLINICAL CHEMISTRY (SERUM PLASMA, URINE)

Test	Normal Range
Alanine aminotransferase (ALT)	8–36 units/L 8–78 units/L (children 0–2 mos)
Albumin	3.2–5 g/dl
Alkaline phosphatase	33–131 (adults 25–60 yrs) 51–153 (adults >60 yrs)
Amylase	30–110 units/L
Aspartate aminotransferase (AST)	5–35 units/L
Bilirubin (direct)	0–0.3 mg/dl
Bilirubin (total)	0.1–1.2 mg/dl
BUN	7–20 mg/dl
Calcium, ionized	2.24–2.46 mEq/L

Test	Normal Range
Calcium (total)	8.6–10.3 mg/dl
Carbon dioxide (CO_2) total	23–30 mEq/L
Chloride	95–108 mEq/L
Cholesterol (total) HDL cholesterol LDL cholesterol	Less than 200 mg/dl 40–60 mg/dl <160 mg/dl
Creatinine	0.5–1.4 mg/dl
Creatinine clearance	M: 80–125 ml/min/1.73 m^2 F: 75–115 ml/min/1.73 m^2
Creatinine kinase (CK) isoenzymes CK-BB CK-MB (cardiac) CK-MM (muscle)	 0% 0%–3.9% 96%–100%
Creatine phosphokinase (CPK)	8–150 units/L
Ferritin	13–300 ng/ml
Glucose (pre-prandial)	<115 mg/dl
Glucose (fasting)	60–110 mg/dl
Glucose (non-fasting, 2 hr postprandial)	<120 mg/dl
Hemoglobin A_{1c}	<8
Iron	66–150 mcg/dl
Iron-binding capacity, total (TIBC)	250–420 mcg/dl
Lactate dehydrogenase (LDH)	56–194 units/L
Lipase	23–208 units/L
Magnesium	1.6–2.5 mg/dl
Osmolality	289–308 mOsm/kg
Oxygen saturation	90–95 (arterial) 40–70 (venous)
pH	7.35–7.45 (arterial) 7.32–7.42 (venous)
Phosphorus, inorganic	2.8–4.2 mg/dl
Potassium	3.5–5.2 mEq/L
Protein (total)	6.5–7.9 g/dl
Sodium	134–149 mEq/L
Thyroid-stimulating hormone (TSH)	0.7–6.4 milliunits/L (adults ≤20 yrs) 0.4–4.2 milliunits/L (adults 21–54 yrs) 0.5–8.9 milliunits/L (adults 55–87 yrs)
Transferrin	Greater than 200 mg/dl
Triglycerides (TG)	45–155 mg/dl
Urea nitrogen	7–20 mg/dl
Uric acid	M: 2–8 mg/dl F: 2–7.5 mg/dl

Appendix K

ORPHAN DRUGS

The term *orphan drug* refers to either a drug or a biologic that is intended for use in a rare disease or condition. A rare disease or condition is one that affects less than 200,000 people in the United States or, if more than 200,000 people, in which there is no reasonable expectation that the cost of developing the drug or biologic and making it available would be recovered from the sales of that product.

A drug or biologic becomes an "orphan drug" when it is so designated from the Office of Orphan Products Development (OOPD) at the FDA. Orphan drug designation allows the sponsor of the drug or biologic to receive certain benefits from the government in exchange for developing the drug.

The drug or biologic must go through the FDA approval process like any other drug to evaluate it for both safety and efficacy. Since 1983, over 1,400 drugs and biologics have been designated orphan drugs, with over 250 products approved for marketing. After the orphan drug has been approved by the FDA for marketing, it becomes available through normal pharmaceutical supply channels. If not approved by the FDA, the product may be made available on a compassionate use basis. Contact information can be obtained from the OOPD at the FDA.

Office of Orphan Products Development
Food and Drug Administration
5600 Fishers Lane
Rockville, MD 20857
http://www.fda.gov/orphan/

Examples of orphan drugs:

Drug Name	Proposed Use	Sponsor
Amrubicin	Treatment of small cell lung cancer	Celgene
AMT-080	Gene therapy for treatment of Duchenne muscular dystrophy	Amsterdam Molecular Therapeutics
Atacicept	Treatment of systemic lupus erythematosus (SLE)	Merck Serono
Belimumab (Benlysta)	Treatment of SLE	Human Genome Sciences/ GlaxoSmithKline
Carfilzomib	Treatment of multiple myeloma	Proteolix
CBLB502	Prevention of death after full-body exposure to potentially lethal dose of radiation	Cleveland BioLabs
CPP-115	Treatment of infantile spasms	Catalyst
Darinaparsin (Zinapar)	Treatment of peripheral T-cell lymphoma	Ziopharm Oncology
Ensituximab	Treatment of pancreatic cancer	Neogenix Oncology
Migalastat (Amigal)	Fabry disease	Amicus Therapeutics/Shire
MP4CO	Treatment of acute sickling crises in sickle cell disease	Sangart
Naloxone	Topical lotion for treatment of pruritus accompanying cutaneous T-cell lymphoma	Elorac
Palifosfamide	Treatment of soft tissue sarcoma	Ziopharm Oncology
SF1126	Treatment of B-cell chronic lymphocytic leukemia	Semaphore Pharmaceuticals
Terguride	Treatment of pulmonary arterial hypertension	Ergonex
Velaglucerase alfa	Type 1 Gaucher disease	Shire

Appendix L

Cytochrome P450 (CYP) Enzymes

Most drugs are eliminated from the body, at least in part, by being changed chemically to a less lipid soluble product (i.e., metabolized) and thus more likely to be excreted from the body via the kidney or bile. Drugs may go through two different metabolic processes: Phase 1 and Phase 2 metabolism.

In Phase 1 metabolism, hepatic microsomal enzymes found in the endothelium of liver cells metabolize drugs via hydrolysis and oxidation and reduction reactions. These chemical reactions make the drug more water soluble. In Phase 2 metabolism, large water-soluble substances (e.g., glucuronic acid, sulfate) are attached to the drug, forming inactive, or significantly less active, water soluble metabolites. Phase 2 processes include glucuronidation, sulfation, conjugation, acetylation, and methylation.

Virtually any of the Phase 1 and Phase 2 enzymes can be inhibited, and some of these enzymes can be induced by drugs. Inhibiting the activity of metabolic enzymes results in increased concentrations of the drug (substrate), whereas inducing metabolic enzymes results in decreased concentrations of the drug (substrate).

The term "cytochrome P450" (CYP enzymes) refers to a family of over 100 enzymes in the human body that modulate various physiologic functions. First identified in the 1950s, the CYP enzyme system contains two large subgroups: steroidogenic and xenobiotic enzymes. Only the xenobiotic group is involved in the metabolism of drugs. The xenobiotic group includes 4 major enzyme families: CYP1, CYP2, CYP3, and CYP4. The primary role of these families is the metabolism of drugs. These families are further subdivided into subfamilies designated by a capital letter and given a specific enzyme number (1, 2, 3, etc.) according to the similarity in amino acid sequence it shares with other enzymes (e.g., CYP1A2).

The key CYP450 enzymes include CYP1A2, CYP2C9, CYP2C19, CYP2D6, and CYP3A4 and may be responsible for metabolism of 75% of all drugs, with the CYP3A subfamily responsible for nearly half of this activity.

The CYP enzymes are found in the endoplasmic reticulum of cells in a variety of human tissue but are primarily concentrated in the liver and intestine. CYP enzymes can be both inhibited and induced, leading to increased or decreased serum concentration of the drug (along with its effects).

The following tables of CYP substrates, inhibitors, and inducers provide a perspective on drugs that are affected by, or affect, cytochrome P450 (CYP) enzymes. **CYP substrate** includes drugs reported to be metabolized, at least in part, by one or more CYP enzymes. **CYP inhibitor** includes drugs reported to inhibit one or more CYP enzymes. **CYP inducer** contains drugs reported to induce one or more CYP enzymes.

P450 ENZYMES: SUBSTRATES, INHIBITORS, INDUCERS

CYP1A2 ENZYME

CYP1A2 SUBSTRATES	CYP1A2 INHIBITORS	CPY1A2 INDUCERS
Caffeine	Cimetidine (Tagamet)	Barbiturates
Clozapine (Clozaril)	Ciprofloxacin (Cipro)	Carbamazepine (Tegretol)
Mirtazapine (Remeron)	Fluvoxamine	Rifampin (Rifadin)
Olanzapine (Zyprexa)	Zileuton (Zyflo)	Smoking
Ramelteon (Rozerem)		
Ropinirole (Requip)		
Tizanidine (Zanaflex)		

- CYP1A2 enzyme is increasingly involved in drug interactions.
- More potent inhibitors include cimetidine, ciprofloxacin, and fluvoxamine.
- Smoking is most important inducer, but rifampin and barbiturates also can increase enzyme activity.
- Example of reaction: Tizanidine plasma concentrations increased over 30-fold when the inhibitor fluvoxamine was given concurrently.

CYP2C9 ENZYME

CYP2C9 SUBSTRATES	CYP2C9 INHIBITORS	CYP2C9 INDUCERS
Candesartan (Atacand)	Amiodarone (Cordarone)	Barbiturates
Celecoxib (Celebrex)	Clopidogrel (Plavix)	Carbamazepine (Tegretol)
Diclofenac (Voltaren)	Fluconazole (Diflucan)	Rifampin (Rifadin)
Glipizide (Glucotrol)	Metronidazole (Flagyl)	St. John's wort
Glyburide (DiaBeta)	Sulfamethoxazole	
Ibuprofen (Advil, Motrin)	Valproic acid (Depakote)	
Irbesartan (Avapro)		
Meloxicam (Mobic)		
Warfarin (Coumadin)		

- More potent inhibitors include amiodarone, metronidazole, and sulfamethoxazole.
- All of the inducers can substantially increase enzyme activity.
- Both warfarin and oral hypoglycemics are of serious concern with regard to drug interactions. Substrates warranting attention include warfarin and oral hypoglycemics.

CYP2C19 ENZYME

CYP2C19 SUBSTRATES	CYP2C19 INHIBITORS	CYP2C19 INDUCERS
Citalopram (Celexa)	Cimetidine (Tagamet)	Barbiturates
Diazepam (Valium)	Clopidogrel (Plavix)	Carbamazepine (Tegretol)
Escitalopram (Lexapro)	Esomeprazole (Nexium)	Rifampin (Rifadin)
Omeprazole (Prilosec)	Fluconazole (Diflucan)	St. John's wort
Pantoprazole (Protonix)	Fluvoxamine	
Sertraline (Zoloft)	Modafinil (Provigil)	

- Inhibition by itself does not frequently cause adverse effects compared to other CYP enzymes because many of the substrates do not have serious toxicity.
- Inhibition or induction of the enzyme nonetheless may result in an adverse drug interaction.
- Racial background is important in the likelihood of being deficient in this enzyme (e.g., 3%–5% of Caucasians and 12%–23% of Asians are poor metabolizers of this enzyme).

CYP2D6 ENZYME

CYP2D6 SUBSTRATES	CYP2D6 INHIBITORS	CYP2D6 INDUCERS
Amitriptyline (Elavil)	Amiodarone (Cordarone)	See comment below
Atomoxetine (Strattera)	Bupropion (Wellbutrin)	
Duloxetine (Cymbalta)	Fluoxetine (Prozac)	
Fluoxetine (Prozac)	Paroxetine (Paxil)	
Metoclopramide (Reglan)		
Metoprolol (Lopressor)		
Paroxetine (Paxil)		
Risperidone (Risperdal)		
Tamoxifen (Nolvadex)		
Tolterodine (Detrol)		
Tramadol (Ultram)		
Venlafaxine (Effexor)		

- Potent inhibitors include fluoxetine and paroxetine.
- Evidence suggests that this enzyme is not very susceptible to enzyme induction.
- Genetics, rather than drug therapy, accounts for most ultra-rapid metabolizers (e.g., Greeks, Portuguese, Saudis, and Ethiopians have high enzyme activity).

CYP3A4 ENZYME

CYP3A4 SUBSTRATES	CYP3A4 INHIBITORS	CYP3A4 INDUCERS
Alfuzosin (Uroxatral)	Amiodarone (Cordarone)	Carbamazepine (Tegretol)
Alprazolam (Xanax)	Clarithromycin (Biaxin)	Efavirenz (Sustiva)
Budesonide (Entocort EC)	Diltiazem (Cardizem)	Phenobarbital
Carbamazepine (Tegretol)	Erythromycin (Ery-Tab)	Rifampin (Rifadin)
Cyclosporine (Neoral)	Fluconazole (Diflucan)	St. John's wort
Fluticasone (Flovent)	Fluoxetine (Prozac)	
Lovastatin (Mevacor)	Itraconazole (Spoiranox)	
Repaglinide (Prandin)	Ketoconazole (Nizoral)	
Sildenafil (Viagra)	Verapamil (Calan, Isoptin)	
Simvastatin (Zocor)		
Tadalafil (Cialis)		

- This enzyme metabolizes about half of all medications on the market.
- Drug toxicity of CYP3A4 substrates due to inhibition of CYP3A4 is relatively common.
- This enzyme is very sensitive to induction, tending to lower plasma concentrations of substrates, resulting in reduced efficacy of the substrate.
- Most potent inhibitors include clarithromycin, itraconazole, and ketoconazole.
- Rifampin is a potent inducer and may reduce serum concentrations of substrates by as much as 90%.

Appendix M

POISON ANTIDOTE CHART

Poisoning Agent	Antidote	Dosage
Acetaminophen	Acetylcysteine (Acetadote, Mucomyst)	PO: ADULTS, CHILDREN: Loading dose: 140 mg/kg, then 70 mg/kg q4h for a total of 18 doses. Total dose delivered: 1,330 mg/kg. IV: ADULTS, CHILDREN: Loading dose: 150 mg/kg over 60 min, then 50 mg/kg over 4 hrs, then 100 mg/kg over 16 hrs. Total dose delivered: 300 mg/kg.
Anticholinergic agents (e.g., atropine)	Physostigmine	IM/IV/SUBCUTANEOUS: ADULTS: Initially, 0.5–2 mg, then repeat q20 min until response occurs or adverse effects occur. Repeat 1–4 mg q30–60 min as life-threatening symptoms recur. IV: CHILDREN (Reserve for life-threatening situation only): 0.01–0.03 mg/kg/dose. May repeat after 15–20 min to maximum total dose of 2 mg, or until response occurs or adverse cholinergic effects occur.
Arsenic	Dimercaprol (BAL in oil)	Mild Poisoning IM: ADULTS, CHILDREN: 2.5 mg/kg/dose q6h for 2 days, then q12h for 1 day, then once daily for 10 days. Severe Poisoning IM: ADULTS, CHILDREN: 3 mg/kg/dose q4h for 2 days, then q6h for 1 day, then q12h for 10 days.
Benzodiazepines (e.g., midazolam)	Flumazenil (Romazicon)	IV: ADULTS: 0.2 mg over 30 sec. May give 0.3-mg dose after 30 sec if desired LOC not obtained. Additional doses of 0.5 mg can be given over 30 sec at 1-min intervals up to cumulative dose of 3 mg. CHILDREN: 0.01 mg/kg (**Maximum:** 0.2 mg) with repeat doses of 0.01 mg/kg (**Maximum:** 0.2 mg) given every minute to maximum total cumulative dose of 1 mg.
Beta-blockers (e.g., propranolol)	Glucagon	IV: ADULTS: 5–10 mg over 1 min, followed by infusion of 1–10 mg/hr.
Calcium channel blockers (e.g., verapamil)	Glucagon	IV: ADULTS: 5–10 mg over 1 min, followed by infusion of 1–10 mg/hr.

(continued)

Poisoning Agent	Antidote	Dosage
Carbamate pesticides	Atropine	IV: ADULTS: Initially, 1–5 mg doubled q5min until signs of muscarinic excess abate. IV INFUSION: ADULTS: 0.5–1 mg/hr. IM: ADULTS (Mild symptoms): 2 mg. If severe symptoms develop after first dose, 2 additional doses should be repeated in 10 min. (Severe symptoms): Immediately administer three 2-mg doses. IV: CHILDREN: 0.02–0.05 mg/kg q10–20 min until atropine effect observed, then q1–4 h for at least 24 hrs. IM: 0.5–2 mg/dose based on weight (0.5 mg: 15–40 lb, 1 mg: 41–90 lb, 2 mg: greater than 90 lb). (Mild symptoms): 1 injection. (Severe symptoms): 2 additional injections given in rapid succession 10 min after receiving first injection.
Digoxin (Lanoxin)	Digoxin immune FAB (Digibind)	**ADULTS** Unknown amount of ingestion: 800 mg IV infusion if acute ingestion, 240 mg IV infusion if chronic ingestion. **Dosing for Ingestion of Single Large Dose** Dose (in no. of vials) = (Total digitalis body load in mg)/(0.5 mg of digitalis bound per vial). Total digitalis body load in mg = (No. of tablets/capsules ingested) × (mg strength of tablet/capsule) × (bioavailability of tablet/capsule). Digoxin tablets and elixir are 80% bioavailable. Digoxin capsules and injection are 100% bioavailable. **Dosing Based on Serum Level** Digoxin: Dose (in no. of vials) = (Serum digoxin level in ng/mL) × (weight in kg)/(100). Digitoxin: Dose (in no. of vials) = (Serum digitoxin level in ng/mL) × (weight in kg)/(1,000). **CHILDREN** **Dosing for Ingestion of Single Large Dose** Dose (in no. of vials) = (Total digitalis body load in mg)/(0.5 mg of digitalis bound per vial). Total digitalis body load in mg = (No. of tablets/capsules ingested) × (mg strength of tablet/capsule) × (bioavailability of tablet/capsule). Digoxin tablets and elixir are 80% bioavailable. Digoxin capsules and injection are 100% bioavailable. WEIGHING 20 kg or less: Dilution of reconstituted vial to 1 mg/ml may be desirable for doses of 3 mg or less. Dose (in no. of mg) = Dose (in no. of vials) × 38 mg/vial. Dose (in no. of vials) = (Serum digoxin level in ng/ml) × (weight in kg)/(100).

Poisoning Agent	Antidote	Dosage
Ethylene glycol	Fomepizole (Antizol)	IV: ADULTS, CHILDREN: Loading dose 15 mg/kg, then 10 mg/kg q12h for 4 doses, then 15 mg/kg q12h thereafter until ethylene glycol levels reduced to less than 20 mg/dl and patient is asymptomatic with normal pH.
Extravasation vasoconstrictive agents (e.g., dopamine)	Phentolamine (Regitine)	ADULTS, CHILDREN: Infiltrate area with small amount of solution made by diluting 5–10 mg in 10 ml 0.9% NaCl within 12 hrs of extravasation. In general, do not exceed 0.1–0.2 mg/kg (5 mg total).
Heparin	Protamine	IV: ADULTS, CHILDREN: Dosage is determined by most recent dosage of heparin or low molecular weight heparin (LWH): 1 mg protamine neutralizes 90–115 units of heparin and 1 mg (100 units) of LWH. **Maximum dose:** 50 mg.
Iron	Deferoxamine (Desferal)	Acute IM: ADULTS: Initially, 1,000 mg, then 500 mg q4h for 2 doses. Additional doses of 0.5 g q4–12 h. **Maximum:** 6 g/24 hrs. CHILDREN 3 YRS AND OLDER: 90 mg/kg/dose q8h (not to exceed 1 g/dose). **Maximum:** 6 g/24 hrs. IV: ADULTS, CHILDREN: 15 mg/kg/hr. **Maximum:** 6 g/24 hrs. Chronic IM: ADULTS: 500–1,000 mg/day. IV: ADULTS, CHILDREN: 15 mg/kg/hr. **Maximum:** 12 g/24 hrs.
Isoniazid	Pyridoxine (vitamin B_6)	IV: ADULTS, CHILDREN: Total dose of pyridoxine equal to amount of isoniazid ingested as first dose of 1–4 g IV, then 1 g IM q30min until total dose completed. If not known, give 5 g at rate of 1 g/min. May repeat q5–10min.
Lead	Calcium EDTA	Symptomatic Treat for 3–5 days; give in conjunction with dimercaprol. IM: ADULTS, CHILDREN: 167 mg/m² every 4 hrs. IV: ADULTS, CHILDREN: 1 g/m² as 8- to 24-hr infusion or divided q12h. Lead Encephalopathy Treat for 5 days; give concurrently with dimercaprol IM: ADULTS, CHILDREN: 250 mg/m² every 4 hrs. IV: ADULTS, CHILDREN: 50 mg/kg/day as 24-hr continuous infusion.
Lead	Dimercaprol (BAL in oil)	Mild IM: ADULTS, CHILDREN: Loading dose 4 mg/kg, then 3 mg/kg/dose q4h for 2–7 days. Begin calcium EDTA with second dose. Severe and Lead Encephalopathy IM: ADULTS, CHILDREN: 4 mg/kg/dose q4h for 3–5 days. Begin calcium EDTA with second dose.

(continued)

Poisoning Agent	Antidote	Dosage
Lead	Succimer (Chemet)	PO: ADULTS, CHILDREN: 10 mg/kg/dose q8h for 5 days, then q12h for 14 days. **Maximum:** 500 mg/dose. Note: For children younger than 5 yrs, dose based on mg/m^2.
Methanol	Fomepizole (Antizol)	IV: ADULTS, CHILDREN: Loading dose 15 mg/kg, then 10 mg/kg q12h for 4 doses, then 15 mg/kg q12h thereafter until ethylene glycol levels reduced to less than 20 mg/dl and patient is asymptomatic with normal pH.
Opioids (e.g., morphine)	Naloxone (Narcan)	IV/IM/SUBCUTANEOUS: ADULTS: 0.4–2 mg/dose. May repeat every 2–3 min as needed. Therapy may need to be reassessed if no response is seen after cumulative dose of 10 mg. CHILDREN (5 YRS OR OLDER or WEIGHING 20 KG OR GREATER): 2 mg/dose IV/IM/subcutaneous. May repeat every 2–3 min as needed. Therapy may need to be reassessed if no response is seen after cumulative dose of 10 mg. CHILDREN (WEIGHING LESS THAN 20 KG): 0.1mg/kg/dose. May repeat every 2–3 min as needed.
Organophosphate pesticides	Atropine	IV: ADULTS: Initially, 1–5 mg doubled q5min until signs of muscarinic excess abate. IV INFUSION: ADULTS: 0.5–1 mg/hr. IM: ADULTS (Mild symptoms): 2 mg. If severe symptoms develop after first dose, 2 additional doses should be repeated in 10 min. (Severe symptoms): Immediately administer three 2-mg doses. IV: CHILDREN: 0.02–0.05 mg/kg q10–20 min until atropine effect observed, then q1–4h for at least 24 hrs. IM: 0.5–2 mg/dose based on weight (0.5 mg: 15–40 lb, 1 mg: 41–90 lb, 2 mg: greater than 90 lb). (Mild symptoms): 1 injection. (Severe symptoms): 2 additional injections given in rapid succession 10 min after receiving first injection.
Organophosphate pesticides	Pralidoxime (Protopam)	IM/IV: ADULTS: 1–2 g. Repeat in 1–2 hrs if muscle weakness has not been relieved, then at 10- to 12-hr intervals if cholinergic signs recur. CHILDREN: 20–50 mg/kg/dose. Repeat in 1–2 hrs if muscle weakness is not relieved, then at 10- to 12-hr intervals if cholinergic signs recur.
Warfarin (Coumadin)	Phytonadione (vitamin K)	PO/IV/SUBCUTANEOUS: ADULTS: 2.5–10 mg/dose. May repeat in 12–48 hrs if given PO, 6–8 hrs if given by IV or subcutaneous route. CHILDREN: 0.5–5 mg depending on need for further anticoagulation, severity of bleeding.

Appendix N

PREVENTING MEDICATION ERRORS AND IMPROVING MEDICATION SAFETY

Medication safety is a high priority for the health care professional. Prevention of medication errors and improved safety for the pt are important, esp. in today's health care environment when today's pt is older and sometimes sicker and the drug therapy regimen can be more sophisticated and complex.

A medication error is defined by the National Coordinating Council for Medication Error Reporting and Prevention (NCC MERP) as "any preventable event that may cause or lead to inappropriate medication use or pt harm while the medication is in the control of the health care professional, pt, or consumer."

Most medication errors occur as a result of multiple, compounding events as opposed to a single act by a single individual.

Use of the wrong medication, strength, or dose; confusion over sound-alike or look-alike drugs; administration of medications by the wrong route; miscalculations (esp. when used in pediatric pts or when administering medications intravenously); and errors in prescribing and transcription all can contribute to compromising the safety of the pt. The potential for adverse events and medication errors is definitely a reality and is potentially tragic and costly in both human and economic terms.

Health care professionals must take the initiative to create and implement procedures to prevent medication errors from occurring and implement methods to reduce medication errors. The first priority in preventing medication errors is to establish a multidisciplinary team to improve medication use. The goal for this team would be to assess medication safety and implement changes that would make it difficult or impossible for mistakes to reach the pt. Some important criteria in making improved medication safety successful include the following:

- Promote a nonpunitive approach to reducing medication errors.
- Increase the detection and the reporting of medication errors, near misses, and potentially hazardous situations that may result in medication errors.
- Determine root causes of medication errors.
- Educate about the causes of medication errors and ways to prevent these errors.
- Make recommendations to allow organization-wide, system-based changes to prevent medication errors.
- Learn from errors that occur in other organizations and take measures to prevent similar errors.

Some common causes and ways to prevent medication errors and improve safety include the following:

Handwriting: Poor handwriting can make it difficult to distinguish between two medications with similar names. Also, many drug names sound similar, esp. when the names are spoken over the telephone, poorly enunciated, or mispronounced.

- Take time to write legibly.
- Keep phone or verbal orders to a minimum to prevent misinterpretation.
- Repeat back orders taken over the telephone.
- When ordering a new or rarely used medication, print the name.

- Always specify the drug strength, even if only one strength exists.
- Print generic and brand names of look-alike or sound-alike medications.

Zeros and decimal points: Hastily written orders can present problems even if the name of the medication is clear.

- Never leave a decimal point "naked." Place a zero before a decimal point when the number is less than a whole unit (e.g., use 0.25 mg or 250 mcg, **not** .25 mg).
- Never have a trailing zero following a decimal point (e.g., use 2 mg, **not** 2.0 mg).

Abbreviations: Errors can occur because of a failure to standardize abbreviations. Establishing a list of abbreviations that should never be used is recommended.

- Never abbreviate unit as "U"; spell out "unit."
- Do not abbreviate "once daily" as OD or QD or "every other day" as QOD; spell it out.
- Do not use D/C, as this may be misinterpreted as either discharge or discontinue.
- Do not abbreviate drug names; spell out the generic and/or brand names.

Ambiguous or incomplete orders: These types of orders can cause confusion or misinterpretation of the writer's intention. Examples include situations when the route of administration, dose, or dosage form has not been specified.

- Do not use slash marks—they may be read as the number one (1).
- When reviewing an unusual order, verify the order with the person writing the order to prevent any misunderstanding.
- Read over orders after writing.
- Encourage that the drug's indication for use be provided on medication orders.
- Provide complete medication orders—do not use "resume preop" or "continue previous meds."

High-alert medications: Medications in this category have an increased risk of causing significant pt harm when used in error. Mistakes with these medications may or may not be more common but may be more devastating to the pt if an error occurs. A list of high-alert medications can be obtained from the Institute for Safe Medication Practices (ISMP) at www.ismp.org.

Technology available today that can be used to address and help to solve potential medication problems or errors include the following:

- Electronic prescribing systems—This refers to computerized prescriber order entry systems. Within these systems is the capability to incorporate medication safety alerts (e.g., maximum dose alerts, allergy screening). Additionally, these systems should be integrated or interfaced with pharmacy and laboratory systems to provide drug–drug and drug–disease interactions alerts and include clinical order screening capability.
- Bar codes—These systems are designed to use bar-code scanning devices to validate identity of pts, verify medications administered, document administration, and provide safety alerts.
- "Smart" infusion pumps—These pumps allow users to enter drug infusion protocols into a drug library along with predefined dosage limits. If a dosage is outside the limits established, an alarm is sounded and drug delivery is halted, informing the clinician that the dose is outside the recommended range.
- Automated dispensing systems–point of use dispensing system—These systems should be integrated with information systems, esp. pharmacy systems.
- Pharmacy order entry system—This should be fully integrated with an electronic prescribing system with the capability of producing medication safety alerts. Additionally, the

system should generate a computerized medication administration record (MAR), which would be used by the nursing staff while administering medications.

Medication reconciliation: Medication errors generally occur at transition points in the pt's care (admission, transfer from one level of care to another [e.g., critical care to general care area], and discharge). Incomplete documentation can account for up to 60% of potential medication errors. Therefore, it becomes necessary to accurately and completely reconcile medication across the continuum of care. This includes the name, dosage, frequency, and route of medication administration.

Medication reconciliation programs are a process of identifying the most accurate list of all medications a pt is taking and using this list to provide correct medications anywhere within the health care system. The focus not only is on compiling a list but on using the list to reduce medication errors and provide quality pt care.

Additional Strategies to Reduce Medication Errors

The Institute for Safe Medication Practices (ISMP), FDA, and other agencies have identified high-risk areas associated with medication errors. They include the following:

At-risk population: Increased awareness of at-risk populations primarily includes pediatric and geriatric pts. For both, this risk is due to altered pharmacokinetic parameters with little published information regarding medication use in these groups. Additionally, in the pediatric population, the risk is due to the need for calculating doses based on age and weight, lack of available dosage forms, and concentrations for smaller children.

In a USP report, more than one third of medication errors reaching the pt occurred in pts 65 yrs of age and older. More than 50% of fatal hospital medication errors involve seniors. In the senior population, decreased renal function can reduce drug elimination and lead to drug accumulation in the body.

Avoid abbreviations and nomenclature: The confusion caused by abbreviations has prompted the ISMP to develop a list of abbreviations that should be avoided (see back cover of handbook).

Recognize prescription look-alike and sound-alike medications: The ISMP has developed an extensive list of confused drug names (see www.jointcommission.org). See individual monographs for **DO NOT CONFUSE** information.

Focus on high alert medications: High alert medications are medications that bear a heightened risk of causing significant pt harm if incorrectly used. High alert medications in the handbook have a colored background for the entire monograph.

Look for duplicate therapies and interactions: Drug interactions and duplicate therapies can increase risk of adverse reactions. Refer to individual monographs for significant interaction information (drug, herbal, food).

Report errors to improve process: This action plays an important role in preventing further errors. The intent is to identify system failures that can be altered to prevent further errors.

Appendix O

RECOMMENDED CHILDHOOD AND ADULT IMMUNIZATIONS

Recommended Adult Immunization Schedule by Vaccine and Age Group—United States, 2011

VACCINE ▼ AGE GROUP ▶	19–26 yrs	27–49 yrs	50–59 yrs	60–64 yrs	≥65 yrs
Influenza[1,*]	1 dose annually				
Tetanus, diphtheria, pertussis (Td/Tdap)[2,*]	Substitute 1-time dose of Tdap for Td booster; then boost with Td every 10 yrs				Td booster every 10 yrs
Varicella[3,*]	2 doses				
Human papillomavirus (HPV)[4,*]	3 doses (females)				
Zoster[5]				1 dose	
Measles, mumps, rubella (MMR)[6,*]	1 or 2 doses		1 dose		
Pneumococcal (polysaccharide)[7,8]	1 or 2 doses				1 dose
Meningococcal[9,*]	1 or more doses				
Hepatitis A[10,*]	2 doses				
Hepatitis B[11,*]	3 doses				

*Covered by the Vaccine Injury Compensation Program.

For all persons in this category who meet the age requirements and who lack evidence of immunity (e.g., lack documentation of vaccination or have no evidence of previous infection)

Recommended if some other risk factor is present (e.g., based on medical, occupational, lifestyle, or other indications)

No recommendation

These schedules indicate the recommended age groups and medical indications for which administration of currently licensed vaccines is commonly indicated for adults ages 19 yrs and older, as of January 1, 2011. For all vaccines being recommended on the adult immunization schedule, a vaccine series does not need to be restarted, regardless of the time that has elapsed between doses. Licensed combination vaccines may be used whenever any components of the combination are indicated and when the vaccine's other components are not contraindicated. For detailed recommendations on all vaccines, including those used primarily for travelers or that are issued during the yr, consult the manufacturers' package inserts and the complete statements from the Advisory Committee on Immunization Practices (http:// www.cdc.gov/vaccines/pubs/acip-list.htm).

Report all clinically significant postvaccination reactions to the Vaccine Adverse Event Reporting System (VAERS). Reporting forms and instructions on filing a VAERS report are available at http://www.vaers.hhs.gov or by telephone, 800-822-7967.

Information on how to file a Vaccine Injury Compensation Program claim is available at http://www.hrsa.gov/vaccinecompensation or by telephone, 800-338-2382. Information about filing a claim for vaccine injury is available through the U.S. Court of Federal Claims, 717 Madison Place, N.W., Washington, D.C. 20005; telephone, 202-357-6400.

Additional information about the vaccines in this schedule, extent of available data, and contraindications for vaccination also is available at http://www.cdc.gov/vaccines or from the CDC-INFO Contact Center at 800-CDC-INFO (800-232-4636) in English and Spanish, 24 hrs a day, 7 days a wk.

Use of trade names and commercial sources is for identification only and does not imply endorsement by the U.S. Department of Health and Human Services.

1. **Influenza vaccination**

Annual vaccination against influenza is recommended for all persons aged 6 mos and older, including all adults. Healthy, nonpregnant adults aged less than 50 yrs without high-risk medical conditions can receive either intranasally administered live, attenuated influenza vaccine (FluMist), or inactivated vaccine. Other persons should receive the inactivated vaccine. Adults aged 65 yrs and older can receive the standard influenza vaccine or the high-dose (Fluzone) influenza vaccine. Additional information about influenza vaccination is available at http://www.cdc.gov/vaccines/vpd-vac/flu/default.htm.

2. **Tetanus, diphtheria, and acellular pertussis (Td/Tdap) vaccination**

Administer a one-time dose of Tdap to adults aged less than 65 yrs who have not received Tdap previously or for whom vaccine status is unknown to replace one of the 10-yr Td boosters, and as soon as feasible to all 1) postpartum women, 2) close contacts of infants younger than age 12 mos (e.g., grandparents and child-care providers), and 3) healthcare personnel with direct patient contact. Adults aged 65 yrs and older who have not previously received Tdap and who have close contact with an infant aged less than 12 mos also should be vaccinated. Other adults aged 65 yrs and older may receive Tdap. Tdap can be administered regardless of interval since the most recent tetanus or diphtheria-containing vaccine.

Adults with uncertain or incomplete history of completing a 3-dose primary vaccination series with Td-containing vaccines should begin or complete a primary vaccination series. For unvaccinated adults, administer the first 2 doses at least 4 wks apart and the third dose 6–12 mos after the second. If incompletely vaccinated (i.e., less than 3 doses), administer remaining doses. Substitute a one-time dose of Tdap for one of the doses of Td, either in the primary series or for the routine booster, whichever comes first.

If a woman is pregnant and received the most recent Td vaccination 10 or more yrs previously, administer Td during the second or third trimester. If the woman received the most recent Td vaccination less than 10 yrs previously, administer Tdap during the immediate postpartum period. At the clinician's discretion, Td may be deferred during pregnancy and Tdap substituted in the immediate postpartum period, or Tdap may be administered instead of Td to a pregnant woman after an informed discussion with the woman.

The ACIP statement for recommendations for administering Td as prophylaxis in wound management is available at http://www.cdc.gov/vaccines/pubs/acip-list.htm.

3. **Varicella vaccination**

All adults without evidence of immunity to varicella should receive 2 doses of single-antigen varicella vaccine if not previously vaccinated or a second dose if they have received only 1 dose, unless they have a medical contraindication. Special consideration should be given to those who 1) have close contact with persons at high risk for severe disease (e.g., healthcare personnel and family contacts of persons with immunocompromising conditions) or 2) are at high risk for exposure or transmission (e.g., teachers; child-care employees; residents and staff members of institutional settings, including correctional institutions; college students; military personnel; adolescents and adults living in households with children; nonpregnant women of childbearing age; and international travelers).

Evidence of immunity to varicella in adults includes any of the following: 1) documentation of 2 doses of varicella vaccine at least 4 wks apart; 2) U.S.-born before 1980 (although for healthcare personnel and pregnant women, birth before 1980 should not be considered evidence of immunity); 3) history of varicella based on diagnosis or verification of varicella by a healthcare provider (for a patient reporting a history of or having an atypical case, a mild case, or both, healthcare providers should seek either an epidemiologic link with a typical varicella case or to a laboratory-confirmed case or evidence of laboratory confirmation, if it was performed at the time of acute disease); 4) history of herpes zoster based on diagnosis or verification of herpes zoster by a healthcare provider; or 5) laboratory evidence of immunity or laboratory confirmation of disease.

Pregnant women should be assessed for evidence of varicella immunity. Women who do not have evidence of immunity should receive the first dose of varicella vaccine upon completion or termination of pregnancy and before discharge from the healthcare facility. The second dose should be administered 4–8 wks after the first dose.

4. **Human papillomavirus (HPV) vaccination**

HPV vaccination with either quadrivalent (HPV4) vaccine or bivalent vaccine (HPV2) is recommended for females at age 11 or 12 yrs and catch-up vaccination for females aged 13 through 26 yrs.

Ideally, vaccine should be administered before potential exposure to HPV through sexual activity; however, females who are sexually active should still be vaccinated consistent with age-based recommendations. Sexually active females who have not been infected with any of the four HPV vaccine types (types 6, 11, 16, and 18, all of which HPV4 prevents) or any of the two HPV vaccine types (types 16 and 18, both of which HPV2 prevents) receive the full benefit of the vaccination. Vaccination is less beneficial for females who have already been infected with one or more of the HPV vaccine types. HPV4 or HPV2 can be administered to persons with a history of genital warts, abnormal Papanicolaou test, or positive HPV DNA test, because these conditions are not evidence of previous infection with all vaccine HPV types.

HPV4 may be administered to males aged 9 through 26 yrs to reduce their likelihood of genital warts. HPV4 would be most effective when administered before exposure to HPV through sexual contact.

A complete series for either HPV4 or HPV2 consists of 3 doses. The second dose should be administered 1–2 mos after the first dose; the third dose should be administered 6 mos after the first dose.

Although HPV vaccination is not specifically recommended for persons with the medical indications described in Figure 2, "Vaccines that might be indicated for adults based on medical and other indications," it may be administered to these persons because the HPV vaccine is not a live-virus vaccine. However, the immune response and vaccine efficacy might be less for persons with the medical indications described in Figure 2 than in persons who do not have the medical indications described or who are immunocompetent.

5. **Herpes zoster vaccination**

A single dose of zoster vaccine is recommended for adults aged 60 yrs and older regardless of whether they report a previous episode of herpes zoster. Persons with chronic medical conditions may be vaccinated unless their condition constitutes a contraindication.

6. **Measles, mumps, rubella (MMR) vaccination**

Adults born before 1957 generally are considered immune to measles and mumps. All adults born in 1957 or later should have documentation of 1 or more doses of MMR vaccine unless they have a medical contraindication to the vaccine, laboratory evidence of immunity to each of the three diseases, or documentation of provider-diagnosed measles or mumps disease. For rubella, documentation of provider-diagnosed disease is not considered acceptable evidence of immunity.

Measles component: A second dose of MMR vaccine, administered a minimum of 28 days after the first dose, is recommended for adults who 1) have been recently exposed to measles or are in an outbreak setting; 2) are students in postsecondary educational institutions; 3) work in a healthcare facility; or 4) plan to travel internationally. Persons who received inactivated (killed) measles vaccine or measles vaccine of unknown type during 1963–1967 should be revaccinated with 2 doses of MMR vaccine.

Mumps component: A second dose of MMR vaccine, administered a minimum of 28 days after the first dose, is recommended for adults who 1) live in a community experiencing a mumps outbreak and are in an affected age group; 2) are students in postsecondary educational institutions; 3) work in a healthcare facility; or 4) plan to travel internationally. Persons vaccinated before 1979 with either killed mumps vaccine or mumps vaccine of unknown type who are at high risk for mumps infection (e.g. persons who are working in a healthcare facility) should be revaccinated with 2 doses of MMR vaccine.

Rubella component: For women of childbearing age, regardless of birth yr, rubella immunity should be determined. If there is no evidence of immunity, women who are not pregnant should be vaccinated. Pregnant women who do not have evidence of immunity should receive MMR vaccine upon completion or termination of pregnancy and before discharge from the healthcare facility.

Healthcare personnel born before 1957: For unvaccinated healthcare personnel born before 1957 who lack laboratory evidence of measles, mumps, and/or rubella immunity or laboratory confirmation of disease, healthcare facilities should 1) consider routinely vaccinating personnel with 2 doses of MMR vaccine at the appropriate interval (for measles and mumps) and 1 dose of MMR vaccine (for rubella), and 2) recommend 2 doses of MMR vaccine at the appropriate interval during an outbreak of measles or mumps, and 1 dose during an outbreak of rubella. Complete information about evidence of immunity is available at http://www.cdc.gov/vaccines/recs/provisional/default.htm.

7. **Pneumococcal polysaccharide (PPSV) vaccination**

Vaccinate all persons with the following indications:

Medical: Chronic lung disease (including asthma); chronic cardiovascular diseases; diabetes mellitus; chronic liver diseases; cirrhosis; chronic alcoholism; functional or anatomic asplenia (e.g., sickle cell disease or splenectomy [if elective splenectomy is planned, vaccinate at least 2 wks before surgery]); immunocompromising conditions (including chronic renal failure or nephrotic syndrome); and cochlear implants and cerebrospinal fluid leaks. Vaccinate as close to HIV diagnosis as possible.

Other: Residents of nursing homes or long-term care facilities and persons who smoke cigarettes. Routine use of PPSV is not recommended for American Indians/Alaska Natives or persons aged less than 65 yrs unless they have underlying medical conditions that are PPSV indications. However, public health authorities may consider recommending PPSV for American Indians/Alaska Natives and persons aged 50 through 64 yrs who are living in areas where the risk for invasive pneumococcal disease is increased

8. **Revaccination with PPSV**

One-time revaccination after 5 yrs is recommended for persons aged 19 through 64 yrs with chronic renal failure or nephrotic syndrome; functional or anatomic asplenia (e.g., sickle cell disease or splenectomy); and for persons with immunocompromising conditions. For persons aged 65 yrs and older, one-time revaccination is recommended if they were vaccinated 5 or more yrs previously and were aged less than 65 yrs at the time of primary vaccination.

9. **Meningococcal vaccination**

Meningococcal vaccine should be administered to persons with the following indications:

Medical: A 2-dose series of meningococcal conjugate vaccine is recommended for adults with anatomic or functional asplenia, or persistent complement component deficiencies. Adults with HIV infection who are vaccinated should also receive a routine 2-dose series. The 2 doses should be administered at 0 and 2 mos.

Other: A single dose of meningococcal vaccine is recommended for unvaccinated first-yr college students living in dormitories; microbiologists routinely exposed to isolates of *Neisseria meningitidis;* military recruits; and persons who travel to or live in countries in which meningococcal disease is hyperendemic or epidemic (e.g., the "meningitis belt" of sub-Saharan Africa during the dry season [December through June]), particularly if their contact with local populations will be prolonged. Vaccination is required by the government of Saudi Arabia for all travelers to Mecca during the annual Hajj.

Meningococcal conjugate vaccine, quadrivalent (MCV4) is preferred for adults with any of the preceding indications who are aged 55 yrs and younger; meningococcal polysaccharide vaccine (MPSV4) is preferred for adults aged 56 yrs and older. Revaccination with MCV4 every 5 yrs is recommended for adults previously vaccinated with MCV4 or MPSV4 who remain at increased risk for infection (e.g., adults with anatomic or functional asplenia, or persistent complement component deficiencies).

10. **Hepatitis A vaccination**

Vaccinate persons with any of the following indications and any person seeking protection from hepatitis A virus (HAV) infection:

Behavioral: Men who have sex with men and persons who use injection drugs.

Occupational: Persons working with HAV-infected primates or with HAV in a research laboratory setting.

Medical: Persons with chronic liver disease and persons who receive clotting factor concentrates.

Other: Persons traveling to or working in countries that have high or intermediate endemicity of hepatitis A (a list of countries is available at http://wwwn.cdc.gov/travel/ contentdiseases.aspx).

Unvaccinated persons who anticipate close personal contact (e.g., household or regular babysitting) with an international adoptee during the first 60 days after arrival in the United States from a country with high or intermediate endemicity should be vaccinated. The first dose of the 2-dose hepatitis A vaccine series should be administered as soon as adoption is planned, ideally 2 or more wks before the arrival of the adoptee.

Single-antigen vaccine formulations should be administered in a 2-dose schedule at either 0 and 6–12 mos (Havrix), or 0 and 6–18 mos (Vaqta). If the combined hepatitis A and hepatitis B vaccine (Twinrix) is used, administer 3 doses at 0, 1, and 6 mos; alternatively, a 4-dose schedule may be used, administered on days 0, 7, and 21–30, followed by a booster dose at mo 12.

11. **Hepatitis B vaccination**

Vaccinate persons with any of the following indications and any person seeking protection from hepatitis B virus (HBV) infection:

Behavioral: Sexually active persons who are not in a long-term, mutually monogamous relationship (e.g., persons with more than one sex partner during the previous 6 mos); persons seeking evaluation or treatment for a sexually transmitted disease (STD); current or recent injection-drug users; and men who have sex with men.

Occupational: Healthcare personnel and public-safety workers who are exposed to blood or other potentially infectious body fluids.

Medical: Persons with end-stage renal disease, including patients receiving hemodialysis; persons with HIV infection; and persons with chronic liver disease.

Other: Household contacts and sex partners of persons with chronic HBV infection; clients and staff members of institutions for persons with developmental disabilities; and international travelers to countries with high or intermediate prevalence of chronic HBV infection (a list of countries is available at http://wwwn.cdc.gov/travel/contentdiseases.aspx).

Hepatitis B vaccination is recommended for all adults in the following settings: STD treatment facilities; HIV testing and treatment facilities; facilities providing drug-abuse treatment and prevention services; healthcare settings targeting services to injection-drug users or men who have sex with men; correctional facilities; end-stage renal disease programs and facilities for chronic hemodialysis patients; and institutions and nonresidential day-care facilities for persons with developmental disabilities.

Administer missing doses to complete a 3-dose series of hepatitis B vaccine to those persons not vaccinated or not completely vaccinated. The second dose should be administered 1 mo after the first dose; the third dose should be given at least 2 mos after the second dose (and at least 4 mos after the first dose). If the combined hepatitis A and hepatitis B vaccine (Twinrix) is used, administer 3 doses at 0, 1, and 6 mos; alternatively, a 4-dose Twinrix schedule, administered on days 0, 7, and 21 to 30, followed by a booster dose at mo 12 may be used.

Adult patients receiving hemodialysis or with other immunocompromising conditions should receive 1 dose of 40 μg/mL (Recombivax HB) administered on a 3-dose schedule or 2 doses of 20 μg/mL (Engerix-B) administered simultaneously on a 4-dose schedule at 0, 1, 2, and 6 mos.

12. **Selected conditions for which *Haemophilus influenzae* type b (Hib) vaccine may be used**

1 dose of Hib vaccine should be considered for persons who have sickle cell disease, leukemia, or HIV infection, or who have had a splenectomy, if they have not previously received Hib vaccine.

13. **Immunocompromising conditions**

Inactivated vaccines generally are acceptable (e.g., pneumococcal, meningococcal, influenza [inactivated influenza vaccine]) and live vaccines generally are avoided in persons with immune deficiencies or immunocompromising conditions. Information on specific conditions is available at http://www.cdc.gov/vaccines/pubs/acip-list.htm.

Recommended Immunization Schedule for Persons Aged 0 Through 6 Yrs—United States • 2011

For Those Who Fall Behind or Start Late, See the Catch-up Schedule

Vaccine ▼ Age ▶	Birth	1 mo	2 mos	4 mos	6 mos	12 mos	15 mos	18 mos	19–23 mos	2–3 yrs	4–6 yrs
Hepatitis B[1]	HepB	HepB				HepB					
Rotavirus[2]			RV	RV	RV[2]						
Diphtheria, Tetanus, Pertussis[3]			DTaP	DTaP	DTaP	*see footnote*[3]	DTaP				DTaP
Haemophilus influenzae type b[4]			Hib	Hib	Hib[4]	Hib					
Pneumococcal[5]			PCV	PCV	PCV	PCV				PPSV	
Inactivated Poliovirus[6]			IPV	IPV		IPV					IPV
Influenza[7]								Influenza (Yearly)			
Measles, Mumps, Rubella[8]						MMR			*see footnote*[8]		MMR
Varicella[9]						Varicella			*see footnote*[9]		Varicella
Hepatitis A[10]						HepA (2 doses)				HepA Series	
Meningococcal[11]										MCV	

Legend:
- (light shading) Range of recommended ages for all children except certain high-risk groups
- (dark shading) Range of recommended ages for certain high-risk groups

This schedule includes recommendations in effect as of December 21, 2010. Any dose not administered at the recommended age should be administered at a subsequent visit, when indicated and feasible. The use of a combination vaccine generally is preferred over separate injections of its equivalent component vaccines. Considerations should include provider assessment, patient preference, and the potential for adverse events. Providers should consult the relevant Advisory Committee on Immunization Practices statement for detailed recommendations: http://www.cdc.gov/vaccines/pubs/acip-list.htm. Clinically significant adverse events that follow immunization should be reported to the Vaccine Adverse Event Reporting System (VAERS) at http://www.vaers.hhs.gov or by telephone, 800-822-7967.

1. **Hepatitis B vaccine (HepB).** (Minimum age: birth)
   At birth:
   - Administer monovalent HepB to all newborns before hospital discharge.
   - If mother is hepatitis B surface antigen (HBsAg)-positive, administer HepB and 0.5 mL of hepatitis B immune globulin (HBIG) within 12 hrs of birth.
   - If mother's HBsAg status is unknown, administer HepB within 12 hrs of birth. Determine mother's HBsAg status as soon as possible and, if HBsAg-positive, administer HBIG (no later than age 1 wk).

   Doses following the birth dose:
   - The second dose should be administered at age 1 or 2 mos. Monovalent HepB vaccine should be used for doses administered before age 6 wks.
   - Infants born to HBsAg-positive mothers should be tested for HBsAg and antibody to HBsAg 1 to 2 mos after completion of at least 3 doses of the HepB series, at age 9 through 18 mos (generally at the next well-child visit).
   - Administration of 4 doses of HepB to infants is permissible when a combination vaccine containing HepB is administered after the birth dose.
   - The final (3rd and 4th) dose in the HepB series should be administered no earlier than age 24 wks.
2. **Rotavirus vaccine (RV).** (Minimum age: 6 wks)
   - Administer the first dose at age 6 through 14 wks (maximum age: 14 wks 6 days). Vaccination should not be initiated for infants aged 15 wks, 0 days or older.
   - The maximum age for the final dose in the series is 8 mos, 0 days.
   - If Rotarix is administered at ages 2 and 4 mos, a dose at 6 mos is not indicated.
3. **Diphtheria and tetanus toxoids and acellular pertussis vaccine (DTaP).** (Minimum age: 6 wks)
   - The fourth dose may be administered as early as age 12 mos, provided at least 6 mos have elapsed since the third dose.
4. ***Haemophilus influenzae* type b conjugate vaccine (Hib).** (Minimum age: 6 wks)
   - If PRP-OMP (PedvaxHIB or Comvax [HepB-Hib]) is administered at ages 2 and 4 mos, a dose at age 6 mos is not indicated.
   - Hiberix should not be used for doses at ages 2, 4, or 6 mos for the primary series but can be used as the final dose in children aged 12 mos through 4 yrs.
5. **Pneumococcal vaccine.** (Minimum age: 6 wks for pneumococcal conjugate vaccine [PCV]; 2 yrs for pneumococcal polysaccharide vaccine [PPSV])
   - PCV is recommended for all children aged younger than 5 yrs. Administer 1 dose of PCV to all healthy children aged 24 through 59 mos who are not completely vaccinated for their age.
   - A PVC series begun with 7-valent PCV (PCV7) should be completed with 13-valent PCV (PCV13).
   - A single supplemental dose of PCV13 is recommended for all children aged 14 through 59 mos who have received an age-appropriate series of PCV7.
   - A single supplemental dose of PCV13 is recommended for all children aged 60 through 71 mos with underlying medical conditions who have received an age-appropriate series of PCV7.
   - The supplemental dose of PCV13 should be administered at least 8 wks after the pervious dose of PCV7. See *MMWR*. 2010:59(No. RR-11).
   - Administer PPSV at least 8 wks after last dose of PCV to children aged 2 yrs or older with certain underlying medical conditions, including a cochlear implant.
6. **Inactivated poliovirus vaccine (IPV)** (Minimum age: 6 wks)
   - If 4 or more doses are administered prior to age 4 yrs, an additonal dose should be administered at age 4 through 6 yrs.
   - The final dose in the series should be administered on or after the fourth birthday and at least 6 mos following the previous dose.
7. **Influenza vaccine (seasonal).** (Minimum age: 6 mos for trivalent inactivated influenza vaccine [TIV]; 2 yrs for live, attenuated influenza vaccine [LAIV])
   - For healthy children aged 2 yrs and older (i.e., those who do not have underlying medical conditions that predispose them to influenza complications), either LAIV or TIV may be used, except LAIV should not be given to children aged 2 through 4 yrs who have had wheezing in the past 12 mos.
   - Administer 2 doses (separated by at least 4 wks) to children aged 6 mos through 8 yrs who are receiving seasonal influenza vaccine for the first time or who were vaccinated for the first time during the previous influenza season but only received 1 dose.
   - Children aged 6 mos through 8 yrs who received no doses of monovalent 2009 H1N1 vaccine should receive 2 doses of 2010–2011 seasonal influenza vaccine. See *MMWR*. 2010;59(No. RR-8):33–34.
8. **Measles, mumps, and rubella vaccine (MMR).** (Minimum age: 12 mos)
   - The second dose may be administered before age 4 yrs, provided at least 4 wks have elapsed since the first dose.
9. **Varicella vaccine.** (Minimum age: 12 mos)
   - The second dose may be administered before age 4 yrs, provided at least 3 mos have elapsed since the first dose.
   - For children aged 12 mos through 12 yrs the recommended minimum interval between doses is 3 mos. However, if the second dose was administered at least 4 wks after the first dose, it can be accepted as valid.
10. **Hepatitis A vaccine (HepA).** (Minimum age: 12 mos)
    - Administer 2 doses at least 6 mos apart.
    - HepA is recommended for children aged older than 23 mos who live in areas where vaccination programs target older children, who are at increased risk for infection, or for whom immunity against hepatitis A is desired.
11. **Meningococcal conjugate vaccine, quadrivalent (MCV4).** (Minimum age: 2 yrs)
    - Administer 2 doses of MCV4 at least 8 wks apart to children aged 2 through 10 yrs with persistent complement component deficiency and anatomic or functional asplenia, and 1 dose every 5 yrs thereafter.
    - Persons with human immunodeficiency virus (HIV) infection who ar vaccinated with MCV4 should receive 2 doses at least 8 wks apart.
    - Administer 1 dose of MCV4 to children aged 2 through 10 yrs who travel to countries with highly endemic or epidemic disease and during outbreaks caused by a vaccine serogroup.
    - Administer MCV4 to children at continued risk for meningococcal disease who were previously vaccinated with MCV4 or meningococcal polysaccharide vaccine after 3 yrs if first dose administered at age 2 through 6 yrs.

The Recommended Immunization Schedules for Persons Aged 0 through 18 Yrs are approved by the Advisory Committee on Immunization Practices (**http://www.cdc.gov/vaccines/recs/acip**), the American Academy of Pediatrics (**http://www.aap.org**), and the American Academy of Family Physicians (**http://www.aafp.org**).

Department of Health and Human Services • Centers for Disease Control and Prevention

Recommended Immunization Schedule for Persons Aged 7–18 Yrs—United States • 2011

For Those Who Fall Behind or Start Late, See the Schedule Below and the Catch-up Schedule

Vaccine ▼ Age ▶	7–10 yrs	11–12 yrs	13–18 yrs
Tetanus, Diphtheria, Pertussis[1]		Tdap	Tdap
Human Papillomavirus[2]	*see footnote 2*	HPV (3 doses)(females)	HPV series
Meningococcal[3]	MCV4	MCV4	MCV4
Influenza[4]		Influenza (Yearly)	
Pneumococcal[5]		Pneumococcal	
Hepatitis A[6]		HepA Series	
Hepatitis B[7]		Hep B Series	
Inactivated Poliovirus[8]		IPV Series	
Measles, Mumps, Rubella[9]		MMR Series	
Varicella[10]		Varicella Series	

Range of recommended ages for all children

Range of recommended ages for catch-up immunization

Range of recommended ages for certain high-risk groups

This schedule includes recommendations in effect as of December 21, 2010. Any dose not administered at the recommended age should be administered at a subsequent visit, when indicated and feasible. The use of a combination vaccine generally is preferred over separate injections of its equivalent component vaccines. Considerations should include provider assessment, patient preference, and the potential for adverse events. Providers should consult the relevant Advisory Committee on Immunization Practices statement for detailed recommendations: http://www.cdc.gov/vaccines/pubs/acip-list.htm. Clinically significant adverse events that follow immunization should be reported to the Vaccine Adverse Event Reporting System (VAERS) at http://www.vaers.hhs.gov or by telephone, 800-822-7967.

1. **Tetanus and diphtheria toxoids and acellular pertussis vaccine (Tdap).** (Minimum age: 10 yrs for Boostrix and 11 yrs for Adacel)
   - Persons aged 11 through 18 yrs who have not received Tdap should receive a dose followed by Td booster doses every 10 yrs thereafter.
   - Persons aged 7 through 10 yrs who are not fully immunized against pertussis (including those never vaccinated or with unknown pertussis vaccination status) should receive a single dose of Tdap. Refer to the catch-up schedule if additional doses of tetanus and diphtheria toxoid–containing vaccine are needed.
   - Tdap can be administered regardless of the interval since the last tetanus and diphtheria toxoid–containing vaccine.
2. **Human papillomavirus vaccine (HPV).** (Minimum age: 9 yrs)
   - Quadrivalent HPV vaccine (HPV4) or bivalent HPV vaccine (HPV2) is recommended for the prevention of cervical precancers and cancers in females.
   - HPV4 is recommended for prevention of cervical precancers, cancers, and genital warts in females.
   - HPV4 may be administered in a 3-dose series to males aged 9 through 18 yrs to reduce their likelihood of genital warts.
   - Administer the second dose 1 to 2 mos after the first dose and the third dose 6 mos after the first dose (at least 24 wks after the first dose).
3. **Meningococcal conjugate vaccine, quadrivalent (MCV4).** (Minimum age: 2 yrs)
   - Administer MCV4 at age 11 through 12 yrs with a booster dose at age 16 yrs.
   - Administer 1 dose at age 13 through 18 yrs if not previously vaccinated.
   - Persons who received their first dose at age 13 through 15 yrs should receive a booster dose at age 16 through 18 yrs.
   - Administer 1 dose to previously unvaccinated college freshmen living in a dormitory.
   - Administer 2 doses at least 8 wks apart to children aged 2 through 10 yrs with persistent complement component deficiency and anatomic or functional asplenia, and 1 dose every 5 yrs thereafter.
   - Persons with HIV infection who are vaccinated with MCV4 should receive 2 doses at least 8 wks apart.
   - Administer 1 dose of MCV4 to children aged 2 through 10 yrs who travel to countries with highly endemic or epidemic disease and during outbreaks caused by a vaccine serogroup.
   - Administer MCV4 to children at continued risk for meningococcal disease who were previously vaccinated with MCV4 or meningococcal polysaccharide vaccine after 3 yrs (if first dose administered at age 2 through 6 yrs) or after 5 yrs (if first dose administered at age 7 yrs or older).
4. **Influenza vaccine (seasonal).**
   - For healthy nonpregnant persons aged 7 through 18 yrs (i.e., those who do not have underlying medical conditions that predispose them to influenza complications), either LAIV or TIV may be used.
   - Administer 2 doses (separated by at least 4 wks) to children aged 6 mos through 8 yrs who are receiving seasonal influenza vaccine for the first time or who were vaccinated for the first time during the previous influenza season but only received 1 dose.
   - Children 6 mos through 8 yrs of age who received no doses of monovalent 2009 H1N1 vaccine should receive 2 doses of 2010-2011 seasonal influenza vaccine. See *MMWR*. 2010;59(No. RR-8):33–34.
5. **Pneumococcal vaccines.**
   - A single dose of 13-valent pneumococcal conjugate vaccine (PCV13) may be administered to children aged 6 through 18 yrs who have functional or anatomic asplenia, HIV infection or other immunocompromising condition, cochlear implant or CSF leak. See *MMWR*. 2010;59(No. RR-11).
   - The dose of PCV13 should be administered at least 8 wks after the previous dose of PCV7.
   - Administer pneumococcal polysaccharide vaccine at least 8 wks after the last dose of PCV to children aged 2 yrs or older with certain underlying medical conditions, including a cochlear implant. A single revaccination should be administered after 5 yrs to children with functional or anatomic asplenia or an immunocompromising condition.
6. **Hepatitis A vaccine (HepA).**
   - Administer 2 doses at least 6 mos apart.
   - HepA is recommended for children aged older than 23 mos who live in areas where vaccination programs target older children, or who are at increased risk for infection, or for whom immunity against hepatitis A is desired.
7. **Hepatitis B vaccine (HepB).**
   - Administer the 3-dose series to those not previously vaccinated. For those with incomplete vaccination, follow the catch-up schedule.
   - A 2-dose series (separated by at least 4 mos) of adult formulation Recombivax HB is licensed for children aged 11 through 15 yrs.
8. **Inactivated poliovirus vaccine (IPV).**
   - The final dose in the series should be administered on or after the fourth birthday and at least 6 mos following the previous dose.
   - If both OPV and IPV were administered as part of a series, a total of 4 doses should be administered, regardless of the child's current age.
9. **Measles, mumps, and rubella vaccine (MMR).**
   - The minimum interval between the 2 doses of MMR is 4 wks.
10. **Varicella vaccine.**
   - For persons aged 7 through 18 yrs without evidence of immunity (see *MMWR*. 2007;56[No. RR-4]), administer 2 doses if not previously vaccinated or the second dose if only 1 dose has been administered.
   - For persons aged 7 through 12 yrs, the recommended minimum interval between doses is 3 mos. However, if the second dose was administered at least 4 wks after the first dose, it can be accepted as valid.
   - For persons aged 13 yrs and older, the minimum interval between doses is 4 wks.

The Recommended Immunization Schedules for Persons Aged 0 through 18 Yrs are approved by the Advisory Committee on Immunization Practices (**http://www.cdc.gov/vaccines/recs/acip**), the American Academy of Pediatrics (**http://www.aap.org**), and the American Academy of Family Physicians (**http://www.aafp.org**).

Department of Healthand Human Services • Centers for Disease Control and Prevention

Appendix P

SIGNS AND SYMPTOMS OF ELECTROLYTE IMBALANCE

HYPOGLYCEMIA (excessive insulin)

Tremors, cold/clammy skin, mental confusion, rapid/shallow respirations, unusual fatigue, hunger, drowsiness, anxiety, headache, muscular incoordination, paresthesia of tongue/mouth/lips, hallucination, increased pulse and B/P, tachycardia, seizures, coma.

HYPERGLYCEMIA (insufficient insulin)

Hot/flushed/dry skin, fruity breath odor, excessive urination (polyuria), excessive thirst (polydipsia), acute fatigue, air hunger, deep/labored respirations, mental changes, restlessness, nausea, polyphagia (excessive appetite).

HYPOKALEMIA (potassium level less than 3.5 mEq/L)

Weakness/paresthesia of extremities, muscle cramps, nausea, vomiting, diarrhea, hypoactive bowel sounds, absent bowel sounds (paralytic ileus), abdominal distention, weak/irregular pulse, postural hypotension, difficulty breathing, disorientation, irritability.

HYPERKALEMIA (potassium level greater than 5.0 mEq/L)

Diarrhea, muscle weakness, heaviness of legs, paresthesia of tongue/hands/feet, slow/irregular pulse, decreased B/P, abdominal cramps, oliguria/anuria, respiratory difficulty, cardiac abnormalities.

HYPONATREMIA (sodium level less than 130 mEq/L)

Abdominal cramping, nausea, vomiting, diarrhea, cold/clammy skin, poor skin turgor, tremors, muscle weakness, leg cramps, increased pulse rate, irritability, apprehension, hypotension, headache.

HYPERNATREMIA (sodium level greater than 150 mEq/L)

Hot/flushed/dry skin, dry mucous membranes, fever, extreme thirst, dry/rough/red tongue, edema, restlessness, postural hypotension, oliguria.

HYPOCALCEMIA (calcium level less than 8.4 mg/dl)

Circumoral/peripheral numbness and tingling, muscle twitching, Chvostek's sign (facial muscle spasm; test by tapping of facial nerve anterior to earlobe, just below zygomatic arch), muscle cramping, Trousseau's sign (carpopedal spasm), seizures, arrhythmias.

HYPERCALCEMIA (calcium level greater than 10.2 mg/dl)

Muscle hypotonicity, incoordination, anorexia, constipation, confusion, impaired memory, slurred speech, lethargy, acute psychotic behavior, deep bone pain, flank pain.

Appendix Q

PARENTERAL FLUID ADMINISTRATION

Replacing fluids in the body is based on body fluid needs. Water comprises approximately 60% of the adult body. Approximately 40% is intracellular fluid and 20% is extracellular fluid, of which 15% is interstitial (tissues) and 5% is intravascular. The walls separating these compartments are porous, allowing water to move freely between them. Small particles such as sodium and chloride can pass through the walls, but larger molecules such as proteins and starches usually are unable to pass through the walls.

Hydrostatic and osmotic pressures are forces that move water and regulate the body's water. Intravenous fluid manipulates these two pressures. Hydrostatic pressure reflects the weight and volume of water. The greater the volume, the higher the blood pressure.

Effects of Osmotic Pressure: *Osmosis* is the diffusion of water across a semi-permeable membrane from an area of high concentration to an area of low concentration (water moves into the compartment of higher concentration of particles, or solute). This is similar to the action of a sponge soaking up water. This pull is referred to as *osmotic pressure.* It is the number of particles in each compartment that keeps water where it is supposed to be. By administering fluids with more (or fewer) particles than blood plasma, fluid is pulled into the compartment where it is needed the most.

How do we know where the water is needed? To assess water balance, measure the *osmolality* of blood plasma (number of particles [osmoles] in a kilogram of fluid). *Osmolarity* is the number of particles in a liter of fluid. Normal serum osmolality is approximately 300 milliosmoles (mOsm) per liter.

Crystalloids are made of substances that form crystals (e.g., sodium chloride) and are small, so easy movement between compartments is possible. Crystalloids are categorized by their tonicity (a synonym for osmolality). An isotonic solution has the same number of particles (osmolality) as plasma and will not promote a shift of fluids into or out of cells. Examples of isotonic crystalloid solutions are 0.9% sodium chloride and lactated Ringer's solution. Dextrose 5% in water is another isotonic crystalloid. However, it is quickly metabolized, and the fluid quickly becomes hypotonic. Hypotonic solutions (e.g., D_5W, 0.45% sodium chloride) are a good source of free water, causing a shift out of the vascular bed and into cells by way of osmosis. Hypotonic solutions are given to correct cellular dehydration and hypernatremia. Hypertonic solutions have more particles than body water and pull water back into the circulation, which can shrink cells.

Sodium Chloride

Uses

- Extracellular fluid replacement when chloride loss is greater than or equal to sodium loss
- Treatment of metabolic alkalosis in presence of fluid loss; chloride ions cause a compensatory decrease of bicarbonate ions
- Sodium depletion, extracellular fluid volume deficit with sodium deficit
- Initiation and termination of blood transfusion, preventing hemolysis of RBCs (occurs with dextrose in water solutions)

Side Effects/Abnormalities

- Hypernatremia
- **Acidosis:** 0.9% sodium chloride contains one third more chloride ions than is present in extracellular fluid; excess chloride ions cause loss of bicarbonate, resulting in acidosis

- **Hypokalemia:** Increased potassium excretion at the same time extracellular fluid is increasing, which further decreases potassium concentration in extracellular fluid
- Circulatory overload

Dextrose (Glucose)

Effects

- Provides calories for essential energy
- Improves hepatic function because it is converted into glycogen
- Spares body protein, preventing unnecessary breakdown of protein tissue
- Prevents ketosis
- Stored in the liver as glycogen, causing a shift of potassium from extracellular to intracellular fluid compartment

Uses

- Dehydration
- Hyponatremia
- Hyperkalemia
- Vehicle of drug delivery and nutrition

Note: Once infused, dextrose is rapidly metabolized to water and carbon dioxide, becoming hypotonic rather than isotonic.

Side Effects/Abnormalities

- Dehydration: Osmotic diuresis occurs if dextrose is given faster than the pt's ability to metabolize it
- Hypokalemia (see Effects)
- Hyperinsulinism due to rapid infusion of hypertonic solution
- Water intoxication due to an imbalance based on increase in extracellular fluid volume from water alone

Selected Parenteral Fluids

Solution	Comments
Dextrose 5% in water (D_5W)	Supplies approximately 170 cal/L and free water to aid in renal excretion of solutes Avoid excessive volumes in pts with increased antidiuretic hormone activity or to replace fluids in hypovolemic pts
0.9% Sodium chloride (0.9% NaCl)	Isotonic fluid commonly used to expand extracellular fluid in presence of hypovolemia Can be used to treat mild metabolic alkalosis
0.45% Sodium chloride (0.45% NaCl)	Hypotonic solution that provides sodium, chloride, and free water; sodium and chloride allow kidneys to select and retain needed amounts Free water is desirable as aid to kidneys in elimination of solutes
3% Sodium chloride	Used only to treat severe hyponatremia
Lactated Ringer's solution	Isotonic solution that contains sodium, potassium, calcium, and chloride in approximately the same concentrations as found in plasma Used to treat hypovolemia, burns, and fluid loss as bile or diarrhea

Appendix R

SPANISH PHRASES OFTEN USED IN CLINICAL SETTINGS

Created by Esperanza Joyce

TAKING THE MEDICATION HISTORY

Tomando la Historia Médica
(Toh-mahn-doh lah Ees-toh-ree-ah Meh-dee-kah)

- Are you allergic to any medications? (If yes:)
¿Es alérgico a algún medicamento? (sí:)
(Ehs ah-lehr-hee-koh ah ahl-goon meh-dee-kah-mehn-toh) (see:)

- —Which medications are you allergic to?
¿A cuál medicamento es alérgico?
(ah koo-ahl meh-dee-kah-mehn-toh ehs ah-lehr-hee-koh)

- Do you take any over-the-counter, prescription, or herbal medications?
¿Toma medicamentos sin receta, con receta, o naturistas (hierbas medicinales)?
(Toh-mah meh-dee-kah-mehn-tohs seen reh-seh-tah, kohn reh-seh-tah, oh nah-too-rees-tahs [ee-ehr-bahs meh-dee-see-nah-lehs])

—How often do you take each medication?
¿Con qué frequencia toma cada medicamento?
(Kohn keh freh-koo-ehn-see-ah toh-mah kah-dah meh-dee-kah-mehn-toh)

Once a day?
¿Una vez por día; diariamente?
(Oo-nah behs pohr dee-ah; dee-ah-ree-ah-mehn-teh)

Twice a day? ¿Dos veces por día?
(dohs beh-sehs pohr dee-ah)

Three times a day? ¿Tres veces por día?
(Trehs beh-sehs pohr dee-ah)

Four times a day? ¿Cuatro veces por día?
(Koo-ah-troh beh-sehs pohr-dee-ah)

—Does the medication make you feel better?
¿Le hace sentir mejor el medicamento?
(Leh ah-seh sehn-teer meh-hohr ehl meh-dee-kah-mehn-toh)

—Does the medication make you feel the same or unchanged?
¿Le hace sentir igual o sin cambio el medicamento?
(Leh ah-seh sehn-teer ee-goo-ahl oh seen kam-bee-oh ehl meh-dee-kah-mehn-toh)

—Does the medication make you feel worse?
¿Se siente peor con el medicamento?
(Seh see-ehn teh peh-ohr kohn ehl meh-dee-kah-mehn-toh)

PREPARING FOR TREATMENT WITH MEDICATION THERAPY

Preparando para un régimen de medicamento
(Preh-pah-rahn-doh pah-rah oon reh-hee-mehn deh meh-dee-kah-mehn-toh)

MEDICATION PURPOSE
PROPÓSITO DEL MEDICAMENTO

(Proh-poh-see-toh dehl meh-dee-kah-mehn-toh)

This medication will help relieve:
Este medicamento le ayudará a aliviar:
(Ehs-teh meh-dee-kah-mehn-toh leh ah-yoo-dah-rah ah ah-lee-bee-ahr)

abdominal gas
gases intestinales
(gah-sehs een-tehs-tee-nah-lehs)

abdominal pain
dolor intestinal; dolor en el abdomen
(doh-lohr een-tehs-tee-nahl; doh-lohr ehn ehl ahb-doh-mehn)

chest congestion
congestión del pecho
(kohn-hehs-tee-ohn dehl peh-choh)

chest pain
dolor del pecho
(doh-lohr dehl peh-choh)

constipation
constipación; estrenimiento
(kohns-tee-pah-see-ohn; ehs-treh-nyee-mee-ehn-toh)

cough
tos
(tohs)

headache
dolor de cabeza
(doh-lohr deh kah-beh-sah)

muscle aches and pains
achaques musculares y dolores
(ah-chah-kehs moos-koo-lah-rehs ee doh-loh-rehs)

pain
dolor
(doh-lohr)

This medication will prevent:
Este medicamento prevendrá:
(Ehs-teh meh-dee-kah-mehn-toh preh-behn-drah)

blood clots
coágulos de sangre
(koh-ah-goo-lohs deh sahn-greh)

constipation
constipación; estreñimiento
(kohns-tee-pah-see-ohn; ehs-treh-nyee-mee-ehn-toh)

contraception
contracepción; embarazo
(kohn-trah-sehp-see-ohn; ehm-bah-rah-soh)

diarrhea
diarrea
(dee-ah-reh-ah)

infection
infección
(een-fehk-see-ohn)

seizures
convulciónes; ataque epiléptico
(kohn-bool-see-ohn-ehs; ah-tah-keh eh-pee-lehp-tee-koh)

shortness of breath
respiración corta; falta de aliento
(rehs-pee-rah-see-ohn kohr-tah; fahl-tah deh ah-lee-ehn-toh)

wheezing
el resollar; la respiración ruidosa, sibilante
(ehl reh-soh-yahr; lah rehs-pee-rah-see-ohn roo-ee-doh-sah, see-bee-lahn-teh)

This medication will increase your:
Este medicamento aumentará su:
(Ehs-teh meh-dee-kah-mehn-toh ah-oo-mehn-tah-rah soo):

ability to fight infections
habilidad a combatir infecciones
(ah-bee-lee-dahd ah kohm-bah-teer een-fehk-see-oh-nehs)

appetite
apetito
(ah-peh-tee-toh)

blood iron level
nivel de hierro en la sangre
(nee-behl deh ee-eh-roh ehn lah sahn-greh)

blood sugar
azúcar en la sangre
(ah-soo-kahr ehn lah sahn-greh)

heart rate
pulso; latido
(pool-soh; lah-tee-doh)

red blood cell count
cuenta de células rojas
(koo-ehn-tah deh seh-loo-lahs roh-hahs)

thyroid hormone levels
niveles de hormona tiroide
(nee-beh-lehs deh ohr-moh-nah tee-roh-ee-deh)

urine volume
volumen de orina
(boh-loo-mehn deh oh-ree-nah)

This medication will decrease your:
Este medicamento reducirá su:
(Ehs-teh meh-dee-kah-mehn-toh reh-doo-see-rah soo:)

anxiety
ansiedad
(ahn-see-eh-dahd)

blood cholesterol level
nivel de colesterol en la sangre
(nee-behl deh koh-lehs-teh-rohl ehn lah sahn-greh)

blood lipid level
nivel de lípido en la sangre
(nee-behl deh lee-pee-doh ehn lah sahn-greh)

blood pressure
presión arterial; de sangre
(preh-see-ohn ahr-teh-ree-ahl; deh sahn-greh)

blood sugar level
nivel de azúcar en la sangre
(nee-behl deh ah-soo-kahr ehn lah sahn-greh)

heart rate
pulso; latido
(pool-soh; lah-tee-doh)

stomach acid
ácido en el estómago
(ah-see-doh ehn ehl ehs-toh-mah-goh)

thyroid hormone levels
niveles de hormona tiroide
(nee-beh-lehs deh ohr-moh-nah tee-roh-ee-deh)

weight
peso
(peh-soh)

This medication will treat:
Este medicamento sirve para:
(Ehs-teh meh-dee-kah-mehn-toh seer-beh pah-rah)

depression
depresión
(deh-preh-see-ohn)

inflammation
infamación
(een-flah-mah-see-ohn)

swelling
hinchazón
(een-chah-sohn)

the infection in your ____
la infección en su ____
(lah een-fehk-see-ohn ehn soo)

your abnormal heart rhythm
su ritmo anormal de corazón
(soo reet-moh ah-nohr-mahl deh koh-rah-sohn)

your allergy to ____
su alergia a ____
(soo eh-lehr-hee-ah ah)

your rash
su erupción; sarpullido
(soo eh-roop-see-ohn; sahr-poo-yee-doh)

ADMINISTERING MEDICATION

Administrando el Medicamento
(Ahd-mee-nees-trahn-doh ehl meh-dee-kah-mehn-toh)

- Swallow this medication with water or juice.
  Tragüe este medicamento con agua o jugo.
  (Trah-geh ehs-teh meh dee-kah-mehn-toh kohn ah-goo-ah oh hoo-goh)

- Do not chew this medication. Swallow it whole.
  No mastique este medicamento. Tragüelo entero.
  (Noh mahs-tee-keh ehs-teh meh-dee-kah-mehn-toh. Trah-geh-loh ehn-teh-roh)

ADMINISTRATION FREQUENCY
FRECUENCIA DE LA ADMINISTRACIÓN
(Freh-koo-ehn-see-ah deh lah Ahd-mee-nees-trah-see-ohn)

English	Spanish	Pronunciation
Once a day	Una vez por día; diariamente	(Oo-nah behs pohr dee-ah; dee-ah-ree-ah-mehn-teh)
Twice a day	Dos veces por día	(Dohs beh-sehs pohr dee-ah)
Three times a day	Tres veces por día	(Trehs beh-sehs pohr dee-ah)
Four times a day	Cuatro veces por día	(Koo-ah-troh beh-sehs pohr dee-ah)
Every other day	Cada tercer día	(Kah-dah tehr-sehr dee-ah)
Once a week	Una vez por semana	(Oo-nah behs pohr seh-mah-nah)
Every 4 hours	Cada cuatro horas	(Kah-dah koo-ah-troh oh-rahs)
Every 6 hours	Cada seis horas	(Kah-dah seh-ees oh-rahs)
Every 8 hours	Cada ocho horas	(Kah-dah oh-choh oh-rahs)
Every 12 hours	Cada doce horas	(Kah-dah doh-seh oh-rahs)
In the morning	En la mañana	(Ehn lah mah-nyah-nah)
In the afternoon	En la tarde	(Ehn lah tahr-deh)
In the evening	En la noche	(Ehn lah noh-cheh)
Before bedtime	Antes de acostarse	(Ahn-tehs deh ah-kohs-tahr-seh)
Before meals	Antes de la comida; Antes del alimento	(Ahn-tens deh lah koh-mee-dah; Ahn-tehs dehl ah-lee-mehn-toh)
With meals	Con los alimentos; Con la comida	(Kohn lohs ah-lee-mehn-tohs; Kohn lah koh-mee-dah)
After meals	Después de los alimentos; Después de la comida	(Dehs-poo-ehs deh lohs ah-lee-mehn-tohs; Dehs-poo-ehs deh lah koh-mee-dah)
Only when you need it	Solo cuando la necesite	(Soh-loh koo-ahn-doh lah neh-seh-see-teh)
When you have ______ pain	Cuando tiene ______ dolor	(Koo-ahn-doh tee-eh-neh ______ doh-lohr)

50 COMMON SIDE EFFECTS
CINCUENTA EFECTOS SECUNDARIOS COMÚNES
(Seen-koo-ehn-tah Eh-fehk-tohs Seh-koon-dah-ree-ohs Koh-moo-nehs)

English	Spanish	Pronunciation
Abdominal cramps	Retorcijón abdominal	(Reh-tohr-see-hohn ahb-doh-mee-nahl)
Abdominal pain	Dolor abdominal	(Doh-lohr ahb-doh-mee-nahl)
Abdominal swelling	Inflamación abdominal	(Een-flah-mah-see-ohn ahb-doh-mee-nahl)
Anxiety	Ansiedad	(Ahn-see-eh-dahd)
Blood in the stool	Sangre en el excremento	(Sahn-greh ehn ehl ehx-kreh-mehn-toh)
Blood in the urine	Sangre en la orina	(Sahn-greh ehn la oh-ree-nah)
Bone pain	Dolor de hueso*	(Doh-lohr deh oo-eh-soh)
Chest pain	Dolor de pecho	(Doh-lohr deh peh-choh)
Chest pounding	Palpitación; latidos fuertes en el pecho	(Pahl-pee-tah-see-ohn; lah-tee-dohs foo-ehr-tehs ehn ehl peh-choh)
Chills	Escalofrío	(Ehs-kah-loh-free-oh)
Confusion	Confusión	(Kohn-foo-see-ohn)
Constipation	Constipación, estreñimiento	(Kohns-tee-pah-see-ohn, ehs-treh-nyee-mee-ehn-toh)
Cough	Tos	(Tohs)
Depression, mental	Depresión mental	(Deh-preh-see-ohn mehn-tahl)
Diarrhea	Diarrea	(Dee-ah-reh-ah)
Difficulty breathing	Dificultad al respirar	(Dee-fee-kool-tahd ahl rehs-pee-rahr)
Difficulty sleeping	Dificultad al dormir	(Dee-fee-kool-tahd ahl dohr-meer)
Difficulty urinating	Dificultad al orinar	(Dee-fee-kool-tahd ahl oh-ree-nahr)
Dizziness	Mareos; vahídos	(Mah-reh-ohs; bah-ee-dohs)
Dry mouth	Boca seca	(Boh-kah seh-kah)
Easy bruising	Fragilidad capilar; le salen moretones con facilidad	(Frah-hee-lee-dahd kah-pee-lahr; leh sah-lehn moh-reh-toh-nehs kohn fah-see-lee-dahd)
Faintness	Desvanecimiento; sintió un vahído	(Dehs-bah-neh-see-mee-ehn-toh; seen-tee-oh oon bah-ee-doh)
Fatigue	Fatiga, cansancio	(Fah-tee-gah, kahn-sahn-see-oh)
Fever	Fiebre	(Fee-eh-breh)
Frequent urination	Orina frecuente	[illegible]

Headache	Dolor de cabeza	(Doh-lohr deh kah-beh-sah)
Impotence	Impotencia	(Eem-poh-tehn-see-ah)
Increased appetite	Aumento en el apetito	(Ah-oo-mehn-toh ehn ehl ah-peh-tee-toh)
Increased gas	Flatulencia	(Flah-too-lehn-see-ah)
Increased perspiration	Aumento en el sudor	(Ah-oo-mehn-toh ehn ehl soo-dohr)
Indigestion	Indigestión	(Een-dee-hehs-tee-ohn)
Itching	Comezón	(Koh-meh-sohn)
Loss of appetite	Pérdida en el apetito	(Pehr-dee-dah ehn ehl ah-peh-tee-toh)
Menstrual changes	Cambios en la menstruación; Cambio en el ciclomenstrual	(Kahm-bee-ohs ehn la mehns-truh-ah-see-ohn; Kahm-bee-oh ehn ehl see-kloh mehns-truh-ahl)
Mood changes	Cambio en el humor; Cambio en la disposición	(Kahm-bee-oh ehn ehl oo-mohr, Kahm-bee-oh ehn lah dees-poh-see-see-ohn)
Muscle aches	Achaques musculares	(Ah-chah-kehs moos-koo-lah-rehs)
Muscle cramps	Calambre muscular	(Kah-lahm-breh moos-koo-lahr)
Muscle pain	Dolores musculares	(Doh-loh-rehs moos-koo-lah-rehs)
Nasal congestion	Congestión nasal	(Kohn-hehs-tee-ohn nah-sahl)
Nausea	Nausea	(Nah-oo-seh-ah)
Ringing in the ears	Zumbido en los oidos	(Soom-bee-doh ehn lohs oh-ee-dohs)
Skin rash	Erupción en la piel	(Eh-roop-see-ohn ehn lah pee-ehl)
Swelling on the hands, legs, or feet	Hinchazón en las manos, piernas, o pies	(Een-chah-sohn ehn lahs mah-nohs, pee-ehr-nahs, oh pee-ehs)
Vaginal bleeding	Sangrado vaginal	(Sahn-grah-doh bah-hee-nahl)
Vision changes	Cambios en la visión; cambios en la vista	(Kahm-bee-ohs ehn lah bee-see-ohn; cahm-bee-ohs ehn lah bees-tah)
Vomiting	Vomitando	(Boh-mee-tahn-doh)
Weakness	Debilidad	(Deh-bee-lee-dahd)
Weight gain	Aumento de peso	(Ah-oo-mehn-toh deh peh-soh)
Weight loss	Pérdida de peso	(Pehr-dee-day deh peh-soh)
Wheezing	Resollar; respiración sibilante	(Reh-soh-yahr; rehs-pee-rah-see-ohn see-bee-lahn-teh)

*h is silent.

Appendix S

TECHNIQUES OF MEDICATION ADMINISTRATION

OPHTHALMIC

Eye Drops

1. Wash hands.
2. Instruct pt to lie down or tilt head backward and look up.
3. Gently pull lower eyelid down until a pocket (pouch) is formed between eye and lower lid (conjunctival sac).
4. Hold dropper above pocket. Without touching tip of eye dropper to eyelid or conjunctival sac, place prescribed number of drops into the center pocket (placing drops directly onto eye may cause a sudden squeezing of eyelid, with subsequent loss of solution). Continue to hold the eyelid for a moment after the drops are applied (allows medication to distribute along entire conjunctival sac).
5. Instruct pt to close eyes gently so that medication is not squeezed out of sac.
6. Apply gentle finger pressure to the lacrimal sac at the inner canthus (bridge of the nose, inside corner of the eye) for 1–2 min (promotes absorption, minimizes drainage into nose and throat, lessens risk of systemic absorption).
7. Remove excess solution around eye with a tissue.
8. Wash hands immediately to remove medication on hands. Never rinse eye dropper.

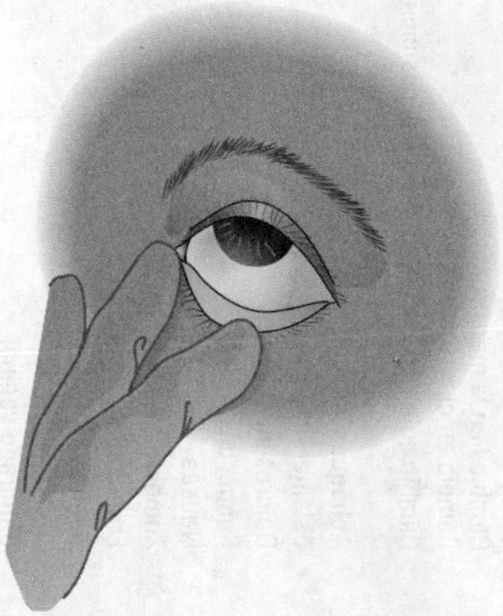

Eye Ointment

1. Wash hands.
2. Instruct pt to lie down or tilt head backward and look up.

3. Gently pull lower eyelid down until a pocket (pouch) is formed between eye and lower lid (conjunctival sac).
4. Hold applicator tube above pocket. Without touching the applicator tip to eyelid or conjunctival sac, place prescribed amount of ointment (¼–½ inch) into the center pocket (placing ointment directly onto eye may cause discomfort).
5. Instruct pt to close eye for 1–2 min, rolling eyeball in all directions (increases contact area of drug to eye).
6. Inform pt of temporary blurring of vision. If possible, apply ointment just before bedtime.
7. Wash hands immediately to remove medication on hands. Never rinse tube applicator.

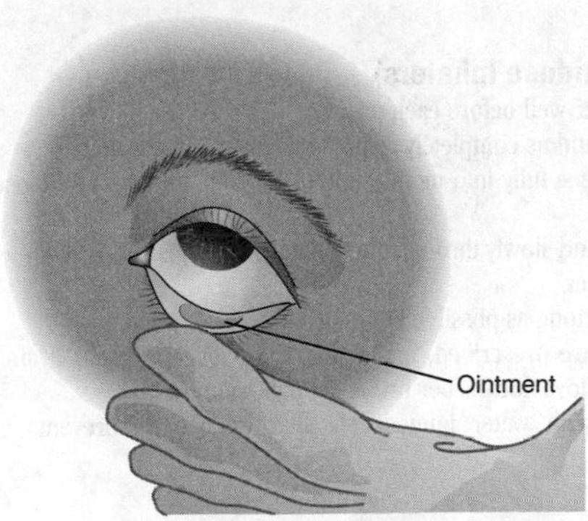

OTIC

1. Ear drops should be at body temperature (wrap hand around bottle to warm contents). Body temperature instillation prevents startling of pt.
2. Instruct pt to lie down with head turned so affected ear is upright (allows medication to drip into ear).
3. Instill prescribed number of drops toward the canal wall, not directly on eardrum.
4. To promote correct placement of ear drops, pull the auricle down and posterior in children (A) and pull the auricle up and posterior in adults (B).

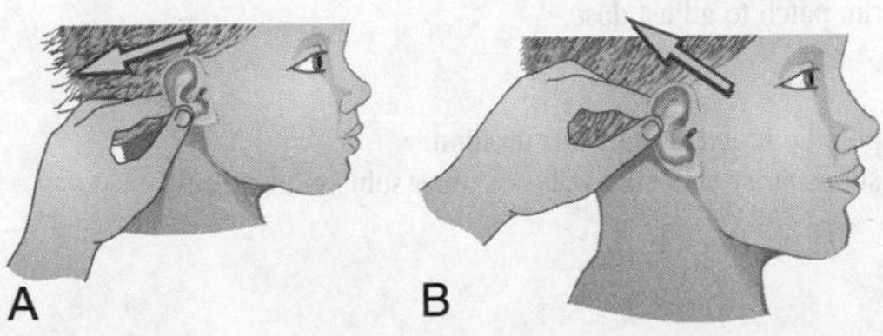

NASAL

Nose Drops and Sprays

1. Instruct pt to blow nose to clear nasal passages as much as possible.
2. Tilt head slightly forward if instilling nasal spray, slightly backward if instilling nasal drops.
3. Insert spray tip into 1 nostril, pointing toward inflamed nasal passages, away from nasal septum.
4. Spray or drop medication into 1 nostril while holding other nostril closed and concurrently inspire through nose to permit medication as high into nasal passages as possible.
5. Discard unused nasal solution after 3 mos.

INHALATION

Aerosol (Multidose Inhalers)

1. Shake container well before each use.
2. Exhale slowly and as completely as possible through the mouth.
3. Place mouthpiece fully into mouth, holding inhaler upright, and close lips fully around mouthpiece.
4. Inhale deeply and slowly through the mouth while depressing the top of the canister with the middle finger.
5. Hold breath as long as possible before exhaling slowly and gently.
6. When 2 puffs are prescribed, wait 2 min and shake container again before inhaling a second puff (allows for deeper bronchial penetration).
7. Rinse mouth with water immediately after inhalation (prevents mouth and throat dryness).

SUBLINGUAL

1. Administer while seated.
2. Dissolve sublingual tablet under tongue (do not chew or swallow tablet).
3. Do not swallow saliva until tablet is dissolved.

TOPICAL

1. Gently cleanse area prior to application.
2. Use occlusive dressings only as ordered.
3. Without touching applicator tip to skin, apply sparingly; gently rub into area thoroughly unless ordered otherwise.
4. When using aerosol, spray area for 3 sec from 15-cm distance; avoid inhalation.

TRANSDERMAL

1. Apply transdermal patch to clean, dry, hairless skin on upper arm or body (not below knee or elbow).
2. Rotate sites (prevents skin irritation).
3. Do not trim patch to adjust dose.

RECTAL

1. Instruct pt to lie in left lateral Sims position.
2. Moisten suppository with cold water or water-soluble lubricant.

3. Instruct pt to slowly exhale (relaxes anal sphincter) while inserting suppository well up into rectum.
4. Inform pt as to length of time (20–30 min) before desire for defecation occurs or less than 60 min for systemic absorption to occur, depending on purpose for suppository.

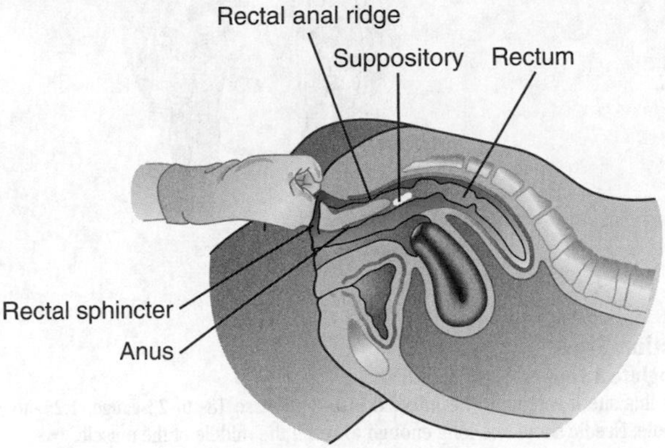

SUBCUTANEOUS

1. Use 25- to 27-gauge, ½- to ⅝-inch needle; 1–3 ml. Angle of insertion depends on body size: 90° if pt is obese. If pt is very thin, gather the skin at the area of needle insertion and administer also at a 90° angle. A 45° angle can be used in a pt of average weight.
2. Cleanse area to be injected with circular motion.
3. Avoid areas of bony prominence, major nerves, blood vessels.
4. Aspirate syringe before injecting (to avoid intra-arterial administration), except insulin, heparin.
5. Inject slowly; remove needle quickly.

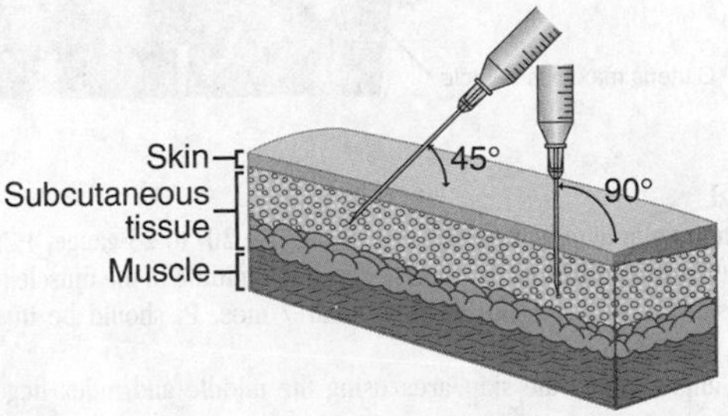

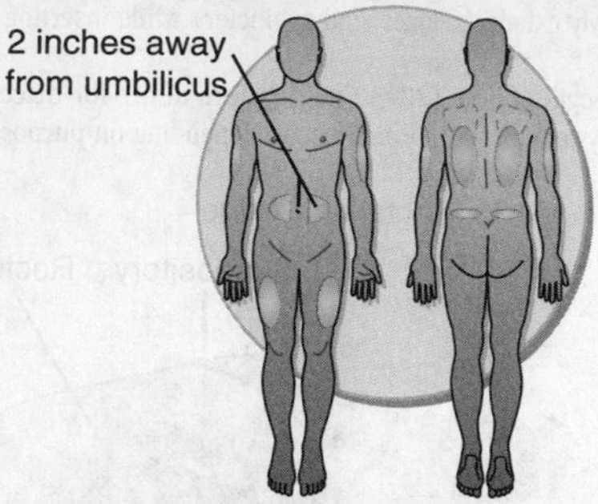

Subcutaneous injection sites

IM

Injection Sites

Dorsogluteal (upper outer quadrant)

1. Use this site if volume to be injected is 1–3 ml. Use 18- to 23-gauge, 1.25- to 3-inch needle. Needle should be long enough to reach the middle of the muscle.
2. Do not use this site in children younger than 2 yrs or in those who are emaciated. Pt should be in prone position.
3. Using 90° angle, flatten the skin area using the middle and index fingers and inject between them.

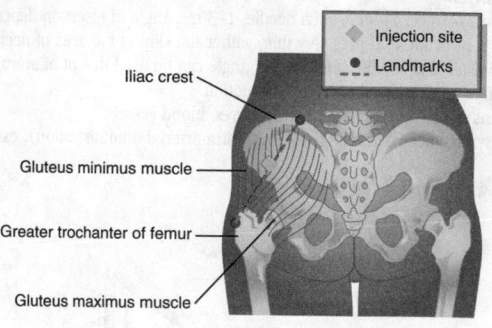

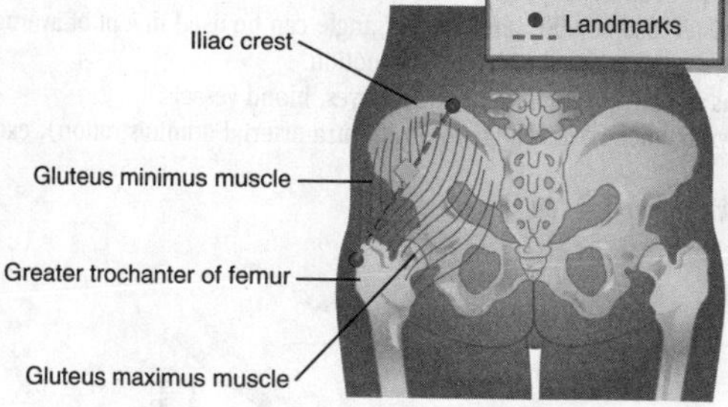

Ventrogluteal

1. Use this site if volume to be injected is 1–5 ml. Use 20- to 23-gauge, 1.25- to 2.5-inch needle. Needle should be long enough to reach the middle of the muscle.
2. Preferred site for adults, children older than 7 mos. Pt should be in supine lateral position.
3. Using 90° angle, flatten the skin area using the middle and index fingers and inject between them.

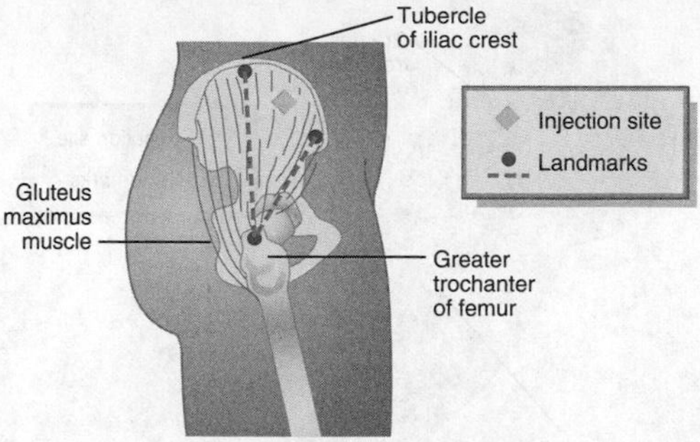

Deltoid

1. Use this site if volume to be injected is 0.5–1 ml. Use 23- to 25-gauge, ⅝- to ½-inch needle. Needle should be long enough to reach the middle of the muscle.
2. Pt may be in prone, sitting, supine, or standing position.
3. Using 90° angle or angled slightly toward acromion, flatten the skin area using the thumb and index finger and inject between them.

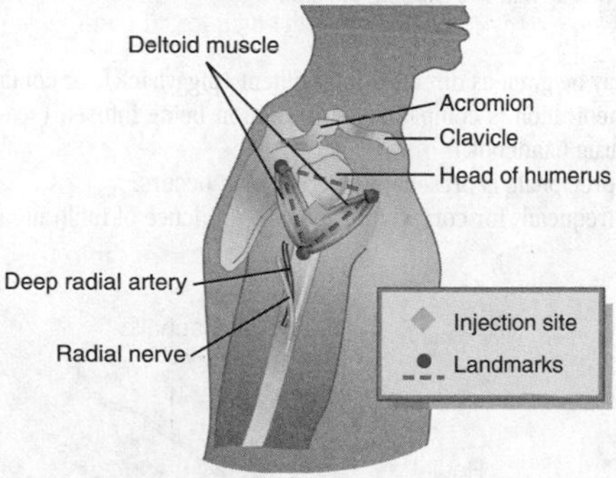

Anterolateral Thigh

1. Anterolateral thigh is site of choice for infants and children younger than 7 mos. Use 22- to 25-gauge, ⅝- to 1-inch needle.
2. Pt can be in supine or sitting position.
3. Using 90° angle, flatten the skin area using the thumb and index finger and inject between them.

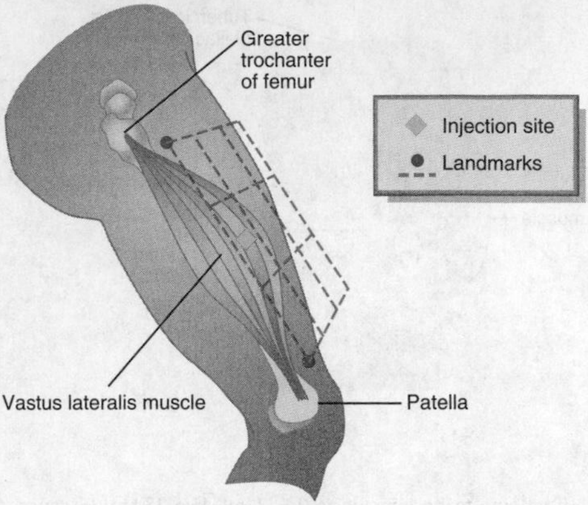

Z-TRACK TECHNIQUE

1. Draw up medication with one needle, and use new needle for injection (minimizes skin staining).
2. Administer deep IM in upper outer quadrant of buttock only (dorsogluteal site).
3. Displace the skin lateral to the injection site before inserting the needle.
4. Withdraw the needle before releasing the skin.

IV

1. Medication may be given as direct IV, intermittent (piggyback), or continuous infusion.
2. Ensure that medication is compatible with solution being infused (see IV compatibility chart in this drug handbook).
3. Do not use if precipitate is present or discoloration occurs.
4. Check IV site frequently for correct infusion rate, evidence of infiltration, extravasation.

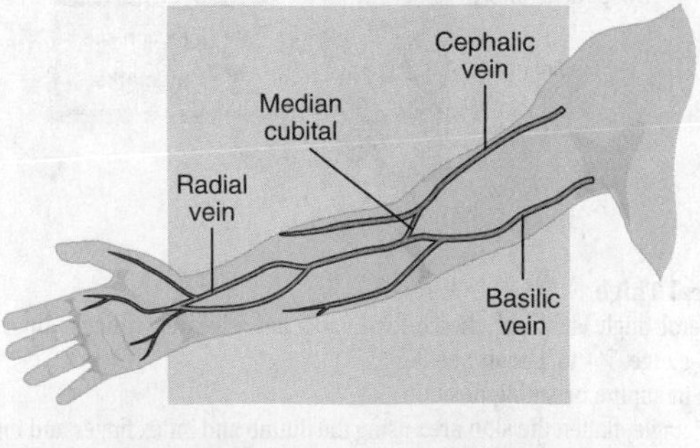

Intravenous medications are administered by the following:

1. Continuous infusing solution.
2. Piggyback (intermittent infusion).
3. Volume control setup (medication contained in a chamber between the IV solution bag and the pt).
4. Bolus dose (a single dose of medication given through an infusion line or saline lock). Sometimes this is referred to as an IV push.

Adding medication to a newly prescribed IV bag:

1. Remove the plastic cover from the IV bag.
2. Cleanse rubber port with an alcohol swab.
3. Insert the needle into the center of the rubber port.
4. Inject the medication.
5. Withdraw the syringe from the port.
6. Gently rotate the container to mix the solution.
7. Label the IV, including the date, time, medication, and dosage. The label should be placed so that it is easily read when hanging.
8. Spike the IV tubing and prime the tubing.

Hanging an IV piggyback (IVPB):

1. When using the piggyback method, lower the primary bag at least 6 inches below the piggyback bag.
2. Set the pump as a secondary infusion when entering the rate of infusion and volume to be infused.
3. Most piggyback medications contain 50–100 cc and usually infuse in 20–60 min, although larger-volume bags take longer.

Administering IV medications through a volume control setup (Buretrol):

1. Insert the spike of the volume control set (Buretrol, Soluset, Pediatrol) into the primary solution container.
2. Open the upper clamp on the volume control set and allow sufficient fluid into volume control chamber.
3. Fill the volume control device with 30 cc of fluid by opening the clamp between the primary solution and the volume control device.

Administering an IV bolus dose:

1. If an existing IV is infusing, stop the infusion by pinching the tubing above the port.
2. Insert the needle into the port and aspirate to observe for a blood return.
3. If the IV is infusing properly with no signs of infiltration or inflammation, it should be patent.
4. Blood indicates that the intravenous line is in the vein.
5. Inject the medication at the prescribed rate.
6. Remove the needle and regulate the IV as prescribed.

Appendix T

CHRONIC WOUND CARE

Introduction

A chronic wound is one that has not healed completely after 4–6 wks. The most common chronic wounds include pressure ulcers (also called *decubitus ulcers* or *bedsores)*, diabetic ulcers (diabetes causes neuropathy, which inhibits the perception of pain and may cause repeated injury), and venous ulcers, primarily occurring in legs, most likely affecting the elderly.

Causes of chronic wounds include the following:

- **Diseases:** Diabetes, cancer, liver/kidney conditions may slow the healing process
- **Poor blood supply/oxygen:** Decreased blood flow may be due to low blood pressure, blocked or narrow blood vessels; low oxygen may be due to heart or lung disease
- **Repeated trauma:** May be due to swelling, increased pressure in tissues, constant pressure on the wound area
- **Impaired immune system:** May be due to radiation, poor nutrition, medications (e.g., steroids)
- **Infection or presence of foreign objects:** May delay wound healing

Treatment

Treatment is based on the severity of the wound, the location of the wound, and whether other areas are affected. Staging of ulcers and other chronic wounds is common practice and relates to the depth and severity of the wound.

Stage 1: Wound is seen as nonblanching redness of intact skin
Stage 2: Ulcer extends through the epidermis or dermis
Stage 3: Ulcer extends through the full thickness of the skin into the subcutaneous tissue, creating a crater
Stage 4: Tissue necrosis with muscle, bone, or underlying structural damage

Treatment of chronic wounds involves maintaining appropriate moisture levels, preventing/treating infections, debridement (removal of necrotic or fibrous tissue, which may include surgical debridement for pts with sepsis or advancing cellulitis), cleansing the wound, eliminating or minimizing pain, and protecting the surrounding skin.

During the healing process, wounds progress through three, sometimes overlapping, phases:

- **Inflammatory phase:** Redness, heat, pain, swelling
- **Proliferative phase:** Migration of fibroblasts into the wound, cellular proliferation, granulation
- **Maturation phase:** New collagen production, deposition and migration of epithelial cells

Products used for treatment of chronic wounds include antimicrobials, debriding agents, dressings, and wound cleansers. **Note:** Papain-containing products are no longer available. These products have historically been marketed without approval. Also, adverse events with use of these products raise serious safety concerns (reported to produce hypersensitivity reactions, anaphylactic reactions, hypotension, tachycardia). Pts allergic to latex may be allergic to papaya, the source of papain.

Wound Care Products

Description	General Uses	Comments
Alginate dressings: Spun fibers of brown seaweed that act as ion exchange mechanisms to absorb serous fluid or exudate, forming a gel-like covering that conforms to the shape of the wound. Facilitate autolytic debridement and maintain a moist wound environment. **Products:** AlgiDERM, Curasorb, Sorbsan. Available as ropes, pads.	Abrasions/lacerations/skin tears Arterial/venous ulcers Deep and tunneling wounds Diabetic ulcers Pressure ulcers Second-degree burns Odorous wounds Contaminated and infected wounds	Good for moderately to heavily exudative wounds and hemorrhagic wounds Can be left in place until soaked with exudate Requires a secondary dressing (e.g., transparent film, foam, hydrocolloids) Do not moisten prior to use Nonadhesive, nonocclusive Contraindicated in third-degree burns; not recommended for dry or minimally exudative wounds
Collagenase ointment: Sterile enzymatic debriding ointment that possesses the ability to digest collagen in necrotic tissue. **Products:** Santyl.	Eschar or necrotic tissue in wound bed Diabetic foot ulcer Pressure ulcers, stages 2–4 Varicose ulcers	Can be used for infected wounds Gauze is used as a secondary dressing Discontinue when granulation tissue is present Optimal pH for enzymatic action is 6–8 Avoid acidic agents for cleansing; avoid detergents and agents containing heavy metal (e.g., mercury or silver), which may adversely affect enzymatic activity
Trypsin, castor oil, Peru balsam: Trypsin is a mild debriding agent that helps shed damaged skin cells. **Castor oil** acts as a lubricant to protect tissue. **Peru balsam** increases blood flow to a wound area, reduces wound odor. **Products:** Granulex, Xenaderm. Available as gel, ointment, spray.	Eschar or necrotic tissue in wound bed Pressure ulcers, stages 1–4 Varicose ulcers	Can be used for infected wounds Avoid concurrent use of silver-containing products (may reduce efficacy) Promotes healing and relieves pain caused by bed sores and other skin ulcers
Hydrophilic polyurethane foam: Also called open cell foam dressings. Sheets of foamed solutions of polymers containing variably sized open cells that can hold wound exudate away from wound bed. Maintains moist wound environment. **Products:** Biopatch, Curafoam, Flexzan. Available as sheets in a wide variety of formulations.	Moderate to heavy exudative wounds with or without a clean granular wound bed Diabetic ulcers, pressure ulcers, venous stasis ulcers Draining surgical incisions Superficial burns Tube and drain sites	Contraindicated for use in third-degree burns Not recommended for wounds with little to no exudate or when tunneling is present Good for cavitating wounds Highly absorbent, semi-occlusive dressing Usual dressing change is up to 3 times per wk

(continued)

Description	General Uses	Comments
Hydrocolloids: Formulations of elastomeric, adhesive, and gelling agents; the most common absorbent ingredient is carboxymethylcellulose. Most hydrocolloids are backed with a semi-occlusive film layer. The wound side of the dressing is adhesive, adhering to a moist surface as well as to dry skin but not to the moist wound bed. As wound fluid is absorbed, the hydrocolloid forms a viscous gel in the wound bed, enhancing a moist wound environment. **Products:** Aquacel, Curaderm, DuoDerm. Available as dressings, granules, patches, paste.	Minimal to moderate exudate in partial and full thickness wounds Cuts and abrasions First- and second-degree burns Pressure ulcers Stasis ulcers	Not for wounds producing heavy exudate, infected wounds, dry eschar-covered wounds May provide pain relief Good for chronic wounds that are epithelializing Can be left in place for up to 7 days Contraindicated for third-degree burns
Hydrogels: Glycerin- or water-based dressings designed to hydrate the wound. May absorb small amounts of exudate. **Products:** Curasol, Tegaderm, Flexderm, Vigilon. Available as gel, sheets, gauze.	Partial and full thickness wounds Dry to minimal exudate Cuts and abrasions First- and second-degree burns Pressure ulcers Stasis ulcers	Not for wounds producing moderate to heavy exudate Not for infected wounds May provide pain relief Good for wounds that are debriding Good for keeping a dry wound moist Can be left in place for 1–3 days
Iodine compounds: **Cadexomer iodine:** Iodine is complexed with a polymeric cadexomer starch vehicle, forming a topical gel or paste. The cadexomer moiety absorbs exudate and debris and releases iodine for antimicrobial activity. **Products:** Iodosorb, Iodoflex. Available as gel, dressing, ointment, powder.	Chronic nonhealing, exuding wounds including pressure or leg ulcers and exuding, infected wounds	Requires use of a secondary dressing Contraindicated in pts with iodine sensitivity, Hashimoto's thyroiditis, nontoxic nodular goiter, children Dressing to be changed when it turns white, indicating that the iodine has been depleted
Silver compounds **Silver sulfadiazine cream:** Silver possesses bactericidal properties. Has been shown to reduce bacterial density, vascular margination, migration of inflammatory cells. Enhances rate of re-epithelialization.	Prevent infection in second- and third-degree burns Prevent or treat infection in chronic wounds	May have cytotoxic effects that could delay wound healing Allergic reactions may occur Use should be limited to a 2- to 4-wk period Bacteria may become resistant with prolonged use Avoid use with collagenase- or trypsin-containing debriding agents

Description	General Uses	Comments
Transparent film dressings: Polyurethane sheets coated on one side with an adhesive that is inactivated by moisture and will not adhere to a moist surface such as the wound bed. Have no absorbent capacity and are impermeable to fluids and bacteria but are semi-permeable to oxygen and water vapor. **Products:** Bioclusive, CarraFilm, Tegaderm HP. Available in a variety of sizes and features.	Prophylaxis on high-risk intact skin Superficial wounds with minimal or no exudate Eschar-covered wounds when autolysis is indicated Clean, closed surgical incisions Pressure ulcers, stage 1 or 2 Second-degree burns	Prevents wound desiccation and contamination by bacteria Contraindicated in third-degree burns Promotes autolysis of necrotic tissue in the wound; maintains moist environment Avoid in arterial ulcers and infected wounds requiring frequent monitoring Do not use as primary dressing on wounds with depth or tunneling May provide pain relief Leave in place for up to 7 days or until fluid leaks
Becaplermin gel: Recombinant formulation of platelet-derived growth factor that promotes cell mitogenesis and protein synthesis for granulation tissue granulation. **Products:** Regranex.	Diabetic foot ulcers that extend into subcutaneous tissue or beyond	Usually applied daily Adequate blood supply and absence of necrotic tissue are needed for efficacy Repeated use (3 or more tubes) may increase risk of cancer-related death Use cautiously in pts with known malignancy

Appendix U

QT-INTERVAL PROLONGATION AND MEDICATION SAFETY

The QT interval is a measure of time between the start of the Q wave and the end of the T wave in the heart's electrical cycle. An abnormal prolonged QT interval may be due to long QT syndrome (LQTS). LQTS can be inherited or acquired, often as a side effect of certain medications.

A prolonged QT interval is a marker for ventricular tachyarrhythmias, including torsade de pointes, which can cause cardiac arrest. Torsade de pointes is a rare occurrence. Risk factors for torsade de pointes include advanced age, female gender, heart disease, renal/hepatic impairment, low potassium, magnesium, and/or calcium levels, diuretic use, and use of one or more QT-prolonging medications.

Below is a list of medications that prolong the QT interval and/or induce torsade de pointes. The list does not include every medication. Additionally, some medications are more likely than other medications to cause QT prolongation.

Antiarrhythmics
Amiodarone (Cordarone)
Disopyramide (Norpace)
Dofetilide (Tikosyn)
Dornedarone (Multaq)
Flecainide (Tambocor)
Ibutilide (Corvert)
Procainamide
Propafenone (Rythmol)
Quinidine
Sotalol (Betapace)

Antibiotics
Azithromycin (Zithromax)
Ciprofloxacin (Cipro)
Clarithromycin (Biaxin)
Erythromycin
Levofloxacin (Levaquin)
Moxifloxacin (Avelox)
Norfloxacin (Noroxin)
Ofloxacin

Antineoplastics
Arsenic trioxide (Trisenox)
Dasatinib (Sprycel)
Lapatinib (Tykerb)
Nilotinib (Tasigna)
Sunitinib (Sutent)
Tamoxifen (Nolvadex)

Antidepressants
Amitriptyline (Elavil)
Citalopram (Celexa)
Desipramine (Norpramin)
Desvenlafaxine (Pristiq)
Fluoxetine (Prozac)
Sertraline (Zoloft)
Trazodone (Desyrel)
Venlafaxine (Effexor)

Antipsychotics
Aripiprazole (Abilify)
Asenapine (Saphris)
Haloperidol (Haldol)
Iloperidone (Fanapt)
Paliperidone (Invega)
Quetiapine (Seroquel)
Risperidone (Risperdal)
Thioridazine (Mellaril)
Ziprasidone (Geodon)

Antivirals
Atazanavir (Reyataz)
Foscarnet (Foscavir)
Lopinavir/ritonavir (Kaletra)

Miscellaneous Agents
Alfuzosin (Uroxatral)
Chloroquine (Aralen)
Fosphenytoin (Cerebyx)
Galantamine (Razadyne)
Methadone (Dolophine)
Octreotide (Sandostatin)
Solifenacin (Vesicare)
Tacrolimus (Prograf)
Tizanidine (Zanaflex)
Tolterodine (Detrol)
Vardenafil (Levitra)

General Index

A
5-aminosalicylic acid, 736–737
5-ASA, 736–737
5-FU, 495–497
abacavir, 1–2
Abacavir, 67C–70C, 114C–118C
Abacavir/lamivudine, 114C–118C
abatacept, 2–3
abciximab, 4–5, 30C–33C
Abelcet, 61–63, 46C
Abenol, 9–12
Abilify, 76–78, 64C–66C
Abilify Discmelt, 76–78
abobotulinum toxin A, 6–7
Abraxane, 886–889
Acai, 1257–1269
acamprosate, 7–8
acarbose, 8–9, 42C–44C
Accolate, 1224–1225, 73C–76C
AccuNeb, 25–27, 73C–76C
Accupril, 991–993, 9C, 59C–62C
Accuretic, 571–573, 991–993
Accutane, 639–641
Acebutolol, 16C–18C, 71C–72C
Aceon, 9C
Acephen, 9–12
Acetadote, 13–15
acetaminophen, 9–12
acetazolamide, 12–13, 50C–52C
acetylcysteine, 13–15
acetylsalicylic acid, 86–88
Acid, 1248–1254
Acilac, 658–659
Aciphex, 996–998, 148C
Aclasta, 1232–1233
Aclovate, 99C–100C
Actemra, 1144–1146
Actimmune, 624–625
Actiq, 472–475
Activase, 41–43, 30C–33C
Activella, 440–443
Actonel, 1021–1022, 143C–144C
Actonel with Calcium, 1021–1022
Actoplus Met, 741–743, 934–935
Actos, 934–935, 42C–44C
Acular, 652–654
Acular LS, 652–654
Acular PF, 652–654
acyclovir, 16–19, 67C–70C
Adalat, 77C–78C
Adalat CC, 831–833, 59C–62C
Adalat XL, 831–833
adalimumab, 19–20
Adam, 1248–1254
Adcirca, 1092–1093
Adderall, 339–341, 1248–1254
Adderall-XR, 339–341
adefovir, 20–21, 67C–70C
Adenocard, 21–23
Adenoscan, 21–23
adenosine, 21–23
Adoxa, 387–389
Adrenalin, 415–417, 158C
Adriamycin, 384–387, 79C–89C
Adrucil, 495–497, 79C–89C
Advair, 505–507
Advair Diskus, 505–507, 1041–1042, 73C–76C
Advair HFA, 505–507, 1041–1042, 73C–76C
Advate, 71–73
Advicor, 710–711, 825–827
Advil, 590–593, 127C–128C
Advil Children's, 590–593
Advil Cold, 983–984
Advil Infants', 590–593
Advil Junior, 590–593
Advil Migraine, 590–593
Advil PM, 360–362
Aerius, 326–328
AeroBid, 493–495, 73C–76C, 97C–98C
AeroBid M, 493–495
Aerospan HFA, 73C–76C
Afinitor, 456–457, 79C–89C
Afrin, 4C
Aggrastat, 30C–33C
Aggrenox, 86–88, 364–365
AHF, 71–73
ail, 534–535
Airomir, 25–27
AK-Dilate, 927–929

Akne-Mycin, 433–435
AK-Pred, 140C
AK-Tob, 1141–1144
Alamast, 139C
Alavert, 705–706
Alavert Allergy and Sinus, 705–706
Alaway, 139C
Albert, 919–920
Albumarc, 23–24
albumin, human, 23–24
Albuminar-5, 23–24
Albuminar-25, 23–24
AlbuRx, 23–24
Albutein, 23–24
albuterol, 25–27, 73C–76C
Albuterol/ipratropium, 73C–76C
Alcaftadine, 138C
Alclometasone, 99C–100C
Alcomicin, 540–543
Aldactazide, 571–573, 1078–1080
aldactone, 1078–1080, 101C–102C
aldesleukin, 625–627, 79C–89C
Aldomet, 59C–62C
Aldoril, 571–573
alefacept, 27–28
alemtuzumab, 28–30, 79C–89C
alendronate, 30–31, 143C–144C
Alertec, 785–786
Aleve, 811–813
alfuzosin, 31–32
Alimta, 910–912, 79C–89C
Alinia, 837–838
aliskiren, 33–34, 59C–62C
Alitretinoin, 79C–89C
Alkeran, 729–730, 79C–89C
Alkeran IV, 729–730
Allegra, 480–481, 53C–54C
Allegra D 24 Hour, 983–984
Allegra-D, 983–984
Allegra-D 12 Hour, 480–481
Allegra-D 24 Hour, 480–481
Allerdryl, 360–362
Allergic Rhinitis Nasal Preparations, 2C–4C
AllerNaze, 1171, 3C
all-heal, 1185–1186
Alli, 871–872
allium, 534–535
allopurinol, 34–36
almotriptan, 36–38, 63C
Alocril, 139C
Aloe, 1257–1269
Alomide, 139C
Alophen, 129–130
Aloprim, 34–36
Alora, 440–443
Aloxi, 892–893
Alphagan, 50C–52C
Alphanate, 71–73
Alplenzin, 151–153
Alprazolam Intensol, 38–39
alprazolam, 38–39, 13C–14C
alprostadil, 40–41
Alrex, 140C
Alsuma, 1087–1088
Altace, 1001–1003, 9C, 59C–62C
alteplase, 41–43, 30C–33C
Alti-Sulfasalazine, 1083–1085
Altoprev, 710–711
Altretamine, 80C
Aludrox, 715, 1058–1059
Aluminum hydroxide, 11C–12C
Alupent, 739–740
Alu-Tab, 11C–12C
Alvesco HFA, 232–234, 73C–76C
alvimopan, 43–45
amantadine, 45–46, 67C–70C
amantilla, 1185–1186
Amaryl, 547–548, 42C–44C
Amatine, 769–771
amber, 2850
Ambien, 1235–1236, 149C–150C
Ambien CR, 1235–1236, 149C–150C
AmBisome, 61–63, 46C
ambrisentan, 46–48
Amcinonide, 99C–100C
Amerge, 813–814, 63C
american dwarf, 1046
Amevive, 27–28
Amicar, 50–51
Amidate, 5C
amikacin, 48–50, 21C
Amikin, 48–50, 21C
Amiloride, 101C–102C
aminocaproic acid, 50–51
Aminoxin, 988–989
amiodarone, 51–54, 16C–18C
Amitiza, 711–712
amitriptyline, 54–55, 37C–40C
amlodipine, 56–57, 16C–18C, 77C–78C
Amnesteem, 639–641
Amoclan, 59–61
amoxicillin, 57–59, 28C–29C

amoxicillin/clavulanate, 59–61, 28C–29C
Amoxil, 57–59, 28C–29C
Amphetamine, 1248–1254
Amphojel, 11C–12C
Amphotec, 61–63, 46C
amphotericin B, 61–63, 46C
Amphotericin B lipid complex, 46C
Amphotericin B liposomal, 46C
Amphotericin colloidal dispersion, 46C
ampicillin, 63–65, 28C–29C
ampicillin/sulbactam, 65–67, 28C–29C
Ampyra, 298–299
Amrix, 285–287
Amturnide, 33–34
Anafranil, 258–259, 37C–40C
anakinra, 67–68
Anandron, 834–835
Anaprox, 811–813, 127C–128C
Anaprox DS, 811–813
Anaspaz, 585–587
anastrozole, 68–69, 79C–89C
Ancef, 190–192, 22C–24C
Andriol, 1114–1116
Androderm, 1114–1116
AndroGel, 1114–1116
Andropository, 1114–1116
Anectine, 124C
Anestacon, 689–691
Anesthetics: General, 4C–5C
Anesthetics: Local, 6C–7C
Anesthetics: Local Topical, 7C–8C
Anexate, 491–493
Anexsia, 573–575
Angel dust, 1248–1254
Angiomax, 133–134, 30C–33C
Angiotensin-Converting Enzyme (ACE) Inhibitors, 8C–9C
Angiotensin II Receptor Antagonists, 10C
anidulafungin, 69–71, 46C–47C
Ansaid, 502–503, 127C–128C
Antacids, 11C–12C
Antagon, 104C–106C
Antara, 467–469, 56C–58C
Antianxiety Agents, 12C–14C
Antiarrhythmics, 15C–18C
Antibiotic: Aminoglycosides, 21C
Antibiotic: Cephalosporins, 22C–24C
Antibiotic: Fluoroquinolones, 25C
Antibiotic: Macrolides, 26C
Antibiotic: Penicillins, 27C–29C
Antibiotics, 19C–20C
Anticoagulants/Antiplatelets/Thrombolytics, 30C–33C
Anticonvulsants, 34C–36C
Antidepressants, 37C–40C
Antidiabetics, 41C–44C
Antidiarrheals, 45C
Antifungals: Systemic Mycoses, 46C–47C
Antifungals: Topical, 48C–49C
Antiglaucoma Agents, 50C–52C
antihemophilic factor, 71–73
Antihistamines, 53C–55C
Antihyperlipidemics, 55C–58C
Anthypertensives, 59C–62C
Antimigraine (Triptans), 62C–63C
Antipsychotics, 64C–66C
Antivert, 722–723
Antivirals, 67C–70C
Anusol HC, 575–578
Anzemet, 373–374
Apache, 1248–1254
aphrodien, 1223–1224
Apidra, 615–619, 42C–44C
Apo-Acetaminiphen, 9–12
Apo-Acetazolamide, 12–13
Apo-Acyclovir, 16–19
Apo-Alendronate, 30–31
Apo-Alfuzosin, 31–32
Apo-Allopurinol, 34–36
Apo-Alpraz, 38–39
Apo-Amiodarone, 51–54
Apo-Amitriptyline, 54–55
Apo-Amlodipine, 56–57
Apo-Amoxi, 57–59
Apo-Ampi, 63–65
Apo-Atenol, 90–92
Apo-Azathioprine, 101–102
Apo-Azithromycin, 104–106
Apo-Baclofen, 109–111
Apo-Beclomethasone, 113–114
Apo-Benazepril, 114–116
Apo-Benztropine, 119–120
Apo-Bicalutamide, 127–128
Apo-Bisacodyl, 129–130
Apo-Bisoprolol, 131–133
Apo-Bromocriptine, 144–145
Apo-Buspirone, 154–155
Apo-Butorphanol, 157–158
Apo-Cal, 163
Apo-Calcitonin, 162–163
Apo-Capto, 172–174

Apo-Carbamazepine, 174–176
Apo-Carvedilol, 183–185
Apo-Cefaclor, 187–188
Apo-Cefadroxil, 188–190
Apo-Cefoxitin, 199–201
Apo-Cefprozil, 203–205
Apo-Cefuroxime, 212
Apo-Cephalex, 216–218
Apo-Cetirizine, 219–220
Apo-Chlordiazepoxide, 226–227
Apo-Cimetidine, 237–239
Apo-Ciproflox, 240–243
Apo-Citalopram, 245–247
Apo-Clarithromycin, 248–250
Apo-Clindamycin, 254–256
Apo-Clomipramine, 258–259
Apo-Clonazepam, 259–261
Apo-Clonidine, 261–263
Apo-Clorzepate, 264–266
Apo-Clozapine, 268–269
Apo-Cromolyn, 282–284
Apo-Cyclobenzaprine, 285–287
Apo-Desipramine, 325–326
Apo-Desmopressin, 328–330
Apo-Dexamethasone, 331–334
Apo-Diazepam, 342–344
Apo-Diclo, 344–347
Apo-Digoxin, 351–353
Apo-Diltiaz, 354–357
Apo-Dipyridamole FC, 364–365
Apo-Divalproex, 1187–1190
Apo-Docusate, 371–372
Apo-Doxazosin, 380–382
Apo-Doxepin, 382–384
Apo-Doxy, 387–389
Apo-Enalapril, 407–409
Apo-Erthro Base, 433–435
Apo-Etodolac, 450–452
Apo-Famciclovir, 461–463
Apo-Famotidine, 463–465
Apo-Fenofibrate, 467–469
Apo-Ferrous Gluconate, 475
Apo-Ferrous Sulfate, 475
Apo-Flavoxate, 486–487
Apo-Fluconazole, 487–489
Apo-Flunisolide, 493–495
Apo-Fluoxetine, 497–499
Apo-Fluphenazine, 499
Apo-Flurazepam, 2535
Apo-Flurbiprofen, 502–503
Apo-Flutamide, 503–504
Apo-Fluvoxamine, 508–510
Apo-Folic, 510–511
Apo-Fosinopril, 519–520
Apo-Furosemide, 526–528
Apo-Gabapentin, 528–530
Apo-Gain, 776–778
Apo-Gemfibrozil, 537–538
Apo-Glimepiride, 547–548
Apo-Glyburide, 552–554
Apo-Haloperidol, 564–566
Apo-Hydralazine, 569–571
Apo-Hydro, 571–573
Apo-Hydroxyquine, 581–582
Apo-Hydroxyurea, 582–584
Apo-Hydroxyzine, 584–585
Apo-Ibuprofen, 590–593
Apo-Imipramine, 603–605
Apo-Indapamide, 608–609
Apo-Indomethacin, 611–613
Apo-Ipravent, 628–629
Apo-ISDN, 637
Apo-ISMO, 637
Apo-K, 945–947
Apo-Keto, 650–652
Apo-Ketoconazole, 648–650
Apo-Ketorolac, 652–654
Apo-Labetalol, 654–656
Apo-Lactulose, 658–659
Apo-Lamotrigine, 661–664
Apo-Lansoprazole, 665–667
Apo-Leflunomide, 669–670
Apo-Levetiracetam, 681–683
Apo-Levocarb, 176–178
Apo-Lisinopril, 696–698
Apo-Lithium, 698–700
Apo-Loperamide, 701–703
Apo-Lorazepam, 706–708
Apo-Lovastatin, 710–711
Apo-Medroxy, 723–725
Apo-Megestrol, 725
Apo-Meloxicam, 727–729
Apo-Metformin, 741–743
Apo-Methotrexate, 747–749
Apo-Methylphenidate, 752–754
Apo-Metoclop, 756–758
Apo-Metoprolol, 760–762
Apo-Metronidazole, 763–765
Apo-Midazolam, 767–769
Apo-Midodrine, 769–771
Apo-Minocycline, 775–776
Apo-Mirtazapine, 778–779

Apo-Misoprostol, 780–781
Apo-Modafinil, 785–786
Apo-Nabumetone, 800–801
Apo-Nadol, 801–803
Apo-Naproxen, 811–813
Apo-Nifed, 831–833
Apo-Nitrofurantoin, 838–839
Apo-Nizatidine, 844–845
Apo-Norflox, 847–848
Apo-Nortriptyline, 848–850
Apo-Oflox, 856–858
Apo-Ofloxacin, 856–858
Apo-Olanzapine, 858–860
Apo-Omeprazole, 866–867
Apo-Ondansetron, 867–869
Apo-Orciprenaline, 739–740
Apo-Oxaprozin, 875–877
Apo-Oxybutynin, 878–880
Apo-Paclitaxel, 886–889
Apo-Pantoprazole, 898–899
Apo-Paroxetine, 899–901
Apo-Pentoxifylline SR, 919–920
Apo-Pen-VK, 916–917, 28C
Apo-Pioglitazone, 934–935
Apo-Piroxacom, 937–939
Apo-Pramipexole, 949–951
Apo-Pravastatin, 954–956
Apo-Prazo, 956–957
Apo-Prednisone, 959–960
Apo-Primidone, 962–963
Apo-Procainamide, 965–967
Apo-Prochlorperazine, 968–970
Apo-Propranolol, 978–981
Apo-Quetiapine, 989–991
Apo-Quinidine, 993–995
Apo-Ramipril, 1001–1003
Apo-Ranitidine, 1003–1005
Apo-Risperidone, 1023–1025
Apo-Salvent, 25–27
Apo-Selegiline, 1049–1051
Apo-Sertraline, 1052–1054
Apo-Simvastatin, 1059–1061
Apo-Sotalol, 1076–1078
Apo-Sucralate, 1082–1083
Apo-Sulfatrim, 279–282
Apo-Sulin, 1085–1086
Apo-Sumatriptan, 1087–1088
Apo-Tamox, 1094–1095
Apo-Temazepam, 1100–1102
Apo-Terazosin, 1107–1109
Apo-Terbinafine, 1109–1110
Apo-Tetra, 1117–1119
Apo-Ticlopidine, 1129–1131
Apo-Timol, 1133–1136
Apo-Timop, 1133–1136
Apo-Tizanidine, 1140–1141
Apo-Topiramate, 1149–1151
Apo-Trazodone, 1166–1167
Apo-Trifluoperazine, 1175–1177
Apo-Trihex, 1177–1178
Apo-Trimethoprim, 1178–1179
Apo-Valacyclovir, 1183–1185
Apo-Verap, 1200–1202
Apo-Warfarin, 1221–1223
Apo-Zidovudine, 1227–1229
Apraclonidine, 50C–52C
aprepitant, 73–74
Apresazide, 569–573
Apresoline, 569–571, 59C–62C
Apri, 92C–96C
Apriso, 736–737
Aptivus, 1138–1140, 114C–118C
Aquachlroal Supprettes, 223–224
AquaMEPHYTON, 1217
Aquasol A, 1211–1212, 161C–162C
Aquasol E, 1216, 162C
Ara-C, 291–293, 79C–89C
Aranelle, 92C–96C
Aranesp, 305–307
Arava, 669–670
Aredia, 893–895
Arformoterol, 73C–76C
argatroban, 74–76, 30C–33C
Aricept, 374–376
Aricept ODT, 374–376
Arimidex, 68–69, 79C–89C
aripiprazole, 76–78, 64C–66C
Aristocort, 99C–100C
Aristospan, 1171
Arixtra, 511–512, 30C–33C
armodafinil, 78–79
Armour Thyroid, 159C
Aromasin, 457–458, 79C–89C
Arranon, 818–819, 79C–89C
arsenic trioxide, 79–81, 79C–89C
Artane, 1177–1178
Arthrotec, 344–347, 780–781
Artichoke, 1257–1269
Arzerra, 854–856
ASA, 86–88
Asacol, 736–737
Asaphen E.C., 86–88

ascorbic acid, 81–82, 161C–162C
Ascriptin, 86–88
asenapine, 82–84, 64C–66C
asian ginseng, 545
Asmanex Twisthaler, 787, 73C–76C
asparaginase, 84–86, 79C–89C
aspirin, 86–88, 30C–33C, 127C–128C
Astaxanthin, 1257–1269
Astelin, 102–104, 3C
Astepro, 102–104
Astragalus, 1257–1269
Astramorph PF, 791–794
Atacand, 169–170, 10C, 59C–62C
Atacand HCT, 169–170, 571–573
Atarax, 584–585, 13C–14C, 53C–54C
Atasol, 9–12
atazanavir, 88–90, 114C–118C
atenolol, 90–92, 59C–62C, 71C–72C
Atgam, 714–715
Ativan, 706–708, 13C–14C
atomoxetine, 92–93
atorvastatin, 93–95, 56C–58C
atovaquone, 95–96
Atralin, 1169–1171
Atriance, 818–819
Atripla, 401–402, 405–407, 1106–1107, 114C–118C
AtroPen Auto Injector, 96–98
atropine, 96–98
Atropine-Care, 96–98
Atrovent, 628–629, 3C, 73C–76C
Atrovent HFA, 628–629
Augmentin, 59–61, 28C–29C
Augmentin ES 600, 59–61
Augmentin XR, 59–61
ava, 646
Avalide, 571–573, 629–631
Avandamet, 741–743, 1036–1037
Avandaryl, 547–548, 1036–1037
Avandia, 1036–1037, 42C–44C
Avapro, 629–631, 10C
Avastin, 124–126, 79C–89C
Avelox, 794–796, 25C
Avelox IV, 794–796
Aventyl, 848–850, 37C–40C
Aviane-28, 92C–96C
Avinza, 791–794
Avita, 1169–1171
Avocado, 1257–1269
Avodart, 396–397
Avonex, 621–623
Avonex Prefilled Syringe, 621–623
Axert, 36–38, 63C
Axid, 844–845, 107C–108C
Axid AR, 844–845
Axiren, 1114–1116
azacitidine, 99–101, 79C–89C
Azactam, 106–108
Azasan, 101–102
AzaSite, 104–106
Azatadine, 53C–54C
azathioprine, 101–102
azelastine, 102–104, 3C, 139C
Azilect, 1007–1008, 146C
azithromycin, 104–106, 26C
Azmacort, 1171, 73C–76C, 97C–98C
Azo-Gesic, 921–922
Azopt, 50C–52C
Azor, 56–57, 860–862
Azo-Standard, 921–922
AZT, 1227–1229
AZT/3TC, 114C–118C
AZT/3TC/ABC, 114C–118C
aztreonam, 106–108
Azulfidine, 1083–1085
Azulfidine EN-Tabs, 1083–1085
Azurette, 92C–96C

B
bachelor's button, 479–480
Baciguent, 108–109
Baci-Rx, 108–109
bacitracin, 108–109
baclofen, 109–111, 151C–153C
Bactocill, 28C
Bactrim, 279–282, 1178–1179
Bactrim DS, 279–282
Bactroban, 796–797
Bactroban Nasal, 796–797
Balacet 325, 9–12
Balminil Decongerstant, 983–984
Balziva, 92C–96C
baneberry, 134–135
Banophen, 360–362
Banzel, 1039–1040
Baraclude, 413–415
Barbiturates, 1248–1254
Barbs, 1248–1254
basiliximab, 111–113, 119C
Bayer, 86–88
Baza Antifungal, 766–767
BCG, 79C–89C

beclomethasone, 113–114, 2C, 73C–76C, 97C–98C
Beconase, 97C–98C
Beconase AQ, 113–114, 2C
Bellergal-S, 426, 923–925
Benadryl, 360–362, 53C–54C
Benadryl Children's Allergy, 360–362
benazepril, 114–116, 9C, 59C–62C
bendamustine, 116–117, 79C–89C
Benicar, 860–862, 10C, 59C–62C
Benicar HCT, 571–573, 860–862
Bentyl, 347–349
Bentylol, 347–349
Benuryl, 964–965
Benzodiazepines, 1248–1254
benzonatate, 118–119
Benzphetamine, 137C
benztropine, 119–120
beractant, 120–121
Beta-Adrenergic Blockers, 71C–72C
Betacaine, 689–691
Betaderm, 121–123
Betagan, 50C–52C
Betaject, 121–123
Betaloc, 760–762
betamethasone, 121–123, 97C–98C
Betamethasone dipropionate, 99C–100C
Betamethasone valerate, 99C–100C
Betapace, 1076–1078, 16C–18C, 71C–72C
Betapace AF, 1076–1078
Betaseron, 623–624
Beta-Val, 121–123
Betaxin, 1122–1123
Betaxolol, 50C–52C, 71C–72C
bethanechol, 123–124, 90C–91C
Betimol, 1133–1136, 50C–52C
Betnesol, 121–123
Betnovate, 121–123
Betoptic, 50C–52C
Betoptic-S, 50C–52C
bevacizumab, 124–126, 79C–89C
bexarotene, 126–127, 79C–89C
Bexxar, 1156–1158, 79C–89C
Biaxin, 248–250, 26C
Biaxin XL, 248–250
bicalutamide, 127–128, 79C–89C
Bicillin, 28C
Bicillin CR, 914–915
Bicillin LA, 914–915, 28C
BiCNU, 182–183, 79C–89C
BiDil, 569–571, 637
Bifidobacteria, 1257–1269
Bilberry, 1257–1269
Bimatoprost, 50C–52C
BioQuin Durules, 993–995
Bio-Statin, 850–852
bisacodyl, 129–130, 121C–122C
bismuth, 130–131, 45C
bisoprolol, 131–133, 71C–72C
Bitter orange, 1257–1269
bivalirudin, 133–134, 30C–33C
black cohosh, 134–135, 1257–1269
black ginger, 530
black susan, 399
Black tar, 1248–1254
Blackberry, 1257–1269
Blenoxane, 135–137, 79C–89C
bleomycin, 135–137, 79C–89C
Blephamide, 957–959
Blocadren, 71C–72C
Boldo, 1257–1269
Bonamine, 722–723
Bondronat, 587–589
Bonine, 722–723
Boniva, 587–589, 143C–144C
Bontril, 137C
Boomers, 1248–1254
bortezomib, 137–139, 79C–89C
bosentan, 139–140
Botox, 140–142
Botox Cosmetic, 140–142
botulinum toxin type A, 140–142
botulinum toxin type B, 142–143
Bravelle, 104C–106C
Brethine, 1110–1112
Brevibloc, 437–439, 16C–18C, 71C–72C
Brevicon, 92C–96C
Brevital, 5C
Bricanyl, 1110–1112
Brimonidine, 50C–52C
Brinzolamide, 50C–52C
bromocriptine, 144–145, 42C–44C, 146C
Brompheniramine, 53C–54C
Bronalide, 493–495
Bronchodilators, 73C–76C
Brovana, 73C–76C
Brovex, 53C–54C
Budeprion SR, 151–153
Budeprion XL, 151–153
budesonide, 145–147, 2C, 73C–76C, 97C–98C
Bufferin, 86–88

bugbane, 134–135
bugwort, 134–135
bumetanide, 147–149, 101C–102C
Bumex, 147–149, 101C–102C
Buminate, 23–24
Bupivacaine, 6C
Buprenex, 149–151
buprenorphine, 149–151
Buproban, 151–153
bupropion, 151–153, 37C–40C, 154C–156C
Burinex, 147–149
BuSpar, 154–155, 13C–14C
Buspirex, 154–155
buspirone, 154–155, 13C–14C
Bustab, 154–155
busulfan, 155–157, 79C–89C
Busulfex, 155–157
Butenafine, 48C–49C
butorphanol, 157–158, 141C–142C
Butrans, 149–151
Butterbur, 1257–1269
Buttons, 1248–1254
Byetta, 459–460, 42C–44C
Bystolic, 817–818

C
C.E.S., 275–277
c7E3 Fab, 4–5
cabazitaxel, 159–161, 79C–89C
cabbage palm, 1046
Cactus, 1248–1254
Caduet, 56–57, 93–95
Caelyx, 384–387
Cafcit, 161
Cafergot, 426
caffeine citrate, 161, 1257–1269
Caladryl, 360–362
Calan, 1200–1202, 16C–18C, 77C–78C
Calan SR, 1200–1202, 59C–62C
Calciferol, 161C–162C
Calcijex, 1212–1215
Calcimar, 162–163
calcitonin, 162–163, 143C–144C
Cal-Citrate, 163
calcitriol, 1212–1215
calcium acetate, 163
calcium carbonate, 163, 11C–12C
Calcium Channel Blockers, 77C–78C
calcium chloride, 163
calcium citrate, 163
calcium glubionate, 163
calcium gluconate, 163
Calculation of Doses, 1240
Caldecort, 575–578
Caldesene, 48C–49C
Caldolor, 590–593, 127C–128C
Calendula, 1257–1269
calfactant, 166–167
CaloMist, 284–285
Caltine, 162–163
Caltrate, 163
Caltrate 600, 163, 11C–12C
Camalox, 715
Cambia, 344–347
Camilia, 92C–96C
Campath, 28–30, 79C–89C
Campral, 7–8
Camptosar, 631–632, 79C–89C
canakinumab, 167–169
Canasa, 736–737
Cancidas, 185–187, 46C–47C
candesartan, 169–170, 10C, 59C–62C
Candy, 1248–1254
Canesten, 266–268
capecitabine, 170–172, 79C–89C
Capital with Codeine, 9–12, 269
Capoten, 172–174, 9C
Capozide, 172–174, 571–573
Capsicum, 1257–1269
captopril, 172–174, 9C
Carac, 495–497
Carafate, 1082–1083
Carbachol, 50C–52C
carbamazepine, 174–176, 34C–36C
Carbatrol, 174–176, 34C–36C
carbidopa/levodopa, 176–178, 146C
Carbocaine, 7C
carboplatin, 178–180, 79C–89C
Cardene, 827–829, 77C–78C
Cardene IV, 827–829
Cardene SR, 2020
Cardizem, 354–357, 16C–18C, 77C–78C
Cardizem CD, 354–357, 59C–62C
Cardizem LA, 354–357
Cardura, 380–382, 59C–62C
Cardura XL, 380–382
Carimune NF, 605–607
carisprodol, 180–182, 151C–153C
carmustine, 182–183, 79C–89C
Carteolol, 50C–52C
Cartia XT, 354–357

carvedilol, 183–185, 71C–72C
Casodex, 127–128, 79C–89C
caspofungin, 185–187, 46C–47C
Cat's claw, 1257–1269
Cataflam, 344–347
Catapres, 261–263, 59C–62C, 154C–156C
Catapres-TTS, 261–263, 154C–156C
Cathflo Activase, 41–43
Catnip, 1257–1269
Caverject, 40–41
Caverject Impulse, 40–41
Cayston, 106–108
Caziant, 92C–96C
Ceclor, 187–188, 22C–24C
Cedax, 208–210, 22C–24C
Cedocard SR, 637
CeeNU, 700–701, 79C–89C
cefaclor, 187–188, 22C–24C
cefadroxil, 188–190, 22C–24C
cefazolin, 190–192, 22C–24C
cefdinir, 192–194, 22C–24C
Cefditoren, 22C–24C
cefepime, 194–196, 22C–24C
cefixime, 196–197
Cefizox, 22C–24C
cefotaxime, 197–199, 22C–24C
Cefotetan, 22C–24C
cefoxitin, 199–201, 22C–24C
cefpodoxime, 201–203, 22C–24C
cefprozil, 203–205, 22C–24C
ceftaroline, 205–206
ceftazidime, 206–208, 22C–24C
ceftibuten, 208–210, 22C–24C
Ceftin, 212, 22C–24C
Ceftizoxime, 22C–24C
ceftriaxone, 210–212, 22C–24C
cefuroxime axetil, 212
cefuroxime sodium, 212
Cefuroxime, 22C–24C
Cefzil, 203–205, 22C–24C
Celebrex, 214–216, 127C–128C
celecoxib, 214–216, 127C–128C
Celestone Soluspan, 121–123
Celestone, 121–123, 97C–98C
Celexa, 245–247, 37C–40C
CellCept, 797–799, 119C
Celsentri, 721–722
Cenestin, 275–277
cephalexin, 216–218, 22C–24C
Cerebyx, 520–522, 34C–36C
certolizumab, 218–219
Cerubidine, 311–314, 79C–89C
Cervidil, 358–360
Cesia, 92C–96C
cetirizine, 219–220, 53C–54C
Cetrorelix, 104C–106C
Cetrotide, 104C–106C
cetuximab, 220–222, 79C–89C
C-Gram, 81–82
Cha de bugre, 1257–1269
chamomile, 222–223, 1257–1269
Champix, 1195–1196
Chantix, 1195–1196, 154C–156C
Chastberry, 1257–1269
Chemotherapeutic Agents, 79C–89C
Children's Advil Cold, 590–593
China girl, 1248–1254
China white, 1257–1269
chinese angelica, 376–377
chinese ginseng, 545
chloral hydrate, 223–224
chlorambucil, 224–226, 79C–89C
chlordiazepoxide, 226–227, 13C–14C
Chloroprocaine, 6C
Chlorothiazide, 101C–102C
Chlorpheniramine, 53C–54C
chlorpromazine, 227–230, 64C–66C
Chlorpropamide, 42C–44C
Chlorthalidone, 59C–62C, 101C–102C
Chlor-Trimeton, 53C–54C
Chlorzoxazone, 151C–153C
cholestryamine, 230–231, 56C–58C
Cholinergic Agonists/Anticholinesterase, 90C–91C
chorionic gonadopropin, 231–232, 104C–106C
Chronic Wound Care, 1320–1323
Chronovera, 1200–1202
Cialis, 1092–1093
Cibalith-S, 698–700
ciclesonide, 232–234, 2C, 73C–76C
Ciclopirox, 48C–49C
cidofovir, 234–235, 67C–70C
cilostazol, 235–236
Ciloxan, 240–243
cimetidine, 237–239, 107C–108C
Cimzia, 218–219
cinacalcet, 239–240
Cipralex, 436–437
Cipro, 240–243, 25C
Cipro HC Otic, 240–243
Cipro I.V., 240–243

Cipro XR, 240–243
CiproDex Otic, 240–243, 331–334
ciprofloxacin, 240–243, 25C
Cisatracurium, 123C
cisplatin, 243–245, 79C–89C
citalopram, 245–247, 37C–40C
Citracal, 163
Citrate of Magnesia, 121C
Citroma, 715
Citro-Mag, 715, 121C
citrovorum factor, 676–677
Citrucel, 121C
cladribine, 247–248, 79C–89C
Claforan, 197–199, 22C–24C
Claravis, 639–641
Clarinex, 326–328
Clarinex D 24 Hour, 983–984
Clarinex RediTabs, 326–328
Clarinex-D 12 Hour, 326–328, 983–984
Clarinex-D 24 Hour, 326–328
clarithromycin, 248–250, 26C
Claritin, 705–706, 53C–54C
Claritin-D, 705–706, 983–984
Clavulin, 59–61
clemastine, 250–252, 53C–54C
Cleocin, 254–256
Cleocin Pediatric, 254–256
Cleocin T, 254–256
Cleocin Vaginal, 254–256
clevidipine, 252–253
Cleviprex, 252–253
Climara PRO, 440–443
Climara, 440–443
Clindagel, 254–256
Clindamax, 254–256
clindamycin, 254–256
Clindesse, 254–256
Clindets Pledget, 254–256
Clinoril, 1085–1086, 127C–128C
Clioquinol, 48C–49C
Clobetasol, 99C–100C
clofarabine, 256–257
Clolar, 256–257
Clomid, 104C–106C
Clomiphene, 104C–106C
clomipramine, 258–259, 37C–40C
Clonapam, 259–261
clonazepam, 259–261, 34C–36C
clonidine, 261–263, 59C–62C, 154C–156C
clopidogrel, 263–264, 30C–33C
clorazepate, 264–266, 13C–14C
Clotrimaderm, 266–268
clotrimazole, 266–268, 48C–49C
Cloxacillin, 28C
clozapine, 268–269, 64C–66C
Clozaril, 268–269, 64C–66C
Cocaine, 1248–1254, 7C
Codeine, 1248–1254, 141C–142C
Codeine Contin, 269
Codeine Phosphate Injection, 269
codeine phosphate, 269
codeine sulfate, 269
Co-enzyme Q-10, 1259–1271
Cogentin, 119–120
Coke, 1248–1254
Cola, 1257–1269
Colace, 371–372, 121C
colchicine, 271–273
Colcrys, 271–273
Colesevelam, 56C–58C
Colestid, 56C–58C
Colestipol, 56C–58C
Colocort, 575–578
CoLyte, 941–943
comb flower, 399
Combigan, 1133–1136
Combi-patch, 440–443
Combipres, 261–263
Combivent, 25–27, 628–629, 73C–76C
Combivir, 659–661, 1227–1229, 114C–118C
Combunox, 590–593, 880–882
Commit, 829–831, 154C–156C
Compazine, 968–970
Compro, 968–970
Comtan, 412–413, 146C
Concerta, 752–754
conivaptan, 273–274
conjugated estrogens, 275–277
Conjugated linoleic acid, 1257–1269
Constulose, 658–659
Contraception, 91C–96C
Controlled Drugs (United States), 1241
Copaxone, 546
Copegus, 1014–1015
Cordarone, 51–54, 16C–18C
Cordran, 99C–100C
Coreg, 183–185, 71C–72C
Coreg CR, 183–185
Corgard, 801–803, 71C–72C
Corlopam, 470–472
Cortaid, 575–578
Cortef, 575–578

Cortenema, 575–578
Corticosteroids, 97C–98C
Corticosteroids: Topical, 99C–100C
cortisone, 277–278, 97C–98C
Cortisone-10, 575–578
Cortisporin, 575–578
Cortone, 277–278, 97C–98C
Cortrosyn, 279
Corvert, 16C–18C
corynine, 1223–1224
Corzide, 801–803
Cosopt, 1133–1136
cosyntropin, 279
co-trimoxazole, 279–282
Coumadin, 1221–1223, 30C–33C
Covera-HS, 1200–1202
Cozaar, 708–710, 10C, 59C–62C
Cranberry, 1257–1269
Crank, 1248–1254
Creon, 895–896
Crestor, 1037–1039, 56C–58C
Crinone, 970–972
Crixivan, 610–611, 67C–70C, 114C–118C
Crolom, 282–284, 139C
cromolyn, 282–284, 3C, 139C
Cruex, 266–268, 48C–49C
Cryselle-28, 92C–96C
Crystal, 1248–1254
Crystal meth, 1248–1254
Crystapen, 915–916
Cubes, 1248–1254
Cubicin, 304–305
Cultivate, 505–507, 99C–100C
Cuprimine, 912–914
Curosurf, 943–944
cyanocobalamin, 284–285, 161C–162C
Cyclamen, 301–302
Cyclessa, 92C–96C
cyclobenzaprine, 285–287, 151C–153C
Cyclocort, 99C–100C
cyclophosphamide, 287–289, 79C–89C
Cycloset, 144–145, 42C–44C
cyclosporine, 289–291, 119C
Cymbalta, 394–396, 37C–40C
Cyproheptadine, 53C–54C
cytarabine, 291–293, 79C–89C
Cytochrome P450 (CYP) Enzymes, 1284–1286
Cytomel, 159C
Cytosar, 79C–89C
Cytosar-U, 291–293
Cytotec, 780–781
Cytovene, 531–534, 67C–70C
Cytoxan Lyophilized, 287–289
Cytoxan, 287–289, 79C–89C

D

D.H.E. 45, 426
d4t, 1081–1082
dabigatran, 294–295
dacarbazine, 295–296, 79C–89C
daclizumab, 296–297, 119C
Dacogen, 314–316
Dalacin, 254–256
Dalacin C, 254–256
dalfampridine, 298–299
Dalmane, 500–502, 149C–150C
dalteparin, 299–300, 30C–33C
danazol, 301–302
dang gui, 376–377
Danocrine, 301–302
Dantrium, 302–304, 151C–153C
Dantrium Intravenous, 302–304
dantrolene, 302–304, 151C–153C
daptomycin, 304–305
darbepoetin alfa, 305–307
darifenacin, 307–308
darunavir, 308–310, 67C–70C, 114C–118C
dasatinib, 310–311, 79C–89C
daunorubicin, 311–314, 79C–89C
DaunoXome, 311–314, 79C–89C
Dayhist Allergy, 250–252
Daypro, 875–877, 127C–128C
Daytrana, 752–754
DDAVP, 328–330
DDAVP Nasal, 328–330
DDAVP Rhinal Tube, 328–330
Decadron, 331–334, 97C–98C, 99C–100C
decitabine, 314–316
Declomycin, 321–322
deferasirox, 316–317
deferoxamine, 317–318
degarelix, 318–320
Delatestryl, 1114–1116
delavirdine, 320–321, 67C–70C, 114C–118C
Delcid, 715
Delestrogen, 440–443
Demadex, 1154–1156, 101C–102C
demeclocycline, 321–322
Demerol, 732–734, 141C–142C

demon chaser, 1080–1081
Demulen 1/35, 92C–96C
denileukin, 322–323, 79C–89C
denosumab, 323–324, 143C–144C
Deop-SubQ-Provera 104, 723–725
Depacon, 1187–1190
Depade, 809–811
Depadene, 34C–36C
Depakene, 1187–1190
Depakote, 1187–1190, 34C–36C
Depakote ER, 1187–1190
Depakote Sprinkle, 1187–1190
Depen, 912–914
Depo-Cyt, 291–293
DepoDur, 791–794
Depo-Estradiol, 440–443
Depo-Medrol, 754
Depo-Provera Cl, 92C–96C
Depo-Provera Contraceptive, 723–725
Depo-Provera, 723–725
Depo-SubQ Provera 104, 92C–96C
Depotest, 1114–1116
Depo-Testosterone, 1114–1116
Dermatop, 99C–100C
Desenex, 48C–49C
Desferal, 317–318
desipramine, 325–326, 37C–40C
desloratadine, 326–328
desmopressin, 328–330
Desogen, 92C–96C
Desonide, 99C–100C
Desoximetasone, 99C–100C
Desoxyn, 1248–1254
desvenlafaxine, 330–331, 37C–40C
Desyrel, 1166–1167, 13C–14C, 37C–40C
Detrol, 1146–1147
Detrol LA, 1146–1147
Devil's claw, 1257–1269
Dexacidin, 331–334
Dexamethasone Intensol, 331–334
dexamethasone, 331–334, 97C–98C, 99C–100C
Dexchlorpheniramine, 53C–54C
Dexedrine, 1248–1254
DexFerrum, 632–634
Dexiron, 632–634
dexlansoprazole, 334–335, 148C
dexmedetomidine, 335–336
dexmethylphenidate, 336–338
DexPak TaperPak, 331–334
dexrazoxane, 338–339
dextroamphetamine and amphetamine, 339–341
DHEA, 341–342, 1257–1269
DiaBeta, 552–554, 42C–44C
Diabinese, 42C–44C
Dialume, 11C–12C
Diamode, 701–703
Diamox, 12–13, 50C–52C
Diamox Sequels, 12–13
Diarr-Eze, 701–703
Diastat, 342–344
Diazemuls, 342–344
diazepam, 342–344, 13C–14C, 151C–153C
Diazepam Intensol, 342–344
Dibucaine, 7C
diclofenac, 344–347, 127C–128C
Dicloxacillin, 28C
dicyclomine, 347–349
didanosine, 349–351, 67C–70C, 114C–118C
Didrex, 137C
Diethylpropion, 137C
Diflucan, 487–489, 46C–47C
Diflunisal, 127C–128C
Di-Gel, 715
Digibind, 353–354
DigiFab, 353–354
Digitek, 351–353
digoxin, 351–353
digoxin immune FAB, 353–354
dihydroergotamine, 426
Dilacor XR, 354–357
Dilantin, 929–931, 34C–36C
Dilantin with PB, 923–925
Dilatrate-SR, 637
Dilaudid HP, 578–581
Dilaudid, 578–581, 141C–142C
Dilt-CD, 354–357
Diltia XT, 354–357
diltiazem, 354–357, 16C–18C, 77C–78C
Diltiazem CD, 59C–62C
dimenhydrinate, 357–358, 53C–54C
Dimetapp ND, 705–706
dinoprostone, 358–360
Diocto, 371–372
Diodex, 331–334
Diotame, 130–131
Diovan, 1190–1191, 10C, 59C–62C
Diovan HCT, 571–573, 1190–1191
Dipentum, 862–863
Diphen, 360–362

Diphenhist, 360–362
diphenhydramine, 360–362, 53C–54C
diphenoxylate with atropine, 362–363, 45C
Diprivan, 976–978, 5C
Diprolene, 121–123, 97C–98C
Diprolene AF, 121–123
dipyridamole, 364–365, 30C–33C
disopyramide, 365–367, 16C–18C
Ditropan, 878–880
Ditropan XL, 878–880
Diuretics, 101C–102C
Diuril, 101C–102C
Divigel, 440–443
Dixarit, 261–263
dobutamine, 367–368, 158C
Dobutrex, 367–368, 158C
docetaxel, 368–371, 79C–89C
docusate, 371–372, 121C
Docusoft-S, 371–372
dofetilide, 372–373, 16C–18C
dolasetron, 373–374
Dolobid, 127C–128C
Dolophine, 743–745, 141C–142C
donepezil, 374–376
dong quai, 376–377, 1257–1269
Donnatal, 96–98, 585–587, 923–925, 1048–1049
dopamine, 377–379, 158C
Doral, 149C–150C
Doribax, 379–380
doripenem, 379–380
Doryx, 387–389
Dorzolamide, 50C–52C
Downers, 1248–1254
Doxacurium, 123C
doxazosin, 380–382, 59C–62C
doxepin, 382–384, 37C–40C
doxercalciferol, 1212–1215
Doxil, 384–387, 79C–89C
doxorubicin, 384–387, 79C–89C
Doxy-100, 387–389
Doxycin, 387–389
doxycycline, 387–389
Dramamine, 357–358, 53C–54C
Dramamine Less Drowsy Formula, 722–723
Drip Rates for Critical Care Medications, 1242–1247
Drisdol, 1212–1215
dronab inol, 389–390
dronedarone, 390–392, 16C–18C
droperidol, 392–393
drotrecogin alfa, 393–394
Droxia, 582–584
Drugs of Abuse, 1248–1254
DTIC, 295–296, 79C–89C
Duetact, 547–548, 934–935
Dulcolax, 129–130, 121C–122C
Dulcolax Balance, 129–130
Dulera, 512–514, 787
duloxetine, 394–396, 37C–40C
Duocet, 573–575
Duoneb, 25–27, 628–629, 73C–76C
Duraclon, 261–263
Duragesic, 472–475
Duralith, 698–700
Duramorph PF, 791–794
Duricef, 188–190, 22C–24C
dutasteride, 396–397
Duvoid, 123–124
Dyazide, 571–573, 1173–1175
Dynacin, 775–776
DynaCirc, 641–642, 77C–78C
DynaCirc CR, 641–642
Dynapen, 28C
Dyrenium, 1173–1175, 101C–102C
Dysport, 6–7
Dytan, 360–362

E

Ebixa, 730–732
ecallantide, 397–399
echinacea, 399, 1257–1269
Echothiophate, 50C–52C
EC-Naprosyn, 811–813
Econazole, 48C–49C
Ecotrin, 86–88
Ecstasy, 1248–1254
Ectosome, 121–123
eculizumab, 400–401
Edex, 40–41
Edex Refill, 40–41
Edluar, 1235–1236, 149C–150C
Edrophonium, 90C–91C
EES, 433–435, 26C
efavirenz, 401–402, 67C–70C, 114C–118C
Effexor, 1198–1200, 13C–14C, 37C–40C
Effer-K, 945–947
Effexor XR, 1198–1200
Effient, 953–954, 30C–33C
Efudex, 495–497, 79C–89C
E-Gems, 1216

Elavil, 54–55, 37C–40C
Eldepryl, 1049–1051, 146C–147C
Elderberry, 1257–1269
Elestat, 139C
Elestrin, 440–443
eletriptan, 403–404, 63C
Elidel, 933–934
Eligard, 677–679
Elixophyllin, 1120–1122
Ellence, 418–419, 79C–89C
Elocon, 787, 99C–100C
Eloxatin, 873–875, 79C–89C
Elspar, 84–86, 79C–89C
eltrombopag, 404–405
Eltroxin, 687–689
Embeda, 791–794, 807–809
Emcyt, 444–445, 79C–89C
Emend, 73–74
Emend for Injection, 73–74
EMLA, 689–691
Emsam, 1049–1051
emtricitabine, 405–407, 114C–118C
Emtricitabine/efavirenz/tenofovir, 114C–118C
Emtricitabine/tenofovir, 114C–118C
Emtriva, 405–407, 114C–118C
Emu oil, 1257–1269
Enablex, 307–308
enalapril, 407–409, 9C, 59C–62C
Enbrel, 447–449
Endantadine, 45–46
Endocet, 9–12, 880–882
Endometrin Vaginal Insert, 970–972
enfuvirtide, 409–410, 114C–118C
Enjuvia, 275–277
enoxaparin, 410–412, 30C–33C
Enpresse, 92C–96C
entacapone, 412–413, 146C
entecavir, 413–415
Entereg, 43–45
Entocort EC, 145–147
Entrophen, 86–88
Enulose, 658–659
Ephedrine, 158C
Epinastine, 139C
epinephrine, 415–417, 158C
EpiPen, 415–417
EpiPen Jr, 415–417
epirubicin, 418–419, 79C–89C
Epitol, 174–176
Epivir, 659–661, 67C–70C, 114C–118C
Epivir-HBV, 659–661
eplerenone, 419–421
epoetin alfa, 421–424
Epogen, 421–424
Eprex, 421–424
eprosartan, 424–425, 10C
eptifibatide, 425–426, 30C–33C
Epzicom, 1–2, 659–661, 114C–118C
Equetro, 174–176
Equianalgesic dosing, 1255
Eraxis, 69–71, 46C–47C
Erbitux, 220–222, 79C–89C
ergocalciferol, 1212–1215
Ergomar, 426
ergotamine, 426
eribulin, 428–430
erlotinib, 430–431, 79C–89C
Errin, 92C–96C
Ertaczo, 48C–49C
ertapenem, 431–433
Erybid, 433–435
Eryc, 433–435, 26C
EryDerm, 433–435
Erygel, 433–435
EryPed, 433–435, 26C
Ery-Tab, 433–435, 26C
Erythrocin, 433–435, 26C
erythromycin, 433–435, 26C
Eryzole, 433–435
escitalopram, 436–437, 37C–40C
Esclim, 440–443
esmolol, 437–439, 16C–18C, 71C–72C
esomeprazole, 439–440, 148C
Espsom salt, 715
Estazolam, 149C–150C
Estrace, 440–443
Estraderm, 440–443
estradiol, 440–443
estramustine, 444–445, 79C–89C
Estrasorb, 440–443
Estring, 440–443
Estrogel, 440–443
estropipate, 445–446
Estrostep Fe, 92C–96C
eszopiclone, 446–447, 149C–150C
etanercept, 447–449
ethambutol, 449–450
ETH-Oxydose, 880–882
Etibi, 449–450
etodolac, 450–452, 127C–128C
Etomidate, 5C
Etopophos, 452–454

etoposide, 452–454, 79C–89C
Etrafon, 54–55
etravirine, 454–456, 67C–70C, 114C–118C
Euflex, 503–504
Euglucon, 552–554
Eulexin, 503–504, 79C–89C
Evamist, 440–443
Evening primrose oil, 1257–1269
everolimus, 456–457, 79C–89C
Everone, 1114–1116
Evista, 998, 143C–144C
Exalgo, 578–581
Exelon, 1028–1030
exemestane, 457–458, 79C–89C
exenatide, 459–460, 42C–44C
Exforge, 56–57, 1190–1191
Exforge HCT, 56–57, 571–573, 1190–1191
Exjade, 316–317
Ex-Lax, 1051–1052
Extavia, 623–624
Extina, 648–650
Extra Strength Maalox, 1058–1059
ezetimibe, 460–461, 56C–58C
Ezetrol, 460–461

F
Factive, 538–540, 25C
factor VIII, 71–73
fairy candles, 134–135
famciclovir, 461–463, 67C–70C
famotidine, 463–465, 107C–108C
Famvir, 461–463, 67C–70C
Fanapt, 597–598, 64C–66C
Fareston, 1153–1154, 79C–89C
Faslodex, 525–526, 79C–89C
FazaClo, 268–269, 64C–66C
FDA Pregnancy Categories, 1256
featherfew, 479–480
febuxostat, 465–466
Feldene, 937–939, 127C–128C
felodipine, 466–467, 59C–62C, 77C–78C
Femara, 674–675, 79C–89C
Femcon Fe, 92C–96C
Femhrt, 440–443
Femiron, 475, 109C
Femring, 440–443
Femtrace, 440–443
fenofibrate, 467–469, 56C–58C
fenofibric, acid, 469–470, 56C–58C
Fenoglide, 467–469
fenoldopam, 470–472
Fenoprofen, 127C–128C
fentanyl, 472–475, 1248–1254, 141C–142C
Fentora, 472–475
Fenugreek, 1257–1269
Feostat, 109C
Feraheme, 477–478
Fergon, 475, 109C
Fer-In-Sol, 475, 109C
Fer-Iron, 475
Ferrlecit, 1069–1070
Ferro-Sequels, 475
ferrous fumarate, 475, 109C
ferrous gluconate, 475, 109C
Ferrous sulfate exsiccated, 109C
ferrous sulfate, 475, 109C
Fertility Agents, 103C–106C
ferumoxytol, 477–478
fesoterodine, 478–479
Feverall, 9–12
feverfew, 479–480, 1257–1269
fexofenadine, 480–481, 53C–54C
Fiberall, 984–985
Fibricor, 469–470
filgrastim, 481–483
finasteride, 483–485
fingolimod, 485–486
Fioricet, 9–12
Fiorinal, 86–88
Firmagon, 318–320
FIRST-Testosterone, 1114–1116
FIRST-Testosterone MC, 1114–1116
Fish oils, 1257–1269
Flagyl, 763–765
Flagyl 375, 763–765
Flagyl ER, 763–765
Flamazine, 1057–1058
flavoxate, 486–487
Flaxseed/flaxseed oil, 1257–1269
Flebogamma, 605–607
Flecainide, 16C–18C
Flector, 344–347
Fleet Bisacodyl Enema, 129–130
Fleet Enema, 931–933
Fleets Phospho-Soda, 931–933, 121C–122C
Flexbumin, 23–24
Flexeril, 285–287, 151C–153C
Flexitec, 285–287
Flexmid, 285–287
Flomax, 1095–1096
Flonase, 505–507, 2C, 97C–98C

Florinef, 97C–98C
Flovent Diskus, 505–507, 73C–76C
Flovent, 97C–98C
Flovent HFA, 505–507, 73C–76C
Floxin, 856–858, 25C
Floxin Otic, 856–858
fluconazole, 487–489, 46C–47C
Fludara, 489–491, 79C–89C
fludarabine, 489–491, 79C–89C
Fludrocortisone, 97C–98C
Flumadine, 1020–1021
flumazenil, 491–493
flunisolide, 493–495, 2C, 73C–76C, 97C–98C
Flunitrazepam, 1248–1254
Fluocinolone, 99C–100C
Fluocinonide, 99C–100C
Fluoroplex, 495–497
fluorouracil, 495–497, 79C–89C
fluoxetine, 497–499, 37C–40C
Fluphenazine, 64C–66C
fluphenazine decanoate, 499
fluphenazine hydrochloride, 499
Flurandrenolide, 99C–100C
flurazepam, 500–502, 149C–150C
flurbiprofen, 502–503, 127C–128C
flutamide, 503–504, 79C–89C
fluticasone, 505–507, 2C, 73C–76C, 97C–98C, 99C–100C
fluvastatin, 507–508, 56C–58C
fluvoxamine, 508–510, 37C–40C
Focalin, 336–338
Focalin XR, 336–338
Folacin-800, 510–511
folic acid, 510–511
folinic acid, 676–677
Follistim AQ, 104C–106C
Follitropin alpha, 104C–106C
Follitropine beta, 104C–106C
Folotyn, 947–949
Folvite, 510–511
fondaparinux, 511–512, 30C–33C
Foradil, 73C–76C
Foradil Aerolizer, 512–514
Forget me pill, 1248–1254
formoterol, 512–514, 73C–76C
Formoterol/budesonide, 73C–76C
Formulex, 347–349
Fortamet, 741–743
Fortaz, 206–208, 22C–24C
Forteo, 1113–1114, 143C–144C
Fortical, 162–163, 143C–144C
Fosamax, 28–29, 143C–144C
Fosamax Plus D, 28–29
fosamprenavir, 514–516, 114C–118C
fosaprepitant, 73–74
foscarnet, 516–518, 67C–70C
Foscavir, 516–518, 67C–70C
fosfomycin, 518
fosinopril, 519–520, 9C
fosphenytoin, 520–522, 34C–36C
fospropofol, 522–523
Fosrenol, 667
fossil tree, 544–545
Fragmin, 299–300, 30C–33C
Froben, 502–503
Froben SR, 502–503
Frova, 523–525, 63C
frovatriptan, 523–525, 63C
fulvestrant, 525–526, 79C–89C
Fungizone, 61–63
Fungoid, 48C–49C
Furadantin, 838–839
furosemide, 526–528, 101C–102C
Fuzeon, 409–410, 114C–118C

G

gabapentin, 528–530, 34C–36C
Gabitril, 1128–1129, 34C–36C
galantamine, 530–531
Gammagard Liquid, 605–607
Gammagard S/D, 605–607
Gammahydroxybutyrate, 1248–1254
Gamunex, 605–607
ganciclovir, 531–534, 67C–70C
Ganirelex, 104C–106C
Garamycin, 540–543, 21C
garden heliotrope, 1185–1186
garlic, 534–535, 1257–1269
Gastrocom, 282–284
Gas-X, 1058–1059
Gaviscon, 715
GCSF, 481–483
Geftinib, 79C–89C
Gelnique, 878–880
Gelusil, 715
gemcitabine, 535–537, 79C–89C
gemfibrozil, 537–538, 56C–58C
gemifloxacin, 538–540, 25C
Gemtuzumab, 79C–89C
Gemzar, 535–537, 79C–89C
Genahist, 360–362

Genapap, 9–12
Genapap Infant, 9–12
Genaphed, 983–984
Genasyme, 1058–1059
Generlac, 658–659
Gengraf, 289–291
Genotropin, 1072–1075
Genotropin Miniquick, 1072–1075
Genpril, 590–593
Gentak, 540–543
gentamicin, 540–543, 21C
Gentasol, 540–543
Gen-Timolol, 1133–1136
Gentlax-S, 1051–1052
Gen-Warfarin, 1221–1223
Geodon, 1231–1232, 64C–66C
german chamomile, 222–223
GHB, 1248–1254
Gianvi, 92C–96C
Gib, 1248–1254
Gilenya, 485–486
ginger, 543–544, 1257–1269
Ginkgo, 1257–1269
ginkgo biloba, 544–545
ginseng, 545, 1257–1269
GlucGen Diagnostic Kit, 550–551
glatiramer, 546
Gleevec, 599–601, 79C–89C
Gliadel Wafer, 182–183
glimepiride, 547–548, 42C–44C
glipizide, 548–550, 42C–44C
GlucaGen, 550–551
glucagon, 550–551
Glucagon Diagnostic Kit, 550–551
Glucagon Emergency Kit, 550–551
Glucobay, 8–9
GlucoNorm, 1009–1010
Glucophage, 741–743, 42C–44C
Glucophage XR, 741–743
glucosamine/chondroitin, 551–552, 1257–1269
Glucotrol, 548–550, 42C–44C
Glucotrol XL, 548–550
Glucovance, 552–554, 741–743
Glu-K, 945–947
Glumetza, 741–743
glyburide, 552–554, 42C–44C
Glycon, 741–743
glycopyrrolate, 554–555
Glynase, 552–554
Glynase Pres-Tab, 552–554
Glyset, 42C–44C
GM-CSF, 1044–1046
goatweed, 1080–1081
Goldenrod, 1257–1269
Goldenseal, 1257–1269
golimumab, 555–557
GoLYTELY, 941–943
Gonal-F, 104C–106C
Goodfellas, 1248–1254
goserelin, 557–558, 79C–89C, 104C–106C
Gotu kola, 1257–1269
granisetron, 558–560
Granisol, 558–560
granulocyte macrophage colony-stimulating factor, 1044–1046
Grapefruit, 1257–1269
Grass, 1248–1254
Green tea, 1257–1269
Grifulvin V, 560–561
griseofulvin, 560–561
Gris-PEG, 560–561
guaifenesin, 561–562
guanfacine, 562–563
Guarana, 1257–1269
Guggul, 1257–1269
Guiatuss, 561–562
Gymnema, 1257–1269
Gyne-Lotrimin, 266–268

H

H_2 Antagonists, 107C–108C
Habitrol, 829–831
Halaven, 428–430
Halcion, 1248–1254, 149C–150C
Haldol, 564–566, 64C–66C
Haldol Decanoate, 564–566
Haley's MO, 715
Halfprin, 86–88
Halobetasol, 99C–100C
haloperidol, 564–566, 64C–66C
hardhay, 1080–1081
Hashish, 1248–1254
Hawthorn, 1257–1269
hCG, 231–232
Hectorol, 1212–1215
Helidac, 763–765
Hematinic Preparations, 108C–109C
Hemegon, 104C–106C
Hemofil M, 71–73
Hepalean, 566–569
Hepalean Leo, 566–569

heparin, 566–569, 30C–33C
Hep-Lock, 566–569
Hepsera, 20–21, 67C–70C
Heptovir, 659–661
Herbal Therapies and Interactions, 1257–1269
Herceptin, 1164–1166, 79C–89C
Heroin, 1248–1254
Hexalen, 79C–89C
Hexilate FS, 71–73
Hivid, 67C–70C, 114C–118C
Hizentra, 607–608
Hoodia, 1257–1269
Hormones, 109C–112C
Horse chestnut, 1257–1269
Horse, 1248–1254
Humalog, 615–619, 42C–44C
Humalog Mix 75/25, 615–619
Human Immunodeficiency Virus (HIV) Infection, 113C–118C
Humate-P, 71–73
Humatrope, 1072–1075
Humira, 19–20
Humulin 70/30, 615–619
Humulin Mix 50/50, 615–619
Humulin N, 615–619, 42C–44C
Humulin R, 615–619, 42C–44C
Hycamtin, 1151–1153, 79C–89C
Hycet, 9–12, 573–575
Hycodan, 573–575
Hycotuss, 573–575
hydralazine, 569–571, 59C–62C
Hydrea, 582–584, 79C–89C
hydrochlorothiazide, 571–573, 59C–62C, 101C–102C
Hydrocil, 984–985
hydrocodone, 573–575, 141C–142C
hydrocortisone, 575–578, 97C–98C, 99C–100C
HydroDIURIL, 571–573, 59C–62C, 101C–102C
Hydromorph Contin, 578–581
hydromorphone, 578–581, 141C–142C
hydroxychloroquine, 581–582
hydroxyurea, 582–584, 79C–89C
hydroxyzine, 584–585, 13C–14C, 53C–54C
Hygroton, 59C–62C, 101C–102C
hyoscyamine, 585–587
Hyosine, 585–587
Hyper-RHO S/D Full Dose, 1012–1013
Hyper-RHO S/D Mini Dose, 1012–1013
Hypotears, 853–854
Hytone, 575–578, 99C–100C
Hytrin, 1107–1109, 59C–62C
Hyzaar, 571–573, 708–710

I

ibandronate, 587–589, 143C–144C
ibritumomab, 589–590, 79C–89C
Ibu-200, 590–593
ibuprofen, 590–593, 127C–128C
Ibutilide, 16C–18C
Ice, 1248–1254
Idamycin PFS, 593–595, 79C–89C
idarubicin, 593–595, 79C–89C
Ifex, 595–597, 79C–89C
ifosfamide, 595–597, 79C–89C
IL-2, 625–627, **870–871**
Ilaris, 167–169
iloperidone, 597–598, 64C–66C
iloprost, 598–599
imatinib, 599–601, 79C–89C
Imdur, 637
imipenem/cilastatin, 601–603
imipramine, 603–605, 37C–40C
Imitrex, 1087–1088, 63C
immune globulin IV, 605–607
immune globulin subcutaneous, 607–608
Immunosuppressive Agents, 118C–119C
Imodium, 701–703, 45C
Imodium A-D, 701–703
Imodium Advanced, 701–703
Implanon, 92C–96C
Imuran, 101–102
Inapsine, 392–393
indapamide, 608–609, 101C–102C
Inderal, 978–981, 16C–18C, 71C–72C
Inderal LA, 978–981
Inderide LA, 978–981
indinivar, 610–611, 67C–70C, 114C–118C
Indocid, 611–613
Indocin, 611–613, 127C–128C
Indocin-IV, 611–613
indomethacin, 611–613, 127C–128C
Infant Mylicon, 1058–1059
Infasurf, 166–167
Infed, 632–634
infliximab, 613–615
Infufer, 632–634
Infumorph, 791–794
Innohep, 1136–1137, 30C–33C

InnoPran XL, 978–981
Inspra, 419–421
insulin, 615–619
insulin aspart, 615–619, 42C–44C
insulin detemir, 615–619, 42C–44C
insulin glargine, 615–619, 42C–44C
insulin glulisine, 615–619, 42C–44C
insulin lispro, 615–619, 42C–44C
Insulin regular, 42C–44C
Intal, 282–284
Integrilin, 425–426, 30C–33C
Intelence, 454–456, 67C–70C, 114C–118C
interferon alfa-2b, 619–621, 79C–89C
interferon beta-1a, 621–623
interferon beta-1b, 623–624
interferon gamma-1b, 624–625
interleukin-2, 625–627, 870–871
Intron-A, 619–621, 79C–89C
Intropin, 377–379, 158C
Intuniv, 562–563
Invanz, 431–433
Invega Sustenna, 890–891
Invega, 890–891
Invirase, 1042–1043, 67C–70C, 114C–118C
Ionamin, 137C
Iopidien, 50C–52C
ipratropium, 628–629, 3C, 73C–76C
Iquix, 684–687
irbesartan, 629–631, 10C
Iressa, 79C–89C
irinotecan, 631–632, 79C–89C
iron dextran, 632–634
iron sucrose, 634–635
Isentress, 999–1000, 67C–70C, 114C–118C
ISMO, 637
Isochron, 637
isoniazid, 636–637
Isoptin, 16C–18C, 77C–78C
Isoptin SR, 1200–1202, 59C–62C
Isopto Atropine, 96–98
Isordil, 637, 125C–126C
Isosorbide, 125C–126C
isosorbide dinitrate, 637
isosorbide mononitrate, 637
Isotamine, 636–637
isotretinoin, 639–641
Isotrex, 639–641
isradipine, 641–642, 77C–78C
Istalol, 1133–1136, 50C–52C
Istodax, 1031–1033
itraconazole, 642–644, 46C–47C
IVIG, 605–607
ixabepilone, 644–646, 79C–89C
Ixempra, 644–646, 79C–89C

J
Jantoven, 1221–1223
Janumet, 741–743, 1063–1065
Januvia, 1063–1065, 42C–44C
Jevtana, 159–161, 79C–89C
johimbi, 1223–1224
Jolessa, 92C–96C
Jolivette, 92C–96C
Junel 1/20, 92C–96C
Junel 1.5/30, 92C–96C
Junel Fe 1/20, 92C–96C
Junel Fe 1.5/30, 92C–96C

K
Kadian, 791–794
Kalbitor, 397–399
Kaletra, 703–705, 67C–70C, 114C–118C
Kaolin (with pectin), 45C
Kaon-Cl, 945–947
Kaopectate, 130–131, 45C
Kapidex, 334–335, 148C
Kariva, 92C–96C
kava kava, 646, 1257–1269
Kay Ciel, 945–947
Kayexelate, 1070–1071
K-Dur, 945–947
Keets, 1248–1254
Keflex, 216–218, 22C–24C
Keftab, 22C–24C
Kefurox, 22C–24C
Kelnor 1/35, 92C–96C
Kenalog, 1171, 97C–98C, 99C–100C
Kenalog in Orabase, 1171
Kenalog-10, 1171
Kenalog-40, 1171
Kepivance, 889–890
Keppra, 681–683, 34C–36C
Keppra XR, 681–683
Kerlone, 71C–72C
Ketalar, 647–648, 1248–1254, 5C
ketamine, 647–648, 1248–1254, 5C
ketoconazole, 648–650, 46C–47C, 48C–49C
ketoprofen, 650–652, 127C–128C
ketorolac, 652–654, 127C–128C
Ketotifen, 139C
kew, 646

Key-E, 1216
Key-E Kaps, 1216
Kidrolase, 84–86
Kineret, 67–68
Kit-kat, 1248–1254
Klean-Prep, 941–943
Klonex, 1070–1071
Klonopin, 259–261, 34C–36C
Klonopin Wafer, 259–261
K-Lor, 945–947
Klor-Con, 945–947
Klor-Con EF, 945–947
Klor-Con M10, 945–947
Klor-Con M20, 945–947
K-Lyte, 945–947
K-Lyte DS, 945–947
Koate-DVI, 71–73
Kogenate FS, 71–73
Kombusha,1257–1269
Konakion, 1217
Konsyl, 984–985
K-Phos MF, 931–933
K-Phos Neutral, 931–933
Kristalose, 658–659, 121C–122C
Krystexxa, 908–909
Kuric, 648–650
Kytril, 558–560

L

labetalol, 654–656, 71C–72C
lacosamide, 656–658
Lacrilube, 853–854
lactulose, 658–659, 121C–122C
Lamictal, 661–664, 34C–36C
Lamictal ODT, 661–664
Lamictal XR, 661–664
Lamisil, 1109–1110, 48C–49C
Lamisil AT, 1109–1110
Lamisil Oral Granule, 1109–1110
lamivudine, 659–661, 67C–70C, 114C–118C
lamotrigine, 661–664, 34C–36C
Lanoxin, 351–353
lanreotide, 664–665
lansoprazole, 665–667, 148C
lanthanum, 667
Lantus, 615–619, 42C–44C
lapatinib, 668–669, 79C–89C
Largactil, 227–230
Lasix, 526–528, 101C–102C
Lastaceft, 138C
Latanoprost, 50C–52C
Latuda, 713–714
Laxatives, 120C–122C
Laxilose, 658–659
l-carnitine, 1257–1269
Leena, 92C–96C
leflunomide, 669–670
lenalidomide, 670–673
lepirudin, 673–674, 30C–33C
Lescol, 507–508, 56C–58C
Lescol XL, 507–508
Lessina, 92C–96C
Letairis, 46–48
letrozole, 674–675, 79C–89C
leucovorin calcium, 676–677
Leukeran, 224–226, 79C–89C
Leukine, 1044–1046
leuprolide, 677–679, 79C–89C, 104C–106C
Leupron, 79C–89C
Leustatin, 247–248, 79C–89C
levalbuterol, 679–681, 73C–76C
Levaquin, 684–687, 25C
Levate, 54–55
Levbid, 585–587
Levemir, 615–619, 42C–44C
levetiracetam, 681–683, 34C–36C
Levitra, 1194–1195
Levlite, 92C–96C
Levobunolol, 50C–52C
levocetirizine, 683–684, 53C–54C
Levo-Dromoran, 141C–142C
levofloxacin, 684–687, 25C
Levophed, 845–847, 158C
Levora, 92C–96C
Levorphanol, 141C–142C
Levothroid, 687–689, 159C
levothyroxine, 687–689, 159C
Levoxyl, 687–689, 159C
Levsin, 585–587
Levsin S/L, 585–587
Lexapro, 436–437, 37C–40C
Lexiva, 514–516, 114C–118C
Lexxel, 407–409, 466–467
Lialda, 736–737
Librax, 226–227
Librium, 226–227, 1248–1254, 13C–14C
Licorice, 1257–1269
Lidex, 99C–100C
lidocaine, 689–691, 6C, 7C, 16C–18C
Lidocaine with epirnephrine, 689–691

Lidoderm, 689–691
LidoSite, 415–417
Lifespan and Cultural Aspects of Drug Therapy, 1270–1273
Limbitrol, 54–55, 226–227
linezolid, 691–693
Lioresal, 109–111, 151C–153C
Liotec, 109–111
Liothyronine, 159C
Liotrix, 159C
Lipitor, 93–95, 56C–58C
Lipofen, 467–469
Lipsovir, 16–19, 575–578
Liquid ecstasy, 1248–1254
Liquid X, 1248–1254
liraglutide, 693–694, 42C–44C
lisdexamfetamine, 695–696
lisinopril, 696–698, 9C, 59C–62C
lithium carbonate, 698–700
lithium citrate, 698–700
Lithobid, 698–700
Livalo, 939–940, 56C–58C
Lo/Orval-28, 92C–96C
Lodine, 450–452, 127C–128C
Lodine XL, 450–452
Lodoxamine, 139C
Loestrin 1/20 Fe, 92C–96C
Loestrin Fe 1.5/30, 92C–96C
Loestrin-24 Fe, 92C–96C
Lofibra, 467–469, 56C–58C
Lomine, 347–349
Lomotil, 96–98, 362–363, 45C
lomustine, 700–701, 79C–89C
Loniten, 776–778, 59C–62C
Lonox, 362–363
Loperacap, 701–703
loperamide, 701–703, 45C
Lopid, 537–538, 56C–58C
lopinavir/ritonavir, 703–705, 67C–70C, 114C–118C
Lopressor, 760–762, 59C–62C, 71C–72C
Lopressor HCT, 571–573
Loprox, 48C–49C
Loradamed, 705–706
loratadine, 705–706, 53C–54C
lorazepam, 706–708, 13C–14C
Lorazepam Intensol, 706–708
Lorcet, 573–575
Lortab, 9–12
Lortab Elixir, 9–12, 573–575
Lortab/ASA, 86–88, 573–575
losartan, 708–710, 10C, 59C–62C
Losec, 866–867
Lotemax, 140C
Lotensin, 114–116, 9C, 59C–62C
Lotensin HCT, 114–116, 571–573
Loteprednol, 140C
Lotrel, 56–57, 114–116
Lotrimin, 266–268, 766–767, 48C–49C
Lotrisone, 121–123, 266–268
lovastatin, 710–711, 56C–58C
Lovaza, 865–866
Lovenox, 410–412, 30C–33C
Low-Ogestrel-21, -28, 92C–96C
Loxapine, 64C–66C
Loxitane,64C–66C
Lozide, 608–609
Lozol, 608–609, 101C–102C
LSD, 1248–1254
lubiprostone, 711–712
Ludes, 1248–1254
Lumigan, 50C–52C
Luminal, 923–925
Lunelle, 440–443
Lunesta, 446–447, 149C–150C
Lupron, 677–679, 104C–106C
Lupron Depot, 677–679
Lupron Depot-Ped, 677–679
lurasidone, 713–714
Lusedra, 522–523
Lutera, 92C–96C
Luvox, 508–510, 37C–40C
Luvox CR, 508–510, 37C–40C
Luxiq, 121–123
Lybrel, 92C–96C
lymphocyte immune globulin N, 714–715
Lyrica, 960–962, 34C–36C
Lysodren, 79C–89C
Lysteda, 1161–1162

M

Maalox, 715
Maalox Plus, 715
Maalox Total Stomach Relief, 130–131
MabCampath, 28–30
Macrobid, 838–839
Macrodantin, 838–839
Mag-Delay, 715
Magic mushroom, 1248–1254
Magnacet, 9–12, 880–882
magnesium, 715

magnesium chloride, 715
magnesium citrate, 715, 121C
magnesium hydroxide, 715, 11C–12C, 121C
magnesium oxide, 715, 11C–12C
magnesium protein complex, 715
magnesium sulfate, 715
Magnesium sulfate injection, 715
Mag-Ox 400, 715, 11C–12C
maidenhair tree, 544–545
Mangosteen, 1257–1269
mannitol, 719–720
Mapap, 9–12
maraviroc, 721–722, 67C–70C, 114C–118C
Marcaine, 6C
Marijuana, 1248–1254
Marinol, 389–390
Matulane, 967–968, 79C–89C
Mavik, 1160–1161, 9C
Maxalt, 1030–1031, 63C
Maxalt RPD, 1030–1031
Maxalt-MLT, 1030–1031, 63C
Maxide, 571–573
Maxidex, 331–334
Maxipime, 194–196, 22C–24C
Maxitrol, 331–334
Maxzide, 1173–1175
MDMA, 1248–1254
Meadowsweet, 1257–1269
Mechlorethamine, 79C–89C
meclizine, 722–723
Medrol, 754
medroxyprogesterone, 723–725
Medroxyprogesterone Acetate, 92C–96C
Mefoxin, 199–201, 22C–24C
Megace, 725, 79C–89C
Megace ES, 725
Megace OS, 725
megestrol, 725, 79C–89C
melatonin, 726–727, 1257–1269
Mellaril, 1123–1125, 64C–66C
meloxicam, 727–729, 127C–128C
melphalan, 729–730, 79C–89C
memantine, 730–732
Menopur, 104C–106C
Menostar, 440–443
Menotropins, 104C–106C
Mentax, 48C–49C
meperidine, 732–734, 141C–142C
Mephyton, 1217
Mepivacaine, 7C
Mepron, 95–96
Mercaptopurine, 79C–89C
Meridia, 137C
meropenem, 734–736
Merrem IV, 734–736
mesalamine, 736–737
Mesasal, 736–737
Mescaline, 1248–1254
M-Eslon, 791–794
mesna, 737–739
Mesnex, 737–739
Mesoridazine, 64C–66C
Mestinon, 987–988, 90C–91C
Mestinon SR, 987–988
Mestinon Timespan, 987–988
Metadate CD, 752–754
Metadate ER, 752–754
Metadol, 743–745
Metaglip, 548–550, 741–743
Metamucil, 984–985, 121C
metaproterenol, 739–740
metaxalone, 740–741, 151C–153C
metformin, 741–743, 42C–44C
Meth, 1248–1254
methadone, 743–745, 141C–142C
Methadone Intensol, 743–745
Methadose, 743–745
Methamphetamine, 1248–1254
Methaqualone, 1248–1254
Methergine, 749–750
methocarbamol, 745–746, 151C–153C
Methohexital, 5C
methotrexate, 747–749, 79C–89C
Methylcellulose, 121C
Methyldopa, 59C–62C
Methylenedioxymethamphetamine, 1248–1254
methylergonovine, 749–750
Methylin, 752–754
Methylin ER, 752–754
methylnaltrexone, 751–752
methylphenidate, 752–754, 1248–1254
methylprednisolone, 754, 97C–98C
methylprednisolone acetate, 754
methylprednisolone sodium succinate, 754
Methylsulfonylmethane, 1248–1254
Metipranolol, 50C–52C
metoclopramide, 756–758
metolazone, 758–760, 101C–102C
metoprolol, 760, 59C–62C, 71C–72C

Metozolv ODT, 756–758
Metro-Cream, 763–765
MetroGel, 763–765
MetroGel-Vaginal, 763–765
metronidazole, 763–765
Mevacor, 710–711, 56C–58C
Mexiletine, 16C–18C
Mexitil, 16C–18C
Mg-PLUS, 715
Miacalcin, 162–163, 143C–144C
Miacalcin Nasal, 162–163
Micaderm, 766–767
micafungin, 765–766, 46C–47C
Micardis, 1099–1100, 10C
Micardis HCT, 571–573, 1099–1100
Micatin, 766–767, 48C–49C
miconazole, 766–767, 48C–49C
Micorgestin 1/20 Fe, 92C–96C
Micozole, 766–767
Microgestin 1.5/30, 92C–96C
Microgestin Fe 1.5/30, 92C–96C
MICROhoGAM, 1012–1013
Micro-K, 945–947
Micronase, 552–554, 42C–44C
Micronor, 92C–96C
Microzide, 571–573
Midamor, 101C–102C
midazolam, 767–769, 5C
midodrine, 769–771
midsummer daisy, 479–480
Mifeprex, 771–772
mifepristone, 771–772
Miglitol, 42C–44C
Migranal, 426
Milk of Magnesia, 11C–12C
Milk thistle, 1257–1269
Millipred, 957–959
milnacipran, 772–773
Milophene, 104C–106C
milrinone, 773–775
Minipress, 956–957, 59C–62C
Minirin, 328–330
Minitran, 839–842, 125C–126C
Minocin, 775–776
minocycline, 775–776
Minox, 776–778
minoxidil, 776–778, 59C–62C
Miostat, 50C–52C
MiraLax, 941–943, 121C–122C
Mirapex, 949–951, 146C
Mirapex ER, 949–951
Mircette, 92C–96C
Mirena, 92C–96C
mirtazapine, 778–779, 37C–40C
misoprostol, 780–781
Miss Emma, 1248–1254
Mister blue, 1248–1254
Mithracin, 79C–89C
mitomycin, 781–783
Mitomycin-C, 79C–89C
Mitotane, 79C–89C
mitoxantrone, 783–785, 79C–89C
Mitrazol, 766–767
Mivacron, 123C
Mivacurium, 123C
Mobic, 727–729, 127C–128C
modafinil, 785–786
Modecate, 499
Modicon, 92C–96C
Moduretic, 571–573
moexipril, 786–787, 9C
mometasone furoate, 787
mometasone, 787–789, 3C, 73C–76C, 99C–100C
Monarc M, 71–73
Monistat, 766–767, 48C–49C
Monistat 3, 766–767
Monistat 7, 766–767
Monoclate-P, 71–73
Monocor, 131–133
Monodox, 387–389
Monoket, 637
Mononessa, 92C–96C
Monopril, 519–520, 9C
montelukast, 789–791, 73C–76C
Monurol, 518
Morinda, 1257–1269
morphine, 791–794, 1248–1254, 141C–142C
Motrin, 590–593, 127C–128C
Motrin Children's, 590–593
Motrin Cold, 983–984
Motrin IB, 590–593
Motrin Infants', 590–593
Motrin Junior Strength, 590–593
Moxatag, 57–59
moxifloxacin, 794–796, 25C
Mozobil, 940–941
MS Contin, 791–794, 1248–1254, 141C–142C
MSIR, 791–794
MSM, 1248–1254

Mucinex, 561–562
Mucinex D, 561–562
Mucinex DM, 561–562
Mucomyst, 13–15
Multaq, 390–392, 16C–18C
mupirocin, 796–797
Muro 128, 1067–1069
Muse, 40–41
Mustargen, 79C–89C
Mutamycin, 781–783, 79C–89C
Myambutol, 449–450
Mycamine, 765–766, 46C–47C
Mycelex, 266–268, 48C–49C
Mycobutin, 1015–1017
Myco-II, 1171
Mycolog, 850–852
Mycolog II, 1171
mycophenolate, 797–799, 119C
Mycostatin, 850–852, 48C–49C
Myco-Triacet, 850–852, 1171
Mydfrin, 927–929
Myfortic, 797–799
Mylanta, 715, 1058–1059
Mylanta Gas, 1058–1059
Myleran, 155–157, 79C–89C
Mylocel, 582–584
Mylotarg, 79C–89C
Myobloc, 142–143
Myrac, 775–776
Mysoline, 962–963, 34C–36C

N

nabumetone, 800–801, 127C–128C
N-acetylcysteine, 13–15
nadolol, 801–803, 71C–72C
nafarelin, 803–804, 104C–106C
nafcillin, 804–805, 28C
nalbuphine, 805–807, 141C–142C
Nalfon, 127C–128C
Nallpen, 804–805
naloxone, 807–809
naltrexone, 809–811
Namenda, 730–732
Namenda XR, 730–732
Naphazoline/pheniramine, 138C
Naphcon-A, 138C
Naprelan, 811–813
Naprosyn, 811–813, 127C–128C
naproxen, 811–813, 127C–128C
naratriptan, 813–814, 63C
Narcan, 807–809
Nardil, 922–923, 37C–40C
Naropin, 7C
Nasacort AQ, 1171, 3C
Nasal Moist, 1067–1069
Nasalcrom, 282–284, 3C
Nasalide, 493–495, 97C–98C
Nasarel, 493–495, 2C
Nascobal, 284–285
Nasonex, 787, 3C
natalizumab, 814–815
Natazia, 92C–96C
nateglinide, 815–817, 42C–44C
Natrecor, 822–824
Natulan, 967–968
Nature Throid, 159C
Navane, 1127–1128, 64C–66C
Navelbine, 1208–1210, 79C–89C
Nebcin, 21C
nebivolol, 817–818
NebuPent, 917–919
Necon 0.5/35, 92C–96C
Necon 1/35–28, 92C–96C
Necon 1/50, 92C–96C
Necon 7/7/7, 92C–96C
Necon 10/11, 92C–96C
nectar of the gods, 534–535
Nedocromil, 139C
nelarabine, 818–819, 79C–89C
nelfinavir, 820–821, 67C–70C, 114C–118C
Nembutal, 1248–1254
Neomycin, 21C
NeoProfen, 590–593
Neoral, 289–291, 119C
Neosporin, 108–109
neostigmine, 821–822, 90C–91C
Neo-Synephrine, 927–929, 4C, 158C
Nephro-Fer, 475
Nesacaine 6C
nesiritide, 822–824
Neulasta, 903–904
Neumega, 870–871
Neupogen, 481–483
Neuromuscular Blockers, 123C–124C
Neurontin, 528–530, 34C–36C
Neut, 1065–1067
Neutra-Phos, 931–933
Neutral-Phos K, 931–933
nevirapine, 824–825, 114C–118C
Nexavar, 1075–1076, 79C–89C
Nexium, 439–440, 148C
niacin, 825–827, 56C–58C, 161C–162C

Niacor, 825–827, 56C–58C
Niaspan, 825–827, 56C–58C
nicardipine, 827–829, 77C–78C
NicoDerm, 829–831
NicoDerm CQ, 829–831, 154C–156C
Nicorette, 829–831, 154C–156C
Nicorette Plus, 829–831
nicotine, 829–831
Nicotine gum, 154C–156C
Nicotine inhaler, 154C–156C
Nicotine lozenge, 154C–156C
Nicotine nasal spray, 154C–156C
Nicotine patch, 154C–156C
nicotinic acid, 825–827, 56C–58C
Nicotrol. 829–831, 154C–156C
Nicotrol Inhaler, 829–831
Nicotrol NS, 829–831, 154C–156C
NidaGel, 763–765
Nifediac CC, 831–833
Nifedical XL, 831–833
nifedipine, 831–833, 59C–62C, 77C–78C
Nilandron, 834–835, 79C–89C
nilotinib, 833–834, 79C–89C
Nilstat, 850–852, 48C–49C
nilutamide, 834–835, 79C–89C
Nimbex, 123C
nimodipine, 835–837, 77C–78C
Nimotop, 835–837, 77C–78C
Nipent, 79C–89C
Nipride, 842–844
Niravam, 38–39
nitazoxanide, 837–838
Nitoman, 1116–1117
Nitrates, 125C–126C
Nitro-Bid, 839–842, 125C–126C
Nitro-Dur, 839–842, 125C–126C
nitrofurantoin, 838–839
nitroglycerin, 839–842, 125C–126C
Nitrolingual, 839–842
Nitropress, 842–844
nitroprusside, 842–844
NitroQuick, 839–842
Nitrostat, 839–842, 125C–126C
Nitro-Time, 839–842
nizatidine, 844–845, 107C–108C
Nizoral, 648–650, 48C–49C
Nizoral AD, 648–650
Nizoral Topical, 648–650
Nolvadex, 79C–89C
Non-Crushable Drugs, 1274–1279
Nonsteroidal Anti-Inflammatory Drugs (NSAIDs), 126C–129C
Nora-BE, 92C–96C
Norco, 9–12, 573–575
Norcuron, 124C
Nordette, 92C–96C
Norditropin, 1072–1075
norepinephrine, 845–847, 158C
Norethin 1/35–28, 92C–96C
Norflex, 151C–153C
norfloxacin, 847–848, 25C
Norfloxacine, 847–848
Norinyl 1+50, 92C–96C
Noritate, 763–765
Normal Laboratory Values, 1280–1281
Normodyne, 654–656
Normozide, 571–573, 654–656
Noroxin, 847–848, 25C
Norpace, 365–367, 16C–18C
Norpace CR, 365–367, 16C–18C
Norpramin, 325–326, 37C–40C
Nor-QD, 92C–96C
Nortrel 0.5/35, 92C–96C
Nortrel 7/7/7, 92C–96C
nortriptyline, 848–850, 37C–40C, 156C
Norvasc, 56–57, 77C–78C
Norventyl, 848–850
Norvir, 1025–1027, 67C–70C, 114C–118C
Norvir-SEC, 1025–1027
Novaldex-D, 1094–1095
Novamoxin, 57–59
Novantrone, 783–785, 79C–89C
Novarel, 231–232
Novasen, 86–88
Novo-Alendronate, 28–29
Novo-Amiodarone, 51–54
Novo-Amlodipine, 56–57
Novo-Ampicillin, 63–65
Novo-Aprazol, 38–39
Novo-Atenol, 90–92
Novo-Azathioprine, 101–102
Novo-Azithromycin, 104–106
Novo-Bicalutamide, 127–128
Novo-Bisoprolol, 131–133
Novo-Buspirone, 154–155
Novocaine, 6C
Novo-Captopril, 172–174
Novo-Carbamaz, 174–176
Novo-Carvedilol, 183–185
Novo-Cefaclor, 187–188
Novo-Cefadroxil, 188–190

Novo-Chlorpromazine, 227–230
Novo-Cholamine, 230–231
Novo-Cimetidine, 237–239
Novo-Ciprofloxacin, 240–243
Novo-Citalopram, 245–247
Novo-Clindamycin, 254–256
Novo-Clonazepam, 259–261
Novo-Clonidine, 261–263
Novo-Clopate, 264–266
Novo-Cycloprine, 285–287
Novo-Desmopressin, 328–330
Novo-Difenac, 344–347
Novo-Diltiazem, 354–357
Novo-Dipam, 342–344
Novo-Divalproex, 1187–1190
Novo-Docusate, 371–372
Novo-Doxazosin, 380–382
Novo-Doxepin, 382–384
Novo-Doxylin, 387–389
Novo-Enalapril, 407–409
Novo-Famotidine, 463–465
Novo-Fenofibrate, 467–469
Novo-Fentanyl, 472–475
Novo-Fluconazole, 487–489
Novo-Fluoxetine, 497–499
Novo-Flutamide, 503–504
Novo-Fluvoxamine, 508–510
Novo-Fosinopril, 519–520
Novo-Furantoin, 838–839
Novo-Gabapentin, 528–530
Novo-Gemfibrozil, 537–538
Novo-Glimepiride, 547–548
Novo-Glyburide, 552–554
Novo-Hydrazide, 571–573
Novo-Hydroxyzin, 584–585
Novo-Hylazin, 569–571
Novo-Indapamide, 608–609
Novo-Ipramide, 628–629
Novo-Ketoconazole, 648–650
Novo-Keto-EC, 650–652
Novo-Ketorolac, 652–654
Novo-Lamotrigine, 661–664
Novo-Lansoprazole, 665–667
Novo-Leflunomide, 669–670
Novo-Levocarbidopa, 176–178
Novo-Levofloxacin, 684–687
Novolexin, 216–218
Novolin 70/30, 615–619
Novolin N, 615–619, 42C–44C
Novolin R, 615–619, 42C–44C
Novo-Lisinopril, 696–698
Novolog Mix 70/30, 615–619
Novolog, 615–619, 42C–44C
Novo-Loperamide, 701–703
Novo-Lorazem, 706–708
Novo-Lovastatin, 710–711
Novo-Medrone, 723–725
Novo-Meloxicam, 727–729
Novo-Metformin, 741–743
Novo-Methacin, 611–613
Novo-Metoprolol, 760–762
Novo-Minocycline, 775–776
Novo-Mirtazapine, 778–779
Novo-Misoprostol, 780–781
Novo-Nabumetone, 800–801
Novo-Nadolol, 801–803
Novo-Naprox, 811–813
Novo-Nifedin, 831–833
Novo-Nizatidine, 844–845
Novo-Norfloxacin, 847–848
Novo-Nortriptyline, 848–850
Novo-Ofloxacin, 856–858
Novo-Olanzapine, 858–860
Novo-Ondansetron, 867–869
Novo-Oxybutynin, 878–880
Novo-Pantoprazole, 898–899
Novo-Paroxetine, 899–901
Novo-Pen-VK, 916–917
Novo-Peridol, 564–566
Novo-Pioglitazone, 934–935
Novo-Pirocam, 937–939
Novo-Pramine, 603–605
Novo-Pramipexole, 949–951
Novo-Pravastatin, 954–956
Novo-Prazin, 956–957
Novo-Prednisolone, 957–959
Novo-Prednisone, 959–960
Novo-Profen, 590–593
Novo-Quetiapine, 989–991
Novo-Quinidine, 993–995
Novo-Rabeprazole, 996–998
Novo-Ramipril, 1001–1003
Novo-Ranitidine, 1003–1005
Novo-Risperidone, 1023–1025
Novo-Selegiline, 1049–1051
Novo-Semide, 526–528
Novo-Sertraline, 1052–1054
Novo-Simvastatin, 1059–1061
Novo-Sotalol, 1076–1078
Novo-Spiroton, 1078–1080
Novo-Sucralate, 1082–1083
Novo-Sumatriptan, 1087–1088

Novo-Sundac, 1085–1086
Novo-Tamoxifen, 1094–1095
Novo-Tamsulosin, 1095–1096
Novo-Temazepam, 1100–1102
Novo-Terazosin, 1107–1109
Novo-Terbinafine, 1109–1110
Novo-Ticlopidine, 1129–1131
Novo-Timol, 1133–1136
Novo-Topiramate, 1149–1151
Novo-Trazodone, 1166–1167
Novo-Trifluzine, 1175–1177
Novotrimel, 279–282
Novo-Tryptyn, 54–55
Novo-Venlafaxine, 1198–1200
Novo-Veramil SR, 1200–1202
Novo-Warfarin, 1221–1223
Noxafil, 944–945, 46C–47C
NPH, 615–619, 42C–44C
Nplate, 1033–1034
Nu-Ampi, 63–65
Nu-Baclo, 109–111
Nubain, 805–807, 141C–142C
Nucynta, 1096–1097
Nu-Ipratropium, 628–629
NuLytely, 941–943
Nu-Metop, 760–762
Nu-Naprox, 811–813
Nu-Pen VK, 916–917
Nupercainal Hydrocortisone Cream, 575–578
Nupercainal, 7C
Nu-Propranolol, 978–981
Nuromax, 123C
Nu-Tetra, 1117–1119
Nutrition: Enteral, 130C–133C
Nutrition: Parenteral, 134C–136C
Nutropin AQ, 1072–1075
Nutropin, 1072–1075
NuvaRing, 92C–96C
Nuvigil, 78–79
nystatin, 850–852, 48C–49C
Nystat-Rx, 850–852
Nystop, 850–852
Nytol, 360–362

O

Obesity Management, 137C
Ocean, 1067–1069
Ocella, 92C–96C
Octagam 5%, 605–607
Octostim, 328–330
octreotide, 852–853
Ocufen, 502–503
Ocuflox, 856–858
ocular lubricant, 853–854
Ocupress, 50C–52C
ofatumumab, 854–856
ofloxacin, 856–858
Ogen, 445–446
Ogestrel 0.5/50–28, 92C–96C
olanzapine, 858–860, 64C–66C
Oleptro, 1166–1167
Olfloxacin, 25C
olmesartan, 860–862, 10C, 59C–62C
Olmetec, 860–862
Olopatadine, 3C, 139C
olsalazine, 862–863
omalizumab, 863–865
omega-3 acid ethyl esters, 865–866
Omega-6 fatty acid, 1257–1269
omeprazole, 866–867, 148C
Omnaris, 232–234, 2C
Omnicef, 192–194, 22C–24C
Omnitrope, 1072–1075
Oncaspar, 79C–89C
Oncovin, 79C–89C
ondansetron, 867–869
Onglyza, 1046–1048, 42C–44C
Onsolis, 472–475
Ontak, 322–323, 79C–89C
Onxol, 886–889
Opana, 882–884, 141C–142C
Opana ER, 882–884, 141C–142C
Opana Injectable, 882–884
Opcon-A, 138C
Ophthalmic Medications for Allergic Conjunctivitis, 138C–140C
Opioid Analgesics, 141C–142C
oprelvekin, 870–871
Optimine, 53C–54C
OptiPranolol, 50C–52C
Optivar, 102–104, 139C
Oracea, 387–389
Oramorph SR, 791–794
Orapred ODT, 957–959
Orapred, 957–959
OraVerse, 925–927
Oravig, 766–767
Orencia, 2–3
Organidin, 561–562
orlistat, 871–872, 137C
Orphan Drugs, 1282–1283
Orphenadrine, 151C–153C

Ortho Evra, 92C–96C
Ortho-Cept, 92C–96C
Ortho-Cyclen, 92C–96C
Ortho-Est, 445–446
Ortho-Novum 1/35–28, 92C–96C
Ortho-Novum 7/7/7, 92C–96C
Ortho-Tri-Cyclen Lo, 92C–96C
Ortho-Tri-Cyclen, 92C–96C
Orudis KT,127C–128C
Oruvail, 650–652
Os-Cal 500, 163
OsCal, 163
oseltamivir, 872–873, 67C–70C
Osmitrol, 719–720
Osteocit, 163
Osteoporosis, 143C–144C
Ovcon-35, 92C–96C
Ovcon-50, 92C–96C
Ovol, 1058–1059
Oxacillin, 28C
oxaliplatin, 873–875, 79C–89C
oxaprozin, 875–877, 127C–128C
Oxazepam, 13C–14C
oxcarbazepine, 877–878, 34C–36C
Oxeze, 512–514
Oxiconazole, 48C–49C
Oxistat, 48C–49C
Oxy, 1248–1254
oxybutynin, 878–880
oxycodone, 880–882, 1248–1254, 141C–142C
OxyContin, 880–882, 1248–1254
OxyIR, 880–882
Oxymetazoline, 4C
oxymorphone, 882–884, 141C–142C
oxytocin, 884–886
Oxytrol, 878–880
Oyst-Cal, 11C–12C

P

Pacerone, 16C–18C
Pacerone, 51–54
paclitaxel, 886–889, 79C–89C
Palafer, 475
palifermin, 889–890
paliperidone, 890–891
palivizumab, 892
Palmitate A, 1211–1212
palonosetron, 892–893
Pamelor, 848–850, 37C–40C, 154C–156C
pamidronate, 893–895
Pamprin, 811–813
Pancreaze, 895–896
pancrelipase, 895–896
Pancuronium, 124C
panitumumab, 896–897, 79C–89C
Panretin, 79C–89C
Panto, 898–899
pantoprazole, 898–899, 148C
Pantothenic acid, 161C–162C
Parafon Forte, 151C–153C
Paraplatin, 178–180, 79C–89C
Paraplatin-AQ, 178–180
Parcopa, 176–178, 146C
Parenteral Fluid Administration, 1302–1303
paricalcitol, 1212–1215
Pariet, 996–998
Parkinson's Disease Treatment, 145C–147C
Parlodel, 144–145, 146C
Parnate, 1162–1164, 37C–40C
paroxetine, 899–901, 13C–14C, 37C–40C
Parvolex, 13–15
Patanase, 3C
Patanol, 139C
Pathocil, 28C
Pavulon, 124C
Paxil, 899–901, 13C–14C, 37C–40C
Paxil CR, 899–901
pazopanib, 901–903
PCE Dispertab, 433–435
PCE, 26C
Peace pill, 1248–1254
Pediapred, 957–959
Pediazole, 433–435
Pedi-Dri, 850–852
Pegaspargase, 79C–89C
Pegasys, 904–906
PEG-ES, 941–943
pegfilgrastim, 903–904
peginterferon alfa-2a, 904–906
peginterferon alfa-2b, 906–907
PEG-Intron, 906–907
pegloticase, 908–909
Peglyte, 941–943
pegvisomant, 909–910
pemetrexed, 910–912, 79C–89C
Pemirolast, 139C
penicillamine, 912–914
penicillin G benzathine, 914–915, 28C
penicillin G potassium, 915–916, 28C
penicillin V potassium, 916–917, 28C
Pennsaid, 344–347

Pentam-300, 917–919
pentamidine, 917–919
Pentasa, 736–737
Pentostatin, 79C–89C
Pentothal, 5C
pentoxifylline, 919–920
Pentoxil, 919–920
Pepcid, 463–465, 107C–108C
Pepcid AC, 463–465
Pepcid AC Maximum Strength, 463–465
Pepcid Complete, 463–465
Peppermint, 1257–1269
Pepto-Bismol, 130–131, 45C
Percocet, 9–12, 880–882
Percodan, 86–88, 880–882
Perforomist, 512–514, 73C–76C
Periactin, 53C–54C
Peri-Colace, 371–372
Peridol, 564–566
Perindopril, 9C
Periostat, 387–389
Persantine, 364–365, 30C–33C
Pexeva, 899–901
Pexi-cam, 937–939
Pfizerpen, 915–916, 28C
PGE1, 40–41
Phanasin, 561–562
Pharmorubicin, 418–419
Phazyme, 1058–1059
Phellodendron, 1257–1269
Phenadoz, 972–975
Phenazo, 921–922
phenazopyridine, 921–922
Phencyclidine, 1248–1254
Phendimetrazine, 137C
phenelzine, 922–923, 37C–40C
Phenergan VC, 972–975
Phenergan VC with codeine, 972–975
Phenergan, 972–975, 53C–54C
Phenergan with codeine, 972–975
Phennies, 1248–1254
phenobarbital, 923–925, 34C–36C
Phenteramine, 137C
phentolamine, 925–927
phenylephrine, 927–929, 4C, 158C
Phenytek, 929–931
phenytoin, 929–931, 34C–36C
Phillips Milk of Magnesia, 715
PhosLo, 163
phosphates, 931–933
Phospholine Iodide, 50C–52C
phytonadione, 1217
Pilipine HS, 50C–52C
Pilocarpine, 50C–52C
pimecrolimus, 933–934
Pindolol, 71C–72C
pineal hormone, 726–727
pinheads, 222–223
pioglitazone, 934–935, 42C–44C
piperacillin sodium/tazobactam sodium, 935–937, 28C–29C
piroxicam, 937–939, 127C–128C
pitavastatin, 939–940, 56C–58C
Pitocin, 884–886
Pitressin, 1196–1198
plam tree, 1046
Plan B, 92C–96C
Plaquenil, 581–582
Plasbumin, 23–24
Platinol-AQ, 243–245, 79C–89C
Plavix, 263–264, 30C–33C
Plendil, 466–467, 59C–62C, 77C–78C
plerixafor, 940–941
Pletal, 235–236
Plicamycin, 79C–89C
PMS-Amantadine, 45–46
PMS-Chloral Hydrate, 223–224
PMS-Clarithromycin, 248–250
PMS-Docusate, 371–372
PMS-Ipratropium, 628–629
PMS-Isoniazid, 636–637
PMS-Methylphenidate, 752–754
PMS-Norfloxacin, 847–848
PMS-Pseudoephedrine, 983–984
PMS-Salbutamol, 25–27
PMS-Sertraline, 1052–1054
PMS-Sodium Polystyrene Sulfonate, 1070–1071
PMS-Sotalol, 1076–1078
PMS-Temazepam, 1100–1102
PMS-Timolol, 1133–1136
PMS-Tobramycin, 1141–1144
PMS-Trazodone, 1166–1167
PMS-Trifluoperazine, 1175–1177
Poison Antidote Chart, 1287–1290
Polaramine,53C–54C
Policosanol, 1257–1269
Polocaine, 7C
Polyethylene glycol, 121C–122C
polyethylene glycol-electrolyte solution, 941–943
Polysporin, 108–109

Pomegranate, 1257–1269
Pontocaine, 8C
poor man's treacle, 534–535
poractant alfa, 943–944
Portia, 92C–96C
posaconazole, 944–945, 46C–47C
Posanol, 944–945
Pot, 1248–1254
potassium acetate, 945–947
potassium bicarbonate/citrate, 945–947
potassium chloride, 945–947
potassium gluconate, 945–947
Pradaxa, 294–295
pralatrexate, 947–949
pramipexole, 949–951, 146C
pramlintide, 951–952, 42C–44C
PrandiMet, 741–743, 1009–1010
Prandin, 1009–1010, 42C–44C
prasterone, 341–342
prasugrel, 953–954, 30C–33C
Pravachol, 954–956, 56C–58C
pravastatin, 954–956, 56C–58C
Pravigard, 86–88, 954–956
prazosin, 956–957, 59C–62C
Precedex, 335–336
Precose, 8–9, 42C–44C
Pred Forte, 957–959
Pred Mild, 957–959
Prednicarbate, 99C–100C
prednisolone, 957–959, 97C–98C, 140C
prednisone, 959–960, 97C–98C
Prednisone Intensol, 959–960
pregabalin, 960–962, 34C–36C
Pregnyl, 231–232, 104C–106C
Prelone, 957–959, 97C–98C
Premarin, 275–277
Premphase, 275–277, 723–725
Prempro, 275–277, 723–725
Preparation H Hydrocortisone, 575–578
Prepidil, 358–360
Pressyn, 1196–1198
Pressyn AR, 1196–1198
Prevacid, 665–667, 148C
Prevacid NapraPac, 665–667, 811–813
Prevacid Solu-Tab, 665–667
Prevalite, 230–231, 56C–58C
Preventing Medication Errors and Improving Medications Safety, 1291–1293
Previfem, 92C–96C
Prevpac, 665–667
Prezista, 308–310, 67C–70C, 114C–118C
Prickly pear cactus, 1257–1269
Prilosec, 866–867, 148C
Prilosec OTC, 866–867
Primacor, 773–775
Primacor IV, 773–775
Primatene Mist, 415–417
Primaxin, 601–603
primidone, 962–963, 34C–36C
Primsol, 1178–1179
Principen, 28C–29C
Prinivil, 696–698, 9C, 59C–62C
Prinzide, 571–573, 696–698
Pristiq, 330–331, 37C–40C
Privigen, 605–607
ProAir HFA, 25–27, 73C–76C
ProAmatine, 769–771
probenecid, 964–965
procainamide, 965–967, 16C–18C
Procaine, 6C
Procanbid, 965–967
Procan-SR, 965–967, 16C–18C
procarbazine, 967–968, 79C–89C
Procardia, 831–833, 77C–78C
Procardia XL, 831–833, 59C–62C
Prochieve, 970–972
prochlorperazine, 968–970
Procrit, 421–424
Proctocort, 575–578
Procytox, 287–289
Profasi HP, 104C–106C
Proflavanol C, 81–82
progesterone, 970–972
Prograf, 1090–1092, 119C
Proleukin, 625–627, 79C–89C
Prolia, 323–324, 143C–144C
Prolixin, 499, 64C–66C
Prolixin Decanoate, 499
Proloprim, 1178–1179
Promacta, 404–405
promethazine, 972–975, 53C–54C
Promethegan, 972–975
Prometrium, 970–972
Pronestyl, 16C–18C
Pronestyl-SR, 965–967
Propaderm, 113–114
propafenone, 975–976, 16C–18C
Propecia, 483–485
propofol, 976–978, 5C
propranolol, 978–981, 16C–18C, 71C–72C
propylthiouracil, 981–982
Propyl-Thyracil, 981–982

Proquin XR, 240–243
Proscar, 483–485
ProSom, 149C–150C
prostaglandin E1, 40–41
Prostigmin, 821–822, 90C–91C
Prostin E2, 358–360
Prostin VR Pediatric, 40–41
protamine, 982–983
Protamine sulfate, 982–983
Proton Pump Inhibitors, 147C–148C
Protonix, 898–899, 148C
Protonix IV, 898–899
Protopic, 1090–1092
Provenge, 1061–1062, 79C–89C
Proventil HFA, 25–27, 73C–76C
Provera, 723–725
Provigil, 785–786
Prozac, 497–499, 37C–40C
Prozac Weekly, 497–499
Prudoxin, 382–384
pseudoephedrine, 983–984
Psilocybin, 1248–1254
psyllium, 984–985, 121C
Pulmicort, 97C–98C
Pulmicort Flexhaler, 145–147, 73C–76C
Pulmicort Respules, 145–147, 73C–76C
Pulmicort Turbuhaler, 73C–76C
Purinethol, 79C–89C
Purple passion, 1248–1254
Pylera, 763–765, 1117–1119
pyrazinamide, 985–987
Pyridium, 921–922
pyridostigmine, 987–988, 90C–91C
pyridoxine, 988–989, 161C–162C

Q
QT-Interval Prolongation, 1324
Quaalude, 1248–1254
Quasense, 92C–96C
Quay, 1248–1254
Quazepam, 149C–150C
Quelicin, 124C
Questran Lite, 230–231
Questran, 230–231, 56C–58C
quetiapine, 989–991, 64C–66C
Quinaglute, 16C–18C
quinapril, 991–993, 9C, 59C–62C
Quinidex, 16C–18C
Quinidex Extentabs, 993–995
quinidine, 993–995, 16C–18C
quinupristin-dalfopristin, 995–996
Quixin, 684–687
Qvar, 113–114
QVAR HFA, 73C–76C

R
rabeprazole, 996–998, 148C
race ginger, 530
Ralivia ER, 1158–1160
raloxifene, 998–999, 143C–144C
raltegravir, 999–1000, 67C–70C, 114C–118C
ramelteon, 1000–1001, 149C–150C
ramipril, 1001–1003, 9C, 59C–62C
Ranexa, 1005–1007
Raniclor, 187–188
ranitidine, 1003–1005, 107C–108C
ranolazine, 1005–1007
Rapaflo, 1056–1057
Rapamune, 1062–1063, 119C
rasagiline, 1007–1008, 146C
Rasilez, 33–34
Razadyne, 530–531
Razadyne ER, 530–531
Reactine, 219–220
Rebetol, 1014–1015
Rebetron, 619–621, 1014–1015
Rebif, 621–623
Reclast, 1232–1233, 143C–144C
Reclipsen, 92C–96C
Recombinate, 71–73
Recommended Childhood and Adult Immunizations, 1294–1300
Red clover, 1257–1269
red ginseng, 545
red sunflower, 399
Red yeast, 1257–1269
Reefer, 1248–1254
Refacto, 71–73
Refissa, 1169–1171
Refludan, 673–674, 30C–33C
Regitine, 925–927
Reglan, 756–758
Regonol, 987–988
regular insulin, 615–619
Regulex, 371–372
Rejuva-A, 1169–1171
Rela, 151C–153C
Relafen, 800–801, 127C–128C
Relenza, 1226–1227, 67C–70C
Relistor, 751–752
Relpax, 403–404, 63C

Remeron Soltab, 778–779
Remeron, 778–779, 37C–40C
Remicade, 613–615
Reminyl, 530–531
Reminyl ER, 530–531
Remodulin, 1167–1169
Renagel, 1054–1055
Renedil, 466–467
Renova, 1169–1171
Renvela, 1054–1055
ReoPro, 4–5, 30C–33C
repaglinide, 1009–1010, 42C–44C
Reprexain CIII, 573–575, 590–593
Repronex, 104C–106C
Requip, 1034–1036, 146C
Requip XL, 1034–1036
Rescriptor, 320–321, 67C–70C, 114C–118C
Restasis, 289–291
Restoril, 1100–1102, 149C–150C
Retavase, 1010–1012, 30C–33C
reteplase, 1010–1012, 30C–33C
Retin-A, 1169–1171
Retin-A Micro, 1169–1171
Retin-A Regimen Kit, 1169–1171
Retrovir, 1227–1229, 67C–70C, 114C–118C
Revatio, 1055–1056
ReVia, 809–811
Revitalose C-1000, 81–82
Revlimid, 670–673
Reyataz, 88–90, 114C–118C
Rheumatrex, 747–749, 79C–89C
Rhinalar, 493–495
Rhinocort Aqua, 145–147, 2C
Rhinocort, 97C–98C
rho (D) immune globulin, 1012–1013
Rhodis, 650–652
RhoGAM, 1012–1013
Rhophylac, 1012–1013
RibaPak, 1014–1015
Ribasphere, 1014–1015
ribavirin, 1014–1015, 67C–70C
Riboflavin, 161C–162C
rifabutin, 1015–1017
Rifadin, 1017–1019
Rifadin IV, 1017–1019
Rifamate, 636–637, 1017–1019
rifampin, 1017–1019
Rifater, 636–637, 985–987, 1017–1019
rifaximin, 1019–1020
rimantadine, 1020–1021
Riomet, 741–743
Riopan, 715
Riphenidate, 752–754
risedronate, 1021–1022, 143C–144C
Risperdal, 1023–1025, 64C–66C
Risperdal Consta, 1023–1025
Risperdal M-Tabs, 1023–1025
risperidone, 1023–1025, 64C–66C
Ritalin, 752–754, 1248–1254
Ritalin LA, 752–754
Ritalin SR, 752–754
ritonavir, 1025–1027, 67C–70C, 114C–118C
Rituxan, 1027–1028, 79C–89C
rituximab, 1027–1028, 79C–89C
Rivanase AQ, 113–114
rivastigmine, 1028–1030
Rivotril, 259–261
rizatriptan, 1030–1031, 63C
Robaxin, 745–746, 151C–153C
Robidone, 573–575
Robidrine, 983–984
Robinul, 554–555
Robitussin, 561–562
Robitussin AC, 561–562
Robitussin DM, 561–562
Rocaltrol, 1212–1215
Rocephin, 210–212, 22C–24C
Rock, 1248–1254
Rocket fuel, 1248–1254
Rocuronium, 124C
Rofact, 1017–1019
Rogaine, 776–778
Rogaine Extra Strength, 776–778
Rogitine, 925–927
Rohypnol, 1248–1254
Romazicon, 491–493
romidepsin, 1031–1033
romiplostim, 1033–1034
Romycin, 433–435
Roofies, 1248–1254
Rope, 1248–1254
Rophies, 1248–1254
ropinirole, 1034–1036, 146C
Ropivacaine, 7C
rosiglitazone, 1036–1037, 42C–44C
rosin rose, 1080–1081
rosuvastatin, 1037–1039, 56C–58C
Rowasa, 736–737
Roxanol, 791–794, 1248–1254, 141C–142C
Roxicet, 9–12, 880–882
Roxicodone, 880–882, 141C–142C

Roxicodone Intensol, 880–882
Rozerem, 1000–1001, 149C–150C
Rubex, 384–387
rufinamide, 1039–1040
Rythmodan, 365–367
Rythmodan LA, 365–367
Rythmol, 975–976, 16C–18C
Rythmol SR, 5570
Ryzolt, 1158–1160

S
sabal, 1046
Sabril, 1202–1204, 34C–36C
Saizen, 1072–1075
sakau, 646–647
Salazopyrin, 1083–1085
Salazopyrin EN-Tabs, 1083–1085
SalineX, 1067–1069
salmeterol, 1041–1042, 73C–76C
Salmeterol/fluticasone, 73C–76C
Salofalk, 736–737
Sal-Tropine, 96–98
Salty water, 1248–1254
SAMe, 1257–1269
Samsca, 1147–1149
Sanctura, 1181–1182
Sanctura XR, 1181–1182
Sancuso, 558–560
Sandimmune, 289–291, 119C
Sandostatin, 852–853
Sandostatin LAR Depot, 852–853
santa marla, 479–480
Saphris, 82–84, 64C–66C
saquinavir, 1042–1043, 67C–70C, 114C–118C
Sarafem, 497–499
sargramostim, 1044–1046
Savella, 772–773
saw palmetto, 1046, 1257–1269
saxagliptin, 1046–1048, 42C–44C
Schisandra, 1257–1269
Schoolboy, 1248–1254
Scoop, 1248–1254
scopolamine, 1048–1049
scurvy root, 399
Seasonale, 92C–96C
Seasonique, 92C–96C
Seconal, 1248–1254
Sectral, 71C–72C
Sedative-Hypnotics, 149C–150C
Selax, 371–372
selegiline, 1049–1051, 146C–147C
Selfemra, 497–499
Selzentry, 721–722, 67C–70C, 114C–118C
Senexon, 1051–1052
senna, 1051–1052, 121C–122C
Senna-Gen, 1051–1052
Sennatural, 1051–1052
Senokot, 1051–1052, 121C–122C
Senokot-S, 371–372, 1051–1052
Sensipar, 239–240
Sensorcaine, 6C
Septra, 279–282, 1178–1179
Septra DS, 279–282
Serax, 13C–14C
Serentil, 64C–66C
Serevent, 1041–1042
Serevent Diskus, 1041–1042, 73C–76C
Serophene, 104C–106C
Seroquel, 989–991, 64C–66C
Seroquel XR, 989–991
Serostim, 1072–1075
Sertaconazole, 48C–49C
sertraline, 1052–1054, 37C–40C
sevelamer, 1054–1055
Shark cartilage, 1257–1269
Sibutramine, 137C
Signs and Symptoms of Electrolyte Imbalance, 1301
sildenafil, 1055–1056
Silenor, 382–384
silodosin, 1056–1057
Silvadene, 1057–1058
silver sulfadiazine, 1057–1058
Simcor, 825–827, 1059–1061
simethicone, 1058–1059
Simponi, 555–557
Simulect, 111–113, 119C
simvastatin, 1059–1061, 56C–58C
Sinemet, 176–178, 146C
Sinemet CR, 176–178, 146C
Sinequan, 382–384, 37C–40C
Singulair, 789–791, 73C–76C
sipuleucel-T, 1061–1062, 79C–89C
sirolimus, 1062–1063, 119C
sitagliptin, 1063–1065, 42C–44C
Skelaxin, 740–741, 151C–153C
Skeletal Muscle Relaxants, 151C–153C
Skelid, 1132–1133
Slo-Niacin, 825–827
Slow-Fe, 475, 109C
Slow-Mag, 715

Smoking Cessation Agents, 154C–157C
Snow, 1248–1254
sodium bicarbonate, 1065–1067
sodium chloride, 1067–1069
sodium ferric gluconate complex, 1069–1070
Sodium phosphate, 121C–122C
sodium polystyrene sulfonate, 1070–1071
Soflax, 371–372
Solaraze, 344–347
Solia, 92C–96C
solifenacin, 1071–1072
Soliris, 400–401
Solodyn, 775–776
Soltamox, 1094–1095
Solu-Cortef, 575–578, 97C–98C
Solu-Medrol, 754, 97C–98C
Soma, 180–182
Soma Compound, 180–182
somatropin, 1072–1075
Somatuline Depot, 664–665
Somavert, 909–910
Somnote, 223–224
Sonata, 1225–1226, 149C–150C
sorafenib, 1075–1076, 79C–89C
Sorine, 1076–1078
sotalol, 1076–1078, 16C–18C
Sotret, 639–641
Soy, 1257–1269
Soybean oil, 1257–1269
Spanish Phrases Often Used in Clinical Settings, 1304–1311
Special K, 1248–1254
Spectazole, 48C–49C
Spectracef, 22C–24C
Spectral, 16C–18C
Speed, 1248–1254
Spiriva, 1137–1138, 73C–76C
spironolactone, 1078–1080, 101C–102C
Sporanox, 642–644, 46C–47C
Sprintec, 92C–96C
Sprix, 652–654
Sprycel, 310–311, 79C–89C
SPS, 1070–1071
Sronyx, 92C–96C
SSD, 1057–1058
SSD AF, 1057–1058
St. john's wort, 1080–1081, 1257–1269
Stadol, 157–158, 141C–142C
Stadol NS, 157–158
Stalevo, 176–178, 412–413
Starlix, 815–817, 42C–44C
stavudine, 1081–1082, 67C–70C, 114C–118C
Stavzor, 1187–1190
Staxyn, 1194–1195
Stelara, 1182–1183
Stelazine, 1175–1177, 64C–66C
Stemetil, 968–970
Sterapred, 959–960
Sterapred DS, 959–960
Stimate, 328–330
stinking rose, 534–535
STP, 1248–1254
Strattera, 92–93
Streptomycin, 21C
Streptozocin, 79C–89C
Striant, 1114–1116
Sublimaze, 472–475, 1248–1254, 141C–142C
Suboxone, 149–151
Subutex, 149–151
Succinylcholine, 124C
sucralfate, 1082–1083
Sudafed, 983–984
Sudafed 12 Hour, 983–984
Sudafed 24 Hour, 983–984
Sudafed Children's, 983–984
Sudafed PE, 927–929
sulfamethoxazole-trimethoprim, 279–282
sulfasalazine, 1083–1085
Sulfatrim, 279–282
sulindac, 1085–1086, 127C–128C
sumatriptan, 1087–1088, 63C
Sumavel DosePro, 1087–1088, 63C
sunitinib, 1088–1090, 79C–89C
Super acid, 1248–1254
Super K, 1248–1254
Supeudol, 880–882
Suprax, 196–197
Surfak, 371–372, 121C
Survanta Intratracheal, 120–121
Sustiva, 401–402, 67C–70C, 114C–118C
Sutent, 1088–1090, 79C–89C
Symax, 585–587
Symax SL, 585–587
Symax, SR, 585–587
Symbicort, 145–147, 512–514, 73C–76C
Symbyax, 497–499
Symlin, 951–952, 42C–44C
Symmetrel, 45–46, 67C–70C

Sympathomimetics, 157C–158C
Synagis, 892
Synalar, 99C–100C
Synarel, 803–804, 104C–106C
Synera, 689–691
Synercid, 995–996
Synthroid, 687–689, 159C
Syntocinon, 884–886

T
Taclonex, 121–123
tacrolimus, 1090–1092, 119C
tadalafil, 1092–1093
Tagamet, 237–239, 107C–108C
Tagamet HB 200, 237–239
Tambocor, 16C–18C
Tamiflu, 872–873, 67C–70C
Tamofen, 1094–1095
tamoxifen, 1094–1095, 79C–89C
tamsulosin, 1095–1096
tanakan, 544–545
tang kuei, 376–377
tapentadol, 1096–1097
Tarceva, 430–431, 73C–76C
Targretin, 126–127, 73C–76C
Tarka, 1160–1161, 1200–1202
Tasigna, 833–834, 73C–76C
Tasmar, 146C–147C
Tavist Allergy, 250–252, 53C–54C
Tavist ND, 705–706
Taxol, 886–889, 73C–76C
Taxotere, 368–371, 73C–76C
Tazicef, 206–208, 22C–24C
Tazidime, 22C–24C
Tazocin, 935–937
Taztia XT, 354–357
Tears Naturale, 853–854
Tebrazid, 985–987
Techniques of Medication Administration, 1312–1319
Teczem, 354–357, 407–409
Teflaro, 205–206
Tegopen, 28C
Tegretol, 174–176, 34C–36C
Tegretol XR, 174–176, 34C–36C
Tekamlo, 33–34, 56–57
Tekturna, 33–34, 59C–62C
Tekturna HCT, 33–34, 571–573
telavancin, 1097–1099
telmisartan, 1099–1100, 10C
Telzir, 514–516
temazepam, 1100–1102, 149C–150C
Temodal, 1102–1103
Temodar, 1102–1103, 79C–89C
Temovate, 99C–100C
temozolomide, 1102–1103, 79C–89C
Tempra, 9–12
temsirolimus, 1103–1105, 79C–89C
tenecteplase, 1105–1106, 30C–33C
Teniposide, 79C–89C
tenofovir, 1106–1107, 67C–70C, 114C–118C
Tenolin, 90–92
Tenoretic, 90–92
Tenormin, 90–92, 59C–62C, 71C–72C
Tensilon, 90C–91C
Tenuate, 137C
Terazol, 1112–1113
Terazol 3, 1112–1113
Terazol 7, 1112–1113
terazosin, 1107–1109, 59C–62C
terbinafine, 1109–1110, 48C–49C
terbutaline, 1110–1112
terconazole, 1112–1113
teriparatide, 1113–1114, 143C–144C
Tessalon Perles, 118–119
Testim, 1114–1116
Testopel, 1114–1116
testosterone, 1114–1116
tetrabenazine, 1116–1117
Tetracaine, 8C
tetracycline, 1117–1119
Teveten, 424–425, 10C
Teveten HCT, 424–425, 572
thalidomide, 1119–1120
Thalomid, 1119–1120
Theo-24, 1120–1122
Theochron, 1120–1122
theophylline, 1120–1122
TheraCys, 79C–89C
Thermazene, 1057–1058
thiamine, 1122–1123, 161C–162C
Thioguanine, 79C–89C
Thiopental, 5C
Thioplex, 1125–1127, 79C–89C
thioridazine, 1123–1125, 64C–66C
thiotepa, 1125–1127, 79C–89C
thiothixene, 1127–1128, 64C–66C
Thorazine, 227–230, 64C–66C
Thrive, 829–831, 154C–156C
Thyroid, 159C
Thyroid dessicated, 159C

Thyrolar, 687–689, 159C
tiagabine, 1128–1129, 34C–36C
Tiazac, 354–357
Ticarcillin/clavulanate, 28C–29C
Tice BCG, 79C–89C
Ticlid, 1129–1131, 30C–33C
ticlopidine, 1129–1131, 30C–33C
tigecycline, 1131–1132
Tikosyn, 372–373, 16C–18C
Tilia, 92C–96C
Tilia Fe, 92C–96C
tiludronate, 1132–1133
Timentin, 28C–29C
Timolide, 571–573, 1133–1136
timolol, 1133–1136, 50C–52C, 71C–72C
Timoptic, 1133–1136, 50C–52C
Timoptic OccuDose, 1133–1136
Timoptic XE, 1133–1136, 50C–52C
Tinactin, 48C–49C
tinzaparin, 1136–1137, 30C–33C
tiotropium, 1137–1138, 73C–76C
tipranavir, 1138–1140, 114C–118C
tipton weed, 1080–1081
Tirofiban, 30C–33C
Titralac, 163
tizanidine, 1140–1141, 151C–153C
TNKase, 1105–1106, 30C–33C
TOBI, 1141–1144
TobraDex, 1141–1144
tobramycin, 1141–1144, 21C
Tobrex, 1141–1144
Tocainide, 16C–18C
tocilizumab, 1144–1146
Tofranil, 603–605, 37C–40C
Tofranil-PM, 603–605
toki, 376–377
Tolcapone, 146C–147C
Tolect, 338–339
Tolectin, 127C–128C
Tolmetin, 127C–128C
Tolnaftate, 48C–49C
tolterodine, 1146–1147
tolvaptan, 1147–1149
tonga, 646
Tonocard, 16C–18C
Topamax, 1149–1151, 34C–36C
Topicort, 99C–100C
topiramate, 1149–1151, 34C–36C
Toposar, 452–454
topotecan, 1151–1153, 79C–89C
Toprol XL, 760–762, 59C–62C
Toradol, 652–654, 127C–128C
toremifene, 1153–1154, 79C–89C
Torisel, 1103–1105, 79C–89C
torsemide, 1154–1156, 101C–102C
tositumomab and iodine131I-tositumomab, 1156–1158
Tositumomab, 79C–89C
Toviaz, 478–479
Tracleer, 139–140
tramadol, 1158–1160
Trandate, 654–656, 71C–72C
trandolapril, 1160–1161, 9C
tranexamic acid, 1161–1162
Tranks, 1248–1254
Trans-Derm Scop, 1048–1049
Transderm-V, 1048–1049
Tranxene, 264–266, 13C–14C
Tranxene SD, 264–266
Tranxene SD Half-Strength, 264–266
Tranxene T-Tab, 264–266
tranylcypromine, 1162–1164, 37C–40C
trastuzumab, 1164–1166, 79C–89C
Travatan, 50C–52C
Travoprost, 50C–52C
trazodone, 1166–1167, 13C–14C, 37C–40C
Treanda, 116–117, 79C–89C
Trelstar Depot, 1179–1181
Trelstar LA, 1179–1181
Trental, 919–920
treprostinil, 1167–1169
Tretin X, 1169–1171
tretinoin, 1169–1171, 79C–89C
Trexall, 747–749
Treximet, 811–813, 1087–1088
Tri Lo Spriutec, 92C–96C
Triacetin, 48C–49C
triamcinolone acetonide, 1171
triamcinolone hexacetonide, 1171
triamcinolone, 1171, 73C–76C, 97C–98C, 99C–100C
triamterene, 1173–1175, 101C–102C
Triavil, 54–55
Triazolam, 149C–150C
Tribenzor, 56–57, 571–573
Tricor, 467–469, 56C–58C
Triderm, 1171
Tridesilon, 99C–100C
Tridural, 1158–1160
trifluoperazine, 1175–1177, 64C–66C
Triglide, 467–469, 56C–58C

trihexyphenidyl, 1177–1178
Tri-Legest Fe, 92C–96C
Trileptal, 877–878, 34C–36C
Trilipix, 469–470, 56C–58C
Tri-Lyte, 941–943
trimethoprim, 1178–1179
Trimox, 28C–29C
Tri-Nasal, 1171
Trinessa, 92C–96C
Trinipatch, 839–842
Tri-Norinyl, 92C–96C
Triostat, 159C
Tri-Previfem, 92C–96C
triptorelin, 1179–1181
Trisenox, 79–81, 79C–89C
Tri-Sprintec, 92C–96C
Trivora, 92C–96C
Trizivr, 1–2, 659–661, 1227–1229, 114C–118C
Trosec, 1181–1182
trospium, 1181–1182
Trusopt, 50C–52C
Truvada, 405–407, 1106–1107, 114C–118C
Tubocurarine, 124C
Tums, 163, 11C–12C
Turmeric,1257–1269
Tussend, 573–575
Twinject, 415–417
Twinsta, 56–57, 1099–1100
Tygacil, 1131–1132
Tykerb, 668–669, 79C–89C
Tylenol, 9–12
Tylenol Arthritis Pain, 9–12
Tylenol Children's Meltaways, 9–12
Tylenol Extra Strength, 9–12
Tylenol Junior Meltaways, 9–12
Tylenol with Codeine, 9–12, 269
Tylox, 9–12, 880–882
Tyrosine, 1257–1269
Tysabri, 814–815
Tyvaso, 1167–1169

U
Uloric, 465–466
Ultracet, 9–12, 1158–1160
Ultradol, 450–452
Ultram, 1158–1160
Ultram ER, 1158–1160
Ultravate, 99C–100C
Unasyn, 65–67, 28C–29C
Undecylenic acid, 48C–49C
Unidel, 1146–1147
Unipen, 804–805, 28C
Uniphyl, 1120–1122
Uniretic, 571–573, 786–787
Unithroid, 687–689, 159C
Univasc, 786–787, 9C
Uppers, 1248–1254
Urecholine, 123–124, 90C–91C
Urispas, 486–487
Uristat, 921–922
Urofollitropin, 104C–106C
Uro-KP-Neutral, 931–933
Uro-Mag, 715
Uromitexan, 737–739
Uroxatral, 31–32
ustekinumnab, 1182–1183

V
Vagifem, 440–443
valacyclovir, 1183–1185, 67C–70C
Valcyte, 1186–1187, 67C–70C
valerian, 1257–1269, **1185–1186**
valeriana, 1185–1186
valganciclovir, 1186–1187, 67C–70C
Valium, 342–344, 1248–1254, 13C–14C, 151C–153C
valproic acid, 1187–1190, 34C–36C
Valrubicin, 79C–89C
valsartan, 1190–1191
Valstar, 79C–89C
Valtrex, 1183–1185, 67C–70C
Valturna, 33–34, 1190–1191
Vancocin, 1191–1193
vancomycin, 1191–1193
Vandazole, 763–765
Vantin, 201–203, 22C–24C
Vaprisol, 273–274
vardenafil, 1194–1195
varenicline, 1195–1196, 154C–156C
Vaseretic, 407–409, 571–573
Vasocidin, 957–959
vasopressin, 1196–1198
Vasotec, 407–409, 9C, 59C–62C
Vectibix, 896–897, 79C–89C
Vectical, 1212–1215
Vecuronium, 124C
Velban, 1204–1206, 79C–89C
Velcade, 137–139, 79C–89C
Velivet, 92C–96C
venlafaxine, 1198–1200, 13C–14C, 37C–40C

Venofer, 634–635
Ventavis, 598–599
Ventolin HFA, 25–27, 73C–76C
VePesid, 452–454, 79C–89C
Veracolate, 129–130
Veramyst, 505–507, 3C
verapamil, 1200–1202, 16C–18C, 77C–78C
Verapamil SR, 59C–62C
Verelan, 1200–1202
Verelan PM, 1200–1202
Versed, 767–769, 5C
Vesanoid, 1169–1171, 79C–89C
VESIcare, 1071–1072
Vfend, 1218–1220, 47C
Viadur, 677–679
Viagra, 1055–1056
Vibativ, 1097–1099
Vibramycin, 387–389
Vibra-Tabs, 387–389
Vicodin, 9–12, 573–575
Vicodin ES, 9–12, 573–575
Vicodin HP, 9–12, 573–575
Vicoprofen, 573–575, 590–593
Victoza, 693–694, 42C–44C
Vidaza, 99–101, 79C–89C
Videx, 349–351, 67C–70C, 114C–118C
Videx-EC, 349–351
vigabatrin, 1202–1204, 34C–36C
Vigamox, 794–796
Vimovo, 811–813
Vimpat, 656–658
vinblastine, 1204–1206, 79C–89C
Vincasar PFS, 1206–1208
vincristine, 1206–1208, 79C–89C
vinorelbine, 1208–1210, 79C–89C
Vioform, 48C–49C
Viracept, 820–821, 67C–70C, 114C–118C
Viramune, 824–825, 114C–118C
Virazole, 1014–1015, 67C–70C
Viread, 1106–1107, 67C–70C, 114C–118C
Virilon IM, 1114–1116
Visine-A, 138C
Visken, 71C–72C
Vistaril, 584–585, 13C–14C
Vistide, 234–235, 67C–70C
Vita-C, 81–82
vitamin A, 1211–1212, 161C–162C
vitamin B_1, 1122–1123, 161C–162C
vitamin B_{12}, 284–285, 161C–162C
Vitamin B_2, 161C–162C
Vitamin B_3, 161C–162C
Vitamin B_5, 161C–162C
vitamin B_6, 988–989, 161C–162C
vitamin C, 81–82, 161C–162C
vitamin D, 1212–1215, 161C–162C
vitamin E, 1216, 161C–162C
vitamin K, 1217
vitamin K_1, 1217
Vitamins, 160C–162C
Vitrasert, 531–534
Vitussin, 573–575
Vivaglobulin, 607–608
Vivelle, 440–443
Vivelle Dot, 440–443
Vivitrol, 809–811
Vivomo, 439–440
Volibris, 46–48
Voltaren, 344–347, 127C–128C
Voltaren Gel, 344–347
Voltaren Ophthalmic, 344–347
Voltaren XR, 344–347
voriconazole, 1218–1220, 46C–47C
vorinostat, 1220–1221, 79C–89C
VoSpire ER, 25–27
Votrient, 901–903
VP-16, 452–454
Vumon, 79C–89C
Vytorin, 460–461, 1059–1061
Vyvanse, 695–696

W
warfarin, 1221–1223, 30C–33C
Welchol, 56C–58C
Wellbutrin, 151–153, 37C–40C
Wellbutrin SR, 151–153
Wellbutrin XL, 151–153
Wes Throid, 159C
Westcort, 575–578
Whey protein, 1257–1269
White girl, 1248–1254
Wigraine, 426
Wild yam, 1257–1269
Willow Bark, 1257–1269
Winpred, 959–960
WinRho SDF, 1012–1013

X
Xalatan, 50C–52C
Xanax XR, 38–39
Xanax, 38–39, 1248–1254, 13C–14C
Xatral, 31–32

Xeloda, 170–172, 79C–89C
Xenazine, 1116–1117
Xenical, 871–872, 137C
Xifaxan, 1019–1020
Xigris, 393–394
Xodol, 9–12, 573–575
Xolair, 862
Xolegel, 648–650
Xopenex, 679–681, 73C–76C
Xopenex HFA, 679–681
Xylocaine, 689–691, 16C–18C
Xyntha, 71–73
Xyzal, 683–684, 53C–54C

Y

yagona, 646
Yasmin, 92C–96C
Yaz, 92C–96C
Yellow jackets, 1248–1254
Yellow sunshine, 1248–1254
yohimbe, 1223–1224, 1257–1269

Z

Zaditor, 139C
zafirlukast, 1224–1225, 73C–76C
Zalcitabine, 67C–70C, 114C–118C
zaleplon, 1225–1226, 149C–150C
Zanaflex, 1140–1141, 151C–153C
Zanaflex Capsules, 1140–1141
zanamivir, 1226–1227, 67C–70C
Zanosar, 79C–89C
Zantac, 1003–1005, 107C–108C
Zantac EFFERdose, 1003–1005
Zantac-75, 1003–1005
Zantac-150, 1003–1005
Zaroxolyn, 758–760, 101C–102C
Zazole, 1112–1113
Zebeta, 131–133, 71C–72C
Zegerid, 866–867
Zegerid Powder, 866–867
Zelapar, 1049–1051, 146C–147C
Zeldox, 1231–1232
Zemplar, 1212–1215
Zemuron, 124C
Zenapax, 296–297, 119C
Zenchent, 92C–96C
Zenpep, 895–896
Zerit, 1081–1082, 67C–70C, 114C–118C
Zestoretic, 571–573, 696–698
Zestril, 696–698, 9C, 59C–62C
Zetia, 460–461, 56C–58C
Zevalin, 589–590, 79C–89C
Ziac, 131–133, 571–573
Ziagen, 1–2, 67C–70C, 114C–118C
zidovudine, 1227–1229, 67C–70C, 114C–118C
Zidovudine/lamivudine, 114C–118C
Zidovudine/lamivudine/abacavir, 114C–118C
zileuton, 1229–1231, 73C–76C
Zinacef, 212, 22C–24C
Zinecard, 338–339
zingiber, 530
ziprasidone, 1231–1232, 64C–66C
Zipsor, 344–347
Zirgan, 531–534
Zithromax, 104–106, 26C
Zithromax TRI-PAK, 104–106
Zithromax Z-PAK, 104–106
Zmax, 104–106
Zocor, 1059–1061, 56C–58C
Zofran, 867–869
Zofran ODT, 867–869
Zoladex, 557–558, 79C–89C, 104C–106C
Zoladex LA, 557–558
zoledronic acid, 1232–1233, 143C–144C
Zolinza, 1220–1221, 79C–89C
zolmitriptan, 1234–1235, 63C
Zoloft, 1052–1054, 37C–40C
zolpidem, 1235–1236, 149C–150C
Zometa, 1232–1233
Zomig, 1234–1235, 63C
Zomig Rapimelt, 1234–1235
Zomig-ZMT, 1234–1235, 63C
Zonalon, 382–384
Zonegran, 1237–1238, 34C–36C
zonisamide, 1237–1238, 34C–36C
Zorbitive, 1072–1075
ZORprin, 86–88
Zortress, 456–457
Zosyn, 935–937, 28C–29C
Zotrim, 279–282
Zovia, 1/35, 92C–96C
Zovia 1/50–28, 92C–96C
Zovirax, 16–19, 67C–70C
Zuplenz, 867–869
zuzhong, 1046
Zyban, 151–153, 154C–156C
Zydone, 573–575
Zyflo, 73C–76C
Zyflo CR, 1229–1231
Zylet, 1141–1144

Zyloprim, 34–36
Zyprexa, 858–860, 64C–66C
Zyprexa Intramuscular, 858–860
Zyprexa Relprevv, 858–860
Zyprexa Zydis, 858–860
Zyrtec, 219–220, 53C–54C
Zyrtec D 12 Hour Tablets, 219–220
Zyrtec-D, 983–984
Zyvox, 691–693
Zyvoxam, 691–693

COMMONLY USED ABBREVIATIONS

ABG(s)—arterial blood gas(es)
ACE—angiotensin-converting enzyme
ADHD—attention deficit hyperactivity disorder
AIDS—acquired immunodeficiency syndrome
ALT—alanine aminotransferase, serum
ANC—absolute neutrophil count
aPTT—activated partial thromboplastin time
AST—aspartate aminotransferase, serum
AV—atrioventricular
bid—twice per day
B/P—blood pressure
BSA—body surface area
BUN—blood urea nitrogen
CBC—complete blood count
Ccr—creatinine clearance
CHF—congestive heart failure
CNS—central nervous system
CO—cardiac output
COPD—chronic obstructive pulmonary disease
CPK—creatine phosphokinase
CSF—cerebrospinal fluid
CT—computed tomography
CVA—cerebrovascular accident
D_5W—dextrose 5% in water
dl—deciliter
DNA—deoxyribonucleic acid
EEG—electroencephalogram
EKG—electrocardiogram
esp.—especially
g—gram
GGT—gamma glutamyl transpeptidase
GI—gastrointestinal
GU—genitourinary
H_2—histamine
Hct—hematocrit
HDL—high-density lipoprotein
Hgb—hemoglobin
HIV—human immunodeficiency virus
HMG-CoA—3-hydroxy-3-methylglutaryl-coenzyme A (HMG-CoA) reductase inhibitors (statins)
hr/hrs—hour/hours
HTN—hypertension
I&O—intake and output
ICP—intracranial pressure
ID—intradermal
IgA—immunoglobulin A
IM—intramuscular
IOP—intraocular pressure
IV—intravenous
K—potassium
kg—kilogram
LDH—lactate dehydrogenase
LDL—low-density lipoprotein
LOC—level of consciousness
MAC—*Mycobacterium avium* complex
MAOI—monoamine oxidase inhibitor
mcg—microgram
mEq—milliequivalent
mg—milligram
MI—myocardial infarction
min—minute(s)
mo/mos—month/months
N/A—not applicable
Na—sodium
NaCl—sodium chloride
NG—nasogastric
NSAID(s)—nonsteroidal anti-inflammatory drug(s)
OD—right eye
OS—left eye
OTC—over the counter
OU—both eyes
PCP—*Pneumocystis jiroveci* pneumonia
PO—orally, by mouth
prn—as needed
PSA—prostate-specific antigen
pt/pts—patient/patients
PT—prothrombin time
PTCA—percutaneous transluminal coronary angiography
q—every
qid—four times daily
RBC—red blood cell count
REM—rapid eye movements
RNA—ribonucleic acid
SA—sinoatrial node
sec—second(s)
SSRI—selective serotonin reuptake inhibitor
tbsp—tablespoon
tid—three times daily
TNF—tumor necrosis factor
tsp—teaspoon
UTI—urinary tract infection
VLDL—very-low-density lipoprotein
WBC—white blood cell count
wk/wks—week/weeks
yr/yrs—year/years